Medical–Surgical Nursing Practice

Medical–surgical nursing practice is defined as the nursing care of adults with known or predicted physiological alteration, with trauma, or with disability. Nursing care includes the care and treatment necessary to provide comfort; to assist individuals in the promotion and maintenance of health and the prevention, detection, and treatment of illness; to promote restoration to highest possible productive capacities; and to assist with a peaceful death. Medical–surgical nursing practice encompasses patient assessment, planning, implementation, and evaluation. It takes into account the interrelatedness of biological, psychological, and social components of the patient's response or adjustment to the physiological alteration, trauma, or disability.

The field of medical–surgical nursing makes use of theories that address ethics, stress/adaptation, learning and communication, behavioral change, disease, and systems. A body of knowledge for practice is emerging from scholarly conceptualizations and research findings generated from intra- and inter-disciplinary studies.

Medical–surgical nursing encompasses the following elements:

1. Maintenance or restoration of normal patterns of functioning in areas such as sleep, rest, ventilation, activity, nutrition, elimination, sexuality, and skin integrity
2. Pain and discomfort
3. Emotional problems related to illness and treatment, such as grief, loss, anxiety, and depression
4. Knowledge for maintenance of health
5. Self-care
6. Decision making and exercise of personal choice
7. The dying process and death

From "*A Statement on the Scope of Medical–Surgical Nursing Practice,*" American Nurses' Association, Division on Medical–Surgical Nursing Practice. Kansas City, MO: 1980. Reprinted with permission.

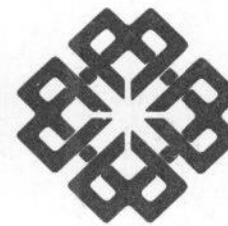

Essentials of Adult Health Nursing

SueAnn Wooster Ames, RN, MS, ANP-C

Carol Ren Kneisl, RN, MS

Addison-Wesley Publishing Company

Health Sciences Division, Menlo Park, California

Reading, Massachusetts ■ Menlo Park, California ■ New York

Don Mills, Ontario ■ Wokingham, England ■ Amsterdam ■ Bonn

Sydney ■ Singapore ■ Tokyo ■ Madrid ■ Bogota ■ Santiago ■ San Juan

This book is dedicated to clients and the nurses who care for them

Sponsoring Editor: Nancy Evans
Production Supervisors: Anne Friedman, Wendy Earl
Interior Designer: Paul Quin
Cover Designer: Rudy Zehntner
Copyeditor: Melissa Andrews
Illustrators: Susan Strawn, Stephanie McCann, Steve Beebe
Proofreaders: Helene Harrington, Jenny Pulsipher, Steve Sorensen
Indexer: Katherine Pitcoff
Compositor: Graphic Typesetting Service, Inc.

Library of Congress Cataloging-in-Publication Data

Ames, Sue Ann.
Essentials of adult health nursing.

Includes index.

1. Nursing. 2. Holistic medicine. 3. Humanistic psychology. 4. Physiology, Pathological. I. Kneisl, Carol Ren. II. Title. [DNLM: 1. Nursing Care. WY 100 A513e]
RT42.A44 1988 610.73 87-27529

ISBN 0-201-12667-2

ABCDEFGHIJ-VH-891098

The authors and publishers have exerted every effort to ensure that drug selection and dosage set forth in this text are in accord with current recommendations and practice at the time of publication. However, in view of ongoing research, changes in government regulations and the constant flow of information relating to drug therapy and drug reactions, the reader is urged to check the package insert for each drug for any change in indications of dosage and for added warnings and precautions. This is particularly important where the recommended agent is a new and/or infrequently employed drug.

Addison-Wesley Publishing Company
Health Sciences Division
2725 Sand Hill Road
Menlo Park, California 94025

CONTENTS IN BRIEF

CONTENTS IN DETAIL

Rapid technologic advances in health care have radically altered the delivery of health care services. The skills and knowledge nurses must possess to use the technology have also undergone radical transformation. However, the focus of the technology—the client—remains stable. Technologic advances have not obviated the interpersonal needs of people. In fact, in some instances, the technology may have made these needs more visible.

Communicating the science of caring challenges nurse educators in every subject area. Nowhere is the challenge greater than in medical–surgical nursing. As the focus of health care shifts from hospital to home and community and a rapidly increasing aged population, courses and textbooks must respond. *Essentials of Adult Health Nursing* was developed to meet the changing needs of today's student in medical–surgical nursing. Focusing on the essentials of safe, competent, holistic care of adults, the text synthesizes nursing process, pathophysiology, and clinical nursing practice in a humanistic context.

This new text reflects the same philosophy and approach as *Adult Health Nursing: A Biopsychosocial Approach.* Health and illness are not one-dimensional phenomena but the result of interacting physiologic, cultural, psychologic, sociologic, developmental, economic, and lifestyle factors. These biopsychosocial factors are the antecedents of health and illness.

Central themes in this text encompass the holistic nature of humans: the importance of individuality, self-worth, and dignity, and the essentially humanitarian nature of nursing. Family and lifestyle implications of health and illness are emphasized throughout. The text focuses uncompromisingly on nursing care, using a nursing process format.

In addition to traditional medical–surgical content, this text discusses such often-neglected topics as physiologic and psychosocial/lifestyle implications of illness for the client; malnutrition, obesity, and eating disorders; and the care of clients with problems of substance abuse who are seen in non-psychiatric settings.

A Contemporary Perspective

Essentials of Adult Health Nursing acknowledges our beliefs about the nature of nursing, the meaning of health and illness, and the role of the healthcare consumer. Many nurse educators have indicated through their response to the larger text that they share these beliefs and that their teaching is based on the following concepts:

- It is essential for nurses to understand the biopsychosocial influences on health and illness.
- Adult health nursing focuses on the health care needs of persons who are well, who are ill, or who are at risk.
- Nurses have a major impact on health status because of broad access to clients in all age groups, in all settings, and during all phases of their lives.
- Health care consumers are clients. Clients participate in health care decision-making and self-care to the fullest extent possible and assume primary responsibility for their own health.
- Positive health practices can reduce many health risks. Teaching lifestyle modification is a critical role in nursing.

Special Features

Accessibility of information has been a primary goal in developing this new text. To help students apply the concepts outlined above, we have used many special features throughout the text.

- This special logo alerts students to important considerations in caring for elderly clients. For example, students are cautioned not to overlook atypical symptoms and signs of pneumonia in the frail elderly, page 383.
- This special logo signals information about home care, such as advising clients with respiratory disorders to monitor air quality reports and rely on home air conditioning to decrease exposure to pollutants and maintain temperature control, page 398.
- This special logo highlights client education information integrated into discussion of nursing care. Highlighted tables and boxes also feature health teaching guidelines, page 407.
- Resource lists, such as those on page 337, describe self-help groups and other organizations, telephone hotlines, and health education material for client/family teaching and self-care.
- Generic nursing care plans are included in each nursing process chapter; case studies incorporating specific nursing care plans are included in each body system unit, page 317.
- Tables summarize both the physiologic and the psychosocial/lifestyle implications of specific surgical procedures for clients and their families, page 344.
- Nursing research notes annotate current and relevant research from the nursing literature, such as on page 347.
- Cross reference boxes are placed in certain chapters to indicate where discussion of related topics can be found. We have used this device to remind readers that material in other chapters can further amplify the content.

Consistent Organization

The text comprises 13 units. Unit 1 orients the student to the shared experience of health and illness—changing health care in a changing society, basic pathophysiologic concepts and processes, and how people cope with the experience of illness.

Unit 2 discusses multisystem stressors affecting the client, such as malnutrition, obesity and eating disorders, substance abuse, infection, cancer, surgery, and burns.

Units 3 through 13 focus on caring for clients with dysfunction of specific body systems. Because nursing practice uses a nursing model parallel to, rather than instead of, a medical model, each of these units presents a clear classification in the familiar language of body systems, as follows:

- A review of anatomy, physiology, pathophysiology, and psychosocial/lifestyle influences and effects.
- The nursing process for clients with health care needs related to the body system.
- The nursing care unique to clients with specific disorders of the body system, whether their treatment is medical or surgical.

All units include 1986 NANDA-approved nursing diagnoses.

Superbly Illustrated Two-Color Format

More than 600 photographs and drawings enliven the content and facilitate understanding. The two-color format enhances the teaching value of both text and illustrations. Boxes and tables, highlighted in red, and the liberal and consistent use of headings help the student locate important information. The typographic design makes the book inviting to look at and easy to read. The clear, lively style of writing makes the subject matter interesting and meaningful to students and faculty.

Full-Color 16-Page Insert

Sixteen pages of outstanding full-color art graphically depict the anatomy and physiology of each body system. In addition, these color plates portray some of the major pathophysiologic processes that can disrupt each system.

Acknowledgments

We acknowledge and thank the contributors to the first edition of *Adult Health Nursing* whose work formed the nucleus of this text. They are:

- JANIS P. BELLACK, RN, MN Content related to CPR and the Heimlich maneuver
- LINDA RAE BELSKY, RN, MSN Content related to the care of clients with disorders of the blood and blood forming organs
- SHEILA BITTLE, RNC, PhD Content in the substance abuse chapter
- JOYCE M. BLACK, RN, MSN Content in the infection and burn chapters
- MARGARET A. BRADY, RN, MS, CPNP Nursing care plan for clients with acne
- PENNY BRESNICK, RN, MS Content related to fluid and electrolyte balance and acid–base balance
- PATRICIA ANN BROWN, RN, PhD Content in the surgery chapter and content related to the care of clients with gastrointestinal dysfunction
- PATRICIA A. BURNS, RN, MS Content related to fluid and electrolyte balance and acid–base balance
- JEANETTE K. CHAMBERS, RN, MS, CS Content related to the care of clients with kidney and urinary system dysfunction
- RITA A. COLLICHIA, RNC, MS Content related to the care of clients with musculoskeletal dysfunction
- JANICE LECH DUSEK, RN, MS Content related to the care of clients with vascular dysfunction
- ELIZABETH SCHEIDT FARREN, RN, MSN Content related to the structure and function of the male reproductive system
- JANICE COOKE FEIGENBAUM, RN, MS Content in the substance abuse chapter
- MARY LYN FIELD, RN, MSN Content related to the structure and function of the female reproductive system
- THERESA M. FLAHERTY, RN Content related to the care of clients with visual dysfunction
- MARION J. FRANZ, RD, MS Content related to the care of clients with disorders of glucose regulation
- CAROLYN GORCZYCA, RN, MS Content related to the care of clients with disorders of the integument
- VICKY ROSE HARTWELL-IVINS, RN, MSN Content related to the care of clients with respiratory dysfunction
- BRENDA P. HAUGHEY, RN, PhD Content related to health risk appraisal
- JANE ESTHER HOKANSON HAWKS, RN, MSN Content related to the care of clients with hepatic–biliary and kidney and urinary dysfunction
- PHYLLIS FOSTER HEALY, RN, MS Content related to the care of men with reproductive dysfunction
- PATRICIA HORRIGAN-CREAHAN, RNC, MS Nursing Research Notes
- DOROTHY KAMINSKI, RN, CNRN, CNOR Content related to the care of clients with nervous system dysfunction and content on hypophysectomy
- LESLIE S. KERN, RN, MS, CCRN Content related to the care of clients having cardiac surgery
- NANCY NUWER KONSTANTINIDES, RNC, MS Content related to malnutrition and the care of clients with gastrointestinal dysfunction
- DOMINICA ANN LIMBURG, RN, MS Content related to auditory dysfunction
- MARTHA FIRTH MARKARIAN, RN, MS Content related to the care of clients with nervous system dysfunction

- LYN MARSHALL, RN, MSN Content related to eating disorders
- CAROLYN FRITZ McCAIN, RN, MSN Content related to the care of women with reproductive dysfunction
- LINDA HEIM McCAUSLAND, RN, MS Content related to the care of clients with musculoskeletal dysfunction
- LeANN ANDERSON McNEILL, RN, MS Content related to the care of clients with disorders of glucose regulation
- MARDY NORD MEADOWS, RN, BS Content related to the care of clients with visual dysfunction
- CAROLYN CZECH MONTGOMERY, RNC, MSN Content related to the care of clients with musculoskeletal dysfunction
- SUSAN KATHLEEN NEVINS, RN, MA Content related to the care of clients with nervous system dysfunction
- THOMAS E. OBST, MS, CRNA Content in the surgery chapter related to anesthesia
- ROSEMARY CAROL POLOMANO, RN, MSN, CS Content in the cancer chapter
- YVONNE KRALL SCHERER, RN, EdD Content related to the care of clients with respiratory dysfunction
- SANDRA E. SEFF, RN, PhD Content related to the care of women with reproductive dysfunction
- CONSTANCE A. SETTLEMYER, RN, PhD Content related to the care of clients with cardiovascular dysfunction
- BARBARA TOBIAS SHIRK, RN, MS Content related to obesity
- ANNE HERRSTROM SKELLY, RNC, MS Content related to the care of clients with endocrine dysfunction
- FRANCES L. STIER, RNC, MSN Content related to the care of clients with heart and blood vessel dysfunction
- DIANE WIND WARDELL, RNC, MS Content related to the care of women with reproductive dysfunction
- DEE WONCH, RN, MSN Content in the cancer chapter

We would also like to mention others who have helped significantly with *Essentials of Adult Health Nursing:*

- JANET REISS LEDERER, RN, MN and GAIL L. MARCULESCU, RN, MSN, co-authors of *Care Planning Pocket Guide: A Nursing Diagnosis Approach,* 2nd edition, provided invaluable assistance in keeping us current with the growing and changing concept of nursing diagnosis in our nursing process chapters and our nursing care plans.
- JOYCE M. BLACK, RN, MS provided valuable consultation in updating the cosmetic and reconstructive surgery section of the skin disorders chapter.
- BARBARA OOT-GIROMINI, RN, an enterostomal therapist at Lourdes Hospital in Binghamton, N.Y., developed the pressure ulcer care plan, Table 55–2.
- LINDA A. TOWNSEND, RN, of HomeMed, Mill Valley, CA; GAIL ZIMMERMAN, RN, of HomeMed, Los Angeles, CA; and JULIE LARSON, RN, of HomeMed, Menlo Park, CA; experts in home health care, contributed valuable and very specific information for nurses and for families on the care of acutely ill clients in the home.
- IRENE RUSSO, RN, MS spent endless hours working and reworking the Instructor's Manual and Test Bank for *Essentials of Adult Health Nursing,* for which we are eternally grateful.
- Special thanks to SANDY SHERER of Sherer Word Processing Service, Buffalo, NY for her enthusiasm, energy, and high quality work on this project.

We are grateful to all the nurses who reviewed and critiqued this manuscript. They are Eda Adams, Felicitas Alfaro, Lois Caldwell, Mary Chartier, Virgien Clark, Elaine Crabtree, Juanita Z. Flint, Sr. Ann Loretto Fraas, Judy Hammond, Christine Harper, Carolyn Harvey, Carol Haug, Cheryl Kieffer, Priscilla LeMone, Brenda Lyon, Maxine Mann, Toni McDonald, Janet R. Miller, Joan Paulson, Janet Pratt, Desma Reno, Laguita Showen, Kathleen Higgins Streckler, Martha Sullivan, Pamela L. Swearingen, Margaret Taylor, Elizabeth Wajdowicz, Judith Anne Walker, Elaine Gilligan Whelan, and Rose Wilcox.

Many wonderful people at Addison-Wesley were responsible for making *Essentials of Adult Health Nursing* a reality. We especially want to thank Nancy Evans and Anne Friedman who offered tremendous help, encouragement, and support throughout this project.

Our husbands and children, who have very busy lives of their own, put up with the aggravations a project such as this entails. So to our spouses, Steve Ames and Ed Kneisl; our daughters, Kevi Ames and Heidi Kneisl; and our sons, Greg Ames and Kyle Kneisl—we say thank you for being who you are and for hanging in there with us. You are the most important part of our lives.

SueAnn Wooster Ames
Carol Ren Kneisl

HOW TO USE THIS BOOK

We believe that the biopsychosocial approach of *Essentials of Adult Health Nursing* will prove uniquely effective in preparing nurses who will base their practice not only on clinical and pathophysiologic knowledge, but also on an understanding of the whole person and the nurse's role as health teacher and client advocate.

Essentials of Adult Health Nursing has been organized with readers' needs clearly in focus. Information is presented from unit to unit and from chapter to chapter in a systematic way so that readers will be able to easily find what they need.

The body system units, Units 3–13, are organized according to a specific pattern. The first chapter of each unit is divided into four sections, with general discussions covering the structural and functional interrelationships of the system in question, the pathophysiologic influences and effects, the related system influences and effects, and finally, psychosocial/lifestyle influences and effects.

The second chapter of each unit uses and examines the nursing process. The nursing assessments required in establishing a data base are discussed, including specific components of the health history, physical examination, and relevant diagnostic studies. The nursing diagnoses are then presented, followed by planning, implementation, and evaluation of related nursing care.

The following chapter(s) focus on the care of clients with specific health problems. Clinical disorders of multifactorial origin; degenerative, immunologic, infectious, neoplastic, or traumatic diseases are covered as relevant. For each disorder, the clinical manifestations, medical measures, and specific nursing measures are explained. Surgical management of specific health problems is included. For each surgical procedure, the implications for the client (physiologic and psychosocial/lifestyle), as well as the nursing implications, are discussed.

BODY SYSTEMS AND RELATED PATHOLOGIES

PLATE 1

The Circulatory System

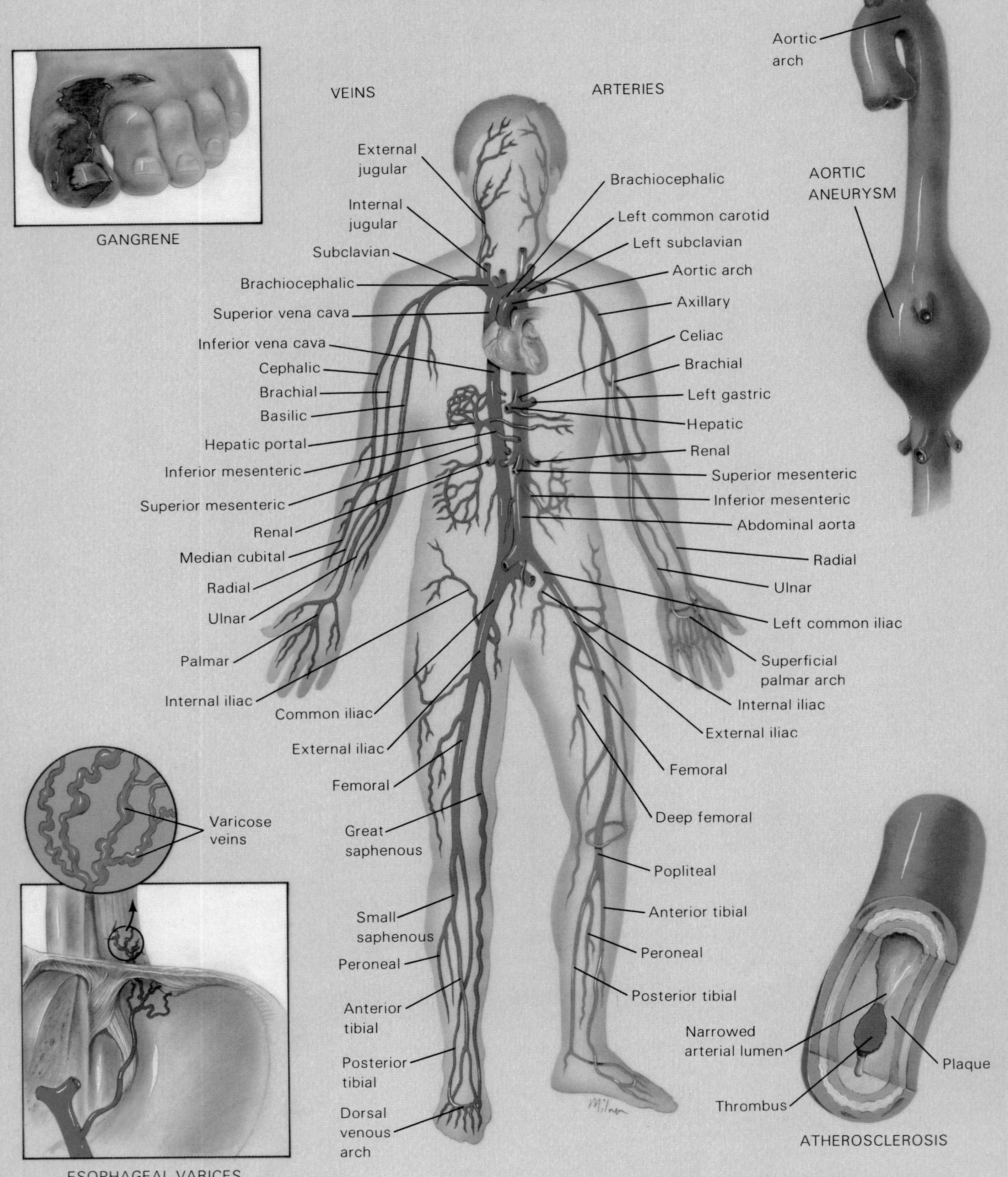
VEINS
ARTERIES
External jugular
Internal jugular
Subclavian
Brachiocephalic
Superior vena cava
Inferior vena cava
Cephalic
Brachial
Basilic
Hepatic portal
Inferior mesenteric
Superior mesenteric
Renal
Median cubital
Radial
Ulnar
Palmar
Internal iliac
Common iliac
External iliac
Femoral
Great saphenous
Small saphenous
Peroneal
Anterior tibial
Posterior tibial
Dorsal venous arch
Brachiocephalic
Left common carotid
Left subclavian
Aortic arch
Axillary
Celiac
Brachial
Left gastric
Hepatic
Renal
Superior mesenteric
Inferior mesenteric
Abdominal aorta
Radial
Ulnar
Left common iliac
Superficial palmar arch
Internal iliac
External iliac
Femoral
Deep femoral
Popliteal
Anterior tibial
Peroneal
Posterior tibial
Aortic arch
AORTIC ANEURYSM
Varicose veins
Narrowed arterial lumen
Plaque
Thrombus

GANGRENE

ESOPHAGEAL VARICES

ATHEROSCLEROSIS

PLATE 2

The Lymphatic System

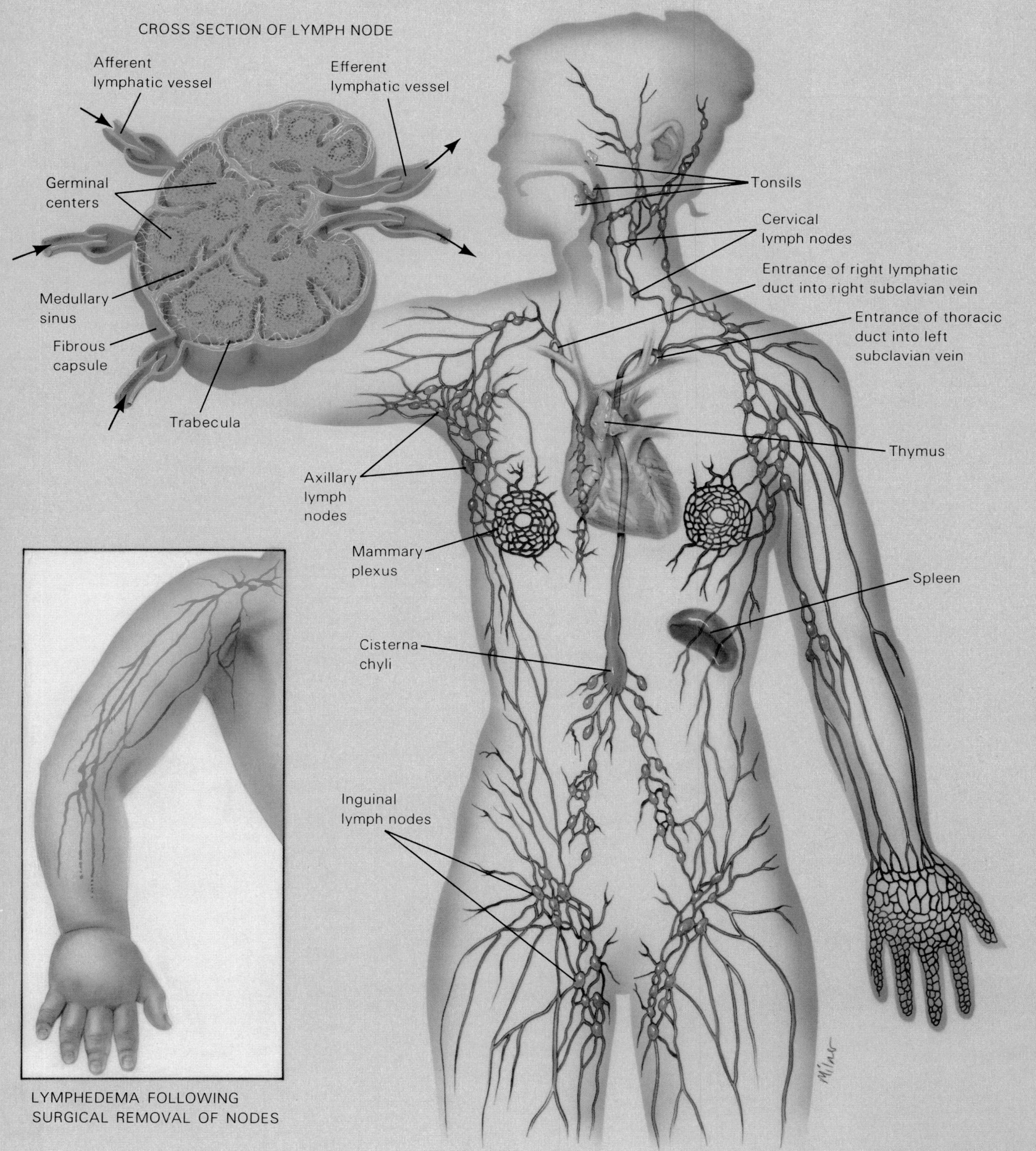

LYMPHEDEMA FOLLOWING SURGICAL REMOVAL OF NODES

PLATE 3

The Cardiovascular System

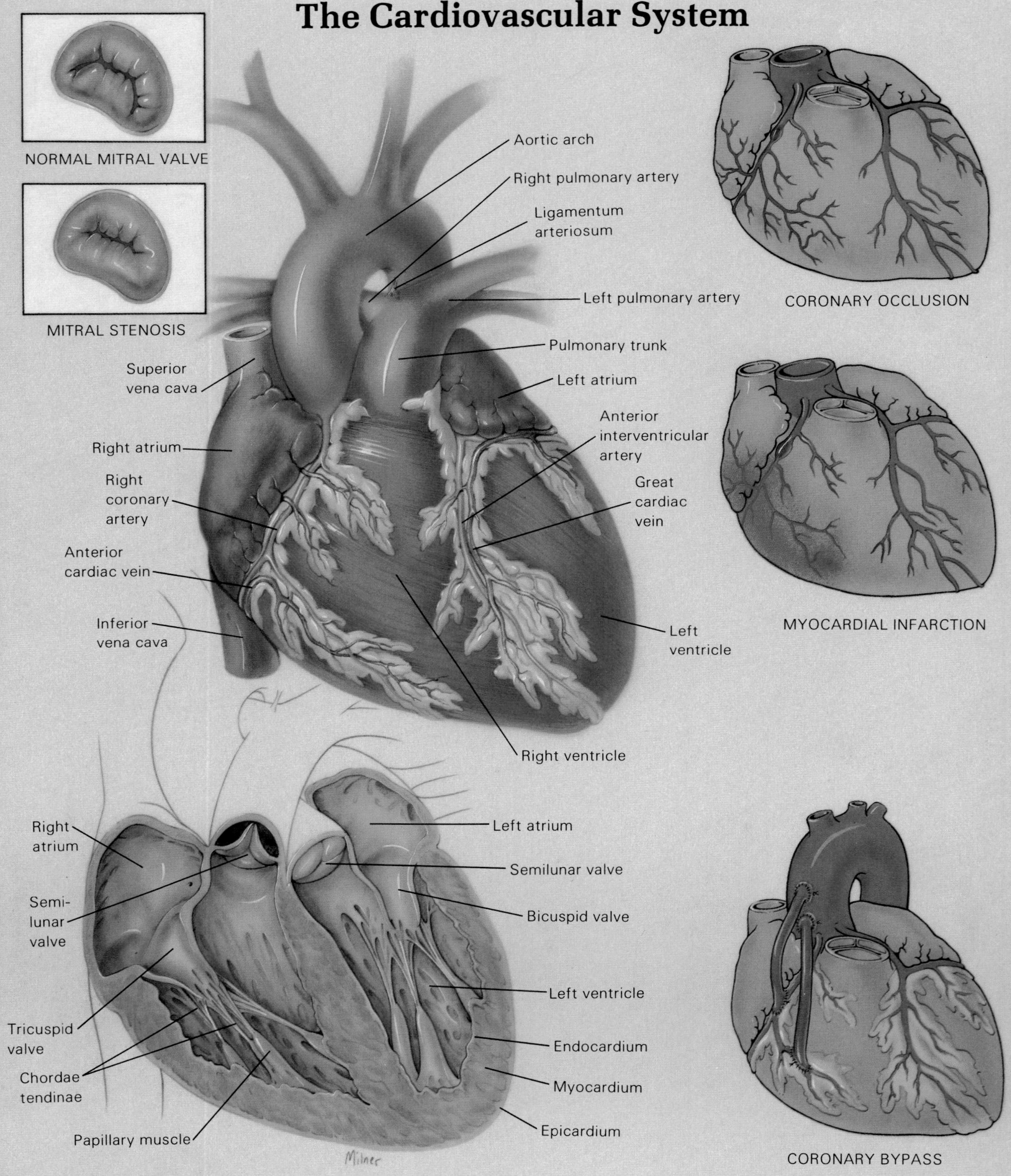
NORMAL MITRAL VALVE
MITRAL STENOSIS
Aortic arch
Right pulmonary artery
Ligamentum arteriosum
Left pulmonary artery
Pulmonary trunk
Superior vena cava
Left atrium
Anterior interventricular artery
Right atrium
Great cardiac vein
Right coronary artery
Anterior cardiac vein
Inferior vena cava
Left ventricle
Right ventricle
CORONARY OCCLUSION
MYOCARDIAL INFARCTION
Right atrium
Left atrium
Semilunar valve
Semi-lunar valve
Bicuspid valve
Left ventricle
Tricuspid valve
Endocardium
Chordae tendinae
Myocardium
Papillary muscle
Epicardium
Milner
CORONARY BYPASS

PLATE 4
The Respiratory System

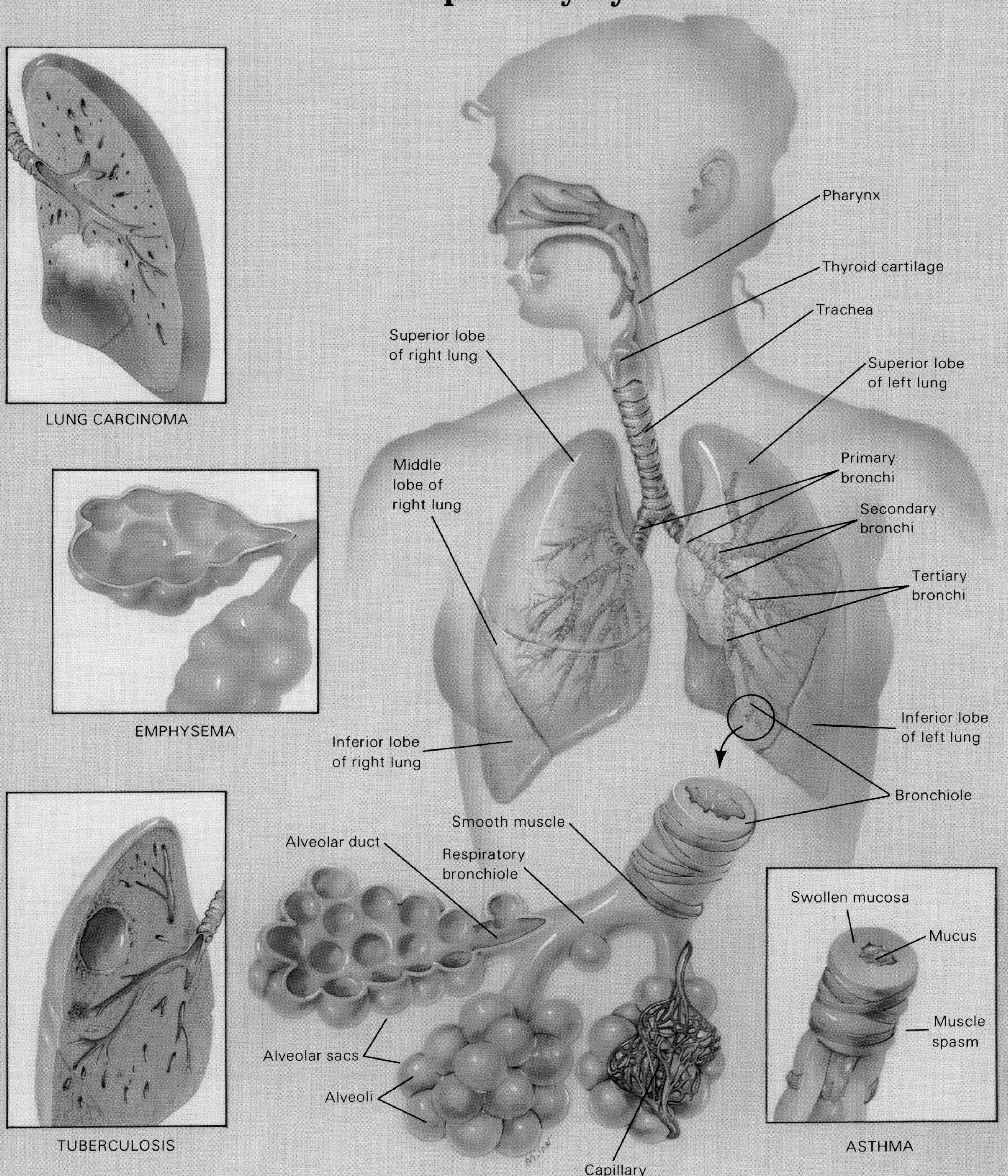

LUNG CARCINOMA

EMPHYSEMA

TUBERCULOSIS

ASTHMA

PLATE 5

The Digestive System

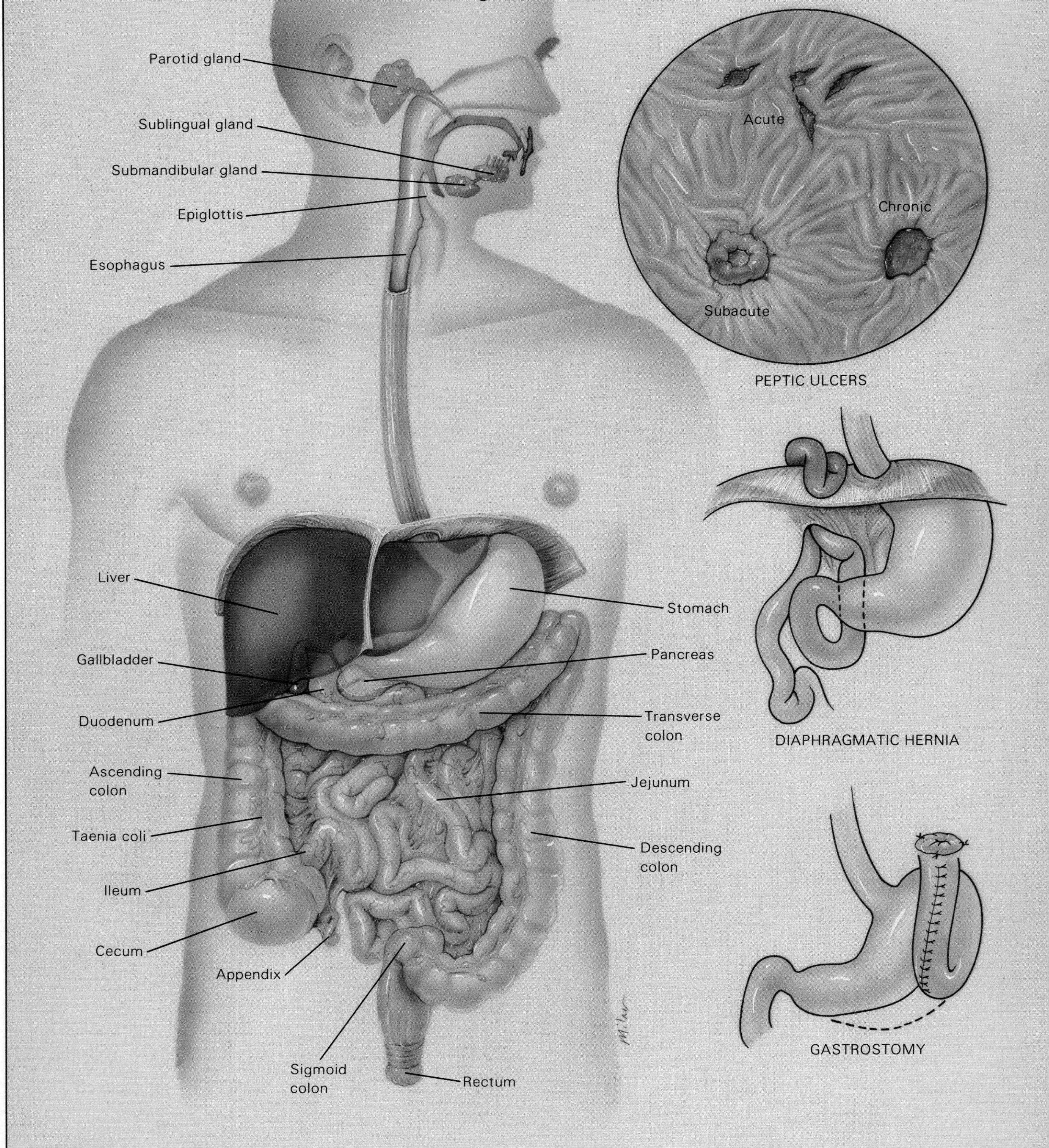

Parotid gland
Sublingual gland
Submandibular gland
Epiglottis
Esophagus
Liver
Gallbladder
Duodenum
Ascending colon
Taenia coli
Ileum
Cecum
Appendix
Sigmoid colon
Rectum
Stomach
Pancreas
Transverse colon
Jejunum
Descending colon

Acute
Chronic
Subacute

PEPTIC ULCERS

DIAPHRAGMATIC HERNIA

GASTROSTOMY

Miler

PLATE 6

Pathologies of the Digestive System

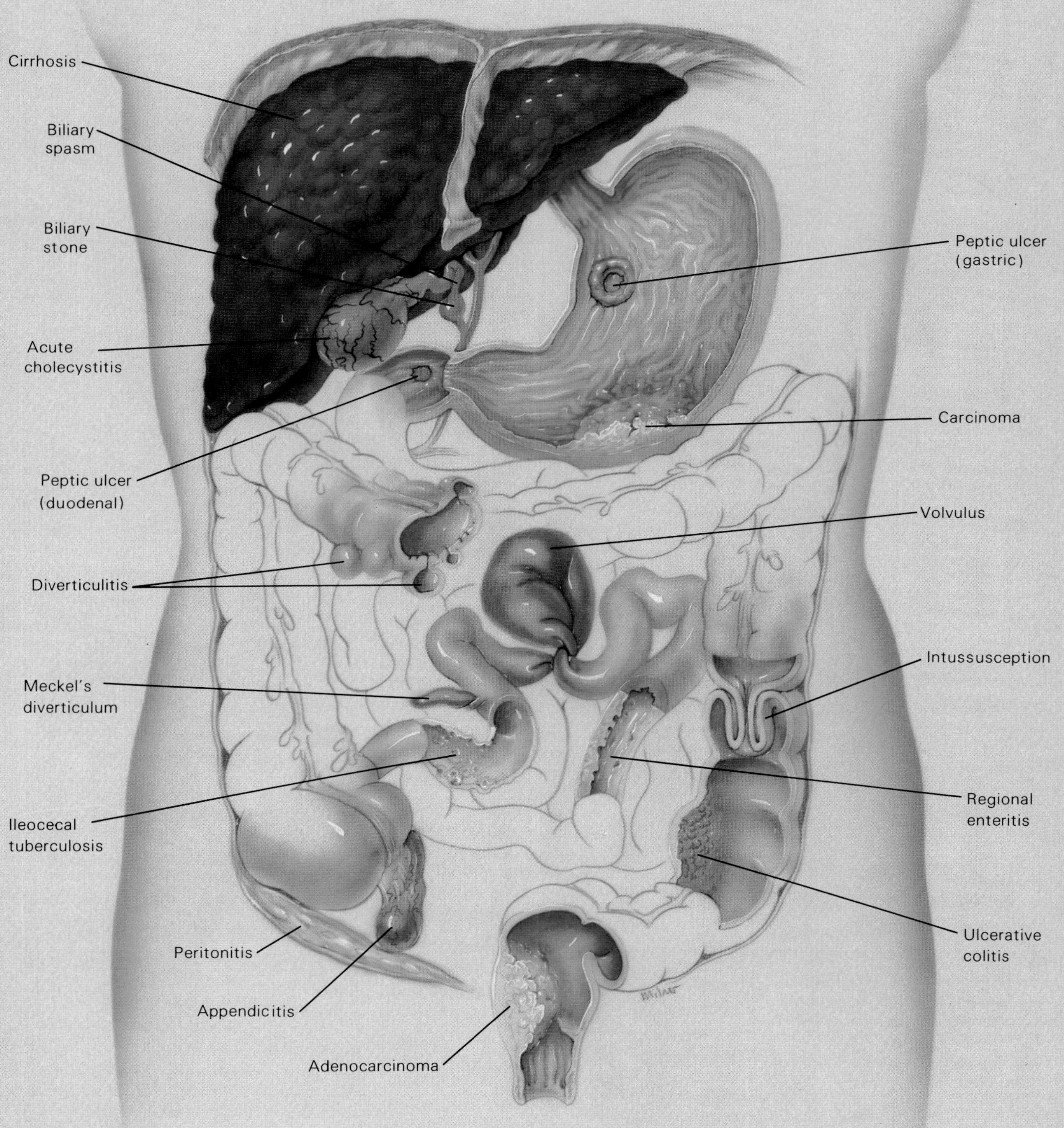

PLATE 7

The Urinary System

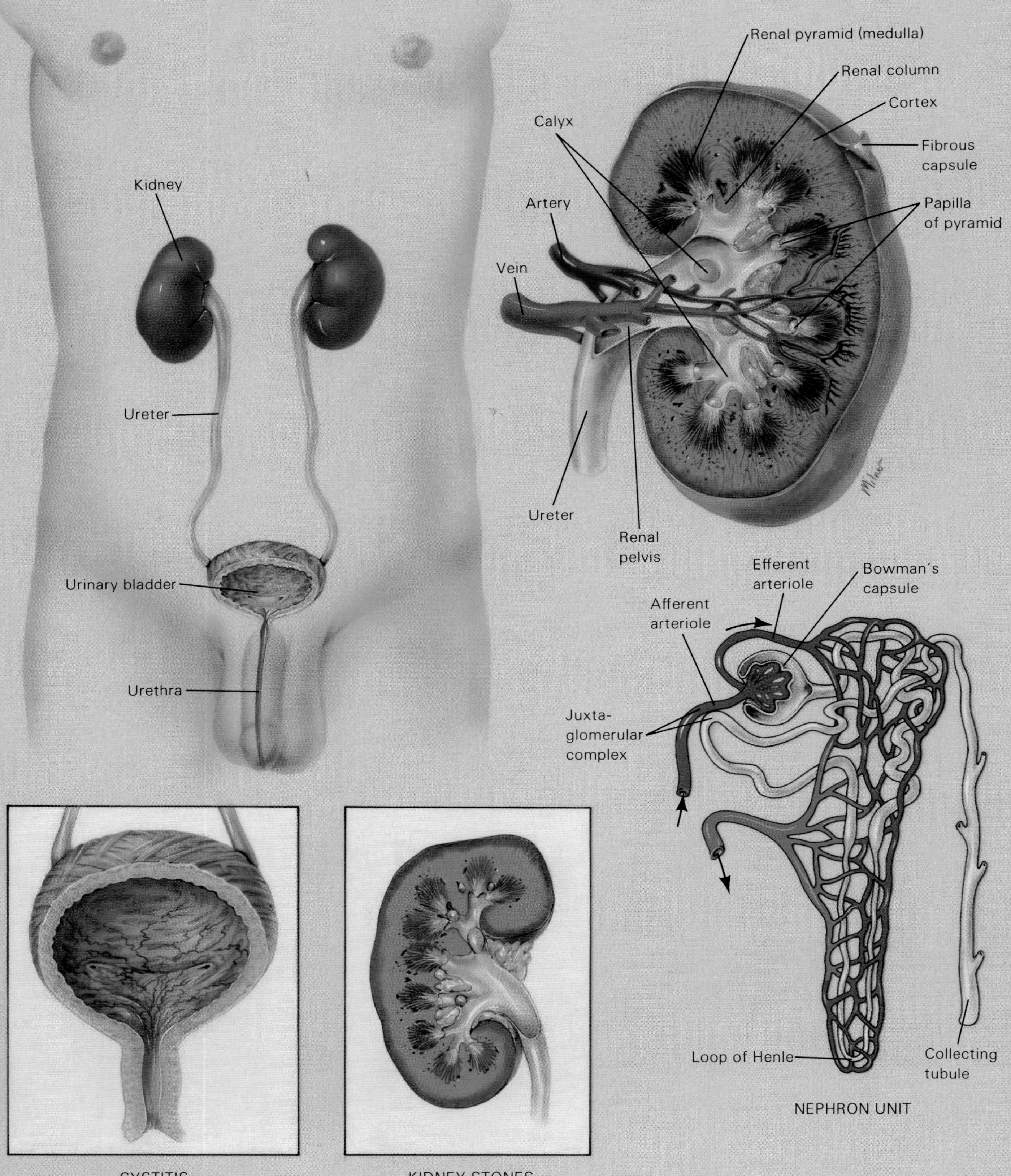

NEPHRON UNIT

CYSTITIS

KIDNEY STONES

PLATE 8

The Reproductive System

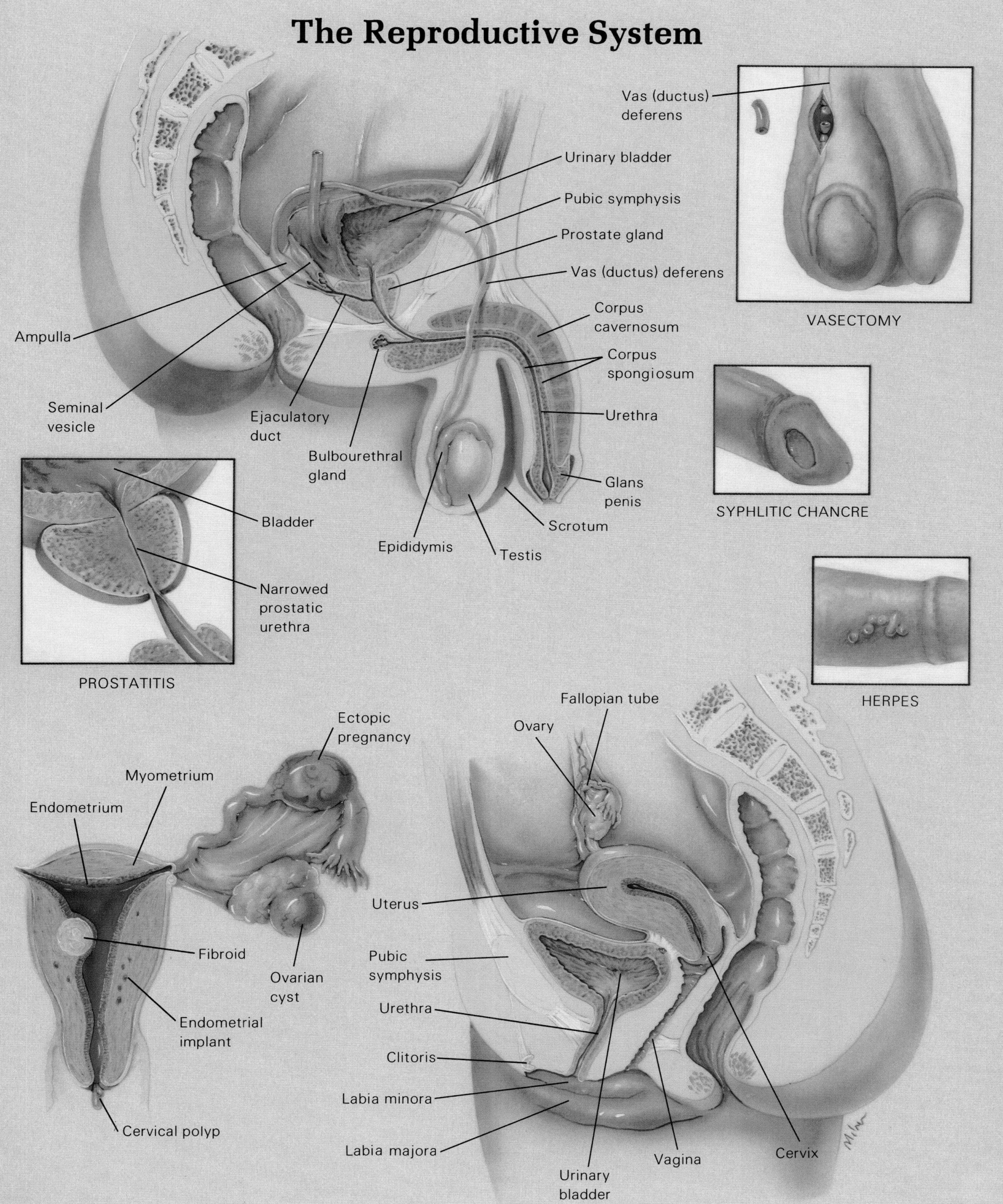

Vas (ductus) deferens
Urinary bladder
Pubic symphysis
Prostate gland
Vas (ductus) deferens
Corpus cavernosum
Corpus spongiosum
Urethra
Glans penis
Scrotum
Testis
Epididymis
Bulbourethral gland
Ejaculatory duct
Seminal vesicle
Ampulla
VASECTOMY
SYPHLITIC CHANCRE
HERPES
Bladder
Narrowed prostatic urethra
PROSTATITIS
Ectopic pregnancy
Myometrium
Endometrium
Fibroid
Ovarian cyst
Endometrial implant
Cervical polyp
Fallopian tube
Ovary
Uterus
Pubic symphysis
Urethra
Clitoris
Labia minora
Labia majora
Urinary bladder
Vagina
Cervix

PLATE 9

The Central Nervous System

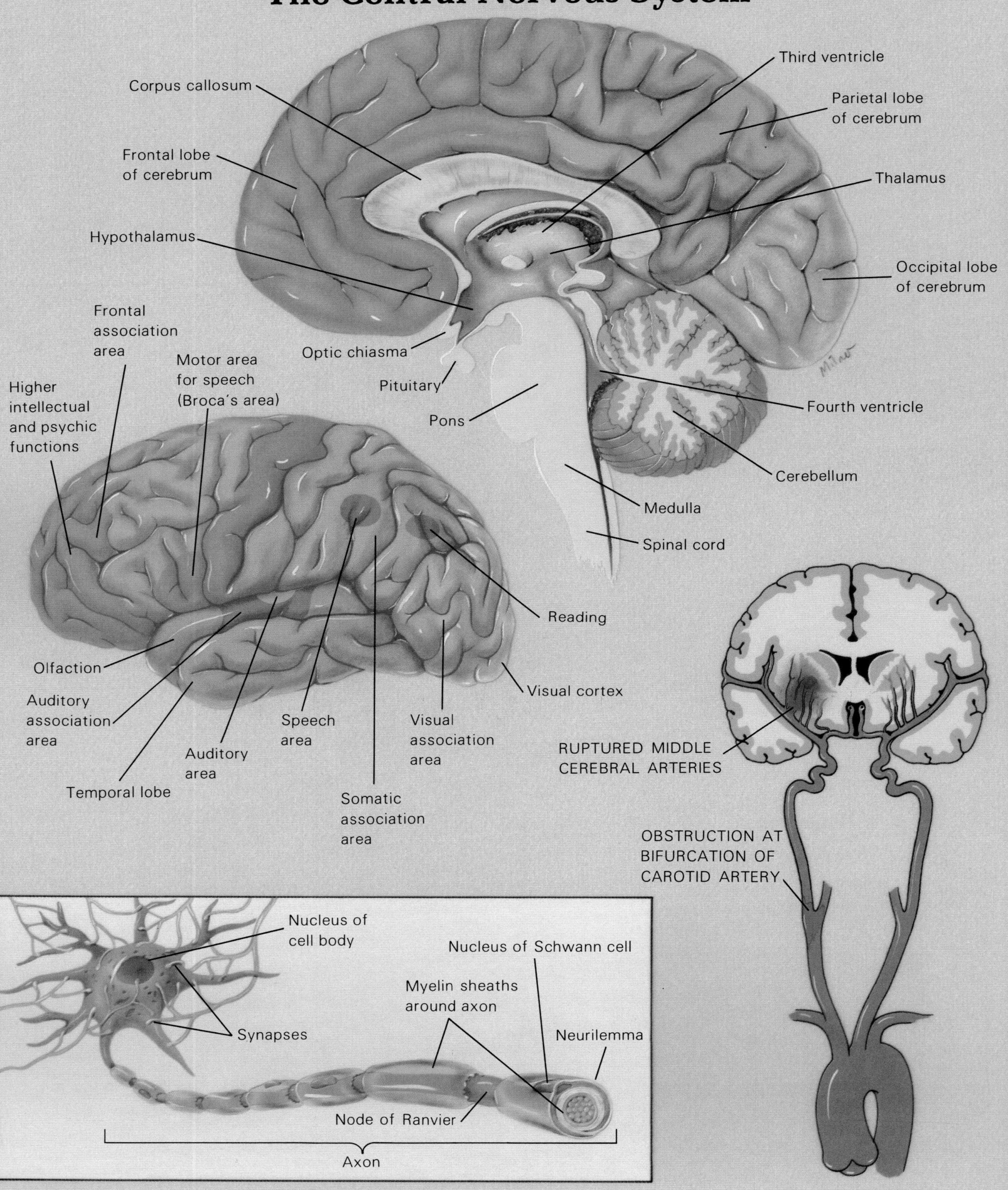
Third ventricle
Corpus callosum
Parietal lobe of cerebrum
Frontal lobe of cerebrum
Thalamus
Hypothalamus
Occipital lobe of cerebrum
Frontal association area
Optic chiasma
Motor area for speech (Broca's area)
Pituitary
Higher intellectual and psychic functions
Fourth ventricle
Pons
Cerebellum
Medulla
Spinal cord
Reading
Olfaction
Visual cortex
Auditory association area
Speech area
Visual association area
RUPTURED MIDDLE CEREBRAL ARTERIES
Auditory area
Temporal lobe
Somatic association area
OBSTRUCTION AT BIFURCATION OF CAROTID ARTERY
Nucleus of cell body
Nucleus of Schwann cell
Myelin sheaths around axon
Synapses
Neurilemma
Node of Ranvier
Axon

MOTOR NEURON

PLATE 10

The Autonomic Nervous System

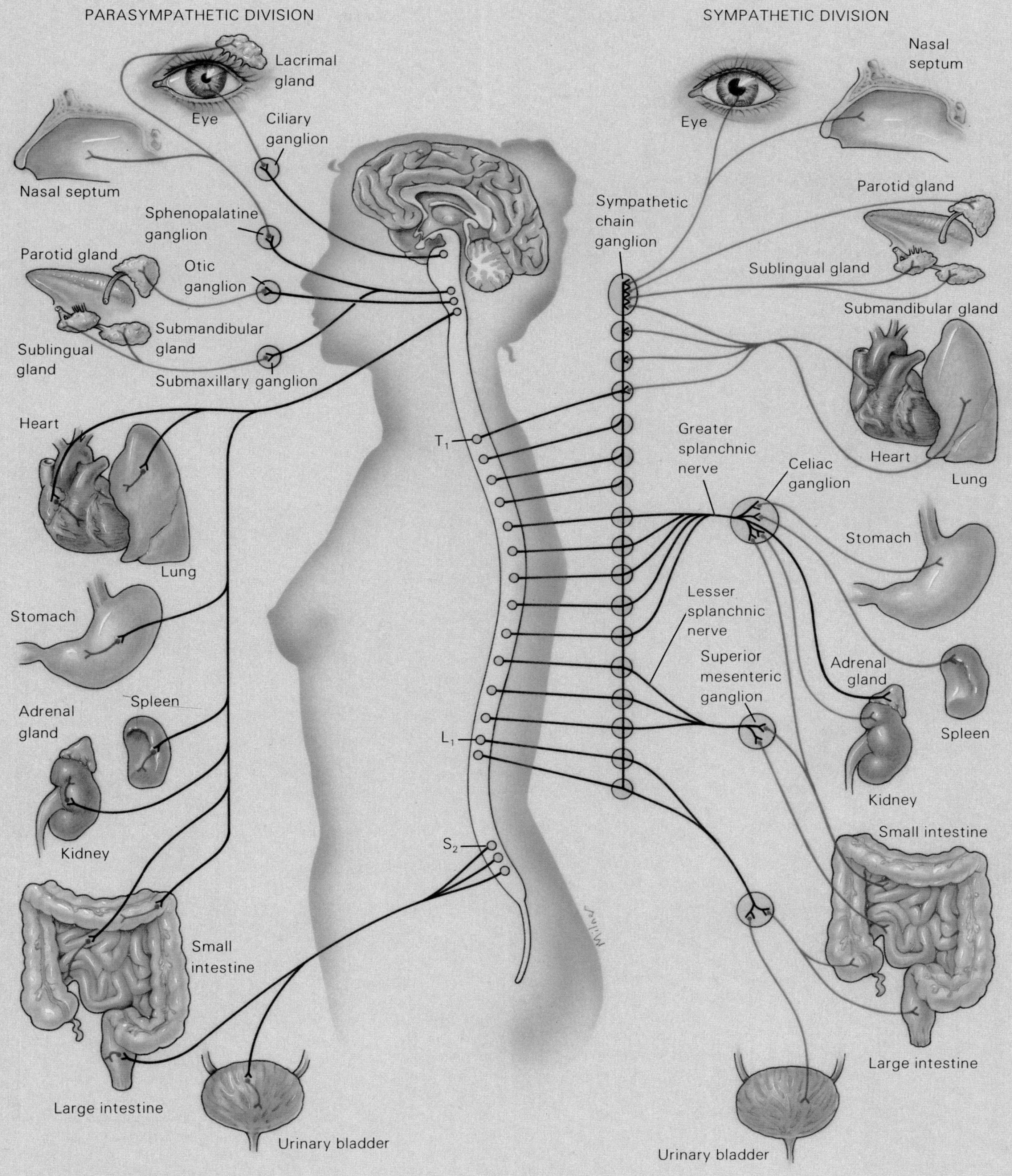

PLATE 11

The Skeletal System

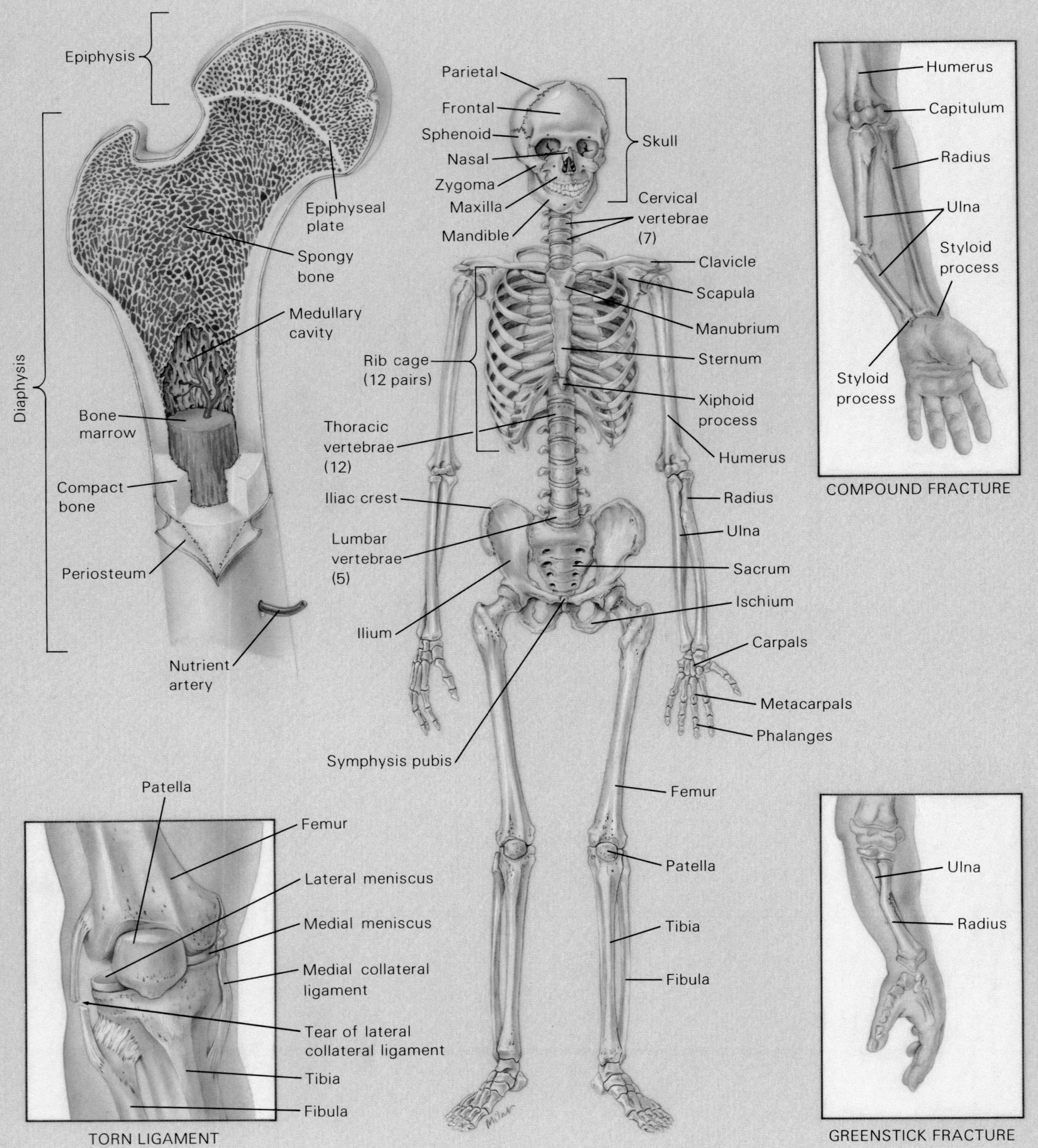
Epiphysis
Diaphysis
Epiphyseal plate
Spongy bone
Medullary cavity
Bone marrow
Compact bone
Periosteum
Nutrient artery
Parietal
Frontal
Sphenoid
Nasal
Zygoma
Maxilla
Mandible
Skull
Cervical vertebrae (7)
Clavicle
Scapula
Manubrium
Sternum
Xiphoid process
Rib cage (12 pairs)
Thoracic vertebrae (12)
Humerus
Radius
Ulna
Iliac crest
Lumbar vertebrae (5)
Sacrum
Ischium
Ilium
Carpals
Metacarpals
Phalanges
Symphysis pubis
Femur
Patella
Tibia
Fibula
Humerus
Capitulum
Radius
Ulna
Styloid process
Styloid process
COMPOUND FRACTURE
Patella
Femur
Lateral meniscus
Medial meniscus
Medial collateral ligament
Tear of lateral collateral ligament
Tibia
Fibula
TORN LIGAMENT
Ulna
Radius
GREENSTICK FRACTURE

PLATE 12

Pathologies of the Skeletal System

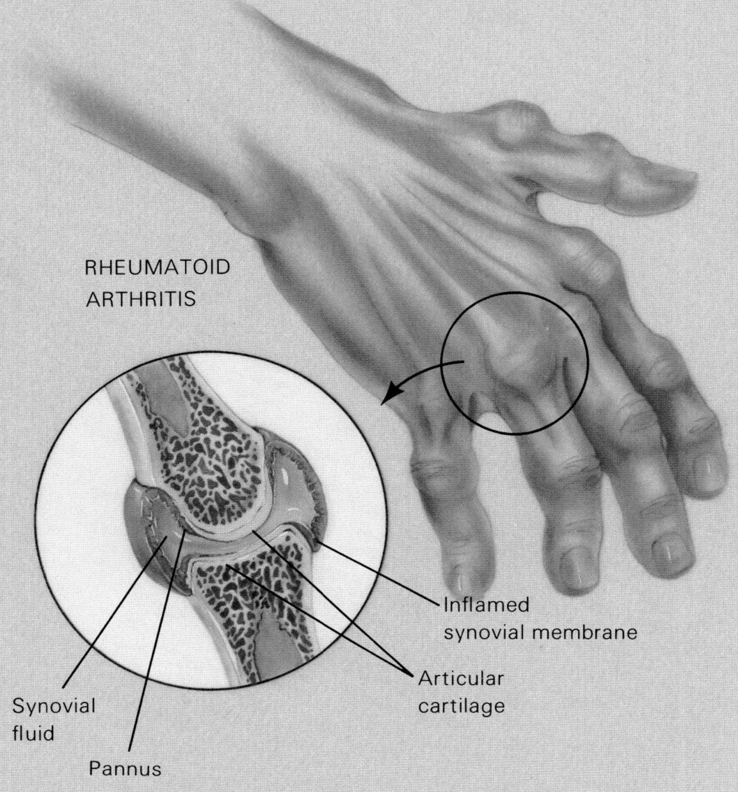

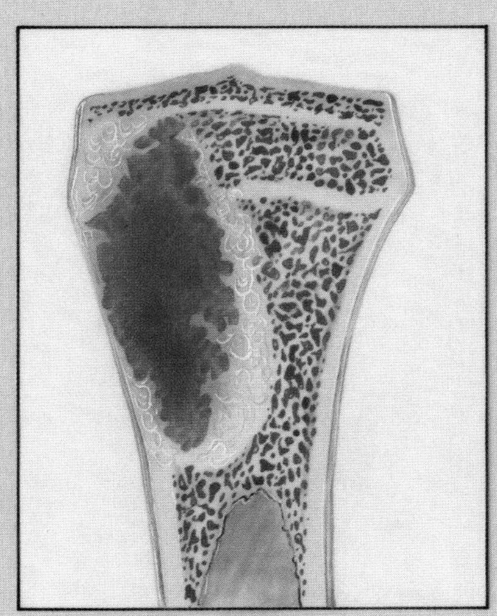

BONE CANCER

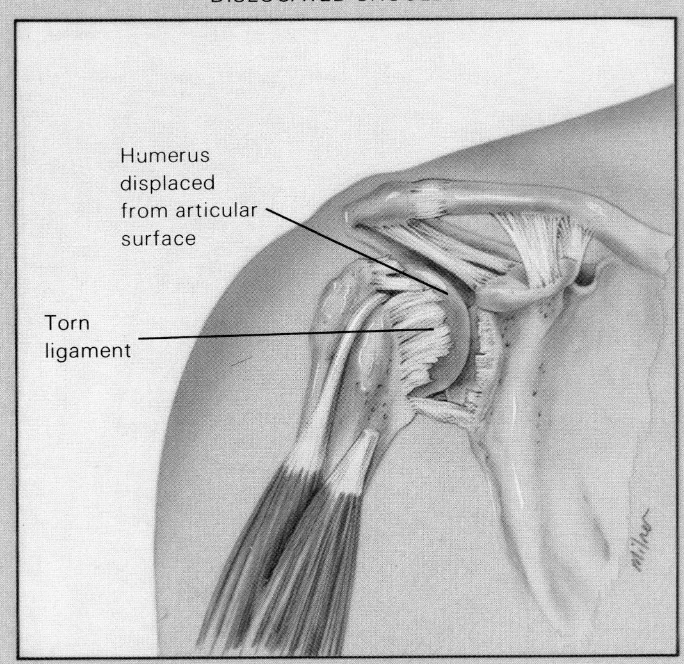

DISLOCATED SHOULDER

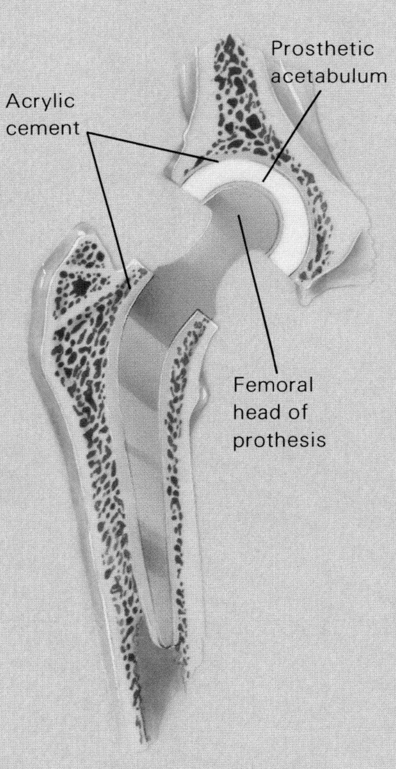

HIP REPLACEMENT

PLATE 13

The Muscular System

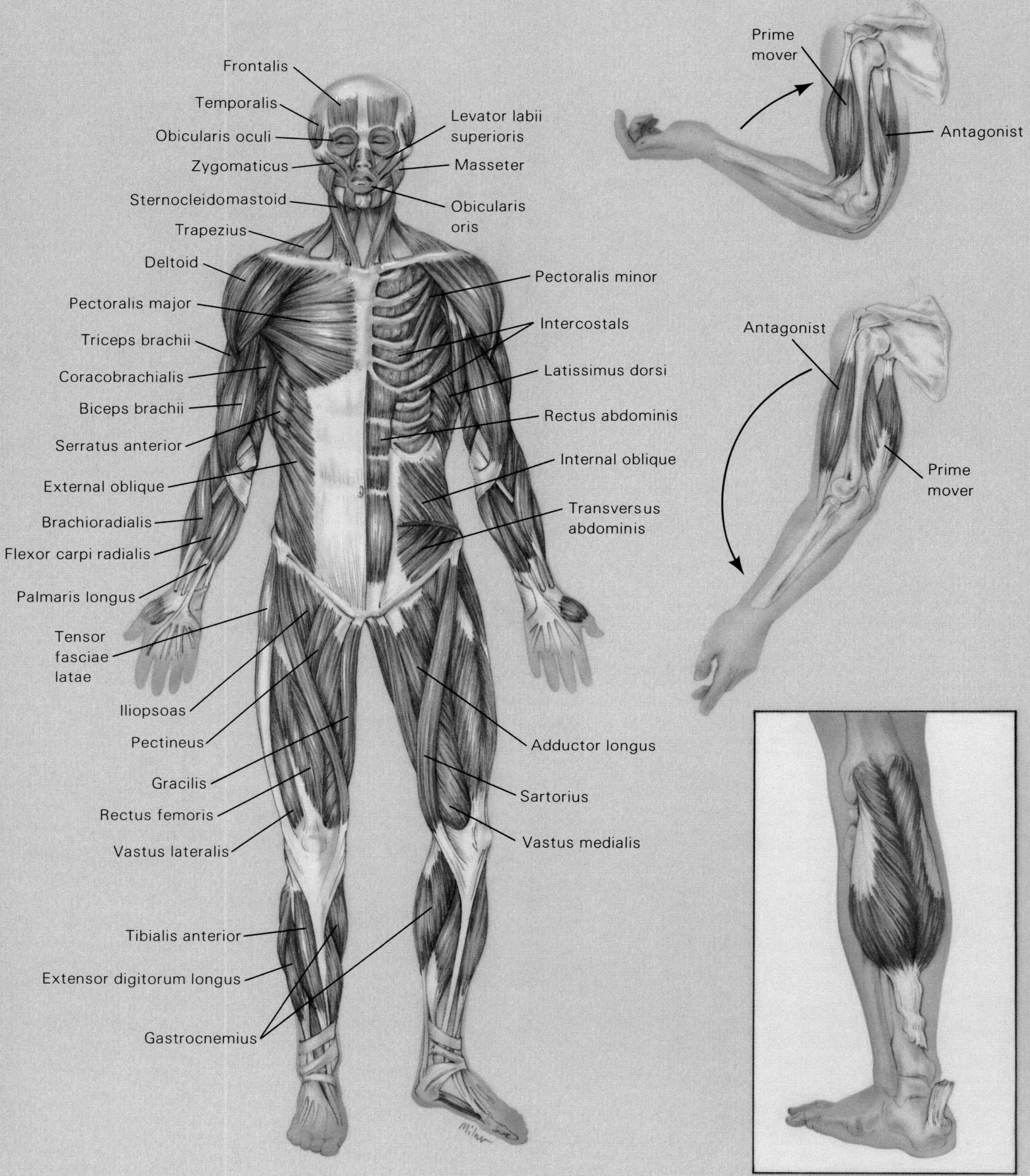
MUSCLE ACTIONS
Prime mover
Antagonist
Antagonist
Prime mover
Frontalis
Temporalis
Obicularis oculi
Zygomaticus
Sternocleidomastoid
Trapezius
Deltoid
Pectoralis major
Triceps brachii
Coracobrachialis
Biceps brachii
Serratus anterior
External oblique
Brachioradialis
Flexor carpi radialis
Palmaris longus
Tensor fasciae latae
Iliopsoas
Pectineus
Gracilis
Rectus femoris
Vastus lateralis
Tibialis anterior
Extensor digitorum longus
Gastrocnemius
Levator labii superioris
Masseter
Obicularis oris
Pectoralis minor
Intercostals
Latissimus dorsi
Rectus abdominis
Internal oblique
Transversus abdominis
Adductor longus
Sartorius
Vastus medialis

ACHILLES TENDON TEAR

PLATE 14

The Integumentary System

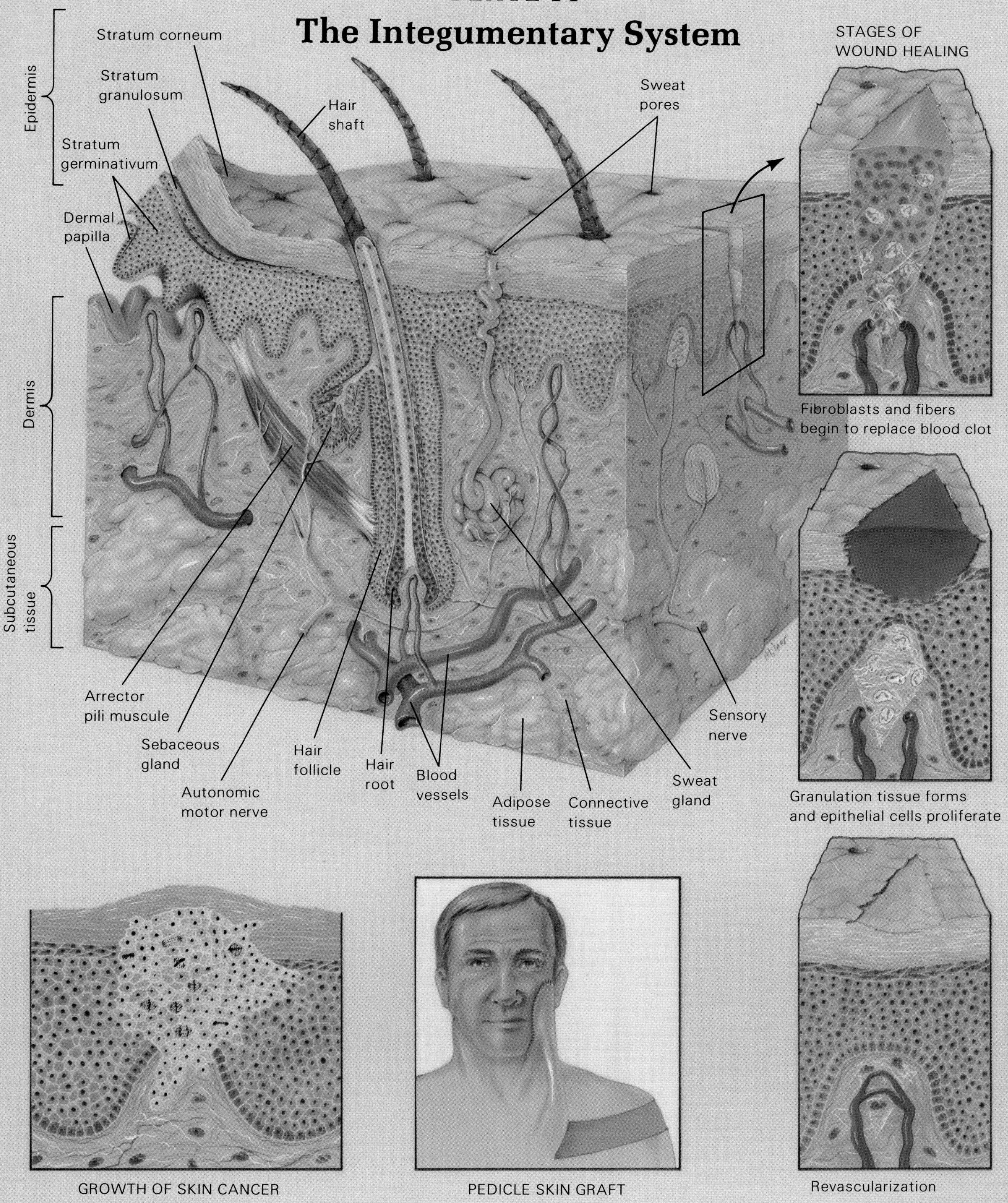

Epidermis
Stratum corneum
Stratum granulosum
Stratum germinativum
Dermal papilla
Dermis
Subcutaneous tissue
Hair shaft
Sweat pores
Arrector pili muscule
Sebaceous gland
Autonomic motor nerve
Hair follicle
Hair root
Blood vessels
Adipose tissue
Connective tissue
Sweat gland
Sensory nerve
STAGES OF WOUND HEALING
Fibroblasts and fibers begin to replace blood clot
Granulation tissue forms and epithelial cells proliferate
Revascularization
GROWTH OF SKIN CANCER
PEDICLE SKIN GRAFT

PLATE 15

The Eye and the Ear

Canal of Schlemm
Choroid
Sclera
Retina
Blood vessels
Optic nerve
Conjunctiva
Optic disc
Cornea
Macula
Pupil
Suspensory ligaments
Lens
Ciliary muscles
Iris
Ora serrata
Flow of vitreous through tear in retina
DETACHED RETINA
Blocked exit for drainage of aqueous humor
Increased intraocular pressure
GLAUCOMA

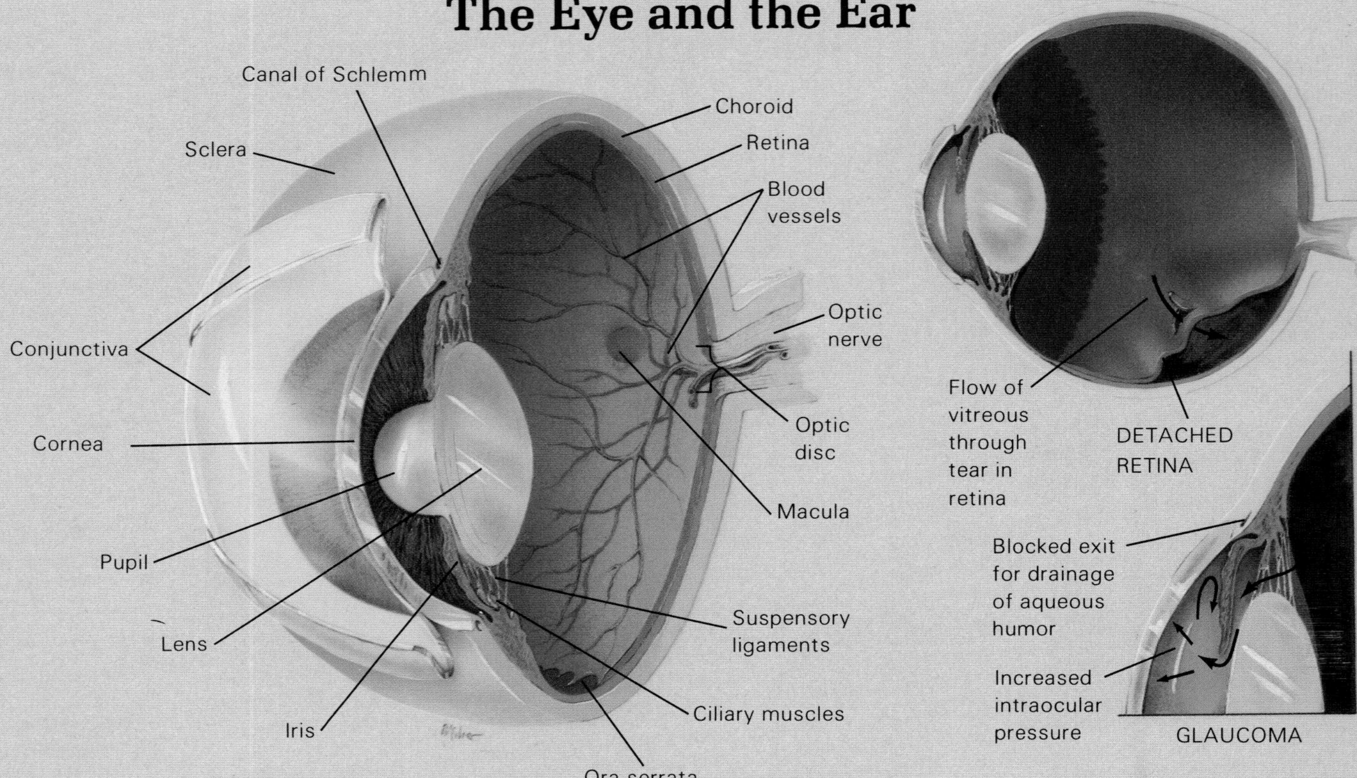

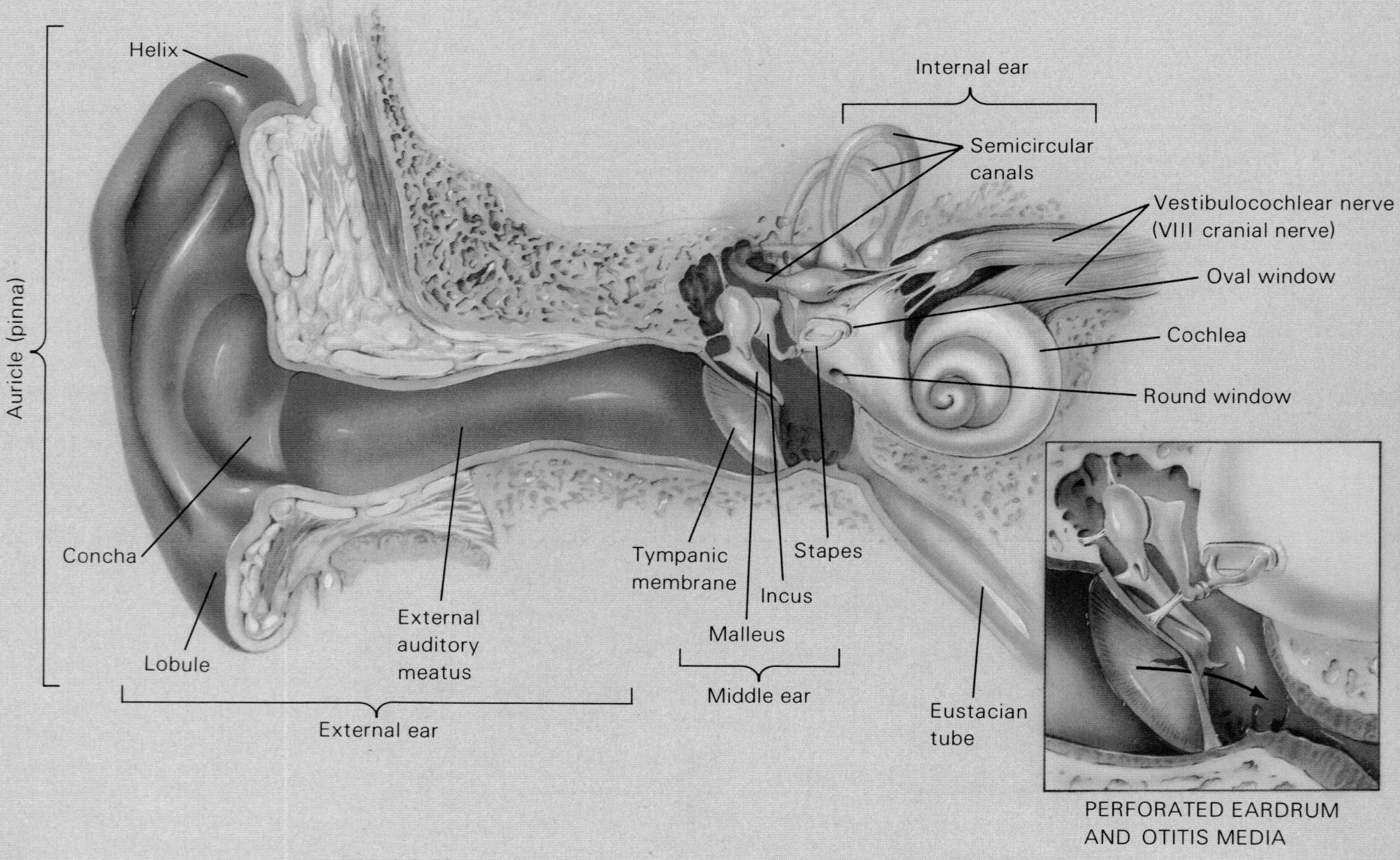

Helix
Internal ear
Semicircular canals
Vestibulocochlear nerve (VIII cranial nerve)
Oval window
Auricle (pinna)
Cochlea
Round window
Concha
Tympanic membrane
Stapes
Incus
Malleus
External auditory meatus
Lobule
Middle ear
External ear
Eustacian tube
PERFORATED EARDRUM AND OTITIS MEDIA

UNIT

1

The Shared Experience of Health and Illness

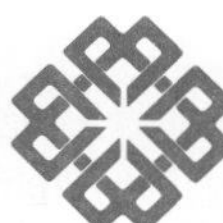

CHAPTER 1

Changing Health Care in a Changing Society

Objectives

When you have finished studying this chapter, you should be able to:

Describe the effects of changes in family structure, life expectancy, environment, values, cultural diversity, and health patterns on health care.

Delineate the economic factors responsible for spiraling health care costs.

Discuss the technologic developments affecting health care.

Identify the changing patterns of health and their effects on the focus of health care.

Compare lifestyles favorable to health with lifestyles unfavorable to health.

Differentiate among primary, secondary, and tertiary health care.

Explore the personal responsibility of each individual in maintaining health.

Advocate risk-reducing lifestyle modification and increased health consciousness.

Describe the nursing role in activating clients to take steps to protect and maintain their own health.

Explain the importance of the nursing process and nursing research in clinical nursing practice.

Transplants, implants, artificial organs, laser surgery, birthing rooms, trauma centers, hospices—health care continually changes and is changed by practices of birth, life, and death. Because all change is stressful, changes in lifestyles, economics, technology, and values affect health. Meeting the challenge of caring in the computer age means understanding not only sociologic, economic, and technologic changes as well as changing patterns of health, but also how they affect the health care consumer, the health care system, and the roles and responsibilities of nurses.

SECTION 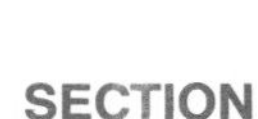

Social Change and Health Care

Sociologic Changes

During the second half of the twentieth century, many aspects of society have undergone dramatic and rapid change. Family structure, life expectancy, environment, values, cultural diversity, and health patterns have all been affected.

Family Structure

The character and mobility of the American family have changed markedly during the past three decades. For many years, the family provided care, stability, and support for its members in both health and illness. Families lived in the same geographic area for generations. Today, 17% of Americans move every year (Louis Harris, 1982). Reliance on the extended family for support and help is not always possible. In 1982, married couples were only 59% of total households, a decrease of 12% since 1970. Couples who marry may choose to remain childless or to delay first pregnancy until the wife is past 30.

Divorce and greater acceptance of children born outside marriage have led to an increase in the number of single-parent families. More than 9 million families (11% of all households) are headed by women, an increase of 72% since 1970. A serious illness and hospitalization could create major financial and logistical problems for a single mother unless she has family or friends available to help.

In many parts of North America, the number of homosexual couples is increasing. Generally, the health care system does not acknowledge these or other nontraditional relationships as legitimate, recognizing only the rights of "immediate family," even though the partner may be the most important "significant other" to the ill person.

In the midst of this affluent society, in which a higher standard of living is potentially health-promoting, homelessness is epidemic. More Americans are homeless than at any point since the Great Depression of the 1930s. Some are welfare mothers who have been evicted from tenement rooms. Many are former mental hospital clients who, after release from the institution, have fallen through the cracks of an inadequate system of follow-up and become society's rejects. At least 20% of the homeless are over age 65. Although much media attention has been focused on the plight of the homeless, only short-term solutions to the problem have been proposed, such as food and shelter.

Life Expectancy

Nearly 80% of all babies born will live to be old. There are now more Americans over 65 than there are teenagers. This growing population of persons over 65—more than 27 million—presents one of the greatest health care challenges. Of the $1 billion America spends each day on health care, more than 30% is allocated to meet the needs of this group. Chronic illness such as arthritis, impairments in hearing and vision, hypertension, and cardiovascular problems, is a fact of life for more than 85% of persons over age 65. Their chronic physical problems may be combined with loneliness and depression, conditions that can lead to poor nutrition or excessive use of alcohol or other drugs. Poor nutrition can also result from living on a fixed income in an age of inflation and can lead, in turn, to a myriad of other health problems. Because female life expectancy exceeds that of males, a majority of these older persons are women, often widows.

The fastest growing segment of the population is the group over age 85, the *oldest old,* also referred to as the *frail elderly.* Now numbering more than 2.6 million, this group is expected to increase to 5 million by the year 2000. As their numbers increase, the oldest old will find health care a growing financial burden.

It is important to remember that persons over age 65 are a diverse group emotionally, physically, behaviorally, economically, socially, and politically. Only 5% are institutionalized because of health problems. Even in the oldest old, many persons work and live independently.

Life expectancy also reflects health problems and how they are dealt with. Among blacks, life expectancy is 69.3 years, 6 years less than for whites. Black infant mortality in 1983 was 22.1 deaths per 1000 live births, almost double the rate for whites. These differences reflect, at least in part, differences in income, nutrition, and health education plus limited access to health care.

Environment

Since the 1950s, awareness has grown of the air and water pollution that threatens life and health throughout the world. Industrial and agricultural wastes have found their way into the water supply of many communities. Families in such communities may experience an unusually high number of infertility problems, spontaneous abortions, birth defects, malignancies, and neurologic disorders. Many cities publish a daily *air quality index* so persons with respiratory complications will know whether the outside air is safe to breathe.

On a less spectacular but equally dangerous level, the daily hazards of the work environment require further research to arrive at definitive answers about their effects. Black lung in coal miners, brown lung in textile workers, and asbestosis in construction workers have been acknowledged as occupationally related disorders. Other potential hazards in the work environment include anesthetic gases, video display terminals (VDTs), airport security machines, and other radiation-emitting devices.

Values

The uncertainty of living in a nuclear age seems to have altered the emphasis in society from living carefully and planning for the future to living for the present and experiencing as much as possible in the time allotted. This emphasis on the experience-packed present, plus the stresses of modern life, has fostered escapism. Escapism is made easier by mobility and relative affluence.

More liberal attitudes about sex have led to increased promiscuity and, with it, the problems of sexually transmitted diseases (STD), now second in incidence only to the common cold. Another outcome of escapism is the growing use of mood-altering drugs, including alcohol. One of the most popular recreational drugs is cocaine, second only to marijuana in its widespread use. Despite its devastating effects on health and life, cocaine continues to attract new users, as does alcohol.

Culture

Long considered a cultural "melting pot," the United States continues to attract immigrants from all over the world. The 1980 census showed more than 77% of the United States population as white; the remainder is grouped as follows: blacks, 12%; Hispanics, 6%; American Indians, Eskimos, Aleuts, Asians, and Pacific Islanders, 5% (Spain, 1983). Each group has its own beliefs and values that may differ markedly from those of the dominant white culture. Recent immigrants to North America, particularly those from developing countries, experience a kind of culture shock when they are thrust into the high-tech health care system. Culture determines how illness and health are perceived and therefore how they are thought to exist, what causes illness, how it should be diagnosed, what symptoms of illness are, how it should be treated, and who should do the treating. This perception may be the basis for decisions about where health care will be sought, and even if health care will be sought. Suggestions for incorporating cultural values are in Chapter 5.

Economic Changes

Economic factors are playing an increasingly important role in modern life. The growing incidence of poverty plus escalating health care costs are creating a revolution in the health care system.

Poverty and Health

Poverty goes hand in hand with health problems, an increased need for health services, and an inability to pay for them. Persons living below the poverty level often do not have health insurance or a regular source of health care, either because of their financial problems or lack of information. An example of poverty's impact on health is the disproportionately high number of black males who die from lung cancer each year even though they smoke at about the same rate as white males. Cooper and Simmons (1985) attribute the difference to occupational hazards and various consequences of poverty.

Health Care Economics

Health care is big business, the second largest industry in the United States, exceeded in size only by the automotive industry. America spends $1 billion a day on health care and the price is going up. During the two decades between 1965 and 1985, medical care costs increased more than 429%, an increase far above the general rate of economic inflation. Four fundamental factors that have been responsible for this tremendous increase are: inflation, improved and costly techniques and technologies, an increase in the number of persons who use health services, the way in which physicians and hospitals have been paid (Lee, Estes, & Ramsay, 1984).

Until recently, hospitals were reimbursed according to their costs. Insurers have traditionally paid a large percentage of those charges, no matter how high. In an effort to stem the upward spiral of health care costs, Congress passed prospective payment legislation in 1983 to limit the amount paid to hospitals by Medicare. This legislation uses a classification system known as diagnosis-related groups (DRGs). Hospitals are paid a predetermined amount for a client with a given medical diagnosis rather than being reimbursed for the cost of services. This system has forced hospitals to take steps to reduce the cost of client care. Savings from this new system of hospital payment are projected at $20.4 billion by 1988 (Coleman, Dayani, & Simms, 1984).

Among the effects of this prospective payment system on client care is earlier discharge of clients (which also means greater need for nursing care at home, creating a surge in home care agencies), reduction of services, and reduction of staff, particularly LPN/LVN staff and nurse's aides. Many hospitals are changing to all-RN staffs, nurses able to deliver the broadest range of care.

The DRG system has caused concern among health professionals that the quality of care will be sacrificed for the sake of cost reduction. A study by Sovie and colleagues (1985) showed that professional nursing care (using a staff composed of 92% RNs) is both safe and cost effective. Many nursing leaders think that the prospective payment system is an opportunity to demonstrate the importance of nursing care and its cost effectiveness.

Technologic Changes

Health care today is *high tech* and *high ticket.* Modern technology makes it possible to medicate, monitor, and maintain most body functions for extended periods with little human intervention. In this atmosphere, care can become routine and depersonalized unless it is also *high touch.* The same technology that saves lives also raises questions about the quality of lives saved. What is the quality of a solitary, pain-filled life? In human terms, what purpose is served by such a delay if the remaining life is without reasonable freedom, comfort, or dignity? Questions such as this will arise more frequently as technology increases in sophistication.

Improved technology and growing clinical knowledge have provided another source for chronic health problems. Persons with disorders such as cerebral palsy or cystic fibrosis who would not have lived beyond adolescence in the 1940s have received treatment sufficient for survival into adulthood. Early diagnosis and more effective treatment have meant cancer is not always a terminal diagnosis. Hundreds of thousands of persons are living reasonably normal lives despite surgery to remove a malignancy of the colon, larynx, or breast.

For more than two decades, the skilled technology of newborn intensive care units has kept alive severely compromised premature infants, many of whom survive with moderate to severe central nervous system damage and other chronic problems. The long-term sociologic and economic effects of this technology are unknown and will be difficult to measure.

Computers

Modern health facilities are highly computerized; from accounting to intensive care, information is managed by computer. These sophisticated systems are part of the life support equipment that sustains the critically ill when they cannot sustain themselves. Computers are literally the heart of pacemakers, the commonplace devices that regulate the pulses of thousands of Americans.

Transplants

New developments in pharmacologic and bioengineering technology have offered new hope to persons who can benefit from an organ transplant or an artificial implant. Transplant surgery is now possible to replace the pancreas, heart, lungs, veins, pituitary gland, kidneys, liver, cornea, and bone marrow.

Although increasingly common, transplant surgery is still high in risk and some transplant surgeries can cost in excess of $200,000. Though many insurance companies do cover these costs, others consider transplant surgery to be experimental and not generally accepted.

Shortage of donor organs continues. New laws in some states require hospitals to ask the families of all deceased clients for organ donations. The intent of the law is to provide support for physicians in requesting organ donation, so they will not be perceived by families as insensitive toward the death of their loved ones. Sponsors of this law also hope it will make more hearts, livers, and kidneys available

Implants

Far more common than transplant surgery, implant surgery to replace damaged body parts is highly sophisticated. Approximately 900,000 intraocular lens implants are performed each year (American Intraocular Implant Society, 1985). Replacement of joints damaged by arthritis with plastic or metal prostheses has brought increased mobility and pain relief to hundreds of thousands since the early 1960s. Pacemakers, another kind of implant, can now transmit information to physicians by home-based monitoring systems.

Home-Based Technology

As hospital cost cutting pushes health care back into the home, and as individuals assume greater responsibility for their own health, home-based technology is certain to follow. Already, many homes have apnea monitors for infants at risk for sudden infant death syndrome. Persons with diabetes are using insulin pumps and performing blood glucose testing at home. Bioengineering experts are working to simplify the operation of medical instrumentation and the reading of basic laboratory results at home.

SECTION 

Changing Patterns of Health

Patterns of health and disease change over time. Diseases that once decimated whole populations (eg, bubonic plague) may become so rare that a modern health professional in the United States or Canada would scarcely recognize their symptoms. It is highly unlikely that the typical American health professional of today has ever seen a client with typhoid fever—a disease that regularly reached epidemic proportions only 50 years ago. Among the US population in the last few decades, the relative importance of specific causes of death has shifted significantly.

Shifts in Leading Causes of Death

Some diseases that were major killers in 1900 no longer rank as fatal: gastroenteritis (once ranked third), chronic nephritis (once ranked sixth), and diphtheria (once ranked tenth). Tuberculosis, the second leading cause of disease in 1900, now ranks 19th.

Conversely, some diseases have gained in importance. The death rate for malignancies is nearly three times that for 1900, and cardiovascular disease, once ranked fourth, now ranks first. Changing lifestyle patterns doubtless affect specific causes within the more general categories: the "all accidents" category for 1900 had virtually no automobile fatalities; the current situation is quite different.

The leading three causes of death in 1900—influenza and pneumonia, tuberculosis, and gastroenteritis—were infectious disorders. The current "top three"—cardiovascular disease, malignancies, and cerebrovascular disease—are not. These diseases primarily affect adults of middle age or older—especially persons over 65.

Remember also that the elimination of a disease as a cause of early death may mean that people are *living* with the disease or illness. For example, trauma units and health care facilities designed to treat acute life-threatening situations may have reduced the number of deaths from accidents while increasing the number of clients in need of long-term rehabilitation. Before the development of insulin, most persons with Type I (insulin-dependent) diabetes mellitus died in early adulthood; now clients with Type I diabetes form a significant part of any health care professional's practice. And Type II (noninsulin-dependent) diabetes is becoming a major health concern, in part because more persons are living to its age of onset. Diabetes is one example of a trend that is having major effects on health care in the United States: long-term illnesses, often related to lifestyle, are becoming the significant health problems of Americans.

Long-Term Disease and Lifestyle

Among the major characteristics of the long-term disorders that are now the principal causes of death in the United States are: They are relatively irreversible (ie, there is no specific "cure"); they have multiple causes; they tend to develop over long periods; and many show a strong association with lifestyle. Moreover, studies have suggested that, for persons aged 40 to 64, current medical practices have less potential for saving lives than significant reductions in inactivity, overnutrition, alcoholism, and hypertension (Pender, 1982). No wonder, then, that lifestyle is receiving increasing attention for its potential for prevention of illness.

Of the various causes of disease mentioned at the beginning of this section, lifestyle is uniquely subject to each individual's control. Individual life patterns such as eating, exercise, drinking, coping with stress, and using substances such as tobacco and drugs are known to be modifiable causes of illness. Environment is sometimes, though not always, subject to societal control or modification.

An individual's lifestyle is a unique composite of thoughts, feelings, customs, and habits that often have cultural and historical roots. Just as each person's health status ranges along a continuum from optimum health through illness to death, so lifestyles range along a continuum from health enhancing to self-destructive.

Lifestyles Favorable to Health

A major advance in establishing a connection between lifestyle, well-being, and longevity is a study of adults residing in Alameda County, California, begun in 1965. Many studies of **morbidity** (illness) and **mortality** (death) are based on hospitalized populations. In this study, however, members of a general community population were studied to determine the relation, if any, among health status and seven favorable health practices:

- Never having smoked
- Limiting alcohol consumption
- Controlling weight
- Sleeping 7 to 8 hours a night
- Engaging in physical activity
- Eating breakfast almost daily
- Not eating between meals

These practices showed a positive association with health status that was cumulative (the more practices followed, the healthier the individual) and independent of age, sex, and economic status (Belloc & Breslow, 1972).

When the study was followed up, the data collected showed a positive association among the first five practices and the health status of the surviving subjects. Moreover, mortality rates were lower for those who had reported favorable health practices in 1965 than for those who had not (Breslow & Enstrom, 1980). A national survey conducted in 1979 and 1980 indicates that the results of the Alameda study are applicable to the general population of the United States (Wilson & Elinson, 1981).

Lifestyles Unfavorable to Health

Relations between lifestyle and disease have also been documented. For example, the following lifestyle factors have been identified as risks to health:

- **Cigarette smoking:** cancer of the lung, oral cavity, larynx, urinary bladder, and pancreas have been linked to this practice. Cigarettes have been linked to more cancer incidence and mortality than any other carcinogenic agent. Smoking has also been linked to coronary artery disease and chronic obstructive pulmonary disease.
- **Alcohol consumption:** increased risk of cancer of the mouth, pharynx, larynx, esophagus, and liver has been linked to alcohol consumption. Motor vehicle accidents, cirrhosis of the liver, suicide, homicide, and falls are also related to alcohol consumption.
- **Dietary factors:** various dietary substances have been linked to either increased or decreased risk of cancer: dietary fiber, vitamins A and C, fats, minerals (eg, selenium), nonnutritive sweeteners, and food additives and contaminants. A rich diet (high in saturated fat, cholesterol, sugar, calories, and salt) can put one at risk for coronary artery disease, hypertension, obesity, and diabetes.
- **Sexual practices:** higher risk for cancer of the cervix has been associated with multiple sexual partners and early age at first intercourse. A high incidence of Kaposi's sarcoma, a relatively rare form of malignancy, has been seen among victims of AIDS (acquired immune deficiency syndrome), many of whom are homosexual men.
- **Sedentary lifestyle:** coronary artery disease and obesity are risk factors associated with a sedentary lifestyle.

Driving habits also have a significant effect on injury, disability, and death in the United States. Indeed, automobile accidents are a major cause of death for persons up to middle age. Although wearing seat belts has been shown to reduce death or injury, studies indicate that only 10% to 15% of drivers and passengers use them (Fielding, 1982).

SECTION 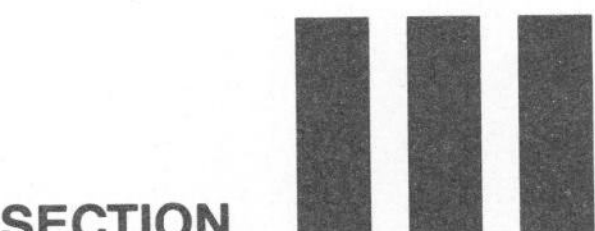

Change and Health Care Delivery

A study for the American College of Hospital Administrators (1984) predicted that the following trends will continue into the 1990s:

- Shift to outpatient care
- Sharing of costs between consumers and third-party payers
- Self-care
- Competition among health care providers
- Cutbacks in Medicare and Medicaid

Individually and collectively, these trends have significant implications for both consumers and providers of health care.

Primary Care

Primary care—comprising health maintenance, health promotion, and disease prevention—holds the greatest hope for reducing costs and improving health. Settings for primary care include homes, schools, community clinics, physicians' offices and increasingly, business and industry. Many corporations, alarmed by the cost of health care (20 cents for every dollar of salary paid), are initiating primary care programs to help employees lose weight, stop smoking, reduce stress, and improve their overall fitness. In addition, many offer free medical screenings. Through client education and self-care, primary care will no doubt expand remarkably during the next decades.

Health Maintenance Organizations

One of the largest, most influential types of primary care organizations, the *health maintenance organization* (HMO), offers a comprehensive range of services in exchange for a fixed periodic payment. By encouraging preventive care and ambulatory visits, HMOs have helped reduce the hospitalization rate of members. The total cost of premiums plus out-of-pocket expenses are less to employees covered through an HMO plan than to employees covered by traditional health insurance plans. HMO participants appear satisfied with their care, which seems to equal, and in some cases, improve on that received in the traditional fee-for-service system. Members seem satisfied despite the fact that participants' choice of health care providers is, in many HMOs, limited to those employed by the HMO. By introducing competition into the health care marketplace, HMOs have helped reduce the cost of conventional health insurance.

Preferred Provider Organizations

In response to the growing surplus of physicians and the competition offered by HMOs, another health care innovation has emerged, the *preferred provider organization* (PPO). The providers, hospitals and physicians, negotiate discounted fee-for-service rate schedules with insurers. These rates usually amount to 80% to 85% of the "usual and customary" rates in return for quick, guaranteed claims payment. Physicians can contract with one or several PPOs, and consumers can choose among the PPO physicians or ask their own physicians to join. Consumers receive complete coverage for services rendered by the PPO and reduced coverage for services rendered elsewhere. Hospitals, physicians, and insurance companies are the principal sponsors of PPOs, usually in response to requests from companies or unions.

Secondary Care

Secondary care, interventions that prevent complications of disease conditions, is no longer exclusively the province of the hospital. Ambulatory care clinics, outpatient surgical centers, and home health agencies offer clients an alternative to hospitalization.

Ambulatory Care Clinics

Ambulatory care clinics (also called freestanding emergency clinics), designed to handle a variety of minor emergencies, have proliferated since the first one opened in 1973. Clients often prefer these facilities rather than hospital emergency rooms or formal appointments with health care providers because the clinics are conveniently located, no appointment is necessary, and the average charge is about $50—less than half the cost of a hospital emergency room visit.

Outpatient Surgical Centers

New technology and the growth of freestanding surgical centers have created a boom in less expensive one-day outpatient surgery. The number of freestanding surgical centers doubled between 1980 and 1985 and is expected to reach 600 by 1988. Forced to compete with these innovative facilities, many hospitals have opened their own centers for outpatient surgery, boosting the outpatient surgery rate while inpatient operations fall. Initial fears that clients would develop complications that could not be handled at home have proven unfounded.

Hospitals

Once the unchallenged controllers of secondary care, hospitals are undergoing cataclysmic changes. The trends toward outpatient care in freestanding clinics and HMOs, reduced government support, and competition among themselves have forced hospitals to adopt business methods and strategies to survive. Some experts think that by 1990, 20% of the nation's hospitals will either close, merge, or sell out to large multihospital for-profit corporations. Firms such as Humana Inc, Hospital Corporation of America, American Medical International, and National Medical Enterprises now own approximately one-sixth of hospitals in the United States.

To replace revenue formerly supplied by Medicare and Medicaid payments, hospitals are marketing innovative services to consumers. Services may include fitness and nutrition classes, day-care for the elderly, gifts or discounts, candlelight, gourmet dinners, or taxi service for persons who have been drinking. Some hospital management experts question the value of these services, believing that a better way to compete is by developing low-cost products and services.

As economic forces are changing hospitals' methods of operation, demographic forces are changing the very nature of hospitals. Despite the trend toward ambulatory care, the chronically ill and older segments of the population are increasing the demand for acute care. All but the most seriously ill persons are treated in one or more outpatient facilities, and only the most acutely ill enter the hospital. The American Hospital Association predicts a 15% increase in the number of inpatient days between 1980 and 1990; 89% of that increase will be attributable to those over 65. With this development, former general hospitals are fast becoming large intensive care centers.

Home Health Care

Home care is not a new idea but an old one enjoying unprecedented popularity. Growth is so rapid that accurate statistics are difficult to obtain. Earlier discharge from hospitals and high-tech client support systems used in treating chronic illness have fueled an explosion in home care. Home care agencies are providing services for sicker persons: clients on respirators, oxygen, intravenous therapy, total parenteral nutrition (TPN), chemotherapy, and dialysis. In addition to skilled nursing care, home care clients may require a host of other services such as a homemaker, home attendant, or Meals-on-Wheels.

Once considered strictly long-term or tertiary care, home health care today spans both secondary and tertiary care. Many types of agencies and services exist, ranging from one- or two-service providers to large, multiservice agencies (offering both professional and nonprofessional services, and extended as well as intermittent care). Some agencies are nonprofit, either private or voluntary (such as traditional visiting nurse associations); some are proprietary (for profit), either extensions of hospital services or national home care corporations. These agencies may be owned by physicians, nurses, business persons, or pharmaceutical companies.

Professional intermittent care might include such activities as teaching a client and family a procedure or skill, providing ongoing assessment of a client's condition, changing dressings, and administering medication. Professional extended care can range from 4 to 24 hours per day and requires experienced, highly skilled nurses to care for clients with acute health problems, such as those requiring respiratory support or parenteral nutrition, and to teach family members how to assist in this care. Paraprofessionals, such as certified nurses' aides, home health aides, and homemakers, can be employed when skilled care is not needed. Their services include bathing or feeding the client and relieving family members, at least briefly, from the stress of constant care. Also known as respite care, these services can make it possible for families to care for a chronically ill or disabled family member at home by supplementing the family's caregiving capabilities. Home care not only offers a more humane alternative to institutionalized care and a more therapeutic environment for restoration of health but enormous cost savings as well.

Tertiary Care

Also called rehabilitation or long-term care, tertiary care consists of helping to restore maximum function and/or helping the client live with illness, whether chronic or terminal. Home health care, discussed earlier as secondary care because it often involves care of the acutely ill, is the largest segment of the tertiary care delivery system. Other institutions involved in tertiary care include rehabilitation centers, nursing homes and other extended care facilities, and hospices. Rehabilitation centers and nursing homes have been part of the health care delivery system for decades. With the increase in physical trauma from auto accidents and other vehicular accidents and a burgeoning population over 65, their numbers can only increase.

Hospice, another form of tertiary care, is a concept relatively new to this country. Initiated in England largely through the efforts of Dame Cicely Saunders, hospice care offers either intermittent or extended palliative care for the dying and their families, either at home or in the hospice facility. The National Association for Home Care has begun development of a hospice service to meet the needs of persons with remittent or progressive cancer.

SECTION 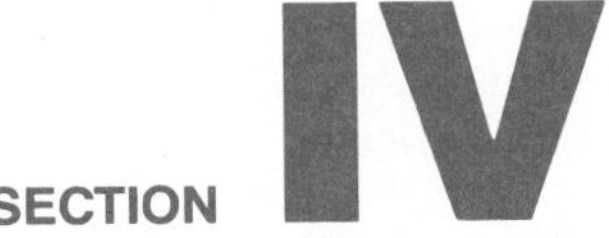

Change and the Health Consumer's Responsibility

This society is health conscious, spending billions of dollars on health and fitness activities and equipment and billions more on health care. Health and health care are regarded as a right. Too few persons think of health as a personal responsibility, however, even though the leading health problems—cardiovascular disease, cancer, cerebrovascular disease, accidents, homicides, and suicides—result from how persons live and the environments they create.

The language used to discuss health care—for example, "the health care delivery system"—reflects a concept of health that has been generally accepted for many years. Health care is regarded as a product that can be "delivered" to each person if the system functions properly; in fact, the product is illness care. The most significant health care is what individuals do for themselves in the way they live, eat, exercise, manage stress, and avoid excessive use of alcohol and other drugs.

Deterrents to Lifestyle Modification

Most persons still think of health in terms of "not being sick." As long as people do not feel ill, they may be disinclined to change their ways—especially when change means giving up enjoyable foods, walking instead of driving, and otherwise sacrificing present pleasures for a vague promise of "better health" on some future day. Many persons say or feel that living 10 years less but doing what they want is preferable to the "penal servitude" that a life of self-control and moderation suggests to them. They are especially likely to take this view when the "10 years less" is not a clear and present danger.

Habits and attitudes are formed over many years, and these practices embrace all dimensions of life. Changing lifestyles is difficult; it takes concentration and dedication, especially when others urge "just one more" drink, piece of pie, or cigarette; when the seat belts in friends' two-year-old cars are still wrapped in plastic; when it is hot outside and sitting by the television with a cold beer seems far more appealing than taking a two-mile walk. In the absence of an overt threat to health—and even if a threat is present—motivation may be lacking.

Many other psychosocial considerations are undoubtedly involved in determining who will readily take positive health action and who will not. Social support networks, coping style, social class, health status, self-esteem, educational level, age, and religion may all be partial predictors of individual health behaviors.

Models for Lifestyle Change

Individual motivation to initiate change is probably the most significant factor in successful lifestyle change. The health consciousness of Americans is apparently rising, but widespread apathy toward health remains. Once a threshold of concern has been reached, however, lifestyle modification is best approached in stages. According to Milsum (1980), these states consist of:

- Being aware of risk and accepting that the risk applies to one personally (eg, "*I* might develop cancer if I continue to smoke").
- Integrating the knowledge; that is, making the desired modification part of the self-image (eg, "*I* am, or at least can be, a nonsmoker").
- Making the effort to change (deciding how to modify behavior and then sustaining the effort).

Plunging into change without informed motivation is unlikely to bring long-term improvement.

The Consumer Movement in Health Care

Since the mid-1900s, a national movement has grown to protect the rights of consumers through legislation mandating such practices as truth in advertising, honest packaging, fair pricing, and improved safety standards. This movement has broadened to include health care, partly as a result of dissatisfaction with the present system. The public is aware that professional care is less than perfect. Indeed, professional care is regarded as about 10% effective overall and 10% ineffective or even dangerous (Levin, 1981). Reports of incompetent treatment and lack of sensitivity have tarnished the image of all health care workers, including nurses.

Evidence of the consumer movement in health care is everywhere—in the more than 3500 health and medical self-help books; in newsletters, conferences, and workshops related to health promotion and management of acute and chronic disease; and in the more than 500 national self-help or mutual support groups. It is readily apparent that individuals want more control over their primary health care needs. In the case of chronic health problems, they recognize that an increased level of involvement in self-care is essential. At the end of each nursing process chapter in this text is a list of self-help groups and health education material that can be used in health promotion.

Mutual support groups such as Alcoholics Anonymous, Reach for Recovery, and Make Today Count, were formed by persons who felt their needs were not being met by existing institutions and health professionals. Today, more than 17 million persons have joined these groups for mutual support and education in dealing with their health problems.

There is a mutual support group for nearly every major health problem or life crisis. Although most are helpful, some may be less than effective or even harmful. For this reason, nurses who may wish to refer clients to these groups or perhaps participate as an advisor or group leader must be able to assess the probable effectiveness of a particular self-help group and its appropriateness for a particular client and family (Newton, 1984). The National Self-Help Clearinghouse can provide information on current support groups plus guidelines on how to start a self-help group.

SECTION 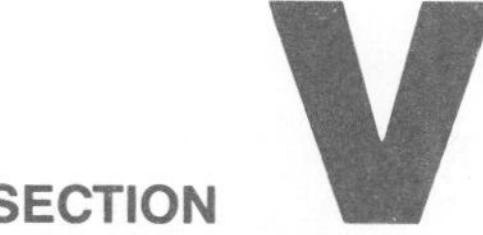

Change and the Nurse's Responsibility

Cost containment, assertiveness of health care consumers, an aging population, and increasing chronic health problems are rapidly reshaping the health care system. The changes are creating new opportunities for nurses. Concern for the client, clinical and technical skills, and sound clinical judgment are only the beginning requirements for a successful nursing career in today's health care system. Nurses need to understand the economics and the politics of health care; they need to gain a voice in shaping health policy at every level. They need to be computer literate and share a universal professional language based on the nursing process and nursing diagnoses.

Nursing Process

Since the 1960s, the term *nursing process* has been used to describe nurses' overall function. First outlined in four steps, then further delineated as five in 1982, the nursing process comprises assessment, analysis (or nursing diagnosis), planning, implementation (or intervention), and evaluation.

Nursing diagnosis has greatly contributed to standardizing the terms that define client characteristics and actual or potential nursing care needs. In 1982, a list of nursing diagnoses approved by the North American Nursing Diagnosis Association (NANDA) was published. These nursing diagnoses are tested, discussed, periodically refined, and updated in the nursing literature (Kim, McFarland, & McLane, 1984).

Nursing diagnoses may or may not relate to the client's medical diagnosis; they do relate to the actual purpose of nursing as defined by the American Nurses' Association (ANA): "the diagnosis and treatment of human responses to actual or potential health problems" (ANA, 1980). Nursing diagnoses help nurses to describe thoughtfully the phenomena that are the human responses to illness as they apply to the special and unique characteristics of each client. Understanding and using nursing diagnoses appropriately help nurses to separate nursing care from "room and board" in hospital cost accounting and also help refine the client classification system on which prospective payment depends.

Client/Family Advocacy and Education

The traditional nursing roles of client advocate and health teacher assume new importance in today's health care climate. As cost containment threatens to erode the quality and even the safety of care, nursing must assert its rights to protect the rights of the client and family. To support the important self-care trend, nursing needs to reemphasize one of its central roles, that of client teacher. Since Nightingale, nurses have recognized the importance of teaching the client about health and illness. Today teaching is even more important because clients want and need to learn about their own health, how to maintain and improve it, and how to help restore it when accident or illness occurs.

None of this is possible without nursing acknowledging and exercising its power, what Benner (1984) describes as the "power of caring." One of the qualities of this power is *advocacy power,* "the kind of power that removes obstacles or stands alongside and enables." When clients cannot understand medical jargon or negotiate the seemingly mysterious workings of the health care system, the nurse can make a positive difference.

The power of caring as Benner defines it is not a dominating, coercing, or controlling kind of power. Instead, it is a power that nurses can and do use to empower their clients. Some nurses are uncomfortable with the concept of being powerful and using power (Dumas, 1985); however, nurses need to assert their power not only to protect the rights of the clients and families they care for but also to preserve and protect the profession.

Helping Clients Take Charge of Their Health

Nurses are readily available to clients in industry, homes for the aged, hospitals, physicians' offices, clinics, schools, community agencies, and health maintenance organizations. Their accessibility offers unlimited potential for developing health-protective behaviors. Assisting clients to understand their potential susceptibility or helping clients acknowledge that they are exposing themselves to potentially health-damaging situations are opportunities for developing health-promoting strategies. When the long-term impact of the nurse's role is considered, stressing wellness instead of illness is perhaps the most significant contribution nursing can make to improving the quality of life and decreasing the cost of health care.

Nurses are often present when clients and families are especially vulnerable. It is the nurse who establishes a relationship with the daughters of a woman who has just had a mastectomy. The nurse naturally spends the most nursing time in the postoperative care of the mother and helping the family become involved in supportive care. But the nurse also recognizes that the daughters are at increased risk for breast cancer. The nurse is in an excellent position to help them understand that risk, to teach them breast self-examination, and thus to enhance their future health and the health of all women born into that family.

The nurse in the college health center has access to a population potentially at high risk for motor vehicle accidents, alcohol and drug abuse, sexually transmitted diseases, sports injuries, and cancer of the testicle. The nurse can help these young adults, who are concerned with developing independent lifestyles, to be aware of how these risks threaten their future; to work out approaches to combat the risks; and to assist in developing alternative health-promoting lifetime patterns.

Clearly, lifestyle modification has vast potential for raising national and individual levels of health. Nurses can identify exciting possibilities for teaching their clients about health risks and working with their clients in developing healthier lifestyles. Nevertheless, altering customary practices and attitudes is always a formidable task.

Activating Clients

Participation in self-help groups can be valuable in motivating clients and helping clients assume responsibility for their own health. These groups provide both emotional and informational support.

Reading material is another avenue for assisting the consumer to assume more personal autonomy for positive

Nursing Research Note

Dixon J: Group self-identification and physical handicap: Implications for patient support groups. *Nurs Health* 1981; 4:299–308.

The relation between attitudes toward self and attitudes toward general types of handicapped and nonhandicapped persons were examined. Data were collected from subjects who had no handicaps and from individuals with one of the following physical impairments: amputation, arthritis, emotional disturbances, spinal cord injuries, or stroke. The subjects were tested for willingness to associate with handicapped persons and evaluated themselves with reference to handicapped and nonhandicapped individuals.

The results indicated a strong identification between subjects and their own handicap group for amputees, clients with spinal cord injuries, and stroke subjects. Subjects with arthritis and emotional disturbances did not strongly identify with their own handicap group but identified with the average person. The nonhandicapped had a significant association between self and concepts associated with the handicapped.

The study suggests that some individuals may benefit from self-help groups but not all. Nurses should assess each client individually and determine if group identification would help or hinder psychological adjustment.

health practices. Bookstores are filled with books on diet, exercise, first aid, medication, self-improvement, and a host of other topics. Besides giving consumers valuable information about how to avoid illness and care for themselves, these books also assist in developing clients who are better informed and who know what to ask when they enter the health care system. Browsing in the self-help section of the bookstore or library and using the health education material included in the resources list in this text can contribute to the nurses' own knowledge as well as client referral.

Remember that lifestyle modification is often triggered by a factor external to the health care system. Clients spend the majority of their lives outside of health facilities in environments that have far greater impact on their health. A woman with mild hypertension whose sister just had a stroke might be motivated to take action after hearing a nurse speak on high blood pressure at her church women's group. Picking up a pamphlet on diet and heart attack at the YMCA could be the trigger factor for an overweight man whose business partner just suffered a coronary. Often, the well-publicized illness of a celebrity is the impetus for taking health action. For example, the practice of breast self-examination rose markedly following First Lady Betty Ford's mastectomy in 1974.

Setting short-term and long-term goals helps activate the client. Remember that *the goals should be the client's.* The nurse's part is making sure the client has enough information to understand fully the health risks associated with any behavior that is to be changed, knows the options available for reducing those risks, and acknowledges the personal benefits associated with the planned changes. For example, Mrs T, an obese, hypertensive client, will probably agree that decreasing salt intake, losing weight, and reducing blood pressure consistently to acceptable levels are desirable goals. But she may *not* agree. Further exploration may reveal barriers to communication or learning or perceived short-term disadvantages that, to the client, may outweigh the long-term benefits.

Appreciating Uniqueness

The educational, cultural, religious, personal, and philosophical barriers to incorporating new practices into one's lifestyle would fill an entire volume. By being sensitive to each client's uniqueness—including a set of beliefs and values that may be quite different from the nurse's—the nurse can gradually develop a trusting relationship with the client that will enable asking the right questions. Much effort is wasted in health education activities because unique elements of each client's lifestyle are never discovered.

Consider Mrs T again. What kinds of foods does she eat now? Does she eat at home? In a restaurant? Do time pressures necessitate her using many prepared foods? Many prepackaged, frozen, or "fast" foods are high in sodium; "fast" foods are also high in fat. Does she use canned foods, perhaps because they are inexpensive? Canned foods are usually very high in sodium. Does she cook for a family? What foods are they used to? Are ethnic foods among her or her family's favorites? Soy sauce—much used in Oriental cooking—is very high in sodium. Lox, a favorite of many Jews, has a high sodium and fat content; so does smoked fish. Lists of "foods to avoid" often include ethnic favorites; lists of "foods to eat" often ignore ethnic preferences. Neither list will help the client if it is not related to what, where, and how the client eats. Moreover, many foods—especially ethnic foods or childhood favorites—have "comfort value" that transcends their food value. Remember that asking the client to change her eating habits means also asking for a lifestyle change that the client may perceive as unpleasant. Should the client be asked to forgo all such foods, or can compromises be arranged? In their zeal to bring clients to optimum health, professionals often forget that any change is better than no change, and a small change faithfully followed is better than a major "remake" that is soon abandoned.

It is not easy to modify one's lifestyle, as those who have tried can testify. Some are successful and some are not. For those who are successful, was it because they were psychologically ready? Because they perceived themselves as vulnerable? Because they entered into a behavior modification program that fit their needs? Because they are women? Men? Young? Old? The best answer is probably that at that particular point in their lives, all factors came together, and the internal factors combined with the external factors to motivate them to act in a positive way.

Lack of family support, lack of money, lack of transportation—and lack of self-esteem, feeling "unworthy to be well"—all may underlie a client's resistance to beginning or continuing a plan of care (see Chapter 4). Unrealistic goal setting may also be at fault. These problems, in turn, point to inadequate history taking at the initial stages of the client's care (see Chapter 5).

Research and Theory in Nursing

Nurses are actively engaged in scholarly inquiry into the very nature of nursing. The purpose of research and theory construction in nursing is to move the profession away from an intuitive base toward an intellectual base. Several conceptual models or theories of nursing have been proposed, each with its proponents and critics. Although these models of nursing are diverse, they share several themes: the holistic nature of humans; the importance of individuality, self-worth, and dignity; and the essentially humanitarian nature of nursing. These commonalities undergird the framework of this text.

Just as every scientific discipline uses research as a primary tool to broaden and deepen its understanding of the world, nursing uses research to enhance its understanding of health and illness and human responses to actual or potential health problems." For example, while the Centers for Disease Control in Atlanta study the AIDS virus, nurses in San Francisco, New York, and other major cities are studying the impact of this epidemic on clients and families, their relationships, and their abilities to cope with a potentially fatal illness.

Nursing research must belong to all nurses, not just the academicians and the career nurse scientists. As Wilson (1985) stated: "If nursing is to build a scientific body of knowledge and if nursing practice is to be shaped by research findings rather than tradition, intuition, or habit, then the investigative skills of all nurses, regardless of their educational level, must be as integral to their repertoire as communication skills and sterile technique."

Priorities for future research identified by ANA (1981) focus on health care and illness prevention, development of cost-efficient systems for delivery of nursing care, and strategies for effective care of high-risk groups. Equal in importance to these priorities is making nursing research visible, both within and outside the profession. For nursing research to change the practice of nursing, it must be disseminated. More potential avenues for its publication exist today than ever before—four journals exclusively devoted to nursing research and dozens of others actively seeking articles based on research but written in a less formal style. The Nursing Research boxes throughout this text demonstrate the integral role of nursing research within nursing practice.

Chapter Highlights

One of the greatest health care challenges is being posed by the growing population of persons over 65. Unfortunately, health policy and the health care system often categorize and stereotype older persons.

Environmental pollution and occupational hazards threaten life and health throughout the world.

The United States, a traditional cultural "melting pot," continues to attract immigrants from a variety of other cultures; their cultural blueprints affect their health care needs.

The health care business is the second largest industry in the United States; health care costs have spiraled far above the general rate of economic inflation.

Implementing the DRG system for prospective payment concerns health professionals who worry that quality will be sacrificed to cost consciousness.

Highly technologic health care is expensive; it also runs the risk of becoming depersonalized care.

The leading causes of death in the United States have shifted over the past century. Long-term illnesses, often related to lifestyle, are becoming the significant health problems of Americans.

Lifestyles range along a continuum from self-enhancing to self-destructive. Many aspects are under an individual's control; some are not.

Favorable health practices—never having smoked, limiting alcohol consumption, controlling weight, sleeping 7 to 8 hours a night, engaging in physical activity, eating breakfast almost daily, and not eating between meals—are positively associated with health status independent of age, sex, and economic status.

Increasing numbers of individuals are asserting their rights in health care and assuming the responsibilities that accompany those rights.

Self-help groups are important sources of support for clients and help clients assume responsibility for their own health.

The nursing roles of client advocate and health teacher assume new importance in today's health care climate. These roles help nurses balance high technology with human response.

Nurses can have a major impact on general health because of their broad access to clients

in all age groups and in all phases of their lives. To affect health, nurses must make every individual and group encounter with clients an opportunity for teaching lifestyle modification. Stressing wellness instead of illness is perhaps the most significant contribution nursing can make to improving the quality of life and decreasing the cost of health care.

Bibliography

American College of Hospital Administrators, 1984, 840 N Lakeshore Drive, Chicago, IL 60611.

American Intraocular Implant Society, 3700 Pender Drive, Suite 108, Fairfax, VA 22030.

American Nurses' Association Commission on Nursing Research: *Research Priorities for the 1980s.* Kansas City, MO: ANA, 1981.

Belloc NB, Breslow L: Relationship of physical health status and health practices. *Prev Med* 1972; 1:409–421.

Benner P: *From Novice to Expert: Excellence and Power in Clinical Nursing Practice.* Menlo Park, CA: Addison–Wesley, 1984.

Breslow L, Enstrom JE: Persistence of health habits and their relationship to mortality. *Prev Med* 1980; 9:469–483.

Coleman JR, Dayani EC, Simms E: Nursing careers in the emerging systems. *Nurs Management* (Jan) 1984; 15:19–27.

Cooper R, Simmons BE: Cigarette smoking and ill health among black Americans. *Am J Nurs* (July) 1985; 85(7): 344–347.

Curtin L: Nursing: High-touch in a high-tech world. *Nursing Management* (July) 1984; 15:7–8.

DeCrosta T: Megatrends in nursing: 10 new directions that are changing your profession. *Nurs Life* (May–June) 1985; 5:17–19.

Dumas R: Two perspectives on power: Women and power. In: *Political Action Handbook for Nurses: Changing the Workplace, Government, Organizations, and Community.* Mason D, Talbott S (editors). Menlo Park, CA: Addison–Wesley, 1985.

Faber MM, Reinhardt AM (editors): *Promoting Health Through Risk Reduction.* New York: Macmillan, 1982.

Fielding JE: Risk reduction goals throughout life. In: *Promoting Health Through Risk Reduction.* Faber MM, Reinhardt AM (editors). New York: Macmillan, 1982.

Griffith H: Who will become the preferred providers? *Am J Nurs* 1985; 85(5):538–542.

Kim MJ, McFarland GK, McLane AM: *Pocket Guide to Nursing Diagnoses.* St. Louis: Mosby,, 1984.

Lederer JR et al: *Care Planning Pocket Guide: A Nursing Diagnosis Approach.* Menlo Park, CA: Addison–Wesley, 1986.

Lee PR, Estes CL, Ramsay NB: *The Nation's Health,* 2nd ed. San Francisco: Boyd & Fraser, 1984.

Levenstein A: Storm clouds on the horizon. *Nurs Management* (April) 1985; 16:52–53.

Levin LS: The role of the individual in health care. In: *The Nation's Health,* 2nd ed. Lee PR, Estes CL, Ramsay NB (editors). San Francisco: Boyd & Fraser, 1984.

Louis Harris & Associates: National access survey, 1982. In *Special Report.* Princeton, NJ: Robert Wood Johnson Foundation, 1983.

Marchewka AE: When is paternalism justifiable? *Am J Nurs* 1983; 83:1072–1073.

Mason DJ, Talbott SW: *Political Action Handbook for Nurses: Changing the Workplace, Government, Organizations, and Community.* Menlo Park, CA: Addison–Wesley, 1985.

Miller A: When is the time ripe for teaching? *Am J Nurs* 1985; 85:801–804.

Milsum JH: Health, risk factor reduction and life-style change. *Fam Commun Health* 1980; 3:1–13.

Nelson JP, Carlstrom JA: A new confrontation: Nursing education and computer technology. *Image* (Summer) 1985; 17(3):86–87.

Newton G: Self-help groups: Can they help? *J Psychosoc Nurs* (July) 1984; 22:27–31.

Pender NJ: *Health Promotion in Nursing Practice.* Norwalk, CT: Appleton–Century–Crofts, 1982.

Sovie MD, Tarcinale MA, Vanputee AW, Stunden AE: Amalgam of nursing acuity, DRGs and costs. *Nurs Management* (March) 1985; 16:22–42.

Spain D: Country profile: The United States: Just the facts. In: *American Demographics, Inc, Special Report. Ithaca, NY: American Demographics,* June 1983.

Swearingen PL: *Manual of Nursing Therapeutics: Applying Nursing Diagnoses to Medical Disorders.* Menlo Park, CA: Addison–Wesley, 1986.

Wilson HS: *Research in Nursing.* Menlo Park, CA: Addison–Wesley, 1985.

Wilson RW, Elinson J: National survey of personal health practices and consequences: Background, conceptual issues, and selected findings. *Public Health Report* 1981; 96:218–225.

Resources

SELF-HELP GROUPS AND OTHER ORGANIZATIONS

National Self-Help Clearinghouse
Graduate School University Center
City University of New York
33 W 42nd St
New York, NY 10036

This organization monitors the activity of hundreds of self-help organizations throughout the United States and Canada and will supply referrals to appropriate groups.

Self Help Center
1600 Dodge Avenue
Evanston, IL 60204
Phone: (312) 328–0470

Another self-help clearinghouse, it, too, provides information on self-help groups in the United States and Canada and provides referrals.

HOT LINES

National Health Information Center
PO Box 1133
Washington, DC 20013
Phone: (800) 336–4797

Provides health and medical information, lists of other toll-free numbers, referrals to appropriate organizations, and researches answers to health questions. Also provides government-produced pamphlets such as *Healthstyle: A Self Test.* A service of the Office of Disease Prevention and Health Promotion (ODPHP), US Department of Health and Human Services.

Tel-Med Telephone Tape Library
Phone: Check local telephone directories

Free health information on audiotapes is available in over 200 communities in the United States. Check the local telephone directory for the number for more than 300 recorded messages on health-related topics.

HEALTH EDUCATION MATERIAL

Specific health education material is identified in appropriate chapters. Of interest might be the *Self-Care Catalog,* published and distributed free by:

Medical Self-Care Magazine
PO Box 717
Iverness, CA 94937

This catalog provides information on home-based medical equipment at affordable prices. *Medical Self-Care Magazine* is also of interest to those involved in health self-help.

The following softcover books on client advocacy and informed health care consumerism should be of interest to both clients and nurses and can be obtained at local bookstores.

Berman H, Burhenne D, Rose L: *The Complete Health Care Advisor.* New York: St. Martin's, 1983. (The authors are a physician, a psychologist, and a medical writer.)

Hogan NS: *Humanizing Health Care: Task of the Patient Representative.* Oradell, NJ: Medical Economics, 1980. (The author is a founder and former president of the Society of Patient Representatives of the American Hospital Association.)

Huttman B: *The Patient's Advocate: The Complete Handbook of Patient's Rights.* New York: Penguin, 1981. (The author is a nurse committed to the concept of client advocacy.)

Nierenberg J, Janovic F: *The Hospital Experience: A Guide for Patients and Their Families,* 2nd ed. New York: Berkley, 1985. (The authors are a nurse and a medical writer.)

CHAPTER 2

How Illness Develops

...ext advocates, bridges ...tween mind and body, between "illness" care delivery and "health" care delivery—acknowledging that disease is directly related to the sum of all factors affecting a person's life.

...rsus Illness (Dis-ease)

...l theory, which has traditionally emphasized ... subsystem level of the cell, the organ, or ...em, nursing theory has its roots in holistic ...re 2–1). Nurses base their practice on the ...on theory of health alterations, considering ...n problems as unemployment, racism, urban ...lution, and stressful living patterns as ...ts in explaining why persons become ill. ...*illness,* while recognizing that biological ...rs contribute to disease, is strongly re... individual and the individual's family, so...ironment, and culture. Disease is mere... health. *Illness is the human experience of*

...word *disease* derives from the prefix *dis* ... French *aise* (ease)—literally meaning ... ease,"—disease is usually discussed ...e abnormality in an organ or organ sys...tem that results in certain symptoms and signs. Disease may be further described by such terms as *acute* or *chronic, communicable, congenital, degenerative, functional, malignant, psychosomatic,* or *idiopathic.* The causation of a disease is called its etiology, and often a disease is discussed as if there were one specific etiology. But whenever dis-

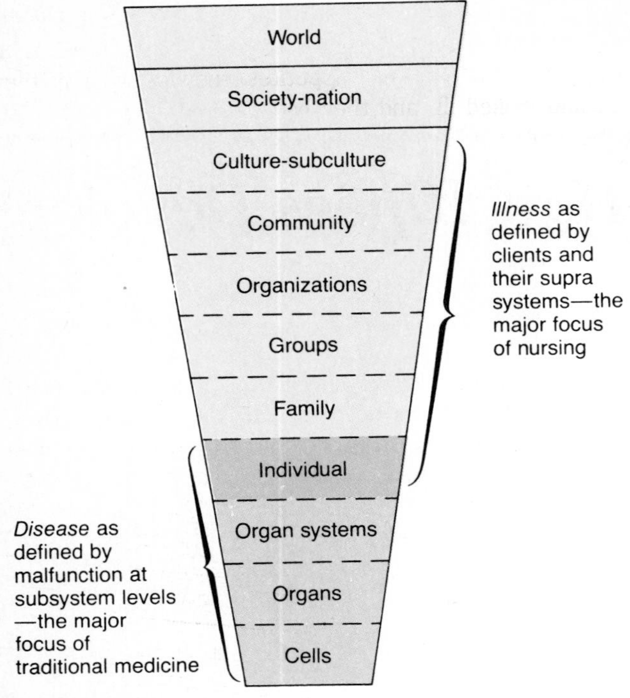

Figure 2–1

A systems hierarchy differentiating illness from disease and nursing from traditional medicine. SOURCE: *Adapted from Ames SA, Gelein J, Humphrey E, Mason-Kaufman J, Osborne JE: A systems approach to curricula in primary health care nursing. In* Approaches to Teaching Primary Health Care, *Knopke HJ, Diekelmann NL (editors). St. Louis: Mosby, 1981.*

ease exists, a *whole person* is involved—not only an organ or organ system.

Consider Mrs W, who has a urinary tract infection (UTI). The organism *Escherichia coli* is cultured, and appropriate antibiotic therapy is begun. The infectious agent may not entirely account for the illness, however. In women, *E. coli* is always present in the perineal region, yet women do not continuously have UTIs. Perhaps before the onset of the UTI, Mrs W inadvertently wiped her perineal area from back to front during toileting. Perhaps she reduced her fluid intake from her usual eight glasses of water a day, or perhaps she neglected to void after intercourse. To carry the analysis further, perhaps she was upset over losing her job, so she neglected perineal hygiene or forgot to consume enough fluids. This brief example points out the multifactorial origin of *dis-ease,* or illness. Regarding disease, the cause of this woman's urinary tract infection is the bacterium *E. coli.* But the origin or cause of the illness (dis-ease) was multifactorial.

In this text, all illness is considered multifactorial; in the fundamental sense, all disease is illness. Nevertheless, a nurse must understand certain basic internal and external mechanisms of disease or degeneration that influence the onset and duration of illness. These factors, which closely interrelate with psychosocial and environmental influences, are stress, the immune system and immune response, infection and inflammation, genetic predispositions, neoplasia, aging, and trauma. As an overview of these factors, this chapter reviews concepts discussed in earlier courses and lays the foundation for the more extensive discussions of each of these factors in the specific disorders chapters in each body systems unit.

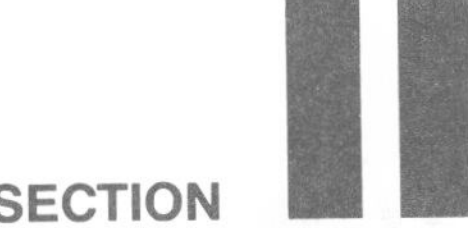

SECTION II

Stress: A Cause and an Effect of Illness

Stress is a part of being alive. Standing erect stresses the musculoskeletal system (muscles and bones must work together to keep the body erect), eating stresses the digestive system (enzymes must be produced and nutrients absorbed), and breathing stresses the respiratory system (carbon dioxide and oxygen must be exchanged). In unseen ways, the immune system is constantly engaged in a war with the bacteria in the body. The interaction and eventual balance among these various forces constitute the routine stress with which all humans contend. According to Selye (1956), stress is the amount of wear and tear on the human body.

However, stress is both a physiologic and a psychosocial experience. More broadly and holistically, stress designates a broad class of experiences in which a demanding situation taxes a person's resources or coping capabilities causing a negative effect (Lazarus & Folkman 1984). This definition more closely approximates the holistic perspective on which this textbook is based. In this view, stress is a person–environment interaction. The source of the stress, the demanding situation, is known as a stressor. The internal state the stress produces is one of tension, anxiety, or strain.

While there is no universally accepted definition of stress among stress theorists and researchers, an interactional view of stress, such as the one given above, is consistent with how nurses view human experiences. The ideas about stress that follow are some of the perspectives in common use. While they do tell us a great deal about responses to stressful situations, they fail to explain why individual responses to stress vary. Such factors as cause, the situational context in which the stressful event occurs, and the psychological interpretation of the demanding situation are all important in a holistic approach to client care.

Stress as a psychologic event and the ways in which people cope with stress are discussed in psychiatric nursing texts.

The Fight–Flight Response to Stress

Humans can encounter undesirable or excess stress that threatens well-being and may even be life threatening. They cope with such threats through either a *fight* (aggression) or *flight* (withdrawal) response. The fight–flight response was first discussed by Walter Cannon, a physician, in 1932 when he identified stress as an actual cause of disease. Consider the following situation of extreme stress: A woman is walking down a dark, deserted street when a man with a knife emerges from the shadows just in front of her. Does she try to defend herself? Does she run away? Whichever action she takes has been enabled by a variety of physiologic responses to extreme danger. According to Mason (1980), when a person faces such a situation:

- The heartbeat increases.
- As the heart rate increases, the blood pressure rises.
- Breathing becomes rapid and shallow.
- Epinephrine and other hormones are released into the blood.
- The liver releases stored sugar into the blood to meet increased energy needs for survival.
- The pupils dilate to let in more light; all the senses are heightened.
- Muscles tense for movement, either for flight or protective actions.
- Blood flow to the digestive organs is constricted.
- Blood flow increases to the brain and major muscles.
- Blood flow to the extremities is constricted, and the hands and feet become cold.
- The body perspires to cool itself, because increased metabolism generates more heat.

The General Adaptation Syndrome

Hans Selye, a Canadian endocrinologist and the most well known and widely recognized stress researcher, developed another framework for understanding how persons respond to stress. Each person has a limited amount of energy to use in dealing with stress. How quickly it is used and, therefore, how quickly one adapts to stress depend on several factors such as heredity, mental attitude, and lifestyle, among others.

Stress can be appraised by measuring the structural and chemical changes it produces in the body. These changes are called the *general adaptation syndrome* (GAS) because when stress affects the whole person, the whole person must adjust to the changes.

While a medical student, Selye made an interesting and important observation that became the cornerstone of his stress-adaptation theory. He observed that, regardless of the diagnosis, most clients had certain symptoms in common—they lost their appetites, they lost weight, they felt and looked ill, and they had aches and pains in their joints and muscles. He introduced his observations and the general adaptation syndrome concept in 1936 in a letter to the editor of *Nature*.

A long series of experiments (1956) led to more objective evidence of actual body damage—enlargement of the adrenal glands; shrinkage of the thymus, spleen, and lymph nodes; and the appearance of bleeding gastric ulcers. These symptoms, he said, were part of the body's *alarm* reaction to disease, the first stage in the general adaptation syndrome. In the second stage, the stage of *resistance*, the body tries to return to equilibrium despite continuing disease. If the stress persists, the person becomes exhausted from the wear and tear required by constant adjustment. This third stage is appropriately named the stage of *exhaustion*. In this stage, the ability to resist stress is lost because the body's resources are depleted.

Life Changes as Stressful Events

Although most persons readily recognize undesirable or traumatic life experiences as stressful, fewer recognize that stress is also associated with what is normally viewed as positive—graduating from nursing school, being promoted on the job, getting along better with the boss. The cumulative effect of both positive and negative life changes may reduce a person's ability to handle stress and may even promote subsequent illness.

Holmes and Rahe (1967) explored life changes and developed a scale that assigned value rankings to 43 life events associated with stress. According to this theory, each life event was assigned a value determined by the degree of stress involved. These rankings are called life-change units (LCU). The higher the total score of a person's life-change units, the more likely the person is to become ill within the next year.

This model is based on several assumptions that a review of the recent stress research (Lyon & Werner 1987) shows to be faulty. These assumptions are: a person is a passive recipient of stress; events affect all persons in the same way, regardless of how an individual perceives the event; the same amount of adaptation is required for each event among all persons; and, there is a common threshold beyond which disruption occurs.

Thoughtful nursing care requires identifying what each individual perceives as stressful in order to understand the effects of life changes on health. Scales for identifying stressful life events can then be used to help people become aware of the stress they face in their lives.

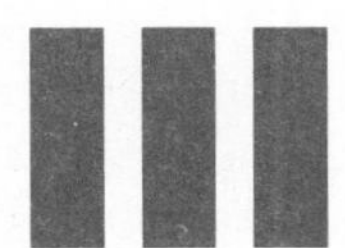

SECTION III

The Immune System and Immune Response

The immune system is one of the body's principal defenses against disease; however, disturbances of the immune system or, in some cases, dysfunctional immune responses, can themselves cause illness. The system consists of a complex group of organs, tissues, and cells located in various parts of the body. The thymus, bone marrow, lymph nodes, spleen, tonsils, appendix, and the Peyer's patches of the small intestine constitute the organs of the immune system. Lymphocytes, plasma cells, and macrophages are its principal cells.

The function of the lymphocytes (a specific type of white blood cell or leukocyte) is the key factor in all immune responses. Lymphocyte cells migrate through tissues, circulate in blood and lymph, and accumulate in the spleen and lymph nodes. The two major types of lymphocytes are B cells and T cells. **B-lymphocytes** mature in the bone marrow. When triggered by an antigen, they differentiate into antibody-producing cells. **T-lymphocytes** are a heterogeneous group of cells that mature in the thymus gland and differentiate into a variety of **effector T cells,** namely killer cells, helpers, and suppressors. These cells are essential in regulating the intensity of the body's fight against invasive organisms and in summoning antibody production.

Macrophages, derived from monocytes (large leukocytes), are cells of the reticuloendothelial system that can engulf foreign particles. This process is called **phagocytosis.** The uptake of antigens by the macrophages is the first step in the processing of antigen leading to antibody production.

The Immune Response

The essence of an immune response is the capacity of the host to recognize and react to foreign substances. Antigens signal the host that a "nonself" invader is within.

An **antigen** is a foreign protein or protein complex capable of stimulating a specific immune response when it is present in the body. An antibody is a specialized plasma protein called an **immunoglobulin** (Ig) produced by the B-lymphocytes in response to the presence of an antigen. The five major classes of immunoglobulins are IgG, IgM, IgA, IgD, and IgE (Table 2–1).

The complement system is a group of at least 15 plasma proteins activated in an ordered sequence when an antibody couples with its antigen, producing substances that participate in inflammation and host defense. IgG and IgM can activate the complement system, which in turn enhances phagocytosis, vascular permeability, and cellular lysis (destruction of the cell).

When an antigen enters the body, the B-lymphocyte system is stimulated to begin gradual production of antibodies. This *primary response* sensitizes the immune system of the host so subsequent exposure to the antigen stimulates a rapid outpouring of antibodies (Figure 2–2). This *secondary response* depends on a specific subgroup of B cells called **memory cells,** which signal the system that previous exposure to an antibody has occurred.

Mechanisms of Immunity

Cell-Mediated and Humoral Immunity

Immunologic responses are classified as either humoral or cell-mediated. **Humoral immunity** is mediated by antibodies that circulate in the blood and are present in the body fluids. The action of those antibodies occurs at a

Table 2–1
Characteristics of Antibodies (Immunoglobulins = Ig)

Name	Major Area of Concentration	Pertinent Information
IgG	Principal Ig in serum	Only Ig that crosses the placental barrier; major Ig for secondary immune responses
IgM	Present in moderate amounts in serum	Major Ig for primary immune response
IgA	Present in colostrum; saliva; tears; secretions of GI, GU, and respiratory tracts	Protects mucosal surfaces of GI, GU, respiratory tracts
IgD	Present in small amounts in serum	Specific activity unknown
IgE	Present in small amounts in serum	Mediates immediate hypersensitivity reactions and anaphylaxis

distance from the B cells that produce them. **Cell-mediated immunity** depends on the local action of the T-lymphocyte when it becomes sensitized by contact with a specific antigen.

Natural and Artificial Immunity

Specific immunity to an antigen may be acquired naturally or through artificial introduction. **Active immunity** occurs when the host produces antibodies in response to antigenic stimulation. **Passive immunity** is essentially "borrowed." It is acquired when antibody and complement are transferred to a person without the active participation of the body. For example, *natural active immunity* can be acquired by having a disease and recovering successfully from it or by being exposed to an antigen for a long time without actually developing the disease. *Natural passive immunity* occurs when a child receives antibodies from the mother across the placental barrier or through colostrum. *Artificial active immunity* is achieved through immunization with an antigen—as in routine childhood immunization against diphtheria, pertussis, tetanus, rubella, measles, mumps, or polio. *Artificial passive immunity* involves injection of serum that contains antibodies from a sensitized donor—as when immune globulin is given to persons exposed to viral hepatitis. Immunization is discussed further in Chapter 9.

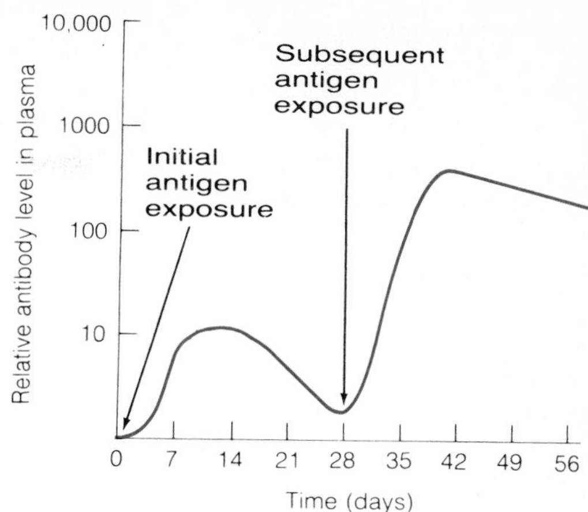

Figure 2–2

Antibody production following initial exposure to an antigen and subsequent exposure to the same antigen. SOURCE: *Spence AP, Mason EB:* Human Anatomy and Physiology, *3rd ed. Menlo Park, CA: Benjamin/Cummings, 1987, p. 631.*

Immune Reactions That Produce Tissue Damage

Autoimmunity

When the immunologic system of the host attacks normal cellular components within the host, *autoimmune disease* may result. Viruses may be the initiating factor in the pathogenesis of autoimmunity. Diseases currently considered to have autoimmune involvement include lupus erythematosus, rheumatic fever, scleroderma, ankylosing spondylitis, rheumatoid arthritis, multiple sclerosis, and thyroiditis among others.

HLA Complex

Recently, studies have shown that individual differences in surface antigens of human lymphocytes are related to susceptibility to certain diseases. Understanding of the role of human leukocyte antigen (HLA) complex in human immune responses is limited.

Apparently, **HLA antigens** are implicated in rejection of transplanted organs, as Figure 2–3 illustrates. HLA studies may also be of value in genetic counseling for certain rare genetic diseases. In addition, diseases such as Type I diabetes mellitus, lupus erythematosus, myasthenia gravis, and multiple sclerosis show HLA associations. A highly significant HLA association has been found with HLA antigen B27 and ankylosing spondylitis.

Hypersensitivity or Allergy

Hypersensitivity or **allergy** is an altered bodily state in which an exaggerated response occurs with exposure to an antigen. Substances capable of inducing hypersensitivity are called **allergens.** The individual's initial exposure to the allergen—called the sensitizing dose—does not cause a reaction. Subsequent exposure to the allergen does cause a hypersensitivity reaction, however.

Immediate hypersensitivity reactions such as urticaria, anaphylaxis, and allergic rhinitis (hay fever) are mediated by immunoglobulins—a humoral response. *Delayed hypersensitivity* reactions, such as a reaction to a tuberculin skin test, are mediated by the T-lymphocytes—a cell-mediated response. An example of a hypersensitivity response requiring immediate nursing action is anaphylaxis, which is discussed in Chapter 3.

Factors That Affect Immune Response

Stress

Many studies have investigated the association of psychosocial stress with immune system dysfunction. Autoimmune, hypersensitivity, infectious, and malignant disease all may be somehow related to life stress.

Studies such as those by Riley (1981) lend credence to the idea that emotional, psychosocial, or anxiety-stim-

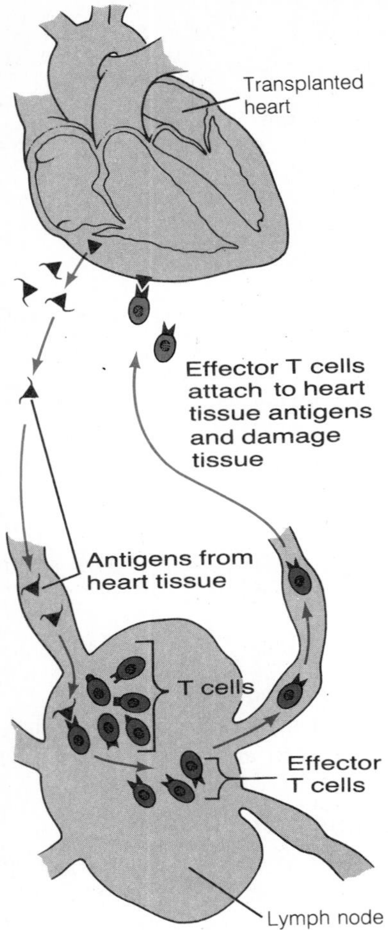

Figure 2–3

Role of cell-mediated immune responses in transplant rejection. SOURCE: *Spence AP, Mason EB:* Human Anatomy and Physiology. *Menlo Park, CA: Benjamin/Cummings, 1983, p. 565.*

ulated stress can produce an increase in plasma concentration of certain hormones associated with injury to parts of the immune system. The individual then may be vulnerable to the action of latent oncogenic (tumor-inducing) viruses (see Chapter 10), newly transformed cancer cells, or other pathological processes that would normally be checked by a heathy immune system.

Age

Developmental factors may also play a role in vulnerability to immune system dysfunction. Levels of immunoglobulin reserve—especially IgG and IgA—are highest between ages 20 and 60. The idea that children and adults over 60 are more susceptible to health problems directly related to the immune system seems plausible considering the major health problems of the very young and the elderly. Infections (eg, otitis media and tonsillitis) and allergy are common in the young. Infections, autoimmune problems, and malignancy are common problems of the elderly. All these disorders are related to immune-system dysfunctions.

SECTION IV

Infection and Inflammation

Infection occurs when the body is invaded by a pathogen that multiplies and produces injurious effects. *Inflammation* is the bodily reaction to injury. Although the terms *infection* and *inflammation* are sometimes used synonymously, they are not interchangeable. Inflammation is a nonspecific response of the body to any tissue injury. Infectious agents are only one of many possible initiators of the inflammatory response.

Infection

Preventing foreign microorganisms from entering the body is the easiest way to avoid infection. The skin and mucous membranes, when intact, are impermeable to most infectious agents. A variety of bacteria inhabit the normal skin but are kept in check by the secretions of the sweat and sebaceous glands. The mucous membranes secrete mucus that entraps small particles, which can then be swept away by the action of cilia, expelled by coughing or sneezing, or engulfed by phagocytic cells. Many of the secreted bodily fluids contain bactericidal components (eg, lysozymes in tears and acids in gastric juice).

The washing action of tears, saliva, and urine also helps protect epithelial surfaces. The nurse who instructs a woman to void after intercourse to prevent urinary infections is applying this principle. Passing urine helps wash out any organisms that have been milked into the urethra and bladder during sexual intercourse.

When host defenses against infection are impaired, the individual becomes susceptible to microbial agents; such a client is called a **compromised host.** Often, the alteration in the defense mechanisms is incompletely understood. From the nurse's standpoint, however, knowing what predisposes the alcoholic client to infection is less important than knowing that the client is a compromised host and at risk. A comprehensive history and physical assessment should always include specific attention to the possibility of infection in any client who could be considered a compromised host. The principle of the compromised host is further discussed in Chapter 9.

Inflammation

The inflammatory response is the body's response to cell injury. Many factors can initiate the process of inflammation, including invasion of the body by microorganisms, mechanical trauma, chemical agents, heat, and cold. The inflammatory response is essentially the same, regardless of the damaging agent. Inflammatory reactions can be local or systemic. *Pain, heat, erythema,* and *edema* are the cardinal subjective and objective findings with local inflammation. Systemic inflammation is associated with *fever* and *leukocytosis.*

How Inflammation Occurs

The vasoconstriction immediately after injury is followed by vasodilation, increasing the blood flow to the area and thereby delivering phagocytes and plasma proteins. Erythema and increased warmth are related to this increased localized blood volume. The permeability of capillaries and venules increases, and plasma fluid and solutes leak from the blood vessels into the inflamed tissues, producing edema. Pain is thought to be secondary to localized pressure from the swelling as well as to action of chemicals on the nerve endings.

Blood viscosity increases as fluid and solutes are lost, and clumping of the red blood cells (erythrocytes) slows the blood flow to the area. Fibrinogen moves from the blood to the tissue spaces and is converted to fibrin, creating a clot that walls off the injured area. Leukocytes enter the damaged tissue and phagocytize invading organisms and cellular debris.

Chemical Mediators of Inflammation

Many chemical substances are activated when tissue damage takes place. *Histamine,* which is present in most tissues, is released when injury occurs, leading to vasodilation and vascular permeability. The *kinins,* a group of polypeptides, also increase vascular permeability and induce pain. In addition, the complement system is involved in enhancing vasodilation, vascular permeability, and phagocytosis. Other substances thought to increase vascular permeability are the *prostaglandins* (a specialized group of fatty acids).

Interferon is a protein produced by T-lymphocytes and many other cells in response to the presence of viruses and other parasites. Interferon seems to protect the body initially against invading viruses until the slower-acting immune response is activated. The possible role of interferon in protecting the body against some cancers is receiving considerable research attention. Use of injected interferon as an anticancer agent has been promising in some clinical studies (see Chapter 10). Generalized stress, which can alter the immune response, may also reduce interferon production by the body.

SECTION 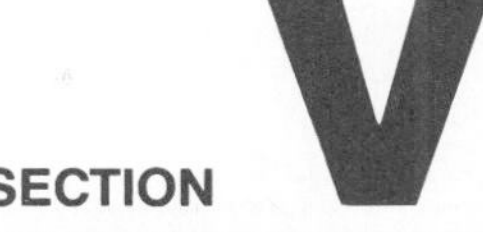

Genetic Influences

Heredity is the transmission of certain characteristics from parent to offspring through *genes*—specific sections of molecules of deoxyribonucleic acid (DNA) carried in the chromosomes within the nucleus of each cell. Genes are arranged linearly along the chromosome, with each gene occupying a specific position, or locus, on a particular chromosome. Each human cell is estimated to contain enough genes to govern about 50,000 traits.

The nucleus of every healthy human cell contains 46 threadlike strands of genetic material (*chromosomes*) arranged in 23 pairs, one of each pair derived from each parent. Of the 23 pairs of chromosomes, one pair is sex chromosomes, and the other 22 pairs are called autosomes. In the female, the sex chromosome is made up of two X chromosomes, and in the male, the sex chromosome contains one X and one Y. The Y chromosome of the male combines with the X chromosome of the female to produce a boy. An X chromosome from each parent produces a girl.

A given gene (eg, hair color) can exist in one of several different states. Alternative forms of the same gene (blond hair versus brown hair) are called *alleles.* The **homozygous** individual has two identical alleles of the gene determining the characteristic under consideration. That is, the person with two identical alleles for blond hair will have blond hair. A person who is **heterozygous** has two different alleles (an allele for blond hair from one parent and an allele for brown hair from the other) at the same locus. In the heterozygous state, one gene may mask or suppress the effect of the other. The brown hair allele will mask or suppress the blond hair allele. The gene characteristic that is expressed (brown hair) is said to be *dominant,* and the one that is masked (blond hair) is called *recessive.* When both alleles of a pair are expressed in the heterozygous state, the genes are said to be *codominant.* Sickle cell anemia, sickle cell trait, and blood type AB are examples of a codominant mode of inheritance.

Genotype is a term that refers to the actual genetic constitution or make up of the individual. Phenotype refers to the way in which the genetic information is expressed as particular traits or characteristics; in other words, the individual's appearance, or what can be observed about that person. Phenotype is influenced by environment as well as by genes. For example, a child may have the genetic capacity for great intelligence but may not achieve that potential because of inadequate nutrition, lack of stimulation, residual defects from birth injury, or diseases of infancy and childhood.

Inheritance Patterns: Some Examples

If an individual who is heterozygous for a dominant gene (Gg) conceives a child with someone who is not carrying the dominant gene, the probability is that half of their children will be affected by the dominant trait. This probability is illustrated in the pedigree pattern (a schematic method for classifying inheritance) in Figure 2–4A. If both individuals are heterozygous for the dominant gene, the probability is that one-fourth of the children will be homozygous dominant (GG), half will be heterozygous (Gg), and one-fourth will be unaffected (Figure 2–4B).

Remember that chance plays a major role in these probability levels, which are based on a large population. For example, in Figure 2–4B where both parents are heterozygous for the trait, the assumption is that if four children are born, two will be Gg, one will be GG, and one will be gg. All four could be GG, or gg, or Gg, however. The probabilities are based on the hypothesis that if these two people could manage to produce a sample size of 100 or so offspring, 50% would be Gg, 25% would be GG, and 25% would be gg.

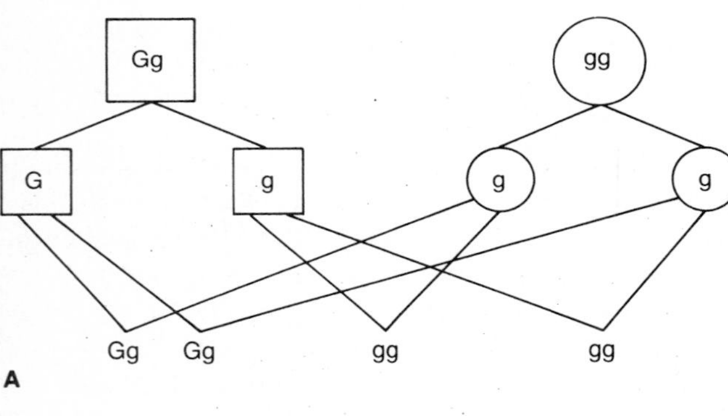

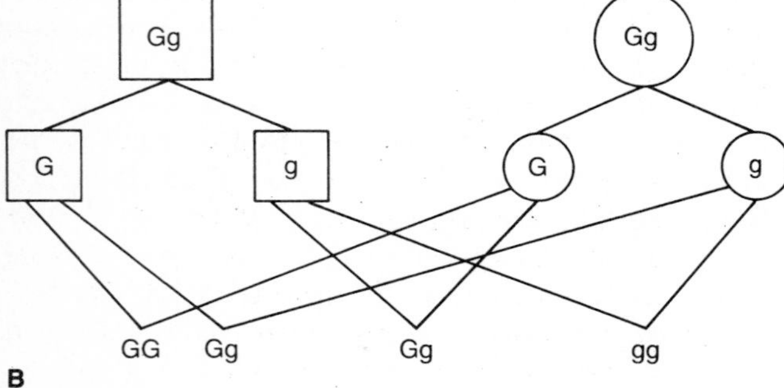

Figure 2–4

Inheritance patterns. **A.** One parent heterozygous, one parent homozygous. **B.** Both parents heterozygous.

Genetic Disorders

Genetic disorders can be classified into three categories:

- Chromosome disorders
- Single-gene disorders
- Multifactorial disorders and their interaction with environmental influences

Chromosomal Disorders

Chromosomal disorders are related to the lack, excess, or abnormal arrangement of one or more chromosomes or segments of the chromosome. These chromosomal aberrations are rarely hereditary and usually affect only a single pregnancy in the family history. Many spontaneous abortions are thought to be related to chromosomal abnormalities.

Cytogenic analysis of chromosomes by banding techniques has been a major breakthrough in the study of chromosomal disorders. A small sample of heparinized blood is all that is required for analysis. Special staining techniques create alternating patterns of light and dark bands, which are highly characteristic for each chromosome, so individual chromosomes may be recognized. Photographs of an individual's banded chromosomes may then be assembled to show a picture of that person's karyotype, or chromosomal arrangement. Down's syndrome is the most common chromosomal disorder.

Single-Gene Disorders

A single mutant gene is the cause of single-gene disorders. The types of inheritance patterns with single-gene traits are: autosomal dominant, autosomal recessive, codominant, and sex linked or X-linked.

Autosomal dominant disorders often have a delayed age of onset and usually vary considerably in clinical expression. Examples of autosomal dominant disorders are Huntington's chorea, adult polycystic kidney disease, familial hypercholesterolemia, and Marfan's syndrome. In autosomal dominant disorders, the abnormal allele is dominant, and the normal allele is recessive.

With *autosomal recessive* disorders, the parents appear to be unaffected by the disorder but are carriers of the disease. The abnormal allele is recessive. The trait must be inherited from *both* parents for it to be expressed. Examples of these diseases include Tay–Sachs disease, cystic fibrosis, and phenylketonuria.

The genes responsible for *sex-linked* disorders are located on the X chromosome and affect men more than women. The complex nature of X-linked inheritance makes it possible for the disease to be passed down through several generations of a family without manifesting itself. Among the most common X-linked disorders are hemophilia A, color blindness, and glucose-6-phosphate dehydrogenase (G-6-PD) deficiency.

The effect of certain drugs on clients with some single-gene disorders can be life threatening. For example, clients with G-6-PD deficiency may develop a hemolytic anemia when given analgesics, sulfonamides, or antimalarials.

Multifactorial Disorders

Multifactorial disorders are a diverse group of genetic diseases in which genetic susceptibility combines with environmental factors to produce a variety of disorders. Although these traits tend to cluster in families, they are not clearly predictable. They include common birth defects such as cleft lip and palate, spina bifida, and congenital heart disease. They also include diseases with an inherited susceptibility such as diabetes mellitus, hypertension, coronary artery disease, peptic ulcer, thyroid disease, and schizophrenia.

SECTION 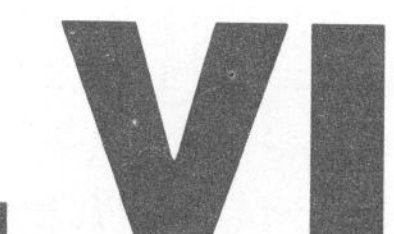

Neoplasia

The word neoplasia means "new growth" (*neo* + *plasia*), and **neoplasm** is generally used synonymously with tumor.

Benign Versus Malignant Neoplasia

Neoplasms are classified as *benign*—meaning the dividing cells adhere to each other and the tumor remains circumscribed—or *malignant*—meaning that the tumor cells invade surrounding tissue. The cells of malignant tumors (cancers) also may enter natural channels such as the blood vessels or the lymphatics and spread from their original site to other parts of the body. There they produce secondary growths called *metastatic lesions*.

Tumor nomenclature is not entirely consistent, so it is sometimes difficult to determine from the name of a tumor whether it is benign or malignant. Generally, the suffix "oma" combined with the name of the affected tissue designate a benign tumor (eg, a lipoma is a benign tumor of the lipid (fat) tissue). Malignant tumors are first differentiated according to the cellular structure from which they arise. Malignant tumors arising from epithelial tissue are called carcinomas. Those arising from connective tissue are called sarcomas.

Benign neoplasms do not invade surrounding tissue or metastasize, but they can cause injurious local and systemic effects. For example, pressure from a benign tumor can be life threatening if the tumor is located in the brain where there is no room for expansion. A benign tumor can also cause obstruction (eg, within the intestine or in a bronchus) leading to potentially serious sequelae. Some benign tumors secrete hormones that have injurious effects (eg, an adenoma of the islets of Langerhans in the pancreas leads to an oversupply of insulin and thereby to hypoglycemia).

Because malignant neoplasms can infiltrate surrounding tissues and metastasize to distant structures, their potential for destruction is immense. Like benign tumors, cancers can cause pressure and obstructive problems as well as overproduction of hormones if a gland is involved. Among the devastating effects associated with cancer are the following: hemorrhage, anemia, ulceration, infection, pathological fractures, pain, and **cachexia** (a term denoting the progressive weakness, malnutrition, weight loss, and emaciation that sometimes occurs with advanced cancer).

Much remains to be learned about what causes cells to overproliferate, forming tumors. Research on malignant neoplasms has generated a number of theories, including genetic composition of the host, immunologic factors, viruses, environmental and occupational exposures, drugs and radiation effects, diet, and stress. Because all persons exposed to known carcinogens do not develop cancer, host factors are thought to play a major role in the process. Therefore, a multifactorial approach seems the most promising in finding a cancer cure. See Chapter 10 for a full discussion of cancer and care of the client with malignant neoplasia.

Early Detection and Prevention of Cancer

Cancer of the cervix, breasts, bowel, oral cavity, and testes can be detected early by relatively noninvasive techniques practiced by health care providers or in some cases, by clients themselves. Self-examination of the mouth, the breasts, and the testicles requires that the client receive careful instruction initially and understand the importance of routine self-assessment (eg, monthly). In their ability to detect disease early, the value of yearly Pap smears for women, digital rectal examinations for both men and women, and testing of stool for occult blood outweigh the possible embarrassment they may cause.

Until recently, efforts at cancer prevention have primarily included cessation of smoking, reduction of exposure to the sun, and protection of workers against known carcinogens in the workplace. Currently, there is considerable interest in evidence that high-fat diets are implicated in cancer of the colon, rectum, breast, and perhaps prostate. Cancer of the colon and rectum have also been linked to diets low in fiber. In light of current evidence on the connection between diet and cancer, it appears sensible to increase the fiber content and decrease the fat content in the average daily diet.

The link between stress and cancer is somewhat more nebulous. Part of the human stress response involves an increased production and release of adrenocorticotropic hormone (ACTH) from the pituitary, which in turn stimulates production of glucocorticoids in the adrenal cortex. Elevations of ACTH and glucocorticoids suppress immunocompetence by causing involution of the thymus and lymphatics and reducing the number of circulating lymphocytes. Some researchers believe that this stress-produced alteration in the immune response may be a contributing component in the development of cancer. Incorporating stress-reduction approaches in daily living may therefore be another way to reduce the risk of cancer.

Nursing Research Note

Chang BL et al.: Adherence to health care regimens among elderly women. *Nurs Res* 1985; 34:27–31.

After viewing videotaped interactions between nurse practitioners (NPs) and clients, 26 older adults rated components of the NPs' care according to whether the measures would affect the client's intent to adhere to the care plan. The components—technical quality, psychosocial care, and client participation—were not found significant. Significant factors included widowhood, religion, perceived importance of the exam, social network, and pre-existing satisfaction with health care. These results reinforce the necessity of identifying a client's supportive networks and previous health experiences in determining intent to adhere to a plan of care.

SECTION **VII**

The Aging Process and Degeneration

Why do humans age? What degenerative changes are invariably associated with aging? These questions are the focus of a great deal of research. Physiologic theories of aging center on the immune system, genetic programming, metabolic changes, and a lifetime of wear and tear. Immune system research suggests that the decrease in size and function of the thymus gland and the resulting decline in T cell activity with age impair the body's ability to fight off infection. An autoimmune process may also occur in which the body begins to attack its own cells. Another theory suggests that aging is caused by cumulative damage from environmental insults to the genetic information systems of the cell—DNA and RNA. Degenerative theories speculate that the body's ability to reproduce new cells or repair damaged ones decreases over time and eventually cannot keep up with the years of destruction. Other theories suggest that cellular aging is programmed to produce tissue death and that chemical substances called "free radicals" are active in the aging process.

As persons age, they are at greater risk for certain types of diseases and injuries. The degree of disability from these disorders appears to increase with age, yet many elderly persons are never afflicted with serious health problems. Of problems that do occur, many are preventable (eg, falls), most are treatable (eg, hypertension), and the majority can be compensated for in one way or another (eg, decreased auditory or visual acuity).

Being aware of the normal physiologic changes associated with aging is important for nurses so they can help clients cope with the changes. Using the approach of *promoting* health and *preventing* disease, nurses can do much to offset the effects of aging. The most common changes related to aging are summarized in Table 2–2.

Muscle groups generally weakened in the elderly (pectorals, abdominal muscles, pelvic and hip extensors) can be firmed by muscle-strengthening activities. Swimming, riding a stationary bicycle, and performing regular stretching exercises make both muscles and joints more flexible. Walking, swimming, and dancing are excellent ways to improve cardiopulmonary function and to combat fatigue. Clients can learn that avoiding quick head movements or rapid change in position can help them avert falls. Yearly visual examinations with tonometry aid in detecting glaucoma early and preventing blindness.

Homes can be made safer with support rails in the bathtub and on stairways, rubber mats or nonskid strips on the tub or shower floor, smoke detectors, assistance with proper footwear, and precautions with heating pads and hot water bottles. The client can be encouraged to plan dietary changes, such as increasing fiber consumption to prevent constipation or reducing fat and sugar intake to prevent weight gain. Dietary measures can also assist in controlling or preventing Type II diabetes mellitus and hypertension. Dental problems and periodontal disease can be minimized by avoiding sugars, brushing and flossing the teeth thoroughly each day, and having them cleaned professionally twice a year. Dentures or partial plates should be worn for proper chewing, and discomfort or sores secondary to their use should be evaluated immediately. Malignancies in the elderly can be detected early through oral self-examinations, breast self-examinations, testing stools for occult blood, mammography, and Pap smears.

The aging process is not merely a function of physiology. Social factors are crucial to how the aged view their health, and, in fact, to how healthy they actually are. The

Table 2–2
Physiologic Changes Associated With Aging

Organ or System	Physiologic Change
Skin	• Becomes thinned and dry; ↓ in subcutaneous fat; ↓ in activity of hair follicles, sweat glands, and sebaceous glands • Atrophy of melanocytes with graying of hair • Thickening of nails
Eyes	• Pupil loses its ability to dilate fully, contributing to ↓ in vision and development of glaucoma • Lens gradually loses elasticity, resulting in presbyopia • Lens gradually yellows, altering color vision • Lens may opacify causing ↓ in vision, falls • Lifetime exposure of rods and cones to light results in damage, contributing to ↓ in vision, falls
Ears	• ↓ Elasticity of tympanic membrane, impaired articulation of ossicles, resulting in ↓ hearing • Degenerative cochlear changes and loss of cells from the organ of Corti, causing ↓ hearing • Possible degeneration in vestibular function contributing to loss of balance
Respiratory system	• ↑ Rigidity of chest wall; ↓ elasticity of lungs, resulting in ↓ in vital capacity • ↓ In phagocytic activity of macrophages and ↓ in efficiency of cilia lining the respiratory tract, resulting in susceptibility to respiratory infections
Cardiovascular system	• ↓ Stroke volume, ↓ heart rate, resulting in ↓ cardiac output • Sinus node dysfunction, contributing to atrial dysrhythmia • Thickening of the intima of the arterial wall with gradually increasing rigidity of vessels, contributing to hypertension and aneurysm formation
Kidneys	• ↓ Blood flow, resulting in ↓ glomerular filtration rate and ↓ urea clearance • ↓ In renal tubule function, resulting in ↓ ability to concentrate urine
GI system	• Atrophy of taste buds and ↓ salivary flow • Enamel loss, ↑ pigmentation of teeth and recession of gums • ↓ Motility, resulting in constipation • ↓ Intestinal blood flow, which may affect drug absorption
Muscles	• ↓ Skeletal muscle mass with resultant ↓ strength and ↓ agility, ↑ in falls
Bones	• Loss of calcium from bones (more severe in postmenopausal women), resulting in osteoporosis • Bone matrix breaks down, resulting in brittleness.
Joints	• Progressive loss of cartilaginous joint surface, resulting in degenerative joint disease
Neurologic system	• ↓ Velocity of nerve conduction • ↓ In memory • Alterations in circadian rhythms, sleep patterns • ↓ In brain size and weight; ↓ cerebellar function resulting in loss of balance, falls
Endocrine system	• Decline in glucose tolerance • Menopause with ↓ estrogen secretion and thermoregulation alterations in women • ↓ Testosterone, ↑ estrogen in males resulting in prostatic hyperplasia, possible gynecomastia
Immune system	• ↓ Thymus activity, ↓ T cell function • ↓ B cell response • ↑ Susceptibility to infection, autoimmune disease, and malignancy

traditional, disease-oriented health care system tends to view the older person with degenerative joint disease and decreased hearing as diseased. Yet the elderly person who has adjusted well to the gradual limitations imposed by age may be content with life, may participate fully in social roles, and may feel healthy both physically and psychologically. Some research has shown that elderly persons who maintain active social contact with others are more satisfied with life and are more likely to view themselves as healthy than those who are socially isolated. Although it is clear that as aging progresses, the body gradually loses its capacity for peak performance, it is also clear that much can be done to maximize health and the quality of life as persons grow older.

SECTION 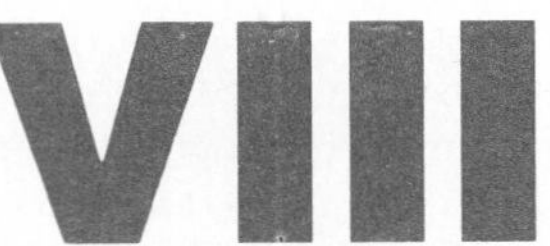

Trauma

Injuries rank as the fourth leading cause of death in the United States for all age groups (*Morbidity and Mortality Weekly Report,* May 14, 1982). Considering years of life lost prematurely, injuries rank first. The risk of injury from motor vehicle accidents, falls, burns, accidental poisoning, drowning, sports activities, and occupational accidents is inherent in daily living. Certain groups are at higher risk for specific types of trauma; for example, motor vehicle collisions are a major cause of disability and death for children aged 1 to 14, whereas for the elderly, falls are the most likely to bring about permanent or fatal injury. Reducing traumatic injury depends upon efforts of heath care providers, employers, legislators, equipment designers and manufacturers, and individuals to monitor policies and practices that promote health and safety. Groups such as MADD (Mothers Against Drunk Driving) have been effective in introducing tougher legislation on drunk driving, a major factor in senseless injury and death for thousands each year.

Traumatic injuries can affect a single body part or may involve several body parts (multiple trauma). Trauma may be categorized as blunt, penetrating, contrecoup, or crushing. *Blunt trauma* occurs when a blunt object forcibly hits the body, such as a steering wheel, fist, or the ground in a fall. *Penetrating injuries* involve actual penetration of the body by a foreign object, such as a knife or bullet. When the velocity of impact against a blunt object causes internal organs to bounce forcefully against the internal body wall or bony structures surrounding the organs, a *contrecoup injury* results. Severe head and chest injuries often involve this "shifting" type of trauma. *Crushing trauma* results when body parts are literally crushed or smashed. This type of injury may occur in falls from high places or motor vehicle accidents where the force of impact collapses or crushes body structures. Accidents involving equipment such as farm tractors or industrial machinery often cause crushing injuries.

Motor Vehicle Accidents

Occupants of motor vehicles sustain the largest percentage of fatal injuries for all ages up to age 75. Risk of injury and death is highly correlated with amount of highway travel, road characteristics, speed of vehicle, vehicle size, and use of restraint systems. Alcohol use is a major contributing factor.

For a number of years, efforts have been under way to require automobile manufacturers to design systems that provide passive (automatic) crash protection, especially for those in the front seat who tend to receive the most serious injuries. Active restraint systems, such as seat belts and infant/child car seats, have been shown to reduce drastically the likelihood of serious injury and death. But these systems require individuals to participate actively in protecting themselves and others. Unfortunately, knowing about the benefits of such systems is not enough to induce people to use them.

Pedestrian deaths from motor vehicles are also a major problem. Those most likely to be killed are the aged, the very young, or individuals impaired by alcohol or drugs. Efforts to protect pedestrians include better illumination, traffic lights timed to favor pedestrian traffic, and placing bus stops farther from intersections.

Many states have raised the legal drinking age to 21 to reduce motor vehicle accidents and have imposed severe penalties on those who are apprehended for driving while intoxicated. Comprehensive driver education programs for teenagers and raising the legal driving age are other approaches to preventing vehicle-related injuries and death.

Motorcycles, mopeds, and bicycles are responsible for a significant number of head injuries each year as well as for other traumatic injuries such as fractures of the long bones of the extremities. The use of helmets has been the most effective approach to reducing severe head injury and death in motorcyclists.

Falls

Fatal falls occur most often in the home. Falling is also a major factor in occupational deaths, especially among construction workers. The elderly are at high risk of falling; moreover, sequelae of fractures from falls prevent many elderly victims from resuming independent lives after their injuries.

Reducing the distance a person in a high-risk situation can fall or modifying the surface on which a fall is likely to occur can effectively reduce the impact. Hospital beds, diving boards, and high chairs can be lowered; floors and stairs can be carpeted or padded. Padded clothing and helmets may be worn by those at particular risk. Falls can be prevented by providing proper illumination, installing window guards and handrails, using nonslip surfaces in bathtubs, removing clutter of furniture and toys, and wearing shoes that properly support the foot and provide sufficient friction between the shoe sole and the walking surface.

Burns

Residential fires are a leading cause of accidental death and an important source of disability and disfigurement. Injuries and deaths related to house fires can be reduced by installing smoke detectors, providing alternative exit routes, using drapes and clothing made of flame-retardant fabric, and using flame-retardant paint and construction materials. Tap water scald injuries can be prevented by keeping the water heater temperature no higher than 120° F (48.9° C). Having fire extinguishers readily accessible and in good working order, not smoking in bed, and not overloading electrical circuits are all important fire and burn prevention measures. The nursing care of the burned client is discussed in Chapter 12.

Accidental Poisoning

Nurses have many opportunities to teach clients how to avoid accidental poisoning. Among the toxic substances that pose a hazard are household cleaning products, medications, pesticides, cosmetics, alcohol, poisonous indoor and outdoor plants, and lead paint. Many cities have poison control centers that can give information quickly about most toxic substances and provide protocols for treatment for clients of any age.

Nurses should be aware of folk remedies that may cause lead poisoning. Some Hispanics use fine powders for chronic diarrhea, called greta or azarcón, which have a high lead content. Children from the Hmong tribe in northern Laos now living in Minnesota, were found to have lead poisoning secondary to the use of pay-loo-ah, a red and orange powder used to treat fever or rash (*Morbidity and Mortality Weekly Report,* Oct 28, 1983). Elevated blood levels of lead secondary to inhalation and ingestion are an occupational hazard among workers involved in smelting; recovery of scrap; cutting of steel; and manufacture of batteries, lead pigment, and stained glass (*Morbidity and Mortality Weekly Report,* April 29, 1983).

Drowning and Aquatic Injuries

Spinal cord injuries from diving and sliding into the water head first permanently paralyze many teenagers and young adults each year. Surfing and water skiing are also implicated in spinal cord trauma. Drowning and serious trauma are more likely when alcohol or drug use are part of aquatic recreational activities.

Sports Injuries

Athletic safety depends on the physical conditioning of the participant, proper protective equipment, and control of the sports environment. Informal sports and recreation, in which there are little physical preparation and use of protective equipment, may be an even greater threat to personal health and safety than organized sports. The rate of sports-related injury and illness can be reduced by wearing face masks and helmets; designating obstacle-free zones around playing fields; eliminating common injury-producing maneuvers from the sport; preventing heat cramps, heat stroke, hypothermia, and frostbite; and doing warming-up exercises before vigorous activity.

Work-Related Injuries

On-the-job injuries are common in construction, manufacturing, mining, and agriculture. Types of wounds include abrasions, lacerations, contusions, fractures, concussions, crushing injuries, and traumatic amputations. More work time is lost from low-back pain than any other related injury; low-back pain also is the main category of workers' compensation payments. Injury from inhaled gases, vapors, and smoke is not uncommon in firefighters and those involved in manufacturing synthetic materials such as plastics and polyurethanes.

The preemployment history and physical can be helpful in identifying persons who might be at increased risk for on-the-job injury (eg, those with impaired sight, hearing, or balance or those taking medications that produce drowsiness, such as antihistamines). The occupational health nurse can be instrumental in preventing accidents on the job by referring employees at risk—such as those with visual or hearing loss—to appropriate health care providers and recommending appropriate jobs.

The nurse in industry is also responsible for employee education programs dealing with risk reduction. Occupational trauma may be prevented, or at least reduced, by teaching workers how to bend and lift properly, how to care for the machinery they use, and how to spot potential hazards. Workers should be encouraged to use such safety equipment as earplugs, protective goggles, and respirators. Constant vigilance—assessing the work area and work practices continually for potential hazards—is crucial to preventing injury.

Chapter Highlights

Illness (dis-ease) is directly related to the sum of all factors affecting a person's life.

Nursing practice is based on holistic concepts and a multifactorial view of illness.

Stress, with its physiologic and psychosocial concomitants, causes wear and tear on the whole person. Continued and unabated stress may even cause death.

Common human events, both joyous and catastrophic, are likely to cause stress when they occur in clusters.

Internal and external factors affecting physiology, such as stress, immune response, infection and inflammation, genetic predispositions, neoplasia, aging, and trauma, are closely interrelated with psychosocial and environmental influences on the individual.

The immune system is one of the body's principal defenses against disease. Disturbance or

dysfunction of the immune system itself can cause disease, however.

Microbial agents can produce injurious effects in the body. Inflammation is the body's response to cell injury.

Inherited disorders can result from a defect in a chromosome or chromosomal segment, a defect in a single gene, or an interaction between genetic susceptibility and environmental factors.

Neoplasms can cause both injurious local and systemic effects.

Degenerative changes, usually associated with aging or the cumulative effects of wear and tear on a body part, can have a major impact on lifestyle.

Traumatic injuries are a leading cause of death for all age groups. The incidence of traumatic injury can be reduced through public education and legislation.

Bibliography

Allen JC: *Infection and the Compromised Host,* 2nd ed. Baltimore: Williams & Wilkins, 1981.

Ames SA, Gelein J, Humphrey E, Mason–Kaufman J, Osborne JE: A systems approach to curricula in primary health care nursing. In: *Approaches to Teaching Primary Health Care.* Knopke HJ, Diekelmann NL (editors). St Louis: Mosby, 1981.

Atchley RC: *Aging: Continuity and Change.* Belmont, CA: Wadsworth, 1983.

Beard MT: Trust, life events, and risk factors among adults. *ANS* (July) 1982; 4:26–43.

Dohrenwend BS, Dohrenwend BP (editors): *Stressful Life Events and Their Contexts.* Brunswick, NJ: Rutgers University Press, 1984.

Flynn ME: Influencing repair and recovery. *Am J Nurs* 1982; 82:1550–1558.

Flynn ME, Rovee DT: Wound healing mechanisms. *Am J Nurs* 1982; 82:1543–1550.

Folk remedy-associated lead poisoning in Hmong children—Minnesota. *MMWR* (Oct 28) 1983; 32:555–556.

Gold EB: *The Changing Risk of Disease in Women: An Epidemiologic Approach.* Lexington, MA: Collamore, 1984.

Holmes TH, Rahe RH: The social readjustment rating scale. *J of Psychosom Res* 1967; 11:213–218.

Kenney RA: *Physiology of Aging: A Synopsis.* Chicago: Yearbook Publishers, 1982.

Lazarus RS, Folkman S: *Stress, Appraisal, and Coping.* New York: Springer, 1984.

Lead poisoning from Mexican folk remedies—California. *MMWR* (Oct 28) 1983; 32:554–555.

Leiberman MA, Tobin SS: *Experience of Old Age.* New York: Basic Books, 1983.

Lyon BL, Werner J: Stress: Ten years of practice-relevant research. In: Werley H, Fitzpatrick J (editors): *Annual Review of Nursing Research.* New York: Springer, 1987.

Mason LJ: *Guide to Stress Reduction.* Culver City, CA: Peace Press, 1980.

Pelletier KR: *Healthy People in Unhealthy Places: Stress and Fitness at Work.* New York: Doubleday, 1984.

Porcino J: *Growing Older, Getting Better.* Reading, MA: Addison–Wesley, 1983.

Ramsey JM: *Basic Pathophysiology: Modern Stress and the Disease Process.* Menlo Park, CA: Addison–Wesley, 1982.

Reed P: Implications of the life-span developmental framework for well-being in adulthood and aging. *ANS* (October) 1983; 5:18–25.

Results of blood lead determinations among workers potentially exposed to lead—United States. *MMWR* (April 29) 1983; 32:216–219.

Richter MA: *Clinical Immunology: A Physician's Guide,* 2nd ed. Baltimore: Williams & Wilkins, 1982.

Riley V: Psychoneuroendocrine influences on immunocompetence and neoplasia. *Science* 1981, 212:1100–1109.

Selye H: *The Stress of Life.* New York: McGraw–Hill, 1956.

Unintentional and intentional injuries—United States. *MMWR* (May 14) 1982; 31:240, 245–248.

Walter JB: *An Introduction to the Principles of Disease,* 2nd ed. Philadelphia: Saunders, 1982.

Resources

SELF-HELP GROUPS AND OTHER ORGANIZATIONS

Mothers Against Drunk Driving (MADD)
5330 Primrose, Suite 146
Fair Oaks, CA 95628
Phone: (916) 537–9045

An organization that acts as a voice for victims of drunk driving accidents and their families. The group is active in supporting highway patrol programs and lobbying for state and federal legislation for reform of drunk driving laws. MADD also provides counseling services for victims and families and publishes brochures and a newsletter aimed at widespread public education.

National Center for Human Genetic Diseases
38th and R St, NW
Washington, DC 20057
Phone: (202) 625–8400

Provides information on prevention, diagnosis, and treatment of genetic diseases.

National Institute of Mental Health
Public Inquiries Branch
Room 15C05
5600 Fishers La
Rockville, MD 20857
Phone: (301) 443–4517

This division of the federal government provides information on stress control programs and resources throughout the country.

National Clearinghouse for Poison Control Centers
US Department of Health and Human Services
Public Health Service
5401 Westbard Ave
Bethesda, MD 20016

Provides a list of Poison Control Centers in the United States. Publishes a news bulletin and distributes poison information cards (Poison Control Cards).

National Foundation for Jewish Genetic Diseases
250 Park Ave, Suite 1000
New York, NY 10017
Phone: (213) 371–1030

Publishes information on Jewish genetic diseases, their prevention, diagnosis, and treatment.

National Institute for Occupational Safety and Health (NIOSH)
Centers for Disease Control
Robert A. Taft Laboratory
4676 Columbia Pkwy
Cincinnati, OH 45226
Phone: (513) 684–8326

This arm of the Centers for Disease Control serves as a clearinghouse for information and research on occupational safety and health.

National Safety Council
425 N. Michigan Ave
Chicago, IL 60611
Phone: (312) 527–4800

This organization gathers and distributes information to the public and to professionals concerning the causes of accidental death and disability with a focus on methods of prevention. The goal is to reduce the number and severity of all types of accidents and occupational illnesses.

Occupational Safety and Health Administration (OSHA)
Office of Public and Consumer Affairs
US Department of Labor (Room N3637)
200 Constitution Ave, NW
Washington, DC 20210
Phone: (202) 523–8148

This federal agency is responsible for overseeing and enforcing safety practices and regulations in occupational and industrial work settings.

HOT LINES

Information Clearinghouse on Aging
(National Geriatrics Society)
212 W Wisconsin Ave
Milwaukee, WI 53203
Phone: (414) 272–4130

Poisoning Information Hotline
Pittsburgh Children's Hospital
3705 Fifth Ave
Pittsburgh, PA 15213
Phone: (412) 681–6669 (24 hours)

Provides information to aid victims of accidental poisoning, supplies the address of the nearest poison treatment center, and calls the center while the victim is en route to ensure prompt attention. Sponsored by the National Poison Center Network at Pittsburgh Children's Hospital.

HEALTH EDUCATION MATERIAL

From: US Department of Health and Human Services
National Institutes of Health
Bldg 31, Room 7A32
Bethesda, MD 20205

Free booklet entitled *Understanding the Immune System,* 1983.

NURSING ORGANIZATION

Emergency Nurses' Association (ENA)
230 E Ohio
Suite 600
Chicago, IL 60611
Phone: (312) 649–0297

This professional association for nurses who work in emergency nursing or are interested in the field is concerned with establishing standards for optimum emergency care. Provides public education and continuing education in emergency nursing and conducts a certification program. Also publishes the *Journal of Emergency Nursing.*

CHAPTER 3

How the Body Maintains and Protects Homeostasis

Objectives

When you have finished studying this chapter, you should be able to:

Explain the terms isotonic, hypertonic, and hypotonic.

Specify how the body normally maintains fluid equilibrium.

Compare and contrast the major electrolyte imbalances.

Describe the major buffer systems for maintaining the pH of the extracellular fluid.

Summarize the acid–base changes that occur in both acidosis and alkalosis.

Compare and contrast hypovolemic shock, cardiogenic shock, and distributive shock.

Anticipate the common clinical manifestations of shock and identify clients at risk for shock.

Describe how gate control theory and theories about the role of endorphins and enkephalins explain the phenomenon of pain and pain control.

Distinguish between acute pain, chronic pain, referred pain, and phantom pain.

Specify how the nurse can individualize nursing approaches to keep clients pain free.

The human body maintains its homeostatic balance through the complex interaction of all bodily systems. This chapter is concerned with the processes that normally preserve a state of equilibrium—the balance of fluids, electrolytes, acids, and bases. In addition, this chapter considers processes that protect the body from internal and external insults—the phenomena of shock and pain. Although these processes are often considered physiologic, it is clear that the mind has a significant influence on these bodily responses.

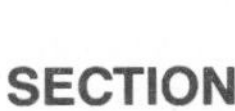

SECTION I

Fluid and Electrolyte Balance

Proper fluid and electrolyte balance in the body is essential for good health and for life itself. This balance of fluid and electrolytes must be maintained within a normal range and is an essential component of the body's homeostatic processes. The body's physiologic processes maintain this balance in health, but almost all illnesses or states of disequilibrium threaten the balance. The young, the old, and those with chronic illness are the most susceptible to imbalances.

Proportions and Distribution of Body Fluids

Water is the largest single constituent of the body, composing 55% of the average healthy woman's weight and 57% of an average man's weight. This volume of body fluid remains relatively constant in health, varying less than 0.2 kg (0.5 lb) in 24 hours, regardless of the amount of fluid ingested. The percentage of total body fluid varies with a person's sex, age, and amount of total body fat. An early human embryo is 97% fluid. This percentage decreases with age; an elderly adult is composed of approximately 45% fluid. Body fat is essentially water-free, and persons with less body fat have a greater proportion of water to body weight. Women after puberty have proportionately more fat than men and, therefore, have a smaller percentage of fluid in relation to total body weight.

Fluid Compartments

Body water is divided into two major compartments: intracellular and extracellular. Intracellular fluid (ICF), also referred to as cellular fluid, is within the cells and makes up two-thirds to three-quarters of total body fluid, or about 25 L. Extracellular fluid (ECF), fluid outside the cells, makes up the remainder of the body's fluid, about 15 L. ECF is subdivided into interstitial fluid and intravascular fluid, or plasma. Interstitial fluid surrounds the cells and contains lymph, providing the cells with the external medium for cellular metabolism. Intravascular fluid, the liquid part of the blood, is found within the vascular system. Plasma contains colloids (plasma proteins), and in conjunction with the red blood cells, maintains vascular volume.

The fluids in the ICF and ECF compartments are not static and move freely among the cells, tissue spaces, and plasma. ECF serves as the transportation system of the body via two mechanisms: the movement of blood through the circulatory system and the movement of fluid between the cells and the blood capillaries. Plasma carries nutrients, water, and electrolytes to the cells and removes the waste products of cellular metabolism from them. Additionally, plasma carries oxygen from the lungs to the capillaries and removes carbon dioxide, returning it to the lungs. The lymph component of interstitial fluid also transports wastes from the cells, ultimately entering the vascular circulation through the thoracic duct.

Transcellular fluids, or the body's secretions and excretions, are also part of the ECF volume. A *secretion* is the product of a gland, such as saliva, gastrointestinal secretions, cerebrospinal fluid, and synovial fluid. *Excretions* are waste products produced in the body, such as urine and feces. These transcellular fluids must remain in balance for effective bodily function. Excessive excretions deplete the ECF volume and then the ICF volume. Inadequate or excessive secretions may also interfere with digestion and elimination. Eventually, these imbalances alter homeostasis.

Electrolytes

Extracellular and intracellular body fluids contain both electrolyte and nonelectrolyte particles. *Electrolytes* are substances, often salts or minerals, whose molecules dissociate in water. When the molecules dissociate, they disintegrate into electrically charged ions (*ionization*) that are capable of conducting a weak electrical charge, hence the term *electrolyte*. Nonelectrolyte substances, such as glucose and urea, do not dissociate in water, nor do they develop electrical charges. When a salt such as sodium chloride dissociates and ionizes, the particles develop either a positive charge, becoming *cations*, or a negative charge, becoming *anions*. Sodium is always a cation with one positive charge (Na^+), and chloride is an anion with a negative charge (Cl^-). Body water contains both cations and anions, maintaining electrolyte balance. Thus, each cation is balanced chemically by an anion: for example, sodium chloride (Na^+Cl^-).

The common cations with one electrical charge (*monovalent* cations) are sodium (Na^+) and potassium (K^+); the common cations with two electrical charges (*bivalent*) are calcium (Ca^{2+}) and magnesium (Mg^{2+}). The commonovalent anions are chloride (Cl^-) and bicarbonate (HCO_3^-), whereas the bivalent anions are sulfate (SO_4^{2-}) and hydrogen biphosphate (HPO_4^{2-}).

Measurement and Distribution of Body Electrolytes

Electrolytes exist in both fluid compartments of the body in differing concentrations and compositions. They are measured according to numbers of particles, osmotic activity, or chemical activity. The number of particles per unit of volume is expressed as moles or millimoles (1/1000 of a mole). This unit of measure, expressed as grams or milligrams per 100 mL, gives no direct information about the number of ions or about the numbers of electrical charges the particles carry. For this reason, this measurement is seldom used in referring to electrolyte concentrations.

Osmols and milliosmols (1/1000 of an osmol) are the units of measurement based on osmotic activity. They are the measures of the amount of work dissolved particles can do in drawing fluid through a semipermeable membrane. *Osmotic activity* depends on the number of actual particles in solution irrespective of any charge they may carry; even nonionizable charges such as glucose and urea exert an osmotic effect.

Electrolytes are usually measured in milliequivalents per liter of water (mEq/L). The term *milliequivalent* means 1/1000 of an equivalent, with an equivalent referring to the chemical combining power of a substance. The chemical combining power of a substance is the power of cations to unite with anions to form molecules and is measured in relation to the chemical combining power of hydrogen (H^+). Sodium and chloride ions are equivalent because they combine equally (eg, 1 mEq of Na^+ = 1 mEq of Cl^-). The milliequivalent system is used most often clinically because the reacting capacity and number of solute particles are known, and electrical imbalances and shifts are easier to evaluate and follow.

The predominant electrolytes in the ECF are sodium and chloride, whereas the major electrolytes in the cells or ICF are potassium and phosphate. The ion composition of the two major subdivisions of ECF (plasma and interstitial fluid) are similar; the main difference is that plasma has a higher concentration of protein. Electrolyte levels are measured in the intravascular portion of the ECF. The plasma is relatively easy to sample, but the electrolyte composition of cellular fluid is difficult to measure and varies somewhat from tissue to tissue. Therefore, the "normal range" of electrolyte values used clinically is a *serum measurement*, which is only an approximate measurement for the cellular fluids. The normal ranges for the four most commonly measured electrolytes are: Na^+, 136–145 mEq/L; K^+, 3.5–5.0 mEq/L; Ca^{2+}, 4.3–5.3 mEq/L; and Cl^-, 100–106 mEq/L. The transcellular fluids such as urine, bile, and saliva each has its distinct electrolyte composition, which tends to be stable in health.

Movement of Body Fluid and Electrolytes

Substance transport and fluid movement within the body can be described in three phases. First, nutrients and fluids are absorbed by the plasma from the lungs and gastrointestinal tract and carried within the circulatory tract. Second, the interstitial fluid and its components move between the capillaries and cells, carrying the nutrients from the plasma. Third, fluid and its solutes move from the interstitial fluid into the cells. The process then reverses itself, ending with the kidneys receiving the by-products of cellular metabolism carried by the plasma. Fluids and their carried substances move by diffusion, active transport, and osmosis.

Diffusion

Diffusion is the mixing of molecules caused by the tendency of molecules to move continuously and randomly in a solution or a gas. Particles move from an area of greater concentration to an area of lesser concentration. The greater the difference in concentration, the faster the rate of diffusion. Two other factors affect the rate of diffusion: molecule size and temperature of the solution. The larger the molecule, the slower the process because larger molecules need more energy to move. Also, higher temperatures increase the rate at which molecules move and, therefore, increase the rate of diffusion. When discussing the diffusion of electrolytes, remember that the particle's electrical charge also affects the process, because ions are pulled toward ions with opposite charges. Body electrolytes diffuse between the membrane pores in the capillaries and the interstitial fluid.

Active Transport

Active transport is the movement of small particles across cell membranes from an area of lesser concentration to greater concentration. This movement requires energy from an outside source (ie, metabolic energy provided by enzymes) and, therefore, differs from osmosis and diffusion. Other substances requiring transport combine with their specific carrier outside the cell membrane to enter the cell. Once inside the cell, they separate, releasing the substance. This active transport system is used within the body to help maintain the proper concentrations of sodium and potassium ions in their appropriate fluid compartments.

Osmosis

Osmosis is the movement of water through a semipermeable membrane, such as a cell wall, from an area where there is more water to where there is less water. An area with a greater percentage of water contains a smaller percentage of particulate matter; therefore, osmosis can also be described as the movement of water from an area of lesser concentration of particles to an area of greater concentration of particles. The osmotic process continues until an equilibrium in the concentration of particles is reached on each side of the semipermeable membrane.

Two terms are used when discussing the concentration of particles in solution—osmolality and osmolarity. **Osmolality** refers to the number of osmols (particles in solution) per liter of solvent. **Osmolarity** refers to the number of osmols per liter of solution. Osmolality is approximately equal to osmolarity when the concentration of solute is small. Therefore, the two terms are used interchangeably in this text, with a preference for the term *osmolality* because it is more precise.

Osmosis occurs when two solutions have different osmolalities, and water moves from a solution of lesser osmolality to a solution of greater osmolality. **Osmotic pressure** is the force exerted by particles in the solution to stop osmosis. Osmotic pressure is exerted by molecules or ions that cannot penetrate the semipermeable membrane and is directly proportional to the concentration or degree of osmolality of the solution. The greater the degree of osmolality on one side of a semipermeable membrane, the greater the osmotic pressure and attraction for water on that side. Because of osmotic pressure, water flows toward the solution of greater concentration until the osmolality of the solutions is equalized.

Clinical Application

The administration of intravenous solutions is a clinical example of osmosis. Usually, intravenous solutions, such as 0.9% NaCl, are **isotonic**; they have the same osmolality as blood plasma, preventing shifts of fluids and electrolytes. This type of intravenous therapy simply replaces fluid and maintains the normal electrolyte balance in the body. A **hypertonic** solution, such as 50% glucose, has a greater osmolality than blood plasma and causes a rapid influx of water from the cells and interstitial spaces into the plasma. Glucose is sometimes used to reduce cerebral edema temporarily. **Hypotonic** solutions have a lower osmolality than blood plasma, causing water to move from the plasma into the cells (Figure 3–1).

Body Homeostasis

Body homeostasis is a dynamic equilibrium that maintains the body's fluid balance in a relatively constant state. This homeostasis is based on the amount of fluid taken in a normal diet and the volume of fluid excreted daily. Clini-

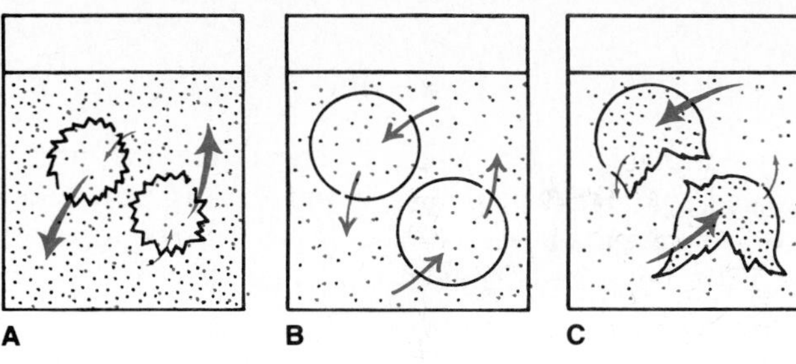

Figure 3–1

Osmosis. **A.** Hypertonic solution. Osmotic pressure is greater in the solution than in the cell, causing water to move out of the cell, with destruction or crenation of the cell. **B.** Osmotic pressure in the solution is the same as that in the cell, therefore the movement of solution is equal. **C.** Hypotonic solution. Osmotic pressure is greater in the cell than in the solution, causing water to move into the cell, with eventual rupturing or hemolysis of the cell.

Table 3–1
Twenty-Four-Hour Fluid Balance in a Healthy Client

Intake	mL	Output	mL
Oral fluid intake	1500	Urine	1500
H_2O in food	700	Insensible loss:	
H_2O from oxidation	300	Respiration	350–400
		Perspiration	350–400
		Feces	200
	2500		2400–2500

cally, a healthy adult eating a normal diet satisfies the need for electrolytes and fluid and, with the help of the body's regulating mechanisms, excretes an appropriate amount of fluid to maintain this critical balance. Illness and interference with normal intake and output can seriously derange the electrolyte and fluid balance. The client can become critically ill in a matter of days and in some instances, hours.

Homeostatic regulation of the body is maintained by lungs, kidneys, cardiovascular system, pituitary gland, adrenal glands, and parathyroid glands. These organs and their regulating mechanisms control the body's fluid volume, electrolyte concentration, and the electrolyte composition of body fluids.

Normal Intake and Output

The body maintains fluid equilibrium by equalizing its intake and output in a state of health. A healthy body in moderate temperatures needs about 2500 mL of water daily, but only 1500 mL is ingested in oral liquids. The remaining 1000 mL is acquired in solid food (700 mL) and from the oxidation of these foods during the metabolic processes (300 mL). The primary regulator of fluid intake is the body's thirst mechanism. The thirst center in the brain's hypothalamus is highly sensitive to changes in body fluid osmolality. Thirst may result from decreased water intake, excessive water loss, excessive sodium intake, and excessive infusion of a hypertonic solution. Thirst usually occurs when the water loss is equal to 2% of the body weight. These circumstances result in cellular dehydration, reduced blood volume, and hyperosmolality of the ECF. In dehydration, the increased osmolality of the serum stimulates the thirst center via neurologic impulses, and the person feels thirsty. Conversely, overhydration diminishes the drive to drink.

Fluid intake is balanced by the body's water losses. The major organs of fluid loss are the kidneys, which are responsible for approximately 1500 mL of urine produced daily. This volume approximates the daily oral fluid intake of an adult. Two other ways that the body normally excretes fluid are through insensible loss and feces. Insensible losses occur through the skin and lungs and cannot be measured accurately. The fluid is exhaled in expired air and diffused through the skin. Insensible losses account for 800 mL, and fluid in feces, for 200 mL in 24 hours (Table 3–1).

Fluid and Electrolyte Imbalances

Fluid and electrolyte imbalances can be categorized into two types of conditions according to causes: (1) a deficit or excess of essential body substances, such as water, sodium, hydrogen, potassium, calcium, or magnesium or (2) an abnormal shift of fluid from one compartment to another, or volume imbalances. Almost every hospitalized client is susceptible to water and electrolyte imbalances. Illness upsets the delicate state of body homeostasis, and certain conditions, diseases, and treatments make a client even more vulnerable to fluid and electrolyte imbalance. Diseases and conditions such as kidney disease; burns; congestive heart failure (CHF); diabetes; cirrhosis of the liver; pulmonary disease; and treatments such as surgery, diuretic therapy, low-sodium diets, and intravenous therapy may all cause serious threats to body homeostasis. A client suffering from any of these conditions or therapies requires careful recording of intake and output and careful observation for symptoms and signs of imbalance.

Water–Sodium Imbalances

Osmolar imbalances involve disturbances in osmolality and, therefore, water distribution in the fluid compartments in the body. Water always moves from an *area of lesser solute concentration* to an *area of greater solute concentration* until both are equal. A clinical measure of osmolality in the body is the measurement of the solute sodium in the serum. An elevated serum sodium level or *hyper-*

natremia (high solute concentration), indicates hyperosmolality. A lowered serum sodium level, or *hyponatremia* (low solute concentration), indicates hypo-osmolality.

HYPEROSMOLAR IMBALANCES Hyperosmolar imbalances or water deficit syndromes result from either water depletion or extracellular solute excess. In water depletion, the amount of solute is correct, but the solute is dissolved in too little water. With solute excess, there is an excess of solute per unit of water. Either condition leads to hyperosmolality, which causes cell shrinkage and dehydration. The ECF becomes hypertonic in relation to the ICF, causing water to leave the cells and enter the ECF, causing cellular dehydration. The causes of hyperosmolar imbalances are shown in Table 3–2.

The symptoms and signs of hyperosmolar states, regardless of cause, stem from dehydration. The client may have a dry mouth; dry, furrowed tongue; and be thirsty. The eyeballs are soft and sunken in severe cases. Decreased skin turgor, especially over the forehead and chest, and elevated temperature are seen. The client becomes restless and apprehensive. Untreated, this condition can progress to delirium, convulsions, and death. As a compensatory mechanism, the kidneys concentrate the urine produced, and eventually, oliguria and anuria occur. Laboratory findings include a high urine specific gravity (> 1.030), elevated hemoglobin, and hypernatremia (> 150 mEq/L).

The treatment for hyperosmolar disturbances is to administer water. In mild dehydration, oral fluid replacement is sufficient. In severe dehydration, intravenous solutions of isotonic glucose (5% glucose) are administered in proportion to the degree of dehydration, adjusted for each client. Water should not be replaced too quickly, or water intoxication may result.

Table 3–2
The Causes of Hyperosmolar Imbalances

Water Deficit	Solute Excess
Decreased intake: NPO Water unavailable Coma Severely ill or immobilized Sense of thirst impaired Increased output: GI: Diarrhea, vomiting, suction Renal: Inability to concentrate urine Excessive urine output (ie, diabetes insipidus) Lungs: Hyperventilation, tracheostomy Skin: Excessive perspiration, burns, high fever	• Infusions of hypertonic solutions • Excessive IV glucose administration • Excessive IV sodium bicarbonate administration • Uncontrolled diabetes mellitus with hyperglycemia

HYPO-OSMOLAR IMBALANCES Hypo-osmolar imbalances, or water-excess syndromes, result in either fluid overloads or solute deficits. Water intoxication is an excess of water in the extracellular compartment with a normal amount of solute. Solute-deficit imbalances result when the solute concentration is normal but is diluted in too much water. Either situation results in swollen cells. The causes of hypo-osmolar imbalances are shown in Table 3–3.

The symptoms and signs of all hypo-osmolar states are due to cellular edema. The client may gain considerable weight in the presence of anorexia, nausea, and vomiting. Signs of fluid overload such as peripheral and periorbital edema, a bounding pulse, pulmonary rales, and shortness of breath without exertion may also be seen. Neurologic abnormalities due to cerebral edema can be observed, especially when the hypo-osmolar state has occurred suddenly. These include headache and personality changes that progress to confusion and delirium, muscle weakness, twitching, and decreased reflexes. ADH secretion is decreased, and healthy kidneys attempt to excrete as much urine as possible; therefore, polyuria with a decreased specific gravity will be observed. Hemodilution also produces decreased hemoglobin and hematocrit values, as well as decreased Na^+ and K^+ values.

The treatment for hypo-osmolar imbalances is to restrict water until homeostasis is achieved. In moderate fluid excess, oral fluids are restricted for 24 hours, and administration of intravenous solutions is decreased or discontinued. More severe fluid excesses caused by underlying disease processes must be treated appropriately (ie, CHF may be treated with digoxin and diuretic therapy).

Volume Imbalances

Volume imbalances occur in the ECF compartment only as a result of the movement of sodium and water between the plasma and interstitial fluid. It is important to note that, in fluid shifts, both the solvent (H_2O) and solute (Na^+) move in equal proportions, creating isotonic fluid imbalances. This condition is in contrast to osmolar imbalances, in which the solute and solvent move disproportionately, as previously described.

Table 3–3
The Causes of Hypo-osmolar Imbalances

Water Excess	Solute Deficit
Excessive H_2O ingestion in a short time Excessive infusions of isotonic IV solutions Malfunction of the homeostatic mechanisms: • Pituitary: ADH secretion • Renal: ↑ aldosterone, water retention in kidney failure • Adrenal: hyperaldosteronism; excessive administration of adrenal cortical hormones	Inadequate salt intake (ie, diuretics, low-salt diet) Replacement of Na and H_2O losses with only water (ie, replacing vomitus losses [which contain Na+] with plain H_2O)

EXTRACELLULAR VOLUME DEPLETION/HYPOVOLEMIA Extracellular volume depletion, or hypovolemia, is caused by a shift of Na^+ and H_2O from the plasma to the interstitial fluid. Any condition that results in large acute losses of salt and water can precipitate hypovolemia. Severe burns, hemorrhage, diarrhea and vomiting, fever, and kidney disease are examples. Symptoms and signs of hypovolemia are those of shock: pallor, decreased blood pressure, tachycardia, weakness, restlessness, and unconsciousness. The client's red blood cell count is increased in hypovolemia because of the concentration of the plasma. Extracellular volume depletion can be treated quickly, once recognized, by intravenous administration of isotonic solutions.

EXTRACELLULAR VOLUME EXCESS/HYPERVOLEMIA Extracellular volume excess, or hypervolemia, is caused by a shift of Na^+ and H_2O from the interstitial fluid to the plasma. Excessive increases in proportionate amounts of H_2O and Na^+ can cause hypervolemia. Causes include excessive infusions of normal saline; cortisone therapy; and disease states such as cardiac, renal, or hepatic failure. Symptoms of hypervolemia include a bounding pulse, weight gain and pitting edema, engorged peripheral veins, and pulmonary edema. The treatment of hypervolemia includes fluid restriction and diuretic therapy.

Electrolyte Imbalances

Each of the major electrolytes—sodium, potassium, calcium, and magnesium—performs specific roles in bodily function. Their normal concentrations must be maintained to sustain life.

SODIUM Sodium (Na^+) is the major cation of the extracellular fluid. Two important facts about sodium are: (1) the sodium ion moves rapidly between the plasma and the interstitial fluid within the ECF, and (2) sodium and water move together. Therefore, sodium is the primary regulator of ECF volume and concentration. Sodium affects not only the fluid balance in the body but also is responsible for the osmotic pressure of the ECF. Additionally, sodium establishes the electrochemical state necessary for muscle contraction and transmission of nerve impulses. Imbalances of sodium, therefore, affect fluid volume, blood volume, and the nervous system.

HYPONATREMIA Hyponatremia is a sodium deficiency of the ECF, reflected in a serum sodium level of less than 135 mEq/L. This deficiency may be a result of a loss of sodium or a gain in water but is always due to proportionately greater amounts of water than sodium. It is always a hypo-osmolar state. The hypo-osmolar state causes a shift of fluid from the extracellular compartment into the intracellular compartment and results in cellular swelling. The causes of hyponatremia are summarized in Table 3–4.

The clinical symptoms and signs of hyponatremia directly depend on the cause, severity, and rapidity with which inadequate serum sodium level develops. With gradual loss of sodium, the client feels apathetic and weak. GI symptoms can occur, such as anorexia, nausea, vomiting, and abdominal cramping. As the serum sodium level becomes progressively lower, neurologic signs such as confusion, muscle twitching, seizures, and coma develop, which are directly related to brain swelling. Laboratory findings include a serum sodium level of less than 135 mEq/L, sometimes as low as 100 mEq/L; a low urinary specific gravity, usually 1.002–1.004; a decreased blood volume; and increased hemoglobin and hematocrit values.

Treatment of sodium loss is sodium replacement, usually by the parenteral route. If the client's fluid volume is low, an isotonic salt solution (0.9% NaCl) may be used; however, a small amount of hypertonic saline can be used if the plasma volume is normal or excessive. If excessive fluid volume is the cause for hyponatremia, fluid restriction and diuretic therapy are indicated.

SYNDROME OF INAPPROPRIATE ANTIDIURETIC HORMONE Syndrome of inappropriate antidiuretic hormone (SIADH) is a type of hyponatremia associated with water excess or hypo-osmolality. The urine of SIADH clients is either hypertonic or not maximally dilute. Sodium continues to be excreted by the kidneys. Although hyponatremia is

Table 3–4
Causes of Hyponatremia

Fluid Gain	Na^+ Loss
• Excessive administration of intravenous solutions (usually 5% dextrose in water) • Excessive ingestion of H_2O • Syndrome of inappropriate antidiuretic hormone (SIADH) secretion • Renal failure	• Diuretic therapy, especially thiazide diuretics • Low-salt diets • Loss of GI secretions, ie, vomiting, diarrhea, GI suction or drainage, excessive sweating • Addison's disease (decreased aldosterone causes Na^+ loss) • Extensive burns • Sequestering of Na^+ in body cavities (ie, peritonitis)

present and there is no edema, the physiologic disturbance in SIADH stems from excessive ADH activity, resulting in water retention and consequent hyponatremia. The syndrome is termed "inappropriate" because ADH production continues in spite of hypotonic plasma; hypotonic plasma normally serves as a regulatory mechanism for antidiuretic hormone secretion. Sodium continues to be lost in the urine because aldosterone does not conserve it; the normal renin–angiotensin system for stimulation of aldosterone production is not functioning in SIADH.

The causes of SIADH are either sustained secretion of ADH by the hypothalamus or aberrant ADH production from a malignancy. See Unit Seven for more information on SIADH.

The symptoms and signs of SIADH are similar to those previously described for hyponatremia. Nursing measures to monitor for SIADH include recognizing clients at high risk for the syndrome because it is potentially fatal if not recognized and treated. Other measures are careful monitoring of the client's weight, intake and output, serum sodium levels, and GI symptoms and/or neurologic changes. Treatment of SIADH centers on correcting the cause of excessive ADH secretion and alleviating excessive water retention.

HYPERNATREMIA Hypernatremia is a sodium excess of the ECF, reflected in a serum sodium level of greater than 145 mEq/L. This excess may be a result of a gain of sodium or a loss of water but is due to a disproportionate amount of sodium to water; it is a hyperosmolar state. This hyperosmolar state causes a shift of fluid from the intracellular space to the extracellular space, causing shrinking or dehydration of the cells. The causes of hypernatremia are summarized in Table 3–5.

The clinical symptoms and signs of hypernatremia are related to the central nervous system (CNS) and are directly correlated to the degree and rapidity of the rise of serum sodium. The client may at first note a dry, red, sticky tongue and mouth and become restless and irritable. This condition progresses to delirium, twitching, seizures, and coma. Accompanying these CNS signs are increased muscle tone, hyperactive deep tendon reflexes, metabolic acidosis, and death. Laboratory findings include an elevated serum sodium level (greater than 145 mEq/L), an increased serum osmolality greater than 295 mOsm/kg (normal = 280–295 mOsm/kg), and a urine specific gravity of greater than 1.015.

The treatment of hypernatremia is to lower the serum sodium, primarily by infusing a hypotonic electrolyte solution, often 0.3% NaCl. The gradual reduction of serum sodium over 48 hours has been recommended to lower the risk of cerebral edema and brain damage.

POTASSIUM Although found in all the body compartments, potassium (K^+) is the major intracellular cation, with 98% of the body's potassium contained within the cells. That remaining 2% of potassium helps regulate the proper functioning of the entire body's neuromuscular system. In addition, potassium regulates intracellular osmolality and promotes cellular growth; in fact, any condition that disrupts cell wall integrity produces a potassium shift. Finally, potassium promotes proper heart muscle function and assists with acid–base balance.

Although the movement of potassium within the body is complex, it is important in understanding potassium's functions. Potassium is essential to life yet cannot be stored in the body, so a daily dietary intake of potassium is required. The average adult dietary intake ranges from 50 to 100 mEq per day, with 40 mEq essential for life. Eighty percent of the daily excretion of potassium is by way of the distal renal tubules in the urine. The remaining 20% is lost through the bowels and sweat glands. Potassium is dynamic in that it is constantly moving through the cell walls in reaction to the body's needs. The amount of potassium in a cell at a given time depends on the integrity of the cell wall, the ability of the kidney to conserve some K^+ when the cells are depleted, and the sodium–potassium pump.

The *sodium–potassium pump* is a mechanism by which Na^+ is actively excluded from the cells, allowing K^+ to be present in the cells. Glucose metabolism and alkalosis are

Table 3–5
Causes of Hypernatremia

Fluid Loss	Na^+ Gain
• Diabetes insipidus, uncompensated • Excessive perspiration and other insensible losses • Copious diarrhea • Impaired renal function (ie, polyuria in nephritis) • Decreased fluid intake (common in elderly, young, confused, or comatose clients; also in clients on ventilators or with tracheostomies) • Peritoneal dialysis with glucose solutions	• Parenteral administration of salt solutions (hypertonic saline, sodium bicarbonate, isotonic saline) • Hypertonic saline abortions • Excessive intake of table salt • Partial drowning in salt water • Homeostatic mechanism failures: CHF, ↓ cardiac output, ↓ renal flow, ↑ Na^+ retention Nephrotic syndrome and cirrhosis: ↑ Aldosterone production ↑ Na^+ retention

both conditions in which potassium moves into the cells. Potassium moves out of the cells during any cellular destruction or impairment of cellular metabolism, during acidosis, or after strenuous exercise. Potassium balance is also affected by aldosterone. When the renin–angiotensin mechanism is stimulated, usually by decreased blood flow through the kidneys, aldosterone is produced by the adrenal cortex. Increased aldosterone production conserves Na^+ and, therefore, promotes K^+ excretion by the kidneys.

HYPOKALEMIA A potassium deficit, or hypokalemia, associated with a serum potassium level of less than 3 mEq/L, can be serious. Hypokalemia results from decreased K^+ intake, excessive K^+ loss, and excessive use of K^+ within the body. See Box 3–1 for causes of hypokalemia.

The clinical symptoms and signs of hypokalemia include disturbances of the neuromuscular, cardiovascular, gastrointestinal, and respiratory systems as well as H^+ balance (see section on acid–base balance). Neuromuscular symptoms include general weakness, diminished or absent deep tendon reflexes, weak leg muscles, and leg cramps. Cardiovascular changes such as a weak pulse, low blood pressure, and faint heart sounds are seen. In the ECG, ST segment depression, varying degrees of heart block, and depressed T waves are common. There is an increased sensitivity to digitalis, and premature atrial and ventricular beats may be seen in hypokalemic clients with digitalis toxicity. The client may also have a marked decrease in blood pressure on assuming an upright position (postural hypotension). Gastrointestinal symptoms such as vomiting and decreased bowel motility often occur and can progress to an ileus (intestinal muscle paralysis). Respiratory changes include shortness of breath and shallow respirations.

Treatment of hypokalemia begins with the correction of the underlying cause of the hypokalemia. Mild hypokalemia can be corrected by oral replacement of potassium. Hypokalemia with serum levels of less than 2.0 mEq/L requires parenteral replacement. The replacement amount is usually 40 mEq of K^+ in 1000 mL of IV solution over 8 hours. Faster replacement of potassium requires constant ECG monitoring in a coronary care unit.

Box 3–1
Causes of Hypokalemia

Inadequate K^+ Intake

Poor nutrition
NPO with IV fluids without K^+
Nausea, anorexia, acute alcoholism, starvation

Excessive Use of K^+ Within the Body

Healing phase of burns
Hyperinsulinism
Recovery from diabetic acidosis

Loss of K^+ from the Body

Medical treatments:
- Diuretics, especially thiazide and furosemide
- Low-/or no-salt diets
- High-dose corticosteroid therapy
- Prolonged administration of K^+-free IVs and hyperalimentation fluids

Parenteral administration of insulin and glucose (causes glycogen formation with a shift of K^+ into the cells)

Gastrointestinal disturbances:
- Excessive vomiting, diarrhea
- Fistula drainage
- Ulcerative colitis
- Surgical treatments such as ileostomy, colostomy

Excessive perspiration

Metabolic disease:
- Diabetes mellitus
- Hyperaldosteronism
- Adrenal tumor, cirrhosis, CHF

Renal disease:
Particularly tubular necrosis/acidosis

Box 3–2
Causes of Hyperkalemia

Retention of K^+ Within the Body

Renal failure, with an inability of the kidneys to excrete potassium

Adrenocortical insufficiency

Release of K^+ from the Cells

Burns

Massive trauma and crushing injuries

Potassium "Overdose"

Excessive administration of intravenous infusions containing K^+

HYPERKALEMIA Hyperkalemia is less common than hypokalemia but can be more life threatening. The condition is unusual in clients with normal kidney function and is reflected by a serum potassium level of greater than 5.5 mEq/L. See Box 3–2 for the causes of hyperkalemia.

The clinical symptoms and signs of hyperkalemia include musculoskeletal, GI, and cardiac symptoms. Muscular symptoms including weakness, paresthesia, cramps, and pain are common. Indications of gastrointestinal hyperactivity include nausea, intermittent GI colic, and diarrhea. Cardiac changes on the ECG include tented T waves, small to nonvisible P waves, widened QRS complexes, and life-threatening dysrhythmias. Supraventricular and/or ventricular tachycardias, premature ventricular beats, and ventricular fibrillation may all lead to cardiac arrest.

Treatment for hyperkalemia includes restricting both parenteral and oral K^+ intake and reducing serum K^+ by administering cation-exchange resins such as Kayexalate. Intravenous administration of glucose and insulin may be ordered to facilitate movement of K^+ into the cells. Severe hyperkalemia is an emergency and should be treated in an intensive care unit.

CALCIUM Calcium (Ca^{2+}) exists in two forms in the body: ionized calcium and nonionized calcium. Nonionized calcium is in the serum and is bound to proteins, primarily albumin. Ionized serum calcium is physiologically active and plays a role in muscle contraction, neural function, and the formation of prothrombin for blood coagulation. There is a reciprocal relation between ionized and nonionized calcium, with a rise in one causing a decrease in the other. The calcium level routinely measured is the total serum calcium level; the ionized portion is estimated according to simultaneous measurement of serum protein (ie, albumin). Because serum albumin levels and serum calcium levels fall and rise together, it is important to evaluate them together. Changes in the arterial pH cause more calcium to become bound to protein ($\uparrow$ pH = alkalosis) or less calcium to be bound ($\downarrow$ pH = acidosis), whereas the total serum calcium remains unchanged.

The release of calcium into the serum is primarily controlled by the parathyroid glands. Parathyroid hormone (PTH) promotes a transfer of calcium from bones to the plasma, stimulates intestinal resorption of calcium, and enhances renal reabsorption of calcium. Conversely, calcium is moved from the serum back into bones by the action of calcitonin, produced by the thyroid gland, thus lowering the serum calcium. Finally, calcium levels are influenced by phosphorus levels. As calcium levels rise, phosphorus levels decrease and vice versa.

HYPOCALCEMIA Hypocalcemia can be due to an acute loss of calcium from the body secondary to acute diarrhea, acute pancreatitis, hypoparathyroidism, and renal disease. Additionally, if there is an increased need for calcium, as in pregnancy and lactation, calcium deficiencies can occur unless dietary intake is increased.

Symptoms and signs of hypocalcemia include increased neuromuscular irritability, which causes tetany-type muscle spasms; fatigue; and laryngospasm, sometimes with airway obstruction.

A prolonged QT interval is seen on the ECG due to decreased cardiac contractility. Laboratory findings include a serum Ca^{2+} level of less than 4.5 mEq/L and an elevated serum phosphorus level.

Treatment of hypocalcemia consists of re-establishing the normal plasma level of ionized calcium by correcting the underlying clinical problems. If the Ca^{2+} deficit is acute, 10 to 20 mL of calcium gluconate (10%) is administered intravenously over 10 to 15 minutes. In nonacute cases, oral calcium supplements (calcium lactate) and a high-calcium diet are prescribed. Vitamin D is also a part of treatment for hypocalcemia because it facilitates the absorption of calcium supplements. Dosage usually ranges from 50,000 to 250,000 units per day.

HYPERCALCEMIA Hypercalcemia may result from excessive calcium or vitamin D intake (increases calcium absorption in the intestines), including overuse of antacids. Hypercalcemia may also result from conditions that increase calcium absorption or prevent renal excretion of calcium. Hyperparathyroidism or a tumor of the parathyroid glands increases Ca^{2+} catabolism and increases the amount of ionized Ca^{2+} in the serum. When bone destruction is greater than bone production, as in Paget's disease or osteolytic metastasis, serum calcium is elevated as well.

Symptoms and signs of hypercalcemia are opposite those of hypocalcemia, with decreased muscle tone and decreased neuromuscular irritability. Reflexes are hypoactive, and there is generalized muscle weakness and fatigue. Bone pain, osteoporosis, and eventual pathologic fractures can occur. Gastrointestinal symptoms include constipation, anorexia, nausea, and vomiting. Neurologic manifestations usually begin with decreased memory and attention span and can progress to psychosis, if untreated. Cardiac changes on ECG show shortened ST segments, resulting in a shorter QT segment and a widened and rounded wave. Hypercontractility of heart muscle can lead to cardiac arrest in systole if hypercalcemia is severe. Laboratory findings indicate a serum calcium level of greater than 5.8 mEq/L or 10.5 mg/dL.

Treatment of mild to moderate hypercalcemia begins with correcting the underlying cause and restricting calcium intake. If a hypercalcemic crisis occurs, the first treatment is to provide adequate hydration. Rehydration is with a normal saline infusion, usually 1000 mL every 4 to 6 hours. If diuresis does not occur, additional loop diuretics such as furosemide should be given. Oral phosphates are administered because they are successful in treating both acute and chronic hypercalcemia. Phosphate is usually given orally as sodium phosphate solution (Fleet Phospho-Soda) 5 mL three to four times daily.

Corticosteroids and mithramycin are also used to treat high serum levels of calcium. Doses of steroids range to 40 mg per day and require several days for maximal effect. Mithramycin is given by IV push for 2 days. Its use is reserved for treating hypercalcemia secondary to the side effects of cytotoxic drugs.

MAGNESIUM Magnesium (Mg^{2+}) is the second most abundant intracellular cation, but its importance in helping maintain proper bodily function has only recently been investigated. Consequently, its role is poorly understood, and it is still not routinely ordered when an electrolyte balance is being evaluated. The normal adult body contains approximately 20 to 25 g of magnesium, about 70% of which is stored with calcium and phosphorus in the bones. The remainder is divided intracellularly (28%) among the soft tissues of the liver, heart, skeletal muscles, and body fluids and extracellularly (2%) mostly in the cerebrospinal fluid. The normal dietary requirement of magnesium for adults is 200 to 300 mg daily, with an increase of up to 400 mg for lactating mothers. Dietary sources of magnesium include nuts, soybeans, seafood, and whole grains.

About half the magnesium ingested is absorbed in the GI tract, and the rest is excreted in the feces. Urinary excretion of magnesium is minimal because the kidneys efficiently conserve Mg^{2+}. Calcium and magnesium are both regulated by the parathyroid glands and appear to have a mutually suppressive effect. Calcium in abundance will be absorbed over magnesium and vice versa. Additionally, if the body's magnesium level is low, the kidneys will excrete more potassium, and hypokalemia may result. Therefore, with any imbalance of calcium, phosphorus, or potassium, a parallel magnesium imbalance may also exist and warrants investigation.

Magnesium is essential for neuromuscular integration, regulation of the blood phosphorus level, and in activating multiple enzymatic reactions. Magnesium is especially important in the generation and use of adenosine triphosphate (ATP).

HYPOMAGNESEMIA Magnesium deficiency, the most common magnesium disorder, develops when the serum concentration of Mg^{2+} is below the normal range of 1.5 to 2.5 mEq/L. Causes of magnesium depletion include conditions in which there is an inadequate magnesium intake or an excessive magnesium loss. Chronic states of malnutrition or malabsorption predisposing clients to hypomagnesemia are chronic alcoholism, intestinal bypass surgery, starvation, hyperalimentation without replacement of magnesium, and simple inadequate dietary intake. Magnesium loss occurs by several means including diarrhea, prolonged nasogastric suctioning, diuretic therapy, primary aldosteronism (causing increased urinary and fecal losses of Mg^{2+}), hypoparathyroidism, and the diuretic phase of acute renal failure.

The clinical symptoms and signs of magnesium depletion are predominantly neuromuscular and cardiac. Nervous system irritability results in coarse tremors, hyperreflexia, muscle cramps, generalized convulsions, and paresthesia of the hands and feet. Stimulation of the CNS causes visual and/or auditory hallucinations, intense confusion, and disorientation. Ventricular dysrhythmias (including ventricular premature contractions and ventricular fibrillation), tachycardia, and hypotension (due to decreased cardiac function) are signs of cardiac irritability. ECG findings include tall T waves and widening QRS complexes in mild magnesium deficiency to prolonged P-R intervals (first-degree block); wide QRS complexes; and/or broad, flat or inverted T waves in severe hypomagnesemia associated with hypocalcemia and hypokalemia (usually 0.2 to 0.6 mEq/L).

Magnesium deficiencies are treated by the administration of magnesium by oral, intramuscular, or intravenous routes, depending on the severity of the clinical situation. Intramuscular administration of magnesium sulfate is painful. If it must be given IM, it should be given deep in the gluteal muscle. In severe hypomagnesemia, 5 g or 40 mEq of magnesium sulfate may be added to 1L of 5% dextrose in water and given as a slow infusion. A too-rapid infusion of magnesium sulfate can cause cardiac arrest. In an acute neurologic crisis such as convulsions, 1 to 2 g of magnesium sulfate can be given by direct IV push. Nurses should be alert for cardiac abnormalities during magnesium therapy and should be certain that adequate urine output (at least 100 mL every 4 hours) is maintained to allow renal elimination of magnesium.

HYPERMAGNESEMIA Excess serum magnesium, a rare imbalance, can be caused by renal insufficiency, excessive magnesium administration during replacement therapy, excessive use of magnesium-containing antacids by clients in renal failure, and severe dehydration causing oliguria and retention of Mg^{2+}.

The main clinical symptoms and signs result from a marked decrease in neuromuscular irritability. They include a warm sensation, hyporeflexia leading to flaccid paralysis, hypotension, lethargy progressing to coma, depressed respirations, and cardiac arrest. Laboratory findings include a serum magnesium level in excess of 3 mEq/L.

Treatments of hypermagnesemia include eliminating the source of excessive magnesium intake and offsetting the toxicity of the condition. Calcium gluconate can be administered to antagonize the action of magnesium, and hemodialysis or peritoneal dialysis can be done as an emergency.

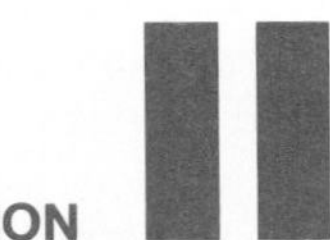

SECTION II

Acid–Base Balance

Acid–base balance depends on the homeostasis of the hydrogen (H^+) ion concentration in body fluids. Hydrogen ion concentration determines the acidity and alkalinity of body fluids concentration. An *increase* in hydrogen ion (H^+) makes a solution more acid, and a *decrease* makes it more alkaline. The concentration of hydrogen ions, as indicated by the symbol pH, denotes the power of the hydrogen ion. The weight of the H^+ ion is about .0000001 g/L and is expressed as 10^{-7}, or a *pH of 7*. This hydrogen ion concentration is usually expressed as the negative logarithm of the weight of ionized hydrogen in water. Because of the *negative* logarithm, *a higher H^+ ion* concentration *means a lower pH* (ie, 6.5, 6.0, 5.0), and a *lower H^+ ion* concentration indicates a *higher pH* (ie, 7.5, 8.0).

A solution having a pH of 7 is neutral because at that time, the hydrogen (acid) ions (H^+) equal the hydroxyl (base) (OH^-) ions. Therefore, an *acidic* solution has a *pH below 7.0*, and a base or *alkaline* solution has a *pH above 7.0*. These facts are important to health care providers because *extracellular fluid* is slightly alkaline, having a *pH of 7.35 to 7.45*. For life to be maintained, the pH of the extracellular fluid must be between 6.8 and 8.0 (Figure 3–2). Slight changes in the pH or H^+ ion concentration cause marked changes in the cellular chemical reactions. If the body is in acidosis or increased H^+ ion concentration, the client can die in a coma. Conversely, if the client has a decrease in H^+ ion concentration, alkalosis and tetany or convulsions may result.

The following facts are necessary to understand and relate the chemical principles previously discussed to basic bodily physiology:

- Basic physiologic processes produce an excess of acid.

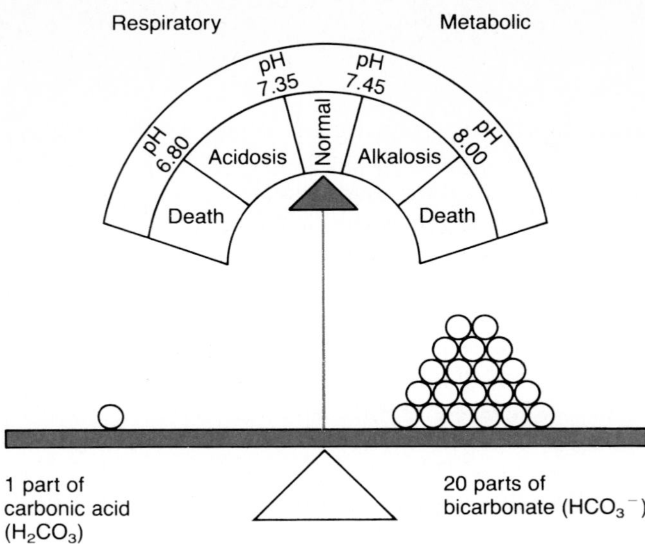

Figure 3–2

Normal acid-base balance.

- Two major types of acids are produced: (1) carbonic acid (H_2CO_3) and (2) nonvolatile acids.
- The renal, respiratory, and circulatory (blood buffer) systems act as part of the body's response as it attempts to rid itself of these acids.

Normally, the body maintains the pH between *7.35 and 7.45*. This body pH is stabilized by the buffering capacity of the body fluids. Three defense mechanisms are used to maintain the body's acid–base balance: the circulatory (blood buffer) system, respiratory system, and renal system.

Defense Mechanisms

A buffering system maintains the pH of ECF within the normal range. A *buffer* is a substance that has the ability to bind or release hydrogen H^+ in solution, keeping the pH of the solution relatively constant despite the addition of considerable quantities of acid or base. A buffer system consists of a weak acid in combination with one of the salts of that acid.

The Bicarbonate Blood Buffer System

The blood buffer system reacts within less than a second to prevent excessive changes in the H^+ ion concentration. Although the body has several blood buffer systems, the most important in the ECF is the carbonic acid (H_2CO_3)–sodium bicarbonate ($NaHCO_3$) system. Normally, to maintain acid–base balance, the ratio of carbonic acid to sodium bicarbonate is 1:20 (see Figure 3–2). There are also small amounts of potassium bicarbonate, calcium bicarbonate, and magnesium bicarbonate. The symbol $BHCO_3$ is used to indicate any of these base bicarbonates. The bicarbonate buffer system is not an exceedingly powerful buffer for two reasons: (1) it does not operate at its fullest buffering capacity at the normal ECF pH of 7.4, and (2) there are small concentrations of bicarbonate in the blood buffer system. Yet the system is important and effective because the concentrations of the two elements (CO_2 and HCO_3^-) of the bicarbonate system can be easily regulated, carbon dioxide (CO_2) by the respiratory system and the bicarbonate ion (HCO_3^-) by the kidneys. As a result, the pH of the blood can be shifted up or down by the respiratory and renal regulatory systems. The respiratory system activates rapidly within 1 to 3 minutes to eliminate excess carbon dioxide formed from the dissociation of carbonic acid to carbon dioxide and water ($H_2CO_3 \longrightarrow H_2O + CO_2$). In contrast, the kidneys, the most powerful control mechanism, require several hours to a complete day to effect hydrogen ion concentration changes.

The Phosphate Buffer System

The phosphate buffer system is important in red blood cells and other body cells, especially in the kidney tubule cells where it enables the kidney to excrete hydrogen ions. The buffer acts similarly to the bicarbonate buffer system but is composed of the following elements: sodium dihydrogen phosphate (NaH_2PO_4) and sodium monohydrogen phosphate (Na_2HPO_4). When a strong acid is added to a mixture of these two substances, the following reaction occurs:

$$\begin{gathered} HCl \text{ (hydrogen chloride)} + \\ Na_2HPO_4 \text{ (sodium monohydrogen phosphate)} \longrightarrow \\ NaCl \text{ (sodium chloride)} + \\ NaH_2PO_4 \text{ (sodium dihydrogen phosphate)} \end{gathered}$$

In other words, a strong acid is converted to a neutral salt (sodium chloride) by a phosphate buffer salt. Similarly, if a strong base such as sodium hydroxide (NaOH) is introduced into the body, the following reaction occurs:

$$NaOH + NaH_2PO_4 \longrightarrow Na_2HPO_4 + H_2O$$

A strong base is converted into water, and the phosphate buffer salt sodium dihydrogen phosphate (NaH_2PO_4) is converted from a mild acid to a mild base, sodium monohydrogen phosphate (Na_2HPO_4).

The Protein Buffer System

Three-quarters of all the chemical buffering power of the body fluids is inside the cells and results from intracellular proteins. These proteins act as anions in the alkaline pH of the body. Existing as either acids or alkaline salts, they can operate in both acidic and basic buffering systems, binding or releasing hydrogen ions as needed.

The Respiratory System

Carbon dioxide is constantly formed in the body by different intracellular metabolic processes. CO_2 is then transported to the lungs and exhaled. If the rate of metabolic formation of carbon dioxide increases, the concentration of carbon dioxide in ECF increases. Excretion of carbon dioxide is directly related to respiration; therefore, extracellular CO_2 *decreases* as the respiratory rate *increases.* Conversely, if the respiratory rate *decreases,* the amount of carbon dioxide in the ECF *increases.*

The respiratory center in the medulla responds when the hydrogen ion concentration increases because of the ability of carbon dioxide to combine with water to form carbonic acid:

$$\underset{\text{(carbonic acid)}}{H_2CO_3} \underset{\text{(carbonic anhydrase)}}{\overset{CA}{\rightleftharpoons}} \underset{\text{(water)}}{H_2O} + \underset{\text{(carbon dioxide)}}{CO_2}$$

The respiratory center stimulates the respiratory system to increase the rate and depth of respiration to give off carbon dioxide. This respiratory mechanism operates *within a minute* with a 75% efficiency partially to restore the pH level.

The Renal System

Normal metabolism produces an excess of acids. The kidneys compensate for this acidity by excreting acids and returning bicarbonate to the plasma and extracellular water. This process is accomplished by the following mechanisms: (1) reabsorption of bicarbonate, (2) acidification of phosphate buffer salts, and (3) secretion of ammonia.

In *acidosis,* all of these renal mechanisms are exaggerated. The excretion of acids and chloride is increased, and the absorption of bicarbonate into the plasma to correct the acidosis is increased. Conversely, in *alkalosis* these mechanisms slow or cease. Although the renal system requires more time to correct the pH than other systems (10 to 20 hours), it is more powerful, removing up to 500 mmol of acid or alkali daily.

Changes in Acid–Base Balance

Deficits or excesses of base bicarbonate or carbonic acid are designated as acid–base imbalances. A normal balance consists of a ratio of 1 part carbonic acid (H_2CO_3) to 20 parts bicarbonate (HCO_3^-) (1:20) (see Figure 3–2). An acid–base imbalance may occur as an increase (3:20) or a decrease (0.5:20) in carbonic acid or an increase (1:25) or decrease (1:15) in bicarbonate.

Acidosis occurs whenever a disturbance in the acid–base balance results in an increase in H^+ concentration. That is, the 1:20 ratio is altered, and the proportion of carbonic acid to bicarbonate is greater than 1:20. This can be caused by an increase in carbonic acid (ie, 2:20) or a decrease in bicarbonate (ie, 1:18) (Figure 3–3).

Alkalosis is a disturbance in acid–base balance that results in a decrease in the hydrogen ion concentration. The normal ratio of 1:20 is altered as the proportion of

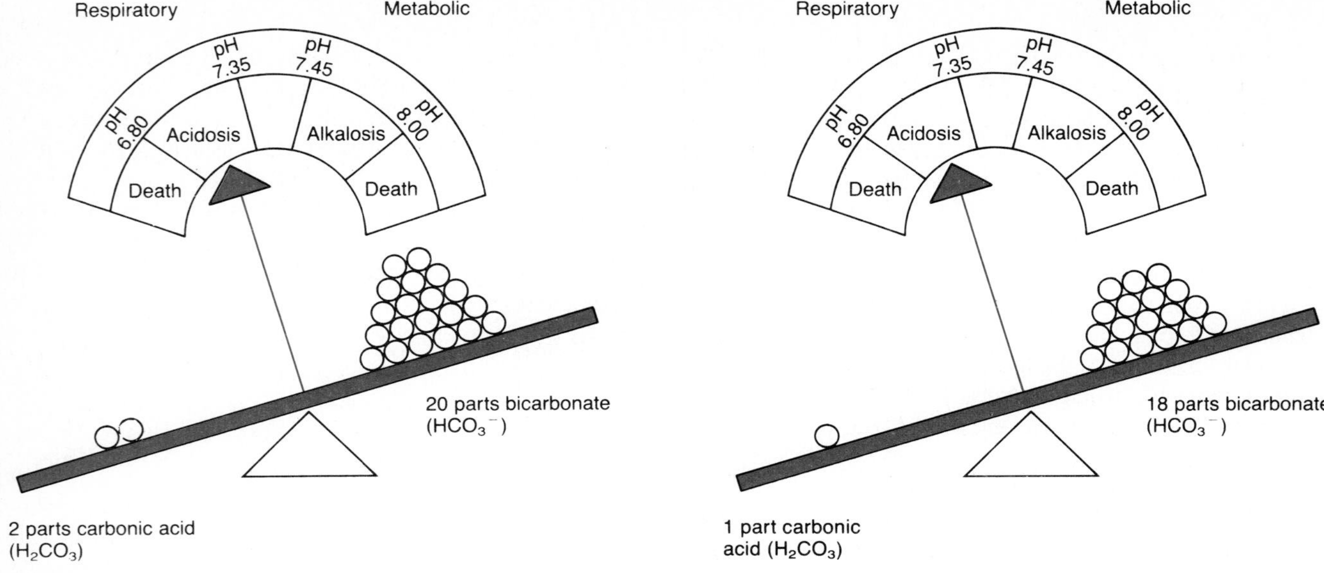

Figure 3–3

Left. Respiratory acidosis. **Right.** Metabolic acidosis.

carbonic acid to bicarbonate changes to less than 1:20. The cause may be either a decrease in carbonic acid (ie, 0.6:20) *or* an increase in bicarbonate (ie, 1:24) (Figure 3–4). The ratio of carbonic acid to bicarbonate in the ECF determines the concentration of hydrogen ions. This balance can be altered by either a metabolic or a respiratory disorder.

Metabolic disorders affect the base bicarbonate by either adding to the base or subtracting from it. Consequently, either a *metabolic acidosis* (subtracting HCO_3^-) or *metabolic alkalosis* (adding HCO_3^-) occurs (see Figures 3–3, 3–4).

Respiratory disturbances affect carbonic acid by adding to the carbonic acid or subtracting from it. Consequently, either a *respiratory acidosis* (adding H_2CO_3) or *respiratory alkalosis* (subtracting H_2CO_3) occurs (see Figures 3–3, 3–4).

Respiratory Acidosis

Respiratory acidosis occurs whenever there is an accumulation of carbon dioxide and therefore carbonic acid due to an interference with the alveolar exchange of oxygen and carbon dioxide. This condition may develop from prolonged overbreathing of carbon dioxide; hypoventilation secondary to paralysis of the respiratory muscles—for example, poliomyelitis; upper airway obstructions due to emphysema or asthma; and depression of the medullary respiratory centers from head trauma, brain tumor, narcotic or barbiturate poisoning, or spinal cord injury.

Interference with ventilation is often classified as either acute or chronic respiratory acidosis. Acute respiratory acidosis results in a severe change in an acidotic state. The most common causes include atelectasis, pneumothorax, respiratory paralysis, or drug-induced respiratory suppression.

Clients with acute respiratory acidosis do not benefit greatly from the body's compensatory mechanisms because of the limited time mechanism. The only buffer systems that react quickly enough to effect a change in an acute respiratory problem are the blood buffer systems. Unfortunately, they require normal blood circulation and efficient tissue perfusion. Therefore, for normal treatment to be effective, respiratory function must be improved as quickly as possible.

Clients in chronic respiratory acidosis are continuously in a moderate degree of acidosis. This state is usually secondary to chronic obstructive pulmonary disease (COPD) or lung carcinoma. Chronic respiratory acidosis responds well to renal compensation. The kidneys have enough time to retain bicarbonate and can maintain a 1:20 ratio by increasing the bicarbonate portion to offset the high acid. The oxyhemoglobin blood buffer system does not function efficiently in chronic respiratory acidosis because of the decreased blood oxygen content.

COMPENSATORY MECHANISMS Compensatory mechanisms to correct respiratory acidosis begin within seconds as blood buffers react with an increase in carbon dioxide to reestablish the ratio from 2:20 to 1:20. Within hours, the kidneys attempt to excrete the hydrogen ion and compensate the acid–base imbalance through:

- Formation and excretion of the ammonium ion (NH_4)
- Retention of HCO_3^- (bicarbonate ions) and excretion of chloride (Cl^-)
- A shift in electrolytes as hydrogen (H^+) and sodium ions (Na^+) move into the cells, and potassium (K^+) ions are exchanged and move from the ICF into the ECF, causing the serum potassium level to rise.

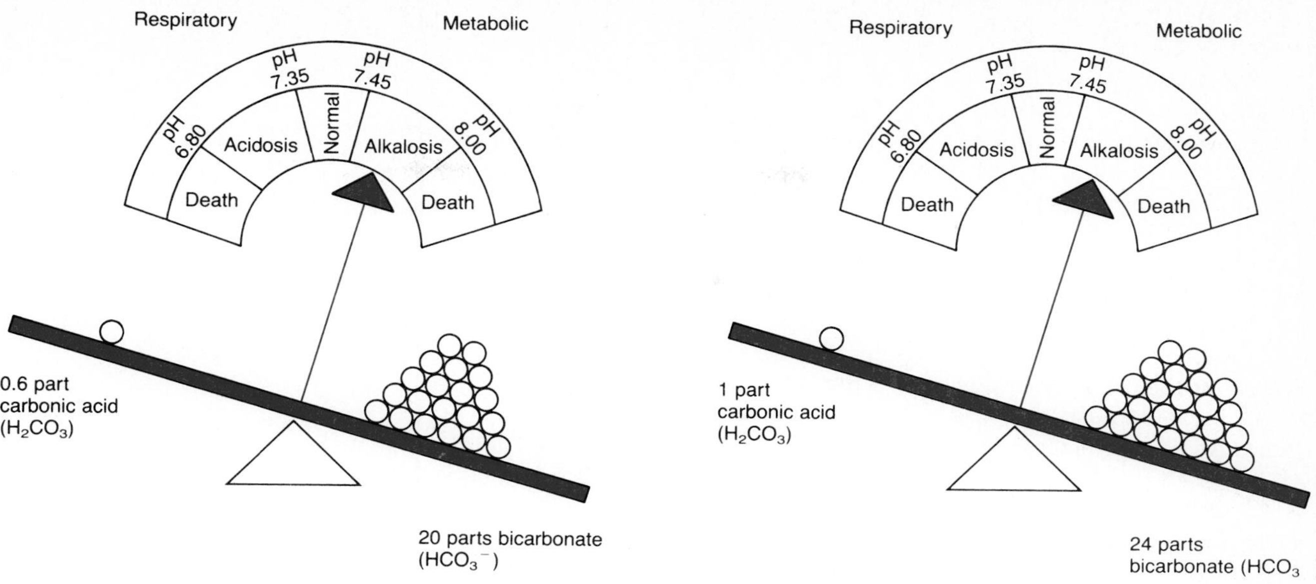

Figure 3–4

Left. Respiratory alkalosis. **Right.** Metabolic alkalosis.

As a result of these compensatory mechanisms, the bicarbonate concentration and pH rise toward normal to produce a partially compensated respiratory acidosis. Compensation is apparently always incomplete in clients with severe respiratory acidosis when PCO_2 is 80 mm Hg or greater.

Unfortunately, these clients usually stretch their compensatory mechanisms to the fullest because of the chronic long-term nature of their disease. They are extremely vulnerable to rapid changes that precipitate acidosis, such as an upper respiratory infection. These clients also have persistent cyanosis of varying severity, seen as lip or nail-bed cyanosis. Nurses should recognize that any surgical procedure or respiratory infection can precipitate acute or severe acidosis.

SUBJECTIVE AND OBJECTIVE FINDINGS The symptoms and signs of respiratory acidosis include: weakness, irritability, restlessness, tachycardia, and ventricular fibrillation secondary to increased potassium. Nursing care for clients with respiratory acidosis is critical within the first 24 to 48 hours. Providing an adequate airway and ventilation is the first priority. An endotracheal tube or tracheostomy may be needed to provide a patent airway to remove excess carbon dioxide. Suctioning is important to maintain a patent airway. Giving fluids to thin secretions, with pulmonary physiotherapy to loosen secretions, is also necessary. Postural drainage adds gravity to remove loosened mucus. Normally, increased levels of carbon dioxide stimulate the respiratory center to increase respirations and increase the inhalation of needed oxygen. In clients with chronic respiratory acidosis, sustained high levels of carbon dioxide lose their effect to stimulate the respiratory center, and an oxygen deficit is the only stimulus to breathe. The oxygen deficit is maintained by giving 1 to 2 L of oxygen per minute via cannula unless arterial blood gases and client symptoms indicate that higher levels are warranted and will be beneficial.

Respiratory Alkalosis

Respiratory alkalosis occurs when there is an excess loss of H_2CO_3 (carbonic acid) and therefore a decrease on the carbonic acid side of the carbonic acid–bicarbonate ratio. This condition is not as frequent as respiratory acidosis and is usually the result of hyperventilation secondary to hypoxia at high altitudes, encephalitis, or fever and an excessive loss of carbon dioxide. Salicylate poisoning (aspirin overdose) also causes a direct stimulus to the respiratory center and, in early stages, alkalosis. Alkalosis may also occur from rapid mechanical ventilation and hysterical hyperventilation, both of which increase the exhalation of carbon dioxide. Acute respiratory alkalosis can also be a compensatory reaction due to the sudden increase in alveolar ventilation in clients with respiratory acidosis who have a tracheostomy.

COMPENSATORY MECHANISMS Compensatory mechanisms to restore the normal pH are carried out by the renal system. The normal excretion of acid urine by the kidneys decreases. The kidneys reduce ammonia formation (NH_4), excretion of hydrogen (H^+) and chloride (Cl^-), and no longer conserve bicarbonate (HCO_3^-). In addition, potassium moves from the extracellular water into the cells in exchange for hydrogen and sodium ions in an attempt to add acid (H^+) to the extracellular fluid. As a result of all of these changes, a compensatory metabolic acidosis develops.

SUBJECTIVE AND OBJECTIVE FINDINGS The clinical picture of respiratory alkalosis includes: light-headedness, circumoral paresthesia, numbness and tingling of the fingers and toes, tinnitus, dyspnea or air hunger, palpitations, diaphoresis, panic, muscle cramps, and/or lower abdominal pain. The signs of tetany such as carpopedal spasms also occur due to the decreased availability of calcium. As the pH rises in an alkalotic state, calcium binds to protein, and its availability for cellular functions decreases.

Treatment is aimed at increasing the PCO_2 and decreasing the pH. If hyperventilation is the cause, having clients breathe into a paper bag and rebreathe their own carbon dioxide may improve the symptoms.

Clients with cerebral lesions can breathe a combination of 5% carbon dioxide and 95% oxygen until the condition improves. Mechanical ventilation should be adjusted to decrease the respiratory rate and/or increase the dead space on the ventilation tubing to reduce excessive loss of CO_2.

Nursing care should center on:

- Restoring a normal respiratory breathing pattern
- Encouraging appropriate breathing techniques
- Providing emotional support and being alert to iatrogenic causes of respiratory alkalosis
- Assessing for symptoms and signs of other disease processes that could be masked by respiratory alkalosis

Metabolic Acidosis

Metabolic acidosis develops because of an increased amount of acid or a decreased amount of base in the body. The normal bicarbonate-to-acid ratio of 20:1 is decreased, and the pH falls *below 7.35*.

Clients with metabolic acidosis can be divided into two categories, related to the concentration of unmeasured anions: (1) normal anion gap (delta) (*16 mEq or less*) and (2) abnormally large anion gap (*22 mEq or more*). The anion gap is determined by subtracting the values of the major anions in the ECF (HCO_3^-, Cl^-) from the values of the major cations (Na^+, K^+). Examples of a normal anion gap and an abnormal anion gap are shown in Box 3–3.

A metabolic acidosis in which the anion gap is normal results from inappropriate wasting of bicarbonate (as in diarrheal states) or failure of the kidney to excrete the normal endogenous acids (ie, renal tubular acidosis). In either situation, the bicarbonate concentration is reduced and replaced by an increase in the chloride (Cl^-) concentration.

In the secondary category of metabolic acidosis, the anion gap is increased or abnormal because of the circulating residual anions that are the result of the acids dissociating. These abnormal anions accumulate in lactic acidosis (lactate anions present), in diabetic ketoacidosis (unmeasured aceto-acetic acids), in salicylate poisoning (organic acid anions), and in azotemia or renal failure (phosphoric, sulfuric, and organic acid anions). See Figure 3–5 for further etiologic factors of normal and abnormal anion gap metabolic acidosis.

Box 3–3
Anion Gaps

Normal Anion Gap

Na^+ = 142 mEq/L
K^+ = 4 mEq/L
HCO_3^- = 27 mEq/L
Cl^- = 103 mEq/L

Anion gap = (Na^+ + K^+) − (HCO_3^- + Cl^-)
(delta) (142 + 4) − (27 + 103)
146 − 130 = 16 mEq/L (normal anion gap)

Abnormal Anion Gap

Na^+ = 142 mEq/L
K^+ = 4 mEq/L
HCO_3^- = 27 mEq/L
Cl^- = 90 mEq/L

Anion gap = (Na^+ + K^+) − (HCO_3^- + Cl^-)
Anion gap = (142 + 4) − (27 + 90)
146 − 117 = 29 mEq/L (increased anion gap)

COMPENSATORY MECHANISMS As the pH decreases in metabolic acidosis, the respiratory center is stimulated. Repirations increase in rate and depth in an attempt to lower carbonic acid concentration $H_2CO_3 \longrightarrow H_2O + CO_2$ (exhaled) and thereby restore the normal pH. Pulmonary compensation is usually not complete and is markedly inadequate with chronic pulmonary disease and respiratory acidosis (eg, a client with severe emphysema and in diabetic acidosis).

If the renal compensatory mechanism is operational (ie, not involved in the cause of the metabolic acidosis), the following mechanisms develop:

- Secretion and excretion of hydrogen ions increase.
- Hydrogen is excreted in the form of ammonium ions.
- The negative anion bicarbonate (HCO_3^-) is retained, and chloride (Cl^-) is excreted instead.

As a result of acidosis and the increase of hydrogen ion concentration, an electrolyte shift develops. Hydrogen and sodium move into the cells, and potassium moves into the ECF. This may cause an abnormally high potassium level in acidotic clients, leading to ventricular fibrillation and death.

The aims of treatment are to correct the metabolic disturbance and restore the electrolyte balance. In clients with diabetic acidosis, insulin is necessary to restore normal glucose metabolism and return glucose to the cells.

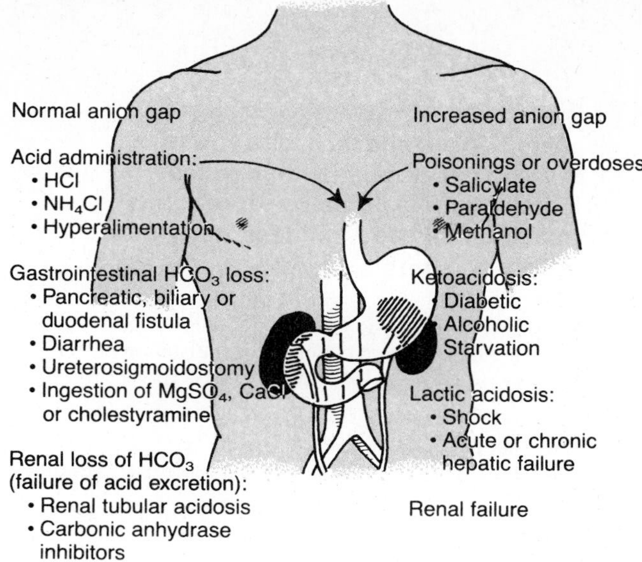

Figure 3–5

Etiologic factors in metabolic acidosis.

Treatment of metabolic acidosis due to loss of intestinal fluids is aimed at restoring sodium, potassium, water, and other electrolytes through administration of intravenous fluids. As treatment progresses, potassium re-enters the cells, and hypokalemia may result. Administration of potassium chloride with monitoring of potassium levels is necessary. Correction of acidosis from renal failure requires peritoneal or hemodialysis and a low-protein, high-calorie diet.

Normally, alkalinizing solutions (sodium bicarbonate) are reserved for the seriously ill. The quickest method to overcome life-threatening acidosis is to replenish the supply of bicarbonate buffer by giving intravenous bicarbonate (1 to 3 ampules of sodium bicarbonate, with 44.6 mEq per ampule).

SUBJECTIVE AND OBJECTIVE FINDINGS A mild metabolic acidosis may be asymptomatic. As the acidosis increases in severity, the client may experience weakness, malaise, or dull headache. Nausea, vomiting, and/or abdominal pain can also be present. Deep respirations (Kussmaul's breathing) are more often present in clients with acute metabolic acidosis rather than chronic metabolic acidosis. When the pH falls below 7.0, respiratory depression may occur.

The cause of the acidosis has a major effect on the client's clinical picture. Clients in diabetic acidosis may have a fruity, acetone breath odor and signs of severe water loss, eg, thirst, dry mucous membranes, and signs of sodium loss such as loss of skin turgor and shock. In addition, there are high glucose levels in the blood and urine and ketonemia (ketones in the blood and urine). Uremic clients may share these symptoms and have a fruity breath odor with signs of water or sodium loss (eg, loss of skin turgor).

Nursing care is directed toward prevention and early detection of life-threatening situations. Diabetic clients should be taught to monitor their blood glucose levels and to manage their diets and insulin correctly.

Metabolic Alkalosis

Metabolic alkalosis results from a loss of hydrogen (and chloride) ions or an excess of base bicarbonate ions.

Metabolic alkalosis can occur in the following situations:

- With the excessive oral or parenteral administration of sodium bicarbonate or other alkaline salts such as sodium or potassium acetate, lactate, or citrate.
- With the excessive use of milk and antacids in ulcer treatment, producing alkalosis and severe hypercalcemia (*milk–alkali syndrome*).
- When hydrochloric acid (hydrogen ions) is lost because of vomiting and gastric suction, the bicarbonate ion passes into the bloodstream unneutralized and the pH rises, leading to alkalosis.
- Whenever excessive potassium ions are lost through diarrhea, vomiting, or diuretic therapy.

COMPENSATORY MECHANISMS When the hydrogen ions are lost, the bicarbonate ions are retained. The bicarbonate–carbonic acid ratio increases, and the pH rises. The kidneys respond by suppressing hydrogen ion formation and ammonia formation, and they cease conservation of bicarbonate. The respiratory system responds by decreasing the rate and depth of respirations and allowing the PCO_2 to rise so a respiratory acidosis develops to compensate for the metabolic alkalosis.

The most important electrolyte shift involves the potassium and hydrogen ion exchange. With a *potassium deficit*, the hydrogen (H^+) ion, instead of the potassium (K^+) ion, is exchanged for *sodium* in the distal convoluted tubule. This exchange is an effort to preserve and increase potassium levels, thus depleting the H^+ concentration and increasing the level of bicarbonate (HCO_3^-), and promoting alkalosis. In addition, hydrogen moves into the cells so intracellular potassium (K^+) can enter the ECF to raise the potassium concentration.

Conversely, metabolic alkalosis promotes the development of potassium deficit (K^+). In alkalosis, K^+ enters the cell in exchange for H^+. In addition, K^+ rather than the hydrogen ion is exchanged for sodium in the distal tubules. Therefore, *metabolic alkalosis* causes a potassium deficit, or *hypokalemia,* and *hypokalemia* causes a reciprocal *metabolic alkalosis*.

SUBJECTIVE AND OBJECTIVE FINDINGS Recognition of metabolic alkalosis strongly depends on recognition of the underlying causes of this acid–base imbalance, especially if the client also has signs of hypokalemia. Anorexia, nausea, and vomiting occur after an excessive amount of antacids has been ingested for a prolonged period. The client may have sensorium changes (eg, confusion) and be mentally unreliable. Tetany is also a common sign of metabolic and respiratory alkalosis, because tetany is caused by an elevation of the pH, which decreases the ionization of calcium.

Nursing care focuses on observation of the client's state of consciousness, restlessness, and respiratory signs. It is also important to monitor replacement of fluids in clients in alkalosis, especially potassium replacement. Because chloride is still being excreted by the kidneys and being lost in HCl through the GI tract, replacement therapy should be given using potassium chloride (KCl).

Clinical Determination of Acid–Base Balance

A client's acid–base balance can be assessed through an arterial blood gas (ABG) determination. This measurement provides specific information about the acid–base imbalance and crucial clues for early intervention. Blood gas analysis measures:

- Acidity or alkalinity, as determined by the pH.
- The partial pressure of carbon dioxide in the blood. The dissociation of H_2CO_3 (carbonic acid) forms CO_2 and H_2O. The lungs regulate CO_2 levels; therefore, an increase or decrease in CO_2 represents respiratory acid or base problems.
- The bicarbonate level in the blood, which can be plotted on a nomogram to determine levels of compensation. The bicarbonate ratio is regulated by the kidneys and is affected by metabolic acid or base disturbances.

Blood gas changes in respiratory acidosis, respiratory alkalosis, metabolic acidosis, and metabolic alkalosis are shown in Table 3–6.

Table 3–6
Blood Gas Changes in Uncompensated Acid–Base Imbalances

Acid–Base Imbalance	pH	HCO_3^- (Bicarbonate)	PCO_2 (Carbon Dioxide)
Respiratory acidosis	7.3 (decreased)	Normal	Increased
Respiratory alkalosis	7.5 (increased)	Normal	Decreased
Metabolic acidosis	7.3 (decreased)	Decreased	Normal
Metabolic alkalosis	7.5 (increased)	Increased	Normal

SECTION III

The Client in Shock

Shock is a state of widespread reduction in tissue perfusion resulting in inadequate oxygenation and nutrition of vital organs. The three major classifications of shock are shown in Box 3–4. Regardless of whether shock results from hypovolemia, myocardial damage, or altered distribution of blood volume, inadequate tissue perfusion is the common denominator in all types.

Classification of Shock

Hypovolemic Shock

When the normal compensatory mechanisms following extensive fluid loss are inadequate to maintain effective tissue perfusion, hypovolemic shock occurs. Cardiac output falls, arterial blood pressure drops, and blood flow through tissues becomes inadequate to meet metabolic requirements. Tissue cells are damaged from progressive hypoxia and from the accumulation of waste products, leading to acidosis.

Hypovolemic shock is usually caused by multiple trauma, gastrointestinal bleeding, or severe burns. The goal of care with these clients is prompt replacement of intravascular volume to reestablish perfusion of vital organs, resulting in adequate oxygenation at the cellular level.

Box 3–4
Classification of Shock

Hypovolemic shock:

- Hemorrhage secondary to trauma (accidental or surgical), GI bleeding, coagulation disorders, childbirth, carcinoma
- Plasma loss secondary to burns, dehydration, excessive diuretic use

Cardiogenic shock:

- Myocardial damage secondary to myocardial infarction, prolonged dysrhythmias, pericardial tamponade

Distributive shock (Altered distribution of blood volume):

- Neurogenic shock secondary to general or spinal anesthesia, spinal cord injury resulting in decreased peripheral resistance
- Septic shock secondary to gram-negative bacilli (and occasionally other organisms) resulting in increased capillary permeability and hypovolemia
- Anaphylactic shock secondary to antigen–antibody reaction resulting in bronchoconstriction, peripheral arteriolar dilation, and increased capillary permeability

Shock is called reversible when the client recovers following rapid, effective treatment, such as blood transfusion. Sometimes blood pressure continues to drop in spite of vigorous efforts, the client deteriorates, and death ensues. This process is called irreversible or decompensated shock.

Cardiogenic Shock

Cardiogenic shock occurs when the heart is unable to pump adequately (pump failure). The most common cause is myocardial infarction. Other etiologies include disturbances of heart rate or rhythm, trauma to the heart, rupture of the interventricular septum, pericardial tamponade, or any insult compromising the heart's ability to pump (eg, congestive heart failure). With myocardial infarction, the infarcted area is nonfunctional, and the surrounding area may only contract weakly. The resultant poor cardiac pump activity and decreased cardiac output are reflected by hypotension, diaphoresis, clammy skin, reduced urinary output, and altered levels of consciousness. Cardiogenic shock is the most lethal variety of shock. The goal of care is to maintain coronary perfusion by raising the arterial blood pressure with vasopressor drugs and adequate volume replacement.

Distributive Shock

Distributive shock is a result of abnormal distribution of blood volume due to altered vessel resistance. Neurogenic, septic, and anaphylactic shock are included in this category.

NEUROGENIC SHOCK Neurogenic shock occurs with a loss of vasomotor influences from the medulla, resulting in peripheral vasodilation. Circulating blood volume is sequestered in the capillary system, and blood pressure falls. Venous return to the heart is decreased, leading to reduced cardiac output that is inadequate to maintain tissue perfusion. Brain damage, spinal cord injury, severe pain, drugs, and general or spinal anesthesia may cause neurogenic shock. Fainting is considered a transient form of neurogenic shock.

SEPTIC SHOCK Septic shock is usually associated with gram-negative bacteremia, although gram-positive bacilli and viruses can also be the cause. It is unclear whether the bacteria themselves or the toxins released by the bacteria are the causative factor in septic shock.

Clients most susceptible to septic shock are those with in-dwelling catheters, venous and arterial cannulation, postpartum infection, peritonitis, burns, or immunosuppression. Any client having instrumentation or surgery of the genitourinary, gastrointestinal, or biliary tracts is also at risk. Toxic shock syndrome (TSS) is septic shock secondary to use of tampons or the vaginal contraceptive sponge. Nasal packing can also cause TSS.

ANAPHYLACTIC SHOCK Anaphylactic shock is a life-threatening immediate hypersensitivity response of a previously sensitized person to an antigen—a foreign protein or drug. The response is caused by a damaging antigen–antibody reaction occurring on the surface of certain cells, which causes histamine, slow-reacting substance of anaphylaxis (SRS-A), and other mediators to be released. IgE antibodies predominate in the anaphylactic response.

The major causes of systemic anaphylaxis are injections of therapeutic drugs, diagnostic contrast media, and insect stings. Penicillin is perhaps the most common drug implicated, although many drugs—even vitamins—are capable of eliciting a systemic anaphylactic reaction.

In septic and anaphylactic shock, vasodilation and increased capillary permeability occur. One goal of care in all types of distributive shock is replacement of circulating volume.

Identifying Clients at Risk for Shock

Nurses must be fully aware of clients at risk for shock, and that risk should be emphasized in the plan of care. The health history is crucial in documenting risk factors. Has the client recently had invasive diagnostic testing of the gastrointestinal, biliary, or genitourinary tracts (eg, endoscopy or cystoscopy)? Has the client recently had a baby? A miscarriage? An abortion? Does the client have a known malignancy or coagulation disorder? Does the client take excessive diuretics? These clients may be at risk for hypovolemic shock.

Has the client had an MI in the past? Has the client had any previous cardiac problems such as dysrhythmias? These clients may be at risk for cardiogenic shock.

Has the client ever had an adverse reaction to drugs? To anesthesia? If the client is a menstruating woman, does she use tampons during the menses? Does she use a diaphragm or the contraceptive sponge? Is the client on immunosuppressants? These clients may be at risk for distributive shock.

Nurses caring for postoperative clients must be constantly vigilant for signs of hypovolemic shock. Nurses in coronary care units must be equally observant for signs of cardiogenic shock. Emergency room nurses should consider any client a potential candidate for shock.

Clinical Manifestations

Careful client assessment is the best way to monitor clients at risk for shock. The common clinical manifestations of shock are in Table 3–7. Heart rate and rhythm and an estimate of arterial pressure and stroke volume are best gauged by palpation of the carotid or femoral pulses. Evaluation of skin temperature and peripheral pulses (brachial, radial, posterior tibial, and dorsalis pedis) give an estimate

Table 3–7
Clinical Manifestations of Shock

Organ or System	Objective Data
Skin*	Pallor, cyanosis, sweating; altered temperature of fingers, toes, ears, nose
Brain	Restlessness, disorientation, confusion, coma
Cardiovascular*	Tachycardia, ↓ BP, ↓ cardiac output, dysrhythmias, ischemic ECG changes
Pulmonary	Increased respiratory rate
Renal*	Reduced glomerular filtration, low urine output (< 30 mL/h)
Blood	Agglutination of platelets, leukocytes, and erythrocytes; sludging (red cells flowing in clumps), contributing to poor perfusion of tissues
Metabolic	Acidosis, hypoglycemia

*In septic shock, some clients go through an early phase called "warm shock" in which they have warm extremities, high or normal cardiac output, normal blood pressure, and normal urinary output; later, "cold shock" occurs with the findings in the table.

of cardiac output and peripheral vasoconstriction. For example, cardiac output is high if the fingers, toes, ears, and nose are warm. These structures are cold and blue with vasoconstriction and reduced cardiac output.

Blood pressure readings are not particularly helpful in monitoring shock because of the client's markedly altered hemodynamics. True arterial pressure is usually underestimated when peripheral resistance is high. Use of vasoconstrictors in this circumstance can dangerously elevate the arterial pressure. Palpating the central arteries (carotid or femoral pulses) is a better gauge of arterial pressure, and the discrepancy between full bounding pulses and a blood pressure of 80/50 tells the nurse that the blood pressure is inaccurate.

Diminished cerebral perfusion is indicated by confusion, disorientation, restlessness, convulsions, or coma. Oliguria is evidence of reduced glomerular filtration. Mental status and urine output are extremely important parameters in evaluation of shock. Nursing diagnoses applicable to the client in shock are listed in Box 3–5.

In anaphylactic shock bronchospasm may occur within seconds to minutes after introduction of the antigen. Respiratory distress and hypoxemia result. Urticaria, a cutaneous eruption of well-circumscribed, intensely pruritic wheals with erythematous raised borders and blanched centers, may appear. These wheals (also known as hives) can coalesce into localized or well-distributed giant wheals.

Angioedema, edema of the subcutaneous tissue and mucous membranes, may occur, leading to mechanical obstruction of the epiglottis and larynx. Widespread vasodilation results in hypotension, circulatory insufficiency, lowered cardiac output, and decreased perfusion of the brain and coronary arteries. Death results from asphyxiation or circulatory failure. Table 3–8 summarizes the subjective and objective findings in anaphylaxis.

Box 3–5
Nursing Diagnoses Applicable to the Client in Shock

Diagnoses Directly Related to Shock

- *Tissue perfusion, decrease in*, related to loss of circulating volume
- *Tissue perfusion, decrease in*, related to impaired myocardial contractility
- *Tissue perfusion, decrease in*, related to altered distribution of blood volume
- *Gas exchange, impaired*, related to ventilation/perfusion imbalance
- *Urinary elimination, decrease in*, related to impaired renal perfusion
- *Thought processes, alteration in*, related to impaired cerebral perfusion

Additional Potential Nursing Diagnoses

- *Anxiety*, related to change in health status
- *Powerlessness*, due to illness-related regimen
- *Comfort, alteration in*
- *Injury, potential for*, related to invasive treatment

Diagnostic studies useful in evaluating the possible physiologic alterations in shock are found in Table 3–9. Many of these studies are invasive, involving inserting a venous or arterial line for client monitoring. The client's already tenuous situation may be aggravated by complications from the tests. The nurse must be alert for the possibility of thrombus formation, embolism, hemorrhage, dysrhythmia, or infection.

Table 3–8
Anaphylaxis: Subjective and Objective Data

Subjective Data	Objective Data
Pruritus	Skin eruptions: Wheals, giant wheals
Sensation of a lump in the throat	Localized skin edema of face, neck, hands
Shortness of breath, tightness in chest	Dyspnea, wheezing, cough, laryngeal stridor, hoarseness, cyanosis
Abdominal cramps, nausea	Diarrhea, vomiting
Extreme apprehension	Rapid weak pulse, drop in blood pressure

Table 3–9
Diagnostic Studies for Clients in Shock

Diagnostic Study	Physiologic Dysfunction
Central venous pressure (CVP) Pulmonary artery wedge pressure Intra-arterial blood pressure Hematocrit, electrolytes	Volume depletion or volume overload
ECG, CVP, pulmonary artery wedge pressure, intra-arterial pressure	Altered cardiac function
Creatinine, BUN, urinalysis	Altered renal function
Arterial blood gases (ABG)	Altered acid–base balance
Blood lactate levels	Altered cellular metabolism
White blood cell count and differential; blood cultures	Sepsis
Coagulation studies	Disseminated intravascular coagulation (DIC)

Medical and Specific Nursing Measures

Hypovolemic Shock

With multiple trauma, basic life support is the first priority. The client is placed in a horizontal position. Airway, breathing, and circulatory status are evaluated. The client is then checked for signs of external hemorrhage. As soon as the client has a patent airway, is being ventilated with oxygen, and has a discernible pulse, attention is directed toward control of further blood loss. Intravenous lines are established, and crystalloid solutions containing electrolytes and water, such as lactated Ringer's solution, are administered until blood can be typed and cross matched. Blood transfusion is generally required when the estimated blood loss exceeds 25% of the circulating volume. Colloids containing large molecular weight molecules, such as albumin, hetastarch, or high-molecular-weight dextran, may also be used. Use of colloids in initial management of shock is somewhat controversial, although clients with burns may need them early.

Volume replacement and cardiac function are monitored by central venous pressure (CVP) or pulmonary artery occlusive pressure measurement. The CVP line is placed by threading a long polyethylene catheter into the superior or inferior vena cava. The catheter tip is located at the junction of the vena cava and right atrium. The CVP reflects the pressure in the right atrium and systemic veins but does not reliably reflect left ventricular pressures.

Pulmonary artery wedge pressure approximates left ventricular pressure. A flow-directed, balloon-tipped catheter (eg, Swan–Ganz catheter) is placed similar to a CVP line but is advanced through the right heart to wedge into a branch of the pulmonary artery. This pressure reflects left atrial pressure and thus, left ventricular pressure, if there are no mitral valve problems. Using the CVP or pulmonary artery wedge pressure, a fairly accurate assessment can be made of volume depletion, volume overload, and myocardial function, helping to determine the need for additional volume replacement or cardiac support drugs.

Antishock trousers (Figure 3–6) provide for rapid treatment of hypovolemic shock in emergencies. The trousers were developed for use with military casualties and are now being used in emergency departments with some success. Sometimes called a MAST (military antishock trouser) suit, the inflatable nylon garment is applied from below the 12th rib to the ankles to compress bleeding sites in the pelvis and extremities. The feet are exposed so circulation can be monitored. Box 3–6 lists indications for use of antishock trousers.

Pulmonary edema is an absolute contraindication to use of antishock trousers. Other possible contraindications include pregnancy, increased intracranial pressure, decreased ventilation, pneumothorax, and cardiac tamponade.

When the client is stabilized, antishock trousers may be removed by gradual deflation, beginning with the abdominal compartment. Blood pressure measurement guides the rate of deflation. Shock, dysrhythmia, and death can occur with too rapid removal of the MAST suit.

Other approaches to management of hypovolemic clients include continuous ECG monitoring to alert care providers

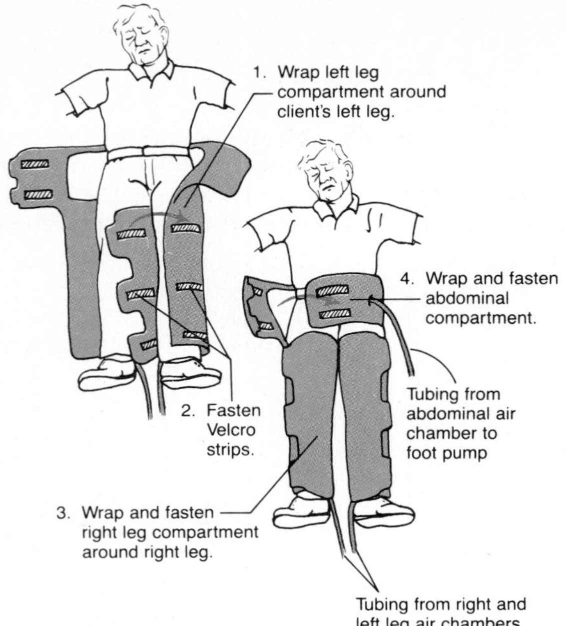
1. Wrap left leg compartment around client's left leg.
2. Fasten Velcro strips.
3. Wrap and fasten right leg compartment around right leg.
4. Wrap and fasten abdominal compartment.
Tubing from abdominal air chamber to foot pump
Tubing from right and left leg air chambers

Figure 3–6

Antishock trousers

Box 3–6 Indications for Antishock Trousers

Hypovolemic shock:

- Trauma
- GI hemorrhage
- Ruptured spleen
- Leaking aortic aneurysm
- Postpartum hemorrhage
- Ruptured ectopic pregnancy
- Postoperative shock
- Hemorrhage in the lower extremities

Stabilization of fractures of the pelvis or lower extremities

May aid in venous access for IV lines in the upper extremities by increasing venous pressure

to impending dangerous dysrhythmias, insertion of an indwelling catheter to measure hourly urine output for assessment of renal perfusion, and arterial blood gases, especially if oxygen or ventilatory therapy is needed.

Cardiogenic Shock

Basic management of clients with cardiogenic shock is similar to care in hypovolemic shock—establishment of an airway, ventilation, oxygenation, correction of acidosis, and pain relief. Another major treatment objective in cardiogenic shock is increasing cardiac output. Output is increased by increasing the cardiac preload (the volume in the ventricle just prior to systole), improving myocardial contraction with drugs, and lowering the afterload against which the heart must pump (blood pressure and vascular system).

Volume expansion with colloids, use of antishock trousers, or leg elevation will increase the preload, which results in an amplification of left ventricular stroke work. CVP or pulmonary artery wedge pressure measurement are necessary to guide fluid management to avoid the complication of pulmonary edema. Myocardial contractility can be improved with drugs such as dopamine (Intropin), dobutamine (Dobutrex), isoproterenol (Isuprel), or digitalis.

Coronary artery perfusion can be improved using the intra-aortic balloon pump, which is inserted into the descending aorta via the femoral artery. The balloon inflates during diastole and deflates during systole. Because the coronary arteries are filled during diastole, the inflated balloon increases diastolic filling and coronary blood flow while decreasing afterload and the work of the heart. Vasodilators may also be used to reduce afterload by decreasing peripheral vascular impedance.

Distributive Shock

NEUROGENIC SHOCK Nursing care of clients with neurogenic shock is directed toward maintaining the client in a supine position and administering IV fluids to restore normal blood pressure. Other nursing activities involve specific client care related to the cause of shock (eg, spinal cord injury or postoperative sequelae).

SEPTIC SHOCK Preventing septic shock through prevention of infection is a major nursing responsibility. Clients who are to give themselves injections or change their own dressings at home must be taught good sterile technique. Women should be cautioned to avoid superabsorbent tampons and to change all tampons frequently. Vaginal contraceptive sponges and diaphragms should not be left in longer than eight hours after intercourse.

Nurses working on burn units, in the operating room, on the IV team, in the cystoscopy laboratory, in the coronary care and intensive care units, and anywhere injections are given, blood is drawn, and dressings are changed must be impeccable in their use of asepsis and vigilant about breaks in technique. Handwashing for both client and care provider is basic to maintaining a safe environment. Overuse of antibiotics in illness care has resulted in drug-resistant bacterial strains, particularly in the hospital. As a result, hospital-acquired (nosocomial) infections are more difficult to treat.

Before beginning antibiotic treatment, obtain all needed specimens and send them for culture. Culture specimens may include blood, urine, sputum, cerebrospinal fluid, or purulent aspirates or drainage. Antibiotics are then selected and started according to the suspected microorganism, the source of the organism, the site of the infection, and the underlying disease of the client. Antibiotics are generally given intravenously because decreased perfusion makes the intramuscular and oral routes less reliable. It is difficult for antibiotics to penetrate an area that is sealed off, such as an abscess. Surgical incision and drainage of abscesses are essential to remove the septic focus.

ANAPHYLACTIC SHOCK Early recognition of an anaphylactic reaction is essential. Urticaria and pruritus can be controlled with subcutaneous injection of 0.2 to 0.5 mL of 1:1000 epinephrine, which can be repeated at 3-minute intervals in the event of a severe reaction. If the reaction was secondary to an insect sting or drug injection, a tourniquet applied proximal to the site of injection may reduce absorption of the antigenic material. When an insect stinger remains, it should be removed without compression. Epinephrine 0.2 mL is administered into the sting or injection site.

When the reaction takes place in a clinical setting, in addition to the previous treatment, an IV is started to provide a route for IV administration of epinephrine if needed as well as for volume expanders and vasopressors, if extreme hypotension occurs. Oxygen is administered, and endotracheal intubation or tracheostomy may be necessary. Additional possible therapeutic agents include diphenhydramine for urticaria and angioedema and aminophylline for bronchospasm.

Individuals with a known hypersensitivity should wear a Medic-Alert bracelet and have an emergency kit on hand for self-administration of epinephrine. Persons with allergy to insect stings should always carry epinephrine during seasons when contact with insects is possible.

Complications of Prolonged Shock

Shock lung, or adult respiratory distress syndrome (ARDS), is a serious pulmonary complication that may follow shock from all causes. Initially, there seems to be an increased permeability of the alveolar capillaries to plasma proteins with development of interstitial edema. Tracheobronchial secretions, tachypnea, and cyanosis increase. As the condition progresses, arterial blood gases show a decreasing PaO_2 and an increasing $PaCO_2$. Later, atelectasis, microthrombosis, hemorrhage, and fibrosis occur.

Acute tubular necrosis (ATN) is another possible complication from any type of shock. ATN results from destruction of tubular epithelial cells secondary to impaired perfusion, which can lead to renal failure and death.

Disseminated intravascular coagulation (DIC) is a serious complication of septic shock. Stasis of blood in capillary beds leads to uncontrolled microcirculatory clotting with widespread organ ischemia and necrosis.

SECTION IV

Understanding and Caring for the Client in Pain

Pain is a universal experience. Everyone has known pain to some degree. Pain is often a useful protective signal because it is a warning of potential health problems (eg, the dysuria caused by a bladder infection or the earache of otitis media). Pain is also a consequence of some normal bodily functions (eg, mild dysmenorrhea or the pain of childbirth). Pain can also warn of emotional or stress-related problems (eg, the headache, gastritis, or low-back pain caused by tension, anxiety, or the stress of daily living).

Pain is a totally subjective personal experience. No one can fully appreciate the pain of another. No two persons feel the same degree of pain in the same way. Pain is a complex perceptual phenomenon. There is no direct relation between pain stimulus and individual response.

Fortunately for most, pain is transitory. Often cuts and bruises, a fleeting gas pain, discomfort following sports activity, or a few days of postoperative pain are the only identification persons have with the pain experience. Consider what it must be like to have persistent, unrelenting, immobilizing chronic pain. Every day is disrupted, and lives are crippled, controlled by the fine balance between activity and pain exacerbation.

Despite the universality of pain, much is still unknown about what actually causes a sensation to be perceived as painful. The reappraisal of theories of pain by Melzack and Wall in 1965 stimulated great interest in pain research. The following brief review of pain physiology and pain theories provides a background for caring for the client in pain.

Pathways of Pain

Pain signals in peripheral nerves are transmitted by small-diameter, thinly myelinated A-delta fibers and unmyelinated C fibers. The A-delta fibers are slightly larger and transmit information rapidly, whereas C fibers have a slow conducting velocity. Pain produced by A-delta fibers is a sharp, well-localized pricking pain called **epicritic** (discriminating) pain. C fiber pain is a slower, diffuse, burning or aching pain that is poorly localized. It is called **protopathic** (undiscriminating) pain.

Sensory nerve fibers enter the spinal cord via the dorsal root of a spinal nerve. They synapse in the substantia gelatinosa, a functional unit of densely packed cells that extends the length of the spinal cord. The substantia gelatinosa is located in the dorsal horns on either side of the cord. The impulses cross over and ascend contralaterally in the lateral spinothalamic tracts to the thalamus and then move on to the cerebral cortex. The sensations of pain and temperature ascend the spinal cord in the same fiber tracts.

Previously, it was thought that **nociceptive impulses**, impulses giving rise to sensations of pain, were transmitted straight through to the brain without modulation. It is now known, however, that pain can be inhibited all along the course of transmission. The dorsal horn has been found to be a complex structure anatomically, physiologically, and biochemically. Its synaptic arrangements permit reception and transmission as well as local integration and selection.

Although the spinothalamic tract has been considered the specific pain and temperature tract, there is evidence that it may have other functions as well. In addition, there are probably other ascending systems that play some role in transmitting nociceptive information to the brain.

The limbic system, which includes the thalamus, hypothalamus, hypocampus, amygdala, and various other structures, plays a major role in the complex phenomena of emotion and motivation. Input from the limbic system is also thought to account for the motivational and emotional components of pain.

Theories of Pain

Specificity Theory

Prior to the work of Melzack and Wall, specificity theory was the accepted explanation for the mechanism of pain. This theory assumed that the intensity of the nociceptive impulse and the perception of pain were directly related. Specificity theory failed to account for the broad range of individual responses to similar pain stimuli (eg, why two persons undergoing uncomplicated appendectomy experience postoperative pain so differently).

Gate Control Theory

The gate control theory, introduced by Melzack and Wall (1965) and subsequently modified by them and others, suggests that nociceptive impulses can be modulated in the spinal cord, brainstem, or cerebral cortex. These authorities postulate that neural mechanisms in the substantia gelatinosa in the dorsal horns act as a gate that can increase or decrease the flow of nerve impulses from peripheral fibers to the spinal cord cells that transmit these impulses to the brain.

A few brief clinical applications of the theory may more fully explain its usefulness. The theory suggests that activity in large-diameter nerve fibers closes the gate and decreases or eliminates the pain. Transcutaneous electrical nerve stimulation (TENS), in which electrodes are applied to the skin, has been used for pain relief with some success. TENS is thought to stimulate the large rapid-velocity fibers, which effectively closes the gate. Reducing clients' anxiety also often reduces their pain. It is thought that inhibiting impulses from the cerebral cortex and thalamus closes the gate. Analgesic drugs act on the central nervous system, essentially reducing or abolishing the integration of the pain experience.

Although the gate control hypothesis may only partially explain the pain phenomenon, this theory has made major contributions to the understanding and treatment of pain. The concept of a gate mechanism is a scientific explanation for the uniqueness of each pain experience and the multidimensional influences on that experience.

Endorphins and Enkephalins

The discovery of the endorphin system in the mid-1970s added an entire new dimension to pain research. Endorphins, literally meaning the "morphine within," are opioidlike substances in the brain, spinal cord, and gastrointestinal tract. The endorphins apparently combine with specific receptors to produce analgesic activity similar to that of the drug morphine.

Enkephalins, part of the endorphin system, are central nervous system neurotransmitters that mediate the transmission of pain information. Enkephalins may inhibit the release of substance P, a peptide released in the dorsal horn with nociceptive stimulation. Substance P seems to function as a sensory neurotransmitter for relay of pain signals.

Stress and pain both activate the endorphin system. Endorphin release is also thought to accompany other pain-relief measures such as acupuncture and TENS. Naloxone, an opiate antagonist drug, has been found to reverse the analgesic effects of the endorphins.

Pain as Defined by the Health Professional

Acute Pain

Acute pain is usually of rapid onset, varies in intensity from mild to severe, is self-limiting, and is of less than 6 months' duration. Common examples of acute pain are dental pain, postsurgical or postpartum pain, and pain from injury or infection. Acute pain is usually successfully treated with analgesic medications or hypnosis, or it may require no specific intervention. If tissue damage was the cause of pain, pain declines steadily as the tissue heals.

Chronic Pain

Chronic pain is an ongoing pain experience of 6 months or longer that fails to resolve naturally and does not respond to traditional medical intervention. Chronic pain is now thought to be a specific disease in its own right rather than a symptom of disease.

Referred Pain

Referred pain is felt in a part removed from the pain's point of origin. One explanation for this phenomenon is that sensory neurons that transmit pain signals from a particular body surface area enter the same spinal segment as nerve fibers from the diseased internal organ. The ascending neurons carry pain signals to the brain from both locations. Because cutaneous pain is more common than visceral pain, the brain interprets the pain as originating in the skin. Many conditions are diagnosed by the pattern of referred pain. For example, pain radiating into the left shoulder and down the left arm is associated with myocardial infarction.

Phantom Pain

Phantom pain is a sensation in a body part that has been amputated. Even though the nerves supplying the amputated part were severed, the remaining neurons may continue to send impulses to the same area of the brain as before. Some time may elapse before the brain stops interpreting impulses from the severed neurons as if the part were still present.

Pain as Expressed and Acted on by Clients

Persons in pain react in a wide variety of ways. Some attempt to keep their pain hidden and say nothing. Others verbally express their discomfort using descriptive words and phrases. Sometimes body language tells the story. How individuals express their pain and attempt to deal with it depends on a myriad of factors including family tradition and upbringing, culture, religion, previous pain experience, bodily part involved, and beliefs about health and illness—to name a few.

Approaches to pain relief are highly individual. The use by North Americans of over-the-counter (OTC) analgesics containing acetylsalicylic acid, acetaminophen, or ibuprofen has spawned a multimillion-dollar drug industry geared toward relief of common human discomforts. Think for a moment about how persons learn to deal with aches and pains when growing up. Perhaps they are told to "grin and bear it," to take two aspirin and go to bed, or to use ice or heat. Perhaps a child is given a piece of candy or distracted when complaining of a minor discomfort. More severe pain may be dealt with in the same way, or perhaps a physician is called or the person is taken immediately to the emergency room. Perhaps a knowledgeable neighbor, a grandmother, a nurse in the family, or a healer associated with the cultural or religious beliefs of the family is consulted. If the treatment suggested by the consultant is not effective, further information probably is gathered until an effective approach is found, or the pain goes away by itself.

Most adults, having developed their own approach to pain management from childhood and having lived with their unique aches and pains for some time (eg, tension headaches, tennis elbow), self-treat these discomforts better than the health care system could. Through trial and error, most persons discover what initiates or aggravates their pain. Avoiding these factors becomes part of their lifestyle. When avoidance is not completely possible, early warning signs are recognized and preventive action initiated. When pain occurs despite preventive care, most persons have a routine plan of attack.

For example, the person who has suffered the severe discomfort of constipation has probably learned that whole grains, plenty of fluids, fresh fruits and vegetables, and regular exercise are preventive. When the pattern of a regular morning bowel movement is altered, the client may initiate action such as eating an extra bowl of bran cereal, increasing fluid intake, stepping up an exercise program, or taking a dose of psyllium. Persons usually consult a health care provider only when they have exhausted their own approaches to pain management or when they experience pain unlike any they have had in the past.

Assessment of the Client in Pain

Subjective Data: The Health History

When gathering information from clients about their pain, appreciate that clients know their own bodies better than anyone else. Sometimes a client will describe a pattern of pain or an approach to treatment that sounds implausible. These descriptions must not be minimized. The client's language may not be particularly scientific, but the view of the pain experience is real. The only way the nurse can assess pain accurately and implement an effective plan of care is to understand fully each client's pain experience.

The history should include questions about factors that *provoke* or *palliate* the pain, the *quality* of the pain, the *region* of the body involved, and the *severity* and *timing* of the pain—the PQRST of pain evaluation (see Chapter 5). The history should also attempt to describe any cultural, familial, or religious influences on the client's feelings and beliefs about pain. There may also be specific cultural or religious approaches to managing pain or limitations on types of treatment. Information about previous pain experiences and previous encounters with the health care system are helpful to discuss and document.

Objective Data: Physical Assessment

While taking the health history, especially observe the client's facial expression and body language. Is the client extremely restless or lying rigid in bed? Does the client clutch at or massage a particular body region? Does the client maintain a certain position or pace the floor? What is the skin color? Is diaphoresis present? Are the respirations rapid or shallow? Before beginning a physical examination, obtain as much data as possible by observing the client during history taking.

Specific physical assessment depends on the bodily system involved, although in many instances, this is not known. For example, a client with chest pain could have a disease of the lungs such as pneumonia, arthritic pain from an old rib fracture, premenstrual breast tenderness, angina from coronary artery disease, or a problem associated with the gastrointestinal system such as reflux in hiatus hernia, to name a few. In this example, assessment would include complete evaluation of the thorax and lungs, the breasts, the heart, and the abdomen.

An important point when evaluating the client in pain is to avoid the painful area until the other areas have been accurately assessed. Important clues might be missed if the nurse concentrates on the painful area alone. Consequently, a general assessment should be done first. For example, in a client with a swollen, painful knee, assess the other joints of the body and evaluate the skin and soft tissues of the affected leg before touching the knee itself. Another reason to assess the painful area last is that probing of the area generally elicits more pain, which makes examination difficult or even impossible.

Nonpharmacologic Approaches to Pain Management

Transcutaneous Electrical Nerve Stimulation

Electrical stimulation of peripheral nerves provides an analgesic effect in both acute and chronic pain states. Although the mechanism of action is not exactly clear, TENS is thought to modify the transmission of nociceptive impulses in the central nervous system by improving the function of the large-diameter nerve fibers, closing the pain gate.

Flexible electrodes that are self-adhering or coated with a conductive gel are applied to the skin overlying or proximal to the painful region. The electrodes are activated by a battery-operated device to produce a tingling or vibrating sensation in the painful area.

TENS has been used with varying degrees of success for pain modulation in postoperative clients and in clients with phantom limb pain, stump pain, postherpetic neuralgia, low back pain, arthritis, and pain associated with dysfunction of the temporomandibular joint.

Although TENS is noninvasive and generally safe, certain precautions are indicated. Safety of TENS in pregnancy is not documented, and the electrical stimulation with TENS can interfere with some types of cardiac pacemakers. A pacemaker may also alter the efficacy of TENS. Because TENS can stimulate muscle spasm, electrodes should not be placed in areas such as the upper anterior neck where laryngeal and pharyngeal muscle spasm could cause laryngeal spasm and airway closure. Stimulation of the carotid sinus in the neck at the bifurcation of the common carotid artery should also be avoided, because bradycardia can result. TENS electrodes should not be placed over an incision line or on an area of skin irritation. To prevent skin irritation from TENS use, the electrodes should be removed daily and the skin carefully cleansed and air dried.

Acupuncture

Acupuncture is a 2000-year-old Chinese technique of inserting fine needles into the skin at selected points on the body. The technique is based on the Eastern philosophy of mind–body unity, a concept Westerners are only beginning to appreciate fully. In Eastern healing, disease is thought to be a manifestation of imbalance between yin (female) and yang (male) energy flows. Needle insertion is believed to remove the blocks to energy flow and restore harmony.

One theory about how acupuncture relieves pain is related to the concept of trigger points, hypersensitive areas in muscle that can give rise to localized and referred pain. When the trigger point is stimulated, the effect is not unlike pulling the trigger of a gun (ie, the pain is experienced in the target area, distant from the trigger point). This referred pain does not follow usual dermatome patterns but has a predictable zone of referral. Extinction of the trigger points alleviates the referred pain. Acupuncture points (approximately 800 of them) lie on meridians that are believed to be pathways of energy within the body. When acupuncture charts are compared to descriptions of trigger-point locations, they are similar.

A second theory suggests that acupuncture needle insertion stimulates the endorphin system, releasing the body's natural opiates. Sometimes the needles are wired to stimulate the nerve endings electrically, enhancing the treatment. It is not known whether acupuncture achieves analgesia by extinction of trigger points, by release of endorphins, or even through the stimulation of large-diameter nerve fibers that effectively close the gate, as in TENS.

Acupressure, a less invasive variant of acupuncture, is finger pressure and massage specifically directed to acupuncture points. Acupuncture is practiced in many pain centers in North America, although it has not been widely accepted by practitioners of traditional medicine. Nevertheless, interest is high in use of acupuncture and acupressure for both acute and chronic pain states.

Nerve Blocks

Interrupting nerve function or myofascial trigger points by injecting a local anesthetic such as 1% lidocaine or 0.5% bupivacaine can provide temporary pain relief in some clients with acute or chronic pain. Nerve blocks are also done for severe muscle spasticity, such as that in clients with multiple sclerosis. Neurodestructive agents such as phenol or alcohol can be injected to achieve a longer-lasting effect, although adjacent tissue destruction can be a serious problem. Clients are carefully selected for this more permanent type of blockade.

Biofeedback

Biofeedback is a teaching method that assists clients to tune in to their bodies and eventually learn to control certain visceral responses (eg, muscle tension, hand temperature, heart rate, and blood pressure). A selected physiologic activity is monitored by attaching the client by electrodes or transducers to an electronic instrument that amplifies the bodily response with lights, digital readings, graphs, or auditory signals. The client is thus able to see or hear fluctuations of physiologic activity and develop an awareness of how to reproduce the desired response. Through concentration, the client can learn to shift brain wave activity patterns from the usual beta waves of daily activity to alpha waves, which characterize relaxation and tranquility. Achieving a high degree of alpha rhythm is helpful in controlling certain pain states, particularly those related to muscle tension.

The eventual goal of biofeedback training is to have clients develop skills that can be used outside the clinical setting to achieve the relaxed alpha wave state. Biofeedback is often used in conjunction with stress management techniques such as guided imagery, diaphragmatic breathing, and progressive muscle relaxation. Biofeedback as the sole modality in pain control is not as effective as biofeedback accompanied by other ancillary relaxation techniques.

Hypnosis

Hypnosis is a self-induced state of relaxation and concentration in which cognitive thinking is bypassed, allowing the client to be more susceptible to suggestion. Hypnosis has been used for pain reduction with dental procedures, in labor and delivery, and in clients with cancer. In recent years, hypnosis has increased in popularity as an approach to weight loss and smoking cessation. Although some question whether hypnosis is a sound approach to pain control, the literature reports many dramatic accounts of hypnotic analgesia in a wide variety of acute and chronic pain states (Barber & Adrian, 1982).

Placebo Effect

The relief of pain or other symptoms by a so-called "useless" medication or treatment is called the placebo effect. In the past, clients who responded favorably to a placebo were considered malingerers. More recently, the placebo response has been explained as mind–body interaction; a heightened expectation of positive effects caused those effects to take place. In essence, the placebo worked because the person believed it would. The current thinking is that placebos relieve pain or other symptoms by causing the body to release endorphins, which have analgesic and other opioid properties.

Much is still unknown about the placebo response. Some persons do not seem to respond to placebos at all. Some consistently respond, and others respond only occasionally. Some experts suggest that the degree of placebo response depends on what medication clients believe they are receiving. Others suggest that a care provider the client perceives as honest and convincing can affect the degree of response with a statement such as, "Here is your medication. I believe it will help."

Because the prescribing of placebos seems to involve a degree of client deception, their use is controversial. Research has certainly disproved that persons who respond to a placebo have imaginary symptoms. Until more is understood about the totality of the placebo effect, however, the debate about placebo use will continue.

Pharmacologic Approaches to Pain Management

Aspirin

Acetylsalicylic acid (ASA), or aspirin, is the most frequently used OTC analgesic, antipyretic, and anti-inflammatory drug in North America. Aspirin seems to produce analgesia by a peripheral action on synthesis of prostaglandins, substances generated by tissue damage. Aspirin is absorbed in the stomach and upper intestine, reaching adequate plasma concentration within 30 minutes and peak concentration in 2 hours. The usual adult dose of aspirin is 325 to 650 mg PO q. 4–6 h.

High doses of aspirin, as used in rheumatoid arthritis, or prolonged use of aspirin can cause epigastric distress and occasionally, gastrointestinal bleeding. Excessive doses can also produce tinnitus. Buffered aspirin (a combination of aspirin and antacids) and enteric-coated aspirin reduce the gastric irritation of plain aspirin. Because aspirin affects blood platelets, prolonging bleeding time, clients with peptic ulcer, on anticoagulants, or with bleeding disorders should not take aspirin. Aspirin is a common ingredient in many OTC and prescription drugs. Therefore, clients who cannot take ASA should remind their nurse, physician, and pharmacist when medications are prescribed.

Acetaminophen

Acetaminophen (Tylenol, Datril) is the second most common OTC analgesic, antipyretic drug sold. Acetaminophen does not have the anti-inflammatory properties of aspirin but neither does it interfere with clotting nor produce epigastric distress. The usual adult dose of acetaminophen is the same as aspirin—325 to 650 mg PO q. 4–6 h. Toxicity is uncommon with acetaminophen, although serious hepatic necrosis and death have occurred after large overdoses.

Nonsteroidal Anti-Inflammatory Drugs

Nonsteroidal anti-inflammatory drugs (NSAIDs) have analgesic, antipyretic and anti-inflammatory properties. The therapeutic effects of NSAIDs result from inhibition of prostaglandin synthesis. **Prostaglandins** are a group of compounds synthesized from unsaturated fatty acids that seem to have a role in both acute and chronic inflammatory reactions. There is a known variable clinical response in different clients to the NSAIDs. Therefore, a client who fails to respond to one drug may be helped considerably by another NSAID. Two common NSAIDs are indomethacin (Indocin) and ibuprofen (Motrin, Advil, Nuprin). Advil and Nuprin are available OTC.

Adverse effects of NSAIDs are mainly gastrointestinal. Dyspepsia, heartburn, gastritis, and gastric or duodenal ulcer have been reported. The gastrointestinal side effects seem to be less severe than those of aspirin, however. Renal function in clients with preexisting renal disease can be impaired with NSAIDs. Edema formation, blurring of vision, insomnia, and constipation are other reported adverse effects.

Narcotic Analgesics

Narcotic analgesics produce analgesia by acting directly on the central nervous system. They seem to activate an endorphin-mediated network in the CNS designed to inhibit nociceptive transmission. The central analgesic effect is often accompanied by enhanced feelings of well-being or euphoria and sometimes drowsiness and mental clouding. Respiratory depression and nausea and vomiting may also occur.

Alternative approaches to administering narcotics for pain control have been used with some success. Continuous administration of morphine by IV infusion, titrated to the client's needs, has provided effective analgesia in some clients and decreased the total amount of drug needed for pain relief (Boyer, 1982). Extravascular infusion of meperidine (Demerol) or a local anesthetic such as bupivacaine via a catheter placed in the epidural space for 5 to 7 days has also been effective in some clients with chronic pain. The brachial plexus, celiac plexus, or lumbar sympathetic chain are other areas used for catheter placement and drug infusion (Alberico, 1984).

Patient-controlled analgesia (PCA) is a new drug delivery system that allows clients to administer their own pain medications through a PCA unit connected to an intravenous line. The client presses a button to trigger the medication dose. A timing device on the unit prevents overdose. Nurses working with clients using the PCA unit report that clients seem to achieve better pain relief and use less medication when they have this kind of control over their own medication schedules (Bast & Hayes, 1986).

Other drugs effective for pain relief, alone or in combination with narcotics, include amphetamines and antidepressants. Amphetamines seem to reduce the amount of narcotic required to control pain. Some clients welcome the stimulant effect of amphetamines to counteract the sedative effect of many narcotic analgesics. Tricyclic antidepressants (amitriptyline, imipramine) have been most successful in relieving pain associated with depression. Clients on these drugs should have urinary output monitored carefully because tricyclic antidepressants can cause urinary retention.

Nursing Implications

The effect of pain on the life of the client and loved ones is as variable and unique as each person. Some generalizations can be made that are important for nursing care, however. Clients often reduce their food and fluid intake, so they may become malnourished and dehydrated. Clients may be unable to sleep, resulting in chronic fatigue. Because of their decreased energy, they are unable to participate in strategies to cope with their pain (guided imagery, relaxation techniques, and distraction); consequently, the pain cycle is exacerbated. Social and sexual relationships deteriorate, reinforcing the client's isolation and feelings of frustration, helplessness, and anger in loved ones. Planning and nursing intervention for these problems are discussed in other chapters. This discussion will focus on comfort and pain relief.

Nurses have known for years that certain measures relieve pain in many clients. For example, touch, massage, breathing techniques, repositioning, explanation, and teaching have all been documented by nurses as helpful for promoting comfort and relieving pain. The physiologic reasons for the effectiveness of these approaches are only beginning to be understood. For example, cutaneous stimulation, massage, and pressure may stimulate the large-diameter nerve fibers and close the pain gate. Careful explanation and teaching may decrease anxiety and reduce pain by stimulating release of endorphins. Diversion or distraction, as with relaxation approaches (music, watching TV, Lamaze breathing, guided imagery, and meditation), may also reduce muscle tension and modify pain perception through endorphin release. When the client is also receiving analgesic medications, nursing activities involving touch, explanation, and listening enhance the effect of the drug.

The nurse is the care provider most responsible for evaluating the client's need for analgesic medications. Medications are frequently ordered with variable dosage and variable timing (eg, Demerol 50 to 100 mg q. 3–4 h. p.r.n.). The nurse decides how much of the drug will be given and how soon. Unfortunately, nurses often do not medicate the client soon enough or with a sufficient dose. Consequently, the client never achieves a level of comfort compatible with rest. Anxiety and muscle tension increase, and the pain is exacerbated.

Nurses often worry that a client will become addicted. Clients and families also frequently express the same concern. Addiction can be a problem in some instances, but when responsible health care providers are working with clients in pain, they continually evaluate the client's response, and adjust the medication schedule accordingly. The age and weight of the client, the severity of the health problem, other extenuating factors, and history of response to analgesic medication are considerations in deciding about medication management. Although it could be assumed that a small, elderly person needs less medication than a 25-year-old, 250-lb football player, health care providers should continuously evaluate the client's response to medication. The elderly client might suffer unnecessarily because of insufficient dosing for weight and age but be too stoic to ask for better pain relief. Carefully monitoring the client during the first two to three dose intervals helps the nurse to gauge the efficacy and duration of the analgesic effect as well as any adverse side effects.

Postoperative clients need analgesics for 24 to 72 hours after surgery and perhaps longer, depending on the procedure. Withholding narcotics or encouraging the client to "wait a little longer" in the first postoperative days only increases the client's level of discomfort and may cause feelings of guilt, embarrassment, or weakness in asking for pain relief.

There should be less fear of addiction in terminally ill clients in excruciating pain. It is difficult to justify an attitude that encourages living with unbearable pain while dying. Nurses often feel helpless in working with clients with relentless pain. Their discussions with physicians about more effective pain control measures may lead nowhere, often because physicians are equally frustrated when they are unable to keep a client comfortable. This helplessness and inability to control a situation may cause both physician and nurse unconsciously to withdraw from the client and family.

The hospice movement and the increasing efforts to give clients more control over their lives, whether hospitalized or at home, is a promising development in pain management. Clients on oral medication can easily be given control over their own dosing schedules. Even when on parenteral medications, clients and their families can titrate the dosage and adjust the dose intervals as needed. On some days, clients in pain may feel good and only need oral aspirin and relaxation techniques. On other days, clients may be uncomfortable enough to need sufficient parenteral medication to make them completely unaware of their surroundings or their pain. Individualizing approaches to medication management in the terminally ill client in pain improves the quality of life for the client and family. Health care providers also see the wisdom in giving clients and families more control over decisions that so profoundly affect their lives.

Pain Clinics

Persons with chronic pain are frequently unable to find help in the traditional health care system. Many are now being helped in multidisciplinary pain clinics, of which there are a growing number in North America. Treatment at a clinic begins with a thorough health history, physical examination, and psychologic evaluation. Clients dependent on narcotics are weaned from them, and methadone is substituted, if necessary. Psychologic counseling, physical therapy, hypnosis, biofeedback, TENS, and acupuncture are potential approaches to treatment. The rehabilitation program is individually designed for each client.

Some clinics encourage inpatient treatment, and others favor an outpatient approach. Clients learn new patterns of moving and living that ameliorate the pain. Reduction in pain medication, resumption of more normal activities, and a positive self-image are the eventual goals.

Other centers may meet the needs of individual clients. Holistic health centers usually provide programs to promote relaxation and reduce stress. Hospice programs provide terminally ill clients in pain and their families with thoughtful, supportive, humanistic care. Organizations such as the National Committee on the Treatment of Intractable Pain are valuable resources to clients and families.

Nursing Research Note

Wells N: The effect of relaxation on postoperative muscle tension and pain. *Nurs Res* 1982; 31(4):236–238.

Relaxation has been used to control pain following abdominal surgery. This study examined the effect of relaxation training on muscle tension and subjective reports of pain. Of two groups of subjects who had cholecystectomies, one group received relaxation instruction and the other received standard preoperative instruction.

The results indicated that relaxation training reduced the psychological discomfort associated with pain but had no significant effect on physiologic measures. Muscle tension was not significantly altered by either technique. In applying these findings, nurses can incorporate relaxation training into preoperative teaching and encourage clients to use such techniques postoperatively.

Chapter Highlights

Osmols are the measures of the amount of work dissolved particles can do in drawing fluid through a semipermeable membrane. Osmolality refers to the number of osmols per liter of solvent.

Isotonic solutions have the same osmolality as blood plasma, preventing shifts of fluids and electrolytes.

Hypertonic solutions have a greater osmolality than blood plasma, causing a rapid influx of water from the cells and interstitial spaces into the plasma.

Hypotonic solutions have a lower osmolality than blood plasma, causing water to move from the plasma into the cells.

Fluid and electrolyte imbalances include water–sodium imbalance, volume imbalance, and electrolyte imbalance.

Sodium is the primary regulator of extracellular fluid volume and concentration. Potassium is the major intracellular cation.

Acid–base balance depends on the homeostasis of the hydrogen ion concentration in body fluids. An acidic solution has a pH below 7.0. A base or alkaline solution has a pH above 7.0. Extracellular fluid is slightly alkaline, having a pH from 7.35 to 7.45.

A buffer is a substance that has the ability to bind or release hydrogen in solution, maintaining the pH of the solution relatively constant despite the addition of considerable quantities of acid or base.

Acidosis occurs whenever a disturbance in the acid–base balance results in an increase in hydrogen ion concentration. Alkalosis is a disturbance in acid–base balance that results in a decrease in hydrogen ion concentration.

Respiratory acidosis occurs whenever there is an accumulation of CO_2 and, therefore, carbonic acid due to an interference with the alveolar exchange of O_2 and CO_2.

Respiratory alkalosis occurs when there is an excess loss of carbonic acid and, therefore, a decrease on the carbonic acid side of the acid–bicarbonate ratio.

Metabolic acidosis develops because of an increased amount of acid or a decrease in the amount of base.

Metabolic alkalosis results from a loss of hydrogen and chloride ions or an excess of base bicarbonate.

Shock is a state of widespread reduction in tissue perfusion resulting in inadequate oxygenation and nutrition of vital organs. The three major classifications of shock are hypovolemic shock, cardiogenic shock, and distributive shock.

Clients at risk for hypovolemic shock include those with recent surgery, trauma, burns, invasive diagnostic testing, childbirth, miscarriage, or abortion; clients with a malignancy or coagulation disorder; and clients who take excessive diuretics.

Clients at risk for cardiogenic shock include those in the coronary care unit and those with previous cardiac problems such as myocardial infarction or dysrhythmias.

Clients at risk for distributive shock include those with known or unknown allergy to drugs or anesthesia; women using tampons, diaphragms, or contraceptive sponges; and clients on immunosuppressants.

Pain produced by A-delta fibers is a sharp, well-localized pain called epicritic pain. Pain produced by C fibers is a diffuse, poorly localized pain called protopathic pain.

Chronic pain is pain of 6 months or longer that fails to resolve and does not respond to traditional medical intervention.

Because clients understand their bodies better than anyone else, nurses should listen carefully to the ways in which clients describe their pain experience and approaches they have found helpful.

Bibliography

FLUID AND ELECTROLYTE BALANCE/ACID–BASE BALANCE

Barta MA: Correcting electrolyte imbalances. *RN* (Feb) 1987;30–33.

Collins R, Douglas MD: *Illustrated Manual of Fluid and Electrolyte Disorders,* 2nd ed. Philadelphia: Lippincott, 1983.

Flink E: Nutritional aspects of magnesium metabolism. *West J Med* 1980; 133:304–312.

Goldberger E: *A Primer of Water, Electrolyte and Acid–Base Disorders,* 6th ed. Philadelphia: Lea & Febiger, 1980.

Lane G, Peirce AG: When persistence pays off: Resolving the mystery of an unexplained electrolyte imbalance. *Nurs 82* (Jan) 1982; 12:44–47.

Maxwell MH, Kleeman CR: *Clinical Disorders of Fluid and Electrolyte Metabolism,* 3rd ed. New York: McGraw–Hill, 1980.

Menzel LK: Clinical problems of electrolyte balance. *Nurs Clin North Am* 1980; 15(3)559–576.

Menzel LK: Clinical problems of fluid balance. *Nurs Clin North Am* 1980; 15(3)549–558.

Metheny N, Snively WD: *Nurse's Handbook of Fluid Balance,* 4th ed. Philadelphia: Lippincott, 1983.

Strott V, Lee C, Barrett C: *Fluid and Electrolytes: A Practical Approach,* 3rd ed. Philadelphia: Davis, 1984.

Toto KH: When the patient has hypokalemia. *RN* (March) 1987;38–42.

Urrows ST: Physiology of body fluids. *Nurs Clin North Am* 1980; 15(3):537–547.

Weldy NJ: *Body Fluids and Electrolytes,* 2nd ed. St. Louis: Mosby, 1980.

Witkowski AS: *Pulmonary Assessment: A Clinical Guide.* Philadelphia: Lippincott, 1985.

Zucker AR, Chernow B: Diabetes insipidus and the syndrome of inappropriate antidiuretic hormone release. *CCQ* (Dec) 1983; 6:63–74.

SHOCK

Ayres SM et al: Rescuing the patient in cardiogenic shock. *Patient Care* (July 15) 1983; 17:255–278.

Christopher KL: The use of a model for hemodynamic balance to describe burn shock. *Nurs Clin North Am* 1980; 15(3):617–627.

Gaunder BN, Winkle D: Anaphylaxis: Managing and preventing a true emergency. *Nurse Pract* (May) 1984; 9:17–20.

Houston MC, Thompson WL, Robertson D: Shock: Diagnosis and management. *Ann Intern Med* 1984; 144:1433–1439.

Lamb LS: Think you know septic shock? *Nurs 82* (Jan) 1982; 12:34–43.

McAdams, RC, McClure K: Hypovolemia: When to suspect it. *RN* 1986; Dec:34–37.

McAdams, RC, McClure K: Hypovolemia: How to stop it. *RN* 1986; Dec:38–41.

Nursing care of patients in shock. (Programmed instruction) 1. Pharmacotherapy. 2. Fluids, oxygen, and the intra-aortic balloon pump. 3. Evaluating the patient. *Am J Nurs* 1982; 82:943–964; 1982; 82:1401–1422; 1982; 82:1723–1746.

Purcell JA: Shock drugs: Standardized guidelines. *Am J Nurs* 1982; 82:965–974.

PAIN

Alberico JG: Breaking the chronic pain cycle. *Am J Nurs* 1984; 84:1222–1225.

Barber J, Adrian C: *Psychological Approaches to the Management of Pain.* New York: Brunner/Mazel, 1982.

Bast C, Hayes P: PCA: A new way to spell pain relief. *RN* 1986; Aug:18–20.

Battenfield BL: Suffering: A Conceptual description and content analysis of an operational schema. *Image* (Spring) 1984; 16:34–41.

Boyer MW: Continuous drip morphine. *Am J Nurs* 1982; 82:602–604.

Brown SJ: Morphine: The benefits are worth the risks. *RN* (March) 1987;20–26.

Clark PE, Clark MJ: Therapeutic touch: Is there a scientific basis for the practice? *Nurs Res* 1984; 33:37–41.

Copp LA: Pain coping model and typology. *Image.* Summer 1985; 17(3):69–71.

Ersek RA: *Pain Control With TENS: Principles and Practice.* St Louis: Green, 1981.

Escobar PL: Management of chronic pain. *Nurse Pract* (Jan) 1985; 10:24–32.

Geden E et al: Self-report and psychophysiological effects of five pain-coping strategies. *Nurs Res* 1984; 33:260–265.

Grainger S: No cause, no cure—but he's still in pain. *RN* (Feb) 1987;43–45.

Hendler NH, Long DM, Wise N: *Diagnosis and Treatment of Chronic Pain.* Boston: Wright, 1982.

Horsley JA: *Pian: Deliberative Nursing Interventions.* New York: Grune & Stratton, 1982.

Huhman M: Endogenous opiates and pain. *ANS* (July) 1982; 4:62–71.

Kane RL, Berstein L, Wales J, Rothenberg R: Hospice effectiveness in controlling pain. *JAMA* (May 10) 1985; 253:2683–2686.

Kotarba JA: *Chronic Pain.* Beverly Hills, CA: Sage, 1983.

Levin RF: Choice of injection site, locus of control, and the perception of momentary pain. *Image* (Feb–Mar) 1982; 14:26–32.

McAffery M: Narcotic analgesia for the elderly. *Am J Nurs* 1985; 85:296–298.

McGuire D: The measurement of clinical pain. *Nurs Res* 1984; 33:152–156.

Meinhart NT, McCaffery M: *Pain: A Nursing Approach to Assessment and Analysis.* Norwalk, CT: Appleton–Century–Crofts, 1983.

Melzack R: *Pain Measurement and Assessment.* New York: Raven, 1983.

Melzack R, Wall PD: Pain mechanisms: A new theory. *Science* 1965; 150:971–979.

Miller TW, Jay LL: Cognitive-behavioral and pharmaceutical approaches to sensory pain management. *Top Clin Nurs* (Jan) 1985; 6:34–43.

Moore DE, Blacker HM: How effective is TENS for chronic pain? *Am J Nurs* 1983; 83:1176–1177.

Moulin DE, Coyle N: Spinal relief of cancer pain. *Am J Nurs* 1986; 86:1049–1050.

Panayotoff K: Managing pain in the elderly patient. *Nurs 82* (Aug) 1982; 12:53–57.

Randolph GL: Therapeutic and physical touch: Physiological response to stressful stimuli. *Nurs Res* 1984: 33:33–36.

Taylor AG et al: How effective is TENS for acute pain? *Am J Nurs* 1983; 83:1171–1174.

Taylor AG, Skelton JA, Butcher J: Duration of pain condition and physical pathology as determinants of nurses' assessments of patients in pain. *Nurs Res* 1984; 33:4–8.

Turk DC, Meichenbaum D, Genest M: *Pain and Behavioral Medicine.* New York: Guilford, 1983.

Update on pain. *Female Patient* (Jan) 1985; 10:96–104.

Witt JR: Relieving chronic pain. *Nurse Pract* (Jan) 1984; 9:36–38.

Resources

(See also resources in Chapter 28 for headaches)

SELF-HELP GROUPS AND OTHER ORGANIZATIONS

Biofeedback Society of America
10200 W 44th Ave
Suite 304
Wheat Ridge, CO 80033
Phone: (303) 422–8436

Biogenic Institutes of America
615 S 10th St
LaCrosse, WI 54601

This nonprofit corporation offers client training in pain control through biofeedback, autogenic training, and external electrical stimulation at facilities throughout the United States. Clients must be referred by their own physicians.

Committee on Pain Therapy
American Society of Anesthesiologists
515 Busse Hwy
Park Ridge, IL 60068
Phone: (312) 825–5586

National Committee on the Treatment of Intractable Pain
9300 River Road
Potomac, MD 20854
Phone: (202) 944–8140

This committee of individuals was organized to promote education and research on more effective management of intractable pain. Information on the latest methods of pain management and current research can be obtained by contacting their Pain Control Information Clearinghouse. Referrals to other agencies for pain control information or treatment are available on request.

National Hospice Organization
1901 N Fort Myer Dr, Suite 307
Arlington, VA 22209
Phone: (703) 243–5900

An organization of hospices and individuals that encourages public and professional education on caring for the terminally ill, monitors legislation affecting the hospice movement, and publishes a quarterly newsletter.

HEALTH EDUCATION MATERIAL

Pamphlet available:
Chronic Pain: Hope Through Research, April 1982
NIH Publication No. 82–2406
National Institutes of Health
Bethesda, MD 20892

Booklet available: *Questions and Answers About Pain Control,* 1983

Available through local chapters; if necessary, call national headquarters for location of local chapter: (212) 736–3030.

Paperback books from local bookstores:
Benjamin BE, Borden G: *Listen to Your Pain.* New York: Penguin, 1984.

Olshan NH: *Power Over Your Pain Without Drugs.* New York: Beaufort, 1983.

Smollen B, Schulman B: *Pain Control: The Bethesda Program.* New York: Zebra Books, Kensington, 1982.

CHAPTER **4**

Coping With Illness

Objectives

When you have finished studying this chapter, you should be able to:

Describe constructive and destructive coping strategies in response to the stress of illness.

Discuss the reasons why clients may have difficulty in following treatment plans.

Identify common defense-oriented behaviors.

Assess anxiety, anger, denial, depression, and dependence in clients.

Develop nursing diagnoses for clients who are anxious, angry, denying, depressed, or dependent.

Plan and implement the nursing care of clients experiencing anxiety, anger, denial, depression, or dependence.

Evaluate nursing interventions for clients experiencing anxiety, anger, denial, depression, or dependence.

Illness is difficult to cope with because it alters, sometimes in permanent and irreconcilable ways, both internal and external environments. Instead of feeling safe and secure, a person may feel vulnerable and threatened. A previously stable and predictable existence may become unsettled and inconstant, and a person may lose confidence that events will work out for the best. To make the situation even more complex, being ill may require clients to be more, not less, coherent, in charge, and capable.

SECTION 

The "Noncompliant Patient" Label

Consider the following clinical situation from the perspective of the client as well as the nurse:

Mr J K was well known to the staff of 5 West; this was his third hospitalization within the past 10 months. During his first hospital visit, he was diagnosed as having Buerger's disease; his second admission was prompted by small ulcerations of the feet and ankles; this third hospitalization followed his discovery of black areas around the nails of two toes of his left foot.

Since the original diagnosis of Buerger's disease, Mr K has had complication after complication. The health care professionals working with Mr K have advised him to stop smoking; to keep his extremities warm and reduce exposure to cold weather; to avoid either standing or sitting in one position for too long; and to continue taking a prescribed vasodilator, tolazoline hydrochloride (Priscoline).

One hour after his admission, 5 West was in turmoil. Mr K was standing at the doorway to his room loudly arguing with John Baker, his nurse, who had made another of many attempts to persuade his client to change jobs and stop smoking. Mr K's job as a chairlift handler at a ski resort requires him to stand outdoors all day regardless of temperature to assist skiers into the chairlifts on their way up the mountain. He almost always has a cigarette dangling from his lips. John Baker vented his frustration by delivering an angry lecture on the harm Mr K was doing to himself by not complying with the prescribed medical regimen. Later, at the change of shift report, John said: "If that man really wanted to get better and save his leg, he'd get his act together and do what we tell him. He's getting good advice. Why doesn't he follow it?"

Why don't some clients follow the good advice they get from well-meaning health professionals? In Mr K's case, the reason may be that the required changes seem too overwhelming, or his self-view may not comfortably allow for the necessary lifestyle alterations. Perhaps Mr K does not understand the reasons behind John Baker's suggestions. Possibly John Baker has not been clear enough. It may even be that Mr K cannot afford to change jobs because too many persons depend on the money he earns at the ski resort. On the other hand, Mr K may not really believe he is susceptible to the long-term complications his nurse has identified. It is also possible that he thinks the physical and psychosocial costs outweigh the potential benefits.

Clients like Mr K who do not follow the advice of their caregivers are often labeled resistive or "noncompliant." Sometimes such clients fail to enter a treatment program, or they drop out. Often they do not keep follow-up or referral appointments. At other times, clients do not take prescribed medication, or they do not alter their lifestyles or activities. Implicit in the "noncompliant" label is the belief that these clients are troublemakers who refuse to do what is good for them.

Labels seem to become attached to persons—almost permanently, at times. After the noncompliant label has been "earned" (ie, perceived by health care providers as accurate) it may remain attached to the client regardless of behavior or future compliance. Labels turn nurses into adversaries instead of advocates, and what should be a mutual effort toward recovery becomes a tug-of-war between client and nurse. Being an advocate, rather than an adversary, is much easier when nurses are able to acknowledge that persons face stress differently.

Reasons for Noncompliance

Nurses may be able to avoid labeling clients as "resistive," "noncompliant," or "problem patients" by understanding their social, emotional, cultural, and practical needs. These factors may make it difficult if not impossible for clients to perform exactly as nurses deem proper or appropriate.

Knowledge Deficit

In some cases, a client resists treatment or fails to cooperate because of a knowledge deficit. The client may not know what is happening in his or her body or why the condition is being treated as it is.

Knowledge deficit can exist for a variety of reasons. The health care provider may not have taken the time to explain events to the client. Or perhaps the health care provider's "bedside manner" alienated the client. Misunderstandings may also arise because nurse and client come from different cultural or ethnic groups (see Chapter 5). The client's ability to understand explanations may have been impaired by a cognitive or intellectual deficit or by an emotional state.

Unfortunately, some health care providers (including nurses) mistakenly think they can change clients' behavior by using fear. Lessons from the past dispel the myth that fear encourages adherence to the medical regimen.

In 1967, Leventhal, Watts, and Pagano used a variety of techniques to encourage their cigarette-smoking subjects to stop smoking, including an anxiety-provoking color film of the surgical removal of a lung blackened by smoking and obstructed with cigarette tar. After viewing this film, the smokers feared for their health, expressed their determination to stop smoking, and actually reduced the number of cigarettes they smoked during the following week.

In addition, some smokers received instruction on how to stop smoking, and some did not. The detailed instructions from a booklet used in antismoking clinics included:

- Avoiding conditions conducive to smoking
- Preparing excuses for refusing cigarettes offered by others
- Carrying gum
- Not carrying matches or lighters
- Taking deep breaths when the urge to smoke was strong

By the end of the first week, there was little difference between the two groups—both groups had smoked much less. At one month and again at three months, the instructed group held to their gains, but the uninstructed group moved back toward the original level of smoking. In other words, *the effect of fear petered out.* Effects lasted in those who knew what to do and when to do it. The instruction they received had equipped them with the coping strategies they needed to carry out their intent to stop smoking.

The Cost of Acknowledging Ill Health or Health Risk

The reality of illness or being at health risk may provoke anxiety. Denial (discussed further later in this chapter) offers a certain amount of comfort to most. Illness happens to others, not to oneself—it can be viewed from a safe distance. Adhering to a treatment program is a constant reminder of vulnerability. Being at risk frequently carries duties but seldom offers payoffs.

The Cost of Imposed Lifestyle Burdens

Compliance with a medical regimen may impose unfavorable lifestyle burdens. Medication or treatment regimens and schedules may require a change in work schedule or even a change in jobs. Because of dietary restrictions, dining out may no longer be the simple pleasure it once was. Further, the treatment plan may contradict the values, customs, beliefs, and behaviors of the client's cultural or social group. Duration of treatment—whether an illness is temporary or permanent—affects how drastic the lifestyle change is perceived to be.

The Cost of Painful, Disfiguring, or Hazardous Treatments

Some clients may be faced with risking pain, disfigurement, even death, without assurance that they will feel better or that their health status or lives will be improved. Radical head and neck surgery causes disfigurement, a heart transplant is certainly a hazardous procedure, and treatment with certain hormones may greatly increase one's risk of developing cancer. Although these examples may seem extreme, nurses encounter many clients who face these and similar concerns daily to varying degrees.

The Cost of Financial Burdens

Being ill or being at risk for illness may entail financial burdens. Some medications and treatments and home health care services carry high price tags. Not all insurance coverage is adequate or available to everyone, and the client and the client's family may have to take up the financial slack. Even the cost of staying well may seem exorbitant; consider the ongoing cost of insulin syringes and blood sugar monitoring for a diabetic.

Indirect costs may arise because treatment schedules require clients to change to jobs that pay less but have more convenient hours. Some treatments may be so time consuming or debilitating that it is difficult, or even impossible, for an individual to maintain a job; a nonpaid leave of absence may be necessary.

The Cost of Submitting to Outside Authority

Most clients of the health care system relinquish some control over their lives. Although this loss of control may not disturb some, others may find it anxiety provoking. Clients who fail to follow a prescribed treatment plan may be trying to regain control and autonomy. Being submissive or compliant may be frightening for some persons. They may want to be partners with their nurses and physicians and to participate in health care decisions that involve them. Deprived of this opportunity, they engage in a power struggle with the staff.

The Cost of Burdening Family and Friends

Medical regimens and the costs of health care cause changes not only in the lives of clients but also in the lives of their family and friends. Families and friends may also be called upon for emotional support. Depending on the quality of their own lives, they may or may not have enough energy to provide the client with emotional and practical support. Knowing this, some clients may be reluctant to undertake courses of treatment that add to the problems facing an already-stressed family system. The problem may be particularly severe when there is family instability or disharmony.

Predicting Noncompliance

Research has indicated that, although it is difficult to predict exactly which clients will not follow a treatment plan, noncompliance is more likely for:

- Clients with unstable or disharmonious families
- Clients who live alone and lack the support of family and/or friends
- Clients with a low level of fear about their condition
- Clients with a high level of fear about their condition

One cannot assume that clients will always comply in the absence of these conditions, however. It is important to also consider the many reasons for noncompliance discussed in the preceding section.

SECTION 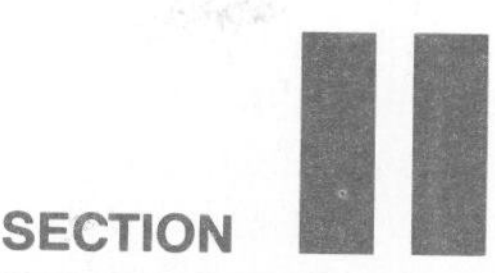

Coping With Illness

Coping strategies are a set of behaviors persons under stress use in struggling to improve their situations. Coping strategies can be thought of simply as ways of getting along in the world.

Ways of Coping

A person can cope on different levels, including the physical, social, cognitive, and emotional levels. Problem solving, daydreaming, drinking or taking drugs, meditating, getting angry, praying, working out, and accepting the situation are common methods of coping.

Most often, individuals use behaviors that have worked well for them in the past. Sometimes they behave in a certain way because it is the only method they have of coping with stress or because other coping strategies failed to work. Some persons learn to turn to others for protection and nurturance; some learn to turn to chemicals or to food; some rely on self-discipline and keeping a stiff upper lip; others feel better after the intense expression of feelings; some withdraw physically and/or emotionally; still others work out or talk the problem out. Coping methods are as varied as individuals. Some work; some don't.

Coping Resources

Recent studies that consider the whole being in interaction with the environment have helped in viewing coping as a dynamic process that involves the demands and restrictions on a client as well as the resources available. According to Antonovsky (1980), persons stay healthy or cope with stress because they possess *generalized resistance resources* (GRRs). A GRR is any factor in the person, group, or organization that helps in managing tension.

Physical and biochemical GRRs are characteristics such as genetic features, levels of immunity, and interactions of the nervous and endocrine systems that help in adaptation (eg, interactions involving adrenocorticotropic hormone or ACTH, thyroid-stimulating hormone or TSH, vasopressin, norepinephrine, and insulin and their influence on human behavior). Not only are individuals different in their genetic and biochemical makeup, but the effects of illness and stress may also alter the person's ability to use physical and biochemical GRRs positively.

Material goods and relative wealth constitute the *artifactual and material* GRRs; having these attributes makes it easier to cope with illness. Money helps to ensure the best health care available. Effective coping is often interrelated with one's socioeconomic status simply because the higher the socioeconomic status, the greater the resources to help the person cope. For example, household help not only relieves an ill person's worries but also reduces the practical burden.

Cognitive GRRs have to do with intelligence and knowledge. When persons know about stressors, they can avoid them. They can also predict when periods of stress are imminent and thus reduce their impact (see the discussion of life changes as stressful events in Chapter 2). Knowing what community services are available is also a cognitive GRR.

Emotional GRRs are possessed by those who are self-aware—who know their own capacities and potentials and have a well-developed sense of themselves. Emotional GRRs determine the extent of psychological hardiness.

Valuative and attitudinal GRRs are the products of a person's culture and environment. Persons are apt to respond in learned ways. The more rational or accurate one's appraisal of a threatening situation and the more flexible one is in approaching the situation and envisioning the consequences, the greater one's resources for coping.

Interpersonal–relational GRRs are available social support systems. The greater a person's social contacts, the greater the social resources available to augment the ability to deal with stress. Love, affection, and nurturance are hallmarks of interpersonal–relational GRRs.

Institutional structures that facilitate coping are called *macrosociocultural* GRRs. These resources include governmental programs such as Aid to Dependent Children as well as cultural institutions such as death and funeral rites, religious rituals, and ceremonies.

According to this model, the ability to stay healthy or to cope with illness is determined by the extent and effectiveness of each person's generalized resistance resources. Yet the actual process of coping remains unclear. Exactly which personal resources should be mobilized and under which conditions still is not fully understood. One nursing study (Ziemer, 1982) found that over 50% of the study population reported that their preferred method of coping was to talk to someone. This finding has profound implications for nursing, because nurses are the health care providers who spend the most time with clients. It also has profound implications for clients whose ability to communicate freely is restricted.

Conscious and Unconscious Modes of Coping

The coping methods discussed earlier are largely conscious strategies. What happens to the client who has no one to talk with, who can't jog 5 miles, or who can't laugh off the problem?

When a person is unable to ward off stress or reduce tension in the usual way, anxiety mounts as the client feels increasingly inadequate to cope with the situation. Under these circumstances, the person is more likely to engage in *defense-oriented behavior.* Rather than specifically attempting to solve a problem, defense-oriented behaviors, often called *defense mechanisms,* are geared toward reducing anxiety regardless of cost.

Defense mechanisms are primarily unconscious and often inflexible coping patterns that protect a person through intrapsychic distortions that are really self-deceptions. The person usually has little awareness of what is happening or even less control over events. Although these reactions may help keep the lid on anxiety, they also limit the ability to grow from the experience, they interfere with rational decision making and the ability to work productively, and they impair and erode interpersonal relationships. Even adaptive devices can go wrong.

Nursing Research Note

Lewis FM: Experienced personal control and quality of life in late-stage cancer patients. *Nurs Res* 1982; 31:113–118

This study examined the relation between personal control and quality of life in terminal cancer clients. Four scales were used and tested—self-esteem, purpose in life, locus of control, and anxiety.

The results suggested that greater personal control over one's life is associated with higher levels of self-esteem, greater purpose in life, and decreased self-report of anxiety. There was a statistically significant relation between higher levels of personal control over health and higher levels of purpose-in-life measures. The relation between personal control over health and anxiety and self-esteem was not significant statistically. It was also found that as length of time since diagnosis increased, the subjects experienced less personal control over their health.

Fostering in clients a sense of personal control over their lives may encourage increased self-esteem and purpose in life. Because personal control in health issues did not enhance self-esteem, nurses may need to assess clients' psychological states in preparing them to take control over health issues. Nurses must determine how each client is coping and plan intervention accordingly.

Common Defense-Oriented Behaviors

Several kinds of defense-oriented behaviors have been identified in the literature. The common ones are discussed in this section.

Denial

The husband is reacting with *denial* when he shouts, "No, it can't be true; there must be a mistake," when told his wife has just died in the trauma unit of injuries from an automobile accident. The person who denies may totally disregard the reality of the situation or may transform the situation into a less threatening one.

Denial can be constructive when it provides temporary protection from a threatening event or an unpleasant reality until an individual has shored up coping ability. Denial can also be harmful or destructive when it interferes with a person's ability to take steps to ensure health.

Regression

Regression is a means of reducing anxiety by retreating from the present to a more pleasant past, to behavior more characteristic of an earlier developmental level. The behavior is less mature but more comforting.

Suppose a nurse who is ill with an upper respiratory infection takes to her bed, enjoys being medicated with Vick's Vaporub, and asks her spouse or children to bring her apricot nectar to drink, as her mother did when she was a girl. She is demonstrating regression—reverting from an independent health care provider to being temporarily dependent on others, a move that provides comfort while she is feeling ill. An extreme form of regression is the infantile behavior of some acutely ill schizophrenic clients. This form of regression is less temporary for the schizophrenic client (who has little control over it) than regression is for the nurse with the cold.

Like denial, temporary regression can help a person to reconstitute defenses. Remember, temporary regression is not harmful. It could be good medicine.

Repression

Repression, the basis of all defense mechanisms, is the dynamic behind much of "forgetting." When persons repress, they unconsciously exclude distressing emotions, thoughts, or experiences from awareness. In this way, they avoid the conflicts these emotions, thoughts, or experiences could bring. The rape victim in the emergency room who cannot recall the circumstances surrounding the rape or what the rapist looks like is repressing.

Suppression

A middle-aged male business executive discovers bright red rectal bleeding the day before he is to leave for a visit to his company's international offices in three European countries. His decision to put off worrying about the bleeding until he returns in 3 weeks is an example of using *suppression* to deal with the emotional discomfort of this discovery. Suppression is an intentional act that helps to keep thoughts, feelings, wishes, or actions that cause anxiety out of conscious awareness.

Rationalization

When a person substitutes "good" or plausible reasons for questionable behavior to justify it, that person is said to be *rationalizing*. Rationalizing helps to avoid social disapproval and to bolster flagging self-esteem. Rationalization appears to be operating, for example, when a nurse who is late in administering a preoperative sedative explains to the head nurse that "it'll probably work out to the good" because the operating suite is busy, and the client's surgery may be delayed anyway.

Displacement

Displacement is the act of transferring unacceptable emotions associated with a threatening person, idea, or object to a less threatening person, idea, or object. For example, a preoperative client shouts at the nurse after an unsatisfying visit from the surgeon. Rather than risk threatening the relationship with the person who will perform the surgery, the client vents his hostility toward the nurse.

Identification and Introjection

Acting or behaving like an admired person is called *identification*. An example is the freshman college student who after hospitalization for minor surgery decides to switch to a major in nursing. *Introjection* is a more intense form of identification in which the person actually assumes the values, beliefs, and attitudes of another and incorporates them into his or her personality. For example, while in nursing school, the college student assumes the gestures, speech mannerisms, and values of an admired nursing instructor.

Fantasy

Fantasy is a way of satisfying a wish that cannot be realized. A client with advanced multiple sclerosis who imagines herself a famous ballerina with complete control of her body is engaging in fantasy. Fantasy and imaging can also be useful tools for reducing stress and promoting health.

Compensation

A young research scientist who has severe scars from facial burns and devotes all his energies to scientific study in his laboratory is *compensating* for his perceived body defect by emphasizing his intellectual strengths. Doing so helps to relieve fears of failure in one area by emphasizing an area in which there is a greater likelihood of success. Compensation can be adaptive for clients who are limited because of the effects of their illness.

The Role of Anxiety in Coping

Anxiety is a state of uneasiness or discomfort experienced to varying degrees. Beyond the mild level, anxiety is often described as a feeling of terror or dread; anxiety is believed to be the most uncomfortable feeling a person can experience. In fact, anxiety is so uncomfortable that most persons try to get rid of it as soon as possible. The coping strategies and defense-oriented behaviors discussed earlier in this chapter are the results of attempts to control or reduce anxiety. Other behavior patterns to control or reduce anxiety commonly seen in clients are discussed later in this chapter.

Sources of Anxiety

Anxiety is an inevitable condition of human existence in the attempt to maintain equilibrium in a changing world. Generally, anxiety stems from two major kinds of threats: threats to biological integrity and threats to the security of the self. It is crucial to understand that either actual *or* impending interference may cause anxiety (ie, actual interference with a biological or psychosocial need is not a necessary condition). All that is necessary for anxiety to arise is the *anticipation* of one of these major threats.

Threats to biological integrity or to the fulfillment of such basic human needs as food, drink, warmth, and shelter are a general cause of anxiety. Threats to the security of self are not as easily categorized. In some instances, they are obvious; in others, they are more obscure because each person's sense of self is unique. To one person, power and prestige may be essential; to another, independence; to a third, being of service to others.

Consider the last category—being of service to others. Suppose that Mrs C, a nurse, is convinced that a particular client would feel much better if he expressed his fears about impending surgery to her. But no matter how often she provides the opportunity, he insists, "This is not the time to talk about it," and thwarts her attempt. She is not able to help him in a way that is important to her sense of self. In addition, she believes that the unit's head nurse expects her to have been successful in this endeavor. When unmet needs or expectations related to essential values (eg, being of service to the client) are coupled with the actual or anticipated disapproval of others who are important (the head nurse), anxiety is generated.

Anxiety as a Continuum

It is helpful to think of anxiety as a continuum. Anxiety is a potent force. At low levels, it may stimulate constructive action. At higher levels, it may become a problem in its own right.

MILD ANXIETY Mild anxiety helps one deal constructively with stress. A mildly anxious person has a broad perceptual field (ie, mild anxiety heightens the ability to take in sensory stimuli). Such a person is more alert to what is going on and can make better sense of what is happening with others and the environment. The senses take in more—the person hears better, sees better, and makes logical connections between events. The person feels relatively safe and comfortable. Because learning is easier when one is mildly anxious, mild anxiety helps clients learn how best to give their own insulin and helps students study for a final examination.

MODERATE ANXIETY In moderate anxiety, a person remains alert, but the perceptual field narrows (Figure 4–1). The moderately anxious person shuts out the events on the periphery while focusing on central concerns. For example, if a nursing student is moderately anxious about the final examination, he may be able to focus so intently on his studies that he is not distracted by an argument between his roommates, loud music on the stereo, and a rousing chase scene on television. He shuts out the chaos in the environment and focuses on what is of central importance to him—preparing for the exam. This process of taking in some sensory stimuli while excluding others is called *selective inattention.*

Selective inattention may also be used to cope with anxiety-provoking stimuli. This phenomenon may account for the anxious preoperative client who fails to remember what the nurse said about postoperative pain or the need to cough and deep breathe after surgery.

Although the perceptual field is narrowed and the person sees, hears, and grasps less, there is an element of voluntary control. The moderately anxious individual can, with direction, focus on what has previously been inattended.

SEVERE ANXIETY In severe anxiety, sensory reception is greatly reduced (see Figure 4–1). Severely anxious persons focus on small or scattered details of an experience. They have difficulty in problem solving, and their ability to organize is also reduced. They seldom have the complete picture. Selective inattention may be increased and may be less amenable to voluntary control. The person may be unable to focus on events in the environment. New stimuli may be experienced as overwhelming and may cause the anxiety level to rise even higher.

The sympathetic nervous system is activated in severe anxiety, causing an increase in pulse, blood pressure, and respiration and an increase in epinephrine secretion, vasoconstriction, and even body temperature. A multitude of physiologic changes may be observed, which are described in the nursing process section that follows.

Many clients in health care settings are severely anxious. An unfavorable diagnosis or prognosis or a painful or disfiguring treatment may threaten both biologic integrity and the security of the self.

PANIC The panic level of anxiety is characterized by a completely disrupted perceptual field (see Figure 4–1). Panic has been described as a disintegration of the personality that is experienced as intense terror. Details may be enlarged, scattered, or distorted. Logical thinking and effective decision making may be impossible. The person in panic is unable to initiate or maintain goal-directed action. Behavior may appear purposeless, and communication may be unintelligible.

Not all those in panic behave alike. At the scene of an

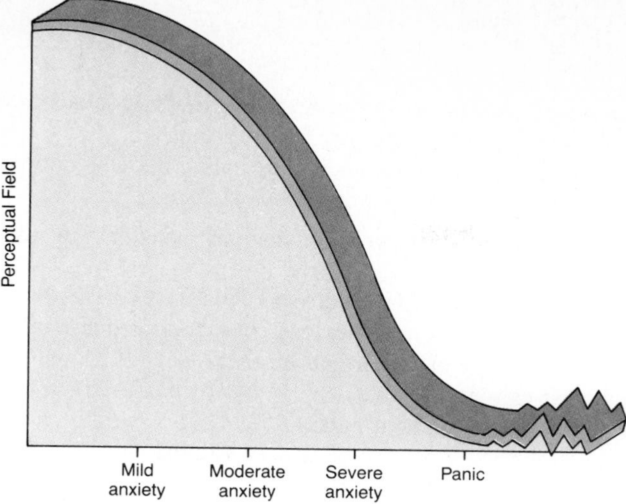

Figure 4–1

The effect of anxiety on the perceptual field.

auto accident in which an elderly couple lost control of the travel trailer they were towing, the husband remained immobile in the driver's seat, hands firmly fixed to the steering wheel, eyes focused on some distant spot despite the threat of explosion from the smoking car. The wife ran around in circles. Having lost her shoes in the accident, she was unaware she was running through the broken glass of the windshield in her bare feet despite numerous bleeding cuts.

Automatic Responses to Anxiety

Because anxiety is such an uncomfortable feeling, persons learn early in life to try to reduce it or diminish its effect as soon as possible. Although individuals use a variety of behaviors described in this chapter, behavior generally falls within a few categories. The most common automatic responses to anxiety are anger, withdrawal, and somatization. Automatic responses are limiting, rigid, and inflexible. Because they are automatic, these responses are called out under anxiety-provoking conditions, preventing a creative response to the threat and inhibiting learning.

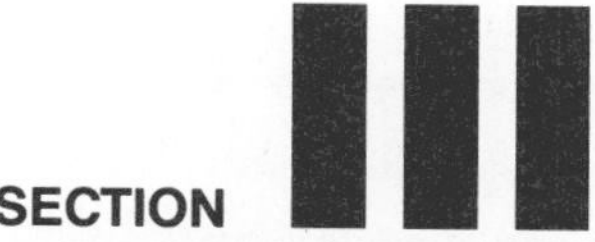

The Nursing Process in Problems of Coping With Illness

Anxiety influences an individual's ability to cope as well as the individual's type of coping strategies. This section begins with a discussion of the nursing process with anxious clients. Other behavior patterns common to anxious clients—anger, denial, depression, and dependence—follow. Keep in mind that this chapter applies to family members and friends as well as clients under direct care.

Anxiety

Anxiety affects a person's thinking, behavior, and feeling. Anxiety may enhance a wellness/illness experience so learning and creativity result, or it may be a destructive force that interferes with the ability to keep well or to get well. For this reason, intervening effectively in clients' anxiety is crucial.

Nursing Assessment: Establishing the Data Base

Anxiety can be assessed in the physiologic, cognitive, and emotional/behavioral dimensions. Objective data, particularly nursing observations, may be critical because of the nature of anxiety. Selective inattention and dissociation interfere with the client's awareness of anxiety and ability to give accurate reports. Families and friends also can contribute data useful to the assessment of anxiety.

PHYSIOLOGIC DIMENSION Observations of the client's physiologic state are likely to indicate autonomic nervous system responses, particularly sympathetic effects. (The autonomic nervous system is discussed in Chapter 30.) Various organs may be affected, such as the adrenal medulla, heart, blood vessels, lungs, stomach, colon, rectum, salivary glands, liver, pupils of the eyes, and sweat glands. Anxious clients may have an increased heart rate, increased blood pressure, difficulty in breathing, sweaty palms, trembling, dry mouth, "butterflies in the stomach" or a "lump in the throat," as well as other symptoms.

Laboratory tests are not routinely done to evaluate anxiety because observation is faster and more accurate, but anxiety affects the results of laboratory tests. Blood studies may show increased adrenal function, elevated levels of glucose and lactic acid, and decreased parathyroid function and oxygen and calcium levels. Urinary studies may indicate increased levels of epinephrine and norepinephrine.

COGNITIVE DIMENSION Assessment of cognitive function may indicate difficulty in logical thinking, narrowed or distorted perceptual field, selective inattention or dissociation, lack of attention to details, difficulty in concentrating, or difficulty in focusing. The extent to which cognitive function is affected is determined by the level of anxiety. Mild, moderate, severe, or panic level of anxiety is assessed according to the descriptions earlier in this chapter.

EMOTIONAL/BEHAVIORAL DIMENSION In the emotional/behavioral dimension, clients may be irritable, angry, withdrawn, restless, or they may cry. The affective response can often be assessed through the client's subjective description. Clients may describe themselves as "on edge," "uptight," "jittery," "nervous," "worried," or "tense." They may feel dizzy or faint and may experience a feeling of impending doom as if something terrible were about to happen.

DETERMINING THE SOURCE OF ANXIETY In the assessment phase, it is essential to determine not only whether the client is anxious and, if so, how anxious, but also to attempt to determine the source of the anxiety. Knowing the source will help in planning and implementing effective care. These two steps can be useful:

1. Help the client to recognize and name the experience as anxiety. The nurse might say something like: "You're trembling. How are you feeling?" Some clients will be able immediately to connect their behavior with feeling anxious. For clients who do not, it is helpful to make the connection: "Often persons tremble because they're feeling anxious (or nervous, uncomfortable, or worried). I was wondering if you could be feeling anxious (or nervous, uncomfortable, or worried) right now."
2. Help the client to discuss the experience more fully by moving into the cognitive dimension. It would be premature to ask the client why he or she feels anxious. Encouraging clients to discuss what they are thinking about is more likely to bring their concerns out into the open. Then the nurse can determine the source of the anxiety and gather data relevant to appropriate nursing diagnoses.

The exception to this general strategy occurs when clients are in panic or are extremely anxious. In this case, formal data gathering is suspended in favor of immediate, direct action to reduce anxiety and maintain the client's safety (see Table 4–1).

Nursing Diagnosis

A number of nursing diagnoses are relevant to anxiety. In addition to the nursing diagnosis of anxiety itself, the most obvious are ineffective individual coping and ineffective family coping. In considering the varying physiologic, cognitive, and emotional effects of anxiety, a variety of other nursing diagnoses may be important.

Alterations in physiologic functioning because of anxiety may prompt nursing diagnoses such as:

- Alteration in bowel elimination: constipation (or, diarrhea)
- Ineffective breathing pattern
- Alteration in nutrition: less than body requirements (or more than body requirements)
- Self-care deficit
- Sleep pattern disturbance
- Alteration in pattern of urinary elimination

Alterations in cognitive functioning because of anxiety may prompt nursing diagnoses such as:

- Knowledge deficit
- Impaired verbal communication
- Alteration in thought processes

Alterations in emotional, social, and behavioral functioning because of anxiety may prompt nursing diagnoses such as fear, noncompliance, and disturbance in self-concepts.

Planning and Implementation

It is important for planning and implementation to take place as soon as possible. Not only does anxiety often escalate, but anxiety is also communicated interpersonally. Other persons, such as the client's family and friends or other clients and staff in the health care setting, may be caught up in the tension as well.

TALKING ABOUT ANXIOUS FEELINGS Many times, simply offering the client the opportunity to acknowledge and discuss feelings of anxiety helps the client to regain control. Having followed the two steps outlined in the section on assessment, the nurse may find the client's anxiety has already abated somewhat. At this point, clients are more likely to share their concerns because the nurse has

Table 4–1
Nursing Intervention Into Severe Anxiety and Panic

Strategy	Rationale
Stay with the client	Being left alone may further increase the anxiety
Maintain a calm, serene manner	Knowing that the nurse is calm and in control may be calming to the client
Use short, simple sentences	Because the client's perceptual field is disrupted, the client will experience difficulty in focusing
Use a firm and authoritative voice	Conveys the nurse's ability to provide external controls
Move the client to a quieter, smaller, and less stimulating environment	Prevents further disruption of the perceptual field by sensory stimuli
Focus the client's diffuse energy on a repetitive or physically tiring task	Repetitive tasks or physical exercise can help to drain off excess energy
Administer antianxiety medications if ordered	Antianxiety medications may help reduce anxiety

already taken the first steps in demonstrating genuine interest and concern in the client's experiences.

It is important to tolerate the client's expression of feelings and concerns once their expression has been encouraged. Clients may express fear, anger, sadness, disappointment, or alienation, and it may be difficult to hear about the client's pain. Some nurses feel helpless in the face of their client's catharsis and think they should be able to provide ready answers. Instead, ready answers are more likely to interfere with and thwart the client's communication. Genuine, concerned listening without judgments is an effective intervention in itself.

PHYSICAL ACTIVITY Simple physical activities often help to reduce anxiety to more tolerable levels. What is important is to encourage adaptive coping mechanisms that work. A client could:

- Soak in a warm bath.
- Listen to soothing music.
- Take a walk or exercise.
- Have a massage or back rub.
- Drink a warm beverage.
- Engage in whatever activity is found relaxing.
- Take slow, deep breaths to counteract the effects of hyperventilation, breathing in harmony with the nurse for support.

STRESS REDUCTION STRATEGIES A nurse could also teach the client a variety of stress reduction strategies and encourage their use. Deep breathing, active progressive relaxation, and imaging techniques are helpful in reducing anxiety. Meditation and biofeedback techniques are other approaches. Teaching clients about these self-management approaches encourages self-care and provides the client with tools to use at home, at school, and on the job as well as in the health care setting.

DECREASING KNOWLEDGE DEFICIT If a knowledge deficit has contributed to anxiety, providing the client with useful information helps reduce anxiety. Explanations should be simple, clear, and concise. Be careful not to overload the moderately or severely anxious person with more information than can be processed. If anxiety has contributed to knowledge deficit, the anxiety level will have to be reduced before trying to teach about health or provide information. Unless the cognitive conditions (such as narrow or disrupted perceptual field) have changed, the client will be unable to assimilate the information.

DIRECTION AND STRUCTURE IN SEVERE ANXIETY OR PANIC Clients who are extremely anxious or in panic require more immediate, direct, and structured intervention. During an acute panic attack, perception and personality are disrupted to such a degree that the client cannot solve problems or discuss the source of anxiety. The first priority is to reduce the anxiety to more tolerable levels (see Table 4–1). The suggested strategies can be applied whenever nurses engage with persons who are extremely anxious or in panic—the emergency room, the trauma unit, or at the scene of a crisis or disaster.

ANTIANXIETY MEDICATION Antianxiety medication may be appropriate for anxious persons. The minor tranquilizers such as chlordiazepoxide (Librium) and diazepam (Valium) are commonly administered. Major tranquilizers, or antipsychotic medications, such as thioridizine (Mellaril), prochlorperazine (Compazine), or chlorpromazine (Thorazine) may be used for extreme anxiety or panic.

Antianxiety medication should be used cautiously. Certain antianxiety medications (diazepam, for one) are among the most prescribed, overprescribed, and abused drugs in the United States and Canada. Valium overreliance is a serious medical problem that has prompted the formation of a self-help group, Valium Anonymous (see the resources list at the end of Chapter 8), to help addicted persons to get off the drug. Certain groups such as the elderly are particularly sensitive to the effects of central nervous system depression associated with diazepam.

Although medications may alleviate the symptoms of anxiety, they do nothing to help clients to understand its source nor to manage their own lives in more comfortable ways. At best, these drugs should be used for the short-term treatment of anxiety—meaning days or even weeks but not months or years.

ANTICIPATING ANXIETY Anticipating anxiety and preparing clients and their families to cope with it ahead of time will often help prevent it. Illness and treatment, because they threaten biological integrity and the security of the self, precipitate anxiety. Nurses can expect clients and their families to become anxious in the face of the unknown or potentially painful, dangerous, or disfiguring events.

Evaluation

Nursing interventions related to anxiety may be considered successful when the client's anxiety has been reduced to a level that the client can more readily manage. Observations verifying this outcome include a broadening of the perceptual field and reduction in sympathetic nervous system effects.

When the client can openly discuss the experience of anxiety, consider its sources, and attempt self-management practices to reduce it, then nursing interventions have helped to attain successful outcomes.

Anger

Anger is an intense emotion of strong displeasure usually linked with antagonism. In fact, the word derives from the Latin *angere*: to strangle. With anger, the feeling of powerlessness stemming from anxiety is converted into power. Anger is one of the learned automatic responses to anxiety.

Because many situations in health care settings can arouse anxiety, there are also many opportunities for anger.

Clients may feel as if they are subject to the whims of health care personnel. Removed from familiar surroundings where they were in charge, clients are forced to deal with unknowns, to wait to have needs met, and to worry about what will happen to them and their families. Their biologic needs and their sense of self-security are threatened from all sides.

Anger is the fight response to anxiety. Unfortunately, even though the angry person may feel restored to power, others who may be the objects of anger feel threatened, frightened, pushed away, or angry in turn.

Nursing Assessment: Establishing the Data Base

Most of the time, anger can be readily assessed. Angry people look tense and tight—the face may be contorted, the jaw tightened, the fists clenched, the cords and veins of the neck protruding, the posture tensed, and the nostrils flared. Angry persons may hold their breath or take deep, rapid breaths with sighing expirations. The pupils may be dilated, and the angry person appears to be glaring. The angry person's voice changes, becoming louder, harsher, and more strident. The person may curse or may be sarcastic, rude, accusatory, or hurtful. The angry person may become physical, pounding one fist into the other palm, pounding on an object, slamming a door, breaking or throwing something, hitting, shoving, pushing, or otherwise striking out. Occasionally, an angry person looks rigid.

Physiologic changes from the autonomic nervous system response to increased secretion of epinephrine may include increased blood pressure and heart rate, decreased gastrointestinal peristalsis and increased hydrochloric acid secretion, increased salivation, and increased urination. Angry persons also become hyperalert and have difficulty relaxing or falling asleep.

As with anxiety, it is essential in the assessment phase to determine not only whether the client is angry but also the source of the anger or the anxiety that preceded it. Knowing the source will help in planning and determining effective care. The following two steps can be useful:

1. Help the client to recognize and name the experience as anger. The nurse might say: "You're shouting. You seem angry." This often helps the client make the connection.
2. Help the client to discuss the experience more fully by moving into the cognitive dimension. Asking the client what the anger is about will encourage open discussion and facilitate the gathering of data relevant to appropriate nursing diagnoses.

Sometimes, anger may be harder to assess. Those who value controlling their angry feelings may have learned to disguise these expressions or to deny their anger. In these instances, cues may be more subtle. Look for mixed messages, in which verbalization and behavior are not consistently matched. Suppose a client says he is "a little upset (or annoyed, or irritated)" because he had to wait 50 minutes before his request for medication to relieve postoperative pain was fulfilled. Do his tone of voice and body actions indicate a more profound anger? If so, adapt step 1. Because the client may not recognize his anger, try to make the client's mixed message evident. Say something such as "You say it doesn't matter, but you look angry."

Nursing Diagnosis

Anger is considered an automatic response to anxiety. Therefore, the nursing diagnoses relevant to anxious clients are also relevant to angry clients.

Planning and Implementation

The first and most obvious action is to reduce the sources of anxiety. This action will indirectly reduce the angry responses resulting from anxiety. Keep in mind that the client is responding to a real or anticipated threat to biologic well-being or self-esteem.

RESPECTING THE CLIENT AS A PERSON Respecting a client's privacy, territory, autonomy, and need for information may help prevent clients from becoming angry with health care providers. In one study (Maagdenberg, 1983), when clients were asked what made them angry with the nursing staff, they identified the following conditions:

- When nursing staff failed to ask permission before touching
- When nurses and physicians inspected incisions or body parts without providing privacy
- When nurses failed to explain beforehand what they planned to do to the client
- When nurses failed to ask permission before performing a nursing task

The study also found that few staff members knew why clients became angry. Being aware of these needs and providing for them in planning and administering nursing care may avoid problems.

PROVIDING FOR THE NONHARMFUL EXPRESSION OF ANGER When anger is situational (ie, a response to the stress and anxiety generated by illness) the nurse can more directly intervene by acknowledging the client's anger and encouraging discussion of the events preceding it. Interventions depend on the source of the anger. Corrective steps can be taken by nursing and medical staff to place clients back in charge and respect their privacy and dignity. The nurse and client can explore alternatives together (eg, discussing the anger rather than throwing the bedpan, working out in the gym, or taking up carpentry or leather working). Occupational therapists will have ideas on how to help angry persons channel their energy in more constructive directions. The objective is to allow the expression of anger in more acceptable and less harmful ways. Review the suggested verbal interventions in the section on anxiety because they also apply in the nursing care of angry clients.

SETTING RATIONAL AND REASONABLE LIMITS Of course, limits must be set on the behavior of angry clients if it endangers the client or others. Limits should be set in a nonjudgmental way. While acknowledging the client's angry feelings, also let the client know that hurting oneself or others or destroying property is not allowed. Although nurses in psychiatric settings may sometimes see violent or assaultive clients, this behavior is not common in most other health settings. Assaultiveness or violence may result from alcohol, drugs, certain medications, and head injury. Nurses in emergency or trauma settings and on neurologic units may encounter such clients.

Under these circumstances, it is wise to seek assistance from other staff to help monitor the client's behavior and enforce limits. Precautions should be taken against physically overwhelming the client and endangering the client's well-being. Training programs in nonviolent management of disruptive, assaultive, or out-of-control behavior (see resource list at the end of this chapter) are useful for staff who are likely to encounter such clients.

REFERRING TO OTHER RESOURCES For some persons, anger, hostility, and even rage are a way of dealing with the world. In addition to the interventions discussed, the nurse might also consider other resources. The assistance of a mental health–psychiatric nurse would be beneficial to the client, family, friends, and the staff.

UNDERSTANDING ONE'S OWN FEELINGS Of crucial importance is that nurses not retaliate or allow themselves to be alienated from angry clients. Remember that anxiety came before anger in the client's experience. Although the nurse may feel angry at the client or frightened, these feelings can interfere with developing realistic goals and effective interventions.

SUPPORTING FAMILY AND FRIENDS Families and friends of angry clients may need the nurse's help as well. They may be embarrassed about the behavior of their family member or friend. They may need help in understanding the behavior and its source and help in dealing with the problems it may bring them. Explain that the client has the need to express both positive and negative feelings about health, illness, and/or hospitalization. Help them to understand when the anger is displaced and when it is not personally directed. Encourage family and friends to accept the angry verbalizations without being judgmental—and acknowledge their efforts.

If their loved one is assaultive or violent, family and friends may also be frightened, confused, or angry. Helping them to understand the client's responses as part of the client's traumatic or toxic condition will also support them in their efforts to manage the situation. They may also need help in setting limits and strategies for reducing the anger.

Evaluation

In evaluating the potential client outcomes, determine whether:

- The client is able to recognize the anger.
- The client is able to discuss the anger and consider the possible sources.
- The client is able to convert the expression of anger to behavior that is not dangerous to the self or to others, preferably in words.
- The client is able to use other more constructive outlets for the expression of anger.
- The client is able to exert greater self-control over the expression of anger.
- The client is able to be increasingly self-directed in managing situations that provoke anger.

In evaluating potential outcomes in relation to family and friends, consider whether:

- Family or friends are able to spend time in the client's company and do not withdraw their presence or their support.
- Family or friends do not personalize the anger and respond defensively.
- Family or friends allow the client to express both positive and negative feelings about what is happening.
- Family or friends are able to accept the client's verbal expressions of anger.
- Family and friends are able to set limits if necessary.
- Family and friends are able to implement strategies for anger reduction.

Do not set overly optimistic expectations. Clients for whom anger has been a lifestyle may have passed an important milestone by simply being able to acknowledge previously unrecognized anger.

Denial

Earlier in this chapter, denial was described as a self-protective measure. Denial helps reduce the anxiety associated with illness, trauma, loss, and other major life changes. Clients or family members may use denial essentially to "buy time" so they will not feel overwhelmed before the associated anxiety abates. Denial is usually limited in time. Persistent denial hinders well-being when it interferes with steps that can be taken to regain health or to prevent further deterioration of health. Persistent denial also drains psychic energy. Denial may also be a factor in noncompliance.

Nursing Assessment: Establishing the Data Base

Clients may be using denial when they give mixed messages to questions about symptoms or how they are feeling (ie, the verbal and nonverbal communications do not match). The grimacing client who denies pain is an example. Denial may also be operating when clients or their families disbelieve the diagnosis, prognosis, or information they are given. This does not mean clients and their families must always unquestioningly accept what the health care provider says or does. In fact, if they did, fewer second opinions would be sought, which would not be in the best interests of health care consumers. Sometimes, however, persons distort information so they can maintain denial without being aware they are doing so. Denial should be suspected when a client refuses to discuss a condition or upcoming surgery; fails to carry out recommended procedures or self-care such as colostomy care; refuses to look at a mastectomy incision or the stump of an amputated limb; or refuses medication, treatment, or diagnostic studies.

Nursing Diagnosis

Nursing diagnoses common in the care of clients who are denying are:

- Anxiety
- Ineffective individual coping
- Ineffective family coping
- Dysfunctional grieving
- Noncompliance

Also consider the diagnoses of self-care deficit, and disturbance in self-concepts.

Planning and Implementation

Interfering with the protective function of denial before the client is ready is usually not helpful and may be harmful. The exception is when the denial is actually causing the client damage.

To ensure denial is not causing harm, monitor the client with this in mind. By spending time with the client and providing opportunities for verbalization, the nurse can begin to create a climate in which the client may feel freer to relax and begin to cope with the anxiety brought on by the threatening situation.

Without pressuring the client, begin introducing reality-based observations and/or health instructions. A comment on how the incision is healing or on what prostheses are available provides an opening for further discussion. Do not support the denial by agreeing with it or by giving false reassurance. Instead, acknowledge that accepting unpleasant or frightening realities can be difficult. Support any progress the client has made in overcoming or reducing the denial. Encourage the client's continuing efforts in this direction.

If family or significant others are denying, the same interventions can be useful in helping them. Remember that the stability of a family system can be threatened by the illness of one of its members. Family and friends can help the client cope with the denial if they understand what is happening and how they can help. Meeting with family and friends to provide health teaching and to enlist their cooperation will help them as well as the client.

As the client begins to accept reality, the anxiety level may again increase. When anxiety rises, consider implementing the strategies discussed earlier in the section on anxiety.

Evaluation

Expected potential outcomes are that the client and/or family and friends will be able to accept reality and give up denial. They will be able to discuss the previously denied prognosis, diagnosis, or body alteration. The client may begin to implement self-care activities. An additional potential outcome might be a temporary increase in anxiety immediately after the denial has been discarded.

Depression

Depression is an alteration of affect or mood to sadness or even despair. The condition has been called "the common cold" of mental health because almost everyone is subject to it at one time or another. Depression is also the next most common condition after cardiovascular and musculoskeletal problems.

An estimated one out of every six Americans is likely to be depressed at some point in life. The condition is most prevalent among women and the elderly (American Psychiatric Association, 1980), but the reasons are unclear. Recent research indicates that heredity, environment, and changes in body chemistry may contribute to depression.

Depression may follow real or perceived loss. Clients who have experienced biologic or self-esteem losses may respond with depression. Nurses are likely to encounter many persons depressed by the stress of illness, surgery, lifestyle changes, and body image alterations.

Nursing Assessment: Establishing the Data Base

Look for the following emotional and behavioral manifestations of depression:

- Looking and feeling sad, despairing, hopeless, or tired
- Loss of interest in work, hobbies, self, and environment
- Inability to experience pleasure or joy
- Lowered self-esteem
- Thoughts of death or suicide

Physiologic manifestations include:

- Loss of appetite usually accompanied by weight loss or, because some people eat more when feeling depressed, weight gain

- Sleep disturbances such as insomnia, early morning awakening, or being unable to get up to face the new day
- Decreased activity level evidenced in slowed speech and movement
- Constipation
- Decrease in sexual activity

Cognitive manifestations include: difficulty in concentrating, slowed thinking, and difficulty in decision making.

History taking should include family and friends. They may be able to share important information about the type and severity of losses the client has recently experienced, the events that led to the client's feeling depressed, and the client's responses to these situations.

Although there are no laboratory tests to diagnose depression, the dexamethasone suppression test (DST) helps determine whether the client's depression is amenable to somatic treatment, such as antidepressant medications.

Nursing Diagnosis

A number of nursing diagnoses are appropriate in caring for persons who are depressed. The primary diagnoses are ineffective individual coping and dysfunctional grieving. Other relevant nursing diagnoses are:

- Alteration in bowel elimination: constipation
- Impaired verbal communication
- Deficit in diversional activity
- Impaired physical mobility
- Alteration in nutrition: less than body requirements (or more than body requirements)
- Self-care deficit
- Sexual dysfunction
- Sleep pattern disturbance
- Distress of the human spirit
- Alteration in thought processes

This list demonstrates the interrelation among the physiologic and psychosocial concerns of depressed persons.

Planning and Implementation

Physiologic needs of depressed clients require special attention to hydration, nutrition, and bowel elimination. A depressed client may not be able to tend to these needs. Because the whole body slows down, the client may be prone to constipation. The client may need more assistance than usual in carrying out personal hygiene and activities of daily living. Comfort measures such as back rubs, a warm drink, a warm bath, or soothing music may promote relaxation and sleep.

Because depressed persons are withdrawn and quiet, they are sometimes forgotten. Be sure to spend time with the client, offering opportunities to express feelings related to the losses the client has experienced. When the client is unable or unwilling to talk, simply being there can demonstrate genuine interest in the client's welfare. Touching the client—a pat on the hand, a touch on the shoulder, or a hug if the client seems open to it and it seems appropriate—is often comforting.

Be careful not to offer empty reassurance to the client. In the client's view, life may look bleak. Attempting to make light of these feelings only demonstrates lack of understanding. Instead, help the client to understand the relation between the client's feelings and recent events that may have provoked the depression. Acknowledge that the client has had a bad time and is going through a period of mourning.

Remember that depressed persons are slowed not only in their motor skills but in their thinking. Allow more time than usual to carry out direct client care activities. The client should be encouraged to undertake self-care activities as able, and allow more time than usual for these activities. The client's activity level can be gradually increased.

Clients who continue to be severely depressed may benefit from mental health intervention by a psychiatric–mental health nurse or other professional. Interventions may include counseling or somatic treatments such as antidepressant medication.

Evaluation

Expected outcomes are that the client's depression will lessen and the client will be able to assume self-care activities. Sleep pattern disturbances should diminish, and the client should feel less fatigued and apathetic. With counseling, the client should be able to identify the events and losses that led to the depression and be able to express the feelings associated with them.

Dependence

Everyone relies on someone or something else at some time for support and to have needs met. As infants, persons learn to rely on parents or other caregivers. As adolescents, they struggle with becoming independent. By the time they reach adulthood, most have learned interdependence—a balance between dependent and independent behavior.

At various times, adults may find that, no matter how independent or how interdependent they usually are, circumstances may require dependence on others. Illness and hospitalization are two of these circumstances. Consider the client whose femur is fractured in an automobile accident. In the early stages, this person will probably have to depend on others to meet physical needs and emotional needs for support and caring. As healing progresses, however, the client begins to meet more of his or her own needs, relying on others to a lesser degree. The behavior is considered *adaptive dependent behavior* because the client was able to be as dependent as necessary to regain health.

In another situation, the client might continue to be

dependent for physical needs even though healing has progressed, and the condition no longer warrants it. This is an example of *maladaptive dependent behavior*. As a method of coping, it is unrealistic and inappropriate. The behavior may come about because the client has not had early needs for dependence met in a satisfying way. These clients fear being left alone and find it difficult to trust that others will take care of them when necessary. Or perhaps the client has learned that anxiety can be reduced by depending on others. Regardless of the reason, the results are problems in the interpersonal relationship between client and nurse that cause obstacles to health care.

Although overly dependent persons may appear helpless, their behavior actually controls others as it becomes demanding. Health care personnel often respond with anger to the client's unrealistic and inappropriate demands. Their anger may only increase the client's anxiety and dependence.

It is important that nurses recognize how their own needs for dependence and independence influence their expectations of clients. Nurses who feel rewarded and fulfilled when clients are overly dependent on them do not assist clients to function at their optimum health level. Nurses who cannot tolerate a client's dependence will not deal effectively with a client's realistic dependence and interfere with the client's return to health. A nurse can help dependent clients most by facilitating adaptive dependent behavior, setting limits on maladaptive dependent behavior, and encouraging eventual independence or interdependence.

Nursing Assessment: Establishing the Data Base

Adaptive dependent behavior is assessed by observing the circumstances under which the dependent behavior occurs. Adaptive dependent behavior is a flexible response to a change in the health situation. Evidence of maladaptive dependent behavior may include:

- The client refuses to participate in self-care.
- The client asks the nurse or other health care personnel to perform tasks that are within the client's capabilities.
- The client frequently uses the call light or calls for nursing personnel.
- The client frequently expresses a lack of confidence, helplessness, and feelings of isolation and alienation.
- The client is reluctant to discontinue treatment or, if hospitalized, to be transferred to a unit, such as an intermediate or ambulatory care unit, that requires greater independence.
- The client refuses to learn to carry out tasks associated with a body change or claims inability to learn.

Also assess how long the maladaptive behavior has been used. Is dependence an ongoing method of coping with life? Or is dependence situational (ie, a method of coping with anxiety brought on by illness [or threat of illness] or hospitalization)? Data relevant to these questions can be obtained from the client as well as from family and friends. Be sure also to identify other coping methods the client has employed.

Nursing Diagnosis

Several nursing diagnoses apply to dependent behavior. Among them are ineffective individual coping, self-care deficit, disturbance in self-concepts, and noncompliance.

Planning and Implementation

The first priority is to initiate frequent contacts with the client. It is essential to demonstrate interest in the client and willingness to spend time with the client other than time the client requests or demands. At the same time, it is important to identify when the client can next expect to see the nurse or another health care worker. Telling the client when a nurse or someone else will return and then doing so helps the client develop trust and may reduce anxiety.

Next, encourage the client to begin self-care activities one step at a time. The intent is to assist the client toward greater independence and not to be punitive. As the client begins to take on self-care activities, provide encouragement and acknowledge the client's efforts. Collaborating with the client in developing a step-by-step plan is likely to result in a more effective plan than one determined solely by the nurse. In some cases, verbal or written contracts between client and nurse assist in establishing common goals and clarify the rights and responsibilities of each party. It goes without saying that adaptive dependence needs are met until the client is physiologically able to participate in self-care.

If dependence has been a lifelong coping strategy for the client, it is probably unrealistic for the nurse to expect to be able to change the behavior. The nurse may not be able to meet the unrealistic and perhaps insatiable demands of such clients. Efforts to encourage self-care activities may not be successful. If that is the case, rational limits may have to be set on the extent to which the client's dependence needs will be met.

Let clients know why their increasing independence is being encouraged. Express interest in helping the client be as self-sufficient as possible and explain that doing everything for the client diminishes autonomy. Criticizing dependent behavior is more likely to increase anxiety than to encourage behavior change.

Family and friends should also participate in the planning and implementation. They often have useful suggestions because they know the client well. They will be in a position to reinforce the client's moves toward greater independence. Family and friends may be helped by explanations that account for the client's dependent behavior. The nurse can help them to learn when to perform activities for the client and when they should encourage independent functioning.

Evaluation

In a successful plan, the client demonstrates an increased ability for self-care. Client requests for help or attention should decrease in frequency. As the client gains greater self-confidence and trusts the nurse to help when necessary, the client will be more interested in greater independence, be pleased with the changes in activity, and be less reluctant to rely more on self than on others. The client's objections to transferring to an intermediate care unit or ambulatory care unit will decrease or cease.

Chapter Highlights

The social, emotional, and practical needs of clients may make it difficult, if not impossible, for them to perform or behave as the nurse thinks appropriate. Labeling such clients "resistive," "noncompliant," or "a problem patient" obstructs effective use of the nursing process.

Clients who fail to follow a treatment program may do so because of knowledge deficit. Assess for this possibility to correct it.

Complying with a treatment regimen may have costs to the client, such as the anxiety of acknowledging the reality of illness or health risk; imposed lifestyle burdens; being subjected to painful, disfiguring, or risky treatments; financial burdens; the need to submit to the authority of health care personnel; and the possibility of burdening family and friends.

Persons cope with stress in a variety of ways that seem to have worked in the past. Some talk it over with others; some jog; others pray or laugh off the problem.

When someone is unable to ward off stress or reduce anxiety in the usual way, tension mounts. Persons may have to rely on largely unconscious and inflexible coping patterns that are self-deceptive.

Anxiety is an uncomfortable feeling that stems from threats to biological integrity and the security of the self.

Quick and accurate assessment and interventions for anxiety are important, because at higher levels, anxiety interferes with a client's ability to get well or to keep well.

Nurses can expect clients and their families to become anxious in the face of unknown or potentially painful, dangerous, or disfiguring events.

Anger is the fight response to anxiety that reduces the powerlessness the anxious client feels. In planning an intervention for anger, the nurse should understand that anger was preceded by anxiety.

Denial helps clients and their families "buy time" as a self-protective measure to reduce the anxiety associated with illness, trauma, loss, and major life changes.

Depression is not uncommon in clients and families under stress. Depression interferes with a person's ability to carry out self-care activities.

Maladaptive dependent behavior exists when a client continues to depend on the nurse to meet physical needs when the client's condition no longer warrants. The behavior creates obstacles to effective health care.

Bibliography

American Psychiatric Association: *Diagnostic and Statistical Manual of Mental Disorders,* 3rd ed. rev. Washington, DC: American Psychiatric Association, 1987.

Antonovsky A: *Health, Stress, and Coping.* San Francisco, CA: Jossey–Bass, 1980.

Barash DA: Defusing the violent patient before he explodes. *RN* (March) 1984; 47:34–37.

Barry PD: *Psychosocial Nursing Assessment and Intervention.* Philadelphia: Lippincott, 1984.

Brigman C, Dickey C, Zegeer LJ: The agitated aggressive patient. *Am J Nurs* 1983; 83:1409–1412.

Davis AJ: *Listening and Responding.* St. Louis: Mosby, 1984.

Hoff LA: *People in Crisis: Understanding and Helping.* 2nd ed. Menlo Park, CA: Addison–Wesley, 1984.

Kneisl CR, Wilson HS: *Handbook of Psychosocial Nursing Care.* Menlo Park, CA: Addison–Wesley, 1984.

Leventhal H, Watts JC, Pagano F: Effects of fear and instructions on how to cope with danger. *J Personal Soc Psychol* 1967; 6:313–321.

Maagdenberg AM: The "violent" patient. *Am J Nurs* 1983; 83:402–403.

Miller JM: Inspiring hope. *Am J Nurs* 1985; 85(1):22–25.

Scarf M: *Unfinished Business.* New York: Simon & Schuster, 1981.

Tavris C: *Anger: The Misunderstood Emotion.* New York: Simon & Schuster, 1983.

Vogel CH: Anxiety and depression among the elderly. *J Gerontol Nurs* 1982; 8:213–216.

Wilson HS, Kneisl CR: *Psychiatric Nursing,* 3rd ed. Menlo Park, CA: Addison–Wesley, 1988.

Yoos L: Compliance: Philosophical and ethical considerations. *Nurse Pract* 1981; 6(5):27+.

Ziemer MM: Coping behavior: A response to stress. *Top Clin Nurs* 1982; 2(4):4–12.

Resource

National Crisis Prevention Institute
Lakewood Building
3315 K N 124th St
Brookfield, WI 53005
Phone: (414) 783–5787
Toll-free number: (800) 558–8976

This organization has offered nonviolent physical crisis intervention programs in health, education, social welfare, security, and correctional facilities since 1972. Staff are trained in the prevention and management of disruptive, assaultive, or out-of-control behavior. The group also offers a quarterly publication, the *CPI National Report,* focusing on current facts and techniques in managing aggressive behavior.

CHAPTER 5

Health Assessment of the Adult

Objectives

When you have finished studying this chapter, you should be able to:

Identify approaches to facilitating nurse–client communication.

Elicit and record a comprehensive health history.

Explain the need for a thorough psychosocial/lifestyle history.

Become comfortable obtaining a sexual health history.

Recognize the importance of a review of the family health history and its implications for the long-term health of the client.

Maintain client dignity and comfort throughout the health assessment process.

Demonstrate techniques of physical assessment and explain appropriate alterations in their sequence depending on the body system being examined and the condition of the client.

Specify areas to be assessed in each bodily system.

Describe common assessment findings that may appear abnormal but are within the wide range of normal.

Anticipate some of the age-related changes often observed during the health assessment process.

To assess the health of adults comprehensively, the nurse must be able to communicate effectively with clients and families, assemble a complete data base, and synthesize the information gathered to form an accurate picture of the client's health. Use of the nursing process is fundamental to the accomplishment of this goal.

The nursing process is a problem-solving approach to the care of clients. The essential steps of the nursing process are:

- Assessment (gathering the subjective and objective client data base)
- Establishing a nursing diagnosis
- Developing a plan of care with the client
- Implementing the plan
- Evaluating the plan and revising it as needed.

The crucial step is the data-gathering phase. If important aspects of the client's life are overlooked or given only cursory attention during the health history, the nursing diagnoses and plan of care will be deficient.

SECTION 

Communicating With Clients

Each client and each nurse bring to the client–nurse interaction unique variables that influence the relationship in a variety of ways. Age and sex, background, culture and life experience, religion or belief system, attitudes and values, expectations, hopes and fears all affect the relationship. Some of these factors enhance communication; others may create barriers.

No matter what their status in the outside world, clients enter the health care system with a perceived loss of status, power, and most of all, control. These losses are often intensified by a system that subtly rewards "good patients" who passively comply with a plan of care devised and directed by health professionals who barely know them. The assertive client who asks pointed questions and demands input into decisions about care is labeled "difficult."

Of the members of the team of health professionals concerned with the client's care, the nurse knows the client and family best. Thus, the nurse often assumes the position of client advocate; reinforcing to the physician the concerns of the client and family; getting answers to unanswered questions; and in general, presenting the case for the client. The nurse also assumes the role of interpreter, restating and explaining the physician's statements to the client in terms appropriate to the client's level of understanding and current emotional state.

Besides functioning as advocate and interpreter, the nurse is responsible for identifying clients' strengths and social resources; evaluating their knowledge of health and illness; becoming acutely aware of sociocultural and religious influences that may affect their responses; and detecting subtle cues of pain, anxiety, emotion, or deteriorating condition. Fulfillment of these numerous responsibilities depends in large part on the nurse's ability to assess a client, blending communication strengths with a systematic approach to history taking and skill in physical assessment.

During the assessment process, nurses integrate their own natural communication style into the communication approaches learned in nursing fundamentals courses. Listening, body language, touch, and silence—as well as verbal approaches like open-ended questions, clarifying, and paraphrasing—are techniques basic to nursing. These must become more than mere techniques; they must be purposefully cultivated so they become "second nature."

When clients come from cultures other than the care provider's, their views of their illness and its cause will be quite unlike the views of the caregivers. Often the client's questions will not be answered satisfactorily because the significance of the query is not clear to the health professional. To provide effective care to clients from different sociocultural backgrounds, the nurse must understand their health beliefs and practices. If a different belief system is interfering with the client's care, it is the nurse's responsibility to investigate these beliefs by asking the client about them in a nonjudgmental manner.

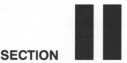

SECTION 

Subjective Health Assessment: The Health History

Whether in an acute care or primary care setting, the nurse, rather than the physician, spends the most time in direct contact with the client. Each interchange, no matter how brief, should strengthen the base on which a nursing diagnosis is made as well as strengthen the nurse–client relationship. The nurse's observation and communication skills can be the key to proper diagnosis and treatment, not only nursing diagnosis but medical diagnosis as well. Consider the following example:

Mrs JS enters the health care system obviously ill with vertigo, malaise, and muscle weakness of sudden onset. She has a number of noninvasive and invasive diagnostic studies. All test results are within normal limits. In talking with the client, the nurse asks her about her life, her habits, how she usually spends her day, and how happy she is in her marriage. At this point, the client bursts into tears and blurts out the story of her husband's extramarital affair. Her symptoms developed shortly after learning of his infidelity. The nurse consults with the physician and arranges for the mental health clinical nurse specialist to see Mrs S. As individual counseling and marital counseling continue, her symptoms gradually resolve.

This example suggests that nurses, who are educated in a holistic mode, find this information essential to a comprehensive picture of the client. Only with such a picture is it possible to make an accurate nursing diagnosis, to consider fully the goals of care, and to develop with the client a mutual plan to achieve these goals.

Approach to the Health History

To depict the health history as an organized whole, history taking will be discussed as though the nurse is taking an initial complete history. Actually, in a clinical situation, history taking continues throughout the nurse–client relationship. A complete history is taken when the client is admitted to an inpatient unit or when the client comes into an ambulatory facility for a complete physical examination or for a health problem. Even so, the history-taking process continues for as long as the nurse and the client are in contact. If the history is viewed as a task to be completed and not thought of again, important data may be missed.

In the initial encounter with the care provider, clients are often anxious, worried, or embarrassed about their health problem. They may simply forget important information or perhaps consciously withhold it. One advantage of an ongoing nurse–client relationship, as in inpatient settings, is that clients can easily share previously withheld information later when they remember it or become more comfortable with the nurse.

The identification of health risk factors is an important part of the health history. A risk factor entails probability; that is, if the risk factor is elevated, more individuals in a given group will be affected by the risk. But not everyone in a high-risk group will inevitably develop a given disorder—and not everyone in a low-risk group will escape it.

How long a person is exposed to a risk and the intensity of exposure affect the probability of that individual's developing the disorder. Moreover, sometimes risk factors are synergistic; that is, if several risk factors are present, the probability that disease will develop is greater than the sum of the individual probabilities associated with the risks. Cardiovascular disease is one example of this effect. Again, remember that the connection between a risk factor and development of disease is not absolute. The association between lung cancer and cigarette smoking is well established—more than 80% of lung cancer among men is attributable to smoking (Gett, Cortese, & Fontana, 1983)—yet only a small proportion of heavy smokers develop cancer of the lung.

Instruments known as health risk appraisals, or HRAs, are sometimes used to gather the data on which risk reduction planning and education are based. HRAs are not a substitute for a complete health history. The basic intention of the HRA is to provide a quantitative measure of lifestyle factors and personal characteristics to estimate an individual's probability of dying from a particular cause within a specified time. Computer-based statistical procedures are used to determine a "risk age" and an "achievable age." The risk age reflects how hazardous behaviors affect the individual's chronologic age. The achievable age delineates the potential improvement in longevity that behavioral change might bring. Presenting these data to the cleint is believed to motivate the client to change.

Format for the Health History

Some portions of the health history are almost self-explanatory (eg, personal data includes such information as name, address, and age). Source of history and reliability of informant refer to circumstances in which the client may not be able to give a clear history (eg, because of a language barrier, aphasia, facial or oral injury, or coma). Identify the person who gave the history (client, parent, spouse, friend) and record a judgment of the overall reliability of the informant. A complete health history appears later in this chapter.

Chief Concern

The chief concern (CC) is the main reason the client sought health care. Usually, the CC is recorded in the client's own words; for example, "[I have had this] severe pounding headache over both eyes for 2 days."

To make the CC more concise, the nurse might translate the client's words into a brief statement. Suppose the client says, "I came to the clinic today because I was in an auto accident a week ago. Since then, I have had aching in both my lower legs and pain in my left arm. My lower back hurts since the accident. I've had low back pain on and off for 10 years, but the accident made it much worse." The CC in this instance might be translated:

CC: Numerous aches and pains both legs, left arm since auto accident 1 week ago.
Low-back pain × 10 years, aggravated by accident.

Box 5–1
Seven Guidelines to Evaluate a Symptom

1. Bodily location
2. Quality
3. Quantity: intensity, volume, number, size or extent
4. Chronology or timing: onset, duration, frequency, course
5. Setting
6. Aggravating and alleviating factors
7. Associated manifestations

SOURCE: Reprinted with permission from Morgan WL Jr, Engel GL: *The Clinical Approach to the Patient*. Philadelphia: Saunders, 1969, p. 35.

Box 5–2
Mnemonic to Evaluate the Symptom of Pain

P: provocative/palliative factors
Q: quality
R: region
S: severity
T: timing

History of the Present Illness

The history of the present illness (HPI) is the heart of the health history. It is a chronologic review of the client's health problem in narrative form. Various approaches to tracking down a symptom have been developed to be certain important historical information is not overlooked (see Boxes 5–1 and 5–2).

For example, when taking the HPI on the client with a CC of severe pounding headache over both eyes for 2 days, the interviewer would initially use the seven guidelines (Box 5–1), or the PQRST mnemonic (Box 5–2) if that is easier to remember. For *bodily location* the nurse might say, "Point to the places on your head where you feel the pain." *Quality* can be evaluated by asking what the pain is like. If the client cannot give an example the nurse might ask, "Does it feel like someone pounding on your head or like a tight band around your head?" To assess *quantity* of the pain, ask the client to describe its severity: "Is it mildly annoying, moderate, severe? Or is it unbearable?"

Chronology begins with the onset of the symptom; for example, "When did these headaches first begin?" Duration, frequency, and course are then reconstructed. "How long do they usually last?" "How often do they tend to recur?" "Have you noticed any pattern to them? For example, are your headaches often associated with your menstrual cycle, or do you seem to develop a headache when you are under stress?"

The *setting* where a symptom is experienced often gives a clue to the diagnosis. Does the client experience headaches only on weekends? Only at work? Only on vacation? Only during allergy season? Or does the setting seem to have no relation at all to the headache?

Conditions that *aggravate* or *provoke* the headache are assessed. "When you have a headache, what seems to make it worse? For example, is the headache made worse by bright lights, potent smells, loud noises, bending over? Factors that *alleviate* or *palliate* the headache are also addressed. "Have you found anything that helps your headache once you have one? For example, is the headache made better by lying down in a dark room? An ice bag? A hot towel? A specific medication?" Any other *symptoms associated* with the headache are also considered. For example, does the client also experience nausea and/or vomiting, photophobia, or vertigo?

Information gathered during the evaluation of the symptom guides the examiner to the next phase of the HPI. For example, if the client associates eating patterns with the headache, the next step is a dietary history. Substances associated with headache are tracked down carefully. Perhaps the headache occurs when the client misses a meal or is secondary to caffeine withdrawal. Any association the client notes should be followed up in the HPI.

With experience and an increasing knowledge base, the nurse also begins to associate symptom complexes and to develop ability to identify information that directly contributes to the client's chief concern. When completed, the HPI should provide a clear picture of the client's problem from onset to the present and should convey an appreciation for how the client's lifestyle has contributed to and been affected by the health problem.

Past Health History

The client's past health is reviewed and recorded as concisely as possible. Childhood illnesses are listed, and specific questions are asked about rheumatic fever, scarlet fever, or any major health problems the client recalls from childhood. An immunization history is obtained. Many adults are unaware that they should have a tetanus–diphtheria (Td) booster every 10 years. Because a booster is given with dog bites or with injuries in which the skin is broken in an unclean manner, the client may be able to associate the most recent Td with such an event.

A review of medical problems and surgical procedures follows. Major diagnostic studies with dates (eg, an intravenous pyelogram) are listed, as are blood transfusions. For the female client, a pregnancy history is obtained, and weight of infants if over 9 lb is noted. A client who has given birth to a large infant may be prediabetic.

Both physical and psychologic trauma are evaluated. A history of fractures or concussions as well as major life stress events that may be unresolved are important to note. Any psychiatric hospitalizations or other hospitalizations not covered under the previous categories are also listed.

An allergy history is obtained, including allergy to pollens, foods, clothing, insects, animals, drugs, diagnostic test contrast media, and anesthetic agents. The client's reaction to the allergen is recorded. Does the client state a penicillin allergy is present because of diarrhea 6 days after beginning the drug, or because of becoming extremely short of breath and cyanotic shortly after taking it? This information may make a major difference in future treatment.

The client's history of medication use is of prime importance. Many clients think of "medicine" as prescription drugs and do not consider over-the-counter (OTC) drugs significant. Yet an OTC medication that the client forgot to mention may interfere with the action of a prescribed drug. For example, antacids inhibit the absorption of tetracycline. OTC drugs may also cause serious side effects if not used carefully. Few clients think of vitamins and oral contraceptives as drugs, so the nurse should ask specifically about them.

Family History

Because many health problems tend to run in families, either through genetic transfer or environmental influence (eg, diet), the nurse gathers a thorough family history (FH). If the client has been adopted and has no knowledge of her/his biologic parents, the genetic aspect will not apply. A discussion of the general health of the entire family is helpful in obtaining an impression of the client and family relationships, however. The family history may be recorded in outline format or in the form of a **genogram,** a diagram of the family tree. Interactional as well as genetic information can be noted on the genogram (Figure 5–1).

The age, health, and cause of death of blood relatives is recorded. Maternal and paternal grandparents, parents, siblings, and children all are included in this history. In addition, ask whether any blood relatives have a history of elevated blood pressure, cerebrovascular accident (CVA), myocardial infarction (MI), hypercholesterolemia, tuberculosis (TBC), alcoholism, cancer of any organ, or diabetes mellitus (DM). It is helpful to follow up with a question such as, "Are there any diseases your family thinks tend to run in the family?" The answer may reveal problems such as migraine headache, cystic fibrosis, or familial polyposis that may not have surfaced during the discussion. Another useful follow-up question is, "Does anyone else in the family have a problem similar to yours?" The response is often revealing and helps put the client's symptoms in perspective. In the client with the headaches, consider what approach to use if the client said, "My best friend who was just my age died last week of a brain tumor. Her symptoms started out just like mine."

The racial and ethnic origins of the family are of great importance when gathering a history. Blacks should be asked about a family history of sickle cell disease or sickle cell trait. Jews should be questioned about Tay–Sachs disease in the family. Uncovering these facts early provides an opportunity to direct the unmarried and/or not-yet-pregnant client to a genetic counselor for counseling and education.

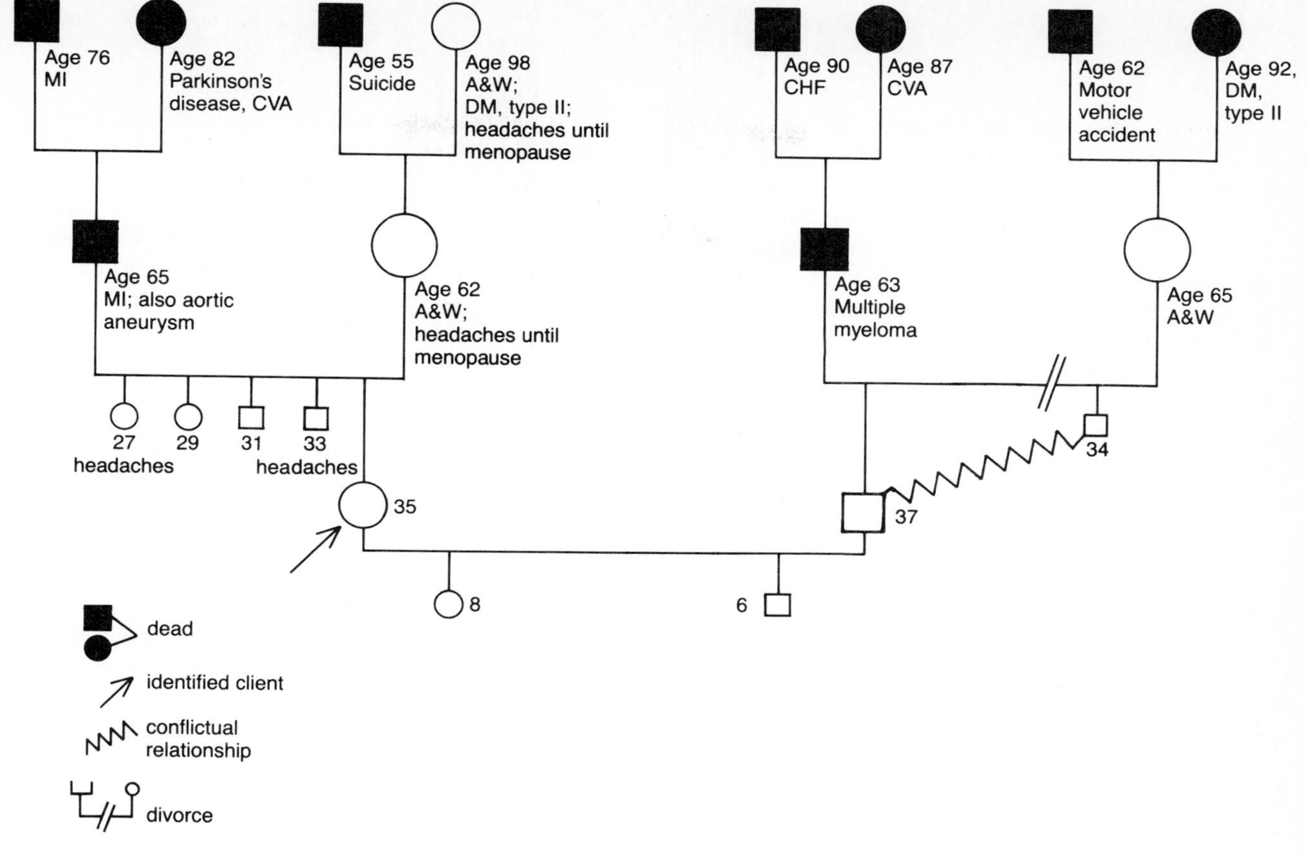

Figure 5–1

Example of a genogram. In this genogram, the identified female client, age 35, is the oldest of five children. Her mother and grandmother are both living. She is married to a 37-year-old man who has some conflict with his younger brother. His parents were divorced. The client and her husband have a daughter and a son. Her family history is positive ⊕ for cardiovascular disease, diabetes mellitus type II, Parkinson's disease, aortic aneurysm, suicide, and headache until menopause. Her husband's family history is ⊕ for cardiovascular disease, diabetes mellitus type II, and multiple myeloma.

Personal/Social History

The personal/social portion of the health history helps the nurse develop a feeling for what clients' lives are like; how they spend an average day; and their interests, beliefs, and habits. Does the client have strong religious beliefs that are a source of hope and spiritual strength? Who are the significant persons in the client's life? Are there persons the client can depend on in times of need? What is the client's social network? What are the client's beliefs about health and illness? What preventive and self-care measures does the client routinely practice?

Sociocultural assessment is an integral component of the health history. Ask about what the client believes may have caused the illness or health problem. Has the client received treatment for the condition elsewhere? Has the client attempted self-treatment or used other healers? What ideas does the client have about how he or she could be helped? What are the health practices of the client's family, friends, and neighbors?

What stresses does the client currently identify? Are there concerns about finances, health, family responsibilities, or social life? Are there multiple changes in the client's life? How does the client usually cope with stress and how does he or she plan to cope with the current stressors?

The client's educational and occupational history are discussed, including future goals. Is the client satisfied with work or school? What occupational or environmental hazards is the client exposed to? Military service and recent travel experiences are reviewed, not only to assess exposure to toxic chemicals of war or to diseases endemic to certain geographic areas but also to consider psychologic consequences of such experiences.

The client should be questioned about practices contributing to poor health such as tobacco, alcohol, and other drug use. Smoking is quantified according to pack years. (One package of cigarettes per day for 1 year equals 1 pack year.) Thus, a client who has smoked 2½ packs per day (PPD) for 20 years has a 50-pack-year smoking history. Alcohol intake should also be quantified, if possible, by the number of ounces of beer, wine, or liquor per day.

A careful dietary history is obtained by asking the client to describe in detail food and fluid intake for a typical 24-hour period. Ask specifically about caffeine, sodium, and fat intake. Does the client make an attempt to incorporate foods from the basic four food groups, or is the eating pattern haphazard? Does the client prepare meals at home or eat out? Are there mobility or transportation problems that prevent the client from shopping for food? What type of restaurants does the client frequent? Are there any restrictions on the client's diet because of finances, religious beliefs, cultural preferences, food intolerance, or health status? Is the client on a weight-reduction diet and, if so, what kind? Is the client a vegetarian? Does the client take vitamin or mineral supplements? (See Chapters 6 and 7 for information on malnutrition, obesity, and eating disorders.)

Review of Systems

The review of systems (ROS) is a verbal rundown from head to toe of the client's overall state of health and the health of each bodily system. The review serves as a memory prod for both the nurse and the client in obtaining missing data. For example if, in questioning the client with headaches, vision was omitted during the HPI, ask under "ROS-Eyes" when the last vision exam was done. The client might respond that it was 3 years ago when glasses were prescribed for reading, but she never wears them. She then talks about how tired her eyes feel at times and states that this probably doesn't help the headaches. In this instance, when recording the history, place the eye information in the HPI because it specifically relates to the CC. If a system has already been reviewed under the HPI, however, do not ask about it again under the ROS unless the review was incomplete.

In each nursing process chapter and in the case studies in this text the important subjective data to be gathered about each system are identified. For example, for the "ROS-GI" ask about appetite, nausea and vomiting, nature and amount of emesis, food intolerance, flatulence, pain such as heartburn or epigastric discomfort, bowel pattern, stool color and consistency, and hemorrhoids.

SEXUAL HISTORY A sexual history is often neglected because both client and care provider may have reservations about discussing this intimate and sensitive subject. If the subject is introduced with ease during the ROS, and the client is questioned about genitourinary function as matter-of-factly as about gastrointestinal function, the sexual history will receive the same emphasis as other physiologic functions.

After a series of questions related to the overall health of the client's genitourinary system, ask an open-ended question about sexual functioning (eg, "How do you feel about the sexual aspects of your life?"). Perhaps the client will not answer. Perhaps nonverbal messages indicate hesitation or discomfort. Suggest that it would be fine to raise the subject some other time, if the client would like to. The subject has been introduced and the client given an opening for discussing possible problems at another time.

If the client has a health problem that may cause concurrent alterations in sexual function, pursue the questioning further. For example, in taking a history from a woman who has a cystocele and rectocele and a concern about stress incontinence, the nurse might say, "Many women who lose urine with coughing or sneezing, as you do, find that the fear of losing urine interferes with their sexual relationship. Has this been true for you?" To a man who is taking an antihypertensive drug that may cause impotence, the nurse might say, "Some men have a problem getting an erection when they are taking certain blood pressure medicines. Has this ever happened to you?" Such approaches also let clients know they are not alone with their problem. That knowledge may encourage them to explore the subject further with the nurse or with their physician.

At the completion of the health history, the nurse should ask, "Do you have any other concerns about your health you would like to discuss?" Perhaps an issue important to the client has not been mentioned or pursued. By now enough rapport has usually been established to make the client comfortable in discussing other matters with the nurse. The concerns shared at this point may be the most significant and should not be taken lightly. The client's deepest worry may be signaled by an off-hand question such as, "By the way, do you think this little lump under my arm means anything?" A sample health history write-up is shown in Box 5–3.

SECTION 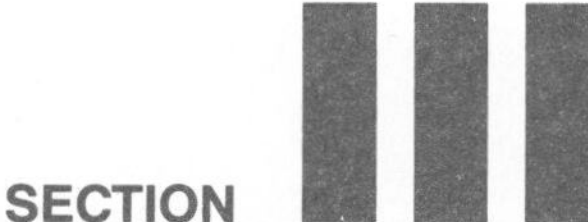

Objective Health Assessment: The Physical Examination

Some of the physical assessment approaches in this chapter may not be a part of a routine nursing assessment (eg, deep palpation, percussion). The level of physical assessment depends on the knowledge and skill of the individual nurse. All nurses, however, should be familiar with the terminology and enough of the examination to be able to prepare clients adequately.

General observations of the client during the history are translated into a brief description, recorded at the beginning of the physical exam; for example:

> Chronically ill, very thin 55-yr-old black male, appears older than stated age, oriented × 3, with scleral icterus, who scratches continuously throughout the history.

General guidelines for approaching the physical examination include:

- Good lighting is essential.

Box 5–3
Sample Health History

Personal data:

Date and time: 3-2-88 1 PM

Full Name: Sarah Harris

ID number (Social Security, insurance number): 000-11-1111

Address: 19 Elmwood, Cassadaga, NY

Telephone: Home: 000-0000; Work: 000-0000

Sex: Female

Age: 35

Birthdate: 1-3-53

Marital status: Married

Race/culture: Caucasian

Religion: Protestant

Occupation: Nurse

Usual health care providers: R. Collins, MD; S. Montgomery, RN, NP

Informant: History given by client, who seems credible

CC: Severe, pounding headache over both eyes for 2 days

HPI: Yesterday, Ms Harris awoke with a pounding headache over both eyes, for which she took two OTC sinus pills with no relief. Later, she tried an ice bag, which had helped headaches she'd had in the past, and ASA, with no relief. The pain, which she described as an annoying pounding gradually increasing to severe pain, remained steady all day. It was made worse by bending over and by bright lights. She continued to work but was unable to eat because the pain made her nauseated. She went to bed early and slept all night but still had the headache on awakening this AM. Her menstrual period began today.

Ms Harris has had similar headaches since she was a sophomore in college. She always got one once a month premenstrually and occasionally at other times, "usually after a stressful experience or when I am overtired." She had no headaches during her two pregnancies. Her mother and grandmother had "sick headaches" similar to hers. Their headaches resolved at menopause.

Ms Harris's headaches are always accompanied by nausea and sometimes vomiting. She feels that at times they may be triggered by foods such as cold cuts or chocolate. Red wine also seems to bring them on. She now avoids these substances. She is a heavy coffee drinker at work and sometimes gets a dull headache at home from "caffeine withdrawal."

Ms Harris states she is a "headachy person" and also tends to get other types of headache that are different from her current symptoms and associated with tension, sinus congestion, or eyestrain. She admits to needing glasses for reading but rarely wearing them.

Ms Harris is not a smoker, is not on oral contraceptives, has no known hx of high BP or hx of head trauma.

She suspects her headaches may be migraines because her younger sister, who has similar headaches, was recently diagnosed as having migraines.

Past Health Hx:

Childhood: Chickenpox; denies rheumatic fever, scarlet fever

Immunization: All childhood immunizations; last Td 1982, stitches for cut on hand while working in the garden

Medical problems: None

Surgeries: Tonsils, age 4, Deaconess Hospital, Buffalo NY

Pregnancies: P_2 G_2

Trauma: Physical, fx rt clavicle, age 9; psychological, father's death, 1981

Other hospitalizations: None

Blood transfusions: None

Allergies: To tomatoes; reaction—hives

Medications: Prescription, none; OTC, sinus medication spring and fall; occasional ASA or acetaminophen for headaches; calcium carbonate 600 mg with vit. D $\div$ q.d.

Family Hx (see Figure 5–1 for genogram format for FHx):

Father: Died age 65, MI; also had aortic aneurysm, benign polyps of colon

Mother: Age 62, A&W; had headaches until menopause

Sisters × 2: Ages 29, 27; A&W; youngest c̄ headache

Brothers × 2: Ages 33, 31; A&W; oldest c̄ headache

Husband: Age 37, A&W

Daughter: Age 8, A&W

Son: Age 6, A&W

PGF: MI

PGM: CVA, Parkinson's

MGF: Suicide

MGM: DM, type II; headaches until menopause
No ⊕ FHx of Ca, HTN, TBC

Personal/Social Hx: Client received a BS in nursing and is currently working toward an MS degree. She works part-time 3 to 11 PM on a surgical unit of a small hospital. Now that both children are in school all day, she is considering taking a full-time 8 to 4 PM job in an HMO close to her home.

She is happily married × 10 years; the family enjoys many activities together, such as bike riding and swimming.

She never smoked and has an occasional glass of white wine on the weekend; she denies ever having used drugs. A typical diet for a 24-hour period includes orange juice, bran muffin, and coffee for breakfast; yogurt for lunch; and a salad and meat such as broiled chicken or fish and roll for dinner. She rarely eats desserts and watches her fat intake because of her father's CV disease.

Reading, biking, sewing, and playing board games or video games with the children are her major leisure activities.

They are financially stable; her spouse owns a small appliance store, which is doing well.

She copes with stress by talking things over with her sisters, with whom she is very close, or by weeding her garden or cleaning a messy closet.

She feels she has many strengths, good support systems, and a positive attitude toward her future.

(continued)

Box 5–3 Sample Health History (continued)

ROS:

General state of health: States she is in excellent health with no lack of energy; weight is stable

Skin/hair/nails: Occasional facial pimple premenstrually

Eyes: Last eye exam, 1985; no probs c̄ eye pain, blurring of vision, or rings around lights; see HPI

Ears: States hearing is excellent; no ear pain or discharge; no dizziness or tinnitus

Nose and sinuses: Occasional sinus headache spring and fall relieved by OTC medicines; no known seasonal allergies; no nasal trauma or epistaxis

Mouth and teeth: Yearly dental exam, no dentures; no problems with gums, tongue, or change in taste

Throat and neck: Rare sore throat; no difficulty swallowing, hoarseness, or neck stiffness

Breasts and axillae: Does monthly BSE; no nipple discharge, no known lumps or lesions

Respiratory: No cough or wheezing; last chest x-ray 15 years ago, wnl; always has ⊕ TB skin test as was given BCG vaccine in nursing school

Cardiovascular: No DOE, PND, orthopnea; no known heart murmur; no ankle edema; has varicose veins since last pregnancy, wears support stockings; no phlebitis hx

Gastrointestinal: No anorexia, n & v except c̄ CC; no food intolerance, flatulence, change in bowel habits; states stools are brown in color; has BM q.d.; no abdominal pain or abdominal surgery; no hx of jaundice or hemorrhoids

Gynecological: Menarche age 14; q. 28–30-day cycle, 5-day flow; currently menstruating; no longer uses tampons since TSS scare; no prob c̄ dysmenorrhea, dyspareunia, or vaginal discharge; no birth control—husband had vasectomy; has intercourse approximately once a week; states sexual aspect of her marriage has "always been good"; see HPI for headaches associated c̄ menses

Urinary: No problems of urgency, frequency, dysuria, nocturia, or hematuria; no hx of stress incontinence, UTI, or renal calculi

Musculoskeletal: No problems c̄ low back pain, muscle weakness, leg cramps, joint pain or stiffness; no foot problems

Neurologic: Headaches—see HPI; no problems c̄ vertigo, tremor, sleep disturbances, memory; no paralysis, numbness and tingling, or decreased sensation to any bodily part

Psychological: No problems c̄ mood swings, paranoid feelings, periods of depression or indecision; no hx of suicidal thoughts or attacks of severe anxiety; saw a nurse mental health counselor monthly for about 8 months after her father's death to sort out her feelings about God and life after death; she found the counseling experience helpful and would return if she felt the need to do so

Endocrine: No polyuria, polydipsia, polyphagia; no changes in skin or hair; no intolerance to heat or cold

Lymphatic: No known enlarged nodes in neck, axillae, or groin

Hematopoietic: No hx of anemia or abnormal bleeding or bruising

- If the examiner is right handed, examine from the client's right side.
- If the client is an inpatient, position the bed to a proper height.
- The environment should be private and as quiet as possible.
- Explain to the client as the examination proceeds.
- Adequately expose areas being examined.

Subjective data gathering continues throughout the physical assessment as each area is examined in sequence (eg, "Tell me about this small scar on your right breast," or "How long have you had this dark mole on your neck?").

Techniques of Physical Assessment

In the usual sequence of physically assessing body organs, inspection always comes first and is followed by palpation, percussion, and auscultation. In assessing the abdomen, this sequence changes slightly. Auscultation is performed after inspection because the intestine is sensitive to touch, and palpation and percussion of the abdomen may alter peristaltic sounds.

Inspection

Careful inspection of the area is the most important part of physical assessment. Placing a stethoscope on the chest before looking at the chest is a common error. Each anatomical region should be inspected carefully *before* it is touched with the examiner's hands or instruments, because valuable information can be obtained by thorough observation.

Palpation

Palpation uses the sense of touch to examine all accessible body parts. Using palpation, the following evaluations are made:

- Size and shape (organs, masses)
- Pulsatility
- Mobility
- Consistency
- Tenderness or pain
- Swelling
- Surface temperature
- Muscle rigidity or spasm
- Presence or absence of masses

Keeping the client comfortable and relaxed facilitates thorough palpation. Muscle tension during examination not only interferes with adequate palpation but may also make the client uncomfortable and reluctant to continue with the examination.

Tender areas should always be palpated last. Suppose the client has pain in the left upper quadrant (LUQ) of the abdomen. Examining the involved area first can create considerable discomfort. The client will guard the abdomen, making it impossible to perform an adequate assessment. Many examiners tend to focus in too quickly on the problem area without thoroughly examining surrounding areas where the problem might actually originate.

The nurse should also be comfortable while palpating, and the hands should be warm. Parts of the hand used during palpation are:

- Fingertips for fine tactile discrimination, lymph nodes, skin texture
- Dorsa of hands for temperature (because dorsal skin is thinner)
- Palmar and ulnar surfaces for vibratory sensation
- Grasping position of fingers for tissue consistency

Light palpation helps to relax and reassure the client. It aids in identifying regions of tenderness and muscle resistance. The pads of the fingertips with the fingers together are used in a gentle dipping motion.

Deep palpation is essentially the same as light palpation except that the examiner is pressing much deeper. The approach can be single handed, or the palpating hand (the dominant hand) can be reinforced with fingers of the other hand (Figure 5–2). In this instance, the underlying hand receives the tactile sensations while the upper hand exerts the pressure.

Rebound is a palpatory technique often used for assessment of peritoneal inflammation with appendicitis. Only experienced examiners should palpate for rebound tenderness. Great caution is necessary. The fingertips are pressed deeply into the abdominal wall and quickly withdrawn. Pain felt after withdrawal of pressure is called **rebound tenderness** and is a reliable sign of peritoneal inflammation.

Bimanual palpation is the use of two hands in assessing an organ or mass. One hand may be placed at either side of the mass, grasping it, or one hand may support an organ to move it upward or more forward to make it more accessible to the examining hand. Bimanual palpation is routinely done in examining the kidneys, liver, spleen, and uterus.

Percussion

Percussion is the technique of striking a body surface lightly but sharply to produce sounds. The sounds enable the examiner to determine position, size, and density of an underlying organ.

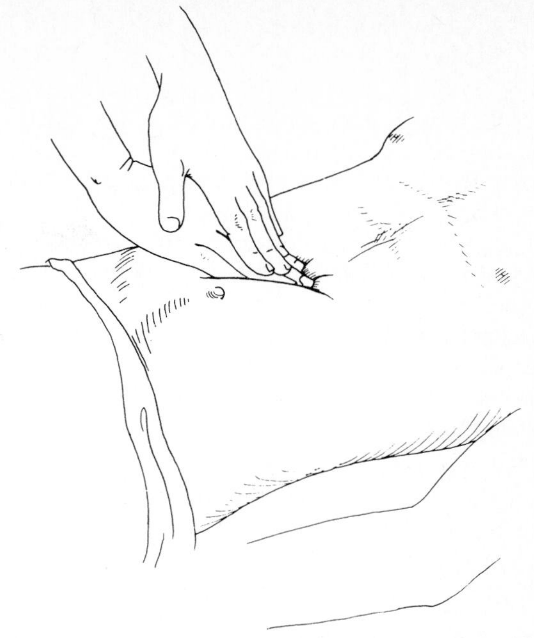

Figure 5–2

Deep palpation. The examiner uses two hands to press deeper into the client's abdomen.

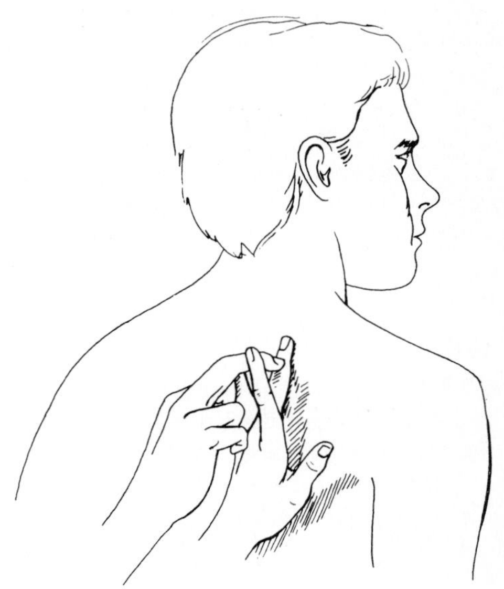

Figure 5–3

Indirect percussion technique to assess the lung sounds.

In *indirect percussion,* the middle finger of the nondominant hand (the **pleximeter**) is placed against the body surface with palms and other fingers raised off the skin. The tip of the middle finger of the dominant hand (the **plexor**) strikes the base of the distal phalanx of the pleximeter in a quick, sharp stroke. A series of two to three quick blows is struck. The pleximeter is then moved to a new site, and percussion continues in symmetrical regions, comparing the sounds from side to side (Figure 5–3). Percussion notes are:

- Resonance: A loud, low note heard over normal lung tissue
- Hyperresonance: A louder, lower, longer note heard over an emphysematous lung
- Tympany: A loud musical note with a drumlike quality, heard over air-filled viscera such as the stomach or bowel
- Dullness: Medium sound heard in areas of increased density (eg, over the liver)
- Flatness: A short, high-pitched sound produced over solid tissue such as the muscles of the thigh

Direct percussion is a gentle direct striking of the body with one or more fingers or with the ulnar surface of the clenched fist. This technique is useful in assessing tenderness in an underlying organ such as a sinus, a kidney, or the liver.

Auscultation

Auscultation is accomplished by use of a stethoscope to evaluate sounds arising from the lungs, the abdomen, and the cardiovascular system. Basic to proper auscultation is a good stethoscope with both a bell and a diaphragm. The stethoscope should be warmed before it touches the client's bare skin. The bell of the stethoscope is used for low-pitched sounds such as murmurs and bruits and is applied lightly to the skin surface. The diaphragm is firmly applied and is used for detecting high-pitched sounds. The bell is also useful on male chests whose hair may scratch against the diaphragm or on a thin client where the diaphragm will not lie flat between the ribs.

Smell

The odor of the breath, sputum, ear drainage, vomitus, urine, feces, vaginal discharge, or pus may be diagnostic. The nurse is exposed repeatedly to these smells, and observations about them may offer important diagnostic clues. For example, foul-smelling sputum may be indicative of a lung abscess or bronchiectasis.

The Physical Examination

A physical examination may be regional (eg, a neurologic assessment), combined (eg, respiratory, cardiac, and abdominal assessment), or a complete physical assessment from head to toe. An organized, sequential approach to the physical examination is important because it saves unnecessary position change for the client and assists the examiner in remembering all parts of the assessment. The approach also saves time. Remember that the skin of every bodily part is carefully inspected during each phase of the examination. A sample physical examination write-up is shown in Box 5–4.

Vital Signs

Body temperature, pulse, respirations, and blood pressure, along with measurement of height and weight are the first assessments taken. Specifics of each are taught in nursing fundamentals courses. The additional important aspects of blood pressure and pulse in total assessment will be mentioned in this section.

Blood pressure should be measured in three positions—supine, seated, and standing—to evaluate the effect of position change. To obtain a baseline supine reading, have the client remain flat for about 10 minutes. Allow 2 to 3 minutes with each position change to assess seated and standing pressures. In orthostatic hypotension, dizziness or even syncope (fainting) occurs when the client stands, associated with a sudden drop in arterial blood pressure. Common causes of *orthostasis* include prolonged immobility, peripheral venous stasis, and use of antihypertensive drugs. In a specific assessment for orthostasis, the standing blood pressure is taken immediately and again after the client has been standing for 3 minutes to note the early drop followed by return to normal.

Blood pressure should also be measured in both arms. Blood pressure normally varies somewhat from arm to arm but should not vary widely. A rudimentary cervical rib or a tight scalene muscle may compress the brachial plexus or subclavian artery on one side. In this circumstance, the blood pressure may not be auscultated or palpated on the affected side. To confirm a suspicion of this problem, which is called *thoracic outlet syndrome,* ask the client to turn the head to the affected side, extend the neck, and take a deep breath. Obstruction of the brachial pulse constitutes a positive *Adson's test* for thoracic outlet syndrome.

Normally, leg blood pressures are somewhat higher than blood pressures in the arm because the muscle mass of the thigh offers greater resistance to arterial compression. Hypertension in the arm pressures of a young client should alert the nurse to the possibility of coarctation of the aorta. To evaluate a client for aortic coarctation:

- Ask the client to assume the prone position.
- Apply a large blood pressure cuff appropriate to the size of the thigh.
- Place a stethoscope over the popliteal artery.

In aortic coarctation, the arm pressures are hypertensive and the leg pressures markedly lower. A comparison of the pulses finds weak femoral pulses with full, bounding brachial and radial pulses.

Assessment of the Skin

The skin is the largest organ of the human body and one of the most visible. Following evaluation of vital signs, begin the physical assessment with inspection of the visible skin. Through inspection and palpation of the skin, the nurse can easily identify cyanosis, icterus (jaundice), fever, dehydration, and edema. Subtle skin lesions may be an

Box 5–4
Sample Physical Examinatiobn Write-Up

Height: 5 ft 4 in

Weight: 125 lb (56.8 kg)

Temperature: 97.8°F (36.6°C)

Pulse: 76

Respiration: 14

BP: Lying, 100/60 right arm, 96/62 left arm; seated, 106/70 right arm, 102/68 left arm; standing, 110/70 right arm, 108/70 left arm

WD/WN pleasant, articulate white female who appears younger than her stated age, wearing sunglasses to protect her eyes from the light

Skin, hair, nails: Pink; good skin turgor, no lesions or changes in pigmentation; hair glossy with appropriate distribution; nails s̄ brittleness, good capillary refill

Head and face: Normocephalic, symmetrical scalp s̄ lesions or areas of tenderness

Eyes: Vision 20/30 OD, OS OU, Snellen's chart; lashes and brows present; conjunctivae clear, sclerae white; PERRLA; EOMs nl, no nystagmus, no lid lag or ptosis; VFs intact; fundi benign

Ears: Hearing intact to whisper test bilat; Weber s̄ lateralization, Rinne AC > BC bilateral; auricles s̄ lesions; ear canals c̄ small amount cerumen; TMs pearly gray and mobile, landmarks visible

Nose and sinuses: Nose symmetrical, both nostrils patent; nasal mucosa slightly edematous and erythematous; watery discharge; frontal and maxillary sinuses s̄ tenderness

Mouth and pharynx: Lips s̄ lesions; teeth in good repair, no dentures or partial plates; buccal mucosa pink s̄ lesions; tongue mobile, s̄ lesions and protrudes midline; uvula rises midline on phonation; gag reflex present; tonsils absent; pharynx not injected; TMJ c̄ full ROM s̄ crepitation

Neck: Symmetrical; no obvious masses or pulsations; thyroid not palpable, trachea midline; one pea-sized freely movable, nontender posterior cervical node on left; full ROM; JVP not elevated; ō carotid bruits

Breasts and axillae: Symmetrical, ō dimpling, ō retraction, ō discharge, ō masses; ō axillary adenopathy

Chest: Expansion = bilat; AP diameter not ↑; tactile fremitus = bilat; resonant to percussion; diaphragmatic excursion = bilat; clear to auscultation; no rales, rhonchi, or wheezes

Heart: PMI visible 5th LICS just medial to the MCL; PMI also palpable; no precordial thrills or lifts; apical rate 66, NSR; S_1S_2 nl, split S_2 at pulmonic area; no murmur, no gallop

Abdomen: Flat, s̄ scars or skin lesions; ō bruits; bowel sounds normoactive; ō tenderness or masses; liver, spleen, kidneys not palpable; liver 8 cm at rt MCL; ō CVA tenderness, ō inguinal adenopathy

Pelvic: External genitalia s̄ lesions; vaginal vault c̄ small amount menstrual blood; cervix pink, s̄ lesions. Bimanual: uterus retroverted, mobile, firm, smooth, not enlarged; adnexae s̄ tenderness; rectal: no external lesions, good sphincter tone; no masses; stool heme ⊖

Extremities: Joints s̄ swelling; full ROM joints and spine; muscle strength intact; no pedal edema; varicose veins bilat, more severe on rt leg

Pulses: (on a 4-point scale)	Radial	Ulnar	Brachial	Carotid	Femoral	Popliteal	Posterior tibial	Dorsalis pedis
Right:	4+	3+	4+	4+	4+	3+	3+	3+
Left:	4+	3+	4+	4+	4+	3+	3+	3+

Neurologic: Oriented ×3; recent and remote memory intact; speech clear; CN II–XII intact; CN I not tested; sensory intact; gait nl; Romberg negative, rapid alternating movements nl

Reflexes: (graded on a 4-point scale)

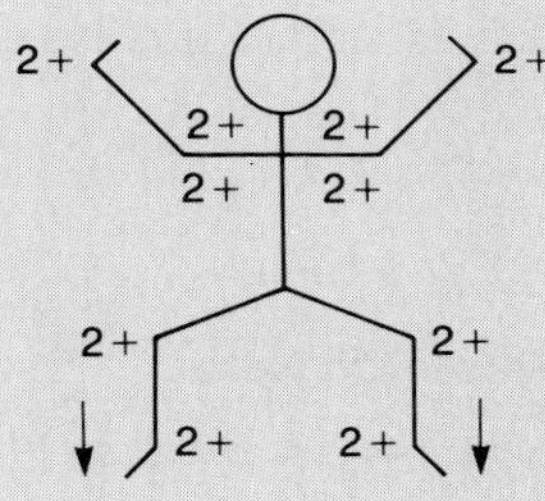

incidental finding during a health assessment. Skin lesions are classified as primary or secondary. A *primary lesion* is an original skin lesion from which a *secondary lesion* may result (eg, from scratching or infection). Skin lesions are discussed in Chapter 55.

The fingernails and skin of the hands and arms are inspected carefully and any visible lesions palpated. The head, scalp, and hair are inspected. The examiner parts the hair with the fingers to examine the underlying skin carefully. Then with each phase of the physical assessment that follows, the exposed skin areas are examined during the inspection and palpatory phases.

Specific skin lesions must be observed systematically, or important information will be overlooked. Description of each lesion and group of lesions includes:

- Type of lesion:
  - Flat (eg, macule)
  - Elevated (eg, papule)
  - Depressed (eg, ulcer)
- Shape of the individual lesion
- Color of the lesion (include dominant hue and color pattern)
- Configuration of groups of lesions:
  - Linear
  - Annular (circular)

Serpiginous (snakelike or creeping)
Iris (bull's eye pattern)
Zosteriform (in the area of a nerve distribution)

- Surface characteristics of the lesions:
  Scaly
  Dry
  Wet
  Greasy
- Anatomical distribution of lesions

Pressure ulcers (also called decubitus ulcers) are a major risk factor for clients who are inactive, immobile, incontinent, or malnourished. Most pressure ulcers develop over the ischial tuberosity, trochanter, sacrum, or calcaneus. The malleoli, elbows, scapulae, patellae, pretibial area, and occiput can also be affected. Inspect these skin areas thoroughly to detect early skin breakdown. Prevention of pressure ulcers is a major nursing responsibility.

Skin turgor, the normal fullness and elasticity of the skin, is assessed by picking up and releasing a small area of skin. This assessment is best done on the forearm, the dorsum of the hand, or over the sternum. Healthy skin springs back into position immediately. Dehydrated skin remains elevated for some time. Skin loses some elasticity in the course of normal aging.

Assessment of the Head and Face

Inspect the head and face for asymmetry, obvious deformities, and areas of erythema. Observe color, character, and distribution of hair. Palpate the head and scalp for lumps, lesions, or areas of tenderness and feel hair for flexibility, brittleness, or dryness.

Two cranial nerves are evaluated during assessment of the face. The trigeminal nerve, or fifth cranial nerve (CN V), is involved with facial sensation and chewing. A mixed nerve with both sensory and motor components, CN V is tested by evaluating the client's ability to open and close the mouth. The sensory portion is checked by touching the client, whose eyes are closed, with a sharp and a dull object in symmetrical areas on the face and by having the client say whether the sensation is sharp or dull.

The facial nerve, or seventh cranial nerve (CN VII), is involved with facial movement, tasting, salivation, and crying. Also a mixed nerve with both sensory and motor components, CN VII is tested by asking the client to wrinkle the forehead, raise the eyebrows, frown, smile, puff out the cheeks, and close the eyes so tightly the examiner is unable to open them forcibly. Observe for any asymmetry, especially in the nasolabial folds.

Nursing Research Note

Tachovsky B: Indirect auscultatory blood pressure measurement at two sites in the arm. *Res Nurs Health* 1985; 8:125–129.

Indirect auscultatory blood pressure measurements at the upper arm (brachial) site and the forearm (radial) site were compared. The forearm site is often recommended for measuring blood pressure on obese clients. For the brachial site, a pressure cuff was applied at the right arm 2.5 cm above the antecubital fossa. For the radial site, a cuff was applied between the middle and distal third of the forearm.

The results, obtained from a sample of 98 female nursing students, indicated a statistically significant systolic difference. The brachial site readings averaged 7.35 mm Hg higher than at the forearm site. There was also a statistically significant difference in diastolic readings. The forearm site had a mean diastolic reading of 14.1 mm Hg higher than the brachial site.

One might ask how clinically significant these findings are. The brachial site remains the site of choice, and pressure should be measured with the appropriate-sized cuff.

Assessment of the Eyes

VISUAL ACUITY Evaluation of visual acuity is an important aspect of health assessment. Snellen's chart is commonly used (see Figure 51–3). Clients stand (or sit) 20 ft from the chart and cover one eye at a time, reading the letters on the chart from the top down. The last row in which the client can read all but one or two of the letters is recorded as the visual acuity for that eye. After the right eye (OD) and the left eye (OS) have been tested individually, both eyes (OU) should be tested together. If the client wears corrective lenses, these should be worn during the exam. In Snellen's chart, the upper number refers to the distance at which the normal eye would see the letter; eg, a notation of 20/50 vision OD indicates that the right eye sees at only 20 ft what a normal eye could see at 50 feet.

Other means to evaluate visual acuity include having clients read from a hand-held card developed for use at the bedside or reading from a newspaper or any printed matter; having them count fingers or, in the case of severe visual problems, checking for perception of light and dark. Assessment of visual acuity is one measure of the function of the optic nerve, or the second cranial nerve (CN II).

ALIGNMENT, LIDS, CONJUNCTIVAE, LACRIMAL APPARATUS The internal structures of the eye are shown in Figure 50–1. The eyes are inspected for symmetry and width of palpebral fissures. The lids are inspected for edema, exudate, scaling, or ptosis. The conjunctivae are evaluated for pallor, vascular injection, edema, and **pinguecula** (yellow raised fatty plaques usually seen nasally).

The lacrimal gland is located in the superior lateral region of the upper eyelid. When swollen, the gland may be visible between the upper lid and eyeball when the lateral upper lid is elevated. The puncta of the lacrimal ducts lie in the medial corner of each upper and lower lid. Excess tears are drained via these ducts into the lacrimal sac and the nasolacrimal duct, which empties into the nasal cavity.

CORNEA Shine a light obliquely on the cornea and note any scars, abrasions, elevations, or ulcers. **Arcus senilis,** a peripheral corneal opacity, is common in clients over age 60. It does not interfere with vision.

PUPILS Evaluate the pupils for shape, size, equality, and position. A pupil size chart is available on neurologic units; a millimeter ruler may also be used. Darken the room and test the pupillary reaction to light by having the client fix on an object in the distance. Then shine a penlight into the client's eye from the side. The pupil should constrict, and consensual constriction should occur in the unexposed eye. Test the other eye in the same manner. The pupils are also tested for **accommodation,** the process by which the eye adjusts for distance, maintaining a clear visual image with a shift in gaze. To assess accommodation, ask the client to look into the distance and then at the nurse's finger, which is held about 12 in from the client's nose. The eyes should converge (move inward), and both pupils should constrict. These pupillary assessments evaluate the oculomotor nerve, or the third cranial nerve (CN III). A normal pupil examination is recorded as PERRLA—pupils equal, round, reactive to light and accommodation.

EXTRAOCULAR MUSCLES Six pairs of extraocular muscles control the motions of the eyeball (globe): the superior, lateral, inferior, and medial rectus muscles and the superior and inferior oblique muscles. Three cranial nerves innervate these muscles: the oculomotor nerve (CN III); the trochlear nerve (CN IV); and the abducens nerve (CN VI). To remember which nerve innervates which muscles, use the mnemonic LR_6SO_4. Translated, it means the lateral rectus is innervated by CN VI and the superior oblique, by CN IV. This leaves CN III to innervate the other muscles.

To test extraocular movements (EOMs), have the client follow the nurse's finger with the eyes in the six cardinal positions of gaze (Figure 50–2). Both eyes should move in unison. At the extremes of lateral gaze, some clients demonstrate an involuntary rhythmic oscillating motion of the eyes called **nystagmus.** A few beats of nystagmus in these extreme positions is considered normal. In disease states, the pattern of nystagmus is helpful in differentiating labyrinthine and brain stem disorders.

LID LAG During evaluation of the EOMs, lid lag is also evaluated. Normally, no portion of the sclera is visible above the iris when the client is gazing straight ahead. With lid lag, the upper lid does not follow the movement of the eyeball when the eyes move from an upward position downward, and rims of sclerae remain visible above the irises. Lid lag is sometimes seen in clients with hyperthyroidism.

VISUAL FIELDS A gross estimate of the visual fields (VFs) is done by confrontation testing, a method of examination in which the VFs of the client are compared to those of the examiner.

- The nurse and the client are at the same eye level, about 3 ft apart.
- Have the client cover the left eye while the nurse covers the right. The client's uncovered eye should be fixed on the nurse's uncovered eye.
- The nurse holds a pencil in the hand midway between nurse and client; the nurse's arm is extended beyond the limits of the field of vision.
- Advance the pencil inward from the periphery toward the center, and ask the client to indicate when the pencil tip appears in the client's field of vision.

The testing should proceed from eight equally spaced directions. The entire procedure should then be repeated with the other eye.

When lesions occur in the optic chiasm, optic tract, or brain, the visual fields are affected, resulting in a variety of possible defects, depending on the specific location of the lesion. (See Figure 29–1.) Glaucoma may also cause visual-field defects.

Assessment of the Ears

AUDITORY ACUITY When evaluating hearing, only one ear is tested at a time. The other ear must be occluded with a finger, either the examiner's or the client's. Whispered and spoken voice tests are common ways of evaluating hearing. Stand 1 to 2 ft from the client's unoccluded ear and whisper in a quiet, medium, and loud tone. Have the client repeat what was heard. Next, check the hearing while speaking in a quiet, medium, and loud voice. Be sure the client is not lip reading. Repeat the tests with the other ear.

INSPECTION AND PALPATION The position, size, color, and symmetry of both ears are assessed. Sebaceous cysts, the tophi of gout, or infection of the puncture site of pierced ears all are possible findings on the auricle (pinna). The external auditory meatus is carefully inspected for discharge, swelling, or erythema. (Figure 50–4 depicts a cross section of the normal ear.)

Notice the odor of any ear discharge because certain organisms causing external otitis produce a distinctive bad odor. For example, the odor of ear discharge from a Pseudomonas infection is pungent and sweet, whereas the odor from a staphylococcal infection is like overripe cheese.

Assessment of the Nose and Sinuses

THE NOSE The contour of the external nose is examined for symmetry and palpated for areas of tenderness. Patency of each nostril is tested by occluding one while the client inhales through the other. The olfactory nerve, or first cranial nerve (CN I), is tested by having the client identify specific odors (eg, soap, tobacco, alcohol, or cof-

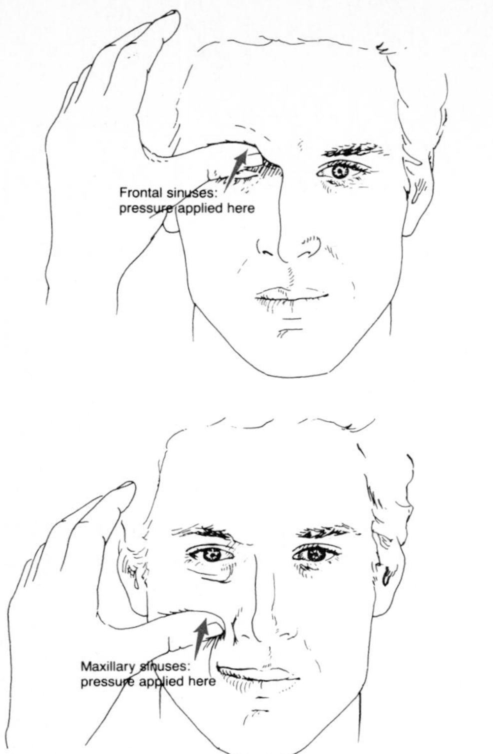

Figure 5–4

Palpation of the frontal and maxillary sinuses.

fee). Each nostril is tested separately while the client's eyes are closed.

THE SINUSES There are four pairs of paranasal sinuses: the frontal, maxillary, sphenoid, and ethmoid. Only the frontal and maxillary sinuses are accessible to evaluation by physical assessment techniques. The ethmoid and sphenoid sinuses must be studied radiographically.

The frontal sinuses are evaluated by palpation of the supraorbital ridge. The maxillary sinuses are assessed by palpation of the maxillary portions of the cheek (Figure 5–4). Firm steady pressure is used during palpation. Tenderness to palpation indicates sinus inflammation.

The frontal and maxillary sinuses are accessible to two additional approaches—*percussion* and *transillumination*. The supraorbital areas and cheeks can be directly percussed for tenderness in the same location where they were palpated. For transillumination of the sinuses, client and examiner must be in a dark room. The client's lips should be closed tightly around a lighted penlight. The two maxillary sinuses should be visible as a reddish glow. To visualize the frontal sinus, place the lighted penlight beneath the inner supraorbital ridge. The outline of the sinus should be visible as a faint glow.

Assessment of the Mouth and Pharynx

INSPECTION The external mouth and lips are carefully observed for color, symmetry, lesions, inflammation, and fissures. Normally, the lips are moist, smooth, and symmetric. Their color varies from pink to more darkly pigmented depending on the client's race.

For inspection of the internal mouth, a penlight and tongue blade are needed. If the client is wearing dentures, the bite and the general fit of the dentures are evaluated. The dentures are then removed so that the entire oral cavity can be carefully inspected. The buccal mucosa is assessed for color, ulcers, areas of pigmentation, and leukoplakia. The gums are inspected for inflammation, edema, pigmentation, retraction, or bleeding. Loose, missing, and carious teeth are noted. Normally, adults have a total of 32 permanent teeth. The color of the teeth may vary. Coloration may indicate conditions such as chronic smoking (yellow brown). Brownish pigmentation may indicate exposure to tetracycline in utero or having received tetracycline before age 7.

The tongue is carefully inspected for size, color, lesions, mobility, and symmetry. The client is asked to stick out the tongue, which should appear symmetrical, should protrude midline rather than deviate laterally, and should be movable from side to side. **Fasciculations** (fine twitchings) should not be present. These observations evaluate the hypoglossal nerve (CN XII). The lateral surfaces of the tongue are carefully inspected while the client's tongue is protruded. To facilitate careful observation, grasp the client's tongue with a piece of gauze and apply gentle traction to pull the tongue outward, exposing the posterior lateral surfaces. Also ask the client to touch the roof of the mouth with the tongue so that the undersurface of the tongue and the floor of the mouth can be inspected. The opening of Wharton's duct, the duct of the submandibular salivary gland (also called the submaxillary gland), is visible at the base of the frenulum of the tongue. The orifice of Stensen's duct, the duct of the parotid gland, is visible as a small papilla opposite the second upper molar.

The palate has two distinct divisions—the anterior two-thirds, or hard palate, and the posterior third, the soft palate, to which the uvula is attached. An unusual-appearing but relatively common finding on the hard palate is a midline bony outgrowth called **torus palatinus.** The uvula varies in width and length, occasionally becoming edematous with upper respiratory infections (URI), causing greater irritation in the throat. The glossopharyngeal nerve (CN IX), and the vagus nerve (CN X), are partially tested by inspecting for midline position of the uvula and rise of the soft palate when the client says "ahhh." Stimulation of the gag reflex by touching the pharyngeal wall with a tongue blade is also a test of CN IX and CN X. The vagus nerve has a broader distribution than any of the other cranial nerves, not restricted to the head and neck regions. The tonsillar pillars, the tonsils, and the posterior pharynx are easily evaluated while holding the tongue down with a tongue blade and using a penlight for visualization. In a client with a URI, there may be considerable mucus on the posterior pharyngeal wall and enlarged erythematous tonsils with or without exudates.

PALPATION The lateral surfaces of the tongue, the floor of the mouth, and any lesions on the lips or in the mouth should be palpated. The examiner wears a glove for this part of the assessment. Lesions should be described according to their size, shape, consistency, location, and tenderness.

The temporomandibular joint (TMJ), which is moved when the jaw is opened and closed, is one of the most active joints in the body. Whenever a person talks, chews, yawns, or swallows, the TMJ is exercised. Estimates are that the TMJ opens and closes 1500 to 2000 times a day. The TMJ must not be neglected when the mouth is assessed, because malocclusion or arthritic problems may damage the joint.

The TMJ is best palpated by placing the index fingers in the external auditory meatus and pressing anteriorly while the client slowly opens and closes the mouth. The joint is assessed for crepitation, clicking, pain, and range of motion (ROM).

Assessment of the Neck

The sternocleidomastoid muscles divide the neck into one anterior and two posterior triangles. Structures within the anterior triangle include the larynx, trachea, and thyroid. The internal jugular veins and carotid arteries lie partially beneath the sternocleidomastoid muscle. Their pulsations are often visible in the anterior triangle (Figure 5–5).

TRACHEA AND THYROID The anterior neck is carefully inspected for asymmetry, masses, abnormal pulsation, limitation in ROM, and tracheal deviation. The lower half of the anterior triangle is observed for enlargement of the thyroid gland. To inspect the thyroid, offer the client a glass of water and watch the neck during swallowing, looking for any ascending mass in the midline or arising from behind either sternocleidomastoid muscle. Thyroid tissue ascends during swallowing.

The trachea is normally seen in the midline and should be palpable at the suprasternal notch. Localized disease or disease within the cardiopulmonary system may cause tracheal deviation.

THE LYMPH NODES Lymph nodes of the head and neck are shown in Figure 5–6. Normally, these lymph nodes are not palpable. They enlarge secondary to a variety of disease processes, the most common being a URI. Most

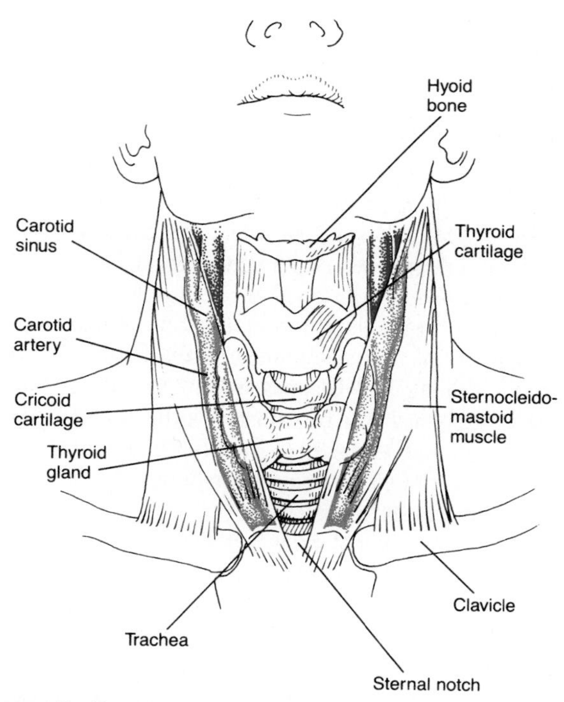

Figure 5–5

Anterior triangle of the neck, showing proximity of structures to carotid artery.

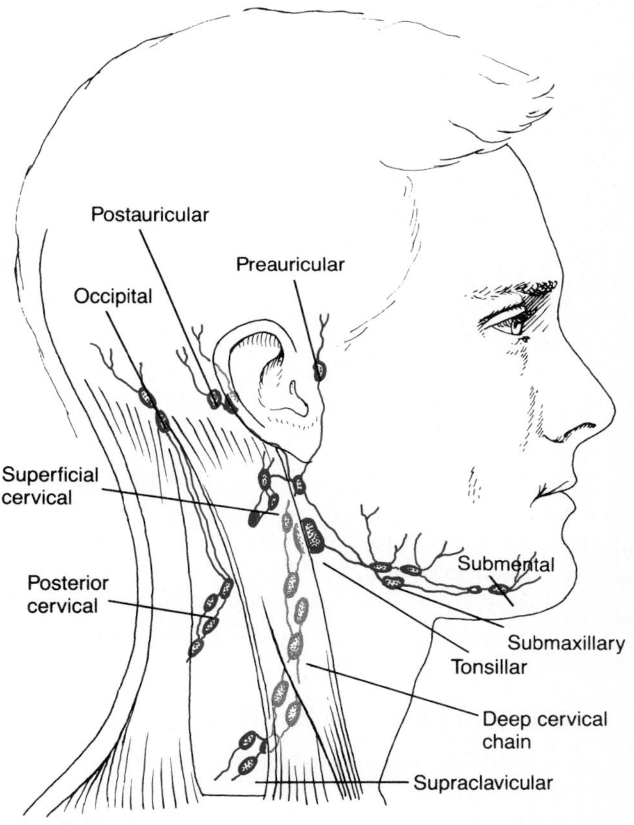

Figure 5–6

Lymph nodes of the head and neck. Palpate for each lymph node group with the fingertips.

persons have had these so-called "swollen glands" at one point or another in their lives. Occasionally, an individual will have an isolated persistently enlarged lymph node in the neck. One isolated node that does not change in size or consistency is not abnormal. In fact, instructors often look for these in their students so others can learn what an enlarged lymph node feels like. They are called "teaching nodes."

The fingertips are used to evaluate the cervical lymph nodes. The neck is palpated sequentially in the areas of the various lymph node groups, beginning with the preauricular node slightly anterior to the tragus. The posterior auricular, occipital, tonsillar, submaxillary, submental, superficial cervical, posterior cervical chain, deep cervical chain, and supraclavicular nodes are examined in sequence. Any palpable nodes should be described in terms of their location, size, shape, consistency, mobility, tenderness, and whether they are discrete or clumped.

An isolated node in the supraclavicular region may be an ominous sign. The *sentinal node* or *Virchow's node,* usually seen in the left supraclavicular group, indicates metastasis from a carcinoma in the upper abdomen (DeGowin & DeGowin, 1981).

NECK RANGE OF MOTION AND THE ELEVENTH CRANIAL NERVE To check ROM of the neck, have the client touch chin to chest (anteflexion), tilt the head backwards (dorsiflexion), touch the chin to each shoulder (rotation), and touch the ear to each shoulder (lateral flexion). The accessory nerve (CN XI) is a motor nerve that supplies the trapezius and sternocleidomastoid muscles. (CN XI was formerly called the spinal accessory nerve.) To test its function, ask the client to shrug the shoulders against resistance. Note the strength of the trapezius muscles. Then have the client turn the head to each side while the examiner resists with pressure against the client's chin. Observe the prominence of the opposite sternocleidomastoid muscle and the strength of the client's movement against resistance.

THE CAROTID ARTERIES Inspect the neck carefully for any pulsations. The carotid pulsations may be visualized just medial to the sternocleidomastoid muscles. Palpate the carotid pulses individually, comparing one side with the other. Take care to avoid the carotid sinus, located below the upper level of the thyroid cartilage; pressure on the carotid sinus can slow the heart.

Assessment of the Breasts

Although this discussion of breast assessment focuses on the female breasts, men also develop breast problems, including malignancy. Consequently, the male breast and axilla should be examined routinely in physical assessment. The approach to examination is identical for both sexes.

INSPECTION The client is seated and exposed from the waist up for adequate visualization. The breasts are inspected for symmetry, skin dimpling, nipple retraction, nipple inversion, lesions, or masses. One breast may be slightly larger than the other, and sometimes there is a marked difference between the size of the breasts. Asymmetry is a normal finding if it has existed since breast development and abnormal if it is recent.

The breasts are then inspected while the client places hands on hips and tenses the chest muscles and while raising the arms over the head. The breasts are assessed again for size and shape, skin alterations, and changes in nipples and areolae. Also note whether both breasts elevate symmetrically when the arms are raised. If the breasts are extremely pendulous have the client assume alternative positions to visualize adequately sections of the breast tissue. Having the client lean forward with hands on the back of a chair for support will demonstrate whether the breasts fall away from the thorax as they should. The axillary, supraclavicular, and infraclavicular regions should also be inspected for evidence of bulging, retraction, edema, or asymmetry.

PALPATION Initial palpation of the breast and surrounding areas is done with the client seated. The supraclavicular and infraclavicular regions are assessed for enlarged lymph nodes. Having the client elevate the shoulders permits deeper palpation in the supraclavicular region. During axillary palpation, the examiner supports the client's arm, keeping it quite close to the chest to relax the axillary muscles. This enables the examiner to reach deeply into the axilla. The examiner's fingers should be close together with the palm of the hand facing the chest wall. After palpation of the axillary region, move the fingers down along the surface of the ribs feeling for enlarged lymph nodes.

Actual palpation of the breast tissue is usually done with the client in a supine position. In several instances, it is also important to palpate while the client is seated. Certainly, if a suspicious sign is seen on inspection, such as a dimpling of the skin on one breast, this area should be palpated with the client in both seated and supine positions. In addition, the area should be marked with a pen, because the finding may disappear when the client is supine. Very large breasts should be palpated with the client seated as well as supine, because positive findings may be concealed, and palpation in various positions offers the best chance of locating early lesions.

Begin systematic palpation with the client supine and the arm on the side to be examined raised over the head to flatten the breast tissue. The pads of the fingertips of the middle three fingers are used for palpation. Peripheral breast tissue is composed of adipose tissue held in place by connective tissue. Centrally, the breast contains approximately 20 lobes of glandular tissue, each of which is drained by a single duct that opens onto the nipple (see Figure 47–4). There is a wide variation in how normal breast tissue feels. Age, stage of menstrual cycle, weight,

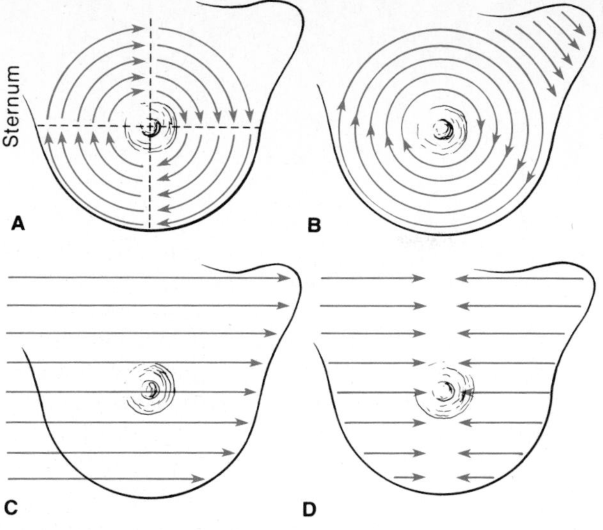

Figure 5–7

Four approaches to breast palpation. **A.** Quadrant-by-quadrant approach. **B.** Concentric-circle approach. **C.** From sternum to AAL. **D.** From AAL to midline; from sternum to midline.

pregnancy, and diet all affect the consistency of the tissue. During palpation, keep in mind the normal structures of the breast and the information gathered about the client when the history was obtained.

The breasts are palpated in a rotary motion with the pads of the fingers, compressing the breast tissue against the chest wall. Systematic palpation is imperative so a section of tissue will not be overlooked. Four approaches have been recommended (Figure 5–7):

- A quadrant-by-quadrant approach
- A concentric-circle approach beginning at the nipple and working outward or beginning at the clavicular region and working inward
- From the sternum to the anterior axillary line
- From the anterior axillary line to midline; from sternum to midline

Regardless of the sequence, the objective is a complete assessment of the breasts. The axillary tail, a section of breast tissue extending into the axilla, must not be overlooked. Throughout the assessment, teach the client the importance and proper technique of breast self-examination. In most instances, the examination sequence should be consistent with what is taught and with any printed information given to the client. If it is not, explain why the examination was conducted in one way, but the printed pamphlet suggests another. For example, say, "The pamphlet I gave you shows a woman examining her breasts in concentric circles. Because you are a large-breasted woman, I can feel your breast tissue better by starting at your breast bone, moving to your nipple, and then repositioning your breast and examining from under your arm across to the nipple. Let's see which approach works best when you examine yourself."

Palpation of the breast is completed by palpating the nipple and then by squeezing it to look for nipple discharge.

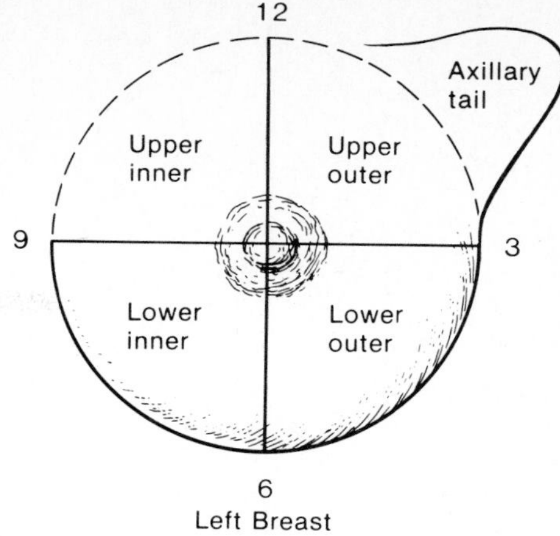

Figure 5–8

Quadrant and face-of-clock method of recording breast findings.

Any discharge obtained may be wiped on a glass slide and sent for a Pap smear or a Gram's stain if infection is suspected. Bilateral milky or watery discharge may not be problematic. Unilateral bloody discharge deserves immediate attention. Many women have inverted nipples or nipples that invert and evert regularly. A unilateral, fixed nipple inversion of recent onset suggests malignancy.

Any lesions are described according to their location, size, shape, consistency, and mobility. In recording the location of findings, use either the four quadrants of the breast or the face-of-the-clock approach (Figure 5–8).

Assessment of the Thorax and Lungs

To locate certain anatomical areas and describe chest findings adequately, the nurse must be familiar with common reference points on the chest. The manubrium of the sternum, the sternal angle or angle of Louis, the intercostal spaces, the costochondral junctions, and the xiphoid process all are important anterior landmarks (Figure 5–9). Addi-

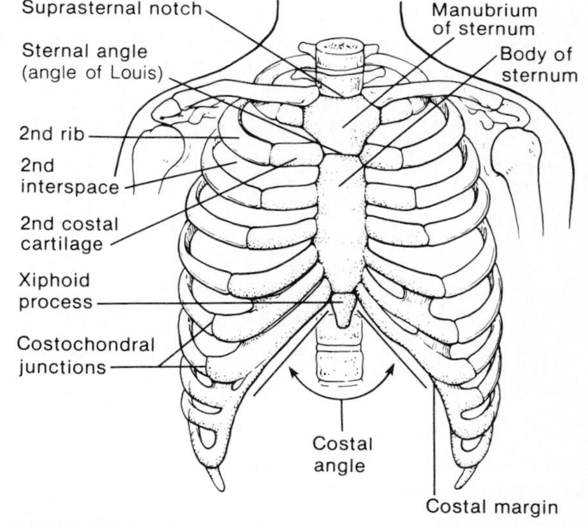

Figure 5–9

Anatomic landmarks on the anterior chest.

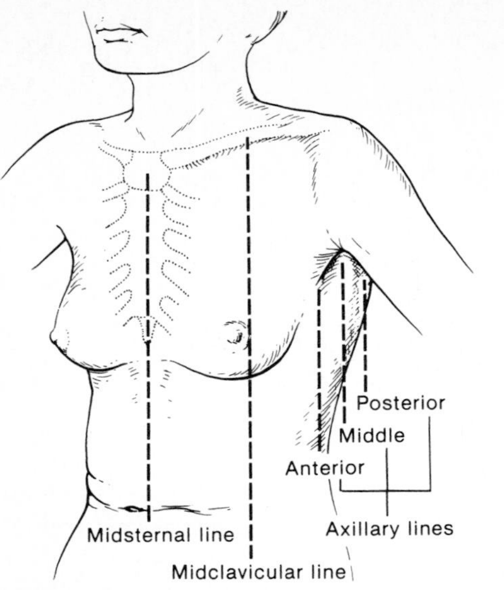

Figure 5–10

Reference points on the chest for describing the location of physical findings.

tional reference points are a series of imaginary lines drawn on the anterior, lateral, and posterior thorax (Figure 5–10). These include the:

- Midsternal line (MSL)
- Midclavicular line (MCL)
- Anterior axillary line (AAL)
- Midaxillary line (MAL)
- Posterior axillary line (PAL)

POSTERIOR CHEST

INSPECTION AND PALPATION Standing behind the client, who is seated and exposed from the waist up, the examiner inspects the posterior chest. The following assessments are made:

- Note skeletal deformities such as scoliosis, a lateral curvature of the thoracic spine, or increased anteroposterior (AP) diameter of the chest as seen in pulmonary emphysema (also called barrel chest).
- Inspect the skin for lesions and surgical scars. Note the respiratory movements and any retraction or bulging of the interspaces during respiration.
- Position the hands on the lateral lower rib cage with thumbs close to the spine, with a loose fold of skin between them. With normal respiratory excursion, the entire thorax should move as a unit. Therefore, as the client inhales, the examiner's hands should move in synchrony and the thumbs should diverge equally from the midline.

The posterior chest is palpated for tenderness and areas of crepitation. **Crepitation,** a coarse crackling sensation, is caused by escape of air from the lungs into the subcutaneous tissue, usually as a result of thoracic trauma or surgery. This condition is called *subcutaneous emphysema.*

Assess the chest for **tactile fremitus,** a palpable vibration of air through the airways as a person speaks. Have the client say "99" repeatedly while the examiner places the palmar bases of the fingers of the dominant hand on the interspaces. Some examiners find the ulnar surface of the hand more sensitive for assessing vibratory palpation. The examining hand is moved in sequence while symmetrical chest areas are compared side to side. If fremitus is faint, ask the client to lower the pitch of the voice. Increased fremitus is normally found anteriorly over the parasternal regions and posteriorly in the interscapular areas because these areas lie closest to the main-stem bronchi. Increased lung density transmits air vibrations better than the healthy air-filled structures of the lungs. Therefore, any condition that increases lung density (eg, the consolidation that occurs in pneumonia) increases the vibration and thus palpatory fremitus. With pleural thickening, fluid in the pleural space, or bronchial obstruction, tactile fremitus is decreased or absent.

The level of the diaphragm on each side may also be estimated by vibratory palpation. The ulnar surface of the hand is placed on the interspaces, parallel to the diaphragm, beginning in the midlung fields and working downward to the costovertebral angle. The diaphragmatic level is approximated in the area where fremitus is no longer palpable.

AUSCULTATION The lungs are auscultated with the diaphragm of the stethoscope placed firmly on the interspaces. The client is asked to breathe slowly and deeply through the mouth. Because some clients may hyperventilate and others may find deep breathing painful and/or exhausting, be conscious of how the client is responding during the examination. It may be necessary to offer the client opportunities to rest between auscultatory assessments.

Auscultation begins at the apices and continues down the chest wall. Symmetrical areas are compared. Keep in mind the anatomy of the right and left lung while auscultating so important areas will not be overlooked. Remember that the right lung has three lobes and the left has only two. The lower lobes are divided from the upper lobes by an oblique fissure (Figures 5–11 and 5–12). This information is important when percussing and auscultating the chest because the lateral or axillary lung fields may be inadvertently omitted during routine anterior and posterior assessment. Significant findings may be missed without special attention to lateral assessment. For example, pathologic conditions in the right middle lobe can be detected only in the right axilla and anterior thorax.

Normal breath sounds are of three types: vesicular, bronchovesicular, and bronchial (see Table 5–1). Abnor-

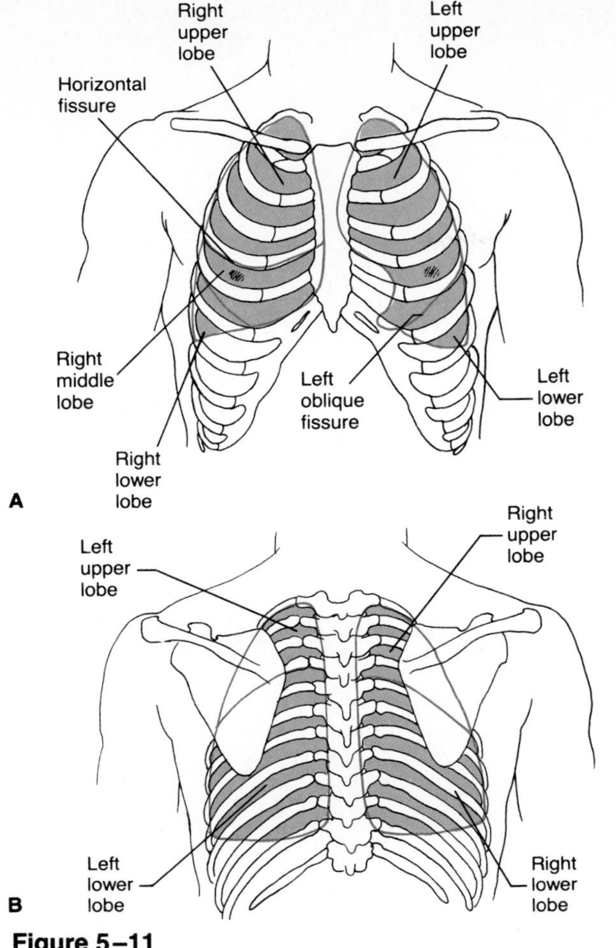

Figure 5–11

Major lung fissures and lobes projected on the anterior and posterior surfaces of the chest. **A.** Anterior. **B.** Posterior.

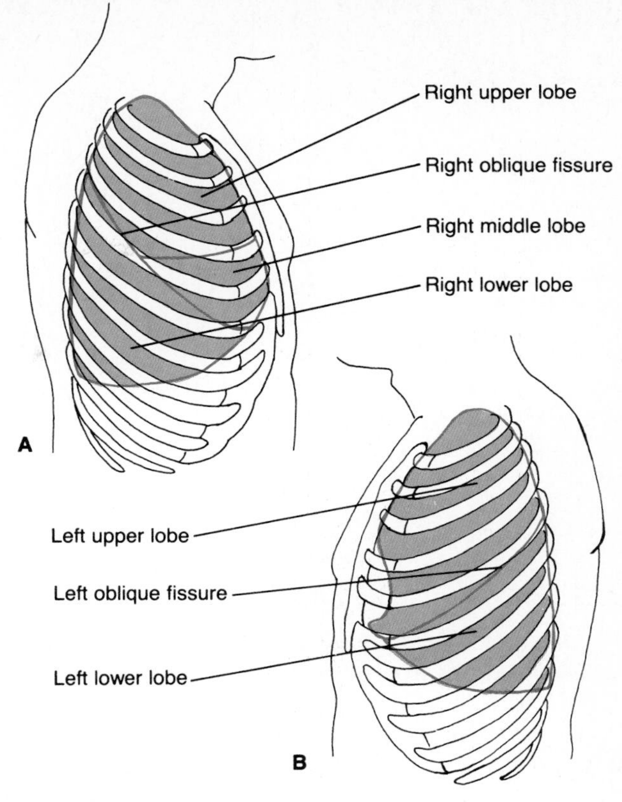

Figure 5–12

Major lung fissures and lobes projected on the lateral surfaces of the chest. **A.** Right. **B.** Left.

mal breath sounds *(adventitious sounds)* often auscultated with pulmonary disease include:

- **Inspiratory crackles** (rales)—noncontinuous sounds that occur when previously closed airways reopen resulting in equalization of pressure. Early inspiratory crackles are heard in clients with airway obstruction (eg, COPD). Late inspiratory crackles, heard mainly at the lung bases, occur when lung compliance is reduced (eg, CHF).
- **Rhonchi**—gurgling sounds originating in the larger air passages; these are also called *coarse rales.*
- **Wheezes**—whistling sounds resulting from the narrowing of respiratory passages.
- **Pleural friction rub**—leathery, grating sound produced when inflamed or roughened pleural surfaces rub together.

Table 5–1
Normal Breath Sounds and Their Characteristic Patterns

Description of Normal Breath Sounds	Characteristic Pattern
Vesicular: Have a long inspiratory phase and short expiratory phase and are heard over most of the lung surface.	Inspiration / \ Expiration — Vesicular
Bronchovesicular: Have equal inspiratory and expiratory phases and are heard over the main-stem bronchi.	Inspiration / \ Expiration — Bronchovesicular
Bronchial or tubular: Have a short inspiratory phase and long expiratory phase; bronchial sounds are not normally heard over the lung but are the normal sounds heard when listening over the trachea.	Inspiration / \ Expiration — Bronchial

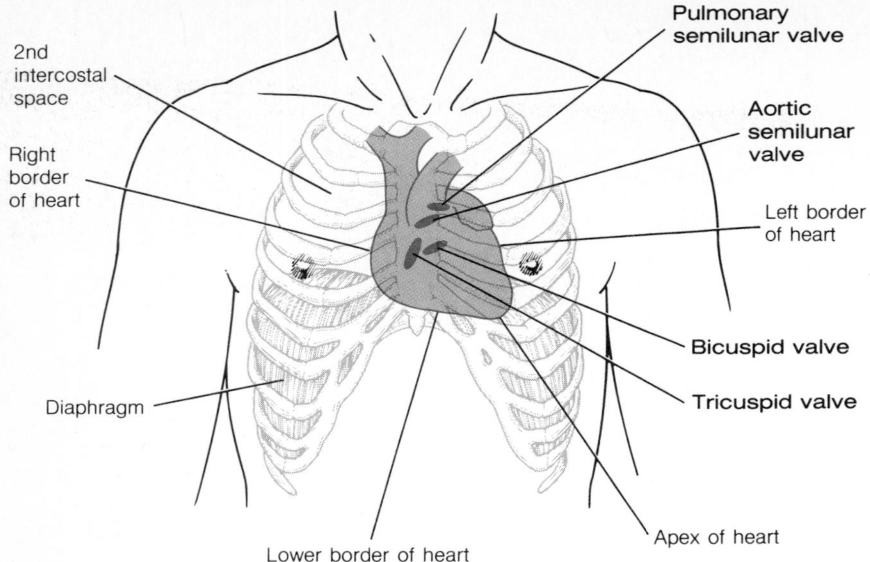

Figure 5–13

Anterior view of the thorax showing the position of the heart and the heart valves in relation to the ribs, sternum, and diaphragm. SOURCE: *Spence AP, Mason EB:* Human Anatomy and Physiology, *3rd ed. Menlo Park, CA: Benjamin/Cummings, 1987.*

ANTERIOR CHEST Assessment of the anterior chest proceeds in the same sequence. Anterior assessment may be done with the client seated or supine. In the female client, the breast tissue is flattened or displaced during auscultation.

Assessment of the Heart

INSPECTION AND PALPATION With the client supine, the **precordium,** the area of the anterior chest overlying the heart (Figure 5–13) is inspected for visible pulsations and areas of retraction. Tangential lighting is helpful. The **point of maximal impulse** (PMI) is specifically sought. The PMI represents the systolic thrust of the cardiac apex, which is sometimes visible in the fifth left intercostal space (LICS) at or just medial to the left MCL. Left ventricular hypertrophy displaces the PMI downward and to the left, lateral to the left MCL.

Palpate for the PMI in the fifth LICS at the MCL whether or not it is visible. Then palpate over the entire precordium, using the palmar bases of the fingers, which are most sensitive to vibration. Evaluate the precordium for **thrills** (palpable vibrations similar to those felt on the throat of a purring cat), thrusts, or lifts. A lifting motion of the lower left parasternal area during systole is indicative of right ventricular hypertrophy.

THE CARDIAC CYCLE AND RELATED HEART SOUNDS A review of the normal events in the cardiac cycle may help in understanding the heart sounds and what they mean. During diastole, pressure in the left atrium, which has been filled by blood returning through the pulmonary veins, slightly exceeds pressure in the left ventricle; therefore, blood flows across the open mitral valve from left atrium into the left ventricle. Just before the onset of ventricular systole, the atrium contracts (the *atrial kick*), forcing more blood into the ventricle. As the ventricle begins to contract, the pressure within it rises rapidly, exceeding the pressure in the atrium, forcing the mitral valve closed. The rising ventricular pressure soon exceeds the pressure in the aorta, causing the aortic valve to open. As the blood is ejected, ventricular pressure continues to rise and then drops off when most of the blood has been emptied. The aortic valve closes when left ventricular pressure drops below aortic pressure. As left ventricular pressure continues to drop, it falls below left atrial pressure; the mitral valve opens and ventricular filling begins anew. The same events also occur on the right side of the heart, almost simultaneously, but events on the left side occur a little sooner.

HEART SOUNDS Closure of the valves causes normal heart sounds. The most important sounds are the *first heart sound* (S_1) and the *second heart sound* (S_2) because they divide the cardiac cycle into systole and diastole. The first heart sound (S_1) is synchronous with the apical impulse (PMI) and corresponds to the onset of ventricular systole. Closure of the mitral and tricuspid valves produces S_1, which sounds like the syllable "lub."

The second heart sound (S_2) occurs at the termination of systole and corresponds with the onset of ventricular diastole. Closure of the aortic and pulmonic valves produces S_2, which sounds like the syllable "dup." Both S_1 and S_2 are clearly audible over all valve areas in healthy persons and together sound like "lub dup."

The third heart sound (S_3), if present, occurs in early diastole during the phase of rapid ventricular filling, as blood flows from left atrium to left ventricle. Phonetically S_1, S_2, and S_3 together sound like LUB duppa. An S_3 is considered normal when heard in children and young adults. The fourth heart sound (S_4), if present, occurs late in diastole or just prior to S_1 and is caused by atrial contraction (atrial kick). Phonetically S_4, S_1, and S_2 together sound like da-LUB dup. An S_4 is often heard in healthy persons. An S_3 may indicate ventricular failure in older adults. An S_4 may suggest cardiac disease such as aortic stenosis or hypertension.

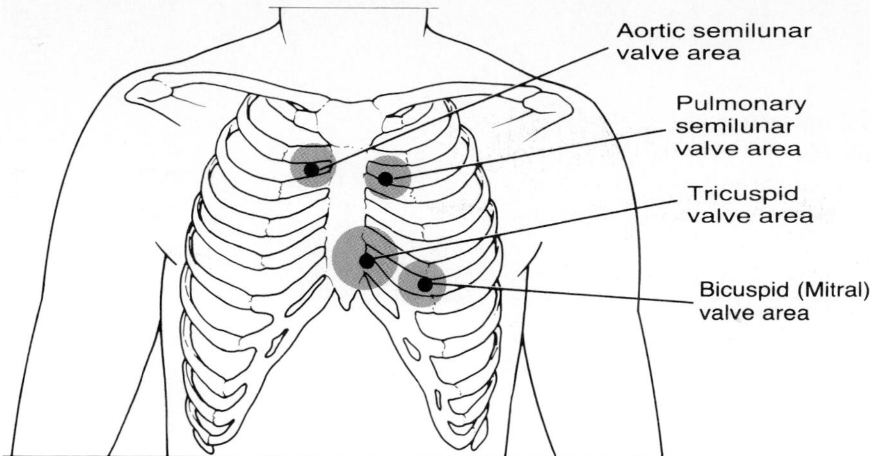

Figure 5–14

Normal heart sounds. Areas of the chest where sounds associated with the heart valves can best be heard. SOURCE: *Spence AP, Mason EB:* Human Anatomy and Physiology, *3rd ed. Menlo Park, CA: Benjamin/Cummings, 1987.*

RELATION OF HEART SOUNDS TO THE CHEST WALL The precordial areas where the heart sounds are most audible do not correspond to the anatomical valve locations as seen in Figure 5–13 but to the following auscultatory areas (Figure 5–14):

- Mitral (or apical or bicuspid) area—fifth LICS at, or just medial to, the MCL
- Tricuspid area—fifth LICS at the LSB
- Pulmonic area—second LICS at the LSB (base of the heart)
- Aortic area—second RICS at the RSB (base of the heart)

The first heart sound (S_1) is louder than S_2 at the cardiac apex and fainter than S_2 at the pulmonic and aortic areas. Because S_1 has two valvular components, mitral and tricuspid closure, and because events in the left heart occur slightly before events on the right, the sound of S_1 is occasionally split. The split of S_1 may be heard better in the tricuspid area, whereas a single component of S_1 is usual in the mitral area.

The second heart sound (S_2) also has two valvular components, the pulmonic and the aortic. S_2 is louder than S_1 at the base of the heart. The aortic component of S_2 is audible in all auscultatory areas, but the pulmonic component, which is weaker, is usually heard only in the second LICS at the LSB. Splitting of S_2 is considered normal only in the pulmonic area (DeGowin & DeGowin, 1981).

If audible, S_3 and S_4 are both heard best at the apex (mitral area). Because they are both low-pitched sounds, they are best heard with the bell of the stethoscope. The term **gallop rhythm** refers to auscultation of an S_3 or S_4 or both, along with S_1 and S_2, which altogether resemble the canter of a horse.

HEART MURMURS Heart **murmurs** are sounds resulting from vibrations produced by turbulence of blood flow in the heart or great vessels. Mechanisms of murmur production include increased velocity of blood flow; constriction or dilation of a cardiac valve, cardiac chamber, or great vessel; or shunting of blood through an abnormal opening. Murmurs are described according to their:

- Location (where best heard on the precordium)
- Radiation
- Timing (systolic or diastolic; early, middle, or late)
- Quality
- Intensity (grade 1 to 6)

The location on the precordium where a cardiac murmur is heard best and the areas to which it radiates are helpful in identifying the origin of the murmur. For example, the murmur of aortic valve stenosis is usually loudest in the second RICS at the RSB and often radiates into the neck.

Whether a murmur occurs in systole or diastole is also important in diagnosis. Systolic murmurs are much more common than diastolic murmurs, and many are benign. Diastolic murmurs are almost always pathologic. Holosystolic or pansystolic murmurs are heard throughout systole. If the murmur occurs during a certain phase of systole, it is recorded as early systolic, midsystolic, or late systolic.

The quality of a murmur describes whether it is harsh, blowing, or musical; its pitch (high or low); and its configuration. If the pitch increases, the pattern is crescendo. If the pitch decreases, the pattern is decrescendo. A diamond pattern is a murmur whose pitch increases and then decreases, called a crescendo–decrescendo murmur.

Murmurs are graded on a scale of 1 to 6:

- Grade 1—so faint it can be heard only with special effort
- Grade 2—quiet but easily recognized
- Grade 3—moderately loud
- Grade 4—loud
- Grade 5—very loud; may be heard with the stethoscope partially off the chest
- Grade 6—audible with the stethoscope entirely off the chest

A palpable thrill is often associated with grade 5 and 6 murmurs. When a murmur is recorded, note that a scale of 6 was used. For example, a grade 2 murmur would be recorded as "grade 2/6."

PERICARDIAL FRICTION RUB A pericardial friction rub arises from the rubbing together of the pericardial surfaces secondary to inflammation of the pericardial sac. The rub may be heard over the entire precordial region. The sound is usually described as scratchy, grating, or squeaky and may be heard through both systole and diastole. The rub may disappear and reappear. Having the client change position may alter the audibility of the rub.

AUSCULTATION When inspection and palpation have been completed, begin auscultation by placing the diaphragm of the stethoscope on the mitral area (apex) and identifying the sounds of S_1 and S_2. Count the apical rate for 1 minute. *Pulse deficit* is the difference between the apical rate and the peripheral pulse rate. Listen carefully for any rhythm irregularity. **Normal sinus rhythm** (NSR) is the orderly rhythm of the healthy heart, whose rate at rest is between 60 and 100 beats per minute.

Then move the stethoscope sequentially to the tricuspid, pulmonic, and aortic areas, listening for S_1, S_2, and any extra sounds in systole or diastole. Turn to the bell of the stethoscope and repeat the listening sequence in all auscultatory areas.

Ask the client to turn onto the left side while auscultating at the apex with the bell of the stethoscope. Murmurs and other sounds may be accentuated in this position, called the left lateral decubitus (LLD) position. Cardiac sounds can be further evaluated by having the client sit up and lean forward. The squatting position may intensify some heart murmurs.

Assessment of the Abdomen

Within the abdomen lie numerous organs and blood vessels, all of which must be considered during the assessment process. In description of examination findings, two topographic divisions of the abdomen are used. Figure 5–15 depicts the abdomen divided into four quadrants, probably the most common divisions. Figure 5–16 shows the abdomen sectioned into nine regions. This system is useful because of its three central areas—the epigastric, umbilical, and suprapubic. For example, it is clearer to describe the bladder as being in the suprapubic region than as being split between the right and left lower quadrants. Many clinicians use the four quadrant descriptions except for centrally located findings. During abdominal assessment, remember the organs found in each quadrant (see Box 5–5).

INSPECTION With the client supine and the entire abdomen exposed, look carefully at sequential areas of the abdomen and note:

- Skin color and lesions
- Striae (stretch marks)
- Scars
- Engorged veins
- Visible pulsations
- Visible peristalsis
- Umbilical position
- Herniation
- Abdominal profile

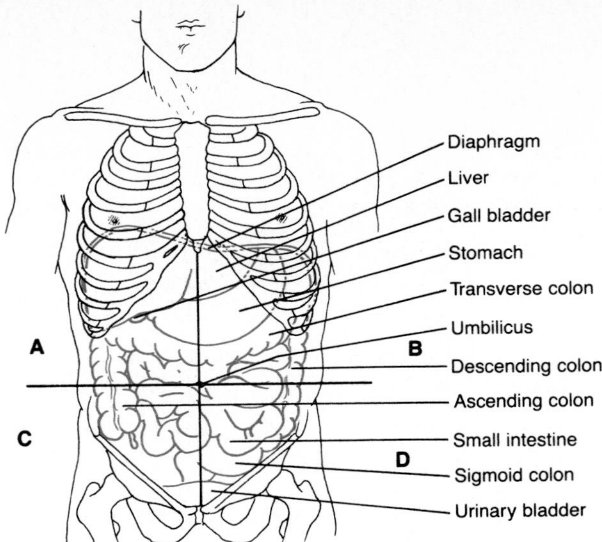

Figure 5–15

The four abdominal quadrants. **A.** Right upper quadrant (RUQ). **B.** Left upper quadrant (LUQ). **C.** Right lower quadrant (RLQ). **D.** Left lower quadrant (LLQ).

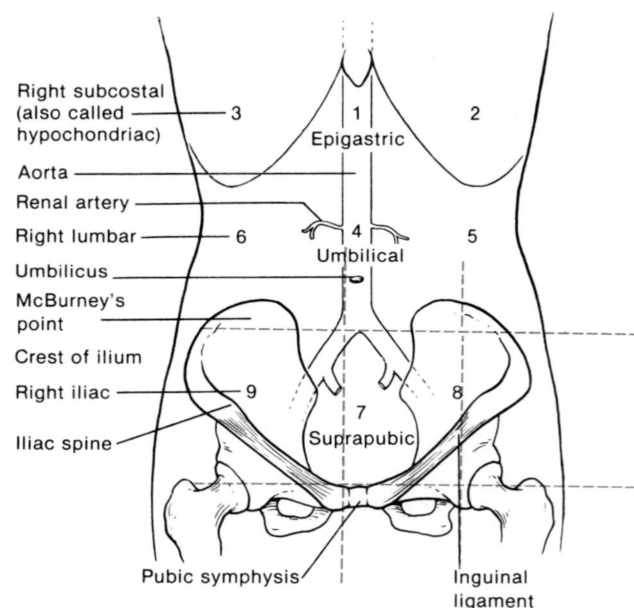

Figure 5–16

The nine abdominal regions: **1.** Epigastric region. **2** and **3.** Right and left subcostal or hypochondriac regions. **4.** Umbilical region. **5** and **6.** Right and left lumbar regions. **7.** Suprapubic or hypogastric region. **8** and **9.** Right and left inguinal or iliac regions.

Abdominal distention is frequently seen when observing the abdominal profile. A mnemonic, the 6 Fs, aids in remembering the six common causes of a distended abdomen:

- Fat
- Fluid
- Feces

Box 5–5
Abdominal Organs Located in the Four Abdominal Quadrants and the Suprapubic Region

Right Upper Quadrant	**Left Upper Quadrant**
Liver and gallbladder	Left lobe of liver
Pylorus	Spleen
Duodenum	Stomach
Head of pancreas	Body of pancreas
Right adrenal gland	Left adrenal gland
Right kidney	Left kidney
Hepatic flexure of colon	Splenic flexure of colon
Ascending colon and portions of transverse colon	Transverse colon and portions of descending colon
Right Lower Quadrant	**Left Lower Quadrant**
Cecum and appendix	Portion of descending colon
Portion of ascending colon	Sigmoid colon
Right ovary ♀	Left ovary ♀
Right fallopian tube ♀	Left fallopian tube ♀
Right spermatic cord ♂	Left spermatic cord ♂
Right ureter	Left ureter
Suprapubic Region	
Bladder	
Pregnant uterus ♀	

NOTE: Portions of the small intestine are located in all quadrants.

- Flatus
- Fetus
- Fatal mass

Another common finding on visual inspection is an abdominal hernia. Incisional hernias (herniations adjacent to old surgical scars) and umbilical hernias are the most usual. **Diastasis recti,** a separation of the two rectus abdominis muscles, is sometimes mistaken for a hernia. No muscle separation is seen when the client is completely flat, but when the abdominal muscles are tensed while the head and shoulders are raised, a separation and midline bulge may be seen from xiphoid to pubis. The condition may be congenital or acquired secondary to pregnancy or obesity. It does not affect the client's health.

Although surgical interventions were discussed when taking the client's history, abdominal scars from surgery the client did not mention may be noted. Often clients who have had a number of operations simply forget about one, or the surgery may have been so long ago that they have forgotten. Asking about scars as they are observed jogs the client's memory, adding information important to the client's health record. If the client deliberately avoided discussing the surgery, that is also important to know. Follow up this information later at an appropriate time in the plan of care after completing the initial data gathering.

AUSCULTATION Although percussion and palpation usually follow inspection, auscultatory findings may be altered by these techniques. Thus, auscultation precedes them in abdominal assessment.

Listen for the normal peristaltic sounds (gurgles) below and to the right of the umbilicus. High-pitched sounds may be indicative of early intestinal obstruction or severe diarrhea. The complete absence of peristaltic sounds is seen in paralytic ileus. To establish that the abdomen is silent, however, the examiner must listen for 5 minutes.

Another auscultatory sound is the peritoneal friction rub indicative of peritonitis. The rub sounds much like the leathery pleural friction rub in the chest and often emanates from the splenic or hepatic region.

A *bruit,* an audible murmer in a blood vessel secondary to turbulent blood flow, is best heard with the bell of the stethoscope. An abdominal aortic aneurysm, renal artery stenosis, or partial occlusion of any major blood vessel can cause a bruit. In young, thin, healthy clients, a bruit over the abdominal aorta is sometimes heard; this is not considered pathologic. See Figure 5–17 for the areas where abdominal sounds are best heard.

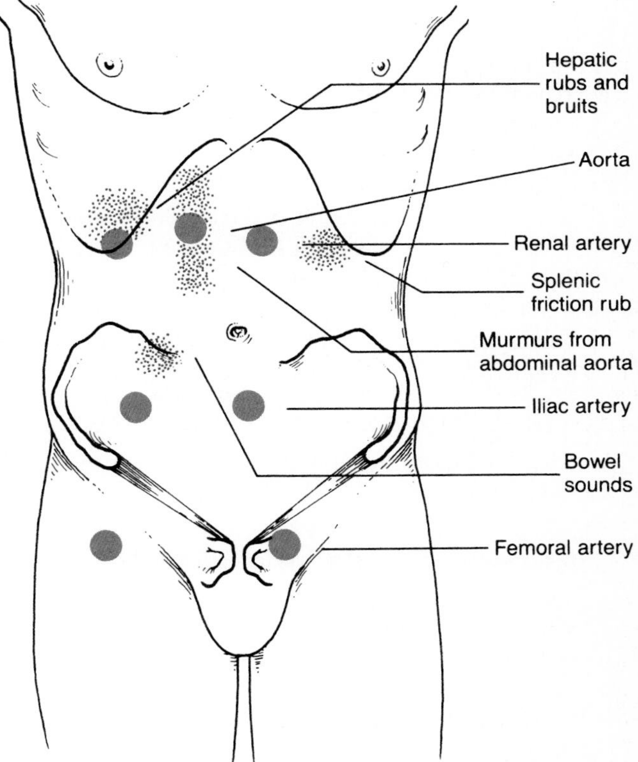

Figure 5–17

Areas for listening to sounds in the abdomen.

PALPATION Most abdominal structures cannot be felt in the healthy abdomen. Structures that may normally be palpable include the:

- Abdominal aorta
- Lower pole of the right kidney
- Liver edge as it descends on inspiration
- Ascending colon } when they contain stool
- Descending colon and sigmoid } when they contain stool
- Distended bladder
- Pregnant uterus

The abdomen is palpated using a gentle dipping motion of the fingertips, keeping the fingers together. All four quadrants are examined. In the ticklish client, placing the client's hand on top of the examiner's during palpation will help in desensitizing the client.

Palpation is then repeated in the same way, with the examiner feeling deeper into the abdomen. Watch the client's face during the examination to detect areas of tenderness the client does not verbalize. Clients deny having pain for many reasons (culture, fear, past experience), but careful observation can reveal what the client does not. If any areas of tenderness were noted during gentle palpation, these areas should be examined last. With the obese client, two hands may be used for deep palpation, one reinforcing the other. Sometimes a mass is located in the abdominal wall rather than in the abdominal cavity. Ask the client to raise the shoulders off the examining table. In this position, an abdominal wall mass remains palpable, but an internal mass is obscured by muscle tension. Any masses or lesions should be described in terms of their location, size, shape, consistency, tenderness, and mobility.

The aortic pulsation is often visible slightly to the left of the midline, above the umbilicus. To palpate the aortic pulsation, press into the middle of the upper abdomen. The normal aortic pulsation is in an AP direction. An examiner who palpates a pulsatile mass with lateral as well as AP movement should suspect an abdominal aortic aneurysm.

The inguinal region of the lower abdomen must not be overlooked. The femoral pulses are palpated, graded, and compared side to side. Palpation is also useful in detecting enlarged inguinal lymph nodes. Enlarged nodes may be secondary to regional infections such as vaginitis or urinary tract infections (UTI).

Assessment of the Male Genitalia

Although a complete examination of the male genitalia may not be part of a routine nursing assessment, nurses should be familiar with the importance of teaching testicular self-examination. Testicular self-examination is an important health maintenance technique that adolescent boys and men should know and practice routinely. The male who is familiar with how his testes normally feel will discover early changes in the tissue more readily. The client grasps his testicle and rolls it between the thumb and forefinger, which is the same technique the examiner uses (Figure 5–18). Self-examination is facilitated by having the scrotal skin relaxed; for example, after a warm shower.

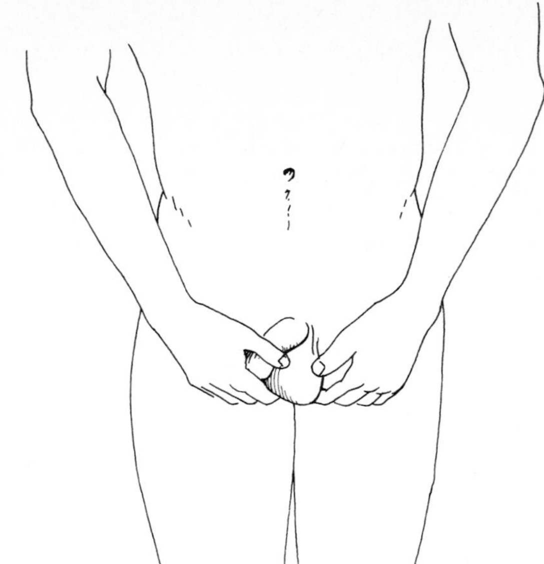

How to do TSE: Testicular self-examination is a simple procedure that all young men should learn to do. Palpation, or feeling, of the testicles is best done using two hands as illustrated in the figure. Explore each testicle individually. Using both hands, gently roll the testicle between the thumbs and fingers. If pain is experienced, too much pressure is being applied.

The examination should be done at least once each month, preferably after a warm bath or shower when the scrotal skin is most relaxed.

What to look for: A normal testicle is egg-shaped, somewhat firm to touch, and should be smooth and free of lumps. When doing TSE, you should be looking for any changes in the size or consistency of the testicle. If you do find something abnormal, most likely it will be an area of firmness or small lump on the front or on the side of the testicle. Do not confuse the epididymis (the soft tubelike structure at the back of the testis) with a tumor. If you do find something abnormal, you should have the condition checked immediately by a physician.

What happens if cancer is found? When detected early enough, testicular cancer is one of the most curable types of cancer. Most early tumors are confined to one testicle. Surgical removal of one testicle does not leave a person impotent; the remaining testicle is capable of maintaining sexual fertility, erection, and orgasm.

Figure 5–18

Teaching the client about testicular self-examination (TSE). *Courtesy of Department of Cancer Control and Epidemiology, Roswell Park Memorial Institute, Buffalo, NY.*

In clients who are confined to bed, the scrotum often becomes edematous, excoriated, and inflamed. The skin of the scrotum should be inspected carefully, lifting it to view the posterior surface.

Assessment of the Female Genitalia

The pelvic examination is one that many women dread. A female nurse often remains with the client during a pelvic exam when the examiner is male. The nurse has an important role in assisting women to understand why the embarrassing lithotomy position is needed for an adequate pelvic exam. The woman in the lithotomy position has her buttocks partially hanging over the edge of the examining table to facilitate distensibility of the inferior vaginal wall.

This position makes the pelvic exam more comfortable because pressure on the superior structures (eg, the urethra) causes pain. Elevating the client from a flat to a semiseated position and providing a properly placed mirror allows her to see what is being visualized. Although some women prefer not to look, many women are pleased to see their own cervix so clearly. This experience greatly enhances their appreciation of the importance of the exam.

Assessment of the Musculoskeletal System

THE SYNOVIAL JOINTS Range of motion (ROM) of many of the joints has already been observed and tentatively assessed to some extent. For example, shoulder motion was noted when the client raised the arms in the air during assessment of the breasts. Mobility of the knees and hips of the woman was partially evaluated when she was assisted into the lithotomy position. All joints are now inspected for swelling, erythema, deformity, symmetry, ROM, and condition of surrounding skin. General joint palpation includes assessment for increased warmth, tenderness, crepitation (a palpable grating sensation produced by joint movement), or bogginess caused by a thickened synovium.

THE HANDS, FINGERS, AND WRISTS Note the number of digits on each hand. Inspect the distal and proximal interphalangeal joints (DIP, PIP). Heberden's nodes, a bony enlargement of the DIP joint, and Bouchard's nodes, a bony enlargement of the PIP joint, are often seen in degenerative joint disease (DJD). Clubbing of the fingers, a bullous enlargement of the distal segment of a digit, should alert the examiner to the possibility of cardiac or pulmonary disease, although the condition may be hereditary (Petersdorf et al., 1983). Ask the client to make a fist and then to extend and spread the fingers of the hand. Have the client flex, extend, hyperextend, abduct, and adduct both wrists. Palpate the metacarpals, the metacarpophalangeal joints, and the PIP and DIP joints. Palpate the wrist.

THE ELBOWS AND SHOULDERS Ask the client to flex, extend, supinate, and pronate both elbows. Palpate the elbow, noting any pain or tenderness over the lateral epicondyle of the humerus, which is suggestive of tendinitis or "tennis elbow." Palpate the ulnar nerve in the groove in the posterior aspect of the medial epicondyle of the humerus. Tenderness in this area indicates nerve irritation, often secondary to direct trauma or to fracture of the elbow. This nerve is commonly called the "funny bone" because of the pain and tingling that occurs when it is struck.

To assess ROM of the shoulder, ask the client:

- To raise both arms to a vertical position at the sides of the head (flexion)
- To place the hands behind the neck with the elbows out to the side (external rotation)
- To place the hands behind the small of the back (internal rotation)

In addition, assess abduction, adduction, extension, and circumduction. Place a hand on the joint to note any crepitation with motion. Palpate the sternoclavicular joint, the acromioclavicular joint, and the greater tubercle of the humerus. The rotator cuff, which is composed of four muscles, inserts into the greater tuberosity of the humerus and is a common site of abduction problems.

THE HIPS Observe the client's gait carefully, because many problems in the hip are readily seen during ambulation. ROM of the hip includes flexion and extension, abduction, adduction, circumduction, and internal and external rotation. Have the client bring the knee to the chest while supine (hip flexion). The thigh of the other leg should remain flat on the table. If flexion contracture of the hip is present on the unflexed side, the thigh does not remain flat but pulls up into flexion when the opposite knee and hip are fully flexed. This is called the *Thomas test* for flexion contracture of the hip.

Shortening of one leg can be caused by a number of problems including disorders of the hip. With the client supine, measure leg length with a flexible tape measure from the anterosuperior iliac spine to the medial malleolus (see Figure 43–1). The leg measurements are compared. A leg-length discrepancy of as little as ¼ in can cause low back pain or greater trochanteric bursitis on the side of the longer leg.

THE KNEES The knee joint is the largest joint in the body and is poorly protected by fat or muscle mass. The joint is especially vulnerable to sports injuries, although knee problems occur in persons of all age groups, whether athletic or not. Inspect the knees for the common knee deformities of *genu varum* (bowed legs), *genu valgum* (knock knees), and *genu recurvatum* (back knee or hyperextension of the knee).

Full ROM includes flexion, extension, and internal and external rotation. Internal and external rotation are gauged by having the client rotate each foot medially and laterally. With a normal knee, there should be about a 10° rotation of the foot to either side.

THE ANKLES AND FEET Note dorsiflexion and plantar flexion of the ankle. Test the stability of the joint in inversion and eversion by grasping the tibia around its distal end to stabilize it and then alternately inverting and everting the heel. Then stabilize the heel and evert and invert the forefoot. Have the client flex and extend the toes.

Inspect the skin of the foot for thickened areas on the sole (calluses), thickened areas on the toes (corns), and plantar warts. Note any toe or toenail abnormalities.

THE BACK AND SPINE There are 33 vertebrae in the vertebral column and 31 pairs of spinal nerves exiting above or below the corresponding vertebrae. Viewed laterally, three curves are normally noted in the vertebral column.

- The cervical curve—slightly concave
- The thoracic curve—convex
- The lumbar curve—concave

Observe the spine for any abnormal curvatures. An accentuation of the thoracic convexity is called *kyphosis,* and an accentuation of lumbar concavity is called *lordosis* (sway back). *Scoliosis* is a lateral deviation of the spine. Normally, no lateral deviation should be seen. Also observe any difference in height of the shoulders and symmetry of the scapulae and iliac crests.

ROM of the lower spine includes flexion and extension, lateral bending, and rotation. Ask the client to bend forward and touch the toes, bend backward, bend from side to side, and rotate from side to side. Clients who have pain should not be asked to go beyond the point of initial pain. In children and adolescents, watch the scapulae as the client returns from forward flexion. An elevation of the scapula on one side may indicate scoliosis.

Palpate over each spinous process and note any tenderness. Then palpate the paraspinal muscle mass on each side, noting tenderness and/or muscle spasm (sustained muscle contractions causing the muscle to feel hard to palpation).

Assessment of the Nervous System

Evaluation of the nervous system includes:

- The mental status exam as a test of general cerebral function
- Assessment of cranial nerves I through XII
- Assessment of the sensory system
- Assessment of the motor system
- Assessment of the reflexes
- Tests for cerebellar function

THE MENTAL STATUS EXAM The mental status exam begins during history taking when the examiner is noting general appearance and grooming, language use, thought processes, emotional state, attention span, and memory. A problem suspected in any area is followed up carefully during the neurologic assessment. If the client's ability to understand and communicate in words is impaired, the sequence of examination is reordered. Vision and hearing are evaluated first. Then a specific assessment of language deficits is begun.

LANGUAGE The examiner points to common objects and asks the client to name them. The client is asked to read some words and to match the printed and written words with pictures. Simple commands such as "point to your toes" can be written out for the client to perform, and simple verbal commands can be offered such as "raise your right arm." As the client speaks, note the loudness, flow, speed, quantity, and logic of the words.

ORIENTATION AND MEMORY Assess whether the client seems relatively trusting, granting the normal suspiciousness many clients have about health professionals. Note excessive evasion and suspicion. Evaluate the client's orientation to time, place, and person, which can be done naturally with questions during the history about specific dates, places, and persons. Ask the client about any difficulty with memory. Question specifically about the day of the week, date of the month, and the year.

Immediate recall and concentration can be tested by giving the client a series of three digits to repeat. The number of digits is gradually increased until the client fails to repeat the series correctly. Start again with a series of three digits, gradually increasing the number. This time ask the client to repeat them backwards. The average person can repeat a series of seven digits in order and four digits in reverse order.

Recent memory is assessed by assigning the client three facts to remember such as an address, a color, and an object. Have the client repeat all three and request that he or she remember them. Later in the interview, ask the client to recall all the items. Remote memory is evaluated by asking the client to describe an event several years in the past. An example might be the Watergate cover-up.

INTELLECT Much of the assessment of intelligence is derived from the detail and subtleties of clients' accounts of themselves and their health problems. In addition, a number of testing techniques are helpful in evaluating higher intellectual functions. Some approaches include asking the client to count backwards from 100 by subtracting 7s, naming the last four presidents and their political affiliations, or calculating the cost of three eggs if a dozen costs 92 cents.

Evaluate abstract reasoning by giving the client a proverb to interpret. Examples would be "a stitch in time saves nine" or "people who live in glass houses shouldn't throw stones." Concrete interpretations may indicate a problem or may simply indicate level of education. Normally, an abstract or semiabstract interpretation is expected. Asking the client to explain how two things are alike such as "an orange and an apple" or how two things are different such as "climate and season" also assists in evaluating abstract thinking.

The client's judgment has already been assessed to some degree during the personal/social part of the health history. If that portion of the history was done well, examples of the client's coping patterns and response to interpersonal conflict are known in detail. Judgment can be further assessed by asking a question such as, "What would you do if you found a wallet with money and owner identification in it?"

THE CRANIAL NERVES Assessment of cranial nerves I through XII is part of the physical examination of the face, eyes, ears, nose, mouth, throat, neck, and shoulders. See Table 5–2 for a summary of the cranial nerves.

ASSESSMENT OF SENSORY FUNCTION Loss or change in somatic sensation is an important manifestation of neurologic disease. Assessment of the sensory system is difficult, however, because the tests are somewhat crude, and interpreting them is quite subjective.

Response to light touch is assessed by lightly touching the client's skin with a wisp of cotton while the client's eyes are closed; ask the client to say "yes" when the cotton is felt. Start from the toes and move up the body symmetrically, comparing the client's response from side to side.

Because pain and temperature fibers run together in the spinal cord, testing of pain sensation alone is satisfactory for general assessment. If pain sensation is altered, temperature sensation is then evaluated. A pin is used to assess pain. Clients close their eyes and say "yes" whenever they feel the pinprick. Symmetrical areas are evaluated.

Position (proprioceptive) sense is tested by passive movement of the client's fingers and toes. With the client's eyes closed, the examiner grasps a finger or toe and flexes or extends it. The client must state what position the digit is in ("down" or "up"). Several digits are checked on each hand and foot.

ASSESSMENT OF MOTOR FUNCTION Evaluation of the motor system includes careful attention to muscle atrophy, muscle tone, muscle strength, and involuntary muscular movements. For inspection of muscles for atrophy or hypertrophy, the client must be exposed well enough for good visualization of major muscles. Corresponding muscle areas in the extremities are measured and compared side to side. The client's occupation must be considered. For example, professional tennis players would be expected to have disproportionate muscle hypertrophy in the dominant arm.

Muscle tone is the tension in the resting muscle—the slight resistance felt when the relaxed limb is passively moved. In a client with upper motor neuron disease, the

Table 5–2
Summary of the Cranial Nerves and Their Functions

Nerve	Name	Type of Nerve	Function
I	Olfactory	Sensory	Smell
II	Optic	Sensory	Vision and visual fields
III	Oculomotor	Motor	Extraocular eye movement (EOM) and movement of sphincter of pupil and ciliary muscles of lens
IV	Trochlear	Motor	EOM, specifically moves eyeball downward and laterally
V	Trigeminal	Motor and sensory	
	Ophthalmic branch	Sensory	Sensation of cornea, skin of face, and nasal mucosa
	Maxillary branch	Sensory	Sensation of skin of face and anterior oral cavity (tongue and teeth)
	Mandibular branch	Motor and sensory	Muscles of mastication; sensation of skin of face
VI	Abducens	Motor	EOM, moves eyeball laterally
VII	Facial	Motor and sensory	Facial expression; taste (anterior tongue)
VIII	Vestibulocochlear (acoustic)		
	Vestibular branch	Sensory	Equilibrium
	Cochlear branch	Sensory	Hearing
IX	Glossopharyngeal	Motor and sensory	Gag reflex, tongue movement, taste (posterior tongue)
X	Vagus	Motor and sensory	Sensation of pharynx and larynx; swallowing and phonation
XI	Accessory	Motor	Head movement; shrugging of shoulders
XII	Hypoglossal	Motor	Protrusion of tongue

SOURCE: Adapted with permission from Kozier B, Erb G: *Fundamentals of Nursing: Concepts and Procedures*, 3rd ed. Menlo Park, CA: Addison–Wesley, 1987, p. 885–886.

tone of the passively moved muscle is increased (spasticity). In lower motor neuron disease, the tone of the passively moved muscle is decreased (flaccidity). Muscle strength is tested as shown in Table 5–3; a grading scale is found in Box 43–2.

Involuntary muscle movements may be normal in some instances. Many healthy persons have an exaggeration of normal physiologic tremor secondary to caffeine intake or situational anxiety. A few types of tremor are recognized as related to certain disease processes. For example, a coarse, rhythmic tremor reduced or eliminated by voluntary movement (intention tremor) is characteristic of Parkinson's disease. A combined rest and intention tremor is often seen in multiple sclerosis.

Clonus, a series of involuntary muscle contractions precipitated by a sudden passive stretch of muscle, is most often elicited at the knee and ankle joints. This sign of disease in the central nervous system may be elicited by dorsiflexion of the foot with the knee flexed.

ASSESSMENT OF CEREBELLAR FUNCTION The cerebellum modulates and coordinates skeletal muscle activity and maintains body posture and muscle tone. A person with cerebellar damage experiences muscle weakness, a loss of muscle tone, and difficulty standing erect and walking. Testing for cerebellar function involves evaluating coordination and the ability to perform rapid alternating movements in both upper and lower extremities.

The upper extremities are tested by having the client alternately supinate and pronate the hand as rapidly as possible and pat the leg with the hand as fast as possible. Then the client is asked to touch the tips of the fingers to the thumb in rapid sequence. Each hand is tested and compared with the other. Instruct the client to touch the index finger of the extended arm to the nose and then return the arm to the extended position. This is done repeatedly, first with the eyes open and then with them closed (finger-to-nose test). With eyes open, the client touches a finger to the nose and then to the examiner's finger while the examiner changes the position of that finger. This activity is repeated with increasing speed. These tests are performed bilaterally.

The lower extremities are tested by having the client tap a foot against the floor or against the examiner's hand as rapidly as possible. While supine, the client places the heel of one foot on the opposite knee and slides the heel slowly down the shin (heel-to-knee test). Both legs are tested. Abnormal findings in these tests include tremor; slow, jerky movements; and breaks in rhythm.

Equilibrium is assessed by asking the client to stand erect with feet together and eyes open. Then assess the client's ability to maintain an upright position with the eyes closed. A loss of balance with the eyes closed is called a positive Romberg's sign. Obviously, the examiner should remain close to support the client who begins to sway or fall. Ask the client to walk across the room to assess the

Table 5–3
Testing Muscle Strength

Muscle	Client/Examiner Activity
Deltoid	Client holds arm up and resists while examiner tries to push it down.
Biceps	Client fully extends each arm and then tries to flex it while examiner attempts to hold arm in extension.
Triceps	Client flexes each arm and then tries to extend it against the examiner's attempt to keep arm in flexion.
Wrist and finger muscles	Client spreads the fingers and then resists as examiner attempts to push the fingers together.
Grip strength	Client grasps the index and middle fingers of the examiner while the examiner tries to pull the fingers out.
Hip muscles	Client is supine, both legs extended; client raises one leg at a time while the examiner attempts to hold it down.
Hip abduction	Client is supine, both legs extended. Examiner's hands are on the lateral surface of each knee; client is asked to spread the legs apart against the examiner's resistance.
Hip adduction	Client is in same position as for hip abduction; the examiner's hands are now placed between the knees; client is asked to bring the legs together against the examiner's resistance.
Hamstrings	Client is supine with both knees bent. Client resists while examiner attempts to straighten them.
Quadriceps	Client is supine with knee partially extended; client resists while examiner attempts to flex the knee.
Muscles of the ankles and feet	Client resists while examiner attempts to dorsiflex the foot back and again resists while examiner attempts to flex the foot.

normal gait. Then have the client walk as if walking a tightrope (heel to toe) in a straight line. Clients with cerebellar disease will lose their balance after two or three steps and will place one foot to the side to avoid falling.

Assessment of the Peripheral Vascular System

The examiner inspects the legs for obvious swelling and checks for pitting edema by applying thumb pressure over the bony prominences in the lower-leg and ankle regions. Pitting edema in an adult indicates at least 10 lb (4.5 kg) of fluid accumulation (DeGowin & DeGowin, 1981). In pitting edema, a depression occurs where thumb pressure against the bone has been applied, and the depression persists for a short time. The depth of the pit is estimated and recorded. The distribution of edema is noted. Bilateral edema indicates a systemic problem, whereas unilateral edema indicates local disease.

Inspect the legs for signs of venous thrombosis, looking for swelling and duskiness of the calf and pitting edema on the ankle of the affected side. The calf is often warmer to the touch and may be tender to gentle palpation. The calf should be measured and its circumference compared with the other leg. *Homans' sign,* pain in the calf or popliteal region when the foot is sharply dorsiflexed with the knee slightly flexed, is a nonspecific but well-known test for deep vein thrombophlebitis.

With the client standing, the legs are carefully inspected for varicosities. *Varicose veins* are dilated, tortuous superficial veins in the saphenous system of the lower limbs. Any suspicious veins are palpated for hardness or tenderness.

Palpation of the peripheral arterial pulses in the upper and lower extremities is essential for assessment of the adequacy of arterial blood flow to the systemic circulation. The pulses are palpated in the following sequence, and their volume is compared (Figure 5–19):

- Radial
- Ulnar
- Brachial
- Carotid
- Femoral
- Popliteal
- Posterior tibial
- Dorsalis pedis

Pulses are classified on a scale of 0 to 4, with 4 being normal:

- 0 = completely absent
- 1+ = barely palpable
- 2+ = moderately impaired
- 3+ = slightly impaired
- 4+ = normal; full and bounding

The popliteal pulses are often difficult to palpate. To facilitate assessment, flex the knee to relax the popliteal fossa and palpate deeply, lateral to the midline.

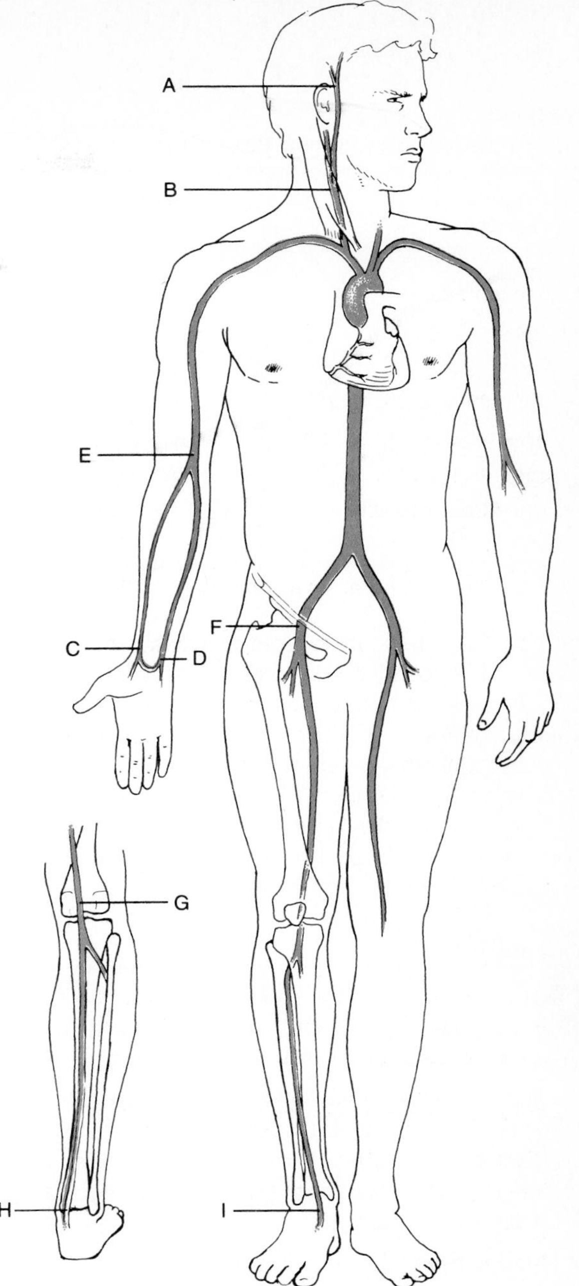

Figure 5–19

Peripheral pulses give important clues to the client's cardiovascular status. Some are more difficult to locate than others, so practice is necessary. Pulses to be evaluated include the temporal (**A**), carotid (**B**), radial (**C**), ulnar (**D**), brachial (**E**), femoral (**F**), popliteal (**G**), posterior tibial (**H**), and dorsalis pedis (**I**).

Completing the Data Base

A review of previous client records, if available, and the results of diagnostic studies completes the data base. Many nations record laboratory data with an international system

Table 5–4
International System (SI) Base Units

Physical Quantity	Base Unit	Symbol
Length	Meter	m
Mass	Kilogram	kg
Time	Second	s
Amount of substance	Mole	mol
Thermodynamic temperature	Kelvin	K
Electric current	Ampere	A
Luminous intensity	Candela	cd

SOURCE: Reprinted with permission from *SI Manual in Health Care*, 2nd ed. Ottawa, Canada: Metric Commission, 1982.

of units (SI), the most current metric system of measurement. SI is founded on seven units called "base units" (Table 5–4). All traditional units of measurement from calorie counts to radiation doses are converted to a new language and new system with SI. Canada is currently converting to this system. A listing of SI units applicable to health is found in the Appendixes. In the future, laboratory tests will probably be listed with both traditional values and SI equivalents.

Chapter Highlights

Nurses play a key role in helping clients to understand their rights and the need for them to exercise their rights.

Clients from various sociocultural backgrounds may not understand questions and often find it difficult to cooperate with examinations and procedures that contradict their belief systems.

Nurses must be aware of the universal potential for cultural, religious, age, socioeconomic, racial, sexual, and lifestyle differences and develop communication skills that facilitate an understanding of these differences to improve client care.

An organized, sequential approach to health assessment is important in gathering a complete data base.

Obtaining a comprehensive data base is the most important phase of the nursing process because all subsequent client care depends on this information.

The most significant step in physical assessment is careful visual inspection.

Nurses should understand the complete physical assessment process so they can adequately prepare clients for examination, even though they may not be doing some components of the assessment themselves.

Bibliography

Bates B: *A Guide to Physical Examination,* 3rd ed. Philadelphia: Lippincott, 1983.

Bramwell L: Use of the life history in pattern identification and health promotion. *ANS* 1984; 6:37–44.

Davis AJ: Informed consent: How much information is enough? *Nurs Outlook* 1985; 33(1):40–42.

DeGowin EL, DeGowin RL: *Bedside Diagnostic Examination,* 4th ed. New York: Macmillan, 1981.

Delancy VL, North C: Skin assessment. *Top Clin Nurs* (July) 1983; 5:5–10.

Gett JR, Cortese DA, Fontana RS: Lung cancer: Current concepts and prospects. *Ca* 1983; 33:74–86.

Ginnetti J, Greig AE: The occupational health history. *Nurse Pract* (Nov–Dec) 1981; 6:12–13.

Heart sounds and common murmurs. *Am J Nurs* 1983; 83(12):1680–1689.

Konikow NS: Alterations in movement: Nursing assessment and implications. *J Neurosurg Nurs* (Feb) 1985; 17:61–65.

Kreps GL, Thornton BC: *Health Communication.* New York: Longman, 1984.

Lindberg SC: Periodic preventive health screening schedule for adult men and women. *Nurse Pract* (Sept–Oct) 1980; 5:9–13, 21.

Malasanos L et al: *Health Assessment,* 3rd ed. St. Louis: Mosby, 1985.

Meyer LS: Untangling communication lines to connect consumers and providers. *Nurs Health Care* (Sept) 1985; 6:367–368.

Ozuna J: Alterations in mentation: Nursing assessment and intervention. *J Neurosurg Nurs* (Feb) 1985; 17:66–70.

Petersdorf RG et al: *Harrison's Principles of Internal Medicine,* 10th ed. New York: McGraw–Hill, 1983.

Pickwell S: Health screening for Indo-Chinese refugees. *Nurse Pract* (April) 1983; 8:20–25, 35.

Primrose RB: Taking the tension out of pelvic exams. *Am J Nurs* 1984; 84:72–74.

Stoneberg C, Pitcock N, Myton C: Pressure sores in the homebound: One solution. *Am J Nurs* 1986; 86(4):426–428.

Taylor DL: Clinical applications: Assessing heart sounds. *Nurs 85* 1985; 15(1):51–53.

Resources

SELF-HELP GROUPS AND OTHER ORGANIZATIONS

InterHealth
2970 Fifth Ave
San Diego, CA 92103

This preventive health organization was founded in 1913 by former president William Howard Taft and other leading citizens. It provides a health risk appraisal called the Interhealth Risk Profile that can be used in health care programs.

Wellness Associates
PO Box 5433
Mill Valley, CA 94942
Phone: (415) 383–3806

An organization that publishes the Wellness Inventory, a broad-based paper-and-pencil questionnaire that individuals can use to determine stress levels and to promote wellness. It does not require laboratory testing or computer analysis, as other more detailed health risk appraisals do, and its results are more general. It can be used without interpretation by a health care provider.

UNIT 2

Multisystem Stressors

CHAPTER 6

Malnutrition

Other topics relevant to this content are: Anorexia nervosa, **Chapter 7;** Bulimia, **Chapter 7;** Enteral feedings, **Chapter 36;** Pressure ulcers, **Chapter 55.**

Objectives

When you have finished studying this chapter, you should be able to:

Define malnutrition.

Identify the incidence of and reasons for malnutrition in hospitalized clients.

Discuss the physiologic and psychosocial causes of malnutrition.

Describe the multisystem effects of malnutrition.

Identify clients at high risk for developing malnutrition.

Discuss subjective and objective data collection in nutritional assessment.

Develop a plan of care for the client with malnutrition.

State nursing responsibilities in administering and monitoring tube feedings and total parenteral nutrition (TPN).

Although more people are making informed choices about what they eat, malnutrition remains a worldwide problem. Chronic malnutrition has tragic consequences. It depletes energy and capacity for work; decreases resistance to infectious disease; and adversely affects concentration, motivation, and learning ability.

That malnutrition is prevalent in third-world countries is well known. But malnutrition is also a serious problem in industrialized nations, especially for the poor and the elderly. The affluent may not be aware of the principles of good nutrition or may ignore them. A person may enter the hospital well nourished only to leave malnourished. Clients with devastating illnesses and inherited disease also suffer from malnutrition. Even health professionals do not always have an adequate background in nutrition.

SECTION 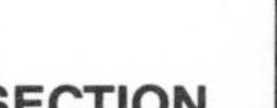

The Problem of Malnutrition

Nutrition is the process of taking in and utilizing necessary nutrients. These nutrients must be consumed (ingested), digested (broken down to basic particles), absorbed (transported into cells or the bloodstream), and used by the body. Good nutrition is the daily ingestion of adequate amounts of essential nutrients including protein, carbohydrates, fats, vitamins, minerals, and water. Each of these nutrients is important in either providing energy for body processes, structural material for tissues, or regulation of biochemical processes. The overall role of good nutrition is to promote growth and development, maintain health, prevent illness, and treat disease.

Malnutrition is a serious consequence of continued poor nutrition. Growth, development, and cognition may be impaired and disease can develop. Malnutrition can prolong disease and complicate treatment, perhaps extending hospitalization.

The term **malnutrition** describes a condition of reduced intake or utilization of nutrients, particularly protein and calories, in relation to requirements. Calories, or heat energy, are supplied primarily by carbohydrates and fats. (A calorie is the unit of energy necessary to raise the temperature of 1 kg of water by 1°C or 33.8°F.) Malnutrition can be defined as an inappropriate reduction in the lean body mass, which consists of skeletal muscle made up primarily of protein. The term **nutrient deficiency** generally refers to specific vitamin and mineral deficiency states.

Incidence in Hospitalized Clients

Even with recent advances in nutritional support, malnutrition among hospitalized clients continues to be a serious problem. In a study of 134 medical clients, researchers found that the 48% who were malnourished when admitted had prolonged hospitalizations and a high mortality rate. In 75% of those admitted with normal nutritional values, nutritional parameters worsened during their hospitalizations (Weinsier & Butterworth, 1981). Another expert reports that 25% to 50% of clients are malnourished upon admission (Cerra, 1984). Of those well nourished when entering the hospital, 25% to 30% will develop malnutrition. Cerra estimates that 69% of all hospitalized clients will demonstrate declining nutritional status, whether they are admitted well nourished or malnourished.

Types of Malnutrition

There are several types of malnutrition. A client may be deficient in a specific nutrient such as vitamin A or have severe protein or calorie deficiency requiring several months of treatment before repletion takes place.

Specific nutrient deficiencies cause related physical changes. For example, a diet with few fruits and vegetables may lead to a vitamin C deficiency, causing bleeding gums. (Objective and subjective data related to nutrient deficiencies are discussed later in this chapter in Table 6–2.) Often several simultaneous deficiencies are found. The diet lacking in fruits and vegetables will also result in deficiencies of a number of other vitamins, such as A and B. Most nutrient deficiency states are easily reversed by providing the necessary nutrient.

Marasmus, or simple starvation, refers to protein and calorie malnutrition, generally occurring as the result of a chronic reduction of protein and calorie intake. It is associated with severe depletion of fat stores and muscle wasting. Those with marasmus will require adequate protein and calories over several months to replace muscle loss.

Kwashiorkor is protein malnutrition resulting from a protein-poor diet or from protein loss due to physiologic stress. The client may not appear malnourished because although fat stores may be depleted, edema maintains the weight level. Malnutrition occurring with obesity is of this type. Persons with kwashiorkor are given protein with adequate calories to improve the protein status.

Causes of Malnutrition

Clients may be malnourished because of starvation, because a disease state has altered their metabolism, or because of treatment (*iatrogenic malnutrition*).

Starvation

Starvation is a state of insufficient intake of necessary calories to supply the body's energy needs. Insufficient intake can occur because of physiologic, psychologic, or socioeconomic factors.

PHYSIOLOGIC CAUSES Physiologic causes of starvation include disease factors, drug–nutrient interactions, or dietary restrictions. Disease-induced starvation results from disorders that impair nutrient intake, prevent nutrient absorption, or promote nutrient losses. Nutrient intake may be impaired because of difficulty in chewing, or disease-induced generalized weakness. With oral lesions or inflammation of the throat or esophagus, chewing and swallowing can be painful, difficult, or impossible. Constriction of the throat and esophagus may cause difficulty in swallowing. Some disorders, such as hiatal hernia with reflux esophagitis, result in pain upon swallowing from lower esophageal inflammation. Cancer in the upper gastrointestinal tract may also make eating difficult because of pain or obstruction.

Disease states may prevent nutrient absorption. Malabsorption, the defective absorption of ingested nutrients, can result from various causes. Diarrhea may speed the passage of nutrients through the intestines, decreasing the time for nutrient absorption. Any gastrointestinal surgery in which the small intestine is removed or bypassed will cause some degree of reduced nutrient absorption.

Several conditions promote nutrient losses. Among these are open draining wounds, fistulas, abscesses; renal dialysis; severe burns; and major blood loss. With prolonged, unreplaced nutrient depletion, starvation may develop. Some gastrointestinal diseases, such as celiac sprue, scleroderma, and regional enteritis cause protein excretion into the stool.

Drug therapy may be associated with starvation or nutrient deficiencies. Drugs that cause a decreased hunger drive (eg, amphetamines), decreased nutrient absorption (eg, antibiotics), or decreased metabolism (eg, barbiturates), can contribute to malnutrition or nutrient deficiency states. Many drugs such as caffeine, amphetamines, and chemotherapeutic drugs, can reduce the appetite and induce nausea. Drugs causing malabsorption of some nutrients include antacids containing aluminum hydroxide (Maalox, Gelusil, Mygel, Gaviscon); antigout preparations such as colchicine; antibiotics such as neomycin; and some laxatives such as mineral oil. Drugs that alter metabolism of nutrients by affecting biochemical processes include some anticonvulsants and steroids.

The elderly are particularly prone to poor dietary intake. The physiologic changes of aging and the presence of disorders significantly affect appetite and ability to ingest and absorb nutrients. Taste perception is impaired, making food less appetizing. Salivation decreases with aging, so eating and swallowing are more difficult. Age-related dental changes, such as osteoarthritis and dentures that fit poorly, impair chewing. Gastrointestinal changes of aging, such as decreased secretions and decreased absorption, alter nutrition status. Constipation, common to the elderly, may diminish appetite. Altered cardiac and respiratory functions may contribute to fatigue or shortness of breath during eating. Some elderly persons are unable to prepare meals because of poor vision, strength, balance, and coordination, and reduced mobility can make food shopping difficult. Limited finances may be another problem.

PSYCHOSOCIAL CAUSES Some poor dietary habits contribute to starvation and the development of malnutrition or nutrient deficiencies. Fad diets and religious or cultural limitations may provide insufficient amounts of nutrients. Dieters often attempt to lose weight by fasting or eliminating foods that contain important nutrients. Bad eating habits may provide sufficient caloric intake but insufficient nutrients, such as in a diet consisting solely of high sugar starchy foods (cakes, breads, etc). Other diets may have enough protein but not enough vitamins. Alcohol intake may be a substitute for food for some people, resulting in malnutrition. Teenagers often prefer to skip mealtimes, choosing instead to satisfy hunger with snack foods such as chips, french fries, soda pop, candy, or ice cream. Such a diet may result in overnutrition yet be deficient in vital nutrients. A teenager's intake may need to be recorded to evaluate diet.

The nurse should also be familiar with psychologic conditions that may result in starvation from inadequate intake of nutrients (anorexia nervosa) or from induced vomiting following eating (bulimia). Psychosis may precipitate psychogenic malnutrition. The psychotic person may have delusions of food poisoning and fear eating foods purchased or prepared by others. Severe depression or apathy may reduce the hunger drive. Psychologic stress precipitated by an anxiety-provoking event or work or family pressures may reduce appetite and interfere with mealtimes. The stress of loss through death, divorce, or separation often reduces appetite to a point where rapid weight loss jeopardizes health.

Socioeconomic factors may contribute to poor nutritional status. Persons in lower socioeconomic groups may not be able to afford an adequate diet. The poorly educated may not know what constitutes a proper diet, although lack of nutritional knowledge occurs at every socioeconomic level. Poor refrigeration or cooking facilities may affect nutritional intake or contribute to food contamination. Environmental sanitation and water supply will affect the quality of nutrient intake. A water supply deficient in minerals such as iodine or fluoride may contribute to nutrient deficiencies or dental problems. At any socioeconomic level, drug and alcohol abuse interfere with good nutrition.

Nursing Research Note

Heitkemper M, Marotta S: Role of diets in modifying gastrointestinal neurotransmitter enzyme activity. *Nurs Res* 1985; 34(1):19–23.

This study examined the effects of fasting on the synthesis and degradation of acetylcholine and norepinephrine, neurotransmitters in the gastrointestinal tract. The study also examined the effects of choline-deficient diets on neurotransmitter enzyme activity. Dietary deficiencies in choline intake occur with total parenteral nutrition (TPN), self-imposed food restriction, inadequate oral intake, starvation, and anorexia.

Starvation decreased adrenergic enzyme activity and increased cholinergic activity. The stress of starvation also resulted in increased plasma and adrenal cortisol levels. Choline-deficient diets decreased adrenergic enzyme activity but did not alter cholinergic enzyme activity.

Nurses might apply these findings in nursing assessment of dietary alterations and the effects on the GI tract. Because the adrenergic and cholinergic neurotransmitters affect the entire central nervous system, behavior as well as physiology can be altered. Fasting clients, clients on TPN, and clients receiving medications such as lecithin or choline are likely to exhibit disequilibrium in parasympathetic/sympathetic activity and experience GI symptomatology. These symptoms must be evaluated and interventions planned to reduce discomfort.

Altered Metabolism

Conditions that cause physiologic stress, such as fever, infection, trauma, hyperthyroidism, and burns, increase metabolism. This increased metabolism, or hypermetabolism, increases the demand for nutrients. At the same time, many of these conditions diminish appetite. A paradox results: increased demand and decreased supply. Malnutrition may develop if the stress state is severe and prolonged and the person does not receive nutritional support.

Chronic disease states may also contribute to poor nutritional status. Diabetes alters the metabolism of carbohydrates, fats, and protein while decreasing circulation to areas where some nutrients are metabolized. Diseases that alter oxygenation of tissues, such as hypertension, coronary artery disease, and chronic obstructive lung disease, reduce the supply of oxygen to cells that need it to metabolize nutrients. Cancer increases the need for calories and protein while depressing the appetite and altering taste perception. The wasting process is accelerated because the body's fat and protein are broken down to meet metabolic demands. Cirrhosis—progressive liver failure—alters metabolism of fat, protein, and carbohydrates, in part because the liver is a major center of nutrient metabolism. The liver's ability to produce protein from amino acids and to store glucose as glycogen is impaired.

Iatrogenic Malnutrition

Treatment-induced malnutrition is a serious problem for hospitalized clients. Failure to observe and record food intake means poor nutritional intake will not be identified. Withholding meals for diagnostic tests further lowers nutritional intake for clients who may already be at risk for malnutrition. Providing low glucose and saline intravenous solutions as the sole nutrient intake over several days also promotes development of malnutrition. Nutritional needs may be unmet if there is inappropriate use of nutrient products through ignorance or carelessness. Similarly, failure to recognize increased nutritional requirements from injury and illness and failure to determine whether nutritional status is satisfactory before performing surgery may also result in unmet needs. Delays in initiating appropriate nutritional support until clients are seriously malnourished exposes them to its results until treatment can take effect.

Multisystem Effects of Malnutrition

Malnutrition affects all body systems. Early identification and prevention of malnutrition will prevent a multitude of physical, emotional, social, and economic problems.

With starvation, the body will use reserves of carbohydrates and fats to meet energy demands. There are no true reserves of protein; therefore, in starvation, functional protein tissue is broken down to meet protein demands. Eventually, the metabolic rate decreases, along with body temperature. Weight loss and a wasted appearance ensue.

In a malnourished client, resistance to infection is poor because of lowered body temperature and decreased ability to produce antibodies, which require protein. Higher morbidity and mortality rates are especially evident in malnourished clients undergoing surgery. When preoperative nutritional repletion is overlooked, the risks of surgery and anesthesia multiply. Following abdominal surgery, the incidence of wound infection, pneumonia, major complications, and mortality is increased in malnourished clients, especially if nutritional support continues to be poor (Muller et al., 1982). Surgical recovery may be prolonged. Malnutrition compounded by illness or stress can lead to apathy, depression, irritability, poor appetite, fatigue, low energy levels, and skin breakdown.

In acute starvation, organ efficiency is reduced with no change in organ mass. With progressive malnutrition, organs are reduced in size (mass) and in function (efficiency). The nurse should be familiar with the response to malnutrition of the major organs or organ systems (Table 6–1).

Drug absorption is impaired in malnutrition because of the gastrointestinal effects. Drug metabolism will be altered when malnutrition affects the organs involved in metabolizing drugs. Some drugs depend on blood proteins to prevent toxic effects. When a person is malnourished, blood proteins are reduced, increasing the chance of toxicity with normal doses. Drug doses must be altered according to the degree of malnutrition.

Table 6–1
Multisystem Effects of Malnutrition

System	Effect
Neurologic	
Temperature regulation	Decreased metabolism causes decreased baseline temperature
Mental changes	Apathy, depression, irritability, depressed cognitive function, impaired reasoning and judgment
Immune	
White blood cell (WBC) production	Very sensitive to protein status resulting in decreased antibody formation; increased risk of developing infection also enhanced because of decreased temperature
Musculoskeletal	Decreased muscle mass, agility, and coordination
Cardiovascular	
Heart	Decreased muscle mass and decreased pumping efficiency; increased dysrhythmias
Red blood cells	Decreased synthesis of red blood cells
WBCs	Decreased production of WBCs
Respiratory	Muscle atrophy; increased pneumonias
Gastrointestinal	Decreased mass; decreased enzymes for digestion; decreased absorption; impaired motility; shortened transit time; increased bacterial overgrowth; diarrhea
Hepatic–biliary	Altered metabolism; reduced ability to store glucose; reduced ability to produce glucose from amino acids; reduced protein synthesis; reduced clotting factors
Integumentary	Easy breakdown of skin
Urinary	Kidney atrophy; altered efficiency in filtration, fluid and electrolyte balance, and acid–base balance

SECTION 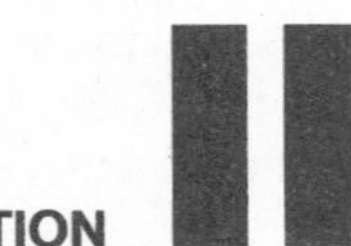

Nursing Process in Malnutrition

Assessment: Establishing the Data Base

The nursing approach to malnutrition includes an assessment of nutritional status to provide information essential for devising an appropriate plan of care. The nutritional assessment includes gathering subjective and objective data from a detailed dietary history, a physical assessment, and diagnostic studies. No single physical finding, measure, or index indicates a definitive diagnosis of malnutrition.

Subjective Data

The subjective data obtained from nutritional assessment should reflect the potential physiologic and psychosocial causes of malnutrition with special attention to identifying the high-risk client (Box 6–1). Ask the client about any disorder that would decrease food ingestion or absorption, increase nutrient losses, or alter nutrient metabolism. (These have been identified in the preceding section.)

Obtain information on recent and current drug therapy to determine whether the client is taking drugs that decrease the appetite or alter nutrient absorption or metabolism. Information on usual and current nutrient intake is also essential. When gathering subjective data for nutritional assessment, determine the client's dietary history as outlined in Box 6–2. A thorough diet history will reveal eating habits including recent changes. It is preferable to request a 3-day record or a 24-hour recall from the client or client's family, if appropriate. The client or family should record time, food, and amount ingested using household measures. For the hospitalized client, the nurse should observe what is eaten at meals and what is brought in by family members.

Ask if the client is following a fad diet, such as a liquid protein diet or diets that consist only of "nutritious" pills. A vegetarian diet may be deficient in protein, especially when milk and eggs are omitted. Review diet information with a nutritionist to determine nutritional content and any gross inadequacies.

Ask the elderly client about problems with eating, such as constipation, disinterest in food, decreased taste, or ill-fitting dentures. A poor appetite, especially with loss of taste acuity, may be associated with illnesses, especially cancer. Poor intake or no intake for 10 days or more is of concern. The time span is even less for extremely malnourished individuals.

Explore any psychosocial causes for decreased intake. The client should be asked why food intake is decreased to determine if the reason is delusions, depression, psychologic stress, or a recent loss. Is the client under pressure at school, at work, or at home? Does the client use alcohol to excess? Ask the client if obtaining food is a financial burden or a serious inconvenience. If appropriate, ask about refrigeration and cooking facilities. The interview should also provide an opportunity for the client to ask about nutrition practices.

Box 6–1
Identifying the High-Risk Client

Grossly underweight: Weight-for-height below 80% of standard

Grossly overweight: Weight-for-height above 120% of standard (risk due to tendency to overlook protein and calorie requirements in the acutely obese patient)

Experiencing recent weight loss: 10% or more of usual body weight

Alcoholic

Taking nothing by mouth: More than 10 days while being given simple IV solutions

Experiencing protracted nutrient losses: Malabsorption syndromes; short-gut syndromes/fistulas; renal dialysis; draining abscesses, wounds

Experiencing increased metabolic needs: Extensive burns, infection, trauma; protracted fever

Taking drugs with antinutrient or catabolic properties: Steroids, immunosuppressants, antitumor agents

SOURCE: Morgan J: Nutritional assessment of critically ill patients. *Focus on Critical Care* 1984; 11(3):30. (Adapted from Weinsier RL, Butterworth CE: *Handbook of Clinical Nutrition.* St. Louis: Mosby, 1981, pp. 7–8.)

Box 6–2
Elements of a Dietary History

Frequency of intake of each food group: milk, meat, fruit, vegetable, and grains

Current nutritional intake versus usual nutritional intake (if it varies)

Meal and snacking patterns

Nutritional supplements

Nutritional preferences and intolerances

Weight history

Food acquisition and preparation habits

Special diet as monitored by health care provider or by client

Cultural or religious dietary considerations

Smoking, caffeine, and alcohol intake

Physical activity

Objective Data

PHYSICAL ASSESSMENT In the physical assessment, look particularly for signs that support or rule out the suspected nutritional disorders. The physical signs of malnutrition and nutrient deficiencies may not always be obvious. Many signs do not appear until the deficiency is advanced. Multiple deficiencies may exist, making the determination of a specific deficiency difficult. Some physical signs of malnutrition such as dry, flaking skin have nonnutritional causes. Obesity may mask protein malnutrition because wasting is not apparent. Since no single sign is diagnostic, the best approach to physical assessment is also to consider the subjective data and laboratory results when drawing conclusions.

The clinical findings of malnutrition and nutrient deficiencies are outlined in Table 6–2. When examining the hair, ask the client if hair collects on the client's pillow, brush, or comb. If any skin lesion is observed, note the body distribution. When examining the mouth, note the status of the teeth. Poor dentition will contribute to poor intake. Muscle mass is assessed by feeling the calves and/or the upper arms. In severe muscle wasting, a decrease in mass is noted throughout the body so the outline of bones is visible. Decreased muscle mass of the hands and the upper chest is seen in advanced protein malnutrition.

In clients where malnutrition has progressed, signs of multisystem effects, as described earlier in Table 6–1, can be observed. Baseline temperature in chronic malnutrition can be as low as 96°F (35.5°C). Record the baseline because elevations may indicate a fever even when below the usual normal of 98.6°F (37°C). Mental changes such as apathy or depression may be detected in advanced malnutrition. Shortness of breath, fatigue, pallor, peripheral edema, and heart rhythm abnormalities may be observed.

As the nurse progresses through the physical assessment, signs of preexisting disorders should also be observed, especially if possibly related to malnutrition. For example, an enlarged thyroid gland may occur with hyperthyroidism, which is associated with increased metabolism.

DIAGNOSTIC TESTS Information from diagnostic tests sensitive to nutritional intake is another aspect of objective data. Diagnostic tests include body measurements, skin testing, and laboratory tests.

Laboratory tests are used primarily to assess protein status because protein is sensitive to nutritional status. Other than protein status indicators, blood levels of minerals and vitamins can be determined when nutrient deficiencies are suspected.

ANTHROPOMETRIC MEASUREMENTS Body measurements, or *anthropometric measurements,* are useful for nutritional assessment because they are altered by states of nutrition. The measurement of body weight, skinfold thickness, and certain body circumferences are the most useful in assessing malnutrition.

Body weight and height should be obtained with the initial nutritional assessment, as a basis for comparison, and at regular intervals thereafter. Ideally, repeated weights should be taken on the same scale. Some clients need a chair or bed scale if their medical condition limits their ability to stand. The present weight should be compared to the reported usual weight and the history of weight gains and/or losses. The present weight should also be compared to the ideal or desired weight. The Metropolitan Life Insurance Company periodically publishes standard weight-to-height tables that are widely used.

Skinfold measurements (measurements of a fold of skin and subcutaneous fat) are used to estimate body subcutaneous fat to determine total body fat (or calorie) stores. These measurements can be obtained in the triceps, biceps, subscapular, suprailiac, and thigh areas and then compared to a table of standards available in most clinical nutrition texts. The result indicates the degree of increased or decreased body fat stores. Directions for obtaining accurate skinfold measurements can be found in nursing fundamentals texts.

The value of anthropometric measurements is questioned in some situations, such as acute starvation because anthropometric changes may lag behind the immediate changes; altered hydrational status from dehydration or overhydration because they also alter the measurement, yielding false high or false low measures; and in the elderly because standard tables were determined on younger people. The results are most useful when observing trends in serial measurements. The trend may indicate an improvement or a decline in nutritional status.

SKIN TESTING FOR DELAYED CUTANEOUS HYPERSENSITIVITY Another diagnostic test useful in nutritional status is skin testing for delayed cutaneous hypersensitivity. Skin testing with various substances (recall antigens) can provide gross information on immune response to those substances. Immune function is particularly sensitive to nutritional status because lymphocytes and antibodies are produced from proteins. Poor protein and/or calorie intake alter the body's ability to produce lymphocytes and antibodies needed to fight infections. In essence, skin tests create a localized infection by introducing antigens that the immune system should recognize and respond to. Malnutrition impairs this response.

Common antigens used for this purpose include *Candida*, mumps, and tuberculin purified protein derivative (PPD). Because many variables—recent surgery, trauma, radiation therapy, immunosuppressive drug therapy, and cancer—can cause false negative responses, it is important to observe trends in serial assessments to determine improving or potentially worsening nutritional status.

NITROGEN BALANCE DETERMINATION One assay of protein and nutrition status is nitrogen balance, since protein is made of nitrogen. *Nitrogen balance* is determined by subtracting the nitrogen intake from the nitrogen output during the same 24-hour period. *Nitrogen intake* is determined by recording the protein intake, from which the

Table 6–2
Clinical Findings of Calorie and Nutrient Deficiencies

Deficiency	Subjective Data	Objective Data
Calorie deficiency	Inadequate dietary intake; weakness; listlessness	Subcutaneous fat loss (especially spine, dorsum of hand, and temporal area); decreased cardiac output; small heart; muscle wasting
Protein deficiency	Inadequate dietary intake; apathy	Flag sign (transverse depigmentation of hair); easily pluckable, thin, or sparse hair; dark hair turns red; flaking skin; enlarged parotid glands; hepatomegaly; edema
Vitamin A deficiency	Inadequate dietary intake; night blindness; disorder of fat malabsorption; altered taste and smell	Dry, scaling, rough skin; shrinking mucous membranes; swelling and redness of eyelids; clouded cornea; Bitot's spots
Thiamine (B_1) deficiency (beriberi)	Inadequate dietary intake; malabsorption; chronic alcohol abuse; apathy; confusion; recent memory loss; nausea, vomiting, anorexia	Cardiomegaly, dyspnea; increase or absence of deep tendon reflexes; peripheral edema; muscle cramps; muscle wasting; pallor; ophthalmoplegia; nystagmus; paresthesia; neuropathy; ataxia
Riboflavin (B_2) deficiency	Inadequate dietary intake; chronic alcoholism; taking oral contraceptives; dimness of vision	Cheilosis, stomatitis; conjunctivitis; edema; neuropathy; seborrheic dermatitis in nasolabial folds; generalized dermatitis; purplish-red tongue; glossitis
Niacin deficiency (pellagra)	Inadequate dietary intake; carcinoid syndrome; chronic alcohol abuse; headache; confusion; muscle weakness; diarrhea	Reddened mouth, tongue, and lips; dermatitis, especially in sun-exposed area(s); glossitis; loss of memory
Pyridoxine (B_6) deficiency	Alcohol abuse; inadequate dietary intake; taking of oral contraceptives	Dermatitis; neuritis; glossitis; convulsions; mild scleral icterus
Cobalamin (B_{12}) deficiency	Strict vegetarian diet; malabsorption from gastrectomy or ileal resection; history of pernicious anemia; hand and feet paresthesia	Lemon-yellow pallor; bright red tongue; pale conjunctivas; glossitis; peripheral neuropathy
Vitamin C (ascorbic acid) deficiency (scurvy)	Inadequate dietary intake; pain and swelling of limbs and joints; easily fatigued	Swollen, bleeding gums; loosening teeth; delayed wound healing; anemia; petechiae; ecchymoses; depression; weakness; easily bruised

Deficiency	Subjective Data	Objective Data
Vitamin D deficiency (adult rickets; osteomalacia)	Inadequate dietary intake; malabsorption; inadequate sunlight exposure	Bone malformations; low serum calcium levels
Vitamin K deficiency	Prolonged use of anticoagulants or antibiotics; malabsorption; biliary obstruction	Bleeding tendencies, especially into gastrointestinal tract, muscles, and joints; petechiae and ecchymoses
Iron deficiency	Inadequate dietary intake; iron malabsorption such as with diarrhea or gastrectomy; blood loss; anorexia, flatulence, constipation; paresthesias in extremities; pregnancy; fatigue	Brittle spoon-shaped nails; cracked corners of the mouth; smooth tongue; tachycardia; dyspnea; listlessness; irritability; pallor; pale conjunctivas; decreased serum iron
Iodine deficiency	Inadequate dietary intake; poor memory; chills; amenorrhea; anorexia	Hoarseness; thick tongue; hearing loss; decreased blood pressure; enlarged thyroid gland

nitrogen intake is derived. (There is approximately 1 g of nitrogen in 6 g of protein.) *Nitrogen output* is determined by analyzing a 24-hour urine collection, with allowances for estimated stool and insensible nitrogen losses. A negative nitrogen balance is an indication of protein breakdown exceeding protein intake, which occurs more in acute malnutrition or in acute stress with chronic malnutrition. With chronic malnutrition, muscle mass is minimal, minimizing the amount of protein available to break down into nitrogen. A nitrogen balance near zero or greater reflects good use of ingested protein.

SERUM ALBUMIN, TRANSFERRIN, AND PREALBUMIN Protein status is also assessed by evaluating the liver's production of transport proteins including albumin, transferrin, and prealbumin. Albumin, a serum protein, has a long half-life of about 20 days. Albumin is not a sensitive indicator of nutrition status because it takes about 20 days to respond to nutritional depletion or repletion. Therefore, it is not reliable in acute starvation. Transferrin has a half-life of 8 to 10 days, making this test more sensitive to changes in nutrition status. Prealbumin, another transport protein, with a half-life of 2 to 3 days, is highly sensitive to nutritional status.

LYMPHOCYTE COUNT Lymphocyte production is sensitive to protein availability because lymphocytes are made of protein. With depressed serum protein levels, lymphocyte production decreases.

Nursing Diagnosis

The nursing diagnoses commonly related to malnutrition are discussed below.

Nutrition, Altered

Malnutrition has many detrimental effects, described earlier in this chapter. As the severity increases, the body's overall health declines.

Bowel Elimination, Altered

Bowel surface area is reduced in malnutrition because of atrophy of the intestinal lining. With a reduced surface area, nutrients and fluids are absorbed less efficiently, causing diarrhea. Also, excess fluids and electrolytes may be lost, leading to a fluid deficit.

Fluid Volume Deficit, Potential

Since many foods contain fluid or water, a reduction in food intake may result in reduced fluid intake. Fluids can also be displaced, causing a deficit. Fluid lost in diarrhea is a good example. Reduced plasma protein from malnutrition alters the vascular compartment osmotic gradient. Edema may result, especially in dependent areas such as the extremities, buttocks, or abdomen, because of the reduced gradient to maintain the fluids in the circulatory system. This fluid imbalance will result, in part, in poor skin turgor.

Injury, Potential for
Mobility, Impaired Physical

Malnourished clients experience easy fatigue and loss of strength, affecting the client's ability to move quickly to avoid danger or trauma. Tasks requiring physical strength may become difficult if not impossible to carry out. Decrease in tissue nourishment also places the client at risk for tissue injury and prolongs healing.

Knowledge Deficit

Some clients may be malnourished because they do not realize that their diets may be lacking in nutrients, that malabsorption may also cause malnutrition, or that medications they are taking may adversely affect their nutritional status. Fad diets used for weight control and "fast food" diets also contribute to inadequate dietary intake.

Self-Concept, Disturbance in

Malnutrition can result in disturbances in self-concept related to body image, self-esteem, and role performance. Those with severe wasting may see themselves as deformed and helpless. Time away from work or the inability to carry on a usual line of work may further intensify feelings of helplessness. The client's role in the family may change because of physical limitations, placing a strain on established relationships. Other family members may need, as a result, to take on additional responsibilities and burdens.

Sexuality Patterns, Altered

As malnutrition progresses, sexual functioning may become impaired because of fatigue and decreased strength and muscle mass. Body changes from malnutrition lessen feelings of sexual attractiveness. Libido may be decreased and, in the woman, decreased vaginal lubrication may cause dyspareunia (painful intercourse).

Skin Integrity, Altered

Skin integrity is sensitive to the state of nutrition. Malnutrition predisposes the client to alterations in skin integrity because the skin relies heavily on good nutrition. Pressure areas on the skin, especially the buttocks, will be prone to skin breakdown. Infection occurs easily in broken-down skin because malnutrition impairs the infection-fighting ability of the body.

Planning and Implementation

Improving Nutritional Intake

Reinforcing instructions from the dietitian regarding good eating habits contributes to dietary counseling. Determining food preferences and taking measures to obtain these foods encourage eating. Removing foul odors from drainage and bedpans will provide a pleasant environment at mealtime. Encouraging or providing oral care before and after meals helps to make food more appetizing. Involving family members in mealtime activities may help improve nutrient intake. If oral supplements are ordered, provide them as the client prefers (eg, on ice, served cold, flavored, or mixed with foods). Encourage good nutritional intake especially prior to surgery and during infections. It is also important to be knowledgeable about nutrient contents of tube feedings, nutrition supplements, and multivitamins. Some elderly persons with limited physical abilities and income require support systems such as communal dining or Meals on Wheels to maintain good nutritional intake.

Some clients require sophisticated nutritional therapy to supply calories, protein, and other nutrients specific to their needs. Nutritional support refers to the administration of oral supplements and enteral and parenteral feedings. Many institutions have nutrition support teams consisting of a multidisciplinary group (physician, dietitian, pharmacist, and nurse specialist). Nursing participation in the team is essential to assure proper identification of client candidates and optimal administration and monitoring of those receiving nutritional support. Some factors that influence the selection of a nutritional therapy route are listed in Figure 6–1.

The nutrition support team can help the nurse in recognizing clients who may suffer from metabolic problems associated with rapid refeeding. In the presence of chronic malnutrition, the body adapts to the state of poor nutrition. If the body is suddenly overwhelmed by nutrients, they are handled poorly. Blood sugar is poorly controlled because of chronic low insulin production. The malnourished heart will be stressed with refeeding because of the high demand for oxygen in the tissues where nutrients are metabolized. Electrolyte imbalances occur because of increased cellular activities related to nutrient metabolism. In nutritional therapy for chronic malnutrition, measures must be taken to replete nutrients slowly.

TUBE FEEDINGS Tube feedings may be necessary for those suffering from malnutrition or those at high risk for developing malnutrition who cannot obtain an adequate oral intake. Tube feedings are given directly into the gastrointestinal tract when the client is unable to eat by mouth, such as after massive head and neck surgery or when swallowing is impaired. Tube feedings are administered through nasogastric tubes or through tubes inserted directly into the gastrointestinal tract during surgery (esophagostomy, gastrostomy, and jejunostomy).

With malnutrition, diarrhea will develop if feedings are given too rapidly. When feedings are first initiated, the nutrients should be diluted in water and administered very slowly over 1 hour or continuously by a feeding pump. It may take 4 to 7 days before the client can tolerate the full amount of tube feeding necessary to meet nutritional requirements.

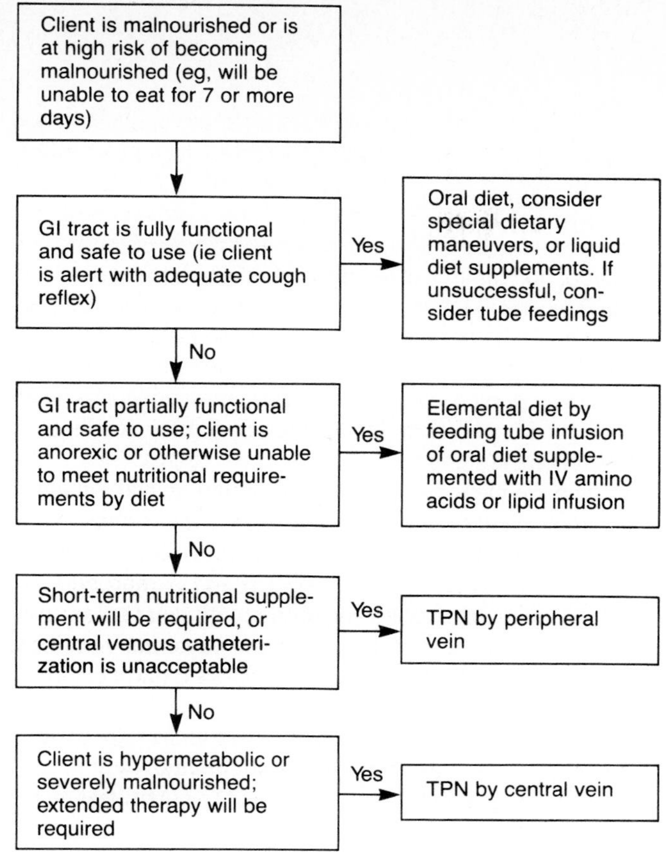

Client is malnourished or is at high risk of becoming malnourished (eg, will be unable to eat for 7 or more days)
GI tract is fully functional and safe to use (ie client is alert with adequate cough reflex)
Yes
Oral diet, consider special dietary maneuvers, or liquid diet supplements. If unsuccessful, consider tube feedings
No
GI tract partially functional and safe to use; client is anorexic or otherwise unable to meet nutritional requirements by diet
Yes
Elemental diet by feeding tube infusion of oral diet supplemented with IV amino acids or lipid infusion
No
Short-term nutritional supplement will be required, or central venous catheterization is unacceptable
Yes
TPN by peripheral vein
No
Client is hypermetabolic or severely malnourished; extended therapy will be required
Yes
TPN by central vein

Figure 6–1

Factors in selection of nutritional therapy route. *SOURCE: Willard MD:* Nutrition for the Practicing Physician. *Baltimore, MD: Williams & Wilkins, 1982.*

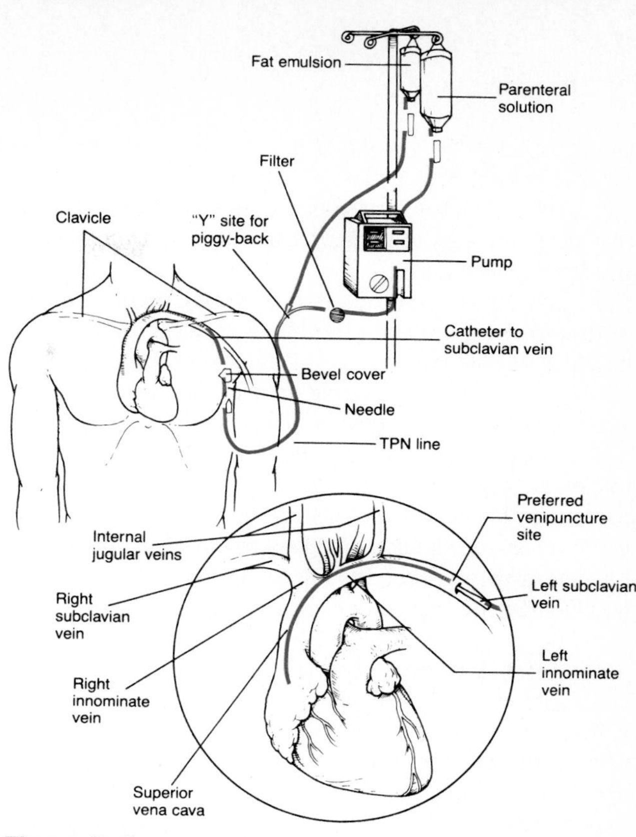

Figure 6–2

Total parenteral nutrition (TPN) through a central vein. The left subclavian vein is most commonly used because of its gentle arch.

TOTAL PARENTERAL NUTRITION When gastrointestinal conditions such as major surgery, obstruction, or inflammation impair the ability to digest and absorb nutrients adequately, the gastrointestinal tract cannot be used to maintain good nutritional status. When this occurs, nutrients can be administered directly into a vein on a short-term or long-term basis. Nutritional status can be maintained indefinitely by the intravenous route.

Total parenteral nutrition (TPN), also referred to as *hyperalimentation,* consists of the intravenous infusion of all necessary nutrients. Carbohydrates in the form of dextrose, protein in the form of crystalline (synthetic) amino acids, electrolytes, vitamins, and minerals are mixed in a container. Intravenous fat emulsions, containing primarily essential fatty acids, are administered from a separate container because of problems with stability when mixed with the other components of the parenteral nutrition solution. The amount of parenteral nutrition and fat delivered varies with the individual nutritional needs.

The nurse plays an important role in the safe and effective administration of parenteral nutrition. Parenteral nutrition is administered by the nurse into peripheral or central (major) veins. Figure 6–2 illustrates a client receiving TPN through a central venous catheter. Because the peripheral veins are easily irritated by high concentrations of dextrose, the amount of dextrose (or carbohydrate calories) that can be infused in the parenteral nutrition solution is limited. The peripheral veins can only tolerate up to a 10% dextrose solution (10 g dextrose per 100 mL of solution). Central veins tolerate dextrose better because of the high volume of blood flow. Usually, central parenteral nutrition solution contains 15% to 25% dextrose, allowing for a greater carbohydrate caloric intake.

Because of the dextrose concentration, parenteral nutrition is administered by an infusion pump to precisely regulate the rate. The proper rate of intravenous dextrose infusion will help regulate glucose homeostasis and cause an appropriate insulin response. Monitor blood and urine glucose to assess for blood glucose imbalances.

Also monitor fluid and electrolyte balance when administering parenteral nutrition. Initial weight gain is common because of the fluid intake. Weight should be monitored daily and daily records kept of fluid intake and output. Electrolyte balance is best assessed by monitoring serum levels.

Take measures to prevent contamination of the parenteral nutrition solution and the infusion catheter. Fungi grow readily in the parenteral solution and bacteria in the fat emulsion. Solutions and infusion tubing should be handled carefully, especially when setting up or changing the tubing. An inline filter, connected at the end of the parenteral nutrition tubing, can be used to collect small organisms that enter the system. These filters also collect small particles of rubber or glass that may have entered in the mixing process. Fat emulsions are too thick to go through the filter, so they are piggybacked to the tubing beyond the filter (see Figure 6–2).

Use aseptic technique in performing regular changes of the dressing covering the infusion catheter to prevent infection at this site. Ideally, gloves and masks are used for dressing changes. The old dressing is removed and the site observed for redness or purulent drainage. An antiseptic solution such as povidone–iodine (Betadine) is used to cleanse the skin around the site, and an antiseptic ointment may be applied at the site to prevent infection. A sterile dressing should be applied to cover and protect the infusion catheter site. Modifications for home parenteral nutrition are discussed in Chapter 36.

The client receiving TPN is at risk for a variety of complications. Some complications resulting from the procedure itself are air embolism, catheter misplacement, circulatory overload, pneumothorax, and hemothorax. Infection (both systemic and at the infusion site) is possible. Metabolic complications are possible, such as acidosis; hyperkalemia; hyperglycemia or hypoglycemia; HHND (hyperosmotic, hyperglycemic, nonketotic dehydration); hypermagnesemia, and deficiencies of sodium, magnesium, calcium, and phosphate; as well as prerenal azotemia.

Improving Bowel Elimination

Bowel elimination can be improved by an adequate dietary intake. Foods high in fiber content, such as bran cereals and muffins, whole grain breads and cereals, fruits, and vegetables add bulk to stool. Antidiarrheals, such as diphenoxylate hydrochloride (Lomotil) or kaolin–pectin mixture, may relieve diarrhea, especially during tube feedings.

Improving Volume Deficit

With potential dehydration, fluids should be administered to replace excess fluid loss and maintain fluid balance. Daily weights and fluid intake-and-output records will help to assess the client's fluid needs and response to fluid replacement.

Improving Self-Concept

Help the client's self-concept by facilitating an understanding of the physical changes of malnutrition. Emphasizing the positive effects of good nutrition may motivate the client to improve nutritional intake. The client should be allowed to ventilate feelings related to body image change.

Improving Skin Integrity

Frequent position changes will prevent undue pressure at points where skin breakdown can occur. Measures should be taken to prevent infection at any skin breakdown sites. If skin excoriation develops from diarrhea, good hygiene should be encouraged following each loose stool.

Evaluation

Malnutrition and/or nutrient deficiency have been corrected when laboratory results normalize and physical signs improve. Malnutrition, especially severe malnutrition, may take months to reverse. Along with reversing malnutrition, another expected outcome is maintaining adequate nutritional intake, whether by oral feeding, tube feeding, or intravenous feeding.

The frequency of bowel movements should diminish, and stools should approach a semisolid state. Bowel movements should assume a regular pattern. This problem may take time to reverse as nutritional status is improved.

Balanced fluid intake and output with good skin turgor and absence of edema are an expected outcome. The client should express knowledge of fluid balance and necessary intake.

Self-concept should improve in response to positive body changes as nutritional status improves.

Skin integrity should improve as the nutritional intake improves. Skin should be healthier and free of breakdown or infection.

Chapter Highlights

Malnutrition is a condition that results from a prolonged reduction of the supply of nutrients or improper utilization of nutrients in relation to demand. It affects all body systems.

Malnutrition is present in 25% to 50% of clients upon admission to the hospital; of those admitted well nourished, 25% to 30% will develop malnutrition during the hospitalization.

Malnutrition significantly contributes to the incidence of morbidity, mortality, and prolonged hospitalizations.

Malnutrition can result from physiologic and psychosocial causes.

The incidence of infection greatly increases with malnutrition.

Chronic malnutrition results in decreased mass and efficiency of organ systems.

Identifying clients at risk for malnutrition as well as assessing those with overt malnutrition or nutrient deficiencies are important nursing responsibilities.

The plan of care for clients with malnutrition should include the correction of the cause of malnutrition when possible.

Rapid refeeding of the client with chronic malnutrition can lead to severe metabolic complications.

Nutritional support (tube feeding and total parenteral nutrition) requires special precautions by nurses.

Bibliography

Anderson L et al: *Nutrition in Health and Disease.* Philadelphia: Lippincott, 1982.

Baker DJ: Ten years of TPN at home. *Am J Nurs* 1984; 84:1248–1249.

Cerra FB: *Pocket Manual of Surgical Nutrition.* St. Louis: Mosby, 1984.

Forlaw L, Bayer LM (editors): Nutrition. *Nurs Clin North Am* 1983; 18:1–128.

Forlaw L, Bayer L, Grant J: *Introduction to Nutritional and Physical Assessment of the Adult Patient for the Nurse.* (Monograph.) Washington, D.C.: American Society of Parenteral and Enteral Nutrition, 1983.

Friedman JD, Cerra FB: Impact of nutritional derangement on organ function. *Infections in Surgery* 1984; 217–221.

Hennessy K: HHNK dehydration. *Am J Nurs* 983; 83:1425–1426.

Heymsfield SB: Metabolic changes associated with refeeding. *Aspen Update* 1982; 4(3):1–2.

Hickler RB: Nutrition and the elderly. *Am Fam Pract* (March) 1984; 29:137–145.

Hui YH: *Human Nutrition and Diet Therapy.* Monterey, CA: Wadsworth, 1983.

Hutchison M McG: Administration of fat emulsions. *Am J Nurs* 1982; 82:275–277.

Konstantinides NN: Home parenteral nutrition: A viable alternative for patients with cancer. *Oncol Nurs Forum* 1985; 12:23–29.

Morgan J: Nutritional assessment of critically ill patients. *Focus Crit Care* 1984; 11(3):28–34.

Munro–Black J: The ABC's of total parenteral nutrition. *Nurs 84* 1984; 14:50–56.

Nurses quick guide to nutritional disorders. *Nurs 83* 1983; 13:56–57.

Roe DA: *Geriatric Nutrition.* Englewood Cliffs, NJ: Prentice-Hall, 1983.

Rogers BL: Home Parenteral Nutrition: Principles and Management. *Nurs Pract* (March) 1984; 9:42–52.

Strotts NA, Friesen L: Understanding starvation in the critically ill patient. *Heart Lung* 1982; 11:469–478.

The Treatment and Management of Severe Protein–Energy Malnutrition. Geneva: World Health Organization, 1981.

Weinsier RL, Butterworth CE: *Handbook of Clinical Nutrition.* St. Louis: Mosby, 1981.

CHAPTER 7

Obesity and Eating Disorders

Other topics relevant to this content are: Anxiety, anger, dependence, and depression, **Chapter 4;** Malnutrition and nutrient deficiency, **Chapter 6;** Physical assessment of the malnourished client, **Chapter 6;** Surgery for morbid obesity, **Chapter 38.**

Objectives

When you have finished studying this chapter, you should be able to:

Differentiate between obesity and overweight.

Define anorexia nervosa and bulimia.

Explain how environment, biology, and psychosocial aspects interact in the development of obesity.

Identify three theories of development related to eating disorders.

Cite the major health problems caused by obesity.

State the physical effects and psychologic disturbances of anorexia and bulimia.

Collect appropriate subjective and objective data for nursing assessment.

Select appropriate nursing diagnoses.

Outline a comprehensive treatment program.

Use the problem-solving method to guide the client through the implementation and evaluation processes.

Eating is the focus of our physical, emotional, and social lives. Food means more than sustenance. It is an expression of love and comfort and a means of reward and punishment.

The emphasis on food is strong, but the value placed on physical appearance is equally strong, particularly for women. Although the ideal form for men has changed little since the ancient Greeks, the ideal female form has shifted with fashion. Slim and ample figures have been in and out of vogue. In contemporary Western society, thin is the ideal.

Until recently, obesity received only perfunctory attention from health professionals. Now this pervasive problem is known to be a high risk factor for a variety of disorders such as diabetes and coronary artery disease. Considerable attention has also been focused on two unusual eating disorders—anorexia nervosa and bulimia—both of which seem to be on the increase.

SECTION 

Obesity

A problem for all age groups, obesity is not limited by social, economic, or ethnic boundaries. The terms *obesity* and *overweight* are not synonymous. **Obesity** is an excess of relative body fat; **overweight** is an excess in body weight. *Morbid obesity* is the maintenance of 100 lb over ideal body weight for 1 year.

In the United States, an estitmated 7 million men (13%) and 14 million women (22%) between the ages of 20 and 74 are obese and overweight. More women are classified as obese across all age groups. The incidence of obesity rises for women between the ages of 34 and 44 years and for men between the ages of 20 and 34 years (Abraham et al., 1983). Demographic studies have shown obesity to be correlated with lower social economic groups, particularly for women, but not with either race or culture in North America or in western Europe.

Classification

Obesity is classified according to adipose tissue morphology (structure and form); age of onset; and definition. The terms describing tissue morphology are **hypertrophy,** an increase in the size of a fat cell, and **hyperplasia,** an increase in the number of fat cells. Hyperplasia–hypertrophy is an increase in both the size and number of fat cells. The terms *juvenile* and *adult* refer to the age at onset. Juvenile-onset obesity begins between the ages of 32 weeks' gestation and 15 years. Adult-onset obesity begins after age 15. There is a correlation between age of onset and tissue morphology. Juvenile-onset obesity is also known as hypertrophy–hyperplasia; adult-onset obesity is denoted as hypertrophy. By definition, individuals are classified as overweight–not obese, obese–overweight, obese–not overweight, and other combinations suitable to specific conditions. For example, a well-conditioned athlete may weigh far more than the norm for his ideal body weight but have less body fat content than normal. He would be termed overweight–not obese. A young mother's weight may be near her ideal body weight, but her body may contain a larger percentage of fat. She would be classified as obese–not overweight.

Causes of Obesity

Obesity is a complex, multidimensional problem. Vigorous investigation of the obesity problem in the past 20 years has generated considerable controversy. The etiology of obesity is central to this debate because effective classification and treatment depend on its determination.

Physiologic Causes

GENETICS Heredity and environment are so closely intertwined in the developmental process that it is difficult to discern which component is dominant. In rare instances, single gene defects and other genetic deficiencies cause obesity. More prevalent causes are lineage (family genes) and somatotype (body configuration). Succeeding generations within a family follow similar patterns of weight gain and body fat accumulation.

Differences in somatotype are genetic and sex specific. Males generally have a larger muscle mass and larger bones than females. In the android body configuration, characteristic of males, fat is deposited in the arms, chest, and abdomen where they also surround the viscera. In the gynoid configuration of females, the fatty deposits are found in the breasts, hips, upper thighs, and gluteal regions.

HUNGER AND SATIETY *Hunger* is defined as a physiologic response to the lack of food, characterized by distressful sensations in the epigastric area coinciding with contractions of the stomach. *Appetite* is more cerebral and can be present without hunger sensations. The thought of food results in a pleasant sensation. *Satiety* is a sense of physiologic fullness.

Until recently, it was thought that hunger and satiety centers were located solely in a specific area of the hypothalamus (the hunger center in the lateral hypothalamus and the satiety center in the ventromedial nuclei) and that stimulation of the hunger center initiated food-seeking behaviors, whereas stimulation of the satiety center inhibited feeding. Other areas of the brain such as the brainstem are now known to be involved. The mechanical aspects of feeding, chewing, salivation, and swallowing are controlled by the brainstem. These movements also occur when the limbic area, contiguous with the hypothalamus, is stimulated. Stimulation of the cortical area of the limbic system perpetuates food-seeking behaviors, without regard to either hunger or satiety. Stimulation of the amygdaloid body induces autonomic nervous system responses of gastrointestinal motility and both inhibition and excitation of gastric secretions.

Hunger and satiety are stimulated and inhibited by other biologic factors such as fluctuations in blood serum levels of glucose, amino acids, and free fatty acids; blood temperature; insulin; and gastrointestinal secretions. The level of free fatty acids in the serum is thought to be the most influential long-term regulator.

Current neuroendocrine research proposes that the hunger and satiety areas serve only as integrating sites for neurologic and hormonal input. The neuroreceptors, neu-

Nursing Research Note

Salter E, Golden M: Obesity in lower and middle socioeconomic status mothers and their children. *Res Nurs Health* 1985; 8(2): 147–153.

The relation between child and maternal obesity, socioeconomic status, maternal nutritional knowledge, and locus of control were studied. Two socioeconomic groups, middle and lower status, were compared by examining maternal obesity, child obesity, maternal locus of control, and maternal nutritional knowledge.

The results demonstrated that mothers of lower socioeconomic status on the average were significantly heavier than middle-class mothers. Children from lower socioeconomic levels were not significantly more overweight than the middle-class group; however, there was a trend toward obesity in the lower-status sample. The amount of adiposity in mothers and children from the lower socioeconomic group was significantly correlated. This was not the case for the middle-class sample. Mothers of lower socioeconomic status scored lower on nutritional knowledge tests and were found to be more external in their locus of control.

This study suggests that in lower-status families, there is a greater trend toward obesity. Nursing intervention for clients of lower socioeconomic status may need to center on nutritional education, developing clients' beliefs that they can control their own body weight, and guidance for nutritional planning for the entire family.

rotransmitters, and neuromodulators affect food-seeking behaviors. Although the physiology of hunger and satiety are not clearly understood, evidence suggests that these endogenous components have a major role.

ENERGY BALANCE In the energy equation, energy intake equal to energy output yields a stable body weight. Any change in caloric intake or caloric expenditure will affect body weight. Weight is gained when caloric intake is increased, energy expenditure is decreased, or both. Conversely, weight is lost when caloric intake is decreased, caloric expenditure is increased, or both. Energy balance is sensitive to small changes. A pound of body fat contains 3500 calories. Elimination of 250 calories from the daily caloric intake while holding the energy expenditure constant will result in a weight loss of 1 lb in 14 days ($3500 \div 250 = 14$).

SETPOINT THEORY This theory proposes that the body has an internal control mechanism, called a *setpoint,* located in some yet-to-be-determined portion of the brain. Exactly how the setpoint is established is unknown. The essential element of the theory is that each person has a set amount of body fat mass determined by genetic and biologic factors. Whenever the body fat mass changes above or below the setpoint, the body adjusts its metabolic rate to keep the percentage of fatty tissue the same. The setpoint may be altered, or reset permanently, if the changed body mass is maintained over an extended period of time.

Psychosocial Causes

PSYCHOLOGIC CAUSES The psychologic causes of obesity have not been delineated. No specific personality pattern or personality disorder seems to characterize obese persons. On the other hand, one psychiatrist (Bruch, 1973), in a now classic work, considers juvenile-onset obesity to be developmental, a response to flawed family relationships. Bruch sees adult-onset obesity as a response to a crisis or trauma.

Many obese people have low self-esteem and a poor self-concept, reflecting societal opinion and family and peer pressure. They may be socially isolated, unable and unwilling to subject themselves to society's ridicule. They may participate minimally in life and have low-paying jobs. They may feel ashamed. They may believe they have a disease. Some find self-destruction the answer. In contrast, other obese persons have a positive attitude, viewing themselves as powerful, important, sensuous, attractive, intelligent, and affectionate. The National Association to Aid Fat Americans has as its motto, "Fat is beautiful."

Overeating is categorized as an addictive behavior similar to alcoholism and drug addiction. The discovery that food metabolism causes release of natural opiates supports this contention. The intake of alcohol, drugs, and food elicits the same set of physiologic responses. The person feels warm, relaxed, and euphoric. Such pleasure is difficult to deny one's self. In addition, eating may be a means of maintaining emotional equilibrium. Obese people report eating because of feelings of loneliness, frustration, boredom, guilt, depression, anxiety, insecurity, and changes in their personal relationships. They eat to cope with life's stresses. Therefore, some theorists suggest that moderately obese people who are emotionally stable and happy should not be urged to lose weight unless they are at risk for a life-threatening disease.

ENVIRONMENTAL CAUSES The diet consumed by many overweight people is higher than recommended in fats, proteins, and simple carbohydrates and lower than recommended in complex starches. Although the actual amount of food consumed may have decreased, the caloric content has increased. Excessive caloric intake and a sedentary lifestyle promote obesity.

Cues for eating are the availability, the sight, the smell, and the taste of food. Inability to resist these stimuli results in inappropriate eating behaviors. Highly palatable, high-calorie foods are available everywhere in supermarkets, fast food restaurants, gas stations, and laundromats. Advertising in magazines, newspapers, and particularly television commercials, emphasizes the desirability of preparing and eating foods. Cookbooks are often among the ten best sellers.

CULTURAL CAUSES Behaviors, beliefs, and attitudes are influenced by social, cultural, and family mores. Eating is a central social activity throughout society and across cultures. Religious and national holidays are celebrated with feasts. In some cultures, a fat wife confers social status on the husband, and obesity is an acceptable condition.

Certain beliefs such as "a fat baby is a healthy baby" and "carbohydrates give energy" promote overfeeding. Adults who require children to clean their plates, and offer food as a comfort or reward, teach children to eat when they are not hungry and to respond to life situations by eating. Children also learn family eating patterns, food preferences, and food preparation. These learned behaviors are retained in adulthood and passed to the next generation.

Sedentary lifestyles have developed over the past 30 years with automation. Labor-saving devices in the home and workplace as well as passive entertainment and spectator sports have reduced energy expenditure and replaced active participation for many. The fitness revolution seems to have attracted those persons who tend to be active participants regardless; it has not significantly increased the overall number of active people.

Obesity as a Multisystem Stressor

Obesity is a stressor to all body systems. An obese person is at greater risk for health-related problems than a person of normal weight. The major health problems associated with obesity are discussed here. These and other health-related problems are listed in Box 7–1.

Cardiovascular and Respiratory Systems

ATHEROSCLEROSIS Obesity is well documented as a risk factor for atherosclerosis, the major cause of coronary artery disease. Atherosclerosis is characterized by narrowing of the lumen of a coronary artery or by total obstruction. Degenerative arterial changes are followed by deposits of fibrous materials and fat, composed primarily of cholesterol. Over time the plaque formation accumulates, decreasing the diameter of the lumen, increasing peripheral resistance, and reducing blood flow (Guyton, 1985).

In the obese state, high-density lipoprotein (HDL) serum levels are reduced. The primary role of HDL is to transport cholesterol from the peripheral tissue to the liver. A deficiency of HDL promotes high serum levels of cholesterol. In addition, ingestion of a high-carbohydrate, high-fat diet promotes low-density lipoprotein (LDL) production in the liver. Because LDL serves as the transport system for cholesterol from the liver to the peripheral tissues, additional cholesterol is provided for plaque formation. Excessive caloric intake also causes overproduction of very low-density lipoproteins (VLDL) from the breakdown of excessive triglycerides. Large quantities of circulating VLDL also contribute to plaque deposits (Morlin, 1984).

Box 7–1
Health-Related Problems in Obesity

- Arteriosclerosis
- Arthritis
- Atherosclerosis
- Cancers of the breast, uterus, prostate, and colon
- Cardiac enlargement
- Cholecystitis and cholelithiasis
- Chronic renal failure
- Congestive heart failure
- Diabetes mellitus, Type II
- Hiatus hernia
- Higher incidence of postoperative complications such as pneumonia, atelectasis, wound dehiscence or evisceration, thrombosis, embolism
- Hypertension
- Impaired pulmonary function
- Kidney enlargement
- Low back pain
- Muscle sprains and strains
- Pregnancy-induced hypertension
- Prolonged labor and delivery
- Stress incontinence
- Thrombophlebitis
- Varicosities

HYPERTENSION There is no direct correlation between obesity and high blood pressure; as many obese persons have hypertension as those who do not. In the massively obese, the heart and the kidneys enlarge. This compensatory enlargement facilitates normotension. Often the diagnosis of hypertension is based on inaccurate measurements made by using an inappropriately sized cuff and by placing the cuff incorrectly on the upper arm.

Elevated blood pressure indicates increased peripheral resistance. It is unclear if the increased peripheral resistance is in response to the expanded intravascular volume accompanying the enlarged body mass or if it is secondary to increased cardiac output and other autoregulatory mechanisms. Some studies are finding that a decrease in body weight results in a decrease in blood pressure.

CONGESTIVE HEART FAILURE In obese persons, the highly vascular fat mass, with the increased metabolic activity of the hypertrophied fat cells, increases demand for cardiac output. As the stroke volume increases, the left ventricle dilates, causing the myocardium of the posterior walls and septum to thicken. Eventually, left ventricle function is impaired, progressing to congestive heart failure.

RESPIRATORY PROBLEMS Obese persons often experience shortness of breath upon exertion. The extra fat and concomitant decrease in mobility hinder ventilation and increase susceptibility to postoperative complications such as atelectasis and pneumonia.

Endocrine System

Truncal obesity (obesity of the trunk of the body), hypertrophied fat cells, genetic predisposition, and the lack of exercise are factors in the development of adult-onset non-insulin-dependent (Type II) diabetes. These conditions, combined with a high-fat, high-carbohydrate intake, create higher than normal serum plasma levels of triglycerides, glucose, and insulin. This produces overt symptoms of glucose intolerance.

Thyroid hormone, cortisol, and growth hormone are also factors in obesity. Both cortisol and growth hormone are decreased during the weight-gaining phase and during maintenance of massive obesity. Less growth hormone promotes fat storage by inhibiting lipolysis. In addition, evidence suggests that low cortisol levels cause an increase in gluconeogenesis, lipogenesis, and fat storage while depressing fat utilization.

Overeating a high-carbohydrate diet causes an increase in triiodothyronine (T_3) and a decrease in reverse-triiodothyronine (rT_3). When food is restricted, T_3 values decrease and rT_3 values increase. During weight loss, adaptation to lower levels of T_3 slows the basic metabolic rate, and energy requirements decrease. Therefore, lipolysis is slowed, and weight loss slows or reaches a plateau. The body uses calories far more efficiently; fewer need to be taken in to maintain weight, and more must be cut back to achieve weight loss.

Treatment of Obesity

The treatment of the obese person is rewarding when the client successfully loses weight and frustrating when the client is unable to do so. Throughout their lives, many persons gain and lose weight on a regular cycle (the yo-yo syndrome). The problem often seems insurmountable. A variety of treatments have been used with minimal success. Presently, bariatric specialists (health professionals who focus on the problems of obesity) recommend a lifestyle that incorporates changes in food intake and physical activity. A comprehensive program includes an eating plan for weight loss and long-term maintenance, physical exercise, behavioral change, social support, and cognitive restructuring.

Motivation

Many persons cite health problems as reasons for losing weight. Others are motivated by psychologic or emotional problems (eg, feelings of embarrassment, social isolation, shame, and guilt). Still others find motivation in the wish to purchase fashionable clothing, wear bathing suits, or attract the opposite sex. During the weight-loss process, additional motivators must be found to meet the long-term goals of achieving ideal body weight and weight maintenance. Assisting clients to develop awareness of their needs is helpful. At the beginning of their weight-loss program, ask them to list reasons for losing weight and to add to this list as they proceed through the program. Clients should review motives daily, particularly when tempted and when making difficult choices.

Regulation of Food Intake

The regulation of food intake is the cornerstone of a weight-loss program. Weight is lost when energy intake is less than energy expenditure. In this text, the term *dieting* is avoided because it connotes short-term behaviors that usually have little success. In fact, it may be that repeated dieting causing the yo-yo effect causes the greatest health risk.

The variety of weight-loss plans is almost unlimited. Restricted food plans proliferate in popular magazines and books. Most of these fad diets lack nutrients and, therefore, are detrimental when followed for more than a few weeks. In the 1970s, a liquid protein diet consisting of hydrolized gelatin and collagen but deficient in essential amino acids, caused more than 50 deaths (almost all of which were linked to cardiac dysrhythmias). Usually, these plans are found to be boring and unsatisfying and are discontinued quickly. This perpetuates the yo-yo syndrome and reinforces feelings of failure and inadequacy. Nutritional instruction focused on long-term weight maintenance assists a client to view changes in behavior as permanent. Patience and persistence are required for long-term adherence to an eating plan. A brief discussion of various eating plans is summarized in Table 7–1.

The balanced deficit diet is the eating plan advocated by most authorities. The food exchange system developed jointly by the American Diabetes Association and the American Dietetic Association outlines a balanced nutritional food plan using household measurements that can be used as a weight reduction regimen. Divided into six food groups, designating food quantities of equal equivalence, this plan permits unlimited variations. Cookbooks and exchange lists for fast food restaurants, frozen food, and other commercially prepared foods are available. Instructional material, food models, and booklets are also available. Nutritional eating behaviors learned during the weight loss period are used for lifelong maintenance.

Exercise

Many authorities believe obesity is related more to inactivity than overeating (Bjorntorp, 1983). Studies show the obese move less and expend less energy than lean persons. (A conditioned muscle requires more energy for movement than an unconditioned muscle.) In most activities, only low-level energy is expended (eg, a 150-lb male walking for approximately 10 minutes expends only about 25 calories). The rate of loss is accelerated with calorie restriction. Elevating the resting heart rate between 40% and 60% of maximum will use stored fat for energy.

An exercise program is designed in progressive steps with a goal of 20 to 30 minutes of continuous activity three to four times per week. The basic exercise program includes flexibility exercises (bending and stretching), muscular strengthening, muscular endurance, and cardiovascular conditioning. Each session consists of a warm-up, the activity, and a cool-down period. Calisthenics and flexibility exercises are done in the warm-up and the cool-down portions. Calisthenics using 3- to 5-lb weights, aerobic dancing, running, rowing, bicycling, and cross country skiing produce muscle strengthening and muscle endurance along with cardiovascular conditioning. For an exercise program to be effective, it must be practical, pleasurable, and an activity the client will perform.

For the morbidly obese, a low-level walking program or merely an increase in the activities of daily living will facilitate weight loss. A walking program consists of flexibility exercises and walking 10 to 15 minutes per day, 7 days a week, progressing to 1 hour per day. All persons should be encouraged to increase routine activities by using the stairs instead of the elevator, parking further from store entrances, and increasing bending and stretching during household chores.

Exercise has added physiologic and psychologic benefits. With conditioning, changes occur in the cardiovascular system—the pulse rate is lowered, the stroke volume increases, and peripheral vascular resistance is lessened. Muscle work promotes increased cellular metabolism, suppresses hunger, and increases lipid utilization. Individuals develop self-confidence, improve their perceptions of themselves, develop a more positive attitude toward their bodies, feel more in control, and recognize the body as a source of pleasure. These new attitudes foster improved interpersonal relationships and social interactions.

Behavioral Change

In the healthy person, most behavior related to food seeking and food intake are the result of habits learned throughout life. According to behavioral therapists, the

Table 7–1
Types of Restricted Diets Used for Weight Reduction *(Note that most of the diets are not safe or effective)*

Diet Type	Description	Possible Health Effects
Balanced diets of 1200 kcal or more	Usually consist of ordinary, readily available, high-nutrient-density foods in limited amounts; often moderate in protein and carbohydrate and most restricted in fat	Can meet the RDA if carefully chosen; weight loss is usually 1–2 lb per week; can be liberalized to stabilize weight for safe lifetime use
Diets of fewer than 1200 kcal	Usually composed of ordinary, readily available, high-nutrient-density foods in very limited amounts; often moderate in protein and very restricted in fat and carbohydrate	Diet often fails to meet the RDA for many nutrients; ketosis may occur; weight loss is often 3 or more pounds per week, much due to water loss; regain is more likely than with slower weight loss
High-carbohydrate, high-fiber diets	Emphasize whole grain breads, cereals, raw fruits and vegetables, moderate amounts of animal proteins, dairy products, avoidance of highly processed foods; supplemental fiber is sometimes recommended	Calculated nutrient intake is nearly adequate, but fiber (especially if supplemented) may reduce availability of minerals
Formula low-kcal diets	Powders, liquids, or wafers constitute diet of 1000 kcal with supplemented vitamins and minerals; provide 20% protein, 30% fat, and 50% carbohydrate	Adequate in vitamins and minerals; may be constipating; ketosis may occur; requires no food choice decisions or contact with food; often discontinued due to monotony or unpalatability; weight regain is likely because old eating habits remain; more acceptable as one meal per day within a low-kcal diet plan
Low-carbohydrate, high-protein, high- or moderate-fat diets	Emphasize high-protein foods, severely limit carbohydrate to 50 g; usually low in kcal because allowed foods become unappealing	Diet may meet RDA if chosen carefully; ketosis occurs, causing fluid loss; can cause increase in blood fat and cholesterol levels; may cause menstrual dysfunction, dehydration, osteoporosis, aggravation of gout, kidney failure or stones; much of lost weight due to water loss
One-food diets	Emphasize one food or food type, such as fruit, rice, or ice cream, as mainstay of the diet	Inevitably deficient in some nutrients, excessive in others; discarded quickly because of monotony; lost weight regained
Fasting	Water and no-kcal beverages allowed; vitamin and mineral supplements given; person usually hospitalized for monitoring	May result in nutrient deficiencies, low blood pressure, ketosis, emotional disturbances; death may result if prolonged; causes weight loss of 3–5 lb per week; regain begins when person begins eating again but has not learned new eating behaviors; former weight usually regained in time
Protein-supplemented fasting	Like fast, but with protein supplement of up to 1.5 g/kg of ideal body weight; protein in form of lean animal products, liquid protein isolates, or amino acids	May result in ketosis, nausea and vomiting, diarrhea or constipation, weakness, muscle cramps, mineral imbalance, irritability; former weight usually regained in time; over 50 deaths attributed to use of over-the-counter liquid protein products

SOURCE: Christian JL, Greger JL: *Nutrition for Living*. Menlo Park, CA: Benjamin/Cummings, 1985, pp. 248–249.

"cure" for obesity lies not solely in dieting, but rather in behavioral change. Behavior modification, a process characterized by the conscious alteration of responses to stimuli, combined with the action-oriented problem-solving approach, can help to change or modify learned behaviors.

First, the client's specific problems and goals are defined. Then the client's life history is obtained and analyzed. Identification of the "triggers" or stimuli for inappropriate food seeking and food intake is the next step in the process. Appropriate alternate behaviors are then identified. The individual selects the most suitable alternate behavior and plans ways for implementation. After the plan is implemented, progress is monitored and the outcomes are evaluated. If results are satisfactory, the behavior is repeated. When unsatisfactory results occur, an alternative strategy is selected, and the process begins again until a solution is found.

Each success contributes to feelings of control and progress. Gaining control encourages the setting of short-term and long-term goals, which structure the arduous process of weight loss. Thus encouraged, the individual develops patience and persistence.

Due to the complexity of food-seeking behaviors, changes in responses to the environment and physiologic and psychosocial stimuli are required. The examples of behavioral strategies listed in Box 7–2 are not inclusive. Additional suggestions are found in the literature and are only limited by the creativity of the individuals involved.

Box 7–2
Strategies for Behavioral Change

Methods for controlling the environment are:

1. Purchase low-calorie food.
2. Shop from a prepared list and on a full stomach.
3. Keep all foods in the kitchen.
4. Store all foods in the refrigerator or in cabinets in opaque containers.
5. Prepare exact portions of food to eliminate leftovers.
6. Become an expert on preparing low-calorie foods.
7. Eat all foods in the same place, avoiding the kitchen.
8. Avoid eating when watching television or reading a book.
9. Reduce the frequency of eating out at restaurants, parties, picnics, etc.

Methods for controlling physiologic responses to food are:

1. Eat slowly in small bites, allowing 20 minutes for a meal.
2. Eat a salad or drink a hot beverage before a meal.
3. Chew each bite thoroughly and slowly.
4. Put eating utensils or food down between bites.
5. Concentrate on the eating process; savor the food.
6. Lengthen the time between courses.
7. Stop eating with the first feelings of fullness.

Methods of controlling psychologic responses to food are:

1. Appreciate the aesthetic experience of eating.
2. Use attractive dinnerware and prepare a formal setting for eating.
3. Use small plates and cups to make servings of food look larger.
4. Concentrate on conversations and socialization during the meal.
5. Use nonfood rewards for meeting a goal.
6. Acknowledge small successes and improvements in all behavior.
7. Substitute other activities for eating (eg, reading, exercise, hobbies).
8. Problem-solve.
9. Identify feelings.
10. Use assertive behavior.

Social Support

The direct involvement of selected family members in the program will often foster understanding and cooperation. Group programs may also produce positive effects as members learn from one another, identify with each other, and develop feelings of belonging. A variety of self-help and mutual support groups are described in the resources list at the end of this chapter.

Cognitive Restructuring

Cognitive restructuring means to change beliefs, attitudes, and thoughts by interpreting reality in new and different ways. The origins of beliefs and attitudes are embedded in lifelong psychologic development. Therefore, change requires conscious, sustained effort. Focusing on changes in eating behaviors and on implementing an exercise program helps identify areas for change. Introspection and discussion with a therapist, in groups, and with family or friends will facilitate the process.

Language changes are also required because thinking is the use of language. Perceptions of self and the world depend on words used. Many obese people use negative words and phrases when speaking of themselves, thus reinforcing negative feelings. They need to change these word choices and thought patterns. For example, compare these phrases: "I am bad," "I have no will power," "I cheated," with "I choose to" and "I ate an apple." Positive statements reflect an objective, in-control attitude that is conducive to building self-esteem.

Surgery

Surgery can be used to treat obesity in difficult cases. Criteria for surgical candidates include morbid obesity, a stable personality, failure to lose weight by conventional methods, age between 25 and 50 years, and medical clearance. Surgery is effective only if the client also changes lifestyles and restricts food intake. Ingestion of high-calorie foods and fluids will cancel the benefits of surgery.

Not considered effective in controlling weight are jaw-wiring and ear-stapling. The once-popular ileojejunal bypass loop is no longer widely used because of serious complications, including death.

Currently, the most widely accepted surgical procedures involve compartmentalizing the stomach.

Drug Therapy

Because of the many causes of obesity, no single drug is effective. Diuretics have numerous side effects and are essentially not effective since the weight lost through diuresis is body water, not fat. Drugs containing cellulose produce a feeling of fullness by absorbing water and expanding the stomach; their effectiveness is unknown. Thyroid hormones have also been administered in attempts to increase body metabolism. However, they must be used in high doses that cause hazardous cardiovascular symptoms, and the effect is transitory.

In the past, the primary anorectic drugs (hunger suppressants) were amphetamines. These addictive drugs have a number of serious side effects such as hypertension, allergy, blood disorders, and paranoid reactions. A newer drug, fenfluramine (Pondimin), derived from amphetamines, may act peripherally by mediating adipocyte cellular metabolism. The basic action of fenfluramine is believed to be on the brain neuroregulators, but the exact mechanisms for its actions are unknown.

For weight loss, appetite-suppressing drugs are usutally prescribed only for the first few weeks and are used in conjunction with a low-calorie eating plan. Research shows these drugs promote quick weight loss. Unfortunately, study results also showed the weight was regained over the long term.

Gastric Bubble

A recent technique developed for the treatment of obesity is the gastric bubble. In this procedure, an acid-resistant balloon is inserted into the stomach and inflated. Although it does not interfere with digestion, it does reduce the amount a person can eat comfortably. Gastric bubbles are used for eight months or more, with new ones inserted every four months. Their use is being recommended in only life-threatening cases because of complications.

Nursing Process With Obese Clients

To be effective in assisting obese clients, nurses must examine their own beliefs, attitudes, and feelings about obese persons. Preconceived notions and prejudices will affect the total therapeutic plan. Health professionals may have negative perceptions of obese persons, viewing them as lazy, undisciplined, neurotic, and lacking in character. The physical difficulties in providing care reinforce these negative feelings. Obtaining reliable data from the physical assessment is difficult and often requires special skills and equipment. The thickened subcutaneous fat interferes with auscultatory techniques and percussion, obscures abnormalities detectable by inspection, and inhibits palpation. Attempts to give physical care, such as bathing, repositioning, ambulating, and venipuncture, are impeded. A clear understanding of this problem is required to circumvent negative views and promote a positive therapeutic milieu.

Nursing Assessment: Establishing the Data Base

SUBJECTIVE DATA The weight history elicits data about:

- Chronologic development of obesity
- Familial attitudes, beliefs, and lifestyle, including ethnic and cultural influences
- The individual's self-perceptions: self-esteem, self-concept, and body image
- Motivation
- Participation in other weight-loss programs
- Food intake and physical activity

More accurate than the weight history is an evaluation of food intake and activity from a recorded analysis because people tend to overestimate their activity levels and underestimate their food intake. Record forms are available or may be developed for individual situations. These records integrate the biopsychosocial areas associated with food-intake behavior. The self-analysis includes recording the time of eating; length of time required to eat; eating site (kitchen, bedroom, den); physical position (sitting, standing); companion; mood (happy, sad, bored); hunger level; amount and types of food intake; and types of meal (meal, snack). Also recorded are the type, amount (repetitions), and time spent in physical activity.

OBJECTIVE DATA Determining the degree of obesity or overweight is accomplished both by gross and precise methods. The gross methods include the simple inspection of the individual body, preferably in the nude, for marked fat deposits. The *pinch test* is performed by grasping the skin between the forefinger and thumb. If the skinfold is greater than an inch, the area contains excessive fat deposits.

Overweight and obesity can be estimated by comparing a person's height and weight with standard tables. The tables do not indicate the amount of body fat, nor do they consider age factors (many people over 40 are overweight); therefore, these weights should be used only as guidelines. Another method, the Hamwi method, calculates the ideal body weight for women of medium frame as 100 lb for the first 5 ft and 5 lb for every inch over 5 ft. Weights for men of medium frame are calculated at 106 lb for the first 5 ft and 6 lb for every inch over 5 ft. Although adjustments for large and small frames are made, this method is subject to the same drawbacks as the standard tables.

More precise methods for determining obesity and overweight are skinfold measurements and calculating the body mass index (BMI). Skinfold measurements using skin calipers yield relative body fat values. The normal body fat content is approximately 15% for men and 18% to 25% for women. The BMI is thought by many experts in obesity research to be a more reliable indicator of obesity than the height–weight table ranges. It can be calculated by dividing a person's body weight (in kilograms) by the person's height (in meters) squared.

Also useful in assessment are laboratory values for serum plasma levels of glucose, triglycerides, cholesterol, cortisol, T_3 and T_4, as well as skull x-rays and an ECG. More sophisticated assessment methods used by researchers are underwater weighing, also known as water displacement; ultrasound; computerized tomography (CT) scanning; and measurement of total body electrical conductivity.

Nursing Diagnosis

Nursing diagnoses related to the obese and overweight client are listed in Box 7–3. The complexity of this disorder may require development of additional diagnosis or alteration of standard diagnoses.

Planning and Implementation

In some instances, the identified problems are outside the scope of the nurse's practice and are referred to an appropriate resource; examples are counseling for severe psychologic dysfunction and the medical treatment of physical problems. The plan depends on the care setting: inpatient, clinic, or private practice. Depending on available resources and the client's needs, the nurse might recommend group sessions or individual counseling. Also influencing the plan is the availability of ancillary support from dietitians and activity assistants and physical facilities. Time constraints for both the nurse and the client must also be considered. Since there will be frequent appointments over a long period, they must be scheduled to avoid conflicts with employment. The cost of the program and reimbursement must also be considered. Some insurance policies cover weight loss associated with high-risk health problems. Prepaid health plans, such as health maintenance organizations (HMOs), emphasize health promotion and therefore are more liberal in benefits.

Generally, a treatment plan prescribes a change in lifestyle through goal setting, problem solving, and information exchange. Specific techniques are recommended for food intake, exercise, behavior, and cognitive restructuring. These techniques are discussed in the section on treatment.

The implementation of the plan may be negotiated by the nurse or other health care provider and the client. The nurse is responsible for providing information and guiding problem solving and goal setting. The client and his or her support systems are responsible for implementation and evaluation.

Box 7–3
Nursing Diagnoses Commonly Related to Obesity

Diagnoses Directly Related to Obesity

Activity intolerance

Breathing pattern, ineffective

Coping, ineffective individual

Knowledge deficit, related to nutrition, exercise

Mobility, impaired physical

Nutrition, altered: more than body requirements

Self-concept, disturbance in

Other Potential Diagnoses

Cardiac output, altered: decreased

Coping, ineffective family

Gas exchange, impaired

Powerlessness

Self-care deficit

Skin integrity, impaired

Social isolation

Evaluation

Although the treatment plan will be individualized, evaluation can be based on several common outcomes. The client can be expected to:

- Maintain normal weight for height, age, sex, and body structure as determined by the assessment tool
- Modify food-intake behaviors
- Participate in an exercise program
- Demonstrate positive cognitive restructuring
- Maintain optimal nutritional status
- Apply principles of nutrition to food choices and food preparation
- Demonstrate an improvement in health problems and develop no additional problems

SECTION 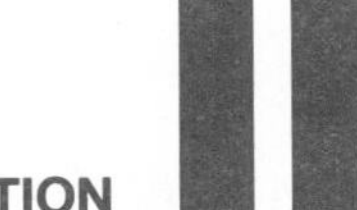

Eating Disorders

Within the past several years, anorexia nervosa and bulimia have captured the attention of both scientists and the general public. There seem to be several reasons for the interest and concern. First, incidence seems to be increasing among the group that is primarily affected—women in adolescence and young adulthood. Also, the etiology is not fully understood even though anorexia nervosa was first described in the clinical literature nearly 300 years ago. Until recently, bulimia was included with anorexia, and researchers are only starting to define and explain its specific aspects. Finally, there is a fascination with the symptomatology. The willpower and denial exercised by emaciated anorexia clients can be astounding even to experts. The numbers of calories ingested by the bulimic client and the vomiting and laxative abuse seem horrifying.

The symptoms are more than just bizarre phenomena. Prolonged starvation, repeated vomiting, and laxative abuse may lead to a life-threatening situation. The body is simply not equipped to withstand starvation and the complications of the extreme weight-loss methods. The mortality rate has been variously estimated in the range of 5% to 21%, with the higher percentage having relevance for anorexia. Worse yet, both disorders have proven difficult to treat.

Anorexia nervosa is a complicated disorder involving self-inflicted starvation that may be accompanied by vomiting, laxative abuse, and hyperactivity. The term *anorexia* is misleading because the individual does not initially experience a loss of appetite. Rather, intake is purposefully reduced to achieve and maintain goal weight well below the minimum norm for body size. In most cases, the target weight continues to drop until weight loss reaches life-threatening proportions. The drive to be thin is propelled by a distorted belief that one's body is "too fat" despite extreme emaciation. Although the disorder may begin as simply a conscious effort to lose weight, weight loss eventually becomes the primary focus in the individual's life. Not eating can be viewed as an attempt to cope.

Anorexia nervosa may be distinguished from bulimia, sometimes called bulimarexia or bulimia nervosa. The word *bulimia* comes from the Greek word meaning "ox hunger." It is characterized by episodic and frenzied binging on large quantities of usually soft-textured, easily eaten, highly caloric food, consumed in a brief period of time, followed by purging with vomiting, laxatives, or diuretics. In some cases, people with bulimia will follow binging behavior with a period of restricted intake and/or rigorous exercising. Binge–purge cycles are usually followed by self-deprecation, a depressed mood, and the realization that the eating pattern is abnormal. Clients with bulimia are usually striving to maintain weight and do not have the distortions in body image common to anorexics. They may in fact be at or above normal weight for their body size, varying from about 10 to 15 lb in either direction at any given time. For the bulimic, eating becomes an uncontrolled, embarrassing, and frightening impulse.

Diagnostic Criteria

Currently, the DSM-IIIR (Diagnostic and Statistical Manual, 1987) diagnostic criteria for anorexia nervosa and bulimia are the most widely used (Table 7–2). There is a

Table 7–2
Diagnostic Criteria for Anorexia Nervosa and Bulimia

Anorexia Nervosa	Bulimia
Intense fear of becoming obese, which does not diminish as weight loss progresses	Recurrent episodes of binge eating (rapid consumption of a large amount of food in discrete period of time, usually less than 2 hours)
Disturbance of body image (eg, claiming to "feel fat" even when emaciated)	1. Consumption of high-calorie, easily ingested food during a binge
Weight loss of at least 25% of original body weight (if under 18 years of age, weight loss from original body weight plus projected weight gain expected from growth charts may be combined to make the 25%)	2. Inconspicuous eating during a binge
Refusal to maintain body weight over a minimal normal weight for age and height	3. Termination of such eating episodes by abdominal pain, sleep, social interruption, or self-induced vomiting
No known physical illness that would account for the weight loss	4. Repeated attempts to lose weight by severely restrictive diets, self-induced vomiting, or use of cathartics or diuretics
	5. Frequent weight fluctuations greater than 10 lb due to alternating binges and fasts
	Awareness that the eating pattern is abnormal and fear of not being able to stop eating voluntarily
	Depressed mood and self-deprecating thoughts following eating binges
	Bulimic episodes not due to anorexia nervosa or any known physical disorder

uing effort to refine diagnostic criteria for both eating disorders. Controversies about symptomatology and etiology may create confusion for nurses who encounter these clients. There are similarities between features present in eating disorders and other psychiatric diagnoses such as depression, schizophrenia, and obsessive–compulsive behavior. For example, symptoms such as depressed affect, sleep disturbances, decreased ability to concentrate, and low self-esteem may occur in both eating disorders and depression. Sometimes clients qualify for more than one diagnosis concurrently. In addition, symptoms of anorexia nervosa and bulimia tend to overlap. There are individuals who alternate between extended periods of restricted intake and periods of bulimia and who reach extremely low body weights. These clients are sometimes referred to as "bulimic-anorexics" or "bulimic-restrictors."

Etiology

A variety of theories have been used to explain the etiology of eating disorders. Most experts agree that anorexia and bulimia develop from an interaction of biologic, psychologic, and sociocultural factors. Theories relating to the early psychologic development of these clients pertain primarily to anorexia nervosa, since bulimia has only recently been considered as a separate phenomenon. Even the earliest descriptions of anorexia stressed a psychologic component. Recent trends, however, explore the influence of hereditary and physiologic factors. Few would deny that society's current norms for thinness play a role in the increasing incidence of eating disorders, but a complete understanding of the interplay of all these factors has not yet been achieved.

Developmental Theory

Hilde Bruch thinks that eating disorders result in part from faulty learning beginning at infancy. That is, the parents of these individuals did not respond appropriately or at least consistently to their infant's cues for physical and emotional needs. A pattern of erratic reinforcement laid the groundwork for the child's inability to identify and satisfy his or her own bodily needs. Faulty communication between parent and infant was the precursor to the development of a sense of ineffectiveness. Instead of developing a sense of ownership of their own bodies and feelings of competence in communicating and satisfying their needs, these children learned instead to respond to the parent's needs and emotions. Bruch believes that this background leads to the compliant behavior characteristic of these clients during their latency years (Bruch, 1973).

Psychoanalytic Theory

Traditional psychoanalytic theorists believe, like Bruch, that problems in early childhood contribute to personality development that predisposes the individual to eating disorders. The belief is that during the toddler years, the child fails to develop a sense of an independent, complete self separate from the caretaking parent. The parent rewards the child with affection for clinging, dependent behavior but withdraws emotional support when the child demonstrates assertive, autonomous behavior. This theory is complex but in essence describes a child who fears emotional displays that may drive away the parent and other important figures. This leads to a quality of relating to others characterized by the desire to please. Problems arise later during adolescence when there is a pull toward increasing autonomy and independence from the family. The child may experience this as a threat of loss of emotional support. Rather than risk the loss of emotional support that could result from increased autonomy and independence, these adolescents remain overly compliant and pleasing. A sense of control and autonomy is achieved through the eating disorder by restricting food intake or engaging in vigorous exercise, for example.

Family Systems Theory

In 1974, Minuchin identified several interaction patterns that are still considered characteristic in families of anorexic children. *Enmeshment* refers to a lack of clear boundaries between the generations as well as between individual members. Members become overly sensitive to one another. Emotions and needs of one individual are shared by the other members of the system, and the members feel endangered by conflict. There is a tendency to avoid conflict, become overprotective of one another, and maintain a facade of harmony. Since every marital system or family has conflict, problems are in effect deflected onto the child, who becomes symptomatic. The family becomes focused on the child with anorexia, freeing the parents and the other family members from addressing their own problems. This system becomes self-perpetuating, and the families become locked into a rigid, unchanging pattern.

Eating Disorders as Multisystem Stressors

Eating disorders have adverse physiologic effects on many different body systems. They are discussed briefly below and listed in Table 7–3.

Physiologic Effects of Starvation

Many symptoms of anorexia nervosa are actually a direct result of the starvation process. Features such as obsessive thinking about food, mixing unusual combinations of foods, hoarding food-related items, and depressed affect have been observed in victims of starvation. The physical effects of anorexia nervosa are often a result of both poor dietary intake and fluid depletion secondary to vomiting or inadequate intake. Typically, the client is dehy-

Table 7–3
Health Consequences of Eating Disorders

Anorexia Nervosa	Bulimia
Abdominal bloating	Constipation because of bowel atony
Amenorrhea	Dehydration
Bradycardia	Difficulty in retaining food even in small amounts (spontaneous regurgitation)
Constipation	Dysphagia
Dehydration	Erosion of stomach lining
Edema	Esophageal irritation, erosion, or bleeding
Fatigue and pain when sitting and lying down	Excessive tooth decay and erosion of tooth enamel
Gastrointestinal intolerance to food	Gum disorders
Hormonal imbalances	Hemorrhage of blood vessels in the eyes
Hypokalemia resulting in fatigue, seizures, cardiac dysrhythmias, nephropathy related to chronically low levels of potassium	Hormone imbalances
Impaired circulation	Hypokalemia
Infertility	Lightheadedness
Loss of hair	Menstrual irregularity
Muscle wasting	Swelling, pain, and tenderness in the salivary glands
Susceptibility to infection	
Vitamin and mineral deficiencies	

drated with poor circulation. Muscle breakdown and lack of padding of the bones and nerves contribute to fatigue and pain when sitting and lying down. A common yet serious complication of starvation is amenorrhea. Researchers have found that in some cases amenorrhea may precede weight loss; however, it is generally thought that cessation of menstruation accompanies loss of body fat. Numerous hormonal changes may occur secondary to changes in the hypothalamic–pituitary axis.

Physiologic Effects of Binging and Purging

The most severe medical complications may occur in clients who engage in repeated vomiting and laxative abuse. Loss of fluid and electrolytes, especially potassium, along with the already compromised nutritional status may lead to renal dysfunction and cardiac dysrhythmia. A less serious though more common complication of vomiting is dental caries and inflammation and erosion of the gums caused by the hydrochloric acid from the stomach. Mild to severe cases of constipation may occur, either because the client's food intake is below the level necessary to provide intestinal bulk or because of bowel atony resulting from prolonged laxative abuse. Esophageal and gastric problems may potentially become severe. Clients may even experience spontaneous regurgitation—difficulty in retaining food when they want to.

Eating Disorders as Psychosocial Stressors

Not only do eating disorders result from psychosocial stress; they may be psychosocial stressors as well.

Body Image, Self-Esteem, and Self-Confidence

The body image and self-image are closely intertwined concepts. For the individual with an eating disorder, the two become centered around the achievement of thinness. The person believes that in becoming thin, all problems will be solved and happiness found. This notion is supported by both internal and external feedback. The process of dieting is inherently rewarding in its measurable successes. Beyond this, friends and family members often congratulate early successes in dieting. Certainly, society equates thinness with success and happiness. The potential anorexic is vulnerable to all these influences because of an already poor sense of self-worth and a belief that she or he has little to offer as a unique individual. Many clients will say they are "nothing" if they are not thin.

In view of their low self-worth and of social influences, it is not surprising that clients with eating disorders persist in a self-destructive pattern. The harmful aspects of starvation elude them. Instead, they are boosted by the self-discipline involved in restricting intake and in long hours of study, work, and exercise. Discipline and success in weight loss become the core of the individual's self-esteem and self-confidence.

In many ways, the anorexic individual fears developing the primary symptom of bulimia—uncontrolled binging. These clients fight the loss of control involved in a binge. Persons with bulimic symptoms may have tried to accomplish the self-discipline of anorexia and in succumbing to the binge, feel deeply humiliated. They share the anorexic's desire to be thin and the low feelings of self-worth, but harbor their symptoms in secrecy from friends and family. At the same time, the binging behavior itself may become a source of pleasure because it is often used to soothe tension or to create a sense of euphoria, similar to that of drug or alcohol abuse. Consequently, their symptoms are a complicated blend of pleasure and pain, and thus difficult to relinquish.

Autonomy, Independence, and Isolation

Often, individuals who develop eating disorders appear to be healthy and functioning well, aside from their symptoms. This facade may have been long-standing. These clients have frequently assumed the role in their families of the "least needy" child. That is, they have been problem-free and have won the love of their parents through a kind of pseudoindependence. They appear to take care of themselves and often assume the role of caring for others. An internal dilemma arises, however, because they deny their own needs for nurturance and support. The symptoms serve as a kind of symbolic representation of their own neediness. In developing a thin body, they take on a childlike quality and receive the care and attention they are often ill-equipped to ask for directly.

The style of relating begun with the family is continued in relationships with others. These clients become kind, supportive friends and are good "listeners," but they seldom identify problems for themselves. They feel guilty asking others to support them. On the surface, clients with bulimia may appear more outgoing and engaging than clients with anorexia, who may appear more reserved and aloof. Beneath the external appearance, however, both types are focused more on others' needs and wants than on their own. The symptoms become a means of coping with the resulting frustrations. The client with anorexia denies neediness and withdraws from others. The bulimic client may remain superficially engaged with others but uses the symptoms to soothe inner tensions from unexpressed anger.

Treatment of Eating Disorders

Treatment of eating disorders usually combines behavior modification and psychotherapy in an interdisciplinary approach. In many settings, the physician, nurse, dietitian, psychotherapist, social worker, and occupational therapist, among others, work as a team in development of a treatment plan. Communication among members is essential in this system, and often the primary nurse will coordinate among team members.

Antidepressant drugs may be helpful; their effectiveness is the focus of a number of current research studies.

Behavior Modification

In most cases, some principles of behavior modification will be incorporated into treatment for clients with eating disorders. Although specific interventions may vary, anorexic clients will usually be reinforced for weight gain. Reinforcements might include increased time for diversional activities, less time under direct supervision of staff, visiting privileges, increased exercise, or passes to leave the unit. Outpatients might be told they must gain weight to avoid hospitalization. Inpatients often will be given liquid protein supplements to drink or receive tube feedings for uneaten portions of meals. These interventions should not be presented as punishment but rather as life-saving measures.

The behavioral principles of desensitization and response prevention are frequently used. The inpatient may be desensitized to eating by beginning a low-calorie diet using stated food preferences. Gradually, calories are increased, and foods are introduced that the client fears (such as spaghetti). Staff supervision after meals to prevent vomiting or laxative abuse allows the client gradually to tolerate the feeling of fullness. It is important to include the opportunity to talk about feelings generated by eating, such as fear, anger, or guilt.

Behavioral techniques such as cognitive restructuring may be particularly helpful. The nurse can provide didactic information on the harmful effects of binging and purging and remind the client that vomiting and laxative abuse are not effective means of weight control. Alternatives to binging may be suggested, such as taking a walk or calling a friend. Helping the client plan a daily mealtime regimen may help relieve anxiety concerning control of eating. This is an important element in treatment because many clients will not eat all day, adding hunger to the precipitating factors of a binge. All of these techniques work to help change the client's thinking about the usefulness of the symptoms.

Psychotherapy

Most behavioral programs are used in conjunction with individual psychotherapy, family therapy, or both. The goal of individual therapy is to increase the client's understanding of the reasons for the symptomatic behavior and to increase self-esteem. Family therapy can assist the family members to cope with the feelings generated by the client with the eating disorder. It may also be helpful in sorting out other problems in family relationships that may affect the family group as a whole.

Nursing Process for the Client With an Eating Disorder

Caring for clients with anorexia nervosa and bulimia is challenging. Not only do clients with eating disorders have complex physiologic and emotional problems, but they may resist treatment. The disorder may be life threatening and require long-term treatment. The nurse sets the tone for treatment by conducting a thorough assessment and establishing a supportive therapeutic relationship.

Nursing Assessment: Establishing the Data Base

SUBJECTIVE DATA When the client is admitted to a hospital unit for severe malnutrition or serious electrolyte abnormalities, it may be difficult to gather subjective data from the client. The client's condition may preclude accurate reporting, and family members may need to supply additional information. Determine the circumstances of the admission, such as whether the client entered treatment voluntarily. If not, the client may deny the severity of the condition and give incomplete data regarding the history of symptoms.

The nurse may need to alter the approach to data gathering depending on the client's age and previous experience with hospitalization. A young client in an initial hospitalization may be frightened and need reassurance before feeling comfortable offering a history. The initial interaction with the client can be extremely important in setting the tone for the course of the hospitalization.

The initial history should include a detailed description of the previous dieting behavior. The goal will be to assess the chronology, nature, and severity of symptoms as well as the client's investment in them. In particular, the nurse will need to know the client's previous high and low weights, the ideal or goal weight, the age of onset of dieting and/or binging, the frequency of use of vomiting or purgatives, the amount of time spent exercising, and percentage of time spent thinking about food and weight control. In addition, ask about the reasons for initiating a diet, such as having been teased about increasing weight or pubertal development. If the client has binging episodes, assess the client's ability to identify what factors trigger a binge.

The interview should illuminate the extent to which the eating disorder interferes with other areas of functioning. Open-ended questions are often helpful. For example, the nurse might ask the client to describe a typical day, detailing all activities including eating. Many clients will spend hours working, studying, or exercising to avoid thinking about food. It is important to elicit information about time spent with friends or family members and the client's response to that time. Individuals may avoid activities with friends that might include a meal and eventually withdraw from relationships altogether.

OBJECTIVE DATA Physical assessment of the malnourished client has been discussed in Chapter 6. The nurse monitors electrolyte values both initially and regularly thereafter to determine if the client is continuing with vomiting or laxative abuse. It is also important to observe the client's affective state. Although the client may be unable to identify depressed feelings, facial expression, posture, eye contact, and tone of voice provide information about internal states. (See also Table 7–2.)

Nursing Diagnosis

Identification of client problems relating to the effects of malnutrition is outlined in Chapter 6. Specific nursing diagnoses for clients with anorexia nervosa or bulimia are listed in Box 7–4.

Planning and Implementation

The nurse working closely with the client will want to establish reasonable short-term goals that will ultimately increase the client's ability to manage independently yet to be able to recognize the need to seek assistance and support when necessary. Many anorexic persons require

Box 7–4
Nursing Diagnoses Commonly Related to Eating Disorders

Diagnoses Directly Related to Eating Disorders

Bowel elimination, altered: constipation, related to insufficient intake of food or laxative abuse

Coping, ineffective individual

Fluid volume deficit, actual or potential, related to diuretic abuse

Injury, potential for

Mucous membrane, alteration in, related to induced vomiting

Nutrition, altered, less than body requirements

Self-concept, disturbance in, body image, self-esteem

Tissue perfusion, altered

Other Potential Diagnoses

Cardiac output, altered: decreased, related to dysrhythmia from electrolyte imbalance

Coping, ineffective family

Injury, potential for, related to dehydration and lightheadedness

Nutrition, altered: potential for more than body requirements, related to binging

Sexuality, altered patterns

Skin integrity, impairment of

Social isolation

inpatient treatment, while outpatient treatment is usually manageable in bulimia.

INPATIENT CARE: STRATEGIES FOR CLIENT AND FAMILY Nursing interventions are aimed at the goal of restoring weight and adequate nutrition within a supportive emotional context. In the treatment of severe emaciation, the client's condition may necessitate intravenous infusions to correct electrolyte imbalance, nasogastric tube feedings, and in some cases, total parenteral nutrition. It is crucial not to overload the client's circulatory system, risking congestive heart failure from the body's inability to handle fluid overload. Too rapid administration of food and the calories the client has been attempting to avoid may result in a sudden and severe escalation of the client's anxiety level to the extent of panic. The process of weight restoration should be initiated slowly, preferably with a balanced diet of 1200 calories with no added salt, incorporating the client's food preferences.

Ideally, the client should be monitored closely for at least 1 hour during and after meals. Clients with anorexia may experience anxiety, guilt, and panic after eating because of the distorted belief that all food is "bad" and will lead to excessive weight gain. This belief leads to desperate behavior, such as hiding food during meals or postmeal vomiting. If the patient refuses food, liquid protein supplements may be given in caloric amounts equivalent to uneaten food portions.

Eating after prolonged periods of starvation or chronic laxative abuse can lead to edema, abdominal distention, and constipation. The nurse will need to monitor such potential problems, keeping in mind that clients with anorexia frequently complain of feeling "bloated" after meals because of their psychologic discomfort with eating.

Weights are usually taken daily at the same time with the client wearing the same clothing. Clients should void before weigh-ins because they may attempt to increase their weights by drinking large quantities of water. To promote weight gain, activity should be restricted to a minimum. In some cases, bed rest may be necessary initially.

In most cases, clients will resist treatment despite an initial sense of relief that the treatment team has assumed responsibility for their decisions. Although anorexic clients usually are not attempting to commit suicide, they are overwhelmed with fear at the idea of gaining weight. The difficulties that arise during eating may surprise staff because of the client's generally pleasing, compliant facade. It is not unusual for some nurses to feel angry and avoid the client because of the apparent refusal to accept treatment. Remember during this stressful time that clients are not maliciously attempting to sabotage efforts of the staff, but rather need to maintain some sense of control.

It is good practice to consult with a psychiatric nurse specialist when caring for clients with eating disorders. Staff members often need assistance in implementing a consistent, firm approach to eating. Clients will need encouragement to explore their feelings after eating, without being given false reassurances. Avoid power struggles with the client about particular food items or portions. Make an effort to see that one nurse is not identified as more strict or more lenient than another. In general, firm limits combined with genuine emotional sensitivity and support will be most helpful to the anorexic client.

Planning and implementation involve both clients and their families. Although dysfunctional family interactions might contribute to the development of eating disorders, it is important that the nurse not make judgments about the client's family. Remain sensitive to the fact that the family members of anorexic clients may have been struggling for many months to force the client to eat. The distress of watching a family member willfully starve may be enough to cause chaos in a household. Parents, siblings, friends, and spouses will likely feel guilty, ineffective, and depressed about the situation and will need support from the nurse with regard to these feelings. At the same time, be aware that family and friends may inadvertently collude in obstructing the client's treatment. For example, clients may complain that the nurse is cruel and punitive, leading families into taking them home before it is medically safe. Forewarn them about this phenomenon and encourage them to discuss this with the nurse. Instruct them also not to discuss eating and weight with the client but to let the staff handle this aspect of care.

OUTPATIENT CARE: STRATEGIES FOR CLIENT AND FAMILY If the client's condition is not severely compromised medically, it may be preferable to attempt outpatient treatment. The nurse may play a key role in establishing a relationship with the client. Often the nurse will be required to make highly skilled judgments in responding to the client. At times, firm limits may need to be set on the symptomatic behavior. At other times, empathy and supportive statements can motivate the client to continue treatment.

The nurse will probably work closely with a physician and perhaps a dietitian in establishing weight goals with the client. Usually, the nurse weighs the client weekly. Some clients who have not achieved their goal weight attempt to hide this fact to avoid hospitalization. Others may actually hide objects on their bodies to increase weight. The nurse who discovers such techniques should avoid acting punitive, angry, or shocked. It is preferable to use a matter-of-fact approach in reweighing the client and later trying to elicit feelings about the difficulty of giving up the symptoms.

It may be helpful to have clients with either anorexia or bulimia complete weekly food diaries as well. The bulimic individual may discover patterns or trends to the binging behavior. The anorexic client may be able gradually to introduce additional food items with encouragement from the nurse. The nurse can provide nutritional teaching and include information about the harmful effects of inadequate nutrition.

A number of organizations offer mutual support groups for individuals with anorexia and bulimia. Some clients may be interested in using a peer group as an adjunct to other treatment. Most individuals will need to continue medical follow-up, however, to monitor side effects of the symptoms. Strategies relevant to the family have been discussed under inpatient care.

Evaluation

The nurse can be helpful in determining the psychologic readiness to manage diet and weight. Decisions might be based on the client's ability to plan menus and tolerate eating without direct supervision. For the client in the hospital, physical stability and weight gain are two critical variables. Many clients will return to the symptoms and begin to lose weight upon discharge. Recovery from anorexia and bulimia can be a long, complicated process, and some persons will require multiple hospitalizations. Most individuals will need some form of follow-up treatment to include ongoing therapy as well as routine monitoring of weight and electrolytes.

Chapter Highlights

Obesity is an excess of relative body fat; overweight is an excess in body weight.

In obesity, both sides of the energy equation—intake and expenditure—are of equal importance.

Obesity is a stressor to all body systems.

Understanding the causes of obesity is central to development of an effective, individualized treatment plan.

Effective treatment of obesity is based on long-term motivation, a nutritious eating plan, and a practical activity program.

Weight loss and long-term weight maintenance are accomplished only with a permanent life-style change.

Anorexia nervosa is a disorder of self-inflicted starvation often resulting in extreme emaciation.

Bulimia is a disorder involving episodes of binging on food, usually followed by purging by vomiting or laxatives.

Prolonged starvation and purging can result in general malnutrition, dehydration and electrolyte imbalances, hormonal changes, and multiple effects on all systems.

Clients with eating disorders base their self-esteem on ability to lose weight.

Treatment of eating disorders can be a long, complicated process because it involves both weight restoration and psychologic changes.

Nursing goals for eating disorders promote weight gain and adequate nutrition in a supportive emotional context.

Bibliography

Abraham S et al: Obese and overweight adults in the United States. *Vital Health Statistics* 1983; 230:1–93.

Bjorntorp P: Physiological and clinical aspects of exercise in obese persons. *Exercise and Sports-Science Reviews* 1983; 11:159–180.

Boskind–White M, White WC: *Bulimarexia: The Binge/Purge Cycle.* New York: Norton, 1983.

Brownell K: The psychology and physiology of obesity: Implications for screening and treatment. *J Diet Assoc* 1984; 84(4):406–413.

Bruch H: *Eating Disorders: Obesity, Anorexia Nervosa and the Person Within.* New York: Basic Books, 1973.

Bruch H: Four decades of eating disorders. In: *Handbook of Psychotherapy for Anorexia Nervosa and Bulimia*, pp. 7–18. Garner D, Garfinkel P (editors). New York: Guilford, 1984.

Cozens RE: Obesity in the aged: Not just a case of overeating. *Nurs Clin North Am* 1982; 17(2):227–232.

Diagnostic and Statistical Manual of Mental Disorders, 3rd ed. (DSM-IIIR). Washington, DC: American Psychiatric Association, 1987.

Friemer N, Echenberg D, Krutchmer N: Cultural variation—Nutritional and clinical implications. *West J Med* 1983; 139(6):928–933.

Garner D, Garfinkel P: *Anorexia Nervosa: A Multidimensional Perspective.* New York: Brunner/Mazel, 1982.

Greenwood MRC: *Obesity.* New York: Churchill Livingstone, 1983.

Guyton AC: *Textbook of Medical Physiology.* Philadelphia: Saunders, 1985.

Harris MB: Eating habits, restraint, knowledge and attitudes toward obesity. *Int J Obes* 1983; 7:271–286.

Minuchin S: *Families and Family Therapy.* Cambridge, MA: Harvard University Press, 1974.

Morlin RJ: Atherosclerosis: Advances in prevention and treatment. *Geriatric Consultant* 1984; (Nov–Dec):11–17, 31.

Pasulka PS, et al: The risks of surgery in obese clients. *Ann Intern Med* 1986; 104(4):540–546.

Sanger E. Cassino T: Eating disorders: Avoiding the power struggle. *Am J Nurs* (Jan) 1984; 84:31–33.

Stunkard AJ, Stinnett JL, Smoller JW: Psychological and social aspects of the surgical treatment of obesity. *Am J Psychiatry* 1986; 143(4):417–429.

Wagner PL, Kirsch ER: Obesity complications in critical care. *Dimensions Crit Care Nurs* 1985; 4(2):81–91.

Resources

SELF-HELP GROUPS AND OTHER ORGANIZATIONS

American Anorexia-Bulimia Association, Inc.
133 Cedar Lane
Teaneck, NJ 07666
Phone: (201) 836–1800 weekdays, 10 AM to 2 PM EST

This national organization will give the names of physicians and treatment centers. On Wednesdays from 10 AM to 2 PM a recovered person takes calls.

Anorexia Nervosa and Related Eating Disorders, Inc. (ANRED)
PO Box 5102
Eugene, OR 97401
Phone: (503) 344–1144

A nonprofit organization that responds to requests for information and referrals.

National Association to Aid Fat Americans, Inc. (NAAFA)
PO Box 43
Bellerose, NY 11426
Phone: (516) 352–3120

In existence since 1969, the group fights prejudice and discrimination against obese people and promotes self-acceptance and societal acceptance.

National Association of Anorexia Nervosa
and Associated Disorders (ANAD)
Box 7
Highland Park, IL 60035
Phone: (312) 831–3438

This mutual support association was founded by Vivian Meehan, a nurse recognized for her achievement by the American Nurses' Association. It will provide advice on joining a self-help group or forming one.

Overeaters Anonymous (OA)
PO Box 92870
Los Angeles, CA 90009
Phone: (213) 542–8363

In Canada:
Overeaters Anonymous
Central Ontario Intergroup
175 St Clair Ave W, Suite 25
Toronto, Ontario, Canada M4V 1P7
Phone: (416) 929–5361

Patterned after the philosophy of Alcoholics Anonymous, this self-help organization views compulsive eating as a disease that can be arrested but not cured. No dues or fees. Literature available upon request. Over 100,000 members.

UNIVERSITY- AND HOSPITAL-AFFILIATED EATING DISORDERS PROGRAMS

Health Psychology Clinic
University of Minnesota Hospital
420 Delaware St., SE
Box 731 Mayo
Minneapolis, MN 55455
Phone: (612) 624–9646
Director: Dr. Manfred Meier

Eating Disorders Program
New York Hospital-Cornell University Medical Center
Westchester Division
21 Bloomingdale Rd.
White Plains, NY 10605
Phone: (914) 682–9100
Director: Dr. Katherine Halmi

Eating Disorders Program
Northwestern Memorial Hospital
Superior Street and Fairbanks Court
Chicago, IL 60611
Phone: (312) 908–7850
Director: Dr. Craig Johnson
Clinical Nursing Manager: Lyn Marshall, RN, MSN

Eating Disorders Program
UCLA Neuropsychiatric Institute
760 Westwood Plaza
Los Angeles, CA 90024
Phone: (213) 825–0173

Eating and Weight Disorder Clinic
Adolph Mayer Bldg
Johns Hopkins Hospital
600 N. Wolfe St.
Baltimore, MD 21205
Phone: (301) 955–3863
Director: Dr. Arnold E. Anderson

These sources will supply information and may be able to recommend local specialists.

CHAPTER 8

Substance Abuse

Other topics relevant to this content are: Cirrhosis, **Chapter 41;** Malnutrition and nutrient deficiencies, **Chapter 6;** Neurotransmitters and nervous system, **Chapter 27;** Programs to help smokers give up the habit, **Chapter 14;** Risk to substance-abusing clients of contacting acquired immune deficiency syndrome (AIDS), **Chapter 23;** Smoking and lung cancer, **Chapter 16.**

Objectives

When you have finished studying this chapter, you should be able to:

Identify the scope of substance abuse problems.

Discuss general theories related to etiology of substance abuse problems.

Define psychologic and physical dependence and tolerance.

Compare and contrast the effects of major drugs of abuse.

Use the nursing process with clients who have problems related to substance abuse.

The use and abuse of prescription, over-the-counter (OTC), and illicit drugs is a problem of staggering proportions in America. Many people use a variety of substances to relax, induce sleep, alleviate pain, relieve depression, increase energy and alertness, alter mood, and heighten fun. Alcohol, sedative-hypnotics, stimulants, and antianxiety drugs are being consumed more often and by more people than ever before.

The history of using mind-altering drugs to excess, or in a manner disapproved by society, is as old as the human race. Fermented beverages were probably used by prehistoric humans, who depicted their effects on cave walls. The Bible and the writings of the ancient Egyptians described their effects. Opium and marijuana have been in worldwide use for centuries, and the Indians of South America recognized the stimulant properties of the coca plant long before the Spanish conquest.

Each society develops rules and guidelines for the use of drugs. In some cultures, men may drink fermented beverages to intoxication; women and children who do so may be punished. Alcohol use is widely accepted in Western society, but its use is prohibited and condemned in Moslem cultures that often tolerate marijuana. In the Eastern world, opium was once a widely accepted recreational drug. In the United States and England, it was available on grocery store shelves until the late nineteenth century. Cocaine, the ingredient that was responsible 75 years ago for making Coca-Cola "the pause that refreshes," is now an illegal drug in the United States.

SECTION 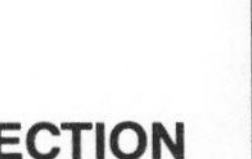

The Problem of Substance Abuse

Drugs are being produced in increasing numbers, making them more readily available through both legal and illicit channels. A drug culture lifestyle with its own jargon supports and maintains its members in their drug-seeking behavior and helps to make the illicit market profitable.

Substance abuse is a major social and public health problem. The abuse of one drug—alcohol—currently is the third major cause of death in the United States, ranking only behind coronary diseases and cancer. Substance abuse costs the American economy billions of dollars a year in lost productivity, health care and treatment costs, and crime.

Nurses have frequent contact with individuals who abuse drugs—clients, friends, neighbors, and colleagues. It has been estimated that 25% of all hospitalized clients experience problems related to substance abuse. Each person who is a substance abuser will have an adverse effect on the health and well-being of family members, friends, and work associates. They, in turn, become clients in the broadest sense, needing assistance in learning how to cope with their substance-abusing relative, friend, or colleague. In addition, nurses have a high rate of substance abuse within their own ranks.

What Constitutes Substance Abuse

Substance abuse or misuse is not easily defined, and the parameters are not clear-cut. The definition also depends on one's perspective. **Substance abuse** can be defined as the continued use of chemical agents despite the emotional, social, legal, and health problems their use creates. One of the hazards of using mind- and mood-altering drugs is dependence.

Drug dependence develops with the repeated use of certain chemical agents; a person requires the effects of a specific drug to function. Two forms of dependence—psychologic and physical—may develop. Some substances cause one form of dependence, whereas others generate both types. **Psychologic dependence** occurs when a person has a compulsion to continue using the substance, craving its effects to experience a sense of self-esteem and well-being. In **physical dependence,** an individual experiences physiologic symptoms of withdrawal when the drug is discontinued. The time from the last ingestion of the substance to withdrawal, as well as the withdrawal symptoms, are drug-specific and depend on the type and amount of drug taken. Diazepam (Valium) causes both psychologic and physical dependence. Besides severe physical symptoms accompanying withdrawal, the diazepam user has a craving to resume using the drug. Imipramine hydrochloride (Tofranil), used to treat depression, is a good example of a drug causing physical dependence but not psychologic dependence. When Tofranil is discontinued after prolonged administration, the client may experience nausea, vomiting, muscle aches, anxiety, and difficulty in sleeping but does not feel compelled to resume its use.

Tolerance is the result of the body's attempts to adapt to repeated exposure to specific chemical agents. Tolerance means that, with repeated use of the drug, the user requires increasingly larger amounts to produce the same effects previously attained with smaller amounts. Another dangerous aspect is that tolerance does not develop uniformly to all of a drug's effects. For example, users of alcohol and barbiturates develop tolerance to the intoxicating effect of the drug, but the potentially lethal dose does not change appreciably. The amount the user then needs to feel good may be nearly enough to cause death.

A concurrent state of **cross-tolerance** may also develop. This condition occurs when the person has developed a tolerance to one agent and then requires larger doses of pharmacologically similar drugs to achieve the desired effect. For example, an alcoholic client admitted for an appendectomy will probably require larger dosages of meperidine (Demerol) to experience relief from postoperative pain than another client who is not dependent on alcohol. An individual tolerant to methaqualone (Quaalude) will also be tolerant to sodium pentobarbital (Nembutal).

Addiction is another term often applied to substance abuse. Although it has been deleted from the diagnostic classifications of the American Psychiatric Association and the World Health Organization, the term continues to be used by professionals and clients to describe psychologic dependence, physical dependence, and both. To avoid confusion, this chapter will use the term *dependence.*

At any given time, some chemicals may be more popular among substance users than others. Preferences change, and some substances become either more or less available. A current trend is toward polydrug use, using many different drugs at the same time. Many drinkers combine alcohol with marijuana, cocaine, and amphetamines. Clients taking prescribed antipsychotic agents, antianxiety agents, and antidepressants often use them concomitantly with alcohol.

Polydrug use may result in the following interactions, depending on which drugs are used simultaneously:

- Additive effect. When two or more drugs that produce the same effects by the same physiologic mechanism are used together, the effects are greater than would be expected from one drug alone. Effects do not exceed what would be expected from simple addition of the drug effects, however.
- Potentiation effect. When one drug enhances the effects of another drug taken in combination with it by intensifying or prolonging its effect, it is said to have a potentiative (synergistic, supraadditive) effect. The drug actions may be much greater than with simple addition. Central nervous system (CNS) depressants, such as barbiturates, benzodiazepines, and opioids, are examples of drugs that have a synergistic effect with alcohol.
- Antagonistic effect. When drugs are combined, one drug may inhibit (lessen or block) the effects of the other. Caffeine, a weak antagonist, is often added to antihistamine drugs to counter the drowsiness they cause. Alcohol and barbiturates are often taken by amphetamine abusers to "take the edge off" their anxiety and agitation.

Polydrug use is a hazardous practice leading to serious medical emergencies and physiologic crises. Be aware that some health problems of clients could be related to drug interactions from polydrug use. The ultimate effects of ingesting many different drugs together remain unknown.

Etiology of Substance Abuse

Despite the hundreds of studies focused on the problem of substance abuse, the cause (or causes) remains unknown. No one physical, social, developmental, psychologic, cultural, or genetic factor can be singled out.

No matter why a person becomes a substance abuser, once dependent on a chemical agent, the person will be motivated to continue its use to experience a sense of self-esteem and worth, to prevent or relieve withdrawal symptoms, or both. Although the question of why one person becomes dependent on a drug while another does not remains unanswered, several explanations have been offered.

Availability and Encouragement

Sedatives and antianxiety agents are not only produced in massive numbers, but they are also excessively prescribed. One of them, diazepam (Valium), is the best-selling drug of all time. Others are easily available on the street through illegal sources. Vigorous advertising campaigns make many chemical substances seem appealing and socially acceptable. The combination of availability and mass media influence is thought to contribute to substance use and abuse. Peer pressure is another strong motivator.

Adverse Social Conditions

Poverty, unemployment, racial discrimination, and lack of social and educational opportunities have been correlated with high rates of substance abuse. Some people may abuse substances as a means of coping with these adverse social conditions. The social conditions themselves may also result from substance abuse: Substance abusers who are unable to function on the job or to keep up with the demands of an educational program may find themselves without employment (and without money).

Developmental Factors

Developmental theorists propose a link between substance abuse and parental loss (either through death, abandonment, or divorce) or the inability of parents to form satisfying emotional relationships with their children. Parents are important role models for their children's behavioral and emotional development; thus, children of substance-abusing parents are at greater risk for developing substance abuse problems.

Psychologic Factors

Psychoanalytic theory links substance abuse with fixation at the oral stage of development. Substance abuse is viewed as self-destructive behavior that stems from lack of adequate self-love and aggression that is turned inward. Other psychologic causes are thought to be unfulfilled dependence needs, depression, low self-esteem, and hostility; thus, substance abusers depend on chemicals to fill emotional needs.

Genetic Predisposition

Recent research has suggested that substance abusers (particularly alcoholics) have a genetic predisposition to dependence. Researchers suspect that alcoholism is caused by a genetically transmitted biochemical defect, resulting in a lack of production of certain enzymes or hormones. This creates a particular kind of homeostatic balance that can only be maintained by ingestion and metabolism of alcohol. Although conclusive evidence is yet to be found, it is anticipated that identification of biologic causes will enhance the treatment and rehabilitation of alcoholics and other substance abusers.

Neurotransmitter Defects

An exciting aspect of current neurochemical and physiologic research is the study of neurotransmitters and their relationship to substance abuse. Neurotransmitters are chemicals in the nerve endings (axons) that are important in the transmission of nerve impulses to the next cell by way of the synapse, the microscopic space between the axon and the receptor of the next nerve cell (dendrite).

Depressant drugs (such as alcohol and antianxiety agents) appear to depress the nerve cell action by inhibiting or interfering with neurotransmitters. Stimulants increase the synthesis and release of neurotransmitters by mimicking the neurotransmitter or inhibiting its reuptake.

SECTION 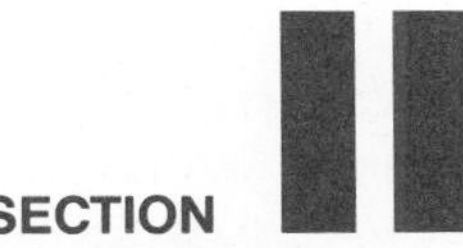

Substances of Abuse

Abused drugs are categorized based on their effects on the CNS. The five primary classifications are: depressants (including alcohol and anxiolytic agents), narcotics, stimulants, hallucinogens, and CNS toxins.

All of the drugs in these five groups have one point in common: Each drug can produce a pleasurable state by either elevating the mood and creating a "high" feeling or decreasing anxiety or tension.

Depressants

The drugs in this category have a depressant effect on the CNS; they include alcohol and the prescription medications known as anxiolytic agents because they reduce anxiety. In addition to decreasing anxiety, anxiolytic drugs also have sedative (promoting relaxation) or hypnotic (producing sleep) effects. Anxiolytic agents include, among others, the barbiturates such as phenobarbital, sodium pentobarbital, and secobarbital (Seconal) and nonbarbiturate drugs such as chlordiazepoxide (Librium) and diazepam. Many people, including nurses, use these agents rather than problem-solving methods to help them cope with the pressures of life. Worldwide, the anxiolytic agents are the most frequently prescribed group of medicines for symptoms of sleeplessness and anxiety (Gilman, Goodman, & Gilman, 1984).

Alcohol

Alcohol is one of the most easily available and frequently abused drugs in America. Of the adult population 18 years and older who report drinking behavior, the average daily consumption is about three drinks per day. Of course, a smaller proportion of people drinks more than average, and a larger proportion drinks much less. Of those who drink, 1 in 10 will become alcoholic (alcohol-dependent). Alcoholism is also a serious problem in the Soviet Union, France, and Sweden.

Alcoholism costs the economy an estimated $50 billion annually because of lost productivity, property damage, medical expenses, rehabilitation programs, family disruptions, alcohol-related illnesses, alcohol-related violence, and neglect and abuse of children. The estimated 13 million Americans who are believed to be alcoholics or problem drinkers are associated with an annual toll of 50,000 traffic fatalities (Chiras, 1985), 15,000 suicides and homicides, most of the family violence, and half of the 5 million arrests each year (Wilson & Kneisl, 1988). Alcohol is cited in a high percentage of other accidental deaths such as drownings, fires, suicides, and homicides.

Although some may have a hereditary predisposition to alcoholism, for others, environmental stresses are important. Cultural factors also play a role. In some countries where drinking wine is a regular practice among youth and adults at family gatherings, incidence of alcoholism is lower. Certain other cultural groups are at high risk for alcoholism. Persons at risk are identified in Box 8–1.

Jellinek's (1952) classic model with an insightful description of the phases of alcoholism, is outlined in Table 8–1. Although widely accepted, Jellinek's model does not hold true in every circumstance. Not all symptoms are present in alcoholics, and the sequence may vary. Women may also progress through the phases more rapidly than men.

EFFECTS AND ABSORPTION Alcohol is rapidly absorbed from the stomach and small intestine and becomes evenly distributed throughout the body. Absorption from the stomach can be slowed by ingesting food or milk. Absorption rate and blood alcohol level are affected by the amount and concentration of alcohol ingested, the rate of drinking, and body weight. For example, a large man can usually tolerate more alcohol than a small woman, provided the large man's size is not from excess fat.

Box 8–1
Persons at High Risk for Developing Alcoholism

The potential for alcoholism is high when the following factors exist:

A family history of alcoholism

A family history of abstinence or strong moral controls

A family history with a high incidence of depression among female relatives

A history of divorce or parental disorder in the family of origin

Being a member of certain cultural groups (Irish, Scandinavian, Native American)

Being a heavy smoker

The level of concentration of alcohol in the blood (the blood alcohol level, or BAL) determines the extent of the psychophysiologic effects. A person who weighs 160 lb would have a BAL of 0.1% (the legal criterion for alcohol intoxication in almost all states) after drinking, in a 2-hour period, 6 beers (12 oz each), 24 oz of table wine, 15 oz of fortified wine, or 6 glasses of liquor (1.3 oz each, 80 proof). Although caloric content varies, a "drink" of each type of beverage contains about the same total amount of alcohol. As tolerance to alcohol develops, these figures are no longer accurate; persons addicted to alcohol may reach higher blood alcohol levels without significant changes in their ability to control motor and CNS functions.

Menstrual cycle is sometimes said to affect the absorption rate of alcohol, although the actual mechanism has not yet been scientifically established. Women with premenstrual syndrome (PMS) have alcohol cravings and feel intoxicated after drinking even small amounts (one or two beers or one or two drinks of hard liquor) during peak PMS symptoms.

The body metabolizes 90% to 98% of the ingested alcohol, mostly in the liver. The rest is excreted by the kidneys through the urine, by the lungs through exhalation, and by the skin through perspiration. The elimination of progressively higher concentrations of alcohol requires progressively longer periods of time. For example, in a person of average size, the average rate of alcohol metabolism is about 10 mL/h. Thus, it requires 5 to 6 hours to metabolize the amount of alcohol contained in 120 mL (4 oz) of whiskey or 1.2 L of beer.

This relatively slow and constant metabolic rate is responsible for the limits on the amount of alcohol that can be consumed over a period of time before a person becomes intoxicated. *Intoxication* occurs when more alcohol is consumed than can be metabolized. Various other factors, such as diet, hormones, and medications, may alter the metab-

Table 8–1
Jellinek's Phases of Progressive Alcoholism

Phase	Description
Phase I Prealcoholic phase	Use of alcohol for relaxation and relief of tension and anxieties. Results in gradual increase in physiologic tolerance.
Phase II Early alcoholic phase	Ushered in by first "blackout" (brief period of amnesia during or directly after drinking). Followed by further blackouts, sneaking of drinks, growing preoccupation with drinking situations, defensiveness about drinking, rationalizations and excuses, guilt about drinking, and increased denial of the problem.
Phase III Crucial phase	Frank addiction occurs, and physiologic dependence is evident, with loss of control over drinking. Social and interpersonal difficulties result in job loss, marital disruption, and increased aggressive behavior. Life goals are replaced by goal to continue drinking.
Phase IV Chronic phase	Alcoholic goes on "benders," has decrease in tolerance, develops physiologic deterioration and illnesses. With abrupt cessation, may experience alcohol withdrawal. Severe depression and other psychologic and emotional symptoms become pronounced.

SOURCE: Adapted from Jellinek EM: Phases of alcohol addiction. Reprinted by permission from *Quarterly Journal of Studies in Alcohol,* 1952; 13:673–684. Copyright Journal of Studies on Alcohol, Inc., Rutgers Center of Alcohol Studies, New Brunswick, NJ 08903.

olism of alcohol. For example, severe malnutrition lowers the rate of alcohol metabolism, but insulin raises it.

MULTISYSTEM EFFECTS Alcohol use can impair health; its abuse leads to many life-threatening, chronic physical and emotional illnesses. Alcohol abuse is, in reality, a potentially fatal illness.

The immediate effects of alcohol on all systems are relatively minor. Difficulties develop with prolonged use of large amounts of alcohol and the development of tolerance.

Excessive consumption of alcohol often results in a reaction popularly known as the *hangover,* with headache, nausea and vomiting, dizziness, tremor, diaphoresis, thirst, and gastritis. Other disturbances associated with hangover are alterations in liver function, acid–base balance, and electrolyte homeostasis.

Even though the symptoms and signs of hangover are well recognized, their possible biochemical background is not well understood. The pathogenesis of hangover has been associated with the accumulation of lactic acid and acetaldehyde in the blood and with hypoglycemia. Experimental evidence is varied and contradictory, however. Ordinarily, alcoholic drinks (such as gin) rich in congeners (various substances such as methanol, esters, and aldehydes) induce a more severe hangover than those that are nearly pure alcohol (such as vodka). It is probable, however, that alcohol alone in large doses is capable of inducing severe hangovers.

HEPATIC SYSTEM Although nearly every body system is eventually affected by prolonged use of alcohol, the system most often affected is the hepatic system, specifically the liver. A major effect of ethanol includes the development of fatty liver, which leads to Laennec's cirrhosis if the individual continues to ingest alcohol. If alcohol ingestion is stopped before the onset of cirrhosis, the fatty liver can return to normal, and cirrhosis is avoided. It may take from 5 to 20 years of chronic alcohol ingestion for cirrhosis to result.

NERVOUS SYSTEM Alcohol has an immediate CNS depressant effect, causing less efficient functioning. Although people often refer to alcoholic beverages as stimulating, the apparent stimulation results from the depression of the brain's inhibitory control mechanisms. The effects are increased impulsive behavior and unrestrained activity that often occur early in progressive intoxication. Alcohol eliminates the usual ability to repress such behavior.

Chronic excessive use of alcohol is directly associated with serious neurologic consequences. Although this is partially because of the toxic effects of alcohol itself, it is also a by-product of the nutritional problems of most heavy drinkers, who prefer alcohol to food. The serious nutritional deficiencies may lead to anemias, beriberi, heart disease, Wernicke–Korsakoff syndrome (associated with thiamine deficiency), and peripheral neuropathy (associated with vitamin B deficiency). Cerebellar degeneration and other rare neurologic disorders may also occur.

Alcoholic peripheral neuropathy is slow, insidious, and progressive. It is the most common form of peripheral neuropathy and results from multiple nerve degeneration because of nutritional deficiency, principally of the B vitamins. Although thiamine is important for its role in the conversion of glucose (needed for nerve cell function), deficiencies of niacin, pantothenic acid, and pyridoxine may also be present.

In some persons, the syndrome may occur rapidly over a few days, but in others, symptoms may go unnoticed. The person may first experience pain or tenderness in the calf muscles or feet or tingling, burning, prickling, or numbness in the lower extremities. Varying degrees of sensory, motor, and reflex loss typically occur in the feet before they do in the hands and arms. As the degenerative process continues, muscle weakness, wasting, and diminished sensation characterized by an ataxic, wide-based gait may occur. Recovery, which depends on the degree of nerve degeneration, may be rapid for those whose condition was diagnosed early but longer for those requiring extensive nerve regeneration. Treatment includes abstinence from alcohol, correction of nutritional deficiencies, and high doses of supplemental B vitamins.

The *Wernicke–Korsakoff syndrome* is an extreme on the continuum of cognitive impairment resulting from alcohol-induced brain damage. Wernicke's encephalopathy is a degenerative brain condition involving lesions in several areas of the brain. It is caused by a deficiency of B complex vitamins, particularly thiamine and Vitamin B_{12}. Symptoms are a global confusional state, somnolence and disinterest, ataxia (lack of muscular coordination), ophthalmoplegia (ocular muscle paralysis), and nystagmus (rhythmic jerking motion on horizontal gaze). In addition, polyneuropathies may be present (pain, loss of sensation, and weakness of legs and arms).

A typical person with these symptoms is likely to be a chronic alcoholic between 40 and 60 years of age in a confused and excited state. Within a few days, this person develops diplopia from palsy of the abducens nerve (CN VI). Diplopia is a critical diagnostic criterion of Wernicke's encephalopathy because many alcoholics may appear confused, excited, or delirious without actually having Wernicke's. Once diplopia develops, the client's mental state may progress from quietness to stupor. Treatment with thiamine must be initiated immediately to prevent fatal midbrain hemorrhage and the onset of Korsakoff's psychosis.

The most striking and common symptoms of Korsakoff's psychosis are severe amnesia, confabulation, and remarkable personality changes. Memory disorder involves two forms of amnesia: anterograde (difficulty in remembering new information since the onset of the illness) and retrograde (difficulty in recalling events prior to the brain damage).

Treatment with high doses of thiamine and other vitamin supplements should be started as soon as possible and abstinence from alcohol encouraged. After 2 or 3 weeks of IV thiamine therapy, the ocular symptoms, ataxia, and global confusion disappear or improve greatly. Recovery is usually slow and incomplete. Unfortunately, clients who suffer severe neurologic alterations have the poorest and most incomplete recovery; they may require supervisory care (usually in an institution) for the remainder of their lives.

CARDIOVASCULAR SYSTEM Alcohol has both direct and indirect effects on the cardiovascular system. In low doses, alcohol increases heart rate and cardiac output. With increased consumption, however, heart rate and cardiac output are decreased. Eventually, with prolonged excessive use of alcohol, the efficiency of the cardiac muscle, valves, conduction system, blood supply, and neural mechanisms is reduced. Impairment of the heart's pumping function eventually results in alcoholic cardiomyopathy.

Alcoholic cardiomyopathy is a syndrome of cardiac dysfunction primarily involving the heart muscle, with relatively little effect on the rest of the cardiovascular system. Clinical symptoms have a slow, insidious onset and are similar to those in congestive heart failure and cardiac dysrhythmias. Treatment includes absolute, continuous abstinence from alcohol and management of congestive heart failure symptoms.

Other indirect effects of excessive alcohol ingestion on the cardiovascular system result from hypokalemia hypomagnesemia, hyperlipidemia, and altered fluid balance (from decreased circulating levels of antidiuretic hormone or diuresis). Beriberi heart disease (from marked thiamine deficiency) is another complication. In contrast to alcoholic cardiomyopathy, beriberi heart disease is characterized by increased cardiac output and decreased circulation time due to marked reduction in peripheral vascular resistance. Treatment includes vigorous thiamine replacement, general nutritional improvement, and abstinence from alcohol.

HEMATOPOIETIC SYSTEM A variety of hematologic abnormalities occur with alcohol ingestion. Inhibition of folate metabolism induces megaloblastic hematopoiesis, ineffective cell production, anemia, leukopenia, and thrombocytopenia. These conditions can be corrected by improving the client's nutritional status or administering folate as a dietary supplement.

MUSCULOSKELETAL SYSTEM Excessive alcohol use has a damaging effect on the skeletal muscles in three clinical forms: acute alcoholic myopathy, subclinical alcoholic myopathy, and chronic alcoholic myopathy. The exact mechanism by which alcohol induces muscle damage has not been completely established. Muscle damage seems to be related to the direct toxic effects of alcohol; these toxic effects cause alterations in muscle cell permeability and interfere with the normal electrochemical and metabolic functions of the cell.

In acute alcoholic myopathy, clients have muscle pain, tenderness, and edema following an episode of excessive alcohol intake. These symptoms are most common in the proximal muscles of the arms and legs, the pelvic and shoulder girdle, and the thoracic cage. In subclinical alcoholic myopathy, clients actually have acute alcoholic myopathy, but the symptoms are masked by the symptoms of concurrent acute intoxication or withdrawal. With appropriate treatment, including alcohol abstinence, balanced nutrition, and vitamin supplementation, symptoms gradually become less severe and abate within a few weeks.

Symptoms may return, however, with a future episode of excessive drinking. In chronic alcoholic myopathy, clients have slow, insidious muscle wasting and weakness in the same muscles affected in acute alcoholic myopathy but without pain and tenderness. Treatment is the same as for acute alcoholic myopathy.

GASTROINTESTINAL SYSTEM Alcohol stimulates the secretion of gastric acid, irritates the gastric mucosa, and causes gastritis. It aggravates preexisting peptic disorders or may even cause them. Alcoholics are prone to esophagitis because of increased gastric secretions and frequent vomiting. Severe vomiting may also lead to the development of lacerations of the mucosa at the gastroesophageal juncture, or the more serious rupture of the lower portion of the esophagus. Excessive alcohol intake may lead to acute and chronic pancreatitis. Insufficient food and bulk intake and malabsorption of fat, xylose, folic acid, B vitamins, and minerals in the digestive tract lead to nutritional deficiency diseases. Alcoholics also suffer from nausea, abdominal pain, erratic bowel function (constipation and diarrhea), gastrointestinal hemorrhage, and jaundice.

Although the exact reason is unknown, alcoholics have a high incidence of digestive tract cancers. This may be because of carcinogenic substances in alcoholic beverages and the possibility that ethanol itself acts as a carcinogen. That many alcoholics are also chronic smokers is also related to their susceptibility to cancer. Because cigarette smoking alone is known to increase the risk of cancer in some of the same body areas, separating the two factors is difficult. One theory is that alcohol increases the metabolizing enzymes in the liver, thereby speeding the conversion of noncarcinogens to carcinogens. In clients with cirrhosis of the liver, the liver may not be able to detoxify carcinogens such as tobacco.

REPRODUCTIVE SYSTEM Sexual problems result from the ineffective and deteriorating relationships common in alcoholism. Early use of alcohol may lessen inhibitions on sexual behavior, and some users may experience a psychologic sexual arousal. Excessive alcohol use generally reduces performance ability, however. In fact, in men, chronic use of alcohol may lead to impotence, sterility, and gynecomastia (excessive development of the mammary glands). Women also become anorgasmic. Recovery from alcoholism is usually paralleled by recovery from sexual dysfunction.

Fetal alcohol syndrome (FAS), one of the three leading causes of birth defects, occurs in infants born to mothers who chronically ingest large amounts of alcohol. Because alcohol rapidly crosses the placenta and affects the developing fetus, FAS babies have growth deficiencies, characteristic clusters of facial deformities, a variety of minor and major abnormalities, intellectual impairments, and psychomotor retardation. At birth, the infant may need to be gradually withdrawn from alcohol just as the infant born to a heroin addict must be withdrawn from heroin. It is not known exactly how much alcohol consumption causes FAS or during which stage of pregnancy the fetus is most likely to be affected. Although light social drinking does not appear to produce FAS, it is wise to advise pregnant women to refrain completely from drinking alcohol.

Anxiolytic Agents

The initial agents used to reduce anxiety were the barbiturates. Because of their ability to reduce anxiety and tension, their use, misuse, and abuse became extensive. Other dangers soon became apparent. The barbiturates create tolerance and cross-tolerance to other depressant drugs, dependence, severe life-threatening withdrawal symptoms, and death from overdose. These problems stimulated the search for a replacement. The drugs that emerged to replace the barbiturates for daytime sedation and treatment of anxiety symptoms were the benzodiazepines. Unfortunately, these drugs possess dangers similar to the barbiturates: tolerance, dependence, and overdose.

EFFECTS AND ABSORPTION The benzodiazepines, first prescribed in the 1950s, are currently used to reduce anxiety, induce sleep, promote relaxation of the skeletal muscles, and to produce an anticonvulsant effect. These agents are thus also prescribed for clients experiencing withdrawal symptoms.

All the benzodiazepines are absorbed and metabolized similarly. They are rapidly absorbed when administered orally. Then, metabolism proceeds according to two phases. Initially, a portion of the drug is quickly eliminated within a few hours. The rest is converted to active metabolites. Since these drugs are lipid-soluble, they are then widely dispersed throughout the body's fat tissues. The accumulation of these metabolites may produce a cumulative effect resulting in oversedation and/or ataxia.

Since the benzodiazepines tend to precipitate in muscle, they are poorly absorbed when administered intramuscularly. If it is necessary to administer a benzodiazepine intramuscularly, however, the injection should be given slowly and deeply into the gluteus muscle.

The barbiturates are basically salts or derivatives of barbituric acid. They produce sedative effects with low dosages or hypnotic effects with high dosages. Since they are derived from the same source, all of the barbiturates possess the same mechanisms of action, problems, and side effects. Very high doses of the barbiturates will produce a feeling of euphoria or a "high" similar to alcohol-induced states.

Barbiturates produce all degrees of depression of the CNS, ranging from mild sedation to general anesthesia. When barbiturates are given in sedative or hypnotic doses, there is little effect on skeletal, cardiac, or smooth muscle. If depression is severe, however, as in acute barbiturate intoxication, serious deficits in cardiovascular and peripheral functions occur. The barbiturates alter the stages of sleep and depress respiration. In hypnotic doses, depressant effects on respiration are minor; however, when clients have pulmonary insufficiency or overdose, severe respiratory depression may occur. In small doses, barbiturates have a hyperanalgesic effect and may increase the client's reaction to pain. Thus, in the presence of pain, barbiturates may produce a paradoxical effect: overexcitement rather than the usual sedation (Gilman, Goodman, & Gilman, 1984).

The barbiturates are readily absorbed and metabolized in the liver. A dangerous side effect of barbiturates is their capacity to increase the synthesis of porphyrins (nitrogen-containing compounds necessary for heme biosynthesis in hemoglobin); thus, they should not be given to clients with acute intermittent porphyria. Since cirrhosis increases both the half-life of some barbiturates and the client's sensitivity to the drug, barbiturates should also not be administered to clients with cirrhosis. Clients receiving anticoagulant therapy should also be monitored carefully since barbiturates decrease the action of anticoagulant drugs.

The barbiturates continue to be used for analgesia and anesthesia and for the treatment of some gastrointestinal disorders, hypertension, asthma, cardiovascular disease, insomnia, and epilepsy. Therefore, they continue to be available for illicit drug use and are often used by amphetamine ("speed") abusers to counter the agitated effects of "overamping" (overuse). Infants born to women who are physically dependent on depressants have symptoms similar to those in infants born to women addicted to heroin. Postnatal withdrawal syndromes vary in severity (see section on narcotics).

PATTERNS OF ABUSE WITH ANXIOLYTIC AGENTS Three patterns of abuse with anxiolytic agents have been identified:

- An individual, usually a middle-class woman between the ages of 30 and 60, gradually begins to increase the prescribed dose without consulting her physician. She may begin to "shop" around, procuring a number of prescriptions from various other physicians for sleep disturbance or anxiety. Several months may pass before a pronounced dependence occurs, bringing the consequences of withdrawal and other complications of high-dose maintenance.
- In periodic recreational intoxication, usually by teenagers or young adults, the pattern is becoming "high" at concerts, social functions, or any event that provides the motivation for use. Risks associated with this pattern include obtaining drugs on the black market that may be "mixed" or have unreliable content, accidents occurring during an intoxicated or out-of-control state, overdose danger because of the trend to mix drugs with alcohol or other depressants, and the potential for addiction.
- A third pattern is specific to the intravenous use of barbiturates. The "barb freak" is characteristically a young adult who has experimented or abused many and various drugs and chooses barbiturates for the "rush" experienced with intravenous injection. Serious health risks include overdose, infections, allergic reactions from contaminants, and accidental injection into an artery.

Physiologic and psychologic dependence and tolerance develop quickly with these drugs. If untreated, withdrawal usually produces serious medical consequences resulting in coma, respiratory depression, and death. When tolerance develops, accidental overdose can easily occur because the upper limit of tolerance is close to the lethal dose. Overdose occurs when the client accidentally takes more medication than is therapeutically indicated or purposefully attempts suicide.

Narcotics

Throughout history, the narcotics have been used for medicine or pleasure. They continue to be used as analgesics in treating both acute and chronic pain. Because of their rapid action and propensity for physical dependence, however, the abuse of these drugs poses a major problem for society. This class of drugs refers to the natural derivatives from the oriental poppy *(Papaver somniferum)*—opium, morphine, codeine—as well as synthetic chemicals that have morphinelike action such as heroin, meperidine (Demerol), and methadone (Dolophine). Narcotics cause mood changes, mental clouding, pain reduction, and drowsiness. Addicts describe a state of euphoria with the use of narcotics similar to that experienced during orgasm.

Codeine is more commonly abused than heroin because it is less expensive and more readily available in cough elixers and syrups or analgesic tablets. Codeine withdrawal is similar to morphine withdrawal though less severe.

All narcotics create psychologic and physical dependence and tolerance and have similar properties and mechanisms of action. Dependence occurs in individuals who take drugs as a way of life rather than in those who use drugs during a specific traumatic time in their lives or for a short-term medical reason.

Heroin was first introduced at the end of the nineteenth century as a cough suppressant and a cure for opium and morphine dependence. By various estimates and depending on the availability of heroin on the illicit market, there are between 400,000 and 750,000 heroin addicts in the United States at any time. Heroin abuse is not confined to large metropolitan areas. It can be found in medium-sized communities and small cities, and the drug is abused by persons from all socioeconomic and ethnic segments of the population.

In addition to having a high annual mortality rate, approximately 10 per 1000 heroin-addicted persons are subject to multiple health and personal hazards (American

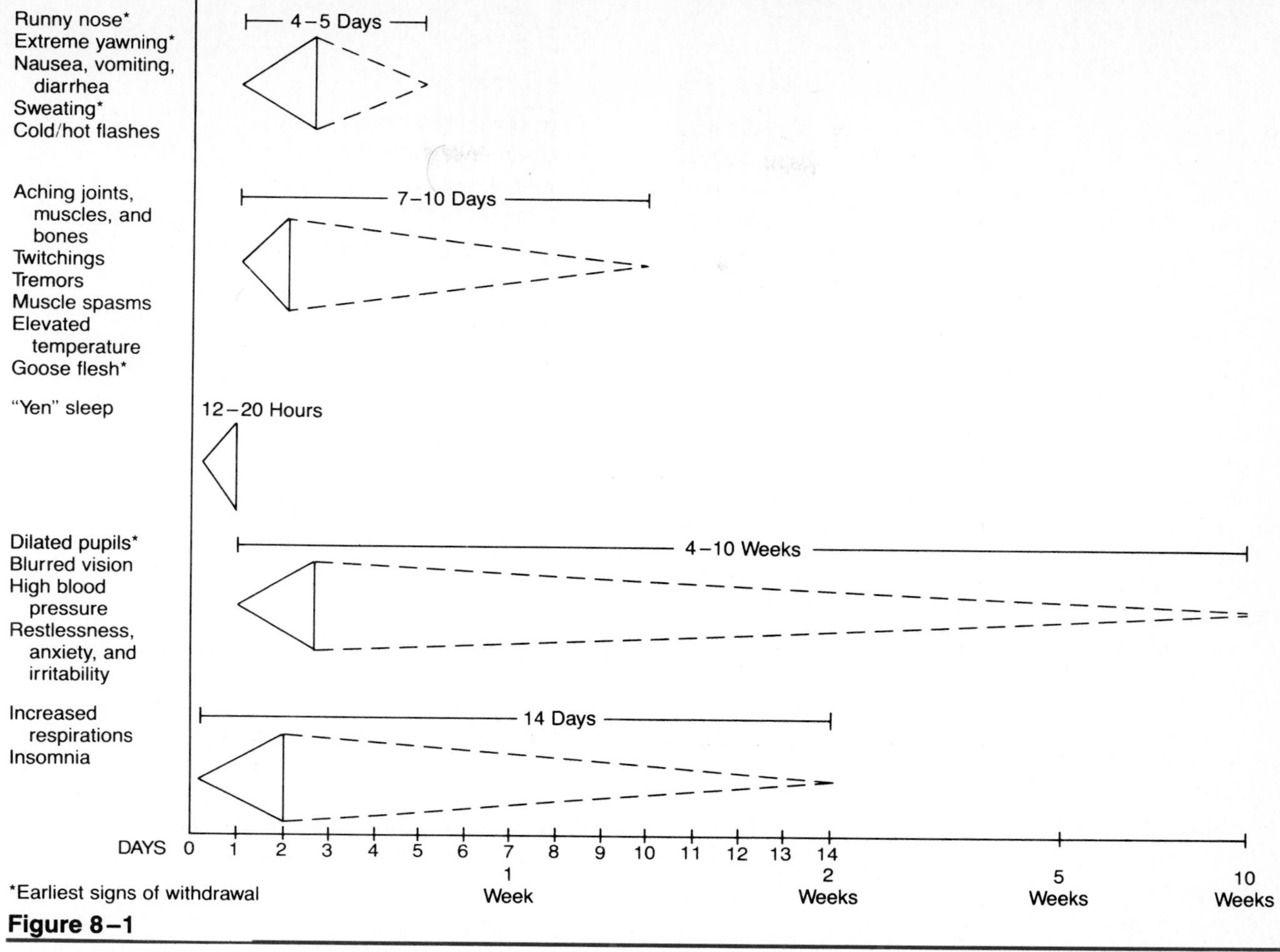

Figure 8–1

Signs and symptoms of morphine withdrawal. *SOURCE: Woolf D: Opioids. In Bennett G, Vourakis C, Woolf DS (editors),* Substance Abuse: Pharmacologic, Developmental, and Clinical Perspectives. *New York: Wiley, 1983.*

Psychiatric Association, 1980). The heroin user is at high risk for hepatitis and other infections from contaminated equipment. Heroin addicts are also one of the high-risk groups for contracting acquired immune deficiency syndrome (AIDS). The drug often contains impurities because of carelessness in manufacture or the purposeful addition of impurities to "cut" the heroin or extend it, increasing bulk and profit for the seller. These impurities also put the addict at high risk for poisoning, inflammation, and a variety of other disorders. The heroin user is also at risk for overdose and death and for chronic undernutrition. Social, work, and family relationships are often disrupted. Pregnant women who have been taking opioids regularly will deliver infants who are physically dependent.

Because heroin is rapidly converted to morphine in the bloodstream, the actions as well as the withdrawal pattern are essentially the same, except withdrawal symptoms may occur earlier with heroin than morphine. The severity of withdrawal is determined by two factors: (1) the amount of the dose and (2) the method of administration. Symptoms are more severe in persons who take high doses or administer the drug intravenously.

Abrupt morphine abstinence produces the pattern of withdrawal signs and symptoms shown in Figure 8–1. Following the last dose, withdrawal generally begins within 8 to 12 hours becoming most intense by 36 to 48 hours. After the onset of early symptoms, there is a period of "yen," or fretful sleep. Upon wakening, symptoms worsen. The acute phase lasts 10 to 14 days. Prolonged irritability, anxiety, inability to cope with minor problems, and physical complaints are symptoms of chronic withdrawal and are associated with the compulsion to obtain more drugs.

Stimulants

Stimulants include two major categories—amphetamines and cocaine—as well as other substances such as caffeine and nicotine contained in some antihistamines and cold preparations. Stimulants are sympathomimetic amines that act on the cerebral cortex and the reticular activating system, elevating mood and decreasing fatigue and appetite.

Millions of legal prescriptions are written each year for these drugs despite their high propensity for psychologic dependence and abuse. Stimulants are used to treat the common cold (Benzedrine inhalers), narcolepsy, hyperactivity in children, and mild depression. Because of their recognized potential for abuse and the speed with which tolerance develops (8 to 12 weeks), current accepted medical use is generally limited to treating narcolepsy and hyperkinesis in children.

Amphetamines

Athletes and entertainers have long been known to abuse stimulants to increase performance and endurance. The stimulant effects falsely signal to athletes that they are "up" and ready to compete. A danger is that the effects of amphetamines mask signs of fatigue and alter judgment. Thus, athletes who use them may perform beyond the safety level in endurance events such as bicycle marathons and risk cardiovascular collapse and death.

Amphetamines as "diet pills" were once popular for weight control. Although they do suppress appetite, they lose their anorexic effects within about 4 to 8 weeks. Beyond this point, the dieter is in danger of developing tolerance and using amphetamines to ward off depression.

PHYSIOLOGIC EFFECTS Although ordinarily taken by the oral route, amphetamines can also be administered intravenously. In this case, the immediate response is a euphoric sensation called a "flash" or "rush," accompanied by feelings of extreme adequacy, self-confidence, unlimited energy, and complete well-being. Frequency of use increases as tolerance develops; eventually, the dose must be increased to obtain the same results. The time between "runs" (injections) must be shortened to avoid intense fatigue and depression.

When abused in high doses, the amphetamines produce symptoms mediated by the autonomic and central nervous system. Cardiovascular symptoms of toxicity include tachycardia, headache, and when taken in sufficiently high doses, life-threatening dysrhythmias. Hypertension may be followed by hypotension when cardiovascular function becomes impaired. Cerebrovascular accident may also occur. Gastrointestinal symptoms include nausea, vomiting, diarrhea, and cramping. Diaphoresis may occur, or in some cases, hyperthermia may develop, and death may follow. Amphetamines produce irritability and jitteriness in high doses, and users may begin to take barbiturates or other sedative-hypnotics to reduce these unpleasant feelings. Dependence on both "uppers" and "downers" results.

Although no physical withdrawal syndrome follows the abrupt discontinuation of amphetamine use, a combination of physical and psychologic symptoms are prominent and may last for several months. They include:

- Long periods of sleep
- Irritability
- Extreme lethargy and apathy
- Marked depression
- Disorientation
- Suicidal tendencies

Clients who abuse barbiturates simultaneously will experience barbiturate withdrawal.

TOXIC PSYCHOSIS A toxic psychosis from amphetamine abuse may occur in chronic abusers. Amphetamine psychosis closely resembles the clinical picture of paranoid schizophrenia with the following symptoms:

- Paranoid ideation with well-formed delusions
- Stereotyped compulsive behaviors such as agitated pacing
- Visual, auditory, tactile, and olfactory hallucinations
- Increased libido
- Severe to panic levels of anxiety with potential for violent behavior

It is important to note that although the two psychoses appear similar, the client with an amphetamine psychosis does not experience the thought disorders common in schizophrenia. Also, the schizophrenic client seldom has tactile and olfactory hallucinations but is more likely to have visual or auditory hallucinations. Rather than the flat, bland affect common in schizophrenia, the client with an amphetamine psychosis appears highly anxious.

Cocaine

Since the mid-1970s, hospital emergency rooms have reported sharp increases in cocaine-related visits. Moreover, the general trend indicates that cocaine use is increasing more rapidly than that of any other drug. Life-threatening dangers from cocaine use and abuse are also on the rise, probably because of changing patterns of administration such as injecting and smoking as well as an overall increase in prevalence and frequency of use, either alone or in combination with other drugs. Recently, deaths from cardiac dysrhythmia have been reported, in some instances from the first dose.

Cocaine, an alkaloid substance extracted from the South American coca shrub, *Erythroxylon coca,* is a powerful CNS stimulant. The medical use of cocaine is limited because of its high potential for abuse and because of the availability of other compounds with less abuse potential. Its two main medical uses today are in nose and throat surgery as an effective local anesthetic that also constricts blood vessels and reduces bleeding at the operative site and as an ingredient in Brompton's cocktail given to clients with terminal cancer.

Because of its ability to produce intense euphoria and a profound sense of well-being, cocaine is a favorite drug for social and recreational use among those who can afford it. Users believe it enhances sociability and talkativeness, elevates mood, and reduces fatigue without clouding the sensorium or causing disorientation. Although the biologic mechanisms responsible for cocaine's effects have not been clearly identified, the drug is thought directly to affect cortical cells or the ascending reticular activating system and to alter catecholamine levels.

The question of whether cocaine causes physical dependence requires further study. Recent studies indicate that cocaine does cause psychologic dependence, however. Among those who develop a pattern of chronic, high-dose use, the abrupt cessation of cocaine use produces symptoms of craving for the drug, prolonged sleep, fatigue, hunger, and depression.

The usual or preferred method of administration is "snorting" or inhalation for absorption through the nasal mucosa. Prolonged use of cocaine by this method can damage and erode the nasal mucosa, with eventual perforation of the nasal septum. "Freebasing" is a method of making cocaine more palatable for smoking by removing water-soluble adulterants from street-grade cocaine to obtain a white talclike powder. Overdosing can occur when cocaine is smoked or injected subcutaneously or intravenously, and death can occur from respiratory paralysis and cardiovascular collapse.

"Crack", or "rock" cocaine, is an inexpensive but potent form of cocaine that is mixed with baking soda and water, heated, allowed to harden, and then cracked or broken into very small pieces that can be smoked in cigarettes or glass pipes. This is the most insidious, addictive, and toxic form of cocaine.

Cocaine psychosis may result from high doses of the drug or prolonged use. The psychosis is characterized by symptoms similar to those of schizophrenia. A specific type of tactile hallucination known as *formication*—the sensation of insects or bugs crawling on the skin or burrowing under the skin ("cocaine bugs")—may lead to scratching, gouging, and excoriation of skin. Nurses may see the cocaine abuser in the withdrawal state, which is similar to amphetamine psychosis except that symptoms are less severe, of shorter duration, and transient.

Caffeine

Caffeine—a methylxanthine derivative from coffee beans, tea leaves, cocoa, and cola nuts—is the most popular CNS stimulant in America. Caffeine is found in a variety of beverages such as coffee, tea, cocoa, and cola drinks; approximately 90% of American youth and adults use coffee and other caffeine-containing beverages. It is also found in a number of OTC preparations—analgesics such as Anacin, Bromo Seltzer, and Midol; stimulants such as NoDoz and Vivarin; cold preparations such as Dristan; and weight-control aids such as Dexatrim. Caffeine is misused and abused when taken excessively for its stimulating effects or when it continues to be used in the face of uncomfortable symptoms or health hazards. These are identified later.

In addition to its mild CNS stimulant effects, caffeine has diuretic properties. It is rapidly absorbed in the gastrointestinal tract, reaching maximum plasma concentrations within 1 hour of ingestion. Stimulant effects are noticeable within 30 minutes after ingestion and last for 3 to 5 hours.

The degree to which caffeine stimulates an individual varies with the amount taken and the development of tolerance. Although some people claim caffeine does not interfere with their sleep after five to six evening cups of coffee, an individual sensitive to its effects may become restless, agitated, and unable to sleep after only one cup. Other effects that vary among users are increased respirations, tachycardia, relaxed smooth visceral muscles, decreased peristalsis, nervousness, gastrointestinal upset, and fine tremors. Toxicity causes insomnia, restlessness, excitement, muscle twitching, increased respirations, tachycardia, and extrasystoles. Mild sensory disturbances such as ringing in the ears and flashes of light (at higher doses) are known to occur.

Caffeine produces acid indigestion, and because it stimulates gastric acid and pepsin, it may cause or aggravate peptic ulcers. In clients with unregulated glaucoma, caffeine can produce increased intraocular pressure. Cardiac clients are advised against using substances containing caffeine because it increases myocardial contractions, causes tachycardia, and increases plasma glucose and lipid levels. The relationship between caffeine and myocardial infarction is currently being investigated.

An abstinence syndrome occurs when a person who regularly ingests more than five cups of coffee (or equivalent) per day ceases regular use. The main signs of the abstinence syndrome are nausea, lethargy, and headache.

Hallucinogens

Hallucinogens, also called psychedelics, are the "mind expanders" that gained notoriety in the United States in the 1960s and continue to be used but to a lesser extent. Hallucinogens are capable of altering time and space perception; changing feelings of self-awareness, body image, and emotions; increasing sensitivity to textures, shapes, sounds, and taste; and bringing on visions of luminescence, flashes of light, kaleidoscopic patterns, and landscapes. They can also induce hallucinations and feelings of having had a religious experience.

Many natural and synthetic hallucinogens are in use today. Naturally occurring hallucinogens include mescaline (which can be found in buttons of the peyote cactus and can also be produced synthetically), psilocybin (known as "God's flesh," from the "divine" mushroom; actually found in about 100 mushroom species), morning glory seeds, nutmeg, jimsonweed, and a great many more. The most commonly used hallucinogenics—lysergic acid diethylamide (LSD) and phencyclidine (PCP)—are both synthetics. PCP is included in this discussion because it causes hallucinations; however, it has a number of other effects not shared by hallucinogenics such as LSD. LSD is the most potent by weight, and also the best researched, of all the hallucinogenics. Other synthetic hallucinogenics include 5-methoxy-3,4 methylenedioxyamphetamine (MMDA), dimethyltryptamine (DMT), paramethoxyamphetamine (PMP), and trimethoxyamphetamine (TMA).

LSD

LSD, first developed in the late 1930s, was used in research to investigate its mystical and creative potential as well as the biochemical etiology of schizophrenia. Its illicit use overshadowed its clinical experimental use in the early 1960s. LSD use reached its peak in the late 1960s and has since declined, stabilizing at a low level.

The usual method of taking LSD is oral; the clear liquid is placed on sugar cubes or other materials and ingested. With rapid absorption in the stomach, it appears to concentrate in the visual cortex, limbic system, and reticular formation. The mechanism by which LSD produces its hallucinogenic effect—called a "*trip*"—remains largely unknown. Autonomic nervous system effects include dizziness, hot and cold flashes, dry mouth, dilated pupils, elevated body temperature, and increased blood pressure. Sometimes excessive salivation occurs. CNS effects include labile mood; synesthesia (stimulation of one sense is perceived as another sense, for example, a sound produces a sensation of color); visual hallucinations; and abnormal color, time, and space perception. Feelings of possessing unusual power or having the ability to perform impossible feats or acts may lead the individual into impulsive actions such as jumping off a building to fly.

Although the hallucinogens do not create physical or psychologic dependence, tolerance develops rapidly. Cross-tolerance also occurs between LSD, mescaline, and psilocybin but not between these and other hallucinogens. Adverse reactions are the panic reaction, aggressive outbursts, overt psychosis, the "bad trip," and the "flashback." Panic reactions are acute anxiety attacks, usually brought on because the person fears not being able to regain control and return from the "trip." Overt psychosis occurs as the person loses touch with reality; it is more likely in individuals who are vulnerable to personality disorganization. A person having a "bad trip" experiences anxiety, panic, and paranoid feelings magnified by the distortion of time perception. Because time seems to have no end, terror sets in, and the individual may be subject to aggressive, violent, or unpredictable self-destructive or grandiose behavior. Flashbacks are frightening recurrences of the LSD "trip" weeks or months after ingesting the drug. They are unpredictable, but may be more pronounced when a person is under stress or lacking sleep. They vary with frequency and eventually decrease when hallucinogen use is discontinued.

PCP

Also known as "angel dust," "rocket fuel," and "horse tranquilizer," PCP is rapidly increasing in popularity in America. It is relatively inexpensive and is readily manufactured in small basement or garage laboratories, making it easily available to persons with limited funds. It was developed in 1959 as the first in a class of new dissociative anesthetics but was quickly abandoned for human use because it caused agitation, delusions, and irrational behavior. Approved only for veterinary use, PCP is still used for immobilizing animals.

In its pure form, PCP is a water-soluble crystalline powder. It is sold on the street in a variety of colors and forms. PCP can be taken as a pill; snorted as a powder; or sprayed as a liquid on parsley, mint, or other leafy substances to be smoked. Because it has so many street names and has often been misrepresented as another drug (mescaline, psilocybin, methaqualone, or cocaine), some users may not even know they have used PCP. Because the dose sold on the street varies widely, the effect is difficult to predict.

The effects of PCP are experienced quickly—usually within 5 minutes of smoking it. Initially, users tend to experience an active fantasy life and focus inward while appearing oblivious to others. Feelings of euphoria, peace, floating, warmth, and tingling are experienced. Users may also experience depersonalization; hallucinations; and distortions of time, space, and body image. Anxiety and labile affect (alternating moods) have also been reported (Kaplan & Sadock, 1985). The "high," which lasts for 4 to 6 hours, may be followed by a mild depression.

Adverse effects and overdoses may be treated in emergency departments, usually because in addition to the above, the client also demonstrates suicidal or aggressive behavior. In some instances, the symptoms abate as the PCP is absorbed. At other times, the symptoms worsen and may require hospitalization. Clients with PCP intoxication may have hypertension, nystagmus, hyperthermia, ataxia, seizures, and other symptoms of neurologic involvement. Respiratory arrest is also possible. The most dramatic of PCP's effects is its ability to mimic acute schizophrenia. In fact, some unusually long, severe, and treatment-resistant initial episodes of what was thought to be schizophrenia have turned out to be responses to PCP. The user may experience delusions and hallucinations (usually auditory, sometimes visual), irrational behavior, blocked speech, body image alteration, and violent behavior. Because PCP also has anesthetic effects, the user's sensations of touch and pain are dulled, making the user unusually resistant to outside control.

Central Nervous System Toxins

Included in this category are nicotine and cannabis, two chemical agents that have mixed effects including toxic effects, on the CNS and, thus, are difficult to categorize elsewhere.

Nicotine

Europeans and Asians discovered tobacco after it was brought back to Spain from the Caribbean islands by one of the early Spanish explorers. By the early 1600s, tobacco was smoked in pipes and cigars, chewed, and sniffed by men, women, and children and used as a medicinal herb. Not until 250 years later in the mid-nineteenth century did tobacco appear in cigarettes, its most widely used form today.

Nicotine is isolated from leaves of tobacco, *Nicotiana tabacum,* and has no therapeutic application. Nicotine is a colorless, volatile base that turns brown and acquires the odor of tobacco when exposed to air. Nicotine use usually begins in adolescence or early adulthood.

Nicotine dependence is recognized by the American Psychiatric Association's *Diagnostic and Statistical Manual* (DSM-IIIR) as a substance use disorder. An individual is considered tobacco dependent who has used tobacco continuously for at least 1 month, has unsuccessfully attempted to quit or significantly reduce the amount of use, has developed nicotine withdrawal, or continues to smoke in the presence of a serious physical disorder that is directly linked to smoking (American Psychiatric Association, 1987).

EFFECTS AND ABSORPTION Although many people begin tobacco use for psychosocial reasons (identification with peers and response to stress and tension), nicotine appears to have specific stimulant properties. It increases alertness, relaxes muscles, and decreases appetite and irritability. Nicotine is quickly absorbed from the lungs, usually bypasses the liver, and reaches the brain within 8 seconds after inhalation—more rapidly than an intravenous dose of heroin. Chewing tobacco is absorbed through the buccal mucosa and snuff through the nasal mucosa. Pipe and cigar tobacco is usually puffed and not inhaled, so it, too, is absorbed through the buccal mucosa.

Cessation of use may lead to the tobacco withdrawal syndrome, which varies in intensity, duration, and symptoms and signs. The onset of symptoms may begin within hours of the last cigarette or may be delayed for several days. Symptoms last from a few days to several months. The symptoms of tobacco withdrawal syndrome are:

- Craving for tobacco
- Restlessness
- Irritability
- Anxiety
- Sleep disturbance
- Drowsiness
- Headache
- Impaired concentration
- Gastrointestinal disturbances

Although this syndrome alone is not life threatening, the added stress and anxiety associated with the symptoms may place the medical or surgical client at a higher risk for complications.

MULTISYSTEM EFFECTS Cigarette smoke contains some 4000 chemical substances, including at least 15 different types of known carcinogens and a number of toxic hydrocarbons or solvents. Nicotine, carbon monoxide, and tar are the three toxic components in tobacco most likely to contribute to health hazards of smoking. Each year approximately 320,000 deaths occur from lung and other cancers, chronic pulmonary disease, and cardiovascular diseases directly linked to smoking. Smoking is considered the major etiologic factor in emphysema and bronchitis. Since pipe and cigar smokers do not ordinarily inhale, they are considered at lower risk than cigarette smokers for developing serious health complications. They are also less likely to develop dependence on nicotine and find it easier to quit when advised to do so.

The potential for developing health problems linked to smoking increases with exposure, but cessation of smoking reduces this potential. For example, 5 to 10 years after quitting, former smokers are at only slightly higher risk than nonsmokers.

Smoking has been directly correlated with prematurity and low-birth-weight infants. Offspring of smoking mothers have a higher incidence of upper respiratory problems and pneumonia in the first 2 years of life. Nicotine is excreted in the milk of lactating mothers, which may contain 0.5 mg/L.

In addition to smokers' high mortality rate from diseases cited earlier in this section, smokers are at higher risk for peptic ulcers and cirrhosis. In addition, women smokers over 35 who take birth control pills are at risk of hemorrhage, especially cerebral hemorrhage. Accidental deaths from fires started by people who smoke in bed or fall asleep while smoking are a major hazard. The incidence is higher with alcoholism.

Physiologic changes from smoking cessation include electroencephalographic changes such as decreased high-frequency activity (characteristic of arousal) and increased low-frequency activity (characteristic of drowsiness and hypoarousal), lowered heart rate and blood pressure, and increased peripheral blood flow. The appetite increases, and weight gain is common over time. Coughing and other respiratory symptoms improve. It is not completely known how many people successfully quit smoking on their own. Of those who seek formal help, about 66% actually quit for a few days, but only 10% to 40% remain abstinent for 1 year (Bennett, Vourakis, & Woolf, 1983).

Cannabis

Cannabis sativa, the Indian hemp plant, produces a strong fibrous material that has been used to make clothing and rope. It is also used as a mind-altering drug by large numbers of persons. Cannabis use is not limited to any specific age, social, economic, or educational group.

The primary psychoactive agent is delta^6-3,4-tetrahydrocannabinol (THC), which is concentrated in the resin secreted from the flowering tops and leaves of the cannabis plant and acts as a CNS depressant. The three most common forms of cannabis in street use are:

- Marijuana, the most prevalent, which is the dried leaves, stems, and flowers of the cannabis plant and has a THC content of 5% to 6%
- Hashish, or hash, which is more potent because it has a higher THC concentration (up to 10%), from the flowering tops of the plant
- Hashish oil, which has the most concentrated THC (may reach 63%) and is produced by boiling hashish in a solvent to filter out the solid material

EFFECTS OF MARIJUANA Marijuana is usually smoked but can be eaten or taken in pill form, and the effects last for a few hours. Blood levels of THC in chronic users have been detected for up to 6 days following the last inhalation. Chronic marijuana smokers are at risk for developing asthma, chronic bronchitis, and adverse pulmonary effects. The "tar" produced by marijuana is considered more carcinogenic than the tar produced by tobacco (1 marijuana cigarette, or joint = 5.0 mg tar; 1 tobacco cigarette = 1.2 mg tar); thus, chronic users are considered at high risk. The harmful effects of one joint a day on the lungs has been compared to the effect of smoking 20 tobacco cigarettes per day because marijuana smokers usually inhale more deeply and hold the smoke in the lungs longer to obtain a heightened effect.

The effects of marijuana that account for its popularity as a recreational drug include:

- The "high"—euphoria, relaxation, reduced anxiety, feelings of well-being
- A sense of hilarity and excitement
- Increased clarity and sensitivity
- Heightened sense of awareness
- Feeling pleasantly detached, floating
- Having ideas that flow freely

Other less pleasurable effects may cause problems in thinking, motor performance, and interpersonal relationships. They are:

- Impaired logical thinking, irrelevant thoughts, and gaps in thoughts or memory
- Rapid, slurred, or otherwise impaired speech and loose associations
- Difficulty in concentrating or making decisions
- Impaired reality testing (auditory and visual hallucinations are possible) that make operating machinery or driving a car dangerous
- Altered sense of time and space
- Increased suggestibility
- Alteration in libido and sexual performance (either increased or decreased)
- Altered body image and self-identity
- Increased anxiety and panic
- Apathy with prolonged use

In addition, cannabis overdose may cause fear, anxiety, panic, suspiciousness, agitation, ataxia, tremors, acute depression, disorientation, and distorted perceptions.

An amotivational syndrome may also occur in the chronic user. It is characterized by apathy; a lack of concern for the future; decreased effectiveness at school or work; and difficulty in completing complex tasks, performing routines, or mastering new experiences. Whether this is a consequence of chronic marijuana use, or a manifestation of personality disorganization that occurred before its use, is difficult to study and continues to be somewhat controversial.

Marijuana may also have medically therapeutic effects. It is being used in selected health centers, on a limited experimental basis, to help alleviate the nausea associated with cancer chemotherapy and to help reduce the intraocular pressure in clients with open-angle glaucoma.

MULTISYSTEM EFFECTS While the illegal status and the harmful effects continue to be debated, national concern is growing over the large number of young people who regularly use and abuse marijuana. Long-term use and cannabis accumulation in the body may cause a high incidence of birth defects in offspring and a high risk of disease due to lowered resistance to infection. Other hazards of cannabis use are associated with the unpredictability of other chemicals (such as PCP) found in cannabis preparations and the health hazards associated with cigarette smoking.

WITHDRAWAL Although infrequent, tolerance and physical dependence have been reported in the chronic marijuana user. Tolerance depends on the dose and duration of use, but as tolerance develops, mild physical dependence also occurs. Mild withdrawal symptoms, which may occur within hours of the last dose, include restlessness, anxiety, insomnia, excitability or irritability, nausea, vomiting, anorexia, and diarrhea. Acute psychotic episodes may occur in certain vulnerable individuals. Mild to moderate adverse symptoms ameliorate within a few hours in a quiet supportive environment. Psychotic episodes may last from 1 to 6 weeks or longer.

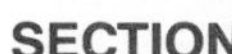
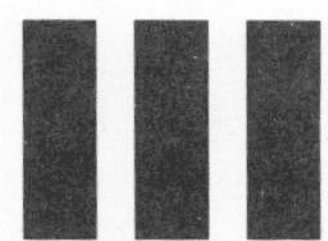

SECTION III

The Nursing Process for Clients Who Abuse Substances

Be aware of the possibility that many clients, regardless of their diagnosis, have problems related to the abuse of chemical agents either because they themselves abuse substances or because significant others do. Nurses in general hospitals, ambulatory care facilities, schools, industry, and community environments are often unaware that clients they are seeing for one reason—to have a broken leg set, an emergency appendectomy, a nose and throat culture, a scoliosis check, a preemployment physical, or a home visit after hospital discharge—may also be substance abusers.

Some of the most dangerous situations occur when misdiagnoses are made: the client in a diabetic coma is mistakenly thought to be drunk and is left to "sleep it off" rather than given insulin; an intoxicated client is mistakenly thought to be a diabetic and receives insulin that further reduces an already extremely low blood sugar level not uncommon in clients in alcoholic coma; a client with a heroin overdose fails to receive naloxone (Narcan) to counteract the respiratory depression. In these situations, immediate appropriate action is imperative. Being alert to these possibilities facilitates early intervention and helps to prevent complications arising from substance abuse.

Historically, nurses' untoward reactions to substance abusers have followed two patterns. Both reactions appear to stem from nurses' own anxieties about substance abuse and their fear of it. These feelings come about, in part, because many nurses feel helpless in the face of substance abuse.

The first reaction pattern is one of disgust and revulsion. This stems from the nurse's belief that substance abuse is irreversible and the substance abuser is helpless and hopeless. Some nurses who react this way tend to withdraw from the client, feeling less responsible for the client's care. Other nurses try to inspire the client to give up the drug, preaching to them about willpower or providing information designed to frighten clients into abstinence. These behaviors only increase the client's feelings of low self-esteem and futility.

The second reaction pattern is one of enabling. Enabling is defined as supporting condoning, or covering up an individual's continued use of the substance or protecting the person from the ultimate consequences of substance abuse. In effect, the nurse, family member, or friend assumes responsibility for the client's actions. The nurse who enables:

- Encourages the substance abuser's use of denial by concurring that the client is only an infrequent "social drinker" or that the client only uses drugs when a "little nervous"
- Apologizes for asking questions about the person's substance use habits
- Ignores cues to possible substance abuse
- Emphasizes repeatedly that the problem can be overcome if the client will only use "willpower"
- Counsels the person to seek psychiatric help for anxiety or depression, yet overlooks the underlying problem of substance abuse
- Sympathizes with the client's reasons (work, financial, and family problems) for using the substance, denying the reality that the difficulties are often the result, and not the cause, of substance abuse

The result of both reaction patterns is that the client fails to receive the needed help; the ultimate result with some drugs, such as alcohol, is death. The ability to analyze one's own feelings and reactions to substance abusers regularly helps avoid withdrawing from, preaching to, or enabling the substance abuser. The questions in Box 8–2 will help in analyzing feelings, beliefs, and attitudes toward substance abuse.

Nursing Assessment: Establishing the Data Base

Assessing for substance abuse requires a cautious, objective, holistic approach. No one sign or symptom definitely and exclusively pinpoints substance abuse. Consider all cues carefully to be able to intervene effectively, but avoid jumping to hasty and stigmatizing conclusions.

Subjective Data

While completing the health history, simultaneously observe for cues of substance abuse. Begin by collecting data about ingestion of alcohol. To determine the frequency, ask the client: "How often do you drink alcoholic beverages?" The magnitude can be determined by asking: "When you do drink, how much do you drink?" Remember to ask about the conditions under which the client drinks. Asking: "When do you tend to drink alcohol?" and "Under what circumstances?" and "With whom?" will help to gather specific facts. Remember also to ask, "When was your last drink?" to be able to anticipate the onset of symptoms of withdrawal in an alcoholic.

Also explore the client's current and past use of drugs, including prescription and nonprescription medications to assess the client's pattern of drug use. Ask the client what drugs are being taken. It may be useful to tell the client:

Box 8–2
Guide to Analyzing Personal Responses Toward Substance Abusers

Analyze your responses to the following questions:

1. What thoughts and feelings does the term *alcoholic* evoke in me?
2. What thoughts and feelings does the term *addict* evoke in me?
3. Do I believe that substance dependence occurs out of moral weakness?
4. Do I believe that substance dependence is an illness that can be treated?
5. Is the person who abuses substances deliberately destroying his or her life and the lives of significant others?
6. Who in my personal life has abused drugs, alcohol, or other chemicals?
7. How does my experience with relatives, friends, colleagues, or clients who have abused substances affect my attitude toward caring for a substance-abusing client?
8. Is substance abuse a social problem, an emotional–psychologic problem, or a physical abnormality?
9. How do I view the family, spouse, or friends of the substance abuser? Do they encourage the abuse, or otherwise "enable" the person to continue their abuse? Or are they victims?
10. How does my own personal use of nicotine, caffeine, drugs, or alcohol affect my attitude toward clients?

"I need to know all the drugs/medications that you are taking because it may be dangerous to abruptly stop taking some of them," or "I need to know all the drugs/medications that you have been taking because it is important not to mix certain chemicals, and some stay in the body for a long time." Since it is not unusual for the client to know only the drug's street name, be prepared to correlate street names with pharmacologic names (no easy task, since the street names frequently change).

Determine how much is being taken, how often, and for how long. Ask how it has affected the client's social, work, and sexual relationships. Carefully observe the nonverbal cues, acknowledging that the topic of substance abuse may be difficult for both nurse and client to discuss.

Anticipate that if the person is abusing chemical agents, particularly illicit ones, this information is not likely to be offered voluntarily. Sometimes family members verbalize their concerns about the client's substance abuse; others tend to conceal this data.

Objective Data

OBSERVATION OF PHYSICAL AND BEHAVIORAL SYMPTOMS Objective data can be gathered during the physical assessment or more indirectly when interacting with the client for other reasons. The client may have dilated or constricted pupils, needle tracks from intravenous administration, or ulcerations in the nares. Note whether the client appears intoxicated, agitated, stuporous, assaultive, severely anxious, or panicky. Any one, or a combination, of these physiologic or behavioral cues may indicate substance use or abuse, untoward reactions, or drug overdose (see a pharmacology text for specifics).

In monitoring vital signs, observe for respiratory depression. Fluctuations in pulse and blood pressure for no seemingly plausible reason can indicate that the client is in the process of withdrawal from a depressant, narcotic, or stimulant. Signs of withdrawal for specific substances have been discussed earlier. Withdrawal from alcohol is discussed in the section on planning and implementation.

Does the client demonstrate the anticipated physiologic response to analgesics, anesthetics, or sedative-hypnotics? If the response is "less than expected," this may be a cue to cross-tolerance. The client may require larger than usual doses of the medication to achieve the desired response. If the response is greater than expected, the client may be unknowingly or surreptitiously taking medications similar to those administered by the nurse.

DIAGNOSTIC STUDIES Routine laboratory studies may provide indirect cues to undiagnosed substance abuse. For example, unexplained abnormal liver function studies may suggest the need to evaluate a client for possible alcohol or heroin abuse. On the whole, routine studies point to complications of long-term abuse. Once a client is identified as a substance user, laboratory and diagnostic studies such as complete blood count (CBC), serologic studies, chest x-ray, ECG, EEG, and others suggested by the history or physical examination help to uncover related health problems and complications.

Blood and urine specimens, and sometimes gastric specimens, may be collected for forensic or legal purposes, especially in the investigation of drug or alcohol abuse, suicide, and intentional poisoning. It is crucial that in medicolegal investigations, the chain of possession remains unbroken from the time the specimen is collected until courtroom testimony is completed. Each person obtaining or handling such specimens should be sure that each step in the collection, processing, and handling of a medicolegal specimen is witnessed and properly documented. Certain precautions will help to ensure the legal credibility of laboratory test results. The nursing responsibilities in relation to these precautions are outlined in Box 8–3.

DRUG SCREENING A toxicologic screen of 100 mL of urine and 20 mL of blood may indicate the presence of a variety of drugs of abuse. Although a toxicologic screen can identify use, it cannot identify abuse (how long and how often the individual uses the drug). Negative results may mean either that the individual does not use drugs or that the drug is no longer detectable. For example, cocaine traces last for only a relatively brief time, but heroin can

Box 8–3
Nursing Responsibilities in Ensuring the Legal Credibility of Toxicology Reports

1. Obtain a signed consent form before collecting the specimen.
2. Collect the specimen in the presence of a witness, using appropriate collection containers and equipment.
3. Have the witness sign the laboratory request slip, noting the time the specimen was collected.
4. Seal the collection container with tape to prevent tampering.
5. Label the container with the date, contents, and subject's name. Be sure to sign the label.
6. Complete the laboratory request slip, including the type, source, and weight or volume of the specimen, data obtained, and test requested. Sign the laboratory request slip.
7. Maintain a continuous record of the chain of possession for the specimen. Each person who receives the specimen must sign the laboratory request slip, recording the exact time and date the exchange took place. Keep the number of people who handle each specimen to a minimum.
8. Seal the specimen and laboratory request slip in a package and label it "Medicolegal Case" on all sides.
9. Deliver the specimen to the laboratory immediately. If transportation is delayed, lock the specimen in a container and refrigerate the entire container and its contents.

SOURCE: Byrne JC et al: *Laboratory Tests: Implications for Nursing Care,* 2nd ed. Menlo Park, CA: Addison–Wesley, 1986, pp. 357–358.

often be detected in the urine as long as 48 hours after use. Sometimes a toxicology screen gives negative results except for the presence of quinine (frequently used as a diluent with many drugs of abuse), which can be detected as long as 5 to 6 days after use. The presence of quinine is not definitive for drug abuse, however, since quinine is also found in some cold remedies and soft drinks.

While the results of a toxicologic screen are often useful in guiding long-term treatment, they may not always be available soon enough to aid in the management of emergency situations such as coma or respiratory depression. In these emergencies, health care providers will need to rely on subjective data and the specific physical findings discussed earlier in this chapter when giving immediate treatment. Specific toxicologic tests for barbiturate levels and blood alcohol levels are discussed below.

BARBITURATE LEVELS The measurement of barbiturate levels requires the collection of a venous blood specimen. Since each barbiturate varies in its duration of action and rate of absorption, different barbiturates produce coma at different blood levels. Short-acting barbiturates such as pentobarbital and secobarbital are more toxic and produce coma at low concentrations. Long-acting barbiturates such as phenobarbital (Luminal) are absorbed more slowly and do not produce coma until higher concentrations are reached.

High concentrations of several drugs can falsely elevate barbiturate levels. Some of these are:

- Glutethimide (Doriden)
- Phenytoin sodium (Dilantin) and other hydantoins used to treat epilepsy
- Meperidine
- Methyprylon (Noludar)
- Nitrazepam
- Salicylamide
- Theophylline and its derivatives

An accurate medication history will help to avoid treatment based on falsely elevated toxicology reports.

BLOOD ALCOHOL LEVELS Laboratory analysis of blood alcohol level (BAL) is used to identify the presence of alcohol intoxication, to establish its degree, and to help determine appropriate treatment. It is essential to differentiate between alcohol intoxication and other conditions such as diabetic coma, cerebral trauma, and drug overdose. For example, the fruity breath odor of a person in diabetic

Nursing Research Note

Forchuk C: Cognitive dissonance: Denial, self-concepts and the alcoholic stereotype. *Nurs Papers* 1984; 16(3):57–67.

Using a sample of 116 men and women in an alcoholic treatment program, the author measured acceptance of the alcoholic stereotype (the alcoholic is not worthwhile and is "weak" and "bad"), denial, and self-concept. The results indicated that 61% accepted their alcoholism, 28% felt they had a drinking problem but denied alcoholism, 6% denied alcoholism, and the remaining 5% did not answer the denial questions. There was a positive relation between improving self-concept and self-esteem and denial. As denial increased so did self-esteem. The subjects consistently rated alcoholics as more negative than themselves. Similarly, for those denying their alcoholism, there was a greater distance between self-rating and ratings for alcoholics. Problem drinkers and those accepting their alcoholism rated themselves more closely to alcoholics in their traits. On the average in this study, alcoholics accepted the alcoholic stereotype and rated other alcoholics more negatively than themselves, supporting the cognitive dissonance theory (if a person's knowledge, opinions, or beliefs [cognitions] are inconsistent with those of important others, the individual will be motivated to change and hold similar beliefs and opinions).

Health teaching and counseling are necessary to encourage alcoholic clients to reject the alcoholic stereotype. The client must accept the problem but not accept the social stigma attached to the disease. In addition, when treating the alcoholic, nurses must focus on the client's positive qualities and enhance the self-image.

Nurses must also become aware of their own feelings regarding alcoholics and alcoholic stereotyping. Alcohol problems are not limited to the psychiatric setting but are present in all health care settings. Therefore, all nurses must become familiar with alcoholism, treatment modalities, and nursing interventions.

coma, caused by the excretion of accumulated ketones by the lungs, can be mistaken for the breath odor of alcohol intoxication caused by congeners. An error in diagnosis can have serious consequences for the client. The concentration of alcohol in the blood or urine is the major reliable indicator of alcohol intoxication.

Because blood alcohol concentration levels may be used for medicolegal purposes, strict requirements for specimen collection must be followed. For example, alcohol should not be used for cleansing the client's arm, and the exact times when the specimen was collected and sent to the laboratory should be noted. Be sure to also follow the guidelines outlined in Box 8–3.

Nursing Diagnoses

As has become evident in this chapter, the abuse of chemical substances has complex physiologic and psychosocial ramifications. Nursing diagnoses may be relevant to the usual physical or behavioral effects of the substance, alterations due to overdose, alterations due to withdrawal, or alterations due to health complications. Nursing diagnoses relevant to the plan of care for substance-abusing clients span this wide range. The list of nursing diagnoses in Box 8–4 is by no means all-inclusive and needs to be individualized for each client.

Box 8–4
Nursing Diagnoses Commonly Related to Substance Abuse

Anxiety

Breathing patterns, ineffective, related to respiratory depression

Coping, ineffective individual

Coping, ineffective or disabled family

Gas exchange, impaired

Injury, potential for, related to substance abuse

Knowledge deficit, related to polydrug abuse

Mobility, impaired physical, related to perceptual or neuromuscular impairment

Nutrition, altered: less than body requirements, related to lack of interest in food

Powerlessness, related to drug dependence

Self-concept, disturbance in: body image, self-esteem, role performance, personal identity

Sensory–perceptual alterations: visual, auditory, kinesthetic, tactile, related to chemical alterations from alcohol or drugs

Sexuality, altered patterns

Skin integrity, impairment of, related to parenteral administration of drugs

Thought processes, altered

Tissue perfusion, altered: cerebral

Violence, potential for, related to amphetamine overdose

Planning and Implementation

Nurses become involved in planning and implementation for the substance-abusing client at a variety of different levels.

INTOXICATION Clients in intoxication or overdose need prompt emergency treatment. The nursing care plan focuses on alleviating the effects of the substance.

Drug and alcohol intoxication is usually self-limiting. In a physiologic emergency, hospitalization is needed. Attending to any secondary complications, such as those related to falls, infections, and physical injuries, is a priority once the emergency is under control.

Intoxication occurs when an individual has consumed a drug in excess of the body's ability to metabolize it. Maladaptive behaviors resulting from intoxication may include aggressiveness; altered judgment; and other social, personal, or work-related impairment. Psychologic characteristics include euphoria, irritability, impaired attention or concentration, loquacity, and emotional lability. Physiologic characteristics include flushed face, slurred speech, lack of coordination, unsteady gait, and nystagmus. Intoxicated persons must be supervised to make sure they do not mistakenly assume that they can drive safely.

Intoxication may alter or accentuate the individual's usual behavior. Shy or inhibited persons may become outgoing and gregarious, whereas a person who tends to be mistrustful may become extremely suspicious. In the early stage of intoxication, individuals may experience an increased sense of well-being and confidence. They may talk as if they are experts who can solve the problems of the world, or they may become overbearing and opinionated, demanding that those around them agree with their point of view. The early behavioral manifestations of intoxication may appear uninhibited. In later stages, however, persons may become depressed, speech and thoughts are slowed down, and they may become withdrawn and even lose consciousness, or "pass out."

The duration of intoxication depends on the amount of the drug ingested over what period of time and whether food was taken at the same time. Weight, height, age, and sex also affect the rate of alcohol metabolism. The individual's tolerance for alcohol also affects the length of intoxication, as do individual variations and susceptibility.

The usual manifestations of alcohol intoxication require no specific nursing intervention or medical treatment. There are no proven methods to speed up the metabolism of a drug. Such time-honored remedies used for alcohol intoxication as a warm shower followed by a cold one, strong coffee, forced activity, or induced vomiting may provide some comfort but should not be suggested as a means for increasing the rate of dissipation of alcohol from the blood. Pathologic intoxication, characterized by increased excitement and combativeness, may require restraints and administration of sedatives such as sodium luminal 100 mg subcutaneously, or amobarbital sodium (Amytal) 500 mg IM, repeated once in 30 or 40 minutes.

Intoxicated persons in an emergency room may cause a critical nursing situation. Some medical and nursing personnel may see them as a nuisance and may refuse them entry to the ER or call the police department. Instead, the astute nurse evaluates the person for level of intoxication, determines the drug history, and evaluates the potential for physiologic complications and medical emergency (pathologic intoxication, alcoholic coma, or potential for alcohol withdrawal) to determine the need for treatment.

COMA Coma from a drug overdose such as heroin is a medical emergency requiring an immediate assessment of the physical state and depth of coma. Important information frequently can be obtained from those accompanying the client. When the coma is profound, the immediate danger is death from respiratory depression. For respiratory depression from a narcotic overdose, a narcotic antagonist agent such as naloxone hydrochloride (Narcan) counteracts the respiratory depression. The response to naloxone is dramatic: the client's respiratory rate increases, pupils dilate, and level of consciousness improves.

Once emergency measures are established and the client is stable, assess the client for the common acute complications of heroin addiction and overdose such as cardiac dysrhythmias, sepsis, and pulmonary edema. The following measures must also be taken:

- Maintain a clear airway (an endotracheal tube may be necessary).
- Prevent aspiration of secretions and vomitus. (If no injury to head or neck is obvious, place the client in a semiprone position.)
- If the client is in shock, immediate medical treatment will include fluids, vasopressor drugs, and steroids.
- Empty the bladder and institute drainage if urinary retention occurs.
- Measure vital signs frequently.
- Remove accumulated mucus by suction; turn the client to the side.
- Provide mechanical ventilation in case of respiratory paralysis.

If the client is in an alcoholic coma, an intravenous infusion of 5% glucose to reduce hypoglycemia is often begun. The client should be assessed and treated for other injuries and complications such as subdural hematoma, pneumonia, meningitis, hepatic failure, and gastrointestinal bleeding. Gastric lavage is unnecessary because alcohol is rapidly absorbed in the stomach and because there is a danger of aspiration of gastric contents. Gastric lavage or hemodialysis may be undertaken if a large number of pills has been swallowed.

WITHDRAWAL Whether withdrawal is gradual or "cold turkey" (all at once) depends on the specific substance being abused. Regardless of whether withdrawal is gradual or abrupt, the goals of nursing are:

- Preventing death
- Preventing serious complications related to withdrawal
- Keeping the use of other chemical agents to a minimum
- Helping the client understand the withdrawal experience as the result of substance abuse

The care plan for individuals withdrawing from a depressant, narcotic, or stimulant incorporates similar principles. The specific withdrawal symptoms and the anticipated time of their onset differ depending on the category of drug, however. With some drugs, especially narcotics, the dosage is gradually decreased to avoid dangerous withdrawal states. Withdrawal is best carried out by skilled staff in a substance abuse treatment program.

REACTIONS TO HALLUCINOGENS Hallucinogens often cause high levels of anxiety and panic. The goals of intervention should be to reduce anxiety to a mild to moderate level and to prevent suicide or violence. Environmental stimuli must be reduced. Helpful measures include lowering the volume of televisions and radios and turning off bright lights. Do not leave the client alone. Speak slowly and calmly in sentences limited to five to six words so the client can follow them. Monitor vital signs every 2 hours while the client is awake.

Watching a client experiencing panic from a hallucinogen may be frightening. It is important to recognize and attempt to control these feelings so as not to increase the client's anxiety. Have another staff member stand close by but not near enough to overwhelm or threaten the client. Once the client's level of anxiety has decreased, carefully assess suicide potential. A psychiatric nursing textbook will provide guidelines for intervening into hallucinations.

PROMOTING MORE HEALTHFUL COPING After the withdrawal symptoms have decreased, or the panic level of anxiety has been reduced, focus on promoting more healthful methods of coping. The client will have to decide whether to learn to live without the chemical agent.

Recognize that the drug has become like a best friend to the client and empathize with how difficult it will be to live without its effects. The client who is serious about wanting to refrain from drug use may experience grief over the loss of the valued drug. Anticipate, however, that many clients will continue to minimize and deny the gravity of the situation. Instead, they will focus energy on reasons for using the drug. Avoid being caught up in this topic. Focus instead on how the client will avoid using chemical agents from this point on.

INPATIENT TREATMENT PROGRAMS Community agencies that provide intensive 2- to 4-week inpatient treatment programs following withdrawal are often useful referrals. Encouraging the client to investigate and use such a program stresses the seriousness of the problem. These programs usually involve a number of treatment modalities, including individual, group, and family psychotherapy; psychodrama; recreational therapy; lectures on substance abuse; and support groups. These programs seem to be successful in helping individuals cope with all forms of substance abuse, including polydrug abuse.

SELF-HELP GROUPS The importance of self-help groups should also be emphasized. Most, but not all, support groups are modeled after the Alcoholics Anonymous program. Encourage clients to investigate and attend a number of different groups to identify which ones will best suit their needs. Some, such as Women for Sobriety, are particularly suited to women. Others more directly focus on adolescents or young adults, on polydrug users, or on cocaine abusers. These and other resources are briefly described in the resources section at the end of this chapter. Emphasize that, for the initial year of recovery, the client should attend as many meetings as possible. A supportive network, particularly during the initial year of recovery, is especially important.

METHADONE MAINTENANCE PROGRAMS Methadone maintenance programs were developed in the 1960s in response to heroin addiction. Methadone (Dolophine) is a synthetic compound, which in moderate or high doses, blocks the effects of heroin.

Although methadone is the most frequent treatment for heroin addiction in the United States, controversy surrounding its use has both physiologic and psychosocial implications. Those who support methadone maintenance programs say that methadone:

- Effectively reduces the craving for heroin
- Has long-lasting effects
- Has few known side effects
- Can be administered orally
- Is cost effective compared to other forms of treatment
- Reduces criminal heroin-seeking behaviors
- Allows clients to return to their jobs, decreasing the number of heroin addicts receiving governmental assistance

Those who argue against this form of treatment make the following claims:

- Dependence on methadone is merely substituted for dependence on heroin.
- Methadone treatment is simply a chemical solution; it fails to encourage finding solutions to the complex problems that led to drug abuse in the first place.
- The majority of heroin addicts are not attracted to methadone maintenance programs.
- Many clients who enter methadone programs leave before treatment is completed.
- A significant proportion of clients either begin to abuse or continue to abuse a wide spectrum of other drugs, including alcohol, tranquilizers, and barbiturates.

One hazard of prolonged methadone maintenance is, in fact, dependence. Methadone withdrawal is similar to morphine withdrawal except the symptoms develop more slowly and are prolonged. Acute symptoms last for 2 to 3 weeks but may continue until 4 to 6 weeks after abstinence. Other symptoms, such as irritability, fatigue, lethargy, and a variety of physical discomforts, may last up to 6 months (Bennett, Vourakis, & Woolf, 1983). Although it is clear that methadone is not the best or final answer to heroin dependence, it is recognized as one approach to a complex socioeconomic, psychologic, and physical problem.

DISULFIRAM (ANTABUSE) TREATMENT Disulfiram is used in the treatment of alcoholism as a deterrent to drinking. The usual dose is 250 mg/day. By inhibiting the action of acetaldehyde dehydrogenase, disulfiram causes an accumulation of toxic acetaldehyde when alcohol is ingested. If an individual drinks even a small amount of alcohol within a 2-week period after taking disulfiram, a reaction occurs: nausea, vomiting, flushing, dizziness, and tachycardia. Cardiovascular collapse and potential death are possible, depending on how much alcohol is ingested.

While disulfiram can be a powerful deterrent to drinking, the risks to the client must be carefully and individually assessed. Disulfiram is contraindicated in clients with myocardial disease because of the cardiovascular effects that occur in a disulfiram reaction. It is also contraindicated in those who are taking metronidazole (Flagyl) because it can cause a disulfiram reaction. Clients should be clearly instructed, verbally and in writing, against using alcoholic beverages or paraldehyde and to avoid preparations such as cough and cold medicines or mouthwashes that contain alcohol. As little as 1 tablespoon of some of these preparations is enough to cause a disulfiram reaction.

Evaluation

Initially, identifying whether the physiologic and behavioral effects of abused substances have abated helps the nurse determine the effectiveness of the intervention. Long-term evaluation of whether the individual has achieved the goal of living life without the drug (if the client has chosen to) is difficult. The nurse may never again see the client who successfully achieves this goal. On the other hand, the person who does not achieve this goal or who chooses not to give up drugs, may return to the health care setting frequently. Nurses may feel discouraged, helpless, angry or frustrated, and hopeless when clients return to the health care setting; they may feel they have somehow failed the client. It is important to acknowledge these feelings and examine how they affect the nursing care of clients who are substance abusers.

Nurses need to assume the attitude that drug abuse is a long-term, chronic problem that can be altered. When an individual has a relapse, focus on the present and future instead of on the past. Also take the view that the current episode is possibly the right time and situation to motivate the person to be successful in recovering from the drug problem. In effect, focus on one day at a time when caring for clients with substance abuse problems.

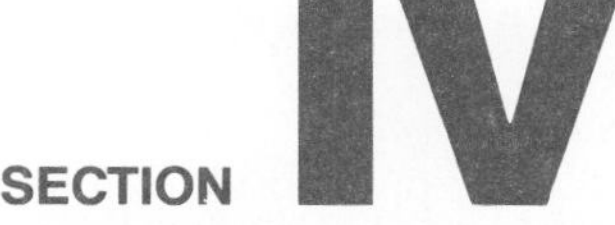

Chemical Dependence Among Health Care Professionals

Health professionals live and work in an environment that puts them at high risk (15% to 20%) for developing substance abuse problems. Nurses, physicians, and other health care professionals are at risk because of:

- Easy access to substances that might be abused
- Knowledge of the health care system, which makes it easier to obtain drugs for personal use
- Stressful and tiring work
- Professional, ethical, and personal conflicts inherent in the care provider role

Alcohol, meperidine, and morphine are the substances most commonly abused by health providers. Fentanyl (Sublimaze) is fast approaching similar levels of abuse among anesthesiologists and nurse anesthetists (Bissell & Haberman, 1984).

Although professionals and the general public have increased knowledge and awareness about alcohol and drug abuse problems, many professionals continue to deny the existence of an obvious problem in their ranks. Covering for a substance-abusing colleague, avoiding confrontation, and ignoring negligent performance result in situations often dangerous for both clients and the abusing professional. Terminating the employment of a nurse or other health care provider without a referral for treatment not only allows the nurse to seek other employment and continue potentially hazardous nursing practice but also perpetuates the nurse's substance abuse problem. Each nurse should be prepared to intervene effectively with a substance-abusing coworker.

Consider the following situation:

Ann, a 35-year-old registered nurse, worked in the operating room of a large hospital and was also on the trauma triage team in the emergency room. She was suspected of using narcotics while working in the operating room but was never detected taking drugs by the other staff. Her colleagues and supervisor failed to discuss their suspicions with her, and she was eventually fired from her job in the OR for "chronic absenteeism."

She continued to work on the triage team and was considered an effective trauma nurse. Again, her peers began to suspect drug use, but were unable to detect that she was abusing narcotics. Soon, both clients and staff reported a number of valuables missing. Rather than confront her directly, the staff informed the administration of their suspicions. The narcotic drawer was dusted by security personnel, and she was apprehended when the dye was revealed on her hands under ultraviolet light. She admitted to having had a narcotic drawer key made and to taking morphine and replacing it with saline.

Ann was fired and informed that she should admit herself to a drug rehabilitation program. No formal charges were filed, however, and she was not reported to the licensing board. Like many of her chemically dependent colleagues in similar circumstances, Ann did not seek treatment on her own. Instead, she found employment in another hospital and continued to abuse morphine, placing herself and her clients in jeopardy.

To avoid control by the government and other authorities over professional practice, nursing and other professions have assumed responsibility for governing professional practice, protecting the public, and providing active assistance to the abusing professional. The American Nurses' Association has issued a policy statement regarding responsibility of the nursing profession to promote education, early identification, and recovery for chemically dependent nurses. Many state nurses' associations have adopted model programs to address the problem and offer support. These programs include telephone hot lines, or crisis information and treatment referral; volunteer peer assistance to aid the nurse in receiving help; and self-help peer support groups to assist in the recovery process. In some states, boards of nursing and state nurses' associations have collaborated on methods for taking disciplinary action and encouraging treatment. The aim of intervention is to protect the client and keep the nurse in active practice, perhaps with certain limitations. If suspension of professional practice is indicated, the aim is to return the nurse to full practice as soon as feasible.

In a state where a peer assistance program is operating, or where legislation allows for alternatives to the customary revocation of a chemically dependent nurse's license, the outcome of Ann's case might have been quite different. Her colleagues could have requested intervention by a peer assistance team usually comprised of two nurses, one of whom is a chemically dependent recovering nurse. Ann's coworkers' observations would have been presented in a manner intended to assist Ann in seeking treatment. Alternatives to being fired would be negotiated, a leave of absence or sick leave arranged, and revocation of licensure avoided. Peer support groups provide the opportunity for discussion and consideration of re-entry into practice and alternatives to working in settings with ready access to controlled substances. The recovering nurse is encouraged to continue after-care treatment or psychotherapy as well as involvement in other support groups such as those in the resource list.

Chapter Highlights

Substance abuse is a problem of major proportions. The abuse of only one drug—alcohol—is the third major cause of death in the United States and is a major health problem in many other countries.

Substance abuse has far-reaching effects on individuals, families, friends, work associates, and neighbors.

One in four hospitalized clients is estimated to have problems related to substance abuse.

Dependence—requiring the effects of a specified drug to function—can be physiologic, psychologic, or both.

Tolerance to drugs develops with repeated use and requires increasingly higher, and potentially lethal, doses.

A nursing care problem develops in clients who develop a cross-tolerance to drugs that are pharmacologically similar.

Substance abuse affects all the systems of the body, and with chronic abuse, results in debilitating physical and emotional illness.

Nurses may not always know that a client is a substance abuser; being alert to this possibility helps to prevent complications and promotes opportunities for appropriate treatment referral.

Analyzing their own feelings, beliefs, and attitudes toward substance abuse will help nurses to implement the nursing process effectively.

States of intoxication, coma, and overdose require immediate and accurate assessment and emergency measures.

Nurses and other health professionals are at high risk for developing substance abuse problems. The professions are assuming active responsibility and promoting programs of prevention, education, intervention, and peer assistance.

Bibliography

American Psychiatric Association. *Diagnostic and Statistical Manual of Mental Disorders,* 3rd ed. Washington, DC: American Psychiatric Association, 1987.

Bennett G, Vourakis C, Woolf E: *Substance abuse: Pharmacologic, Developmental, and Clinical Perspectives.* New York: Wiley, 1983.

Bissell L, Haberman P: *Alcoholism in the Professions.* New York: Oxford, 1984.

Bry B: Substance abuse in women: etiology and prevention. *Issues Ment Health Nurs* 1983; 5(1–4):253–272.

Byrne CJ et al: *Laboratory Tests: Implications for Nursing Care.* 2nd ed. Menlo Park, CA: Addison–Wesley, 1986.

Chiras DC: *Environmental Science: A Framework for Decision Making.* Menlo Park, CA: Benjamin/Cummings, 1985.

Chychula NM: Screening for substance abuse in a primary care setting. *Nurs Pract* 1984; 9:15–24.

Estes NJ, Heinemann ME (editors): *Alcoholism: Development, Consequences, and Interventions,* 2nd ed. St. Louis: Mosby, 1982.

Estes N, Smith–DiJulio K, Heinemann M: *Nursing Diagnosis of the Alcoholic Person.* St. Louis: Mosby, 1980.

Folkers BL: Recognition and management of the alcohol dependent trauma patient. *Ortho Nurs* 1985; 4(2):34–36.

Gilman AG, Goodman LS, Gilman A: The Pharmacological Basis of Therapeutics, 7th ed. New York: Macmillan, 1984.

Gold M: *800–Cocaine.* New York: Bantam Books, 1984.

Jellinek EM: Phases of alcohol addiction. *Q J Studies Alcohol* 1952; 13:673–684.

Kaplan HI, Sadock BJ: *Comprehensive Textbook of Psychiatry,* 4th ed. Baltimore: Williams & Wilkins, 1985.

Malin H et al: An epidemiologic perspective in alcohol use and abuse in the United States. In: *Alcohol Consumption with Related Problems.* Alcohol and Health Monograph No. 1. National Institute on Alcohol Abuse and Alcoholism, 1984.

Naegle M: The nurse and the alcoholic: Redefining a historically ambivalent relationship. *J Psychosoc Nurs Ment Health Serv* 1983; 21(6):17–23.

Pierce RO, Pierce GW: The effect of alcohol on the skeletal system. *Ortho Rev* 1985; 14(1):45–49.

Pilette W: Caffeine: Psychiatric grounds for concern. *J Psychosoc Nurs Ment Health Serv* 1983; 21(8):19–24.

Solomon J: *Alcoholism and Clinical Psychiatry.* New York: Plenum, 1982.

Wilson HS, Kneisl CR: *Psychiatric Nursing,* 3rd ed. Menlo Park, CA: Addison–Wesley, 1988.

Resources

SELF-HELP GROUPS AND OTHER ORGANIZATIONS

(Programs to help smokers give up the habit are in the resources list at the end of Chapter 14.)

Alcoholics Anonymous World Services, Inc. (AA)
PO Box 459
Grand Central Station
New York, NY 10163
Phone: (212) 686–1100

The organization is composed of people who share experiences with alcoholism and provide support for each other in overcoming alcoholism. Pamphlets useful for health professionals are *If You Are a Professional, Alcoholics Anonymous Wants to Work with You* and *Alcoholics Anonymous and the Medical Profession.*

In Canada write to:
Alcoholics Anonymous, Intergroup Office
272 Eglinton Ave., West
Toronto, Ontario, Canada M4R 1B2

Al-Anon Family Group Headquarters
PO Box 862
Midtown Station
New York, NY 10018–0862
Phone: (212) 302–7240

This organization for relatives and friends of alcoholics includes Alateen for children of alcoholics. The organization functions separately from Alcoholics Anonymous and publishes several pamphlets, books (catalog available), and a monthly newsletter *Forum.* Write for a catalog of pamphlets. No dues or fees; donations at meetings.

Nar-Anon Family Group
PO Box 2562
Palos Verdes Peninsula, CA 90274
Phone: (213) 547–5800

An organization for the partners and families of persons who abuse narcotics. No dues or fees; donations appreciated. There are groups in both the United States and Canada (check local telephone book).

Narcotics Anonymous
PO Box 622
Sun Valley, CA 91352
Phone: (818) 997–3822

A worldwide fellowship of recovered narcotics addicts who meet regularly to help one another stay off drugs, this organization is based on the Alcoholics Anonymous philosophy. Membership is open to all; no dues or fees. Local chapters publish the *Narcotics Anonymous Newsletter.*

National Association of Recovered Alcoholics
PO Box 95
Staten Island, NY 10305

Members are recovered alcoholics who help one another deal with economic, legal, social, and vocational problems. Sponsors a job-placement service and a job-opportunities newsletter.

National Clearinghouse on Alcohol and Drug Information
PO Box 2345
Rockville, MD 20852
Phone: (301) 468-2600

This branch of the National Institute on Alcohol Abuse and Alcoholism makes available current information on alcohol use and abuse. They will conduct computerized searches for specific materials, provide bibliographies, provide referrals to local alcohol abuse programs, and give notification of newly published research results. Several pamphlets and books on alcohol are available at no charge or minimal charge.

National Council on Alcoholism, Inc.
12 W 21st St, 7th Fl
New York, NY 10010
Phone: (800) NCA–CALL

This national voluntary health agency consists of state and local affiliates as well as the American Medical Society on Alcoholism and National Nurses Society on Alcoholism (see listing under Nursing Organization). It cooperates with, and supports, self-help groups. The NCA Library Information Service invites questions by telephone or letter.

Drugs Anonymous
PO Box 243, Ansonia Station
New York, NY 10023
Phone: (212) 874–0700

Modeled after AA, this organization has the goal of helping people live a drug-free life. Most members have or had dependence problems with tranquilizers, sedatives, or analgesics. No dues or fees; contributions at meetings.

Salvation Army
National Information Service
799 Bloomfield Ave
Verona, NJ 07044
Phone: (201) 239–0606

Sponsors both alcohol and drug rehabilitation programs, halfway houses, drop-in centers, and family service bureaus.

Therapeutic Communities of America, Intl.
54 W. 40th St.
New York, NY 10018
Phone: (212) 354–6000

This organization monitors the activities of drug-free therapeutic communities throughout the United States and will make referrals to those that meet its standards. Referral resources do not include methadone maintenance programs.

Women for Sobriety, Inc.
PO Box 618
Quakertown, PA 18951
Phone: (215) 536–8026

This is a network of over 200 self-help groups for women alcoholics only. It is supported by contributions and donations at group meetings. Monthly newsletter.

HOT LINES

Alcoholics Anonymous

Local phone books in the United States and Canada list the number of the closest 24-hour answering service.

Federal Drug Administration
Bureau of Drugs
See local listings

Offers information on drug interactions and side effects.

National Cocaine Helpline
Phone: 800–COCAINE

This 24-hour nationwide referral and information service is a resource for cocaine users, nonuser victims, and health care professionals, who can request information on cocaine research. It is based at Fair Oaks Hospital in Summit, NJ.

National Institute on Drug Abuse—Cocaine
Phone: (800) 662–HELP

HEALTH EDUCATION MATERIAL

From: Koala Center
1404 S. State Ave.
Indianapolis, IN 46203
Phone: (317) 783–4084

A free brochure listing the alcohol content of 145 products. Send a large self-addressed, stamped envelope.

NURSING ORGANIZATIONS

National Nurses Society on Addictions (NNSA)
2506 Gross Point Rd
Evanston, IL 60201
Phone: (312) 475–7300

This organization for nurses working in the addiction field publishes a newsletter four times a year. It also provides information on treatment and research in addiction, certification for nurses working in the field, and a chemically dependent nurse network.

CHAPTER **9**

Infection

Other topics relevant to this content are: Aseptic technique for laryngotracheal suctioning, **Chapter 14**; Immune system and immune response, **Chapter 2**; Nursing care of clients with specific infections, *see specific disorders chapter(s) in appropriate body system unit*; Preventing postoperative wound infection, **Chapter 11**; Strategies nurses can use to minimize clients' risk of nosocomial urinary tract infection, **Chapter 25**; White blood count and differential, and significance of "left shift", **Chapter 17**.

Objectives

When you have finished studying this chapter, you should be able to:

Describe the sequence of events necessary for transmission of infection.

Identify persons who are likely to be susceptibile to infection.

Discuss the physiologic and psychosocial/lifestyle factors that can compromise the immune system.

Describe the assessment of the potentially infected client.

Employ direct measures to prevent or limit nosocomial infection.

Educate clients regarding immunization, hygiene and sanitation, food handling, and the administration of antimicrobial medications.

Discuss principles of infection prevention and control in the nursing care of all clients.

Infectious diseases have aroused fear from the time of the ancient Greeks and Chinese to the present. During the Middle Ages, an estimated three-fourths of the population of Europe contracted smallpox. Many died or were left with disfiguring scars. At about the same time, the black death, or bubonic plague, destroyed about one-fourth of the total population of Europe. Yellow fever endangered the successful completion of the Panama Canal. Poliomyelitis terrorized the United States in the late 1940s and early 1950s; many children and adults were left to cope with its paralyzing effects. More recently, legionellosis, or legionnaires' disease, a pneumonialike illness, frightened the citizens of Philadelphia in 1976 when 182 American Legion conventioneers became ill, and 29 of them died. Women who used superabsorbent tampons in the early 1980s feared toxic shock syndrome. And, entire populations fear contracting what is proving to be an exceptionally insidious and lethal disease, acquired immune deficiency syndrome (AIDS).

An infection occurs when potentially pathogenic (disease-producing) organisms invade the body, or host. Not all contact with these microorganisms is harmful, and therefore, not all infections cause disease. In fact, people live in constant contact with infectious agents that normally inhabit their bodies. Usually, a balance between the host's immune system and the *virulence* of the organism (its ability to produce disease) keeps the host healthy. But when the balance is tipped, such as when the immune system is penetrated or when the organism is particularly pathogenic, infectious disease occurs. All body systems are vulnerable to infectious disease; therefore, infection is a multisystem stressor.

This chapter provides a general overview of infection, its prevention and control, and nursing measures relevant to infectious disease. Selected diseases such as botulism, tetanus, and rabies, among others, are also discussed here. Other infectious diseases and related nursing measures are discussed in each of the specific disorders chapters in the units on body system dysfunction.

Infectious disease affects health care and human behavior at many different levels. It can influence or be influenced by culture, economics, religion, environment, and various lifestyle factors. Because all body systems are vulnerable to infectious disease, the thread of infection is woven throughout the fabric of this text.

SECTION 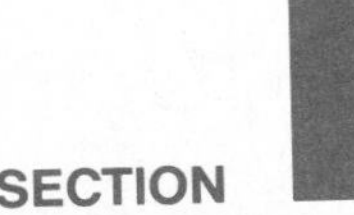

The Problem of Infection

Despite the development of antimicrobials and methods of infection prevention and control, infectious diseases remain a major cause of illness and death, especially in third world countries. It has been estimated that pathogenic microorganisms cause at least half of all human diseases.

Host and Microbe

The relationship between host and microbe varies from mutually beneficial to seriously harmful, depending on the condition of the host and the virulence of the microbe. The relationship between a healthy person and that person's *normal flora* (the microorganisms that normally inhabit the inside as well as the outside of the human body) is called *symbiosis*.

When a human and a microorganism mutually benefit from their symbiotic relationship, the term is *mutualism.* Normal intestinal microbes such as *Escherichia coli* live on ingested food; in return, they aid in synthesis of vitamin K, vitamin B_{12}, thiamine, and riboflavin.

In *commensalism,* one organism is benefited and the other is unaffected. The corynebacteria that live on sloughed-off cells and secretions on the surface of the eye apparently neither benefit nor harm their human host. On the other hand, lactobacilli in the vagina help maintain a vaginal pH of 4.0 to 4.5, inhibiting yeast infection from *Candida albicans.*

The relationship is known as *parasitism* when one organism benefits at the expense of the other (eg, in a serious infection, microbes benefit at the expense of a human). Many microorganisms causing disease are parasites.

Under certain circumstances, a relationship of peaceful coexistence can change, and organisms such as *E. coli* may become harmful. If the client is ill for another reason, or if the integrity of the skin or mucous membranes has been compromised (accidentally or purposefully through an invasive procedure such as surgery or diagnostic testing), allowing the organism access to a body site in which it is not normally found, a normally harmless organism can become pathogenic. For example, when *E. coli* invades the urinary bladder or a surgical wound, it can cause infections or abscesses. Even hygienic measures or drug therapy sometimes disrupts peaceful coexistence. When lactobacilli in the vagina are eliminated through douching, vaginal deodorants, or treatment with wide-spectrum antibiotics or immunosuppressive drugs, *C. albicans* flourishes, causing infectious vaginitis (see Chapter 49). These potentially pathogenic organisms are called **opportunists.**

It is important to keep this concept in mind when delivering hands-on nursing care or teaching clients and their families. Alert clients and health care providers can reduce the risk of opportunistic organisms becoming harmful ones. Specific nursing measures are discussed in Section III.

In addition to the normal flora, other microorganisms usually regarded as pathogenic may be present on or in the body without causing disease. For example, the varicella-zoster virus, a member of the herpesvirus group that causes chickenpox, can remain latent in nerve cells after recovery. Serious illness, trauma, or psychologic stress are factors thought to reactivate the virus, causing a related disease known as herpes zoster, or shingles. The poliovirus also remains latent in the anterior horn cells of the upper spinal cord where it can be reactivated decades later. Some adults who had polio as children are discovering new paralytic symptoms similar to those of the original poliomyelitis 30 and 40 years after having had the disease.

The Spread of Infectious Disease

Until scientists established that specific organisms caused specific diseases, infections were thought to be caused by foul odors from sewage, poisonous swamp vapors, the night air, or by the gods who brought illness down upon a person, family, or community as a punishment for misdeeds. The germ theory of disease was first proven a little over a century ago in 1876 when Robert Koch, a young German physician, first proved that bacteria caused the cattle disease, anthrax.

Now it is known that a sequence of events is necessary for infection to spread. First is a *disease-producing agent*—a bacterium, virus, fungus, rickettsia, protozoan, or helminth. Second, the organisms must have a source, called a *reservoir,* in which the organism survives but may or may not multiply. Although the human body is the most common reservoir for the microorganisms that cause human disease, a reservoir can also be animal or inanimate. Amazingly, about 150 diseases can be transmitted to humans by animals, birds, or insects. Inanimate reservoirs include soil and water as well as other substances or objects not normally considered reservoirs of infection (eg, *Salmonella* organisms can multiply in contaminated turkey at a family gathering, and *Pseudomonas* organisms can multiply in nebulizers, eye drops, and cosmetics). A *portal of exit* is the organism's escape route from the reservoir. Common portals of exit from human reservoirs are the gastrointestinal system (through saliva or feces), the respiratory system (through coughing, sneezing, and even laughing or talking), the urinary system (through the urine), the reproductive system (through the semen or secretions from the penis or vagina), and skin or wound infections (through wound drainage).

Next is a *mode of transmission* from the reservoir to the host. Organisms are transmitted by direct contact, indirect contact, and arthropod vectors. Infection might spread by direct body contact when a nurse accidentally sticks herself with a needle from a hepatitis B client or handles a contaminated wound dressing and forgets to wash her hands before rubbing her eyes. The common cold and venereal diseases are also spread directly from one person to another through such close associations as handshaking, kissing, and sexual intercourse. Droplet spread from talking, coughing, and sneezing, usually limited to 3 ft or less, is another form of direct contact (Figure 9–1).

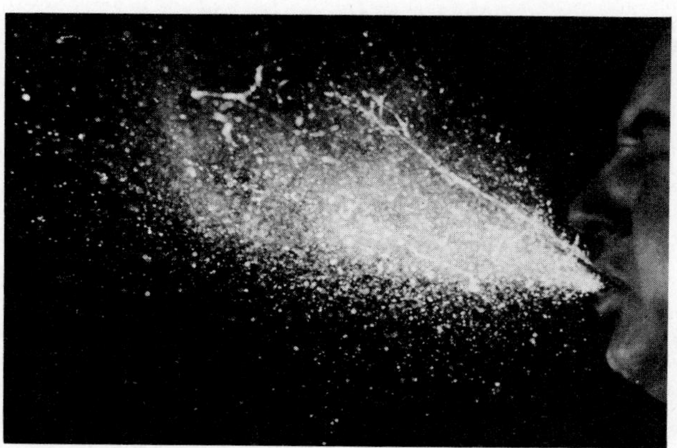

Figure 9–1

This high-speed photograph shows the spray of small droplets that comes from the mouth during a sneeze. SOURCE: *Tortora GJ, Funke BR, Case CL:* Microbiology; *2nd ed. Menlo Park, CA: Benjamin/Cummings, 1986.*

Nonliving objects provide for indirect contact; these objects are called fomites. A contaminated suction catheter used for endotracheal suctioning is an example of an object that provides for indirect contact; another is the contaminated turkey at the family gathering. Because many more steps are involved in indirect transmission, it is a less likely mode of transmitting infectious agents than direct contact. Consider this scene in a dialysis unit: (1) A hemodialysis nurse gets blood on her hands from a client with hepatitis B. (2) The nurse handles the dialysis machine knobs, transferring the hepatitis B virus to them. (3) A second nurse also handles the knobs, picking up the hepatitis B virus. (4) The second nurse starts an intravenous infusion on a second client. (5) On palpating the second client's vein, the nurse transfers the virus to the access route.

Airborne transmission, an indirect method that spreads diseases such as tuberculosis, covers greater distances than droplet spread. Some organisms that live in dry desert soil are transmitted by the wind or in dust storms.

Arthropod vectors include the insects that carry disease and transmit it either mechanically or biologically. Houseflies carry infectious organisms on their feet and transfer them mechanically to food that is later swallowed. In malaria and yellow fever, pathogens reproduce in mosquitoes, which transmit them biologically by injecting them through the skin.

A pathogen gains access to the body by a *portal of entry.* Common portals are the respiratory and gastrointestinal tracts. Pathogens can also enter the body through broken skin, mucous membranes, or by the parenteral route—injections, blood transfusions, wounds, surgery, punctures, cuts, and bites. Finally, to cause an infection, the pathogen must find a *susceptible host,* one whose body defenses are ineffective against the pathogen. The susceptible host is discussed in greater detail later in this chapter.

The Nature and Scope of Infectious Disease

Infectious diseases are classified and understood according to their nature and scope. A disease that can be transmitted from one person to another is a *communicable disease.* Gonorrhea and influenza are communicable diseases. A *noncommunicable disease* is one that is not transmitted from one person to another. Noncommunicable diseases are caused by organisms normally inhabiting the body that only occasionally cause disease, or by organisms that reside outside the body causing disease when introduced into it. Tetanus is an example of a noncommunicable disease. Diseases, such as measles and chickenpox, that can be easily spread from one person to another are termed *contagious diseases.* The initial infectious disease is called a *primary infection.* When an opportunist organism causes a different infection in a body already weakened by a primary infection, the condition is called a *secondary infection.* A person can also have a *subclinical infection* in which there are no apparent symptoms.

A variety of terms describes the frequency of infectious diseases. An *endemic* disease is usually present within a certain population or within a geographic area. For example, yellow fever is endemic in Africa and Central and South America, and coccidioidomycosis is endemic in the American Southwest (especially the San Joaquin Valley of California) and northern Mexico. Whenever there is an excess incidence of a disease over that expected within an area in a relatively short time, a disease is said to be *epidemic.* Measles, smallpox, and poliomyelitis historically have occurred in epidemics. Some sexually transmitted diseases are thought to have reached epidemic proportions. A *pandemic* is an epidemic disease that affects several countries or occurs worldwide. Influenza and bubonic plague have been pandemic.

Infectious diseases may also be classified according to the extent to which the body is affected. For example, in a pimple or an abscess, the infection is confined to a limited area of the body. This is called a *local infection.* A *systemic infection* is generalized rather than limited. The disease is spread throughout the body by the blood and the lymphatics. Typhus and typhoid fever are examples of systemic diseases. A *focal infection* is one that had its beginnings as a local infection but spread to another part of the body. Infections in the teeth and sinuses may spread to the brain via the lymphatics and blood supply.

Susceptibility to Infection

Although everyone has frequent contact with potentially infectious organisms, most persons do not often become ill. They remain well either because the organism's *virulence* (ability to produce disease) is low or because the host's resistance to disease is high. Resistance to disease depends on an equilibrium among these factors. When there is an imbalance, infection is more likely.

The virulence of an organism is influenced by a variety of factors. The first factor is the number of organisms involved; the likelihood of disease increases with the number of pathogens. A second influencing factor is an organism's *invasiveness,* its ability to colonize and multiply in a host and interfere with body function. A third factor is the organism's ability to produce poisonous substances called **toxins.** A fourth factor is the organism's ability to cause changes in cells themselves that result in cell death.

In the past, organisms were considered the dominant factor in infection. Now the role of the host figures as prominently. From experience with chemotherapeutic agents, immunosuppressants, and antimicrobials, it is known that any organism can cause an infection if the host's resistance is sufficiently suppressed. A person with impaired resistance is referred to as a **compromised host.** Factors compromising the host's ability to resist infectious disease are discussed below and listed in Table 9–1.

Table 9–1
The Compromised Host

Conditions Placing Clients at Risk for Infection	Altered Defense Mechanism
Severe burns, extensive trauma	Skin and mucous membranes
Malnutrition	Cell-mediated immunity
Diabetes mellitus	Microcirculation, inflammatory response
Leukemia, lymphoma, multiple myeloma, sarcoidosis	Immune system
Immunosuppressive drugs	Immune system
Broad-spectrum antibiotics	Normal bacterial flora
Glucocorticosteroids	Cell-mediated immunity
Anatomic defects (eg, scoliosis)	Respiratory function
Chronic heavy alcohol use	Normal cough and glottal closure; humoral and cell-mediated immunity
Heavy tobacco smoking	Normal ciliary function, oxygen level, platelet responses
Stress	Immune system

Age and General Health

Infants are born with passive immunity from their mothers that protects them from illness for a short time. After the first few weeks of life, infants must be protected from unnecessary exposure to contagious illness and immunized on schedule because they have not developed their own immunity. The infant's immunity can be extended by breast feeding because the mother passes antibodies to her infant in the breast milk.

As children grow older, their immune systems mature. Although young children are easily infected, they recover from most infections without problems. They build immunity against many diseases through exposure and immunization. Young adults are less easily infected than children and normally recover readily from local infections. For middle-aged adults in good health, minor contagious diseases are the primary infection problem.

By the later years, however, susceptibility to infection increases because of a variety of factors. Chronic diseases, such as diabetes and pulmonary and cardiovascular diseases, which are most common in the elderly, reduce the ability to fight infectious disease. During the winter many elderly persons die from influenza, in part because of their debilitated state.

Nutritional Status

Poor nutritional status increases the risk of infection. Insufficient protein in the diet reduces the numbers of antibodies formed because antibodies are a protein substance. This reduces host resistance. Because caloric and protein needs increase during illness, the malnourished person with an infection may become trapped in a cyclical disease state. Malnutrition exacerbates infection and vice versa, so a minor infection may have serious consequences. A person without normal serum protein levels can sometimes even acquire a disease from the small dose of antigens given in an immunization. Hospitalized clients are at particular risk for malnutrition and consequently for infection.

Immune System Defects

Conditions affecting the production, lifespan, or function of white blood cells reduce the host's ability to fight infection. When the blood neutrophil count drops below

1000 μL, particularly if the count falls below 100 μL, the risk of infection is greatly increased. Low neutrophil counts (neutropenia) occur with leukemia, agranulocytosis, and aplastic anemia.

Other acquired diseases specifically affecting the immune system are multiple myeloma, Hodgkin's disease, Crohn's disease, and sarcoidosis. Of growing concern is AIDS, an infectious disease that involves a defect in cell-mediated immunity and for which there is, as yet, no known cure.

Persons can also be born with a variety of congenital immune abnormalities that affect the production of antibodies, complement, or cellular immunity. A few children with severe congenital combined immune deficiencies have been placed in clear plastic "bubbles" to protect them from pathogens, but such precautions are extremely expensive.

Chronic Disease

Among chronic diseases suppressing the immune system are uremia and diabetes. Studies have shown that persons with uremia from chronic renal failure have a decrease in the number of circulating lymphocytes as well as malnutrition and other factors that impair the body's defenses. Diabetics have an increased incidence of infection, although research has not demonstrated that their immune response is reduced. The increased risk of infection probably results from vascular damage and neurovascular changes. Deficits in sensation place the client at risk of injury, and impaired circulation to the injured area delays healing, increasing the risk of infection. It is also possible that elevated levels of blood glucose and ketones impair the inflammatory response.

Injury to Integumentary and Respiratory Systems

The skin and mucous membranes provide the first barrier to invading organisms. The body is protected by the skin's tough outer layer, the stratum corneum, and by antimicrobial substances produced by the sweat and oil glands.

In the respiratory tract, mucus and other substances prevent organisms from colonizing or invading. Cilia lining the respiratory tract sweep mucus upward on a so-called "ciliary escalator," taking bacteria along so they can be expelled. The sneeze and cough reflexes also expel foreign matter from the airway. Urine, tears, and saliva wash infectious organisms away from body orifices.

Injuries to these protective mechanisms increase a person's infection risk. Burns, pressure ulcers, and extensive trauma are examples of injuries that leave the skin raw and vulnerable to infectious organisms. These wounds often become infected. Persons with diabetes or atherosclerosis can develop ulcers on the legs and feet that are prone to infection.

Damage to the respiratory tract from inhalation burns, mechanical ventilation, or infection can alter the normal resistance of lung epithelium, increasing the risk of pneumonitis and pneumonia. Intubation and tracheostomy with or without mechanical ventilation also increase the risk of pulmonary infection because the normal protective barriers are interrupted or bypassed. These procedures provide direct communication between the environment and underlying tissues.

Psychosocial/Lifestyle Factors

Host resistance is also influenced by psychosocial and lifestyle factors such as finances, environment, occupation, avocation, recreation, and stress. When finances are limited, a common tendency is to delay purchasing health services such as immunizations for preventable diseases. Tuberculosis is a good example of how psychosocial and lifestyle factors influence the development of disease. In the United States, tuberculosis is most prevalent among the poor where overcrowding facilitates the airborne transmission of the causative organism, and malnutrition and stress are likely. Yet, large numbers of the population have a positive reaction to tuberculosis skin testing, indicating previous exposure to the causative organism, without developing active disease.

Where one lives can also make a person more susceptible to certain infectious diseases. Histoplasmosis, a fungal disease of the respiratory system, is essentially limited in the United States to states surrounding the Ohio and Mississippi Rivers, where the moisture and pH provide ideal growing conditions for the fungus. Recall also that coccidioidomycosis is more likely to be found in the San Joaquin Valley of California and the desert regions of Arizona where the dry, highly alkaline soils favor the growth of the fungus that causes it.

Travel exposes persons to infectious diseases that, although rare in one part of the world, are common in another. Travelers have contracted Asiatic cholera in India, schistosomiasis (infestation by a flatworm parasite in contaminated water) in Africa and the Caribbean, and yellow fever in Brazil.

Occupation and avocation may place people at risk for infection. For example, farmers are susceptible to organisms that tend to use animals, the earth, and water as reservoirs. Lifestyle is yet another influencing factor. A person who values health and fitness is more likely to stay away from situations of risk. A person with multiple sex partners is at greater risk for contracting a sexually transmitted disease. A street person who lives on a park bench or seeks shelter in an abandoned building is more likely to become undernourished and exposed to a wide variety of organisms.

Splenectomy

Persons who have their spleens removed, usually because of traumatic injury, seem to have a greater incidence of infectious diseases. Pneumococcal infections are the most common. The increased infection risk after splenectomy is related to a defective production of immunoglobulins and delayed mobilization of macrophages.

Drug Therapy

Antibiotics, glucocorticoids, and immunosuppressants can alter normal resistance to infection. Antibiotics change the normal balance of flora, especially when broad-spectrum agents are given in combination with other antibiotics. With alteration in normal flora, a **superinfection** (secondary infection resulting from overgrowth of normal flora during antibiotic treatment) can occur. An organism responsible for many superinfections is *Pseudomonas aeruginosa*. This organism is resistant to many antibiotics and is often the cause of hospital-acquired respiratory infections in already compromised clients. Superinfections are discussed further in Section III.

Steroids reduce the body's response to infection by reducing inflammation. In the laboratory, it has been observed that steroids decrease mobilization of neutrophils to the site of infection, decrease the killing of microbes by monocytes, and interfere with cell-mediated immune response. Clients with a disease requiring long-term steroid therapy have a high incidence of infection. It is difficult to diagnose these infections because steroid treatment may inhibit the signs of inflammatory response—heat, redness, pain, and swelling.

Immunosuppressive drugs are commonly administered to clients with cancer and those who have had organ transplants. These agents reduce the ability to produce white blood cells. Immunosuppressants also impair the growth of new cells in other body sites. One result is damage to the mucous membrane epithelium, which is normally repaired rapidly. Breakdown of mucous membranes also provides entry for microorganisms.

Nosocomial Infections

According to the Centers for Disease Control (CDC), 5% to 15% of all clients admitted to acute care hospitals in the United States develop a nosocomial (hospital-acquired) infection. With certain operations such as surgery of the large intestine and amputations, the infection rate approaches 30% (Tortora, Funke, & Case, 1986). It is estimated that fully one-third of all infections in hospitalized clients are nosocomial (Kochar, 1983) and about 20,000 die annually of nosocomial infections (Tortora, Funke, & Case, 1986).

Hospitalized clients are more vulnerable to infectious diseases than outpatients or healthy persons. Catheters, intravenous lines and devices, and endotracheal tubes are some of the invasive objects used in hospitals that disturb the normal barriers to infections. In some instances, reusable devices are not properly cleaned and disinfected or sterilized between use in one client and the next. In addition, many clients have coexisting conditions that alter the body's ability to combat organisms that have entered the bloodstream or tissues. (See discussion of the compromised host.)

Table 9–2
Six Bacteria That Account for Over 60% of All Nosocomial Infections

Bacterium	% of Infections
Escherichia coli	18.6
Staphylococcus aureus	10.8
Enterococci	10.7
Pseudomonas aeruginosa	10.6
Klebsiella species	7.4
Coagulase-negative Staphylococci	6.1

SOURCE: From Tortora GJ, Funke BR, Case CL: *Microbiology*, 2nd ed. Menlo Park, CA: Benjamin/Cummings, 1986, p. 389.

The majority of nosocomial infections are caused when an organism normally present in a client overwhelms an impaired immune system. Common examples are *E. coli* causing urinary tract infections and *Klebsiella* causing pneumonia. These and other bacteria that account for the majority of nosocomial infections are listed in Table 9–2.

The remainder of nosocomial infections is acquired from organisms within the hospital environment. Inhalation therapy and hemodialysis equipment are reported to have been sources of infection from gram-negative organisms. The source of most nosocomial infections caused by *Streptococcus* and *Staphylococcus aureus* is usually the client. These infections can also be acquired from other clients or hospital personnel and sometimes from contaminated equipment or inanimate objects. Nurses are also at risk for hospital-acquired infections. A nurse who is not wearing gloves, but has a fresh cut on a finger, can be at risk when suctioning a client. For example, if the client harbors the herpesvirus in oral secretions, the nurse could develop herpetic whitlow from the transfer of the virus from the client's oral secretions to the cut, even though there are no obvious lesions on the client's lips.

Because many nosocomial infections are caused by organisms from the client's normal flora, nosocomial infections cannot be completely eliminated. An active infection control program, however, can be effective in identifying interventions that can reduce nosocomial infection risk and in teaching personnel to use these interventions in their client care activities (discussed later in Section III).

SECTION II

Epidemiology and Disease Control

Epidemiology is the study of the occurrence, distribution, and determinants of disease and other health conditions in populations. When an outbreak of disease occurs, such as salmonellosis, or when a new disease appears, such as toxic shock syndrome, epidemiologists go to work analyzing the incidence and transmission patterns.

Almost all hospitals in the United States have infection prevention and control programs and infection control practitioners or nurse epidemiologists who are responsible for the day-to-day infection prevention and control activities for the hospital. About 85% of these practitioners are nurses. These programs receive their direction from the hospital's infection control committee.

Infection control personnel are responsible for monitoring hospitalized clients for development of nosocomial infections, detecting and investigating infection outbreaks, monitoring isolation precautions for clients admitted with infection and clients who develop infection while hospitalized, educating hospital personnel about infection control risks and prevention strategies, and developing hospital infection control policies and procedures consistent with the latest information. Infection control practitioners can be a valuable resource to the nursing staff.

Epidemiology is also an important function of government at all levels. By gathering information and sharing resources, state, federal, and international agencies can spot trends and recommend disease control measures.

State law specifies which communicable diseases must be reported to the state health department. The lists may vary slightly from state to state. State health departments, in turn, report outbreaks to the federal government. Infection control personnel often provide the link between the hospital and the local or state health department. Nurses who work in other types of health care settings such as a community clinic or a physician's office may be responsible for reporting these diseases.

The CDC in Atlanta is the federal agency charged with disease prevention and control. The CDC administers national programs for the prevention and control of communicable and vector-borne diseases as well as other preventable conditions, such as lead-based paint poisoning and urban rat infestations. The CDC also participates with other national and international agencies in this endeavor.

The World Health Organization (WHO), a division of the United Nations, assists with international cooperation for improved health conditions. WHO has been directed to promote attainment of the highest possible level of health for all people. For infectious disease, WHO sponsors measures for disease prevention and control by promoting vaccinations, sanitation, and use of antibiotics and insecticides. The agency has also standardized quarantine measures.

This section discusses selected infectious diseases not discussed elsewhere in this text. Other infectious diseases are discussed in the specific disorders chapters. A comprehensive summary of the epidemiology and prevention of infectious diseases is in Table 9–3.

Bacterial Diseases

Of the multitudes of bacteria species, relatively few cause human disease. Bacterial diseases are a major health problem, however, especially in developing countries. In industrialized countries, bacterial infections are the most common fatal infectious diseases.

Pathogenic bacteria cause disease in two basic ways: by invasion and by producing toxins. Invading bacteria establish residence in the host and, through metabolism and multiplication, interfere with phagocytosis, damage cells, and interfere with metabolism. There are two types of toxins: exotoxins and endotoxins. **Exotoxins** are particularly lethal substances, usually produced by gram-positive bacteria, that are released by the bacteria. When transported by the blood or the lymph, exotoxins can cause cellular damage far from the site of infection. They are disease specific and are responsible for producing the signs and symptoms of that particular infectious disease. Exotoxins are produced in gas gangrene, tetanus, botulism, diphtheria, and scarlet fever. **Endotoxins,** although toxic, are not as lethal as exotoxins in the same amount; that is, their lethal dose is considerably larger. Endotoxins are actually part of the outer cell wall, usually of gram-negative bacteria, and are released only upon destruction of the cell wall. They are not disease specific; rather, they produce generalized symptoms such as fever, weakness, generalized aches, and shock, regardless of which bacterium is involved. Endotoxins are produced in shigellosis (bacillary dysentery), tularemia, and epidemic meningitis.

Selected bacterial diseases such as bacteremia, septicemia, staphylococcal and streptococcal infection, bacterial food poisoning, botulism, tetanus, and gas gangrene are discussed here.

Bacteremia

Asymptomatic bacteremia (the presence of bacteria in the blood) often occurs following tooth extraction and in up to 10% of clients who have barium enema, sigmoidoscopy, cystoscopy, and tracheal suctioning (Kochar, 1983). The organisms involved are not usually virulent enough to cause problems, and the client's own defenses can usually

Table 9–3
Summary of Epidemiology and Prevention of Selected Infectious Diseases in Adults

Disease	Causative Agent	Mode of Transmission	Incubation Period	Communicable Period	Isolation Precautions	Prevention
Acquired immune deficiency syndrome (AIDS)	Human T-cell lymphoma virus, type III (HTLV-III)	Sexual contact; blood and blood product transfusion; contaminated needles; possible transplacental transfer	Believed to be a few months to 5 yr or more	Unknown; carrier state possible	Blood/body fluid precautions	Public education about risk factors; caution in handling blood and needles; testing of donor blood for HTLV-III antibody
Amebiasis (amebic dysentery)	Protozoa: *Entamoeba histolytica*	Water or food contaminated with *E. histolytica* cysts	Variable, but may be 2–4 wk	As long as individual has cysts in stools (may be years)	Enteric precautions	Handwashing after defecating and before eating or handling food; sanitary disposal of human feces; thorough cooking of foods; treating water with 8 gtt of tincture of iodine per quart when camping or whenever contamination is suspected or possible; removal of carriers from food handling
Anthrax	Bacteria: *Bacillus anthracis*	Contact inhalation or ingestion of heavy spore concentrations from infected animals (cattle, goats, sheep, etc) or infected materials such as hides, wool, and animal hair (especially in imported handicrafts); cutaneous infection from contaminated tissues of animals	1–7 d	Contaminated articles and soil can remain infective for years; not transmitted person to person	Drainage/secretion precautions during illness for cutaneous or inhalation anthrax	Immunization of high-risk persons; early detection and control of disease in animals; importation restrictions on possibly contaminated animal products
Botulism	Bacteria: *Clostridium botulinum*	Ingestion or contact with infected food or soil	12–72 h	Not applicable	Enteric precautions	Public education on home canning, food preservation; avoiding foods suspected of spoilage; proper industrial canning techniques; avoiding giving honey to infants under 1 yr of age

Disease	Causative Agent	Mode of Transmission	Incubation Period	Communicable Period	Isolation Precautions	Prevention
Brucellosis (undulant fever)	Bacilli of Brucella genus: *B. abortus, B. canis, B. melitensis, B. suis*	Ingestion of or contact with unpasteurized dairy products, meat, blood, or aborted fetuses and placentas of infected animals (cattle, goats, pigs, dogs)	5–30 d; may be several mo	Not transmitted person to person	None	Pasteurization of milk and milk products; early detection of disease in animals; education of animal and meat handlers
Cat-scratch fever	Not yet established; may be a gram-negative bacterium	Cat scratch or bite	3–14 d	Unknown; not transmitted person to person	None	Declawing of domestic cats; teaching cats not to claw or bite; thorough cleansing of scratches or bites
Chancroid	Bacteria: *Hemophilus ducreyi*	Direct contact, especially sexual contact	2–5 d; up to 14 d	While lesions are present; usually weeks	None	Treatment of infection; prophylactic treatment of contacts; avoid sexual contact with infected person
Cholera	Bacteria: *Vibrio cholerae*	Fecal–oral route; contaminated water and food	1–5 d (usually less than 3 d)	While organism is present; carrier state may persist for several months	Enteric precautions	Protection of water and food from fecal contamination; vaccination for travelers to endemic areas not required in US but is required in a few countries
Cytomegalovirus infection	Cytomegalovirus (CMV) (Herpesvirus family)	Placental transfer, blood transfusion, skin or mucus membrane contact with infectious tissues, secretions, or excretions, and possibly passage through infected birth canal	Unknown	Unknown but may be several years	None; secretion precautions for hospitalized clients excreting the virus	Isolation of infected persons from pregnant women and newborns
Encephalitis	Arbovirus: St. Louis, western equine, eastern equine, Californian, Venezuelan, Japanese Enterovirus: Coxsackievirus, echovirus, poliovirus Herpesvirus: Herpes simplex Myxovirus: Mumps Rabies virus	Mosquito bite; tick bite or ingestion of infected milk or food	2–21 d, depending on specific organism	Not transmitted person to person; mosquitoes and ticks remain infective for life	Enteric precautions (unless known not to be caused by enteroviruses)	Mosquito and tick control; other measures depend on organism

(Continued)

Table 9–3, *(continued)*
Summary of Epidemiology and Prevention of Selected Infectious Diseases in Adults

Disease	Causative Agent	Mode of Transmission	Incubation Period	Communicable Period	Isolation Precautions	Prevention
Food poisoning, bacterial	*Clostridium perfringens*	Contaminated food and drink	8–24 h	Not applicable	Enteric precautions	Proper refrigeration and cooking of food; infected persons should not prepare food; proper sanitation and handwashing during food preparation
	Salmonella	Inadequate cooking of food; infected food handlers; ingestion of contaminated food and drink; pet turtles, chicks, and ducklings	6–72 h	Throughout the course of infection; temporary carrier state may exist for months	Enteric precautions	As above
	Staphylococcus	Contamination of food by infected food handlers; improperly refrigerated food	30 min–7 h (usually 2–4 h)	Not applicable	None	As above
Giardiasis	Protozoan: *Giardia lamblia*	Ingestion of contaminated water; asymptomatic carriers	4–10 d (may be as long as 25 d)	As long as individual has cysts in stools	Enteric precautions	Avoid drinking tap water or using ice made from tap water in areas with high incidence of giardiasis; avoid drinking untreated wilderness water
Gonorrhea	Bacteria: *Neisseria gonorrhoeae*	Mucous membranes of genitourinary tract and conjunctiva through sexual transmission or direct contact during vaginal delivery	2–5 d (symptoms may not appear for 3 mo)	As long as organism is present; usually until 4 d after onset of antibiotic therapy	None	Treatment of infection; prophylactic treatment of contacts; prophylaxis in eyes of newborns
Granuloma inguinale	Bacteria: *Calymmatobacterium granulomatis*	Probably sexual contact	Unknown; may be from 1 wk to almost 3 mo	Unknown; probably while lesions are open	None	Treatment of infection; prophylactic treatment of contacts

Disease	Causative Agent	Mode of Transmission	Incubation Period	Communicable Period	Isolation Precautions	Prevention
Hepatitis						
Type A	Hepatitis A virus	Direct or indirect contact with feces of infected individual; ingestion of contaminated water or food, particularly shellfish, meat, and milk; blood transfusion possible but rare	2–4 wk but may be as long as 7 wk	1–2 wk before onset of symptoms to a few days up to a week after onset of jaundice	Enteric precautions	Proper handwashing; enteric precautions; passive immunization with immune globulin possible if instituted before anticipated contact (eg, travel to highly endemic areas) or soon after but before disease has developed
Type B	Hepatitis B virus	Parenteral route: transfusion of whole blood or plasma; contaminated equipment that pierces the skin (needles, dental, or medical instruments); sexual contact	45–180 d (usual 60–90 d)	From weeks before the onset of symptoms through chronic carrier state (may last for years)	Blood/body fluid precautions	Avoid unnecessary needle piercing or blood transfusion; careful screening of potential blood donors; hepatitis B vaccine for individuals at risk; hepatitis B immune globulin for prophylaxis after exposure
Non-A, Non-B	Specific viruses unknown	Contaminated water; fecal–oral route possible	14–64 d	Probably similar to hepatitis A	Blood/body fluid precautions	Same as hepatitis A
Herpes simplex	Herpesvirus (herpes simplex virus): Type I ("cold sores"), Type II (genital herpes)	Direct contact (Type I), sexual intercourse (Type II)	2–12 d	Up to 7 wk (Type I), 4–7 d (Type II)	Contact isolation	Avoid contact with infected person; cesarean section delivery of Type II infected pregnant woman
Histoplasmosis	Fungus: *Histoplasma capsulatum*	Inhalation of spores in caves inhabited by bats and in soil nourished by dried bird droppings	5–18 d	Not transmitted person to person	None	Minimize exposure to dust or dried soil in contaminated environments
Hookworm	Helminth: *Ancylostoma duodenale* (hookworm: Old-World type); *Necator americanus* (hookworm: tropical type)	Skin, usually feet; possibly mouth (larva)	Unknown; could be a few weeks to many months	Not transmitted person to person; untreated infected person could contaminate soil	None	Wear shoes while walking in soil; use sanitary disposal systems
Infectious mononucleosis	Epstein–Barr virus (herpesvirus)	Oral–pharyngeal direct contact via saliva; possibly parenteral (transfusions, syringes, etc)	4–6 wk	Unknown; may persist for a year as a latent infection	None	None known

(Continued)

Table 9–3, *(continued)*
Summary of Epidemiology and Prevention of Selected Infectious Diseases in Adults

Disease	Causative Agent	Mode of Transmission	Incubation Period	Communicable Period	Isolation Precautions	Prevention
Influenza	Myxovirus: Myxovirus influenzae hominis types A, B, and C; types A and B include variants or subgroups; type A subgroups cause the following influenzas: Asian, Hong Kong, Russian, swine, Texas, Victoria, among others	Direct or indirect contact with contaminated respiratory droplets	Variable: 18–36 h the most common	Probably 3 d from onset of symptoms	Contact isolation	Limit smoking and provide environmental humidity for susceptible persons during flu season; specific vaccines available
Legionnaires' disease (legionellosis)	Bacteria: *Legionella pneumophila*	Aerosols from contaminated air-conditioning cooling tower water; contaminated hot and cold water systems; soil and water from creeks and ponds	2–10 d	Not transmitted person to person	None	Disinfection of environmental air system
Leprosy (Hansen's disease)	Bacteria: *Mycobacterium leprae*	Transfer of exudates from lesions through breaks in skin or mucous membranes	Variable but usually 3–5 yr; may be 1½–10 yr	Unknown; infectiousness usually lost with regular treatment	Contact isolation	Early detection of infectious cases; protection of contacts not necessary
Lymphogranuloma venereum	Chlamydia: *Chlamydia trachomatis*	Direct contact, especially sexual contact	3–12 d; may be as long as 30 d	While lesions are active (from weeks to years)	None	Use of condoms; treatment of infected person; prophylactic treatment of contacts
Malaria	Protozoa: *Plasmodium vivax, P. falciparum, P. ovale, P. malariae*	Bite of infected female Anopheles mosquito; infected blood transfusions; contaminated needles and syringes	12–30 d, depending on specific organism; *P. vivax, P. falciparum,* and *P. ovale* 12–14 d and *P. malariae* 30 d	3–14 d after symptoms appear; may last for years, depending on organism and treatment; mosquito remains infective for life	Blood/body fluid precautions	Prophylactic therapy for travelers to endemic areas; mosquito control; screening of blood donors; prompt and effective treatment of cases
Meningococcal meningitis	Bacteria: *Neisseria meningitidis*	Contact with a healthy carrier or infected person via respiratory tract; droplet	2–10 d (usually 3–4 d)	As long as organism present in discharges from nose and mouth	Respiratory isolation	Vaccine for population at high risk

Disease	Causative Agent	Mode of Transmission	Incubation Period	Communicable Period	Isolation Precautions	Prevention
Plague	Bacteria: *Yersinia pestis*	Bite of infected flea from rats and other rodents; airborne droplets of persons with pneumonic form of the disease (bacteria carried by blood to lungs)	2–6 d	As long as organism present; fleas remain infective for months	Strict isolation	Flea and rat control; vaccination for high-risk persons and travelers to endemic areas
Pneumococcal pneumonia	Bacteria: *Streptococcus pneumoniae*	Healthy carriers; droplet spread; direct oral contact; indirect contact with respiratory discharges; primarily a disease following viral respiratory infection or other stress	Variable; believed to be 1–3 d	As long as organism present	None; if organisms are antibiotic resistant, then contact isolation	Vaccine available for those at high risk
Poliomyelitis	Poliovirus, an enterovirus; serotypes include 1, 2, and 3	Direct contact: contaminated saliva, vomitus, and feces	3–35 d but usually 7–14 d	Uncertain; virus persists in pharynx for at least 1 wk and in feces for a minimum of 3–6 wk or more	Enteric precautions	Immunization
Rabies	Rabies virus (a rhabdovirus)	Bite of a rabid animal; sometimes virus is transmitted by saliva or a break in the skin	10 d to 1 yr (usually 2–8 wk)	Not usually transmitted person to person	Contact isolation	Vaccination of domestic animals; vaccine for persons at risk or those who have been exposed
Rocky Mountain spotted fever	Rickettsia: *Rickettsia rickettsii*	Bite of infected wood or dog tick (4–6 h of attachment required)	3–12 d	Not transmitted person to person; tick remains infective for life	None	Wear protective clothing in tick-infested areas; check body and clothing for ticks; remove ticks carefully and promptly; inspect dogs for ticks
Shigellosis (bacillary dysentery)	Bacteria: *Shigella* genus: *S. dysenteriae, S. flexneri, S. boydii, S. sonnei*	Direct or indirect contact with feces of infected individual; ingestion of contaminated water, milk, and food	24–48 h but may be as long as 7 d	Until stool cultures are negative; usually 1–4 wk but may be as long as 1 yr	Enteric precautions	Proper handwashing and personal hygiene; treatment of water supply; infected persons should not be food handlers
Smallpox* (variola)	Variola virus	Direct contact with infected person, crustations of lesions, or contaminated articles; may be airborne	7–14 d	1–2 d before rash until shedding of crusts (usually 3–4 wk); most communicable during first week	Strict isolation until all scabs have separated	Vaccination may be required for international travel or exposure to infected person; routine vaccination no longer justified

(Continued)

Table 9–3, *(continued)*
Summary of Epidemiology and Prevention of Selected Infectious Diseases in Adults

Disease	Causative Agent	Mode of Transmission	Incubation Period	Communicable Period	Isolation Precautions	Prevention
Syphilis	Bacteria: *Treponema pallidum*	Sexually, parenterally, transplacentally (after fifth month); by direct contact with body fluids, chancre, or secretions of individuals during the infectious primary and secondary stages	10–90 d (usually 3–4 wk)	Variable; extremely infectious during primary and secondary stages; usually not infectious about 2 yr after start of latent stage; noncontagious during tertiary stage	Blood/body fluid precautions in primary and secondary stages (in hospitals)	Avoid sexual contact with infected person; use condom; treatment of infected person; prophylactic treatment of contacts
Tetanus	Bacteria: *Clostridium tetani*	Skin penetration (usually via puncture) of clostridium endospores, usually from soil contaminated with animal fecal wastes	3–21 d	Not transmitted person to person	None	Thorough wound cleansing and debridement; immunization; immune globulin to exposed nonimmunized persons
Toxoplasmosis	Protozoa: *Toxoplasma gondii*	Ingestion of oocysts of the organism, which are found in contaminated meat and feces of many birds and animals, especially cats; inhalation; transfusions; transplacental	Usually 10–23 d but may be months	Not transmitted person to person except in utero	None	Avoid eating undercooked foods; avoid inhaling dried feces of cats while cleaning litter box; pregnant women should not clean litter box
Trichinosis	Helminth: *Trichinella spiralis*	Ingesting cysts in insufficiently cooked contaminated pork	10–14 d; can be as long as 45 d	Not transmitted person to person	None	Cook all pork and pork products thoroughly; garbage for hogs should be cooked; eat only inspected meat
Tuberculosis	Bacteria: *Mycobacterium tuberculosis* (acid-fast bacillus)	Droplet or sputum of infected human; infected unpasteurized dairy products; dust containing organism; reinfection can occur endogenously years after the primary infection by release of viable bacilli from old tuberculous Ghon's lesions	4–12 wk	While sputum, secretions, and urine contain causative organism	AFB isolation	BCG immunization in endemic areas; avoid unpasteurized dairy products; prophylactic treatment for close contacts

Disease	Causative Agent	Mode of Transmission	Incubation Period	Communicable Period	Isolation Precautions	Prevention
Tularemia	Bacteria: *Francisella tularensis*	Handling infected animals (ground squirrels, rabbits); bites of infected deer flies, ticks, or lice; ingestion of contaminated water or undercooked meats; droplet spread has occurred in laboratory workers	2–7 d	Not directly transmitted person to person	Drainage/secretion precautions for open lesions	Avoid contact with infected animals; cook meats thoroughly; vaccine available for high-risk laboratory workers
Typhoid fever	Bacteria: *Salmonella typhi*	Water or food, usually raw fruits and vegetables, shellfish, and milk contaminated by urine and feces of infected individuals or carriers	Usually 5–14 d; may be up to 21 d	Until three consecutive negative cultures of feces taken at least 24 h apart; may be as long as 3 mo or for life if the individual becomes a chronic carrier	Enteric precautions	Vaccination for travelers to endemic areas and those with intimate exposure to the infected person; good personal hygiene; thorough washing and cooking of foods; proper sewage disposal; decontamination of water sources; infected person or carrier should not handle food; pasteurization of milk
Typhus	Rickettsia: epidemic typhus: *Rickettsia prowazekii;* murine typhus: *Rickettsia typhi*	Bites of infected fleas or lice	1–2 wk	While infested	Not required after delousing	Sanitary living conditions; rat control; vaccine for travelers to endemic areas

*Although smallpox has been eradicated from the world, the occurrence of even a single case in a non immune population could result in a major disaster. Therefore, all health professionals should be familiar with it.

combat the organisms. On the other hand, bacteremia in hospitalized clients can be a serious problem. The organisms are often more virulent, and the client's defenses to combat the invasion are often reduced. The nurse should be alert for symptoms such as fever, tachycardia, hypotension, tachypnea, and confusion. Specific diagnosis is by positive blood cultures. Cultures are also collected from possible sites of infection, such as the urinary tract, lungs, abdomen, or skin. Antibiotics and antipyretics may be prescribed.

Nursing actions include monitoring the client for response to the bacteremia. Vital signs should be checked frequently. Antibiotics should be administered only after blood cultures are collected, because they can disguise or destroy the organism. Urine output and mental status should also be monitored.

Septic Shock

Approximately 40% of clients with bacteremia develop septic shock or septicemia (Kochar, 1983), sometimes called "blood poisoning" by the public. In septicemia, the organisms in the blood multiply rapidly. Although many organisms can cause septic shock, gram-negative bacilli are the most common cause. The endotoxin these bacteria produce increases capillary permeability. Circulation of endotoxin stimulates complement activation and may cause disseminated intravascular coagulation (DIC), a derangement in the clotting mechanism. DIC is discussed in Chapter 23.

Symptoms of gram-negative septic shock are fever, hypotension, and oliguria. Peripheral vascular resistance is usually decreased, so the extremities are warm. Clients are confused because of reduced blood flow to the brain, and acid–base imbalances often occur.

A specific diagnosis is made from cultures collected from blood, urine, and possible infected sites. Clients are generally cared for in an intensive care unit because they are physiologically unstable. These clients often require respiratory assistance, parenteral antibiotics, blood products, vasoactive drugs, and acid–base imbalance correction. Nurses monitor the client's response to therapy by frequently checking vital signs and urinary output. Cardiac, respiratory, and mental status must be closely observed. Even with appropriate therapy, the mortality for septic shock is 50% (Kochar, 1983).

Staphylococcal Infection

Of the several *Staphylococcus* organisms, *S. aureus* is the most common cause of infections, ranging from mild to severe. *Staphylococcus epidermidis,* a normal resident of the skin, is usually not pathogenic, but it may cause disease under certain circumstances. The organisms are spread by direct contact. Many persons, including hospital personnel and clients, carry *S. aureus* in the nares, axilla, and rectum.

Frequent sites of staphylococcal infections are furuncles, carbuncles, chalazia, cellulitis, and wounds. Staphylococcal pneumonia is most common in clients with influenza or chronic bronchopulmonary disease and in newborns; it often ends in abscess formation or empyema. *S. aureus* may cause osteomyelitis and septic arthritis, particularly in children. Toxin or proteases from certain strains of *S. aureus* and *S. epidermidis* are leading causes of bacterial endocarditis. Intravenous drug users and persons with prosthetic heart valves are at highest risk for staphylococcal endocarditis. Narcotic users have an increased incidence of *S. aureus* colonization on the skin; prosthetic valve clients are vulnerable to staphylococcal contamination of the implant site. Staphylococcal food poisoning is caused, not by the organism itself, but by protein toxins produced during the growth of *S. aureus* in food. Food poisoning is discussed later.

Staphylococcal infections are usually treated with penicillinase-resistant penicillins. Many strains are resistant to penicillin G, ampicillin, carbenicillin, streptomycin, and the tetracyclines. Seriously ill clients may require parenteral treatment. Food poisoning usually does not require antibiotic treatment.

Clients with staphylococcal infections are often placed in contact isolation. Hospital personnel with staphylococcal infections such as boils should not be allowed to care for clients until personnel have begun antibiotic treatment.

Streptococcal Infection

Among the *Streptococcus* organisms, group A *Streptococcus* is responsible for many diseases, including pharyngitis, scarlet fever, nephritis, rheumatic fever, impetigo, and puerperal infection. Streptococci are a major cause of subacute bacterial endocarditis, urinary tract infections, neonatal sepsis, and meningitis.

Infections by group A streptococci and *S. viridans* are treated with penicillin. Enterococcal species, which may be resistant to penicillin, are also treated with an aminoglycoside. Symptomatic treatments are also prescribed.

Because streptococcal infections are spread by personal contact, infected clients should be placed in contact isolation until they have received antibiotic treatment and are deemed noninfectious. Assess for complications such as otitis media, nephritis, abscesses, arthritis, pneumonia, and septicemia.

With respiratory infections, the client's room should have good ventilation and high humidity to prevent drying of the mucous membranes of the upper respiratory tract. The nose and throat should be kept clean to ease breathing and reduce the risk of sinus infections. Vital signs and urinary output should be assessed frequently.

Bacterial Food Poisoning

Food poisoning may be caused by *Staphylococcus, Salmonella, Shigella,* and many other less common agents. Some organisms, such as *Staphylococcus,* cause illness by producing **enterotoxins,** exotoxins that impair intestinal absorption and provoke secretion of electrolytes and water. In contrast, some *Salmonella* and *Shigella* species invade the mucosa of the small bowel or colon, producing microscopic ulceration, bleeding, and secretion of electrolytes and water.

Staphylococcal food poisoning often begins with a food preparer who is a carrier; the organism is transferred to the food, where the enterotoxin is produced. Animals are the reservoir for *Salmonella,* and the organisms are transmitted through animal-derived food and feces. Common food reservoirs are meat, poultry, eggs and egg products, and unpasteurized milk and dairy products. Outbreaks have also been associated with household pets such as turtles. *Shigella* organisms are found in infected human feces. The organism is spread from person to person by the fecal–oral route or indirectly through food, such as shrimp, milk, eggs, and cheese.

Staphylococcal food poisoning is an acute gastroenteritis typically occurring suddenly in a group of people who have eaten in the same place, such as at a picnic or wedding reception. The incubation period is from 1 to 6 hours, with diarrhea lasting from 8 to 24 hours. Symptoms include nausea with explosive vomiting, abdominal cramps, diarrhea, and sweating and chills; usually, there is no fever. With salmonella gastroenteritis, there are chills and fever, nausea and vomiting, abdominal pain, and diarrhea, which may be bloody. The incubation period is 8 to 72 hours, with diarrhea for 5 to 7 days.

Symptoms of shigellosis are similar to those for other types of food poisoning: fever, abdominal cramps, nausea and vomiting, and watery diarrhea, which may contain blood and mucus. Symptoms appear in 1 to 3 days, with diarrhea lasting for 3 to 7 days. Some cases of "tourist diarrhea" may actually be milder forms of shigellosis.

Usually, gastroenteritis from food poisoning resolves by itself, and treatment is symptomatic. Most persons recover without complications, although the fluid loss from vomiting and diarrhea may be dangerous for infants and children, the elderly, and debilitated clients.

Strict hand-washing procedures and proper handling of food (see the food handling section later in this chapter) are the keys to reducing transmission. Nurses can contribute to disease control by educating their clients about hand-washing and the proper preparation and handling of foods. For specific nursing measures for clients with infectious gastroenteritis, see Chapter 38.

Botulism

Botulism is a particularly severe type of food poisoning that may lead to death. The disease is usually contracted from home-canned foods with a high pH (low-acid foods such as beans and corn), which have been inadequately sterilized. These foods provide an anaerobic condition for the growth of the spore-forming organism, *Clostridium botulinum.* The toxin produced by this bacterium is highly lethal; 1 mg is enough to kill 1 million guinea pigs. Death can occur from simply tasting, not swallowing, a contaminated food. Cases involving commercially prepared foods are rare.

Wound and infant botulism are other forms of the disease. In wound botulism, the organism grows in infected tissue. Infant botulism occurs when ingested spores colonize in the gastrointestinal tract. One possible cause is honey, which may contain *C. botulinum* spores; honey should not be given to infants under 1 year. Adults do not acquire botulism from honey.

Food-borne botulism usually occurs 18 to 36 hours after ingesting the contaminated food, although onset varies from 4 hours to 8 days. Initial symptoms are nausea, vomiting, dry mouth, dilated pupils, diplopia, and dysphagia. Neurologic symptoms appear later, with a bilateral symmetrical descending paralysis. With wound botulism, there are no GI symptoms, but neurologic symptoms are the same as with the food-borne variety. Infant botulism is marked by constipation and neuromuscular paralysis.

Management of respiratory failure is the first priority. The disease progresses rapidly, so those who are suspected to have botulism should be hospitalized in case a tracheotomy and mechanical ventilation are required. Antitoxin should be given as soon as botulism has been diagnosed before neurologic impairment occurs because it cannot reverse neurologic impairment. Antitoxin is available through the CDC.

Because foods and materials contaminated with *C. botulinum* are highly toxic, they require special handling. Specimen-handling instructions are available from the CDC.

Public education is the major preventive measure. For more information on prevention, see the discussion of food handling in the section on prevention.

Tetanus

Tetanus is caused by *Clostridium tetani,* an anaerobic spore-forming organism with reservoirs in the soil and animal feces. The spores of the bacteria usually enter the body through deep wounds or foreign bodies. A puncture wound from an object lying in the dirt provides a perfect avenue for infection. However, *C. tetani* may also enter the body through what appear to be relatively minor wounds such as abrasions or insect stings or through dental surgery. Intravenous drug users are also vulnerable, as are those with surgical and burn wounds. The organism produces a neurotoxin, which causes generalized muscle spasms followed by contraction of the muscles of the jaw. This explains the popular term, "lockjaw." Eventually, opisthotonos, abdominal rigidity, and other symptoms of increased sympathetic nervous system activity occur. Tetanus is usually severe and is difficult to treat, even for experts. The mortality rate is 50%, but when recovery occurs, it is complete (Kochar, 1983).

Wounds should be cleaned and debrided as soon as

possible because dirt and necrotic tissue provide a medium for growth of *C. tetani*. Depending on the immunization status and the nature of the wound, prophylaxis may be administered. Most persons receive tetanus toxoid immunization during the DPT (diphtheria, pertussis, tetanus) series of immunizations given in childhood; boosters are given every 5 to 10 years. With a serious wound, immunity should be renewed with a booster dose of tetanus toxoid. Tetanus toxoid is not effective after an injury, however, if the person has not been immunized. When immunization is inadequate or uncertain, tetanus immune globulin is an alternative that provides temporary immunity lasting for about 1 month.

Clients with tetanus are usually treated in intensive care units. Treatment includes supportive care as well as antitoxins and sedative–relaxant drugs for seizures or convulsions. Mechanical ventilation may be needed. Aseptic technique should be used when disposing of drainage and respiratory fluids.

Although tetanus is difficult to treat, it can be prevented effectively with tetanus toxoid. Immunization is more effective than prophylaxis at the time of injury.

Gas Gangrene

Gas gangrene can be caused by several species of *Clostridium*, but *Clostridium perfringens* is the most common. The organisms are introduced into traumatic and surgical wounds from the soil or from the person's own intestinal or vaginal flora. Devitalized or necrotic tissues that have lost their blood supply provide the perfect conditions for the growth of the anaerobic organisms.

As the organisms multiply, they ferment carbohydrates in the tissues and actually produce gases (carbon dioxide and hydrogen) that cause the tissue to swell. Combined with the exotoxins and enzymes produced by these microorganisms, these conditions cause further necrosis and spread of the infection. Severe toxemia and death result without immediate and aggressive treatment.

Treatment includes penicillin and aggressive surgery, such as debridement and amputation. Hyperbaric oxygen therapy is sometimes used, especially for gas gangrene in the abdominal cavity, although experts disagree about its effectiveness. Therapy is administered in a hyperbaric chamber that provides an oxygen-rich atmosphere under pressure. Immediate and thorough cleansing of all serious wounds along with prophylactic antibiotic therapy are the best preventive measures.

Viral Diseases

Unlike living cells that contain both nucleic acids DNA and RNA, viruses contain a core of only one (never both) surrounded by a protein coat and sometimes by an additional lipid membrane, called an envelope. Because viruses contain only one nucleic acid, they are unable to carry out chemical reactions or to reproduce unless within living cells. In other words, viruses are inert when outside living cells. For this reason, it is unclear whether viruses are living microorganisms whose essential characteristics differ fundamentally from other living microorganisms, or whether viruses are exceptionally complex nonliving chemicals.

When viruses invade the body, they attach to receptor sites on a host cell surface. The virus and host cell fuse, allowing the virus to penetrate the host cell. Viruses can also be taken into host cells by phagocytosis. Once inside the cell, viruses replicate either in the cytoplasm or the nucleus; mature viruses escape through the cell wall and invade other cells.

Among the wide variety of infections caused by viruses are herpes simplex and zoster, hepatitis, influenza, mononucleosis, and rabies. Only influenza and rabies will be discussed in this chapter. Complete information about the other viral diseases that affect adults is found in other chapters. For information on viral infections during childhood, consult a pediatric nursing textbook.

Influenza

Influenza, or "the flu," is a viral infection as well known as the common cold. Epidemics of influenza spread rapidly through large geographic areas almost annually and have been pandemic at various times. The pandemic of 1918–1919 caused 20 million deaths, many of them from secondary bacterial infections rather than the viral disease itself. One of these bacteria was mistakenly determined to cause influenza and named *Hemophilus influenzae* to link it with the disease. It is now known that *H. influenzae* was one of several secondary invaders responsible for many of the deaths but was not a cause of the disease. (*H. influenzae* causes bacterial meningitis and acute epiglottitis.)

The symptoms of influenza include fever, chills, headache, and general muscular aches, followed by coldlike symptoms after the fever subsides. If not complicated by a secondary bacterial infection, influenza runs its course in a few days. Treating the symptoms will help clients feel more comfortable. For secondary bacterial infections, antibiotic treatment is appropriate. Because of the availability of antibiotic treatment today, a pandemic such as the one of 1918–1919 is unlikely to have such a high mortality rate. Amantadine (Symmetrel), an antiviral drug, can reduce the severity of the symptoms of influenza caused by the Influenza A virus if treatment is begun immediately. Amantadine has also been used as a prophylactic measure to reduce the rate of Influenza A infection and illness. It is not effective against the Influenza B virus.

Vaccines consisting of killed viruses are available against influenza. Vaccinations are administered in the fall before the winter flu season and are used primarily for the elderly and other high-risk individuals. Immunity is effective in about 10 days and lasts 3 to 6 months; thus, yearly immunization is required. Influenza vaccines are not completely effective for several reasons. First, in years when a new strain or subtype appears, vaccine cannot be produced fast enough to be available. Minor antigen changes occur every 2 to 4 years, and there is a major shift about every 10 years. Different strains of the Influenza A and B viruses (and the less common C virus) are often named for the location in which they are first identified (eg, Hong Kong flu, Russian flu). Also, not everyone develops immunity after vaccination, and some persons will not seek out or accept immunization.

Local skin reactions can occur with vaccination. Persons allergic to egg or egg products may develop anaphylactic reactions. A rare complication of the swine influenza vaccine administered during the swine influenza vaccine program in 1976 was Guillain–Barré syndrome, an acute, rapidly progressive form of polyneuropathy. Subsequent influenza vaccines have not been associated with increased risk of this disorder.

Rabies

Rabies (sometimes called hydrophobia), a viral disease transmitted through saliva, is virtually 100% fatal if untreated. The few who do survive experience severe neurologic damage. Fortunately, human rabies is rare in the United States with only one to four cases per year (Tortora, Funke, & Case, 1986). The disease is usually transmitted through an animal bite. The most common animal reservoirs in this country are wild animals including skunks, bats, foxes, and raccoons. Domestic dogs are less often sources of the disease because of canine rabies vaccination. Rabbits and rodents are rarely infected with rabies.

Infection occurs when the rabies virus comes in contact with mucous membranes or the dermal layer of the skin, almost always through a penetrating bite. The virus can also enter through minute abrasions in the skin. Cave explorers have also contracted rabies by inhaling aerosols of the virus in bat caves, as have laboratory workers exposed to these aerosols during laboratory accidents.

Rabies symptoms usually appear 18 to 60 days after exposure although there have been instances up to a year or more before the onset of symptoms. Among the early symptoms are fever, headaches, anorexia, nausea, and paresthesias in the area of the bite. Over the next 2 weeks, neurologic symptoms progress to coma. One characteristic symptom is painful pharyngeal spasms when attempting to swallow liquid or sometimes merely at the sight or thought of water (the basis for the term *hydrophobia,* fear of water). Finally, flaccid paralysis develops, and death follows.

As soon as possible after the bite, the wound should be cleaned thoroughly with soap and water. This is a highly effective first aid measure. Vaccinated domestic animals should be observed for rabies symptoms for 10 days; this may be a legal requirement. If an unvaccinated domestic animal develops rabies symptoms, it should be captured and examined for the presence of rabies antigens in the cornea, skin, saliva, or brain (through flourescent antibody screening). Wild animals should be killed at once and the brain examined for the presence of rabies antigens or the rabies virus in brain smears. If the laboratory test is negative, the client does not require prophylaxis.

The client is given rabies prophylaxis if the animal is rabid, suspected to be rabid, or has escaped before rabidity has been determined. Postexposure treatment begins with passive immunization with human rabies immune globulin (HRIG) followed by active immunization with five doses of human diploid cell vaccine (HDCV). Reactions with HDCV are less frequent than with the former duck embryo vaccine, which required a series of 23 painful subcutaneous injections. Because the series of immunizations must continue, any reactions are treated symptomatically.

Animal vaccination is the best method of rabies control. Nurses can assist in educating the community about the importance of having pets vaccinated. A rigid quarantine program has kept islands such as Australia, New Zealand, and the Hawaiian chain free of the disease.

Rickettsial Diseases

Rickettsia organisms are smaller than bacteria and many viruses. Like viruses, they can reproduce only within a living cell. However, they are classified as bacteria because they more closely resemble bacteria in their structure and biochemistry. They are nonmotile and often parasites of insects. The microbes usually invade by an insect bite, producing a rash and a generalized inflammatory and antibody response. Examples of rickettsial diseases are Rocky Mountain spotted fever, Q fever, and typhus.

Rocky Mountain Spotted Fever

Despite its name, Rocky Mountain spotted fever is most common in the southeastern United States and Appalachia. Its name is derived from the fact that it was first identified in the Rocky Mountain area. The disease is caused by *Rickettsia rickettsii,* a parasite of ticks, and usually spreads to humans by tick bites. Most cases occur in children, and the disease is most common in spring and summer.

The symptoms appear suddenly about 7 days after the bite by a dog tick or wood tick. Initial symptoms are severe headache, high fever, chills, prostration, and muscular pain. About 4 days after exposure, a rash appears on the palms and soles, spreading to the face and neck, buttocks, and trunk. DIC may occur. The mortality rate is 5% to 10%.

Antibiotic therapy with tetracycline and chloramphenicol is effective in the early stages of the disease. Supportive care is required for vasculitis, the distinguishing pathologic characteristic of Rocky Mountain spotted fever.

The client needs management for inadequate blood volume, circulatory collapse, fluid and electrolyte imbalance, and renal insufficiency. Hematologic values must be monitored for signs of DIC.

No vaccine is commercially available, but research is continuing. The best preventive measure is to prevent ticks from attaching to the skin or removing them promptly. Persons frequenting tick-infested areas should use repellent, dress in clothes that inhibit tick attachment (eg, boots and coveralls), and inspect their bodies (and the bodies of domestic animals) daily, especially hairy areas, for ticks. Ticks usually do not transmit infection until they have been feeding for at least several hours.

An attached tick can be removed with gentle traction of a forceps on the mouth parts; if possible, wear a gown and gloves for protection. Try not to crush the tick, because this can contaminate the bite. Wash the bite thoroughly with soap and water. Take care when removing an engorged tick from an animal by hand, because the infection can be transmitted into small abrasions on the skin.

Protozoal Diseases

Protozoa are single-celled animals that can move about independently. They are equipped with structures enabling them to feed, breathe, excrete waste, and attach themselves to other objects. Protozoal infections are not limited to third world countries; they also occur in the United States. Persons who have traveled to other countries and those who have emigrated from countries with endemic protozoal infections may bring the diseases to the United States.

Common examples of protozoal diseases are malaria and toxoplasmosis, which are discussed in this section. *Pneumocystis carinii,* which causes an often fatal pneumonia in compromised hosts and may be endemic in hospitals and institutions (Benenson, 1985), is a protozoan.

Malaria

Caused by four protozoans classified as *Plasmodium,* malaria causes more disability and economic strain worldwide than any other parasitic disease. Carried by mosquitoes, malaria occurs mainly in the tropics, although it has been transmitted by blood transfusions and unsterilized syringes. The disease affects 200 million people throughout the world. In Africa, it is estimated that one-fourth of adults have malaria at one time or another. Malaria remains a serious problem in tropical Asia, Africa, and Central and South America. Malaria is rare in the United States, but occasional small epidemics have been caused by returning military personnel; travelers and emigrants may also bring the disease into the country.

Four types of the *Plasmodium* organism *(P. vivax, P. falciparum, P. malariae,* and *P. ovale)* cause malaria, with varying patterns. Most cases (95%) are caused by *P. falciparum* and *P. vivax.* Depending on the type of malaria, there may be an abrupt onset or a prodromal phase with symptoms including intermittent fever, malaise, headache, myalgia, and chills. The disease is characterized by episodes of shaking chills with fever. Untreated vivax malaria subsides spontaneously in 10 to 30 days but may recur; untreated falciparum malaria has a high mortality rate.

Treatment depends on diagnosis of the *Plasmodium* species. Acute attacks for all except drug-resistant *P. falciparum* are treated with chloroquine. The resistant strains of *P. falciparum* are treated with a combination of quinine, pyrimethamine, and a sulfonamide. For *P. falciparum,* treatment must be prompt and immediate, because the disease progresses rapidly and may lead to coma and death.

Drug treatment for the acute attack will cure the disease. Some strains, particularly those in Southeast Asia and Latin America, are also resistant to pyrimethamine and sulfonamides. In this case, treatment is with quinine sulfate and a tetracycline.

Clients may require oxygen for anemia and tissue hypoxia. Fluid status should be monitored. Other nursing care centers on control of fever, myalgia, and headache. Precautions should be used in disposing of blood and body fluids.

The best prevention in high-risk areas is destroying mosquito breeding places and avoiding exposure to mosquito bites with repellent, screens, and mosquito nets. Drug prophylaxis is used but may be unreliable in areas of Southeast Asia and Latin America because of resistant strains. For nonresistant strains, prophylaxis is with chloroquine phosphate. For resistant strains, pyrimethamine and sulfadoxine are also taken; there is no reliable protection against strains also resistant to these drugs. The drugs are taken 2 weeks before arrival in the area and for 6 weeks after leaving.

Toxoplasmosis

Toxoplasmosis is an insidious disease because infected adults are often asymptomatic. A pregnant woman can transmit the disease through the placenta to the fetus. The result may be abortion, stillbirth, or the birth of a child with congenital disease, which can be severe.

Toxoplasma gondii, the protozoan responsible for the disease, is a parasite of warm-blooded animals. Adults usually acquire the infection by eating raw or undercooked meat containing cysts or by being exposed to cat feces with cysts, often while cleaning a litter box. A large number of cats in urban areas have been shown to be infected with the organism, although they apparently are not ill.

Adults with symptoms usually have lymphadenopathy, fever, and malaise.

Mild infections usually do not require treatment. Newborns, pregnant women, and immunosuppressed clients receive drug therapy with pyrimethamine in combination with trisulfapyrimidines or sulfadiazine.

Nurses can assist in educating the public, particularly pregnant women and immunocompromised clients, about the dangers of toxoplasmosis. These persons should:

- Avoid contact with any area that might have cat feces, such as litter boxes and sand boxes.
- Wash all fruits and vegetables before eating.
- Cook meat to at least 150°F (66°C) and not eat raw meat.
- Wash hands after handling raw meat.

Helminthic Diseases

Three major types of helminths (worms) invade the human intestines: nematodes (roundworms), cestodes (tapeworms), and trematodes (flukes). The life cycle of parasitic helminths is complex and often involves a succession of hosts such as humans, domestic animals, fish, and snails. Enterobiasis, or infestation by pinworms *(Enterobius vermicularis),* which causes perianal itching, is the most common worm infection in the United States. It occurs principally in children. Consult a pediatric nursing textbook for more information on this condition. A disease caused by nematodes—trichinosis—is discussed in this chapter.

Trichinosis

Trichinosis (trichinellosis) is caused by ingesting encysted larvae of the nematode *Trichinella spiralis,* usually in pork. The larval cysts are imbedded in pork muscle; if pork is undercooked, the cysts may remain intact. When the meat is eaten, gastric juices digest the cyst wall, and the larvae burrow into the intestinal mucosa, where they multiply. The new larvae are carried into the bloodstream and disseminated throughout the body, but only those imbedding skeletal muscle survive. There they mature, encyst, and eventually calcify; the organisms may live for several years.

Many of those infected are asymptomatic. There may be initial symptoms of gastrointestinal distress and fever, or the disease may first appear as edema of the upper eyelids on about the eleventh day after infection. Other ocular symptoms including hemorrhage, pain, and photophobia may follow. Shortly thereafter, systemic symptoms appear, including muscle pain, chills, fever, weakness, sweating, urticaria, and eosinophilia. Most likely to be involved are muscles of the diaphragm and tongue as well as the pectoral, eye, and intercostal muscles. The inflammatory reaction to the disseminated larvae may produce a variety of other systemic symptoms. Within about 3 months, most symptoms subside, although the client may feel weak for months.

Symptomatic and supportive care focuses on relief of pain and fever as well as nutrition and fluid replacement. Corticosteroids may be given. Thiabendazole is effective in destroying organisms, but its use is controversial because of possible hypersensitivity response.

Public education is important in prevention. Pork and pork products should always be thoroughly cooked until no longer pink in the center. Less obviously, ground beef may be contaminated by a meat grinder that was not cleaned after grinding pork. Thus, eating raw hamburger meat is to be avoided.

SECTION III

Nursing Measures in Infectious Disease

Since Florence Nightingale outlined her principles and practices of "fever nursing" in 1863, nursing interventions in infection have traditionally been directed toward the care of the already infected client. Since Nightingale's day, scientific discoveries have radically changed the principles and practices of caring for the already infected client.

Contemporary health care often involves exposing uninfected clients to potentially infective agents or altering the normal flora. Thus, prevention of infection and protection of the immunocompromised client are also significant nursing responsibilities. Keep these important principles in mind when planning care for *all clients:*

- Health care personnel and the health care environment harbor many organisms—normal flora and potentially pathogenic organisms.
- All secretions and tissues (of clients, their families, and health care personnel) contain organisms that are potentially harmful to others.
- Many clients are compromised hosts and are therefore at greater risk from these organisms.
- *The single most important preventive strategy is adequate handwashing.*
- Knowledge of the methods of transmission of microorganisms is the basis for developing strategies to protect clients from infection.

This section discusses nursing measures for the prevention of infection as well as the treatment of infection. The nursing measures for specific infectious diseases can be found in the specific disorders chapters in the units on body systems.

Public Education and Prevention

Wherever they work, nurses can educate people about disease prevention and promote immunization. In addition, nurses are often the first to see signs of infection. By recognizing infection, nurses can refer clients for medical care leading to early arrest of the disease; they can also take measures to prevent its spread. Nurses should be well informed about these subjects so they can counsel clients as well as friends and neighbors about preventive measures.

Immunization

Immunization with a vaccine induces a state of immunity in a host. Most vaccines consist of attenuated (living but weakened) organisms or killed organisms. Many diseases, such as poliomyelitis, tetanus, diphtheria, pertussis, measles, and rubella, can be prevented by immunization. The immunologic agents currently available for the prevention and treatment of infectious disease are discussed in pharmacology texts.

Home Health Care

Nurses are in a position to teach the public about the advantages of immunization and to encourage participation in immunization programs. The nurse should explain:

- What disease the immunization is for
- Why immunization is recommended
- When booster doses are needed
- The relative safety and advantages of immunization

Clients should also be instructed to keep up-to-date vaccination records, which may be required when entering school or applying for a passport. Public health clinics often provide immunizations at little or no cost.

International travel may also require immunization. The Bureau of Epidemiology of the CDC distributes a weekly "blue sheet" to health departments, physicians, and public and private health agencies that lists countries infected with diseases requiring quarantine. A toll-free hot line is available to provide the traveler with immediate health information. (Both are listed in the resources section at the end of this chapter.) Travelers arriving from these countries may be required to provide evidence of vaccination. If immunizations are necessary, travelers should allow enough time for a full course of treatment and for discomfort or reactions to subside.

Assess clients before immunization because there are contraindications to vaccination as well as contraindications to the use of certain substances. Before using any immunologic product, read the package insert carefully for indications, precautions, and side effects. Vaccines prepared in chicken or duck embryos may cause an allergic reaction in clients allergic to eggs. Hypersensitivity to horse serum can cause serum sickness. Testing for hypersensitivity should precede immunization whenever possible.

Attentuated virus vaccines should not be given to clients with altered immune status because viral replication after administration might be unchecked. Because trivalent oral poliovirus vaccine (TOPV) viruses are excreted by an immunized person, clients living with an immunocompromised person should not receive TOPV. Attenuated virus vaccines also should not be given to a client who has a cold or other infection because the inflammatory reaction may be greater than usual. Use of these vaccines is also avoided in pregnant women because of the theoretical risk to the fetus. Attenuated virus vaccines should not be given at the same time as passive immunization because passively acquired antibodies can interfere with the response to the live vaccine. All vaccines should be withheld from clients with acute severe febrile illness until the illness is over.

Before leaving the clinic, the client or family members should be instructed about the expected effects of the inoculation. They should be told to contact the physician or go to an emergency room if unexpected symptoms develop. These might include severe headache, palpitations, paresthesias, pruritus, difficulty breathing, nausea and vomiting, urticaria, and joint pain. When antitoxins, antisera, and antivenoms are given, the client is observed for 20 to 30 minutes because symptoms of severe allergic response, as described earlier, usually appear within that time.

Some persons refuse immunization because of religious beliefs. Others hesitate to be immunized or to have their children immunized because of fear about potential side effects. The nurse might explain when the benefits of immunization far outweigh risk of side effects. In the United Kingdom, for instance, the incidence of pertussis and pertussis-related deaths significantly increased after immunization was suspended from 1974 to 1978. On the other hand, a national campaign in the United States of preventive inoculations for swine influenza in the 1976–1977 flu season caused an incidence of Guillain–Barré syndrome five to six times higher in vaccinated than unvaccinated persons. In retrospect, this campaign seems to have been ill advised because the anticipated outbreak of swine influenza did not materialize. This situation points out a serious problem with large-scale inoculation programs against a new strain of flu virus—the immunization program must begin as soon as possible to be effective, often before the new vaccine has been thoroughly tested and before it is known whether the epidemic would actually occur.

Adult clients need to be reminded to complete an immunization series, such as for polio, and to keep tetanus immunization up to date. Those employed in health care should maintain immunity against poliomyelitis, diphtheria, and tetanus. More information can be obtained from the Public Health Service Advisory Committee on Immunization Practices listed with the resources at the end of this chapter.

Hygiene and Sanitation

Public health depends on adequate community sanitation. A clean water supply, sewage treatment, and garbage disposal are the fundamental means of controlling disease in a society. In general, communities in the United States do an adequate job in these areas. On the other hand, precautions must be taken in areas where sewage disposal might not be adequate. An example is rural areas where residents have their own wells and septic tanks. Contamination of drinking water is possible if proper measures are not taken.

With the renewed interest in outdoor recreation, persons may also be vulnerable to infectious organisms. Campers may drink water from streams or lakes without adequate attention to sanitation. Nurses can encourage outdoor enthusiasts to seek the latest information from local authorities before drinking from these water supplies. They can also instruct campers and hikers to boil their water or carry effective water purification tablets.

Personal hygiene is also a factor in preventing disease. Thorough and frequent handwashing by hospital personnel is an important means of preventing the spread of nosocomial infections. Food handlers in the home, restaurants, and institutions must also be conscientious about handwashing and personal care. Specific measures to limit the spread of infectious diseases in health care settings or in the home are discussed later in this chapter.

Food Handling

Proper food handling is an important means of preventing food poisoning and infection spread. Foods that are improperly prepared, preserved, or stored provide an ideal growth medium for microorganisms.

Nurses can help raise public awareness of appropriate food handling regardless of the setting where they practice. General principles for food handling are:

- Wash hands before preparing food.
- Keep hot foods hot and cold foods cold.
- Cook all meat thoroughly.

If there is any question about spoilage, the food should be discarded without tasting. Commercial food preservation is highly sophisticated, and commercial products are rarely contaminated. Home canning, on the other hand, can cause food poisoning, especially in low-acid foods. Home canners should be instructed to purchase jars and lids intended specifically for home canning and follow the manufacturer's directions exactly.

Travelers to foreign countries often have their trips interrupted by gastroenteritis characterized by diarrhea, abdominal cramps, nausea and vomiting, and occasional headache and fever. Known by various colorful names such as "Montezuma's revenge," "Rangoon runs," "Casablanca crud," and "Delhi belly," this condition was thought to be due to changes in diet or the use of cooking oils with a laxative effect. Evidence now shows that an enterotoxin produced by *E. coli* is the most common cause (Rodman & Smith, 1984). Although the use of prophylactic antimicrobial drugs such as doxycycline (Vibramycin) for travelers is controversial, nurses can advise travelers about food and water precautions. For example, fresh fruits and vegetables should be peeled before they are eaten. It is generally not safe to eat lettuce or green salads unless they have been washed in a chlorinated solution. Another good piece of advice is to recommend drinking bottled beverages. Drinking water, water used to make ice cubes, and milk should be boiled before drinking. Using antidiarrheal agents once diarrhea has begun is also controversial; it may be best to let the diarrhea run its course and rid the body of the offending organisms. Clients should be sure to seek health care if symptoms are severe or if they persist, if they become dehydrated, if they are very young or old or have a chronic illness, or if they are a compromised host.

Assessment of the Potentially Infected Person

A comprehensive assessment is essential in planning the care for a potentially infected person. A comprehensive assessment will help determine:

- Whether infection exists
- The most probable primary source of infection
- Which organisms are most likely to be responsible
- Which antimicrobials are indicated
- Whether special procedures such as isolation measures or measures for controlling the spread of the suspected disease should be instituted
- What information and health teaching are needed for client and family

The health history, physical assessment, and diagnostic studies are all part of the assessment phase.

Subjective Data

Collection of a detailed history is essential to the diagnosis of infectious disease. Most infectious diseases begin with nonspecific symptoms such as headache, anorexia, fatigue, and joint and muscle pain. A thorough history may help in pinpointing the diagnosis. Asking where and what a client has eaten in the last few days might aid in reaching a diagnosis of food poisoning. For example, has the client attended a banquet or a company picnic? Are others attending also ill? Has the client eaten pork or raw meat? Some questions to ask during history taking are in Table 9–4.

The client with an infectious disease may harbor feelings of inadequacy or inferiority. Some infectious diseases are stigmatized, especially sexually transmitted diseases, tuberculosis, and AIDS. Clients may feel "dirty" and blame themselves for acquiring the disease. They may shun social contact. Depending on the severity of the disease, they may also fear long-term disability or death. If the disease

Table 9–4
Questions to Ask When Infectious Disease Is Suspected

Questions	Rationale
1. What are the symptoms? When did they begin?	Provides data about duration of illness and specific information to assist with diagnosis
2. Is there fever? With or without chills? What is the pattern: intermittent, recurrent, or constant?	Fever patterns vary with the organism; pattern may help in identifying microbe
3. Is there a stiff neck? Pain when knee and hip are flexed and knee is straightened?	May indicate meningitis
4. Is there back pain?	May indicate kidney infection
5. Is there dysuria?	May indicate bladder infection
6. Is there diarrhea?	May indicate gastrointestinal infection
7. Are there draining wounds?	May indicate wound infection
8. Is there use of prescription, over-the-counter, or illegal drugs?	Identifies client's routine drug use as well as potential problems with self-medication or blood-transmitted infections (eg, hepatitis)
9. Does the client have a chronic disease (eg, diabetes)? Is the client taking an immunosuppressant?	Identifies increased risk for infection through impaired immune response
10. Has the client traveled recently, especially outside the country?	Identifies exposure to foreign diseases
11. Has the client been bitten by an animal, insect, or human? Has the client been in contact with animals?	Identifies exposure to diseases transmitted by bites

carries a social stigma, the nurse must be particularly perceptive in assessing the client's attitude toward the illness, and eliciting the client's concerns. Inquire about the attitudes of family members and friends to determine the client's social support and to help develop a plan of care that considers the psychosocial needs of clients, family members, and friends.

Objective Data

After a history is obtained, a physical assessment should be performed. Particular findings that might indicate an infectious process are:

- Dehydration
- Neck rigidity
- Open or draining lesions
- Inflamed throat
- Enlarged lymph nodes
- Rashes
- Elevated temperature

The absence of a finding may also be important. The absence of a fever might indicate a particular kind of infection, or it might indicate that the infection is improving. For example, there is usually no fever with staphylococcal food poisoning, but there may be with other types.

A variety of diagnostic studies is useful in determining the causative organism and identifying the appropriate antimicrobial drug therapy. One of the most general and most important is the total white blood cell count with differential (WBC with Diff). The total WBC is elevated in most infections. In addition, the Diff shows an increase in the number of immature white blood cells (segmented and banded neutrophils) the body produces to fight infection. This phenomenon, called the left shift, is discussed in Chapter 17.

The nurse's role includes teaching the client about the planned procedure, obtaining cultures and specimens, assisting with diagnostic procedures, and providing emotional support to the client. Gram's stain and culture and sensitivity tests are briefly described because they are the principal means of diagnosis in infection.

Gram's stain, a laboratory procedure performed on a specimen, is one of the most useful and most important procedures for identifying bacteria. If the test is negative, no organisms were identified, indicating the specimen was not infected with bacteria. If the test is positive, signifying a bacterial infection, the Gram's stain indicates whether the bacteria are gram-positive or gram-negative. The Gram's stain reaction provides important information for treatment. Because it requires no incubation of the organism, results can be obtained faster than by a laboratory culture, meaning antimicrobial treatment can begin sooner.

Laboratory cultures of specimens may also be done to identify organisms. Urine, spinal fluid, and blood are normally sterile, and a culture will not reveal organisms in the absence of infection. In contrast, stool has a normal population of bacteria. Interpretation of culture results must consider whether the material is normally sterile. Cultures may be done on all of the specimens discussed in Box 9–1. Results may take 3 or more days. The specimen for culture should be obtained before antimicrobial therapy is begun for more accurate results. The laboratory also can determine the sensitivity and resistance of an organism to antimicrobials. This information is used in selecting an antimicrobial to which the organism is sensitive.

An exception to first obtaining a specimen for culture is the emergency treatment of septicemia. In this situation, a combination of an aminoglycoside-type antibiotic such as gentamicin and a penicillin-type drug such as ampicillin or carbenicillin may be administered without delay because of the seriousness of septic shock (Rodman & Smith, 1984). The organisms primarily responsible for septic shock are usually sensitive to one or both of these classes of drugs.

Preventing Nosocomial Infection

Precautions to prevent nosocomial infections and to avoid becoming infected oneself begin with the recognition that unrecognized or subclinical infections are prevalent and that prevention begins before a diagnosis of infection is made. (Recall the earlier example of the nurse who developed herpetic whitlow.) Nurses should incorporate the recommendations in Box 9–2 in caring for any client. Hospital staff should seek prompt medical attention for upper respiratory problems and breaks in the skin; direct client care should be avoided if these conditions exists. Be especially cautious when caring for clients whose immune systems are suppressed. Additional environmental protection such as protective isolation or the use of patient-isolator units, although recommended by some, does not appear warranted for most compromised clients. Instead, routine techniques such as handwashing should be emphasized and enforced, and these clients should be in private rooms whenever possible and away from other clients who may make infection transmission likely.

The urinary tract is the most common site of nosocomial infections, and urinary tract instrumentation is the most common cause. See Chapter 25 for nursing strategies that minimize the client's risk.

Bacteremias that occur in hospitalized clients with no underlying site of infection are likely to have resulted from contaminated intravenous fluids or from the intravenous delivery system. Check all IV fluid containers and the IV infusion system itself for cracks and holes before using them and inspect the fluid for visual evidence of contamination. Do not use any suspect fluid or equipment and notify infection control personnel who should notify the appropriate agencies and take remedial action. Limiting the need for and use of intravenous infusions is the primary preventive strategy. When IV infusions are unavoidable:

- Maintain scrupulous aseptic technique.
- Use steel needles whenever possible.
- Change the site of a peripheral IV infusion every 48–72 hours.
- Avoid the use of glucose solutions for long-term, slow-running infusions whenever possible.
- Change IV fluid every 24 hours, and tubing every 48 hours.

Respiratory instrumentation and respiratory therapy are major risk factors in hospital-acquired pneumonia. Other risk factors are ineffective coughing, smoking, other infection, and tracheal suctioning. Adequate sterilization and disinfection of all respiratory equipment and frequent changes of respiratory therapy equipment is an important preventive measure. Nurses should focus on encouraging deep breathing and effective coughing in postoperative clients as well as in any clients at risk. Aseptic technique should be used for laryngotracheal suctioning.

Preventing surgical wound infection requires concerted effort during the entire perioperative period because many factors can cause infection. During the preoperative period, nurses can ensure that the client's skin is kept intact and that preoperative preparation such as enemas and antibiotic administration before bowel surgery is carried out. The circulating nurse acts as the client's advocate during surgery by monitoring the surgical team and the operating room environment for adherence to standards of surgical asepsis. Aseptic postoperative care of wounds is another important measure.

Nursing Research Note

Nichols E, Barstow R, Cooper D: Relationship between incidence of phlebitis and frequency of changing IV tubing and percutaneous site. *Nurs Res* 1983; 32(4): 247–251.

This study examined the development of phlebitis related to IV tubing change and changing IV sites percutaneously. No statistically significant difference was found in phlebitis development when tubing was changed at 24 hours and 48 hours. There was not a statistically significant difference in phlebitis development when tubing was changed at 48 hours and 72 hours. Subjects who had tubing changed every 24 hours had less clinical evidence of phlebitis, however.

When IV sites were rotated, there was no statistical significance between site rotation at 48 hours and 72 hours. Clinically, however, 48-hour site rotation coupled with 24-hour tubing change resulted in a trend toward less phlebitis development.

Nurses are responsible for maintaining IV therapy and assessing clients' IV sites for infection. Monitoring sites and regular tubing changes may result in lower incidence of phlebitis formation. More research is needed to determine scientifically what nursing approaches are most effective.

Box 9–1
Guidelines for Obtaining Specimens for Cultures

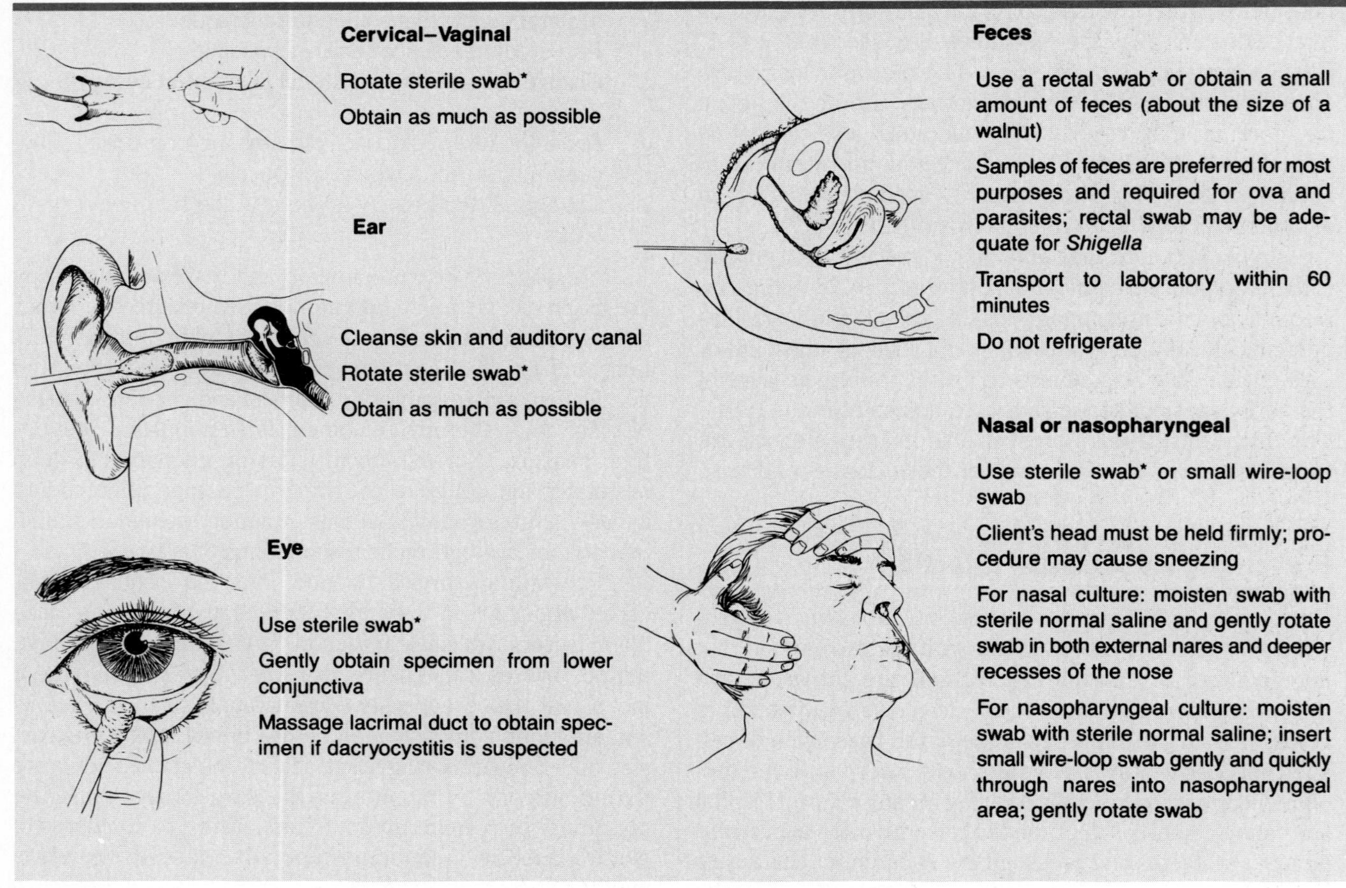

Cervical–Vaginal
Rotate sterile swab*
Obtain as much as possible
Ear
Cleanse skin and auditory canal
Rotate sterile swab*
Obtain as much as possible
Eye
Use sterile swab*
Gently obtain specimen from lower conjunctiva
Massage lacrimal duct to obtain specimen if dacryocystitis is suspected
Feces
Use a rectal swab* or obtain a small amount of feces (about the size of a walnut)
Samples of feces are preferred for most purposes and required for ova and parasites; rectal swab may be adequate for Shigella
Transport to laboratory within 60 minutes
Do not refrigerate
Nasal or nasopharyngeal
Use sterile swab* or small wire-loop swab
Client's head must be held firmly; procedure may cause sneezing
For nasal culture: moisten swab with sterile normal saline and gently rotate swab in both external nares and deeper recesses of the nose
For nasopharyngeal culture: moisten swab with sterile normal saline; insert small wire-loop swab gently and quickly through nares into nasopharyngeal area; gently rotate swab

*Chemicals on cotton swabs are bactericidal and may affect the culture; use specially prepared swabs for cultures.

Providing Physiologic Support

Clients with infectious disease should have vital signs assessed at least every 4 hours. Even afebrile clients should have their temperature documented to establish any fever pattern. Arterial blood pressure monitoring may be required for clients in septic shock.

Tepid water baths may be used to reduce high fever. Be careful not to cause shivering, which only increases temperature. In some situations, alcohol baths bring temperatures down more quickly; however, they are more likely to cause shivering and dry the skin. Both methods are controversial. In critical situations, hypothermia blankets may be used. Antipyretic drugs are usually given.

The profuse diaphoresis, vomiting, and diarrhea that accompany many infectious diseases may cause dehydration and fluid and electrolyte imbalance. Monitor the client's state of hydration, encourage oral fluids, and administer intravenous fluids as indicated. Measure and record intake and output and weigh the client at regular intervals.

Promoting Comfort

Weakness and generalized aches often accompany infectious diseases. Physical activity should be reduced to avoid further fatigue and weakness. Pillows, pads, frequent position changes, and back rubs often help to reduce the discomfort associated with aching. Analgesics may also be useful.

Bathing and frequent linen changes reduce the discomforts associated with diaphoresis. For clients with skin rashes, bathing with sodium bicarbonate, applying antipruritic lotions, or administering antipruritic medications can help reduce the itching associated with skin rashes. Dehydration, fever, and coughing adversely affect the mucous membranes. Frequent oral hygiene is impor-

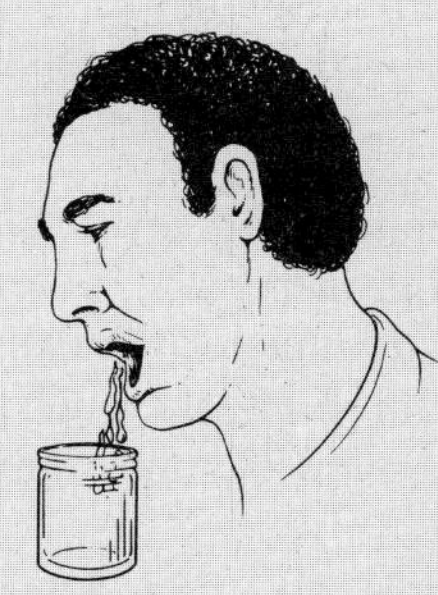

Sputum

Morning samples preferred

Client should rinse mouth thoroughly before raising sputum from deep within the bronchi and expectorating into sterile container

Use sterile suction catheter and aseptic technique for tracheal aspiration

Obtain 2 to 3 mL of sputum (not saliva)

Transport to laboratory within 60 minutes

Do not refrigerate

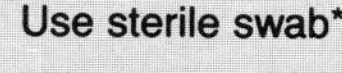

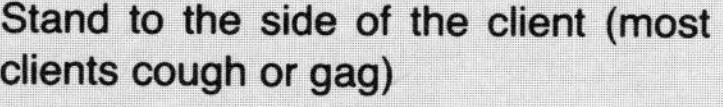

Throat

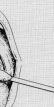

Use sterile swab*

Stand to the side of the client (most clients cough or gag)

Depress client's tongue with tongue depressor

Avoid touching the lips or tongue

Rotate swab firmly and gently over both tonsils, back of the throat, and any areas of inflammation, ulceration, or exudation

Obtain as much as possible

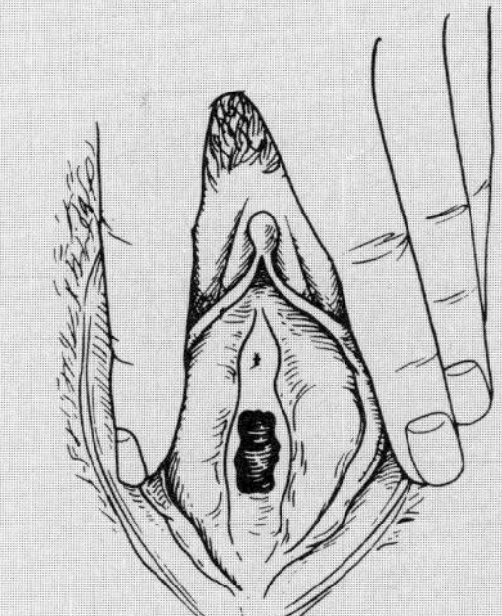

Urine

Early morning specimens are best because bacterial counts are highest then

Females: cleanse vulvar area; client collects midstream specimen while holding labia apart

Males: cleanse glans penis; obtain midstream specimen

Use aseptic technique when aspirating specimens from in-dwelling catheter with sterile needle and syringe

Obtain at least 1 mL for culture (5 mL for urinalysis) in a sterile container

Transport to laboratory immediately; refrigerate if not cultured immediately but transport within 2 hours

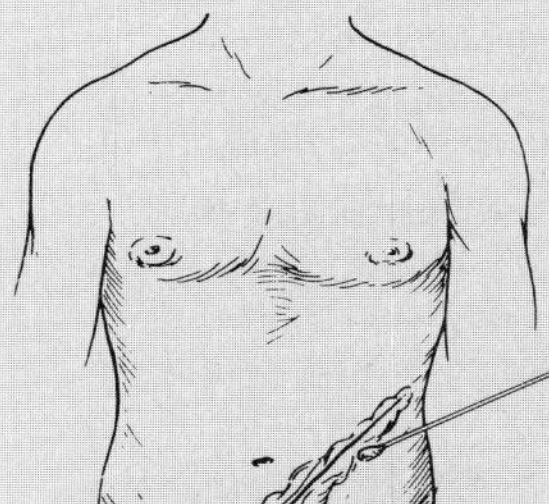

Wound

Cleanse wound with sterile saline to remove skin flora

Use sterile swab* or syringe

Obtain as much as possible

Take care not to contaminate surrounding tissue

Transport within 60 minutes

tant. Warm gargles are often comforting, as is providing warm, humidified air.

Monitoring Antimicrobial Therapy

Antimicrobial drugs are available to control most microbes and parasites, but as yet, few are effective against viruses. Most infections can be quickly controlled. If an organism is resistant to the drug, the drug may have to be discontinued, and an alternative drug or combination of drugs may be tried. If the client is immunosuppressed, antimicrobial therapy alone may not be enough to control or treat the infection. In other situations, clients may even be made worse by drug-induced adverse effects such as direct tissue toxicity, hypersensitivity reactions, and superinfections.

Direct-tissue toxicity takes a number of forms. Some oral antimicrobials irritate the mucosa of the gastrointestinal tract, causing nausea, vomiting, and diarrhea. Others cause local pain when administered intramuscularly, and some cause phlebitis when administered intravenously. The most severe effects result in nephrotoxicity (kidney damage) and neurotoxicity (damage to cranial nerve VIII, the vestibulocochlear nerve). Aminoglycosides and polymyxins are more likely to cause nephrotoxic effects. Monitor the results of laboratory reports of kidney function for signs of drug-related renal impairment. Aminoglycosides can also cause neurologic impairment; monitor the client for dizziness, vertigo, and impaired hearing.

Hypersensitivity reactions, common with penicillin-type antibiotics, can occur immediately after administration of an antimicrobial, or they can be delayed. Hypersensitivity is more likely in persons having other allergies and in those who have been treated with these agents frequently. This is a good reason for not using antibiotics to treat minor upper respiratory tract infections, because most are caused by viruses not sensitive to these drugs. Health care pro-

Box 9–2
Recommended Nursing Measures When Infection Is Unrecognized or Subclinical

Assess what you are going to do for the client *before* you begin an episode of care. When you anticipate coming in contact with body substances, glove your hands. When care is completed, *wash your hands.* Soap, running water, and about 10 seconds of friction are usually enough.

Is the client bleeding or is your care likely to include exposure to blood? If the answer is yes, wear gloves for direct care. Is bleeding enough to soil your uniform? If yes, wear a cover gown and change your uniform if it becomes soiled. (Scrub clothes are available in all hospitals, and this is an appropriate use for them.)

Is the wound draining? If yes, wear gloves for direct care. Is drainage copious? If yes, wear a cover gown.

Is the client incontinent? If yes, wear gloves for contact with urine or stool and a cover gown if you are changing the client's bed linen or if a great deal of soilage is likely.

Will you be suctioning the client? If yes, glove both hands to avoid skin contact with sputum or oral secretions.

It is not always possible to anticipate contact with body substances. When such episodes of care are completed, it is essential to wash hands well before continuing with client care.

The same logic applies to handling linen and trash soiled with body substances. If linen or trash from any client is likely to expose personnel to direct contact with body substances, it should be securely bagged and marked for careful handling.

SOURCE: Adapted from Jackson MM, Lynch P: Infection control: Too much or too little? *Am J Nurs* 1984; 84:208–210.

viders have reportedly developed hypersensitivity reactions because of careless handling of antibiotics (eg, spilling a liquid preparation on the hands; handling tablets; or inadvertent injection of parenteral antibiotics during preparation, administration, or disposal of equipment).

Superinfections are often more serious than the original infection being treated. Superinfections are often associated with various procedures and equipment such as intravenous catheters, parenteral nutrition, heparin locks, arterial catheters and angiographic procedures, hemodialysis and peritoneal dialysis, cerebrospinal fluid shunts, pressure transducers, nebulizers, and endotracheal intubation or tracheostomy. Clients who have undergone these invasive procedures should be carefully monitored for infection. Prosthetic valves, cardiac pacemakers, total hip and knee prostheses, vascular grafts, intraocular lens implantation, and breast implants are devices that are associated with superinfection. With some devices such as cerebrospinal fluid shunts, 50% of the infections occur within the first week. With total hip and knee protheses, it may take as long as 2 years before infection occurs (Sen et al, 1982). Clients with prostheses must not only be monitored by nurses during the postoperative period in the hospital, but must also be instructed to observe for superinfection on discharge.

Nurses must be able to administer antimicrobials properly as well as to advise clients and their families on how to administer them and how to avoid their misuse. The proper administration of antimicrobials will be facilitated by following these guidelines:

- Determine whether the client is allergic to any drugs, especially penicillin or other antimicrobials, before administering them; if so, do not administer the drug.
- Monitor the client closely for adverse effects, such as drug-induced toxicity or hypersensitivity, and report them immediately.
- Maintain therapeutic blood levels of antibiotics by administering them at the appropriate intervals.
- Administer oral antibiotics with food to diminish any unpleasant gastrointestinal symptoms, but check first to be sure food will not interfere with the absorption of the antibiotic.
- Report nausea and vomiting immediately so oral administration can be changed to parenteral administration if necessary.
- Observe the client closely to determine the effect of the drug; report signs of continuing or worsening infection.
- Handle needles and syringes with extreme care to protect oneself from inadvertent infection with contaminated equipment.
- Avoid careless handling of antibiotics.

Advising clients and their families on how to administer antimicrobials safely and avoid misuse will help to ensure that clients are not deprived of the use of a valuable drug when needed. The following guidelines will help to achieve these goals:

- Inform clients that using antimicrobials to treat trivial infections may not only be useless, but it may also render the drug ineffective in a future illness.
- Advise clients to continue taking the drug for the recommended length of time, even if symptoms seem to have abated. (This prevents relapses.)
- Instruct clients to take the drug in the recommended dose. (This prevents chronic infection because of undertreatment as well as the later emergence of resistant strains because of less-than-optimal doses.)
- Caution clients about any special adjunctive measures such as taking sulfonamides with large amounts of fluid; avoiding alcohol when taking moxalactam disodium (Moxam) and other cephalosporin-related drugs; and avoiding dairy products, antacids, and iron salt preparations with tetracyclines.
- Remind clients not to treat themselves with antimicrobials left over from another illness.

Keep in mind there are many different types of antimicrobials, all with different effects and precautions. Consult a pharmacology text for information on specific antimicrobials.

Implementing Isolation Precautions

Health care institutions have isolation procedures to prevent transmission of infectious organisms to clients, visitors, and personnel. In 1983, the CDC issued new recommendations for isolation precautions. Under this system, clients with infections are assigned to the appropriate category. For example, clients with a wound infection are placed in contact isolation because wound infections are spread by contact. The seven isolation categories are:

- Strict isolation
- Respiratory isolation
- Tuberculosis (AFB) isolation
- Enteric precautions
- Contact isolation
- Drainage/secretion precautions
- Blood/body fluid precautions

Refer to the CDC guidelines (see resources at the end of the chapter) to determine appropriate isolation precautions for specific infectious diseases. Each category includes specific information, such as whether a private room is indicated, whether protective clothing must be worn, and the proper handling of contaminated articles. Refer also to a nursing fundamentals text for a discussion of the principles of protective asepsis. The CDC also offers the option of disease-specific isolation precautions as well as the option for hospitals to develop their own system. Health care facilities may differ from one another in this regard. The infection control practitioner should be consulted regarding specific institutional procedures.

Clients assigned to isolation precautions have a variety of psychosocial needs that require sensitive handling. First, client and family need thorough explanations about the disease, the planned treatment, and the rationale for isolation. Although the initial explanation is probably given by the physician, the nurse reinforces, clarifies, and provides additional information as needed.

Depending on the isolation category, the client may be in a private room, perhaps with the door closed. Isolation may lead to withdrawal and possibly even sensory deprivation because the normal sources of stimulation are removed. Assess the client's need for stimulation regularly. Spending time with the client when not providing physical care is one way to provide stimulation. See that the client has means of diversion, such as television, a telephone, books and magazines, craft projects, and other forms of entertainment. Try to provide as much variety in activities as the isolation requirements allow. Friendly conversation that provides opportunities for the client to talk and demonstrates the nurse's interest is perhaps the most important stimulation measure. These measures also help in reducing withdrawal.

Chapter Highlights

The relation between host and organism varies from mutually beneficial to seriously harmful, depending on the host's condition and the type of organism.

A series of events is necessary for an infection to occur: a disease-producing agent, a reservoir, a portal of exit, a mode of transmission, a portal of entry, and a susceptible host.

Although susceptibility is not entirely understood, it depends on several factors, including virulence and number of organisms, age and general health, nutritional status, and the immune system's ability to destroy the invading organisms.

Susceptibility to disease is also influenced by psychosocial/lifestyle factors such as finances, environment, occupation, avocation, recreation, and stress.

The majority of nosocomial (hospital-acquired) infections occur when an organism normally present in a client overwhelms an impaired immune system; the remainder is acquired from organisms in the hospital environment.

Nurses have a major role in infectious disease control through promoting prevention and public education.

Because most infections begin with nonspecific symptoms, a thorough history and physical assessment can help in arriving at a diagnosis.

Assessing the client's and family's attitudes toward the infectious disease is essential in determining psychosocial needs.

Clients with infectious disease often feel inadequate or inferior and shun social contact. Because of the stigma attached to infectious disease, clients may be shunned by others.

Gram's stain and laboratory cultures of specimens are two common diagnostic studies. Sensitivity determinations are often made to select an appropriate antimicrobial.

In addition to providing physiologic support and promoting comfort, monitoring antimicrobial therapy is an important nursing responsibility.

Advising clients and their families on how to administer antimicrobials safely and avoid misuse helps to ensure that clients are not deprived of the use of a valuable drug when needed.

Because isolation may lead to withdrawal and sensory deprivation, the nurse must meet the client's need for stimulation.

Bibliography

Baron S (editor): *Medical Microbiology,* 2nd ed. Menlo Park, CA: Addison–Wesley, 1986.

Benenson AS (editor): *Control of Communicable Diseases in Man,* 14th ed. Washington, DC: American Public Health Association, 1985.

Brooks PM et al: Problems of antibiotic therapy in the elderly. *J Am Geriatr Society* (March) 1984; 32:36–41.

Carroll M: Infection control in long-term care. *Geriatr Nurs* (March) 1984; 5:100–103.

Centers for Disease Control: *Guideline for Handwashing and Hospital Environmental Control.* Atlanta: USDHHS, 1985.

Centers for Disease Control: *Guidelines for the Prevention and Control of Nosocomial Infections.* Atlanta: USDHHS, Public Health Service, 1984.

Corman LC: The relationship between nutrition, infection, and immunity. *Med Clin North Am* 1985; 69(3):519–531.

Garner J, Simmons B: CDC guidelines for isolation precautions in hospitals. *Infect Control* 1983; 4:245–325.

Jackson MM, Lynch P: Isolation practices: A historical perspective. *Am J Infect Control* (Feb) 1985; 13:21–31.

Jackson MM, McPherson DC: Infection control: Keeping current. *Nurse Educator* (July–Aug) 1986; 25:111–114.

Keithley J: Infection and the malnourished patient. *Heart Lung* 1983; 12:23–27.

Kochar M: *Textbook of General Medicine.* New York: Wiley Medical, 1983.

Kottra C: Infection in the compromised host: An overview. *Heart Lung* 1983; 12:10–14.

Quinn T: Precautions for patients hospitalized with acquired immunodeficiency syndrome. *Infect Control* 1983; 4:79–80.

Rodman MJ, Smith DW: *Clinical Pharmacology in Nursing,* 3rd ed. Philadelphia: Lippincott, 1984.

Sen P et al: Superinfection: Another look. *Am J Med* 1982; 73:706–717.

Soule B (editor): *The APIC Curriculum for Infection Control Practice.* Dubuque, IA: Kendall/Hunt, 1983.

Tortora GJ, Funke BR, Case CL: *Microbiology,* 2nd ed. Menlo Park, CA: Benjamin/Cummings, 1986.

Williams WW: Guidelines for infection control in hospital personnel. *Infect Control* 1983; 4:326–349.

Resources

(Resources for AIDS are in Chapter 22 and resources for sexually transmitted diseases are in Chapter 48.)

ORGANIZATIONS

Bureau of Epidemiology
Centers for Disease Control
US Public Health Service
Atlanta, GA 30333

This arm of the CDC distributes weekly "blue sheets," updates on quarantinable diseases worldwide. It also publishes *Morbidity and Mortality Weekly Report* (MMWR), which contains data on the incidence of specific notifiable diseases and the deaths from these diseases (usually organized by state).

Canadian Hospital Infection
Control Association
McMaster University
Medical Centre
1200 Main St W
Hamilton, Ontario, Canada L85 4J9

Pan American World Health Organization
525 23rd St., NW
Washington, DC 20037
Phone: (202) 861–3200

This is the World Health Organization Regional Office for the Americas. It coordinates international health efforts in North, Central, and South America.

Public Health Service Advisory Committee
on Immunization Practices (ACIP)
Centers for Disease Control
US Public Health Service
Atlanta, GA 30333
Phone: (404) 329–2572

A resource for the latest information on immunization, available vaccines, and ongoing research. Will provide current recommendations regarding specific infectious diseases.

World Health Organization (WHO)
Palais de la Santé
Geneva, Switzerland

The organization responsible for coordinating international health efforts according to international health regulations.

SPECIALTY ORGANIZATION

Association for Practitioners in
Infection Control (APIC)
505 E. Hawley St.
Mundelein, IL 60060
Phone: (312) 949–6050

APIC is open to physicians, nurses, and others concerned with infection control problems. APIC holds an annual meeting in the spring.

HEALTH EDUCATION INFORMATION

Copies of the two-volume *The APIC Curriculum for Infection Control Practice* (1983) can be obtained from the Association for Practitioners in Infection Control (see Specialty Organization).

Copies of *CDC Guideline for Isolation Precautions in Hospitals* (1983), can be obtained for $5.50 from:

Superintendent of Documents
US Government Printing Office
Washington, DC 20402
Phone: (202) 783–3238
In ordering, ask for GPO #017-023-00148-5.

Copies of *Control of Communicable Diseases in Man* by A. S. Benenson (14th ed., 1985) can be obtained for about $10 from:

American Public Health Association
1015 15th St., NW
Washington, DC 20005
Phone: (202) 789–5600

From: Channing L. Bete, Inc.
200 State Road
South Deerfield, MA 01373
Phone: (413) 665–7611

Isolation, a booklet explaining why isolation is sometimes necessary, including common rules and procedures in isolation. To help further understanding of clients, their families, and friends.

CHAPTER 10

Cancer

Other topics relevant to this content are: Bone marrow transplant, **Chapter 23;** Immunosuppression and infection, **Chapter 9;** Isolated regional limb hyperthermic perfusion (RLHP), **Chapter 55;** Nursing care of clients with cancers of specific organs, *see specific disorders chapter(s) in appropriate body system unit;* Oral self-examination, **Chapter 38;** Pap smear, **Chapter 48;** Psychophysiologic mechanisms of pain and pain relief measures, **Chapter 3;** Self-examination of breasts and testes, **Chapter 5;** Surgical procedures for cancer, *see surgical approaches chapter in appropriate body system unit.*

Objectives

When you have finished studying this chapter, you should be able to:

Summarize the impact of recent trends in cancer care on survival rates.

Differentiate between characteristics of benign and malignant neoplasia.

Compare various theories of cancer causation.

Discuss the nurse's role in primary and secondary prevention.

Describe the basic principles of each major treatment modality: surgery, chemotherapy, radiation therapy, and immunotherapy.

Analyze the biologic and psychosocial responses to cancer in the early and late phases of illness.

Identify the common side effects of chemotherapy and radiation therapy, appropriate nursing interventions, and expected client outcomes.

Explain the assessment parameters and associated nursing implications of oncologic emergencies.

Discuss the nurse's role in the psychosocial aspects of cancer care.

In 1987, an estimated 965,000 Americans faced a diagnosis of cancer. Of these, about 385,000 or four out of ten could expect to still be alive 5 years after the diagnosis (American Cancer Society, 1987). Although these statistics may seem discouraging, great strides continue to be made in cancer treatment and research. In the past, some forms of leukemia, testicular cancer, and lymphomas were almost always fatal. Today, with effective combination chemotherapy regimens and advancements in radiotherapy techniques, the potential for long-term cure of these cancers has improved.

Nevertheless, pessimistic perceptions about cancer remain. Many clients still perceive a cancer diagnosis to be a sentence to a painful, lingering death—a series of mutilating surgeries accompanied by therapies "worse than the disease." When caring for a newly diagnosed client, be sensitive to fears and concerns while stressing the individual nature of this disease and its response to therapy.

Oncology nursing is a specialty. Yet every nurse encounters and cares for clients with cancer in all phases from diagnosis to the end stage of the disease. Nurses see the woman in the surgeon's waiting room who has just been instructed to arrange for a biopsy for the lump she found in her breast, the client on a medical unit receiving chemotherapy or radiation therapy in hopes of controlling or arresting the disease, and the client at home in the terminal phase of illness.

By becoming thoroughly familiar with the neoplastic process, its physiologic and psychosocial effects, its forms and their prognoses, its treatments and their side effects, the nurse can help clients participate actively in the management of their disease and avoid the despair that so often accompanies it. Comprehensive care of the client with neoplastic disease meets the needs of the body while offering solace and encouragement to the human spirit.

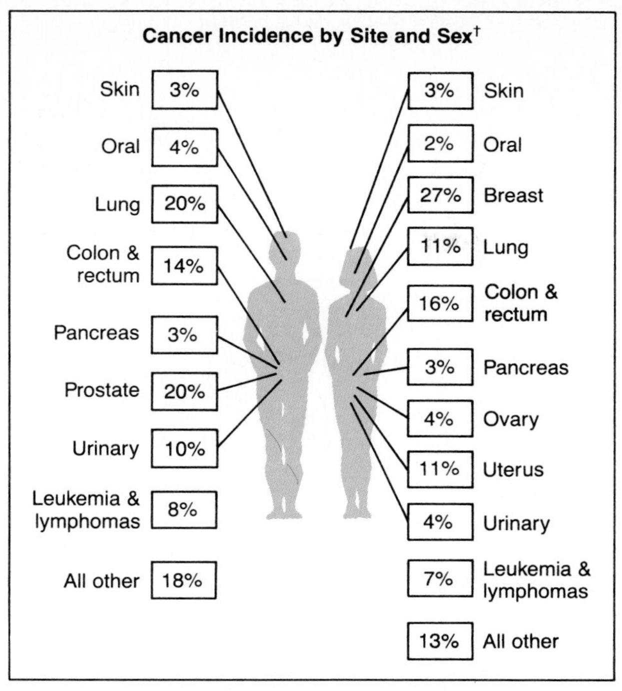

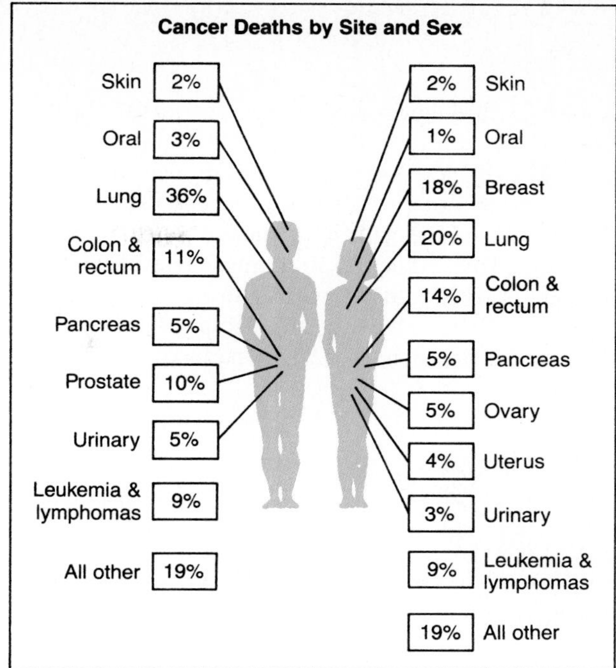

†Excluding nonmelanoma skin cancer and carcinoma in situ.

Figure 10–1

Estimates of cancer incidence and deaths by site and sex, 1987. SOURCE: *American Cancer Society:* Cancer Facts and Figures. *New York: American Cancer Society, 1987.*

Helping clients to understand their disease, maximize their potential for living, cope with the effects of therapy, live with the fear of recurrence, and face imminent death with dignity and comfort makes oncology nursing a special challenge.

SECTION

Incidence and Trends

The poor survival rate at least partially explains the extreme apprehension a diagnosis of cancer evokes. Yet survival has improved over the long prevailing rate of one in three. The improvement in percentages may not seem significant (40.0% compared to 33.3%, a difference of only 6.7%). Yet, for 1987 alone, the improved survival rate means that 65,000 more persons will survive beyond the fifth year.

It is important to remember that 5-year survival is not synonymous with cure. Moreover, cancer, the second leading cause of death in the United States, is not one disease but many. Some forms of cancer are far more common than others (Figure 10–1), and survival rates vary widely, from far better than the overall average to far worse. The 5-year survival rate for cancer of the lung, the most common cancer affecting men, is only 13%. And for cancer of the pancreas, a relatively rare disease accounting for only 3% of male and female cancers, the 3-year survival rate is only 4%.

These differences reflect many factors, including the etiology and course of the various forms of neoplasia, the effectiveness of screening techniques in early detection of particular forms of cancer, and the efficacy of treatment modes. The general psychologic and physical health of the individual client are also factors affecting survival. These issues will be discussed later in this chapter.

Cancer accounts for nearly 21% of all deaths in the United States: about 483,000 persons in 1987. Although the probability of a 5-year survival after a diagnosis of cancer is better than in the past, the national rate of deaths from cancer has gradually but steadily risen since 1930. While the mortality rates for some cancers have been declining (eg, gastric and uterine cancers), the mortality rate for lung cancer has increased. In fact, it has risen so steeply that the overall increase in mortality for the entire category of cancer may be attributed to lung cancer alone.

The incidence of cancer is higher in men than in women. Moreover, both incidence and mortality rates for men are increasing, and those for women—except for lung cancer—are decreasing. When age is considered, however, the picture is altered. The incidence of cancer in women aged 20 to 40 is three times that for men in the same age group.

Both incidence and mortality are higher for black Americans than for whites. Cancers of the lung, colon, rectum, prostate, and esophagus have increased slightly in the black population. Studies attribute this higher rate to socioeconomic and environmental factors rather than biologic factors.

The relation of age, sex, and cultural groups to both the incidence and mortality statistics are useful indicators for identifying high-risk populations, monitoring the success of prevention and detection programs, and evaluating the effectiveness of educational efforts and cancer treatment modalities. These statistics are also helpful in suggesting the future direction of oncology nursing.

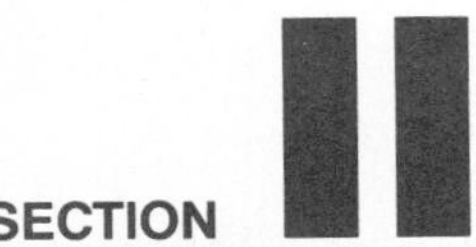

SECTION II

The Oncologic Process

Oncogenesis (from the Greek word *onkos,* meaning mass or bulk) is the process by which neoplasms (new growths or tumors) are produced. Oncology is the study of this process, about which much remains to be learned. Neoplasia (from the Greek words meaning "new" and "formation") is essentially a progressive multiplication of cells that occurs when the cellular "signals" that normally inhibit mitosis are absent, altered, not received, or not properly translated by the target cells. (The neoplastic process was initially defined and explained in Chapter 2.) Although benign (noncancerous) neoplasia occur, the focus of this chapter is malignant (cancerous) neoplasia.

The Cancer Cell

The cell is the basic unit of life—an entity so complex that hundreds of researchers have not discovered all of its secrets. Understanding the similarities and differences between normal and neoplastic cells is essential to comprehend the overall effects of neoplastic disease on the body.

The life cycle of both normal and neoplastic cells is referred to as the *cell cycle.* It comprises five phases described below and illustrated in Figure 10–2:

- The G_0 (gap 0), or resting phase
- The G_1 (gap 1) phase, in which RNA and protein are synthesized in preparation for DNA synthesis
- The S (synthesis) phase, during which DNA is synthesized
- The G_2 (gap 2) phase, poorly understood, in which preparation for mitosis (splitting) continues, RNA is synthesized, and chromosomes condense
- The M (mitosis) phase, during which two new cells are formed by the splitting of the original cell

These phases and their durations are critical to the treatment of cancer by chemotherapy. Some chemotherapeutic

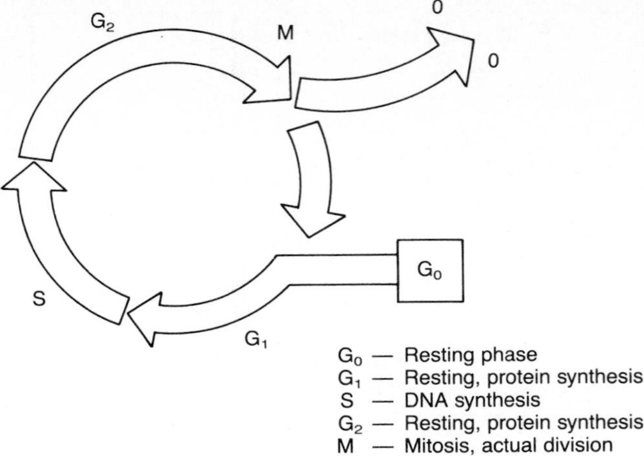

Figure 10–2

The cell cycle.

agents are only effective in a specific phase or phases of the cell cycle.

Malignant cells behave much differently than normal cells because of their selective growth advantages and abilities to invade and spread. These distinguishing features are unique and characteristic of the cancer process and are summarized in Table 10–1.

The growth control mechanisms of normal cells are not clearly understood. It is believed, however, that cells stop growing because of cell-to-cell surface contact or "contact inhibition" and because certain locally active substances (not yet identified) act as signals to regulate cell division or replication. Somehow, malignant cells either do not appropriately receive these messages or are unable to respond to them, allowing progressive growth. Keep in mind that both cancer and normal cells divide at comparable rates (not all cells dividing with equal frequency), meaning that cell cycle growth time is somewhat similar. The loss of effective regulatory control mechanisms is primarily what permits growth in excess of body demands.

In general, once the neoplastic tumor cells outgrow the available blood supply, malignant cells tend to revert to the resting phase (G_0) or die. The overall tumor growth slows. Moreover, inactive cells are less responsive to some forms of treatment, strongly supporting the concept that the tumor response to chemotherapy is invariably poorer with large tumor masses than with smaller ones.

Another unique feature, the highly invasive property of malignant cells, results from the production of proteolytic enzymes, one of which may be hyaluronidase, released at the margin of the tumor and normal tissue (Nowell, 1982). These enzymes literally digest surrounding tissue—a phenomenon reflected in the popular phrase, "eaten up by cancer." A benign tumor is usually clearly delineated from normal tissue, whereas a malignant tumor has no boundaries.

A final characteristic of cancer is the ability to spread or metastasize. **Metastasis** occurs when malignant cells detach from the parent tissue and migrate to other body tissues. These malignant cells colonize into a new cancer cell mass that grossly reflects the primary tissue of origin. Benign cells do not spread, but malignant cells can do so early in the oncogenic process, often negatively influencing the client's chance for recovery.

Metastasis occurs through four mechanisms:

- By direct extension
- By way of the arteriovenous circulatory system
- By way of the lymphatic system
- By implantation or seeding of a body cavity

Strictly speaking, direct extension is not metastasis to a distant site; rather, it is invasion of surrounding tissue. As the mass of a tumor increases, it inevitably extends into adjacent areas. Muscle tissue and connective tissue initially act as barriers to extension, but in time, these, too, are invaded by the neoplasm.

A convenient route for migration of malignant cells is the arteriovenous circulatory system (Figure 10–3). Neoplastic microemboli migrate to the small capillary beds, where growth of a new mass begins. Research has shown that a subpopulation of malignant cells is shed into the bloodstream when a tumor reaches a critical size.

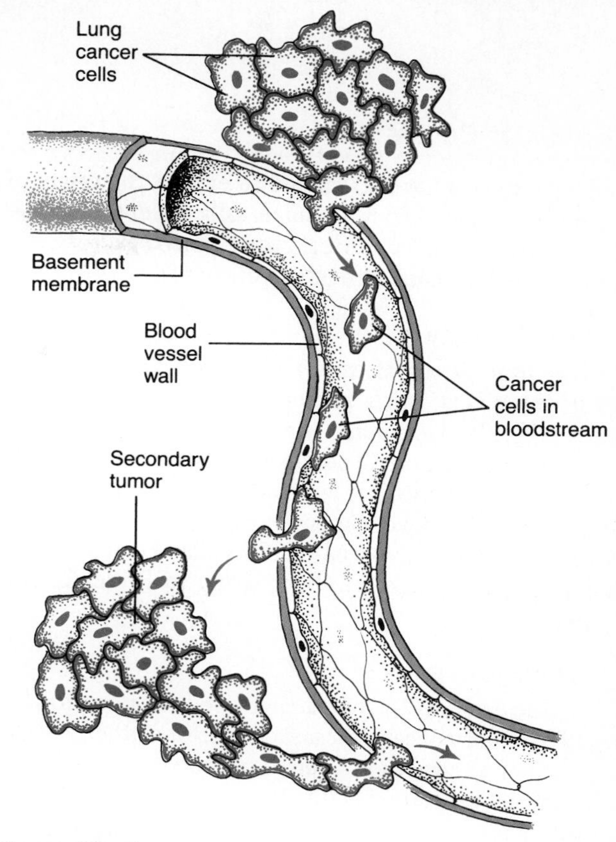

Figure 10–3

Metastasis through the circulatory system. Tumor cells secrete protein-digesting enzymes that cut a path to the basement membrane (the elastic barrier between tissues) and eventually dissolve the membrane. The tumor cells invade the blood vessel walls, creating an opening to slip through. Once in the circulating blood, most tumor cells are killed by the immune system. Survivors grip the wall of the blood vessel, erode the basement membrane, and settle and multiply in the tissue, causing secondary tumors. The secondary tumors eventually metastasize to other locations.

Table 10–1
Characteristics of Benign and Malignant Neoplasms

Benign Neoplasms	Malignant Neoplasms
Grow slowly	Grow rapidly or very rapidly
Usually are encapsulated	Rarely are encapsulated
Grow by expansion causing minor tissue damage	Grow by expansion as well as infiltration of surrounding tissue, causing marked changes, inflammation, ulceration, and necrosis
Show little or no tendency to recur when surgically removed	Show a strong tendency to recur when surgically removed if residual tumor remains
Do not spread, remain localized	Spread or metastasize to adjacent and distant structures by direct extension, lymphatics, blood, and implantation
Microscopically resemble tissue of origin	Usually differ in appearance from tissue of origin in varying degrees
Produce little or no generalized symptoms unless affecting the endocrine glands	Produce generalized symptoms such as cachexia and weight loss
Generally do not cause death unless pressure or obstruction of vital structures occurs	Usually cause death from spread to vital organs

The process of embolization is also the mechanism by which cancer spreads through the lymphatic system. Although lymphatic metastasis is slower than vascular metastasis, it is noteworthy especially because metastasis is often first detected by nodal enlargement.

Cavitary seeding may occur inadvertently during surgery; the surgeon's hand or a surgical implement may transfer tumor cells to a new site. Malignant cells may also be implanted as a tumor enlarges and extends. In either event, new colonies of malignant cells begin to multiply in cavities of the body (eg, in the peritoneal cavity). Today precautions are taken during surgery to prevent microembolic seeding and intracavitary spread.

Different forms of cancer have a predilection for metastasis to different sites, depending on such factors as proximity to lymph nodes or blood vessels.

Theories of Causation

Many hypotheses have attempted to explain the origin of cancer. No single theory is universally accepted as the primary explanation for cancer; rather, oncologic research supports the likelihood of multiple etiologies.

Viral Theory

The viral theory of cancer causation was given new impetus by investigators pursuing an earlier theory that cancer might be hereditary. Because viruses have been shown to cause tumors in exposed animals (eg, the feline leukemia virus in cats), it is possible that tumor viruses also influence the development of cancer in humans. The human T-cell leukemia virus (HTLV-I) has been linked to leukemia, and the Epstein–Barr virus, to Burkitt's lymphoma.

Oncogenes

By the early 1970s, researchers were working toward a unifying theory of cancer causation that hypothesized the existence of **oncogenes**—genetic material that can make a normal cell cancerous and is thought to be latent in the chromosomes of some individuals. A variety of mutagenic agents (chemicals, viruses, and high-energy radiation) can activate oncogenes. Oncogenes may be present in the entire population, lying dormant in those who never acquire cancer or becoming activated in the one in four persons who does develop cancer.

Genetics and Heredity

The tendency of specific tumor types to demonstrate patterns of inheritance (eg, breast and colon cancers, and melanoma) led researchers to analyze closely the familial patterns of cancer. The question is whether these patterns are caused by inherited genetic material or by shared environmental exposures among family members. Researchers have already linked chromosomal aberrations to certain cancers (eg, trisomy 21 or Down's syndrome has been linked to leukemia, and the Philadelphia chromosome has been linked to chronic myelogenous leukemia).

Somatic Mutation Theory

The somatic mutation theory rests on the premise that cancer is characterized by qualitative or mutational changes in cellular DNA. These changes are thought to be directly or indirectly related to repeated exposure to carcinogens (ie, a single mutational insult is not sufficient to cause cancer). Rather, successive changes from several mutational insults over the life span create conditions for oncogenesis.

Environmental Theories

Many substances or agents in the human environment can cause cancer or contribute to its development. These include exogenous chemicals such as polycyclic hydrocarbons, dyes, alkylating agents, urethane, nitrosamines, and polymers; endogenous chemicals such as hormones and cholesterol; ionizing and ultraviolet radiation; viruses; irritations from burns and wounds; and substances ingested in foods. Individuals are exposed to these agents through their work, in medical treatments, and in ordinary pursuits. Some types of exposures are avoidable (cigarette smoking being a notable example); others are not.

Immunologic Factors

The immune system (specifically the T-cell lymphocyte responses) is responsible for eradicating cancerous cells as they arise within the body. Failure of the immune system to respond to these tumor cells, either from an inherent defect or intentional suppression from immunosuppressive treatment, may result in cancer. For example, clients receiving immunosuppressive therapy, such as renal transplant clients, have a higher incidence of cancer than the general population, particularly tumors of suspected viral origin.

Psychosocial Factors

The association among psychosocial influences, stress, and cancer is unknown. Studies attempting to detect such a relation have been hampered by difficulties in establishing reliable and valid measurement tools, controlling variables, and interpreting apparent biases. Although research reports are thus far inconclusive, there is general agreement that psychologic determinants affect cancer incidence and survival. Several factors believed to be associated with cancer have been identified. These include unresolved conflicts; personality characteristics; loss of a significant other; feelings of hopelessness, helplessness, powerlessness, and frustration; psychosomatic disturbances, anxiety, and depression; and sexual disturbances.

The relation of stress to cancer is of growing concern. Early reports propose that stress may damage or alter the immune response, creating a favorable environment for the development of cancer. Because of the complexity of stress-related neurologic and immunologic responses, specific stress-induced effects are difficult to ascertain, however.

Recently, investigators have tried to confirm a common observation—cancer clients with a strong will to live and a positive attitude survive longer than those who passively accept and submit to their illnesses. The so-called "fighting spirit," or strong desire to live, has been associated with improved survival rates among clients with breast cancer.

Nutrition and Cancer

Widespread geographic epidemiologic evidence supports the notion that dietary habits play an important role in preventing and causing cancer. For example, the American diet, high in dietary fat, may be linked to the high incidence of breast and colon cancer, which occur at much lower rates in Asian countries, where dietary fat intake is low. However, in Asian countries including Japan, where the consumption of salted and pickled foods is high, gastric cancer is much commoner than in the United States. It is very difficult to confirm a direct cause-and-effect relation between nutrition and cancer because so many preexisting environmental carcinogens are responsible for cancer.

In search of more information, a Committee on Diet, Nutrition, and Cancer was formed under the direction of the National Cancer Institute to review the scientific data and formulate recommendations. The committee concluded that certain dietary factors are possibly linked to cancer:

- Obese persons tend to be at greater risk for cancer.
- A high-fat diet may increase the risk for cancer of the colon, prostate gland, and breast.
- Dietary fiber may protect against colon cancer. This association is a difficult one to assume because high-fiber diets are generally low in fat.
- High caloric intake may increase the risk for cancer in general because obesity and high fat intake are more likely.
- Carbohydrates show no demonstrable effects on carcinogenesis.

In addition, the American Cancer Society advocates avoiding obesity; cutting down on total fat intake; eating more high-fiber foods; consuming foods rich in vitamins A and C; eating cruciferous vegetables (named for their cross-shaped flowers) such as cabbage, cauliflower, broccoli, brussels sprouts, and kohlrabi; eating less salt-cured, smoked, and nitrite-cured foods; and drinking alcohol in moderation (no more than two drinks a day) if one drinks (American Cancer Society, 1984).

Physiologic Effects of the Oncogenic Process

As a malignant neoplasm develops and grows, many physiologic effects ensue, although millions of cancer cells may form before physical symptoms become apparent. Initially, effects may be localized. Eventually, as the tumor grows, becomes established, and metastasizes, systemic symptoms occur. Although the effects of tumor development vary according to the type of lesion and its location, certain effects are generally characteristic of all malignant neoplasms.

Local Effects

The three major local effects of increase in tumor mass are pressure, erosion of adjacent tissue, and obstruction. As the uncontrolled replication of the cancer cells causes the tumor to grow continually, the enlarging mass causes pressure atrophy in surrounding tissue. Necrosis of normal cells ensues, and tumor cells may also become necrotic as the mass enlarges. These effects are related to the sheer bulk of the tumor mass but also result from the invasive properties of cancer previously discussed. To supply the ever-increasing amounts of nutrients, particularly nitrogen, required by the enlarging tumor, an intricate system of collateral circulation develops. As this circulatory network grows, the risk of hemorrhage increases. The tumor mass may also exert pressure on adjacent organs or may obstruct an organ or the flow of blood or lymph.

Systemic Effects

The spectrum of local and systemic effects from cancer is manifested in conditions as diverse as the kinds of tumors and their sites. It is important to remember that during the course of the disease, a client may encounter one, many, or all such common physiologic problems as anemia, hemorrhage, infection, cachexia, and pain. The client may experience psychosocial responses ranging from anxiety or depression to profound changes in body image and lifestyle. Keep in mind that the degree of these problems depends on the type and extent of the tumor as well as treatment implications. Neoplastic disease as it affects specific organ systems is discussed in each specific disorders chapter in the body systems units.

Effects originally manifested locally may have systemic sequelae; for example, pressure of a tumor on the optic nerve can cause blindness; pressure on the spinal cord may cause paralysis; and obstruction of the bronchus interferes with respiration. A tumor may cause hypersecretion or hyposecretion of glandular hormones, leading to life-threatening systemic complications (eg, hypersecretion by the parathyroid glands may lead to hypercalcemia).

Probably the most universal systemic effect is cancer's ability to alter immunologic responses. Early in the development of malignant neoplasia, the immune system attempts to defend the host by attacking and destroying antigens on the surface of tumor cells. Eventually, in advanced malignant disease, the immune response is impaired. It is speculated that billions of tumor cells may deplete or overwhelm the immune system, reducing or destroying its capacity to defend the body from other insults such as trauma or infection.

ANEMIA Anemia, a common problem for clients with cancer, may be related to the neoplastic process itself or to cancer therapies. Recurrent hemorrhage, malnutrition, or infection may be contributing factors.

Several theories have been proposed to account for the anemia associated with cancer; a mild reduction in the survival capacity of erythrocytes, a level of erythropoietin lower than the existing degree of anemia would explain, and poor responsiveness of apparently normal bone marrow are among the mechanisms proposed. This type of anemia is usually mild, and specific treatment may not be indicated unless the client is symptomatic from the anemia or a correctable contributing cause such as hemorrhage or malnutrition can be identified. Anemia in a client with cancer has diagnostic significance because it indicates extensive disease progression.

Another type of anemia in clients with cancer is associated with tumor invasion of the bone marrow, either as a primary or metastatic site of involvement. Erythrocyte precursor stem cells may be impaired in leukemias, or erythrocyte development may be limited because marrow has been replaced with tumor cells (eg, metastasis from breast tumors and lymphomas). This type of anemia may be severe, necessitating blood replacement therapy.

Tumor-associated autoimmune hemolytic anemia is related to the body's immune defense against red blood cell antigens that have been stimulated by the tumor. The exact cause of this tumor-mediated response remains unknown. Autoimmune hemolytic anemia more often develops in clients with non-Hodgkin's lymphoma and chronic lymphocytic leukemia than in clients with other types of malignancies.

Anemia associated with blood loss is common in clients with gastrointestinal, head and neck, urinary, and uterine malignancies. As the tumor invades vascular structures and erodes tissues, bleeding results. Blood loss may be overt, an early symptom of cancer. The client may seek professional health care advice after noticing blood in the urine or stool or because of irregular vaginal bleeding.

Anemia is associated with many conditions other than cancer; however, because of its frequent association with malignant neoplasia, any anemic condition should be thoroughly investigated. When anemia occurs in a client in whom cancer has already been diagnosed, treatment is necessary to provide the optimal state of health consistent with the client's condition.

HEMORRHAGE Spontaneous hemorrhage may occur when a tumor obstructs an organ or blood vessel, impinges on or erodes a blood vessel during growth, or is surgically disrupted or manipulated. Severe bleeding, secondary to thrombocytopenia, may be an initial symptom of some malignancies of blood cells or blood-forming tissues (eg, leukemias, lymphomas, and multiple myeloma). Hemorrhage may be profound and visible or slow and occult. Detection of occult blood in the stool may signal a previously undetected malignancy.

When hemorrhage occurs, it must be diagnosed promptly. The site of hemorrhage must be quickly determined because emergency measures involve local control of bleeding along with replacement of necessary blood constituents (eg, red blood cells and platelets). Regardless of severity, location, or cause, hemorrhage is a potentially life-threatening condition that must be recognized and treated immediately.

INFECTION In clients with cancer, the immune system may be compromised by the disease process, the treatment modality, or both. Any condition that impairs the body's immunologic defenses creates a favorable environment for infection. These infections are usually opportunistic, resulting from overgrowth of normal flora (eg, oral candidiasis) or because flora that normally reside in one location gain access elsewhere (eg, *E. coli* septicemia).

No single agent of infection has been found to have a predilection for cancer clients; therefore, it is assumed that predisposing factors related to the client's physiologic status or surroundings govern infection. Common sites of infection in cancer clients are the lungs, gastrointestinal tract, anorectal area, skin, mouth, pharynx, urinary tract, and bloodstream. Although uncommon, the site of infection may be associated with the site of neoplastic lesion.

Infection related to neutropenia and immunosuppressive therapy is a major cause of mortality in clients with cancer. Because immunosuppression depresses or eliminates some of the usual signs of infection, diagnosis may be delayed. Therefore, the client must be observed carefully to detect signs of local infections such as erythema, induration, swelling (remember pus formation may be absent in severely leukopenic clients), pain, cough, and signs of systemic infections including elevated temperature and chills. Prompt therapy for immunologically suppressed clients with infections is essential to prevent life-threatening consequences such as septic shock. Because most infections are bacterial, antibiotic therapy may be instituted at the first sign of infection, even before identification of the causative organism. When anti-infective therapy is not effective in controlling the infection, granulocyte transfusions may be administered to clients who are neutropenic.

CACHEXIA Weight loss, related primarily to decreased caloric intake and in part to the increased metabolic requirements of the multiplying neoplastic cells, is a common initial symptom of cancer. On the other hand, cachexia related to anorexia is a life-threatening complication that usually develops late in the course of the disease. **Cachexia** is a syndrome characterized by anorexia, weakness, and emaciation—the "wasting away" associated with cancer. Cachexia is known to be related to decreased food intake, impaired absorption of nutrients, and alterations in metabolism, but the pathogenesis of the anorexia has not been clearly determined.

Researchers suspect that anorexia is caused from a combination of factors predominantly related to the tumor, therapy, and psychosocial effects. Among the factors believed to be associated with anorexia in clients with cancer are:

- Pain, fever, nausea, and other nonspecific manifestations
- Intestinal obstruction

- Alterations in metabolism
- Toxins produced by neoplastic tumors
- Ketosis
- Reactions related to treatments such as chemotherapy and radiation therapy
- Alterations in olfactory perceptions
- Psychologic factors (fear, anxiety, depression)

The anorexic client is trapped in a deadly cycle: Caloric (energy) requirements continually increase as the neoplasm grows; nutritional intake continually declines as factors related to the disease and therapy exacerbate the client's anorexia.

The nurse is a crucial participant in the client's struggle to halt or at least slow the life-threatening cycle. Providing small, palatable meals (blenderized if necessary), relieving pain and nausea, offering comfort measures, and removing offensive food odors are part of a multifaceted approach to cancer-related cachexia. At some point in the course of the disease, total parenteral nutrition may become necessary.

PAIN Of all the psychologic manifestations of cancer, pain is undoubtedly the best known and most feared. Ironically, fear and anxiety can potentiate the pain and interfere with therapies offered to relieve or mitigate it. Although pain is almost inevitable with the oncologic processes of invasion, pressure, and tissue erosion, the degree of pain varies greatly among individuals—even among those with similar diseases. As with many other cancer problems, factors such as tumor type, extent of disease, and site of involvement greatly influence the amount of pain.

The psychophysiologic mechanisms of pain are discussed in Chapter 3. In addition, specific physiologic as well as psychologic components of the cancer pain experience must be considered. The physical mechanisms include:

- Tumor destruction of bone
- Venous engorgement
- Arterial ischemia
- Pressure on nerves
- Inflammation, infection, ulceration, and necrosis

Bone pain from cancer is particularly devastating. A possible reason for the pain is that tumor invasion of bone causes the release of *prostaglandins,* hyperalgesic substances that sensitize nerve fibers, making them more vulnerable to painful stimuli (Twycross & Lack, 1983). Nonsteroidal anti-inflammatory agents (eg, Motrin, Indocin), which inhibit prostaglandins, are widely accepted in the treatment of tumor-induced bone pain.

In caring for the client with cancer, as with any client whose illness is accompanied by chronic pain, the nurse must continually explore the individual's perception of the pain and response to it. The site, intensity, and characteristics of pain should be assessed. Because the painful stimuli from cancer generally originate in body tissues that are not well innervated (eg, bone, blood vessels, and organs), the pain may be perceived as diffuse, vague, and poorly localized. The characteristics of the pain, often changing over time, may be difficult to express. The nurse can best help the client describe the pain sensation by asking the client to relate it to a situation or event that may illustrate the feeling. Simply asking a client with cancer pain, "How is your pain?" may be too broad an inquiry. Ask simple and specific questions to elicit information.

For many clients with cancer pain, a cycle of pain, anxiety, and depression leads to frustration, relentless suffering, and mental anguish. The primary goal of managing cancer pain is to prevent the recurrence or worsening of the pain—to interrupt the cycle. Consistent pain relief is usually accomplished through around-the-clock, not p.r.n., medication schedules; usually, a narcotic analgesic is given in accordance with its relief duration. Unfortunately, medication is sometimes withheld because of an unfounded fear that it will lead to drug addiction. In clients experiencing cancer pain, drug addiction is not a serious problem. In fact, very few cancer clients actually become addicted. It seems unnecessary to worry about an uncommon problem.

Continuous intravenous administration of morphine sulfate has been used to relieve cancer pain. This allows the client to control dosage as needed. Continuous interspinal morphine infusion is a method of analgesic therapy that relieves cancer pain without oversedation. In this method, morphine is infused through an infusion pump implanted in the abdomen and a catheter inserted in the interspinal space. In some settings, Brompton's cocktail, an oral mixture of morphine sulfate, cocaine, ethyl alcohol, and flavorings for palatability, may be given on schedule for pain control. Brompton's cocktail allows the client to be pain-free without stupor and oversedation.

Pharmacologic agents as well as other pain-relieving measures must be a part of a holistic approach. Mild diversion and distraction, relaxation therapy, hypnosis, cutaneous stimulation techniques (eg, transcutaneous electrical nerve stimulation, or TENS), and application of heat and cold may be helpful.

Psychosocial Dimensions of the Cancer Experience

The neoplastic process adds an extra dimension to the experience of illness. The client with cancer must cope with a multitude of internal and external stressors, and the client's significant others have their own problems to face.

A pertinent question during initial assessment is, "What problems and coping resources did the client have *before*

Table 10–2
Psychosocial Nursing Care Plan for the Client and Family, by Nursing Diagnosis

Client Care Goal	Plan/Nursing Implementation	Expected Outcome
Anxiety related to fear of death; fear of body mutilation and pain; prevailing attitudes and beliefs about cancer and cancer therapies; fear of social isolation/role alteration; financial concerns		
Minimize or alleviate anxieties associated with diagnosis, treatment, and long-term effects of cancer; provide emotional support to promote effective coping strategies	Acknowledge that anxiety associated with a diagnosis of cancer is normal; assist client and family in expressing concerns; explore attitudes and beliefs about cancer, dispel misconceptions; stress that responses to the effects of cancer and cancer therapies are individual; implement an organized teaching plan with consumer education materials; emphasize the client and family participation; instruct client regarding relaxation exercises; encourage client and family participation in support groups and educational programs, if available; assist client in formulating realistic goals for self-care, participation in therapy, and family and social interactions; allow client to maintain independence to the extent possible; use an open, honest approach for communication; recommend individual and family counseling, if necessary; offer hospice or palliative care, if available, for clients in the terminal phase of illness	Client will express concerns related to cancer; maintain optimal level of self-care, independence, and family and social interactions; use effective coping strategies to deal with effects of cancer
Self-concept, disturbance in body image related to effects of cancer: weight loss, cachexia, and visible changes (eg, skin lesions, ascites, or lymphedema); effects of cancer therapies such as surgery (physical alterations) and radiation and chemotherapy (alopecia, weight loss or gain)		
Promote a positive body image	Develop an honest and trusting relationship with client; explore with the client the perceived body-image changes; assist the client in coping with body-image changes; allow verbalization of feelings, encourage client to discuss feelings with significant others, allow client to focus on body parts that may not be affected, encourage client to look at physical alterations while the nurse or significant other is present to lend support; explore ways of minimizing altered body image (wigs, scarves, prosthesis); encourage adequate nutrition if possible to minimize weight loss	Client will express concerns regarding altered body image; exhibit ways of promoting a more positive body image (eg, taking interest in appearance)
Coping, ineffective individual/family related to role performance expectations; financial concerns; altered communication patterns		
Establish or maintain effective communication patterns between client and family; provide client- and family-centered care	Assess the family system (eg, communication patterns, role expectations, coping patterns); assess previous client and family losses and ways of dealing with these in the past; encourage open, honest communication; include the family in educational activities and encourage participation in client-centered activities; assist client to set realistic expectations for role as part of a family unit; refer client and family for counseling, if necessary; encourage the client to seek financial advice, if necessary	Client will discuss concerns related to illness with family
Self-concept, disturbance in related to role performance, related to inability to maintain personal and social responsibilities		
Assist the client in establishing realistic goals for personal and social role performance; encourage optimal participation in activities of daily living	Assist the client to identify strengths and weaknesses and to set realistic goals; allow the client to verbalize feelings of loss or grief over inability to maintain previous role function; assist the client to identify realistic role expectations that can be achieved and maintained; offer the client means of maintaining control and providing input into the plan of care; positively reinforce goal-oriented behaviors	Client will formulate realistic goals; manifest optimal interactions with family and environment; maintain optimal level of self-care and independence

Client Care Goal	Plan/Nursing Implementation	Expected Outcome
Knowledge deficit related to denial; anxiety; learning disabilities; pain and other discomforts		
Motivate clients and families to learn; encourage optimal client and family participation in care	Assess readiness to learn (usually can be determined by client and family expressing concerns and questions); remember clients who seem disinterested, preoccupied with other thoughts, denying effects of disease or therapy, or extremely anxious may not benefit from teaching plan until motivated and able to concentrate; identify information regarding the disease and effects of therapy that is essential for clients and families for optimal participation in care; prioritize necessary information and formulate a structured teaching plan to coincide with expected effects from disease or therapy; use various teaching methods, such as consumer publications (see resources list); remember teaching does not ensure learning; remember the elderly may need more time to learn; repeat teaching activities as necessary; evaluate the effectiveness of teaching plan; observe behaviors or desired outcomes as a result of teaching; encourage the client and family to write down their questions; for clients whose learning capacities are impaired, be sure to include family members in all teaching activities	Client will be able to repeat or know where to seek information essential to the plan of care; demonstrate behaviors indicative of learning

the cancer was diagnosed?" For example, does the client have a history of depressive illness? How might this affect response to the current diagnosis? To stresses imposed by treatment? To necessary adjustments of lifestyle? What social or environmental stressors might be affecting client or family in addition to those associated with neoplastic disease? Financial problems? Divorce or widowhood? Ill health of a spouse or child? What about attitudes toward cancer in the client's family? Social or cultural group? Work environment?

There is a "cancer mythology" in Western society—beliefs that influence societal attitudes toward persons with cancer and persons' attitudes toward themselves. These myths include:

- The *contagious myth*—the belief that cancer is "catching"
- The *pain myth*—the belief that the pain of cancer is inevitable, immediate, excruciating, unending, and uncontrollable
- The *treatment myth*—the belief that all cancer treatments are lengthy and painful
- The *mutilation myth*—the belief that all cancers cause mutilation and disfigurement and that all treatments cause extensive, permanent disfigurement

The myth of contagion is without foundation. Others carry sufficient truth to account for their longevity—cancer *may* be painful, and treatments *may* be debilitating and temporarily or permanently disfiguring. But myths that make the client's situation seem worse than it is impose unneeded burdens on both the client and society. For example, fear of contagion can isolate clients when they need maximum support from family and friends. Fear of contagion or a partner's unfounded concerns about damaging the client's health can unnecessarily curtail the client's sexual activity. Fear and misunderstanding can underlie societal discrimination against the individual with cancer; clients whose cancer is cured or in remission may lose their jobs or be unable to find employment. Those who have been treated for cancer at any time in their lives find insurance almost impossible to obtain.

Cancer imposes a large financial burden on client, family, and society. Individuals have expended their life savings on treatment; billions have been spent on research aimed at eradicating neoplastic disease. This burden is increased when individuals with cancer are restrained from leading productive lives because of cancer mythology.

Individuals respond to a diagnosis of cancer in themselves or a loved one in individual ways: fear ("Will I die?" "What will happen?"); guilt ("Am I too much of a burden?"); anger ("Why must this happen to *me*?"); despair ("It's no use; I know I'm doomed."). Families have similar reactions, whether directed inward or at the client. Hostility or fear, for example, may engender oversolicitude. Either client or significant others may relieve stress by lashing out angrily at others, including the nurse. Although the cost in time and patience may seem high, the gift of listening may be the greatest the nurse can offer the client. A psychosocial nursing care plan for the client with cancer is in Table 10–2.

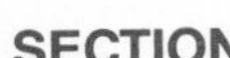

SECTION III

The Diagnosis of Cancer

Diagnosis of cancer has become a specialty in itself. Not only is early detection of malignant neoplasia crucial to the favorable outcome of treatment, but choice of treatment depends on correct identification of the tumor and evaluation of its stage of development. Improper diagnosis and delayed or inappropriate treatment can have fatal consequences.

Symptoms suggesting cancer should be investigated without delay. If the results of initial diagnostic evaluations are even slightly ambiguous, or if precancerous lesions are discovered, the client's progress must be monitored closely and frequently.

Diagnostic Techniques

Initial assessment of the client consists of a physical examination including visual inspection and palpation of the skin, lymph nodes, and organs as well as percussion of underlying body tissues. Often, such an examination is part of a routine physical examination with no prior suspicion of cancer. For female clients, a periodic Papanicolaou (Pap) smear is part of routine health maintenance; a Pap smear may also be ordered if a client reports such symptoms as dysmenorrhea or spotting. Hematologic studies and studies of the urine and stool are also part of the preliminary evaluation. Suspicious findings may be further investigated by x-ray, computerized tomography (CT) scan, ultrasonography, or thermography. Skin tests for immunologic response may also be employed.

Cell and Tissue Examination

Cancer can be diagnosed by microscopic evaluation because the morphology of cancer cells differs significantly from that of normal tissue. *Biopsy* refers to the removal and examination of a sample of tissue; *cytologic diagnosis* is microscopic evaluation of body secretions or body tissues to determine whether abnormal cells are present.

A biopsy may be performed as a separate procedure or during surgery. The specimen may be examined in a laboratory by embedding the tissue in paraffin and sectioning it for diagnosis, although this is time consuming. A faster method is the *frozen section* technique. Within minutes, a pathologist can ascertain whether a lesion is benign or malignant or whether malignancy has spread to lymph nodes or distant parts of the body. A portion of tumor tissue or adjacent tissue is frozen solid and a microtome slices off a thin section, which is prepared, stained, and microscopically examined. A frozen section can be performed during an operation so results are available immediately.

Techniques for obtaining a biopsy specimen include excisional biopsy, incisional biopsy, and needle (aspiration) biopsy. *Excisional biopsy* removes the entire tumor with a wide margin of normal tissue. Depending on the findings, further surgery may be performed. If the tumor is large, an *incisional biopsy* may be performed to remove a small section of the tumor. Incisional biopsy may be done during endoscopic surgery (eg, transurethral resection of the prostate). The amount of tumor and marginal tissue removed must be sufficient to permit a reliable diagnosis. One danger of incisional biopsy is seeding of tumor cells.

Needle or *aspiration biopsy,* a less definitive procedure, does not involve surgery. A hollow needle is inserted into the lesion, twisted, and withdrawn, bringing a core of tissue with it. One drawback of this technique is that, in the case of negative findings, one cannot be certain the appropriate site (the lesion) was sampled. Tumors with increased vascularity (eg, tumors of the thyroid gland) may hemorrhage insidiously after the procedure. The possibility of tumor cell seeding along the needle track is controversial. Needle biopsy has been used, however, in tumors involving the breast, lungs, and lymph nodes. *Punch biopsy,* a method to obtain a superficial sample of skin, is discussed in Chapter 64.

Abnormal cells shed by tumors may also be detected in body fluids and secretions that come into contact with the tumor and in tissue scrapings. Sometimes cytologic examination can detect a tumor when it is still microscopic, long before symptoms develop. One well-known cytologic technique is the Pap smear developed by Dr George Papanicolaou. Its widespread use has played an important role in reducing mortality associated with cervical cancer.

Circulating Tumor Markers

Among diagnostic techniques are tests for circulating tumor markers, blood-borne substances that are diagnostic of some forms of cancer. Human chorionic gonadotropin (HCG) and alpha-fetoprotein are glycoproteins useful in the diagnosis of germ cell tumors such as testicular cancer. Carcinoembryonic antigen (CEA) is a glycoprotein that is being employed as a tumor marker with some success in clients with colorectal adenocarcinoma. Although CEA is generally not detectable in the early stages of cancer, high levels of CEA have been correlated with large tumors or with metastasis. Thus, serial determinations of CEA are a means of monitoring the response of colorectal cancer to surgical removal of the tumor. CEA levels also may be elevated in carcinoma of the breast, prostate gland, lung, and pancreas; in hypothyroidism, liver disease, inflammatory bowel disease, and neuroblastoma; and in smokers (Byrne et al., 1986).

Classification and Staging

Once the existence of a neoplasm has been established, it must be classified and staged before appropriate treatment can be initiated. *Classification* identifies the neoplasm according to type and tissue of origin. *Staging* describes the extent of the disease.

Classification

Benign tumors may be classified as *polyps* if they arise from mucous membrane or *papillomas* if they arise from surface epithelium. Other benign tumors are identified by the suffix *oma* combined with a prefix denoting the cell of origin (eg, a benign tumor arising in neural tissue is called a *neuroma.*) The term *lymphoma* is the exception to this classification since it is used to denote a malignant process.

Malignant neoplasms are generally classified as carcinomas, sarcomas, leukemias, or lymphomas. A cancerous tumor is generally categorized according to the tissue of origin. A carcinoma is a malignant tumor that arises from surface, glandular, or parenchymal epithelium (eg, the outer layer of the skin, the lining of the thyroid gland, the glandular area of the breast, or the parenchyma of the kidney). Malignant tumors arising from surface epithelium are called *squamous cell carcinomas,* and those from glandular or parenchymal tissues are referred to as *adenocarcinomas.* Typically, carcinomas spread first through the lymph system and later through blood.

A *sarcoma* is a malignant tumor originating primarily in connective tissue such as bone, blood vessels, cartilage, muscle, adipose tissue, and neural tissue. In contrast to carcinomas, sarcomas usually spread initially through the blood, with less frequent metastases through the lymphatics.

Although the leukemias, some types of lymphomas, and multiple myeloma constitute their own separate categories, they share a common feature. Unlike carcinomas and sarcomas that generally are solid masses, these tumors proliferate diffusely throughout the blood and blood-forming organs. Because cells are scattered throughout the blood, these tumors are sometimes called *liquid tumors.* Classifications of neoplasms are listed in Table 10–3.

Staging

The American Joint Committee for Cancer Staging has developed a universal system of staging classification, the so-called TNM system. Stages of tumor growth are designated by a combination of letters and subscripts (eg, T designates a primary tumor; N designates lymph node involvement; and M designates metastasis). Numbers from 0 (no evidence) to 4 designate degree of involvement. TIS designates **carcinoma in situ,** or noninfiltrating carcinoma. Most tumors can be staged by this system.

Nursing Implications During the Diagnostic Process

The nurse's role in prevention, education, and early screening procedures is discussed in a later section of this chapter.

Table 10–3
Classification of Benign and Malignant Neoplasms

Origin	Benign	Malignant
Epithelial tissue:	"-oma"	"-carcinoma"
Glandular	Adenoma	Adenocarcinoma
Surface	Papilloma	Carcinoma (squamous cell, basal cell, transitional cell)
Mucous membrane	Polyp	
Connective tissue:	"-oma"	"sarcoma"
Smooth muscle	Leiomyoma	Leiomyosarcoma
Striated muscle	Rhabdomyoma	Rhabdomyosarcoma
Cartilaginous	Chondroma	Chondrosarcoma
Bone osteoblast	Osteoma	Osteosarcoma
Blood vessels	Hemangioma	Angiosarcoma
Lymphatics	Lymphangioma	Lymphangiosarcoma
Fibrous	Fibroma	Fibrosarcoma
Nerve sheath	Neurofibroma	Neurofibrosarcoma
Adipose	Lipoma	Liposarcoma
Embryonic tissue:	"-oma"	"-blastoma"
Kidney	—	Nephroblastoma
Retina	—	Retinoblastoma
Sympathetic ganglia and adrenal medulla	Ganglioneuroma	Neuroblastoma
Germ-cell layers:	Benign teratoma	Malignant teratoma

This section considers care of the client undergoing diagnostic studies after a symptom or sign has suggested the presence of cancer. These clients and their significant others will have many questions, voiced and unvoiced. Underlying all those questions is a fundamental one: What is going to happen to me—right now, in the hospital or outpatient area? How will it affect my life?

The Prediagnostic Phase

Waiting for a definitive diagnosis has been described as "the longest wait in the world." Nurses can best assist clients through this tense and anxious time by first assessing the client's knowledge base, attitudes, and possible misconceptions. Has someone the client knows well died of cancer? What type? What treatments were employed? How did the client view them? As effective? Painful? Palliative? Futile?

Does the client have current information about the suspected type of cancer? Is the information reliable? Or is it a compendium of TV "horror stories" and popular myths? Has the client understood the physician's explanation? (Teaching does not always mean that learning has taken place.) Does the client have at least a general understanding of the tests to be performed? If the tests are painful or uncomfortable, is the client prepared for this?

Are the client's significant others a source of support or of additional concern? Might friends or a spiritual counselor help the client through the waiting period? Or does the client truly prefer solitude? (Some individuals do.)

The prediagnostic phase is a good time to initiate client education about possible outcomes. Once a definite diagnosis of malignancy has been made, the nurse can assist the client in understanding and adjusting to the cancer experience.

The Postdiagnostic Phase

Characteristics of neoplastic disease account for some of the dread and despair the cancer diagnosis frequently evokes in clients and their significant others:

- The onset of cancer is often insidious and difficult to diagnose.
- Cancer metastasizes.
- If not discovered early and promptly controlled, cancer may be incurable; yet even early diagnosis does not necessarily guarantee cure.
- The etiology of the disease is not yet understood; treatment techniques have not been perfected.
- The treatments may be painful or disfiguring.
- No matter how willingly the client cooperates, the treatment regimen may fail, and the client may die.

Each individual confronts the diagnosis of cancer with a unique world view developed over a life span. A young, unmarried man with carcinoma of the testis will have one outlook and set of problems; the mother of three children who has cancer of the breast will have another. The childless widow whose relatives have all died before her will have an entirely different set of questions.

At the beginning of the cancer experience, the client may feel physically strong, yet the prospect of eventual disability must be faced. "Who will take care of me?" asks the client who lives alone. "Who will take care of them?" asks the parent of small children. "Who will support the family and pay my medical bills?" "Will it hurt? How much? For how long?" "Can I work? Garden? Take one last trip to the places I've always wanted to see?" "Will I live? Will I die? Will I live maimed?" A surprising number of persons may ask—or hesitate to ask—"Is it catching?"

Often the nurse is best qualified to address these spoken and unspoken concerns. The client's history and the nursing assessment provide clues on how to begin. Does the client understand the diagnosis and prognosis? If the client's mind is churning with anxieties and concerns, the physician's explanation may not have been absorbed. Was the information given in terms the client can understand? "The probability of metastasis is minimal" may need translation into "the cancer is not likely to have spread." The client's intelligence may be unaffected by the disease process, but the client's level of comprehension is almost certainly diminished by anxiety, pain, debilitation, or the side effects of medication.

Clients often hesitate to question their physicians; the nurse who has established trust and rapport during routine care may seem more approachable. Listening to the client is essential, and listening means attending to the client in several senses. Nonverbal signals may say more than words: the hesitant gesture that heralds a stifled impulse to speak, the slight frown that greets an unfamiliar phrase, the tensed facial muscles that reflect unvoiced pain. The nurse alert to these signals can encourage the client to ask questions about diagnostic studies, treatment options, and lifestyle changes and can encourage both client and family to voice their concerns. In responding, the nurse must be open and honest, engendering neither false hope nor unwarranted despair.

Home Health Care

When the client's concerns have been identified, the nurse may consult other members of the health care team or the community. The dietitian may offer recipes for blenderized meals that can be easily prepared at home; a local church or charitable organization may provide a hospital bed or other equipment for home care. A self-help organization may offer counsel from a member whose cancer has been cured or arrested; the psychiatric nurse specialist may suggest how the client can cope with fears. Simple interventions may do much to alleviate anxiety and offer the client hope. Examples are providing a catalog of wigs for the client undergoing chemotherapy or describing speech aids to the client awaiting a laryngectomy.

To provide this kind of assistance to the client, whether in the hospital, in a physician's office or outpatient facility, or in the client's home, the nurse must be familiar with the therapeutic options available to the client with cancer and those involved in his or her care.

SECTION IV

Primary and Secondary Prevention

Prevention is a concept not formerly associated with cancer; even a decade ago, the word was rarely heard in this connection. Today, cancer prevention offers exciting opportunities for nurses, especially in outpatient and ambulatory care. Community prevention activities are often managed by nurses. Urban and rural cancer detection clinics are gaining wider acceptance. Nurses working in these settings, in physician's offices, and in health maintenance organizations are finding that nursing assessment and education can make a life-saving difference.

Primary prevention of cancer (ie, prevention of its occurrence) presents difficulties because knowledge of the etiology of many forms of cancer is incomplete. Even with known carcinogens, a simple cause-and-effect relation may not have been demonstrated. For example, although cigarette smoking has been clearly associated with lung and laryngeal cancer, not all smokers contract the disease.

Primary prevention is presently directed at eliminating occupational and environmental carcinogens, identifying high-risk populations, and protecting individuals who have been exposed to carcinogenic agents (eg, asbestos). Major risk factors and symptoms and signs of common cancers are in Table 10–4. A painstaking nursing assessment, particularly the health history, can contribute a great deal to identifying individuals at risk and providing follow-up investigation and lifestyle education.

Cancer does not have the infectious properties of other diseases for which prevention programs have been successful. Measures such as isolation of affected individuals or mass inoculation are not applicable to cancer. For this reason, *secondary prevention* (early detection) is significant in reducing cancer-related morbidity and mortality.

For many years, community education has stressed regular checkups and awareness of cancer's seven warning signals (Box 10–1). More recently, self-administered screening such as self-examination of the breasts and testing for blood in the stool, and noninvasive cytologic testing such as the Pap smear have been emphasized. Comprehensive programs of public education directed at both primary and secondary prevention of cancer include:

- Informing the community that some cancers are preventable and explaining preventive measures
- Enhancing public awareness of risk factors, including those related to lifestyle

Table 10–4
Major Risk Factors and Common Symptoms and Signs for Common Cancers

Type of Cancer	Risk Factors, Signs, and Symptoms
Colon–rectum	History of rectal polyps; rectal polyps run in family; history of ulcerative colitis; blood in stool; over age 40
Lung	Heavy cigarette smoker over age 50; started cigarette smoking at age 15 or before; smoker working with or near asbestos
Uterine–endometrial	Unusual bleeding or discharge; late menopause (after age 55); diabetes, high blood pressure, and overweight; aged 50+
Uterine–cervical	Unusual bleeding or discharge; frequent sex in early teens or with many partners; low socioeconomic background; poor care during or following pregnancy
Breast	Lump or nipple discharge; history of breast cancer; close relatives with history of breast cancer; over age 35, especially over age 50; never had children; first child after age 30
Skin	Excessive exposure to sun; fair complexion; work with coal tar, pitch, or creosote
Oral	Heavy smoker and drinker; poor oral hygiene
Ovarian	History of ovarian cancer among close relatives; aged 50+; never had children
Prostate	Aged 60+; difficulty in urinating
Stomach	History of stomach cancer among close relatives; diet heavy in smoked, pickled, or salted foods

SOURCE: Reprinted with permission from *Cancer Facts and Figures 1980*. New York: American Cancer Society, 1980.

Box 10–1
Cancer's Seven Warning Signals

1. Change in bowel or bladder habits
2. A sore that does not heal
3. Unusual bleeding or discharge
4. Thickening or lump in breast or elsewhere
5. Indigestion or difficulty in swallowing
6. Obvious change in wart or mole
7. Nagging cough or hoarseness

SOURCE: Reprinted with permission from American Cancer Society.

- Teaching techniques all persons can use to detect early evidence of neoplasia, eg, breast, testicular, and oral self-examination
- Informing the public of the advantages of early detection (eg, publishing comparative mortality and morbidity data)
- Explaining diagnostic techniques used for early detection of cancer, including information on where to obtain these services

Guidelines for the early detection of cancer are in Box 10–2.

Screening Techniques

Most screening techniques are not designed for diagnosis of specific malignancies. Rather, screening evaluates the well population and detects signs that might indicate neoplasia. Individuals with positive signs are referred for more precise evaluation. Health teaching, including personal hygiene, lifestyle risk factors, and self-examination techniques, may also be part of a screening program.

Noninvasive diagnostic techniques in early detection of cancer include:

- Examination of stool for occult blood
- Ultrasonography, mammography, and thermography for mammary or prostatic cancer
- Injection of radiopharmaceuticals to detect hypervascularization or irregular vascularization of masses (ie, radioisotope scan)
- Cytologic study of serum or body fluids (eg, Pap smear of nipple discharge)

By explaining these techniques, which are painless and relatively simple outpatient procedures, the nurse can encourage clients and the public to seek prompt evaluation of any suspicious symptoms.

Self-Examination Techniques

Self-examination of the breasts and testes is described in Chapter 5, and oral cavity self-examination is described in Chapter 38. Although breast examination has been widely publicized, many women still do not practice it. The nurse can encourage more widespread use of this lifesaving technique by stressing the value of early diagnosis in possibly avoiding the radical dissection that women fear.

Testicular self-examination has been less widely publicized than examination of the breasts. Yet carcinoma of the testis is the third most common tumor in males between ages 20 and 35—the prime reproductive years. Tragically, the usual time between onset of this disease and diagnosis is 6 months; if not detected early, testicular cancer can spread rapidly. Obviously, greater public awareness is needed.

Oral self-examination also has not received as much emphasis as breast self-examination. Yet, because minor lesions in the mouth are common, an early sign of oral cancer may easily be missed. Counsel clients to consult a health professional promptly if a sore in the mouth fails to heal within a few weeks. Regular dental checkups should include a meticulous oral examination; more frequent teaching of oral examination by dentists is encouraging.

SECTION V

Cancer Treatment

The basic treatment modalities for cancer have changed little in the past decade; surgery, chemotherapy, and radiation therapy remain the mainstays of therapy. What has changed are the precision of these techniques and the skill with which they are combined.

Surgery

Surgery, alone or in combination with other therapies, continues to be the preferred treatment for many forms of malignancy. Surgery may be performed for diagnostic purposes, for staging, to control effects of the tumor (eg, pressure, obstruction, or hemorrhage), or for palliation. In some cases (eg, carcinoma in situ), surgery alone may be curative.

Principles of Surgical Treatment

Curative or definitive surgery was performed more frequently before the concept of micrometastasis was fully understood. It was thought that the more extensive the surgery, the better the chance for cure. Traditionally, large masses were excised with a considerable amount of normal marginal tissue, often at great physical and emotional cost to the client. The classic example is the radical Halsted mastectomy, which included extensive surgical removal of

Box 10–2
Guidelines for the Early Detection of Cancer in Persons Without Symptoms 

Age 20–40

Cancer-Related Checkup Every 3 Years
Should include the procedures listed below plus health counseling (such as tips on quitting cigarettes) and examinations for cancers of the thyroid, testes, prostate, mouth, ovaries, skin, and lymph nodes. *Some persons are at higher risk for certain cancers and may need to have tests more frequently.*

Breast
- Exam by health care provider every 3 years
- Self-exam every month
- One baseline mammogram between ages 35 and 40

Higher risk for breast cancer: personal or family history of breast cancer, never had children, first child after 30

Uterus
- Pelvic exam every 3 years

Cervix
- Pap test—after two initial negative tests 1 year apart—*at least* every 3 years, includes women under 20 if sexually active

Higher risk for cervical cancer: early age at first intercourse, multiple sex partners

Age 40 and Over

Cancer-Related Checkup Every Year
Should include the procedures listed below plus health counseling (such as tips on quitting cigarettes) and examinations for cancers of the thyroid, testes, prostate, mouth, ovaries, skin, and lymph nodes. *Some persons are at higher risk for certain cancers and may need to have tests more frequently.*

Breast
- Exam by doctor every year
- Self-exam every month
- Mammogram every year after 50 (between ages 40 and 50, ask your doctor)

Higher risk for breast cancer: personal or family history of breast cancer, never had children, first child after 30

Uterus
- Pelvic exam every year

Cervix
- Pap test—after two initial negative tests 1 year apart—*at least* every 3 years

Higher risk for cervical cancer: early age at first intercourse, multiple sex partners

Endometrium
- Endometrial tissue sample at menopause if at risk

Higher risk for endometrial cancer: infertility, obesity, failure of ovulation, abnormal uterine bleeding, estrogen therapy

Colon and Rectum
- Digital rectal exam every year
- Guaiac slide test every year after 50
- Proctologic exam—after two initial negative tests 1 year apart—every 3 to 5 years after 50

Higher risk for colorectal cancer: personal or family history of colon or rectal cancer, personal or family history of polyps in the colon or rectum, ulcerative colitis

SOURCE: Reprinted with permission from American Cancer Society.

chest wall muscles and axillary lymphatics and resulted in extensive changes in body image and body function (eg, concave chest wall and lymphedema of the affected arm). Recently, studies have shown no significant difference in survival between the Halsted procedure and less radical procedures such as the modified radical or simple mastectomy. The benefits of wide local resections of tumor and normal tissue are questionable now that it is known that tumor cells may spread to distant areas even at an early stage. Radical surgery is still performed, but the trend is toward supplementing less extensive surgical procedures with chemotherapy, radiation therapy, or immunotherapy.

Palliative surgery has the goal of client comfort rather than cure. For example, a tumor may be surgically reduced to relieve invasion of adjacent tissue or remove obstruction, improving the client's condition and allowing time for systemic treatments to take effect. *Ablative* surgery, which involves surgical alteration of the endocrine system, may be employed in clients who have hormone-dependent tumors. Examples of ablative surgery, which is considered palliative, are hypophysectomy, adrenalectomy, oophorectomy, and orchiectomy.

A controversial procedure known as "second-look surgery" is sometimes a part of treatment, usually for gastrointestinal or ovarian cancer. An exploratory laparotomy is performed at the site of a resection to determine whether chemotherapy or radiation treatment has been successful.

Nursing Implications of Surgical Treatment

Underlying all nursing care of the client with cancer must be an awareness of the psychic and physiologic stress imposed by neoplastic disease. The client recovering from first-time surgery asks first, "Will my cancer recur?" After subsequent procedures, the question may be, "Did they get it all this time?" All clients wonder, "What will happen now?"

Surgical treatments for cancer produce changes in body image and lifestyle, some of them profound. No matter how well prepared a client may have been for these changes, the immediate postoperative period may hold surprises, even shocks.

Clients who have had mutilating surgery may fear they are repulsive to others. Habits of a lifetime must be changed; actions taken for granted must be relearned. Significant others, too, must adapt to a changed status. For these reasons, the nurse's continuing assessments, care planning, and evaluation of outcomes must encompass psychosocial as well as physiologic status. As much as possible, the client and the family must be involved in decision making and encouraged to participate in care. (A plan for nursing care related to psychosocial aspects is in Table 10–2.) Nursing implications of specific surgical procedures are described in the specific disorders chapters in Units 3–13.

Chemotherapy

Today a wide range of chemotherapeutic agents is available for treating neoplastic disease. All act in some fashion to destroy cancer cells or inhibit their function. Unfortunately, these agents do not affect cancer cells exclusively; normal cells may be damaged or destroyed as well.

Principles of Chemotherapy

No single drug has been found capable of destroying tumor cells during all stages of the cell cycle. Some kill proliferating cells more effectively than resting cells. These agents are labeled *cell cycle specific* (CCS). *Phase-specific* agents kill or arrest dividing cells during a specific phase of the cell cycle. Others that kill both dividing and resting cells are called *cell cycle nonspecific* (CCNS).

Agents used in treating human cancers generally can be assigned to one of seven categories. *Alkylating agents* bind and brace the double-helix DNA strands, preventing the strands from separating (a necessary step for replication). Although alkylating agents, *nitrosoureas* are classified in a separate category based on their lipid solubility and unique ability to cross the blood–brain barrier.

The chemical structure of *antimetabolites* closely resembles that of normally occurring compounds needed by the tumor cell for functional processes or mitosis. Once the tumor cell has incorporated the "imitation," its function is inhibited or destroyed. Like antimetabolites, *antibiotics* prevent the tumor cell from synthesizing DNA and RNA by interfering with synthesis of nucleic acids.

Plant alkaloids are all strong mitotic inhibitors. *Hormones and steroids* are used in the treatment of hormonally dependent tumors such as some breast and prostate cancers. Hormonal therapy disrupts the hormonal environment, making it unfavorable for the tumor to survive. *Miscellaneous agents* share little or no common properties or mechanisms of action with previously classified drugs. Some antineoplastic agents are listed and classified in Box 10–3.

Chemotherapeutic agents may be administered alone or in combination. *Single-agent therapy* is usually reserved for the treatment of tumors showing little or no response to other agents or for high-dosage chemotherapy (dosages exceeding the normal range of a particular drug) to avoid added toxicities of other drugs.

Combination chemotherapy is preferred to single-agent therapy. The major intent is to optimize "cell kill" and minimize additive side effects or toxicities by combining drugs with varied tumoricidal actions and different side effects. Usually, a drug regimen includes cycle-specific agents or phase-specific agents along with cell cycle nonspecific agents. For example, a phase-specific agent of the vinca alkaloid category causing arrest at the M-phase may be followed by another phase-specific agent from the antimetabolite category causing cell kill at the S-phase (see Figure 10–2).

Clinical Trials of Chemotherapeutic Agents

Investigation of new chemotherapeutic agents and methods of administration continues. Extensive research projects, commonly referred to as protocols, or clinical trials, are underway once a new agent has proved effective in laboratory tests. A protocol is a formal research document with all information necessary to conduct clinical trials, including an informed consent form. A client participating in any investigative protocol should be aware of the risks and benefits of treatment as well as the conventional treatment available. Before being approved by the Food and

Nursing Research Note

Farrel S, Bubela N, Hall–Burlein S: High-volume chemodialysis: A new outpatient program. *Can Nurse* (Feb) 1985; 81:44–47.

This ongoing research is attempting to determine the effectiveness of high-volume intraperitoneal chemotherapy for the treatment of cancer. Chemotherapy is instilled via a Tenckhoff catheter, currently the most widely used catheter for peritoneal dialysis.

Although the efficacy of this procedure for cancer treatment is unknown, the researchers have found many psychosocial benefits. Because the dressing procedure itself is lengthy, it allows for nurse–client interaction. This treatment also has been found to provide additional hope for a response to treatment. The treatment form has reduced hospitalization time and is less disruptive to the client's daily life. It also promotes client participation and reduces feelings of dependence, loss of control, and helplessness.

Drug Administration (FDA), a drug must be subjected to research trials. To ensure valid and reliable findings, the National Cancer Institute has developed strict standards for clinical trials.

Clients undergoing clinical trials should be encouraged to raise questions and discuss concerns about the options at hand. For these clients, the National Cancer Institute's *What Are Clinical Trials All About?* is a helpful client information booklet (see the resources listing at the end of this chapter).

Administration of Chemotherapy

Many nurses care for clients receiving chemotherapy, but only those who are specially trained should administer these drugs intravenously. Chemotherapeutic agents can be irritating to the veins and may cause phlebitis. Therefore, good vein care is essential. Measures include changing IV sites every 48 to 72 hours, flushing the drug through the vein adequately, and applying warm soaks to phlebitic sites.

Other drugs classified as sclerosing agents or vesicants (see Box 10–3) cause severe tissue inflammation and necrosis if **extravasation** (leakage of a drug into the surrounding tissues) occurs. It is generally agreed that only skilled phlebotomists should administer these drugs. Management of extravasation depends on the individual drug and is highly controversial. The Oncology Nursing Society (1984) has developed recommendations for chemotherapy drug extravasations. If extravasation is suspected with drugs *other* than the plant alkaloids, the intravenous needle should remain in place, and ice applied to the area. Steroids or anti-inflammatory agents may be injected through the needle or into the surrounding tissues. For extravasation of plant alkaloids, heat is applied to the area, and hyaluronidase injections are given via the IV needle and subcutaneously into the extravasation site.

Many antineoplastic drugs are mutagenic, and some are carcinogenic, posing hazards for health professionals handling them. Because these drugs can be absorbed through skin and mucous membranes by inhalation and direct skin contact in an unprotected environment, any

Box 10–3
Classification of Selected Antineoplastic Agents

Alkylating agents
Bis (chloroethyl) amines:
*Mechlorethamine, nitrogen mustard (Mustargen)
Cyclophosphamide (Cytoxan, Neosar)
L-phenylalanine mustard, melphalan (Alkeran)
Chlorambucil (Leukeran)

Ethylenimine derivatives:
Thiotepa (Triethylenethiophosphoramide)

Alkyl sulfonates:
Busulfan (Myleran)

Triatenes:
*Dacarbazine, DTIC (DTIC-Dome)

Nitrosoureas
BCNU, carmustine
CCNU, lomustine (CeeNU)
Methyl-CCNU
Streptozocin (Zanosar)

Antimetabolites (inhibitors of nucleic acid biosynthesis)
Folic acid antagonists:
Methotrexate, MTX, amethopterin

Purine antagonists:
6-mercaptopurine, 6-MP (Purinethol)
6-thioguanine, 6-TG

Pyrimidine synthesis inhibitors:
+5-azacytidine
5-fluorouracil, 5FU, fluorouracil (Adrucil)
Cytosine arabinoside, ARA-C (Cytosar)

Antibiotics
*Doxorubicin hydrochloride (Adriamycin)
Bleomycin (Blenoxane)
*Dactinomycin, actinomycin D (Cosmegen)
*Daunorubicin, daunomycin (Cerubidine)
*Mithramycin (Mithracin)
*Mitomycin, mitomycin-C (Mutamycin)
+Mitoxantrone (Novantrone)

Plant alkaloids
+*Vindesine (Eldesine)
+*Teniposide, VM-26
*Vinblastine, VLB (Velban)
*Vincristine, VCR (Oncovin)
Etoposide, VP-16-213 (VePesid)

Hormones
Steroids:
Prednisone
Dexamethasone (Decadron)

Sex hormones:
Diethylstilbestrol (DES)
Conjugated estrogens
Androgens
Progesterones
Antiestrogens:
Tamoxifen

Miscellaneous
+*Amsacrine, M-AMSA
Cisplatin (Platinol)
L-Asparaginase (Elspar)
Procarbazine (Matulane)
Hydroxyurea (Hydrea)

*Vesicant/sclerosing agents
+Investigational (not yet commercially available)

person mixing or giving chemotherapeutic agents should take precautions. The Public Health Service (US Department of Health and Human Services, 1983), the National Study Commission on Cytotoxic Exposure (1984), and the Oncology Nursing Society (1984) have developed guidelines for safe handling of parenteral cytotoxic agents:

- All parenteral chemotherapeutic agents should be prepared by skilled personnel under a vertical laminar flow unit or biologic safety cabinet.
- Personnel mixing should wear a long-sleeved protective garment, surgical latex gloves, and face mask and goggles if a protective glass shield is not available.
- Surgical latex gloves should be worn for all chemotherapy-related preparation, handling, and disposal. (Polyvinyl chloride gloves are permeable and should *not* be worn.)
- All materials used in preparation and administration of antineoplastic drugs should be disposed of as toxic waste.

Toxic Effects of Chemotherapy

Because chemotherapy affects both normal and malignant cells, some normal cellular function is sacrificed. Many of the effects on normal cells are reversible; however, the repair or recovery time of normal cells often determines or limits the dosage, frequency, and total duration of antineoplastic therapy. Each antineoplastic drug has a maximum tolerated therapeutic range beyond which certain toxicities may occur, some irreversible. Constant monitoring is necessary to ensure toxicity does not exceed predetermined limits.

Myelosuppression (suppressive alteration in the function of the bone marrow), a side effect of most antineoplastic agents, is reflected by leukopenia (neutropenia), thrombocytopenia, and less frequently anemia. Usually leukopenia and thrombocytopenia are more pronounced than anemia because the life span of erythrocytes is approximately 120 days, whereas the life span of leukocytes and thrombocytes is much shorter. Because erythrocytes are less affected, anemia associated with chemotherapy is generally mild. Hemorrhage may be a life-threatening consequence of thrombocytopenia associated with bone marrow suppression.

Cytotoxicity is especially likely to affect cells that proliferate rapidly. For example, some cells of the gastrointestinal tract are replaced every 3 days. Drugs that kill cells during the S phase of the cell cycle (eg, antimetabolite drugs) generally cause toxic side effects in the gastrointestinal tract. Diarrhea, mucositis, or stomatitis as well as nausea and vomiting may result from cell damage. Nausea and vomiting probably are caused by central nervous system irritation or excitation, which triggers the vomiting center of the brain.

Integumentary side effects of chemotherapy include alopecia (hair loss), rashes, hyperpigmentation, and altered nail growth. Although these conditions may not be life threatening, they are disturbing to clients, who may already be dealing with severe alterations in body image related to surgical treatment.

Long-term administration of certain antineoplastic agents may produce cumulative effects on the tissue of the lungs, liver, heart, kidney, and nerves. Examples include doxorubicin and daunorubicin cardiotoxicity and bleomycin lung toxicity. Physiologic testing is often used regularly to monitor the status of each organ system. Use of these agents is associated with abnormal sperm production and possibly sterility in males. The ova may be less affected than the sperm, although women may also have temporary or permanent sterility. The drug, dosage, and duration of administration are important variables determining the effects on fertility in any client.

Nursing Implications of Chemotherapy

In addition to their underlying disease, clients receiving chemotherapy experience unpleasant, worrisome, and sometimes life-threatening side effects related to the therapy. Offering emotional support and information on which the client can base decisions is essential.

The nursing care plan in Table 10–5 outlines the nursing diagnoses, goals, interventions, and evaluations related to chemotherapy. Nursing diagnoses related to anxiety, knowledge deficit, and body image changes experienced by clients on chemotherapy are addressed in the psychosocial care plan presented in Table 10–3.

Radiation Therapy

Radiation therapy plays an important role in the treatment of localized malignancies, whether alone or in combination with surgery or chemotherapy. Approximately 60% of clients with cancer receive some form of radiotherapy (Phillips, 1982).

Principles of Radiation Therapy

In radiation therapy, ionizing radiation is delivered in cancericidal doses to destroy tumor cells. Ionizing radiation includes both particulate radiation (alpha and beta particles) and electromagnetic or gamma radiation (x-ray or gamma rays). Alpha radiation has poor penetration ability and is rarely used in therapeutic radiation therapy. Beta radiation, with more penetration potential than alpha radiation, is generally emitted from radioactive isotopes (^{32}P, ^{131}I) and used for internal source radiation. Electromagnetic or gamma radiation penetrates deeper areas of the body.

The dual objectives of radiation therapy are to maximize tumor cell destruction ("cell kill") and minimize destruction or mutation of neighboring normal cells.

Table 10–5
Nursing Care Plan for the Client Receiving Chemotherapy, by Nursing Diagnosis

Client Care Goal	Plan/Nursing Implementation	Expected Outcome
Nutrition, altered related to nausea and vomiting; anorexia; mucositis/stomatitis; diarrhea; constipation		
Prevent or minimize nausea and vomiting; increase nutritional intake during and after treatment; minimize weight loss	Monitor intake and output. Encourage fluids >2 L/day; administer antiemetics as premedication ½–1 h before chemotherapy treatment (eg, Decadron, Compazine, Reglan and continue posttreatment; monitor weights at least weekly; encourage good oral hygiene (see alterations in mucous membranes); encourage high-protein foods such as cheeses, meats, yogurt, milkshakes (be aware lactose intolerance resulting in diarrhea may occur in adults who seldom drink milk); suggest cold foods without strong odors (eg, cottage cheese, cold fruits, cold cuts); consult a dietitian if necessary; institute calorie counts; ask clients at home to keep a diet history; assess for peripheral edema and sacral edema from decreased serum protein	Client will state causes of nausea and vomiting; identify methods of controling nausea and vomiting; modify diet to enhance food and fluid intake; maintain a stable weight during treatment
Nutrition, altered related to adjuvant chemotherapy for breast cancer; steroid therapy; hormonal therapy; estrogens, antiestrogens, androgens		
Prevent or minimize weight gain; assist the client in coping with side effects of therapy	Monitor daily weights; provide dietary counseling for caloric intake control; warn client of potential side effects of steroids (weight gain; increased blood glucose; gastrointestinal upset; acne of face, neck, and chest areas; fluid retention; fat depostion on cheeks, shoulders, and abdomen; emotional changes); warn female clients of potential side effects of androgens (masculinization; fluid retention; weight gain); warn female clients of potential effects of antiestrogens (amenorrhea; hot flashes; weight gain); warn client of potential side effects of estrogens (gynecomastia; fluid retention); instruct client to avoid food high in sodium; assess for edema of hands and ankles and for pedal edema from fluid retention; administer diuretics as ordered; monitor blood and urine glucose for clients on steroid therapy; instruct client in signs and symptoms of hyperglycemia if taking steroids	Client will manifest minimal weight gain (<5 lb) and fluid retention; modify diet appropriately; cope with changes in physical appearance; state signs and symptoms of hyperglycemia if on steroids
Fluid volume deficit, potential related to nausea and vomiting; anorexia; diarrhea; constipation; dehydration; hypokalemia as a result of steroid therapy; hypomagnesemia as a result of cisplatin		
Maintain optimal fluid and electrolyte balance	Encourage fluid intake of greater than 2 L/day; monitor intake and output; assess skin turgor; monitor urine specific gravity if necessary; check blood chemistry studies for Na^+, Cl^-, Mg^{++}; institute measures to control: nausea and vomiting, diarrhea, and constipation to prevent fluid and electrolyte loss and promote fluid intake; administer K^+ and Mg^{++} supplements as ordered	Client will consume more than 2 L/day of fluids with output comparisons ⅔ of intake; laboratory studies will remain within normal limits
Bowel elimination, altered: diarrhea, as a result of cytotoxic effects on intestinal mucosa		
Maintain integrity of the GI mucosa	Assess number and consistency of stools; administer antidiarrhea medications as ordered (Lomotil, Imodium), higher doses of Metamucil (2 tbsp in water or juice q.i.d.) to add bulk to stool; encourage fluids (no fruit juices); instruct client to avoid raw fruit, vegetables, and bran-containing foods high in fiber and to eat a low-residue diet; encourage foods high in potassium; test all stools for occult blood; assess for abdominal pain or distention; observe for signs and symptoms of GI bleeding (black tarry stools, decreased Hct and Hb, hypotension, tachycardia)	Client will state the importance of recording number and consistency of stools; modify diet appropriately; experience none or few problems with diarrhea and/or intestinal ulceration

Continued

Table 10–5 (continued)
Nursing Care Plan for the Client Receiving Chemotherapy, by Nursing Diagnosis

Client Care Goal	Plan/Nursing Implementation	Expected Outcome
Bowel elimination, altered: constipation related to: neurotoxicity from vinblastine and vincristine administration; immobilization and decreased fluid intake		
Prevent or minimize constipation	Administer stool softeners as ordered and laxatives if no bowel movement q 48 h; force fluids and high-fiber diet; encourage ambulation; place client on daily bowel check; instruct client to report frequency of stool	Client will experience no problem with constipation; modify diet and fluid intake appropriately
Tissue perfusion, altered related to direct cytotoxic effects on bone marrow reserves (iliac crests and sternum): leukopenia; thrombocytopenia; anemia		
Leukopenia; prevent and minimize potential risk for infection	Monitor temperature and other vital signs q. 4 h; assess areas of body for signs and symptoms of infection: mouth: lesions, changes in color (pallor vs erythema), soreness, swelling; rectum: tenderness, induration, discoloration, hemorrhoids; GI: constipation/diarrhea daily bowel checks, institute measures to avoid constipation; skin: redness, swelling, induration, lesions, pain; urinary: pain, burning on urination, frequency/urgency, odor; respiratory: pain, cough, secretions (note color and amount). Control environmental factors: strict handwashing, no fresh flowers, fresh fruits, or raw vegetables, screen visitors for colds, viruses (eg, nausea and vomiting, diarrhea, etc), exposure to infectious diseases (eg, chickenpox); avoid invasive procedures: no IM injections; no rectal temperatures, enemas, or suppositories; no urinary catheters; intermittent straight catheter preferred to in-dwelling when necessary; provide client education: instruct client to avoid trauma, use electric razor, wear shoes when out of bed, avoid straining at BM; teach clients signs and symptoms of infection to observe for and report; teach client to take own temperature when at home and report elevations >100.5°F or shaky chills immediately	Leukopenia: client will manifest minimal signs and symptoms of infection; identify signs and symptoms of infection to observe and report; practice appropriate health behaviors to prevent infection
Thrombocytopenia: prevent and minimize potential risk for bleeding	Check platelet counts daily: normal count 150,000–300,000 μL; instruct clients with platelet count <100,000 μL to: use electric razor (no straight-edge blades); use soft toothbrush; report any bruising or bleeding from rectal area, vagina (menstruation), gums, nose; assess daily for signs and symptoms of bleeding; check oral mucosa and dependent parts for petechiae; test all excreta: urine, stool, emesis, sputum; assess neurologic status (headache, blurred vision) for clients with platelet counts <20,000 μL; check skin for ecchymosis, purpura, petechiae; do a pad count for menstruating women; avoid invasive procedures if platelet count < 75,000 μL: no IM injections, rectal temperatures; no urinary catheters, especially if platelet count <50,000 μL; avoid prolonged BP cuff use, or tourniquet application if platelet count <50,000 μL; apply pressure to venipuncture sites 3–5 min; place clients with active bleeding on bed rest; clients with platelet count <20,000 μL should have activity modifications (bed rest, ambulation with assistance); avoid administration of any aspirin-containing compounds; administer platelet transfusions if necessary; assess for fever >101°F, and report to physician because circulating platelet survival time is decreased with fevers	Thrombocytopenia: client will be free from active bleeding; recognize factors that increase risk for bleeding; observe and report early signs of actual or potential bleeding; practice appropriate behaviors to prevent or minimize bleeding
Anemia: adequate tissue perfusion will be maintained	Observe for signs and symptoms of anemia: SOB, H/A, pallor, dizziness, hypotension, tachycardia, palpitations; instruct client to report these symptoms if present; check Hb and Hct; administer blood transfusions as ordered	Anemia: client will state the signs and symptoms of anemia

Client Care Goal	Plan/Nursing Implementation	Expected Outcome
Tissue integrity, impaired: oral mucous membranes related to direct cytotoxic action causing inflammation of buccal and gingival membranes, decrease in saliva, changes in normal flora (usually seen with antimetabolite chemotherapeutic agents); myelosuppression; poor oral hygiene		
Maintain integrity of oral mucosa; foster compliance with good oral hygiene practices	Institute preventive measures; instruct client to: brush teeth in AM and PM with soft brush or oral swabs and mild nonabrasive toothpaste (preferably Crest, Sensodyne); rinse with saline q.i.d. (P.C. and H.S.); avoid commercial mouthwashes; remove ill-fitting dentures between meals; assess for signs and symptoms of early mucositis and alert client to these: swollen, thick mucous membranes; erythematous or pale membranes; increased sensitivity to hot and cold foods; oral discomfort; burning sensation in mouth. Inspect oral mucous membranes daily for ulcerations or lesions, color changes (erythema/pallor), swelling, candidiasis (white opaque lesions), and mouth ulcers. Administer mycostatin mouth rinses or lozenges to prevent or treat oral candidiasis. Institute measures to manage mucositis if present: reinforce preventive measures; soft diet if tolerated; warm, frequent saline rinses or lavage; determine appropriate solution(s) for oral irrigations or rinses with physician (¼–½ strength hydrogen peroxide, modified Dakin's ¼ strength, sodium bicarbonate or other solutions); keep mucous membranes clean and moist (frequent rinses, artificial saliva); teach client to avoid alcoholic beverages, cigarette, pipe, and cigar smoking. Institute comfort measures: administer: local anesthetics if ordered (2% viscous lidocaine, 0.5% dyclonine, and 0.5% dyphenhydramine); milk of magnesia or kaolin mouth rinses to coat oral membranes; systemic pain medication if prescribed by physician. Instruct client with dry mouth to drink fluids frequently, suck on ice chips, and use gravies and sauces on foods	Client will experience minimal or no oral mucous membrane problems as a result of disease or therapy; recognize and report early signs of mucositis; practice appropriate preventive and management measures
Skin integrity, impaired related to alopecia; local effects of intravenous administration of chemotherapy: phlebitis, tissue sclerosis from extravasation or infiltration of vesicant/sclerosing agents (see Box 10–3 for list); photosensitivity, especially from 5-fluorouracil; rashes, urticaria, and pruritus from hypersensitivity reactions; erythema or skin reactions in previously irradiated areas, from chemotherapy-induced "radiation recall"; striae and skin fragility from high doses of steroids		
Prevent or minimize integument toxicities; maintain skin integrity	Teach client that alopecia may occur with certain chemotherapy agents; instruct client that hair loss is temporary and hair will regrow, possibly with a different color or texture; instruct client to keep scalp clean with mild shampoo; encourage client to wear wigs or scarves; be informed about scalp tourniquet and scalp hypothermia, which is only effective in minimizing hair loss with certain IV-push, low-dose medications such as doxorubicin and is not effective with PO or infusion-method chemotherapy; institute measures to prevent phlebitis and preserve veins (eg, change IV sites q. 48–72 h, warm soaks to phlebitic areas, avoid high concentrations of K^+ in IV fluids); be aware that all sclerosing agents should be administered by skilled phlebotomists via a free-flowing IV; instruct clients susceptible to photosensitivity to avoid prolonged exposure to the sun and to use sunscreens; observe for rashes and other skin reactions; be aware that some clients who have had previous radiation may have erythema in the irradiated area after the administration of certain chemotherapy agents (called "radiation recall"); instruct client that striae and skin fragility may occur with long-term high doses of steroids; poor wound healing may also occur with steroids	Client will know alopecia is temporary; care for scalp appropriately; experience little or no skin or vein problems

Continued

Table 10–5 (continued)
Nursing Care Plan for the Client Receiving Chemotherapy, by Nursing Diagnosis

Client Care Goal	Plan/Nursing Implementation	Expected Outcome
Urinary patterns, altered related to: hemorrhagic cystitis from cytoxan administration; oliguria or renal toxicity from cisplatin administration; dysuria secondary to cystitis; renal calculi from hyperurecemia		
Prevent renal and/or bladder toxicities	Force fluids >2 L/day while taking cyclophosphamide (Cytoxan); encourage client to void frequently; dipstick urine for blood for 24 h after PO or IV cyclophosphamide dose; prehydrate with >150–200 mL of fluid/h and ensure urine output is >100 mL/h prior to cisplatin dose; monitor strict input and output post cisplatin administration, urine output should remain >100 mL/h during and at least 4 h post cisplatin; notify physician immediately if urine output decreases below 100 mL/h; check renal function studies; assess for pain in urination, odor of urine, cloudy urine, and frequency and urgency; collect urine for culture and sensitivity if urinary infection suspected; be aware that clients with leukemias and lymphomas may produce increased levels of uric acid from tumor lysis; maintain urine pH at 7.5, force fluids, and administer allopurinal to prevent uric acid formation or sodium bicarbonate or acetazolamide (Diamox) to alkalinize urine	Clients receiving cyclophosphamide will manifest no signs of hemorrhagic cystitis Clients receiving cisplatin will excrete >100 mL/h prior and post cisplatin 4–12 h; manifest renal function studies within normal limits Clients receiving any chemotherapeutic agent will manifest no signs and symptoms of cystitis or increased renal toxicity; maintain a blood uric acid level within normal limits and a urine pH of 7.5 during therapy
Sensory/perceptual alterations: auditory, kinesthetic, tactile, olfactory, related to: cytoxicity from cisplatin; neurotoxicity from vinblastine, vincristine, etopiside, and cisplatin administration; taste and smell changes		
Prevent or minimize alterations in sensory perception	Instruct client to report tinnitus or decreased hearing if receiving cisplatin; baseline audiogram should be done prior to drug; assess for signs and symptoms of neurotoxicity such as numbness and tingling in extremities, decreased sensation, constipation, paralytic ileus, decreased deep tendon reflexes, foot drop, ataxia; place client on daily bowel check; administer stool softener daily and laxatives if no BM in 48 h (for clients on vincristine and vinblastine); monitor BP prior to and q. 15 min during infusion of etopiside, over 30 min to 1 h; instruct clients to avoid foods with strong odors and to eat cold foods such as poultry, cottage cheese, yogurt, milkshakes, cold cuts and cold frutis; be aware that clients may have an aversion to red meats and sweets	Client will experience no hearing loss; state signs and symptoms of neurotoxicity and report if these occur; experience no problems with constipation; experience no hypotension from etopiside; modify diet appropriately
Gas exchange, impaired related to pulmonary fibrosis from bleomycin therapy; atelectasis; pneumonia from myelosuppression		
Maintain adequate respiratory function	Assess for signs and symptoms of respiratory distress: dyspnea, SOB, pallor, cyanosis; auscultate lungs for rales, decreased breath sounds, and stridor; observe for cough, increased sputum production (note amount, color, and consistency) and hemoptysis; monitor temperatures q. 4 h; assess respiratory patterns (eg, rate, depth, and regularity of respirations and use of accessory muscles); check chest x-ray reports, pulmonary function studies, ABGs and blood chemistry; encourage turning, coughing, and deep breathing exercises (diaphragmatic breathing); monitor fluid status input and output; instruct client to avoid strenuous exercise, smoking, and contact with individuals with URIs; encourage frequent rest	Client will experience no respiratory problems during therapy; demonstrate effective breathing exercises; maintain respiratory parameters within normal limits

Client Care Goal	Plan/Nursing Implementation	Expected Outcome
Injury, potential for: related to effects of chemotherapeutic agents on body tissue: cardiotoxicity, usually from dose-related effects of daunorubicin and doxorubicin; phlebitis from chemical irritants: 5-fluorouracil and etopiside; tissue sclerosis from extravasation of sclerosing agents: doxorubicin, daunorubicin, mechlorethamine, mithramycin, mitomycin, vinblastine, vincristine, dacarbazine; hepatotoxicity from cyclophosphamide, methotrexate		
Prevent or minimize potential toxicities	Assess for cardiac toxicity: dysrhythmias, increased cardiac enzymes, signs and symptoms of CHF, chest pain; prevent phlebitis by floating all chemotherapeutic agents through the vein, change IV sites q. 48–72 h; apply warm soaks to phlebitic areas; know that sclerosing agents should only be administered by skilled phlebotomists via a newly started, free-flowing IV; if extravasation is suspected, stop infusion; apply ice to area and notify physician or nurse skilled in management of extravasations; observe for hepatotoxicity, enlarged liver, elevated liver function tests, jaundice, and pruritus	Client will manifest no signs of tissue injury as a result of cardiotoxicity, phlebitis, tissue sclerosis, and hepatotoxicity
Sexuality, altered patterns related to body image; fatigue and other distressing symptoms; changes in hormone levels		
Assist client and sexual partner to understand reasons for sexual changes; promote adaptation to altered body image changes and sexual dysfunction	Discuss with the client sexual concerns; explain changes in sexual desire, responsiveness, and function may occur from fatigue, hormonal changes, and other distressing symptoms (eg, nausea, vomiting, pain, diarrhea); teach female clients who are still menstruating that amenorrhea, irregular menses, hot flashes, and decreased vaginal lubrication may occur; a vaginal lubricant can be suggested; contraception methods should be reviewed because genetic mutation can occur; conception during and shortly after chemotherapy is not recommended; the effects of drug related infertility may be temporary or permanent and will vary according to the drug, dosage, and therapy; instruct female clients receiving chemotherapy who have decreased WBC counts to check with their physician about sexual intercourse; inform male clients that decreased hormone production and decreased spermatogenesis may occur; contraceptive methods should be reviewed; impotence and decreased libido or lack of interest may result from fatigue and/or other discomforts; suggest alternate expressions of physical and sexual contact; refer client for sexual counseling, if necessary; stress the importance of open and honest communication with significant others	Client will express sexual concerns if present; explain reasons for sexual changes; take appropriate actions to cope with sexual changes

Achievement of these goals primarily depends on the differences in radioresponsiveness between normal and malignant cells, whether the tolerance of normal cells has been exceeded, and the capacity of normal cells to repair themselves when damaged. Some tumors are more radioresponsive (a term used to describe tumor regression following radiotherapy) than others. Many lymphomas are exquisitely responsive to radiation; breast, prostate, and lung cancers are responsive to a lesser extent; melanomas and hypernephromas are highly radioresistant.

Normal cells also have some degree of radiosensitivity (cell sensitivity to the effects of radiation) and radioresistance. Radiation has a predilection for rapidly dividing cells such as blood cells (leukocytes, thrombocytes, and to a lesser extent, erythrocytes), cells lining the gastrointestinal tract, and hair follicles. The more radioresistant normal cells include muscle, nerve, and some organ (visceral) cells. Although total dose limitations for certain body tissues have been established, toxicity to normal tissues may still occur. Dose fractionation (ie, dividing the total dose over a period of time) often allows for more efficient normal cell repair.

Methods of Delivery

External beam radiotherapy is the delivery of radiation to a tumor by means of an external machine at a predetermined distance. Selection of the type of x-ray beam is critical in maximizing tumor cell destruction. High-energy or deeper penetrating beams are used for tumors deep within the body; low-energy beams are used for surface lesions. The x-ray beam must be carefully focused to deliver the radiation dose to the tumor.

Internal radiation therapy may be delivered by systemic, interstitial, or intracavitary means. *Systemic radiotherapy* may be administered intravenously or by oral ingestion of radioisotopes. *Interstitial radiotherapy* involves implantation of radioactive needles, wires, or seeds (tiny radioactive particles) into the tissues. Implants may be placed in body cavities to administer *intracavitary radiation.* A surgical procedure may be necessary to place the radioactive material.

Time, Distance, and Shielding Factors

Factors to consider in evaluating the client's exposure to radiation are:

- The radioactive source
- Duration of exposure
- Distance from the source
- Shielding (protecting untreated areas)

These factors are especially important in evaluating exposure hazards from internal radiation sources for those administering the therapy, caregivers, and others such as visitors and family.

Clients receiving external radiotherapy are not radioactive; they pose no risk for caregivers. Personnel in radiation therapy departments (especially those administering treatment) should wear monitoring devices (eg, a film badge) to measure cumulative radiation exposure.

With internal source radiation, the amount of radiation received is directly related to the duration of exposure. Distance is the most effective reducer of radiation, because the amount of exposure is inversely proportional to the distance between the source and receiver. The source must also be considered. For example, a radioisotope such as ^{32}P (phosphorus) emits poorly penetrating beta particles and presents minimal risks to caregivers; whereas ^{137}Cs (cesium) and ^{192}Ir (iridium) emit both beta and gamma rays (higher penetrating rays), which pose greater risks for radiation exposure. Care of the client must not be compromised because of fear. Risk can be substantially lowered with specific information and guidelines for exposure for the individual client; there is no one overall standard guideline. For specific information on radioisotopes, guidelines for time and distance exposure, and methods of collecting and isolating body secretions, consult a radiation safety officer or radiation therapy department personnel.

Shielding or preventing unnecessary exposure is an important factor in handling displaced radiation sources and bodily wastes contaminated by radiation. If dislodged from the body, the radiation source should never be directly handled without forceps. Radioactive wastes should be placed in closed, marked, shielded containers (usually made of lead). The lead aprons usually worn for protection against low-level radiation (eg, dental x-rays) do not provide sufficient protection from high-level radiation from implanted sources.

Goals of Therapy

Response to radiation therapy depends on the type of tumor. Radiation alone may be curative. For example, tumors arising in the hematopoietic system respond favorably to radiation therapy. Radiation is often combined with surgery and/or chemotherapy to effect a cure.

Palliative radiotherapy may also be employed for symptomatic relief when there is no hope of cure. Local radiation to bone metastases may relieve pain. Reduction of tumor size by radiation may also relieve pain, and radiotherapy may reduce distress from obstruction, effusion, spinal cord compression, and superior vena cava syndrome (see discussion of oncologic emergencies).

Side Effects of Radiation Therapy

Radiation therapy invariably destroys or damages both normal and malignant cells. Some cells recover, some die. Certain cells cannot reproduce; others die in the attempt.

Localized effects are generally related to the field of treatment. For example, alopecia from cranial radiation and dysphagia from radiation to the esophagus may occur. Generalized symptoms include fatigue and sometimes nausea and vomiting, both related to cellular breakdown products. The client may experience debilitating fatigue and lassitude. Bone marrow depression can result from radiation to bone marrow reserves (ie, iliac crests, sternum), which may be more pronounced in clients concurrently receiving chemotherapy and may be severe enough to warrant stopping treatment.

Although newer methods of treatment have reduced them, localized skin reactions still may occur. The three stages of skin reaction are:

1. Erythema (usually the only reaction)
2. Dry desquamation with flaking
3. Moist desquamation with shedding of surface epithelium (preventable)

Alopecia caused by epilation occurs at the radiation site and possibly at the site where the radiation exits. Effects at the exit site are usually minimal, however, because as the radiation enters the body, it diverges, and some is absorbed by the underlying body tissues.

Intermediate reactions occur when radiation has been delivered to slowly reproducing cells. Pneumonitis and pericarditis may occur 2 or 3 months after radiotherapy. Late side effects may occur years after treatment. Tissue necroses, fistulas, and pulmonary fibroses are long-term problems. Secondary cancers, such as leukemia, may also arise following radiotherapy.

Nursing Implications of Radiation Therapy

Nursing diagnoses related to radiotherapy are similar to those for chemotherapy. A nursing care plan for the client undergoing radiotherapy is in Table 10–6. Psychosocial aspects are addressed in Table 10–3.

Immunotherapy

Still under investigation, immunotherapy seeks to stimulate specific immune responses or to boost overall nonspecific responses against tumor growth. Conventional treatments (surgery, chemotherapy, and radiation) along with the oncogenic process suppress the body's natural immunologic defenses. (The immune response is discussed in Chapter 2.) Combining immunotherapy with conventional treatments may improve the client's prognosis.

Types of Immunotherapy

In *active immunotherapy,* the client's immune responses are directly stimulated through the use of tumor antigens. In *specific active immunotherapy,* the source of antigenic materials is vaccines. These vaccines contain tumor cell antigens either collected from the client's own tumor or from individuals with the same type of tumor. The antigenicity of these cells may be enhanced by chemicals. To prevent formation of new tumor growths, cells may be irradiated before administration. The vaccine is injected into the client with the hope of stimulating antibody production against the tumor.

Nonspecific active immunotherapy, the most common method, uses antigens and agents that do not originate from tumor cell sources. No attempt is made to stimulate immunity against a specific tumor. Among the common agents are the bacillus Calmette–Guerin (BCG); MER (methanol extraction residue), an extract of BCG; *Corynebacterium parvum;* and levamisole.

Passive immunotherapy uses lymphocytes or serum factors from a healthy person or from a cured client with a similar tumor. These substances are injected into the cancer client to produce an immune response. *Specific passive* or *adoptive immunotherapy* transfers an immune response from a donor to the client. Currently the least used method, passive immunotherapy has the fewest consistent reports of success, perhaps because of its short-lived effect.

Side Effects of Immunotherapy

Generally, the side effects of immunotherapy are much less severe than those of chemotherapy or radiotherapy. Localized erythema or pruritus may occur at the injection site. More severe localized reactions may include pustule formation, necrosis, weeping patches, inflammation at previous injection sites, or regional lymph node involvement. Systemic reactions may include flulike symptoms such as fever, shaking chills, fatigue, arthralgia, or headache. The nurse can reassure the client that these side effects are generally of short duration. Scarring of the injection site persists in some cases.

Allergic responses may also occur. Depending on the individual client's response to a specific immunologic agent, these responses may range from localized urticaria to severe, possible life-threatening anaphylaxis characterized by dyspnea, cyanosis, and convulsions.

Monoclonal Antibodies

One of the most promising leads in immunotherapy is the use of **monoclonal antibodies.** Monoclonal antibodies are specially produced antibodies directed toward the antigens or foreign substances on the cell surface of cancer cells. This antigen–antibody mediated response offers a moderate level of specificity against tumor cells, unlike the generalized normal and malignant cell destruction of chemotherapy and radiation therapy. Some researchers are also studying the possibility of developing a vaccine for cancer from monoclonal antibodies.

Monoclonal antibodies are collected and processed for intravenous administration. Allergic-type reactions such as anaphylactic shock or serum sickness are rare. Close monitoring of the client receiving monoclonal antibodies is warranted, including frequent vital signs and observation for anaphylaxis. Fevers and myalgias a few days after therapy may be early signs of serum sickness.

Nursing Implications of Immunotherapy

By conscientious application of assessment skills and close observation, nurses can make a significant contribution to progress in this promising new field of cancer therapy. Caring for clients during testing of treatment protocols may yield opportunities for nursing research. Thorough familiarity with immunologic agents, treatment techniques, and their side effects is necessary for prompt intervention if complications develop as well as for client education.

Combined Therapies

All treatments have strengths and limitations. In *combination therapy* two or more treatment modalities are used simultaneously or alternately for optimal effect. The idea is not that "more is better"; rather, combined therapy attempts to employ the advantages of each type of treatment. For example, the use of chemotherapy in addition to surgical resection may make it possible to avoid radical and disfiguring surgery. Surgical removal of a portion of a tumor may alleviate pain or obstruction while allowing time for chemotherapeutic measures to take effect, or surgery may enhance the effectiveness of immunotherapy.

Table 10–6
Nursing Care Plan for the Client Receiving Radiation Therapy, by Nursing Diagnosis

Client Care Goal	Plan/Nursing Implementation	Expected Outcome
Nutrition, altered: less than body requirements, related to nausea and vomiting, anorexia as result of: release of cellular waste products; intestinal mucosal alterations from abdominal radiation; direct cranial radiation; delayed smell and taste changes, dry mouth, mucositis from local head and neck radiation; psychologic factors; poor nutritional status		
Prevent or minimize vomiting and nausea; increase nutritional intake during treatment; minimize weight loss	Monitor intake and output; encourage fluids 2 L/day; administer antiemetics ½–1 h before treatment for clients receiving abdominal and cranial radiation if nausea and vomiting after treatment is a problem; clients should be instructed to take antiemetics regularly for nausea and vomiting; encourage good oral care, especially for clients receiving head and neck radiation (see alteration in oral mucosa membranes); monitor weights at least weekly; encourage high-protein foods such as cheeses, meats, nutritional supplements, milkshakes (be aware lactose intolerance may occur in adults who seldom drink milk); suggest cold foods for individuals with taste and smell changes; consult a dietitian if necessary; institute calorie counts if client is hospitalized, or if the client is at home encourage client to keep diet history; assess for peripheral and sacral edema from decreased serum protein; recommend a soft diet with full liquids for clients experiencing esophagitis; thicker fluids are easier to swallow than water or juices; avoid drinking fluids with meals; these can cause bloating, and feelings of fullness; fluids should be encouraged between meals	Client will state causes of nausea and vomiting, identify methods of controlling nausea and vomiting; modify diet to enhance food and fluid intake; maintain a stable weight during treatment
Bowel elimination, altered: diarrhea, related to the effects of radiation on the intestinal mucosa		
Refer to Table 10–5	Refer to Table 10–5	Refer to Table 10–5
Fluid volume deficit, related to nausea and vomiting; anorexia; diarrhea; constipation; dehydration		
Maintain optimal fluid and electrolyte balance	Encourage fluid intake of 2 L/day; monitor intake and output; asess skin turgor; monitor urine specific gravity if necessary; check blood chemistry studies Na^+, K^+, Cl^-; institute measures to control diarrhea and constipation to prevent fluid and electrolyte loss and promote fluid intake	Client will consume 2 L/day of fluid with output comprising approximately ⅔ of intake; laboratory studies will remain within normal limits
Tissue perfusion, altered related to the direct cytotoxic effects on bone marrow reserves (iliac crests and sternum): leukopenia; thrombocytopenia; anemia		
Refer to Table 10–5	Refer to Table 10–5	Refer to Table 10–5
Tissue integrity, impaired: oral mucous membranes related to direct result of mucosal damage from head and neck radiation, causing inflammation of buccal and gingival membranes, decrease in saliva, changes in normal flora		
Refer to Table 10–5	Refer to Table 10–5	Refer to Table 10–5
Skin integrity, impaired related to the local effects of radiation on the skin		
Maintain skin integrity; institute measures to prevent skin discomfort during and after treatment	Instruct client to avoid the use of soaps, ointments, creams, cosmetics, powder, and deodorants on treated skin area during treatment unless prescribed by physician: avoid washing off markings; keep skin area dry; use Ivory soap for bathing, and do not wash or wet the treated area; check skin area for increased erythema, dryness, burning, discomfort, dry or wet desquamation; instruct client to: report changes in skin; avoid tight-fitting clothing against treated area (100% cotton clothing is recommended); avoid using applications of heat (hot water bottle, heating pads, heat lamp) to treated area during or after treatment; protect skin from sunlight during a few	Client will experience minimal skin changes or problems during and after treatment; state appropriate skin care measures necessary to prevent skin problems on the treated areas

Client Care Goal	Plan/Nursing Implementation	Expected Outcome
	months after treatment; institute comfort measures if skin discomfort is present: use cool air to affected area by fan or blow dryer; administer pain medication; avoid pressure to the area; apply cold Vigilon (C.P. Bard, Inc.) dressing during and after treatment if allowed by physician; encourage the use of wigs and scarves for alopecia from cranial radiation; reassure client that hair will regrow after therapy, usually slowly (3–4 months)	
Gas exchange, impaired related to the effects of radiation to lung fields, potentially resulting in: pulmonary fibrosis; interstitial pneumonitis; atelectasis		
Refer to Table 10–5	Refer to Table 10–5	Refer to Table 10–5
Sexuality, altered patterns related to body image; fatigue and other distressing symptoms; changes in hormone levels		
Refer to Table 10–5	Refer to Table 10–5 Also, instruct female clients who are receiving radiation in the pelvic and genital organs to check with their physician about sexual intercourse	Refer to Table 10–5

Adjuvant therapy (auxiliary therapy), combined with surgery, is intended to eradicate any microscopic spread of tumor, prolonging a disease-free state. This type of therapy is of little or no benefit for certain tumors (eg, colon cancers). Adjuvant therapy has improved overall survival for breast, testicular, and head and neck cancers, however. Adjuvant therapy may involve chemotherapeutic, radiologic, or immunologic approaches.

Nutrition and Treatment

The role of nutrition in cancer therapy is controversial. It is generally agreed that enteral or parenteral nutritional support has no demonstrable effects on stimulating tumor growth in humans, although it has in animals. On the other hand, there is agreement that nutritional repletion may increase tumor responsiveness to chemotherapy and radiation therapy, while minimizing side effects such as nausea and vomiting, mucositis, and diarrhea. Adequate nutrition is also necessary for promoting healing after surgery and enhancing effective immunologic responses.

The client with cancer often experiences anorexia from causes previously discussed. The net result of decreased food intake is malnutrition and cachexia. Enteral hyperalimentation via oral, nasogastric, gastrostomy, and jejunostomy feedings (see Chapter 36) as well as intravenous hyperalimentation (see Chapter 6) may be indicated to restore adequate nutrition and prevent the progressive cachexia associated with cancer. Box 10–4 has helpful eating tips for cancer clients that can be incorporated into the nursing care plan as well as shared with the client and family.

Oncologic Emergencies

The oncologic emergencies are potentially life-threatening disorders occurring either as a direct effect of malignant tumors or as a consequence of therapy.

All nurses caring for clients with cancer should be familiar with these oncologic emergencies, know who is at risk, and be able to recognize and assess the signs and symptoms. Although each condition requires a specialized approach, emotional support and comfort are an essential part of any nursing plan of care. The conspicuous physical alterations, coupled with immediate initiation of therapy, can be alarming to clients and families. Their overwhelming fear can be alleviated to some degree by client education. Explanations of procedures and treatments must be directed toward the client's and the family's levels of comprehension.

Septic Shock

Septic shock associated with a malignancy is often a result of an overwhelming infection in an immunologically compromised host. Because the normal immunologic controls are impaired, individuals at risk include clients with neoplastic invasion of the bone marrow from leukemias, lymphomas, or solid tumors; bone marrow suppression from chemotherapy or radiation therapy; or advanced malignant disease. The clinical manifestations and nursing implications are discussed in Chapter 9.

Disseminated Intravascular Coagulation

Acute *disseminated intravascular coagulation* is a pathologic state of abnormal coagulation secondary to another

Box 10–4
Helpful Eating Tips for Cancer Clients

Eat smaller meals more frequently throughout the day. Chew food slowly. Eat whenever you feel hungry.

Keep snacks handy for nibbling. People tend to eat more when food is easily available.

Try eating a snack before you go to bed in addition to your other meals.

If morning is your best mealtime, try to eat as much as you can then without overstuffing yourself.

Rely on food you really love, especially during your not-so-hungry periods. But remember what sounds unappealing today may sound good tomorrow.

Vary the color of foods served on the plate. Make the meal eye appealing. Serve it on a small plate, adding garnishes—an orange or tomato slice or a sprig of parsley.

Make your mealtime a relaxing experience with attractive table settings, bright surroundings, music, and good company.

Stay away from high-fat and greasy foods.

Try resting before a meal. Stop and pause while eating.

Make sure your liquids are nutritious. Do not take a beverage with your meal. Take your beverage between meals to reduce the volume of material in your stomach at eating time.

If protein foods, such as red meat, don't taste right, try eating protein foods cold or at room temperature. Try chicken.

Extra salt may improve the taste of food if you are not on a salt-restricted diet. Try cold cuts.

To enhance taste, meats may be marinated in wine, teriyaki sauce, soy sauce, or Italian dressing.

Tart foods may enhance flavors. Orange juice, pickles, lemonade, vinegar, and lemon juice may be used as seasonings.

Sweeter protein foods may not taste bitter, eg, ice cream, milkshakes, puddings.

Consider using different seasonings, eg, mint, basil, curry, oregano.

When foods taste sweet, use unsweetened (water-packed) fruits and more bland-tasting foods, or rinse canned fruits with water.

If you have an aversion to sweet-tasting foods, try adding a lot of cream to your milkshakes.

Stimulate your appetite with light exercise, such as walking. Check with your doctor about trying wine, dry sherry, or beer before a meal.

Experiment with a diet low in meat but high in other protein foods.

Good odors, such as freshly baked bread or cakes baking, can take your mind off a slumping appetite. If food odors are a problem, don't eat in the room where the food is prepared. And if you feel up to it, try going to a restaurant. Avoid foods that have a strong smell, such as fish.

You can sometimes take away that strange taste in your mouth by eating foods that leave their own tastes in the mouth, such as fresh fruit or hard candies.

In addition to your regular diet, a nutritional supplement containing the needed vitamins, minerals, and nutrients may be used. Ask your doctor about such supplements.

If you wear dentures, make sure they fit properly. Have your dentist rule out dental problems causing bad taste.

Practice good mouth care. Brush teeth gently with a soft toothbrush.

If your mouth is sore, avoid hot spicy foods and eat warm or cool soft, bland foods, eg, cold cuts, cottage cheese, fruits.

If your mouth feels dry, try brushing your teeth before meals or rinsing your mouth with water. Both will stimulate saliva. Also try drinking small sips of fluid with your food.

Consult the American Cancer Society cookbook *Nutrition* and the National Cancer Institute's *Eating Hints: Recipes and Tips for Better Nutrition During Cancer Treatment* (see the resources list at the end of this chapter).

Adapted with permission from American Cancer Society, Philadelphia Division, Cheltenham Unit. Developed in consultation with Rosemary C. Polomano, RN.

underlying process. Thromboplastin, the stimulus for the clotting cascade, is abnormally released from malignant tumors—certain carcinomas, acute promyelocytic leukemia, and neuroblastomas—either as a result of cellular proliferation or lysis, without regard for clotting necessity. In turn, the widespread coagulation stimulates fibrin degradation by the fibrinolytic pathway, breaking down clots as fast as they are formed. The lack of available clotting constituents leads to generalized bleeding. The nurse's role in caring for clients with DIC is discussed in Chapter 23.

Spinal Cord Compression

Spinal cord compression usually results from extradural involvement (outside the cord) as a result of a tumor impinging on the dura mater or from vertebral collapse. This condition can be caused by lymphomas, multiple myeloma, and solid tumors. A less common cause is intramedullary lesions from within the cord itself. Compression may occur at the thoracic, lumbar, or sacral levels. Most clients initially experience either localized or radiating pain (a band or girdle of tightness radiating from the back to the chest or abdomen). Neurologic assessment may find muscle weakness, ataxia, urinary or fecal incontinence, and sensory impairment. Severe or prolonged cord compression can cause progressive paralysis with loss of sphincter control.

Immediate radiotherapy is usually instituted for local control along with high doses of corticosteroids to reduce swelling and inflammation. In some circumstances, a decompression laminectomy is required. Both systemic and intrathecal chemotherapy may be used, depending on the type of tumor and its symptoms.

A primary nursing responsibility is astute observation and follow-up of clients' pain or neurologic deficits to detect spinal cord compression before it progresses to the point where the client is unlikely to become ambulatory again.

Superior Vena Cava Syndrome

Superior vena cava syndrome, characterized by compression of the superior vena cava or intracaval thrombosis of this vessel, obstructs venous blood flow from the head, neck, and upper extremities. Approximately 90% of individuals with this condition are found to have a malignancy. SVCS is most common with bronchogenic carcinomas and, to a lesser degree, with lymphomas and carcinomas of the head and neck, breast, thymus, and testes.

The clinical manifestations of SVCS are those of impaired venous circulation causing fullness in the head and chest, headache, visual changes, dyspnea, cough, wheezing, dysphasia, and syncope. Progression may lead to mental changes; lethargy; and eventually, severe respiratory distress. Obvious signs include distended neck, chest, and arm veins along with facial, neck, and possibly arm edema. Because of this congestion, clients prefer an upright position for effective breathing.

Treatment usually begins with a tissue diagnosis by bronchoscopy or mediastinoscopy to confirm SVCS, because other conditions, such as aortic aneurysm, can cause the same symptoms. For clients requiring a biopsy, be aware of the risk of hemorrhage because of vessel engorgement and the risk of respiratory distress from compression of the trachea. Careful assessment of respiratory and cardiovascular status is essential. Radiotherapy is usually used to achieve a quick response in tumor reduction because death can ensue if the obstruction is not relieved. Capable of effecting a response in drug-sensitive tumors, chemotherapy is used although effects may be somewhat slower. Nursing goals are aimed at promoting comfort by positioning the client in a high Fowler's position and supporting edematous upper extremities, modifying activity, and managing the effects of therapy.

Malignant Pericardial Effusion

Malignant pericardial effusion is an accumulation of fluid between the visceral layer of the pericardium (the lining directly over the heart) and the parietal pericardium (the lining of the pericardial sac) as a result of malignant cell infiltration. As it accumulates, the fluid restricts the heart's expansion capacity during the diastolic or ventricular filling phase. As the heart is compressed, effective cardiac output cannot be maintained; consequently, dyspnea, anxiety, restlessness, chest discomfort, and eventually circulatory collapse may occur. This condition is called *cardiac tamponade.* Physical assessment parameters include jugular vein distention, tachycardia, rapid respiratory rate, decreased blood pressure secondary to decreased cardiac output, and mental status changes.

The condition can be caused by spread of tumor cells from lung and breast cancers, lymphomas, leukemias, and malignant melanoma as well as by high doses of radiation therapy to the heart. Treatment includes the creation of a pericardial window to allow fluid to escape into surrounding lymphatics, and pericardial stripping, removing the fluid-producing membrane layer. Chemotherapy is used if the condition is caused by breast cancers, leukemias, and lymphomas. Radiotherapy may have a general role for all tumor types but not for conditions precipitated by radiation toxicity. Knowledge of the signs and symptoms along with skill in cardiovascular system assessment are important nursing considerations.

Malignant Pleural Effusion

A *pleural effusion* is an accumulation of fluid between the visceral layer (outer lining) of the lung and the parietal layer (lining of the pleural cavity). When caused by a malignancy, the condition is generally secondary to tumor cells in the lung (either primary lung cancer or metastatic disease from other tumor types), seeding or implanting on the parietal lining, or from spread of tumor cells through the blood to the parietal pleura. As the fluid builds up, the area for lung expansion decreases. The severity of symptoms depends on whether there is unilateral or bilateral involvement and on the amount of fluid in the pleural space. Symptoms such as shortness of breath, dyspnea, chest pain, and cough may be present. Usually, a chest tube is inserted to drain the fluid. A sclerosing agent (a drug that causes widespread tissue irritation) may be instilled through the chest tube to initiate a widespread inflammation resulting in fibrosis and scarring and decreasing fluid secretion. Chemotherapy is most frequently used for tumors that are drug sensitive. Local radiation therapy is reserved for drug-resistant tumors.

Hypercalcemia

Hypercalcemia is the most common oncologic emergency. Tumors generally cause calcium elevations by: metastatic tumor invasion of bone (usually from breast cancers), prostaglandin release from tumors, or release of an activating substance associated with multiple myeloma. These mechanisms act on the target osteoclast cells of the bone, causing release of calcium. Uncontrolled excess blood calcium levels may lead to mental status changes (lethargy and confusion), muscle weakness, coma, and eventual cardiac arrest.

The preferred treatment is to eradicate the stimulus for calcium release, usually the tumor. In addition, attempts are made to control the rise in the calcium concentration by increasing renal excretion through fluid diuresis and medications.

Alternative Therapies

Alternative therapies are therapeutic approaches other than the conventional modalities of surgery, chemotherapy, and radiotherapy. (Immunotherapy might be considered a frontier.)

Some alternative techniques supplement conventional therapy, often to improve client comfort (eg, self-hypnosis, psychological counseling, or relaxation techniques). Some researchers are exploring the possibility that nutritional factors underlie the oncogenic process. At present, however, nutritional therapy, including total parenteral nutrition, is used to potentiate conventional therapy.

New drugs or treatment protocols not yet commercially available may be available to selected clients in oncology centers. New drugs or combinations of drugs as well as various forms of high-dose chemotherapy are continually being tested. Other promising techniques that require further study include bone marrow transplantation, interferon, red light (hematoporphyrin) therapy, hyperthermia, visual imagery, and limb salvage surgery techniques.

Bone Marrow Transplantation

Bone marrow transplantation (BMT) is essentially an auxiliary technique that facilitates use of higher doses of chemotherapeutic agents and radiation. In some cases, the dose sufficient to produce tumoricidal effects may suppress bone marrow activity to a life-threatening extent. If transplanted bone marrow can generate the production of new bone marrow to replace what was destroyed, higher doses can be given before the transplant. Either *autologous marrow* (from the client's own body) or *allogeneic marrow* (from a donor) may be used. Bone marrow transplantation has been used with some success in clients with leukemia, anaplastic anemia, and severe immunodeficiency.

Interferon

Essentially, **interferon** is a form of protein produced by the body as a by-product of the physiologic response to a viral infection. When stimulated by interferon, certain body cells produce substances that inhibit the reproduction of viruses. Interferon was initially tested in clients with cancer in the hope it might stimulate body cells to inhibit cancer cell mitosis. It has been found that, in addition to any antitumor activity, interferon may enhance the activity of the client's immune defense system. Any improvement of immune defenses would benefit clients with cancer. Interferon therapy is still being studied.

Photodynamic Therapy

Photodynamic therapy, or red light therapy, uses a light-sensitive drug called hematoporphyrin derivative. When administered intravenously, this drug is quickly washed out by normal cells but is stored by cancer cells. When a fiber-optic beam of red light, usually from a laser, is directed at the hematoporphyrin-containing cancer cells, the drug produces a form of oxygen that is lethal to the cancer cells. Researchers are beginning to report disease regressions with certain kinds of cancers such as lung and esophageal cancer. The treatment has little effect on slow-growing cancers with a poor blood supply and is only effective on tumors that can be visualized. Strictly experimental, phototherapy is available in only a few research centers and has not yet been approved by the FDA.

Hyperthermia

Hyperthermia is based on the premise that certain types of neoplastic cells are more responsive to antineoplastic drugs if they have been exposed to high temperatures. In 1984, the FDA approved a device that uses controlled microwave energy to treat melanoma, squamous cell carcinoma, adenocarcinoma, and sarcoma in clients who have recurrent or regressive cancers of those types despite conventional therapy. A palliative treatment, hyperthermia suppresses cancer growth by heat, or thermal energy. In normal tissue, heat is carried away by the blood that flows through it. Because solid malignant tumors are much less vascular, the heat is not carried away as quickly, and the tumors reach a relatively higher temperature than surrounding normal tissue causing the tumor cells to die. Hyperthermia is an experimental technique available only in a few cancer centers.

Visual Imagery

Visual imagery, a technique developed by the Simontons (Simonton, Matthews–Simonton, Creighton, 1978), stems from the theory that the mind can stimulate the body's natural defenses to withstand neoplastic disease. The theory is not one of "mind over matter"; rather, it is based on advances in understanding of the interrelation of mind and body. The Simonton regimen includes counseling, relaxation, and exercises in visual imagery (eg, clients are encouraged to visualize leukocytes devouring bacteria within the bloodstream or to visualize themselves pursuing a cherished activity). The Simontons advise that this technique be used in conjunction with standard acceptable medical practices. Later work by Stephanie Matthews–Simonton focused on involving the cancer client's family in the creation of a healing environment (1984).

Limb Salvage Surgery

New *limb salvage surgery* techniques allow clients to avoid amputation (eg, in cases of bone cancer). Transplants of bone from cadavers and grafts made of space-age synthetics are being studied.

Unorthodox Therapies

Given the poor prognosis associated with many forms of cancer and the painful and debilitating side effects of some conventional therapies, it is not surprising that cancer victims and their families may be susceptible to unorthodox practitioners who hold out hope—however faint—of cure. To take a recent and well-known example, an estimated 70,000 Americans have tried *laetrile (amygdalin) therapy,* despite the lack of reliable evidence that this compound has an antineoplastic effect (Nixon, 1982).

The principle danger of unorthodox therapies is that conventional treatment may be delayed until it is too late, or treatment may be foregone entirely. Another danger is that clients who have tried unorthodox therapies may be reluctant to inform health care providers of this fact, for fear of scorn and disapproval. Side effects of unorthodox therapy (eg, cyanide poisoning in users of laetrile) may thus go unrecognized and untreated (Nixon, 1982).

Client/Family Teaching

By establishing rapport with the client and responding empathically to expressions of fear and despair, the nurse can caution client and family to be alert for fraudulent claims. Several characteristics suggest unscrupulous practice:

- The treatment regimen is secret.
- Histologic verification of cancer is not required.
- Conventional treatments are denigrated.
- Record keeping is scanty or nonexistent.
- The care provider may have unusual degrees from unfamiliar institutions.
- Treatment is extremely costly compared with conventional therapies.

Proponents of unorthodox therapies may not have mercenary motives and be sincere in their beliefs. The rationale for some therapies may seem plausible (eg, it seems reasonable to believe that nutrition may play a greater role in cellular structure and function than has heretofore been attributed to it). Indeed, the American Cancer Society has recently conducted studies of the relation between cancer and nutrition and made several recommendations listed earlier in this chapter.

Another unorthodox approach to cancer therapy is the macrobiotic diet, introduced into the United States in the 1960s. The predominantly vegetarian diet forbids the ingestion of red meats and dairy products. Proponents of the macrobiotic diet believe that the Western diet promotes carcinogenesis. They believe cancer evolves from an imbalance of yin and yang forces; certain food classifications consumed in excess are believed to have the tendency to cause cancer in the lower or upper part of the body. Because the diet lacks essential nutrients, severe malnutrition may occur. Health care providers do not advocate this diet because scientific evidence shows no benefits in cancer prevention, cure, or control.

Clients must be cautioned to evaluate *all* treatment modalities carefully in the light of the best current thinking about the nature of the neoplastic process and in the light of their personal experience, values, and goals.

Supportive Care

For some clients with cancer, the time comes when nothing further can be done to cure the disease or arrest its course. All treatment options may have been exhausted, or the client may choose not to submit to treatments that might prolong life by sacrificing its quality. Some members of the health care team or the family may find such a decision difficult to accept. In such cases, the nurse may assume the role of client advocate, affirming the client's fundamental right to determine the conditions under which he or she chooses to live.

Supportive care is the palliative treatment of the symptoms and effects of an advancing, incurable, terminal disease process. The underlying premise of supportive care is a shift from the focus on arresting disease and prolonging life to providing the maximum possible quality of life while encouraging the client to cope with and prepare for death.

Control of pain becomes the first priority in supportive care. Nutritional support with emphasis on palatability, control of infection, and comfort measures including emotional support are other important goals. The client may choose to spend the final stage of life at home receiving hospice care, or a hospice facility may seem the best alternative.

Rehabilitation

Because survival among cancer clients has significantly improved, rehabilitation is assuming a new role in oncology as a necessary and integral aspect of cancer care. In recent years, publicity about the cancer experiences of well-known figures such as former First Lady Betty Ford and television personality Betty Rollins has provided a more optimistic view of cancer.

Rehabilitation is a dynamic, holistic process in which the individual with cancer is assisted in achieving optimal function in all areas of life. Rehabilitation for clients with cancer should be similar to that for disabilities and handicaps secondary to other health problems. The rehabilitative process is directed toward maximizing function and fostering psychosocial adaption to lifestyle changes imposed by cancer. Rehabilitation should provide opportunities for the client and family to set new priorities and reformulate realistic goals, all for the purpose of making life more meaningful. Rehabilitation involves clients, significant others, and community support groups, as well as the health care team. Physical rehabilitation includes physical and occupational therapy, nutritional support, and enterostomal therapy as well as reconstructive surgery. Vocational rehabilitation, financial planning, and spiritual and psychologic support care are also essential components of the rehabilitative process.

The type and extent of cancer, the magnitude of physical and emotional impairments, and the available treatment options and response to therapies are important in constructing a rehabilitative program. The clients' and families' motivational levels, availability of social resources, and financial support play equally important roles.

Rehabilitation does not begin with client discharge from a hospital setting. Rehabilitative efforts should start with the initial diagnosis of cancer and continue throughout the period that the client's life is actually or potentially affected by cancer. The process begins with an assessment. Factors to be considered are:

- The pathologic state (Is it progressive or stable?)
- The physical or functional impairments (Are these reversible or irreversible?)
- The client's strengths (motivational, physical, and emotional)
- The family system and supports
- The availability of financial and community resources

Home Health Care

The trend toward greater client involvement in health care planning and treatment regimens is reflected in the growing number of community resources available to clients with cancer and to their families. Some groups offer financial assistance; some offer counseling; some offer mutual support with sharing of the cancer experience. The American Cancer Society offers many kinds of assistance, including homemaker services, blood donors, transportation, equipment, and supplies. Self-help groups such as Reach for Recovery (breast cancer), the International Association of Laryngectomees, and the United Ostomy Association offer the invaluable counsel of those who "have been there." And groups such as Make Today Count offer both practical and emotional support. (A list of support groups is at the end of this chapter.) By informing the client about these services and encouraging the client to use them, the nurse performs the dual service of offering the client practical assistance and reassuring the client that the cancer experience need not be endured alone.

Chapter Highlights

Cancer alters the biopsychosocial environment to such a degree that it disrupts the body's state of equilibrium.

Oncology nursing is a specialty. Because cancer is a widespread health problem, however, nurses from every practice area have the opportunity to care for cancer clients.

The fundamental differences between a benign and malignant cell are the malignant cell's abilities to infiltrate surrounding tissue and metastasize.

The evolution of cancer probably results from a combination of factors. No one theory of causation is universally accepted.

Generalized systemic effects from cancer may include fatigue, anemia, infection, cachexia, organ impairment, hormonal imbalance, and pain. The degree to which these occur depends on the type and extent of the malignant tumor as well as the body area involved.

The client with cancer, and the client's significant others, face a multitude of internal and external stressors.

Self-examination at recommended intervals may lead to early detection of cancers, optimizing chances for cure.

Surgery, chemotherapy, and radiation therapy remain the primary treatments of choice for cancer. These treatments may be used in combination or alone.

Common side effects of chemotherapy include alopecia, bone marrow suppression (leukopenia and thrombocytopenia), and gastrointestinal side effects (mucositis and diarrhea).

Systemic generalized effects of radiotherapy may include fatigue, weakness, anorexia, and perhaps mild nausea. More severe nausea and vomiting may occur from cranial and abdominal irradiation. Local effects are hair loss in the irradiated area and possibly skin toxicity.

Early assessment and recognition and prompt treatment of oncologic emergencies are important factors in reversing or controlling these conditions.

Bibliography

American Cancer Society: *Cancer Facts and Figures.* New York: American Cancer Society, 1987.

American Cancer Society: *Nutrition Common Sense and Cancer.* ACS Publication 84-IMM-No. 2096-LE. New York: American Cancer Society, 1984.

American Joint Committee on Cancer: *Manual for Staging of Cancer,* 2nd ed. Philadelphia: Lippincott, 1983.

Baxley KO et al: Alopecia: Effect on cancer patients' body image. *Cancer Nurs* 1984; 7:499–503.

Bersani G, Carl W: Oral care for cancer patients. *Am J Nurs* 1983; 83:533–536.

Byrne CJ et al: *Laboratory Tests: Implications for Nursing Care,* 2nd ed. Menlo Park, CA: Addison–Wesley, 1986.

Cassileth BR, Cassileth PA (editors): *Clinical Care of the Terminal Cancer Patient.* Philadelphia: Lea & Febiger, 1982.

Chernecky CC, Ramsey PW: *Critical Nursing Care of the Client with Cancer.* Norwalk, CT: Appleton–Century–Crofts, 1984.

Cline BW: Prevention of chemotherapy-induced alopecia: A review of the literature. *Cancer Nurs* 1984; 7:221–228.

Devita V, Hellman S, Rosenburg S (editors): *Cancer: Principles and Practices of Oncology,* 2nd ed. Philadelphia: Lippincott, 1985.

Donaghue M, Nunnally C, Yasko JM: *Nutritional Aspects of Cancer Cure: A Self-Learning Module.* Reston, VA: Reston, 1985.

Donovan MI, Girton SE: *Cancer Care Nursing.* Norwalk, CT: Appleton–Century–Crofts, 1984.

Frank–Stromberg M et al: Psychological impact of the "cancer" diagnosis. *Oncol Nurs Forum* 1984; 11(3):16–22.

Gunn AE: *Cancer Rehabilitation.* New York: Raven, 1984.

Hassey K: Demystifying care of patients with radioactive implants. *Am J Nurs* 1985; 85:788–792.

Higby DJ: *The Cancer Patient and Supportive Care,* 2nd ed. Boston: Martinus Nijhoff, 1985.

Howard–Ruben J, Miller NJ: Unproven methods of cancer management. Part 2: Current trends and implications. *Oncol Nurs Forum* 1984; 11(1):67–73.

Knopf MK, Fischer DS, Welch–McCaffrey D: *Cancer Chemotherapy: Treatment and Care.* Boston: Hall, 1984.

Matje SD: Stress and cancer: A review of the literature. *Cancer Nurs* 1984; 7:399–404.

Maxwell MB: Dyspnea in advanced cancer. *Am J Nurs* 1985; 85:673–677.

Maxwell MB: When the cancer patient becomes anemic. *Cancer Nurs* 1984; 7:321–326.

McNally JC, Stair JC, Somerville ET (editors): *Guidelines for Cancer Nursing Practice.* New York: Grune & Stratton, 1985.

Morton PL, Giuliano AE: Cancer immunology and immunotherapy. In: *Cancer Treatment,* 2nd ed. Haskel, CM (editor). Philadelphia: Saunders, 1985.

National Study Commission on Cytotoxic Exposures: *Recommendations for Handling Cytotoxic Agents.* Syracuse, NY: Bristol Laboratories, March 1984.

Nealon E, Blumberg B, Brown B: What do patients know about clinical trials? *Am J Nurs* 1985; 85:807–810.

Nowell PC: Tumor biology: Evolution toward terminal illness. In: *Clinical Care of the Terminal Cancer Patient.* Cassileth BR, Cassileth PA (editors). Philadelphia: Lea & Febiger, 1982.

Oishi N, et al: Oncology teams. *Nurs Health Care* 1986; 7:447–449.

Oncology Nursing Society: *Cancer Chemotherapy: Guidelines and Recommendations for Nursing Education and Practice.* Pittsburgh, PA: Oncology Nursing Society, 1984.

Pageau MG, Mroz WT, Coombs DW: New analgesic therapy relieves cancer pain without oversedation. *Nurs 85* (April) 1985; 15:46–49.

Patterson WB: Principles of surgical oncology. In: *Clinical Oncology for Medical Students and Physicians: A Multidisciplinary Approach.* Rubin P (editor). New York: American Cancer Society, 1983.

Phillips TL: Principles of radiobiology and radiation therapy. In: *Principles of Cancer Treatment.* Carter SK, Glatstein E, Livingston RB (editors). New York: McGraw–Hill, 1982.

Simonton OC, Matthews–Simonton S, Creighton JL: *Getting Well Again: A Step by Step, Self-Healing Guide to Overcoming Cancer for Patients and Their Families.* New York: Bantam, 1978.

Simonton SM, Shook RL: *The Healing Family.* New York: Bantam, 1984.

Twycross RG, Lack SA: *Symptom Control in Far Advanced Cancer: Pain Relief.* London: Pitman, 1983.

US Department of Health and Human Services, Public Health Service and National Institutes of Health: *Recommendations for the Safe Handling of Parenteral Antineoplastic Drugs.* Publication No. 83-2621, 1983.

Valentine AS, Stewart JA: Oncologic emergencies. *Am J Nurs* 1983; 83:1282–1285.

Yasko JM: *Care of the Client Receiving External Radiation Therapy: A Self-Learning Module.* Reston, VA: Reston, 1982.

Yasko JM: *Guidelines for Cancer Cure: Symptom Management: A Self-Learning Module.* Reston, VA: Reston, 1983.

Resources

In addition to these resources, see the listings in other chapters throughout this text for information about cancer in specific body systems. For example, resources for the client with leukemia are listed in Chapter 22; for the client with a laryngectomy, in Chapter 14; and for the client with a mastectomy, in Chapter 48.

SELF-HELP GROUPS AND OTHER ORGANIZATIONS

American Cancer Society
National Headquarters
19 W 56th St
New York, NY 10019
Phone: (212) 371–2900

This voluntary organization has about 3000 chapters, staffed largely by volunteers, to provide services to cancer clients, educational programs, and research. Sponsors the "I Can Cope" program to address the educational and psychologic needs of clients and families through lecture and group discussion. Also sponsors a number of cancer prevention programs through local units.

Corporate Angel Network (CAN)
Bldg 1
Westchester County Airport
White Plains, NY 10604
Phone: (914) 328–1313

A nationwide service that provides free transportation on corporate aircraft when seats are available. For cancer patients who are ambulatory and stable, to and from established treatment centers. No cost, no financial need must be shown. Especially useful because most insurance plans do not cover medical travel costs. Organized by Priscilla Blum, a pilot and former cancer patient.

National Hospice Organization
1901 N Fort Myer Dr, Suite 902
Arlington, VA 22209
Phone: (703) 243–5900

This is an organization of hospices and individuals that encourages public and professional education on caring for the terminally ill, monitors legislation affecting the hospice movement, and publishes a quarterly newsletter, "National Hospice Organization Newsletter."

HOT LINE

Cancer Information Services
Phone: (800) 4–CANCER (in Hawaii, Oahu (808) 524–1234, neighboring islands call collect; in Washington, DC, and suburbs in Maryland and Virginia (202) 636–5700; in Alaska (800) 638–6070

This service, sponsored by the National Institutes of Health, provides the latest facts on all types of cancers, educational materials available for consumer education, and information on coping with the disease. Spanish-speaking staff members are available to callers from the following areas (daytime hours only); California (area codes 213, 619, 714, 805), Florida, Georgia, Illinois, northern New Jersey, New York City, and Texas.

NURSING ORGANIZATIONS

American Radiological Nurses Association
502 Forest Court
Carboro, NC 27510
Executive Secretary, Elaine Deutsch

An organization of nurses working in radiology, this group has educational and clinical practice goals. In addition to representing the radiology nurse, it serves as a resource to persons in nursing education and acts as client advocate with families, nurses, physicians, and radiology personnel. Dues $25 for RNs; $15 for associate membership for LVNs and LPNs.

Oncology Nursing Society
1016 Greentree Rd
Pittsburgh, PA 15220–315
Phone: (412) 921–7373

A professional organization for RNs interested in oncology or practicing oncology nursing to promote high standards in oncology nursing, provide peer support and networking, encourage specialization by nurses in oncology, develop educational programs, and encourage nursing research.

HEALTH EDUCATION MATERIAL

From: American Cancer Society (the booklets below as well as many others are available from local units)

Cancer Facts and Figures (a booklet of annually updated statistics for health professionals)
I Have a Secret Cure for Cancer! (a booklet on quackery)
Nutrition (a cookbook)

From: Cope Magazine
12600 West Colfax Ave.
Suite B400
Denver, CO 80215

This bi-monthly magazine with the latest cancer news for clients and their families is published by Merrill G. Hastings, Junior, the husband of a cancer client. A medical version for oncology professionals is published ten times a year. For more information, call the toll-free hotline at (800) 343–COPE.

From: "Killer T Cell"
Box 6
M D Anderson Hospital
6723 Bertner
Houston, TX 77030

A computer game, "Killer T Cell" may positively influence the immune system by helping cancer clients visualize cancer cells being destroyed by killer T cells. Available by mail order in Apple II, Commodore 64, and IBM-PC versions, disks cost $20 each, and all proceeds support cancer research.

From: National Cancer Institute
Office of Cancer Communications
Building 31, Room 10A18
Bethesda, MD 20205

Cancer Treatment: An Annotated Bibliography of Patient Education Materials
Chemotherapy and You: A Guide to Self-Help During Treatment
Eating Hints: Recipes and Tips for Better Nutrition During Cancer Treatment
Radiation Therapy and You: A Guide to Self-Help During Treatment
Taking Time: Support for People With Cancer and the People Who Care About Them
What are Clinical Trials All About?
What Black Americans Should Know About Cancer

Available at local bookstores:
The American Cancer Society Cancer Book, edited by Arthur I. Holleb, MD

CHAPTER **11**

Surgery

Other topics relevant to this content are: Atelectasis and pneumonia as postoperative complications, **Chapter 16;** Description and illustration of endotracheal tubes, **Chapter 14;** Effects of drug abuse on analgesia and anesthesia, **Chapter 8;** Effects of malnutrition on surgical client, **Chapter 6;** Fluid and electrolyte balance, **Chapter 3;** Hypertrophic scarring and keloid formation, **Chapter 55;** Measures to assess and relieve postoperative pain, **Chapter 3.**

Objectives

When you have finished studying this chapter, you should be able to:

Discuss the roles and responsibilities of the members of the surgical team.

Anticipate the physiologic and psychosocial factors that influence surgical risk.

Describe the wound-healing process, the factors that influence it, and nursing interventions that foster it.

Formulate nursing interventions aimed at decreasing surgical risk.

Integrate legal aspects, ethical codes, advocacy, and clients' rights into the care of surgical clients.

Apply the nursing process throughout perioperative care.

Identify the components of a comprehensive plan for preoperative care that includes physiologic and psychosocial preparation of the client for surgery.

Discuss the role of the nurse in maintaining the client's safety during surgery and recovery from anesthesia.

Discuss nursing responsibilities in preventing postoperative complications.

Formulate a comprehensive plan for the postoperative recovery and discharge of the surgical client.

The art and science of surgery have been practiced since antiquity. Early practitioners were primarily concerned with repair of wounds caused by trauma. They also attempted to control the spread of infection by means such as amputation, even though the mechanism of infection was not understood. Modern techniques of anesthesia, asepsis, and control of hemorrhage have enabled surgical teams to perform virtual miracles, as sophisticated procedures such as organ transplants and open heart surgery have gradually become commonplace. The early unsterile, crudely equipped operating "theater" has evolved into the technology-dominated operating suite of today in which nurses play major roles.

Although most surgery continues to be performed in hospital operating rooms, this is changing. Ambulatory or outpatient surgery (sometimes called same-day surgery) is becoming increasingly prevalent. The client may enter an outpatient facility, undergo surgery, and return home the same day. The cost of hospitalization and the stresses associated with it are thus reduced.

As techniques advance and as circumstances surrounding surgery change, the nursing knowledge base continues to expand. Cryosurgery, laser surgery, microsurgery, the use of intraoperative hypothermia, and the introduction of client-controlled analgesia are among the innovations that challenge the nurse who provides perioperative care, whether in the operating room, the intensive care unit, or the client's home. This chapter discusses the nursing process as it relates to perioperative care in general. Nursing care for specific surgical procedures, including educating clients about postoperative self-care, is discussed in the surgical approaches chapters in each body system unit.

SECTION I

General Principles of Surgical Treatment

Although surgical procedures vary greatly, both in technique and in the demands they impose on the body, certain fundamental principles are common to all. With a comprehensive understanding of these principles and an empathic attitude, the nurse can assist the client and family in coping with the physiologic and psychosocial stresses of surgery to promote an optimum recovery.

Classification of Surgical Procedures

Surgical procedures may be classified in several ways, according to the purpose, the extent of trauma, or whether the procedure is elective or an emergency (Table 11–1). Knowledge of the type of surgery a client is to undergo as well as the rationale for the procedure are prerequisites for planning nursing care. The client's motivation affects recovery and so does emotional status. For example, a client scheduled for diagnostic or exploratory surgery may be intensely apprehensive about the findings, especially if a diagnosis of malignancy is involved. The client undergoing palliative surgery may feel an overwhelming sense of hopelessness. Conversely, the client anticipating cosmetic surgery may feel joyful expectation of an improved appearance. By knowing the individual client's situation, the nurse can be prepared to offer appropriate psychosocial as well as physical support.

Table 11–1
Classification of Surgical Procedures

Classification	Purpose or Definition
Purpose	
Diagnostic	To determine etiology of client's disorder
Exploratory	To determine a diagnosis and/or to evaluate the extent of a lesion
Curative	
Ablative	To remove diseased tissue or organ(s)
Constructive	To build tissues and/or organs that are absent, anomalous, or have been destroyed or altered by trauma or disease
Reconstructive	To repair or replace tissues or organs (see above)
Palliative	To alleviate symptoms of disease without necessarily altering the disease process
Extent of Trauma	
Major	Imposes extensive trauma and/or is associated with serious risk
Minor	Imposes minimal trauma and is associated with minimal risk
Urgency	
Elective	Recommended, but delay imposes no additional risk on the client
Emergency	Immediately necessary for preservation of life

Surgery as a Multisystem Stressor

Surgery imposes stress on all body systems. It imposes psychologic stresses as well, both on the client and on significant others. The nurse's responsibility includes recognition of these stresses, accurate assessment of their extent, and anticipation and prevention of their consequences to the extent possible. By keeping the client informed of what to expect, reinforcing the physician's explanations in understandable terms, and frankly addressing spoken and unspoken concerns about pain and disability, the nurse can make a major contribution to the client's effort to recover.

Physiologic Stresses

In response to the surgical invasion, the body mobilizes defenses to maintain homeostasis. Most of these mechanisms, which are summarized in Table 11–2, are generally favorable to survival and healing; if uncontrolled or prolonged, however, they may promote the development of complications. Systemic responses to stress and strategies for coping with them are explained in Chapter 2. In addition to systemic responses, local stress reactions also occur in response to tissue injury. These localized effects promote wound healing, which is discussed later in this chapter.

Inactivity related to the surgery also takes its toll on the individual. Although rest aids healing, it may also have detrimental effects on body systems. Hazards associated with immobility are discussed later in this chapter with postoperative care (see also Unit 10). These stresses are superimposed on those related to any existing disease. The specific effects of surgery and anesthesia are discussed later in this chapter.

Psychosocial Stresses

Although physiologic and psychosocial stresses are discussed separately, they are inseparable. The holistic view of health care recognizes that mind and body are inseparable and that mental and emotional states such as fear, anxiety, and uncertainty affect physical as well as psychologic recovery. By minimizing negative responses

Table 11–2
Consequences of Selected Systemic Responses to Surgical Stress

Specific Systemic Responses	Protective Consequences	Negative Consequences
Increase in blood coagulation; peripheral vasoconstriction	Prevention of excessive blood and fluid loss	May increase tendency for postoperative thrombus formation
Increase in the rate and force of the heartbeat, which increases cardiac output and blood pressure; dilatation of coronary arteries	Maintenance of cardiac perfusion and oxygenation when the work load of the heart is increased	Prolonged or repeated effect can promote hypertension and increase work load of the heart, resulting in failure
Increased reabsorption of Na^+ from the kidney, causing retention of Na^+ and water	Maintenance of blood volume, blood pressure, and cardiac output	
Decreased GI peristalsis; increased gastric acidity	Other body functions favored	Paralytic ileus, constipation, stress ulcer
Smooth muscle relaxation promotes dilatation of bronchioles	Improvement of gas exchange and tissue oxygenation	
Increased protein breakdown	Availability of amino acids for tissue repair	If prolonged and uncontrolled, promotes negative nitrogen balance and catabolic effect
Connective tissue proliferation	Promotion of wound healing	
Over a long period, anti-inflammatory effect occurs, with shrinkage of lymphoid tissue		Decreases ability to fight infection
Increase in circulating glucose and mobilization of fat from reserve stores	Provision of needed energy	Chronic increase in glucose and fat stores can promote development of diabetes and atherosclerosis
Increase in basal metabolic rate	Provision of needed energy and tissue nourishment	Sweating in response can be uncomfortable and render the client susceptible to fluid imbalance and decubitus ulcers

and encouraging positive ones, the nurse can assist the client in summoning inherent coping strengths. Coping with the experience of illness is discussed in Chapter 4.

Asepsis and the Care of the Surgical Client

Scrupulous adherence to the principles of infection control is especially important in caring for the surgical client. Once the protective barrier of the integument has been breached, the individual becomes highly susceptible to invasion by pathogenic organisms that may cause local or systemic infections. Moreover, the many invasive procedures associated with surgery create ideal conditions for nosocomial infection.

Nurses have a major responsibility in preventing infections in surgical clients. The principles of asepsis, which are emphasized throughout this chapter, should be conscientiously followed. The general infection control recommendations of the Centers for Disease Control, which are discussed in Chapter 10, should be understood and followed. Specific guidelines for preventing surgical wound infections are reviewed later in this chapter.

Wound Healing

A consequence of surgical manipulation and incision is a localized stress response—the inflammatory process—which contains the tissue injury and promotes wound healing. This process, which is essentially an aggressive response to injury, is discussed in Chapter 2.

The wound-healing process, an outcome of the inflammatory process, involves three phases of repair:

1. The proliferation of epithelial cells to provide a surface covering for incised tissue
2. The formation of pinkish-red granulation tissue, an outgrowth of new tissue and capillaries, to draw wound edges together
3. The synthesis of collagen, which facilitates connective tissue repair and draws wound edges together (scar tissue formation)

Barring complications, the time for normal wound healing depends on the extent of tissue damage from the surgery, the amount of stress and tension placed at the incision, the extent to which wound edges have been approximated, and the client's overall health status. Wound healing generally takes place within 7 to 10 days, although scar tissue contraction continues for some time. Eventually, scar tissue shrinks, but occasionally keloids form. Keloidal tissue is an excessive overgrowth of scar tissue to which dark-skinned persons appear especially susceptible. Keloids can be disfiguring, and although they can be surgically removed, they frequently grow back.

Surgical wounds approximated and closed with clips, staples, sutures, or skin strips heal by **primary intention,** with minimal formation of granulation tissue or scar tissue and minimal loss of function in the affected area. With an infected incision or one that is purposely left open, healing involves greater formation of granulation tissue and contraction from scar tissue **(secondary intention).** Healing by **tertiary intention** involves debridement of large infected or contaminated wounds followed by mechanical skin closure.

A number of factors adversely affect wound healing. Advanced age and nutritional deficiencies are associated with poor healing. Infection also complicates the process, inhibiting tissue repair and perhaps promoting systemic infection or abscess formation. Excessive strain on the incision, from overactivity, for example, can delay union of wound edges. The obese client may have special difficulties with wound healing because adipose tissue has a poor blood supply. The obese client is also prone to dehiscence or evisceration. **Dehiscence** is disruption of the superficial layers of the surgical wound. **Evisceration** is the complete disruption of the wound, with protrusion of the viscera. Often, early signs of these conditions can be detected and measures taken to prevent them. Dehiscence and evisceration are discussed in the section on the later postoperative period.

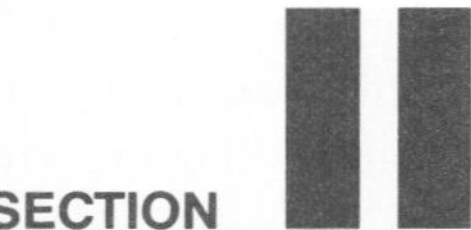

The Scope of Perioperative Nursing Care

During the early days of surgery, nurses had little direct responsibility for the client, and there was little continuity of preoperative and postoperative care. Today the model of care is perioperative nursing, which encompasses care of the client before surgery (preoperative care), during surgery (intraoperative care), and after surgery (postoperative care). The safety and welfare of the client is the nurse's primary concern during all phases of the perioperative period.

Although health care facilities vary, the surgical client is generally cared for by four types of nurses. All share responsibility for the client's well-being throughout the perioperative period, but each has a different focus. *Staff nurses* are responsible for preoperative and postoperative care on the surgical unit, although their responsibility overlaps into the intraoperative period. *Operating room nurses* care for the client primarily during the intraoperative period. Recently, however, the role of operating room nurses has expanded to include preoperative visits to prepare clients for the surgical experience as well as counseling during the postoperative phase. *Nurse anesthetists* (and physician anesthesiologists) develop a plan of anesthesia for the client during the preoperative period, administer the anesthesia during surgery, and evaluate the client's postanesthesia progress.

Postanesthesia recovery room nurses care for the client during the immediate postoperative period, carefully monitoring the client's recovery from anesthesia. Their responsibility for the client is eventually passed back to the staff nurse on the surgical unit. Some clients who require specialized care are taken to the intensive care unit and do not return to the general surgical unit until later, sometimes by way of an intermediate care facility. Recovery room nurses have also become involved with preoperative consultation and postoperative follow-up.

In addition to the basic Standards of Nursing Practice formulated by the American Nurses' Association (ANA), specialized standards pertaining to clients undergoing surgery have been developed. ANA has developed Standards of Medical–Surgical Nursing Practice, and ANA and the Association of Operating Room Nurses (AORN) have jointly issued Standards of Perioperative Nursing Practice. AORN also publishes other recommended practices for operating room nursing and aseptic practice. The American Association of Nurse Anesthetists (AANA) has developed standards of practice for the nurse anesthetist. (See Nursing Organizations in the resource list.)

Nurses who work primarily in the operating room or recovery area require specialized preparation, which may be acquired through inservice education programs or continuing education courses offered through educational institutions and professional organizations. Advanced preparation for surgical nurse practitioners and nurse anesthetists is moving into degree-granting programs at the master's level.

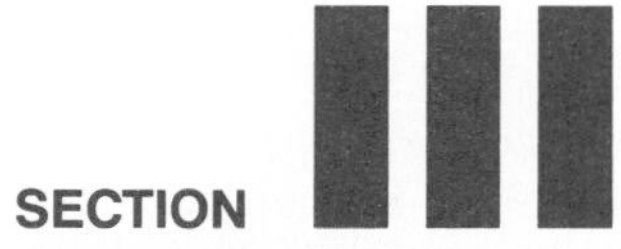

The Nursing Process in Preoperative Care

The preoperative phase of the perioperative period begins when surgery is first considered and ends with the admission of the client to the operating suite. This phase may be long or short, depending on whether surgery is planned or is an emergency.

Nursing Assessment

Before surgery, the nurse participates in assessing the surgical risk, informed consent, and the client's readiness for surgery. These assessments contribute to the formulation of individualized nursing diagnoses and to preoperative planning, implementation, and evaluation.

Surgical Risk

As part of the surgical team, the nurse is involved in determining the client's risk, or potential for complications, associated with the proposed surgery. Assessing risk is important for a number of reasons:

- The client has a legal right to be apprised of all risks before consenting to surgery.
- Identified risks alert health team members to possible complications so they may be considered in planning future care.
- Identified risks can, in some cases, be rectified.

The nurse collects data regarding surgical risk from a number of sources—the health history, the physical examination, and laboratory tests and diagnostic studies. These are discussed later.

By consulting with the surgeon, the nurse can ascertain how extensive the proposed surgery will be. The more extensive the procedure, the greater the surgical risk and the more intensive the nursing care. The nurse can also use the acquired information to clarify the surgeon's instructions to the client and to prepare for postoperative care.

Through ongoing communication with the client, the nurse can encourage expression of feelings about the operation. The client may need more than one explanation, especially if anxiety has impeded comprehension. The client's attitude will greatly influence coping and ultimate recovery, and understanding is likely to improve cooperation with inconvenient or uncomfortable procedures such as NPO status or bowel preparation. All nurses responsible for the client's care throughout the perioperative period should be familiar with the client's risks.

ADVANCED AGE Elderly or aged clients are generally considered poorer surgical risks than younger clients. Cardiac reserve diminishes with advanced age, the heart rate slows, and the individual is less able to adapt successfully to stressful situations such as surgery. Gastrointestinal responsiveness diminishes with age, making the client susceptible to constipation or fecal impaction when surgery also predisposes the client to these problems. The malnutrition common in elderly clients lowers vitality and may interfere with healing. Renal and hepatic function become depressed with advanced age, making it difficult to predict accurately the client's response to medications and anesthetics. One or more degenerative diseases may be present, compromising homeostasis in various ways. Finally, many aged clients—particularly those who are widowed—have lost the support system that contributes to coping with illness.

Nursing Research Note

Faherty B, Grier M: Analgesic medication for elderly people post-surgery. *Nurs Res* 1984; 33(6):369–372.

Analgesic medication prescription and administration to elderly postoperative clients were studied. Elderly clients were compared with younger postoperative clients. The results indicate that less analgesic medication was ordered for postoperative clients aged 54 years and above. Less analgesic medication was administered to clients age 44 years and over. The results also indicate that age more than weight influenced the amount of pain medication administered.

This study demonstrates a need for more research into analgesic use in the elderly population. Nursing assessment must objectively assess the true need for pain medication.

NUTRITIONAL STATUS The success of surgery and the eventual recovery of the client are adversely affected by malnutrition. Malnutrition alters host resistance through depression of the immune response and predisposes the client to wound infection. Laboratory studies have demonstrated a relation between nutritional status and wound repair; deficiencies of protein, vitamins, trace elements, fatty acids, and glucose all have been identified as interfering with the healing process (Flynn & Rovee, 1982). If there is a fluid and electrolyte imbalance before surgery, the client is in serious jeopardy because fluid and electrolyte loss during surgery will compound the problem.

The obese client is at particular risk, because adipose tissue is poorly supplied with blood, is prone to infection, and does not heal well (Flynn & Rovee, 1982). The surgical team may find it harder to position the client appropriately. The surgeon may have greater difficulty in identifying anatomic landmarks during the operation. The anesthetist may have problems inserting and securing peripheral or central intravenous infusion lines, identifying landmarks for regional anesthesia, and securing the airway during surgery.

Finally, surgery itself has a negative effect on nutritional status. Tissue repair and wound healing require energy in excess of that needed for homeostasis; if dietary sources of energy are insufficient, a catabolic effect will occur. Visceral protein depletion (negative nitrogen balance) can significantly increase surgical morbidity and mortality.

UNDERLYING DISORDERS Disorders that alter circulation, such as peripheral vascular disease and atherosclerosis, and those that promote peripheral vascular alteration, such as diabetes, affect tissue perfusion and can inhibit tissue repair. Preexisting anemia can develop into a life-threatening condition when exacerbated by surgical blood loss. Preexisting infections may be spread by surgery and may seriously compromise the ability of the client to fight additional trauma. Unless the purpose of surgery is to treat the infection (ie, by incision and drainage), infection generally contraindicates surgery, at least temporarily. The client with an acute or chronic respiratory disorder may be at greater risk in surgery, because the stress of anesthesia and the surgery can complicate respiratory problems. The cardiovascular system may be particularly taxed during surgery, and the increased work load may overtax the heart of the client with preexisting cardiovascular disease. The client with inadequate renal or hepatic function may be at considerable risk, because the kidneys and liver play a role in wound healing, detoxification and elimination of drugs and anesthetics, and maintenance of fluid and electrolyte balance. If a client has preexisting disorders, a specialist is usually consulted regarding the risks and benefits associated with the intended surgery. Often, measures to reduce risk before surgery are recommended.

MEDICATIONS AND THERAPIES Certain pharmacologic agents and therapeutic regimens increase surgical risk. Examples are chemotherapeutic agents, steroids, anticoagulants, depressants, and radiation therapy. The client receiving chemotherapy, radiotherapy, or steroid treatments is at increased risk of infection and poor tissue healing. Anticoagulants increase the risk of hemorrhage. Central nervous system depressants may cause hypotension or diminished responsiveness. When possible, medications that increase surgical risk are discontinued prior to surgery, but in many cases discontinuing medication may present hazards. This issue is discussed further under planning and implementation.

LIFESTYLE Unhealthy practices such as cigarette smoking or abuse of drugs or alcohol can adversely affect operative risk. The client who smokes has reduced hemoglobin levels and therefore less oxygen available for tissue repair (Flynn & Rovee, 1982). Moreover, increased platelet aggregation in smokers may predispose the client to thrombus formation related to hypercoagulability—a risk superimposed on the risk of thrombosis associated with inactivity.

Clients dependent on alcohol or drugs may experience withdrawal reactions during hospitalization, further complicating recovery. The client who abuses alcohol may have impaired hepatic function as well as nutritional deficiencies. The client who abuses drugs may have untoward reactions to anesthesia and analgesia. In some instances, abused drugs may potentiate the effects, causing dangerous levels of respiratory depression. In other instances, clients may have developed a cross-tolerance to an anesthetic or analgesic agent, increasing the amount of drug needed to achieve the desired effect.

Clients who live a sedentary lifestyle may have poor exercise tolerance and reduced cardiac–respiratory reserve. They may find it difficult to adjust to the physical stresses associated with surgery and recovery.

ATTITUDINAL FACTORS The client who has a high level of anxiety or who lacks confidence in the surgeon or the therapy may also be at greater than normal risk. The highly anxious client experiences greater physiologic and psychologic stress, depleting energy reserves that may be needed in the intraoperative and postoperative periods. Hyperventilation accompanying anxiety may promote a respiratory alkalosis. The client who has lost hope or is depressed may suffer from fatigue, anorexia, and sleep loss, compromising the ability to cope with the stress of surgery and jeopardizing successful recovery.

Health History

The health history provides data about the client's general health and past experiences with surgery. For example, has the client undergone major surgery before? Were there any complications? Hemorrhage? Infection? What type of anesthesia was employed? How rapid or slow was the client's return to normal function? The anesthetist will be particularly interested in the client's prior experience with anesthesia, especially if there were any adverse effects that could influence future anesthesia. In a preoperative visit, the anesthetist will gather these data as well as data about potential intraoperative and postoperative complications.

A thorough history of the client's current and recent but discontinued medication use should be obtained. If the client is taking antihypertensive or antidysrhythmic agents, have they been successful? What drugs could the client be taking that might interact with anesthetic agents? These data help the surgical team plan appropriate perioperative medications. The health history should include all of the factors contributing to risk mentioned previously.

Physical Assessment

In the preoperative physical assessment, pay special attention to the integrity of the respiratory and cardiovascular systems. Wheezes, rhonchi, rales, and decreased or absent breath sounds may indicate the need for more extensive respiratory evaluation or therapy. Assess blood pressure in both arms to gather data concerning possible peripheral vascular disease. Assessment of peripheral pulses should include auscultation for carotid bruits, which indicate impaired cerebral circulation. Any history or physical findings of carotid artery disease indicate that hyperextension of the neck may occlude cerebral blood flow. This is an important finding because the neck is often hyperextended to facilitate various aspects of airway management during endotracheal intubation or when ventilating a client under general anesthesia.

Document the presence of anatomic deformities that may interfere with respiratory or cardiac function (eg, pectus excavatum or severe scoliosis) or indicate the presence of chronic obstructive pulmonary disease (eg, barrel chest). Other musculoskeletal deformities may limit a client's ability to assume various positions during surgery. Hip dysplasia is an example of a musculoskeletal limitation that affects positioning during surgery. Clients with this hip problem will be unable to assume the dorsal lithotomy position. For example, a woman with hip dysplasia may need to have an abdominal hysterectomy rather than a vaginal hysterectomy; a man with hip dysplasia may need to have a suprapubic prostatectomy rather than a perineal prostatectomy. Clients with severe arthritis may be unable to assume even the most routine surgical positions. This information is crucial in planning anesthesia and surgery around the client's limitations, avoiding postoperative complications and unnecessary client discomfort.

LABORATORY TESTS AND DIAGNOSTIC STUDIES Laboratory tests and diagnostic studies help pinpoint possible problems with respiration, circulation, and urinary excretion, as well as other risk factors (eg, previously undiagnosed diabetes or hypertension). Until recently, the client was usually admitted to the hospital for such tests some time—even days—before surgery. The current trend is to perform most tests on an outpatient basis within a week of the scheduled operation. Research has found that the threat of infection is less with shorter preoperative hospital stays (Cruse & Foord, 1980).

Which laboratory tests and diagnostic studies are carried out depends on the findings of the history and physical assessment and the nature of the surgery. Blood type and crossmatch, complete blood count, and urinalysis are commonly performed. Other clients may require an electrocardiogram, liver function studies, a chest x-ray, or other pertinent studies.

Informed Consent

The client usually is requested to sign a form documenting surgical consent. Most hospitals provide standard forms for this purpose. There is a tendency to confuse the mere signing of the form with informed consent. Informed consent is an exchange between the physician and client; the form is a record of the exchange. Informing the client and obtaining consent are the responsibility of the physician. These responsibilities cannot be delegated. The common practice of having nurses obtain consent—or even witness the client's signature—is highly questionable. The nurse who witnesses only the client's signature on the consent form—and who was not present when the physician discussed the treatment or surgery and explained the benefits, risks, or alternatives, to a legally competent individual—should write on the form, "witnessing signature only" (Northrop, 1984).

As a client advocate, the nurse has an important role in assessing whether the client's consent was truly informed. A checklist for information consent, such as the one in Box 11–1, helps the nurse fulfill obligations for informed consent.

If the client does not have adequate information or does not fully understand the procedure, the nurse has a responsibility to refer the problem to the physician. A client has the right to withdraw consent at any time before surgery, and the client should be informed of this right. If the client refuses surgery or withdraws consent, the nurse and physician can cooperate in determining the reason. Often the cause is misinformation or lack of information. Clients who refuse treatment have the right to be fully informed about the consequences of refusal; clients are ultimately responsible for their own bodies, however. Explanations of possible consequences should be given nonjudgmentally.

When surgery is not an emergency, clients should be informed of their right to a second opinion. Information about second opinions might be provided in a printed handout, as shown in Box 11–1. Most insurance carriers, including private insurers, Medicare, and Medicaid, encourage second opinions and will pay for them. Mandatory second opinions are becoming more common.

Client Readiness

Other factors to consider relate to the client's physiologic and psychologic readiness for the experience. Does the client know what to expect during the perioperative period? Is the client familiar with procedures in which he or she must take part (eg, coughing and deep breathing)? Does the client know what tests will be performed? What skin preparation consists of? Whether preoperative medication will be given? Why NPO status is necessary? When the trip to the operating room will take place? What sensory perceptions may be felt during the surgery while under local anesthesia, or upon awakening in the recovery room? Previous experience with surgery does not guarantee that clients are knowledgeable, and the nurse should not neglect to assess their readiness for surgery and to give them preoperative instruction.

Early classic psychologic research demonstrated that a person who knows what to expect is usually better able to tolerate the experience. Most clients fear pain associated with surgery. If the nurse says, "You will have a fair amount of pain during the first 24 hours; then it will abate," the client may be better able to cope because of knowing the pain will soon dissipate. Studies have demonstrated that giving sensory information to clients before a stressful event reduces stress and may even shorten the hospital stay. Other studies have shown that preoperative teaching is associated with less use of pain medication and a lower incidence of vomiting and complications, as well as a shorter stay. An extensive review of such studies documented the potential effectiveness of systematic preoperative teaching; further research is needed to discover the most effective components of such a teaching plan (Devine & Cook,

Box 11–1
Client Checklist for Informed Consent 

To the Client:

Before agreeing to surgical treatment, you have both the right and the responsibility to be sure you understand:

- What your diagnosis is; that is, what is making you ill.
- Why surgical treatment is recommended.
- What the operation will consist of.
- What risks are involved.
- What the probable outcome will be.
- What risks are involved in *not* having surgery.
- What medical (nonsurgical) alternatives there are.

You may want to discuss your operation with your personal physician as well as the surgeon or other specialist who recommended the operation. Here are some questions to ask:

- What is the nature of my illness, in medical terms and in ordinary language?
- What tests have been (will be) done to confirm the diagnosis?
- What risks are associated with the tests?
- What are the test results and what do they mean?

What do the surgery and any additional treatments consist of?

- What will happen during the operation? (Ask for as much detail as *you* need to make a decision.)
- Are there alternative methods of surgery? What are they?
- What additional treatments, if any, will I need after surgery?
- Who will perform the operation? Who will be assisting?
- What are the reasonable risks of the operation?
- Are there any frequent complications of this operation?
- Is this operation experimental or new?

What is the probable outcome of this operation?

- What is the success rate of the operation? (That is, what proportion of the time does it cure my condition?)
- How much pain is involved under normal circumstances?
- Is any long-lasting disfigurement involved? Can it be corrected?
- How long will I be in the hospital?
- How long will I have to stay inactive at home?

What are the alternatives?

- Are there alternative medical (nonsurgical) treatments for my condition? What are they? What are their risks and/or success rates?
- What risks are involved in delaying my decision? How long?
- What is the probable outcome of *not* having surgery?

You are also entitled to obtain a second opinion from a qualified physician. Medicare, Medicaid, and most private insurers will pay for this—check with your insurer. Do not hesitate to seek a second opinion. To find another surgeon or specialist, you may:

- Ask your own doctor.
- Ask a nurse or other health care professional.
- Ask your local medical society or medical school for names of physicians specializing in your condition.
- Call the government's toll-free number to find out how to locate a specialist near you: 800-638-6833 (in Maryland, 800-492-6603).
- If you are covered by Medicare, call your local Social Security office (listed in your telephone directory under US Government, Department of Health and Human Services).
- If you are eligible for Medicaid, call your local welfare office.
- Select a physician who is likely to be most objective and least likely to have a personal relationship with your physician.

1983). Techniques for preoperative teaching are discussed under planning and implementation.

Nursing Diagnosis

Some common nursing diagnoses related to the preoperative client are in Box 11–2.

Planning and Implementation

The preoperative plan of care is based on fundamental principles of preoperative care as they relate to the nursing diagnoses determined for the individual client. Interventions common to all surgical procedures include general physiologic and psychologic preparation, preoperative teaching, and immediate preparation before the surgical procedure.

Physiologic Preparation

MINIMIZATION OF RISK Nursing care before surgery includes assisting with measures to eliminate or minimize identified risks. For example, the condition of the client with cardiac, hepatic, or renal dysfunction or diabetes may need to be stabilized. A client who smokes may reduce his or her risk by giving up smoking 2 weeks before surgery. A client with respiratory difficulties may participate in active respiratory therapy; measures may include coughing and deep breathing, incentive spirometry, and elimination of secretions by postural drainage or intermittent positive pressure breathing (IPPB) therapy. The nurse can encourage the client while assisting in carrying out these measures.

The client with poor nutritional status may be hospitalized for some time before surgery so nutritional deficiencies may be corrected by a well-balanced diet, supplementary feedings, vitamins or minerals, or, in some cases, hyperalimentation. Electrolyte imbalances are also corrected. Nursing measures to maintain and increase the client's appetite may include determining food preferences and providing for them—usually in consultation with the dietitian—by providing small, frequent feedings and by making mealtime pleasant.

The client with potential for infection may be given prophylactic antibiotics before surgery. Preoperative antimicrobial therapy is generally instituted if the wound is dirty or contaminated (eg, a ruptured appendix), with intestinal surgery, or if prosthetic devices are to be inserted. If prophylaxis is to be effective, therapeutic levels of the antibiotic in the tissues must be obtained before surgery.

PREPARATION OF GASTROINTESTINAL TRACT Stress, sedation, general anesthesia, and the inactivity associated with surgery tend to depress gastrointestinal activity, predisposing the client to retention of food and fluids and thereby to abdominal distention and/or vomiting. Besides increasing the client's discomfort, vomiting and distention (often called "gas" by clients) place unnecessary tension on thoracic and abdominal incisions.

Depression of the gastrointestinal tract also predisposes the client to postoperative constipation or fecal impaction. Bowel cleansing by laxative or enema is frequently ordered to help prevent these problems. These measures may be ordered for the evening before surgery or for the day of surgery. For intestinal surgery, however, the bowel may be cleansed for a number of days in advance to minimize the bacterial count in the intestine so contamination of sterile areas is less likely. Cleansing the bowel is especially important in abdominal surgery, because a bowel distended with fecal material may interfere with surgical manipulation of the abdominal organs.

Maintaining NPO status is intended to prevent and alleviate gastrointestinal problems. Allowing ample time for gastric emptying decreases the risk of subsequent pulmonary aspiration of gastric contents, a serious perianesthesia concern discussed later in this chapter. However, preoperative restriction of food and fluids may lead to fluid and electrolyte imbalances in clients who are scheduled for surgery late in the day. When surgery is scheduled in the early afternoon hours, some early morning fluids may be given orally but not within 6 hours of surgery. Minor surgical procedures performed under local anesthesia outside the operating room, as well as those performed in the operating room that do not require the presence of anesthesia personnel, are often performed without dietary restrictions. Many institutions, however, require the presence of the anesthetist to monitor closely, sedate, and support the client even during local anesthesia. In such instances, either client status or the need to anticipate potential problems require the restriction of food and fluids for at least 6 to 8 hours preoperatively in the event that the need for general anesthesia should arise.

MEDICATION STATUS For the client who must be NPO, oral medications are either withheld or administered with a sip of water before surgery; however, the client's physician should be consulted before medications are withheld. Omitting even one dose of certain medications [eg, digoxin (Lanoxin), phenytoin (Dilantin), or various antihypertensives] may place the client in jeopardy. An alternative route of administration such as intramuscular injection may be ordered. The physician may not remember that the client receives routine medication, so be alert to this possibility and be aware of the properties of such medications and the hazards associated with even brief discontinuance.

Box 11–2
Common Nursing Diagnoses Related to Preoperative Care

Anxiety, related to threat to health status

Fear, related to impending diagnostic surgery

Grieving, anticipatory, related to expected loss of body part

Knowledge deficit, related to surgical procedure and associated risks

Self-concept, disturbance in: body image, related to anticipated change in body function

Self-concept, disturbance in: role performance, related to inability to meet usual responsibilities

Also be aware of potential problems associated with routine medications. Clients who receive daily doses of intermediate or long-acting insulins, for example, require a diet that will meet carbohydrate levels to which their insulin dosage has been adjusted. On the day of surgery, when the client is NPO and the principal source of nourishment will be intravenous fluids, carbohydrate levels and insulin requirements are unpredictable. Stress associated with surgery may cause an increase in the client's blood levels of glucose, further complicating the picture. Changes in insulin coverage will be necessary.

PREPARATION OF THE SKIN The area to be incised is usually cleansed before surgery with an antiseptic such as povidone–iodine (Betadine) or tincture of chlorhexidine to minimize the number of microorganisms on the skin (Centers for Disease Control, 1982). Such cleansing reduces the risk of contamination and infection of the wound. The client may be instructed to bathe or shower with antiseptic solutions the night before and/or the morning of surgery.

In the past, the area of the incision was also routinely shaved, because hair was believed to be a potential source of microbial contamination. Recent studies, however, have brought this assumption into question. Several investigators have found that not removing hair at all, clipping hair, or using electric shavers or depilatory agents are associated with lower infection rates than traditional shaving (Cruse & Foord, 1980; Alexander et al., 1983). Fewer infections occurred when hair was removed close to the time of incision (Alexander et al., 1983). The Centers for Disease Control (1982) recommends that hair be removed, if necessary, shortly before surgery. The trend, therefore, is to remove hair immediately before surgery, often in the operating suite. The nurse responsible for hair removal should pay careful attention to preventing skin abrasion or laceration, because skin wounds may harbor microorganisms or provide an entry route for them. See a nursing fundamentals text for further discussion of hair removal before surgery.

REST AND HYGIENE A well-rested client is more relaxed and less anxious. Often, a sedative is ordered to provide a good night's sleep for the hospitalized client the night before surgery. Although clients may protest that the sedative is unnecessary, they should be reminded that this medication is available. A bath or shower may also aid relaxation, ensure that the client is clean and comfortable, and reduce the number of microorganisms.

Psychologic Preparation of Client and Family

Health care professionals, who may see many surgical cases every day, sometimes forget how frightening the prospect of "being cut" is to the client. A procedure that seems minor to the nurse (eg, a dilatation and curettage) may not seem minor to the client. Some clients voice their fears openly; others become withdrawn; still others seem stoic. The prospect of surgery raises many questions, spoken or unspoken, about body image alteration, loss of control, and fear of pain or death. In encouraging the client to discuss fears and in helping to clarify expectations, be careful not to minimize the amount of discomfort the client can expect. Reassure the client that analgesics will be available when needed and that family and friends will be able to visit.

Significant others are usually permitted to visit on the morning that surgery is scheduled, regardless of visiting hours. The presence of a supportive person may greatly aid coping. A visit by a member of the clergy or a spiritual advisor may also be helpful, and the client should be informed that such counsel is available. Insisting on such a visit, however, might suggest to some clients that their condition is more serious than they have been told.

Prepare the family for the experiences they are likely to encounter on the day of surgery and in the postoperative period. Family members and friends may be feeling stressed and anxious, especially in instances where the diagnosis is questionable or the outcome of the surgery is difficult to predict. Be sure to let them know what time to come to the hospital to see the client before surgery and before preoperative sedation is given. Family members and friends should know where to wait while the client is in surgery. Some hospitals permit a family member or friend to accompany the client to the operating room holding area. However, most hospitals require visitors to wait in the client's room or in a waiting area adjacent to the operating room. When surgical procedures are expected to be lengthy, family and friends will probably be more comfortable in an environment other than the hospital and may choose to return home to wait if distance permits.

Family and friends often ask the nurse how long the surgery is expected to take. Predictions about the length of surgery should be made with caution, taking into account the numerous factors (such as the extent of a lesion or even scheduling complications in the operating room itself) that could prolong the amount of time the client spends in the operating room but not necessarily the length of time of the surgery itself. Make sure that predictions are general enough so that visitors do not become unduly concerned if the client does not return to the hospital room exactly when expected.

If a waiting area is provided in the operating suite itself, the operating room nurse or other personnel may give the family and friends periodic updates. If visitors are waiting in the client's hospital room, operating room personnel can inform the staff nurse who can, in turn, relay the messages. Inform the family about the communication system before the client's surgery. Knowing how to go about obtaining information on the progress of the client's surgery is comforting to them.

Preoperative Teaching

Each type of nurse contributes special knowledge to preoperative teaching of the client and family. The surgical staff nurse provides general orientation to the entire perioperative period. The operating room nurse can explain what occurs during the actual surgery. The nurse anesthetist discusses the anesthesia experience. The recovery room nurse concentrates on immediate postsurgical recovery. It may be possible to have the client tour some areas of the operating rooms and recovery rooms and to meet personnel who will be involved in intraoperative and postoperative care. Remember that the client who has same-day surgery also needs comprehensive preparation, with additional teaching about home recovery.

GENERAL ORIENTATION Preoperative teaching generally includes a general orientation to the surgical experience and instruction in specific activities in which the client will participate postoperatively to avoid complications and speed recovery. Explain specific preoperative preparation such as restriction of food and fluids, including the rationale for these measures. Clients who understand the reason for procedures are more likely to remember them and to comply with the regimen. If nasogastric intubation, insertion of an intravenous line, or urinary catheterization has been ordered, prepare the client for these events. "Surprises" of this kind increase the client's apprehension and intensify concerns about control. Also reassure the client and family that the nurse will be available for support and will be concerned for the client's safety throughout the surgical experience.

POSTOPERATIVE MOVING, TURNING, COUGHING, AND DEEP BREATHING Clients should be instructed about the importance of moving and turning, coughing, and deep breathing. Explain that inactivity imposed by surgery makes blood flow sluggish and can predispose the client to thrombosis. Moving and turning help prevent this complication. Inform clients that they will be encouraged to move and turn as soon as possible after surgery. Clients who are able to move without help should be prepared to move their extremities and to turn from side to side within the limits that may be imposed by the surgeon. Tell the client who will be unable to move or turn that the nurse will assist with these activities.

Inactivity, sedation, anesthesia, and pain can cause hypoventilation. The surgical client is susceptible to atelectasis, a condition in which the alveoli collapse and adequate gas exchange cannot occur. Accumulation of mucous secretions can lead to bronchitis and pneumonia. Explain these possible complications and encourage the client to practice deep breathing and controlled coughing, so these procedures will be familiar when they are required after surgery. Recommend the sitting position or Fowler's position because they allow for maximum lung expansion and aeration. Several deep breaths (such as those described in diaphragmatic breathing below) should be followed by a short breath and cough. Or teach the client the *cascade cough:* taking a deep breath, holding it for 3 seconds, and coughing several times while exhaling. These subsequent coughs upon exhalation at successively lower lung volumes prevent small airway collapse (a potential complication of forceful coughing for clients with chronic obstructive pulmonary disease).

Clients should be told that coughing may be painful, especially if a thoracic, lumbar flank, or abdominal incision is involved. Splinting the incision—providing external support—reduces movement of the involved tissues, reduces pain, and thus facilitates coughing and deep breathing. Either the nurse or client can splint the incision by supporting it with a pillow or interlocked hands. Both methods are illustrated in Figure 11–1A and B. The support that splinting provides often helps to alleviate clients' fear of "splitting the stitches." Reassure clients that sutures are strong and able to withstand coughing and deep breathing. Remind the client that analgesics will be available. Coughing and deep breathing, although generally a routine postoperative activity, may be contraindicated in some surgeries, such as eye surgeries, because increased pressure can damage the operative site. These contraindications are discussed in the chapters about surgical approaches to specific disorders.

Deep breathing, or diaphragmatic breathing, uses the diaphragm and abdominal muscles to fully aerate the lungs. The client should relax the abdominal wall by flexing the knees and breathe in deeply and slowly through the nose while pushing the abdomen out. The client can tell if he or she is breathing correctly by practicing with one hand on the chest and the other hand on the abdomen. The hand on the abdomen should rise with inspiration and fall with expiration. The hand on the chest should remain still. Clients with chronic obstructive pulmonary disease should exhale slowly through pursed lips.

Teach clients who are restricting or limiting upper chest movement because of pain (common with clients having chest or kidney surgery or mastectomy) the apical expansion exercises illustrated in Figure 11–1C. Basal expansion exercises, discussed and illustrated in Figure 11–1D, promote and maintain mobility of the lower thorax. They are often helpful for clients after chest surgery when pain on the affected side inhibits bilateral chest movement.

Immediate Presurgical Preparation

In the immediate presurgical period, the nurse on the unit is responsible for ensuring that the client is physically prepared for transport to the operating room and that the appropriate records will accompany the client. Institutional policies regarding these procedures vary, but general considerations include the following measures.

PREPARATION OF THE CLIENT *The importance of appropriate identification cannot be overemphasized.* Asking the client's name is insufficient; check the client's identification bracelet before proceeding with the final preparation and administration of preoperative medications. Vital signs should be monitored immediately before the administration of preoperative medications and transfer to the operating suite. Abnormalities or findings inconsistent with the client's usual values should be reported to the surgeon in case a delay of surgery is appropriate. Allergies and handicaps should also be noted.

Preoperative nasogastric intubation is often ordered for clients having abdominal surgery and those in whom depressed gastrointestinal function may be expected. Foley catheters are usually inserted before genitourinary surgery, before major surgery when careful monitoring of fluid balance will be necessary, and before lengthy procedures that may cause urinary retention and bladder distention. Insertion of an intravenous line is almost always indicated to provide a route for anesthesia, maintenance or replacement fluids, and/or emergency medications. This insertion is usually performed in the operating room, however.

Jewelry, hairpins, prosthetic devices, hearing aids, eyeglasses and contact lenses, and false teeth are removed for the client's safety. The client should be asked about dental caps or bridges that might be dislodged during endotracheal intubation. Agency policy will determine how jewelry is secured; generally, a careful list of the client's belongings is made and security measures are taken. The client should be encouraged to send jewelry home with a relative for safekeeping. A wedding band may occasionally be left on with tape to secure it, depending on institutional

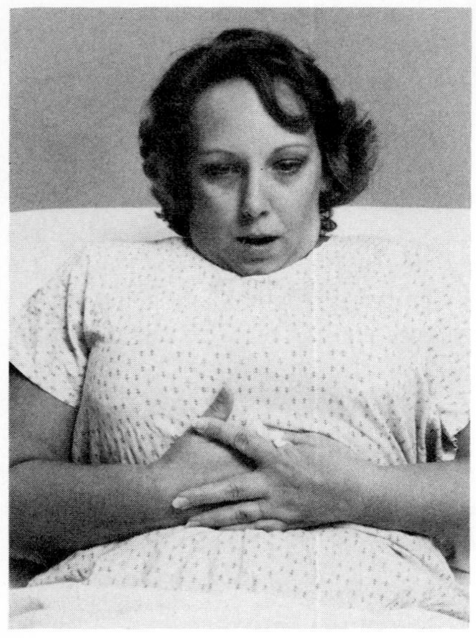

A

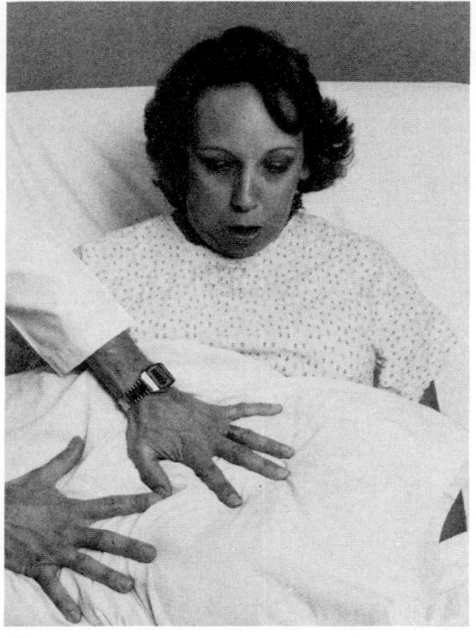

B

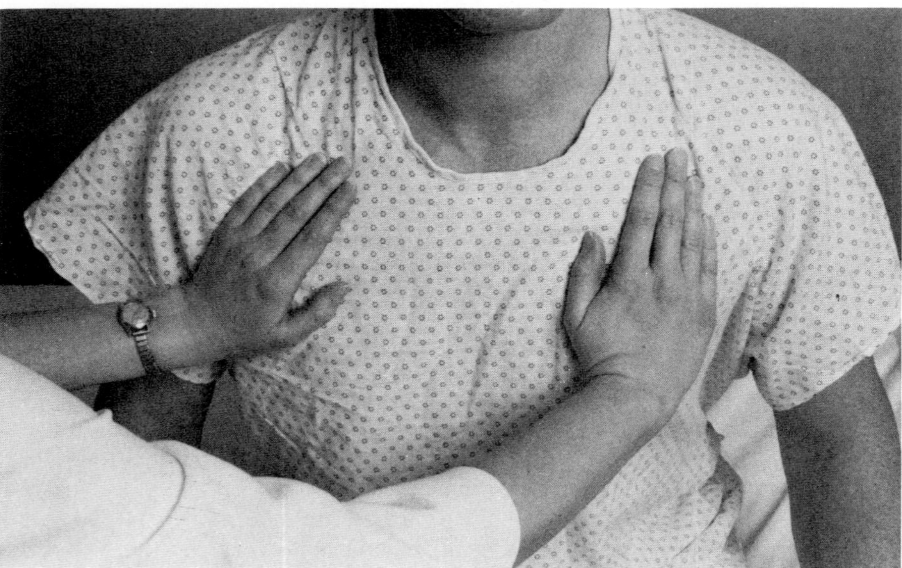

C

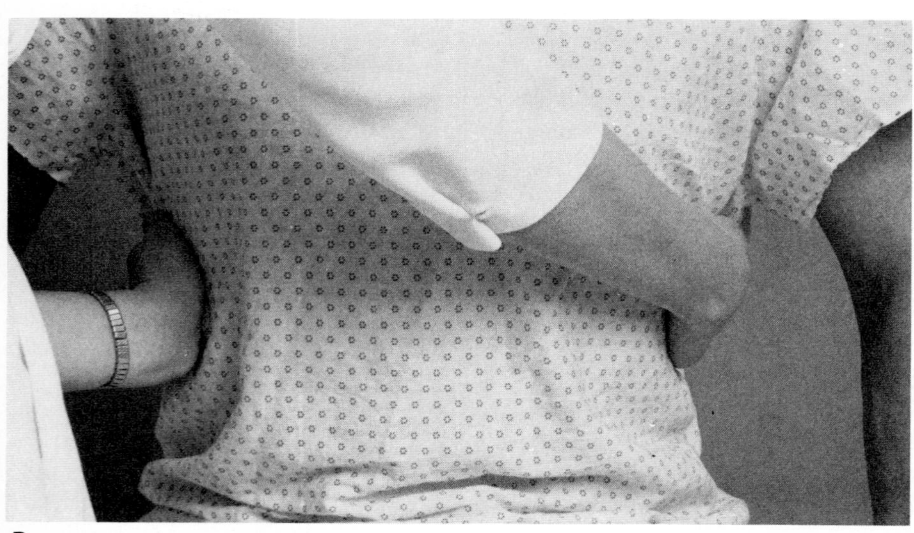

D

Figure 11–1

Splinting the incision for coughing. **A**. Splinting the incision during coughing by supporting it with interlocked hands. An alternative method is to press the arm and hand of the unaffected side against the operative area. **B**. A pillow, pressed against the operative area, can also provide support. Both methods can be done by the client, family member, or nurse. **C**. Apical expansion. The client inhales, pushing the chest upward and outward, against the moderate pressure applied by the nurse. Encourage the client to retain the expansion before exhaling quietly. **D**. Basal expansion. The client inhales, attempting to expand the lower ribs to move the nurse's hands outward. The client may use his or her own hands for both C and D, performing the exercises independently. Encourage the client to retain maximum inhalation for 1 or 2 seconds before exhaling quietly. *SOURCE: Swearingen, PL:* The Addison-Wesley Photo Atlas of Nursing Procedures. *Menlo Park, CA: Addison-Wesley, 1984.*

policy, but this practice can be hazardous. In the event of postoperative edema, jewelry can cut into the skin and obstruct circulation. Generally, any current wound dressings are left in place to prevent cross-contamination of wounds. The nurse should ensure that dressings are clean. Nail polish, lipstick, and other cosmetics can interfere with observations for pallor and cyanosis and should be removed. Instructions to the client about not wearing makeup should include an explanation of the reason.

Clients who have not been catheterized should void before receiving preoperative medications to prevent distention of the bladder during surgery. In abdominal surgery, bladder distention may interfere with the identification of operative landmarks and appropriate surgical technique and may predispose the bladder to trauma. Postoperative bladder distention also contributes to client discomfort. After preoperative medications have been given, the client should not be permitted out of bed to void, because the sedative effects may predispose the client to injury.

Only when these preparations have been completed should preoperative medications be given. Pharmacologic preparation of the client has both physiologic and psychologic objectives. Perhaps the most common objective is to control anxiety and promote a state of calmness. Sedatives are usually ordered the night before surgery to help the client sleep well and may also be given the morning of surgery. Other reasons for preoperative medications are to reduce oral secretions, interrupt vagal nerve impulses that slow the heart, decrease gastric fluid volume, increase gastric fluid pH, and prevent postoperative nausea and vomiting. Clients with preexisting injuries may require narcotics to be able to tolerate movement during transfer to the operating room. Anticholinergics such as atropine or glycopyrrolate may be given to facilitate endotracheal intubation or prevent the accumulation of secretions in a client receiving general anesthesia by a mask technique.

General anesthesia, especially for the client with a full stomach, predisposes the client to the life-threatening risk of aspirating acidic gastric contents into the tracheobronchial tree. This risk may be reduced by decreasing gastric volume or increasing the pH of gastric contents. Several medications (eg, antacids, H_2-antagonists, metoclopramide) used in combination may effect these desired changes in the gastric environment.

The nurse should be familiar with common preoperative medications and their side effects and contraindications. Preoperative medications may be ordered for a specific time or on an on-call basis. Remember to document precisely when these drugs were given. Timely administration of these drugs maximizes the likelihood that they will have the desired effect. After preoperative medications have been given, provide for the safety of the client by raising the siderails of the bed, cautioning the client not to get up, and placing the call device within easy reach.

The client is taken to surgery by stretcher. Verification that preoperative medications have been given and that the client is ready for surgery must be provided, usually in the form of a progress note on the client's chart. A preoperative checklist generally accompanies the client. The checklist serves as a reminder, helping to ensure comprehensive preoperative preparation.

PREPARATION OF THE CLIENT'S RECORD The client's chart accompanies him or her throughout the intraoperative period. Because the client will generally be unable to furnish information to health care providers during this time, the completeness and accuracy of the records are especially important. In addition to any information especially required by agency policy, the chart should be examined for evidence of:

- Signed consent
- Complete health history, including information on allergies, and physical examination records
- Completed consultation report(s), if ordered
- Reports of diagnostic work-up, including laboratory tests and x-rays
- Availability of any blood ordered in preparation for surgery and proof of type and crossmatch
- Identification plate, in case additional chart forms are required

The nurse is responsible for notifying the physician of any abnormal laboratory or diagnostic findings. Results of any ordered consultations should be obtained and reviewed by the physician before surgery.

Evaluation

Goals related to the client's understanding of the surgical experience and postoperative activities may be evaluated by asking the client to repeat the information provided and to demonstrate deep breathing and coughing. Goals related to decreasing surgical risk should be met with evidence of improvement observed through physical assessment and results of laboratory tests and diagnostic studies. The preoperative checklist provides an instrument for evaluating goals of immediate presurgical care.

SECTION 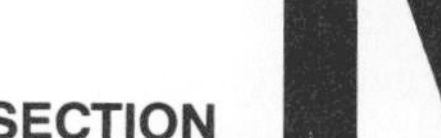

The Nursing Process in Intraoperative Care

The intraoperative phase of the perioperative period begins when the client enters the operating suite and ends with the completion of surgery and transfer of the client to the recovery room. During this period, the operating room nurse, as part of the surgical team, cares for the client. Because many of the routine procedures during this phase compromise the client's safety, comfort, and privacy, nursing care focuses on meeting these needs. Although some specific procedures vary among health care facilities, certain principles and procedures are common to all.

General Intraoperative Procedures

During the intraoperative phase, care of the client is the responsibility of the surgical team. The team is generally composed of the surgeon, one or more surgical assistants, an individual who administers anesthesia (nurse anesthetist or physician anesthesiologist), a scrub nurse or operating room technician, and a circulating nurse. For highly complex operations such as organ transplants or open heart surgery, the team is greatly expanded.

Functions of the Surgical Team

The surgeon performs the actual surgery; surgical assistants retract tissue and suction blood and debris from the surgical site to afford the surgeon clear visualization of the operative field. The physician anesthesiologist or nurse anesthetist maintains the client in a state of adequate surgical anesthesia while monitoring vital functions and providing for physiologic homeostasis. The scrub nurse or operating room technician assists the surgeon by providing instruments and other materials (eg, sponges or sutures) as needed. Finally, the circulating nurse serves the needs of the other team members and the client; the circulator sets up the room, maintains the necessary supply of instruments and materials, and ensures that all equipment is safe and functional. Any required blood, medications, and intravenous solutions are also obtained through the circulating nurse, who also oversees maintenance of sterile technique and alerts team members of any breaks in technique. All members of the surgical team work together to ensure the safety and welfare of the client.

In no other setting is the role of the nurse as client advocate more challenging. During surgery, the client relies entirely on the surgical team to meet physiologic as well as psychosocial needs. The nurse must ensure that the informed consent the client has given is not violated.

The Operating Room Environment

The layout of the operating suite and the procedures performed there are designed to provide for efficiency, safety, and infection control. A typical suite houses operating rooms and scrub areas, clean and dirty linen supply areas, a personnel lounge and dressing room, and a client holding area. A small hospital may have two or three operating rooms, whereas a large surgical suite may have 12 to 15 rooms in a hospital of 500 to 600 beds. Some operating rooms are designed for minor procedures; others, with more sophisticated equipment, are used for major procedures. Regardless of complexity, all operating rooms should contain supplies for emergency care of the client.

Safety and infection control are primary concerns in operating room design. Gruendemann and Meeker (1983) recommend that temperature be maintained between 20°C and 24°C (68°F to 75°F) and humidity at a minimum of 50% to help control bacterial growth and prevent static electricity. The potential for bacterial contamination of the operating room is further reduced by such devices as air filters, positive pressure, and high-flow unidirectional ventilation systems. The operating room is a potentially hazardous environment containing electrical equipment and many materials, such as oxygen, that support combustion.

Operating rooms are generally adjacent to a clean supply area from which sterile supplies can be conveniently obtained. A generous supply of instruments and materials is kept on hand in case of emergency. Soiled and contaminated supplies are removed to a dirty supply area for processing, cleaning, and sterilization.

Scrub Attire

Scrub attire is worn to decrease transport of microorganisms that personnel may harbor on their skin, shoes, and clothing and in their respiratory passages. Attire includes a hat, a pantsuit or dress, shoe coverings, and a face mask. Scrub clothing may be disposable or reusable, and it is clean, not sterile. Individuals who scrub for surgery (the surgeon, assistants, and scrub nurse or OR technician) also wear sterile gowns and gloves that are put on after the surgical scrub and after entering the operating room (Figure 11–2). All scrub apparel should be flame resistant, lint free, cool, and comfortable. Caps are put on first so other attire will not be contaminated by hair. Shoe covers and masks as well as any sterile garb must be changed between procedures and when leaving and reentering the operating room. Other garb may also require changing.

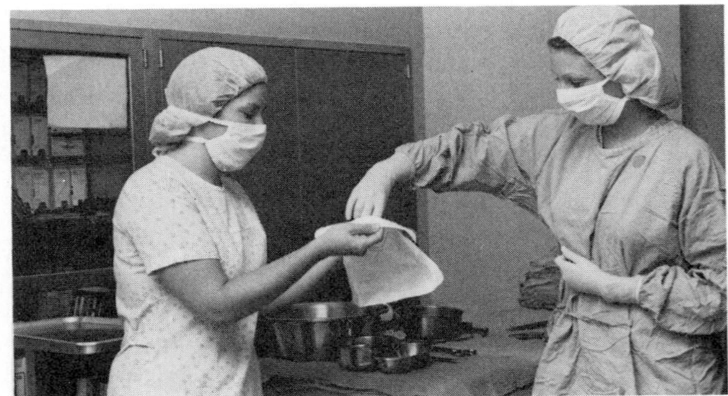

Figure 11–2

Circulating nurse (left) and scrub nurse. *Courtesy of Millard Fillmore Hospital, Buffalo, NY.*

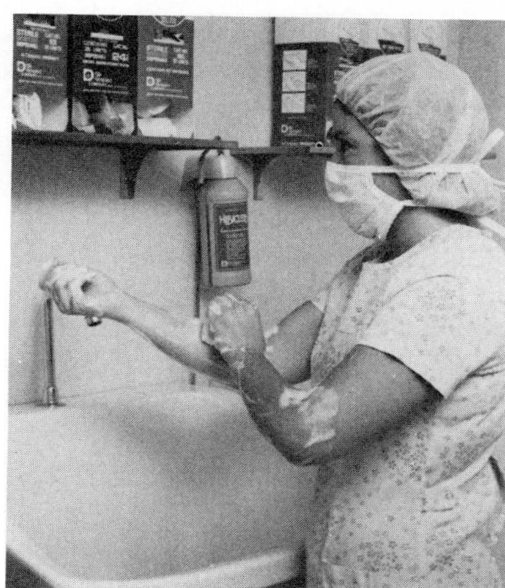

Figure 11–3

The surgical scrub. *Courtesy of Millard Fillmore Hospital, Buffalo, NY.*

The Surgical Scrub

Before entering the operating room, scrub personnel perform a surgical scrub in the area provided for that purpose. The purpose of the surgical scrub is to make the hands and forearms as clean as possible, reducing the number of microorganisms that might contaminate the surgical incision. The procedure takes about 5 minutes. As with routine handwashing, the scrub's effectiveness depends on the application of light friction and the action of an antimicrobial soap or detergent. Hands and forearms are scrubbed with a brush well above the elbows, and the nails are cleaned. The hands are held higher than the elbows for scrubbing and rinsing (Figure 11–3). Hands and forearms are dried with a sterile towel in the operating room, and a sterile gown and sterile gloves are then donned, using aseptic technique.

Anesthesia

Anesthesia is administered to make the client more receptive to surgery and less susceptible to trauma by promoting narcosis (drug-induced unconsciousness), analgesia (pain relief), amnesia (loss of recall), muscle relaxation, and protection from detrimental autonomic reflex responses to surgical stimuli. The anesthetist will have visited the client before the operation to perform a preanesthesia history and physical examination; to help reduce the client's anxiety; participate in preoperative teaching; and obtain information about any previous experience with surgery, associated risks, and contraindications for specific anesthetic agents. Client preferences will have been ascertained, but these are superseded by requirements imposed by the client's health history and the type of surgery to be performed. Anticipated departures from the client's preference will have been explained. Although anesthesia affords freedom from pain, its price is loss of control. Clients feel more comfortable in relegating control after having met and consulted with the anesthetist. The preanesthesia visit can help to establish lines of communication and trust between client and anesthetist.

The person in charge of administering anesthesia also is responsible for preparing necessary equipment and supplies before the operation. Throughout the surgical procedure, this surgical team member monitors all the client's vital functions (temperature, pulse, respirations, blood pressure, and ECG data) and keeps the surgeon continually informed of the client's status. Measures are taken as needed to maintain adequate blood volume, cardiac output, and blood pressure.

General Anesthesia

General anesthetics depress cerebral function and interfere with consciousness, perception of sensations, voluntary motor function, and involuntary reflex action. They are administered by various routes, usually by intravenous administration or inhalation.

ANESTHETIC AGENTS AND ADJUNCTS Inhalation anesthesia requires a mask and/or an endotracheal (ET) tube. The ET tube is frequently employed because it helps maintain a patent airway, provides a route for removal of secretions, prevents aspiration of material into the lungs, and allows for ventilatory assistance if necessary. Only qualified personnel should insert an ET tube because expert appreciation of airway anatomy and placement technique are required to prevent serious complications such as intubation of the esophagus, soft tissue obstruction, and laryngospasm, all of which can interfere with proper oxygenation. (See also Chapter 14 which discusses and illustrates the use of ET tubes.)

Inhalation anesthetics are taken up in the lungs where molecules of the anesthetic vapor cross the alveolocapillary membrane. Once in the blood, the agents induce general anesthesia by affecting the central nervous system (CNS). They also exert many effects (usually depressant) on the cardiovascular, respiratory, urinary, hepatic–biliary, and endocrine systems. Nitrous oxide, halothane (Fluothane), enflurane (Ethrane), and isoflurane (Forane) are common inhalation anesthetics.

Various intravenous drugs are in common use as anesthetic agents and as adjuncts to anesthesia. Barbiturates such as thiopental sodium (Pentothal) are used most frequently to produce rapid, smooth induction of anesthesia before the use of an inhalation agent. Benzodiazepines such as diazepam (Valium), useful because of their sedative qualities, are employed during induction or as preoperative sedation. Narcotics are used during the entire perioperative period. In some circumstances, narcotics may be used to induce anesthesia, and high doses may be used as the sole anesthetic agent throughout the surgical procedure. Etomidate (Amidate) is a new drug useful in producing rapid, smooth induction.

Neuromuscular blocking agents, administered intravenously, are also adjuncts to anesthesia. Succinylcholine chloride (Anectine), pancuronium bromide (Pavulon), and tubocurarine chloride (Tubarine) are examples of this class of drugs. They create optimal conditions for endotracheal intubation and relax skeletal muscles. Relaxation of skeletal muscles serves several important purposes during surgery: facilitating the surgeon's access to the operative area, minimizing retraction trauma against otherwise tense muscles, and preventing client movement while surgery is being performed. Clients receiving neuromuscular blocking agents are closely monitored by the anesthetist because of possible dangerous side effects such as respiratory embarrassment, prolonged apnea, and cardiovascular complications such as hypotension and cardiac dysrhythmias. A number of adjuvant drugs (eg, catecholamines, sympathomimetics, antihypertensives, antidysrhythmics, and sympathetic blockers), although not anesthetics, are used to maintain homeostasis during surgery when the client's own physiologic mechanisms cannot.

During anesthesia, the anesthetist continually monitors and adjusts the client's level of anesthesia. Traditional descriptions of the stages of anesthesia have been based on the signs elicited during ether anesthesia. Today, ether is no longer in use. It has been replaced by inhalation and intravenous agents whose actions vary from those of ether. In addition, the actions tend to be agent-specific; the stages of anesthesia tend to vary with the agent and technique used. Discussion of these stages as they occur with individual anesthetic agents is beyond the scope of this chapter and can be found in textbooks on anesthesia.

COMPLICATIONS OF GENERAL ANESTHESIA The client who has undergone general anesthesia has incurred a neurologic deficit by virtue of the general depression of the CNS by these agents. Many of the complications of general anesthesia are a direct outgrowth of these CNS effects that result in diminution or loss of protective reflexes such as the gag reflex, the corneal reflex, and sympathetic nervous system reflexes. Some potential complications are untoward reactions to drugs, hypoxemia, dysrhythmias, hypothermia, malignant hyperthermia crisis (a hypermetabolic state that presents an acute emergency situation), urinary retention, and nausea and vomiting, among others.

RISKS TO OPERATING ROOM PERSONNEL The operating room environment combines sophisticated technology with the potential for error in its use. Although the hazards of combustion associated with the use of flammable anesthetics has disappeared since the advent of newer nonexplosive agents, dangers such as electrical shock or electrocution have increased. Various measures have been incorporated into the operating room environment to lessen the risk of electrical shock. Laser technology also has certain risks, which are discussed later in this chapter.

Personnel in the operating room are chronically exposed to trace levels of anesthetic gases. Available data suggest that a health hazard may exist in this chronic exposure (Lecky, 1983). Based on the association of trace gas exposure with such phenomena as increased rates of congenital malformations and spontaneous abortion among female personnel and decrements in performance on psychologic tests, steps have been taken to minimize trace gas exposure. Adequate ventilation of operating rooms, closed scavenging of excess gases directly from the anesthesia machine out of the room through the ventilation exhaust or suction, and trace gas monitoring programs may be instituted.

Regional Anesthesia

Regional anesthetics such as lidocaine (Xylocaine), mepivacaine (Carbocaine), procaine (Novocaine), cocaine, and benzocaine block the conduction of nerve impulses to specific sites in the body by blocking nerve pathways, preventing transmission of pain and other sensations, and inhibiting motor function. Because the client remains conscious, psychologic support is necessary throughout.

Spinal anesthesia involves the injection of a local anesthetic agent into the subarachnoid space at the L-3 or L-4 interspace (Figure 11–4A), where it blocks impulse conduction in the spinal nerve roots and the dorsal root ganglia (refer to Chapter 27). In *epidural anesthesia,* a local anesthetic agent is injected into the extradural space, which lies between the dura mater and the body and ligamentous structures of the spinal canal (Figure 11–4B). Epidural anesthesia is usually given in the lumbar region but may also be given in the thoracic epidural space. A *caudal block* is a form of epidural anesthesia that involves injecting the local anesthetic agent in the sacral canal. Although the amount of the anesthetic agent required for spinal anesthesia is small, the amount required in epidural anesthesia and caudal block can be large, meeting or even exceeding toxic levels unless the dose and concentration are carefully monitored.

Peripheral nerve block anesthesia blocks peripheral nerves at specific sites (Figure 11–4C). Brachial, radial, medial, and ulnar nerve blocks are used for the upper extremity. Blocks of the sciatic, femoral, obturator, and lateral cutaneous femoral nerves and nerves of the ankle are used for the lower extremity. Peripheral nerve blocks may also be used for diagnostic purposes and to relieve pain. A *Bier block* is a form of intravenous regional anesthesia to an extremity occluded by a pneumatic tourniquet.

Infiltration anesthesia is the intracutaneous or subcutaneous injection of local anesthetics directly into tissues that are to be surgically cut or sutured, blocking the sen-

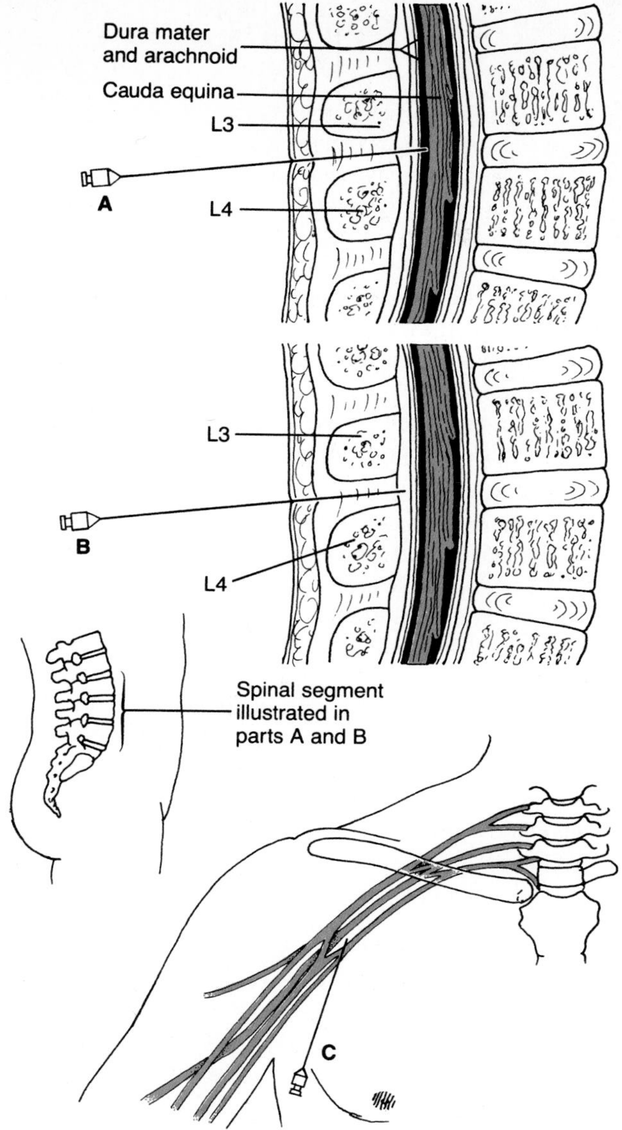

Figure 11–4

Regional anesthesia. **A.** Spinal anesthesia. The anesthetic is injected into the subarachnoid space between L–3 and L–4. **B.** Epidural anesthesia. The anesthetic is injected into the extradural space between L–3 and L–4. **C.** Peripheral nerve block. The anesthetic is injected into the brachial plexus in preparation for surgery on the client's right arm.

sory nerve pathways. This may require a single injection or multiple injections in a ring surrounding the operative area.

Topical, or *surface, anesthesia* involves the direct external application of a local anesthetic in a cream, ointment, drops, spray, or other form. Some forms are used to anesthetize traumatized skin; others are used for mucous membranes.

Regional anesthesia has several disadvantages. Protective motor and sensory functions are lost in the body area of regional anesthesia with consequences similar to general anesthesia. Clients having spinal anesthesia may experience a spinal headache (discussed under immediate postoperative care). In both spinal and epidural anesthesia, hypotension may occur in response to vasodilation. With topical anesthesia of the mucous membranes of the throat (eg, for bronchoscopy), the gag reflex may be suppressed and swallowing affected for about 1 hour after the application of the anesthetic. Compromised cardiopulmonary function may require rapid resuscitation or the administration of supportive medications. The care of a client having a regional anesthetic should be as meticulous as for the client having a general anesthetic.

Other Types of Anesthesia

Other more controversial but potentially less traumatic types of anesthesia are not commonly employed in the United States. *Acupuncture,* an ancient Oriental medical practice that involves the insertion of metal needles at particular body points, is effective in increasing a client's pain threshold and enables most minor surgical and dental procedures to be performed without the use of other anesthetics. Acupuncture is more fully discussed in Chapter 3. *Hypnosis,* another form of anesthesia not fully understood, uses the power of suggestion to control pain. These anesthetic alternatives have advantages because vital functions are not adversely affected, postoperative respiratory and circulatory complications do not occur, and the client's food and fluid intake need not be interrupted.

Surgical Positioning

The dorsal recumbent (supine), prone, and lateral positions are the major ones used for surgery with modification for particular operations. The surgical positions are illustrated in Figure 11–5.

Poor positioning can adversely affect the musculoskeletal, nervous, circulatory, and respiratory systems. Excessive or prolonged pressure on skin, bones, or muscles and/or poor alignment can lead to abrasions, pressure ulcers, and postoperative pain. Pressure on superficial nerves can cause temporary or permanent paresthesia, paralysis, or loss of sensation. Excessive pressure on blood vessels can obstruct the flow of blood, depriving tissues of oxygenation and nourishment. Pressure may also contribute to pooling of blood and formation of thrombi. It is important that all nurses, not only those who work in the operating room, be aware of the inherent potentials for client injury. Damage incurred in the operating room often does not become apparent until the postoperative period.

Although clients should be securely strapped into position on the operating table, check to be sure that the client is not strapped too tightly, that bony prominences are padded, and that supporting pillows, pads, or bolsters do not cause undue pressure on a nerve or a blood vessel, thus risking nerve damage or venous thrombosis. Be sure that the extremity used for the intravenous line is properly supported and positioned to avoid excessive abduction. In

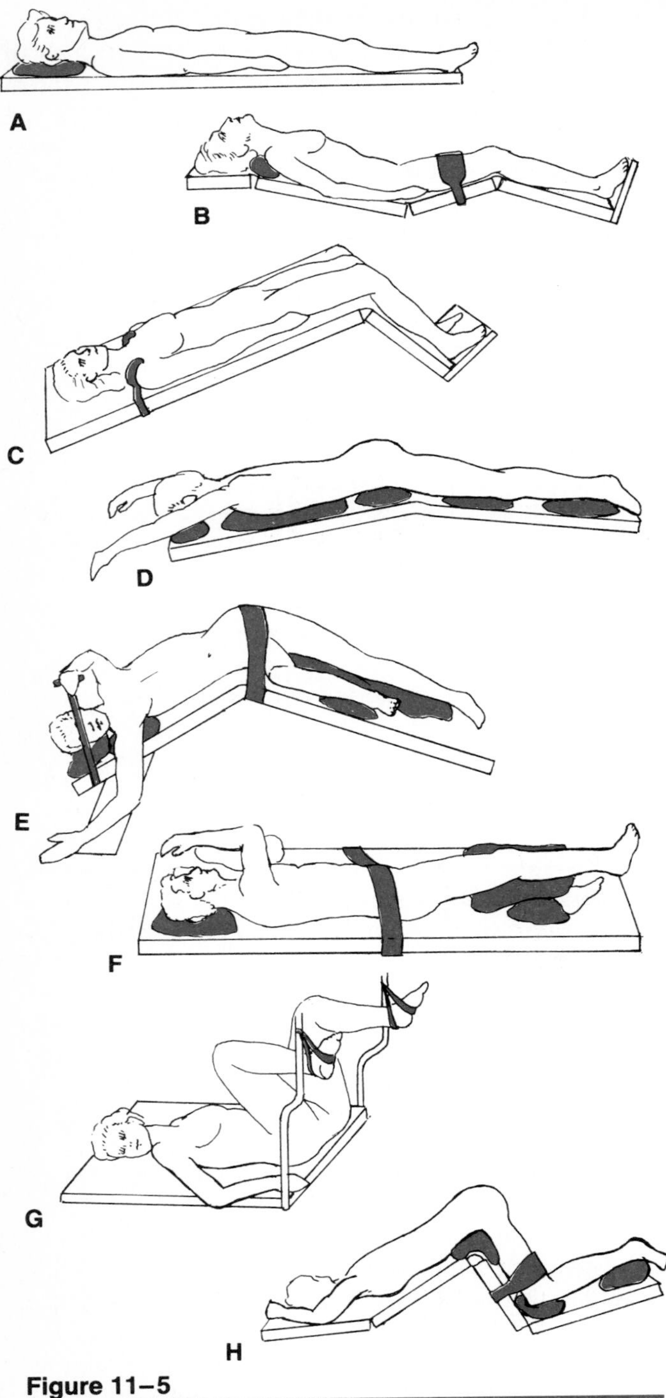

Figure 11–5

Client positions during surgery. **A.** Dorsal recumbent (supine) position for abdominal and thoracic surgery, and surgery on the extremities. **B.** Variation of the dorsal recumbent position for operations on thyroid and neck area. **C.** Trendelenburg's position for pelvic surgery. **D.** Prone position for spinal fusion. **E.** Lateral position for kidney surgery and operations on the upper ureters. **F.** Lateral position for thoracic surgery. **G.** Lithotomy position for vaginal, perineal, or rectal surgery. **H.** Jacknife position for proctologic surgery.

the arm, excessive abduction may damage the brachial plexus causing paralysis and loss of sensation in the arm and shoulder. Radial nerve damage can cause wrist drop; damage to the medial or ulnar nerves causes hand deformities; peroneal nerve damage causes foot drop; and damage to the tibial nerve causes loss of sensation on the plantar surface of the foot. It is possible that the muscle relaxants administered to the client may contribute to the problem by reducing muscle resistance, allowing muscles to become overstretched.

Each surgical position has particular risks. The risks, and the strategies for preventing them, are discussed below.

- Dorsal positioning (used in most abdominal surgery) may cause excessive pressure on posterior bony prominences—sacrum, heels, scapulae—and the back of the head. These areas should be well protected with soft materials. Alterations in circulatory status, however, are less pronounced with the dorsal position than in many of the other positions. Take care that the knees are not flexed with supports even for short periods because vessel compression can lead to sluggish blood flow, thrombus formation, and phlebitis. Avoid internal and external rotation of the hips and shoulders by using trochanter rolls, sandbags, or padding.
- Trendelenburg's position has been known to increase intrathoracic pressure and alter respiration because the weight of the abdominal organs is redistributed. Padded shoulder braces prevent the client from slipping off the surgical table. Take precautions similar to those mentioned for dorsal positioning.
- When the client is in the prone position, the face, knees and thighs, anterior surfaces of the ankles, and the toes sustain the most pressure. Bony prominences should be padded and the feet supported under the ankles. The client's chest and abdomen should be raised off the table and supported on pillows or bolsters to allow for effective respiratory and circulatory function. Be sure that the eyes are closed and that pressure on the eyes is avoided. The arms should be free and not pressed against the surgical table or hyperabducted out to the sides.
- Lateral positioning can create undue pressure on the shoulder, hip, knee, and lateral maleolus on the side on which the client is positioned. In addition, the weight of the upper leg may place excessive pressure on the lower leg causing peroneal nerve injury. Both legs must be padded. Damage to the brachial plexus, medial, radial, and ulnar nerves can be prevented by supporting the shoulder and preventing overextension of the arm. Using an axillary roll (a firm, cushioned pad) prevents undue pressure on the dependent axilla.
- The lithotomy position may compromise respiratory status. Improper padding or positioning in the stirrups

can cause peroneal nerve damage, or damage to peripheral blood vessels. To avoid joint damage, both legs should be simultaneously manipulated into the stirrups. Be especially careful when putting elderly clients into this position.

- The jackknife position requires attention to the respiratory and circulatory status of the client, making sure that the chest and abdomen are free and unrestricted. The greatest pressure is exerted at the bends in the table. The client should be supported by pads at both the groin and the knee areas and under the ankles. Precautions must be taken to avoid pressure on the nerves of the upper arm and on the lower ear and eye, to be sure that the pinna is not folded in on itself, and to avoid kinking of the neck veins.

All of these positions impede maximal inspiration and expiration. Clients having lengthy surgeries are also at risk for pressure ulcers and venous stasis. An operating table air cushion can help prevent problems resulting from pressure. The client's eyes must be protected with all positions. Clients under general anesthesia will have lost the corneal reflex, and the cornea can be damaged by the movement or pressure of the surgical drape if adequate eyelid closure is not ensured. Pressure on the eyeball during surgery has been known to cause blindness resulting from thrombosis of the retinal artery.

Surgical Technique

Surgery necessarily involves a break in the body tissue, compromising the host defenses of the client. As a result of surgical incising, body fluids (blood and serum) are lost. Efforts are made to minimize these consequences, but they occur nevertheless. The more extensive the surgery, the greater the consequences. Various skin closures, dressings, and drainage techniques are used by the surgeon to close the surgical incision, minimize trauma, and encourage wound healing. Nurses who are familiar with these techniques will be better able to provide intraoperative and postoperative care.

Suturing

When surgery is completed, the wound may be closed or left open. Generally, a wound or part of a wound is left open if the probability of infection is high, as with a contaminated wound. An open wound facilitates release of pus and tissue debris and allows for thorough wound cleansing.

In most cases, however, the surgical wound is closed in layers with sutures, clips, staples, skin closure strips, and even zipperlike devices. When closing the skin, the surgeon approximates the wound edges as closely as possible, manipulating the tissue as little as possible. Proper technique promotes healing with minimal scar tissue formation and loss of function.

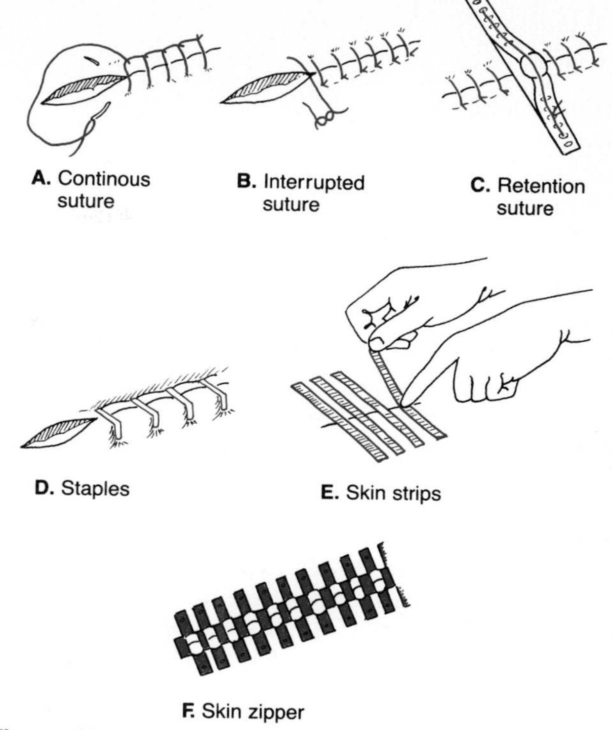

Figure 11–6

Skin closure techniques.

Essentially, suturing is "sewing" tissues together; the popular term for sutures is "stitches" even though alternative closure methods such as staples may be used. Sometimes a single line of sutures is sufficient for external closure. Frequently, however, retention sutures are necessary for closure, especially in abdominal surgery or obese clients. These overlapping sutures, padded with soft material, provide additional support for the wound. Metal clips and staples bind tissue together; the mechanical methods used to apply these sutures reduce manipulation of tissue and generally cause less external scarring than suturing. Finally, skin closure strips, similar to the butterfly type of adhesive bandage, can be applied with tissues closely approximated. These strips also minimize tissue manipulation and scar tissue formation and allow for drainage. When healing has progressed well, sutures, clips, and staples are usually removed within 7 to 10 days. Skin strips usually dry up and fall off as tissue heals. Types of skin closure are illustrated in Figure 11–6.

Drains and Dressings

The surgeon may place a *drain* in the incision line or may insert a drain through a separate incision near the principal wound. A drain provides an exit route for blood, serum, and debris that might otherwise accumulate in the postoperative period, causing tissue edema and pain, interfering with wound healing, and promoting infection. A drain also provides for removal of any infectious debris. The type of drain chosen depends on the depth and breadth of the wound and the need to have a drain held in place by an inflatable device (eg, a Foley catheter balloon). Drains are generally removed when a decrease in secretions indicates they are no longer needed. Types of drains are depicted in Figure 11–7.

Drains may be freestanding or attached to gravity drainage, intermittent suction (eg, Gomco suction), or to a self-contained disposable drainage system that supplies its own suction (eg, Hemovac). A common freestanding rubber drain is the Penrose drain. A sterile safety pin is generally attached to the top of the drain to provide some weight, preventing the drain from slipping into the incision. A Penrose drain is often sutured in place. Other types of drains are also depicted in Figure 11–7.

Drainage should flow freely through the drain's internal lumen. When a small to moderate amount of drainage is expected, a well-padded dressing is generally sufficient for drainage absorption. When larger amounts of drainage are anticipated, bags may be applied to the skin around the drain for drainage collection. Collection bags prevent skin trauma from caustic wound drainage and facilitate the measurement of drainage as fluid output.

A typical wound dressing is sterile gauze pads placed over the incision. The purposes of a dressing are to:

- Protect the wound from physical trauma and potential contaminants in the environment.
- Absorb drainage that might otherwise accumulate, have an odor, excoriate the skin, and provide a medium for bacterial growth.
- Deliver medication, either applied to the gauze (eg, povidone–iodine ointment) or imbedded in the gauze (eg, nitrofurazone).
- Prevent dehydration of exposed wound tissue. Wound dehydration inhibits normal wound healing by promoting unnecessary wound inflammation, discouraging epithelialization, and increasing incisional pain (Flynn & Rovee, 1982).
- Shield the wound from the client's view, especially when an incision may be perceived as a threat to body image.

Recent developments in dressings include foams, gels, and transparent plastic film. The transparency of dressings allows for wound observation, protection, and aeration. Some surgeons prefer to leave a surgical wound completely undressed, avoiding potential irritation from dressings and frequent dressing changes.

Innovative Techniques

Several innovations in biomedical engineering have altered the traditional practice of surgery. The development of instruments such as the binocular operating microscope, the laser, and the cryoprobe have made possible what would once have been impossible surgery, improved the prognosis for surgical clients, decreased the extent of disfigurement the client experiences, and reduced the number of necessary postoperative lifestyle changes.

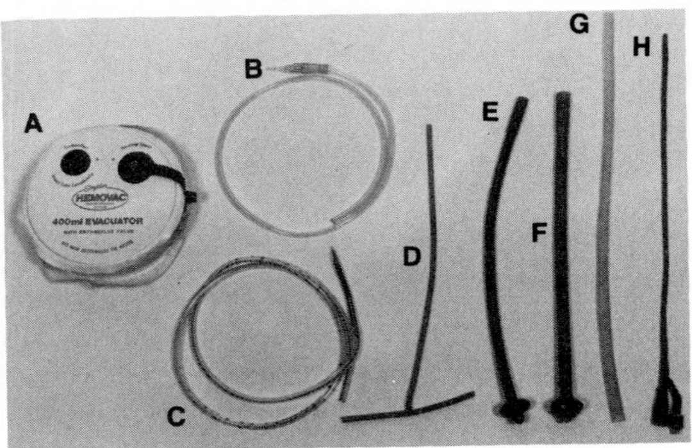

Figure 11–7

Surgical drains. **A.** Disposable suction apparatus. Continuous suction is created by a spring mechanism within the evacuator unit. **B.** Drainage tubes for the Hemovac. **C.** Trochar used to pull the drainage tube from the body cavity to the exterior. **D.** T-tube. **E.** Pezzar, or "mushroom" drain. **F.** Malecot, or "batwing" drain. **G.** Penrose drain. **H.** Foley catheter. *Courtesy of Carol Payne-Zagon, RBP, VA Medical Center, Buffalo, NY.*

BINOCULAR OPERATING MICROSCOPE The binocular operating microscope permits the surgeon to have a brightly illuminated, enlarged three-dimensional view of the operating field. This instrument makes it possible to operate with greater precision on small structures and to visualize structures that are not visible to the naked eye. The subsequent development of microinstruments, microsutures, and microsurgical techniques has made it possible to perform surgeries unheard of a short time ago and to minimize damage to delicate structures. These features are extremely important in eye and ear surgery, in neurosurgery, and in surgery that requires the repair of small blood vessels or the microvascular reattachment of minute blood vessels such as occurs in free tissue flaps.

LASER The **laser** is a device that transforms light of various frequencies into a finely focused, intense beam of light capable of mobilizing great heat and power at close range. As the beam comes into contact with tissue, the light energy is absorbed in the tissue and converted to heat. The heat causes a burn (photocoagulation) that results in a scar. The extent of tissue destruction and the depth of an incision created by the laser depends on how long the laser beam is focused on any given spot. The surgeon must be careful not to cause damage to normal tissue. The main advantage of laser surgery is that incisional surgery can be avoided in many instances. Depending on the type of operation, laser surgery can be performed without anesthesia on an ambulatory basis.

The introduction of optical lasers has produced the need for operating room personnel to wear appropriate eye protection to protect themselves from stray or reflected beams of laser light. The energy from these lasers can cause eye damage, burns, or ignition of endotracheal tubes during microlaryngeal surgery for example.

CRYOSURGERY Cryosurgery involves the freezing and destruction of tissues through a variety of techniques. Liquid nitrogen, Freon 114, or solid carbon dioxide may be applied to tissue by a spray, with a swab, or by a supercooled cryoprobe. Cryosurgery is most commonly used for dermatologic lesions and cataract removal, and in gynecologic surgery.

Assessment and Nursing Diagnosis

Assessment has been discussed earlier in this section. Client assessment during the intraoperative period, an ongoing process that begins with the client's admission to the operating suite, forms the basis for the general nursing diagnoses listed in Box 11–3.

Box 11–3
Common Nursing Diagnoses Related to Intraoperative Care

Anxiety, related to awareness of surroundings during operative procedure in client having regional anesthesia

Fluid volume deficit, potential for, related to altered intake and loss of body fluids during surgery

Gas exchange, impaired, related to inability to move secretions independently

Infection, potential for, related to destruction of skin barrier by surgical incision

Injury, potential for, related to insertion of surgical instruments and supplies, loss of sensation and reflexes while anesthetized, and positioning and use of restraints

Powerlessness, related to anesthesia

Urinary elimination, altered, related to depressant effects of general anesthetic

Planning and Implementation

Planning and implementation during the intraoperative period include measures to ensure emotional well-being, physical safety, and privacy. These measures are discussed in this section.

Promoting Emotional Well-Being

When entering the surgical suite, the client may experience a heightened anxiety. Anxiety may be caused by apprehension about the surgical procedure, concern about safety, and perhaps uncertainty about the diagnosis. The anxiety may bring physiologic, emotional, and intellectual changes. Tachycardia with palpitations and peripheral vasodilation with flushing may occur. With mild and moderate anxiety, the client will be attentive and alert to the surroundings, although the depressive effects of preanesthesia sedation may dull cognitive and problem-solving abilities. With severe anxiety, the client's perception is less acute, tending to focus on details. With panic, the client's perception is completely disrupted; the client has lost control and is unable to understand or communicate intelligibly.

Operating room nurses can alleviate clients' anxiety in a number of ways. Nurses should introduce themselves to the client and explain procedures and activities before and as they are being performed. Reassure the client that the surgical team carefully monitors physiologic status during surgery and that privacy will be maintained. Besides providing verbal reassurance, use touch as a means of communication. Holding the client's hand may be an especially supportive gesture. (See also Table 11–4 later in this chapter.)

If the client is to receive a general anesthetic, physical activity and talking in the operating room must be kept to a minimum until the client is unconscious. Although many activities must be performed at this time, the client should not be ignored. Once the client is unconscious, the surgical team must continue to discuss only matters relevant to the procedure. The client's sense of hearing may be especially acute during this time, and there have been reports of clients recalling conversations and their surgery even while anesthetized. In fact, there is speculation that unconscious learning may occur during anesthesia and that what is learned (eg, a grave prognosis) may influence the postoperative course. On the other hand, listening to relaxing music through headphones is thought to enhance clients' relaxation under general anesthesia.

With a regional anesthetic, the client will remain awake, although usually sedated, during the surgery. As the surgery is performed, keep the client informed of the progress. Touching and talking to the client during the procedure both distracts and supports the client.

Promoting Physical Safety and Privacy

The person accompanying the client to the operating suite (generally a staff nurse) reports to the operating room nurse (generally a circulating nurse), who admits the client to the operating suite. At this time, the preoperative preparation and medical record are again reviewed for completeness and accuracy. In particular, establish that consent has been obtained, that allergies are noted, that preoperative medication has been given if ordered, that the client has been properly identified, that blood is available as ordered, and that risks related to surgery have been identified and corrected if possible.

If the client has been sedated, accident potential is high. While the client remains on the stretcher, ensure that safety straps are secure, that safety rails are in the upright position, and that the client's extremities are kept on the stretcher. Also ensure that the client is transferred from the stretcher to the operating table safely. The client should be safely secured to the table and should remain secured throughout the surgical procedure. Restraint straps should be snug but not too tight, and padding should be provided between the restraint and the client's body unless the restraint itself is padded.

As the client is positioned on the operating table, the circulating nurse should ensure that privacy and warmth are maintained as much as possible, that the body is aligned properly, and that body areas are not subjected to excessive pressure. Only necessary body areas need be exposed; other body areas should be covered to prevent unnecessary heat loss. Reasons for heat loss include a cool temperature in the operating room, the effects of some inhalation anesthetics, and the depressant effects of general anesthesia on heat-regulating mechanisms. Measures to be taken to ensure the client's safety in specific surgical positions have been discussed in the section on surgical positions.

The client's physical safety must be maintained throughout anesthetic administration. The operating room nurse shares responsibility for maintaining the client's safety, although the anesthetist carries the major responsibility. When the intended stage of anesthesia has been reached, the nurse concentrates on monitoring the client's safety and privacy. Be sure there is no excessive pressure on the client's skin, and take corrective measures as necessary. Because of the absent gag reflex and the client's inability to clear accumulated respiratory secretions, the anesthetist will suction the client if necessary. Suctioning is aided by the ET tube, if present, or an oral and/or nasal airway. The anesthetist makes sure these tubes do not place excessive pressure on the mouth or nose and protects the eyes in the absence of the corneal reflex as discussed earlier. If the client has not been catheterized, assess the client for suprapubic distention, which indicates urinary retention and, perhaps, the need for catheterization.

During the procedure, the scrub nurse helps ensure the client's safety by being efficient in anticipating the needs of the surgeon and assistants and providing instruments. Efficiency is increased if the circulating nurse has adequately prepared the room with the appropriate supplies and equipment. The circulating nurse is also responsible for ensuring the sterility of supplies and checking equipment to determine it is in safe working order. All guidelines for the maintenance and use of electrical equipment and flammable substances should be followed.

Although all members of the surgical team use sterile technique, the circulating nurse is responsible for enforcing use of sterile technique throughout surgery. As client advocate, the circulating nurse alerts the surgical team if a break in technique is suspected. If a suspected break or actual break occurs, suspected contaminated clothing or instruments are discarded and replaced with sterile ones. The nurse also helps to protect the client from infection by appropriately disposing of contaminated materials, ensuring that instruments or supplies are cleaned and/or sterilized after surgery, and preparing the room for the next client according to agency policy.

An important aspect of protecting the client's safety is verifying that no surgical instruments, needles, or sponges (gauze pads) remain inside the client's body after suturing. Agency policies vary; most hospitals require sponge counts; needle and instrument counts are more controversial. AORN recommends counting all three. Generally, one scrub person and one circulating person count the items both before surgery and before the surgical incision is closed. Any discrepancy must be accounted for before the incision is closed.

The client's safety is also maintained by administering appropriate fluids, as ordered, to replace body losses and prevent dehydration. Electrolyte solutions (eg, Ringer's lactate) are frequently administered during the operative period, and blood loss is replaced. Agency policy usually requires that two persons make this assessment. The nurse is also responsible for ascertaining that enough blood is on hand for the client's anticipated needs and for ordering more, if needed. In conjunction with fluid replacement, keep an accurate intake and output record, recording all administered intravenous fluids, urinary output (if the client is catheterized), blood loss, emesis (if any), and any other drainage. The intraoperative monitoring and maintenance of homeostasis and vital functions (both traditional nursing functions) are done by the anesthetist.

Evaluation

In evaluating the effectiveness of nursing care throughout the intraoperative period, consider the following:

- Is the client less anxious as a result of the nurse's reassurance?
- Does the client remain free from tissue injury (eg, no reddened areas on the skin) from careful positioning?
- Is the client's privacy maintained by draping?
- Does the client remain free of signs of decreased circulating fluid volume (eg, hypotension) as a result of administered blood and intravenous solutions?
- Was sterile technique maintained?

SECTION 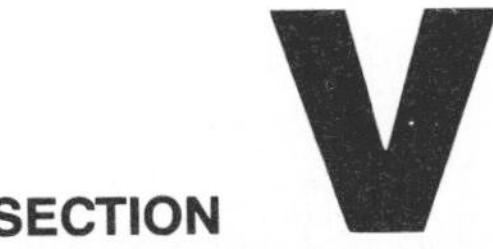

The Nursing Process in Postoperative Care

The central goal of postoperative nursing care is the return of the client to an optimal level of functioning. To accomplish this goal, the nurse must understand factors that affect postsurgical recovery—the expected consequences and potential complications of anesthesia and surgery in the immediate and later postoperative periods.

Nursing Care in the Immediate Postoperative Period

Immediately after surgery, the client is generally cared for in a postanesthesia recovery area close to the operating room. There members of the surgical team can conveniently monitor the client's progress periodically and quickly return the client to the operating room in the event of an emergency. The client is kept there under the care of a recovery room nurse until having recovered from the effects of anesthesia, vital signs are stable, and the wound dressing remains intact with no signs of hemorrhage.

To ensure continuity of care, the surgical team reports to the recovery room nurse about the client's status upon admission to the recovery area. This report includes information about the preoperative status, the kind of surgery performed, the presence and status of drains and dressings, the length of time the client remained in the operating room and under anesthesia, the kind of anesthesia given, the status of the client's vital functions throughout the intraoperative period, the need for oxygen and/or ventilation, the need for monitoring (central venous pressure, arterial pressure), the status of fluid and electrolyte balance and the intraoperative intake and output record, the need for blood transfusions, and the presence and patency of any other tubes (eg, a Foley catheter). Any complications during the intraoperative period (eg, bradycardia, cardiac arrest) should also be communicated, along with appropriate therapies to be instituted if they recur.

Nursing Assessment

Planning appropriate nursing care for the client in the immediate postoperative period is based on thorough understanding of the recovery of persons from anesthesia and surgery and an assessment of each client.

RECOVERY FROM ANESTHESIA AND RESIDUAL EFFECTS In the immediate postoperative period, the effects of anesthesia can be expected to wear off gradually. Until motor and sensory functions return, however, the client remains at risk for injury (as discussed in the intraoperative section). The client may have an altered response to various noxious stimuli that may circumvent normal protective responses.

As the depressive effects of a general anesthetic subside, motor and sensory functions gradually return. The client may begin to feel pain and react to it by moaning or moving around, potentially causing harm to himself or herself and to the incision site. The client with an ET tube or oral airway may fight it as anesthesia wears off and coughing and swallowing reflexes return. Artificial airways are removed once protective airway reflexes return, and once the client's ability to support adequate ventilation and oxygenation has been assessed to be adequate. Afterward, the client should be closely assessed for ability to breathe normally and clear secretions. Often, arterial blood gas determinations and tidal volume assessments are made before removal of the tube; the anesthetist, in conjunction with the recovery room nurse, determines the appropriateness of removing the tube. Premature removal of an ET tube or oral airway can result in obstruction of respiratory passages by the tongue or secretions.

The time it takes a general anesthetic to wear off depends on the length of the procedure (longer procedures produce greater saturation of body tissues with anesthetics, resulting in longer recovery periods); the kind and amount of anesthetic; and the individual client's reaction to the anesthetic. With inhalation anesthetics, recovery is usually rapid; the client may be conscious and able to move when admitted to the recovery area. Nevertheless, the depressive effects of the anesthetic may still affect the client's respiratory function, cognitive and problem-solving abilities, and motor and sensory function for some time, even up to 24 hours. Recovery from intravenous anesthetics is also fairly rapid (within 3 hours), although the client may experience similar prolonged effects.

The return of consciousness and the return of motor and sensory functions, occur in phases. The client who has received a general anesthetic shows signs of arousal when reflex actions, such as the corneal and swallowing reflexes, return. Initially, the client advances from stupor to lethargy and then to drowsiness before becoming fully alert and conscious. The stuporous client responds poorly to verbal and painful stimuli and is still well under the effects of anesthesia. The lethargic, drowsy client demonstrates dull behavior and may fall asleep intermittently. This client may respond to painful stimuli but still be experiencing some effects of anesthesia. The conscious client is alert, awake, fully responsive to verbal stimuli, and has recovered from the effects of anesthesia. As motor functions return, the client may first feel a heaviness in the body, particularly in the extremities, and movements are difficult and uncoordinated. Gradually, the client's sense of self and ability to move become more definite.

Assess level of consciousness by observing the client's behavior and orientation. Does the client respond to pain? Does the client respond to name? Is the client able to carry on a conversation? Does the client know where he or she is? Generally, the client will first respond to pain; then to verbal stimuli; then to the surroundings; and eventually, the client will be able to communicate. At first, the client will be disoriented, but gradually orientation to person, place, and time return. Assess motor ability by asking the client to squeeze the nurse's hand. Motor and sensory function of the affected area can be assessed in the same manner when the client has had a regional anesthetic.

The rate, rhythm, and quality of respirations should

be closely monitored, generally upon admission to the recovery room and every 5 minutes for 15 minutes and then every 15 minutes. Abnormal rate, irregular rhythm, and noisy respirations may indicate an underlying problem and require intervention. As a result of the depressive effects of a general anesthetic, bradypnea (respirations less than 10 per minute) may be noted. Generally, the client will remain in the recovery room until the respiratory rate normalizes (between 10 and 20 breaths/minute). Breath sounds should be assessed for signs of accumulated secretions in respiratory passages and/or for diminution of sounds associated with atelectasis, pneumonia, or pneumothorax. Cyanosis of the nail beds and/or lips should also be observed. Cyanosis may signal a need for the administration of oxygen, although restlessness is an earlier sign of hypoxia. Restlessness may also result from anxiety, pain, or bleeding.

Respiratory obstruction is a serious occurrence in the immediate postoperative period and may occur anywhere along the respiratory tract. The most common cause is soft tissue obstruction of the upper airway. Laryngospasm, a potentially life-threatening event, also must be recognized and treated quickly. While soft tissue obstruction is usually caused by posterior relaxation of the tongue, laryngospasm may be caused by the stimulation of the vocal cords by oral secretions, blood, or vomitus.

Nausea and vomiting are a consequence of some anesthetics, as well as some surgical procedures, making the client uncomfortable and increasing the risk of aspiration. The client may feel chilled because the body temperature may be low, as discussed earlier. The client may shiver in an effort to create body heat, at the same time increasing oxygen needs. Oxygen needs may be greatly increased, compounded by the residual depressive effects of general anesthesia on respiratory function resulting in hypoventilation.

Recovery from regional anesthesia is also gradual. As the client's sensory functions return, pain is perceived, and nursing interventions to promote comfort will be necessary. As motor function returns to the anesthetized area, the client may move inappropriately, causing damage to a surgical area or to an unprotected body part.

RESIDUAL PHYSIOLOGIC AND PSYCHOSOCIAL EFFECTS OF SURGERY Although the body's stress responses generally enhance physiologic and psychologic coping, they may have negative consequences if unchecked. Nursing care is directed at alleviating or minimizing stress to foster a quick recovery.

Being aware of common physiologic sequelae of stress helps the nurse assess an individual client's responses and plan nursing care. Blood pressure, pulse, and respiration commonly increase in the client under stress. These responses may not be apparent, however, until the client emerges from the effects of anesthesia. Hormonal regulation of renal function conserves water and sodium, maintaining circulating fluid volume and blood pressure. To maintain this defensive body action, fluid and electrolyte balance is carefully assessed and fluids are administered in the immediate postoperative period, with attention to preventing fluid overload. Peripheral vasoconstriction accompanying stress may contribute to the pallor commonly observed in the postoperative period. An increase in circulating glucose, as a result of physiologic adaptation to provide for needed energy, can precipitate transient hyperglycemia (elevated blood sugar) and glycosuria (abnormal presence of sugar in the urine).

Table 11–3
Sources of Stress in the Postanesthesia Recovery Period

Physiological	Psychosocial	Environmental
Hypoxia Metabolic changes Electrolyte imbalance Drugs Pain Length of time spent under anesthesia Extent of surgical trauma	Fear of mutilation caused by surgery Fear of death Fear of revealing too much while recovering from effects of anesthesia Fear of complications from anesthesia Separation from family and friends Depersonalization Powerlessness Pain Inability to reduce tension in usual way Physical exposure	Sensory overload because of constant noise, lights, unfamiliar treatments Sensory deprivation because of immobility, restraints, casts, dressings Lack of familiar orienting cues given by clocks, calendars, radio or television, meals, windows, visiting hours Proximity to other clients who may be confused, crying, distressed, or in pain Constant attendance by physicians, nurses, and other health team members Separation from familiar environment

Aside from these generalized stress responses, specific local responses, such as inflammation and bleeding, result from the tissue trauma of surgery. Although blood loss should not be excessive postoperatively, the potential for it requires periodic assessment, especially in the immediate postoperative period.

Finally, the postsurgical client may have other more specific physiologic, psychosocial, and environmental sources of stress in the postoperative period (Table 11–3). These stresses all contribute to anxiety, which may be severe in the immediate postoperative period.

Nursing Diagnosis

An understanding and analysis of these factors enable the nurse to determine nursing diagnoses specific to the care of a client in the immediate postoperative period. Nursing diagnoses common to the client in the immediate postoperative period are listed in Box 11–4 and can be used as general guidelines.

Box 11–4
Common Nursing Diagnoses Related to Immediate Postoperative Care

Comfort, altered, related to pressure on nerve endings caused by surgical incision and recovery from anesthetic

Communication, impaired verbal, related to depressive effects of general anesthetic and/or sedation

Fluid volume deficit, potential for, related to surgical and postsurgical fluid losses

Gas exchange, impaired, potential for, related to respiratory depression associated with general anesthesia, inability to move secretions independently associated with depressed gag reflex, and horizontal positioning for surgery

Impairment of skin integrity, potential for, related to immobility associated with anesthesia and surgery, surgical positioning, and use of restraints

Injury, potential for, related to residual effects of anesthetics and operative sedation

Sensory perceptual alteration, potential for, related to depressive effects of anesthetic, excessive and inappropriate environmental stimuli and separation from significant others and usual surroundings

Urinary elimination, altered, related to depressive effects of general anesthetics (and regional anesthetics affecting the bladder)

Planning and Implementation

The plan of care is aimed at ensuring a safe recovery of the client from the immediate effects of anesthesia and surgery. In addition, postanesthesia nurses plan and implement immediate nursing care specific to the surgical procedure performed such as maintaining the proper position of a client after retinal reattachment surgery or monitoring pedal pulses after vascular surgery to the leg. (See the chapters about surgical approaches to disorders of specific body systems.)

PROMOTING SAFE RECOVERY FROM ANESTHESIA The primary goal of immediate postoperative nursing care is the safe recovery and arousal of the client from the effects of anesthesia. The nurse is responsible for initiating communication with the client, attempting to stir the client from the effects of anesthesia, and providing orienting cues. As the client gradually becomes oriented, alert, and able to move, the recovery room nurse can promote postanesthesia recovery by encouraging the client to breathe deeply and move the arms and legs. These actions encourage elimination from the body of inhalation anesthetics (through exhalation) and other anesthetics (through increased circulation and kidney perfusion and elimination).

If the client has received spinal anesthesia, *spinal headache,* a potential complication of spinal anesthesia, must be prevented. Although the cause of spinal headaches is unclear, a decrease in cerebrospinal fluid (through leakage at the injection site) may be a contributing factor. These headaches are most likely to occur in clients under 60 years of age, and they are more prevalent in pregnant clients. Their incidence is less than 1% when a 25-gauge spinal needle is used. When a 25-gauge (or smaller) needle is used, there may be no reason to limit the client's activity after the return of sensory motor function. If the client experiences a headache upon elevating the head, the client should return to the supine position and increase fluid intake. In some institutions, clients are encouraged to remain supine for 6 to 24 hours after a spinal anesthetic, especially when the spinal needle used is larger than 25-gauge.

Whether the client has received a general or a regional anesthetic, safety precautions must be instituted in the immediate postoperative period. Although the client may feel alert and capable of moving, movements may be uncoordinated, and residual drowsiness and sedation probably persist. Therefore, the client should remain restrained on the stretcher throughout this period. Another aspect of safety is protecting the client from the effects of hypothermia. The client's temperature is generally monitored every 15 minutes. Measures to maintain body warmth, such as covering the client with a warm blanket, should be instituted.

PROMOTING ADEQUATE RESPIRATORY FUNCTION Especially when the client has received a general anesthetic, nursing measures for ensuring adequate respiratory function go hand in hand with measures related to the client's recovery from anesthesia. The first concern is maintaining an adequate airway. If the client arrives in the recovery room with an endotracheal tube, it should be well secured. These devices provide a means for suctioning secretions. Often, the client with an endotracheal tube may require continued ventilatory assistance. The nurse confers with the anesthetist about ventilatory care for the individual client.

The client must be positioned so that a patent airway is maintained, secretions can be suctioned, and oxygen can be administered, if required. Immediately after surgery, the client is usually positioned laterally to discourage pooling of secretions and vomitus. The lateral position also helps prevent the tongue from occluding the pharynx. Remember that the client will not be able to cough or swallow until the gag reflex returns, and any mucous secretions and vomitus must be suctioned by the nurse as required. Take special care in suctioning clients with head or neck surgery, because they are especially susceptible to injury from suctioning. Use proper aseptic technique when suctioning, and assess breath sounds afterward to determine whether suctioning was effective. Likewise, administer oxygen safely and appropriately.

To reverse the depressant effects of anesthetics on respiratory function (hypoxia and hypoventilation with atelectasis), encourage deep breathing to expand the lungs fully and coughing to remove accumulated secretions. Clients are often surprised at the amount of secretions they expectorate postoperatively; secretions accumulate as a result of maintaining one position during surgery and the hypoventilation associated with anesthesia.

PROMOTING ADEQUATE CIRCULATORY FUNCTION Throughout the immediate postoperative period, circulatory function may continue to be compromised by the effects of anesthesia, surgical positioning, fluid and blood losses, and general immobility. Therefore, the nurse generally monitors the client's pulse and blood pressure every 15 minutes for adequate function. An abnormally low blood pressure and increased pulse rate may signify shock and should be reported. Peripheral circulation must also be monitored to ensure adequate perfusion of peripheral tissues and prevent excessive pressure on peripheral vessels. The nurse also monitors the client's fluid balance. Adequate fluid balance is necessary to maintain blood pressure and body tissue perfusion. Fluids and blood should be administered safely and as ordered.

Remember that surgery may impose a great deal of stress on the client's heart. With preexisting cardiac disease (or even without preexisting disease), the heart may be unable to cope with the increased work load; heart failure or myocardial infarction may occur, indicated by changes in pulse, blood pressure, and respiration.

PROMOTING COMFORT As the client recovers from the effects of the anesthetic, he or she will begin to feel incisional pain. Make a thorough pain assessment (including both subjective and objective observations) ascertaining the quality, severity, and location of the client's pain. Do not assume that "pain" necessarily means only "incisional pain." General muscular aches and pains may also occur as a consequence of prolonged surgical immobility and positioning. The client may also describe a sore throat, a residual effect of endotracheal intubation and the drying effects of anticholinergics. Also be alert for unexpected pain, which might indicate a problem such as myocardial infarction.

Nursing comfort measures to alleviate pain, such as turning, positioning, and distraction, may be useful, but pain medication will also be necessary and should not be withheld. Because general anesthetics have residual depressive effects on blood pressure, respiratory status, and circulation, the client usually receives an attenuated dose (usually one-half dose) of an analgesic. (Guidelines for modifying analgesia in the early postoperative period are given later in this chapter.) Before administering a narcotic, especially morphine, carefully assess the client's respiratory status and determine that further respiratory depression will not seriously compromise the client's status. Because these drugs may cause hypotension, blood pressure should also be assessed to ensure that further lowering of the blood pressure will not be dangerous.

Monitor the effectiveness of pain-relief techniques and drugs in relieving the client's pain. Does the client appear more comfortable? Less restless? Does the client state that the pain is less troublesome? In some cases, the nurse may need to confer with the surgeon or anesthetist, advising them that the pain medication dosage needs to be increased to bring relief.

PROVIDING WOUND CARE In the immediate postoperative period, observing for hemorrhage is a major responsibility of the nurse caring for a surgical client. A dressing is generally left in place, and the nurse should carefully monitor wound drainage by circling any drainage and reevaluating drainage spots continually for major increases in bleeding. Check both the dressing and the linen underneath the client. On first inspection, a dressing may look dry because blood is draining to a dependent location by gravity. Dressings are not generally changed but are reinforced as necessary. Unexpected severe bleeding is immediately reported to the surgeon. The client may need to be returned to the operating room for further ligation of bleeding vessels if heavy bleeding persists. Excessive bleeding from drains may be noted and may also signal a need for further surgery.

Drains or other equipment that may be inserted in the surgical wound should be cared for as necessary. A drain might need to be connected to suction or to gravity drainage, or a wound might need to be irrigated as ordered.

REDUCING ANXIETY AND PROMOTING NORMAL SENSORY STATUS Nursing measures should be directed at reducing the client's anxiety level. Orienting the client to the environment as soon as the client is responsive and explaining procedures and equipment are especially helpful. Other nursing actions are suggested in Table 11–4.

Table 11–4
Strategies to Reduce Severe Anxiety and Panic in Postanesthesia Clients

Nursing Action	Rationale
Conduct thorough assessment	Determine whether there is a physiologic basis (eg, hypoxia) for restlessness
Stay with client	Leaving client alone may further increase anxiety
Use short, simple sentences	With high anxiety, there is decreased ability to make sense of sensory input
Use firm and authoritative but kind voice	With high anxiety, internal control is lacking; it is important to convey ability to provide external controls
Minimize environmental stimuli	The client is already overwhelmed by stimuli
Focus the client's diffuse energy on a task such as deep breathing, exercising legs or feet, counting, or other simple activities	Diffuse energy may be drained off until anxiety is more manageable
Consider the need for a sedative or pain medication	Sedatives and narcotic analgesics should be given when warranted, but pronounced depression of the circulatory, respiratory, or central nervous systems may follow. The dose in the recovery room is usually about *one-half* that given after full recovery from anesthesia

PROVIDING PSYCHOSOCIAL SUPPORT The emotional needs of the client, family members, and friends must also be considered in the immediate postoperative period. As soon as possible after surgery, contact the client's family members or significant others and advise them that the surgery is completed and that the client is recovering as anticipated. This action can allay fears and may help to relax the client, who may be concerned that family members are worried.

PROVIDING CONTINUITY OF CARE A postoperative client is generally transferred to the surgical unit when:

- The client has fully recovered from the depressive effects of the anesthetic.
- The surgical wound is intact and without excessive unexpected bleeding or drainage.
- The client is considered stable, with respirations in the normal range, adequate palpable pulses, adequate blood pressure, and temperature approaching normal limits.

With transfer of the client, nurses provide for continuity of care by accurate and thorough written documentation of care and the client's status. The recovery room nurse should also give the surgical unit nurse a thorough oral report; this oral report facilitates the transfer and further promotes continuity of care.

Documentation in the immediate postoperative period may involve the use of flow sheets, progress records, nursing progress notes, and care plans. Whatever the form for documentation, the content is similar, including: vital signs; respiratory and circulatory status assessment; client's level of consciousness and motor and sensory abilities; presence of pain or discomfort; condition of dressing and wound; presence and patency of tubes; urinary output; medications, intravenous fluids, blood ordered and administered; and nursing interventions and client responses to nursing interventions.

Evaluation

During the immediate postoperative period, the nurse continually monitors the effectiveness of nursing interventions. Is the client breathing easier as a result of lying on a side? Is the client more oriented to time, place, and person as a result of the nurse's providing sensory clues? Does the client remain free from injury? Are respirations, blood pressure, pulse, and temperature within the anticipated range? Ongoing evaluation helps the nurse to decide whether particular interventions should continue or whether the nursing care plan should be revised.

Nursing Care in the Later Postoperative Period

In the later postoperative period, the client recovers from the residual effects of the surgical experience, usually on a surgical unit or in an intensive care unit, if necessary. In the final stage of recovery the client is usually at home.

Nursing Assessment

In caring for the postoperative client during recovery, the nurse must be aware of potential complications. Especially important to assess are respiratory and circulatory needs.

ASSESSING RESPIRATORY NEEDS A number of respiratory complications may occur in the later postoperative period. Those associated with anesthesia have been discussed in the previous section. Ventilation of the lungs is inhibited by the horizontal position during surgery and by bed rest after surgery. Mucous secretions may accumulate, leading to pneumonia, bronchitis, respiratory obstruction, or atelectasis.

After the client has been transferred back to the unit from the postanesthesia recovery room, monitoring of respiratory status is generally reduced to every half hour and then to every hour, every 2 hours, and eventually every 4 hours if the client's status is satisfactory. Auscultate the lungs periodically to be sure secretions are not building up. Careful assessment of breath sounds; skin color; and rate, rhythm, and quality of respirations help ensure prompt detection of any complications. Assessment should be continued throughout the postoperative recovery period. *Pulmonary embolism* is a serious potential complication of surgery secondary to thrombus formation. Sudden onset of dyspnea and severe chest pain may indicate this life-threatening condition and should be reported immediately. Pay special attention to clients identified as high risk in the preoperative period—those whose breathing ability has been compromised by cigarette smoking, lung disease, age, or obesity.

ASSESSING CIRCULATORY NEEDS During postoperative recovery, the client is at risk for pooling of blood, thrombophlebitis, and phlebothrombosis. Ongoing assessment is required for prevention and early detection of these conditions.

Venous stasis, a consequence of postoperative bed rest, increases the coagulability of the blood and the client's susceptibility to **phlebothrombosis,** the formation of a blood clot in a vein, usually in the legs. Thrombi that break free from the wall of the vein become emboli, which may be carried to other areas by the bloodstream and cause organ dysfunction. Emboli involving the heart, lungs, or brain can have fatal consequences. Inflammation of the veins **(thrombophlebitis)** may begin in the preoperative or intraoperative periods because of trauma to the veins. Careless transfer of the sedated or anesthetized client to or from the operating table, stretchers, or the client's bed can cause trauma to veins. Prolonged pressure on veins, particularly those on the calf of the leg, may also cause thrombophlebitis and embolus formation. Early signs of thrombophlebitis include calf tenderness, pain with standing, or a positive Homans' sign (pain in the leg when the foot is dorsiflexed).

ASSESSING NUTRITIONAL AND FLUID AND ELECTROLYTE NEEDS If the client remains NPO during the later postoperative period, fluid and electrolyte balance is maintained by intravenous administration. Intake and output must be carefully monitored, and the nurse must be alert for signs of fluid overload or deficit. Careful monitoring and charting of skin turgor, urinary output, and intravenous setups are imperative.

When prolonged fasting is required, detailed nutritional assessment should be ongoing, and the client should be weighed daily. This is particularly important, because malnutrition or nutrient deficiencies prolong wound healing. Fluid balance must be continually assessed for all such clients, and intake and output records should be scrupulously maintained and carefully analyzed. Wound drainage, nasogastric tube drainage, and vomitus must be included in intake and output charting because these may contribute to fluid imbalance. If the threat of fluid imbalance is grave or when imbalance has been identified, an in-dwelling catheter may be inserted to facilitate accurate assessment. Also observe the client for signs of dehydration: thirst, dry skin, or poor skin turgor. The nurse should also be familiar with signs and symptoms of electrolyte imbalance and should observe for them as well.

ASSESSING ELIMINATION NEEDS Surgery may hamper elimination of body wastes (urine and feces). Adequate activity is one of many factors influencing gastrointestinal function; a depressed activity level slows it. The acute stress of surgery itself and the general depressive effects of anesthesia and intraoperative medications also can be expected to alter gastrointestinal and urinary function for some time in the later postoperative period.

Gastrointestinal peristalsis will be depressed, possibly leading to constipation or *paralytic ileus,* a condition in which the intestinal wall is distended and aperistalsis occurs. Paralytic ileus is more likely in the client who has had a general anesthetic and/or abdominal or pelvic surgery with manipulation of organs. Until peristalsis resumes, foods will not pass normally through the gastrointestinal tract. The client will be required to follow a restricted diet that, compounded by fluid losses, may promote constipation and dehydration. Accurate assessment for return of normal peristalsis is an important aspect of postoperative nursing care. The signs of depressed peristalsis are diminished or absent bowel sounds, abdominal distention, and failure to pass flatus or stool. Periodic auscultation for bowel sounds continues until their return is evident.

Similar physiologic effects on the bladder and micturition may result in oliguria (reduced amount of urine) or urinary retention with bladder distention. Although not necessarily a cause for concern, oliguria because of fluid loss and the stress of surgery should be reported. If fluids are being replaced, the amount of urine being excreted should increase. The micturition reflex may be depressed by anesthesia, however, and urinary retention may occur in the client who has had general or spinal anesthesia. If retention occurs, the client will experience suprapubic discomfort, and the nurse may observe evidence of suprapubic distention.

ASSESSING COMFORT AND SAFETY NEEDS Surgery may compromise both comfort and safety. The nurse should continually assess the client's environment for hazardous conditions.

General comfort should also be considered. Poor hygiene, dry mouth, confinement to a single position, and abdominal or suprapubic distention can cause discomfort. Generalized muscular aches and pains may be felt in the later postoperative period as a consequence of intraoperative positioning and the use of restraints. Sore throat may also continue through this period from endotracheal intubation and/or the use of anticholinergics. The surgical incision and the actual cutting or retraction of fascia and muscles may contribute to postoperative discomfort.

Some clients may discuss the comfort problem, but others may not, depending on their cultural orientation or physical condition. Clients having surgery of the chest, anorectum, joints, back, and upper abdomen generally experience the greatest postoperative pain. Observe the client's behavior and inquire about the client's comfort.

The client with postoperative pain appears anxious and restless. To provide medications for pain relief, obtain an accurate description of the pain if the client is able to provide it. What precipitates the pain? What relieves it? What is its quality? Sharp? Dull? Throbbing? Burning? How severe is it? How long does it last? Is it steady or intermittent? Where is it felt? In the incisional area? All over? To avoid oversedating or undersedating the client, determine what intraoperative drugs the client has received. Clients who received a tranquilizer, narcotic, or both, may be pain-free when they first arrive in their room. Those who receive only inhalant anesthesia may have received a parenteral analgesic in the recovery room. If not, they may need relief from pain upon arriving in their room. General guidelines for analgesia are:

- The client may receive a postoperative narcotic analgesic approximately 1 to 1½ hours after the intraoperative administration of meperidine (Demerol) or morphine.
- The client who has received naloxone (Narcan) to relieve respiratory depression may have severe pain in the recovery room or upon return to the unit. The client will need a postoperative narcotic analgesic because naloxone is a quick-acting narcotic antagonist.
- The client who has received intravenous droperidol (Inapsine) during surgery should have the standard dose of a narcotic analgesic reduced by one-third to one-half during the first 8 to 12 hours postoperatively because of the drug's potentiating effects on narcotics.
- The client who has received intravenous diazepam (Valium) or lorazepam (Ativan) during surgery should have the standard dose of a narcotic analgesic reduced by one-third to one-half during the first 2 to 4 hours postoperatively because these drugs also have a potentiating effect on narcotics.

ASSESSING MOTOR AND SENSORY NEEDS During the later postoperative course, the nurse continues to assess vital signs and verbal and nonverbal communication. Is the client oriented to time, place, and person? Is the client grunting, grimacing, or otherwise responding to questions or other stimuli? Is the client showing signs of sensory overload or sensory deprivation. The client is necessarily immobilized during surgery and for some time thereafter. The longer the immobilization during and after surgery, the greater the potential for complications from immobility.

ASSESSING WOUND CARE NEEDS Throughout the postoperative period, assess the wound for evidence of normal healing; expected inflammation; and unexpected complications such as infection, dehiscence, or evisceration. Check to make sure that drainage tubes are patent. A low-grade fever (below 37.8°C or 101°F), associated with the inflammatory process, is generally expected postoperatively and may persist for 2 to 3 days with uncomplicated wound healing. Thereafter, a fever generally signifies an infection.

The wound should be assessed at least daily in the later postoperative period and more frequently if problems are identified. Signs and symptoms of wound-healing problems are often subtle. For example, serous drainage, no matter how small the amount, between the fifth and twelfth postoperative day should alert the nurse to the potential for dehiscence. Reporting the potential for dehiscence before it occurs saves the client pain. Sometimes clients alert the nurse to impending dehiscence or evisceration by describing a "giving" sensation in the operative area. Observing for and reporting signs of redness, induration, or purulent drainage help to prevent or decrease the severity of infection. An infected surgical wound adds about 5 to 7 days to the hospital stay (Curtin, 1984).

ASSESSING PSYCHOSOCIAL NEEDS Faced with body image changes to accept, altered lifestyle patterns to adjust to, and temporary or permanent role change, clients usually continue to be anxious during the later postoperative period. The nurse is responsible for assessing the psychosocial impact of surgery on each client.

Nursing Diagnosis

From a thorough analysis of the assessment factors for the postoperative period, with other factors discussed earlier in this chapter, the nurse formulates nursing diagnoses for the later postoperative period. Some nursing diagnoses common to this period are listed in Box 11–5.

Planning and Implementation

Nursing plans and interventions for the later postoperative period are aimed primarily at meeting needs related to respiration, circulation, nutritional and fluid and electrolyte status, elimination, comfort and safety, motor and sensory status, wound care, and psychosocial status. Continuity of care is provided by adequately preparing the client

Box 11–5
Common Nursing Diagnoses Related to Later Postoperative Care

Airway clearance, ineffective, related to ineffective coughing

Bowel elimination, altered: constipation, related to decreased activity level

Breathing pattern, ineffective, related to incisional pain

Comfort, altered: pain, related to tissue manipulation during surgery

Fluid volume deficit, related to nasogastric and wound drainage

Gas exchange, impaired, related to failure to breathe deeply

Injury: potential for infection, related to incisional disruption of the integument

Nutrition, altered: less than body requirements, related to postoperative NPO status

Self-concept, disturbance in: body image, related to loss of body part

Skin integrity, impaired, related to surgical incision and excessive wound drainage

for discharge. Nursing care for clients having particular surgical procedures is discussed in the units about body systems.

MEETING RESPIRATORY NEEDS Once fully recovered from anesthesia, the client must be properly positioned to facilitate adequate ventilation of the lungs. The client confined to bed should be kept in the high- or semi-Fowler's position as much as possible if the client's condition permits. The client is turned from side to side regularly. Coughing and deep breathing should be encouraged at least every hour in the early postoperative period and periodically thereafter.

The client may be reluctant to cough and deep breathe, because this will be painful. Offer empathic support while reinforcing preoperative explanations of the rationale for coughing and deep breathing. Providing analgesics before deep breathing and coughing will make the client less uncomfortable. Splinting of the incision will provide the client who has an abdominal or thoracic incision with extra support. Incentive spirometry, if ordered, should be encouraged as often as prescribed, and the nurse should assist the client as necessary.

Modify coughing and deep breathing as necessary to meet individual client needs. Elderly, weak, drowsy, or depressed clients may need frequent reminders and assistance with coughing or deep breathing and positioning. Obese clients are also likely to need help with positioning. Smokers are prone to coughing spasms, laryngospasm, and bronchospasm after surgery. In these clients, excessive coughing, as well as insufficient coughing, can cause harm by collapsing alveoli. Teach these clients the cascade cough described earlier in this chapter. Clients with chronic obstructive lung disease should also do pursed-lip breathing exercises to help rid the lungs of high levels of carbon dioxide.

MEETING CIRCULATORY NEEDS The nurse should advise the client to avoid undue pressure on blood vessels and to watch for factors that promote venous stasis, such as immobility and crossing the legs. Turning and moving in bed at least every hour or two should be encouraged, especially while activity is restricted. The nurse should also encourage early ambulation, when permitted, and should assist the client as necessary. Elastic stockings or elastic bandages from toe to midthigh promote venous return to the heart, preventing pooling of blood in the extremities. These supports should be removed at least once daily, skin condition should be checked, and skin care provided. Clean stockings should be provided as necessary.

Bed rest, warm compresses, and anticoagulant therapy are commonly prescribed for clients who develop thrombophlebitis. Massage should be avoided because it might dislodge thrombi.

MEETING NUTRITIONAL AND FLUID AND ELECTROLYTE NEEDS Because of the effects of stress and general anesthesia on the gastrointestinal tract, the postoperative client may be unable to tolerate food or fluids given by mouth. Nausea and vomiting are common sequelae of anesthesia, and antiemetics are often prescribed to relieve these effects. Food and fluids are generally withheld until normal gastrointestinal functioning has returned. In the meantime, the client is nourished by intravenous fluids. Dextrose, saline, and electrolyte solutions are often given, and vitamins are usually added. Routine IV fluids cannot meet long-term nutritional needs, however. Weight loss and nutritional deficiencies may occur.

After minor surgical procedures, intravenous administration may be discontinued soon after surgery and oral feedings may be started. After major procedures normal feeding may be postponed for up to a week. In such cases, hyperalimentation may be indicated. When oral ingestion resumes, the client will generally advance from a clear fluid diet to full fluids and, eventually, to regular foods.

MEETING ELIMINATION NEEDS The client should be instructed to inform the nurse when flatus or stool is passed. Generally, fluids and foods are withheld until normal intestinal peristalsis resumes. The client should be encouraged to ambulate as soon as permitted, and the diet should be adequate in fluids and fiber (roughage) to maintain normal bowel function.

If the client is uncomfortable from the inability to pass flatus, inserting a rectal tube (if allowed) when needed may be helpful. Abdominal distention may indicate that the client is unable to pass stool or flatus (paralytic ileus). Distention may be painful for the client, and a colonic irrigation (or Harris flush) may be prescribed. In this technique, water is instilled into the intestinal tract, as with an enema, and removed by gravity drainage. (Refer to a nursing fundamentals text for a full description of the colonic irrigation technique.)

Nursing measures to promote micturition include rinsing the perineum with warm water, encouraging fluids and ambulation if permitted, and stroking the abdomen. Bedpans and urinals should be kept within easy reach. Many clients find it difficult to void on a bedpan. Providing privacy is essential. A fracture pan may be more comfortable for the client than a regular bedpan. The client should notify the nurse when the first voiding is accomplished, and the specimen should be measured to ensure that the bladder has emptied adequately. Urinary retention with overflow or inadequate emptying may occur. In some cases, the client does not void, and catheterization may be ordered. A one-time catheterization with a straight catheter may be performed, or in-dwelling catheterization may be necessary. Catheterization is usually carried out if the client does not void within 8 hours of surgery.

MEETING COMFORT AND SAFETY NEEDS Plan and implement measures to promote and maintain hygiene to increase the client's comfort. When the client returns to the surgical unit, removal of secretions such as blood and vomitus helps the client relax and rest. Once the client is responsive and receptive, a complete bath may be given. The perineum should be cleansed after urination and defecation. The recovering client can assume increasing responsibility for hygiene, but the nurse must assume this responsibility until the client is able.

Mouth care should be offered frequently. NPO status makes the mouth uncomfortable and can promote cracking of the lips and tongue, xerostomia (excessive dryness of the mouth), and parotitis. The lips and mouth should be lubricated frequently, and ice chips should be offered if permitted.

Nursing measures should be directed at the postoperative pain the client perceives—not the pain the nurse thinks is perceived. Individuals vary greatly in their sensitivity to pain and in pain tolerance. Distraction, relaxation techniques, changes of position, or massage may be employed, and prescribed analgesics should be given as needed. The nurse should not withhold pain medication out of fear of addiction. Pain relief is the first consideration for the surgical client, because pain and fear of pain can induce additional stress, interfering with recovery. The assurance that analgesics have been prescribed and may be requested when needed often relieves anxiety and pain. A relatively recent technique that gives the client some control over postoperative pain is transcutaneous electrical nerve stimulation (TENS). External electrodes are applied near the incision and connected to a control mechanism; the client uses the mechanism to inhibit transmission of pain impulses, inhibiting perception of pain. The TENS device may be kept on continually right after surgery; eventually, the client uses it as necessary.

Bedpans or urinals, call devices, and any supplies the client may need should be kept where the client can easily reach them. Supplies and equipment that are not needed should be removed; a bed table touching the feet of a client who cannot remove it can be extremely uncomfortable. Siderails should be raised while the client is confined to bed or under the effects of anesthesia or narcotics. When the client begins to ambulate, remove obstructing furniture from the path.

MEETING MOTOR AND SENSORY NEEDS Activity will gradually increase as tolerated. As recovery progresses, the client should gradually become capable of a wider range of activity. Clients getting out of bed for the first time may feel dizzy or weak. **Postural hypotension** (a drop in blood pressure when moving from a lying or sitting to a standing position) is often associated with the dizziness or weakness. Having the client dangle the legs off the bed and assisting in a slow, relaxed transfer can minimize these symptoms. If the client appears disoriented, visits by the family may be helpful. The client should be reminded of his or her identity and kept aware of the time, day, and similar facts. Diversion and a change in environment may be helpful. If sensory overload is a problem, try to reduce stimuli.

MEETING WOUND CARE NEEDS When drainage is excessive, either in the recovery room or on the surgical unit, the first postoperative dressing is generally reinforced rather than changed. The amount of drainage or blood loss should be noted. Drainage can sometimes be estimated by drawing a circle around the soiled area on the dressing; to estimate blood loss, note the number of soiled pads or the size of a blood spot.

The first dressing change is usually performed by the surgeon. Subsequently, the nurse may assume responsibility for dressing changes, depending on agency policy. Sterile technique must be maintained during dressing changes. The area around the incision and the area around any drains should be meticulously cleansed. Unless ordered to leave the wound open, protect it from further trauma by applying a clean dressing.

When the client is allowed out of bed, an abdominal binder may be ordered to provide extra support. Clients often describe a feeling that the viscera are dropping or falling out when they first ambulate after abdominal surgery, and a binder provides a sense of security. Binders may also help prevent complications such as dehiscence and evisceration in obese clients.

Should the wound become infected, precautions must be taken to prevent transfer of infection. Drainage and secretion precautions are recommended for minor infections; for major wound infections, contact isolation should be instituted. Wound irrigation is often performed.

If there are indications of dehiscence or evisceration, notify the surgeon immediately. Meanwhile, apply heavily padded pressure dressings soaked with saline. Check vital signs because hypotension and tachycardia may occur, and shock may accompany evisceration.

MEETING PSYCHOSOCIAL NEEDS In general, assisting the client to return to customary functioning helps psychologically. Encourage independence by allowing the client to perform self-care activities, ambulate as soon as possible, and otherwise assume responsibility without endangering recovery. Visits from family members should be permitted and encouraged soon after surgery. Be available so the client can express concerns about the prognosis, body image changes, and changes in lifestyles. The client may need to assume new roles, and the nurse can assist in the transition.

Home Health Care

Throughout the perioperative period, keep in mind the client's eventual return home. What home care needs will the client have? Will the client have drains in place? Catheters? Do the client's significant others understand care of these devices? Will the client's diet or activity be restricted? How will the client get home? Should other agencies be consulted in anticipation of these needs?

Although instructions for postrelease care are often prescribed by the physician, the nurse does the actual teaching, explaining, and clarifying. When possible, ask the client and family to demonstrate any techniques they have been taught, such as dressing changes, and to explain why the procedure must be done in a certain way. Reassurance may also be necessary, because the client may be apprehensive about leaving the protective environment of the hospital. Written instructions will aid the client's memory. Generally, written instructions include: wound care; diet; activity and/or special exercises; medication, including dosages, anticipated effects, and signs of overdose or side effects; date for follow-up visit. If necessary, contact a home care agency to provide for continuity of care. The client may also be furnished with names and addresses of self-help groups. Self-help groups and other resources are listed at the end of each nursing process chapter.

Evaluation

The client who has had surgery may leave the hospital hopeful and eager for rehabilitation, or the client may be apprehensive, angry, or regretful. The quality of nursing care can help make the difference. In all phases of the perioperative period, evaluation provides the data necessary for making decisions about the appropriateness and effectiveness of interventions so they can be continued or modified or so new needs can be addressed.

Chapter Highlights

The role of the nurse as client advocate is especially important for surgical clients, who may be unable to take action on their own.

The prevention of nosocomial infection in surgical clients is a major nursing responsibility throughout the perioperative period.

Surgery has a profound impact on body systems as well as on lifestyle and psychosocial well-being.

Consequences and potential complications of surgery may affect the status of respiration, circulation, nutrition, fluid and electrolyte balance, elimination, safety and comfort, and motor and sensory function.

A preoperative teaching plan should include a general orientation to the surgical experience and instruction in anticipated postoperative activities.

Clients who receive preoperative and postoperative teaching are less anxious, more willing to participate in their own care and to comply with prescribed medical regimens, and have fewer complications.

Excessive and/or prolonged pressure on body tissues, a potential consequence of surgical positioning, can contribute to the development of pressure ulcers, postoperative muscle discomfort, and neurovascular damage.

In caring for the client under anesthesia, the nurse acts as client advocate when ensuring that the client is positioned to protect privacy and with proper body alignment, and that surgical asepsis is maintained.

Clients who have had surgery may have difficulty in coping with body image alterations that may be a consequence of the surgery.

Pain relief and promotion of comfort, which require a variety of medical and nursing measures, deserve high priority in the care of the postsurgical client.

Nursing interventions to promote wound healing include ensuring optimal nutritional and fluid intake, providing aseptic wound care, and avoiding unnecessary stress on the operative area.

Discharge planning for the surgical client should begin at admission. In providing discharge instructions, the nurse should consider the client's acceptance of any surgical alteration of body structure or function, the impact of any imposed limitations on usual lifestyle, the ability for self-care, and the availability of support systems.

Bibliography

Alexander J et al: The influence of hair removal methods on wound infections. *Arch Surg* 1983; 118:347–352.

American Nurses' Association: *Standards of Perioperative Nursing Practice.* Kansas City: ANA, 1981.

Andrews DR, Taylor C: Documenting post-anesthesia recovery. *Am J Nurs* 1985; 85(3):290–291.

Atkinson LJ, Kohn ML: *Berry and Kohn's Introduction to Operating Room Technique,* 6th ed. New York: McGraw–Hill, 1986.

Burns LA: Ambulatory surgery growing at a rapid rate. *AORN J* 1982; 35(2):260–270.

Centers for Disease Control: *Guideline for Prevention of Surgical Wound Infection.* Atlanta: USDHHS, 1985.

Cruse PJE, Foord R: The epidemiology of wound infection. *Surg Clin North Am* 1980; 69(1):17–40.

Curtin L: Wound management: Care and cost—an overview. *Nurs Mgmt* (Feb) 1984; 15:22–25.

Devine EC, Cook TD: A meta-analytic analysis of effects of psychoeducational interventions on length of post-surgical hospital stay. *Nurs Res* 1983; 32:267–274.

Dripps RD, Eckenhoff JE, Vandam LK: *Introduction to Anesthesia: The Principles of Safe Practice.* Philadelphia: Saunders, 1982.

Flynn ME, Rovee DT: Promoting wound healing: Influencing repair and recovery. *Am J Nurs* 1982; 82:1550–1556.

Fraulini KE, Gorski DW: Don't let perioperative medications put you in a spin. *Nurs 83* (Dec) 1983; 13:26–30.

Gruendemann BJ, Meeker MH: *Alexander's Care of the Patient in Surgery.* St. Louis: Mosby, 1983.

Hewitt D: Don't forget your preop patient's fears. *RN* (Oct) 1984; 10:63–68.

Kneedler JA, Dodge GH: *Perioperative Patient Care.* Boston: Blackwell, 1983.

Lecky JH: Problems of trace anesthetic levels. In: Orkin FK, Cooperman LH: *Complications in Anesthesiology.* Philadelphia: Lippincott, 1983, pp. 715–732.

Mattia MA: Hazards in the hospital environment: Anesthesia gases and methylmethacrylate. *Am J Nurs* 1983; 83:73–77.

Mortensen M, McMullin C: Discharge score for surgical outpatients. *Am J Nurs* 1986; 86:1347–1349.

Northrop C: Legal aspects of nursing. In: Flynn J-B, Heffron PB: *Nursing: From Concept to Practice.* Bowie, MD: Brady, 1984, pp. 205–236.

Rosenberg H: Malignant hyperpyrexia. *Am J Nurs* 1981; 81:1484–1486.

Stoelting RK, Miller RD: *Basics of Anesthesia.* New York: Churchill Livingstone, 1984.

Ziemer M: Effects of information on postsurgical coping. *Nurs Res* 1983; 32(5):282–287.

Resources

HOT LINE

Second Surgical Opinion Hotline
(Monday through Friday, 8 AM to 12 noon)
Phone: Nationwide: (800) 638–6833
Maryland: (800) 492–6603

Provides the names of local surgeons who will act as consultants and give a second opinion on nonemergency operations. These surgeons will not treat persons who consult them and thus have no financial interest in whether the client has the operation. Printed information is also available.

HEALTH EDUCATION MATERIAL

From: American Medical Association
535 N. Dearborn St.
Chicago, IL 60610

"Surgery," a booklet explaining what the client will experience before, during, and after surgery.

From: American Society of Anesthesiologists
515 Busse Hwy.
Park Ridge, IL 60068

"Know Your Anesthesiologist," a booklet explaining anesthesia, the role of the anesthesiologist, and the experiences the client will undergo.

From: US Government Consumer Information Center
Pueblo, CO 81009

"Facing Surgery? Why Not Get a Second Opinion?," a booklet describing why a second opinion is important.

NURSING ORGANIZATIONS

American Association of Nurse Anesthetists
216 Higgins Rd.
Park Ridge, IL 60068
Phone: (312) 692–7050

The membership of this organization comprises certified registered nurse anesthetists. The goals are to promote high-quality anesthesia care, to advance the science and art of anesthesiology, and to promote educational standards in the field. Annual dues for active members.

American Society of Post Anesthesia Nurses
Box 11086
Richmond, VA 23230
Phone: (804) 359–3557

Composed of RNs and LPNs who are interested in or working

in postanesthesia care, this organization encourages research, education, and specialization in the care of clients during the immediate postoperative period.

Association of Operating Room Nurses
10170 E. Mississippi Ave.
Denver, CO 80321
Phone: (303) 755–6300
An organization for RNs engaged in supervisory, teaching, or staff positions in operating room nursing. Goals are to improve nursing care, provide educational programs, and encourage study and certification. Annual dues.

National Conference of Operating Room Nurses
% Operating Room
St. Boniface General Hospital
Winnipeg, Manitoba, Canada R2H 2A6

CHAPTER **12**

Burns

Other topics relevant to this content are: Cardiopulmonary resuscitation (CPR), **Chapter 19;** Fluid and electrolyte balance, **Chapter 3;** Helping clients and their families cope with anxiety, anger, dependence, and depression, **Chapter 4;** Keloid formation and hypertrophic scarring, **Chapter 55;** Malnutrition and nutritional support, **Chapter 6;** Skin grafting, **Chapter 55.**

Objectives

When you have finished studying this chapter, you should be able to:

Describe how burns are classified.

Describe the effects of burns on the major body systems, including the cardiovascular, respiratory, renal, gastrointestinal, hepatic–biliary, and integumentary systems.

List priorities in immediate care of burn clients.

State applications of major burn treatments, including debridement, temporary wound coverage, skin grafting, and topical antibiotics.

Apply the nursing process to the care of burn clients in the emergent, acute, and rehabilitative periods.

Discuss psychosocial adjustment of clients with major burns during the three periods of care.

An estimated two million people are treated for burns yearly by physicians, and approximately 70,000 are hospitalized. Burn injuries account for approximately 12,000 deaths per year. Accidents, which include burns, are the major cause of death in children aged 1 to 4.

Burns are among the most devastating injuries a person can sustain. Not only do burns injure the body and leave the skin permanently scarred, but burns also cause severe pain and altered body image. A client's lifestyle may also be affected by lengthy hospitalization, which may alter work patterns and finances. Recovery is likely to be long and grueling, both physically and psychologically. Physical care and emotional support for burned clients and their families require highly developed nursing skills and great sensitivity.

SECTION **I**

The Problem of Burns

Causes of Burns

Approximately 80% of accidental burns occur in the home. Ignorance and carelessness are contributing factors. Burns are common when a person is distracted while cooking or falls asleep smoking.

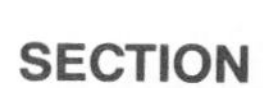

In the elderly, 75% of flame burns happen when they accidentally set their clothing on fire. Bathing is another burn hazard for the elderly because they have decreased sensitivity to temperature and slowed response time. One out of ten burned elderly persons were injured from bath water being too hot. Diabetics are also prone to burn injury from hot water. In the winter, malfunctioning kerosene heaters have caused home fires.

Burns can be described as thermal, chemical, electrical, and radiation. *Thermal burns* include injuries caused by fire, steam, scalding water, and other hot liquids. Children often sustain thermal injuries when they play with matches or pour hot fluids on themselves. Adults are often burned while cooking, trying to ignite a fire with gas, or smoking in bed.

Chemical burns occur most often when caustic chemicals are used in chemistry laboratories and in some industrial settings. Because of this increased risk, eye irrigating fountains and showers should be installed for emergency use. Caustic home-cleaning chemicals, such as oven cleaners and toilet bowl cleaners, are also potentially dangerous.

Electrical burns are possible anywhere there is electrical current. Electrical burns in the home occur most often to children biting on electrical cords or playing with wall sockets. Adults sometimes sustain electrical burns at home while trying to repair outlets or appliances. In the work setting, linemen may sustain electrical burns when electricity in power lines has not been turned off properly.

Radiation burns are caused by overexposure to the sun, x-rays, and nuclear energy. Radiation burns are also seen in clients who have had radiation therapy for cancer.

Prevention of Burns

Much of the suffering and financial burden caused by burn accidents is avoidable. Nurses can help prevent burns by participating in health education programs that stress fire prevention, such as "Learn Not to Burn." Legislation is another avenue in burn prevention, and nurses can work for measures that promote safety in work and home environments. Community health nurses are especially likely to see fire hazards in the home and should assist families to make their homes safe. Occupational health nurses need to be aware of hazards in the work setting and emergency care of burns. Nurses in any setting should also encourage and participate in drills and fire safety inspections. Finally, nurses should set good examples by keeping their homes and work settings free of fire hazards.

Pathophysiology of Burns

The damage from a burn is directly related to the length of exposure and intensity of the burning agent. The same damage to skin will occur in 6 hours at 111°F (43.9°C) as occurs in 1 second at 140°F (60°C).

Burns can be described as first-, second-, or third-degree or as partial-thickness or full-thickness. The depth of burn, according to these classifications, is illustrated in Figure 12–1.

A **first-degree burn** damages only the epidermal layer of the skin. Sunburn is a common first-degree burn. These wounds appear red and dry and blanche with fingertip pressure. First-degree burns are painful because cutaneous nerve endings are injured. These injuries will heal on their own within 1 week if there are no complications.

Second-degree burns, which damage the epidermis and part of the dermis, appear red and blistered. If blisters

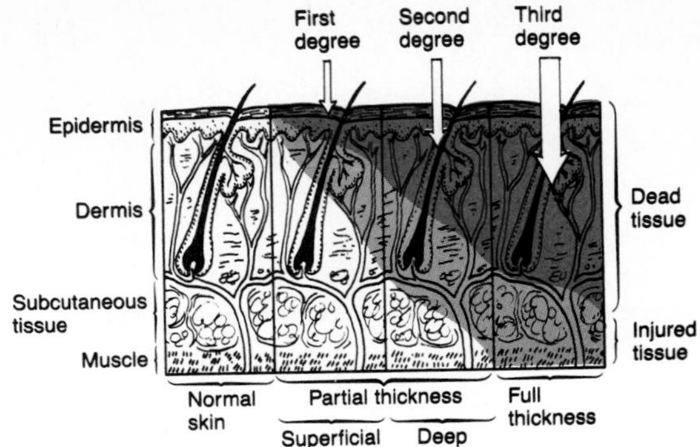

Figure 12–1

Depth of burn. The arrows represent degrees of heat or intensity of burning agent and the duration of contact with skin. The darker shaded area represents dead tissue. The lighter shaded area indicates damaged or injured tissues that will heal with good care.

have broken, the wound will appear wet or crusted. Second-degree burns are painful because cutaneous nerves are exposed to air. Shallow second-degree burns can heal on their own over a few weeks. Deeper second-degree burns can heal on their own but are often skin grafted to speed recovery, reducing the risk of wound infection and minimizing scarring. Second-degree burns will blanche and refill with fingertip pressure.

Third-degree burns damage both epidermal and dermal layers of skin. Subcutaneous tissue, muscle, and bone may also be injured. These wounds appear leathery and may be white, brown, red, or black. The wound will be painless because cutaneous nerve endings have been destroyed and will not blanche with fingertip pressure. Third-degree burns do not heal without skin grafting unless they are small. The deeper the burn wound, the more severe the injury because of pathophysiologic changes.

The term **partial-thickness burn** encompasses first- and second-degree burns. **Full-thickness burns** are equivalent to third-degree burns.

The damage to the body from electrical injury cannot be judged from the size or apparent depth of the skin wound. Severe damage occurs beneath the skin from the electrical current (Figure 12–2). As the electricity travels through the body to an electrical ground, the current causes damage to the structures through which it passes. Blood in the vessels coagulates from the heat, causing necrosis of the tissues those blood vessels formerly supplied. Nerves may be destroyed; muscles may spasm severely enough to fracture bones. In addition, tissue disruption can occur along the active path of the current. These burns are called "exit burns." Exit burns generally appear as quarter-sized red areas that open to expose deeper tissues. Exit burns may appear initially or after many days.

Following a severe burn, all body systems are involved in an attempt to maintain homeostasis. Complications are the rule, not the exception, after burn injury. A client with major burns can be expected to develop four to six major complications in addition to the burn. Complications can

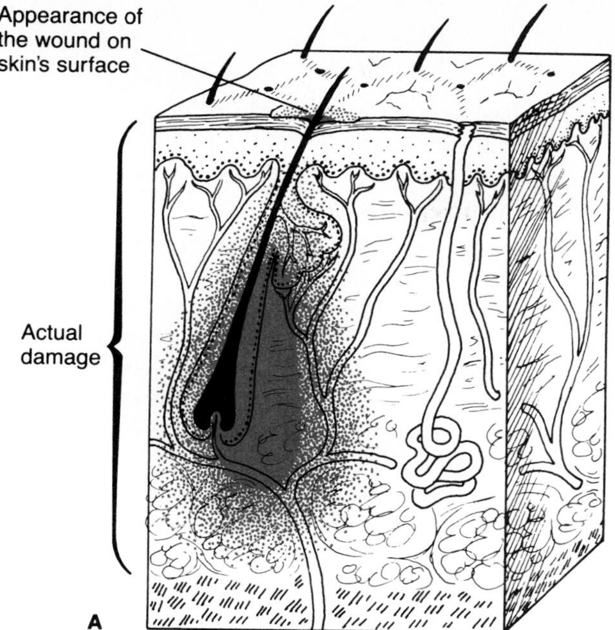

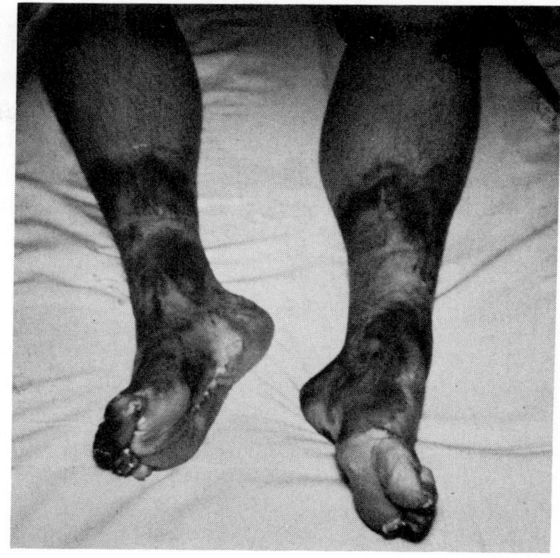

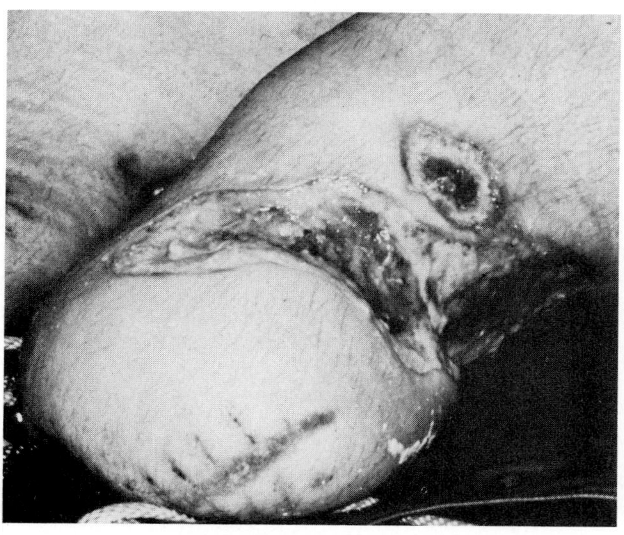
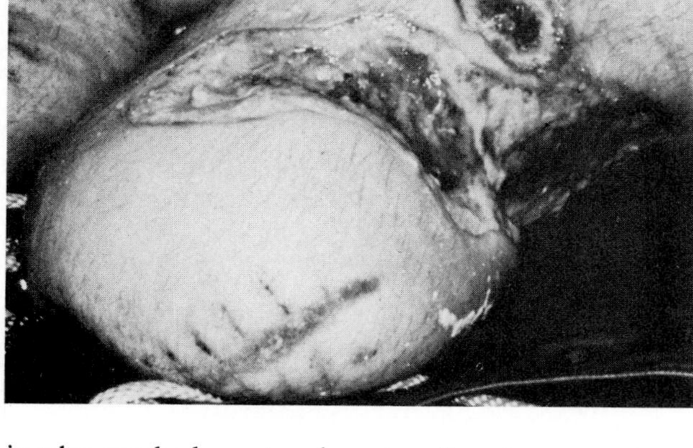
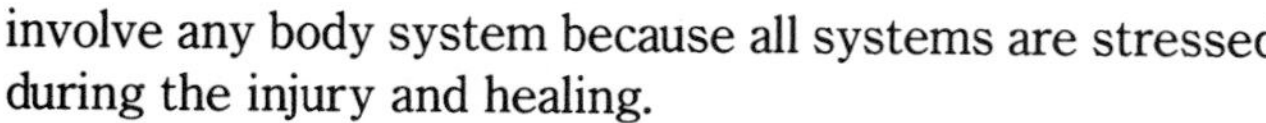

Figure 12–2

Damage to skin from an electrical current. **A.** The damage to the body from an electrical burn cannot be judged by the skin wound. There is extensive damage under the surface of the skin. **B.** Client who sustained electrical burns in an industrial accident. This photograph was taken on admission to the ICU. Note the dark eschar indicating full-thickness injury. **C.** One week after admission the client required bilateral amputation of the legs because of necrosis. Note the exit burns behind the knee; initially, they appeared as blisters.

involve any body system because all systems are stressed during the injury and healing.

Cardiovascular System

Immediately following the burn, the body releases massive amounts of vasoactive substances, such as serotonin and histamine. These substances increase capillary permeability, allowing serum (which contains water), proteins, and electrolytes to escape into both damaged and normal tissues. This loss of serum into the tissues causes hypovolemia, which may lead to massive shock if the injury is severe enough.

Unlike hypovolemia from blood loss, there is no actual fluid loss; instead the fluid is sequestered (isolated) in the tissues where it cannot be utilized. As a result of hypovolemia, cardiac output falls, renal blood flow decreases, blood viscosity increases, and total peripheral vascular resistance increases because of peripheral vasoconstriction. Blood pressure falls because of the fluid shift and local vasodilatation from histamine. The heart rate increases from the low blood pressure and beta-receptor stimulation by epinephrine. Acute renal failure and death may follow unless appropriate measures are taken promptly.

With the fluid shift, blood values change. Hematocrit and hemoglobin values are elevated because of the escape of fluid from the blood. There may be hypernatremia because of dehydration and hyperkalemia because of release of intracellular potassium during the injury. Heat also destroys red blood cells, releasing free hemoglobin into the bloodstream. The client may be disoriented as a result of the decreased cerebral circulation and hypoxia caused by hypotension, dehydration, electrolyte shifts, pain, and shock.

Within 36 to 48 hours of a major burn, capillary permeability returns to normal, and fluids sequestered in body tissues reenter vascular spaces, increasing blood volume. Hemoglobin and hematocrit values will return to normal or below-normal levels. In this phase, clients will exhibit profound diuresis and elevated blood pressure unless fluids were titrated closely to urine output in the emergent phase. They may also develop circulatory overload because of strain on the heart. Cardiovascular complications include congestive heart failure from fluid overload, stroke, disseminated intravascular coagulation (DIC), and suppurative thrombophlebitis from coagulated blood in vessels.

Respiratory System

Pulmonary damage from smoke, super-heated gases, chemical inhalation, and carbon monoxide intoxication is the leading cause of death in fire victims. If the fire occurred in an enclosed space, the victim will have breathed smoke. Chemicals may have been inhaled if petroleum and plastic products were burned (eg, polymer plastics release hydrochloric acid, hydrogen cyanide, and ammonia). The massive fluid shift into extravascular tissues produces massive edema, which may also occlude the airway. Metabolic acidosis is an additional result of fluid shift and hypovolemia. Respirations increase to compensate for the acidosis.

Pulmonary edema may develop from the suddenly increased vascular volume once fluid balance has been normalized. Later pulmonary complications include pneumonia from inhalation injury; pulmonary embolism from immobility; and pulmonary insufficiency, also called adult respiratory distress syndrome (ARDS).

Endocrine System

Burn injury results in hypermetabolism, an increase in the client's basal metabolic rate. In a client with a 40% to 50% body surface burn, the metabolic rate nearly doubles during the first 5 days after the burn and then reaches a plateau. Increased catecholamine production and an endogenous resetting of the body's metabolic rate are the cause of the hypermetabolism.

Burned clients have an elevated core temperature and an elevated skin temperature as part of their hypermetabolism. Their core temperatures average at 38.3°C (101°F). Burned clients feel most comfortable in warmer-than-average rooms at temperatures around 30.6°C (87.0°F), in contrast to the usual room setting temperature of 21.1°C (70°F).

Endocrine system complications following burn injury are adrenal hemorrhage, adrenal insufficiency, diabetes insipidus, and syndrome of inappropriate antidiuretic hormone (SIADH). Adrenal hemorrhage results from increased demands on the adrenal glands to secrete steroids and catecholamines. Symptoms of adrenal hemorrhage are vague; they include upper abdominal pain, cyanotic mottling of unburned skin with cardiovascular collapse, and increased losses of sodium in the urine (over 100 mEq/day). Systemic steroids administered to clients with diagnosed adrenal hemorrhage seem to result in only temporary improvement before death.

Nervous System

Damage to peripheral nerves occurs when tissue is destroyed by any burn. Electrical burns can damage the central or peripheral nerves. If high voltage electrical current comes in contact with the skull, transmitting heat into the brain tissues, brain damage can occur. The spinal cord and peripheral nerves can also be injured by electrical current. Injuries can range from limited areas of weakness to complete paralysis. These neurologic problems sometimes reverse completely, and vigorous therapy must be instituted to maintain full range-of-motion (ROM) in these extremities.

Changes in the client's level of consciousness can occur from hypoxia, hypovolemia, sepsis, electrolyte imbalances, or falling when burned. Burn injuries by themselves do not cause loss of consciousness.

Musculoskeletal System

Severe burns may result in destruction of muscle and connective tissue. Prolonged immobilization following a burn injury can result in muscle atrophy, joint contractures, and loss of calcium from bones. The client may have sustained a related injury, such as a leg fracture that will require special wound care. A fractured burned extremity cannot be casted because infection would quickly result. Therefore fractures are treated by skeletal traction.

Renal System

Urinary output drops in the initial 48 hours because of decreased renal blood flow resulting from hypotension and secretion of antidiuretic hormone and aldosterone. Poor tissue perfusion can progress to renal shutdown if prompt and appropriate measures for fluid replacement are not taken. Free hemoglobin released by destruction of red blood cells or myoglobin released by damaged muscle may pass into the urine through the kidney; if free hemoglobin or myoglobin block the nephrons, renal failure may develop.

Urine output increases with the restoration of intravascular fluid balance, leading to profound diuresis. When diuresis begins, do not assume that fluids are no longer needed, however, because evaporative water loss from the wound can reach 3 to 5 L in 24 hours.

Serum electrolyte values may fall during this period because of the excess body fluids. Most electrolyte changes are from dilution. The only exception is hyperkalemia, which is caused by intracellular potassium leaking into the bloodstream. Potassium leaves the damaged cells after a burn and can reach lethal levels quickly. Serum sodium levels can assist in determining fluid needs. Other indicators of fluid status besides urinary output are the condition of the oral mucosa, skin turgor, body weight, and hemoglobin and hematocrit levels.

Gastrointestinal and Hepatic–Biliary Systems

With the initial insult, ileus often occurs because the stress of the injury shunts blood away from the gastrointestinal tract. The injury also triggers an endogenous reset of metabolism, greatly increasing metabolism over preburn levels. Sympathetic nervous system stimulation mobilizes steroids. Glycogen stores are converted to glucose for energy. The glucose stores are quickly depleted, forcing the body to use fats and proteins for energy.

With catabolism, weight loss following a burn injury can be severe and is directly proportional to the size of the burn. A client with a 40% burn can lose 20% of body weight without nutritional support. A burned client can survive only 3 to 4 weeks without food, compared with a normal, healthy adult who can survive 2 months.

Malnutrition following a major burn is still a serious problem, increasing the client's risk of complications. The increased metabolism continues until clients have less than 20% of the body unhealed. Obviously, closure of the burn wound, which resets metabolism to near normal, is essential in severe cases.

Curling's ulcer, or stress ulcer, is a potential complication with any major trauma. Another complication is hepatic failure caused by sepsis.

Integumentary System

With full-thickness burns, skin loses its elasticity and does not expand to accommodate edema. Therefore, the edema caused by the shift of fluids into interstitial spaces puts pressure on underlying structures such as blood vessels and the airway. In clients with chest burns, **eschar** (thick burned skin or tissue that may be charred or necrotic and may slough) prevents normal chest expansion with breathing. In clients with circumferential burns of the arms and legs, nonexpanding eschar may impair circulation to the distal extremities.

Extensive evaporative water loss from a burn wound contributes to the body's overall fluid imbalance. Burned clients may also lose 30 g of nitrogen per day through the wound, quickly placing them in negative nitrogen balance.

Burn wounds can develop four major problems as they heal: infection, contractures, keloids and hypertrophic scars, and color changes. Infection is the most common complication for burn clients, accounting for 45% of all deaths.

Initially, burn wounds are usually sterile because heat sterilizes the burn surface. After 5 days, all burn wounds are considered contaminated, however. The eschar provides an excellent growth medium for microorganisms because eschar is dark, warm, moist, has the proper pH, and provides ample food. If the microorganisms are limited to the eschar (wound colonization), clients usually are minimally affected by their presence. When pathogens invade deeper structures of the skin, however, clients develop wound infections. When the infection enters normal tissue, sepsis can develop.

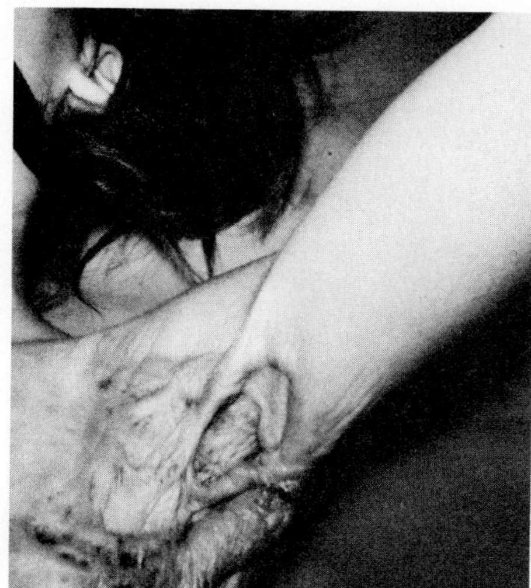

Figure 12–3

Burn wound contracture.

Wound contracture is not the same as wound contraction. Contraction, a normal healing process, can be defined as the drawing together of the edges of the wound by forces within the wound. All wounds undergo some contraction during healing. In contrast, contracture is an abnormal process from excessive wound contraction that causes a fixed deformity (Figure 12–3). Burn wound contracture over joints can become so severe that clients cannot move their extremities. Neck burns can contract, actually pulling the chin down onto the sternum. Mouth burns can contract to the point that clients have only a small hole the size of a dime to eat through.

A keloid is an excessive amount of tumorlike scar tissue that extends far beyond the scar line of the original wound (Figure 12–4A). Hypertrophic scars, on the other hand, are raised scars that do not extend beyond the wound (Figure 12–4B). The cause of keloid formation and hypertrophic scars is unknown. Although excessive scarring tends to occur more often in persons with dark or olive-toned skin, it can occur in fair-skinned people also. Keloids and hypertrophic scars are also more frequent in young people than in adults. In addition to obvious problems with appearance, keloids itch, bleed, and may be painful.

Clients may sustain burns through the melanin layer of skin. During healing, this pigment-forming layer may not be replaced by the body, and the healed areas are paler than the normal pigmentation.

After the wound is healed and grafts are completed,

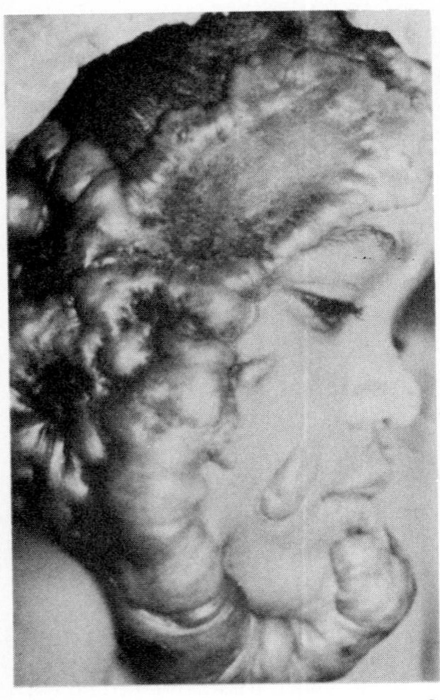

A

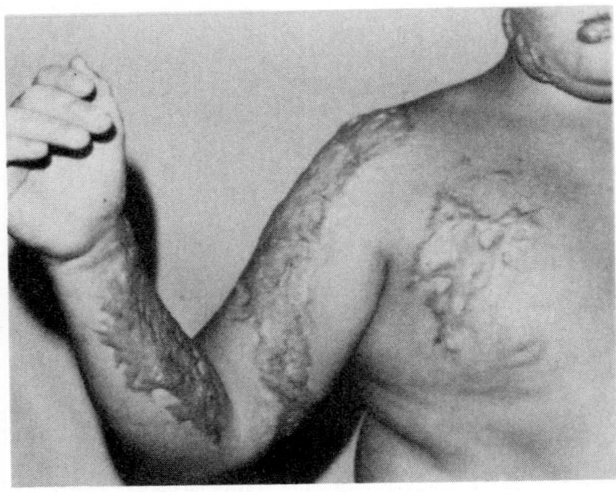

B

Figure 12–4

A. Example of burn wound keloid. **B.** Example of burn wound hypertrophic scarring.

the burn wound scar usually matures over 1 year, changing from angry red to off-white. During this time, aggressive efforts must be taken to minimize scarring and prevent contractures.

Treatment of Burns

The following discussion covers emergency care of the burn victim before transfer to the hospital, as well as outpatient treatment for minor burns. Also discussed are special burn care procedures such as debridement, temporary wound coverage, skin grafting, and topical antimicrobial agents.

Immediate Care of Burns

The first priority in the care of the burned client focuses on one principle: **Stop the burning process.** The specifics for the immediate care of burned clients are discussed below and summarized in Box 12–1.

The rescuer of the burn victim must thoroughly know the immediate plan of care. Burn clients will not always be rational and cooperative because they are frightened and in pain. The rescuer must also be able to execute the plan of care without becoming a second burn victim. It is critical that the rescuer think and remain calm before rushing into a potentially dangerous situation.

Cool, not cold, water can be applied to the burned part if it is less than 20% of body surface (see Figures 12–5 and 12–6 later in the chapter). For example, place a burned finger in cool water until the burning sensation stops. While the burn feels warm and painful, tissue is still being injured. Initial cooling of burns relieves pain, speeds healing, and reduces the need for grafting because the cool temperature stops the injury. **Do not apply ice.** Ice can cause further injury (similar to frostbite) and can cause shock from temperature extremes. Ointments, butter, or grease should not be applied to the wound because ointment keeps the wound warm, potentially increasing the depth of the injury.

The wound should be covered in clean noncotton-filled dressings. In the home, bed sheets work well for severe burns because they are clean and do not have lint. Lint adheres to open wounds and is painful to remove. No dressings need be used on the wound if skin integrity is intact.

Blisters should be left intact, because the skin provides a "biologic dressing," protecting the wound. Large blisters should be covered with sterile gauze and a bulky dressing to absorb the fluid if the blister breaks.

About 95% of burns are minor. Minor burns are superficial wounds (first and second degree), generally not exceeding 10% of the body surface. Minor burns never include electrical burns of any size or burns of the face, feet, perineum, or entire hand. Even though these are small body surface areas, the potential for complication is increased. Burns in these areas, and burns beyond those that would be classified as minor, must be evaluated and usually cared for in a hospital.

Assess the need for analgesia before beginning any wound care. Wash all debris from the wound. Running tap water on the burn or washing it in povidone–iodine solution while cleansing with a gauze pad works well to remove dead skin, dirt, or parts of clothing.

Systemic antibiotics are seldom indicated for minor

burns because they encourage superinfection from resistant organisms. Tetanus prophylaxis should be renewed because burn wounds provide an excellent medium for growth of anaerobic organisms. Use of topical antimicrobials should be considered for burns over 15 × 30 cm. The application of topical antimicrobials and dressings for burn wounds this large is discussed later in the skin integrity section in the acute period. Small wounds can be cared for with ointment or grease-impregnated gauze (Xeroform, Adaptic) applied to the wound. These dressings should be held in place with a gauze wrapping.

The soiled dressing should be removed daily while dry to facilitate debridement of the wound (removal of necrotic tissue). If this is too painful, the dressings can be soaked off. Holding the burn under the shower for 10 to 15 minutes is one effective method. The wound should be examined for signs of infection, which include a foul odor, increased redness at the edges of the wound, increased pain, a lack of healing, or regression of the burn to deeper layers of tissue. Fever need not be present with an infection.

Debridement

Prior to healing or any skin-grafting procedure, the eschar must be removed. There are three types of debridement: natural, mechanical, and enzymatic.

Natural debridement occurs by the body's own processes of phagocytosis. This form of debridement is slow and is not effective to clean and heal a burn over the size of a half-dollar.

Mechanical debridement uses instruments or water to speed wound cleaning. Hydrotherapy is one form of mechanical debridement. Debridement is usually done twice daily in the physical therapy unit in large whirlpool tanks filled with warm saline. Clients are submerged in the tanks after dressings are removed. Dressings should be removed while dry to increase wound debridement. While the client is in the tank, the bubbling water softens and loosens the eschar, allowing it to be clipped off by the physical therapist. No more than a 3-sq-in. area is removed at one time. Removing more eschar increases pain and potential for septicemia. The client is also assisted by the physical therapist to perform ROM while in the water. The hydrotherapy tank does not eliminate the need for personal care. Face, oral, hair, and perineal care must also be completed.

Some burn centers use flat tubs to cleanse burn clients. Clients are cleansed with sprayers instead of being submerged. The rationale for this form of therapy is that spraying can reduce the risk of septicemia because all body parts are not exposed to the contaminated bath water. In either method, the client should be rinsed with clean water after hydrotherapy to reduce residual skin bacteria.

If the client is too physiologically unstable to be transported to the hydrotherapy unit, wound care can be done in the client's room using a sterile basin and sterile saline to wash the wound. The client should be assisted in performing ROM and the wound redressed according to routine.

Box 12–1
Immediate Care of Burn Clients

1. Stop the burning process.

   Thermal burns:

   - Extinguish flames by rolling victim on ground or wrapping in blanket; get victim down on floor or ground to reduce facial burns and airway injury.
   - If burn is less than 20% of body surface area, apply cool water (not cold; no ice). (Do not use ointment, butter, or grease.)

   Chemical burns:

   - Stop burning of liquid chemicals by flushing with large amounts of water. (Phenol is an exception; irrigate with alcohol and *not with water,* which would allow the phenol to penetrate to deeper layers of skin.)
   - Do not attempt to neutralize.
   - Brush dry chemicals off skin or clothing.
   - Carefully remove any clothing containing chemical.

   Electrical burns:

   - Shut off power source or disconnect client from live current.
   - Avoid becoming a second victim.

   Radiation burns:

   - Remove victim from source of heat if possible.
   - Avoid exposure to radiation or nuclear waste during rescue.
2. Assess airway, breathing, and circulation. Establish airway. Perform cardiopulmonary resuscitation if needed.
3. Cover wound with clean, lint-free, noncotton dressing.
4. Assess for other injuries such as fractures or injuries from a fall.

Once the wound is cleaned and requires minimal debridement, bathtubs can be used for wound care. The tub should first be completely filled with hot water and ½ cup of bleach added. The tub should remain filled with this solution for 30 minutes before use. Then the tub should be drained, rinsed, and filled with water and table salt to make normal saline (2 tsp salt per liter of water) for the client's use.

Mechanical debridement can also be performed by peeling or cutting away eschar with a scalpel or dermatome (the instrument used in skin grafting). This form of debridement, an escharotomy, is temporarily painful and may cause bleeding. Pain is caused by stimulation of cutaneous nerves, and excess bleeding is from the loss of engorged blood in the injured area.

Tangential excision is surgical removal of eschar down to bleeding tissues followed by immediate grafting or application of dressings. Tangential excision is completed during the first week after the burn and is used instead of hydrotherapy debridement for more rapid healing of the burn. Compared with more conventional therapy, tangential excision shortens hospitalization, reduces fluid losses and some complications such as sepsis, wound infection, and scarring. The major risk of tangential excision is hemorrhage. Tangential excision is limited by the amount of available skin for grafting and the client's overall condition. Bleeding is often controlled with thrombin solutions.

Enzymatic debridement involves the application of proteolytic enzymes such as sutilains (Travase) to second- and third-degree burns to digest the eschar and dissolve and remove necrotic tissue. This form of debridement causes a burning sensation in the wound and should be limited to 15% of the body surface area at one time. The enzyme action may be inactivated if sutilains ointment is used in conjunction with iodine, nitrofurazone (Furacin), or hexachlorophene.

The ointment is applied in a thin layer over the wound with a sterile gloved hand or a cotton applicator, overlapping onto the unburned skin by about 1/4 in. A moist saline dressing is then applied over the enzyme. This dressing must be kept moist at all times.

Debridement is painful, and clients should be prepared for the experience, either with analgesics, relaxation techniques, or self-hypnosis. General anesthesia may be used when large areas of the wound are debrided in the operating room, but it is not safe for daily wound care. Daily debridement is wearing for clients because they know they will experience pain. Clients quickly fall into a pain–anxiety cycle because of anticipation of pain. Debridement also causes anxiety because the client sees the extent of the burn as wounds are uncovered and sees whether the wound is healing.

Temporary Wound Coverage

Burn wounds can be covered temporarily with homografts (allografts), heterografts (xenografts), or synthetic skin to reduce heat and evaporative water losses. Homografts are skin from other humans, such as cadavers and placental membranes. Heterografts are skin from animals, such as pigskin. Artificial skin includes OpSite and similar products. The only permanent wound coverage is an autograft from the burned person. Advantages and disadvantages of temporary wound covers are described in Table 12–1.

Table 12–1
Temporary Wound Coverage

Preparation	Advantages	Disadvantages
Pigskin	Relief of pain; reduction of water and heat loss; available in several forms; can be meshed	Costly; can provoke rejection
Cadaver skin	Relief of pain; reduction of water and heat loss; can be meshed	Expensive; scarce
Amniotic membrane	Biologic dressing; relief of pain; reduction of water and heat loss; free	Difficult to apply at times
OpSite (transparent polyurethane membrane dressing)	Permeable to air; not permeable to fluid or bacteria; promotes wound healing in moist environment; no scab formation; no debridement necessary; immediate pain reduction; nonpainful removal; transparent; significantly shortens healing time	Time-consuming application; self-adhesive, can be difficult to apply; not suitable for full-thickness burns
Biobrane™ (silicone rubber and nylon with collagen)	Suitable for partial- and full-thickness wounds; semitransparent; flexible, stretchable	Expensive

Skin Grafting

Burn wounds can reepithelialize and heal without skin grafting in 10 days to several weeks if they are not deep dermal burns. Allowing large deep burns to heal is a lengthy process and increases risk of infection and scarring, so these burns are often grafted.

Permanent skin grafting is the movement of skin from an unburned area on the client to a burned area. The burn wound must be clean and granulation tissue present before it is ready to accept a skin graft. Granulation tissue, seen in all clean wounds, is the initial step in healing. It is shiny and pale pink; on close examination, small bumps will be seen.

Burns not requiring skin grafting heal through epidermal cell replication. Hair follicles, which extend into the dermis, are lined with epidermal cells. These epidermal cells grow up into the wound and form "buds" of epidermis. The buds grow together and cover the wound. This is a long process, and problems with wound infection may mandate that a burn wound be grafted to speed healing.

Burn wounds also heal by scarring. Production of scar tissue is normal in the healing of any wound but can cause special problems for the burned client.

Recently, sections of clients' unburned skin have been grown in the laboratory and then used to skin graft burned areas. Laboratory techniques can alter normal skin growth, so the skin grows 150 times faster than normal. This technique permits severely burned clients (90% of body surface area and more) to receive permanent grafts within a shorter time rather than waiting for weeks or months while their burns and donor sites healed and could be used for more grafting. All-cultured skin is still in the experimental stage, and long-term effectiveness has not yet been determined.

Topical Antimicrobial Agents

Topical antimicrobials do not sterilize the burn wound. They simply reduce the number of bacteria so that the client's host defense mechanisms can control bacterial replication. Controlling wound flora merely "buys time" while vigorous efforts are made to change an open, dirty wound to a closed, clean one. If this cannot be accomplished within a reasonable time (approximately 28 days), the bacterial population will grow out of control, and burn wound sepsis will follow.

Silver sulfadiazine (Silvadene), is a white water-soluble cream made from the reaction of silver nitrate and sulfadiazine. Silver sulfadiazine does not cause pain on application, spreads easily over a burn or dressing with a gloved hand, and is easily removed with water. The ointment is effective against a wide range of gram-negative and gram-positive bacteria, as well as yeast. Silver sulfadiazine may cause a greenish-yellow drainage; this is normal and does not indicate infection.

Mafenide acetate (Sulfamylon) is a topical sulfonamide drug in cream form. With intact subcutaneous blood vessels, peak concentrations occur 2 hours after application, or up to 4 hours in avascular areas. The drug is effective against *Pseudomonas aeruginosa, Staphylococcus aureus,* and *Aerobacter aerogenes.* Mafenide acetate is applied in cream form once or twice daily with a gloved hand. It has the consistency of soft butter and burns and stings for 15 minutes to 1 hour following application because it is hydroscopic and draws water out of the tissues.

Silver nitrate ($AgNO_3$) solution has been used as a burn treatment for many years. When used properly, it controls the wound's bacterial population of the superficial tissues and reduces water evaporation. Biochemical abnormalities are the major problem in the use of silver nitrate. Because of the hypotonicity of the distilled water used to carry the silver nitrate, large amounts of distilled water are absorbed into the body, and large quantities of minerals (sodium, potassium, chloride, magnesium, and calcium) are drawn out of the tissues. If clients are burned on more than 20% of their body surface area, they are likely to have a mineral deficiency unless there is regular electrolyte replacement. Daily monitoring of serum and urinary electrolytes may be necessary.

Povidone–iodine (Betadine), also used to help prevent burn wound sepsis, is effective against gram-negative and gram-positive organisms. Povidone–iodine is available in solution, foam, and ointment. It is easily applied to the burn wound with a sterile gloved hand. Gauze dressings are applied over the agent and are kept moist with povidone–iodine solution every 6 hours or as necessary. Because the agent tends to build up a crust, specific care must be given in hydrotherapy to clean the wound thoroughly.

Subeschar Clysis

With this technique, which is a valuable adjunct to topical therapy, appropriate antibiotics are infused directly into the subeschar space. A physician determines the area to be infused, as well as the antibiotic and the amount and type of carrier fluid to be used.

With a 21-gauge needle inserted into the subeschar space at a 45° angle, 25 mL of fluid are infused into a 7.5 cm^2 area (roughly the size of a softball). A new needle is used for each insertion site. This technique is often used for burns of greater than 40% of body surface area.

SECTION 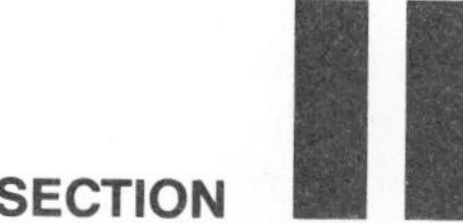

Nursing Process in the Emergent Period

The *emergent period* begins at the time of injury and ends when fluid resuscitation (fluid replacement) is complete, usually within 48 hours. In this phase of care, the focus is on stabilizing the client's physiologic condition and maintaining life.

Assessment: Establishing the Data Base

Depending on the severity of the injury, initial assessment may only consist of a rapid check for a patent airway, respirations, and shock, with a more detailed assessment to be carried out later when the client's condition is stabilized.

Subjective Data

CLIENT'S HISTORY Data about the cause of injury and the time of injury should be recorded. If the client cannot provide this information, ask the family or emergency medical technicians who brought the client to the hospital. Allergies, routine medication, and date of last tetanus immunization should be noted on the medical record.

Take special note of clients who have had chronic illnesses before a burn injury because they have an increased mortality rate. The stress of the burn may exacerbate the disease, making burn management more complex. Examples of such diseases are diabetes mellitus and chronic obstructive pulmonary disease. The stress of injury will cause gluconeogenesis from corticosteroid production. This increased need for glucose will cause irregularities in blood glucose values. Clients with lung disease will be susceptible to pneumonia because they have an ineffective cough reflex for respiratory clearance.

PSYCHOSOCIAL ASSESSMENT The client's immediate adjustment to injury should be assessed. Some clients will be extremely frightened and think they are still burning. Many clients will fear for their lives. Others will be so overwhelmed by the events, they will be irrational. Burned clients will have pain. The pain level and client's coping with pain should be assessed according to the verbal and nonverbal cues and documented.

If possible, learn about the client's pretraumatic coping style from the family members. Clients who normally handle crises by crying, talking, or becoming depressed will continue to use the same methods after their burn. Knowing pretraumatic coping styles allows the nurse to prepare the nursing staff and client's family for these probable behaviors.

One of the most challenging aspects of nursing burn clients is supporting clients' coping as they adjust to their injury and its sequelae. Clients may feel angry at themselves or others for causing or contributing to the accident, guilty for not "being more careful," and victimized if the injury was intentional. They may also be grieving for loss of home, family members who may have died in the fire, appearance changes, or inability to cope with pain. There are also potential losses, such as employment and financial security. All of these feelings are added to feelings of pain and anxiety about the final scarring and altered appearance.

Be aware that these feelings may also arise in family members as they grieve. The client's family must also be assessed for ability to cope with the crisis. While talking with the family, assess for rational and irrational thoughts, stages of grieving, behavior, and general reaction to the client and the injury.

Objective Data

ASSESSMENT OF DEPTH AND SIZE OF BURN Burn depth is assessed according to the guidelines discussed in the section on pathophysiology of burns. Burn size is expressed as a percent of the total body surface area (BSA). There are two methods to calculate burn size. The *rule of nines* divides the adult body into sections: The head is 9% of the total body; the anterior and posterior trunk are each 18%; each leg is 18%; each arm is 9%; and the perineum is 1%, equalling 100%. The rule of nines is a rapid way to estimate burn size in adults (Figure 12–5).

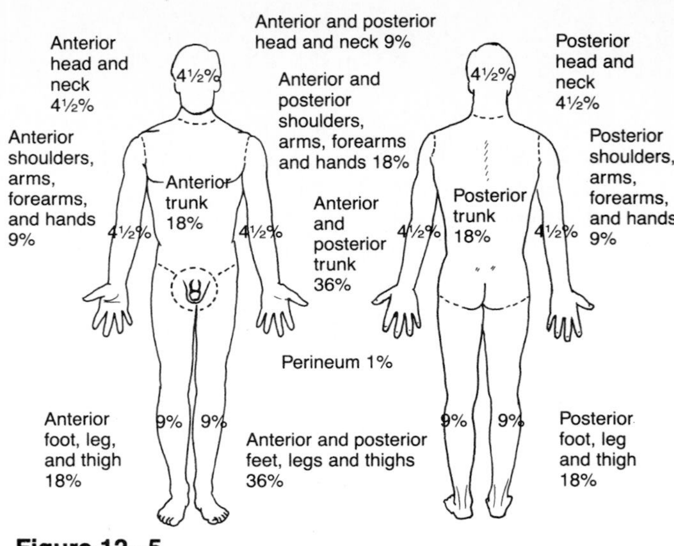

Figure 12–5

Estimating the extent of burns on the body surface area using the rule of nines.

Other methods use charts that allow for changes in body proportion with age. One such method, the *Lund–Browder method,* is illustrated in Figure 12–6. To use the Lund–Browder chart to determine burn size, shade in the area of the burn wound on the diagram for full thickness burns and use slash marks to indicate partial-thickness wounds. The numbers on each body portion indicate the percentage of body surface area for that part. Body areas that change in percentage with growth are marked with letters A, B, C. These areas are calculated by age, using the chart at the bottom of the form. These charts allow a rapid and yet accurate means of determining burn size.

ASSESSMENT OF OXYGENATION Nursing assessments of airway patency and vascular flow to extremities are critical. Edema of the head and neck can become so extensive that the airway swells closed. Blood flow to the foot or hand may be lost because of swelling of a circumferential burn of the arm or leg. Respiratory rate and depth, lung sounds, air hunger, peripheral pulses, and color should be assessed hourly.

Inadequately treated fluid shifts may lead to hypovolemia and shock. Assessments of blood pressure, pulse, skin temperature, urine output, and mental status must be collected frequently—every 15 minutes initially. In the assessment, be alert for:

- Low blood pressure
- Rapid pulse rate
- Absent or weak peripheral pulses
- Elevated hematocrit level
- Cool unburned skin
- Low urine output
- Confusion

These factors indicate hypovolemia caused by fluid shifting into interstitial spaces from the vascular space.

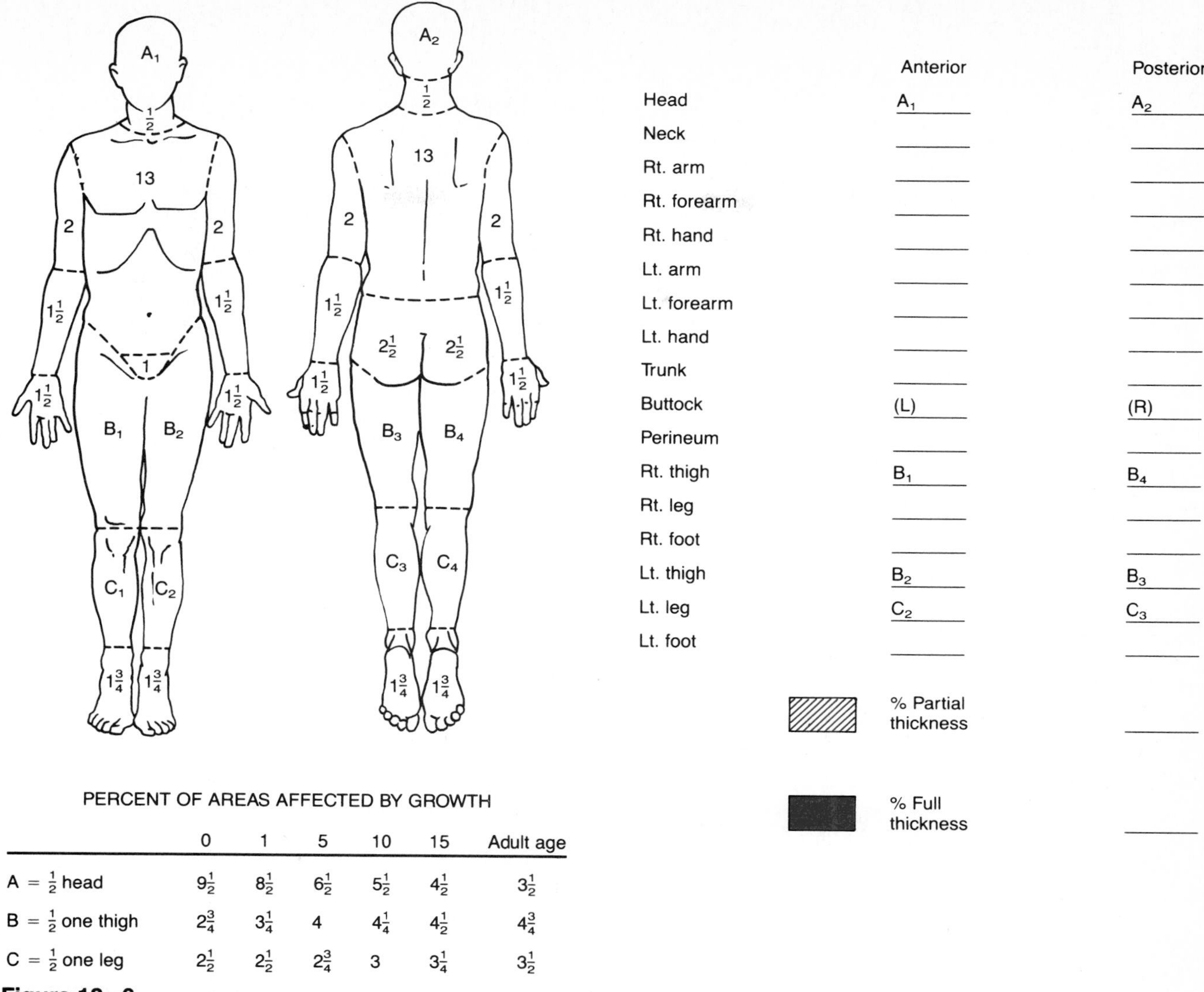

	Anterior	Posterior
Head	A_1	A_2
Neck		
Rt. arm		
Rt. forearm		
Rt. hand		
Lt. arm		
Lt. forearm		
Lt. hand		
Trunk		
Buttock	(L)	(R)
Perineum		
Rt. thigh	B_1	B_4
Rt. leg		
Rt. foot		
Lt. thigh	B_2	B_3
Lt. leg	C_2	C_3
Lt. foot		
% Partial thickness		
% Full thickness		

PERCENT OF AREAS AFFECTED BY GROWTH

	0	1	5	10	15	Adult age
A = $\frac{1}{2}$ head	$9\frac{1}{2}$	$8\frac{1}{2}$	$6\frac{1}{2}$	$5\frac{1}{2}$	$4\frac{1}{2}$	$3\frac{1}{2}$
B = $\frac{1}{2}$ one thigh	$2\frac{3}{4}$	$3\frac{1}{4}$	4	$4\frac{1}{4}$	$4\frac{1}{2}$	$4\frac{3}{4}$
C = $\frac{1}{2}$ one leg	$2\frac{1}{2}$	$2\frac{1}{2}$	$2\frac{3}{4}$	3	$3\frac{1}{4}$	$3\frac{1}{2}$

Figure 12–6

Estimation of size of burn by Lund-Browder chart.

Suspect inhalation injury if the client was burned in an enclosed space or has burns of the face, head, or neck. Also assess for singed nasal hair, hoarseness, voice change, dry cough, soot in sputum, and black coating on the tongue or mouth. See Figure 12–7 for findings in inhalation injury. Acidosis or alkalosis may also be present with hypoventilation or hyperventilation, respectively.

ASSESSMENT OF NUTRITION AND ELIMINATION Bowel sounds should be assessed and recorded. Clients may complain of thirst caused by hypovolemia. Also assess for hemoglobinuria characterized by dark reddish-brown urine. The client's height and weight should be recorded. Monitor nasogastric tube drainage for color and the presence of blood.

Basic hematologic studies, complete blood count, serum electrolytes, and BUN level serve as a baseline for determining hydration status. Hyperkalemia should be noted and reported to the physician.

ASSESSMENT OF OTHER INJURIES OR HEALTH PROBLEMS The health team must suspect internal organ damage, fractures, or head injuries in clients who were victims of explosions or who fell or jumped from a burning building. Existing illness will often be exacerbated by the stress of the burn. For example, diabetics will often have uncontrollable blood glucose levels caused by gluconeogenesis from stress.

Nursing Diagnoses/Planning and Implementation/Evaluation

Nursing diagnoses in the emergent period reflect the priorities of caring for a person with critical and possibly life-threatening injuries. Nursing diagnoses directly related to care of the burn client in all three periods are listed in Table 12–2. The diagnoses for the three phases of care have been prioritized for each phase. Some nursing diag-

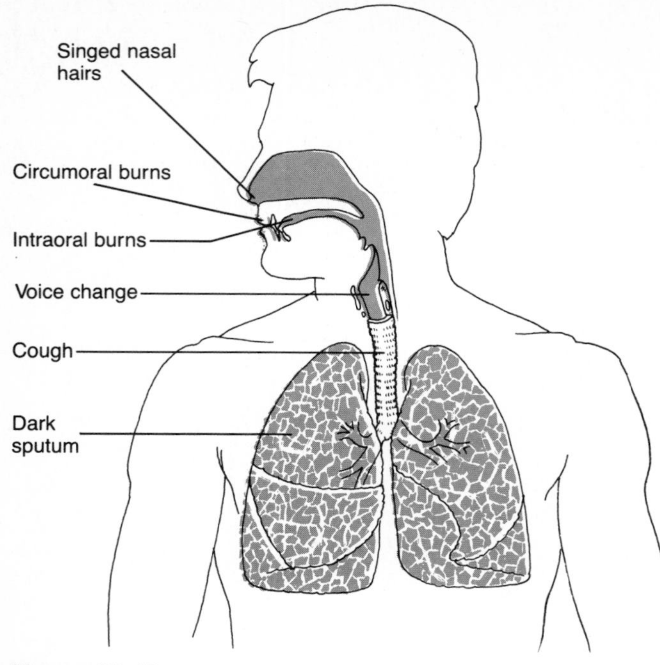

Figure 12–7

Assessment of a client with inhalation injury.

noses are higher priorities in one phase of burn care than in another. A sample nursing care plan for the burn client in the emergent period is in Table 12–3.

Airway Clearance and Gas Exchange

Burns produce a variety of problems that impair oxygenation, as previously described. The combined effects of fluid shift and hypovolemia also produce pulmonary dysfunction. The problem of decreased oxygenation is exacerbated by reactions to pain and fear.

Two immediate goals of treatment are maintenance of the airway and normal blood oxygen levels. Arterial blood gas values are assessed frequently to evaluate oxygenation. The head of the bed is elevated if blood pressure permits. Oxygen can be provided through the appropriate mode. If the airway or normal oxygenation cannot be maintained, tracheotomy or intubation may be performed. Clients may require mechanical ventilation. In this case, nursing responsibilities are the same as for any ventilator-dependent client (see Chapter 14).

Impaired gas exchange will be improved by treating hypovolemia and fluid loss. Nursing interventions for these problems are discussed in the appropriate sections.

Fluid Volume

Untreated, hypovolemia will cause death; therefore, rapid replacement of fluid losses is critical for the burned client. A large-bore intravenous line should be inserted. Major burn clients often have central venous lines. The needle should be placed through unburned skin and proximal to any burns on the extremities.

Ringer's lactate solution is the fluid of choice for resuscitation because it is physiologically similar to blood serum. If Ringer's lactate is not available, use of any other intravenous fluid is preferable to no fluid administration at all. Solutions with glucose should be administered carefully

Table 12–2
Nursing Diagnoses in Burn Care by Priority

Emergent Period	Acute Period	Rehabilitative Period
Airway clearance, ineffective	*Gas exchange, impaired*	*Self-concept, disturbance in,* related to body image
Gas exchange, impaired	*Fluid volume overload, actual or potential*	*Nutrition, altered, potential for more than body requirements*
Fluid volume deficit, actual or potential	*Infection, actual or potential*	*Comfort, altered,* related to pain and pruritus
Skin integrity, impaired, actual and potential	*Comfort, altered,* related to pain	*Coping skills, ineffective individual and/or family*
Tissue perfusion, altered	*Skin integrity, impaired, actual or potential*	*Knowledge deficit,* related to self-care
Comfort, altered, related to pain	*Nutrition, altered, less than body requirements*	*Mobility, impaired physical*
Urinary elimination, altered pattern	*Mobility, impaired physical*	*Skin integrity, impaired, actual or potential*
Coping, ineffective individual and/or family	*Coping, ineffective, individual and/or family*	
Bowel elimination, altered, related to ileus	*Self-care deficit,* related to feeding, bathing/hygiene, dressing/grooming, toileting	
Infection, potential for	*Self-concept, disturbance in,* related to body image	
Mobility, impaired physical	*Knowledge deficit,* related to surgery	

because osmotic diuresis can occur. (Osmotic diuresis is the loss of body water through the urine as the glucose is excreted.) Colloids may be administered after cell membranes have stabilized. Giving colloids too early after the burn can increase edema because the protein leaks through the altered membranes, drawing body water with it.

The volume of fluid replacement is calculated using a formula (Box 12–2). Fluid resuscitation formulas are only guidelines to fluid therapy; the best indicator of fluid balance is the client. Measure vital signs every 15 to 30 minutes and urine output every hour. Signs of continuing hypovolemia should also be noted. When urine output begins to increase, intravenous fluids can be reduced. Physicians may order fluids titrated to maintain a urine output of 30 mL/h. Administer fluids to achieve this urine output, calculating and adjusting the fluid rate every 30 minutes. The client should be weighed daily to determine fluid status. Body weight is more accurate for determining fluid status than intake and output.

Hyperkalemia can be treated with potassium-binding enemas and/or with intravenous glucose and insulin solutions. Glucose and insulin solutions allow potassium to reenter the cells, temporarily reducing the serum levels of the electrolytes.

Skin Integrity

Immediate goals for skin integrity for the burned client are preventing infection and promoting wound healing with minimal scarring. Physiologically stable clients may have their wounds cared for in the emergency room. For unstable clients, wound care is deferred until they are stabilized. Recall that hypothermia can result from loss of skin. Warm the client's room to 94°F + 4 (34°C + 2) and use heat shields, lamps, or blankets to maintain normothermia. Monitor body temperature rectally every 2 hours.

If dressings are used during these initial 48 hours, follow the guidelines in the section on skin integrity during the acute period.

Tissue Perfusion

Tissue perfusion is improved by resuscitative measures to treat fluid loss and hypovolemia. Effects of poor tissue perfusion on the major organ systems are monitored.

Deficits in cardiac output are corrected by providing for oxygenation and fluid replacement, as discussed under airway clearance, ineffective breathing patterns, and fluid volume deficit. The client should have an ECG monitor; electrodes can be placed on burned skin if necessary.

Comfort

Burns cause intense pain. Immediately after the burn, the degree of pain depends on the extent of the burn. First- and second-degree burns are painful because of damage to nerve endings. The third-degree burn victim may not feel pain because cutaneous nerve endings have been destroyed. The client's response to pain varies with the pain threshold and perhaps cultural values.

Clients with severe burns (more than 25% of body surface area) should receive intravenous narcotics. Intravenous administration is used because circulation to the extremities is diminished and therefore, medication given intramuscularly would not be absorbed, pain relief would not be achieved, and the client would require more medication. Then when circulation was restored, all medication pooled in the extremities because of intramuscular administration would flood the body, causing an overdose.

At this early stage, clients are usually unable to participate actively in their own pain control. Alternative pain relief measures are best left for the acute and rehabilitative periods.

Box 12–2
Baxter's Formula for Calculating Fluid Requirements

4 mL × % BSA burned × kilograms = fluid to be administered in the first 24 hours post-burn

Administer one-half of total fluids in 8 hours and one-half in next 16 hours. (Calculate the first 8 hours from the time of injury.) For example, in the first 24 hours, fluid requirements for a 70 kg man with a 50% burn would be calculated as follows:

4 × 50 × 70 = 14,000 mL fluid in 24 hours
(7000 mL in first 8 hours; 7000 mL in next 16 hours)

Urinary Elimination

Measures to improve fluid balance will improve urinary elimination (see previous discussion of fluid volume).

An in-dwelling catheter should be inserted in all clients with major burns and in those with burns of the perineum. Urine should be sent for urinalysis, noting the amount and color. If hemoglobinuria is noted, serial urine samples should be collected until the urine is clear. A sample of 15 to 30 mL should be collected each hour and labeled clearly; the samples are lined up in sequence to monitor the change in color. Notify the physician if hemoglobinuria is noted because unpassed hemoglobin may lodge in the kidney, potentially causing renal damage. Diuretics may be required to open the nephron cell walls, allowing the large hemoglobin molecules to pass through.

Coping

Effective coping can be supported by a variety of interventions. A calm, confident attitude in caring for the client will earn the client's trust. When the client screams or pulls away from a painful procedure, assess the need for safe use of additional analgesia. If no more of the analgesic can be safely administered, the client may need to

Table 12–3
Sample Nursing Care Plan for the Emergent Period, by Nursing Diagnosis

Client Care Goals	Plan/Implementation	Expected Outcome
Airway clearance, ineffective		
Patent airway; adequate oxygen–carbon dioxide exchange	Maintain patent airway through proper positioning, removal of secretions; establish airway if needed	Patent airway and adequate respiration maintained
Gas exchange, impaired		
Adequate oxygen–carbon dioxide exchange	Provide oxygen as appropriate; assess breath sounds and respiration; monitor client on ventilator; observe for signs of respiratory distress or carbon dioxide	No signs of respiratory distress or inadequate oxygenation
Fluid volume deficit		
Restoration of fluid balance	Observe vital signs, urine output, CVP, and sensorium for signs of hypovolemia or fluid overload; maintain IV lines and regulate fluids; observe electrolyte levels and report abnormal values to physician; document input and output (I and O); weigh client daily	No signs of hypovolemia or fluid imbalance
Skin integrity, impaired		
Progress in wound healing; freedom from infection	(See nursing activities for preventing infection)	Progress in wound healing; no signs of infection
Tissue perfusion, altered		
Correction of hypovolemia with increase in cardiac output	Observe vital signs, urine output, CVP, and sensorium for signs of hypovolemia; maintain IV lines and regulate fluids; assess for dysrhythmias	No signs of hypovolemia; cardiac output adequate
Adequate tissue perfusion	Assess peripheral pulses hourly on extremities with circumferential burns; report signs of decreased peripheral circulation or nerve or muscle ischemia to physician; elevate extremities and head of bed (see also nursing activities for fluid volume deficit, cardiac output, and urinary elimination)	No signs of inadequate tissue perfusion
Comfort, altered, related to pain		
Control of pain	Assess pain; differentiate from hypoxia; administer IV narcotics; introduce relaxation techniques, nitrous oxide, and other adjuncts to pain relief; provide emotional support	Adequate control of pain
Urinary elimination, altered pattern		
Adequate urinary elimination	Monitor electrolyte levels; document I and O; weigh client daily; observe urine output for hemoglobinuria (see also nursing activities for fluid volume deficit)	
Coping, ineffective		
Adequate coping skills	Maintain calm, confident manner; provide adequate pain control for painful procedures; prepare family for first visit; provide honest information as client and family seem ready	Demonstration of realistic coping skills

Client Care Goals	Plan/Implementation	Expected Outcome
Bowel elimination, altered		
Adequate bowel function	Maintain NG tube on low intermittent suction until bowel sounds return; auscultate for bowel sounds q. 4 h	Adequate bowel function returns
Infection, potential		
Freedom from infection	Use aseptic technique in client care; support immune response by prevention of shock; maintain isolation; clean client's perineum; administer antimicrobial drugs as ordered; administer tetanus prophylaxis	No signs of sepsis or wound infection
Mobility, impaired physical		
Maintenance of adequate mobility	Prevent client susceptible to neck contracture from sleeping on pillow; assist in ROM exercises; encourage exercise for client with burned hand	Client performs exercises regularly; client describes reason for exercise; ROM is adequate

be restrained to allow a necessary procedure to be completed. Keep in mind the intended outcome and need for the procedure, trying not to be distracted by the client's reaction because this will extend the time needed to complete the task.

Prepare the family for the initial visit with the client. Seeing the client swollen, in pain, covered with dressings, and surrounded by machines may be distressing for them. Before the visit, describe how the client will look, what is temporary (such as swelling), and the reason for unusual behavior, such as confusion or combativeness, especially if the client has been placed in restraints. Often the family will be more concerned initially about the client's future appearance than will the client. A discussion about scarring is best left to the physician because healing is unpredictable.

The health team should be honest with the client and family about expected outcomes. News about unfavorable outcomes should be given gradually, allowing the client and family time for effective coping. Be aware that information may need repeating because stress, fear, pain, and anxiety block clear understanding of information.

Bowel Function

If a nasogastric tube has been placed for ileus, the tube should be attached to suction and the bowel sounds should be auscultated every 4 hours.

Infection

Once transferred to the burn unit, the client will require reverse isolation precautions to reduce the risk of wound infection. In some burn units, each client has a private room; in others, the entire burn unit is isolated from the rest of the hospital.

Aseptic technique must be used for all client care. The client's own intestinal flora is the primary source of infections. For this reason, the nurse must clean the perineal area well, especially after bowel movements. Sterile linens are used if the hospital policy so specifies. The second major source of infection is the environment. The nurse is also responsible for monitoring compliance with isolation precautions by all members of the health care team.

Prophylactic antibiotics are seldom given to burn clients; they cannot penetrate the avascular eschar. The only exception is the administration of penicillin for the first 72 hours to reduce the risk of streptococcal infections. Tetanus prophylaxis is provided or renewed for burn clients. As the eschar separates from the body, an anaerobic environment is left, providing an environment for tetanus organisms to grow. If the client was rolled on the ground to extinguish the flames, risk of tetanus is higher.

Mobility

Some body areas require special attention. With neck burns, the client is susceptible to contractures. Clients with neck burns should not use pillows under the head; this avoids neck flexion. ROM exercises should be performed routinely. Burned hands may also develop contractures with loss of function. Hourly exercises of hands and fingers and elevation to reduce edema are critical. Exercising hands is painful, so clients may be reluctant to do exercises. Encourage the client because hand function is important for long-term recovery. Static splints may be used to maintain a client's hands in a functional position during rest times. They are also helpful when hands are too edematous to exercise. Mobility assumes a higher priority during the acute period.

SECTION 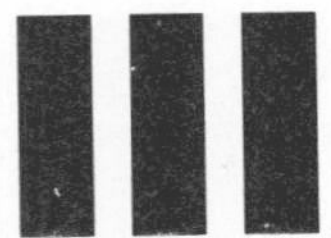

Nursing Process in the Acute Period

The client enters the *acute period* when fluid resuscitation is complete. In this phase of care, the focus is on wound care and promotion of healing. This period, which may last from a few days to many months, ends when less than 20% of the body surface is yet to be healed. As the client's physiologic condition stabilizes, the client faces new physical and emotional challenges.

During this period, the client begins psychologic adjustment by first confronting the extent of the injury and then beginning to come to terms with the possibility of disfigurement. The client may also need to cope with a long series of painful treatments, including debridement and perhaps surgery.

Assessment: Establishing the Data Base

Vigilant monitoring continues for oxygenation and fluid and electrolyte balance. Because of the multisystem impact of burns, complications are a continuing threat. The nurse's assessment is the first line of defense against such potential complications as sepsis, wound infection, stress ulcer, and deteriorating nutritional status.

Subjective Data

Pain continues to be a serious problem in the acute period. Physical pain will be increased by anxiety, creating a pain-anxiety cycle that must be broken by controlling pain. Since pain is subjective, the nurse should not judge whether clients are in pain. Rather, assess the client's reaction to pain and other concurrent factors increasing pain or decreasing pain threshold. Pain may seem exaggerated because of loneliness, and the complaint may signal the need for attention. Anxiety over anticipated procedures that may or may not be painful increases pain. Muscle tension from fear lowers the pain threshold. Sleep deprivation also lowers the client's ability to cope with pain.

Assess clients' behavior to determine not only the coping behavior—withdrawal, denial, anger, dependence, compliance, "a stiff upper lip," or any other of a wide variety of possible responses—but also the psychosocial needs it serves. For example, after seeing the disfigured body, a client may express a desire to abandon it through dying. On the other hand, denial of the injury and its seriousness may be assessed from statements such as, "I'll be home by next weekend," when the nurse is aware the client will be in the hospital many weeks.

Anger following a disfiguring burn can be directed inward or outward. Inwardly directed anger is often manifested as withdrawal; left untreated, it can lead to depression. Outwardly directed anger may be expressed through sarcasm, rudeness, or uncooperativeness. Clients may be angry at themselves or others for causing the accident, killing or maiming other friends or family, or not preventing the accident. Because it is essential that clients and family come to terms with the accident, be observant for cues suggesting a need to work out such feelings.

Burn clients may view their disfigurement as a roadblock to a loving relationship with another person. Clients may feel their scarred appearance makes them untouchable and unlovable. Clients watch others for nonverbal messages about their feelings and are quick to recognize incongruent verbal statements and nonverbal signs.

During the extensive hospital stay, clients are unable to predict future activities and plans realistically. Clients are intensely aware that someone else has had to carry out their roles at home or work. This loss of fulfillment creates anxieties about their capacity to return to previous employment, or whether they are even needed. Continuing psychosocial assessments are crucial to determining an effective plan of care during this period.

Objective Data

Because of the changing condition of all burn clients in the acute stage, thorough head-to-toe physical assessments must be completed on every shift.

ASSESSMENT OF OXYGENATION Oxygenation status is assessed by observing skin color and capillary refill. Lung sounds should be auscultated, listening closely for rales. The ability to cough as well as sputum consistency and color should be noted. Vital signs should be measured at least every 4 hours if the client is stable. Early changes in oxygenation status may be assessed by a change in sensorium because the nervous system is extremely sensitive to small decreases in oxygen levels. Oxygenation assessment assists in early diagnosis of cardiovascular and pulmonary complications from both the burn and immobility.

ASSESSMENT OF NUTRITION AND ELIMINATION Clients should be assessed for nutritional status and signs of weight loss. Calorie counts should be included with daily weight readings. Weight loss may be from poor intake or other problems such as infection. Daily weights should be graphed for ease in evaluation of weight changes. Laboratory values for electrolytes, blood counts, and serum protein should be assessed.

ASSESSMENT OF FLUID BALANCE The client should be assessed for signs of fluid overload during the first few days following fluid resuscitation. Include auscultation of lung and heart sounds, palpation for dependent edema, measuring intake and output, and determining whether weight gain, dyspnea, or orthopnea occur. Symptoms of congestive heart failure may develop if the client cannot excrete the fluid, or if the client receives too much fluid.

ASSESSMENT OF SENSORY–MOTOR FUNCTION Clients can quickly develop flexion contractures of healing burns over both burned and nonburned joints. Flexion and extension of all joints should be assessed, recording the actual degrees of motion. Recording ROM allows for close evaluation of progress or lack of progress. Muscle atrophy can also occur with long-term bed rest and limited activity.

ASSESSMENT OF BURN AREA Integrity of burned and unburned skin must be evaluated daily. Skin over bony prominences may break down from pressure and limited movement. Burned skin must be inspected daily by the same person to evaluate the progress of healing and to recognize infection early. The best time to assess the burn wound is when clients are in the hydrotherapy tub because dressings and ointments are off. Symptoms of burn wound infections are subtle: a change in color of the wound, increased pain, conversion of a partial-thickness wound to full thickness, fever, and signs of sepsis.

Because burn wounds are often infected below the surface of the wound, quantitative cultures and biopsies are a more accurate method for diagnosis of infection than cultures of the wound surface. Quantitative culture differs from other cultures in that the tissue is evaluated for the presence of invasive infection by determining the number of bacteria per gram of tissue. A small clipping or section of burned tissue is excised from the wound. The laboratory liquefies the tissue and cultures it, determining the number and type of each bacteria present. Wound biopsy can show actual organisms invading healthy tissue, indicating invasive infection.

ASSESSMENT OF COMPLICATIONS In burned clients, complications can involve any body system. Complete assessment of all body systems is critical. Sepsis is the leading cause of death in the acute period of burn care. Early signs of sepsis include: fever over 101°F (38°C) or below 98°F (37°C), tachycardia, tachypnea, insidious hypotension, insidious oliguria, confusion, and chills. Blood cultures verify sepsis.

The risk of stress ulcers increases with the size of the burn; ulceration begins immediately following the injury. Drugs that prevent acid secretion (cimetidine) and prompt use of antacids have reduced the incidence of stress ulcer. In assessing clients for this potential complication, look for: occult blood in stool, blood flecks in nasogastric drainage, gastric distension, pallor, and lowered hemoglobin values. Later symptoms include hematemesis, black tarry stools, nausea, vomiting, and abdominal pain.

Nursing Diagnoses/Planning and Implementation/Evaluation

Nursing diagnoses in the acute period shift toward the healing process and the prevention of complications. (Refer to Table 12–2.) A sample nursing care plan for the burn client in the acute period is in Table 12–4.

Gas Exchange

In the acute period, the client's respiration will have been stabilized, although continued respiratory support may be necessary. During this period, promoting adequate gas exchange is largely a matter of monitoring. Also important is continuing assessment for pulmonary complications. The immobile client should be turned every 2 hours and deep breathing and extremity exercises encouraged.

Fluid Volume

Approximately 48 to 72 hours after burn injury, the tissue membranes regain their integrity and fluid is no longer lost into the tissues. When diuresis is noted, intravenous fluid volumes should be lowered to avoid fluid overload. The potential for fluid overload still exists as fluid returns to the bloodstream. Assessing for fluid volume excess is important. Clients with circulatory overload receive similar nursing care as clients in congestive heart failure.

Infection

The prevention of burn wound infection includes proper handwashing prior to all client contact; use of topical antimicrobials; prevention of cross-contamination; removing possible reservoirs of infections; and wearing gowns, gloves, masks, and caps when in direct contact with the wound. Because the most frequent source of wound contamination is the client's own body flora, elimination of infection reservoirs, such as body hair and fecal material, is essential. The early detection of burn wound infection is critical and best accomplished by having the same person evaluate the wound each day.

Sepsis is treated by antibiotics, eliminating the source of infection, and by fluid replacement, steroids, and vasoactive drugs. Clients with sepsis quickly go into shock and are often cared for in intensive care units.

Comfort

After the client's pain is assessed, narcotic analgesics are used to control pain. Many clients will say, "Put me out and get this over with," because the pain seems unbearable. Be honest in explaining the physiologic hazards of excessive narcotics. Antianxiety drugs are not indicated until there is adequate control of pain. Pain should be treated without a fear that the client will become addicted

Table 12–4
Sample Nursing Care Plan for the Acute Period, by Nursing Diagnosis

Client Care Goals	Plan/Implementation	Expected Outcome
Gas exchange, impaired		
Adequate oxygen–carbon dioxide exchange	Monitor respiratory function; be alert for signs of pulmonary complications	No signs of respiratory distress or inadequate oxygenation
Fluid volume overload, potential for		
No signs of fluid overload	Monitor lung and heart sounds; palpate for edema; monitor intake and output and daily weight	Diuresis with stable body weight, clear lung sounds, eupnea
Infection, actual or potential		
Freedom from infection	Wash hands before client contact; cleanse client wound and body daily; apply topical antimicrobials as ordered; prevent cross-contamination; remove possible reservoirs of infection; provide donor site care; monitor graft take	No signs of wound infection or sepsis
Comfort, altered, related to pain		
Control of pain	Assess pain; offer analgesics plus relaxation breathing, transcutaneous electrical nerve stimulation, self-administered nitrous oxide; assess and document response; assist with appropriate means of expressing pain	Adequate control of pain
Skin integrity, impaired		
Progress in wound healing; no further impairment in skin integrity	Maintain appropriate wound care, depending on severity of burn; maintain adequate room temperature and humidity; change dressings as indicated; prevent and/or control infection; take measures to minimize contractures, hypertrophic scarring, and keloids	Client shows progress in wound healing; is free of infection; wound-healing problems are prevented to extent possible
Nutrition, altered		
Adequate caloric intake and tolerance of diet	Consult with dietitian to plan adequate intake; monitor intake and report if inadequate; monitor hyperalimentation, if given; monitor client for input and output (I and O), bowel elimination, abdominal distension	Client eats prescribed number of calories; demonstrates tolerance of diet
Mobility, impaired physical		
Improved ROM and ambulation	Assist with ROM daily; document ROM; position client in open position; assist with ambulation as tolerated	Progress in ROM and ambulation; client cooperates in ROM exercises and ambulation
Coping, ineffective		
Adequate coping skills	Assess client's readiness to express feelings about alteration in body image or lifestyle; provide opportunity to express feelings; maintain positive but honest approach; use other resources, such as counselors, to support coping; employ preventive psychosocial care	Client verbalizes realistic outlook on injury, treatment, and progress

Client Care Goals	Plan/Implementation	Expected Outcome
Self-care deficit		
Increased participation in personal care as able	Provide opportunities to participate in self-care; encourage participation; provide opportunity for client to express feelings of anger and frustration; support appropriate coping skills	Client shows willingness to participate in self-care; expresses feelings; shows improvement in coping skills
Self-concept, disturbance in		
Realistic reaction to changes in body	Assess client's readiness to view burns and express feelings about altered body image; provide opportunity to discuss feelings; tolerate anger and regression that may aid in strengthening coping skills; reinforce feelings of self-worth; encourage family to express positive feelings toward client; refer for psychologic help if appropriate	Client expresses readiness to view burns; discusses feelings about body image; family demonstrates positive attitude toward client; referral made if appropriate
Knowledge deficit, related to surgery		
Accurately describe purpose of treatments, including surgery	Teach client and family about treatment procedures, even if client has had previous procedures	Client accurately describes treatment procedure; asks appropriate questions

to the drug. Research indicates addiction does not occur when drugs are taken to control pain but when drugs are used to produce euphoria. In contrast, antianxiety drugs can produce dependence, and withdrawal from these agents is difficult. In addition to narcotics, other pain control methods such as transcutaneous electrical nerve stimulation (TENS) and relaxation methods have been used in burn care. Self-administered nitrous oxide has also been effective in controlling pain and anxiety. The client holds the mask to the face until relaxation occurs and pain diminishes. If the client falls asleep, the mask is dropped, so overmedication usually is not a concern.

Skin Integrity

Promoting adequate wound healing is a major goal during this phase of recovery. The client's room temperature should be kept at 94°F + 4 (34°C + 2) to prevent heat loss. If the client complains of chilling or body temperature drops, additional heat lamps should be used. The humidity of the room should be between 40% and 50%. If the room is drier, the eschar will crack open and bleed. If the room is too moist, the eschar will soften and separate prematurely. Portable humidifiers or dehumidifiers are effective in maintaining humidity.

Many methods of burn wound care are in use. The method used depends on the size, location, depth, and facilities available for treating the wound. Two or more methods may be used simultaneously, and methods for the same client may change during the course of healing.

OPEN METHOD The open method of burn wound care is the application of antimicrobial ointments without dressings. This technique is used on the face, neck, upper chest, hands, and perineum because these body areas are difficult to dress. Ointments are applied with a sterile gloved hand. The heat of the room and client's skin melts the ointment, so it must be reapplied frequently. The advantages of the open method are that no dressings are required, and antimicrobials hasten eschar separation and reduce infection. The disadvantage of the open method is that frequent reapplication of ointment is necessary.

Burn wounds covered with ointment but not dressed should be kept clean and moist. Normal saline on sterile gauze can be used to clean the wound. Crusts on the wound should also be removed. Crusts harbor bacteria, creating potential for infection and scarring.

SEMICLOSED METHOD In the semiclosed method, topical antimicrobials are applied with dressings and changed once or twice daily. This technique can be used on almost any body part (see discussion of dressing changes for technique). Advantages of the semiclosed method are:

- Wounds are inspected at least daily.
- Infection is reduced by antimicrobials.
- Eschar separation is enhanced through debridement when dressings are removed.
- Body heat loss is reduced.
- Pain is manageable except for dressing changes.

- Body parts are protected because they are not exposed.
- Clients do not continually look at their wounds.

Disadvantages are:

- Dressing changes are required.
- Painful debridement is necessary.
- Dressings can be applied incorrectly, either too tight so they restrict circulation or too loose so they fall off.

CLOSED METHOD The closed method is the occlusive wrapping of a burn with antimicrobials and dressings that are not changed for up to 72 hours. This technique can be used on any body part according to the physician's preference. Precautions must also be taken to wrap the body part in functional body alignment and not to wrap two burned body areas together. Outer dressings should be wrapped distal to proximal. Peripheral circulation and neurologic status are assessed every 4 hours. Advantages of this method are:

- Fewer painful dressing changes.
- Body heat loss is minimized.
- Burned body parts are protected because they are not exposed.

Disadvantages are:

- Wounds cannot be inspected.
- Dressings can be applied incorrectly, either too loose, too tight, or pinning burned parts together.

DRESSING CHANGES Dressings should be removed after the administration of an analgesic. The nurse should don a mask, gown, and gloves before beginning the dressing change. Dressings should be removed while dry to speed debridement because the dried dressing adheres to the wound. Outer dressings should be cut and the dressing spread open and removed. Dressings should be discarded in dressing bags.

After dressings are removed, the wounds should be cleansed either in a hydrotherapy tank or bathtub, or from a basin of sterile water. Once the wound is free of ointment, loose eschar can be clipped off using sterile forceps and scissors. Eschar can be removed to the point of bleeding. If bleeding starts, direct pressure on the area will usually control it. Occasionally, topical hemostatic agents, such as thrombin, or ligation may be required to control large amounts of bleeding.

The wound should be redressed as rapidly as possible following wound care to prevent hypothermia. Dressings should be prepared before or during hydrotherapy. The exact number of dressings for wound care should be a part of each burned client's plan of care. Clients should not be left undressed and alone while nurses are searching for more dressings.

To minimize pain and save time, apply the ointment to the dressing rather than the client. Dressings can be "buttered" with the ointment like a piece of toast and stacked with ointment sides together on a sterile field while waiting for the client. Avoiding touching the wound directly reduces pain and the potential for contamination. Dressings with ointment should be placed on the wound and held in place by outer wrappings of gauze or netting. Remember that on extremities, outer wrappings of gauze must be applied distal to proximal to aid circulation.

To apply silver nitrate dressing, fill a plastic wash basin with warmed 0.5% silver nitrate solution. (Silver nitrate turns everything it touches black. Use caution not to touch the solution to linens or uniforms because the stain is permanent.) Soak precut and rolled dressings in the solution and then apply to all burned areas. The dressings are held in place with a bias-cut stockinette and secured with safety pins; clients are covered with dry sheets and at least one dry cotton blanket. Dry covers are important and must be changed when they become wet. The dressings must be kept soaking wet. If dressings are kept wet, reepithelialization will take place between the fifteenth and fortieth days postburn.

Some areas of the body require special precautions. Ear tissue is primarily cartilage, which has poor circulation. Ear burns heal slowly and become infected easily. Dressings should pad the entire ear well, including the back of the ear, so the ear is not pressed onto the skull. Hands may be dressed in a variety of ways—each finger wrapped separately, the hand placed in a bag with ointment, or the hand placed in a medicated glove. Perineal burns are especially susceptible to infection. Perineal burn wound dressings must be checked after each voiding and bowel movement and changed as needed.

During the first 7 to 14 days, the dressings need to be changed only once daily. After the eschar begins to liquefy and separate, three or four daily dressings may be necessary. As soon as treated parts are exposed to sunlight, the eschar darkens and turns brown, black, or blue, depending on the depth of the burn and the amount of sunlight. Hard blue–black eschar on wounds indicates a probable subdermal burn. Eschars of intradermal burns are brown and begin to separate after 7 to 10 days.

If infection is controlled, eschar will remain in place for weeks until finally separating from the granulating adipose tissue. If the adipose tissue is burned, eschar will begin to separate a few days after the injury. If this occurs, it must be removed promptly because liquefied eschar is an excellent medium for bacterial growth.

BURNED HANDS With some first-degree burns or superficial second-degree burns, hand bags are used to reduce the pain, allow early mobility, and make it possible for clients to use their hands for daily care. A variety of such hand bags have been used including rubber surgical gloves, specially designed bags of semipermeable transparent plastic such as OpSite, and bags filled with liquid silicone. Hand bags are commonly used with topical medications, which are applied to the wound prior to covering the hands with the bags. These bags are easier to change than conventional dressings and are generally well accepted by clients.

Hand bags require several precautions. It is critical that the hand bag be loose enough not to constrict any part of the hand, particularly as the hand becomes edematous. Surgical gloves are often too tight. Precautions must be taken so normal skin does not become macerated from the increased humidity. Bacteria flourish in the moist environment. On the other hand, the bag may adhere to the burn wound if it becomes too dry. Therefore, clients with hand bags require frequent assessment.

Proper positioning of the hand is essential to reduce edema and deformities. The hand should be elevated above the level of the heart, preferably on two pillows. This allows more freedom of movement, and cooperative clients appreciate not being tethered to an IV pole.

PROBLEMS IN BURN WOUND HEALING Wound contractures can be reduced in severity through excellent nursing care and client compliance. Contractures can be surgically treated by a technique known as Z-plasty, which involves rearranging and lengthening the scar tissue. Another surgical treatment is to remove the scar tissue and apply a skin graft in its place to open up the contracture. The best treatment, however, is prevention through nursing care. Applying pressure over healing wounds has been successful in reducing keloid formation.

Keloids have recently been prevented by the use of lathrogen, a drug that interferes with collagen synthesis. (Scar tissue is chiefly collagen fibers.) The drug is still investigational. Steroids have also been injected into keloids but with minimal results in shrinking them. Excision of keloids usually is not successful because clients tend to be "keloid formers" and heal with keloids again. Because the etiology of keloids is unknown, the treatment varies from one physician to another. Constant pressure placed on the wound throughout scar maturation seems to retard growth of scars. Custom-made elastic garments can be measured to fit exactly any burned body part (Figure 12–8). In most hospitals, measurements for these garments are taken by physical therapists.

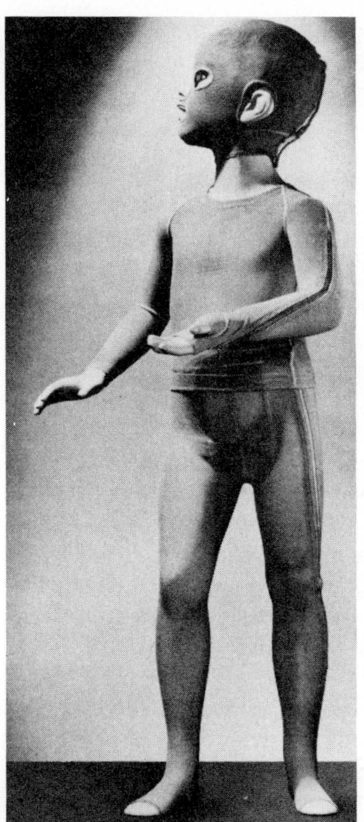

Figure 12–8

Custom-made elastic supports for prevention and correction of postburn hypertrophic scarring.

Nutritional Support

Hypermetabolism following the burn quickly removes body stores of energy. Clients must be given adequate carbohydrates, fats, protein, vitamins, minerals, and fluids to support metabolism, heal the wound, and prevent catabolism and a negative nitrogen balance. Caloric needs are determined for the adult client by the following equation:

25 kcal × kg body weight + 40 kcal × % burn = number of calories

This caloric total may be over 5000 calories a day for major burn clients, and eating that amount of food becomes difficult. In most hospitals, dietitians work with nurses and clients to ensure adequate intake. It is critical that nurses record all that is eaten, so caloric intake can be calculated.

There are many methods to achieve the intake desired. Powdered milk or instant breakfast powder can be added to whole milk, and corn syrup can be added to orange juice; protein supplements can be given in six feedings a day. If oral intake cannot support metabolic needs, and the client loses weight, hyperalimentation or gastrostomy or nasogastric tube feedings may be used. Clients with hyperalimentation lines must be assessed closely for sepsis because the contaminated water from wound care may seep under the dressing at the needle insertion site. Concentrated tube feedings may cause osmotic diuresis and/or diarrhea. Clients should be assessed for their tolerance to their diet. Accurate intake and output, bowel movements, and abdominal distention will be clues to nutrition–elimination tolerance.

As burn wounds heal, clients' caloric needs are reduced. The client should return to a normal diet if all wounds are healed and normal weight has been achieved. The client's eating should be tapered off to allow physical and psychologic adjustments. When burns are grafted, however, the donor sites become a new wound, and caloric requirements may need adjustment.

Mobility

Promoting activity tolerance is an important goal in the acute period. Joints with healing burns as well as other joints should have a ROM performed daily. The degrees of motion should be recorded to document progress or lack of progress. If contractures are forming in healing burns, frequency of ROM should be increased. Splints can be used to support joints in their functional anatomic position while in bed. Clients should be positioned in an open position to decrease flexion in joints.

Assist the client to ambulate as tolerated. After skin grafting to legs, clients will have to increase ambulation slowly.

For a burned hand, physical therapy to maintain ROM should be initiated the first day and continued frequently throughout the healing process, which may take more than a year. ROM exercises for all hand joints will often be performed while the client is in a whirlpool twice daily. Hourly ROM exercises are also essential, however. Exercises can be done actively or passively. Increased motion can be achieved when dressings are changed. If the client has progressed to the point where hand bags can be used, the client can perform active ROM exercises with the hand bags in place. Splints are often necessary, especially during sleep.

Coping

The health care team faces a great challenge in helping the client and family cope with the suffering caused by burns. Coping varies with each client and family, the support provided by the family, and the social and economic status of the client and family. How the family unit is treated throughout the healing will help determine how well they adjust physically and psychosocially.

The repeated debridement, skin grafting, and plastic surgery needed to heal a burn injury may be overwhelming to clients even though they are aware surgery is essential for their survival, function, and appearance. Each operation has inherent risks: anesthesia, postoperative pain and immobility, loss of self-control while anesthetized, and possible death. Healing following a burn is a long, slow process. Daily progress may be measured only by centimeters of wound healing or joint movement. Burn care has an unknown outcome, and the health care team cannot offer empty promises that "you'll be all right."

Preventive psychosocial care will establish a trusting relationship and reduce problems throughout hospitalization. The health care team should be assured that clients and their families understand the burn injury, treatment, and prognosis. In all bedside discussions, speak directly to clients rather than talking about them to others. Allow the client as much control as possible in treatment. Finally, provide adequate analgesia.

It is usually during the acute period that severely injured clients first see the burns and recognize their extent. For clients who fear disfigurement, assist the client and family to maintain hope and allow the client to adapt gradually to the body changes. Support the client's coping methods, such as denial or anger, as long as needed. The nurse will need to be sensitive to the client's reaction and perceptive enough to judge when a coping mechanism has become counterproductive. Help the family understand that the client is attempting to deal with the situation. Clients will offer cues when they wish to see burned body parts or know more about their condition. They will generally ask someone they trust to help support them during their immediate reactions. Clients should not be forced to view their burns. When clients view their burns, especially facial burns, for the first time, be prepared to be supportive because the radical changes may be shocking.

Clients who deny the seriousness of their injury should be assisted to see the reality of their injury and treatment. In some cases, the need for denial may be so extreme that clients will not comprehend what is said. Some degree of denial is acceptable if the client does not cause harm. Families should be repeatedly informed about the true situation so they do not become confused. A firm, kind, nonrejecting approach is needed for clients coping by regression. Embarrassed and worried family members should be informed that regression is a temporary coping method and will resolve as the physical state improves.

For angry clients, the nurse must absorb the brunt of the aggression, realizing that verbal and physical abuses are not personal. The anger is directed at events surrounding the injury and its sequelae. Chemical and physical restraints are punitive; use rational methods instead for dealing with angry clients.

Clients and their families need support and examples of specific improvements to maintain their hope. Sincere, constant praise is needed from family members and the health care team. Clients in later stages of healing can offer much support to others. They offer positive proof that it is possible to be burned and live, boosting morale for other clients.

Self-Care

Clients often struggle against being dependent on others for basic human needs. Not only are they often kept naked for observation of the burn wounds, but severely burned clients require help eating, toileting, and ambulating. Although dependence may be difficult for some clients to accept, others may regress to maintain it.

Supporting the client in developing effective coping mechanisms will assist the client in adjusting to inabilities to provide personal care. As coping mechanisms are strengthened and the self-concept assimilates the changed body image, clients may recover from some of their anger and frustration toward their dependence.

Self-Concept

Recognize that integration of the burn into the person's self-concept may be a long and gradual process. Convey a sense of the client's self-worth despite appearance and treat each client as a unique person. Clients may reject help from the health care team if they sense they are not valued. The family also needs help to develop positive feelings toward the client, even though they may feel repelled. Teach the family to touch the client without causing pain and encourage them to do so. This will help restore a sense of closeness between the family and client.

Preparing the Client for Possible Skin Grafting

For each skin-grafting procedure, clients and families should be taught about the planned procedure and preoperative and postoperative care. Even if a burned client has undergone multiple skin graftings, the nurse should not assume the client and family do not have questions and anxiety about the planned surgery. The nurse can adjust the teaching to the client's needs and anxiety level.

Burn clients should have wound care completed the morning of surgery, with the wounds dressed in clear antibiotic solution or saline dressings. This eliminates the need to clean the wounds of ointment in the operating room. Burn clients are considered contaminated cases and will be the last scheduled for the operating room on the day of surgery. Some institutions use one operating room for the burn surgeries scheduled on that particular day.

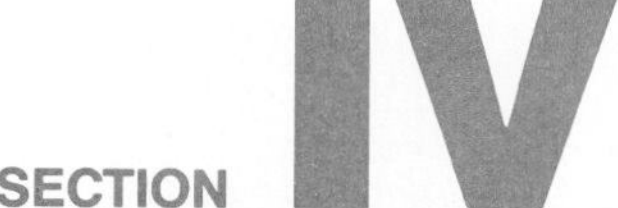

Nursing Process in the Rehabilitative Period

The major focus of the *rehabilitative period* is preparing the client for discharge from the hospital. This period begins when there is less than 20% of the body to be healed and ends with total rehabilitation. In the aftermath of what may have been a life-threatening injury, the client and family begin to focus more on the impact of the burn on their lifestyles. This period may last for years.

Assessment: Establishing the Data Base

Nursing assessment during the rehabilitative phase centers on the final stages of wound healing, psychologic adjustment, and preparations for discharge.

Subjective Data

Clients begin to think about their functional disabilities and appearance during this phase. They begin to internalize their changed body image and often test new behaviors in the safety of the hospital. As clients begin to visualize reassuming responsibilities for self-care in their jobs and lives, anxiety will again rise.

Progressive desensitization—the eventual feeling that the injury is not repulsive—occurs in this stage. The injured body is integrated into the client's self-image with less awareness of the injury. Clients will say, "Yes, I was burned once, but I'm OK now." This change allows the burned client to master body changes and again be in control. See the following sections on self-concept and coping to determine indicators of maladaptive responses.

Objective Data

Burn wounds should be assessed for development of contractures and keloids. Healed burns should be assessed for tightness, dryness, and pruritus. Unhealed wounds must be assessed for continued evidence of healing or lack of healing.

Clients will still have pain during this phase, but it should be less intense. All complaints of pain should be completely assessed before administering medications. Activity tolerance should be assessed to determine the need for ROM exercises and perhaps occupational therapy to accomplish activities of daily living.

Nursing Diagnoses/Planning and Implementation/Evaluation

Nursing diagnoses in the rehabilitative period primarily involve preparing the client for hospital discharge and independent functioning. (Refer to Table 12–2.) Deficits are noted in both physiologic and psychosocial areas so they can be improved before the client leaves the hospital. Especially important during this period is the involvement of family because they will be central to the client's continued rehabilitation at home. A sample nursing care plan for the burn client in the rehabilitative period is in Table 12–5.

Self-Concept

Assisting clients to cope with permanent changes in physical appearance is not easy. In the early stages of burn care, the primary concern was for life, then wound coverage and complications. When the wounds are healed, clients, their significant others, and nursing staff have to come to terms with the permanence of the changed body. In many respects, clients look better than when first burned, but this is the best they probably will look.

Maladaptive adjustments of depression, withdrawal, isolation, and regression may go on for a lifetime. Some clients feel their injury has left them so deformed that they isolate themselves from society. Clients with serious signs of maladaptation need long-term psychologic counseling and when appropriate, referral to a plastic surgeon for possible future plastic surgery. It is important that psychologic problems be addressed because plastic surgery is not a panacea.

If the burn involved the face or hands, the self-concept may be seriously damaged. Burns or grafts to the face obviously alter the appearance. Furthermore, skin grafts

Table 12–5
Sample Nursing Care Plan for the Rehabilitative Period, by Nursing Diagnosis

Client Care Goals	Plan/Implementation	Expected Outcome
Self-concept, disturbance in		
Integration of changed body image	Assess body image and anxiety about returning to home and job; provide information about self-help resources; note signs of maladaptation (see coping skills) and refer for counseling if appropriate	Client expresses realistic self-image; does not seem unduly anxious about hospital discharge; does not show undue signs of maladaptation; accepts referral if made
Nutrition, altered, potential for more than body requirements		
Appropriate adjustment in caloric intake; no unnecessary weight gain	Plan adjustment in calories in consultation with dietitian; explain rationale for adjusting intake; monitor intake and weight	Client explains rationale for adjusted intake; complies with diet; does not gain unneeded weight
Comfort, altered, related to pain and pruritis		
Control of pain and pruritus	Assess pain and document; plan pain management for exercise periods; for pruritus, maintain cool, dry environment; apply lotion and cocoa butter as needed; recommend cotton underwear; use mild soap for bathing	Adequate control of pain; client does not complain of pain while exercising; client does not complain of pruritus; no signs of skin breakdown from scratching
Coping skills, ineffective		
Adequate coping skills for hospital discharge	Assess coping skills; provide teaching about home care; provide information about self-help resources; note signs of maladaptation (depression, withdrawal, isolation, regression) and refer for counseling if appropriate	Client exhibits mastery of self-care skills; discusses feelings about adjustment to return to home and work; expresses interest in self-help resources; does not show undue signs of maladaptation; accepts referral if made
Knowledge deficit, related to self-care		
Demonstrates understanding and mastery of self-care activities needed at home	Teach client about self-care activities to be performed at home: wound care, exercise, and nutrition	Client describes self-care activities accurately and demonstrates them correctly; states understanding of rationale for each activity
Mobility, impaired physical		
Return of ROM and ambulation to near pre-burn levels	Assess joint mobility and ambulation; instruct client in exercises to perform at home; prescribe splints and elastic garments as needed	Client demonstrates exercises and explains rationale
Skin integrity, impaired		
Progress in wound healing; no further impairment in skin integrity	Continue to assess and monitor skin integrity; instruct client and family in wound care to be done at home; teach about susceptibility to skin breakdown, sunburn, and skin cancer	Client continues to show progress in wound healing; demonstrates wound care activities; explains rationale for wound care and skin care

and healed scarred wounds do not allow normal movements. Grafted facial skin does not stretch with expressions, giving a masklike appearance.

Nutrition

The diet should remain high in protein until all wounds have healed. As healing takes place, the diet should be tapered off to normal caloric intake. Burn clients become used to eating a great deal of food and may develop a habit of eating frequently. After healing is complete, metabolism decreases, and the calories are deposited as fat. Clients can gain unneeded weight if the diet and eating habits are not adjusted.

Comfort

Although the client may continue to have pain, it should be diminished. By this time, pain will probably be controlled by mild analgesics and oral narcotics. The majority of pain occurs with stretching and ROM exercises. Clients should receive medication before physical therapy treatments.

The pruritus and skin drying from wound and graft healing can be relieved with the application of heavy lotion and cocoa butter. The environment should be cool and dry. The client may find cotton underwear comfortable, even in bed. Mild soap should be used in bathing to reduce irritation and prevent further drying.

Coping

Coping skills continue to need reinforcement as the client prepares to face the world beyond the hospital. The client should be given an opportunity to discuss fears or ask questions. Arrange for a time when not doing treatments to have such a discussion. Give honest answers to questions, even if the answer is, "We don't know." To assist the client for going home, activities of daily living can be tried in the hospital. Alternative methods to perform activities can be discussed and tried.

Burned clients will frequently express frustration that no one except the health care team knows what they have been through. Clients may need to discuss these feelings. They may need assistance in planning how to react to questions that are meant to be sincere but may sound cold.

Clients who fear the reaction of others should be reminded that they need not discuss every detail of their tragedy with everyone. Clients should be encouraged to be assertive and learn to say they do not care to discuss all aspects of their situation.

Psychiatric nurse clinicians, psychiatrists, or social workers are excellent resources for clients with unresolved problems. The nursing staff in the burn treatment unit does not always have time or preparation to intervene effectively in all aspects of client care. Appropriate referrals for complete and improved client care should be made without hesitation. Other recovered burn victims and the mutual support groups listed in the resource section at the end of this chapter may also be helpful.

Self-Care

Client teaching about care outside the hospital is perhaps the most important activity in preparing the client and family for discharge. Among the subjects on which they may need instruction are skin care, wound care, joint mobility, exposure to sunlight, nutrition, and pain management. Specific teaching activities are discussed under appropriate nursing interventions.

Families are primarily concerned about "doing the right thing" for the client once dismissed to home. Discharge instructions should always include the family because they become the primary caregivers. Instructions should be given in writing because the family may be as anxious as the client and may not absorb oral instructions. Having the family perform a demonstration of wound care is especially helpful in reinforcing teaching. Not only do families need to be taught what to do for clients; they need to be taught what clients can do for themselves. At times, in their zealousness to do everything possible, the family loses sight of the client's need to regain independence. Finally, the family should be reassured that they can call the burn team if questions arise.

Mobility

In the rehabilitation period, wound contractures and ROM are the principal mobility problems. Wound contractures can be minimized with the use of splints to hold joints in extension. ROM exercises are essential, and clients should be encouraged to begin to do their own exercises. Wound contractures cannot be completely prevented because scar

Nursing Research Note

Garts K, Garland S: Marital satisfaction of the post-rehabilitation burned patient. *Occupat Health Nurs* 1983; 31(7):35–37.

A comparative study was conducted of 50 burn clients and 52 general surgical clients to determine marital satisfaction. A highly valid and reliable tool, the Locke–Wallace Marital Adjustment Test, was used to differentiate well-adjusted and maladjusted persons in marriage. Results showed that both groups were equal in marital satisfaction in all areas except for sexual relations, which showed a significant difference. Burn clients' comments about sex referred to altered body image and concern for physical well-being or discomfort. Knowledge that burn clients may have sexual adjustment problems enables nurses to focus interventions on this area and offer alternatives to help the client and spouse cope effectively with their concerns.

contraction is a normal part of healing, but exercising will reduce their severity.

If contractures become so severe that clients cannot move a limb, their necks, or open their mouths, plastic surgery can be performed. Plastic surgical procedures include releasing the scarred tissue and sometimes skin grafting to open up the joint. These procedures are performed throughout the client's life when contractures become unmanageable.

If needed, the client should wear a custom-made elastic garment, such as the Jobst garment illustrated in Figure 12–8, 23 hours a day (1 hour to launder) to prevent keloid formation and hypertrophic scars. The garment is worn until scar maturation is complete, usually 1 year from the time of injury. After the scar has matured, contractures occur more slowly. Jobst garments should be hand washed in a mild soap and air dried.

Skin Integrity

Although healing should be largely completed by the time the client is ready for discharge, the client may still have unhealed areas. The healed burned and grafted skin is tender and will break down more easily than normal skin because it has not formed protective callouses.

Clients and family who will continue wound care at home should be taught how to do the care, including dressing removal, tubbing, debridement, application of medications, and dressings. A shower works well for debridement on small burns because the moving water rather than the client loosens and removes necrotic skin. A return demonstration is critical to evaluate learning.

Clients should be taught to avoid sunlight on burned areas for a full year because burned and grafted skin tans unevenly and unpredictably. One spot may become dark tan, and another may burn. Skin cancers are more frequent in burned skin, especially many years after a burn. Therefore, clients should have frequent physical examinations for the remainder of their lives.

When a burn client leaves the hospital, the health care team feels a sense of accomplishment and joy at the successful recovery; they may also feel sad about the separation, regardless of the problems they faced. Some sadness may be from apprehension about the quality of life for a severely deformed client. Some health team members may be angry to see clients go home to a less-than-ideal environment or to a family that was not supportive during hospitalization. Some of these feelings may be mitigated if the client later returns for a visit, and the staff sees that he or she is functioning and adapting well.

Chapter Highlights

Burns can be classified according to their causes and depth of injury.

A client with major burns can be expected to develop four to six major complications in addition to the burn.

Massive fluid shift, which is the body's immediate response to a burn, has multisystem effects; correction of the fluid deficit is an immediate priority in burn care.

The first step in caring for a burn client is to stop the burning process. The next step is to evaluate the airway, breathing, and circulation. Then initiate care to save the victim's life.

Minor burns never include electrical burns of any size or burns of the face, feet, perineum, or entire hand.

Clients with severe burns generally progress through three stages of treatment: emergent period, acute period, and rehabilitative period.

In the emergent period, initial care is strongly centered on maintaining life and on fluid resuscitation.

In the acute period, emphasis is on continued monitoring for oxygenation and fluid deficit, assessing for development of complications, preventing wound infection, and promoting wound healing.

In the rehabilitative period as the client prepares for hospital discharge, a major focus is self-care instruction for such topics as wound care and nutrition, with continuing assessment of psychosocial adjustment and appropriate referrals as necessary.

Bibliography

Bernstein N: *Emotional Care of the Facially Burned and Disfigured.* Boston: Little, Brown, 1976.

Burns among older Americans aged 70 and over. *National Burn Information Exchange Newsletter* (Aug) 1983; 2.

DeCrosta T: What burn centers want you to know. *Nurs Life* (Jan–Feb) 1984: 4:45–49.

Demling R: Fluid resuscitation after major burns. *JAMA* 1983; 250:1438–1440.

Hill M, Achaver B, Martinez S: Tar and asphalt burns. *J Burn Care Rehab* (July–Aug) 1984; 5:271–274.

Hurt R: More than skin deep. *Nurs 85* (June) 1985; 15:52–57.

Johnson CL, Cain VJ: Burn care: The rehab guide. *Am J Nurs* 1985; 85(1):48–50.

Johnson CL, Cain VJ: Team approach to effective range of motion in burn patients. *J Burn Care Rehab* (Nov–Dec) 1981; 4:218–220.

Kibbee E: Public health nurses: A liaison between home and hospital for burned patients. *J Burn Care Rehab* (Nov–Dec) 1983; 4:427–429.

Leeder C: Focus on burn prevention: A community education program. *Plast Surg Nurs* (Fall) 1983; 3:66–69.

Martyn JA, Greenblatt D, Abernathy D: Increase cimetidine clearance in burn patients. *JAMA* 1985; 253:1288–1291.

Perry S, Heidrich G, Ramos E: Assessment of pain by burn patients. *J Burn Care Rehab* (Nov–Dec) 1981; 2:322–326.

Richard R et al: Autocontamination of the burn patient by hydrotherapy. *Bull Clin Rev Burn Injuries* 1984; 2:40.

Richard R et al: The effect of hydrotherapy on burn wound bacteria. *Bull Clin Rev Burn Injuries* 1984; 2:39.

Robertson K, Cross PJ, Terry JC: Burn care: The crucial first days. *Am J Nurs* 1985; 85(1):29–45.

Rosequist CC, Shepp PH: Burn care: The nutrition factor. *Am J Nurs* 1985; 85(1):45–47.

Surveyer J, Clougherty D: Burn scars: Fighting the effects. *Am J Nurs* 1983; 83(5):746–751.

Tegtmeier R: Nursing care of patients with burned hands. *Plast Surg Nurs* 1983; 3:3–5.

Walkenstein M: Comparison of burned patients' perception of pain with nurses' perception of patients' pain. *J Burn Care Rehab* 1983; 3:233–236.

Zimmerman T, Krizek T: Thermally induced dermal injury: A review of pathophysiologic events and therapeutic intervention. *J Burn Care Rehab* (May–June) 1984; 5:193–201.

Resources

SELF-HELP GROUPS AND OTHER ORGANIZATIONS

National Institute for Burn Medicine
909 E Ann St
Ann Arbor, MI 48104
Phone: (313) 769–9000

National statistics are tabulated here on burn injury. Also provides a burn nurse specialist program.

Society for the Rehabilitation of the
Facially Disfigured
See resources listing in Chapter 54.

HEALTH EDUCATION MATERIAL

From: American Red Cross

(See local listing in telephone directory.) "Red Cross First Aid Module: First Aid for Burns," an 80-page programmed learning manual. Cost: 60¢.

PROFESSIONAL ORGANIZATIONS

American Burn Association
% Dr. Glenn Warder
Shriner's Burn Institute
University of Cincinnati
200 Goldman
Cincinnati, OH 45219

This is a professional organization for the entire burn team. It sponsors many projects to improve burn care.

American Society of Plastic and
Reconstructive Surgical Nurses
See resources listing in Chapter 54.

International Society for Burn Injuries
% Dr. John Boswick
2005 Franklin St., Bldg. 2, Suite 600
Denver, CO 80205

UNIT

3

The Client With Respiratory Dysfunction

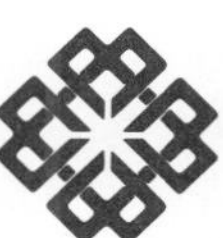

CHAPTER 13

The Respiratory System in Health and Illness

Objectives

When you have finished studying this chapter, you should be able to:

Identify the major structural and functional components of the respiratory system.

Explain the physiologic mechanisms that regulate the activity of the respiratory system.

Describe some pathologic conditions that lead to respiratory dysfunction.

Discuss alterations in other body systems that result from respiratory dysfunction.

Identify and discuss the psychosocial/lifestyle effects of respiratory dysfunction on the client and significant others.

Every cell in the body needs oxygen to carry out its metabolic functions, that is, to live. Likewise, every cell in the body must rid itself of carbon dioxide, a waste product of cellular metabolism. The process of transporting oxygen to the cells and removing carbon dioxide is called respiration. Any disease or trauma that interferes with respiration injures body cells. The body can survive without food for weeks and without water for a few days; without oxygen it dies in a few minutes.

Respiration involves two major body systems, the cardiovascular system and the respiratory system, under regulation of the nervous system. Oxygen and carbon dioxide, which are gases, are conveyed to and from tissues and organs by the cardiovascular system. The respiratory system delivers oxygen from the atmosphere to the bloodstream and delivers carbon dioxide from the blood to the atmosphere. The exchange of oxygen and carbon dioxide, called gas exchange, takes place in specialized structures of the lungs.

SECTION I

Structural and Functional Interrelationships

Although the respiratory airways and the anatomic structures where gas exchange takes place are continuous, their components are classified anatomically and functionally as belonging to either (1) the upper respiratory tract or (2) the lower respiratory tract. The muscles of the chest wall and diaphragm also participate in respiration.

The Upper Respiratory Tract

The upper respiratory tract is primarily an air delivery system: it warms, moistens, and filters inspired atmospheric air on its way to the lungs. Structures of the upper respiratory tract also expel foreign matter and excess secretions from the system. The principal structures of the upper respiratory tract are the nose, the paranasal sinuses, the pharynx, and the larynx (Figure 13–1).

Air enters the system first through the nares, or nostrils—the openings of the two cavities of the nose (nasal fossae). The nasal septum separates the two fossae. The *nose* is composed of both bone and cartilage, and its interior surface has ridges called turbinates. The ridged configuration increases the effective surface of the nasal mucosa. An extensive bed of capillaries transfers body heat to the inspired air. Because of this rich vascularity, bleeding from injured nasal tissue can be profuse.

Mucus secreted by the membrane that lines the nose helps humidify inspired air, which attains a relative humidity of over 90% as it passes through the nares. Hairs that

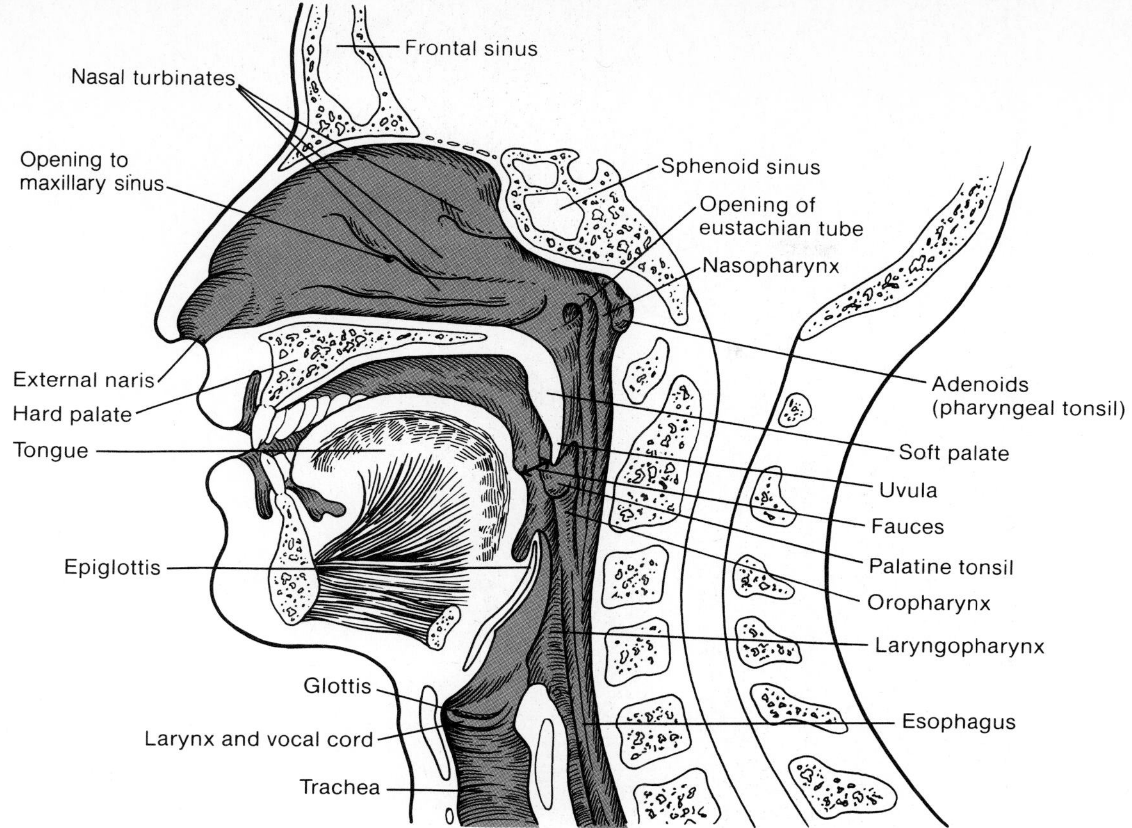

Figure 13–1

Structures of the upper respiratory tract. SOURCE: *Spence AP, Mason EB:* Human Anatomy and Physiology, *2nd ed. Menlo Park, CA: Benjamin/Cummings, 1983.*

line the nose filter out large foreign particles, and a sticky mucus secreted by the serous glands in the mucosa traps finer dirt, dust, and microorganisms. Hairlike structures of the mucous membrane called cilia constantly propel trapped particles toward the pharynx, from which they can be expelled by sneezing or coughing. In addition to its respiratory functions, the nose is the organ of olfaction. Sensory receptors sensitive to various odors are concentrated in the roof of the nasal fossae.

The *paranasal sinuses* are air-filled cavities within bony structures adjacent to the nasal cavity. These sinuses—called the ethmoid, frontal, sphenoid, and maxillary sinuses—drain through the nasal cavity. All are lined with ciliated columnar epithelium that is continuous with the lining of the nose. Because the mucosa is continuous, infection in the nasal passages can readily spread to the sinuses.

The *pharynx* begins at the base of the skull and ends opposite the lowest cartilaginous rings of the larynx. Its three sections, from superior to inferior, are the nasopharynx, the oropharynx, and the laryngopharynx. The nasopharynx contains paired lymphatic structures called adenoids or pharyngeal tonsils, and the eustachian tubes, which maintain appropriate air pressure within the middle ear. Functional eustachian tubes are essential for hearing and crucial to the mechanism by which the body maintains balance. Air and food both enter the body through the oropharynx. The palatine tonsils, which, like the adenoids, are composed of lymphatic tissue, are located there. The laryngopharynx contains the epiglottis, a small flap of tissue that covers the larynx during swallowing to prevent food or liquid from being aspirated into the lower airway.

The *larynx,* often called the voice box, connects the upper and lower airways. The opening of the larynx, called the glottis, closes during swallowing to prevent aspiration. The vocal cords of the larynx, in addition to producing sound, are involved in the cough reflex, which clears the respiratory tract of foreign substances or objects and of accumulated secretions.

The Cough Reflex

The cough reflex is initiated when a foreign substance— (eg, a dust particle)—irritates specialized nerve endings within the larynx, trachea, or major bronchi. Nerve impulses are sent to contract muscles that close the vocal cords and simultaneously contract abdominal muscles and muscle fibers within the respiratory tract itself. Air pressure builds up within the lower airways, and when the vocal cords reopen, a sudden rush of air carries mucus and foreign matter up to be expectorated. Because the vocal cords are crucial to the cough reflex, persons whose larynxes have been removed cannot cough and thus are deprived of an important defense against airway obstruction.

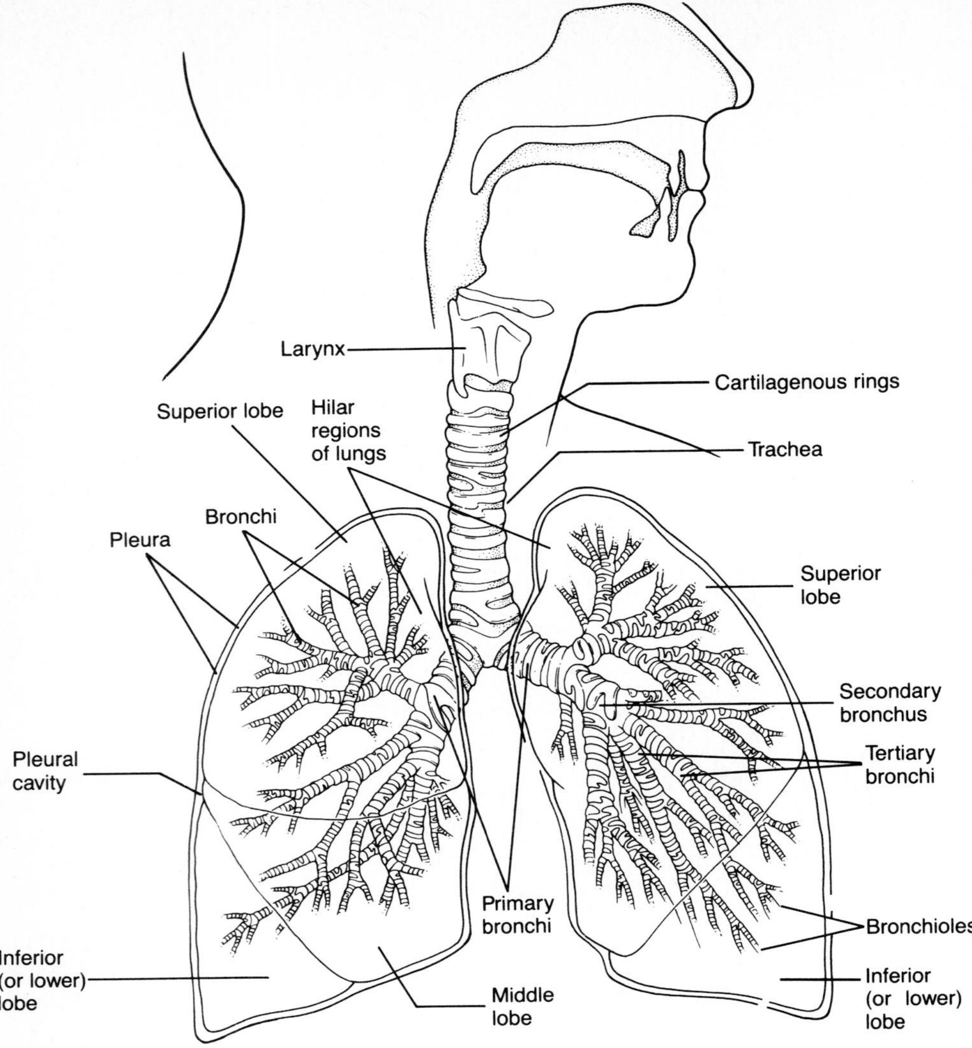

Figure 13–2

The tracheobronchial tree. SOURCE: *Tortora GJ, Funke BR, Case CL:* Microbiology: An Introduction, *2nd ed. Menlo Park, CA: Benjamin/Cummings, 1986.*

The Lower Respiratory Tract

The lower respiratory tract consists of the trachea, the bronchi and their branches, and the various structures of the lungs, which are protected by the chest wall.

The Trachea

The air passage of the trachea, or windpipe, is kept open by C-shaped cartilaginous rings in the tracheal wall, much as the flexible hose of a vacuum cleaner or hair dryer is kept open by rings of plastic or metal (see Figure 13–2). The mucus-bathed ciliary epithelium that lines the trachea sweeps foreign material up into the pharynx, where the cough reflex expels it. The trachea, like the upper respiratory passages, warms and humidifies inspired air.

The Bronchi and Bronchioles

In Figure 13–2, note that the left primary bronchus exits from the trachea at a more acute angle than the right bronchus. The right bronchus might almost be considered an extension of the trachea itself. Because of the angle, foreign material is more often aspirated into the right lung than the left. The cellular structure of the bronchial lining at this point is similar to that of the trachea.

The bronchi contain sensory receptors of the parasympathetic and sympathetic nervous systems. If these nerve endings are stimulated—(eg, by an allergen)—impulses transmitted to the respiratory centers of the brain by cranial nerve X (the vagus nerve) initiate constriction of the bronchi, secretion of mucus, or the cough reflex. Thus, the lungs are protected against foreign particles.

The right primary bronchus divides into three secondary bronchi that supply the three lobes (superior, middle, and inferior) of the right lung. The left bronchus branches (bifurcates), each segment going to one of the two lobes of the left lung. Within the lung, the bronchi branch off into smaller and smaller airways and then into tiny bronchioles.

The primary bronchi, like the trachea, are supported by partial rings of cartilage. As the airways become narrower and narrower, the proportion of smooth muscle to cartilage increases, and the number of serous glands lining the bronchiolar walls decreases. At approximately the point where a bronchiole narrows to 1 mm in diameter, the walls are entirely surrounded by smooth muscle. Thus, when the muscles of the bronchioles undergo spasm—as in an asthma attack—the lack of cartilaginous support causes air passages to collapse, and breathing becomes extremely difficult (Spence & Mason, 1983).

The terminal bronchioles mark the end of the air conduction system and open into the respiratory bronchioles. Each of these in turn branches into several alveolar ducts, which open into grapelike clusters of air-filled sacs called alveoli. The respiratory bronchioles, alveolar ducts, and alveoli form the terminal respiratory units of the lungs, called **acini** (Figure 13–3).

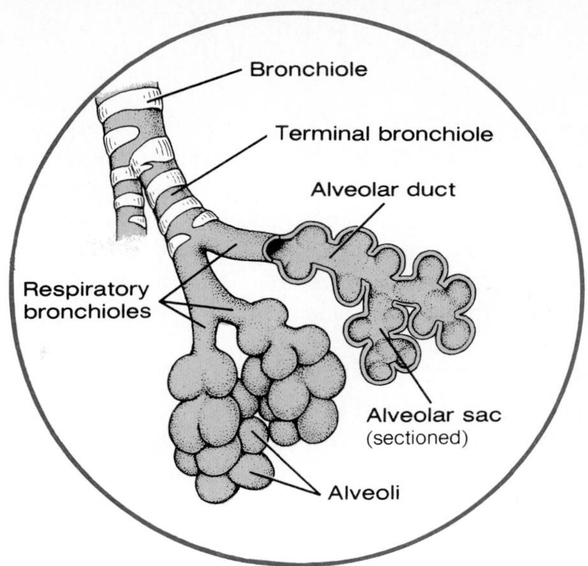

Figure 13–3

An acinus, the terminal respiratory unit of the lung. *SOURCE: Spence AP, Mason EB:* Human Anatomy and Physiology, *3rd ed. Menlo Park, CA: Benjamin/Cummings, 1987.*

The Lungs

The lungs are paired, somewhat cone-shaped structures that lie in the thoracic cavity on either side of the mediastinum, which contains the heart, aorta, venae cavae, and other vital structures. The bases of the lungs rest on the diaphragm. The right lung has three lobes, the left two, and the lobes are further subdivided into smaller bronchopulmonary segments. This segmental structure makes it possible to remove a relatively small portion of the lung if surgical resection is necessary.

The lungs lie free within the pleural cavities of the thorax, except at the hilus, or root, on the medial surface. The bronchi and blood vessels enter and exit through the hilus. The sternum forms the anterior border of the thorax. The lateral boundaries of the thorax are composed of the twelve ribs, or costae, which are attached to the sternum by the costal cartilages anteriorly and the vertebral column posteriorly. This bony thoracic cage protects the vital structures within the mediastinum and the fragile, spongy tissue of the lungs.

The diaphragm, which lies below the lungs, is an important muscle of respiration and separates the thorax from the abdominal cavity. Each half of the diaphragm is innervated by a phrenic nerve. The phrenic nerves originate from the fourth cervical nerve. An injury to one of the phrenic nerves results in a unilateral diaphragmatic paralysis with elevation of half of the diaphragm.

The Pleura

The visceral pleura covering the lungs is continuous with the parietal pleura, which lines the thoracic cavity. Both pleurae are formed of serous membrane that secretes pleural fluid into the extremely narrow pleural cavity between the two layers. This fluid lubricates the two layers, reducing friction as the lungs and thorax move during respiration. The pleural fluid also couples the parietal and visceral pleurae and the structures to which they are attached—much as a drop of water between a laboratory slide and a cover plate will cause the two to adhere.

Inflammation of the pleural membrane (pleurisy) causes the membrane to become dry and fibrous. The ensuing friction makes breathing painful (Spence & Mason, 1983).

INTRAPLEURAL PRESSURE Because of changes that occur when breathing begins after birth, air pressure within the pleural cavity (intrapleural pressure) is lower than air pressure within the lungs (intrapulmonary pressure) (Figure 13–4). This lower pressure keeps the lung expanded because of its tendency to be drawn toward the area of

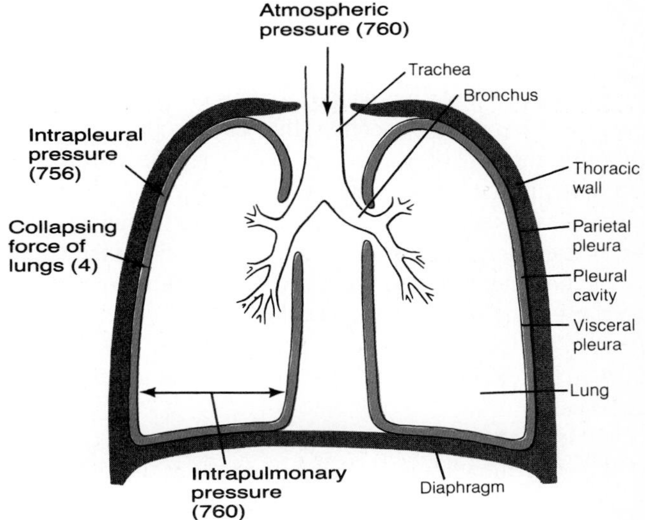

Figure 13–4

Intrapulmonary and intrapleural pressures in resting position (in mm HG). *SOURCE: Spence AP, Mason EB:* Human Anatomy and Physiology, *3rd ed. Menlo Park, CA: Benjamin/Cummings, 1987.*

subatmospheric pressure. If the lung or chest wall is punctured, air rushes into the area of lower pressure, the pleural space, destroying the vacuum that keeps the lung expanded. In severe injury, the amount of air entering the intrapleural space may be sufficient to cause equalization of intrapleural pressure and atmospheric pressure. The result is collapse of the lung on the affected side.

The Pulmonary Circulation

The lungs have a dual blood supply: the tracheal and bronchial circulation, and the pulmonary circulation. The right and left bronchial arteries branch from the descending aorta and supply blood to the trachea and bronchi to the level of the respiratory bronchioles. The terminal respiratory units of the lungs where gas exchange takes place are nourished via the pulmonary circulation.

The pulmonary circulation is where oxygenation of blood occurs. The entire output of the right ventricle leaves the heart via the pulmonary artery, which divides into the right and left pulmonary arteries. This poorly oxygenated blood circulates through the capillaries of the alveoli where gas exchange takes place. Oxygenated blood is then returned to the left atrium via the pulmonary veins.

The Alveoli and Gas Exchange

Each terminal bronchiole supplies its own unit of several alveoli, called the acinus (see Figure 13–3). Exchange of gases takes place here. Essentially, each alveolus is a tiny air space enclosed by a thin wall—the alveolar septum—that consists of a network of pulmonary capillaries held together by connective-tissue fibers and lined with squamous epithelium that contains secretory cells. To appreciate how small alveoli are, consider that the tissue of an adult lung contains over 300 million alveoli.

The secretory glands of the alveolar wall produce a fluid called **pulmonary surfactant.** (A surfactant is a substance that reduces the *surface tension* of a liquid—the attraction between molecules that causes them to form droplets instead of spreading.) Dishwashing detergents contain surfactants so water will spread easily along the surface of dishes. If surface tension were to pull alveolar walls together, expansion of the lungs during inspiration would be hindered, and the alveoli would tend to collapse during expiration as the molecules of fluid cohered. Pulmonary surfactant also contains macrophages that destroy foreign material that has passed through the upper-airway defenses.

Within the alveoli, air is separated from blood by the respiratory membrane, which is formed by the basement membrane of the alveolar and capillary epithelia. This membrane is less than 1 μm thick, and gases move across it in accordance with the principle of diffusion; that is, a gas moves across a membrane from an area of greater partial pressure to one of lesser partial pressure.

The venous blood returning from the tissues is high in carbon dioxide and low in oxygen; the air in the alveolar space is higher in oxygen and lower in carbon dioxide than the blood. Under normal conditions, the approximate partial pressures of oxygen and carbon dioxide in the alveoli and the capillaries are (Spence & Mason, 1983):

	Capillaries	**Alveoli**
Oxygen	PO_2 40 mm Hg	PO_2 105 mm Hg
Carbon dioxide	PCO_2 45 mm Hg	PCO_2 35 mm Hg

Among the prerequisites for efficient gas exchange are:

- *A large number of capillaries must be in contact with the inspired air.* The many-sectioned structure of lung tissue normally provides maximum capillary surface. If alveolar septa are destroyed by a disease process, however, and alveoli coalesce, the surface available for diffusion is reduced.
- *Diffusion of gases must be unimpaired.* If the alveolar membrane becomes fibrous and thickened by scarring, diffusion will be impeded.
- *Pulmonary blood flow must be normal.* If an embolus obstructs blood flow to a portion of the lung, gas exchange will be impaired.
- *Alveoli must be in normal condition.* If alveoli are filled with inflammatory exudate from infection, air cannot reach the respiratory membrane.

In other words, gas exchange, the object of the process of respiration, depends on adequate flow of blood (perfusion) and adequate flow of air (ventilation) to and from alveoli.

The Process of Ventilation

Ventilation is the exchange of air between the atmosphere and the alveoli. At rest, intrapulmonary pressure and atmospheric pressure are equal—760 mm Hg at sea level (Figure 13–4). During inspiration, the muscles of the diaphragm and the intercostal muscles contract, lowering the diaphragm and raising the rib cage. The volume of the intrathoracic space expands, intrapleural and intrapulmonary pressures decrease, until the intrapulmonary pressure is lower than atmospheric pressure. Air moves along the concentration gradient (from higher concentration to lower) into the upper respiratory tract, through the tracheobronchial tree, and into the alveolar tissue of the lungs. Air moves into the lungs until intrapulmonary pressure and atmospheric pressure are equal.

Neuronal receptors sensitive to stretch respond to the expansion of the thoracic cage, stimulating a rebound action of the muscles and connective-tissue fibers of the lungs. The ribs become more vertical and the diaphragm rises, causing intrapulmonary pressure to rise above atmospheric pressure. Air moves passively out of the lungs along the reversed concentration gradient, carrying out carbon dioxide (and other wastes) that have been exchanged for oxygen from the inspired air. This expiration continues until the intrapulmonary pressure is again lower than atmospheric pressure, and the cycle begins again.

During normal inspiration, most of the work is accomplished by the diaphragm, with some participation by the intercostal muscles. Movement of the rib cage may be barely perceptible during quiet respiration, as during sleep. As exertion increases, oxygen demand increases proportionately, and the intercostal muscles are called upon to an increasing extent. During forced or labored respiration, additional chest muscles and even abdominal muscles are used in moving the thoracic cage.

Respiratory Control

The rate and extent of inspiration and expiration are governed by nervous pathways that respond to various stimuli that signal increased or diminished oxygen requirements or carbon dioxide levels. Requirements are greater during exertion and least during sleep. Like other mechanisms vital to survival—(ie, heart action and digestion)—respiration proceeds without conscious control.

Cerebral control of the respiratory mechanisms is believed to be centered in the pons and the medulla oblongata, both located in the brain stem. The apneustic and pneumotaxic centers of the pons apparently control and modify the activities of the medullary center through stimulation and inhibition, respectively. The cerebral centers receive impulses from a wide array of nerve endings (dendrites and axons), some sensitive to chemical stimuli and some to mechanical stimuli.

SECTION 

Pathophysiologic Influences and Effects

Hypoventilation

Ventilation below the level needed to maintain normal arterial carbon dioxide tension (PCO_2) is called hypoventilation. If a client is hypoventilating, arterial blood levels of carbon dioxide (CO_2) will be above normal (**hypercapnia,** sometimes called *hypercarbia*), because alveolar ventilation is not keeping pace with body metabolism. As arterial CO_2 rises, arterial oxygen (PO_2) falls; this condition is called **hypoxemia.** Although hypercapnia can be caused only by hypoventilation, hypoxemia may be caused by several other conditions as well (Broughton, 1982).

Hypoventilation is related to many conditions; airway obstruction is one of the most common. The upper airway, especially the pharynx and larynx, may be obstructed by inflamed, edematous mucosal linings or by hypertrophic tonsils or adenoids. Polyps, tumors, or foreign bodies may partially block the airway. Impairment of the lower respiratory tract or the alveoli can have even more serious effects. Retained secretions, mucosal edema, and bronchospasm can narrow or even collapse some or all of the airways. Obstructive diseases such as emphysema cause hypoventilation because they impair air flow.

Functional alterations in the central nervous system, as well as neuromuscular or skeletal abnormalities, can also play a part in hypoventilation. Hypoventilation often occurs as a consequence of immobility or inappropriate positioning for extended periods. These effects are discussed in the section on related-system alterations.

Diffusion Impairment

Remember that oxygen and carbon dioxide molecules are transported between the alveolar air spaces and the capillary beds of the alveolar septum by diffusion. Significant diffusion abnormalities can interfere with the passage of inspired oxygen from the alveoli into the blood. Because carbon dioxide diffuses readily, the partial pressure of carbon dioxide is generally unaffected by diffusion impairment. Hypoxemia may lead to hyperventilation, however, and this, rather than diffusion impairment itself, may lower PCO_2.

Any condition that thickens the alveolar septum can impair diffusion. Metastatic carcinoma may invade the interstitial spaces. Pulmonary edema also hampers oxygen diffusion because of the increased amount of fluid in the alveoli and the interstitial spaces. If the amount of functioning lung tissue is reduced because of emphysema, pneumonectomy, or tumor growth, diffusion will also be impaired.

In the early stages of diffusion impairment, hypoxemia may occur only during exertion. As the condition progresses, hypoxemia and related symptoms (dyspnea, restlessness, tachycardia) may occur even when the client is resting.

Ventilation–Perfusion Abnormalities

Efficient exchange of carbon dioxide for oxygen requires equality of alveolar ventilation (V) and perfusion (Q). That is, ventilation–perfusion inequality (or V/Q mismatching) is defined as an imbalance of pulmonary ventilation and perfusion. Slight imbalances occur in healthy individuals, but excessive ventilation–perfusion imbalances are the most common cause of hypoxemia. Such abnormalities may be classified as:

- Normal ventilation to no perfusion
- No ventilation and normal perfusion
- No ventilation and no perfusion

Normal Ventilation to No Perfusion (Dead Space Unit)

Without perfusion, gas exchange cannot take place. This condition is called *wasted ventilation,* since ventilation of the alveoli brings about no exchange of carbon dioxide for oxygen. Conditions related to wasted ventilation include a decrease in total blood volume (eg, in hemorrhage or dehydration), pulmonary embolism, and chronic obstructive pulmonary disease (COPD) such as emphysema. Emphysema may also destroy both alveoli and capillaries within portions of the lungs, so neither ventilation nor perfusion can take place. If large areas of the lungs are affected by wasted ventilation, hypoxemia and hypercapnia with related respiratory acidosis can occur.

No Ventilation to Normal Perfusion (Shunt Unit)

In shunting, the alveolus is perfused but not ventilated (wasted perfusion). Any pathologic condition that obstructs the alveoli can lead to a low ventilation-to-perfusion ratio. For example, a client who is in pain from upper abdominal surgery may take shallow breaths, resulting in atelectasis (lung collapse). Then unoxygenated blood from the collapsed area mixes with oxygenated blood from the unaffected areas, lowering the level of oxygen in the arterial blood. This venous admixture represents the shunting phenomenon. In addition, insufficient carbon dioxide is eliminated. Arterial hypoxemia occurs, but hypercapnia may not occur unless the lungs are severely compromised, because of the compensating effect of hyperventilation.

No Ventilation to No Perfusion (Silent Unit)

Conditions leading to diminished or absent ventilation of some alveolar units include pneumonia, atelectasis, pulmonary edema, and COPD. Conditions leading to diminished or absent perfusion of some alveolar units include compression of intrathoracic blood vessels by a neoplasm; occlusion of blood vessels by emboli or thrombi; and collapse of blood vessels because of decreased perfusion pressure, shock, or hypotension. The severity of client symptoms depends on the extent of alveolar units involved.

SECTION 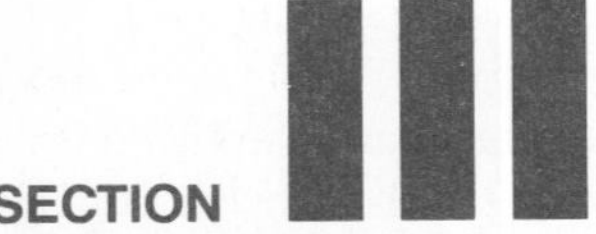

Related System Influences and Effects

In addition to abnormalities of the lungs and upper respiratory structures, pathophysiologic processes involving other body systems can adversely affect respiratory function. Conversely, since oxygen is a primary need of every body cell, dysfunction of the respiratory system can have extensive repercussions in any body system.

Nervous System

Drugs or disease processes affecting the nervous system will inevitably affect respiration to some extent. Anesthetic agents are a major example of drugs having respiratory side effects. Infections, tumors, diseases of the peripheral nervous system, neuromuscular diseases and others, will affect respiration in various ways. The respiratory system may respond to these influences by hyperventilation, hypoventilation, a combination of the two (eg, Cheyne–Stokes respiration), or apnea. If the brain or spinal cord is damaged, respiratory function may be greatly impaired or even totally destroyed, depending on the location and severity of the damage. So closely are the nervous and respiratory systems interrelated that abnormalities in either can have major consequences for both.

Cardiovascular System

The heart must not only move blood to the pulmonary arteries for exchange of oxygen and carbon dioxide but must supply oxygenated blood to the lung tissue itself. Consequently, functional alterations in the cardiovascular system also affect respiratory function. If severe hemorrhage depletes the volume of circulating blood, the supply of oxygen and nutrients for the airways and terminal respiratory units will be diminished. The oxygen and nutrient deficit will be greater in pulmonary tissue because even under normal conditions, pressure in the pulmonary circulation is lower than pressure in the systemic circulation. Because the lungs are adjacent to the heart, little pressure is normally required for pumping blood to them.

Failure of the right side of the heart related to certain disease states may affect the volume of pulmonary blood circulation. Conversely, certain disorders of the respiratory system are closely related to right-sided heart failure. Left-sided heart failure also affects pulmonary function because of backup of blood in the pulmonary vasculature and related pulmonary edema. If the volume of blood circulating either to or from the lungs is compromised for any reason, oxygen, carbon dioxide, and acid–base abnormalities may occur.

Oxygen obtained during gas exchange in the pulmonary circulation must combine with hemoglobin to be transported to the tissues. Normally, the circulation contains approximately 15 g of hemoglobin to carry about 20 mL of oxygen at any given time. If the hemoglobin concentration is below normal, the capacity of the blood to transport oxygen will be reduced.

Other Related Systems

Diseases and deformities of the skeletal system can also alter respiratory function, generally by restricting movement of the thoracic cage. Problems in the gastrointestinal tract such as hiatal hernia can interfere with lung expansion. Extreme obesity can restrict movement of the thoracic cage and places an abnormal load on the respiratory system by increasing the exertion required for ordinary activities.

Surgery of the gastrointestinal tract, especially procedures such as cholecystectomy that have a high abdominal incision, can be associated with pulmonary complications in the postoperative period. Pain in the surgical site inhibits adequate deep breathing and coughing, resulting in inadequate expansion of the lungs. Atelectasis or pneumonia can be the consequence.

SECTION 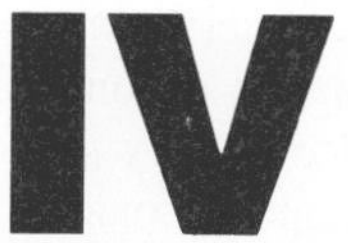

Psychosocial/Lifestyle Influences and Effects

Developmental Influences

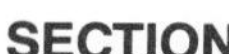 Aging, although not a disease, usually diminishes respiratory capacity as it does cardiovascular function. Cerebral neurons have one of the highest metabolic rates of all body cells, and brain cells are thus the first to be affected by any reduction in respiratory efficiency. Moreover, since neurons (alone among body cells) do not reproduce once mature, destruction of neurons permanently affects cerebral function. The vagueness and forgetfulness often seen in older people can be related to oxygen deficit. These symptoms interfere with personal autonomy and are upsetting to client and family.

Regardless of age, clients react differently when breathing problems develop. A client with supportive friends and family—a support network—will find it easier to cope with disability than a client who is socially isolated. Like many vital body functions, breathing is generally taken for granted. "As natural as breathing" is a common simile for an act that takes virtually no thought or effort. When such an ordinary process becomes a matter of extraordinary concern, many areas of life are inevitably affected.

Cultural Influences

For many people, breathing is intimately related to deep fears about death, and even a slight interference with breathing can mobilize the primitive fear of suffocation. For example, nurses may find that clients have torn off oxygen lines while semiconscious because of a sensation of being smothered.

Masculinity in many cultures is equated with physical performance. When respiratory insufficiency impedes physical activity, self-esteem suffers. American society is work oriented, and inability to do work can have profound effects on self-esteem. Cultural expectations of self-reliance and independence can make the mere admission of illness a threat to the client's sense of self-worth.

In North American culture, the chest is a focal point of sexual identity. The "manly chest" and female breasts are symbols of masculinity and femininity. Disorders that affect the chest area thus threaten not only life but the individual's sexuality.

Lifestyle Factors

Studies have shown that positive lifestyle changes have more potential for improving health than any treatment of an illness once developed. By encouraging lifestyle modification and by setting an example, nurses offer their clients an opportunity for better long-term health. This is especially true in preventing or alleviating respiratory disorders, since smoking has clearly been implicated in cancer of the lung and a multitude of other disorders.

Nursing Research Note

Sexton D, Munro B: Impact of a husband's chronic illness (COPD) on the spouse's life. *Res Nurs Health* 1985; 8:83–90.

When a husband has chronic obstructive pulmonary disease (COPD), the wife assumes new roles and responsibilities and faces new stresses. This research examined the effect of COPD on the life of wives.

The wives of COPD husbands reported new roles and responsibilities, poorer sleeping patterns, less frequent sexual relations, greater financial strain and reported their health status as low. The COPD wives also reported paying greater attention to their husband's health and environment than in the past and giving up social activities because of their husband. The COPD wives said their biggest problems were the husband's condition and symptoms, his attitude and irritability, and the loss of their personal freedom. These women said they live with considerable fear and worry about their husbands and the situation.

Nurses must attend to the care of both husband and wife. Nurses can provide guidance for these women. Support networks and respite care can allow the woman time for herself. Counseling and group meetings can offer the opportunity to talk and share feelings. These women need to have regular physical examinations and follow the advice of their care provider. The woman must be helped to learn to manage her daily activities in less stressful ways to attain some life satisfaction.

Smoking

More than 340,000 Americans die prematurely each year from disorders related to smoking; millions of others lead restricted lives because of pulmonary damage and cardiovascular impairment. The chemical agents in tobacco smoke reduce and eventually destroy ciliary movement in the bronchial mucosa, making the lungs more susceptible to infection. The hot smoke dries out and inflames the delicate tissues of the mouth, larynx, trachea, and lungs. Carbon monoxide in cigarette smoke combines with hemoglobin more readily than does oxygen; this competition reduces the amount of oxygen available to body tissues. Nicotine is a vasoconstrictor that reduces oxygen supply. Sensors in the blood and the tissues thus signal the heart to beat faster to make up the deficit. Tars in cigarette smoke have produced cancerous lesions in the lungs of test animals.

Unfortunately, cigarette smoking starts as early as grade school. Nearly a million teenagers start smoking each year, and the proportion of teenage girls who smoke is higher than the proportion of boys. Smoking by teenagers is often related to peer pressure, but most teenagers who smoke also have parents who do.

Smoking not only endangers the health of the smoker but pollutes the air breathed by nonsmokers. Public awareness of the hazards of smoking has led to requests for "no smoking" areas in restaurants and other public places. Nurses, as health professionals, are well qualified to help publicize the need for such facilities.

Nutrition and Exercise

Nutritional intake has little direct bearing on respiratory disorders, but overall health related to nutrition does affect susceptibility to infection. Individuals who are poorly nourished have a higher incidence of respiratory infections; moreover, they have less capacity to withstand disease or trauma. Nutritional status affects healing in the respiratory system as elsewhere in the body.

Some allergens in food may affect respiratory function, and some clients may have to curtail their intake of dairy products because these foods apparently overstimulate mucus production.

Overweight individuals may suffer from dyspnea because the excess tissue increases oxygen requirements. Movement of the chest wall and diaphragm may be restricted, particularly in clients who are extremely obese.

Clients with dyspnea may become anorectic. The mere act of eating may require more energy than they can summon, and the presence of large quantities of food in the stomach impedes the descent of the diaphragm during inspiration. Foods that stimulate flatus formation—beans, cabbage, cucumbers—may have to be curtailed to avoid excess pressure on the diaphragm. Clients may have to eat smaller meals at more frequent intervals.

Various studies have demonstrated that moderate exercise such as walking, if done regularly, can have beneficial effects on cardiovascular and respiratory capacity, another example of the value of incorporating healthy habits into one's lifestyle.

Environmental Factors

Airborne allergens can cause or aggravate respiratory disease. The most common respiratory disease associated with allergens is extrinsic asthma, which usually affects children but is sometimes seen in adults. Ragweed pollen and animal dander are related to allergic rhinitis and the uncomfortable symptoms associated with "hay fever."

Pollution of air by industrial and agricultural chemicals can increase the severity of numerous respiratory conditions, including long-term obstructive disorders. Individuals who have such conditions as chronic bronchitis may have to change their residence or stay indoors when pollution levels are high. Although increasing public awareness of pollution hazards has stimulated efforts by government and industry to reduce the quantity of pollutants released into the air, new technology is needed and much remains to be done. Nurses experienced in caring for victims of respiratory illness can alert their clients and the general public to the ill effects of air pollution.

Economic and Occupational Factors

Crowded living conditions increase the risk of respiratory disorders. The classic example is tuberculosis. Inadequate knowledge about risk factors and healthful lifestyles increases the likelihood of illness and decreases the likelihood that professional health care will be sought promptly.

Once long-term respiratory disease occurs, treatment can be costly, yet the earning capacity of the client is usually curtailed by disease symptoms such as dyspnea and pain. Frequent hospitalization may be necessary, disrupting employment still further, and home care equipment such as oxygen units or mechanical ventilators may have to be rented or purchased.

Occupation is a significant factor in the development of some respiratory disorders. "Black lung disease," which affects coal miners, is a well-publicized example; asbestosis is another. Solvents in paints and varnishes have also been implicated in respiratory disorders, not only among factory workers and professional painters but among hobbyists. A timely question about recent craft or hobby projects can yield a valuable diagnostic clue about a respiratory ailment. Clerks in dry cleaning establishments and beauticians exposed to permanent wave solutions (ammonia) and hair dyes may also develop respiratory abnormalities.

Existing respiratory problems can be made worse by exposure to chemical pollutants at work. The trend toward tightly insulated buildings brought about by the energy crisis has raised concerns about chemical pollution—eg, photocopying materials—in office environments that formerly were relatively hazard free. By being alert to occupational information in the client's history, the nurse can help identify individuals at risk and can counsel clients with respiratory disorders about possible hazards in their working environments.

Long-term respiratory illness will affect the client's capacity to work, often progressively. The client may have to find part-time work or a new occupation, depending on the kind of work the client does. A bank teller may be able to continue working almost indefinitely; a pneumatic drill operator will not. Loss of occupation will affect not only the client's income but the client's psychologic well-being as well. Thus, occupation, income, and respiratory status are interrelated, and any plan of care for the client must consider them all.

Social Factors

A disease that affects so fundamental an activity as breathing necessarily influences all aspects of the client's life, from intimate relationships to casual social contacts. Fear, anxiety, and anger related to symptoms and restrictions of activity place added burdens on an already compromised respiratory system and on personal relationships. Tensions rise, and depression is common.

As work activities are restricted, people see their position and value in their family and community as being threatened or destroyed. Another family member may have to step in as breadwinner; household chores and gardening must be taken over by others; the client feels displaced and disoriented. When sports or hobbies are abandoned because they require more energy than the damaged respiratory system can supply, the social relationships accompanying these activities are also lost.

Clients with breathing difficulties may avoid sexual contact or their mates may avoid them, fearing to worsen the illness. The depression that so often accompanies long-term illness diminishes sex drive, and some medications can cause or contribute to loss of libido and impotence. Lowered self-esteem, low energy, reduced strength, and easy fatigability also contribute to sexual difficulties. Clients who are unable to bring themselves to discuss these problems with their mates often find the nurse a nonthreatening confidante. Consultation with the psychiatric nurse on the health care team may provide the client sympathetic and helpful advice.

Chapter Highlights

The upper respiratory tract warms, filters, and humidifies inspired air. It consists of the nose, paranasal sinuses, pharynx, and larynx.

The trachea, bronchi, and bronchioles of the lower respiratory tract conduct air to and from the functional lobules of the lungs, where gas exchange takes place. The lobules are composed of respiratory bronchioles, alveolar ducts, and grapelike clusters of alveoli.

The defense mechanisms of the respiratory system include filtration, ciliary movement, mucus secretion, and the cough reflex.

Respiration is regulated by apneustic and pneumotaxic centers in the brain stem in response to chemical and mechanical stimulation of sensors in the bloodstream, tissues, and organs.

The lungs are kept inflated by subatmospheric pressure in the intrapleural space. Loss of normal intrapleural pressure from leakage of air into the intrapleural space can cause the lung on the affected side to collapse.

Excess levels of carbon dioxide in the blood (hypercapnia) stimulate the respiratory centers to increase rate and depth of ventilation.

Insufficient levels of oxygen in the blood (hypoxemia) stimulate chemoreceptors in the aortic arch and carotid arteries, sending impulses to the respiratory centers to increase ventilation.

The basic abnormalities of oxygen/carbon dioxide exchange are hypoventilation, diffusion impairment, and ventilation–perfusion inequality.

Air pollution by industrial and agricultural contaminants is related to a number of respiratory disorders.

Impairment of respiratory status has profound and far-reaching effects on the individual's psychosocial status, including occupation, social and family relationships, emotional state, and self-image.

Bibliography

American Lung Association: *Cigarette Smoking—The Facts About Your Lungs.* New York: American Lung Assn, 1982.

Broughton JO: Pathophysiology of the respiratory system. In: *Critical Care Nursing.* Hudak C, Lohr T, Gallo B (editors). Philadelphia: Lippincott, 1982.

Callahan M: COPD makes a bad first impression, but you'll find wonderful people underneath. *Nurs 82* (May) 1982; 12:68–72.

Crowley LV: *Introduction to Human Disease*. Belmont, CA: Wadsworth, 1983.

D'Alonzo GE, Dantzker DR: Respiratory failure: Mechanisms of abnormal gas exchange and oxygen delivery. *Med Clin North Am* 1983; 67:557–571.

Dudley DL et al: Psychosocial concomitants to rehabilitation in chronic obstructive pulmonary disease. *Chest* 1980; 77:413–420.

George RB, Light RW, Matthay RA: *Chest Medicine*. New York: Churchill Livingstone, 1983.

Petty TL: *Intensive and Rehabilitative Respiratory Care*. Philadelphia: Lea & Febiger, 1982.

Sexton D, Munro B: Impact of a husband's chronic llness (COPD) on the spouse's life. *Res Nurs Health* 1985; 8:83–90.

Spence AP, Mason ER: *Human Anatomy and Physiology*, 2nd ed. Menlo Park, CA: Addison–Wesley, 1983.

Subcommittee of the Research Committee of the British Thoracic Society: Smoking withdrawal in hospital patients: factors associated with outcome. *Thorax* Sept 1984; 39(9):651–656.

Traver GA: *Respiratory Nursing: The Science and the Art*. New York: Wiley, 1982.

CHAPTER **14**

The Nursing Process for Clients With Respiratory Dysfunction

Other topics relevant to this content are: Acid-base balance, **Chapter 3;** The health history and physical examination, **Chapter 5;** Nursing care of the client with tracheotomy or cricothyroidotomy, **Chapter 15**.

Objectives

When you have finished studying this chapter, you should be able to:

Specify the major components of the health history to be obtained from clients with respiratory disorders.

Explain specific assessment approaches in evaluating clients with respiratory disease.

Identify the nursing implications of diagnostic studies commonly used to evaluate clients with respiratory dysfunction.

Determine apppropriate nursing diagnoses for clients with respiratory disease.

Develop, with the client, realistic goals of care.

Anticipate the psychosocial/lifestyle implications of respiratory dysfunction for clients and their significant others.

Develop a nursing care plan for a client with respiratory dysfunction.

Implement nursing interventions specific to clients with respiratory problems.

Evaluate the effectiveness of the nursing care plan and modify it as necessary to meet client needs.

Alterations in the function of the respiratory system not only have localized effects but can alter the client's systemic physiologic function. For example, certain disorders may prevent the client from maintaining a clear airway or alter the mechanics of breathing. This can slowly or rapidly lead to impairment of carbon dioxide and oxygen exchange in the lungs. Nursing diagnoses used frequently when caring for clients with respiratory disorders include: airway clearance, ineffective; breathing pattern, ineffective; gas exchange, impaired; and activity intolerance.

SECTION 

Nursing Assessment: Establishing the Data Base

Subjective Data

Clients with disorders of the upper and lower airway may describe a variety of symptoms. These symptoms vary primarily with the location and severity of the disorder.

When the nasal airway is involved, clients often report a "stuffy nose" or decreased ability to breathe through the nose and sometimes a voice with a nasal quality. Other concerns may be a "runny nose" and a headache or feeling of fullness over the paranasal sinuses. People often say they have a "sinus headache." If nasal discharge is present, the client may report soreness around the nostrils. In some instances, clients may state they have nasal stuffiness but cannot remove secretions when blowing their noses. Reports of postnasal drip are not uncommon. These symptoms may be produced by an infection such as sinusitis or rhinitis. A decrease in the size of the nasal airway may be related to disorders such as nasal polyps, a deviated nasal septum, or a tumor.

The client should be questioned about the use of nose

drops and nose sprays and the frequency and amount of use. Also note if the client has obtained relief from this medication. Remember that rhinitis medicamentosa results from frequent and prolonged use of local vasoconstrictor nose drops and sprays. In this condition, use of nasal preparations causes an immediate vasoconstriction of the mucosal arterioles with temporary improvement in the airway, followed by vasodilation and nasal obstruction.

Dyspnea and Cough

A common symptom in clients with respiratory disorders is difficult breathing **(dyspnea).** Dyspnea is more often caused by disorders of the lower respiratory tract, such as COPD and carcinoma of the lung. Disorders of the upper airway that may cause dyspnea include obstruction of the airway by inflammation or obstruction by a foreign body or tumor. Clients should be asked whether they are short of breath during rest or exertion and, if so, what factors aggravate and alleviate the symptom.

Bronchospasm, retained secretions, edema, and obstruction by foreign objects can result in wheezing. This may be the chief concern of clients with asthma or allergic rhinitis. The client should be questioned about the frequency of wheezing and precipitating factors.

Another common symptom of respiratory disorders is a cough. A cough can result from irritation or from retained secretions that obstruct some part of the airway. Causative disorders in the upper airway may include sinusitis (leading to postnasal drip) and infections of the pharynx. Causative disorders in the lower respiratory tract include bronchitis, bronchiectasis, and pneumonia. Ask the client whether the cough is productive or nonproductive. If the cough is productive, ask about the color, amount, odor, and consistency of the sputum. Ask about precipitating factors and the frequency of the cough.

Chest Pain

Clients with respiratory dysfunction often describe sensations of pain and tenderness. Discomfort of the upper airway can be from an infection such as rhinitis, sinusitis, or pharyngitis. Trauma to the head and neck area can also cause pain in the upper respiratory tract.

Although chest pain is not uncommon for clients with respiratory system dysfunction, chest pain can also result from cardiovascular, gastrointestinal, hepatic–biliary, genitourinary, and musculoskeletal disorders. Difficulty with managing life stresses can also contribute to chest pain.

Use the seven dimensions or PQRST discussed in Chapter 5 as a guide to gathering a complete history of the pain. A careful history and physical examination are necessary to determine the origin of the pain so proper intervention can be carried out. Some disorders that cause chest pain, such as myocardial infarction or a punctured lung, can be fatal if not treated appropriately.

Voice Change and Dysphagia

Infections of the pharynx, vocal nodules, laryngeal paralysis, and laryngeal tumors can cause a voice change. Laryngeal paralysis results from damage to the recurrent or superior laryngeal nerve or the vagus nerve. For example, pressure on the recurrent laryngeal nerve from bronchogenic carcinoma or an aortic aneurysm can lead to paralysis of the vocal cord. Ask the client how long ago the voice change occurred and whether it is associated with pain when speaking or swallowing.

Dysphagia, a decrease in the client's ability to swallow, drink, and eat may result from disorders such as pharyngitis, infectious mononucleosis, peritonsillar abscess, and tumors of the oropharynx and laryngopharynx. Ask clients how long they have experienced the difficulty, if they experience pain when attempting to swallow, and if a sensation of choking or gagging occurs. Determine whether nutritional intake has been affected. Ask specifically how much the client has been able to eat and drink since the problem was noticed.

Fatigue and Weight Change

Clients may also have generalized feelings of fatigue. This may result from respiratory infections or other conditions that alter the normal levels of oxygen and carbon dioxide in the body. Neoplastic disorders also cause fatigue because of increased metabolic demands.

Determine whether the client has had a weight change. A weight loss may be deliberate or may result from a neoplastic process or COPD. A weight gain may indicate fluid retention secondary to pulmonary edema or congestive heart failure. Ask how much weight was lost or gained, over how long, and whether the client's appetite increased or decreased during the change.

Many disorders of the respiratory tract may lead to an alteration in carbon dioxide and oxygen levels in the blood. This imbalance may manifest itself as respiratory acidosis or respiratory alkalosis. Respiratory acidosis and alkalosis are discussed in Section II of this chapter and also in Chapter 3. Clients in an acidotic state may have headache, double vision, weakness, drowsiness, and difficulty in breathing. These symptoms can result from hypoxia and/or hypercapnia. Clients who are in an alkalotic state may report they are dizzy and have a tingling sensation in the fingers and toes. These subjective feelings are the result of hypocapnia.

Habit History

Obtain a detailed smoking history from the client. Cigars, pipes, and chewing tobacco should be included along with cigarettes. Smoking has been implicated as a risk factor in the development of lung cancer, cancer of the head and neck, and COPD. Smoking also aggravates upper respiratory symptoms such as rhinorrhea, sinusitis, and pharyngitis because of damage to the cilia and mucous membranes. The longer the person has smoked and the greater the number of cigarettes, the greater the risk of developing respiratory disorders. Clients who smoke should be asked how many cigarettes they smoke each day? What brand? Filtered or nonfiltered? How many years have they smoked? Do they inhale? Clients who have stopped smoking should be asked the date they quit smoking in addition to the previous questions. The client's smoking history is recorded in pack years (number of packs per day × the number of years they have smoked). For example, the client who has smoked 2 packs per day for 10 years, has a 20 pack-year smoking history.

Clients should also be asked if they use chewing tobacco, since this has been implicated as a factor in the development of cancers of the mouth, larynx, throat, and esophagus (American Cancer Society, 1987). The nurse should determine how long the client has chewed tobacco and how frequently it is used.

An excessive use of alcohol has been implicated as a predisposing factor in the development of tuberculosis, pneumonia, and cancers of the mouth, larynx, throat, esophagus, and liver (American Cancer Society, 1987). Clients should be questioned specifically about what they drink, how much per day, and how long they have been drinking. Clients may tend to minimize their drinking. Therefore, a careful, sensitive, nonjudgmental approach is needed when asking questions related to alcohol intake.

Past Health History

Obtain a thorough history of past respiratory, face, neck, and thoracic problems. Has the client ever had maxillofacial trauma or rib fractures? Is there any history of scoliosis or thoracic deformity? Has the client ever had a positive tuberculosis skin test or abnormal chest x-ray? Has the client ever had respiratory complications following general anesthesia or surgery? A history of any of these could contribute to the current health problem of the client.

ALLERGY AND MEDICATION HISTORY Find out whether the client has any history of allergies. Allergies can cause sinusitis, allergic rhinitis, and asthma. If the client has a history of allergies, ask how long the allergic symptoms have been present, what the symptoms are (severe difficulty breathing? a runny nose? watery eyes?), has allergy testing been done, have specific allergens been identified, whether the client is receiving allergy shots, and what specific medications relieve the symptoms.

Ask clients about all medications they are taking and why. Also ask if clients are using medications as prescribed and if they seem to provide the desired effects.

OCCUPATIONAL AND TRAVEL HISTORY Exposure to certain chemical agents and other irritants can result in respiratory disorders. Therefore, a thorough occupational history is obtained. Two common occupational diseases are asbestosis and silicosis. Clients should be asked if they work or have ever worked in a job that exposed them to chemical fumes, dust, smoke, or asbestos.

Does the client work in an environment with people who smoke? Do the windows open to allow fresh air to enter or is the air recirculated?

The client's recent travel history is important because some infectious disorders affecting the lungs are endemic to certain geographic regions.

Family History

Information should be gathered on respiratory problems in blood relatives. Any family history of allergies, asthma, chronic bronchitis, emphysema, tuberculosis, or malignancy should be documented. Did the client grow up in a family of smokers? Does the client live with a smoker? Does anyone in the home or in the family have symptoms like the client's?

Objective Data

Physical Assesssment

When performing a physical assessment of clients suspected of having a respiratory disorder, the nurse uses the skills of inspection, palpation, and auscultation.

INSPECTION The size and shape of the nose should be noted. An alteration in its shape may be the result of trauma or a tumor in or near the nose. Assess the characteristics of the nasal secretions. They may be watery, mucoid, mucopurulent, purulent, or bloody. Watery discharge is usually of viral origin. Secretions that are mucoid or mucopurulent may result from inflammation, as in acute rhinitis or allergic rhinitis. Mucopurulent secretions often result from infectious processes, as when acute rhinitis progresses. Purulent discharge is usually of bacterial origin. Blood may drain from the nares because of irritation or trauma.

Structures of the oropharynx may be enlarged, reddened, and covered with secretions. The color of the oral mucosa should be noted. White patches or spots on the mucous membrane of the cheek or tongue (leukoplakia) may indicate a premalignant lesion. Observe for inflammation, swelling, bleeding, retraction, or distortion. Inflammation and secretions are often present with infections such as pharyngitis. Bleeding, retraction, or distortion of the area may be from a neoplasm of the oropharynx or an infectious process. Inspect the uvula, fauces, and pharyngeal tonsils as part of the examination. These areas may be distorted in disorders such as peritonsillar abscess, infectious mononucleosis, and tumors of the pharynx.

Examine the neck for enlarged lymph nodes. Enlarge-

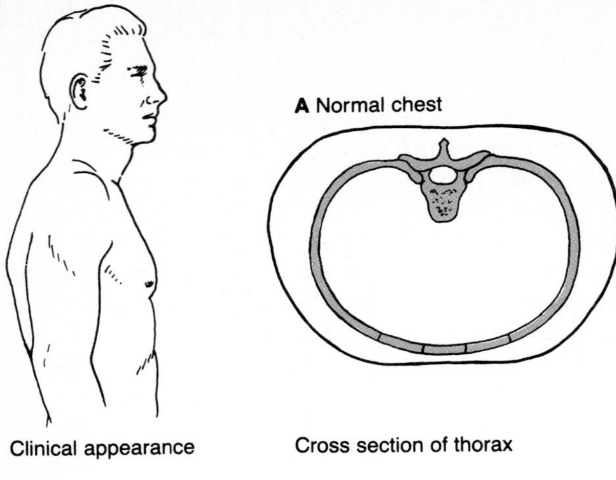

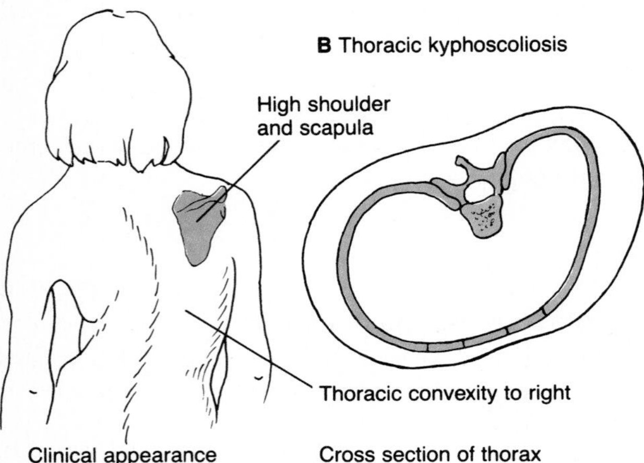

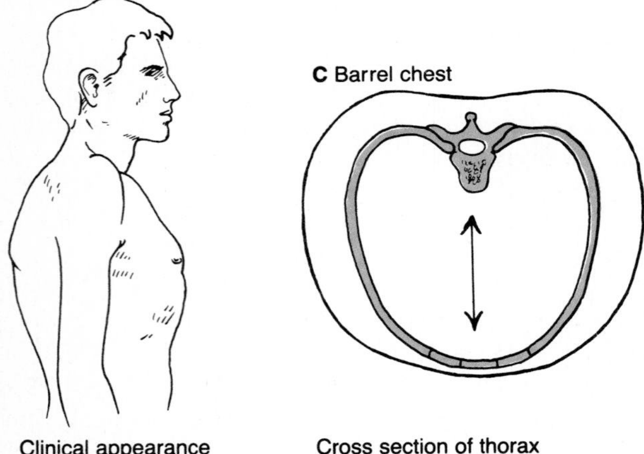

Figure 14–1

Cross section of thorax. **A.** Normal. **B.** Thoracic kyphoscoliosis. **C.** Barrel chest in COPD.

ment may be the result of common upper respiratory infections, mononucleosis, lymphoma, or metastatic cancer.

Inspection of the chest may reveal thoracic deformities such as kyphoscoliosis or an increased anteroposterior (AP) diameter (barrel chest). Kyphoscoliosis reduces thoracic movement and limits lung expansion. "Barrel chest" is a common finding in clients with COPD (Figure 14–1). Asymmetrical chest expansion can result from trauma (pneumothorax, hemothorax, flail chest).

General overall appearance such as facial expression, posture, and ease of movement should be assessed. Clients with COPD may have to sit up to breathe or lean forward in a chair resting their arms on tables for support.

Examination of sputum may reveal thick tenacious secretions; mucus plugs; or purulent, bloody, or blood-tinged sputum (**hemoptysis**). Secretions that are yellow–green or foul smelling may indicate an infectious process. Sputum that is pink or rust-colored may indicate bleeding, which can result from irritation, infection, or neoplasia.

The pattern and character of respirations should be observed. This includes rate and depth of breathing and the presence of labored breathing. Labored breathing may be marked by nasal flaring, the use of neck and accessory chest muscles, asymmetry of chest expansion, and increase in respiratory rate. This occurs in conditions such as airway obstruction by a foreign body, COPD, and mediastinal shift. Pursed-lip breathing, a slow, relaxed expiration against pursed lips, prevents collapse of small bronchioles and reduces the amount of trapped air. It is characteristic of clients with emphysema. Chest trauma may result in subcutaneous emphysema (air under the skin), which can compromise the airway.

When inspecting clients with respiratory disorders, also observe for signs of respiratory acidosis, respiratory alkalosis, and hypoxemia. Disorders that can lead to acidosis are COPD, pneumonia, or respiratory depression due to trauma or drugs. Clinical manifestations of respiratory acidosis or hypercapnia include: confusion, drowsiness, dizziness, tetany, and asterixis. Tachycardia and dysrhythmias may be present. Late signs of hypercapnia are convulsions and coma.

Respiratory alkalosis occurs in conditions resulting in hyperventilation. Disorders that may lead to hyperventilation include brain injury or tumors, gram-negative sepsis, acute asthmatic attacks, and extreme anxiety. Manifestations of respiratory alkalosis are related to stimulation of the nervous system. The nurse may observe muscle spasms, which can be in the form of carpopedal spasm—contractions of the hands and feet. The client's thumb is flexed, wrist and metacarpophalangeal joints are flexed, the interphalangeal joints are hyperextended, and fingers are adducted in the form of a cone. Severe spasms can progress to tetany or continuous muscle contractions. Diaphoresis and cardiac dysrhythmias may occur. The client will be tachypneic and may lose consciousness.

When the respiratory system is affected by disease, the ability to deliver oxygen to the tissues may become impaired, resulting in **hypoxia** (insufficient oxygen to cells) or **hypoxemia** (inadequate blood oxygen levels). Conditions that limit the volume of air entering the lungs result in inadequate amounts of available oxygen at the alveolar level. Disorders leading to hypoxia or hypoxemia include restrictive lung diseases (such as pulmonary fibrosis, occupational lung diseases, and sarcoidosis), obstructive lung diseases (such as asthma, chronic bronchitis, and emphysema), and occasionally, morbid obesity. Any disorder that lowers the oxygen-carrying capacity of the hemoglobin in the blood will also produce tissue hypoxia.

The symptoms manifested by acute hypoxia are reflected in the neurologic, cardiovascular, and respiratory systems. Deprivation of oxygen to the brain causes signs of restlessness, irritability, and mental confusion. Effects on the cardiovascular system include tachycardia, hypertension, and cardiac dysrhythmias. Respiratory manifestations are tachypnea and dyspnea. As the condition worsens, the client may become comatose with a decrease in respiratory rate, heart rate, and blood pressure. Manifestations of chronic hypoxia include exercise intolerance, a general feeling of fatigue, and clubbing of the fingers.

PALPATION Palpation of structures of the upper respiratory tract may reveal swelling, which results from the growth of neoplasms or from an infectious process. Palpate the areas over the frontal and maxillary sinuses. With sinusitis, clients may feel tenderness or pressure. The neck should also be palpated for the presence of enlarged lymph nodes.

With palpation over the chest, tactile fremitus, a palpable vibration of air as the client speaks, will be increased with excessive secretions, tumors, or pneumonia. Fluid-filled or solid structures transmit vibrations better than structures filled with air. A decrease in vocal fremitus is present in pleural effusion, since it slows the transmission of sound.

Crepitation is palpable when small air bubbles are present underneath the skin (subcutaneous emphysema). Touching the area results in a crackling sensation. Intercostal bulging may be noted in a client who has lung abscesses, tumors, or rib fractures. A deviation of the trachea may be palpated in conditions such as tension pneumothorax and neck masses.

AUSCULTATION Auscultation of the lungs is performed to determine the presence or absence of abnormal breath sounds. Bronchial or tracheal, bronchovesicular, and vesicular breath sounds are normal respiratory sounds in certain areas of the lungs. However, auscultation of these sounds in areas where they are not normally heard may indicate pathology. The presence of bronchial or tracheal sounds over the periphery of the lung may be an indication of atelectasis or consolidation. The presence of bronchovesicular sounds over the peripheral lung tissue may also indicate consolidation. Decreased vesicular sounds in the peripheral lung may be present in early pneumonia or emphysema.

Adventitious or abnormal breath sounds may also be heard during auscultation. These can include: fine to medium rales, medium to coarse rales, rhonchi, wheezing, and friction rubs. Fine to medium rales may indicate pneumonia. Medium to coarse rales are heard in bronchitis, pneumonia, bronchiectasis, emphysema, and pleural effusion. Wheezing may be noted in clients with asthma and COPD. Rhonchi indicate an obstructive mass or secretions in the larger airways. A friction rub may be heard in clients with pneumonia, lung cancer, pleurisy, or tuberculosis.

Diagnostic Studies

PULMONARY FUNCTION TESTS Pulmonary function tests measure the functional ability of the lungs. More specifically, they:

- Provide objective evidence of the presence, type, and degree of lung abnormality
- Monitor the course of a disease process over time
- Evaluate the effectiveness of various medications on breathing function
- Determine the risk of respiratory complications of surgical procedures

In routine pulmonary function studies, the client's lung size and breathing ability are compared with values for normal individuals who are similar to the client in age, sex, height, and race. The spirometer is the primary instrument used in this test. Spirometry provides an easy and inexpensive method to measure lung volume with relatively little risk to the client. Several different types of spirometers are used to measure lung volumes; the most common are electronic computerized units and the kymograph.

Pulmonary function study results can show either a restriction or an obstruction to airflow or a combination. Disease conditions that commonly result in a restriction to airflow include certain neuromuscular disorders such as myasthenia gravis, thoracic deformities such as kyphoscoliosis, restriction to lung expansion as occurs in pneumothorax and fibrosis, or infiltrative diseases such as tuberculosis and lung cancer. These restrictive conditions cause a reduction in lung compliance, which decreases chest expansion and therefore decreases the volume of air inspired and expired (Wade, 1982). Disorders that result in pathologic changes of the airways or alveoli obstruct airflow into and out of the lungs. These include chronic bronchitis, emphysema, asthma, and bronchiectasis.

NURSING IMPLICATIONS To allay anxieties, clients should be told how the test will be conducted and what will be expected of them. It is important to explain that the test is not painful or harmful in any way. Some clients may need to be reassured that the degree of exertion necessary to complete the test will not cause injury to their lungs. Others may fear their lungs will burst or that they will be unable to catch their breath. Explain the technique and equipment to clients in terms they can understand. This will aid in lowering client anxiety and increasing cooperation. Clients should be told their noses will be clamped intermittently and they will be asked to breathe in and out through a mouthpiece connected to a machine. The client should understand that accurate results can be obtained only by following instructions carefully. Since gastric distention may impair ability to expand the lungs, tests should be performed before meals. Medications that may alter respiratory function, such as bronchodilators, should be withheld unless otherwise indicated by the physician (Wade, 1982).

Before the test, the client is asked to loosen any constricting clothing that might interfere with chest expansion. The client may be either sitting or standing. The client should be told to seal both lips around the mouthpiece and keep the nose clip on because air leakage would make the test results inaccurate. The client is then asked to breathe as normally as possible through the spirometer and does not begin the next step until comfortable with breathing normally on the machine. At the completion of four or five normal breaths, the client is told to breathe in as much air as possible, to fill the lungs far more than usual, and then to blow out all the air from the lungs. The volume breathed in and that breathed out are the measures, along with the time needed for expiration.

LUNG VOLUMES AND CAPACITIES Lung volumes and capacities as measured by spirometry are shown in Figure 14–2. The values given for pulmonary function tests are average values for a young adult male. Values for women are approximately 10% to 25% less. (Some women, of course, will show higher values than some men.)

- **Lung volumes**
  • Tidal volume (TV) is the amount of air inspired and expired with each normal breath. The normal is approximately 500 mL.
  • Inspiratory reserve volume (IRV) is the additional volume of air that can be inspired beyond the normal tidal volume. It amounts to approximately 3000 mL.
  • Expiratory reserve volume (ERV) is the volume of air that can be forcefully expired at the end of the normal tidal expiration. This is about 1100 mL.
  • Residual volume (RV) consists of the amount of air that remains in the lungs after a forceful expiration. This equals about 1200 mL.
- **Lung capacities.** When discussing the pulmonary cycle, it is often helpful to consider two or more of the pulmonary volumes together. These combinations are referred to as pulmonary capacities. The four capacities include:
  • Inspiratory capacity (IC) is the volume of air that a person can inspire from a resting level. This equals the tidal volume plus the inspiratory reserve volume, and amounts to about 3500 mL.
  • Functional residual capacity (FRC) is the volume of air remaining in the lungs after a normal expiration. It equals the expiratory reserve volume plus the residual volume, and is about 2300 mL.
  • Vital capacity (VC) is the maximum volume of air that can be exhaled forcefully from the lungs following a maximal inspiration. This equals the inspiratory reserve volume plus the tidal volume plus the expiratory reserve volume; it totals about 4600 mL.
  • Total lung capacity (TLC) refers to the maximum volume to which the lungs can be expanded with the greatest possible inspiratory effort. It equals the vital capacity plus the residual volume and is approximately 5900 mL.
- **Pulmonary volumes** measured in time intervals
  • Forced vital capacity (FVC) is the maximal pulmonary volume the client has for ventilation. The client inhales the maximum amount of air and then forcefully exhales as fast as possible. The amount of air the client can forcefully exhale within specific time periods is calculated. The usual time periods are 1, 2, and 3 seconds. Forced vital capacity is also referred to as the forced expiratory volume in 1, 2, or 3 seconds (FEV 1.0, FEV 2.0, FEV 3.0). A healthy individual can usu-

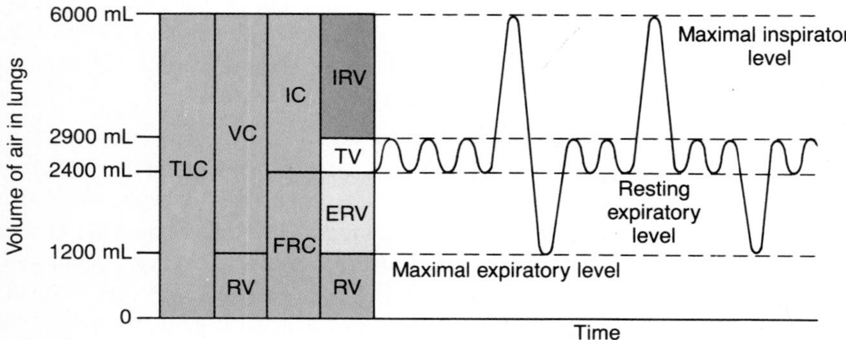

Figure 14–2

Measurement of lung volumes and capacities by spirometry.

ally exhale approximately 75% of vital capacity in 1 second and all of it by 3 seconds (Harper, 1981).

• Minute respiratory volume (MRV) is the amount of air moved into the respiratory passages each minute. This consists of the tidal volume times the respiratory rate. The normal finding is approximately 6 L/min.

PARANASAL SINUS FILMS Clients suspected of having sinusitis may benefit from evaluation with paranasal sinus films. Roentgenographic examination of the paranasal sinuses may also be ordered for clients with head trauma and those suspected of having sinus neoplasms. Traditional x-ray assessment of the paranasal sinuses often necessitates a series of different views.

NURSING IMPLICATIONS The nurse should explain the procedure in terms the client can understand. Clients should be told that x-ray films will be taken of their sinuses from different views, and that the process will not cause them much if any discomfort. Clients will be asked to hold the head in certain positions against the x-ray plate. The nurse might find it helpful to compare the process to a chest x-ray since most clients have had these.

CHEST X-RAY Chest x-ray, one of the most common procedures used to evaluate the lungs, is part of the evaluation of most clients suspected of having pulmonary disease, except during pregnancy. The evaluation should include a posteroanterior (PA) view and at least one lateral film.

In PA views, the upright position is used because the diaphragm is lower and the lungs are larger. The client is asked to take a deep breath and hold it for a few seconds. An x-ray beam is projected from the back to the front of the client. Since the heart and mediastinum are in the front of the thorax, in this position magnification on the x-ray is much less than in an anteroposterior (AP) film. Individuals who are very ill, infants, and young children are usually x-rayed lying down in the supine or anteroposterior (AP) position (George, Light, & Matthay, 1983).

Lateral views add information about areas of the lungs that cannot be viewed well in the PA position, such as the anterior part of the lung close to the mediastinum. Oblique views are beneficial in delineating pulmonary or mediastinal masses or lesions, and pleural effusion that may not be well demonstrated on PA or lateral views. The lateral decubitus view is used to detect a small amount of free pleural fluid, pneumothorax, cavitation, or lung abscess. This view is taken with the client in the side-lying position. General abnormal findings that may be evident on chest x-ray include areas of density (may be related to atelectasis, pneumonia, or a pneumothorax), hypersecretion, presence of masses, and increased vascular markings.

NURSING IMPLICATIONS The procedure should be explained in terms that the client can understand. In a chest x-ray, an x-ray beam passes through the body to a film. The films obtained will provide the radiologist with information about the structure and function of the lungs. Clients may have misconceptions about the physiologic effects of exposure to diagnostic x-rays (eg, fears of cancer). Allow the client to verbalize these fears and then provide correct information. If the client is pregnant, x-rays are avoided unless absolutely necessary. If critical illness of a pregnant woman necessitates a chest x-ray, the abdomen is protected with a lead shield.

For a chest x-ray, clients are asked to remove clothing down to the waist and don an open-backed gown. They will be asked to inhale and hold their breath for a few seconds. If the client is connected to equipment such as a ventilator, the tubing should be placed above the level of the chest. Tubing and jewelry may appear as shadows on the film.

When clients are acutely ill, portable chest x-rays may be necessary. The quality of a chest film taken with a portable x-ray is not as good as the film taken in the x-ray department because the client cannot be positioned for the best view, nor can the x-ray equipment. To increase the quality of these films, the client should be sitting completely upright. Visitors and other staff members should be asked to leave the immediate area. Personnel who must remain in the room while the x-ray is taken should be protected by lead aprons. Pregnant personnel or pregnant visitors should *never* be exposed to x-rays.

BRONCHOGRAPHY On a chest x-ray, a small portion of the bronchial tree beyond the first two major divisions is visible. To diagnose abnormalities of the smaller sections of the bronchial tree, bronchography may be performed. The diagnostic test begins with instillation of radiopaque contrast medium through a catheter into the lumen of the trachea and bronchial tree. Chest x-rays are then taken.

Bronchography is primarily indicated for diagnosing bronchiectasis and determining its location before surgical resection. Bronchography may also aid in diagnosing compression, obstruction, presence of a foreign body, or a lesion in the trachea or larger bronchi.

NURSING IMPLICATIONS Explain the procedure and make sure that the client understands the explanation. This includes informing clients that they will be placed in various positions to aid in distribution of the dye. Question the client and also check the chart for known hypersensitivity to the dye used for the procedure.

Proper visualization requires that the airways be as free of secretions as possible. To achieve this, the nurse may have to carry out bronchial drainage, nasotracheal suctioning, or both. The client should have nothing by mouth for several hours prior to the procedure. A signed consent is necessary.

After completion of the procedure, monitor the client's vital signs. To facilitate removal of the contrast medium, deep breathing and sighing, postural drainage, and nasotracheal suctioning are usually necessary. Before allowing the client to drink, check for return of the gag reflex by stimulating the posterior pharynx with a swab or tongue blade. If the reflex is not yet present, the client will not gag and is vulnerable to aspiration.

TOMOGRAMS Tomograms are views of the area in horizontal, sagittal, and coronal planes. This method is used when conventional x-rays cannot detect the extent of the pathologic process or when the area is obscured by other structures. Tomograms allow visualization of minute structures. The major application of tomography of the nose and paranasal sinuses is in determining the presence of fractures or bone destruction due to a tumor. Tomography of the thorax is indicated when more precise knowledge of the morphologic characteristics of lesions is needed.

NURSING IMPLICATIONS Tell the client that films will be taken of the areas that allow the physician to see different sections of tissue from several angles, to identify changes that traditional x-ray films cannot show. Clients should be told that the procedure will not cause them any discomfort. Some of the equipment may be rather large and noisy, however.

LUNG SCAN A lung scan may be classified as either a perfusion scan or a ventilation scan. To obtain a *perfusion* scan, radioactive dye is administered intravenously. When the dye is injected, the client should be supine and breathing normally to produce a uniform distribution of radioactive particles that are trapped in the pulmonary capillary bed. The scan may begin immediately after injection of the dye. Anterior, posterior, both lateral views, and both posterior oblique views are obtained. An x-ray of the lung should be obtained at the same time so comparisons can be made.

Ventilation scans are usually performed using inert gases. The client should be sitting or supine. Clients will usually wear a tightly fitting facial mask that allows them to breathe radioactive gas for a few minutes. Depending on the type of gas, clients may need only to breathe through a nasal cannula.

Ventilation and perfusion scanning are used to diagnose pulmonary embolism, lung cancer, COPD, pulmonary edema, and pulmonary infections. Unlike most pulmonary function tests, the lung scan can measure regional lung function. This makes possible the diagnosis of pulmonary diseases at an earlier stage, before other parameters of respiratory function become abnormal.

NURSING IMPLICATIONS Explain that the purpose of the test is to determine if all of the client's lung tissue has adequate circulation and if air is reaching areas as it should. Clients should know they will receive radioactive dye IV for a perfusion scan. Any history of an allergic reaction to dye used in diagnostic tests must be documented beforehand and brought to the attention of the physician. The nurse should stress that clients should try to relax and breathe normally during the test. Clients should be told that a machine will move over the chest to obtain different views of the lungs. A conventional chest x-ray will also be taken at that time.

Clients should be informed that during a ventilation scan they will be asked to breathe a mixture of gases through a mask or nasal cannula so that the air flowing in and out of their lungs can be traced. Inhalation of this gaseous mixture should not cause them discomfort. A machine will move over their chest to obtain different views.

ARTERIAL BLOOD GAS ANALYSIS Arterial blood is collected for analysis of the pH, PCO_2, PO_2, oxygen saturation, bicarbonate level, and base excess. These values show how well the client's lungs are delivering oxygen to the bloodstream and eliminating the waste product of cellular metabolism, carbon dioxide. Individual values are discussed below.

pH The normal pH of arterial blood is 7.35 to 7.45. Values below 7.35 indicate acidemia, while those above 7.45 are indicative of alkalemia. The normal pH range is maintained primarily by two buffers—carbonic acid (H_2CO_3) and bicarbonate (HCO_3).

The normal ratio of carbonic acid to bicarbonate (1:20) must be maintained; otherwise, the pH will not be within the normal range. The lungs control the carbonic acid by selectively retaining or ventilating the carbon dioxide (CO_2) that combines with water to form the carbonic acid's hydrogen ion. The bicarbonate portion of the balance is controlled by the kidneys, which excrete either alkaline or acidic urine. Chapter 3 gives a detailed explanation of acid–base balance.

The normal range of PCO_2 in the arterial blood is 35 to 45 mm Hg. An elevation of PCO_2 above 45 mm Hg may be indicative of hypoventilation, which results in respiratory acidosis, or it may result from compensated metabolic alkalosis. A PCO_2 below 35 mm Hg may arise from hyperventilation, which can result in respiratory alkalosis or from compensatory metabolic acidosis.

The normal value of PO_2 in arterial blood is 80 to 100 mm Hg. This value has no direct bearing on the pH but is an important indication of whether adequate oxygen is available for cellular metabolism. A PO_2 elevation may be seen in clients who are receiving a high-liter flow of oxygen. Prolonged elevation in PO_2 levels can result in damage to the pulmonary tissue.

OXYGEN SATURATION The extent of oxygen saturation, the amount of hemoglobin combined with oxygen, is expressed as a percentage of the blood's capacity for full saturation. The normal value is 95% to 98% in arterial blood. Figure 14–3 represents the oxyhemoglobin dissociation curve—the binding capacity that hemoglobin has for oxygen. The flat part of the curve represents strong

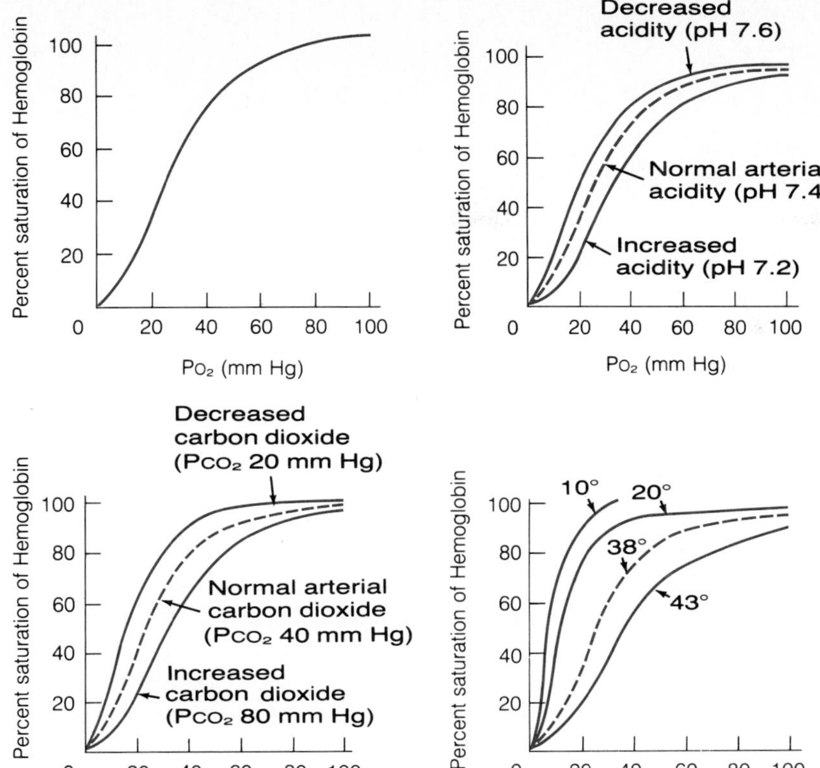

Figure 14–3

Oxyhemoglobin dissociation curves. SOURCE: *Spence AP, Mason EB:* Human Anatomy and Physiology, *3rd ed. Menlo Park, CA: Benjamin/Cummings, 1987.*

hemoglobin binding capacity for oxygen; reduction in the amount of arterial oxygen (PO_2) does not significantly reduce the percentage of saturation of hemoglobin with oxygen. The steep part of the curve represents the situation where oxygen is dissociated or released from the hemoglobin.

A shift of the curve to the *right* means oxygen is released to the tissues more readily. Factors that can cause a shift to the right include acidosis, chronic hypoxemia, hypercapnia, and an elevated temperature. A shift of the curve to the *left* can result from alkalosis, hypocapnia, and a decrease in temperature. These conditions result in increased binding of oxygen to hemoglobin.

BICARBONATE ION Bicarbonate is a negative ion whose normal value in arterial blood is 22 to 26 mEq/L. A lower value is indicative of metabolic acidosis or compensation for respiratory alkalosis. A value above 26 mEq/L is indicative of metabolic alkalosis or compensated respiratory acidosis.

BASE EXCESS The base excess represents an increase or a decrease in the total amount of buffer bases available. The normal range is −2 to +2 mEq/L in arterial blood. This value is considered a more reliable indication of the true metabolic makeup of an acid–base disturbance than the bicarbonate value. An increase indicates metabolic alkalosis or compensated respiratory acidosis. A decrease indicates metabolic acidosis or compensated respiratory alkalosis.

NURSING IMPLICATIONS For arterial blood gas tests, tell the client that a small amount of blood needs to be obtained from an artery to determine how well the lungs are functioning in the transport of oxygen and carbon dioxide. Common sites for obtaining an arterial blood gas sample are the radial, brachial, and femoral arteries.

After the blood gas is drawn, pressure must be applied to the puncture site for at least *5 minutes* or longer, particularly if the client is receiving anticoagulants. This should be followed by application of a dressing, preferably a pressure dressing. The arterial blood sample must be protected from atmospheric oxygen by removing the needle and capping the tip of the syringe. The syringe is then rotated so the blood and heparin are mixed together to prevent clotting. The sample is then immediately placed in ice (to slow down oxygen metabolism) and taken to the lab for analysis.

CULTURES A culture is the growing of bacteria or other microorganisms from a specimen of material obtained in an aseptic manner or using sterile technique. Sterile technique is necessary whenever cultures are needed. The specimen is placed in an environment where organisms can grow. When the microorganisms increase, laboratory personnel can isolate and identify the pathogen. Sensitivity studies are then done to determine which antimicrobial drug is effective against the organism. The organism can be described as sensitive or resistant to specific antibiotics. This helps the physician select the most effective agent for drug therapy.

Specimens are examined in direct smears, stained and unstained. The most frequent staining test is Gram's stain, which distinguishes among bacteria with similar morphology by classifying them as gram-negative or gram-positive. Certain organisms such as the tubercle bacilli and other mycobacteria cannot be stained using this method and require acid-fast staining techniques.

NURSING IMPLICATIONS Obtaining a nose or throat culture rarely causes the client discomfort, but tell the client that a cotton swab will be inserted into the nose or throat to obtain a specimen. Explain the purpose for the specimen—that is, to identify organisms present and which antibiotic will suppress them. Nose and throat cultures are obtained by the following methods:

- For cultures from the nares, introduce the swab as far back as possible without bending it and rotate it gently.
- For cultures from the pharynx (throat), avoid touching the tongue or teeth, which would result in contamination. Depress the tongue with a tongue blade. Swab the posterior wall of the pharynx below the level of the uvula. The swab should be rotated over any involved or inflamed areas. The specimen collected on the swab should be placed in the appropriate container and taken to the laboratory as soon as possible to prevent drying of the organisms.

Sputum cultures are often indicated in problems of the respiratory system. Obtaining sputum specimens is discussed in the next section. Other culture specimens (eg, from abscesses in the lungs) are obtained during bronchoscopy.

SPUTUM CYTOLOGY Sputum cytology involves the detailed examination of the cellular structures of sputum under a microscope. This is primarily done to assist in the identification of malignant cells in individuals suspected of having lung cancer.

NURSING IMPLICATIONS When obtaining a sputum specimen, keep in mind:

- The optimal time for obtaining a specimen is early in the morning. The first sputum expectorated will contain secretions that have pooled in the client's lungs during the night, giving a more productive sample.
- To decrease contamination of the sputum, the client should rinse out the mouth without swallowing, brush the teeth, or both.
- For a true sputum sample (not saliva), the client should take several deep breaths and then cough forcefully.
- If the client cannot cough up a sputum sample, three different techniques can be used to obtain the specimen: postural drainage, inhalation of cold steam or nebulized vapor, and suctioning. If suctioning is used, a sputum collection trap is used to obtain a sterile sample (Figure 14–4).
- When cultures are being obtained, the specimens should be collected in sterile containers using sterile technique.

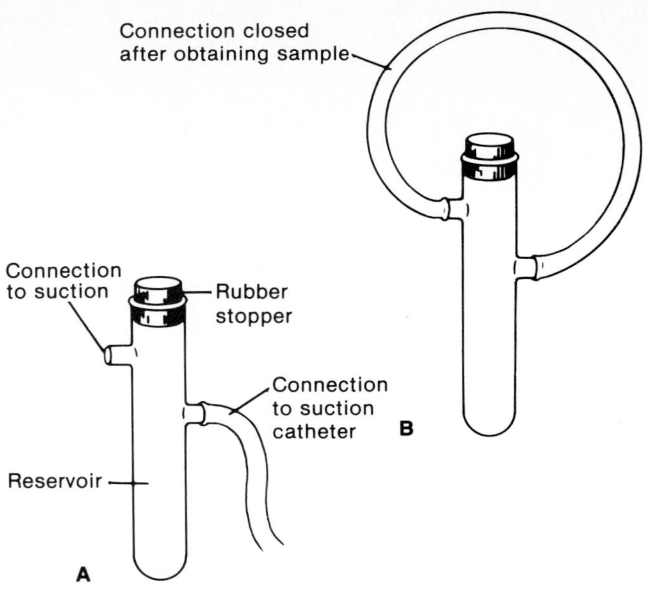

Figure 14–4

A. Sputum trap (Lukin's tube) used when suctioning is necessary to collect a sterile sputum specimen. **B.** Tubing is disconnected from suction catheter and connected to suction orifice to maintain asepsis.

SKIN TESTS

MANTOUX INTRADERMAL SKIN TEST This test is used in the detection of tuberculosis (TBC). Anyone infected with the tubercle bacillus develops hypersensitivity to certain products of the organism. The method of administering the test is to inject 0.1 mL of purified protein derivative (PPD) intradermally on the inner aspect of the forearm, with the bevel of the needle upward. If the fluid is injected properly, a raised area 6 to 10 mm in diameter will appear on the surface of the skin. Anyone who has been previously sensitized will show an induration (hardening) and erythema at the injection site as T-lymphocytes collect there over 48 to 72 hours. It usually requires 2 to 10 weeks after the initial infection with the bacilli for a positive tuberculin test. An induration measuring 10 mm or more within 72 hours is considered indicative of infection with *Mycobacterium tuberculosis* (Figure 14–5). A reading of between 5 and 9 mm of induration is considered doubtful unless there is known exposure to the organism. With 0 to 4 mm of induration, the result is considered negative.

The tuberculin test is not 100% accurate. A positive test merely indicates that tuberculosis exposure occurred at some point in the past. It does not mean active disease is present. Also, a negative reaction does not necessarily rule out TBC. Incorrect results may occur because of errors in the administration and reading of the test, the nature of the test material, or factors related to the test subjects. Clients with certain illnesses, those who are poorly nourished, or those on immunosuppressive drugs can have false negative reactions to the Mantoux skin test. False positive reactions can occur because *Mycobacterium tuberculosis*

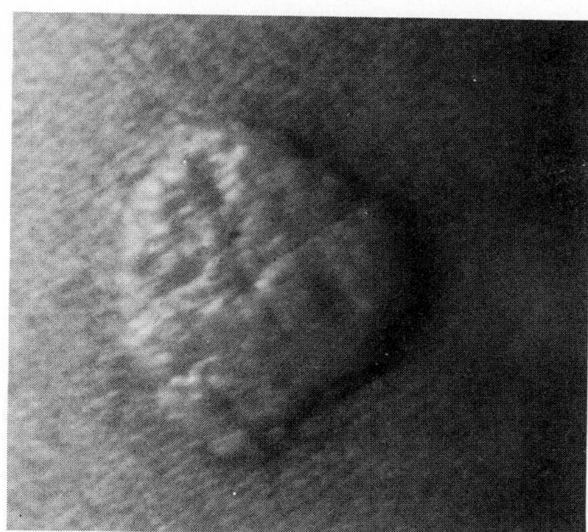

Figure 14–5

Positive Mantoux test. *Courtesy of Millard Fillmore Hospital, Buffalo, NY.*

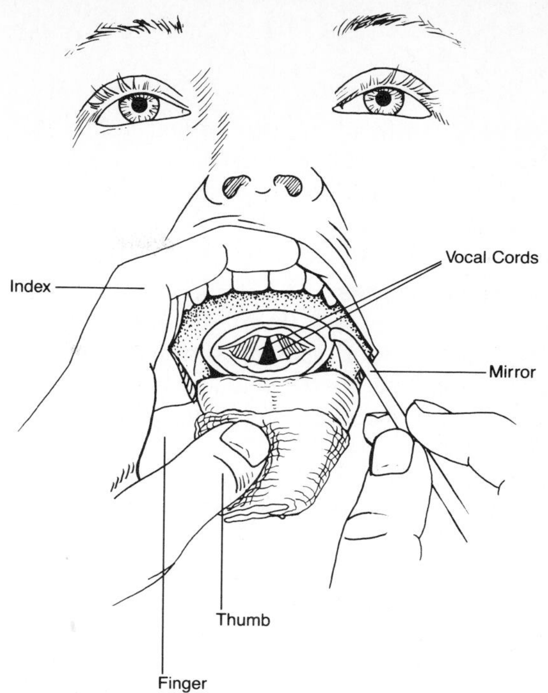

Figure 14–6

The mirror image of the vocal cords in indirect laryngoscopy. The index finger holds up upper lip; client's tongue is grasped with a fold of gauze.

shares numerous antigens with many other Mycobacteria that can also produce a positive skin test.

False positive results may also be due to previous administration of the BCG vaccine. Bacillus Calmette–Guerin (BCG) contains live, attenuated bovine tubercle bacilli. The substance is incapable of producing active disease. In the past, many health care providers received BCG to increase their resistance to TBC. These people will always have a positive tuberculin skin test.

Multiple puncture devices such as the tine test are not recommended for individual screening because they are not as reliable as the Mantoux test. The amount of concentrated tuberculin is not standardized in the multiple puncture technique, which is recommended only in the screening of large groups. Any positive tests should be followed with the Mantoux test.

Nursing implications for the Mantoux intradermal skin test include explaining the procedure carefully because client cooperation is essential. The elderly may have great anxiety about TBC, as may newcomers from third-world countries. Reassure the client that the test is relatively painless and that the solution is injected into the superficial layers of the skin only. Question the client about whether they have had a positive tuberculin skin test in the past, have recently been exposed to anyone with TBC, or have ever received a tuberculosis vaccine (BCG). Remind the client to report back to have the skin test read after 48 hours. Emphasize the importance of returning, since results of this test will indicate whether the client requires further testing and/or treatment for tuberculosis. A chest x-ray is necessary for any client with a positive Mantoux skin test.

INDIRECT LARYNGOSCOPY This standard diagnostic examination allows the examiner to view the vocal cords and other laryngeal structures by inserting a mirror into the oropharynx. Clients are usually positioned so they are sitting all the way back in the chair with the head and shoulders forward. Mirrors of different sizes can be used, depending on the amount of space between the tonsils. The examiner dips the mirror in warm or hot water and dries it with gauze to prevent fogging when the mirror is placed in the client's mouth. The client is asked to stick out the tongue. The examiner grasps the tongue with gauze, pulls it away from the back wall of the pharynx, and places the mirror near (but not touching) the back wall. Touching the tonsils or back of the tongue will cause the client to gag. The desired position is that from which the laryngeal orifice and the epiglottis can be seen (Figure 14–6). The examiner can inspect the area when the client is quiet and when the client says "ah." The mirror image can also be viewed with a magnifying instrument.

Various surgical procedures can be performed using indirect laryngoscopy, but the client must be cooperative. Surgical procedures that can be performed by this method include the injection of Teflon to treat unilateral vocal cord paralysis and removal of vocal nodules.

NURSING IMPLICATIONS This examination is easier and more information is gained if the client is relaxed and knows what to expect. Position the client correctly and explain the importance of remaining in that position. It is helpful if clients know that they will be instructed to say "ah" or make other sounds while being examined. It is important that clients try to relax during the exam.

If surgical procedures are performed using this approach, the client is usually given a sedative. In this case the nurse would assist the client in maintaining the desired position. The nurse also assesses the client for changes in appearance, changes in vital signs, and abnormal bleeding.

DIRECT LARYNGOSCOPY The physician inserts a laryngoscope to be able to view the larynx directly under magnification. A variety of types of instruments can be used. Microlaryngoscopic instruments with binocular magnification allow the physician to view changes that cannot be seen with a mirror.

Direct laryngoscopy is used to investigate symptoms and signs associated with the larynx, such as when a client has hoarseness for more than 2 weeks, but indirect laryngoscopy shows no abnormality. Direct laryngoscopy is frequently used for such surgical procedures as biopsy of a growth on the larynx. This procedure is usually preferred for the removal of laryngeal polyps and vocal cord nodules and is also used for the removal of foreign bodies from the larynx. Trauma victims may require direct laryngoscopy to assess the extent and severity of the injury.

NURSING IMPLICATIONS Direct laryngoscopy can be performed using either local or general anesthesia. Assure clients that they should not experience pain during the procedure and that the airway will be maintained throughout. Preoperative medications may be administered to help the client relax if local anesthesia is used. The client should not drink or eat for several hours before the procedure, and any dentures must be removed.

After the procedure, the client will be allowed to drink soon after waking up. If a local anesthetic is used, be sure the gag reflex has returned and that the client can swallow. A sore or irritated throat is not uncommon from passage of the laryngoscope. The client should be observed for symptoms and signs of respiratory distress from laryngeal edema or spasm. After the removal of laryngeal polyps or vocal cord nodules, the client should rest the voice for several days. Clearing the throat and coughing should be avoided if possible.

BRONCHOSCOPY Bronchoscopy is the direct viewing of the trachea and tracheobronchial tree by means of a rigid or flexible fiberoptic bronchoscope. The flexible fiberoptic bronchoscope is a slender tube with mirrors and a light at the distal end. A brush, biopsy forceps, or catheter may be passed through the bronchoscope to obtain samples for cytologic examination (Hollen, Toomey, & Given, 1982).

Bronchoscopy is used in the diagnosis of such conditions as hemoptysis, lesions, masses, and abnormalities seen on chest x-ray. Bronchoscopy may also be used to treat lung abscesses, pneumonia, aspiration, to debride mucosal eschar resulting from burns and other inhalation injuries, and to remove foreign bodies. Bronchoscopy can aid in removal of excessive tenacious secretions when nasotracheal suctioning is ineffective. Bronchoscopy is performed with the client sitting or supine. The flexible bronchoscope is inserted either through the client's nose or mouth, whereas the rigid bronchoscope is inserted through the mouth.

NURSING IMPLICATIONS Bronchoscopy entails a certain amount of physical discomfort. The client is likely to be anxious not only about pain but also about the findings, especially if the procedure is being performed to confirm the presence of a tumor. Take time not only to explain the procedure but to answer any questions the client may have and allay any anxieties based on misconceptions. Clients should be told that they will receive an intravenous sedative to help them relax, and that a local anesthetic will be sprayed into the nose and mouth to suppress the gag reflex. This will produce the sensation of a dry mouth, swollen tongue, and swollen throat, and will make the client unable to swallow. Clients should be reassured that they will be able to breathe during the procedure. The client takes nothing by mouth 6 to 12 hours prior to the procedure, and any dentures are removed. Occasionally, clients will require a general anesthetic. A signed consent form is necessary.

Following bronchoscopy vital signs are monitored. The conscious client is placed in a semi-Fowler's position, and the unconscious client is positioned on one side with the head of the bed slightly elevated. An emesis basin should be provided and the client instructed to expectorate secretions into the basin rather than swallow them so the nurse can observe them. Clients should be advised that clearing the throat or coughing could dislodge a clot and possibly cause hemorrhage. Watch for subcutaneous emphysema, which may indicate tracheal or bronchial perforation. Foods and fluids are restricted until the gag reflex returns. Hoarseness and a sore throat can be relieved by gargles and throat lozenges. Watch for any breathing difficulty (from laryngeal edema or laryngospasm), hemoptysis, symptoms of a pneumothorax, and bronchospasm (Hollen, Toomey, & Given, 1982).

MEDIASTINOSCOPY This procedure is usually done in the OR. The surgeon makes an incision over the mediastinum and inserts a scope to explore the area. The mediastinum is the area in which the esophagus, trachea, great vessels, and heart are located. Mediastinoscopy is also used to obtain biopsies of lymph nodes or other masses, to determine the presence of lymph node metastases due to bronchogenic carcinoma, and to diagnose intrathoracic sarcoidosis.

NURSING IMPLICATIONS Mediastinoscopy can be performed under either local or general anesthesia. Tell clients that the procedure will leave a small incision with a dressing covering it postoperatively and that the incision site might be somewhat sore for a few days. A signed consent is necessary.

Postoperative nursing care includes monitoring vital signs, observing for bleeding from the incision site, and alleviating discomfort by comfort measures or administering prescribed pain medication as appropriate. Be alert for symptoms and signs of wound infection. Possible complications, in addition to hemorrhage and wound infection, include right recurrent laryngeal nerve paralysis and esophageal perforation.

THORACENTESIS Thoracentesis is performed to identify disease involving the pleura and to remove fluid from the client with a pleural effusion. After the selected area is cleansed, a local anesthetic is injected into the skin, the needle is inserted, and fluid aspirated.

The presence of fluid in the intrapleural space is abnormal. The amount, color, odor, and character of the fluid should be noted in the chart. The fluid may be described as serous, serosanguineous, or turbid. Serous fluid may be obtained from clients who have disorders of nontraumatic origin, including congestive heart failure, pleural effusion due to a malignancy, granulomatous disease, and disorders resulting in inflammation. Blood in the fluid is usually due to trauma to the lungs, but it may be seen in clients with an advanced malignancy. Turbid fluid in the intrapleural space is most commonly from an infectious process. Rarely, hyperalimentation solution may be present in the fluid. This occurs when a central venous line is placed into the intrapleural space instead of the vena cava, and hyperalimentation solution is infused via the intravenous line.

No more than 1000 to 1500 mL of fluid should be removed at any one time because of the danger of hypotension. The specimen is sent to the laboratory where red cell count, white cell count with differential, protein, glucose, lactic acid dehydrogenase, amylase, pH, cultures, bacteriologic stains, and pleural fluid cytology are done.

NURSING IMPLICATIONS Although thoracentesis is a relatively simple procedure, it can be frightening to the client. Explain the basic steps of the thoracentesis to the client calmly and completely. A signed consent is necessary. Nurses must be careful not to transfer their own anxiety about the procedure to clients. Clients should be warned to expect a sensation of pressure or discomfort when the needle is inserted. Premedication is not usually necessary. However, medication may be prescribed to calm a frightened client.

Proper positioning of the client is essential for the procedure. The client should either be leaning over a bedside table (Figure 14–7) or sitting on a chair facing the chairback and leaning against it. These positions give the client support and stability and allow for elevation of the ribs. Clients should be encouraged to remain still to avoid trauma to the lung tissue. If the client has a frequent cough, a cough suppressant may be administered to avoid excessive movement of the needle while it is in the intrapleural space. Depending on which medication is given, the timing is important for maximum effectiveness. Remain with the client throughout the procedure to provide support and monitor vital signs.

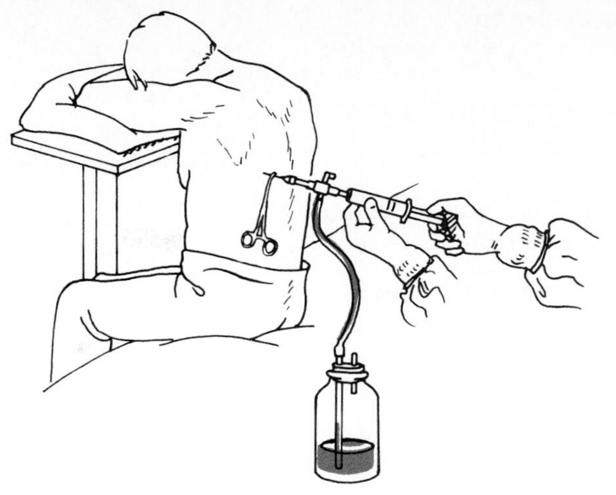

Figure 14–7

Client position for thoracentesis.

Complications of thoracentesis are relatively rare. They include hemorrhage, pain, and pneumothorax. After the procedure, monitor the client's vital signs and respiratory status to detect any adverse reactions. The insertion site should be observed for swelling that could result from bleeding into the area.

LUNG BIOPSY Both open and closed approaches are used to obtain lung tissue for cytologic analysis and culture. Closed approaches include fine needle aspiration, biopsy via a percutaneous cutting needle, and biopsy via flexible bronchoscope. All closed procedures are done under local anesthesia with fluoroscopic guidance. Open lung biopsy requires a thoracotomy. This approach provides the largest volume of tissue, but general anesthesia is needed. Lung biopsy is indicated when the client's diagnosis remains unclear despite a complete work-up.

NURSING IMPLICATIONS Explain the basic procedure. If only local anesthetic is used, clients should be told that the area will be numbed, but they will probably still feel some pressure or discomfort when the biopsy is taken. Clients may be asked not to eat or drink anything for a few hours prior to the procedure. A signed consent is necessary.

When the biopsy is completed, observe the site for swelling or bleeding, and monitor the client for approximately 24 hours for any symptoms and signs of pneumothorax, air embolism, or hemorrhage.

NURSING DIAGNOSES IN
Respiratory Dysfunction

DIRECTLY RELATED DIAGNOSES

- Activity intolerance
- Airway clearance, ineffective
- Breathing pattern, ineffective
- Gas exchange, impaired

OTHER POTENTIAL DIAGNOSES

- Adjustment, impaired
- Anxiety
- Comfort, altered: pain
- Communication, impaired: verbal
- Infection, potential for
- Knowledge deficit
- Nutrition, altered: less than body requirements
- Self-concept, disturbance in: body image

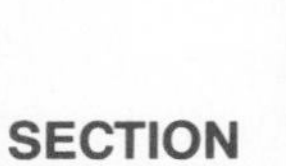

SECTION II

Nursing Diagnosis/Planning and Implementation/Evaluation

Assessment of clients with respiratory dysfunction involves obtaining the history, physical assessment, and reviewing the results of diagnostic studies. The Nursing Diagnoses box above lists diagnoses **directly related** to respiratory dysfunction along with **potential** nursing diagnoses for clients with respiratory problems. A nursing care plan for four major nursing diagnoses—activity intolerance; airway clearance, ineffective; breathing pattern, ineffective; and gas exchange, impaired—is developed in Table 14–1.

Airway Clearance, Ineffective

A variety of nursing interventions are used when the nursing diagnosis is ineffective airway clearance. The most useful include pursed-lip breathing, diaphragmatic breathing, postural drainage, and nasotracheal suctioning. In severe disorders, the client may require intubation and placement on a mechanical ventilator.

Pursed-Lip Breathing

Pursed-lip breathing, a slow, even expiration against pursed lips, prevents collapse of small bronchioles and reduces the amount of trapped air in the lungs. The client should be sitting up. To assume the proper lip position for pursed-lip breathing, have the client pretend to blow out a candle. Clients with emphysema can use pursed-lip breathing to maximize expiration.

Diaphragmatic Breathing

Diaphragmatic breathing (abdominal breathing) facilitates maximum use of the diaphragm in breathing. This is particularly helpful for clients who have had thoracic surgery and those with COPD.

Ask the client in the sitting position to take a deep, slow breath through the nose, concentrating on maximum expansion of the abdomen. Place the client's hand on the abdomen to feel it rise. Then have the client exhale slowly through pursed lips while contracting the abdominal muscles. The client should place manual pressure on the abdomen during expiration. Use of this breathing pattern should be encouraged during daily activities so it can become an automatic approach to breathing during periods of respiratory difficulty.

Postural Drainage

Postural drainage combines the force of gravity with normal ciliary action to move secretions from smaller to larger airways, where they can be removed by coughing or suctioning. Auscultate the client's lungs prior to postural drainage to determine which segments require drainage. Auscultate afterward to determine effectiveness of the therapy. Postural drainage can be directed to any segment of the lung. Figure 14–8 shows client positions for specific pulmonary segments.

Percussion and vibrating techniques are often used with postural drainage. Percussion with a cupped hand (Figure 14–9) helps loosen secretions and stimulate coughing. The client should use diaphragmatic breathing during percussion.

Vibration involves manual pressure on the chest using a vibrating movement of the hand during expiration. The loosening and mobilizing of mucus secretions are increased with vibration. The client should cough after the procedure.

Percussion and vibration are directed to the specific lung segments involved. For example, using Figure 14–8, to loosen secretions in the right middle lobe (position f), percuss over the anterior and lateral right chest from the midaxillary line to the sternum for about 2 minutes. Then perform three to five vibrations over the same area during expiration only.

Extremely ill or elderly clients may not be able to tolerate some of the positions for postural drainage, particularly those with the head lower than the feet. Individual modifications of position will be necessary, based on the client's condition.

Schedule postural drainage exercises before meals because sputum will be minimal and vomiting and aspiration will be prevented. Postural drainage is generally done two to four times a day.

Nasotracheal Suctioning

Clients who are not intubated may require suctioning of the tracheobronchial tree. It is important to explain the

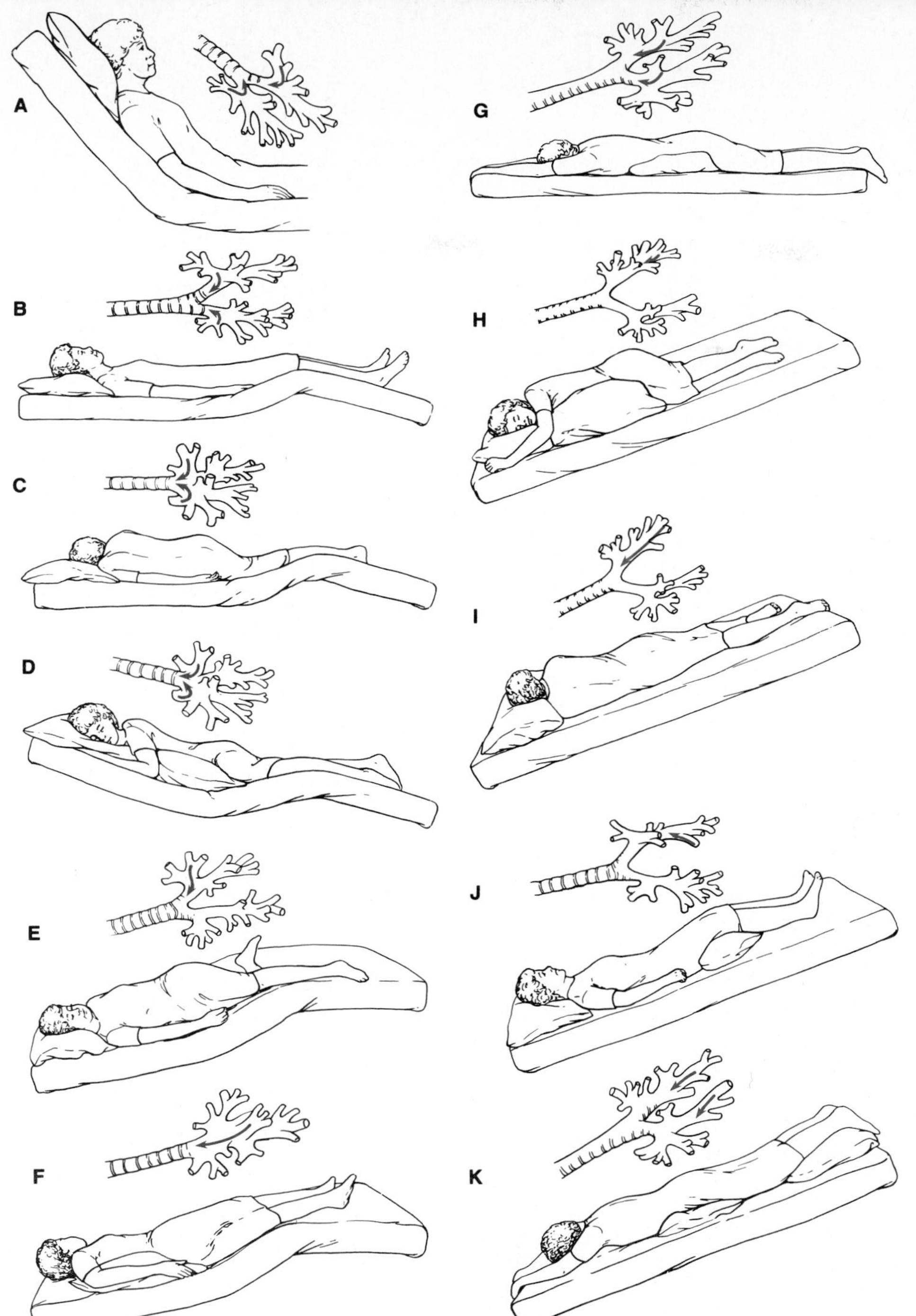

Figure 14–8

Postural drainage positions for specific pulmonary segments. **A.** Left and right upper lobes (apical segment). **B.** Left and right upper lobes (anterior segment). **C.** Right upper lobe (posterior segment). **D.** Left upper lobe (posterior segment). **E.** Left upper lobe (lingular segment). **F.** Middle lobe of right lung. **G.** Lower lobe (superior segment), client lying prone with one pillow under abdomen. **H.** Left lower lobe (lateral basal segment). **I.** Left and right lower lobes (anterior basal segments). **J.** Left and right lower lobes (anterior basal segments). **K.** Left and right lower lobes (posterior basal segments).

procedure to the client to allay anxiety and gain as much cooperation as possible. An explanation is important even if clients are unresponsive, since they may still be aware of activities. The client is positioned at a 45° angle unless contraindicated. Clients should be hyperoxygenated before suctioning; if they are receiving oxygen, the flow rate is increased during the procedure. Box 14–1 on page 323 describes the procedure for insertion of a nasotracheal suction catheter. The procedure and basic principles of suctioning are discussed later in Table 14–3. Oral suctioning is considered a clean procedure, whereas nasotracheal, tracheostomy, and endotracheal tube suctioning are sterile procedures.

Breathing Pattern, Ineffective

Several nursing interventions may be initiated when the nursing diagnosis is breathing pattern, ineffective. Some of these actions are discussed in the nursing care plan (Table 14–1).

Table 14–1
Sample Nursing Care Plan for Clients With Respiratory Dysfunction, by Nursing Diagnosis

Client Care Goals	Plan/Nursing Implementation	Expected Outcomes
Activity intolerance related to imbalance between O_2 supply and demand		
Understand reasons for use of oxygen, medications and/or equipment to increase activity tolerance	Instruct in use of O_2 prior to, during, and after activities; use of medications to enhance breathing; equipment use in the home such as nebulizer, humidifier, and assistive devices during ambulation	Acts to obtain benefits of O_2, medications and/or equipment
Maintain increased tolerance for ADLs.	Reinforce measures to assist with performance of ADLs: instruct in pacing activities to tolerance, breathing techniques during activity, keeping frequently used objects within easy reach, and requesting assistance with activities	Performs ADLs to level of tolerance
Understand limitations in strength and endurance	Encourage client to talk about feelings regarding limited tolerance to activity: need for assistance and assistive devices; and variations in activity tolerance determined by physical and physiologic status	Express feelings about limitations in strength and endurance
Airway clearance, ineffective related to inflammation of the upper airway		
Decrease or eliminate secretions of the upper respiratory tract	Assess for redness and swelling of the upper airway; note amount and characteristics of drainage; assess for discomfort of the nose, paranasal sinuses, and pharynx; monitor vital signs at regular intervals; administer prescribed humidified air or oxygen as appropriate; administer prescribed decongestants/antihistamines as needed; suction nasal or oropharyngeal area using aseptic technique	• Absence of nasal obstruction • Absence of nasal discharge • Absence of nasal stuffiness • Sinus films normal • Absence of inflammation, redness, and tenderness over paranasal sinuses • Absence of headache • Absence of inflammation, redness, and drainage in pharynx • Voice return to normal • Absence of sore throat • Absence of dysphagia • Normal vital signs • Intake of 2000 to 3000 mL of fluid per day
Maintain adequate fluid intake	Encourage fluids, at least 3000 mL/24 h	
Understand measures necessary to avoid spread of infection to others	Instruct in measures to prevent spread of infectious organisms such as decreased personal contact with others, hand-washing, proper tissue disposal, and covering mouth and nose when coughing and sneezing	Acts to prevent spread of infection
Describe the benefits of humidification and adequate hydration	Instruct that humidification and adequate hydration will facilitate removal of secretions; include cold mist or steam humidifier, pans of water around room, fluid intake	Acts to obtain the benefits of adequate hydration and humidification and implements it in the home
Describe how to blow nose and cough to remove secretions effectively	Instruct the client how to blow the nose and cough to remove nasal and pharyngeal secretions effectively	Uses correct method of blowing nose and coughing
Describe how to administer decongestants/antihistamines properly	Instruct client in use of decongestants/antihistamines; include family members when carrying out teaching measures	Follows proper administration of decongestants/antihistamines

Client Care Goals	Plan/Nursing Implementation	Expected Outcomes
Airway clearance, ineffective related to inflammation of the lower airway		
Remove secretions from the lower respiratory tract effectively	Assess the pulmonary status of the client: monitor and record amount, consistency, and color of sputum; auscultate lungs for abnormal breath sounds (rales, rhonchi, wheezing); monitor vital signs at regular intervals; monitor for symptoms and signs of arterial blood gas abnormalities	• Absence of purulent, tenacious sputum • Sputum C&S negative • Lungs clear to auscultation • Chest x-ray normal • Vital signs are within normal limits • Arterial blood gas values within normal limits for the client
Maintain adequate oxygen to tissues	Measures to remove excessive secretions from the lower respiratory tract may include: turning a bedridden client every 2 h; having a client cough and deep breathe at least every 2 h; if appropriate, getting client out of bed three times each shift; pursed-lip breathing, diaphragmatic breathing, and/or postural drainage as prescribed; suctioning using sterile technique; administering IPPB treatments as prescribed; administering prescribed expectorants, bronchodilators, steroids, as appropriate; administering prescribed oxygen as needed	Absence of adventitious breath sounds; absence of symptoms and signs of hypoxemia
Maintain acceptable intake and output	Ensure fluid intake of 2 to 3 L/day (fluid requirement will vary with weight and physical condition; fluid restrictions may be necessary in disease states such as congestive heart failure and renal failure); careful monitoring of intake and output; inspect skin turgor daily; monitor vital signs at regular intervals	• Drinks 2000 to 3000 mL fluid per day • Good skin turgor • Absence of tenacious secretions • Intake and output within acceptable limits
Describe how to cough and perform breathing exercises	Instruct on proper technique used in coughing and breathing exercises	Performs coughing and breathing exercises correctly
Describe how to make use of oxygen and breathing equipment	Instruct client in use and proper placement of oxygen delivery equipment; instruct in correct use of breathing equipment such as incentive spirometer	Uses oxygen and breathing equipment correctly
Discuss proper administration of prescribed medications	Instruct in the actions, side effects, and proper administration of medications	Complies with instructions as to administration of medications, reports side effects, understands actions and reports any ineffective medication
Identify measures to avoid development of a respiratory tract infection	Reinforce measures to prevent spread of infection; instruct in measures to prevent development of a respiratory infection such as avoiding contact with an infected individual, hand washing, and taking precautions to maintain optimal health; include family members when teaching	• Acts to prevent spread of infection • Acts to prevent development of respiratory tract infections • Actions of family members show they understand information
Breathing pattern, ineffective related to inadequate chest expansion from pain or trauma		
Maintain normal respiratory rate and pattern	Assess client for: respiratory rate and depth; symmetrical chest expansion; abnormal breath sounds; fractured ribs; tracheal deviation; fluctuation of vital	• Adequate aeration of lungs as evidenced by: normal breath sounds; normal chest x-ray; normal arterial blood gas values

(continued)

Table 14–1 (continued)
Sample Nursing Care Plan for Clients With Respiratory Dysfunction, by Nursing Diagnosis

Client Care Goals	Plan/Nursing Implementation	Expected Outcomes
	signs; pain on inspiration and on movement, as with a fractured rib	• Vital signs within normal limits • Symmetrical chest expansion (These outcomes hold for all nursing interventions under this problem)
Remain free of complications that can result from trauma	Note signs that may indicate inadequate ventilation: stridor, use of accessory muscles, flaring of nares, dyspnea, asymmetrical chest movement, paradoxical breathing, open chest wound, hemoptysis, subcutaneous emphysema, tracheal deviation, hyperresonance on percussion, dullness on percussion, diminished or absent breath sounds	
Tolerate pain on breathing within limits	Assess client for location, type, and intensity of pain; provide comfort measures: positioning; splinting when coughing and deep breathing; administer prescribed analgesics as appropriate; assess respiratory rate after administration of narcotic analgesic to identify any respiratory depression; assess respiratory rate, depth, and chest expansion; monitor vital signs at regular intervals	• Pain sensation remains within tolerable limits as reported by client • Vital signs within normal limits
Understand reasons for procedures and what to expect during them	Carefully prepare client and family members for procedures: explain reason procedure is performed, length of procedure; discuss steps involved in procedure; inform client about likely sensations during the procedure and that pain medication is available	• Expresses feelings and anxiety about conditions and situation
	Maintain a patent airway: suction as necessary; prepare to assist with intubation or tracheotomy; place in a semi-Fowler's position unless contraindicated	• Adequate ventilation and oxygenation as evidence by: normal lung sounds; normal pulmonary function studies; normal chest x-ray; normal arterial blood gas values
	Maintain optimal pulmonary ventilation: prepare for insertion of chest tube if necessary; monitor for adequate function of the closed chest tube system; encourage client to perform pulmonary hygiene measures such as coughing and deep breathing exercises on a set schedule. Administer humidified oxygen as necessary; administer IPPB treatments as necessary; monitor vital signs at regular intervals as indicated; prepare client for placement on a mechanical ventilator; monitor client who requires mechanical ventilation	• Chest tube system functioning normally • Normal function of the ventilator
Breathing pattern, ineffective related to pathophysiologic conditions (eg, COPD, pulmonary fibrosis, infection, neuromuscular disorders, musculoskeletal disorders, and carcinoma)		
Maintain optimal pulmonary ventilation	Assess for signs of inadequate ventilation: dyspnea, increased respiratory rate, shallow respiration, use of accessory muscles, nasal flaring, pursed-lip breathing, increased	• Improved ventilatory status as evidenced by: improved lung sounds on auscultation; return to baseline levels for arterial blood gas values, chest x-ray, and pulmonary function studies

Client Care Goals	Plan/Nursing Implementation	Expected Outcomes
	anterior–posterior diameter, diminished or absent breath sounds, signs of hypoxia and hypercapnia/hypocapnia; encourage measures to promote pulmonary hygiene such as coughing and deep breathing, chest physical therapy, breathing exercises, and suctioning; administer humidified oxygen as prescribed; administer IPPB treatment as prescribed; administer medications as prescribed: antibiotics, bronchodilators, expectorants, steroids; prepare for intubation and mechanical ventilation when indicated	• Decreased production of sputum
Explain reasons for procedures and pulmonary hygiene measures	Carefully prepare client and family members for necessary procedures: explain reason procedure is performed; discuss steps involved in procedure; inform client what sensations to expect during the procedure and explain that pain medication is available; explain and demonstrate breathing exercises	• Expresses feelings and anxiety about condition and situation; can demonstrate breathing exercises
Understand and able to perform care measures needed for long-term management	Teaching intervention for long-term management should include: avoiding individuals and situations where respiratory tract infections are likely; notifying a care provider at the first sign of development of a respiratory tract infection; avoiding exposure to irritants such as smoking and other air pollutants; performing bronchial hygiene measures such as effective coughing technique, breathing exercises, and bronchial drainage; using respiratory equipment if necessary, such as nebulizers, IPPB machines, and oxygen delivery systems; reporting symptoms indicative of hypercapnia and hypoxia; maintaining adequate hydration and nutrition; following an organized pulmonary rehabilitation program	• Client and family members carry out measures for long-term management
Maintain a positive self-concept	Consultation with social service if change in occupation is required; encourage client to express feelings related to curtailment in social interaction because of disease process	• Copes effectively with physical and psychosocial limitations imposed by disease process
Gas exchange, impaired related to decreased functional lung tissue secondary to hypoxia from problems of diffusion, ventilation, and ventilation–perfusion		
Maintain adequate oxygenation for cellular metabolism	Observe for symptoms and signs of hypoxia: restlessness, irritability, impaired judgment, central cyanosis, diaphoresis, labored breathing, tachypnea, tachycardia, fluctuation in blood pressure, alteration in level of consciousness, clubbing of the fingers; perform pulmonary hygiene measures: deep breathing and coughing exercises; administration of humidified oxygen;	• Decrease in symptoms and signs of cerebral, cardiovascular, and respiratory hypoxemia • Return to baseline normal PO_2 as reflected in arterial blood gas values • Hemoglobin values come to within normal limits • O_2 saturation returns to baseline normal values

(continued)

Table 14–1 (continued)
Sample Nursing Care Plan for Clients With Respiratory Dysfunction, by Nursing Diagnosis

Client Care Goals	Plan/Nursing Implementation	Expected Outcomes
	IPPB treatments as prescribed; chest physical therapy as indicated; perform suctioning as necessary; administer appropriate medication (bronchodilators, expectorants, antibiotics, steroids); prepare to assist with intubation and mechanical ventilation when indicated; monitor client receiving PEEP for effectiveness of therapy	
Maintain orientation to self and surrounding environment	Assess client's degree of orientation; if confused, attempt to reorient to time, place, and person; perform measures to prevent client from self-harm; explain to family members and significant others that confusion may be due to a lowered oxygen level; administer oxygen as prescribed	• Client responds correctly with name, date, time, place • Family members show an understanding of the cause of confusion and how to care for the client • Copes effectively with the limitations of a lowered oxygen level
Understand the physical limitations of hypoxia	Inform client and family members about symptoms and signs of hypoxia such as shortness of breath, fatigue, and confusion	
Understand therapy necessary to correct hypoxia	Instruct in correct use and administration of oxygen in the hospital and at home	• Client and family members respond in ways that show correct knowledge of oxygen therapy
Gas exchange, impaired related to decreased pulmonary blood supply secondary to hypercapnia from hypoventilation		
Maintain a PCO_2 level compatible with a normal pH	Observe for symptoms and signs of hypercapnia: confusion, drowsiness, headache, dizziness, tetany, asterixis, tachycardia, dysrhythmias, convulsion, and coma; perform pulmonary hygiene measures: deep breathing and coughing exercises; administer humidified oxygen; administer IPPB treatments as prescribed; provide chest physical therapy as indicated; perform suctioning as necessary; administer appropriate medication (bronchodilators, expectorants, antibiotics, steroids); prepare to assist with intubation and mechanical ventilation when indicated	• Decrease in symptoms and signs of cerebral, cardiovascular, and respiratory hypercapnia • Return to normal blood pH of 7.35–7.45
Understand reasons for procedures and what to expect during them	Carefully prepare client and significant others for procedures: explain reason procedure is performed; discuss steps involved in procedure; inform client what may be felt during the procedure	• Expresses feelings and anxiety about condition and situation
Gas exchange, impaired related to decreased pulmonary blood supply secondary to hypocapnia from hyperventilation		
Maintain PCO_2 level compatible with a normal pH	Observe for symptoms and signs of hypocapnia: muscle spasm, carpopedal spasm, tetany, diaphoresis, cardiac dysrhythmia, tachypnea, alteration in level of consciousness; carry out measures to decrease client anxiety and to slow the respiratory rate: calm approach to client, reassurance	

Client Care Goals	Plan/Nursing Implementation	Expected Outcomes
	and explanation, administer antianxiety medications as prescribed, administer bronchodilators and expectorants as prescribed, assist client to breathe effectively via breathing exercises Use equipment to increase PCO_2 level as prescribed, such as rebreathing mask (or paper bag), adjustment of ventilator settings	• Decrease in symptoms and signs of cerebral, cardiovascular, and respiratory hypocapnia • Return to normal blood pH of 7.35–7.45 as reflected by arterial blood gas analysis

The Client With an Artificial Airway

The indications for placement of an artificial airway are to relieve obstruction, facilitate suctioning of the lower airway, allow for mechanical ventilation, and to prevent aspiration. Artificial airways include the endotracheal tube, the tracheostomy tube, and the laryngectomy tube.

ENDOTRACHEAL TUBES Endotracheal intubation (by nasal or oral route) is one of the most widely used methods to institute and maintain an open airway. The oral route is most often used when emergency intubation is required because of the relative ease of insertion. When long-term intubation is anticipated, the nasal route is preferred. Nasotracheal intubation is tolerated better by the conscious client and allows for better tube stabilization. Intubation with an endotracheal tube requires the use of a laryngoscope, which permits visualization of the area and facilitates passage of the tube into the trachea (Wade, 1982).

Endotracheal tubes come in various lengths and sizes. The physician or anesthetist intubating will choose a suitable tube size for the route used and the size of the client's airway. Too large a tube can damage the airway structure and mucosal lining, whereas a tube that is too small will not allow adequate ventilation. The tube should be inserted gently to avoid structural damage.

Most tubes used today are disposable and are made of polyvinylchloride or silicone rubber. Nondisposable tubes are used less frequently. Most endotracheal tubes have inflatable cuffs (Figure 14–10). The cuff is inflated by injecting air into the pilot balloon. The amount of air required varies with the type of tube. The specific amount necessary is included in the package directions and may be printed on the tube. The cuff provides a seal so air does not leak around the tube when the client is ventilated. The cuff also prevents aspiration of material into the lungs. The newer endotracheal tubes have a low-pressure cuff that is more compliant and less likely to cause injury to the tracheal mucosa (Petty, 1982). Nursing considerations for the client with a cuffed tube are presented in Box 14–2.

NURSING CARE OF THE CLIENT WITH AN ENDOTRACHEAL TUBE Immediately after intubation, auscultate the lung fields to determine if the tube is placed properly. Since the right bronchus is straighter than the left, the tube is sometimes inserted into the right mainstem bronchus. This permits aeration of the right lung only. If the end of the endotracheal tube rests on the carina, partial or complete obstruction results. (The carina is the area where the trachea bifurcates into the left bronchus and right bronchus.) Inadvertent entry of the tube into the esophagus will result in gastric dilation. A chest x-ray should be obtained to determine the position of the tube. Endotracheal tubes provide a means of suctioning secretions from the lower respiratory tract. Sterile technique is used.

The tube must be stabilized to prevent inadvertent removal (extubation) or change in placement. This is most often accomplished by taping the tube. When the client is intubated nasally, tape is applied at the insertion site. Stabilizing the oral endotracheal tube involves placement of an oral airway to prevent the client from biting down and obstructing the tube. Avoid applying excessive tape at the mouth, which would make inspection of the oral cavity difficult. Plastic devices may be used rather than tape to secure the tube. Meticulous oral hygiene is important for

Box 14–1
Inserting a Nasotracheal Suction Catheter

To find out how far the catheter should be inserted, measure off the amount of catheter needed from the ear lobe to the tip of the client's nose. Lubricate the tip of the sterile catheter using sterile water-soluble lubricant to facilitate passage through the nose. Insert the catheter gently through the client's nostril *without suction*. If the client is alert, ask him or her to stick out the tongue to prevent swallowing the catheter. If the client is not alert, hyperextend the neck and hold the client's tongue forward with a piece of gauze to facilitate catheter entry into the trachea. Entry into the trachea rather than the esophagus is indicated by coughing. If the catheter is in the esophagus, the client may gag or vomit. Avoid frequent suctioning via the same nostril to prevent traumatizing the mucosa. If frequent suctioning is necessary, a flexible rubber nasal pharyngeal airway may be inserted to prevent trauma of the nasal mucosa.

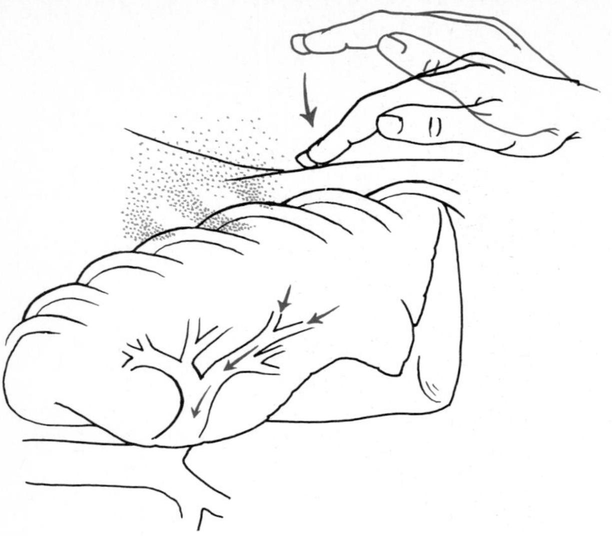

Figure 14–9

Percussion with the cupped hand over the pulmonary segment being drained.

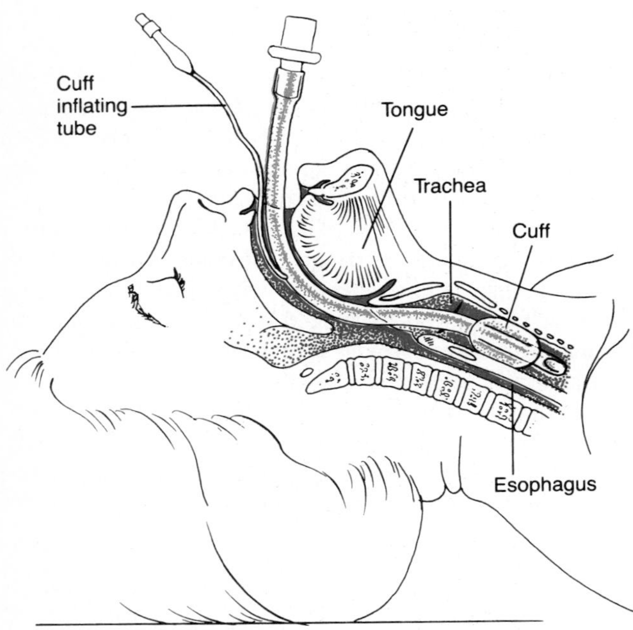

Figure 14–10

Endotracheal tube in position in an anesthetized client.

these clients. The position of the orotracheal tube should be changed daily and the tape replaced at the same time. Care must be taken to avoid skin breakdown, which can result from irritation by the tape.

Assess the client's skin daily when tape is changed. A rash may indicate an allergic reaction to the tape. The use of nonallergenic tape or plastic devices may then be indicated, particularly for clients, such as diabetics, who are likely to have skin breakdown and poor wound healing.

Assess clients with endotracheal tubes daily for complications involving the nose, mouth, pharynx, sinuses,

Box 14–2
Nursing Considerations for the Client With a Cuffed Endotracheal Tube

Effective and safe nursing care of clients with a cuffed endotracheal tube depends on an adequate understanding of the characteristics of the cuff being used. The two basic types of cuffs are air-filled and foam-filled. The newer tubes on the market (such as the Lanz or the Shiley) have a built-in control mechanism to prevent excessive pressure on th tracheal wall.

When using air-filled tubes, realize that once the syringe is removed from the one-way inflation valve, the cuff loses its ability to regulate or readjust for correct cuff pressure. For example, some cuffs are constructed to vent air when the pressure within the cuff exceeds 15 mm Hg on inflation. Once the syringe is removed from the one-way inflation valve, there is no route for escape of excess air. Therefore, an increase in tracheal and intracuff pressure will not be vented, and intracuff pressures may go above 15 mm Hg (Harper, 1981).

With the modern soft-cuff tracheostomy and endotracheal tubes, deflation of the cuffs is not necessary. However, the intracuff pressure must be checked at regular intervals. This reading can be obtained using an aneroid manometer or the Portex pressure gauge, designed specifically for this purpose (Harper, 1981).

Foam-filled cuffs work on a different principle than the air-filled type. The inflation line is left open to the atmosphere to allow the foam inside the cuff to reexpand. Air should never be injected into these cuffs since the pressure would greatly increase (Harper, 1981).

Occasionally, the nurse may care for a client who is intubated with a tube that does not have a soft cuff. To prevent damage, the "minimal leak" technique allows a small amount of air to escape around the cuff. To accomplish this, place a stethoscope on the client's neck over the trachea. During inspiration, inject air into the pilot balloon until the gurgling or hissing of air around the tube is no longer present. Then slowly remove 0.2 to 0.3 mL of air from the pilot balloon. The pressure should then be checked. Cuff pressures should never exceed 15 mm Hg, or 25 cm water.

Regardless of the type of cuff, check and record the pressures at least once each shift. Some clinicians recommend that inflatable cuffs be deflated for a few minutes every hour to relieve pressure on the tracheal lining. The benefit of periodic deflation has not been documented by research. If the cuff is deflated, however, the area above the cuff should be suctioned to prevent aspiration of secretions.

and ears. A nasotracheal tube could obstruct the eustachian tube, causing otitis. Damage to the nasal mucosa may occur from pressure or irritation from the tube.

Other possible complications include damage to the vocal cords, laryngeal edema, and laryngeal ulcers. These complications are caused by traumatic insertion of a tube, improper stabilization of the tube once it is in place, and unnecessary manipulation of the tube. Laryngeal ulcers occur more frequently with oral intubation than with nasal intubation because it is difficult to anchor the endotracheal tube in the mouth, and an unanchored tube exerts pressure on the posterior rim of the glottis.

There is little agreement about how long an endotracheal tube should be left in place. The length of time varies with agency policy and the physician. If the physician suspects that the client will require prolonged intubation, a tracheotomy is performed because the longer the client has an endotracheal tube in place, the greater the risk of complications.

The client should be adequately ventilated, oxygenated, and suctioned before extubation begins. The nurse deflates the cuff and again suctions the client to remove secretions that may have accumulated. The tube is removed, and oxygen is administered. An individual qualified to reintubate the client should be present, and an intubation tray should be at the bedside. Complications that may follow tube removal include laryngeal edema and laryngospasm. Observe the client for any signs of these complications, such as labored breathing, use of accessory muscles, and stridor. Laryngospasm and laryngeal edema can result in upper airway obstruction. If these complications occur, the administration of parenteral corticosteroids and reintubation are necessary (Petty, 1982).

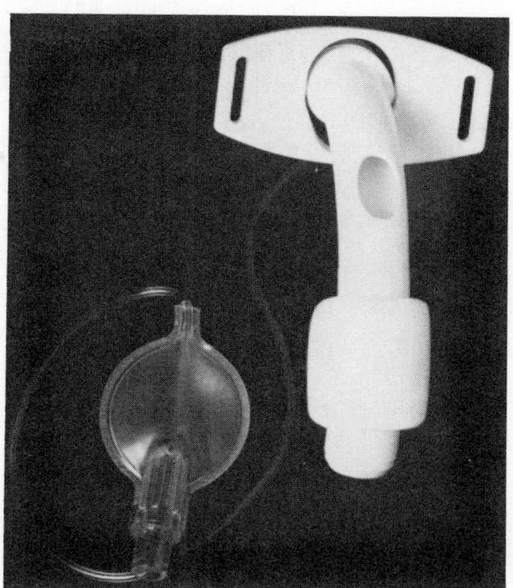

Figure 14–11

Fenestrated tracheostomy tube.

TRACHEOSTOMY TUBES Other methods of establishing an artificial airway include tracheotomy and cricothyroidotomy. (Chapter 15 describes these procedures and indications for their use.) Tracheostomy tubes are placed during these procedures. These are short curved tubes and have a flange that assists in stabilization of the tube on the neck. A variety of types are available, including metal tubes or disposable tubes of polyvinylchloride or silicone. Tubes come in several sizes. Most tubes today have an inner cannula to facilitate cleansing of the inside of the tube. All tubes are packaged with an obturator, which is used to minimize trauma when the tube is inserted.

Fenestrated tracheostomy tubes are sometimes used prior to extubation of the client (Figure 14–11). This tube has an opening, or fenestration, in the outer cannula; it may or may not have a cuff. If the fenestrated tube is cuffed, the cuff should be deflated to allow the client to breathe around, as well as through, the tube. This allows the client to adjust gradually to removal of the tracheostomy tube. It also allows nursing staff to determine how the client will tolerate removal. Covering the tracheostomy tube enables the client to talk, to breathe normally through the upper airway, and to cough up secretions.

Another way of preparing the client for permanent removal of the tracheostomy tube is by applying a tracheostomy button (Figure 14–12). The button extends from the tracheostomy opening to just inside the tracheal wall. If the tracheostomy tube has a cuff, the cuff is deflated before the tracheostomy button is placed to allow the client to breathe around the tube. To determine readiness for decannulation, a tracheostomy button is most effective with a fenestrated tube. Placement of this button facilitates talking, coughing, and normal breathing through the upper airway. If the client has difficulty breathing or expelling secretions, the button is removed, and the client breathes through the tracheostomy tube.

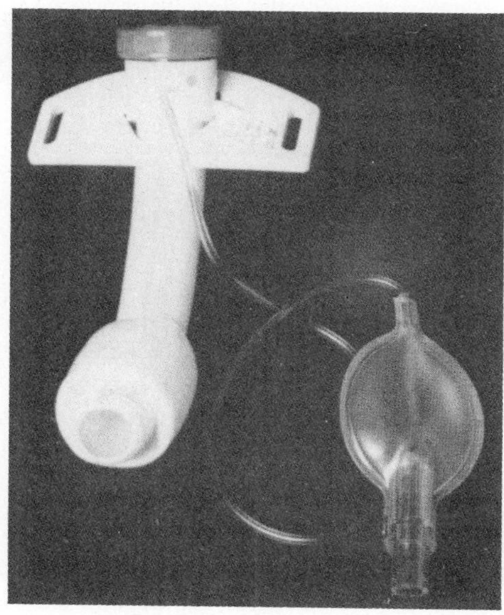

Figure 14–12

Shiley tracheostomy tube with tracheostomy button in place.

TRACHEOSTOMY CARE Tracheostomy care is performed to minimize bacterial contamination and to decrease the possibility of obstruction by secretions. Routine tracheostomy care consists of cleansing of the inner cannula and the area around the stoma. The frequency of cleaning the inner cannula may vary depending on the amount of secretions present. Cleaning may be necessary as frequently as

Table 14–2
Tracheostomy Care—A Sterile Procedure

Nursing Implementation	Rationale
1. Assemble the following equipment: sterile drape; sterile pipe cleaners, brush, swabs, scissors, forceps, gloves; sterile gauze squares; trach ties and trach bib; two sterile basins; sterile normal saline; sterile hydrogen peroxide; paper bag.	With all the equipment at hand, it is easier to carry out the steps in an organized sequence.
2. Wash hands using soap and water.	This removes bacteria from the hands, decreasing the chance of contaminating the client's airway.
3. Explain procedure to the client and provide reassurance, even if the client is unresponsive.	Explanations help to allay the client's anxiety. Explaining the reasons for the procedure and the steps helps to involve alert clients in their own care. Later, clients can be encouraged to help with the procedure. If the tracheostomy will be permanent, it is important that clients learn the procedure and participate actively in their own care.
4. Suction the client as necessary using sterile technique.	Suctioning using strict asepsis prevents airway contamination.
5. Open the sterile drape and place on the bedside stand.	This will serve as a sterile field on which sterile equipment should be placed.
6. Open all equipment using sterile technique.	Since the lung is normally a sterile environment, trach care must be performed using sterile technique.
7. Fill one basin with hydrogen peroxide and one with sterile normal saline.	Pouring the solution before putting on the sterile gloves prevents contamination.
8. Remove the soiled tracheostomy dressing and dispose of it in the paper bag.	Proper disposal prevents contamination of the environment.
9. Loosen the inner cannula.	This facilitates removal.
10. Put on sterile gloves. One hand should be kept sterile and the other clean.	Wearing sterile gloves minimizes contamination of the respiratory tract.
11. Remove inner cannula and place it in the hydrogen peroxide solution. Allow the cannula to soak for a few minutes, then clean with the sterile brush and pipe cleaners.	This facilitates removal of secretions.
12. Rinse inner cannula with sterile saline. Cannula should then be gently shaken and reinserted.	The inner cannula should not remain out longer than 5 to 10 min to prevent the formation of crusts in the outer cannula (Brown, 1982).
13. Maintaining sterile technique, cleanse the skin around the stoma and phlanges of the tube using gauze soaked in a hydrogen peroxide solution. Care must be taken to prevent hydrogen peroxide and lint from entering the stoma.	Hydrogen peroxide facilitates the removal of secretions and crusts, which are a source of bacteria. Cotton applicators should not be used around the stoma since lint from the cotton may be aspirated into the lungs.
14. Rinse area around the stoma with sterile normal saline and dry with sterile gauze.	Hydrogen peroxide is irritating to tissue and should be removed. Drying is important because moisture provides an environment conducive to the growth of bacteria and eventual skin breakdown.
15. Inspect the surrounding area and the stoma site for inflammation, skin breakdown, and presence of secretions. Any abnormalities should be documented and reported.	Signs of impaired wound healing and infection require immediate attention.
16. Make a new tracheostomy dressing by cutting a sterile gauze square (without cotton filler) halfway up the center and place it over the incision under the faceplate of the tracheostomy tube.	Pieces of cotton could inadvertently enter the tracheostomy tube. The dressing will absorb any drainage from the incisional area.

Nursing Implementation	Rationale
17. Apply a new tracheostomy bib and ties. The ties should be tight enough to prevent the tube from being dislodged yet not result in skin irritation. If the ties are fastened appropriately, the nurse should be able to insert one finger underneath the string. Secure with a square knot.	The bib prevents contamination of the airway, and the ties secure the tube.
18. Whenever possible, two people should be present when changing the trach ties. One person can then hold the trach tube securely in place while the other changes the ties. Often clients are able to assist in this way.	This prevents accidental dislodgment of the trach tube.

every half hour or only once a shift. There are two schools of thought regarding care of the inner cannula. Some advocate cleaning the inner cannula as often as necessary. Others believe that proper humidification and suctioning negate the need for cleansing of the inner cannula because frequent cleansing may increase the chance of infection. Table 14–2 presents the steps for routine tracheostomy care (Brown, 1982).

When caring for clients with a tracheostomy or laryngectomy tube, it is wise to have another sterile tube at the bedside in case of accidental decannulation or obstruction of the tube. A clearly labeled obturator for the tube should be in the room because it would be needed to reinsert the tube. Some nurses prefer to keep sterile forceps at the bedside since, in the early period after tube insertion, decannulation may result in closure of the stoma. The forceps would be used to reopen the stoma. Scissors should also be at the bedside to cut the tracheostomy tube ties in case they become too tight or the tube is partially dislodged by coughing.

Prior to removal of the tube, the client is ventilated, oxygenated, and suctioned to remove tracheal and pharyngeal secretions. The cuff is deflated, and the client is again suctioned. The tube is removed, and a moist gauze dressing is placed over the stoma. Normally, the opening closes within 5 days (Petty, 1982).

Home Health Care

Clients with chronic respiratory problems are frequently sent home with tracheostomy tubes. Planning for effective home care includes insuring that the client or a designated household member is familiar with the care and safe maintenance of the airway and the appliance.

The long-term home care of a tracheostomy does not require sterile technique. Clean technique is usually adequate to maintain the client at home safely. Good handwashing before and after the procedure is the most important aspect of safe home care to prevent infection. Pipe cleaners (the tobacco store variety) are acceptable. These may be used to clean the inner cannula. The brush may be reused if washed well with soapy water after each use and left to air dry. Basins need not be sterile, but must be washed well with dish washing detergent, rinsed, dried, and kept covered to protect from dust between uses. Sterile gloves are not necessary, especially if clients are providing self-care. Clean, disposable gloves may be preferable for both client and household members providing care.

When caring for clients with airway appliances at home it is important to have ready access to reputable vendors who are able to provide 24 hour service for supplies and equipment. Lay care givers in the home environment should know the procedure for ordering supplies and equipment. They may need assistance with insurance billing or with obtaining financial assistance.

An important consideration in planning home care for a very dependent client with an airway appliance is the need for respite the primary care giver will inevitably experience. Respite care sources should be worked out prior to hospital discharge.

LARYNGECTOMY TUBES The terms *tracheostomy tube* and *laryngectomy tube* are often used interchangeably. Actually, the laryngectomy tube is shorter. Metal tubes are commonly used, such as the one shown in Figure 14–13. These consist of an obturator, inner cannula, and outer cannula. These tubes are usually placed following a total laryngectomy to provide a route for removal of secretions and to maintain a patent airway.

COMPLICATIONS OF ARTIFICIAL AIRWAYS The insertion of artificial airways can result in a variety of complications. Since inspired air bypasses the nose, air must be humidified to prevent drying of the mucosa of the lower respiratory tract. These clients are more vulnerable to the development of an infection because of altered ciliary function, trauma to the mucosa caused by suctioning and intu-

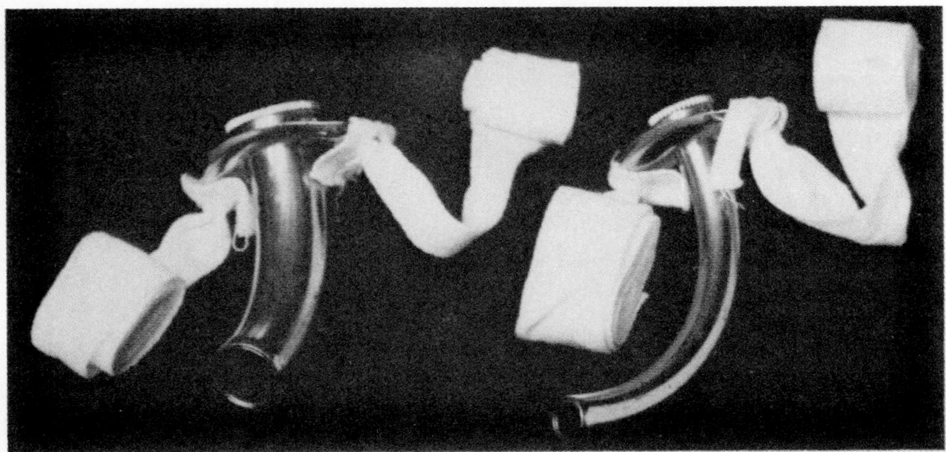

Figure 14–13

Comparison of shorter laryngectomy tube (on left) with tracheostomy tube.

bation, and colonization of the airway with bacteria. Organisms commonly isolated from the respiratory tract in these clients include *Staphylococcus aureus* and *Pseudomonas*.

Excessive pressure on the trachea from the cuff of endotracheal tubes will decrease blood supply to the area and cause tissue necrosis. This may lead to tracheal stenosis or a tracheoesophageal fistula.

Another complication from cuffed tubes is herniation of the cuff over the end of the tube, resulting in partial or complete airway obstruction. Signs include a significant air leak through the stoma, mouth, or nose; the sounding of the high-pressure alarm on the ventilator; and obstruction when attempting to suction the client. An underinflated cuff may be caused by instillation of an insufficient amount of air or a ruptured cuff. An air leak is detected around the stoma, nose, or mouth, and the ventilator indicates a decrease in the expired volume of air with sounding of the low pressure alarm.

Obstruction of artificial airways may occur because of accumulation of secretions or a kink in the endotracheal tube. Obstruction will result in the sounding of a high-pressure alarm. It must be corrected immediately or the client will asphyxiate.

NURSING CARE OF THE CLIENT WITH AN ARTIFICIAL AIRWAY Placement of an artificial airway can be a source of anxiety and apprehension for the client and family members. A major source of anxiety is the client's impaired ability to communicate. This problem is only temporary, except for clients who have undergone a total laryngectomy. To allay the client's anxiety and fear, provide an alternative means of communication. A "magic slate" or a pad of paper and a pencil should be available. The call light should be within reach of the client at all times and should be answered promptly. The intercom at the nurses' station should be marked to indicate that the individual cannot speak. Some clients who cannot communicate by writing might use gesturing as an alternative method. The client who has had a total laryngectomy must adjust to permanent changes.

The ability of the client to remove secretions effectively is also impaired. The artificial airway prevents the client from closing the glottis and generating intrathoracic pressure to dislodge secretions. Thus, the cough is less effective. Also, the artificial airway impairs the effectiveness of the mucociliary mechanism. Secretions that accumulate in the airway may cause the client to fear suffocation. When the client is unable to cough and expel secretions, the uncomfortable and frightening procedure of suctioning must be performed. Table 14–3 describes the procedure for tracheostomy or endotracheal tube suctioning. During this procedure, the client will experience discomfort as well as a feeling of breathlessness. Attempt to allay the client's anxiety by providing an explanation of the artificial airway and the suctioning procedure.

Obviously, the placement of an artificial airway will result in a change in the client's body image. This not only affects the way in which clients view themselves but the way in which they are viewed by family members and significant others. Family members should always be included when providing information and reassurance. Clients should be encouraged to participate actively in their own care as much as possible.

For most clients, an artificial airway is temporary. They should be informed that the airway will be removed after they are able to ventilate adequately.

Home Health Care

For some clients the artificial airway may be permanent. One of the main goals for these clients is developing independence in rendering self care. Household members who will also be involved as care givers should be well informed about the reasoning behind procedures and given time and opportunity to develop competence in all aspects of care.

Table 14–3
Tracheostomy or Endotracheal Tube Suctioning—A Sterile Procedure

Nursing Implementation	Rationale
1. Assemble the following equipment: oxygen source, flowmeter, Ambu bag, connecting tubing; suction source and connecting tubing; sterile suction catheter about half the diameter of the tracheostomy or endotracheal tube; sterile glove; sterile normal saline; 5mL sterile syringe; sterile container to pour saline in; disposable bag.	Because intubated clients may require immediate suctioning, this equipment should be at the bedside at all times. A small catheter will not occlude the tracheostomy or endotracheal tube. Having all needed equipment readily availabe also helps the nurse to carry out the procedure in a more organized manner. This helps to allay client anxiety.
2. Wash hands using soap and water.	Bacteria on the hands could contaminate the clients airway. Hand-washing removes bacteria.
3. Explain procedure to client and provide reassurance even if client is unresponsive.	Explaining helps allay client anxieties.
4. If possible, have the client cough and deep breathe. Postural drainage may be helpful.	Measures that loosen pulmonary secretions or move them toward the major bronchi or trachea facilitate their removal.
5. Hyperoxygenate the client by using an Ambu bag connected to a high liter flow of oxygen. This procedure is more easily performed with two people, one to ventilate the client and another to suction.	Hypoxemia can occur during suctioning and could result in the development of cardiac dysrhythmias.
6. Open all equipment using sterile technique.	The lung is normally a sterile environment.
7. Put on the sterile glove.	
8. Attach the catheter to the connecting tubing. Suction of 80–120 mm Hg should be applied.	Pressure above 120 mm Hg may damage the tracheal mucosa.
9. Insert the sterile catheter carefully into the endotracheal or tracheostomy tube with the suction *off*, taking care not to contaminate the catheter. The catheter is inserted only until resistance is met.	This prevents the introduction of bacteria into the lower respiratory tract. Forcing the catheter can cause trauma to the lower airways.
10. Apply suction intermittently for no longer than 10 sec at a time. Rotate the catheter gently between gloved fingers when withdrawing the catheter.	Short-term suctioning limits the amount of oxygen removed. Suctioning for longer than 10 sec can result in hypoxemia. Continuous suctioning may damage the tracheal mucosa.
11. Turning the client's head from side to side may facilitate suctioning.	The anatomic position of the left main bronchus makes it difficult to enter with the suction catheter. Alteration in client position can facilitate positioning of the catheter.
12. The nurse again hyperoxygenates the client using an Ambu bag and evaluates respiratory status to determine if futher suctioning is necessary.	Hyperoxygenation prior to, between, and after suctioning prevents hypoxemia.
13. The catheter should be inserted in the container of sterile saline and flushed after use in suctioning.	Flushing removes bacteria from the catheter so they are not reintroduced into the respiratory tract.
14. Characteristics of the sputum should be recorded, including amount, color, consistency, and odor. Removal of tenacious secretions may require the instillation of 1–3 mL of sterile normal saline prior to introducing the suction catheter into the airway.	Changes in the sputum indicate alterations in the physiologic status of the client.
15. When suctioning is completed, the catheter is disposed of.	A sterile catheter must be used each time the client is suctioned.
16. The client's tolerance of the procedure is recorded.	This information is important in overall assessment of the client's physiologic and psychosocial status.
17. A fresh container of sterile saline should be obtained every 24 h. When the container is first opened, the date and time should be written on the label. When not in use, the bottle should be tightly capped.	Always assume that if bacteria can grow in the solution, they will. Every effort must be made to prevent introduction of bacteria into the lungs.

Home care professionals should be sensitive to the impact of the client's illness on the lifestyle of all members of the household. Providing opportunities for the client and other household members to express concerns and feelings is an important aspect of care.

As with most home care procedures, suctioning a tracheostomy tube or stoma becomes a clean procedure. Catheters may be reused. They should be washed in soap and water (dishwashing detergent), rinsed well and then soaked in a vinegar water solution or dried and wrapped in clean towels that are lint free. Sterile gloves are not necessary. Clean single-use gloves may be preferred by the care giver. Paper cups may be used to hold the catheter rinsing solution and disposed of after each use. Saline may be made at home. A physiologic solution of saline contains one teaspoon of salt per pint of boiled water. This can be stored in a clean, covered jar and made fresh daily. Careful handwashing before and after the procedure provides the degree of cleanliness required to keep the procedure safe for both client and care giver.

The Client With Chest Tubes

Inspiration and expiration depend partly on the presence of normal intrapleural pressure. Even though this pressure varies with breathing, it remains lower than atmospheric pressure. Disruption of intrapleural pressure by trauma, disease, or surgery will decrease the effectiveness of ventilation. To reestablish normal intrapleural pressure, the insertion of chest tubes may be required.

NURSING CONSIDERATIONS DURING CHEST TUBE INSERTION The insertion of a chest tube is painful. If the procedure is not an emergency, analgesics or pain medications should be given about 30 minutes prior to tube insertion. The nurse may need to request the medication order from the physician. It is of utmost importance that the nurse explain the procedure and equipment used. Clients should be told that the tube (or tubes) will be placed through the chest wall to drain air, fluid, or both, so their lungs can function normally. These tubes will be secured by a dressing and connected to a drainage apparatus.

When chest tubes are inserted at the bedside, the nurse will be responsible for obtaining equipment. The equipment may vary among institutions, but basically the following will be required:

- Local anesthetic, usually 1% lidocaine
- Antiseptic, such as povidone–iodine
- Sterile gloves
- Suture materials
- Collection receptacle
- Chest tube(s)
- Tape and petrolatum gauze for an occlusive dressing

Unless contraindicated, the client is placed in a recumbent position for insertion of the chest tube. If the tube is being inserted to remove air (pneumothorax) the client should be supine. Because air rises, the chest tube is inserted anteriorly in the midclavicular line in the second to fifth intercostal space. If the tube is being placed to remove fluid (hemothorax), the client should be placed in a semi-Fowler's position. Since fluid collects in the dependent area, the tube is inserted in the sixth to eighth intercostal space in the midaxillary line (Figure 14–14). The client who cannot tolerate a semi-Fowler's position should lie on one side with the affected side up.

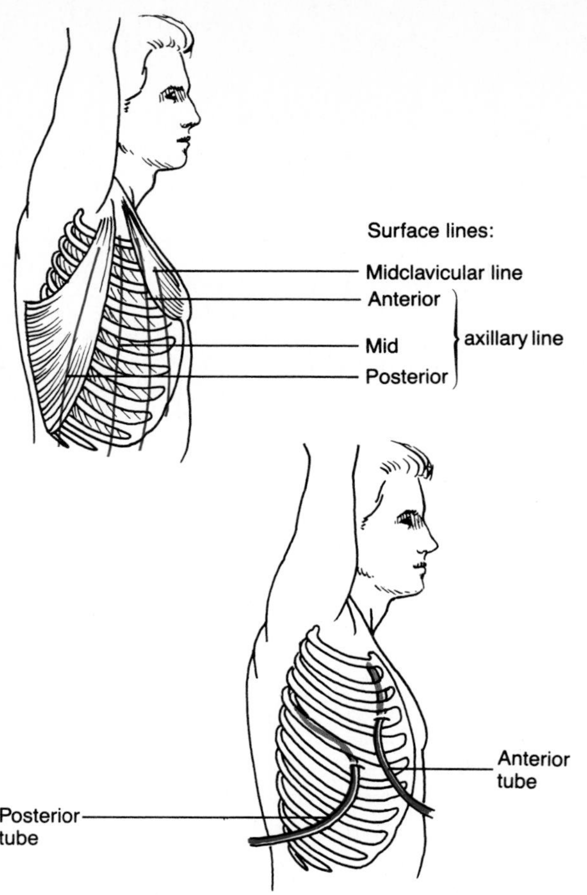

Figure 14–14

Insertion of an anterior or posterior chest tube.

DRAINAGE SYSTEMS FOR CHEST TUBES The chest tube will be connected to approximately 6 ft of tubing that leads to the collection system, which is placed considerably below the client's chest. The tubing should be long enough that it allows the client to move and turn without pulling. A long tube also decreases the chance that a deep breath would cause fluid to be sucked back into the chest.

The collection receptacle is placed below the level of the client's chest to take advantage of gravity flow, facilitating removal of air and fluid from the intrapleural space. This dependent position also prevents the backflow of fluid into the intrapleural space.

To prevent the reentry of air into the intrapleural space, the distal end of the tube must be submerged under water.

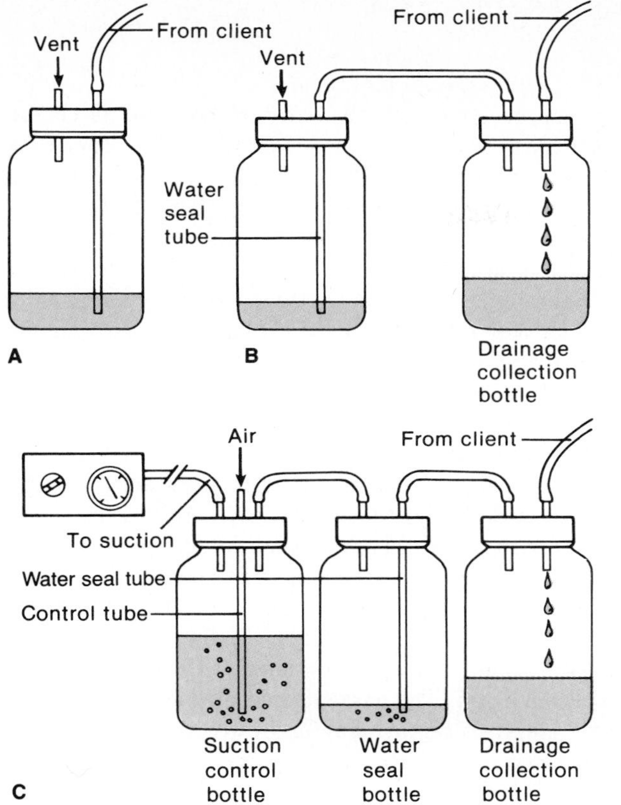

Figure 14–15

Drainage systems for chest tubes. **A.** One-bottle system. **B.** Two-bottle system. **C.** Three-bottle system.

This water seal is a necessary part of any chest drainage unit. During exhalation, the pressure in the lungs forces air out of the pleural space into the tubing, which is submerged under water (as shown by bubbling).

THE ONE-BOTTLE SYSTEM The one-bottle system may be used when a small portion of the lung has collapsed. Fluid or air is drained from the intrapleural space by gravity into the bottle (Figure 14–15). The end of the connecting tube is attached to a rigid tube, which is placed into the bottle. The end of the rigid tube is submerged in about 1 in or 2 cm of sterile saline or water, creating the water seal that prevents reentry of air. As indicated in Figure 14–15A, an open vent releases air into the atmosphere and prevents excessive buildup of air inside the bottle. Water-seal drainage using one bottle is not recommended if the chest drainage is expected to be significant, because any rise in the fluid level increases the pressure the client must exert to expel air and fluid from the chest cavity. If a moderate to a large amount of drainage is expected, a second bottle is added to the system.

THE TWO-BOTTLE SYSTEM In the two-bottle system, the drainage and water-seal bottles are separate, and fluid drains only into the collection bottle (Figure 14–15B). This system allows the water-seal bottle to remain at a fixed level so chest drainage can be more accurately measured. As with the one-bottle system, gravity drives the drainage system. When gravity drainage is not sufficient to remove air or fluid from the lungs, suction may be added.

THE THREE-BOTTLE SYSTEM The three-bottle system is sometimes used when suction is necessary (Figure 14–15C). The first two bottles are as explained above. The third bottle is added to control the amount of suction applied to the intrapleural space. The bottle has three tubes: one tube is connected to a suction source (a wall suction inlet or a portable suction unit); another is connected to the water-seal bottle; the long tube is the suction control manometer and is open to the atmosphere (Figure 14–15C). Suction not only pulls air from the drainage bottles but also pulls air in from the atmosphere through the manometer. If the manometer is submerged in 15 cm of water, the amount of suction necessary to pull atmospheric air to the bottom of the manometer is −15 cm of water pressure. When this amount of suction is obtained, bubbling will occur in the suction control bottle. Increasing the amount of suction applied to the system will result in more bubbling but will not increase the amount of negative pressure applied to the intrapleural space. The depth to which the manometer tube is submerged determines the amount of suction applied to the intrapleural space. Thus, the suction control bottle acts as a breaker system to prevent excessive pressure from being exerted on the intrapleural space.

COMMERCIAL WATER-SEAL UNITS There are a number of variations of chest drainage units available. One of the most popular is the disposable Pleur-Evac (Figure 14–16). The advantages of the Pleur-Evac are: it is lightweight, it takes up a small amount of space, it can be placed on the floor on a stand or hung on the side of the bed to facilitate transporting the client, and it is not breakable. The Pleur-Evac functions like a three-bottle system; it can be used as a water-seal gravity drainage system, or it may be connected to suction.

NURSING CARE OF THE CLIENT WITH CHEST TUBES The major objective of nursing care is to facilitate drainage of fluid and air, fostering lung reexpansion. After insertion of the chest tube, it is often the nurse's responsibility to apply the dressing. Sterile technique is necessary. Petrolatum gauze is wrapped around the insertion site, and wide tape is applied to provide an occlusive dressing. This prevents air from entering the intrapleural space. Even though the chest tube is sutured in place, great care must be taken to secure the tube when applying the tape. If drainage is present on the dressing, the physician should be notified.

Characteristics of the chest tube drainage should be recorded, including amount, color, consistency, and odor. Initially, the drainage characteristics should be noted every 15 to 20 minutes. If the container does not have calibrated markings, apply tape vertically and mark the level of drain-

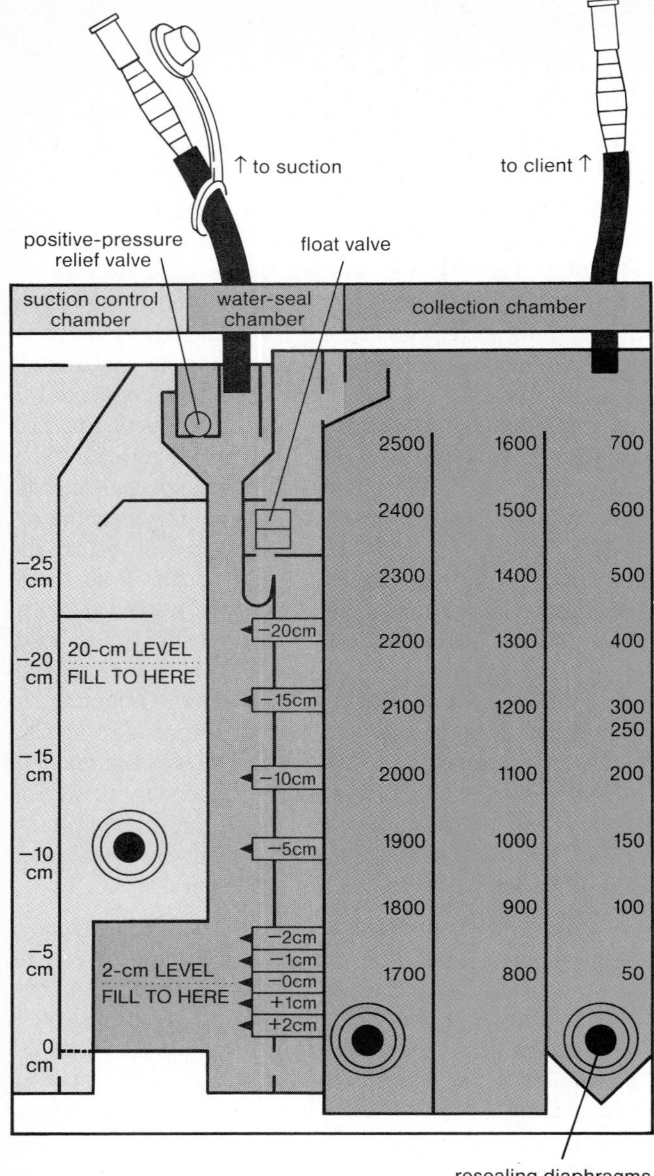

Figure 14–16

Anatomy of a Pleur-Evac.

age on the tape every hour. Persistent drainage of more than 100 mL per hour should be reported to the physician.

An important aspect of care for the client with chest tubes is assessment of the client's respiratory status. Question clients about their level of discomfort and any difficulty in breathing. Auscultate lung fields to determine if all areas of the lungs are being aerated. Watch for symmetrical expansion of the chest when the client breathes, and listen for any adventitious breath sounds. Note the rate, depth, and quality of respirations. To facilitate lung reexpansion and prevent complications, encourage the client to cough and deep breathe every hour.

MAINTAINING THE WATER SEAL It is essential that the water seal be maintained to prevent reentry of air into the pleural space. At least 2 to 2.5 cm of sterile water or normal saline should be placed in the water-seal bottle. Check the fluid level frequently and add sterile water or saline to replace whatever evaporates. It is important that the drainage unit be kept well below the chest level. If any part of the system is lifted above chest level, fluid may reenter the pleural space. When transporting the client, use a stretcher with a bottom shelf and place the collection unit on the stretcher shelf, keeping all of the system below the level of the client's chest. It is recommended that someone familiar with the water-seal system accompany the client.

The water seal can be lost by accidentally disconnecting the tubing or breaking the water-seal bottle. If this happens, air will enter the pleural space. Air may also enter the pleural space if the chest tube is dislodged. Disconnection should be suspected if the nurse notices an absence of fluctuation in the water-seal bottle or chamber. In the event that it becomes disconnected, the end of the disconnected tubing should be cleansed with an alcohol swab and reconnected. The nurse should then ask the client to cough deeply to remove any excessive air that may have accumulated in the intrapleural space.

If the bottle breaks, there is controversy about the actions to take. Some clinicians recommend clamping the tube for a minute or two (no longer). Check with the physician about whether chest tubes may be clamped, and record this on the care plan and in the chart.

If the chest tube is pulled out or falls out of the intrapleural space, the client should be asked to exhale forcefully, and the opening should be immediately covered. Ideally, the wound should be covered with petrolatum gauze and pressure applied until the tube can be inserted. If petrolatum gauze is not available, a gauze 4 × 4 or the palm of the hand or a sheet can be used. (Tissue should not be used because lint may enter the chest cavity.) If the client develops symptoms and signs of a tension pneumothorax, the pressure should be momentarily relieved to allow air to escape (Harper, 1981).

MAINTAINING PATENCY OF THE DRAINAGE SYSTEM The patency of the drainage system must be maintained to facilitate expansion of the lung. Make frequent, systematic observations to determine that the system is patent. Check the system for loose connections and reinforce the dressing as needed. Tape all connections to prevent disconnection of tubes.

Observe for fluctuation in the water-seal bottle or chamber. The water rises and falls with changes in intrapleural pressure. As the client inhales, fluid should be pulled up the water-seal tube or the chest tube, and the level should fall back as the client exhales. Absence of fluctuation may be caused by an obstructed tube, by a disconnected tube, or by reexpansion of the lung.

Bubbling is normally present in the water-seal chamber during exhalation. However, continuous bubbling during both inspiration and expiration may signal an air leak. The air leak can be from the client's lung or from an opening in the tubing or collection receptacle. The physician should be notified of any absence of fluctuation or continuous bubbling.

Inspect the drainage tubing for kinks or dependent loops. Kinking, which can occur along any section of the tubing from the chest tube to the collection bottle, will obstruct the flow of air or fluid. To prevent kinking where the tubing enters the drainage bottle, secure the tubing to a tongue blade with tape. Dependent (hanging) loops, which allow fluid to accumulate and thus alter the pressure within the system, can be avoided by proper positioning of the tubing. The tube should be coiled flat on the bed and should fall in a straight line from the coil to the drainage receptacle. The coiled tubing can be attached to the edge of the bed with a rubber band or tape and a safety pin.

When suction is applied, observe the suction control bottle or chamber for bubbling. Absence of bubbling suggests that the specified amount of suction is not being applied to the intrapleural space, whether because of an obstructed suction control tube, a leak in the system, an obstructed air inlet, or simply setting the suction too low.

Milking or stripping of the chest tubes is sometimes recommended to prevent the formation of clots or remove clots from the tubing. Grip and stabilize the tubing with the thumb and forefinger of one hand. Compress a section of the tubing by sliding the other hand from that point toward the drainage unit (away from the client to the collection receptacle). Release the first hand, and repeat the procedure along the rest of the tubing. This is facilitated by the use of lotion or lubricant. Some nurses prefer to use a special chest tube roller.

PSYCHOSOCIAL CONSIDERATIONS FOR THE CLIENT WITH CHEST TUBES The insertion of a chest tube is a painful, invasive procedure. Explanations and reassurance should be provided for the client, family members, and significant others. During the insertion, remain with the client to provide emotional support.

Clients may restrict their breathing and movement not only to minimize pain but because they fear they may dislodge the tube. Inform clients that the tube is secured with sutures and tape. Encourage movement such as turning, coughing, and deep breathing since this will facilitate reexpansion of the lung. Tell the client that pain medication can be given to decrease discomfort during breathing exercises. Narcotics, however, should be administered judiciously since they can depress the respiratory rate.

Explain the collection receptacle to the client. If suction is necessary, clients should be aware that bubbling and some noise is expected. Encourage clients, family members, and significant others to verbalize fears and ask questions about the procedure and equipment. Be aware that chest tubes may seem far more frightening to visitors than other sorts of tubes.

REMOVAL OF CHEST TUBES Chest tubes are removed when fluid drainage is less than 80 to 100 mL per day, when an air leak is no longer present, or when the tube is occluded. The sutures are cut, and the tube is pulled out quickly. (Thoracic surgeons disagree whether the tube should be removed as the client inhales or exhales.) The area is then covered by petrolatum gauze and a dressing that can be removed in 48 hours. The client may have some discomfort following the procedure, so be sure an analgesic has been ordered by the physician. A chest x-ray is done after removal of a chest tube to evaluate lung expansion.

Gas Exchange, Impaired

Clients with impaired gas exchange often require highly skilled nursing care and may need the assistance of mechanical ventilators. Other nursing measures include: deep breathing and coughing exercises, administration of oxygen, postural drainage, and suctioning.

The Client Requiring Mechanical Ventilation

Mechanical ventilation may be necessary for any client in whom the process of ventilation has been significantly altered. A significant alteration would be caused by a condition that prevents the client from maintaining normal oxygen and carbon dioxide levels in the blood. There are basically three types of positive-pressure ventilators: time-cycled, pressure-cycled, and volume-cycled machines. There are four common ventilation patterns: assist control, IMV, SIMV, and PEEP. Each is discussed here.

In assist control ventilation, the inspiratory phase is initiated by the client. Modern ventilators have a built-in safety feature so that if the client becomes apneic, the machine will deliver the preset volume at the ordered rate. In controlled ventilation, the machine has complete control of the client's rate and depth of ventilation.

IMV, or intermittent mandatory ventilation, delivers a preset tidal volume at a specific rate while also providing a continuous flow of air for spontaneous breaths. IMV was introduced for the purpose of gradually weaning individuals from ventilators.

SIMV refers to synchronized intermittent mandatory ventilation. With this method, air is delivered by the ventilator in synchronization with the client's own ventilatory efforts.

PEEP, or positive end expiratory pressure, prevents the collapse of the airways and alveoli at the end of expiration, facilitating the diffusion of more oxygen from the alveoli into the pulmonary capillaries. PEEP allows for a reduction in inspired oxygen concentrations because oxygen can diffuse during both inspiration and expiration.

NURSING CARE OF THE CLIENT WHO IS MECHANICALLY VENTILATED Accidental disconnection of the client from the ventilator must be prevented. A warning should be placed on all ventilators and on the nursing care plan reminding health care personnel to leave the ventilator alarm on at all times, even during client suctioning. The sound of the alarm is a minor nuisance compared to the brain damage that may occur if someone fails to remember to turn the alarm on and the client is accidentally disconnected from the ventilator.

An Ambu bag should be kept at the client's bedside to be used in the event of a power failure or ventilator malfunction. If the ventilator is not working properly, do not waste time trying to identify the mechanical difficulty. Instead, use the Ambu bag to ventilate the client, and have someone call the maintenance technician.

Clients who are ventilated mechanically often require monitoring of central venous pressure or pulmonary capillary wedge pressure. The positive pressure exerted by the ventilator will alter these readings. It is important that they be taken one way consistently, either with the client connected to or disconnected from the ventilator.

As a rule, respiratory therapists are responsible for checking the function of the ventilator at regular intervals. However, the nurse should also be familiar with the machine and how it functions. There are certain observations that the nurse should make at regular intervals.

The pressure indicator shows the amount of force required to ventilate the client's lungs. If the amount of pressure required increases or decreases significantly, assess the situation. Whenever any alarm sounds on the ventilator, respond immediately. If the reason for the alarm cannot be readily ascertained and rectified, the client should be disconnected from the ventilator and ventilated manually with an Ambu bag until the ventilator can be replaced or fixed. Since the alarms can be frightening to clients and any others in the room, reassure them that the client can be adequately oxygenated.

Check the settings on the ventilator hourly. Also check the ventilator tubing for water condensation. When any is found, the tubing should be disconnected and the water emptied. This will prevent accidental aspiration of water into the trachea or impairment in ventilation.

In addition to checking the ventilator, carefully assess the client. Observe the client for overt signs of hypoxia, hypercapnia, or hypocapnia. In addition, arterial blood gas values are obtained at regular intervals. Assess the client to ensure that both lungs are aerated. This involves auscultating lung sounds and observing for symmetrical expansion of the chest. Carefully monitor the client's vital signs.

Nursing care of the client who is mechanically ventilated also includes position change and skin assessment every hour, putting joints through active or passive ROM every 8 hours, and frequent mouth care. Clients who are comatose will need eye care, including use of artificial tears to keep the eyes moist, removal of crusts on lashes and lids with sterile saline or sterile water-soluble lubricant, and protection from corneal drying, irritation, or trauma by taping the eyelids closed.

A client will occasionally fight the ventilator. (This is also referred to as "bucking the ventilator" or "being out of phase with the ventilator.") The client attempts to exhale actively while the ventilator is still delivering the inspired volume. This conflict must be corrected because it results in decreased volume delivery and excessively high airway pressures. Measures to alleviate the problem include manual ventilation using an Ambu bag to increase volume delivery gradually and decrease the respiratory rate. Altered inspiratory flow rates may be ordered for the ventilator to correct the situation, or medication may be prescribed to sedate the client and allow the ventilator to function more efficiently (Traver, 1982).

A complication of prolonged mechanical ventilation is the development of a stress ulcer. The mechanism of the formation of stress ulcers is not entirely understood. It is related to a combination of hypersecretion of hydrochloric acid and decreased resistance of the gastric mucosal lining. The gastric irritation may lead to bleeding. Therefore, the nurse should assess stool and nasogastric drainage for fresh and occult blood. Gastric dilation may also occur from introduction of air into the esophagus. This may necessitate the insertion of a nasogastric tube.

PSYCHOSOCIAL CONSIDERATIONS FOR THE CLIENT WHO IS MECHANICALLY VENTILATED Mechanical ventilation is frightening for both the client and family. It is important to take the time to explain the equipment, the alarms, and the blinking lights. Assure the client and significant others

Nursing Research Note

Dressler D, Smejkal C, Ruffolo M: A comparison of oral and rectal temperature measurement on patients receiving oxygen by mask. *Nurs Res* 1983; 32:373–375.

These researchers investigated the differences in temperature readings from oral and rectal sites in clients receiving oxygen mask therapy. An IVAC 2000 electronic thermometer was used. The results suggest that both oral and rectal temperatures are stable measures. Rectal temperatures were more stable than oral ones, however. The mean difference between oral and rectal readings was 1.46°F.

The implications for nursing practice are related to clinical judgment. Should a 1.46°F difference in temperature change nursing intervention to a significant degree? Is the difference worth disturbing the client for rectal temperature taking? This study indicates a need for more investigation into temperature measurement and site selection.

that a nurse is always close by and will respond promptly to the client's call light and alarms. Clients should not be left alone in the room until they appear relatively comfortable with the situation. Be careful not to become so involved with monitoring the equipment and performing the procedures that the client is forgotten. Allow time for the client, family members, and significant others to verbalize fears and concerns. These clients are acutely ill and may have realistic fears about being dependent on the machine and the possibility of dying (Traver, 1982).

Mechanical ventilation obviously limits client mobility. Clients confined to their rooms have limited contact with the larger world, which may lead to disorientation. Make a point to interact with the client frequently. Orientation to date, time, and place helps to minimize confusion and prevent anxiety. Clients in an environment with a lot of activity and a high noise level may suffer from sensory overload, so it is important that nursing care be organized to provide periods of uninterrupted rest. Lighting can be controlled to create a day–night change. Sometimes it is helpful to keep a large calendar in the room where the client can see it and cross off days. Suggest that family members bring a few pictures or other articles to the hospital to personalize the environment. As clients improve, encourage them to become actively involved in their care to maintain a sense of control over their lives.

When clients require use of mechanical ventilation after discharge, the client and significant others need extensive instruction. Ancillary health care providers may be needed in the home. The nurse can coordinate activities among health team members (eg, respiratory therapy, social service, public health nurses) to assure the highest quality of care in the home.

Home Health Care

Home care of clients requiring mechanical ventilation poses some unique problems. Most home ventilators require either an AC or DC power source. Some are equipped with their own automatic switching device if the AC source of power is interrupted. Others must be changed over manually.

It is important that care givers have full understanding of the equipment and its capabilities. Local power companies should be made aware that a ventilator is in use and its specific requirements, AC/DC capabilities, hours of stored DC current available, and the client's degree of dependence on ventilator support. These clients are given priority in the event of a serious power failure and, if necessary, portable generators can be provided.

Many companies now specialize in providing equipment and care for the home ventilatory client. Competent companies will provide nurses, respiratory therapists, and other professionals to insure client safety. The client and all care givers should be comfortable using the equipment and in performing all procedures related to care and cleaning. Twenty-four hour phone numbers for service or advice should be readily available. Procedures to follow in the event of an emergency or equipment failure should be clear to all involved in the care of the client.

WEANING THE CLIENT FROM THE VENTILATOR Weaning the client involves reducing both physiologic and psychologic dependence on the ventilator. Criteria that should be met before weaning include acceptable arterial blood gas values on a liter flow of oxygen no greater than 40% to 50%. Additional criteria for weaning include: a stable chest wall, an acceptable chest x-ray, adequate cardiac output, normal temperature, adequate nutritional status, and a generally well rested condition.

Two methods used to wean clients are the T-piece and intermittent mandatory ventilation (IMV). Regardless of the weaning method used, the cuff on the endotracheal or tracheostomy tube is usually deflated. Explain the weaning process to the client before beginning. In T-piece weaning, the client is taken off the ventilator and a T-tube carrying humidified oxygen is attached to the airway (Figure 14–17). Encourage clients to use the breathing exercises taught to them while they were on the ventilator. Weaning is started during the day, scheduled around medications and activities so that the client is not uncomfortable and is not interrupted. The client should be suctioned prior to being disconnected from the ventilator. A semi-Fowler's position will facilitate the weaning process by preventing abdominal contents from pressing on the diaphragm.

Weaning is usually started with 15 minutes off the ventilator and then gradually increased if the client's respiratory status remains stable. The client's vital signs should be checked frequently. Indications that the weaning is being poorly tolerated are: increased respiratory rate and dyspnea, increased pulse rate, cardiac dysrhythmias, change in mentation, increase in fatigue, and decrease in pulmonary

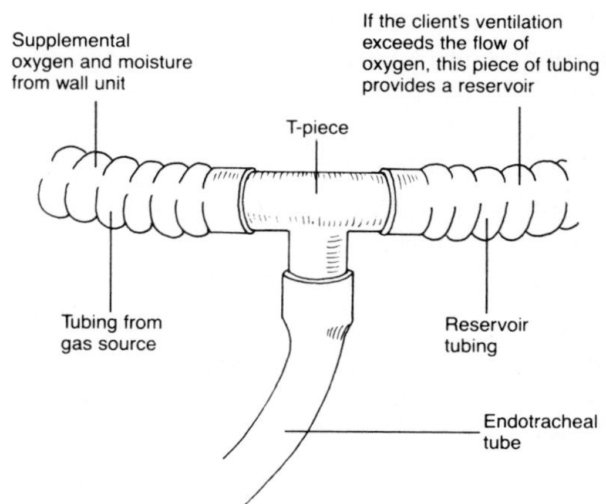

Figure 14–17

T-piece setup for weaning a client from a ventilator.

volumes. Arterial blood gas measurements are obtained for objective evidence of how well the client is ventilating.

PSYCHOLOGIC CONSIDERATIONS WHEN WEANING CLIENTS FROM THE VENTILATOR Clients who are mechanically ventilated for extended periods may develop a psychologic dependence on the ventilator that makes weaning difficult. Factors that can interfere with the weaning process include fear of sudden death, anger from being asked to give up dependence on the ventilator, secondary depression when the illness is chronic, and interpersonal problems such as a resentful or impatient spouse.

Counseling may be necessary for clients, family members, or significant others when attempts to wean the client from the ventilator are resisted. This is particularly true where physiologic parameters clearly indicate that weaning is feasible but difficulties are encountered. Along with counseling, psychotropic drugs may be necessary. For clients who are near panic, antianxiety medications administered prior to weaning have been found helpful. If depression is a problem, the physician may prescribe antidepressants.

Evaluation of the effectiveness of nursing care for clients with respiratory dysfunction includes assessment of the client's physiologic status, psychosocial function, and self-care skills. The evaluation process should include family members or significant others. Expected outcomes for the client with respiratory dysfunction are summarized in Table 14–1. If data collected concerning the client's responses and those of the family or significant others show that the expected outcomes are not being met, the nursing care plan must be revised.

Chapter Highlights

Disorders of the upper and lower respiratory tract can result in ineffective airway clearance, ineffective breathing patterns, and impaired gas exchange.

Pulmonary function tests are used in the diagnosis of lung volume abnormalities, to monitor the course of disease, and to evaluate the effectiveness of treatment.

Arterial blood gas analysis provides an objective measurement of oxygenation, carbon dioxide elimination, and blood pH.

Oxygen is primarily transported in the blood in combination with hemoglobin. The oxygen saturation and the oxygen-hemoglobin dissociation curve are measurements of the amount of hemoglobin combined with the oxygen.

Thoracentesis involves the insertion of a needle into the intrapleural space for the purposes of removing fluid that impairs breathing and to obtain a specimen for laboratory evaluation.

Pulmonary hygiene measures to improve ventilation and enhance the removal of secretions include pursed lip breathing, diaphragmatic breathing, and postural drainage.

Indications for placement of an artificial airway are to relieve obstruction, facilitate suctioning, allow for mechanical ventilation, and prevent aspiration.

Nursing management of the client with an artificial airway involves providing humidification, maintaining airway patency, and observing for complications.

Mechanical ventilation is used for clients who can no longer maintain adequate oxygenation and carbon dioxide elimination on their own.

Nursing management of the client with a chest tube consists of: assessment of respiratory status, ensuring proper function of the closed chest drainage system, assessing level of fluid drainage, and maintaining patency of the chest tube.

Evaluation of the client with a respiratory disorder includes assessment of: physiologic and psychosocial status; effectiveness of teaching; and ability of the client and significant others to cope with the health problem.

Bibliography

American Cancer Society: *1987 Cancer Facts and Figures*. New York: American Cancer Society, 1987.

Brown I: Trach care? Take care: Infection's on the prowl. *Nurs 82* (May) 1982; 12(5):44–49.

Burton GG, Hodgkin JE (editors): *Respiratory Care: A Guide to Clinical Practice*, 2nd ed. Philadelphia: Lippincott, 1984.

Byrne CJ et al: *Laboratory Tests: Implications for Nursing Care*. Menlo Park, CA: Addison–Wesley, 1986.

Chalikian J, Weaver TE: Mechanical ventilation—Where it's at, where it's going. *Am J Nurs* 1984; 84(11):1372–1379.

D'Agostino J: Set your mind at ease on oxygen toxicity. *Nurs 83* (July) 1983; 13(7):55–56.

Ellmyer P, Thomas N: A guide to your patient's safe home use of oxygen. *Nurs 82* (Jan) 1982; 12(1):55–57.

Fromme LR, Kaplow R: Mechanical ventilation: High frequency jet ventilation. *Am J Nurs* 1984; 84(11):1380–1383.

Fuchs P: Before and after surgery, stay right on respiratory care. *Nurs 83* (May) 1983: 13(5):47–50.

George RB, Light RW, Matthay RA (editors): *Chest Medicine*. New York: Churchill Livingstone, 1983.

Hanlon R: Contracting for care. *Am J Nurs* 1984; 84(3):335.

Harper RA: *A Guide to Respiratory Care: Physiology and Clinical Applications*. Philadelphia: Lippincott, 1981.

Harris RB, Hyman RB: Clean vs sterile tracheostomy care and level of pulmonary infection. *Nurs Res* 1984; 33:80–84.

Herrold RK: The drug connection. *Am J Nurs* 1984; 84(11):1389–1391.

Hoffman LA, Maskiewicz RC: The basics of suctioning; the specifics of suctioning; tubes and cuffs. *Am J Nurs* 1987; 87(1)56–58.

Hollen E, Toomey I, Given S: Bronchoscopy. *Nurs 82* (June) 1982; 12(6):120–122.

Irwin MM, Openbrier DR: A delicate balance: Strategies for feeding ventilated COPD patients. *Am J Nurs* 1985; 85(3):274–280.

Irwin MM, Openbrier DR: Feeding ventilated patients safely. *Am J Nurs* 1985; 85(5):544–546.

Janowski MJ: Accidental disconnections from breathing systems. *Am J Nurs* 1984; 84(2):241–244.

Natanson C, Shelhamer JH, Parrillo JE: Intubation of the trachea in the critical care setting. *JAMA* Feb 22, 1985, 253(8): 1160–1165.

Palau D, Jones S: Test your skill at troubleshooting chest tubes. *RN* (Oct) 1986;43–45.

Petty T (editor): *Intensive and Rehabilitative Respiratory Care.* Philadelphia: Lea & Febiger, 1982.

Pfister S, Bullas JB: Caring for a patient with a chest tube connected to the Emerson pump. *Crit Care Nurs* 1985; 5(2):26–32.

Traver G: *Respiratory Nursing: The Science and the Art.* New York: Wiley, 1982.

Treseler K: *Clinical Laboratory Tests: Significance and Implications for Nursing.* Englewood Cliffs, NJ: Prentice-Hall, 1982.

Wade JF: *Comprehensive Respiratory Care: Physiology and Technique.* St. Louis: Mosby, 1982.

Weaver T: Bronchoscopy, laryngography, and their potential complications. *RN* (Dec) 1982; 45:64–65.

Wimsatt R: Unlocking the mysteries behind the chest wall. *Nurs 85* 1985; 15(11):58–63.

Zori SJ: Mechanical ventilation: Bringing the patient into focus. *Am J Nurs* 1984; 84(11):1384–1388.

Resources

SELF-HELP GROUPS AND OTHER ORGANIZATIONS

American Lung Association
1740 Broadway
New York, NY 10019
Phone: (212) 315-8700

Members of this all-volunteer, nonprofit organization have established a mutual support network of self-help groups throughout the US, Canada, and Mexico. Contact a local chapter for information.

Asthma and Allergy Foundation of America
1700 Massachusetts Avenue
Suite 305
Washington, DC 20036
Phone: (202) 265-0265

A national, voluntary health agency that sponsors research, training of asthma and allergy specialists, and information for the public. Also maintains a directory of physicians who specialize in the treatment of these disorders and provides referrals to impatient and outpatient asthma and allergy treatment facilities.

Cystic Fibrosis Foundation
6931 Arlington Rd, Suite 200
Bethesda, MD 20814
Phone: (301) 951-4422

In addition to supporting research, educational and training programs for professionals and the public, and providing referral services, clinical care and counseling for children with cystic fibrosis.

International Association of Laryngectomees
% American Cancer Society, Inc.
4 West 35th St
New York, NY 10001
Phone: (212) 736-3030

This organization is composed of over 325 clubs known as "Lost Chord," "New Voice," or "Anamilo" (depending on geographic area). Members are persons who have undergone laryngectomies and wish to help others who have had this surgery. Local clubs sponsor counseling for clients and their families, self-help meetings, voice rehabilitation services, workshops on esophageal speech and the use of other voice appliances and seminars for health educators on first aid and artificial resuscitation for laryngectomees.

In Canada
Lost Chord Club
% Princess Margaret's Lodge
545 Jarvis St.
Toronto, Ontario, Canada M4Y 2H8
Phone: (416) 924-0671, ext. 4949

Organization for clients who have had laryngectomies, and their families. Provides self-help and mutual support with monthly meetings of group.

STOP SMOKING PROGRAMS

American Cancer Society
4 West 35 St
New York, NY 10001
Phone: (212) 736-3030

American Health Foundation Lifesign
Smoking Cessation System
320 E. 43rd St.
New York, NY 10017
Phone: (212) 953-1900

5-Day Plan to Stop Smoking
Seventh Day Adventist Church
Narcotics Education Division
6840 Eastern Ave. NW
Washington, DC 20012
Phone: (202) 722-6000

SmokEnders
50 Washington St.
Norwalk, CT 06854
Phone: (203) 846-4371 or (800) 828-4357

St. Helena Hospital
Deer Park, CA 94576
Phone: (707) 963-3611
(5-day live-in plan)

HOT LINES

Lung Line Information Service
National Jewish Hospital/National
Asthma Center
Phone: (800) 222-LUNG

Questions about asthma, emphysema, chronic bronchitis, tuberculosis, juvenile rheumatoid arthritis, occupational and environmental lung diseases and other respiratory and immune system disorders are answered by a specially trained nurse.

Asthma and Allergy Foundation of America
Phone: (800) 624-0044
Brochures and referrals are available.

HEALTH EDUCATION MATERIAL

American Lung Association

Provides numerous booklets and pamphlets on a wide variety of respiratory diseases. Contact a local chapter for information.

Asthma and Allergy Foundation of America
"Handbook for the Asthmatic," a booklet explaining treatment approaches and offering advice on how to eliminate household allergens. Many other booklets are available.

The President's Committee on Employment of the Handicapped
1111 Twentieth St., N. W.
Washington, DC 20036
Phone: (202) 653-5044
"Respond to: Workers With Cystic Fibrosis," a booklet for employers and those who work with cystic fibrosis clients.

NURSING ORGANIZATIONS

American Association for Respiratory Care
1720 Regal Row
Dallas, TX 75235
Phone: (214) 630-3540

Society of Otorhinolaryngology Head/Neck Nurses
% Warren Otologic Group
3893 E. Market St.
Warren, OH 44484
Phone: (216) 856-4000
This organization promotes the recognition of ORL and head and neck nursing as a distinct subspecialty. Members are RNs.

CHAPTER **15**

Specific Disorders of the Upper Respiratory Tract

Other topics relevant to this content are: Benign and malignant disease, **Chapter 10;** Care of the intubated client and the client with a tracheostomy, **Chapter 14;** Direct laryngoscopy, **Chapter 14;** The Heimlich maneuver, **Chapter 20;** Skin grafts and flaps, **Chapter 55.**

Objectives

When you have finished studying this chapter, you should be able to:

Identify and discuss the etiology and clinical manifestations associated with disorders of the upper respiratory tract.

List the medical and surgical procedures used for clients with problems of the upper respiratory tract.

Describe the recommended nursing care for clients with upper respiratory disorders.

Specify the role of the nurse in prevention of the spread of upper respiratory tract infections.

Explain the complications of head and neck surgery and related nursing interventions.

Anticipate the psychosocial/lifestyle implications of disorders of the upper respiratory tract on clients and significant others.

Educate the general public about etiologic factors associated with the development of disorders of the upper respiratory tract.

Specific disorders of the upper respiratory system cover a wide spectrum. Some may be considered minor annoyances of short duration. Other upper respiratory disorders can be related to extensive morbidity that may threaten the client's life or may seriously affect the client's lifestyle.

Clients who undergo surgery of the respiratory system are often very ill and very frightened. Their breathing may be compromised, they may be in pain, and they may be anxious. They, and their families and friends, often require a great deal of teaching, support, and encouragement to cope with the enormous alterations in lifestyle faced by some. To be effective, the nurse who cares for these clients must blend technical competence and human sensitivity.

SECTION 

Disorders of Multifactorial Origin

Epistaxis

Epistaxis (bleeding from the nose) is a common problem that occurs in people of all ages. It is an indication of underlying trauma or physiologic abnormality.

Epistaxis is usually related to hemorrhage from the anterior portion of the nose. The most common site of bleeding is the vascular area of the anterior nasal septum known as Kiesselbach's area. Epistaxis originating in this area is commonly observed in young and middle-aged adults. Epistaxis originating from the posterior area of the nasal septum is often quite severe and is observed more commonly in elderly people.

The most frequent cause of epistaxis is trauma. Trauma may be related to an external cause such as a blow to the nose or maxillofacial area, or minor injury such as after

NURSING DIAGNOSES IN
Respiratory Dysfunction

DIRECTLY RELATED DIAGNOSES

- Activity intolerance
- Airway clearance, ineffective
- Breathing pattern, ineffective
- Gas exchange, impaired

OTHER POTENTIAL DIAGNOSES

- Adjustment, impaired
- Anxiety
- Comfort, altered: pain
- Communication, impaired: verbal
- Infection, potential for
- Knowledge deficit
- Nutrition, altered: less than body requirements
- Self-concept, disturbance in: body image

picking of the nose or noseblowing. Epistaxis may be related to lack of humidification, local nasal infections, or tumors of the nose or paranasal sinuses. Some systemic disorders are associated with an increased incidence of nosebleeds (eg, hypertension and arteriosclerosis). Epistaxis may be a manifestation of an underlying blood dyscrasia or it may be related to treatment with anticoagulants.

Clinical Manifestations

Epistaxis is usually unilateral. Sometimes drainage from the posterior portion of the nose may flow behind the septum and out both nares; the nosebleed appears bilateral but is actually unilateral. Bilateral epistaxis may occur after nasal fractures. Clients who have blood dyscrasias may hemorrhage bilaterally from the nasal mucosa; generally, these clients will hemorrhage at other body sites as well.

Clients frequently swallow some of the blood and may report nausea or vomiting. If the swallowed blood passes through the gastrointestinal (GI) tract, the stools will be black, and stool guaiac testing will be positive for blood. Hypertensive clients may report headaches. If a large amount of blood is lost, the client may exhibit symptoms and signs of hypovolemia.

Medical Measures

Vasoconstrictive agents may be applied locally for initial control of hemorrhage from the anterior portion of the nose. A suction catheter is used to remove clots from the nasal cavity, and a sterile cotton ball moistened with a topical vasoconstrictor, such as aqueous epinephrine 1:1000, is inserted into the nostril. Pressure is then applied to the nose for several minutes.

If epistaxis is related to a systemic disorder, measures for correcting the underlying abnormality should be undertaken. For example, antihypertensives may be prescribed, or coagulation abnormalities may be corrected. Blood transfusion and fluid replacement may also be required.

Cauterization using a silver nitrate stick, trichloroacetic acid, or an electric cautery device may be used to promote hemostasis by sealing the vessels with denatured protein. If cauterization does not control the hemorrhage, an anterior nasal pack is placed (Figure 15–1). The material commonly used for this is a long, continuous strip of half-inch petrolatum gauze. Antibiotic ointment may be applied.

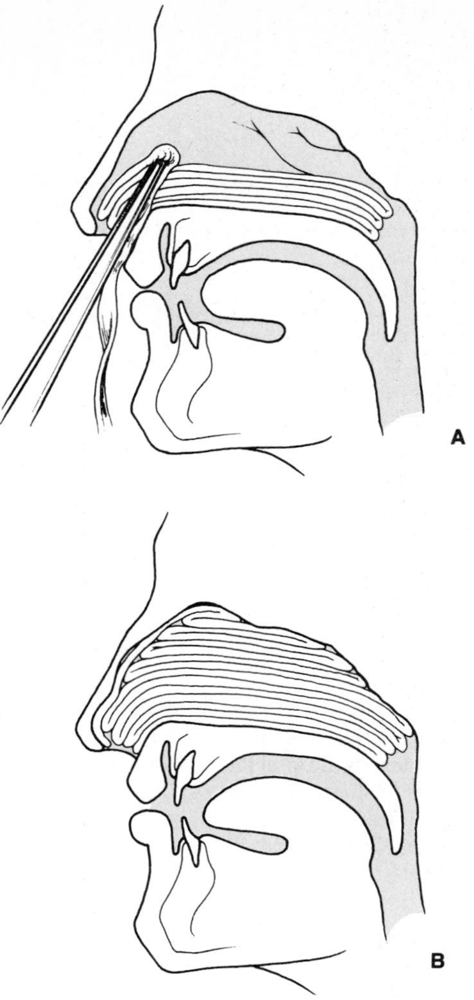

Figure 15–1

Anterior nasal pack. **A.** Gauze is layed in switch-back fashion. **B.** Both nostrils are completely packed with gauze in all crevices.

Hemorrhage from the posterior area of the nose is often more severe than anterior hemorrhage, and the site is more difficult to treat. A posterior nasal pack is inserted to apply pressure to the site of hemorrhage (Figures 15–2A and B). A sedative or analgesic may be prescribed to help calm the client and to reduce the discomfort caused by insertion of the pack. One method of posterior packing uses 4 × 4 gauze rolled up and tied with sutures as a pack. A catheter is inserted through the nostril into the nasopharynx, down into the oral cavity, and out through the mouth. The catheter is clamped, the pack is tied to it by the sutures, and the catheter is then pulled through the nose until the pack is in the appropriate position. Once the

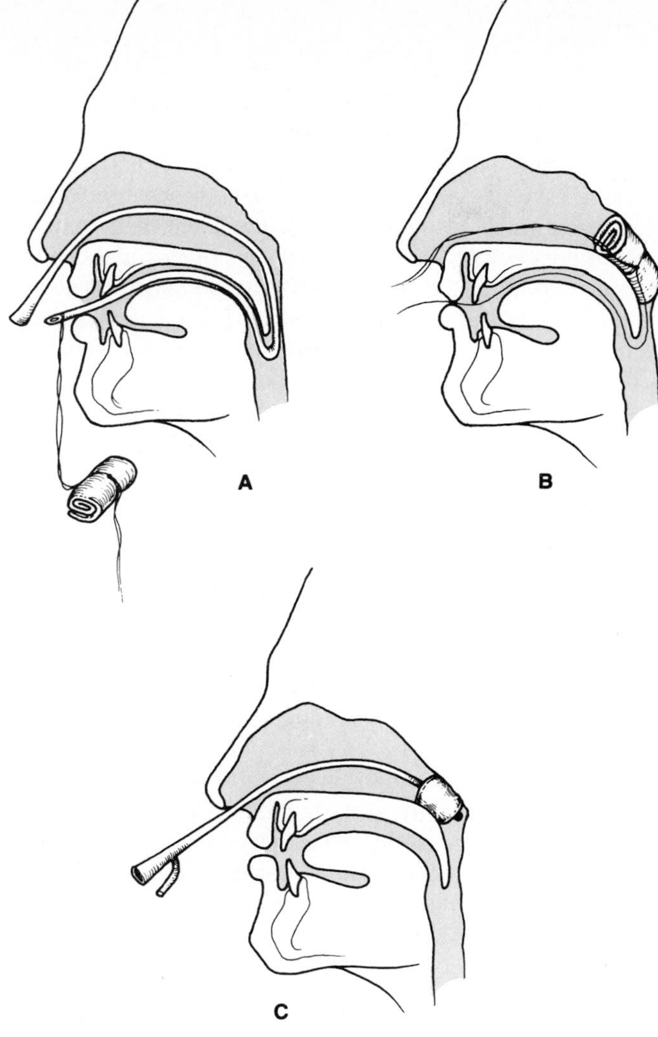

Figure 15–2

Posterior nasal pack with gauze. **A.** Catheter inserted via one nostril, passed into oral pharynx and out through the mouth; a rolled gauze sponge is attached to it. **B.** The sponge is drawn into the nasopharynx. **C.** Foley catheter method of packing the posterior portion of the nose.

pack is in the nasopharynx, an anterior pack may be applied also. An alternative method uses a Foley catheter (Figure 15–2C). The balloon is inflated with water once it is in the nasopharynx; the anterior portion of the nose is packed, and the catheter is secured. The pack is left in place for 3 to 7 days.

Specific Nursing Measures

Seeing large quantities of blood is often frightening to the client. The nurse can offer reassurance to alleviate the client's anxiety. Clients who are not hypotensive should be seated in an upright position with the head slightly flexed forward to prevent blood from dripping into the pharynx. Clients who cannot tolerate the upright position should be placed on their sides or supported with pillows to prevent aspiration. Blowing the nose is contraindicated. Since the client has lost blood, blood pressure and pulse must be monitored. Elevated blood pressure may be related to underlying hypertension or to agitation and anxiety. Clients who have lost a significant amount of blood may be hypotensive and are usually tachycardic.

Clients with anterior packing are usually sent home. Prior to discharge, tell the client to:

- Observe for bloody drainage. If bleeding begins and the gauze becomes blood-soaked, the client should call the physician immediately. When bleeding recurs, the client is usually instructed to return to the office or hospital. If unable to contact a health care provider by phone, the client should go to the emergency room for assistance.
- Avoid picking or unnecessary touching of the packing or nose.
- Apply a lubricant around the nares to prevent drying and crusting of secretions and skin.
- Since mouth breathing is necessary, oral hygiene should be given every 2 hours to prevent drying of the oral mucosa. Lubricants should be applied to the lips to prevent drying or cracking.

Clients who require posterior packing are usually admitted to the hospital because of risk of respiratory obstruction. The client with posterior packing will also mouth breathe and therefore will need good oral care. The posterior pharynx should be inspected often with good lighting, to check for bleeding and to ensure that the packing has not moved. Misplacement of the packing into the oral pharynx could obstruct the upper airway. Tell the client that swallowing may be difficult and causes a sucking sensation in the back of the throat. Because of this, a liquid or soft diet is best tolerated.

Nurse and client should be alert for renewed or increased bleeding. Frequent swallowing may indicate bleeding. Tell the client to report any sensation of fluid draining in the back of the throat or the taste of blood. Monitor vital signs at appropriate intervals, depending on the client's condition. Bleeding may result in tachycardia and hypotension. Stools may be tarry if bleeding has lasted for a few days.

Rhinitis

Inflammation of the nasal mucosa, or rhinitis, has many causes. It is often accompanied by inflammation of the throat and sinuses. Among the different types are acute rhinitis, allergic rhinitis, rhinitis medicamentosa.

Acute Rhinitis

Acute rhinitis, also known as the common cold or coryza, is the most common cause of nasal airway obstruction. Epidemiologists have noted that colds occur in three major waves a year—one in September, a second in midwinter, and another in the spring. Adults average two colds a year. Acute rhinitis is a contagious disorder; one can contract the disorder from aerosol particles spread by infected individuals as they sneeze, cough, or talk. It can also be transmitted by way of contaminated articles.

Acute rhinitis occurs when any of over 100 different viruses infects the upper respiratory tract. A large percentage is thought to be related to the rhinovirus, but other responsible agents include parainfluenza, influenza, respiratory syncytial virus, enterovirus, and adenovirus. One reason more colds occur in the colder months is that people tend to crowd together indoors, facilitating spread of infection; dry, heated indoor air also diminishes the protective function of the nasal mucosa. Evidence concerning predisposing factors is conflicting. Although most people believe chilling of the body and fatigue favor the development of symptoms, well-controlled laboratory studies have failed to corroborate this supposition. Stress, nutritional status, and other factors are thought to be related to colds, but no data presently confirm this.

CLINICAL MANIFESTATIONS Acute rhinitis has a relatively short incubation period. Symptoms begin to appear within 18 to 48 hours after an individual contracts the virus. Initial symptoms include irritation or a burning sensation in the nasopharynx, nasal stuffiness, dry scratchy throat, and headache. A persistent sore throat usually does not accompany the uncomplicated common cold. On examination of the nares with a nasal speculum, the nasal turbinates will be swollen, and a mucoid nasal discharge will be visualized that may become purulent as the infection progresses. Frequent bouts of sneezing are common, and a dry, hacking cough may be present. The client may be febrile and may report malaise. The uncomplicated cold usually resolves in 5 to 6 days. Significant pain or persistent temperature elevation should make one suspect a secondary bacterial infection. Possible complications of acute rhinitis include sinusitis, otitis media, bronchitis, or pneumonia.

MEDICAL MEASURES Aspirin may provide some relief from the feeling of malaise. Initially, decongestants such as pseudoephedrine may provide symptomatic relief; if not, an antihistamine–decongestant combination may be tried. Although vasoconstrictor nose drops may provide relief from nasal congestion, they should be used infrequently to prevent rhinitis medicamentosa, which is discussed later in this section. If secondary bacterial infection occurs, antibiotics will be prescribed.

SPECIFIC NURSING MEASURES Clients who develop acute rhinitis may request antibiotic therapy. The nurse should stress that antibiotics are not indicated, since acute rhinitis is caused by a virus, and antibiotics are not effective against viruses. Remind the client that aspirin, fluids, humidified air, and rest are a proven regimen. Liquids will replace fluid lost through diaphoresis and will loosen secretions. Humidified air, especially in the bedroom during sleep, will maintain moist mucous membranes. Rest will help alleviate fatigue. The nurse should warn clients that antihistamines have side effects such as drowsiness and dry mouth. The nurse might also suggest that the client limit contact with others during the first 2 or 3 days of the infection to reduce spread of the cold. Clients can be taught hygienic measures such as good handwashing technique and covering the nose and mouth when sneezing or coughing. Clients should also be cautioned not to blow their noses too vigorously. They should not close their mouths completely or occlude their nostrils while blowing the nose, since doing so can force nasal discharge into the eustachian tubes.

Allergic Rhinitis

Allergic rhinitis can be classified as an acute (seasonal) or chronic (perennial) allergy. Seasonal rhinitis is often referred to as hay fever. The symptoms last several weeks and recur each year. A person who has perennial allergic rhinitis may experience symptoms throughout all or most of the year.

Seasonal allergic rhinitis is related to sensitivity to pollens from flowers, grasses, or trees. Perennial allergic rhinitis is usually related to sensitivity to such substances as animal danders, wool, feathers, household dust and molds, foods, tobacco, drugs such as aspirin, and a host of other agents present in the environment.

CLINICAL MANIFESTATIONS Clients will often have nasal obstruction, sneezing, recurrent thin nasal discharge, itching of the eyes and nose, increased lacrimation, and frontal headache. If the reaction is severe, the individual may experience dyspnea related to bronchospasm. The nasal mucosa appears pale blue-gray and boggy. Clients who suffer from allergic rhinitis often develop nasal polyps.

MEDICAL MEASURES Antihistamines may relieve symptoms. Short-term administration of systemic steroids may benefit a client with severe allergic rhinitis, but prolonged use of steroids should be avoided because of their side effects. Desensitization may be attempted; this involves injecting gradually increasing quantities of the allergen weekly until a specific level is achieved. The process of desensitization stimulates antibody production against the specific allergen. Sometimes clients are given a series of injections prior to hay fever season to desensitize them.

Some clients will benefit from a submucous resection or a polypectomy to remove excess mucosa or nasal polyps. These procedures are explained below.

SPECIFIC NURSING MEASURES Clients who are undergoing desensitization can benefit from explanations of the purpose and technique of the procedure; the nurse can reinforce the physician's explanation. Clients should be warned about the side effects of antihistamines and cautioned about driving or operating machinery while taking these medications. They should also be cautioned about drinking alcoholic beverages, since antihistamines can potentiate the effects of alcohol.

If the cause of allergic rhinitis is not known, the client can try the following measures to alleviate symptoms:

- Using hypoallergenic cosmetics
- Avoiding wool clothing and blankets
- Limiting chocolate, milk, and eggs in the diet
- Removing domestic animals from the home
- Installing air conditioning or air filtration equipment in the home
- Covering mattresses and pillows with plastic

Clients should be cautioned not to use vasoconstrictor nose drops or sprays frequently.

Rhinitis Medicamentosa

Rhinitis medicamentosa involves a so-called rebound phenomenon related to excessive use of nose drops or sprays. Short-term use of these agents may decrease engorgement of the nasal turbinates, but continued use causes reengorgement and an actual increase in nasal stuffiness. Individuals who use these products initially obtain 1 or 2 hours of relief before nasal stuffiness recurs. Most people apply the medication repeatedly, and the cycle repeats itself, with the severity of the nasal congestion increasing and the duration of relief decreasing as more and more medication is applied more and more often. Eventually, the client becomes a "nose drop addict." Inspection reveals congested, shiny red nasal mucosa. Any client with nasal obstruction that has no apparent cause should be questioned about use of nose drops or nasal sprays.

MEDICAL AND SPECIFIC NURSING MEASURES The client is instructed to discontinue use of all intranasal medications. Recovery usually follows in 2 to 3 weeks, but the client may be uncomfortable during this period because of the mucosal engorgement. An oral antihistamine or decongestant and humidified air may relieve some symptoms.

The nurse should explain the rebound phenomenon to reinforce the client's understanding of why intranasal medication should be discontinued.

Deviated Nasal Septum

The nasal septum, which is composed of cartilage and bone overlaid with ciliated mucosa, is normally thin and straight. A variation from this ideal is called a deviated nasal septum; variations range from a single bulge to S-shaped deviations, sharply angulated deformities, or excessive spurring of the maxillary crest. Most adults have some degree of nasal septal deviation.

In adults, deviation of the septum may be due to either congenital or traumatic factors. Deviation may be related to a single, severe trauma to the area or to a number of insignificant blows to the nose that pass unnoticed over the years.

Clinical Manifestations

Septal deviations may produce no symptoms at all. When symptoms do occur, the most common is nasal obstruction, which may be unilateral or bilateral, intermittent or continuous. Other symptoms are nebulous. Headache is sometimes associated with a septal defect, but no etiologic relationship has been established. Deviation sufficient to cause pressure on other structures may cause pain in the nares, cheeks, or orbit. Hemorrhage can also occur. Inspiration may be obstructed, and continual exposure of the nasal mucosa to unhumidified air may lead to drying and cracking of the mucosa and to epistaxis. Clients who breathe through their mouths may experience dryness and irritation of the throat. The client may be predisposed to sinusitis because drainage from the sinuses is obstructed.

Deviation of the nasal septum is generally apparent upon inspection. If the condition has developed over a period of years, the inferior turbinate on the contralateral side may be hypertrophied. The degree of deviation does not always correspond to the degree of nasal obstruction.

Medical and Specific Nursing Measures

Many individuals require no treatment. If nasal obstruction is present or if drainage from the sinuses is impeded, a submucous resection or septoplasty may be performed. Nursing management is related to preoperative instruction and postoperative care as discussed below.

Submucous Resection of the Nasal Septum

A submucous resection (SMR) is a procedure to correct a deviated nasal septum. An incision is made through the mucosa of the nose to remove cartilage or bone using a special forceps (or, if necessary, a hammer and gouge). Bilateral nasal packing is inserted to prevent postoperative bleeding. The gauze packing may be impregnated with an antibiotic ointment to prevent infection and odor and left in place approximately 24 to 36 hours. This procedure is now more commonly performed as same-day surgery rather than inpatient surgery.

Surgery of the nose can be performed under local or general anesthesia, depending on the preference of the surgeon and client. Local anesthesia consists of topical or injectable medication, or both. This is often accompanied by the administration of a sedative and an analgesic.

The physiologic and psychosocial/lifestyle implications for the client are summarized in Table 15–1.

Nursing Implications

PREOPERATIVE CARE Inform the client about the events that will precede the operation. The client must not

Table 15–1
Nasal Surgery: Implications for the Client 

Physiologic Implications	Psychosocial/Lifestyle Implications
Submucous resection	
Pain in immediate postoperative period; headache possible	Initial anxiety about appearance because of ecchymosis and edema and effect on voice
Ecchymosis (and perhaps black eyes) and edema in early postoperative period causing obstruction and alteration in the sound of the voice	Need to avoid sneezing (or, if impossible, to keep the mouth open while sneezing) and to avoid vigorous nose blowing, sniffing, picking, or feeling the nose
Nasal packing for 24–36 hours may cause sensation of suction in the throat when swallowing and interfere with sleep	Need to avoid cleaning the inside of nose until directed to do so (usually in 10 days); may use cotton-tipped swabs soaked in 3% hydrogen peroxide
Increased nasal discharge from irritation to nasal lining	Numbness in tip of nose and alteration in sense of smell for weeks or months
Possible complications are: hemorrhage, septal hematoma, septal abscess, septal perforation, nasal deformities from removal of too much cartilage or bone, adhesions between septum and turbinates	May return to a desk job within several days; to vigorous physical labor in 1 week
Rhinoplasty	
Nasal packing for 1–2 days and splint for 5–7 days; nose may be taped in place for an additional 5–6 days	Anxiety due to swelling and ecchymosis and fear that results may not be positive
Hemorrhage and infection are potential complications (see also submucous resection above)	May require 2–3 days hospitalization
	Need to limit talking and facial movement
	Eyeglasses should be taped to forehead for 3–6 weeks rather than resting on nose
	Normal activity in 1 week; contact sports should be avoided for 5–6 months
	Need to tolerate 18–24 month period until appearance stabilizes

eat or drink within 6 to 8 hours of surgery, to prevent aspiration of stomach contents. Preoperative medication is usually given about an hour prior to surgery—usually a sedative and/or analgesic.

Explain the procedure and why it is performed under local anesthesia. (Bleeding is less, the operative area is free of equipment necessary in general anesthesia, and the client has some awareness of what is happening.) Tell the client to expect a sensation of pressure during the surgery when local anesthesia is used.

It is sometimes helpful for the client to practice mouth breathing prior to surgery since nasal packing will be in place. Gauze will be folded and taped under the client's nose to catch drainage in the postoperative period. This is referred to as a mustache dressing or a gauze snuffer.

POSTOPERATIVE CARE The major goal of nursing care in the postoperative period is to maintain safety and comfort. Hemorrhage is a potential problem because of the rich vascular supply of the nose. Bleeding is usually controlled by the nasal packing. Observe the gauze *under the nose* frequently and change it as it becomes blood-soaked. Remember to be gentle with dressing changes since the area may be tender. As a rule, the amount of bleeding is small, only enough to color the gauze two or three times a day in the first 24 to 36 hours. The client can be taught to change the gauze. The surgeon should be notified if frank bleeding is present or additional packing needs to be inserted.

After the operation, the client's vital signs should be monitored every 15 minutes until stable and then every 4 hours during the first day. The temperature should be taken rectally. Instruct the client to avoid sneezing and, if that is impossible, to keep the mouth open while sneezing. Frequent swallowing may be an indication of blood dripping into the pharynx. Instruct the client to expectorate postnasal drainage instead of swallowing it. Inspect the back of the throat at regular intervals for bleeding. If the client has swallowed blood, stools may appear tarry for a day or two. Because the client mouth-breathes while the packing is in place, frequent use of a mouthwash and lubrication of the lips are indicated. Because the nasal packing may interfere with sleep, a sedative may be helpful at night.

Edema of the nasal tissues is caused by manipulation

of the nose during any nasal surgery. The edema may cause varying degrees of obstruction. Obstruction of the sinus ostia may result in a headache in addition to the general discomfort caused by the swelling. When the client returns from the operating room, a semi-Fowler's position will increase venous return from the head. (An unconscious client should be turned to the side.) Ice packs can be applied during the first 24 hours to minimize the swelling and discoloration around the eyes.

Some physicians recommend after the nasal packing is removed that clients irrigate the nose with normal saline at regular intervals. Steam inhalations or decongestant tablets such as ephedrine or an antihistamine may help to alleviate the edema. Like nasal packing, edema that obstructs the nasal airway makes swallowing more difficult. The client may benefit from a soft diet and drinking through a straw. Regular diet can be introduced as tolerated.

Postoperative tenderness and pain are generally experienced. Initially, the client may require analgesics such as meperidine, 50 to 100 mg or morphine, 10 mg for one or two doses. Later the discomfort can be relieved by medication such as acetaminophen. Decongestant tablets assist in decreasing the bothersome nasal discharge.

Infections rarely develop after a submucous resection because of the rich vascular supply of the nose. Nevertheless, any temperature elevation should be reported, as should any unusual redness or tenderness of the nasal tissues, which may indicate an infection. Antibiotics may be prescribed.

Septoplasty

Septoplasty, reconstruction of the nasal septum, is used to conserve the nasal septum as much as possible. When too much of the cartilaginous septum is removed during a submucous resection, the tip of the nose can collapse because of lack of support. Septoplasty is an effort to avoid this by straightening rather than removing the deviated piece of septum. The septum is held in place by a suture or nasal packing.

The physiologic and psychosocial/lifestyle implications for the client (see Table 15–1) and nursing implications are the same as for a submucous resection.

Turbinectomy

Turbinectomy refers to a partial or total resection of a nasal turbinate. The procedure is most often performed to correct nasal airway obstruction by the inferior turbinate, but may be applied to the middle turbinate as well. Other surgical methods include electrocautery, cryosurgery, and the injection of sclerosing agents. Since one function of the turbinate is to warm and humidify inspired air, some clients may find this capacity reduced after turbinectomy.

The implications for the client are the same as those mentioned for the submucous resection in Table 15–1, and nursing implications are also the same as those described for a submucous resection.

Nasal Polyps

Nasal polyps are not neoplasms; they are masses of hypertrophied mucosa that may contain fluid. The majority develop as an outpouching of the mucosa covering the maxillary or ethmoid sinuses. They extend from the sinuses into the nasal cavity through the ostium. A polyp that develops in a maxillary sinus and protrudes into the nasopharynx is called an antrochoanal polyp. Polyps are often multiple and may occur bilaterally. Obstruction of the nasal passages develops gradually as the polyps multiply and enlarge.

Polyps form in response to recurrent swelling of the mucosa of the nose or sinuses. They may be related to long-term nasal allergy or to an infectious condition such as rhinitis or sinusitis. Nasal polyps are often observed in clients with allergic rhinitis. They are also found in clients who have aspirin-intolerant asthma, a condition characterized by aspirin sensitivity, nasal polyposis, and asthma.

Clinical Manifestations

Clients with nasal polyps may find that breathing through the nose is impeded. Disturbances of olfaction may be noted, and the voice may have a nasal quality **(rhinolalia).** On inspection, nasal polyps appear as smooth gray or gray-blue masses that can be readily manipulated. Their appearance has been described as that of "skinned white grapes." Infection or irritation causes the polyps to become reddened. Radiologic examination of the sinuses may show changes in the mucosa, since many nasal polyps originate in the sinuses.

Medical and Specific Nursing Measures

Although systemically or locally administered steroids may effect regression of nasal polyps, steroid therapy is contraindicated by the known side effects of steroids and by the fact that regression is frequently only temporary (DeWeese & Saunders, 1982). Polypectomy—surgical removal by one of a number of procedures—is recommended for most clients.

Inspection of the internal nares with a nasal speculum in any client with upper respiratory symptoms or problems with smell is important. Nasal polyps are often missed because this aspect of physical assessment is omitted.

Nasal Polypectomy

A nasal polypectomy, the removal of nasal polyps, is done when polyps result in some degree of nasal airway obstruction. The procedure is not used to remove an antrochoanal polyp or long-standing polyps with secondary infection.

This procedure is often performed in an outpatient

setting with the use of topical anesthesia and premedication. A wire snare is looped around the stalk of the polyp, closing the snare so the polyp is evulsed in one piece. The polyp is removed via suction or forceps and sent to the laboratory for examination.

Nasal polypectomy is often followed by some bleeding. If bleeding is significant, the client will probably be admitted to the hospital for observation. This minor surgical procedure does not usually affect lifestyle, body image, or require psychosocial adjustments.

Nursing Implications

The nurse should make sure the client understands that nasal polyps tend to recur and that decreasing the intensity of any allergy (or avoiding the allergen) may slow polyp recurrence.

Rhinoplasty

Rhinoplasty, reconstruction of the nose, is used to reconstitute and shape the anatomic features of the nose into a more pleasing form without impairing physiologic function. Rhinoplasty may also be performed to improve respiratory function when posttraumatic or developmental deformities result in nasal obstruction. This surgery is often done in conjunction with reconstruction of the nasal septum.

Basically, the operation involves rearranging and remodeling the nasal bones and cartilage. The classic rhinoplasty consists of the following interrelated steps: (1) remodeling the tip of the nose, (2) removing the nasal hump (cartilage and bone), (3) narrowing the nose, and (4) reconstructing the nasal septum. After the surgery is completed, packing is inserted, the nasal tip is strapped into position with tape, and an external splint is applied. The purpose of the dressing is to control the swelling and secure the nose in the desired shape.

The physiologic and psychosocial/lifestyle implications for the client are summarized in Table 15–1.

Nursing Implications

PREOPERATIVE CARE Most clients admitted to the hospital for elective cosmetic surgery are motivated, healthy individuals. Because of this, nurses may think these clients do not need much attention; however, this is not the case. They will be anxious about the procedure and the anticipated alteration in appearance. Some may even feel guilty that they are in the hospital but are not "ill."

POSTOPERATIVE CARE Nursing care is the same as described for the submucous resection, with a few additions. After surgery, the client's nose will be covered by a layered dressing of tape and a splint. Nasal packing will be in place with a mustache dressing. Caution the client not to pick at the dressing and to limit talking and facial movement as much as possible. As with other types of nasal surgery, the client is likely to show edema and ecchymosis. After a rhinoplasty, the eyes may be swollen shut. The nurse may need to reassure the client that this will pass in a matter of hours. Instruct the client to seek assistance immediately if frank bleeding begins, since hemorrhage can occur up to 1 week after surgery. Include the implications discussed in Table 15–1 in discharge teaching.

Laryngeal Polyps

A laryngeal polyp is a growth that arises from the mucous membrane of the vocal cord. Such polyps are usually benign but may become malignant or may be related to other complications. Polyps may have a thin stalk (pedunculated polyp) or they may have a broad base (sessile polyp).

The precise etiology of laryngeal polyps is not clear. Polyps have been known to develop in relation to vocal abuse and other irritative factors such as smoking.

Clinical Manifestations

The principal symptom of laryngeal polyps is hoarseness. The voice assumes a deep quality because the tissue of the larynx cannot resonate properly during phonation. If the polyp is pedunculated, it may drop below the level of the vocal cords occasionally, and hoarseness may be intermittent. Sessile polyps are related to continuous hoarseness. In rare instances, a large polyp may be associated with respiratory distress.

Medical Measures

Laryngeal polyps should be removed for tissue biopsy to rule out the possibility of malignancy. Polyps are generally removed by endoscopy under local anesthesia combined with sedation, but general anesthesia may also be used. Very small polyps may be resected by microlaryngoscopy. Use of a carbon dioxide laser has reportedly been successful in eradicating laryngeal polyps.

Specific Nursing Measures

Following removal of a laryngeal polyp, the client should talk as little as possible for 7 to 10 days. The nurse can provide alternative means for communication and encourage the client to use them. Coughing and clearing of the throat should be avoided for the first few days after the procedure. If the condition has been related to abuse of the voice, the client may benefit from referral to a speech therapist.

Laryngeal Edema

Edema of the laryngeal tissue is seen in both acute and chronic forms. Rapidity of onset varies, depending on etiology and the response of the individual.

Infectious processes that involve the larynx will be related to some degree of edema. Edema may also be related to irradiation of the neck, neoplastic disease involving the region of the neck, or infections that alter the lymphatic drainage of the area. Laryngeal edema may also be secondary to iatrogenic injury in connection with intubation or surgical procedures. In some instances, edema occurs in systemic diseases that alter capillary permeability or disturb the oncotic pressure of the plasma. **Angioneurotic edema** involves an allergic response of the tissue of the larynx. Angioneurotic edema occurs rapidly with an allergic reaction to inhalants, injected substances (including contrast media), transfusions, insect bites, food, or medications.

Clinical Manifestations

The initial symptom of laryngeal edema is hoarseness. As the condition progresses, the person may be barely able to speak. When inspected by indirect mirror laryngoscopy, the laryngeal structures and vocal cords may appear swollen. As obstruction becomes more severe, dyspnea, stridor, tachypnea, and cyanosis may occur. Onset of the edema is usually gradual, involving structures other than the larynx. Onset of angioneurotic edema, however, is usually acute. Symptoms and signs of laryngeal obstruction develop rapidly, and the condition can progress to total obstruction and death.

Medical Measures

Angioneurotic edema is a medical emergency. Intravenous administration of epinephrine usually brings about rapid decrease in inflammation. Corticosteroids are also sometimes used. Tracheotomy or intubation may be required to maintain a patent airway, particularly in cases of acute onset.

Laryngeal edema related to systemic disorders responds to treatments directed at the underlying condition. Serum protein and electrolyte levels may have to be monitored and corrected.

Specific Nursing Measures

Nursing responsibilities involve obtaining a history from the client of known allergies and documenting them well on the nursing care plan and in the client's chart. Clients who have been intubated should be monitored for evidence of laryngeal edema. Emergency drugs and a tracheotomy setup should be at the bedside of clients at risk and generally accessible on the unit for acute laryngeal obstruction.

Tracheotomy/Tracheostomy

Tracheotomy, an incision into the trachea, is performed to obtain a temporary opening into the trachea. If the trachea is brought to the skin and sutured there to make a permanent opening, it is a *tracheostomy.* The procedure is performed to provide access for aspiration of the bronchial tree or to relieve upper airway obstruction. It is often employed when the client is unable to cough effectively and expel secretions. Indications include:

- Mechanical ventilation that will be required for more than 7 to 10 days
- When an artificial airway is required, but the client is not a candidate for orotracheal or nasotracheal intubation (eg, because of severe facial injuries)
- To reduce the work of breathing for a weak or critically ill client by decreasing the amount of dead space
- A neurologic disorder paralyzing the chest muscles and diaphragm
- In conjunction with certain procedures such as a radical neck dissection or laryngectomy
- To bypass an obstructed upper airway caused by a tumor of the trachea or pharynx

A tracheotomy is commonly performed under local anesthesia. A vertical incision is made into the trachea through the second and third or third and fourth tracheal rings (Figure 15–3B), and the tracheostomy tube is inserted. Some surgeons place stay sutures on both sides of the opening to facilitate changing the tube in the early postoperative period. A tracheotomy is not recommended in an emergency; instead, a cricothyroidotomy (described later in this section) should be performed.

The physiologic and psychosocial/lifestyle implications for the client are summarized in Table 15–2. Alterations in anatomy after tracheotomy are illustrated in Figure 15–4B.

Nursing Research Note

Harris RB, Hyman RB: Clean vs. sterile tracheostomy care and level of pulmonary infection. *Nurs Res* 1984; 33:80–84.

The researchers set out to determine if clean tracheostomy care was more effective than sterile technique in preventing postoperative pulmonary infections. Based on laboratory data, they found that clean tracheostomy care was associated with fewer infections. Sterile technique and a mixed technique of clean and sterile procedures resulted in higher infection rates.

The study also found that nurses did not consistently follow written procedures and poor technique was a recurrent problem. This study reinforces the need for additional clinical experimentation in comparing tracheostomy procedures. It also substantiates the need for nurses to follow written policy to provide consistency in care and accurate assessment of the efficacy of the procedure.

Nursing Implications

Prepare the client for the effects of the operation—breathing through the stoma in the neck and loss of ability to speak while the stoma is open.

Frequently assess respiratory rate and breathing pat-

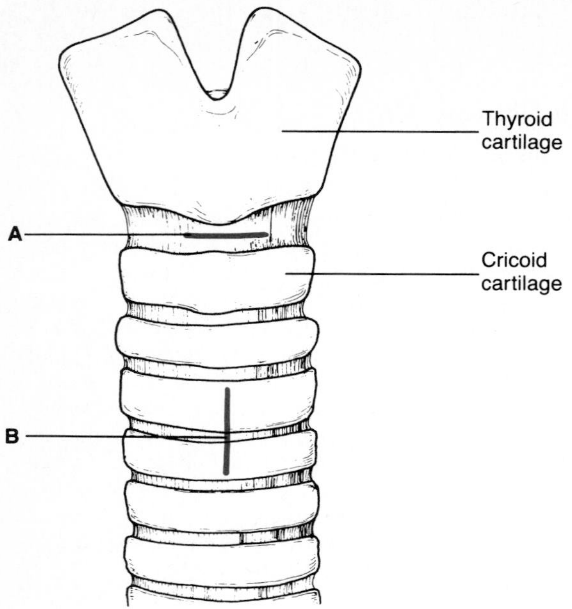

Figure 15–3

Incision sites for openings into the trachea. **A.** Area of incision for cricothyroidotomy. **B.** Area of incision for tracheotomy. (This illustrates incision at the second and third tracheal rings. It can also be performed at the level of the third and fourth tracheal rings.)

terns after the tracheotomy is performed. Humidification may be provided by humidified air or oxygen via a tracheal mask. It can also be achieved by placing a piece of 4 × 4 gauze moistened with sterile normal saline or water over the stoma. Tracheal suctioning should be performed as needed, depending on the status of the client. The nurse determines the need for suctioning by auscultation of lung sounds or by the degree of the client's respiratory distress. Other indications are arterial blood gas results and chest x-rays. Cleansing of the area around the stoma and the tracheostomy tube will be necessary.

Clients with tracheostomy tubes are also prone to complications such as fistula formation and tracheal stenosis that may result from the long-term nature of a tracheostomy. These complications and their associated nursing interventions are discussed in Table 15–3.

Clients who have a tracheotomy will need to learn how to care for themselves at home. The client and at least one family member should demonstrate competence at suctioning and cleansing the tube prior to discharge. Clients should be assured that occlusion of the opening by clothing (as when sleeping) would awaken them. Water poses a risk, however; clients should be reminded to cover the stoma when taking a shower. Some physicians advise against all water sports; others indicate that clients can engage in certain water sports if cautious. Stress that drowning can occur rapidly and that clients must be extremely cautious if they choose to engage in boating or fishing.

Clients may also be concerned about how a tracheostomy will affect sexual activity. Suggest suctioning the stoma beforehand to remove mucus and wearing a stoma cover or other clothing to avoid expelling mucus during sexual activity.

Laryngeal Paralysis

Paralysis of the larynx may be unilateral or bilateral. The nature of the presenting symptoms will depend on whether

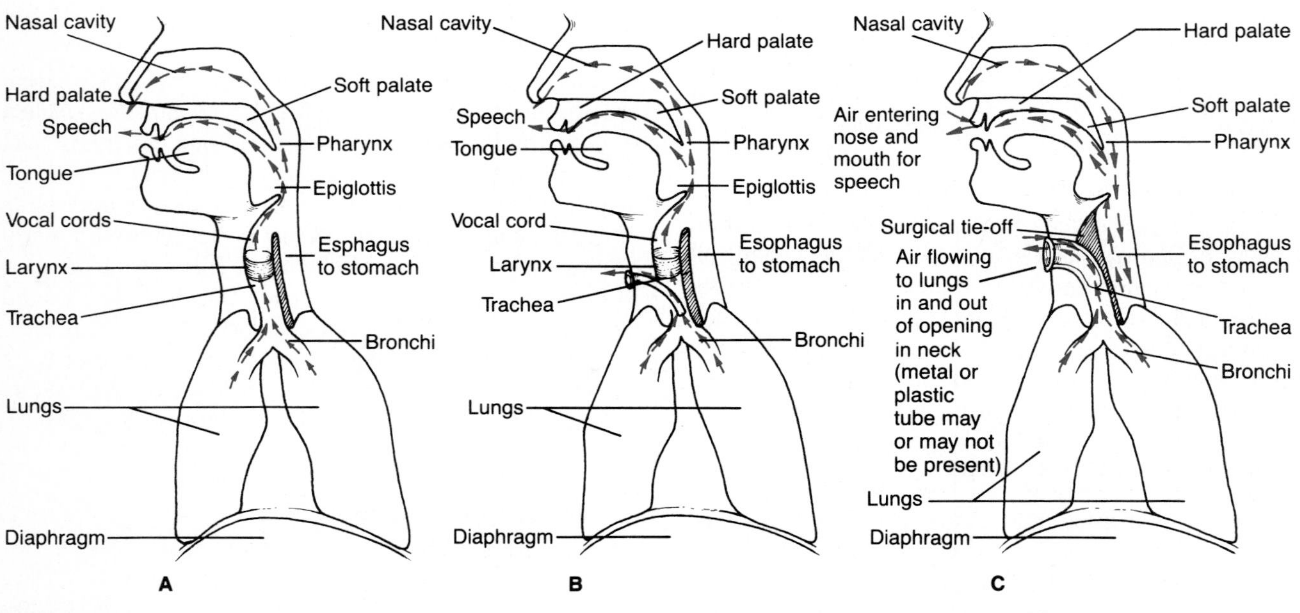

Figure 15–4

A. Normal anatomy. **B.** Anatomy after tracheotomy. **C.** Anatomy after total laryngectomy.

Table 15–2
Tracheotomy/Tracheostomy: Implications for the Client 

Physiologic Implications	Psychosocial/Lifestyle Implications
Discomfort requiring analgesics	Inability to speak unless opening is occluded
Ability to swallow may be impaired requiring nasogastic tube feeding	Fear of suffocation by inadvertent closure of the opening
Lack of humidification, warming, and filtering of inspired air	Body image alteration due to presence of stoma
Potential early complications are hemorrhage, tracheal tear, extratracheal intubation (inappropriate placement of tube anterior to trachea in a false passage), subcutaneous emphysema	Need to carry out self-care if stoma is permanent
Potential later complications are innominate artery-tracheal fistula, tracheal stenosis, tracheoesophageal fistula	Participation in water sports is risky because drowning can occur rapidly

Table 15–3
Nursing Interventions for Complications of Tracheotomy/Tracheostomy

Complication	Nursing Intervention
Innominate artery-tracheal fistula An infrequent but profound complication of placement of a tracheostomy tube is a fistula from the innominate artery to the trachea. A tube that is sharply angled may cause pressure to the tracheal wall and eventual erosion of the innominate artery. Erosion may sometimes be prevented by placement of a shorter tube. Hemorrhage from the artery will cause death if not stopped. Placement of a cuffed endotracheal tube with packing may be used to control bleeding until surgery can be performed.	Notify the physician immediately if a pulsating movement of the tracheostomy tube is noted. Assist with physiologic support of the client if fistulization occurs: • Suction blood from the airway. • Administer oxygen. • Administer replacement intravenous fluids as prescribed. Provide emotional support of client and significant others (refer to carotid artery rupture in Table 15–7).
Tracheal stenosis Tracheal stenosis or narrowing of the tracheostoma is a long-term complication that usually arises as a result of scar tissue at the site of the tracheostomy tube. Treatment consists of tracheal dilation, although surgical removal of the stenosed section and reanastomosis of the trachea may be required.	Prior to discharge, the client should be told to report air hunger as well as obvious narrowing of the tracheostoma.
Tracheoesophageal fistula Tracheoesophageal fistula is an abnormal connection between the trachea and the esophagus. It may occur as a result of pressure from an inflated cuff on a tracheostomy tube. This complication has become less common since the introduction of low-pressure cuffs.	Prevent excessive pressure on the walls of the trachea and esophagus (refer to care of the client with a cuffed endotracheal tube in Box 14–2 in Chapter 14). Report symptoms and signs that might indicate the presence of a fistula: • Food or liquids in tracheal secretions • Decreased exhalation volume when the client is assisted by a mechanical ventilator

one or both cords are affected and on the position of the vocal cords.

Laryngeal paralysis may be related to disease or injury to the recurrent or superior laryngeal nerves (branches of the vagus nerve) or to the vagus nerve itself. Although the underlying cause may be a disorder of the central nervous system, peripheral nerve disorders are more frequently responsible. Since the recurrent laryngeal nerve passes under the aortic arch on the left side, the nerve may be stretched and paralyzed if the client has an aortic aneurysm. Enlargement of the left atrium related to mitral stenosis may damage the nerve. Neoplasms in the chest or neck may stretch or invade the nerve. Laryngeal paralysis may also be related to trauma or to neuritis caused by metallic poisons (eg, lead) or infectious diseases (eg, diphtheria). Iatrogenic injury to the recurrent nerve or one of its branches during a thyroidectomy is a common cause of laryngeal paralysis.

Clinical Manifestations

Hoarseness may be present if vocal cord paralysis is unilateral, but the client's voice may also remain unaffected. Dyspnea does not occur with unilateral paralysis, because the functioning cord abducts to allow for a normal airway. If paralysis is bilateral, the cords are usually adducted. The client's voice will be adequate but weak. The major problem is the compromised airway; the client usually breathes normally during bed rest or minimal activity, but stridor is present upon exertion.

Medical Measures

Treatment of unilateral paralysis of the vocal cords is not mandatory. Some clients are disturbed by the change in voice quality, however. In these clients, injections of Teflon into the paralyzed cord may cause it to swell sufficiently to allow the normally functioning cord to approximate it (Passy, 1982).

Bilateral paralysis of the vocal cords compromises the client's airway, sometimes so severely that a tracheotomy is required to prevent asphyxiation. Arytenoidectomy is the most frequent surgical approach for bilateral paralysis; one or both of the arytenoid cartilages are removed and one of the vocal cords is retracted laterally and sutured, enlarging the glottic opening and improving the airway.

Foreign Body in the Nasal Cavity

Foreign bodies found in the nasal cavity are usually objects small enough to be inserted through the nostril. Occasionally, an insect may be sucked into the nasal cavity during inspiration. Objects inserted into the nares voluntarily—usually by a child but occasionally by a mentally ill or mentally retarded adult—make up a nearly endless list, including stones, dried peas or beans, nuts, beads, and buttons.

Clinical Manifestations

A complex of symptoms and signs including nasal obstruction, edema of the nose or the nasal mucosa, seropurulent nasal discharge, and foul odor are typically associated with a foreign body in the nose. The classic sign is lasting, unilateral foul-smelling discharge. On inspection, the foreign body may be visualized; the nasal mucosa is swollen, and pus may be present. Stasis of nasal discharge may be related to formation of a **rhinolith,** or nasal calculus, when the inorganic salts in nasal secretions collect around the foreign body.

Medical Measures

Usually, the foreign body can be removed with forceps; curved hemostatic forceps may be used if the object is hard and smooth. To increase client comfort and exposure of the object, a topical anesthetic and vasoconstrictor, such as 2% tetracaine and 0.5% phenylephrine hydrochloride, can be used. Soft material may be removed by suction or with a blunt, right-angled hook. An anterior nasal pack may be inserted if hemorrhage occurs after removal.

Specific Nursing Measures

It is dangerous to attempt removal of a foreign body from the nose without proper instrumentation. The object could be accidentally forced into the nasopharynx or could fall into the larynx or trachea, causing airway obstruction. The client should be reassured that it is normal for some bleeding to occur when the object is removed. Nursing measures related to use of nasal packs and to epistaxis are discussed earlier in this chapter.

Foreign Body in the Larynx

Foreign substances lodged in the throat can cause partial or total obstruction of the airway. If total obstruction occurs, the person will asphyxiate in minutes unless the object is dislodged. Foreign bodies may be aspirated in a number of ways. Many people carelessly hold objects in their mouths while working—pins, tacks, nails—and swallow or aspirate them when they are distracted. Intoxicated individuals, or those taking sedative drugs, may aspirate because their protective reflexes are impaired. A bone or other unexpected object contained in food, or a portion of the food itself may be drawn into the larynx because of difficulty in swallowing it. Individuals who talk while eating or eat hurriedly without chewing their food sufficiently are at increased risk, as are elderly people who may have poor dentition and cannot masticate effectively.

Clinical Manifestations

Any foreign body that becomes lodged in the larynx will impair respiration to some extent. If complete obstruction occurs, the victim will be unable to talk and may indicate choking by clutching the neck between the thumb and open palm. The symptoms of choking mimic those of a heart attack; hence the popular term "cafe coronary." If the airway is incompletely obstructed, the victim will exhibit signs of respiratory distress; coughing, choking, or gagging indicates that some air is moving through the respiratory tract.

Medical Measures

Total obstruction of the airway is of course an emergency; the victim can die in minutes if a patent airway is not restored. The Heimlich maneuver is recommended in this situation (see Chapter 19). If the maneuver is unsuccessful, a cricothyroidotomy should be performed. If the obstruction is not total, the individual may seek medical care. No attempt should be made to remove the object, since it might be dislocated in such a way as to obstruct the airway completely. The victim should be accompanied to a health care facility, since the obstruction might shift position at any time. Endoscopic removal of the obstruction should be performed by direct laryngoscopy (see Chapter 14).

Specific Nursing Measures

A person whose airway is partially obstructed will be anxious. The nurse should remain calm and reassure the client. Nurses should be skilled in the Heimlich maneuver and take every opportunity to teach it to the public. The laryngoscopy procedure should be explained to the client and significant others.

Cricothyroidotomy

This procedure consists of making an opening between the thyroid and cricoid cartilages into the trachea to establish an airway. Cricothyroidotomy is the procedure of choice in an emergency when establishment of an airway is necessary and orotracheal or nasotracheal intubation is not possible. Occasionally, it may be done electively for a client who requires the altered route of airflow for a short period of time. *This procedure is not without risk and should not be attempted by an unqualified individual.*

The emergency room of a hospital, the client's bedside, or the scene of an accident are the common settings for this technique, which must often be done without anesthesia because of its emergency nature. If the procedure is elective, local anesthesia is given. A short transverse incision is made in the neck immediately below the thyroid cartilage to expose the cricothyroid membrane. A stab wound is made through this membrane (Figure 15–3A), and a small tracheostomy tube is inserted to establish the airway. If the client will require intubation for more than a few days, the cricothyroidotomy is often converted to a standard tracheotomy.

The implications for the client and the nursing implications are the same as for a tracheotomy.

SECTION 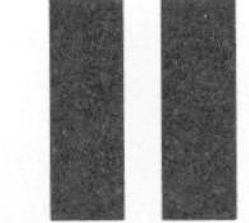

Infectious Disorders

The term *upper respiratory infection* (URI) refers to infections of the nose and paranasal sinuses, nasopharynx, middle ear and eustachian tube, pharynx, and larynx. Upper respiratory infections are among the most common infections found in the adult population; they are responsible for 80% of all school days missed and 40% of all workdays lost (Cluff & Johnson, 1982). Most of these infections are minor and self-limiting; if unattended, however, they may lead to more serious infections.

Sinusitis

Sinusitis is an inflammatory change in the mucosa of the paranasal sinuses. Inflamed, edematous mucous membranes partially or totally occlude the ostia leading from each sinus into the nasal passages. Mucus accumulates in the obstructed passage and exerts pressure against the walls of the sinus. One or all sinuses may be affected.

In strict otolaryngologic terms, sinusitis refers to a suppurative infection involving bacterial invasion of the mucosa. This condition, which may be acute or long term, is relatively common. Clients may report they are suffering from "sinus trouble," however, when the actual condition is allergic rhinitis, postnasal drip, headache related to unidentified causes, or various infections of the upper respiratory tract. Of every 100 persons who consult an otolaryngologist about sinus trouble, fewer than 10 have sinusitis (DeWeese & Saunders, 1982).

Acute suppurative sinusitis often accompanies or follows acute rhinitis. So-called swimmer's sinusitis is related to contaminated water being forced into the nose during swimming or diving. Maxillary sinusitis may be related to dental infection. Certain predisposing factors contribute to development of sinusitis (eg, conditions that impede drainage, such as nasal polyps or a deviated septum). Inflammation related to allergy can also obstruct drainage. Dryness of the mucosa, which may occur in overheated rooms in winter or in chronic smokers, can interfere with mucociliary defenses. Lower resistance related to any of a number of conditions can also contribute to development of sinusitis. Bacteria most often involved in sinus infection are pneumococci, streptococci, and staphylococci.

In chronic suppurative sinusitis, the mucosal lining of one or more of the paranasal sinuses has been irreversibly damaged. Failure to treat acute sinusitis, or repeated episodes of the acute form of the disorder, can lead to chronic suppurative sinusitis.

Clinical Manifestations

ACUTE SUPPURATIVE SINUSITIS Onset of symptoms is gradual, except in the case of swimmer's sinusitis. The initial symptom is nasal stuffiness followed by a sensation of pressure over the infected sinus. The client will experience general malaise and may have a headache. In uncomplicated cases, temperature is only slightly elevated (99°F to 99.5°F, or 37°C to 37.5°C). The leukocyte count is usually normal. During the 48 to 72 hours after onset, the client experiences localized pain and tenderness over the affected sinus. Palpation over the involved area elicits tenderness. Severe, constant headache frequently develops. Maxillary sinusitis will cause pain in the cheek. Pain

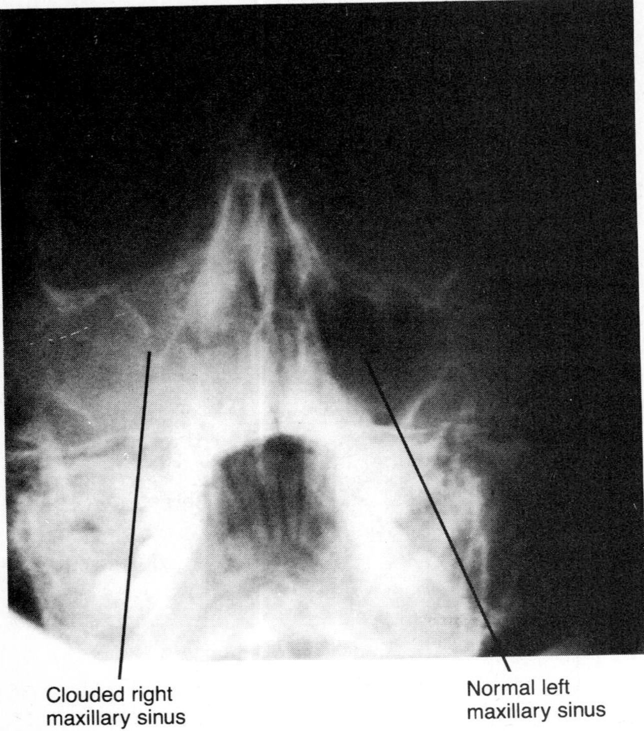

Figure 15–5

X-ray of a client with acute right maxillary sinusitis; the left maxillary sinus is normal. *Courtesy of Health Care Plan, Buffalo, NY.*

in the nasal bridge or around the eyes is related to ethmoid sinusitis, whereas clients with sphenoid sinusitis report deep pain behind the eyes and in the occipital area. Those with frontal sinusitis typically report a frontal headache. Most clients report nasal and postnasal discharge. Nasal discharge may be blood tinged initially, soon becoming copious and purulent. Postnasal drip may be accompanied by sore throat related to irritation. The client may be anorexic and nauseated.

The nasal mucosa on the involved side appears red and edematous. Purulent secretions may be observed in the nares. The face may appear swollen and red in the area over the involved sinuses, and periorbital edema may be noted. On radiologic examination, the involved sinus appears clouded (Figure 15–5); a fluid level may be visible. The affected frontal or maxillary sinus appears dark when examined by transillumination. The ethmoid and sphenoid sinuses cannot be examined in this manner because of their anatomic location.

CHRONIC SUPPURATIVE SINUSITIS Symptoms of chronic suppurative sinusitis vary in intensity. Nasal discharge is a common sign; it may be mucoid, purulent, or mucopurulent. Postnasal drip is frequently present and may be the only problem reported by the client. Related to postnasal drip may be an unpleasant taste in the mouth, frequent cough, and constant need to clear the throat. Some nasal obstruction may occur, particularly if nasal polyps are present. Clients may report headaches, but most do not, and pain in other areas does not generally occur unless a complication develops. Inspection of the nasal mucosa reveals redness and edema. As in acute sinusitis, an involved maxillary or frontal sinus appears dark with transillumination. Mucosal thickening or fluid in the area may appear on x-ray.

Medical Measures

Acute suppurative sinusitis is usually treated medically; surgical intervention is often necessary in chronic sinusitis. Analgesics, including codeine, meperidine, and morphine, may be prescribed. Vasoconstrictor nose drops or sprays may have short-term usefulness in maintaining an open nasal passage; the disadvantages of these agents have been discussed previously. Commonly used decongestants include ephedrine sulfate and phenylephrine HCl (Neo-Synephrine) administered as nasal drops or as inhalants. Antibiotic therapy is prescribed on the basis of culture and sensitivity tests and the duration and extent of the infection.

If the infected sinuses become totally occluded, and conservative measures fail to bring about improvement, surgical drainage and irrigation may be indicated. Generally, surgical intervention is contraindicated during the acute stage because of the risk of spreading the infection.

Specific Nursing Measures

Hot wet packs applied continuously or for 1 to 2 hours four times each day may reduce inflammation. A hot water bottle may also be used for this purpose. Steam inhalation may relieve symptoms. Clients should be instructed to avoid sudden changes in temperature, which may aggravate the condition (eg, entering an air-conditioned room when it is hot outside). Smoking should be avoided, since it causes further irritation of the mucous membranes.

Antral Irrigation

Antral irrigation (lavage) is one of the most common surgical procedures performed on the maxillary sinus. The maxillary sinus may be lavaged either as a diagnostic procedure to confirm chronic sinusitis, or as treatment for subacute sinusitis, to remove purulent secretions.

This procedure is often carried out in the outpatient clinic under local anesthesia. The client should be in a sitting position. The physician either punctures the wall below the inferior meatus with a trocar or inserts a cannula into the ostium of the middle meatus. Sterile normal saline, heated to body temperature (about 98.6°F, or 37°C), is then run through connecting tubing to the cannula. The fluid washes purulent material through the natural ostium, out of the nose, into a receptacle held by the client or

Table 15–4
Surgery of the Sinuses: Implications for the Client

Physiologic Implications	Psychosocial/Lifestyle Implications
Antral irrigation	
May experience a cracking sound and feeling of pressure during instrument insertion through sinus wall Potential complications are bleeding and puncture of the lateral wall or roof of the sinus	Does not significantly alter lifestyle
Caldwell–Luc procedure	
Sinus packing may be necessary for 24–48 h Edema of lip, cheek, and/or eye and ecchymosis for 1–2 weeks Analgesics may be required for discomfort during first week Temporary (for months) or permanent numbness of upper lip, gum, and cheek from damage to infraorbital nerve Potential complications are hemorrhage, osteomyelitis, and meningitis	Anxiety from temporary alteration in appearance Need to avoid irritating incision during oral hygiene Requires 2–3 days hospitalization Liquid diet for several days is tolerated best before progressing to soft foods Need to avoid nose blowing, chewing on the operative side, and wearing an upper denture for 2 week
Maxillectomy	
Postoperative discomfort usually requires narcotics Ability to swallow may be impaired Tube feedings necessary until healing takes place Increased oral secretions that require frequent suctioning Potential complications are hemorrhage, infection, visual problems, and discomfort when opening the mouth (trismus)	Ability to speak may be impaired May require use of dental prosthesis to enable swallowing and speaking Anxiety regarding cancer diagnosis and fear of dying Alteration in body image and function may be extensive if a large amount of tissue was resected May require reconstructive surgery
Ethmoidectomy	
Discomfort, edema, and ecchymosis Bleeding often considerable Diplopia initially, but subsides if superior oblique muscle was not damaged Nasal packing for 1–2 days after intranasal approach; 2–5 days after external approach Potential complications are hemorrhage, osteomyelitis, and meningitis	Anxiety from edema, ecchymosis, and diplopia Alteration in body image initially due to temporary change in appearance Concerns over possible facial scarring

nurse. The irrigation is continued until returning fluid is clear. The physiologic and psychosocial lifestyle implications for the client are summarized in Table 15–4.

Nursing Implications

Inform the client of the experiences he or she is likely to have during insertion of the instrument (see Table 15–4).

Observe the client for at least 30 minutes after completion of the procedure. Most clients will have a slight nosebleed lasting approximately 15 minutes. If epistaxis continues, the client will be admitted to the hospital for observation. Some clients may faint.

Caldwell–Luc Procedure

This radical antrum operation is commonly used to gain access to the maxillary sinus, primarily for treatment of chronic sinusitis, by removal of a part or the entire lining of the maxillary sinus. The Caldwell–Luc approach to the maxillary sinus is also used to remove an antrochoanal polyp; examine and biopsy a suspected sinus-cavity neoplasm; remove a foreign body from the sinus cavity, such as the root of a molar tooth; repair a fistula between the oral cavity and the sinus; perform surgery on a dental cyst that involves the sinus; or reduce a blowout fracture of the eye.

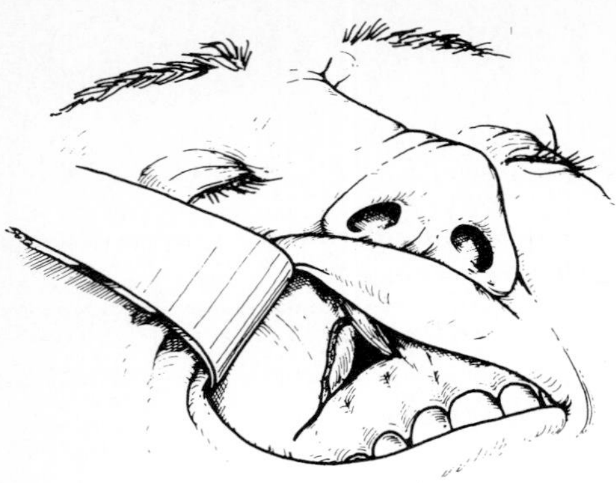

Figure 15–6

Caldwell-Luc antrum surgery.

The procedure may be performed under either local or general anesthesia with the client in a semisitting position. An incision is made under the upper lip (Figure 15–6). The surgeon then removes the infected lining of the sinus, leaving a large nasoantral window through the bone that separates the maxillary sinus from the nose to promote drainage from the antrum. The sinus may be packed with gauze to control bleeding. The physiologic and psychosocial/lifestyle implications for the client are summarized in Table 15–4.

Nursing Implications

Ice packs may be applied to minimize the edema. Ensure that the client has adequate oral hygiene. The upper lip may be quite swollen for several days, making it difficult for the client to brush the teeth. The nurse can assist by providing soft toothbrushes or sponges and mouthwash. Explain the danger of irritating the incision above the teeth, since if the area is numb, the client may not be aware of abrading the surface.

Check for unusual bleeding. When the packing is removed, blood may drip from the nose for approximately 20 minutes. Analgesics such as acetaminophen or codeine may be required during the first week after surgery.

Make sure the client understands the importance of not blowing the nose for 2 weeks. (The pressure could force air from the nose into the maxillary sinus and out the incision.) Inform the client about the other implications discussed in Table 15–4.

Ethmoidectomy

An ethmoidectomy is the removal of one or more of the ethmoidal air cells. An ethmoidectomy may be performed to remove polyps; eradicate chronic infection of the ethmoid cells resulting from impaired nasal drainage; approach tumors of the frontal, ethmoid, and sphenoid sinuses; repair cerebrospinal fluid leaks; as an extracranial approach when performing a hypophysectomy.

Ethmoidal cells can be removed through the nose (intranasally) or through an incision around the inner canthus of the eye (external ethmoidectomy; Figure 15–7).

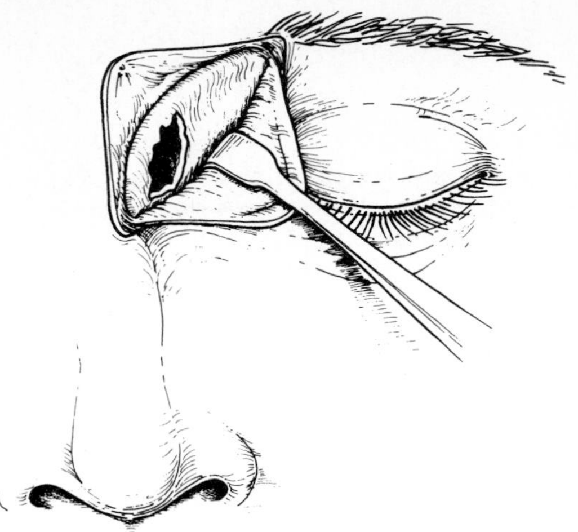

Figure 15–7

External ethmoidectomy. An external ethmoidectomy can be done under better visualization as cell by cell can be carefully removed.

An intranasal ethmoidectomy is usually performed under local anesthesia. An external ethmoidectomy may be performed under local or general anesthesia. After the infected tissue and ethmoid cells are removed, the operative area is packed, and one end of the packing is placed into the nose to assist in removal of the gauze postoperatively. A pressure dressing (eye pads and fluffs held in place by an elastic bandage) is applied from the client's forehead to the cheek for 1 or 2 days. The physiologic and psychosocial/lifestyle implications for the client are summarized in Table 15–4.

Nursing Implications

Make sure that the client's head remains elevated to minimize edema and ecchymosis. Monitor the client for bleeding around the dressing and below the nasal packing. Assess the client's neurologic status with particular attention to visual changes that might occur.

Once the surgeon removes the nasal packing, fibrin clots and mucus are removed frequently until the sinus cavity has healed. The client should be instructed to return for evaluation and removal of fibrin clots to prevent infection and the formation of adhesions. Incorporate the physiologic and psychosocial/lifestyle implications described in Table 15–4 into the teaching plan for the client.

Pharyngitis

Inflammation of the mucous membranes of the pharynx, or pharyngitis, is a common, troublesome disorder causing considerable loss of time from work and school. The three major classifications of this disorder are acute pharyngitis (the most common throat inflammation), acute follicular pharyngitis, and chronic pharyngitis.

Acute pharyngitis is usually related to a viral infection but sometimes to a bacterial infection. Acute follicular pharyngitis is a bacterial infection, most commonly caused by group A beta-hemolytic streptococci. Epidemiologists have found that streptococcal pharyngitis is most prevalent during February, March, and April. The incubation period is 3 days. Staphylococci may also cause pharyngitis, most commonly in debilitated clients. Pharyngitis related to infection with *Neisseria gonorrhoeae* has been reported; the condition appears to occur most often in homosexual males (Sloane, 1982).

Chronic pharyngitis has no clearly defined etiology; one or more factors may be involved. Acute pharyngitis may become chronic if not adequately treated. Irritation of the mucous membranes by postnasal drip associated with chronic infectious disorders or allergies affecting the nose or sinuses can cause pharyngitis. Administration of antimicrobial or antiseptic agents may suppress the normal bacterial flora of the oral cavity, leading to fungal infection and related inflammation. Lack of humidification of inspired air (eg, due to mouth breathing) or impaired production of saliva can lead to dryness of the pharyngeal mucosa, which predisposes it to infection. Xerostomia (dry mouth) is often associated with irradiation and the use of anticholinergic medication. Alcohol and tobacco irritate the pharynx, and environmental pollutants may also be related to pharyngitis. The incidence of chronic pharyngitis is higher among individuals whose tonsils have been removed.

Clinical Manifestations

ACUTE PHARYNGITIS Symptoms and signs of acute pharyngitis include a mild sore throat, slight difficulty in swallowing, and low-grade fever often accompanied by cough, **rhinorrhea** (nasal discharge), and headache. Symptoms remain mild unless complications occur, and the inflammation usually resolves within 4 to 6 days. Edema and redness of the pharyngeal and nasal mucosa can be observed, with visible rhinorrhea. Enlarged lymph nodes in the neck may be palpable.

ACUTE FOLLICULAR PHARYNGITIS Onset of inflammation is usually abrupt. Temperature elevation to 103°F (39°C) or higher may occur, accompanied by chills. The client may report headache, myalgia, and joint pain. Inspection of the throat reveals severe inflammation of the mucosa and edema of the uvula. White or yellow follicles may be observed on the lymphoid areas of the throat. Tonsils (if present) are enlarged and studded with follicles.

CHRONIC PHARYNGITIS Persistent sore throat and a constant desire to clear the throat characterize chronic pharyngitis. This disorder is often referred to as granular pharyngitis because of the presence of prominent granules on the posterior pharyngeal walls. The mucosa appears red and dry.

Medical Measures

Acute pharyngitis is usually treated at home with a combination of rest, oral fluids, warm gargles or throat irrigations, throat lozenges, and aspirin or acetaminophen. The recommended therapy for acute follicular pharyngitis consists of bed rest, throat irrigations, and the administration of antibiotics and analgesics. The majority of clients can be cared for at home. If the throat becomes so painful and swollen that fluids cannot be swallowed, the client must be hospitalized. Intravenous fluid administration may be required for 24 to 72 hours, until inflammation subsides.

Penicillin is generally the drug of choice for acute follicular pharyngitis since streptococci are the usual causative organisms. Erythromycin may be used if the client is allergic to penicillin. The client should be carefully questioned about any history of penicillin sensitivity before it is administered. To prevent recurrence of the infection, antibiotic therapy is continued for a full 10 days even though symptoms and signs of infection usually subside in 5 to 7 days.

Chronic pharyngitis that is allergy related is managed by removal of the allergen from the client's environment, if possible; if not, desensitization treatments are given. If the disorder is not allergy related, silver nitrate 10% may be applied locally by a physician. Throat irrigations are beneficial in treatment of chronic pharyngitis; irrigations are preferable to gargling because the warm fluid reaches the oropharynx.

Specific Nursing Measures

Throat irrigations play an important part in therapy for various forms of pharyngitis. Hot or warm saline is used to cleanse the throat, relieve symptoms, and stimulate vasodilation of the pharyngeal mucosa. Cleansing and vasodilation promote resolution of the infection by washing away irritants and stimulating the body's natural defense mechanisms related to blood flow. In the course of administering irrigations, the nurse teaches the client how to perform them. If the client is to continue irrigations at home, the instructions in Box 15–1 would be helpful. Teach clients with recurrent pharyngitis who also smoke about the damaging effects of smoking on mucous membranes and ciliary effectiveness.

Tonsillitis

The term *tonsillitis* describes inflammation and enlargement of tonsillar tissue with accumulation of leukocytes, dead cells, and bacteria in the crypts. Although the condition may affect either the palatine or the lingual tonsils, only palatine tonsillitis is discussed here because lingual tonsillitis is rare.

Although the tonsils are believed to provide defensive barriers against microorganisms invading the upper respiratory system, these defenses can be overcome by invading organisms. Acute or chronic tonsillitis then develops, either as a localized infection involving only the tonsils, or as part of a generalized pharyngitis.

Acute tonsillitis may begin as a bacterial infection of

Box 15–1
Client Instructions for Throat Irrigation

Use hot or warm saline (110°F to 115°F or 43°C to 46°C) unless it causes discomfort (2 tsp salt to 1 qt water).

Fill an irrigation container with saline and hang it 2 to 3 ft above your head. (A 1-qt douche bag works well.)

Hold a basin under your mouth or stand over a sink to catch fluid as you irrigate.

Direct the tip of the tubing toward the back of your throat.

Hold your breath and allow the saline solution to run into the back of your throat. Stop the flow when you need to breathe or rest. Be careful not to inhale or swallow as fluid comes in contact with mucosa.

Repeat the process several times a day. Frequency of irrigation will vary from every 2 to 3 hours while you are awake, to two or three times a day, depending on how severe your sore throat is.

SOURCE: DeWeese DD, Saunders WH: *Textbook of Otolaryngology,* 6th ed. St. Louis: Mosby, 1982.

the tonsils, or it may be secondary to a viral infection of the upper respiratory system. Group A beta-hemolytic streptococci are the usual etiologic agents. Chronic tonsillitis may follow an acute episode in which the infection lingers.

Clinical Manifestations

The initial symptom of acute tonsillitis is a severe sore throat, often accompanied by fever, chills, headache, and muscular discomfort. The sensations of discomfort and malaise may slowly subside after the first 24 to 72 hours.

Typically, palpation will reveal swollen, tender, cervical lymph nodes. Inspection of the throat reveals enlarged, inflamed tonsils, and inflammation of the pharynx. The uvula and palate are red and edematous. Uncomplicated tonsillitis will usually subside in 7 to 10 days in response to bed rest, throat irrigations, and adequate fluid intake.

If tonsillitis is caused by a streptococcal infection, the tonsils are studded with yellow follicles. This condition may be referred to as acute follicular tonsillitis or "strep throat" (see Figure 15–8). Streptococcal tonsillitis is marked by abrupt onset of fever, often as high as 104°F (40°C). Other symptoms include a sore throat of increasing severity, pain on swallowing, a sensation of fullness in the throat, chills, and joint and muscle pain. The client may experience referred ear pain (otalgia). The breath may smell foul. Leukocyte count and erythrocyte sedimentation rate are elevated. A throat culture is positive for group A beta-hemolytic streptococci. Also, an ASO (antistreptolysin O) titer greater than 125 in adults indicates recent streptococcal infection. Possible complications of acute tonsillitis include peritonsillar abscess, chronic tonsillitis, rheumatic fever, acute glomerulonephritis, cervical adenitis, and otitis media.

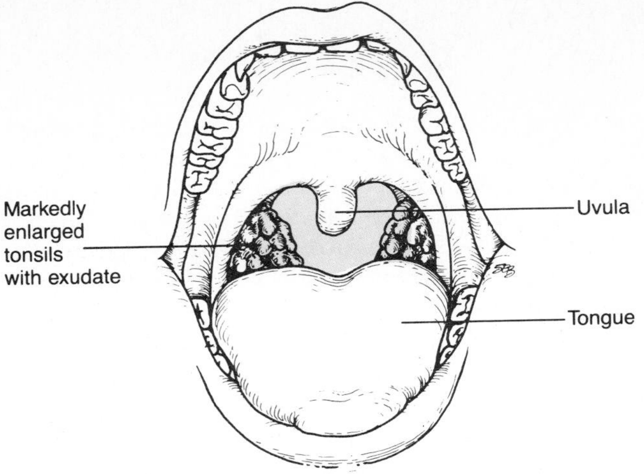

Figure 15–8

"Strep" throat.

Medical Measures

Penicillin is the treatment of choice for "strep throat." Erythromycin may be used if the client has a penicillin allergy. The usual dose for both penicillin and erythromycin is 250 mg q.i.d. for 10 days. Analgesics and antipyretics may improve comfort and reduce temperature. Throat irrigations are helpful. Tonsillectomy may be indicated for chronic tonsillitis.

Specific Nursing Measures

The client should be instructed regarding the need for increased oral fluids, rest, and continuation of medication therapy for the full 10 days. Throat irrigations as described in the section on pharyngitis are helpful. A soft, bland diet will help the client maintain nutritional intake.

Peritonsillar Abscess (Quinsy)

Peritonsillar abscess is an abscess, or collection of pus, between the tonsillar capsule and the superior constrictor muscle of the pharynx. Peritonsillar abscess, or quinsy, occurs as a complication of untreated or improperly treated acute bacterial tonsillitis, usually related to streptococcal or staphylococcal infection. The abscess forms when infection extends through the capsule and invades surrounding tissue. Cultures taken from the abscess may reveal *Streptococcus pyogenes, Staphylococcus aureus,* gram-negative organisms, or anaerobic organisms.

Clinical Manifestations

The client has a sore throat that persists for several days. An apparent improvement may be followed by unilateral increase in severity. Increasing dysphagia is accompanied by pain and spasm of the muscles of the jaw (trismus); inability to swallow saliva may result in drooling. Referred otalgia is not uncommon, and the client is febrile. The client's voice is muffled.

Inspection of the oral cavity reveals edema of the soft

palate on the involved side. This area is often reddened, and there may be fluctuation (a wavy impulse produced by the vibration of fluid) with palpation. The edema causes the uvula to deviate toward the uninvolved side, and the involved tonsil is displaced toward the midline.

Medical Measures

Frequently, the client must be hospitalized so that fluids and antibiotics can be administered intravenously. The abscess is incised and drained under local or topical anesthesia. Analgesics are given to relieve pain, and hot saline irrigations are administered. Once the infection has subsided, or in about 1 month, a tonsillectomy is performed to prevent recurrence.

Specific Nursing Measures

Nursing management of the client receiving throat irrigations is discussed in the section on pharyngitis. The client should receive instruction on how to perform this procedure at home. Clients with quinsy often have difficulty in swallowing until the inflammation has subsided.

Infectious Mononucleosis

Infectious mononucleosis, sometimes called glandular fever, is a viral infection that causes diffuse hyperplasia of lymphoid tissue. It affects children and young adults and rarely occurs in persons over 30. Mononucleosis is most often seen in college students and military recruits.

Infectious mononucleosis is caused by a virus in the herpes family known as the Epstein–Barr virus. The virus is not highly contagious, so roommates and family members rarely contract the disease unless exhaustion or some other factor has impaired their immune systems. The virus can be transmitted by saliva, however; thus, the nickname, "the kissing disease." The incubation period is 2 to 7 weeks. Levels of Epstein–Barr viral antibodies are elevated in persons who have the disorder or who have a history of mononucleosis.

Clinical Manifestations

An episode of infectious mononucleosis may be mild and transient, or the client may be severely ill. Symptoms include fever, sore throat, malaise, generalized weakness, and headache. Clinical findings can include marked cervical lymphadenopathy, especially of the posterior cervical nodes, pharyngitis, splenomegaly, and elevated temperature. Mononucleosis may be suspected in clients with pharyngitis when enlargement of the cervical lymph nodes is disproportionate to the severity of the pharyngitis. The nodes are firm, discrete, and tender on palpation. Lymph glands in the groin and axilla may also be enlarged. The nasal and pharyngeal mucosa appears red and edematous, the tonsils are enlarged, and a gray membrane may cover the tonsillar tissue. Exudate in the pharynx is indicative of secondary infection.

Fever ranges from 100°F to 103°F (38°C to 39°C) and may persist for 7 to 10 days. In more severe cases, the temperature may reach 105°F (41°C). The spleen may be enlarged and palpable. Approximately 10% of clients will have hepatic dysfunction accompanied by jaundice and hepatomegaly. Some clients will have a skin rash, petechiae, and icterus.

Laboratory studies will reveal a leukocyte count of 12,000 to 25,000, with an elevated number of atypical lymphocytes. Heterophil antibody tests and Monospot tests will be positive. Liver function studies are often abnormal.

Mononucleosis generally persists for 2 to 4 weeks, and it is not uncommon for clients with this disorder to develop secondary infections. Complications are rare but serious, including laryngeal edema and airway obstruction, splenic rupture, hepatitis, and hemolytic anemia. Guillain–Barré syndrome has been reported in association with infectious mononucleosis.

Medical Measures

If copious pharyngeal exudate is present, airway obstruction may occur; steroids may be administered to reduce inflammation but will have no effect on the virus. Antibiotics are given only if secondary bacterial infection develops. Ampicillin should be avoided, since this drug is related to development of a rash or hypersensitivity reaction in a high percentage of clients with mononucleosis.

Hospitalization may be required if the client is severely ill with anorexia, airway obstruction, or severe splenomegaly. The abdomen of a person with an enlarged spleen should not be palpated, because splenic rupture could occur. Sudden abdominal pain in a client with splenomegaly may indicate splenic rupture.

Specific Nursing Measures

Usually, the client can be cared for at home. Isolation is not necessary. The client should be on bed rest while febrile and should continue to get ample rest for 4 to 6 weeks after the fever has broken. Warm saline gargles and nonaspirin analgesics will alleviate throat pain (aspirin is contraindicated when hepatic dysfunction is present). Semisolid foods like gelatin, ice cream, or yogurt are more easily swallowed. Intimate contact (eg, kissing) should be avoided until laboratory results are normal.

Young people often are able to continue their routine activities, such as school attendance and homework, after the acute stage has passed. In addition to the need for increased rest, clients should know that avoiding trauma to the abdomen is important during the recovery process to prevent splenic rupture. Contact sports and playful roughhousing are to be avoided. A stool softener may prevent constipation and straining.

Vincent's Angina

Vincent's angina is an acute ulcerative infection of the pharynx that initially involves a tonsil—usually only one, although the infection may spread to the contralateral tonsil, the pharynx, and the gingiva. The disease occurs most often in young adults aged 15 to 35 and rarely occurs in persons who have had a tonsillectomy. Vincent's angina is not uncommon and may occur in epidemic form (Paparella & Shumrick, 1980).

Vincent's angina is related to proliferation of gram-negative organisms, spirochetes *(Borrelia vincentii),* and fusiform bacilli, small numbers of which are normally present in the mouth. Predisposing factors include irritative oral lesions such as decayed teeth, poor oral and dental hygiene, low blood levels of vitamin C, and debilitation.

Clinical Manifestations

The client reports unilateral pharyngitis that increases in severity over several days. Additional symptoms may include referred otalgia on the involved side, an unpleasant taste in the mouth, and a fetid odor. These symptoms are usually accompanied by a generalized malaise and a mildly elevated temperature (99°F to 100°F or 37°C to 38°C). Typical findings include an ulcerated area in one tonsil that does not involve the tonsillar pillar and a gray pseudomembrane covering the affected tonsil. The membrane can be easily rubbed off, and hemorrhage of the ulcerated area usually occurs when the membrane has been removed. Gingivostomatitis (trench mouth) may accompany Vincent's angina; gingival hemorrhage may then be the principal symptom. Cervical lymphadenopathy may be noted, usually unilaterally. Diagnosis is confirmed by a Gram's stain of a specimen from the ulcerated area.

Medical Measures

Penicillin is administered parenterally for approximately 1 week; sodium borate or hydrogen peroxide is applied to the ulcerated area. The therapeutic value of these agents is related to their release of oxygen; the microorganisms involved in Vincent's angina are anaerobic. Vincent's angina generally responds rapidly to treatment; complications are rare.

Specific Nursing Measures

Meticulous oral hygiene is of primary importance. The nurse should instruct the client in the use of mouthwashes and gargles (half-strength hydrogen peroxide has been recommended) and in precautionary measures to prevent spread of the infection. This disorder is transmitted by close contact or by contact with contaminated objects used by the infected person (fomites).

Laryngitis

Laryngitis is an inflammation of the laryngeal mucosa that affects phonation and sometimes respiratory function. It occurs in both acute and chronic forms. The term *chronic laryngitis* describes long-standing inflammatory changes in the laryngeal mucosa. Upper respiratory infections are frequently accompanied by acute laryngitis, and isolated laryngeal infections may also occur. Acute laryngitis may also be related to misuse of the voice, inhalation of hot gases, or aspiration of hot or corrosive substances.

No single etiologic factor is related to chronic laryngitis. In some instances, the disorder is related to recurrent episodes of acute laryngitis, continued vocal abuse, smoking, purulent drainage from chronic sinusitis or bronchitis, or allergies. It is sometimes related to hypometabolic states (eg, hypothyroidism). Alcohol abuse may contribute to laryngitis, since an intoxicated person may misuse or abuse the voice. Rare causes include syphilis and laryngeal tuberculosis.

Clinical Manifestations

ACUTE LARYNGITIS The typical symptom is hoarseness or loss of the voice. The client may report roughness or a tickling sensation in the throat. A dry cough may occur, and there may be discomfort in the laryngeal area that increases during swallowing. Talking tends to aggravate the condition. General symptoms of upper respiratory tract infection will be present; if the inflammation progresses, respiratory obstruction may occur. The client may have no fever, or temperature may be as high as 104°F (40°C) depending on related factors.

When inspected by indirect mirror laryngoscopy, the vocal cords appear red and edematous. The entire larynx may be inflamed, and secretions may be present. A false membrane is not generally associated with simple laryngitis; its presence suggests the possibility of diphtheria, although a membrane may form in response to trauma caused by hot gases or steam.

CHRONIC LARYNGITIS Hoarseness is the principal symptom of chronic laryngitis. The client may be unable to speak for a period of hours. Aching of the throat may be reported; otherwise, there is generally no pain. A dry cough is usually present, unless there are secretions related to an associated infection such as bronchitis. The vocal cords may appear polypoid and edematous or red and thickened. If the false cords are affected, they appear red and thickened.

Medical Measures

Acute laryngitis generally subsides once the accompanying upper respiratory infection is resolved. Antibiotics, steam or aerosol therapy, and voice rest may be prescribed for clients with fever, persistent cough, or stridor. They should be cautioned not to smoke. Throat lozenges containing a topical anesthetic such as benzocaine may provide some relief from hoarseness. Hospitalization and tracheotomy may be required in severe cases.

Chronic laryngitis is best treated by removing the cause, if known (eg, by ceasing to smoke). Total rest of the voice is helpful. A biopsy may be ordered to rule out the possibility of cancer of the larynx.

Specific Nursing Measures

The client should be taught to use humidification to relieve symptoms and prevent aggravation of the condition. Room humidifiers may be used, or the client can inhale steam from a shower or teakettle. Precautions against burns should be emphasized. If purulent sputum is being produced, encourage the client to cough; if the cough is dry and nonproductive, coughing should be avoided. Coughing occasionally becomes a habit after a respiratory infection; such coughing should be discouraged. The nurse can encourage the client to maintain total voice rest by providing alternative means of communicating such as a tablet or a "magic slate," and by stressing the importance of voice rest to significant others. Family members can be shown how to help the client by asking questions that can be answered by nodding or shaking the head. Clients who smoke should be urged to discontinue smoking or at least to reduce the number of cigarettes smoked. *It is important that clients with hoarseness lasting more than 2 weeks be further examined to rule out malignancy.*

Epiglottitis

Inflammation of the epiglottis is considered an emergency because it can rapidly lead to total obstruction of the airway. This serious infection, sometimes called supraglottitis, is now being reported more frequently in adults, possibly because of better recognition of the disorder (Ossoff, 1981). Epiglottitis is more common in young children.

Hemophilus influenzae type B is the organism most frequently implicated in cases of epiglottitis, but the disorder has also been associated with *Staphylococcus aureus,* group A beta-hemolytic streptococcus, *Neisseria catarrhalis,* and *Streptococcus pneumoniae.*

Clinical Manifestations

Typically, epiglottitis is manifested by sore throat of short duration (less than 12 hours) and rapidly increasing severity, pain in the area of the hyoid at the base of the tongue, significant dysphagia, and elevation of temperature that may reach 103°F (39°C). Secretions may be so copious that the client drools. Hoarseness, if any, is minimal, but the client's voice may have a muffled, "hot potato" quality. Respiratory obstruction becomes evident as the inflammation progresses.

The pharyngeal and tonsillar mucosa appears normal, but pooled secretions may be seen in the lower pharynx (hypopharynx). Although the enlarged, cherry red epiglottis may be seen by means of indirect (mirror) laryngoscopy, lateral x-rays of the neck taken with the client in an upright position are a less hazardous means of diagnosis; manipulation can aggravate edema, leading to sudden total occlusion of the airway. Cultures of blood and secretions may be used to isolate the causative organism. A leukocyte count of 18,000 to 24,000 is common.

Medical Measures

The client should be hospitalized and closely monitored for signs of progressive respiratory obstruction. Restlessness, stridor, cyanosis, and retraction of the supraclavicular and intercostal spaces indicate a need for immediate tracheotomy. Endotracheal intubation may be an alternative to tracheotomy. Antibiotic therapy appropriate to the organism identified by culture studies is generally prescribed. Recovery usually follows 24 to 48 hours after treatment is initiated. Failure to recognize the seriousness of the disorder can lead to death in up to 20% of clients with epiglottitis (DeWeese & Saunders, 1982).

Specific Nursing Measures

The importance of continuous monitoring for signs of respiratory obstruction cannot be overemphasized. Onset of obstruction can be extremely rapid. Keep a tracheotomy tray in the client's room, and be prepared to assist in this procedure. If endotracheal intubation is used, the tube should be taped securely in place so the client cannot remove it. Confused clients may require soft wrist restraints. Both client and family are extremely frightened when symptoms of respiratory obstruction occur and the measures to relieve it initiated. Explanation, reassurance, and a caring, confident approach by the nurse are extremely important.

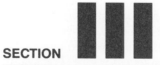

SECTION 

Neoplastic Disorders

Benign and malignant disease is defined and explained in Chapter 10. The discussion in this chapter is limited to specific benign and malignant growths affecting the larynx. The incidence of cancers of the head and neck in women has recently risen; this is thought to be related to their increased use of tobacco.

Cancer of the Larynx

Although benign neoplasms of the larynx do occur—usually small, easily removed papillomas—the following discussion centers on malignant neoplasia. Laryngeal cancers may be classified according to locus of origin; the four major types are:

- Glottic (arising from the vocal cords)
- Supraglottic (arising above the vocal cords)
- Subglottic (arising below the vocal cords)
- Transglottic

Laryngeal cancer has a high rate of cure *when detected early.* But the average client has consulted three physicians about persistent hoarseness over a period of 8 months by the time the condition is diagnosed (DeWeese & Saunders, 1982). The estimated morbidity and mortality for laryngeal cancer in 1985, according to the American Cancer Society, was 11,500 new cases and 3750 deaths.

Heavy cigarette smoking and ingestion of alcohol are believed to be major factors in the development of laryngeal cancer. Environmental pollution, particularly air pollution, occupational exposure to radiation, and chronic pharyngeal infection have also been related to this disorder. Although laryngeal carcinoma has predominantly affected males aged 50 to 70, incidence in women has been rising (McGuirt, 1983).

Clinical Manifestations

The most common symptom of benign laryngeal neoplasms is hoarseness, sometimes accompanied by dysphagia if the lesion is large. Symptoms of laryngeal carcinoma vary according to the type of lesion.

In glottic carcinoma hoarseness occurs early in the course of the disorder. Pain may be felt in the latter stages. Dyspnea and inability to speak (aphonia) are also late signs. With supraglottic carcinoma hoarseness is uncommon. The client may report a sensation of "something in the throat" or a change in voice quality. The throat may burn when hot or acidic liquid is ingested. The client may notice a lump in the neck, which may be the reason for consulting a professional caregiver. Pain unrelated to ulceration may occur, as may referred otalgia. Later symptoms include pain, hoarseness, and dyspnea related to obstruction of the airway. In subglottic carcinoma, dyspnea may be the initial reported symptom. Hoarseness is rare. Transglottic carcinoma refers to tumors that have invaded various sections of the larynx; thus, a variety of the previously described symptoms may occur.

Lesions involving one or both vocal cords may be seen by indirect mirror laryngoscopy, as may supraglottic lesions. The latter are more likely to ulcerate than are glottic lesions. Visualization of the subglottic area requires direct laryngoscopy by a physician. Cervical nodes may be palpable if the lesion has metastasized. Roentgenographic examinations will aid in determining the extent of the disease, and biopsy specimens may be removed under local or general anesthesia.

Medical Measures

Surgical procedures for laryngeal carcinoma include excision via suspension laryngoscopy, laryngofissure with partial laryngectomy, total laryngectomy, and supraglottic laryngectomy. A radical neck dissection may be performed in conjunction with total or supraglottic laryngectomy. Partial laryngectomy has the most favorable prognosis.

In cases of localized carcinomas involving only one vocal cord, radiation may be efficacious and will have less effect on voice quality than will surgical excision. Radiotherapy is least effective with advanced lesions because the level of irradiation required to destroy the neoplasm would cause destruction of surrounding tissues (DeWeese & Saunders, 1982). Sometimes adjuvant chemotherapy is used in an attempt to shrink the tumor and eradicate micrometastases; research is currently in progress to explore this approach.

Specific Nursing Measures

Nurses play an important role in educating the public about the health benefits of not smoking or chewing tobacco and avoiding excessive consumption of alcohol. By becoming familiar with the early symptoms and signs of cancer a nurse can facilitate early diagnosis and refer clients who are at risk.

Treatment of neoplasia involving the face and upper respiratory structures may cause severe disfigurement and loss of the voice. The client may have to wear a facial prosthesis and may have to learn new ways of communicating through artificial devices or esophageal speech. Full knowledge is necessary for decision making. Be careful, however, to avoid imposing values on the client, even if the client asks, "What would you do?" It is the client who must make major adjustments in lifestyle and who may have to cope with a drastically altered appearance or with learning to speak all over again. It is the client who must work through a rehabilitation process that may be painful, tedious, and often discouraging. Thus, it is the client who must make the final decision about treatment. But the nurse can offer information, physical assistance, and emotional support for that decision.

Some clients will refuse therapy altogether, and this decision may be difficult to accept. Yet providing supportive care during the remainder of the client's hospital stay and, in some cases, after the return home, can be a worthwhile challenge to empathy and professional skills.

A case study of a client with cancer of the larynx is presented at the end of this chapter.

Surgery of the Larynx

Laryngeal surgery may be performed to remove benign or malignant neoplasms, or to repair damage resulting from trauma to the neck. Growths such as vocal nodules and laryngeal polyps can be removed using indirect or direct laryngoscopy. Laser surgery to eradicate benign laryngeal lesions and early localized laryngeal neoplasms is increasingly common.

This section will focus on three types of surgical intervention for carcinoma of the larynx: partial laryngectomy using a laryngofissure approach, supraglottic laryngectomy, and total laryngectomy. Excision via suspension laryngoscopy, a form of direct laryngoscopy, may be used for the removal of carcinoma in situ or other lesions that are minimally invasive.

Partial Laryngectomy

Partial laryngectomy using the laryngofissure approach is recommended for clients in whom the cancerous growth is limited. The ideal client is one who has an early growth confined to one vocal cord or to the anterior section of the larynx. This procedure is accompanied by a high cure rate. It has the advantages of preserving the normal airway and the client's ability to speak. As the malignant process advances, the likelihood of obtaining favorable results with this procedure declines.

Either local or general anesthesia can be used. The cancerous tissue and a margin of normal tissue are removed in an attempt to obtain all of the malignant cells. This may include excising only the true cord; however, a larger lesion may necessitate removal of the true cord, ventricle, and false cord on one side. A tracheotomy is performed to ensure a patent airway in the early postoperative period in the event of edema or hemorrhage. Occasionally, a *hemilaryngectomy* may be performed, removing half of the thyroid cartilage and soft tissue on the inside of the larynx.

The physiologic and psychosocial/lifestyle implications are summarized in Table 15–5.

Nursing Implications

Initially, the nurse should direct the most attention to promoting respiratory function. Tracheal suctioning is performed when appropriate.

Since clients may find swallowing difficult, be alert for symptoms and signs of aspiration, such as coughing during or immediately after drinking or eating. Check tracheal secretions for the presence of food and liquids, which may spill over into the trachea and out the opening. If aspiration occurs, perform tracheal suctioning and notify the physician. Some clients will tolerate soft foods better than liquids, since the soft foods do not tend to spill over into the trachea. A client who has aspirated may also become febrile. The client may require intravenous or nasogastric feedings until the swallowing difficulty subsides. The nurse must cleanse the tracheostomy tube and the skin around the area.

Reminding the client that the tracheostomy tube will be removed 2 to 3 days after surgery and that the client will regain the ability to talk helps to reduce anxiety.

Clients should be told to report signs of infection, such as drainage from the incisional area or a persistent temperature elevation, and should be encouraged to return for follow-up examination to assess healing of the area.

Smoking should be discouraged. Remind clients addicted to smoking that the nicotine is now gone from their systems and that not returning to smoking is the one thing they can do that may prevent a recurrence.

Supraglottic Laryngectomy

This procedure, removal of the portion of the larynx above the true vocal cords, is performed on clients who have carcinoma of the epiglottis and adjacent structures above the true vocal cords. The surgical procedure involves a horizontal cut that passes just above the vocal cords to excise the malignant and damaged tissue. A tracheostomy provides an adequate airway. The surgeon often does a unilateral neck dissection in conjunction with this type of laryngectomy. The physiologic and psychosocial/lifestyle implications are discussed in Table 15–5.

Nursing Implications

The nurse is responsible for assisting clients to mobilize and expel secretions, facilitating maximum respiration, and caring for the tracheostomy tube. The tracheostomy will be kept open until adequate healing occurs and the client can learn to swallow effectively.

After approximately 2 weeks of nasogastric tube feeding, healing should be sufficiently advanced to permit the nurse to start instructing the client in how to swallow (Box 15–2). A client can usually swallow best after the tra-

Box 15–2
Learning to Swallow After a Supraglottic Laryngectomy

Instruct the client in the following method of swallowing, which facilitates closure of the epiglottis:

- Take a deep breath and hold it, keeping the neck flexed forward.
- Put the food on the back of the tongue.
- Swallow three times while continuing to hold the breath, and then cough.
- Any food that has been aspirated will be coughed out through the tracheostomy tube or through the opening where the tube had been.

Table 15–5
Laryngeal Surgery: Implications for the Client 

Physiologic Implications	Psychosocial/Lifestyle Implications
Partial laryngectomy	
Tracheostomy for 2–3 days (see Table 15–2)	Hospitalization for 5–7 days
Incisional discomfort and difficulty swallowing during first few days	Anxiety and fear over cancer diagnosis and potential permanent damage to vocal ability
Bleeding is a potential complication	
Scar tissue forms where diseased cord was removed; remaining vocal cord usually close enough to allow voice production	
Supraglottic laryngectomy	
Tracheostomy for about 1 week (see Table 15–2)	Need to learn to swallow effectively
Great difficulty swallowing for 2–3 weeks	Voice usually normal after healing
Normal protective mechanism against aspiration is absent; food and especially fluids tend to flow directly into the trachea	Anxiety and fear over cancer diagnosis
IV or NG feedings for 2–3 weeks	Greater (and perhaps unexpected) alteration in body image if neck dissection also performed
Potential complications are hemorrhage, fistula formation, carotid artery rupture (the latter two are more likely if neck dissection was performed)	
Total laryngectomy	
Permanent tracheostomy results in anosmia and possible permanent alteration of sense of taste	Loss of ability to speak affects body image and may require job change
Mucus secretion often copious	Need to find an alternate means of speech
Initial difficulty in swallowing subsides after healing	Production of mucus and accompanying odor may be offensive to client or significant others
Inability to cough effectively, blow the nose, drink through a straw, or perform glottic Valsalva's maneuver	May find quality of sounds produced by communication aids mechanical or abnormal
Potential complications are infection, hemorrhage, nerve damage, fistula formation, and carotid artery rupture	Need to cope with diagnosis of cancer and fear of dying
	Need to learn self-care (ie, stoma, laryngectomy tube, suctioning)
	Depression not unusual

cheostomy tube and nasogastric tube have been removed. Waiting until the tracheostoma is almost closed before starting means that pressure can build up to assist in swallowing. Start oral feedings with semisolid foods such as custard, gelatin, and mashed potatoes. Avoid fluids initially because they tend to be aspirated. Record the type of food and fluid best tolerated, the amount consumed, the weight pattern of the client, signs of aspiration, and any signs of possible fistula formation. Some clients learn rapidly, whereas others have a great deal of difficulty. Encouragement and patience on the part of the nurse will facilitate the learning process. Supplemental intravenous feeding is often necessary.

The degree of motivation greatly affects client success. Learning and maintaining deglutition (swallowing) after surgical resection require strenuous effort. Debilitated or elderly clients may need considerable time to gain strength before they can swallow effectively. When aspiration continues, the nasogastric tube should be reinserted and the client sent home for several weeks to be maintained on tube feedings. *If a client pulls out the nasogastric tube or it is accidentally removed after a laryngectomy or other type of pharyngeal reconstruction, do not attempt to reinsert it.* Attempts to replace the tube could result in damage to tissue and the creation of a fistula.

Clients who have a great deal of difficulty swallowing may benefit from a therapist who specializes in this type of rehabilitation. The dietitian and nursing staff should reinforce nutritional information. The client should be told to contact the physician if signs of infection occur. Clients should be encouraged in efforts not to smoke and referred to a stop smoking program or to the literature for helpful suggestions. (See the resources list at the end of Chapter 14.)

Total Laryngectomy

This surgical procedure involves the removal of the entire larynx. A person who undergoes this type of surgery is referred to as a *laryngectomee.* Total laryngectomy is appropriate for the removal of neoplasms too extensive to be removed by a partial or supraglottic laryngectomy.

The surgeon generally removes the hyoid bone, the preepiglottic space, the strap muscles, and one or more of the tracheal rings in addition to the larynx. Removing the larynx severs the connection between the trachea and the pharynx, so the trachea is sutured to the skin of the neck, forming a permanent tracheostomy (Figure 15–4C). A radical neck dissection often accompanies this surgery.

The physiologic and psychosocial/lifestyle implications are summarized in Table 15–5.

Nursing Implications

PREOPERATIVE CARE Preparation of the client and family members or significant others for the results of the surgery is of paramount importance. How much the client wants to know varies among individuals; therefore, the members of the health care team must use their judgment. An array of professionals may work with the client to provide comprehensive care, including surgeons, nurses, the speech therapist, social worker, and psychiatrist. Radiologists and chemotherapy specialists may be part of the team, since these clients may receive multimodal therapy. Ideally, the client will be seen by a speech pathologist preoperatively. Sessions usually consist of voice and speech evaluation and tape recording, a hearing evaluation, and time for discussion of the consequences of a laryngectomy. Preoperative teaching will focus on the permanent alterations in breathing and communication. (A case study of a client with cancer of the larynx at the end of this chapter details the preoperative care.) Some clients benefit from a preoperative visit by a well-adjusted laryngectomee, but others may become more anxious. When planning preoperative counseling, consider individual differences.

The room assignment for this type of client is extremely important. See that the client is not assigned to a room with a laryngectomee who is suffering from metastasis or complications from surgery.

POSTOPERATIVE CARE Priority must be given to maintaining a patent airway. The nurse will suction the trachea to remove secretions. Humidified air or oxygen is administered initially. Most surgeons prefer to have the client wear a laryngectomy tube for 1 to 2 weeks or until the stoma maintains its size. The surgeon changes the tube the first time. The nurse then changes and cleans the tube, and teaches the client to do so.

After the tube has been permanently removed, the client should wear a lightweight stoma covering or bib. This allows movement of air into and out of the stoma, yet prevents dust particles or insects from entering the stoma. If the bib is moistened with sterile normal saline, it provides some humidification.

If thick secretions are a problem, the nurse teaches the client to instill a few drops of normal saline into the stoma, followed by suctioning; this will remove tenacious secretions. A mucous plug that obstructs the trachea can usually be removed by suctioning, which stimulates the client to cough. If these measures are unsuccessful, notify the physician.

A nasogastric tube will often be in place after surgery. In the immediate postoperative period, it may be connected to low suction to prevent nausea and vomiting. Initial feedings begin with a small amount of water or dietary supplement to see how well the client tolerates it. If no problems arise, feedings are given every 2 to 3 hours. Moving or disturbing the feeding tube risks trauma to the pharyngeal suture lines, which could result in fistula formation. Intravenous fluids are administered until the client's intake is adequate. Physicians differ about when the feeding tube should be discontinued and the client started on an oral diet. No one who has undergone a total laryngectomy can aspirate easily because there is no longer a connection between the trachea and esophagus. The only way a laryngectomee will aspirate is if a fistula forms to connect the esophagus and trachea or if material is inhaled through the tracheostoma.

Nursing measures should promote wound healing and prevent infection. The nurse observes for drainage from the suture lines, inflammation and redness of the suture lines and surrounding tissue, and a persistent temperature elevation. If dressings are used over suture lines, they are usually removed the first postoperative day. Cleansing may be prescribed. Inspect the stoma closely for inflammation or drainage from either the outer or inner edges.

Oral care is important in the postoperative period, especially until clients are swallowing. Suctioning of oral secretions may be necessary. A mouthwash of half-strength hydrogen peroxide every 2 hours will improve the client's comfort, cleanse the mouth, and reduce breath odor. Since the laryngectomee is unable to blow his or her nose, suctioning of each nostril is useful. Because the sense of smell is altered, the client may need to be reminded to perform normal hygienic measures such as using deodorants and cautioned about the inability to smell smoke and noxious stimuli.

The nursing staff should begin to encourage self-care as soon as the client is stabilized after surgery. This can begin with oral suctioning and progress to removing, cleaning, and replacing the laryngectomy tube. The withdrawn client should be encouraged to walk in the hallway rather than avoid social contact. Include the significant others in the client's care. They will also need a great deal of information and support similar to that given to the family of a client who has had a maxillectomy.

DISCHARGE TEACHING Make certain the laryngectomee understands changes in personal habits that are necessary. For example, the stoma should be covered when taking a shower to avoid aspiration. A shower head below the level of the neck is recommended. When washing the hair, the client should bend over a sink or bathtub and use a spray hose to direct the spray. Some otolaryngologists warn laryngectomees to avoid all water sports, whereas others condone fishing if the client is cautious. Remind the client that drowning can occur rapidly with a laryngectomy. A scarf or high collar can be worn for warmth and for prevention of foreign body aspiration. The client should be encouraged to carry a wallet card or bracelet indicating that he or she is a laryngectomee.

Self-care understanding and technique should be reinforced and checked at intervals. Arrange for the client to demonstrate suctioning, cleansing the stoma, and the like to ensure that the client maintains proper technique. Feedback should be provided for clients concerning their alaryngeal speech. Most clients will return as outpatients for continued instruction and evaluation of the method they choose for voice production. Smoking should be discouraged.

COMMUNICATION AFTER TOTAL LARYNGECTOMY Clients may or may not be exposed to alaryngeal methods of communication prior to surgery. In the early postoperative period, the individual may rely on writing or gesturing. Suggestions for alternate means of communication are given in Chapter 14. A special problem is posed by the client who is blind, deaf, or cannot read or write. The options available to laryngectomees other than nonverbal communication include: esophageal speech, artificial speech aids, and surgical–prosthetic voice restoration. These methods are discussed below.

A patient and understanding nurse can do much to support the client during speech rehabilitation. It is crucial that clients who are trying to communicate by writing or alaryngeal speech not be rushed. Impatience adds to their anxiety and frustration. Explain to others why they should not attempt to finish the sentence for clients or pretend to understand them when they have not. Family members often need guidance in this area so they can be a source of support for the client. Films, slide strips, and written material are available through community resources such as the American Cancer Society. The Lost Chord or Nu Voice Club is sponsored by the American Cancer Society. Clients, family members, and significant others often find affiliation with these resource groups helpful. Specific information is included in the resources list at the end of Chapter 14.

ESOPHAGEAL SPEECH In the past, speech rehabilitation was directed almost exclusively toward learning esophageal speech. The esophageal voice is produced by trapping air inside the mouth and forcing it down the esophagus. Air in the esophagus is quickly forced out, causing the walls of the upper esophagus and lower pharynx to vibrate similar to a belch. The sound is then modified by the tongue, lips, and teeth. Learning this type of speech requires weeks to months, and not all succeed. (It has been suggested that fewer than half of all laryngectomees learn esophageal speech.)

ARTIFICIAL SPEECH AIDS Artificial speech aids are also available. The "artificial larynx" devices can be used to communicate very soon after surgery and may be useful while the client learns to produce an esophageal voice. The device will remain the primary mode of speech for some people. Disadvantages of these devices include the machinelike quality of the voice, the cost of maintenance, the necessity of holding and operating the device with one hand, and the visibility of the device. There are three general types: oral, neck, and pneumatic. They are described and illustrated in Box 15–3.

SURGICAL–PROSTHETIC VOICE RESTORATION Surgical–prosthetic voice restoration consists of the creation of a connection between the esophagus and trachea. Air can then be directed from the lungs and trachea to the esophagus and into the pharynx, resulting in tissue vibration much like that of traditional esophageal speech. This is performed on selected clients who, for one reason or another, were unable to develop adequate esophageal speech. However, food and fluids can flow from the esophagus into the trachea, resulting in aspiration.

One-way valve prostheses have been developed that allow air to pass from the trachea to the esophagus, but prevent aspiration. The Blom–Singer or "duckbill" prosthesis consists of a silicone tube that projects through the stoma into the esophagus. When the stoma is occluded with a finger, air from the lungs passes into the esophagus through a small opening. The opening is closed when the client swallows to prevent aspiration. A disadvantage is that the prosthesis must be worn at all times and must be removed and cleaned every day. The Panje prosthesis, or "voice button," is a small silicone one-way valve prosthesis that can be worn up to several weeks without changing. It is not easily dislodged by coughing or retching.

Various forms of laryngeal reconstruction are also being attempted. In one type, the surgeon uses an arm or leg tendon and rib cartilage to create vocal cords and a thyroid cartilage. The resulting voice is reported to be of good quality.

Maxillectomy

Maxillectomy, the surgical removal of part or all of the maxilla, is primarily performed to remove malignant lesions from the maxillary or maxilloethmoidal sinuses. Benign lesions are occasionally removed via partial or complete maxillectomy.

Maxillectomy is performed under general anesthesia. A *partial maxillectomy* is an individualized operation to remove a specific lesion. The surgeon may remove a part of the palate, a portion of the anterior maxilla, or other areas. A *total maxillectomy* involves the removal of the entire upper jaw and may be accompanied by removal of the orbit (eye) and resection of the cheek. After surgical excision, a split-thickness skin graft is removed from the thigh and used to line the cavity, which is then packed with gauze containing antibiotic ointment. Ideally, a previously manufactured prosthesis is available. Some surgeons prefer to use muscle flaps to reconstruct this area. This can be done in such a way that the client need not wear a removable prosthesis. A nasogastric, gastrostomy, or cervical esophagostomy tube is inserted during the procedure to ensure that the client maintains an adequate diet to promote wound healing. The physiologic and psychosocial/lifestyle implications for the client are discussed in Table 15–4.

Nursing Implications

PREOPERATIVE CARE The client and family members (or significant others) must be informed of the expected change in physical appearance. The extent of the change will vary depending on the location and extent of the neoplasm. Some clients benefit from meeting a well-adjusted client who has experienced the same type of surgery, while others will not.

Make sure that family members, as well as the client, understand that the ability to swallow and speak will be impaired. The client's primary communication immediately after surgery may be via writing or gesturing.

POSTOPERATIVE CARE The nurse's approach to the client, family members, and significant others can make a tremendous difference in their emotional adjustment. Although the client will require extensive nursing care in the early postoperative period, encourage self-care as soon as possible, instructing the client in oral care, oral suctioning, and self-administration of tube feedings. Care must be taken not to damage suture lines when the pharynx has been reconstructed.

Inspect the suture line for any signs of infection, such as inflammation and drainage. Cleansing with a solution of hydrogen peroxide and the application of antibiotic ointment are often prescribed. Nursing care of the recipient and donor sites of skin grafts and flaps is discussed later in Chapter 55. Nursing implications following removal of the orbit of the eye are discussed in Chapter 52.

If extensive portions of oral structures are removed in conjunction with a maxillectomy, a tracheotomy will be performed to ensure a patent airway. Nursing care of the client who has undergone a tracheotomy is discussed later in this chapter.

Interact with these clients in ways that communicate an acceptance of the client's altered appearance. Any surgical intervention of the head and neck can alter the way clients view themselves. Changes may be temporary, as in ecchymosis from nasal surgery, or permanent, as with a maxillectomy or total laryngectomy. Inability to adjust to a temporary change may not pose any problem; inability to adjust to a permanent change will. The reaction of family members and significant others to the client's altered appearance and/or function is important and may influence the client's rehabilitation. Family members may require as much support as the client, or even more.

Box 15–3
Artificial Larynx Devices

Cooper–Rand electrolarynx
The oral device transmits an electronically-produced tone into the mouth by a tube, which is attached to a tone generator. The client introduces the plastic tube 1 or 2 inches into the side of the oral cavity, presses the tone generator, and modifies the tone into meaningful sounds. The oral device does not interfere with suture lines or dressings and can be used as soon as the client is alert after surgery.

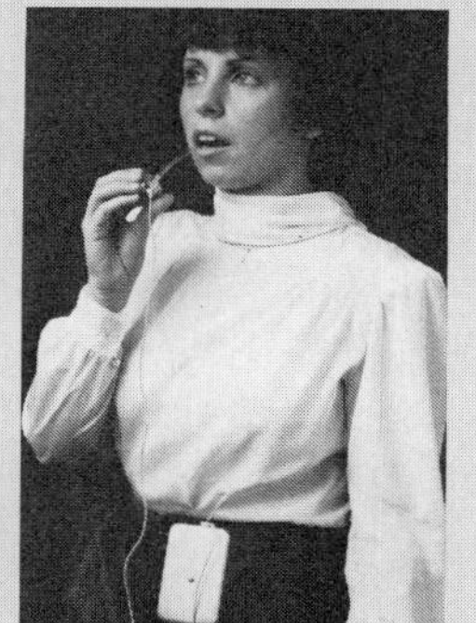

Western Electric electrolarynx
The neck-type aid consists of a diaphragm, circuitry, and a battery. When the client switches the device on, it produces a buzzing sound. The device diaphragm is placed against the neck. The sound is transmitted through the neck tissue and modified by the client into meaningful sounds.

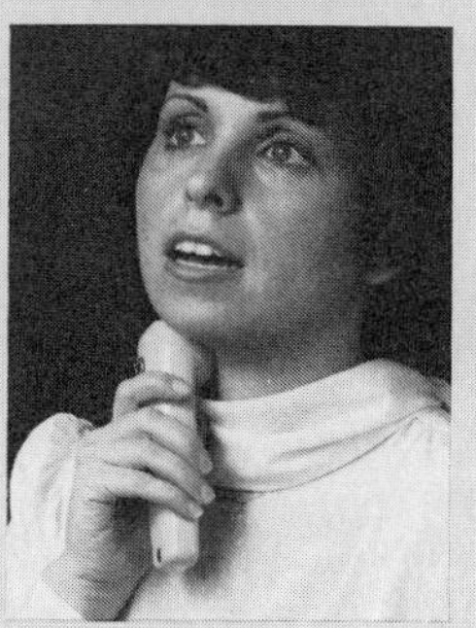

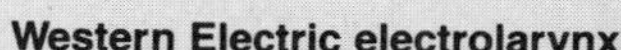

TOKYO speech aid
The pneumatic aid consists of a reed (or diaphragm) in a metal housing. Air from the stoma is directed through a funnel placed over the stoma during voice production. The air then passes into the mouth via the plastic tubing, and sound is modified by the speech musculature. This type of device produces a more natural sound and is relatively inexpensive.

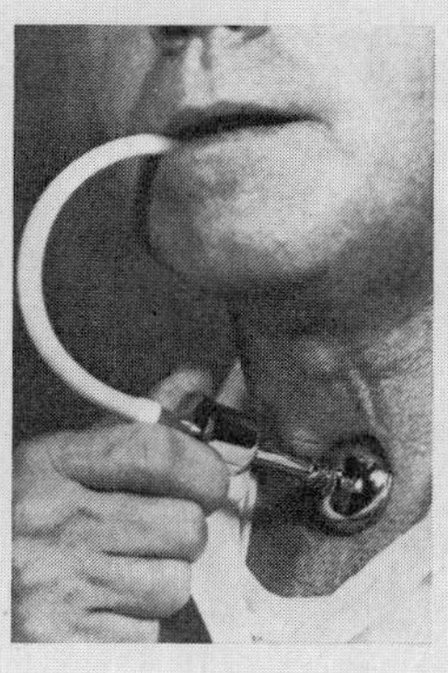

The client will gradually begin to deal with the change. The initial steps may include talking about the disfigurement and taking a first look at it. Clients who continue to refuse to see themselves in a mirror may need specialized professional help in accepting the results of the surgery and the disease process.

The following nursing interventions will provide emotional support and encouragement for the client, family, and friends:

- Approach the client in a manner that indicates acceptance of the disfigurement or altered function.
- Maintain direct eye contact when interacting with the client.
- Spend time with the client and significant others after completing nursing care. This provides nonverbal reassurance that the nurse considers the client, family, and friends important. It also offers a chance to find out about misconceptions and fears.
- Provide honest answers to questions.
- Focus on the client's strengths rather than weaknesses.

Clients using a dental prosthesis need to know how to remove and replace it and how to keep it clean. The removable prosthesis should be removed and cleansed after each meal; if it is not, there is a high probability of irritation of the surrounding tissue. Instruction should include the importance of frequent brushing of teeth and use of mouthwash. Encourage clients to return for follow-up evaluations to assess healing and to check for recurrence of cancer. The dental prosthesis will have to be adjusted as healing continues and the size of the cavity is altered.

Some clients will find speaking difficult even with the dental prosthesis. They should be referred to a speech therapist on an outpatient basis. Mental health counseling can help clients come to terms with altered appearance and function.

Radical Neck Dissection

Lymph from most of the areas in the head and neck where carcinomas may develop drains into the lymph nodes of the neck. These nodes constitute a fairly efficient barrier to malignant cells from the head and neck. Even after cancer spreads to the nodes, distant metastasis may not occur for months. A radical neck dissection, removal of a large portion of the contents of the neck, can be useful because removing the area of "localized metastasis" can often prevent dissemination of the cancer to other parts of the body.

The structures removed include the sternocleidomastoid muscle, the omohyoid muscle, the external jugular vein, and generally the internal jugular vein. The accessory nerve (CN XI) is frequently resected. All of the nodes in the anterior and posterior triangle superficial to the deep fascia are removed.

Depending on the extent of the cancer, the surgeon may perform other procedures in conjunction with the neck dissection, such as a total or supraglottic laryngectomy, hemiglossectomy (removal of a portion of the tongue), or hemimandibulectomy (removal of part of the lower jaw). The otolaryngologist or plastic surgeon will try to remove the diseased tissue, yet leave the client with results that are functionally and cosmetically acceptable.

The use of flaps and grafts enables the surgeon to repair the surgically created defects (eg, for reconstruction around the oral cavity and maxillary sinus).

The physiologic and psychosocial/lifestyle implications are discussed in Table 15–6.

Nursing Implications

PREOPERATIVE CARE Many clients believe that the disfigurement resulting from a neck dissection is much greater than it actually is. This is particularly true when they have seen others who have undergone extensive surgery in conjunction with neck dissection. The nurse should not only explain, but listen to the client and make sure any misconceptions are clarified.

POSTOPERATIVE CARE Ensure that the airway is patent. A hematoma under the skin flaps could compromise the airway, for example. Observe the area for swelling, drainage, and increased redness, and note the amount of fluid from the drains frequently. If a Hemovac unit is used, ensure that it is compressed to apply continuous suction, is emptied every shift, and the amount of drainage is recorded. The amount of drainage expected is approximately 70 to 100 mL of serosanguineous drainage the first day, 30 to 50 mL the second day, and 0 to 30 mL on the third day. Inadequate drainage may result in the formation of a hematoma under the skin, which in turn may delay wound healing. The drainage tubes are removed by the surgeon about the fifth day after surgery.

The client is able to resume oral intake of fluids after having fully recovered from the general anesthesia. The advance to a regular diet can take place the first or second postoperative day. If pharyngeal construction or laryngectomy is performed, the client's intake will be altered as discussed earlier in this chapter.

Prescribed wound care for the suture lines may consist of cleansing with a hydrogen peroxide solution. An antibiotic ointment may also be prescribed. If a tracheotomy or laryngectomy is performed in conjunction with this procedure, care must be taken to avoid trauma to the suture line by the tracheostomy ties.

Assess cranial nerve function to determine the effects of purposeful resection or inadvertent damage to the cranial nerves. (Refer to Chapter 27 for a review of cranial nerves and their functions.)

Nursing measures can assist the client to deal with the loss of the function of the trapezius and sternocleidomastoid muscles. The sternocleidomastoid in conjunction with

Table 15–6
Radical Neck Dissection: Implications for the Client

Physiologic Implications	Psychosocial/Lifestyle Implications
Discomfort less than expected considering extent of tissue removed (the nerves that supply sensation to the cervical neck are resected)	Hospitalization necessary for about 1 week
Pounding and persistent headache due to ligation of jugular vein with resulting increased cerebrospinal fluid pressure	May experience temporary alteration in body image from facial edema and neck incisions
Impaired drainage of venous blood and lymph from the head causes facial edema	Anxiety over extent of disfigurement
Sacrifice of accessory nerve causes atrophy of trapezius muscle	Fear of metastasis and recurrence
Removal of sternocleidomastoid muscle causes shoulder drop, limited abduction, and discomfort in shoulder area for several months	Other psychosocial/lifestyle implications depend upon whether other structures such as the larynx, tongue, or mandible are removed
Potential complications include hemorrhage, facial nerve damage, fistula formation, flap necrosis, carotid artery rupture, chyle leak	Need to perform neck and shoulder exercises to compensate for muscle function loss
	(See also Table 55–8 in Chapter 55 for client implications of skin grafts and tissue flaps)

CN XI is the primary flexor and rotator of the neck. The scalene muscles and the small intrinsic neck muscles are secondary flexors and rotators. These muscles can be strengthened by gentle, gradual neck and shoulder ROM exercises such as neck flexion, lateral bending, and lateral rotation, with and without resistance. Exercises should not be attempted until the surgeon gives permission, usually when the wound is healed. Shoulder exercises are discussed under thoracic surgery.

If the client has a skin flap or graft, the nursing care of both the donor and recipient sites should be directed toward preventing damage and promoting healing. A more comprehensive discussion of the nursing care involved appears in Chapter 55.

Because of the extent and nature of the surgery, as well as the effects of other treatment such as radiation and chemotherapy, the client having a radical neck dissection may experience other severe complications. These complications (carotid artery rupture, chyle leak, and fistula formation) and their related nursing interventions are discussed later in Table 15–7.

SECTION 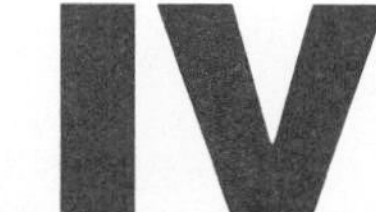

Traumatic Disorders

Maxillofacial Trauma

Trauma to the face may cause extensive damage to soft tissue as well as damage to bone and cartilage. Facial fractures discussed in this section include injury to the nasal bone and septum, the zygomatic bone (malar bone), the maxilla, and the mandible. Because the nose is located in the center of the face and because it protrudes, it is injured more frequently than other areas of the body.

Maxillofacial trauma is related to some kind of direct blow. Nasal fractures are a common aftermath of fistfights; a blow to the cheek may fracture the zygomatic bone. Zygomatic fractures frequently accompany maxillary fractures but may occur alone. Maxillary and mandibular fractures may be related to a variety of causes already discussed; fractures of the mandible occur most often in young adult males (Bailey, 1982).

Clinical Manifestations

NASAL FRACTURES Nasal fractures are accompanied by the classic signs of nasal pain, edema, nasal obstruction, and epistaxis. They are diagnosed most easily 1 or 2 hours after the injury, before maximum edema occurs. Because nasal tissue is richly vascularized, trauma to the nose usually causes extravasation of blood that is manifested as edema and the appearance of a black eye. The nasal bones may appear asymmetrical, the skin may be lacerated, and crepitation may be noted on palpation. The interior of the nose must be examined for additional damage; this can be painful for the client.

ZYGOMATIC FRACTURES Symptoms depend on the location of the fracture, which can be classified according to the LeFort system. A LeFort III fracture involving the zygoma; maxilla; and nasal, orbital, ethmoid, and sphenoid bones is the most serious. Profuse hemorrhage, edema, and hypoesthesia of the middle third of the face are com-

Table 15–7
Nursing Interventions for Complications of Radical Neck Dissection 

Complication	Nursing Intervention
Carotid artery rupture Rupture (blowout) of the external carotid artery occurs after destruction of the outer, middle, and inner layer of the vessel. It is a complication of radical neck dissection, caused by damage from infection, exposure during surgery, and treatment with radiation and chemotherapy. The most common factor contributing to carotid artery blowout is previous irradiation. Carotid artery rupture will rapidly result in death unless the bleeding is stopped, the circulatory volume replaced, and a patent airway maintained. The blood may flow outward, away from the neck, or into the tracheostoma or pharynx. Attempts are not always made to save the terminally ill client who develops a carotid artery rupture. The client, family members, and the physician may have agreed that no heroic measures to save the client are to be performed.	Observe for signs that could indicate the client is at increased risk for carotid artery rupture: • Presence of blood in drainage from overlying area • Exposure of the carotid artery after wound breakdown Control of bleeding when rupture occurs: • Call for assistance and have the physician notified immediately. • Carotid "blowout" tray containing necessary equipment should be kept at the bedside. • Suction source and catheter should be at bedside. • Exert pressure on the point from which bleeding occurs. Bleeding may be controlled by finger pressure at the site. Abdominal pads may be used to absorb blood. • To prevent aspiration from external bleeding, turn client to the side. If the client has a tracheostomy, inflate the cuff. • If bleeding occurs into the pharynx or a tracheostoma, suction via mouth or stoma. Assist with physiologic support of the client: • Administer intravenous fluids and blood as prescribed. • Administer oxygen. • Assist surgeon if ligation of artery is attempted. This may be performed in the client's room or the operating room depending on the situation. Provide psychologic support for the client and significant others: • Remain with the client. • Interact with the client and significant others calmly. • Briefly explain your actions. • Administer sedatives or pain medication as prescribed. • Have clergyman contacted if client wishes.
Chyle leak During a radical neck dissection, the thoracic duct may be damaged; chyle may leak into the underlying tissues, causing wound breakdown. Small lesions may close spontaneously, although drainage may occur for weeks. A firm pressure dressing should be applied to the area for 5–7 days. Suturing of the vessel may be necessary to control the leak.	Report symptoms and signs of a chyle leak: • White, milky secretions (chyle) from drains • Swelling of the area of the clavicle Perform measures to aid in resolution of the leak and support the client's physical condition: • Apply pressure dressing as needed. • Report abnormal electrolyte and protein levels. • Administer prescribed dietary supplements. • Maintain pressure dressing as needed.
Fistula formation Fistula formation is more likely when the client has undergone extensive surgery and has received radiotherapy to the area. It tends to occur about 5–10 days after surgery. An *orocutaneous* fistula is a connection between the oral cavity and the skin. A *pharyngocutaneous* fistula is a connection between some part of the pharynx and the skin. Both types result in drainage of saliva onto the skin. Enzymes in the saliva irritate the skin and can prevent wound healing. If a large fistula is present, a catheter may be placed in the opening and attached to continuous suction.	Report signs of fistula formation: • Drainage from wound • Elevated temperature Prevent secretions from fistula from irritating skin, contaminating suture lines, or entering tracheostoma: • Apply dry gauze dressing. • Maintain suction to catheter placed in opening of fistula (if utilized). • Change gauze frequently to keep area dry and clean.

mon symptoms of zygomatic fractures. Malocclusion may also occur.

MANDIBULAR FRACTURES Common findings include pain on movement, malocclusion, and abnormal mobility. The dental arch will be irregular. Fractures of specific sections are often diagnosed by palpation.

Roentgenograms are usually obtained in all cases of maxillofacial trauma, although nasal fracture is often diagnosed by physical examination alone. If the client has been unconscious or has suffered a significant blow to the head, skull films may be obtained to rule out the possibility of cranial fracture.

Medical Measures

If there is evidence of significant wound contamination, antibiotics are administered to clients with open fractures to avert infection. Tetanus toxoid may be given, depending on the degree of wound contamination and the client's history of tetanus immunization.

Intubation or tracheotomy may be required, hemorrhage must be controlled, and blood replacement may be necessary. Skin lesions are treated by cleansing, debridement, and suturing as indicated, and fractures must be reduced. Open reduction may be necessary for complicated fractures.

In the case of maxillary and mandibular fractures, interdental wiring may be necessary to restore correct alignment of the jaws and teeth. Dental arch bars are placed against the mandibular and the maxillary teeth, and wires or rubber bands attached to hooks on the bars are used to draw the dental structures into proper alignment (Figure 15–9). Maxillomandibular fixation must remain in place for approximately 6 weeks in adults and sometimes longer in elderly people.

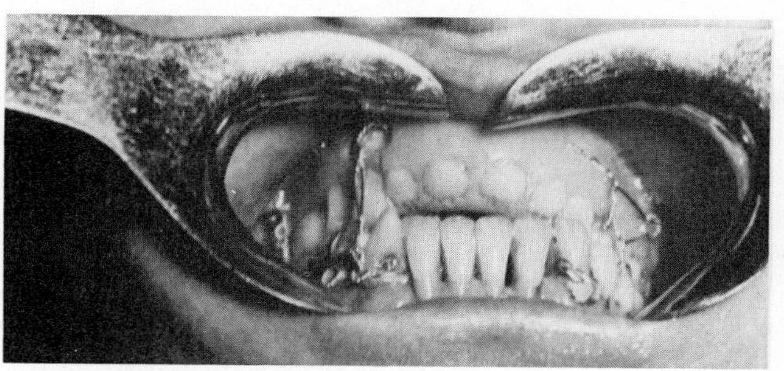

Figure 15–9

A client with wiring in place. *Courtesy of Millard Fillmore Hospital, Buffalo, NY.*

Specific Nursing Measures

Clients with nasal fractures must be given the following instructions:

- Avoid blowing the nose, which could push nasal flora into tissues of the face and orbit, promoting infection.
- Try to sneeze through the mouth instead of the nose.
- Do not use decongestant nasal sprays or drops, as these medications reduce blood supply to the area and impede healing.

The following precautions are important in caring for clients who require interdental fixation. Maintenance of a patent airway is the predominant concern.

- A wire cutter and suction equipment should be at the bedside at all times; taping the cutter to the head of the bed may be a wise precaution. If secretions cannot be removed by suctioning or if the client shows signs of respiratory distress, the rubber bands or wires should be cut.
- If the client vomits, either tip the head forward or turn it to the side (if the client is supine) and use suction to remove the secretions. (The client may be taught how to suction secretions through a space between the teeth.)
- Mark the intercom at the nurses' station to indicate that the client cannot articulate clearly.
- Maintain meticulous oral hygiene by irrigating the oral cavity with saline or an alkaline solution. Lubricate the lips to prevent drying and cracking.
- Provide a high-calorie diet. Clients usually begin with clear liquids and may progress to blenderized soft foods.
- Provide an alternative means of communication such as a writing tablet or "magic slate."

The nurse is responsible for home care instruction because of the length of time the fixation must remain in place. A sample set of instructions that may be reproduced and given to the client appears in Box 15–4. The nurse may consult with the dietitian, who can provide the client with suggestions for palatable and nutritious meals and instructions for preparation.

Laryngotracheal Trauma

Laryngotracheal trauma may be classified as open or closed. It may be accompanied by neural and vascular trauma of the head and neck, and fracture of the cervical spine commonly occurs with this kind of injury.

Automobile accidents in which an individual is thrown against the steering wheel or dashboard at a high rate of speed are the most common cause of laryngotracheal trauma. Some penetrating injuries are caused by sharp objects (eg, stab wounds). Iatrogenic laryngeal injury can occur in relation to endoscopy, endotracheal intubation, or tracheotomy; improper endoscopic technique can dislocate the larynx or tear the laryngeal mucosa. Pressure exerted by the cuff of an endotracheal or tracheostomy tube against the

Box 15–4
Home Care Instructions for Clients With Maxillomandibular Fixation 

Carry wire cutters with you at all times in case of respiratory obstruction. You and your significant others will be shown how to cut the wires before you leave the hospital. Notify your physician immediately if the wires have been cut.

Blenderize your food and maintain a high-calorie diet according to the instructions given you by the dietitian. Losing 10 to 20 pounds while your jaws are wired is not uncommon.

Maintain good oral hygiene. A Water-Pik may be helpful, but do not use too forcible a spray, and do not direct the stream of water over the lacerated area at first. You may use plain water, a mouthwash, or salt water for rinsing the mouth.

Brush your teeth regularly. Rinse your mouth after meals and at bedtime.

Apply paraffin to the ends of the wires, which will help prevent irritation of the inside of your mouth.

Refrain from swimming, because it will be hard for you to clear your throat of water.

Avoid alcoholic and carbonated beverages. Alcohol impairs the reflexes you need to clear your throat. Carbonated beverages produce foam that may make it hard for you to clear your throat.

Notify your physician of any sudden swelling or atypical pain.

SOURCE: Adapted from Black JM, Arnold PG: Facial fractures, *AM J Nurs* (July) 1982; 82(7):1086–1088.

arytenoid cartilage may result in formation of scar tissue (arytenoid stenosis), although this has occurred less frequently since low-pressure cuffs have been employed.

Clinical Manifestations

Depending on the type of injury, clinical findings may include hoarseness, dysphagia, dyspnea, cyanosis, hemoptysis, and edema of the larynx and pharynx. Laryngeal fracture is generally associated with pain on swallowing and speaking and protrusion of the tongue.

An open or closed wound may be apparent on inspection. Edema may occur in the region of the larynx, and the normal prominence of the thyroid cartilage may be absent because of fracture. Subcutaneous emphysema, signs of respiratory distress, and hemoptysis accompany severe injuries. Subcutaneous emphysema is related to any disruption of the integrity of the respiratory tract that allows air to escape into the subcutaneous tissue. The client will feel pain in the affected area, and the skin may appear puffy. On touching the area, the nurse will feel a crackling sensation similar to that of touching wrinkled cellophane. Once the underlying disorder has been treated, subcutaneous air is usually absorbed by the body over a period of several days.

Indirect mirror laryngoscopy may reveal edema and mucosal lacerations of the pharynx and larynx. Direct laryngoscopy and x-ray studies may be ordered for further diagnosis.

Medical Measures

Hemorrhage must be controlled, lost blood must be replaced, and a patent airway must be maintained. As with maxillofacial trauma, antibiotic therapy and tetanus toxoid are administered as indicated. The client is usually intubated not only to maintain respiratory function but also to provide support for (stent) the fractured laryngeal fragments. Tracheotomy may be necessary if severe facial fractures accompany the laryngeal injury. Debridement and cleansing of the wound is followed by repair of mucosal lacerations. Complex fractures may necessitate wiring of cartilaginous fragments.

Specific Nursing Measures

Clients with laryngeal trauma must be assessed for signs of damage to the carotid artery and jugular vein. This includes observing for signs of hemorrhage such as formation of a hematoma and diminution of pulses in the upper extremities. The carotid arteries should be auscultated for bruits. Care of the intubated client and the client with a tracheostomy are covered in Chapter 14.

Chapter Highlights

Clients who undergo nasal surgery should be forewarned about the edema and ecchymosis that may occur.

Packing is inserted after certain surgical procedures of the nose and paranasal sinuses to control bleeding, hold structures in place, and prevent infection and odor.

Clients with a posterior nasal pack require hospitalization because of the risk of respiratory obstruction.

A client who breathes through a tracheostoma does not have the benefit of warming, humidification, and filtering of inspired air by the nose.

Humidification and hydration of the client aid in the thinning and removal of secretions from the upper respiratory tract.

Clients with hoarseness lasting more than 2 weeks should be examined to rule out a malignancy.

Malignant neoplasms of the larynx occur more frequently in individuals who smoke and consume large quantities of alcohol.

Malignant neoplasms of the larynx have a high cure rate if diagnosed early.

The client's voice is spared after a partial laryngectomy and a supraglottic laryngectomy.

A client's ability to produce vocal sounds by normal means is permanently altered by a total laryngectomy.

If complete airway obstruction occurs from aspiration of a foreign body into the larynx, the individual will not be able to speak or cough.

A client who has had a tracheostomy can aspirate food or fluids into the lungs.

It is anatomically impossible for a client who has had a total laryngectomy to aspirate unless a fistula forms between the trachea and esophagus or fluid enters through the stoma.

Neoplastic and traumatic disorders of the upper respiratory tract can be devastating because of physical disfigurement and altered function.

Clients with traumatic disorders of the upper respiratory tract must be assessed for multisystem damage, particularly the neurologic and cardiovascular systems.

Bibliography

A step-by-step workup for neck masses. *Patient Care* (April 30) 1984; 100–131.

Bailey BJ: Management of maxillofacial trauma. *Resident Staff Physician* (Dec) 1982; 28:57–68.

Bertz JE: Maxillofacial injuries. *Clin Symp* 1981; 33(4):2–32.

Black JM, Arnold PG: Facial fractures. *Am J Nurs* (July) 1982; 82(7):1086–1088.

Bumsted RM: Evaluation and therapy of nasal obstruction. *Primary Care* (June) 1982; 9(2):385–400.

Cluff L, Johnson J (editors): *Clinical Concepts of Infectious Disease,* 3rd ed. Baltimore: Williams & Wilkins, 1982.

Denning DC: Head and neck cancer: Our reactions. *Cancer Nurs* 1982; 5:269–273.

DeWeese DD, Saunders WH: *Textbook of Otolaryngology,* 6th ed. St. Louis: Mosby, 1982.

Donlon WC, Jacobson AL: Maxillofacial Pain. *Am Fam Physician* 1984; 30(1):151–163.

Gates G (editor): *Current Therapy in Otolaryngology: Head and Neck Surgery.* Trenton, NJ: Decker, 1982.

Harris LL, Kraege J: After T-E puncture: Relearning to speak. *Am J Nurs* 1986; 86(1):55–58.

Knapp B, Panje E: A voice button for laryngectomees. *AORN J* 1982; 36:183–191.

Larsen G: Rehabilitation for the patient with head and neck cancer. *Am J Nurs* (Jan) 1982; 82(1):119–120.

McCormick GP et al: Artificial speech devices. *Am J Nurs* (Jan) 1982; 82(1):121–122.

McGuirt WF: Head and neck cancer in women: A changing profile. *Laryngoscope* (Jan) 1983; 93(1):106.

Passy V: Hoarseness: Evaluation and treatment. *Primary Care* 1982; 9:337–354.

Pilcher L: Carbon dioxide lasers in laryngeal surgery. *AORN J* (June) 1981; 33(7):1402–1406.

Ryan J: *The Nurse and the Communicatively Impaired Adult.* New York: Springer, 1982.

Saunders W et al: *Nursing Care in Eye, Ear, Nose, and Throat Disorders.* St. Louis: Mosby, 1979.

Saunders WH: Surgery of the inferior nasal turbinates. *Ann Otol Rhinol Laryngol* 1982; 91:445–447.

Saxton D, Pelikan PK, Nugent PM, Hyland PA: *The Addison-Wesley Manual of Nursing Practice.* Menlo Park, CA: Addison-Wesley, 1983.

Silverberg E: Cancer. *Statistics 1983* 1983; 33:9–25.

Sloane PD: Sore throats: They're common but full of surprises. *Consultant* 1982; 22:110–117.

Sumner SM, Eaton P: Emergency! First aid for choking. *Nurs 82* (July) 1982; 12(7):40–49.

CASE STUDY

The Client With Cancer of the Larynx

I. Descriptive Data

James Curtis, age 56, has come to the medical clinic of the county hospital with a concern about hoarseness × 6 mo and recent dysphagia. He is accompanied by his wife.

II. Personal Data

Date and Time: October 7, 1987, 9 AM
Full Name: James S. Curtis
Social Security Number: 000-00-0000
Address: 1613 S. Market St., Buffalo, NY
Telephone: Home: 000-0000
Work: 000-0000
Sex: Male
Age: 56
Birthdate: 10-2-31
Marital Status: Married
Race/Culture: Black
Religion: Baptist
Occupation: Truck driver
Usual Health Care Provider: Company physician

III. Health History

Source of Information: Client and wife
Reliability of Informant: Mr Curtis is moderately reliable. Has difficulty remembering time of onset of symptoms. Mrs Curtis provides detailed information regarding history, symptoms, and time of onset.
Chief Concern: Hoarseness of approximately 6 mo duration, becoming progressively worse; slight difficulty swallowing during the past month.

History of Present Illness:

The client's wife noticed an alteration (deepening) in the quality of Mr Curtis's voice approximately 6 mo ago. He attributed this change to the aftermath of a cold and refused to seek evaluation until this time. According to Mrs Curtis, the hoarseness has progressively worsened. He has not had prolonged upper respiratory problems, postnasal drip, or sinusitis. He has no known allergies. He does not overuse his voice; does not sing—except in the shower.

The client has lost 25 lb during the last 6 mo, going from 200 to 175 lb. He did not experience anorexia and continued to eat his regular diet. He states he has experienced slight difficulty swallowing during the past month. Mr Curtis has noticed feeling more tired than usual during work.

He smokes 1 pack of cigarettes/day × 40 yr (40 pack yr); has a nonproductive cough, mild DOE; no history of TBC or other respiratory problems. Usual alcohol intake includes 2 beers after work and 2 to 4 beers on the weekend. He has had mild hypertension × 12 yr, controlled on hydrochlorothiazide 50 mg q.d. He takes no other medications.

Past Health History:

Childhood: Usual childhood diseases—chickenpox, mumps, and measles
Immunizations: Received immunization during elementary school and in the army
Medical Problems: Mild essential hypertension for 12 yr, which is controlled with medication
Surgeries: 1973—left inguinal herniorrhaphy
1976—hemorrhoidectomy
Transfusions: None

Special Diagnostic
Procedures: None
Trauma: None
Allergies: None known
Medications: Hydrochlorothiazide, 50 mg PO q.d. for hypertension

Family History:

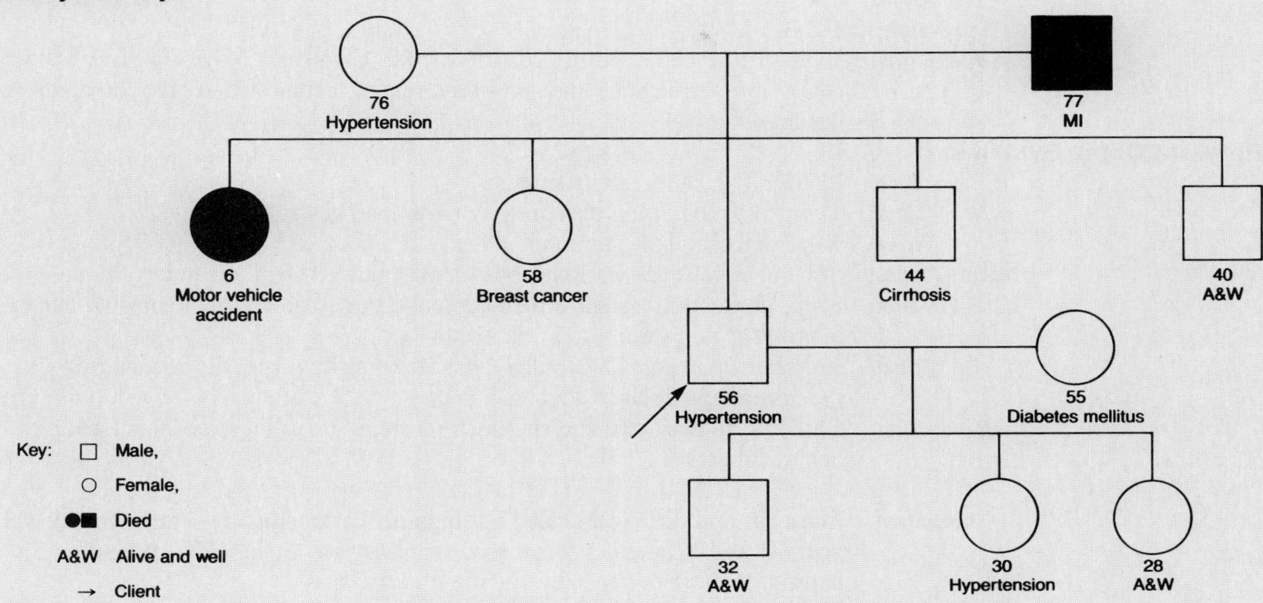

Personal/Social History: The client is married and lives with his wife in their suburban home, which they own. Their three children have their own homes in the surrounding community. His wife works as a school teacher. The client spends 10 to 12 hr a day driving a truck; has worked for the same company for 22 yr; plans to retire in 9 yr; total yearly combined income is $38,000. After work, he stops at the local tavern and visits with his friends. Enjoys working in his garden on weekends. Also enjoys football and horse races. Sleeps approximately 7 hr each night without difficulty. Mr Curtis completed high school. He was a private in the army; remained in the United States through his tour of duty.

Diet: Mr Curtis's physician has instructed him to follow a low-sodium diet. The client states that he eats what he wants. His regular diet is high in fats and carbohydrates. He eats a large proportion of fried foods. He does not add salt at the table, and his wife does not cook with salt.

Review of Systems: Generally feels more tired than usual; 25 lb weight loss over past 6 mo

Throat/Neck/Chest: See history of present illness

Cardiovascular: Experiences headaches when blood pressure is elevated; no chest pain, epistaxis, ankle edema, or claudication; wife takes BP at home. Ranges from high of 160/100 to low of 130/90; average BP 140/92.

Gastrointestinal: No change in appetite or bowel habits; no melena, hematemesis, diarrhea, constipation, or ulcer hx; slight dysphagia during the past month

Genitourinary: No dysuria, UTI, impotence; sexually active without difficulty

Musculoskeletal: Slight aching in knee joints after driving all day in the truck

Psychologic: States that he did not think his symptoms were significant; is now very concerned and fearful about the diagnosis; states he avoided seeing a physician since he thought the symptoms would disappear

(continued)

CASE STUDY (continued)

The Client With Cancer of the Larynx

IV. Physical Assessment

Height: 6 ft 1 in.

Weight: 175 lb

Vital Signs: T. 98^{8}°F (37°C), P. 88, R. 20, BP 150/90. Client is a 56-yr-old black male in NAD; appears anxious and somewhat reliant on his wife to give the details of his illness.

Relevant Organ Systems:

Eyes: PERRLA, bilateral arcus senilis

Ears: Tympanic membrane obscured by cerumen bilaterally

Nose: Nasal mucosa pink, septum midline

Mouth/Throat: Several carious teeth; no lesions on oral mucosa, lips, or under tongue

Neck: Firm, nontender, nonmovable node posterior to sternocleidomastoid muscle in rt neck; no thyromegaly; no bruits

Chest: Breath sounds equal bilaterally c̄ basilar rhonchi; bilaterally resonant to percussion; no axillary adenopathy

Cardiovascular: S_1, S_2 nl; regular rate and rhythm s̄ murmurs or gallops; pedal pulses 2+ and symmetrical

Abdomen: Muscular and flat; well-healed left inguinal herniorrhaphy scar; active bowel sounds; abd. nontender s̄ masses; liver palpable 1 cm below rt costal margin; liver span at MCL, 10 cm by percussion

Genitourinary: Normal uncircumcised male; testes s̄ masses

Rectal: Normal prostate s̄ nodules; no hemorrhoids or masses; stool occult blood test negative

Extremities: No cyanosis, clubbing, or edema; full ROM

Neurologic: Cranial nerves II–XII grossly intact; DTRs 2+ and symmetrical; normal motor and vibratory sense

Psychologic: Appears anxious; has difficulty sitting still; constantly tapping fingers and feet; relies on wife to answer some questions; does not offer information without being questioned specifically

V. Diagnostic Data

Indirect laryngoscopy: mass present on rt vocal cord. Laboratory tests: moderately elevated liver enzymes; mild anemia

VI. Summary

Mr Curtis underwent a direct laryngoscopy with biopsy.

Findings: Mass on right true vocal cord and beneath it, 1 mm subglottic extension; pyriform sinuses clear

Diagnosis: Well-differentiated squamous cell carcinoma of the larynx

Medical Plan: Mr Curtis was scheduled for a total laryngectomy with right radical neck dissection on 10-14-87

VII. Nursing Care Plan, by Nursing Diagnosis

Client Care Goals	Plan/Nursing Implementation	Expected Outcomes
Nutrition, altered: less than body requirements, related to increased metabolism secondary to cancer of the larynx		
Remain well hydrated; understand importance of adequate intake of food and fluids	Encourage client to eat low Na diet including adequate amounts of calories, protein, carbohydrates and fats: 2500 calories daily, 160 g protein; encourage fluids, at least 3000 mL/24 h; initiate a nutritional consult so client receives food he likes and is familiar with, in accordance with his low Na diet; provide environment conducive to eating; administer dietary supplements and vitamins prescribed by physician; stress importance of maintaining present weight by good nutritional intake; explain that cancer increases body's need for intake of adequate calories	Takes in well-balanced low-sodium diet of at least 2500 calories with 160 g of protein; takes in 2000 to 3000 mL of fluid per day; good skin turgor; BP, heart rate wnl; describes what constitutes adequate nutritional and fluid intake
Swallowing, impaired related to mechanical obstruction		
Remain free of foreign objects such as food or liquids in airway; understand importance of taking small bites, chewing food well, and eating in unhurried manner	Encourage client to eat and drink in an unhurried manner, taking small bites and chewing food well; observe for symptoms and signs of choking—grasping throat, difficulty or inability to speak, dyspnea/stridor, use of accessory muscles, nasal flaring, skin color changes; keep suction machine and suction catheter in the room in case he should choke and oral suction becomes necessary	Discusses importance of eating in an unhurried manner, taking small bites, and chewing food well; demonstrates proper eating as described and does not choke
Fear, related to diagnosis of cancer and impending surgery		
Begin to cope effectively with the diagnosis and impending surgery; understand basic information regarding laryngeal cancer and his symptoms	Approach client and significant others in calm, unhurried manner; assess level of understanding of client and family regarding laryngeal cancer and impending surgery; provide atmosphere in which the client and significant others will verbalize fears and anxieties related to the illness and management; explain in basic terms the disease of laryngeal cancer and the relationship of the client's symptoms to the disease; clarify misconceptions	Client will exhibit symptoms and signs of decreased anxiety level (eg, blood pressure, respiratory rate, and pulse wnl); client and family will express their feelings and fears about the diagnosis and impending surgery; they willl be able to say "cancer" when discussing the diagnosis
Knowledge deficit, related to planned surgery		
Understand in basic terms the procedure of a total laryngectomy and radical neck dissection	Provide preoperative teaching and counseling related to a total laryngectomy and a radical neck dissection; administer antianxiety medications when appropriate as prescribed by physician; initiate consultation with speech therapist and psychologist in the preoperative phase; introduce client to a well-adjusted client who has undergone a total laryngectomy; share information about self-help groups and other resources for laryngectomy clients	Describes total laryngectomy and radical neck dissection; discusses his situation and expected outcome of surgery with speech therapist and psychologist; interacts with a well-adjusted laryngectomee; describes available support groups and resources
Understand the surgical procedure and what to expect postoperatively	Explain the procedure of a total laryngectomy and radical neck dissection to the client and significant others in terms they can understand; inform client and signifi-	Explains the surgical procedure in general terms; discusses the postoperative events related to the altered airway

(continued)

CASE STUDY (continued)

The Client With Cancer of the Larynx

VII. Nursing Care Plan (continued)

Client Care Goals	Plan/Nursing Implementation	Expected Outcomes
	cant others that his route for breathing will be permanently altered; include the following information: ■ He will breathe through a stoma (opening) in his lower neck ■ Initially, humidified oxygen will be administered to compensate for loss of humidification by the nose ■ Suctioning through the stoma will be necessary to remove excessive secretions ■ Drains inserted under the skin are connected to a suction source to promote drainage of fluid ■ Suture lines will be inspected frequently to assess the healing process ■ Suture lines will be cleansed, and an antibiotic ointment may be applied ■ Edema (swelling) may be present in the face ■ VS will be monitored at frequent intervals, initially every 15 min, then q.1h, 2 h, and 4 h	
Recognize the parts of a laryngectomy tube; demonstrate interest in becoming involved in his own care	Show client a laryngectomy tube; explain that the tube will remain in the stoma for a period of time (often 2–3 weeks after surgery); explain that the tube is removed every day (after 2 or 3 postoperative days) and a sterile tube reinserted; the inner cannula is removed and cleansed as often as necessary, depending on the amount of secretions that accumulate on inner cannula; initially, this will be done by a nurse; however, soon he will be expected to learn the procedure	Able to identify the three parts of a laryngectomy tube; recognizes that he will be encouraged to participate actively in his care in the early postoperative period (ie, cleansing the laryngectomy tube and stoma)
Know physical limitations that result from the procedure of a total laryngectomy; understand that after surgery he will no longer be able to communicate as he does at the present time	Explain that the client will no longer be able to perform certain actions (eg, swimming, drinking through a straw, blowing his nose, Valsalva's maneuver); also his sense of smell will be diminished or absent, and taste sensation may be altered; inform client and significant others that his ability to communicate will be permanently altered	Verbally describes or lists required alterations in current lifestyle after surgery; will discuss altered communication status and its significance to him
Know that several options are available as methods of communication	If client is receptive, discuss alaryngeal methods of speech he may choose from (ie, esophageal speech and artificial aids such as electrolarynx or Cooper–Rand device); explain that immediately after surgery he can communicate by writing and gesturing; reassure him that he will have a call bell to alert staff; explain that many laryngectomees develop excellent commu-	Verbalizes feelings and emotions regarding loss of ability to produce a natural voice; gives some thought to communication options available following laryngectomy and discusses them with staff and family; expresses interest in communicating with a well-adjusted laryngectomee; copes with impending loss of "natural" voice

Client Care Goals	Plan/Nursing Implementation	Expected Outcomes
	nication skills and return to their previous jobs and activities	
Know method by which he will receive nutrition in the postoperative period	Inform client and significant others that an NG tube will be placed in surgery as a route for providing nutrition in the postoperative period; soon after surgery, he will receive liquid feedings through the tube every 2–3 h; initially, this will be done by a nurse. Then client will be expected to learn the procedure; the NG tube will remain in place approximately 1 to 2 weeks; explain that he will receive fluids through an intravenous infusion for a short time after surgery	Verbalizes an understanding of the liquid diet he will receive via NG tube in the postoperative period
	The client will need to rinse his mouth frequently with a solution that will be provided	Discusses importance of good oral hygiene after surgery
Recognize need for close monitoring postoperatively	Explain that he will be in an intensive care unit for a few days after surgery so he can be monitored closely; take client and significant others through intensive care unit (depending on individual and family)	Expresses feelings and anxiety about the postoperative period; asks questions
Explain necessity of performing ROM exercises to his rt shoulder and arm	Explain that client will experience some discomfort and limited movement of his rt shoulder because of the surgery; teach ROM exercises client will be instructed to perform postoperatively; determine the effectiveness of preoperative instruction; ask client and significant others to repeat information provided	Demonstrates ROM exercises to rt shoulder and arm; client and significant others discuss information presented demonstrating an understanding of the preoperative instruction
Maintain a relatively pain-free state during his postoperative course	Explain that during the first postoperative days, the nursing staff will medicate him for pain q. 3–4 h; after the first few days, he will be medicated for pain as he feels he needs it; inform the client and family that they should not hesitate to request medication when the client feels pain	Client and family both express satisfaction with client's level of comfort in the postoperative period; verbalizes he will not hesitate to ask for pain medication if he feels significant discomfort

CHAPTER 16

Specific Disorders of the Lower Respiratory System

Other topics relevant to this content are: Mantoux intradermal skin testing, **Chapter 14;** Nursing care of the client who is intubated, **Chapter 14;** Nursing care of the client with chest tubes, **Chapter 14;** Basal expansion exercises after chest surgery, **Chapter 11.**

Objectives

When you have finished studying this chapter, you should be able to:

Identify the major respiratory diseases categorized under multifactorial, infectious, neoplastic, obstructive, and traumatic causation.

Describe the appropriate therapeutic measures involved in the medical and surgical management of clients with specific respiratory diseases.

Explain the complications of thoracic surgery and the related nursing interventions.

Explain appropriate nursing interventions based on the nursing diagnoses of clients with specific respiratory diseases.

Specify the appropriate health teaching for clients with specific respiratory diseases.

Anticipate the psychosocial/lifestyle impact that specific respiratory disorders can have on the lives of clients, their families, and significant others.

Demonstrate the role of the nurse in health education by not smoking and by actively teaching others the health dangers of cigarette smoking and exposure to respiratory irritants.

Discuss the significance of and approaches to rehabilitation of clients with chronic respiratory disorders.

Problems of the lower respiratory tract constitute a major concern in health care. These disorders can range from a minor bout of acute bronchitis to major life-threatening conditions such as acute respiratory failure. Many of the disorders are chronic and debilitating, making it necessary for clients and their significant others to make long-term adjustments in lifestyle. Clients admitted to a hospital with other debilitating conditions may develop respiratory difficulties in the form of atelectasis, retained respiratory tract secretions, and pneumonia. A majority of these are preventable with good nursing care.

SECTION 

Disorders of Multifactorial Origin

Occupational Lung Disease (The Pneumoconioses)

The pneumoconioses are lung diseases resulting from inhalation of inorganic dusts. Silicosis, asbestosis, and coal workers' pneumoconiosis fall in this category.

Clinical Manifestations

The clinical manifestations of the pneumoconioses are similar in that these disorders can lead to pulmonary fibrosis. This condition causes the lungs to become stiff and nonelastic, reducing lung volume. Also, the development of a thickened pulmonary membrane can interfere with gas exchange.

Silicosis may occur in various forms. The most common is chronic or classic silicosis, which occurs in individuals who have inhaled relatively low concentrations of dust for 10 to 20 years. Initially, the accumulated dust and tissue reaction result in the development of scattered nodules throughout the lungs and shortness of breath on exertion. Chronic silicosis may become more serious, resulting in increased shortness of breath, cough, and sputum production. In complicated silicosis, fibrosis of the lung occurs, leading to restriction in lung function and right-sided heart failure. Respiratory impairment is severe. Those with silicosis may also develop tuberculosis. Acute silicosis, most commonly due to exposure to high concentrations of silica dust (as in sandblasting), is a rapidly progressive disease leading to severe disability and death within 5 years of diagnosis.

Asbestosis is a diffuse interstitial fibrosis of the lungs resulting from repeated trauma caused by the impact and deposition of asbestos fibers on the alveolar walls. As the fibrosis becomes widespread, the elasticity and compliance of the lung are reduced. Fibrosis results in a thickening of the alveolar walls and interstitial space, which in turn reduces the oxygen diffusion to the pulmonary capillary bed. Pulmonary function studies show a reduced forced vital capacity. X-rays reveal linear opacities, especially in the lower lung fields. Unfortunately, physical findings are few until the disease is relatively advanced. Individuals may see their care provider for symptoms of a productive cough, shortness of breath, and weight loss. Asbestosis has no cure and usually results in death after a period of years. Lung cancer is associated with all types of asbestos inhalation. Mesothelioma, a cancer of the pleura, accounts for 7% to 10% of the deaths of asbestos workers.

Coal workers' pneumoconiosis results from the accumulation of coal dust in the lungs, which accounts for its common name, black lung disease. Simple coal workers' pneumoconiosis, not complicated by other lung conditions, causes no symptoms or respiratory difficulty. A small percentage develop progressive massive fibrosis with large lesions consisting of fibrous tissue, coal dust, and central cavitation. Clients may produce thick, black sputum and suffer from shortness of breath and dyspnea. X-rays reveal large opacities, and pulmonary function studies indicate an obstructive deficit. The large-mass lesions produced may eventually lead to pulmonary hypertension, cor pulmonale, and death from congestive heart failure.

Medical Measures

Pulmonary function studies and chest x-ray assist in the diagnosis and in assessing the degree of lung impairment. Superimposed respiratory tract infections are treated with antibiotics. Antituberculosis medications are administered if tuberculosis develops in clients with silicosis. Bronchodilators may be beneficial when there is evidence of a reversible obstructive component.

Oxygen therapy may be necessary for individuals with low arterial oxygen levels. Cardiotonic drugs may be prescribed if the cardiovascular system has been affected. Bronchial hygiene measures such as deep breathing, coughing, and postural drainage are often indicated. Clients are advised to discontinue exposure.

Specific Nursing Measures

Nursing management is supportive. Stress the importance of avoiding further exposure to the harmful agent. Smoking will aggravate the symptoms. Answering client questions, explaining the disease process, and explaining treatments, will give clients more knowledge about how to cope effectively with their illness.

Be aware that many people will be afraid to leave a job they know how to do. Others, unable to leave a geographic area and with responsibility for a family, will feel their options are limited. They may choose to stay on the job even though it interferes with their health. If nurses acknowledge the reality of the client's situation, their health teaching efforts may be more readily accepted.

Sarcoidosis

Sarcoidosis is a multisystem disorder characterized by noncaseating granulomas in many organs. It is most common in young adults and more prevalent among blacks. Objective findings include bilateral hilar lymphadenopathy, pulmonary infiltration, and skin or eye lesions. Other areas affected can include the liver, spleen, heart, muscles, peripheral lymph nodes, mucous membranes, parotid glands, phalangeal bones, and nervous system.

The etiology of sarcoidosis is unknown, but immune system involvement is suspected. The tubercle bacillus and genetic susceptibility are also under investigation. The illness can vary from self-limiting with spontaneous remission to a progressive widespread granulomatous inflammation and fibrosis. Death is usually from advanced pulmonary disease.

Clinical Manifestations

Intrathoracic lesions are the most common manifestation of sarcoidosis and the most frequent indication for treatment. There is usually dyspnea and a cough that may be severe, incapacitating, and occasionally occurring in paroxysms that lead to vomiting. There is scanty sputum, which occasionally can be blood streaked from straining. Wheezing and pulmonary obstruction also can occur. Physical examination reveals crackling rales that are diffuse or only at the bases of the lungs. Restricted pulmonary excursion and an accentuated or split-second heart sound in the pulmonic area can be heard if pulmonary hypertension is present. Hemoptysis and spontaneous pneumothorax are also possible. Systemic features of sarcoidosis include fever, weight loss, fatigue, and night sweats. Tuberculosis must be ruled out by careful examination. Mediastinal and hilar lymph nodes are most commonly

NURSING DIAGNOSES IN
Respiratory Dysfunction

DIRECTLY RELATED DIAGNOSES

- Activity intolerance
- Airway clearance, ineffective
- Breathing pattern, ineffective
- Gas exchange, impaired

OTHER POTENTIAL DIAGNOSES

- Adjustment, impaired
- Anxiety
- Comfort, altered: pain
- Communication, impaired: verbal
- Infection, potential for
- Knowledge deficit
- Nutrition, altered: less than body requirements
- Self-concept, disturbance in: body image

involved. There also may be peripheral lymphadenopathy that is generalized or localized to axillary or femoral areas. The nodes found are discrete, firm, nontender, and usually symmetrical. Epitrochlear nodes are often palpable.

Other extrathoracic lesions may produce symptoms and signs in any organ system. Skin lesions may range from maculopapular eruptions, plaques, and raised nodules to erythema nodosum. Ocular involvement is possible, including conjunctivitis, retinal lesions, and lacrimal gland enlargement. There may be asymptomatic enlargement of the parotid, sublingual, and submaxillary glands. Granulomas can form in muscles. Although they do not always produce pain, severe weakness and incapacitation can result. Arthralgias and arthritis may also be seen.

Pulmonary function studies demonstrate decreased lung compliance and loss of diffusing surface. Vital capacity and carbon monoxide diffusing capacity also are decreased. These two indexes are indicators of progression of the illness and the client's response to treatment. Significant pulmonary function impairment can remain even after the x-ray is clear. The vital capacity will always be slightly decreased, even after treatment or spontaneous remission of the disease.

Diagnosis is made by clinical features, along with histologic evidence of granulomas composed of epithelioid cells from tissue biopsy. Most biopsied tissue should come from superficial or palpable lesions in the skin or lymph nodes. When the predominant lesions are in the lung, lung biopsy via fiberoptic bronchoscopy or mediastinoscopy with lymph node biopsy can be performed, but these are much more invasive procedures.

Medical Measures

No treatment is required if the client is asymptomatic. Most asymptomatic clients will have spontaneous resolution of the disease within 1 to 2 years. Corticosteroids have a dramatic impact on the symptomatic client by suppressing the active inflammatory reaction.

Sarcoidosis can remain in remission after corticosteroid treatment but can recur in some clients when treatment is reduced. X-rays and pulmonary function tests are used to monitor treatment. Occasional clients may need lifelong treatment.

Chloroquine (Aralen) improves skin and mucosal lesions, but they return when the drug is discontinued. For clients receiving this medication, it is important to monitor the retina for damage.

Specific Nursing Measures

Because sarcoidosis can affect any body system, the nurse must continuously assess the client for new system involvement. For example, the nurse observes the skin for lesions and auscultates the lungs for rales and the heart for dysrhythmias and an abnormal S_2. Record weight and vital signs frequently, and provide comfort measures according to the client's symptoms. Follow laboratory reports closely, especially pulmonary function and x-ray studies.

If the client is taking corticosteroids, check the urine for glucose and acetone, and carefully evaluate the client for other symptoms and signs of side effects. The client taking corticosteroids is vulnerable to infection, so instruction about prevention of infection is important. During and after withdrawal from corticosteroids (which must be gradual), watch for vomiting, orthostatic hypotension, hypoglycemia, restlessness, anorexia, malaise, and fatigue.

Discharge planning includes encouraging clients to avoid working in an environment subject to dust or chemicals because of the continuing pulmonary involvement. Clients should not smoke for the same reason. Clients taking chloroquine should have ophthalmologic examinations every 6 months, and more often if visual symptoms develop. Those with hypercalcemia may benefit from a diet with low calcium levels and decreased vitamin D.

Adult Respiratory Distress Syndrome

Adult respiratory distress syndrome (ARDS) is a pathophysiologic state best recognized in clients with no previous underlying lung disease who have suffered a sudden catastrophic, often multisystem insult, which has led to the development of severe dyspnea, hypoxemia, loss of pulmonary compliance, and noncardiogenic pulmonary edema (Petty, 1982). ARDS is not a clearly defined disease but a name given to a group of conditions of different etiology but having similar manifestations (Burrell & Burrell, 1982). ARDS has also been called shock lung, white lung, DaNang lung, adult hyaline membrane disease, stiff lung syndrome, wet lung, and many other names (Petty, 1982).

Clinical Manifestations

There is often a latent period of 12 to 48 hours between the initial injury or insult and the development of ARDS.

The pathophysiology in ARDS is caused by diffuse damage to either side of the alveolar–capillary membrane. Whether the damage is alveolar or capillary, the result is an increase in vascular permeability with edema and hemorrhage. Fluid and red blood cells leak into the interstitial space and into the alveoli. The resulting pulmonary edema leads to decreased lung volume and impaired oxygenation. The presence of fluid in the alveoli results in a decrease in surfactant activity, causing an increased tendency of the alveoli to collapse. In alveoli that are collapsed or filled with edema fluid, little or no ventilation can take place. Since oxygen-poor blood is still perfused to these nonventilated alveoli, the result is an abnormally low ventilation-to-perfusion ratio with an increased right to left intrapulmonary shunt. This is responsible for the severe hypoxemia that is refractory to increases in inspired oxygen concentrations (Traver, 1982).

The fluid accumulation in the interstitial space and alveoli causes the lungs to become less compliant, or stiff. The functional residual capacity also decreases because of alveolar instability and collapse (Petty, 1982). These destructive factors will increase the work of breathing, causing clients to hyperventilate in an effort to correct the hypoxemia. Initially, the hyperventilation may result in a lower than normal arterial carbon dioxide tension. As the condition worsens, dyspnea will become more severe. Grunting respirations along with intercostal and suprasternal retractions may be present. Cyanosis is present along with tachycardia, diaphoresis, and confusion (Cline & Fisher, 1982). The client may have rales and rhonchi. Chest x-rays usually reveal pulmonary edema without evidence of heart failure. Arterial blood gases reveal hypoxemia, the cardinal feature of ARDS despite the initiation of high liter flows of oxygen. Hypocapnia may be present initially. Unless treatment is begun, the client will eventually no longer be able to hyperventilate, and this may result in CO_2 retention and respiratory acidosis.

Medical Measures

Therapeutic measures begin with anticipating which clients are candidates for ARDS. These clients should be closely monitored for early signs of abnormal lung function so preventive measures can be instituted.

Treatment of ARDS requires that the client's ventilation be supported and adequate inspired oxygen be delivered to correct the life-threatening hypoxemia. The client must be intubated and placed on a mechanical ventilator with supplemental oxygen to maintain an arterial PO_2 between 60 and 70 mm Hg.

Careful monitoring of fluid administration is critical because of the increased pulmonary capillary permeability. Overhydration could increase the existing pulmonary edema, shunting, and compliance abnormalities; underhydration could result in inadequate pulmonary and systemic perfusion. A pulmonary artery catheter is frequently used to aid in determining fluid status and left ventricular function.

The use of corticosteroid drugs in the treatment of ARDS remains controversial. The use of prophylactic antibiotics is not recommended. They are used only for identified infections as revealed by culture and sensitivity tests.

Colloids such as albumin and dextran may be used to draw fluid from the pulmonary interstitial space, but this therapy is somewhat controversial. Diuretics such as furosemide may be given to treat fluid overload when systemic circulation is adequate (Petty, 1982). Nutritional management is essential in these acutely ill clients, and intravenous hyperalimentation is often instituted to maintain an adequate nutritional balance.

Specific Nursing Measures

Nurses need to be alert to the precipitating causes of ARDS and closely monitor individuals at risk, assessing vital signs and any abnormalities of lung function such as atelectasis, rales, shortness of breath, and symptoms of hypoxia. Once ARDS has been diagnosed, nursing care becomes complex. Nursing care of the client's airway requires suctioning, postural drainage, and proper management of the endotracheal or tracheostomy tube.

Monitor the level of arterial oxygen closely to guard against both hypoxemia and oxygen toxicity. Monitor fluid balance by weighing the client daily and keeping accurate intake and output records. Also be alert to the possibility of electrolyte imbalances. Central venous pressure, pulmonary artery pressure, and pulmonary capillary wedge pressure are frequently measured by the nurse in the intensive care setting. The equipment used and procedures performed can be frightening to the client and significant others. Take time to explain what is being done and why.

SECTION 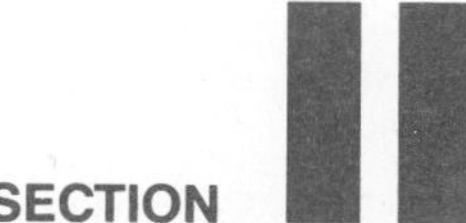

Infectious Disorders

Acute Bronchitis

Acute bronchitis is primarily an infection of the larger bronchi in clients whose airways are otherwise normal. This infection is most commonly viral, and usually starts as an extension of an upper respiratory infection.

Clinical Manifestations

The major symptoms include coughing, a burning substernal sensation (often aggravated by a deep breath), and sputum production. The amount of sputum may be slight initially, but as the infection progresses, the sputum becomes mucoid or purulent. The client may or may not have an elevated temperature. Malaise, muscle aches, and headache are common. Chest auscultation reveals rales, rhonchi, and wheezes. The disease is self-limiting, and the duration depends on the underlying causative organism. Smoking tends to prolong and aggravate the condition.

Medical Measures

Treatment is aimed at relieving the symptoms. Bed rest may be ordered initially. Debilitated clients sometimes require hospitalization. Hot or cold steam inhalation or intermittent positive pressure breathing (IPPB) will liquefy and loosen secretions so they can be more easily expectorated. Antipyretics such as aspirin may be ordered if temperature is elevated; expectorants may be ordered to loosen secretions or antitussives to quiet a chronic nonproductive cough. Lozenges may be used to soothe an irritated throat. Antibiotics are not routinely given unless sputum cultures identify a superinfection with a bacterial agent.

Specific Nursing Measures

Since acute bronchitis is contagious, clients should learn to guard against spreading the infection by properly disposing of tissues, using good hand-washing technique, covering the nose and mouth when coughing or sneezing, and not sharing drinking glasses or towels. Instruct clients about proper deep breathing and coughing techniques. Bronchial drainage may be required in situations where secretions are numerous and the client has difficulty in expectorating them. In more debilitated clients who have a poor cough reflex, suctioning may be necessary. Encourage fluid intake of at least 2 to 3 L/day unless contraindicated to help prevent dehydration and to keep respiratory tract secretions liquid so they can be more easily expectorated.

Nutritional management includes an adequate intake of fluids such as soft drinks and fruit juices. Encourage light meals consisting of toast, gelatin, puddings, and cereals. This type of diet is easily tolerated and digested while helping to meet caloric needs.

Keep the environment warm and dry and free of drafts to prevent chilling. Encourage clients to rest and to avoid becoming overly fatigued. A period of convalescence is usually necessary after the infection. Caution clients to avoid further exposure to infection, to dress warmly, eat properly, get enough rest, avoid people with colds, and avoid environmental irritants such as cigarette smoke and other pollutants.

Table 16–1
Common Types of Pneumonia

Types of Pneumonia	Etiologic Agent
Community-acquired pneumonias	
Pneumococcal pneumonia	*Streptococcus pneumoniae*
Mycoplasmal pneumonia	*Mycoplasma pneumoniae*
Legionnaires' pneumonia	*Legionella pneumophila*
Viral pneumonia	Influenza virus (Type A or Type B)
Hospital-acquired pneumonias	
Staphylococcal pneumonia	*Staphylococcus aureus*
Klebsiella pneumonia	*Klebsiella pneumoniae* (Friedländer's bacillus)
Pseudomonal pneumonia	*Pseudomonas aeruginosa*
Aspiration pneumonia	Aspiration of a foreign body, gastric contents, or bacteria from the upper respiratory tract

The Pneumonias

Pneumonia is an inflammation of the alveolar spaces caused by infection. Many different organisms can cause pneumonia with a resultant variation in symptomatology. Microorganisms can enter the alveolar spaces when infected airborne droplets are inhaled, when food or fluid is aspirated, or when an infection is spread to the lungs by the bloodstream (George, Light, & Matthay, 1983).

Pneumonia is most common in the elderly, but it can occur at any age. Although relatively healthy adults can contract pneumonia, certain predisposing conditions make individuals more susceptible. One predisposing condition is impaired upper airway defense mechanisms such as can occur with cigarette smoking, trauma, or decreased levels of consciousness (eg, impaired gag reflex). Abnormalities of the lungs or thorax, such as those in chronic obstructive pulmonary diseases, are another predisposing factor, as is general debility from heart disease, diabetes mellitus, or chronic alcoholism. Diseases known to impair immunity, such as leukemia or aplastic anemia, can also lower resistance to pneumonia-causing organisms (Mitchell & Petty, 1982). Hospitalized clients may develop pneumonia, especially those who are debilitated and bedridden, those with artificial airways such as tracheostomies, and certain high-risk postoperative surgical clients.

Overall, pneumonia accounts for more than 10% of all hospital admissions and occurs in about 5% of the clients admitted for other reasons (nosocomial pneumonia). During one recent year, over 2 million cases of pneumonia were reported, and pneumonia is listed as the fifth leading cause of death in the United States. As shown in Table 16–1, the pneumonias and their causative organisms can be divided into those commonly acquired in the community and those that are more frequently hospital acquired.

Clinical Manifestations

Pneumococcal pneumonia, caused by *Streptococcus pneumoniae,* is the most common community-acquired bacterial pneumonia. This pneumonia, which may be preceded by an upper respiratory tract infection, is usually lobar or segmental, involving one or two lobes of the lung. The rest of the lung may remain free of infection. The onset is abrupt beginning with shaking chills, severe pleural pain, rapidly rising fever (as high as 106°F or 41°C), and a hacking cough. A cough productive of purulent sputum that is greenish, bloody, or rusty is common. Generalized symptoms such as malaise, weakness, headache, nausea, and vomiting occur frequently. Clients are diaphoretic and generally uncomfortable but usually remain alert. Lobar consolidation is shown on x-ray (Figure 16–1). Laboratory studies usually reveal leukocytosis, respiratory alkalosis, mild hypoxemia, and an elevated erythrocyte sedimentation rate. In those who improve without antibiotic treatment, recovery usually begins between the seventh and fourteenth day. With antibiotic treatment, uncomplicated pneumococcal pneumonia usually responds within 24 hours.

Mycoplasmal pneumonia, caused by *Mycoplasma pneumoniae,* is referred to as an "atypical" pneumonia, primarily to distinguish it from the more common bacterial pneumonias. The atypical pneumonias more closely resemble viral infections, but they usually respond to antibiotic therapy. *Mycoplasma pneumoniae* is a common cause of pneumonia in children and young adults, but can affect all age groups. The organism is not highly contagious, and significant outbreaks usually stem from close interpersonal contact, as in schools or families. The onset is gradual. The most common symptoms, developing over 3 to 4 days, are a low-grade fever, malaise, headache, sore throat, and a cough with minimum sputum production, which is often mucoid. As the illness progresses, earache, tracheal irritation, and chest pain commonly accompany the cough. Clients appear mildly to moderately ill. In most instances, this pneumonia is self-limiting, with recovery beginning in 10 to 14 days. Deaths are extremely rare.

Legionnaires' disease is an atypical pneumonia that received national attention when an outbreak of severe respiratory illness was traced to the 1976 American Legion Convention in Philadelphia. The causative organism was later named *Legionella pneumophila,* a gram-negative bacterium. Although all age groups can be affected, those over 50 are more susceptible. Males are more vulnerable than females, as are those who smoke, are on immunosuppressive therapy, or have an underlying chronic debilitating condition. Outbreaks have been traced to contaminated water and air conditioning systems and to soil at contaminated excavation sites. The general symptoms are weakness, malaise, nausea and vomiting, diarrhea, and headache. The cough is nonproductive but later can become productive of minimally purulent or nonpurulent sputum. As the illness progresses, fever rises to about 104°F (40°C), accompanied by bradycardia. Pulmonary symptoms and signs include dyspnea, rales, bronchial breath sounds, and dullness to percussion. The general course and prognosis depend on the underlying risk factors of clients and appropriate management of care.

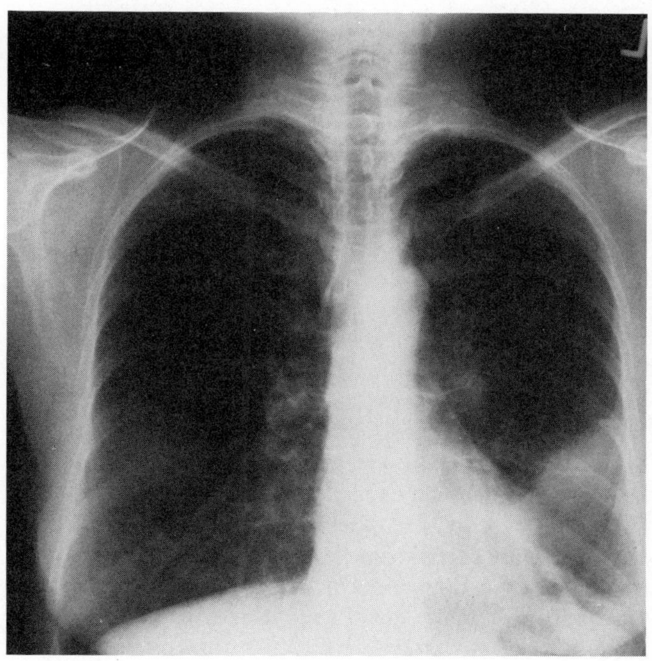

Figure 16–1

A female client with pneumonia. Chest x-ray shows large areas of consolidation in the left lower lobe. *Courtesy of Health Care Plan, Buffalo, NY.*

The cause of viral pneumonia in adults is primarily the influenza virus, either Type A or Type B. Influenza pneumonia is more common in elderly clients who have underlying chronic debilitating disease. Clients appear acutely ill with a sudden onset of chills, malaise, anorexia, headache, and tearing, burning eyes. The cough produces bloody sputum. Belated bronchial involvement occurs, along with dyspnea and cyanosis. Individuals have a high fever accompanied by tachycardia. The duration and outcome of this pneumonia depend on the underlying condition of the client and control of secondary bacterial infections.

Staphylococcal pneumonia is primarily a disease of hospitalized clients or clients with altered defense mechanisms. *Staphylococcus aureus* is normally present in the nose and skin of healthy individuals and can be spread by aerosol or direct contact. Debilitated adults whose resistance to infection is hampered are targets for the development of infections from this organism. The organism can also be spread hematogenously (via the bloodstream) from infected areas to the lungs in clients with bacteremia. Intravenous drug abusers are also susceptible. Staphylococcal pneumonia begins suddenly with chills, diaphoresis, and spiking temperatures. There are dyspnea, pleural pain, hypoxemia, and a cough that produces yellow, blood-tinged sputum. Chest x-rays most commonly show patchy, rapidly spreading areas of bronchopneumonia. Tissue necrosis and abscess formation can occur. The destructive nature of this organism may lead to permanent lung damage in the form of fibrosis or bronchiectasis. The prognosis varies with the age and general condition of those affected.

Klebsiella pneumonia (also known as Friedländer's bacillus) produces an especially lethal form of pneumonia with a predilection for older men who are debilitated by some form of chronic illness, especially alcoholism. The onset is abrupt. Symptoms include marked respiratory distress, high fever, violent chills, pleuritic chest pain, and a cough producing copious amounts of thick grey–green or reddish brown sputum (often described as resembling currant jelly). Rales and rhonchi are present. Chest x-rays show dense lobar consolidation with infiltration. A high mortality is associated with this pneumonia because of the overall debilitated condition of those most likely to contract it and because of the virulence of the organism.

Pseudomonas aeruginosa is an important cause of hospital-acquired infections. Pneumonias caused by this organism usually result from aspiration of organisms indigenous to the upper respiratory tract or inhalation of the organism from contaminated nebulizers. Susceptible clients are debilitated and suffer from underlying chronic lung or heart disease or burns, are on steroids or antibiotics, or are intubated and on nebulizer breathing devices. Initial symptoms include an elevated temperature, chills, dyspnea, cyanosis, and a cough productive of copious amounts of foul smelling yellow or green sputum. Chest x-rays reveal diffuse bronchopneumonia, which is often bilateral, involving several lobes. Abscesses and pleural effusions can develop. The treatment is long and the prognosis poor because of underlying debilitating disease and the lack of responsiveness of the organism to antibiotics.

Aspiration pneumonia usually occurs in clients with impaired gag or swallowing reflexes. Several processes are associated with aspiration. A foreign substance may be aspirated that is large enough to obstruct the airway and cause asphyxiation. A chemical pneumonia can occur secondary to aspiration of gastric contents. Whenever the level of consciousness is depressed, the reflex response preventing aspiration diminishes. Others at risk are those with tracheostomies, elderly and chronically ill bedridden clients, those with nasogastric feeding tubes, and those on antidepressant drugs or under the influence of alcohol. The pH of the aspirated liquid determines the severity of the resulting damage to the lungs. If the pH is above 2.4, the effects are comparable to the aspiration of the same amount of saline. A pH below 2.4 will cause an intense inflammatory response. The presence or absence of food or bacteria also plays a part in the pathophysiology of aspiration pneumonia. Aspiration pneumonia can be caused by the aspiration of bacteria from the upper respiratory tract. The same factors that predispose persons to the aspiration of gastric contents can lead to the aspiration of bacteria. The right upper lobe and the apical segments of the lower lobes are most commonly involved because when the client is supine, the organism has easiest access to these areas. Uncomplicated pneumonitis is rather mild and responds well to treatment with antibiotics. If untreated, pneumonitis may progress to a necrotizing pneumonia or lung abscess.

Medical Measures

The treatment of the bacterial pneumonias centers around selecting the antibiotic or antibiotics to which the infecting organism is most sensitive. Table 16–2 lists the usual antibiotics of choice for the various pneumonias. Most viral pneumonias have no specific therapy. Amantadine has had limited success in the treatment of one specific influenza strain. Polyvalent pneumococcal vaccine can be used to prevent the development of pneumococcal pneumonia, providing protection for at least 3 years against 14 sero-

Table 16–2
Pharmacologic Management of Pneumonia

Types of Pneumonia	Usual Antibiotic(s) of Choice
Pneumococcal pneumonia	Penicillin G or erythromycin
Mycoplasmal pneumonia	Erythromycin or tetracycline
Legionnaires' disease	Erythromycin
Viral pneumonia	Amantadine for prophylaxis (antibiotics useless for a virus)
Staphylococcal pneumonia	Nafcillin, oxacillin, cephalothin, amikacin
Klebsiella pneumonia	Gentamicin or tobramycin with or without cephalothin
Pseudomonal pneumonia	Tobramycin, gentamicin, or amikacin
Aspiration pneumonia	Penicillin G, or nafcillin if client acquires staphylococci while in the hospital

types causing 75% of this type of pneumonia (Mitchell & Petty, 1982).

Antipyretics and analgesics such as acetylsalicylic acid (aspirin) or acetaminophen may be given. Narcotics may be required if chest pain is severe. Codeine is most frequently given. Expectorants are given to reduce the viscosity of pulmonary secretions; examples are terpin hydrate orally or acetylcysteine (Mucomyst) by nebulization. Antitussives may be ordered to treat nonproductive coughs.

Clients are frequently placed on bed rest because of the debilitating nature of pneumonia. Hospitalization is sometimes necessary. IPPB along with other pulmonary hygiene measures such as postural drainage may be ordered. Supplemental oxygen is used if arterial oxygen levels become too low. Hospitalized clients may receive intravenous fluids as well as oral fluids to replace fluid loss caused by an elevated temperature, increased cellular metabolism, tachypnea, and diaphoresis. Electrolytes may also need to be replaced. Between 3 and 4 L of fluid per day are required unless contraindicated. A high-calorie, high-protein diet is ordered to help the body fight the infection. If the client is unable to eat, nasogastric feedings or hyperalimentation may be ordered. If respiratory failure occurs, the client is intubated and placed on a mechanical ventilator. Depending on the infectious agent, clients may be placed in respiratory isolation. If a pleural effusion develops, a thoracentesis may be performed.

Specific Nursing Measures

Although the types of pneumonia vary, the overall nursing care is similar. Since bed rest is frequently needed during the acute phase of pneumonia, nursing care for hospitalized clients should be organized to allow periods of uninterrupted rest combined with turning, coughing, and deep breathing at least every 2 hours. Postural drainage measures may also be needed. If clients are not able to cough up secretions effectively, tracheal suctioning may be required.

Carefully assess the client's respirations and remain alert to the complications pneumonia can cause in the lungs such as pleurisy, pleural effusion, empyema, lung abscess, and pulmonary edema. Monitor the client for systemic complications (septicemia, septic shock, meningitis, endocarditis, and renal and liver involvement) so they can be recognized and treated early (Burrell & Burrell, 1982).

Sputum specimens are important to identify the causative organism. Try to collect an adequate sputum sample and not saliva. Tracheal suctioning may be required for clients who cannot cough effectively. If the client has an elevated temperature and is diaphoretic, provide tepid baths along with frequent changes of bed linen to prevent chilling.

Keep the client hydrated to loosen secretions so they can be more easily expectorated and to prevent dehydration. Closely monitor fluid intake, giving prescribed amounts each shift. Urinary output is a good indicator of hydration. If clients can eat, good mouth care helps to improve the appetite. Clients should cover the nose and mouth when they cough and dispose of tissues in a paper bag to prevent cross-infection. Strict hand-washing by staff, clients, and families will help to reduce the spread of bacteria.

Clients who are acutely ill with pneumonia may suffer from fears or anxiety related to respiratory impairment caused by the infection. This is especially true if the pneumonia is superimposed on another illness such as chronic lung disorders. Symptoms such as shortness of breath, expectoration of blood-streaked sputum, and chest pain can arouse undue anxiety for both client and family. Take time to answer questions and explain procedures. If clients are bothered by chest pain, analgesics may be needed. If narcotic analgesics are ordered however, it is important to observe the client for signs of respiratory depression. Splinting the chest during coughing and deep breathing exercises will help to reduce chest pain. Teach family members to do this, keeping the fingers together to apply firm support.

Discharge planning involves reviewing medications, their actions, and side effects with client and family. Clients should understand how to avoid overfatigue by increasing activities gradually. Teach clients with an underlying chronic debilitating condition about their increased susceptibility to respiratory tract infections and the techniques of avoiding infections (eg, sufficient rest, well-balanced diet, avoiding people with colds, and not getting chilled). Tell clients to contact their physician if they develop a cough, notice a change in the color or amount of sputum they normally produce, or suffer any shortness of breath. Explain to cigarette smokers that they are at higher risk and that the American Lung Association or the American Cancer Society has information on smoking cessation. Alcohol abusers should be aware of their risks and told about Alcoholics Anonymous or other treatment programs for alcoholism. If these measures are not attempted, the chances of the recurrence of pneumonia are greater (Ryan, 1982).

To prevent aspiration pneumonia, semicomatose or comatose clients should be in the side-lying position with the foot of the bed elevated 6 to 9 in unless contraindicated. Support the client with pillows behind the back, between the knees, and in front of the chest. Turn the client q. 2h to prevent formation of decubiti. Elevate the head of the bed at least 30° during feeding and for 1 hour after completion of the feeding. Check gag and cough reflexes before feeding. Before administering a nasogastric feeding, check for proper placement of the tube in the stomach. Aspirate for stomach contents, and if 100 mL or more is withdrawn, withhold the feeding and consult with the physician. Administer the tube feeding slowly over 20 minutes and remain with the client. If the tube feeding is continuous, keep the head of the bed elevated. Frequent mouth care and the removal of secretions that accumulate in the back of the throat will help to prevent the aspiration of organisms into the lower respiratory tract (Ryan, 1982).

Tuberculosis

Mycobacterium tuberculosis is a nonmotile, acid-fast, weakly gram-positive, aerobic bacillus. The organism is transmitted by inhaling invisible infective particles (droplet nuclei) produced when an infected person speaks, coughs, laughs, or sneezes. Larger infected inhaled particles are removed by the mucociliary action of the respiratory airways. Bacteria that land on furniture or other surfaces are not contagious, since they can no longer be inhaled and are usually quickly killed by the ultraviolet rays of sunlight or by drying. Tuberculosis is not highly contagious; transmission generally requires close, frequent, or prolonged contact with the infected individual.

When infected droplet nuclei are inhaled into the alveoli of a susceptible adult, tubercle bacilli begin to multiply slowly. A small area of bronchopneumonia develops at the site, known as the primary focus (or primary disease). In spite of the body's reaction to phagocytize the invading organism, there is little or no resistance to the multiplication of the bacilli. As a result, bacilli are disseminated from the primary site, primarily by the lymphatics with extensive involvement of the regional (hilar) lymph nodes (Figure 16–2). The primary peripheral lesion in the lung and the associated enlarged draining lymph nodes form what is called the Ghon complex. From the lymphatics, the organism drains into the systemic circulation, potentially spreading the bacilli to all the organs and tissues of the body.

The infected individual is usually asymptomatic at this time. Infection with *Mycobacterium tuberculosis* does not necessarily mean developing active TBC. After a few days or weeks the multiplication of the virulent tubercle bacilli usually decreases, the pneumonic process resolves, and there is no further spread of the bacilli by the lymphatics or blood.

This pattern is the same in any other organs infected with tubercle bacilli. The body's defenses can effectively contain the organisms. Macrophages engulf the bacilli, forming clusters of cells that give rise to the granuloma, the characteristic lesion of TBC. This reaction usually occurs over 4 to 10 weeks and results in reactivity to the tuberculin skin test. A relative immunity to exogenous reinfection (reinfection from another active case) by the tubercle bacilli also appears to develop.

In most adults, the healed granulomas remain stable and may calcify. While some of the bacilli are destroyed as the lesions heal, a significant number of bacilli become dormant. Thus, a person infected with the bacilli but not treated with antimicrobial drugs may develop tuberculosis in the future.

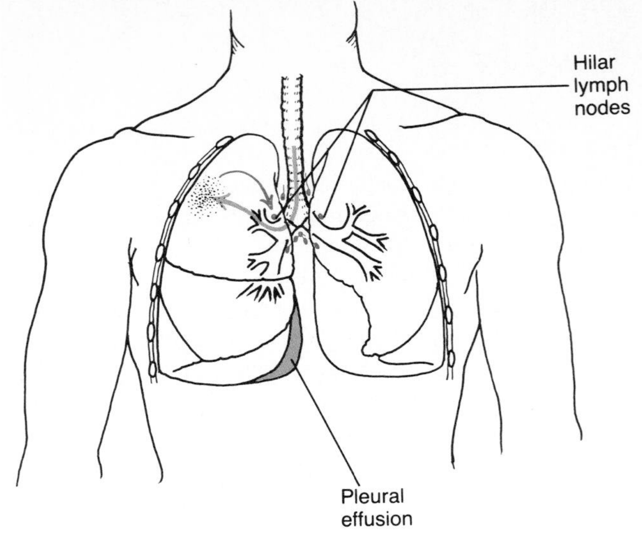

Figure 16–2

Hilar lymph node involvement in TBC. Anatomic relationship of the hilar lymph nodes to the pulmonary structures.

The full-blown disease may never develop; if it does, it may develop weeks or many years after the initial infection. The likelihood of developing the disease diminishes as the time from infection lengthens.

In approximately 5% to 15% of individuals infected with TBC, one of the granulomas in the lung or elsewhere breaks down, the tubercle bacilli multiply, and the individual becomes ill with tuberculosis. The adult can also become reinfected through contact with a host who has active TBC. Because the organism requires oxygen to grow, the apices of the lungs where the concentrations of oxygen are highest, are favored.

The reasons why a person develops active TBC are not clearly understood. Certain factors such as aging, degenerative diseases, malnutrition, diabetes mellitus, silicosis, chronic obstructive pulmonary disease (COPD), and immunosuppressive therapy, all of which lower resistance to infection, promote the development of TBC.

Clinical Manifestations

Tuberculosis of the lung most often develops as a chronic illness, and symptoms appear over weeks or months. Symptoms can include anorexia, weight loss, fatigue, a low-grade fever that usually occurs in the afternoon, irregular menses in women, and night sweats. A cough occurs, which progressively becomes productive of mucoid or sometimes mucopurulent sputum. There may be chest pain or a feeling of tightness in the chest. Caseous material may erode into the pleural space, causing a pleural effusion, which is painful (see Figure 16–2). Hemoptysis occurs and is often the reason the client seeks health care.

A history of possible exposure to TBC is important, but the exposure could have occurred years before, and the client may not even have been aware of it. Making the diagnosis is crucial not only for treatment of the infected individual but also to reduce spread of the disease. Contacts must be screened because they may have become infected with the bacilli and may require treatment to prevent TBC.

A positive Mantoux intradermal skin test (Chapter 14) or a positive tine test may confirm the diagnosis of infection with *Mycobacterium tuberculosis,* but false positive (and false negative) tests occur. The chest x-ray can show active or calcified lesions. The Ghon complex and characteristic cavity in the lung tissue can be seen on x-ray. The problem with making a definitive diagnosis with a chest x-ray is that other diseases of the lungs (pneumonia or malignant tumors) can look like TBC.

A definitive diagnosis of TBC can only be made when *M tuberculosis* is cultured from secretions or tissues. A culture and sensitivity report takes 8 weeks or more because of the slow growth of the bacilli.

Medical Measures

Ten drugs currently available in the United States have been approved for the treatment of tuberculosis. These drugs are divided into three categories: primary, secondary, and tertiary (Table 16–3). The primary drugs, isoniazid and rifampin, are highly effective, especially if used together. The secondary drugs are not as effective and have more toxic side effects. They are usually used in combination with one or both of the primary drugs. Since the organism can develop resistance to any single drug, combining two or three drugs helps to maintain drug effectiveness. The tertiary medications are not as effective as the primary or secondary drugs and have greater toxic side effects.

In individuals who are being treated for TBC for a second time, different drugs should be used than were used for the previous treatment. Response to medication therapy is fairly rapid, and individuals become noninfectious within a period of weeks. To prevent the recurrence of active disease, drug therapy is continued for 18 months to 2 years. Isoniazid has been used alone for 12 months to prevent clinical symptoms in certain individuals with dormant TBC who show a positive skin test, such as household contacts.

Monitoring of clients is required during the course of drug therapy. This monitoring involves sputum smears and cultures, which usually will be negative after 2 months of

Table 16–3
Pharmacologic Management of Tuberculosis

Drug	Dosage	Adverse Side Effects
Primary (highly effective, rarely toxic)		
Isoniazid (INH)	5 mg/kg/day (300–400 mg)	Hepatotoxic; inhibits phenytoin metabolism leading to ↑ blood levels and toxicity; peripheral neuropathy
Rifampin	450–600 mg q.d.	Hepatotoxic; when used with INH, ↑ incidence of liver damage; accelerates catabolism of quinidine, warfarin, corticosteroids, and oral contraceptives
Secondary (less effective, may have more toxic side effects, usually used in combination with one or both primary drugs)		
Ethambutol	15 mg/kg	Optic neuritis
Para-aminosalicylic acid (PAS)	8–12 g/day	GI disturbance
Streptomycin	1 g/day IM for 60 days	Ototoxic (CN VIII); paresthesia; rash; fever; nephrotoxic
Pyrazinamide	20–35 mg/kg (but no more than 3 g/day)	Hepatotoxic; urate retention leading to gout
Tertiary (usually used only when resistance develops to previous drugs)		
Capreomycin	1 g/day IM	Nephrotoxic; ototoxic
Cycloserine	500 mg to 1 g/day in divided doses	Personality changes; convulsions; rash
Ethionamide	500 mg to 1 g/day in divided doses	GI disturbance; peripheral neuritis; hepatotoxic
Kanamycin	15 mg/kg/day IM in two equally divided doses 12 h apart	Ototoxic; nephrotoxic

therapy. If the smears remain positive, a new treatment regimen must be started. Change in the client's symptoms and chest x-rays will also show how well the client is progressing with treatment. Once an adequate course of therapy has been completed, clients can be discharged from further supervision. Since the advent of effective chemotherapy against TBC, surgical intervention is rare.

Specific Nursing Measures

Although TBC can be cured, many clients are fearful when the diagnosis is made. It is important that the nurse explain what TBC is, how it is transmitted, and that it can be cured. Nursing staff may also react with fear toward the client with tuberculosis, leaving the client isolated and ignored. All staff need a proper understanding of the disease.

If clients require hospitalization, they are routinely placed in isolation. The only isolation measures necessary are careful handling and disposal of secretions and the avoidance of direct face-to-face contact. Tissues contaminated with sputum should be discarded in a paper bag and burned. The client's room should be properly ventilated with nonrecirculating air. Laminar flow or ultraviolet lighting will accomplish the same purpose as nonrecirculating ventilation. Masks are not routinely required for persons who come in contact with the client or for clients themselves. Clients should cover the nose and mouth when they cough or sneeze. Clients who are very ill and unable to cover their mouths when they cough should be masked when direct care is given. The mask must be capable of filtering out the small droplet nuclei. No other isolation measures, such as gowning or wearing gloves, are necessary. Within 2 weeks after chemotherapy is begun, the possibility of transmitting the disease is markedly reduced.

Since strict adherence to the medication schedule is required if tuberculosis is to be cured, make certain that clients understand and accept the importance of following the medication schedule. Both clients and family members must give this aspect of care precedence over other needs. Even after the client is discharged from the hospital, many more months of medication therapy are required. The medications are provided by the county health department, and clients must not let their medications run out.

The importance of follow-up must be stressed, not only so progress can be monitored but also to check for possible side effects from the antituberculosis medications and to make sure drug resistance has not developed. Instruct clients to see a physician immediately if symptoms of TBC recur or if side effects from the medication develop. Side effects of common TBC drugs are listed in Table 16–3. The responsibility for client care and education falls not only on hospital nurses but on public health nurses who must continue to monitor clients with tuberculosis and their contacts (Traver, 1982).

Fungal Infections

Fungal infections of the lungs generally are the result of infectious spores that are inhaled into the distal air spaces, multiply, and cause an inflammatory response. The fungi that cause diseases in humans are nonmotile yeasts or molds. The infection can spread from the lungs to other organs, including the skin, bones, and the central nervous system. Many fungi can cause respiratory diseases, all of which have similar pathologic findings, symptomatology, and treatment. Coccidioidomycosis, histoplasmosis, and blastomycosis are three of the most common fungal infections.

Coccidioidomycosis

Coccidioidomycosis is endemic only in the Americas, especially the southwestern United States, including parts of New Mexico, Utah, California, Texas, and Arizona. The growth of the organism is supported by a semiarid hot climate with a short, intense rainy season. Infectious spores are inhaled from spore-laden dust. Person-to-person transmission has not been documented.

CLINICAL MANIFESTATIONS Approximately 50% to 60% of those infected with coccidioidomycosis are only subclinically affected. The rest develop influenzalike symptoms 1 to 3 weeks after infection, including cough, fever, chest pain, headache, and fatigue. Symptoms of infection other than in the lungs include arthralgia, conjunctivitis, and erythema nodosum, a skin rash seen primarily on the lower legs of young women. Chest x-rays can show infiltrates that may occur in any part of the lungs, hilar adenopathy, pneumonia, and pleural effusions. Leukocytosis is present because of the inflammatory response. The cell-mediated response limits the extent of the illness and gives lifelong immunity. Complete clinical and x-ray resolution will occur within 6 to 8 weeks.

MEDICAL MEASURES In the simple primary infection, no antibiotic is required, only symptomatic care. In progressive coccidioidal pulmonary disease and in disseminated coccidioidomycosis, the antibiotic amphotericin B is the treatment of choice.

Histoplasmosis

Histoplasmosis is caused by the dimorphic fungus *Histoplasma capsulatum*. Histoplasmosis is a worldwide infection. In the United States, it is more prevalent in the Mississippi and Ohio River valleys. The organism likes a temperate climate, and its growth is enhanced in soil that contains chicken, starling, or blackbird droppings, or bat guano. The fungi become airborne when the soil is disturbed and can be inhaled, leading to infection. Transmission from person to person does not occur.

CLINICAL MANIFESTATIONS Once the spores are implanted in the lungs, they mature and rupture, releasing yeast forms of the organism. These yeast forms are surrounded and engulfed by macrophages. The pathogenesis of this disease is similar to that of tuberculosis. Caseating granulomas form, and delayed hypersensitivity develops. Invariably, the organism invades the bloodstream, spreading to various organs, especially the liver and spleen. In most cases, the disease is brought under control by the body's defense mechanisms. Histoplasmosis can be asymptomatic, acute, or chronic. Acute histoplasmosis is most common in infants and small children. Acute histoplasmosis in adults is most often a reinfection with a large number of fungi. Symptoms include fever, chills, malaise, dry cough, and muscle aches. Pulmonary infiltrates plus hilar and mediastinal lymphadenopathy are visible on x-ray. This form of histoplasmosis is usually self-limiting, with symptoms persisting for about a week. Lesions on the lung eventually calcify, leaving a so-called "buck shot" appearance (George, Light, & Matthay, 1983). In some cases, a severe pneumonia results that is sometimes fatal.

Chronic histoplasmosis is most common in middle-aged or older white males who have a history of smoking and COPD. Symptoms that usually persist over several months include a low-grade fever, chronic cough, and weight loss. There is a progressive loss of lung tissue.

MEDICAL MEASURES No antifungal medication is required for the primary infection under most circumstances. Amphotericin B is indicated for chronic progressive pulmonary disease.

Blastomycosis

Blastomycosis, caused by the fungus *Blastomyces dermatitidis,* is most common in the southeastern United States and in the Mississippi and Ohio River valleys. It also occurs in Canada, Mexico, and parts of South America and Africa. *Blastomyces* has been found in the soil and is acquired by inhaling the spores into the lungs.

CLINICAL MANIFESTATIONS Once spores are deposited in the lung, the inflammatory response occurs as with coccidioidomycosis and histoplasmosis. Subclinical and mild infections are possible, but more frequently clients have a progressive pulmonary disorder often associated with dissemination. Symptoms include a cough, which is productive of purulent material and sometimes contains blood, a low-grade fever, weakness, and weight loss. Chest x-rays may show diffuse fibronodular infiltration, cavitations, bronchopneumonia, or miliary lesions. The pleura can be affected. The disease may be limited to one lobe or may involve all parts of both lungs. The most common area to be affected by dissemination is the skin, where lesions consist of granulomas surrounding small abscesses. The other two most common sites of spread are the bone and the male genitourinary system. The mortality rate for untreated progressive blastomycosis is high.

MEDICAL MEASURES Amphotericin B, IV is used in the treatment of progressive and disseminated disease. A drug that can be used for isolated cutaneous lesions is hydroxystilbamidine.

Specific Nursing Measures

Nursing care for clients with fungal diseases of the lungs centers around explaining the disease and treatment and monitoring potential side effects of drugs. Clients and their families may be apprehensive that the disease is contagious, so it is important to explain that person-to-person spread does not occur.

Since the primary drug used in the treatment of fungal infections, amphotericin B, can cause kidney damage, liver damage, severe chilling, and malaise, monitor the administration of this IV medication closely. Inquire about any effects experienced by the client, and note results of laboratory tests indicating impaired liver and renal function. The color and consistency of urine should also be observed and urinary output measured. The client's skin should be inspected in natural light to detect any jaundice.

SECTION 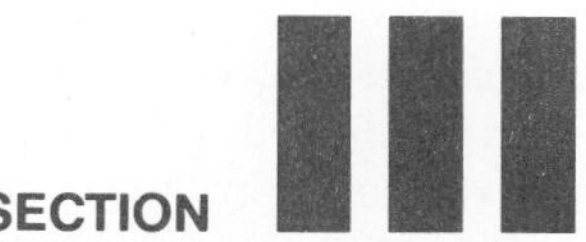

Obstructive Disorders

Obstructive disorders of the respiratory system are lung diseases that cause a persistent obstruction of bronchial air flow. Different names have been applied to this group of diseases. The most common are chronic obstructive pulmonary disease (COPD) and chronic airway obstruction (CAO). Chronic bronchitis and emphysema are the most common diseases associated with COPD, but asthma, bronchiectasis, and cystic fibrosis are also included.

Bronchiectasis

Bronchiectasis is a permanent abnormal dilatation of one or more large bronchi because of the destruction of the elastic and muscular components of the bronchial wall. In the past, bronchiectasis was considered a disease of children, and few individuals lived beyond their third or fourth decade. Before antibiotics, children developed the disease after bacterial pneumonia, which followed such diseases as measles and pertussis. While the number of people developing bronchiectasis as a complication of severe pulmonary infections is decreasing, there are more clients in whom bronchiectasis is a complication of an underlying systemic disorder, particularly cystic fibrosis.

The basic disturbance in bronchiectasis is a weakness of the bronchial wall that may be congenital, acquired, or both. Developmental anomalies of the bronchial system can lead to bronchiectasis by promoting infection in the involved airways. Immotile cilia syndrome, a genetic disorder causing immotility of cilia in the respiratory tract, leads to recurrent sinus and bronchial infections, which eventually result in bronchiectasis. Certain hereditary immune-deficiency diseases are frequently complicated by bronchiectasis because affected clients are predisposed to development of infections of the upper and lower airways. Most forms of bronchiectasis are associated with persistent respiratory tract infections and prolonged bronchial obstruction. Occasionally, bronchiectasis may follow the aspiration of corrosive chemicals or the aspiration of gastric fluid.

The infectious process involved in bronchiectasis destroys parts of the bronchial mucosa. These areas are then replaced by fibrous tissue. Since this scar tissue has no resilience, the dynamics of breathing cause the affected airways to become permanently deformed and dilated. The involved airways can dilate up to four times their normal size and take on cylindrical, fusiform (varicose), or saccular shapes. The cylindrical bronchi are dilated with regular outlines; the dilatation may have a square end because of obstruction by mucus. Fusiform bronchi are irregular in form and size with irregular areas of constriction; the ends of the bronchial tree are bulbous and distorted. In the saccular form, the bronchi increase in diameter progressively and end in large blind sacs (Figure 16–3). These structural changes may be located in one or both lungs. The most severe involvement tends to occur in the smaller bronchi and bronchioles.

The impaired bronchial wall movement and loss of cilia, coupled with nonaerated alveoli distal to the bronchiectatic area, cause secretions to pool, stagnate, and become infected. The retained secretions, along with obliteration of the bronchioles distal to the affected areas, also cause diffuse bronchial obstruction and ventilation–perfusion abnormalities.

Clinical Manifestations

The symptoms and signs of bronchiectasis vary depending on its extent, severity, location, and complications. If only one bronchopulmonary segment is involved, the symptoms may be mild; however, if the bronchiectasis is diffused throughout the lungs, the disease may be incapacitating.

The primary clinical feature of bronchiectasis is a chronic, loose cough that is usually productive of large amounts of mucopurulent, often foul-smelling sputum. Hemoptysis is a frequent occurrence, and recurrent bronchopulmonary infections are common. Clients can suffer from dyspnea, chronic malnutrition, fatigue, and anemia as the disease progresses. Chronic paranasal sinusitis is frequently associated with bronchiectasis. Advanced bronchiectasis is often associated with anastomosis between the bronchial and pulmonary vessels, resulting in right-to-left shunts, which in turn lead to hypoxemia, pulmonary hypertension, cor pulmonale, and clubbing of fingers (Mitchell & Petty, 1982).

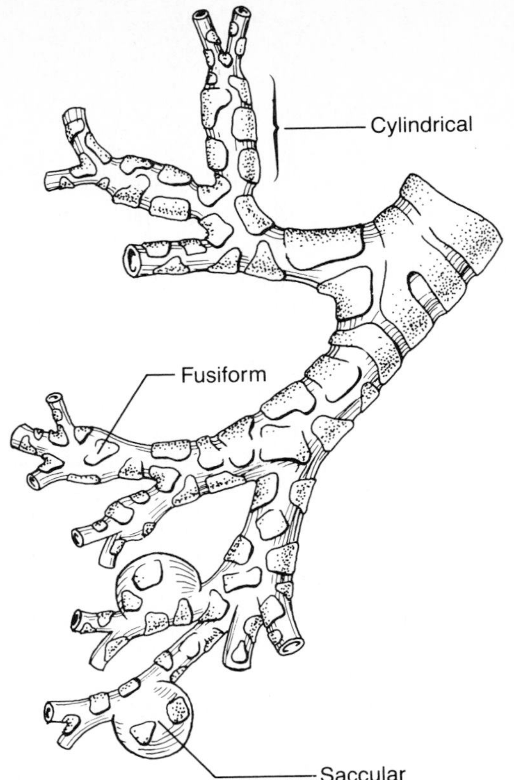

Figure 16–3

Bronchiectasis. Examples of cylindrical, fusiform, and saccular bronchi.

Auscultation of the chest usually reveals rales. Chest x-rays may show chronic inflammatory changes, at times including recognizable dilatations. Pulmonary function studies may be normal if involvement is minimal; however, in diffuse disease, findings similar to those of the other chronic obstructive pulmonary disorders are usually evident. Arterial blood gas values reveal a reduced PO_2 because of perfusion of poorly ventilated alveoli; PCO_2 is often normal. The prognosis of severe untreated bronchiectasis is generally poor, with a survival rate of 10 to 15 years. The use of antibiotics has greatly improved the outlook for this disease, however.

Medical Measures

Bronchiectasis can often be diagnosed from the history alone and sometimes by a routine chest x-ray showing dilated sacs with fluid levels. Often the chest x-ray is normal. Bronchography can confirm the disease by demonstrating the permanent bronchial dilatation. Because of the possible untoward effects of this procedure, it is recommended only for clients with known or suspected bronchiectasis who are being considered for resection of one or more lobes of the lung.

The cornerstone of treatment in bronchiectasis is daily bronchial hygiene with postural drainage, which usually has to be continued for life. Adequate hydration and humidification along with the possible use of IPPB is necessary to assist in the liquefaction of bronchial secretions. Bronchodilators are indicated when bronchospasm compounds the problem. Expectorants may be used but are of questionable value (Petersdorf, 1983).

Antibiotic therapy is used in the treatment of the infection associated with bronchiectasis. The choice of antibiotic is guided by results of sputum culture. If the sputum culture is normal, ampicillin is usually prescribed. Prolonged use of antibiotics, especially multiple antibiotics, should be avoided because it tends to eliminate the drug-susceptible organisms, allowing drug-resistant organisms to multiply (Mitchell & Petty, 1982). Treatment of accompanying sinusitus with decongestants and humidified air is also important.

For the most part, acquired bronchiectasis is considered a preventable disease. Aspirated foreign bodies should be removed immediately by bronchoscopy or surgery. Pneumonia should be appropriately treated with antibiotics to prevent complications that can lead to bronchiectasis. Surgery and resection of the lung are rarely used today as a treatment for bronchiectasis.

Specific Nursing Measures

Since bronchiectasis is a chronic condition, clients and their families need to learn how to perform deep breathing and coughing exercises as well as bronchial drainage. These measures aid in mobilizing and removing bronchial secretions, controlling problems of accumulation and stagnation and preventing pneumonia. Adequate fluid intake and humidified air will also help to liquefy secretions.

Clients must avoid exposure to infections and other situations, such as smoke or heavy smog, that could aggravate their condition. All persons living in the home should know that smoking cigarettes, cigars, or pipes will exacerbate the client's condition. Visitors to the home should be forewarned that smoking of any kind is not allowed. Obviously, the client must not smoke.

Nutritional management should be stressed, because clients with bronchiectasis are anorexic due to coughing and sputum production which leaves a foul taste in the mouth. A nutritious diet is necessary to keep resistance up, so clients are better able to ward off respiratory tract infections.

Clients will be more likely to eat a nutritious diet if they have good oral hygiene before meals and get as much rest as possible. Bronchial hygiene measures before eating may help reduce coughing and expectoration during eating. Clients and families should be aware that any exacerbation in the bronchiectasis warrants immediate attention by the physician so prompt antibiotic therapy can be started. Encourage clients to receive the influenza vaccine yearly and the pneumococcal vaccine every 3 years.

Because of the productive cough and frequent need to expectorate sputum, clients often markedly curtail their social lives, rarely eat out, and many times feel rejected by friends and family. Emotional support is important for both client and significant others as they cope with a disease that does not necessarily alter life expectancy but may interfere with the client's work, sexual relationships, and other important aspects of life.

Asthma

The American Thoracic Society defines asthma as a disease characterized by increased responsiveness of the trachea and bronchi to various stimuli, manifested by a difficulty in breathing caused by generalized narrowing of the airways. This narrowing of the airways changes in degree, either spontaneously or because of therapy. Asthma differs from the other obstructive disorders in that it is a reversible process, and individuals may be asymptomatic for extended periods. When asthma and bronchitis occur together, airway obstruction persists. The condition is then called chronic asthmatic bronchitis.

No single specific factor is recognized as the causative agent of asthma. Asthma is routinely classified according to the type of precipitating factor: extrinsic (exogenous, immunologic, or noninfectious); intrinsic (endogenous, nonallergic, nonimmunologic, or infectious); and mixed (a combination of intrinsic and extrinsic).

Extrinsic asthma develops before the age of 35 with the onset frequently in childhood. Those who develop this type of asthma often have a history of accompanying allergies, such as hay fever or eczema. Individuals with extrinsic asthma are atopic, that is, they are susceptible to hypersensitization from common environmental allergens. An inhaled, ingested, or parenterally introduced allergen results in the formation of sensitizing antibodies (immunoglobulins, particularly IgE). This type of sensitization develops rapidly in response to exposure to allergens occurring in the environment. In extrinsic atopic asthma, IgE is elevated.

Intrinsic asthma occurs in adults. In this form of asthma, no immunologic reaction or reactivity to injected antigens has been demonstrated. Asthmatic symptoms often occur with a respiratory tract infection. IgE levels are normal, and skin tests are nonreactive. This type of nonallergic asthma can be precipitated by various factors, including respiratory tract infections, exercise, cold air, tobacco smoke, polluted air, and emotionally stressful situations.

The pathophysiology behind the symptoms is primarily related to a decrease in the size of the airways because of bronchospasm, inflammation and edema of the bronchial mucosa, and an increase in mucus secretion (Figure 16–4).

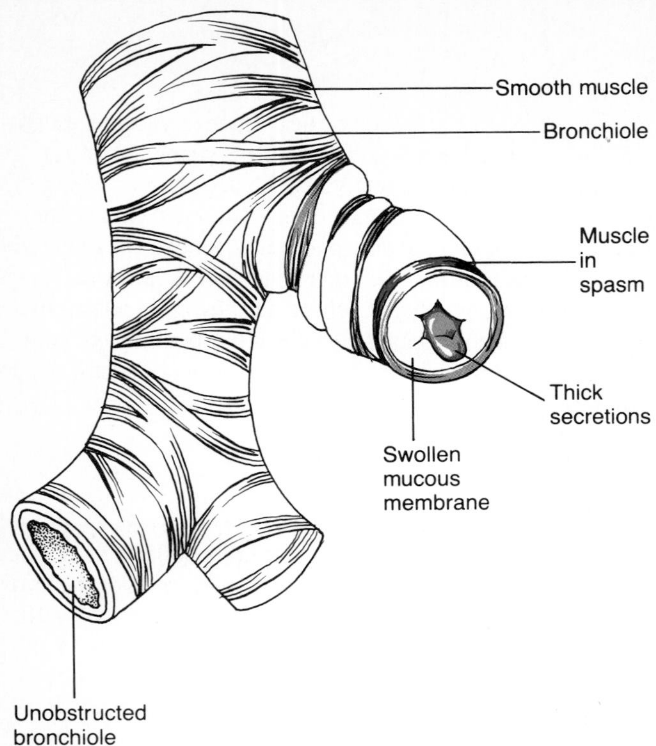

Figure 16–4

Bronchiole obstruction in asthma.

The decrease in airway size is responsible for the primary symptom of asthma—wheezing. Also, the thick, tenacious mucus produced during an asthma attack tends to adhere to the bronchial walls, further obstructing the flow of air. The primary obstruction to airflow occurs during expiration, because the airways normally narrow during this phase of breathing. This physiologic process, along with added bronchial constriction, edema, and mucus plugs, can severely impede or totally obstruct the expiratory flow of air. This can cause alveolar hyperinflation and collapse (Traver, 1982).

Clinical Manifestations

Sporadic paroxysmal attacks characterize bronchial asthma. In extrinsic asthma, symptoms are provoked by seasonal and environmental changes, and response to therapy is generally good. Intrinsic asthma is usually less responsive to pharmaceutical therapy, is more difficult to treat, and requires long-term rather than intermittent therapy (George, Light, & Matthay, 1983).

Individuals having an asthma attack experience chest tightness, shortness of breath, wheezing, difficulty getting air in and out of their lungs, and a cough. The cough is productive of thick mucoid or white tenacious mucus. Asthmatics also experience marked anxiety, profuse diaphoresis, tachycardia, and an elevated blood pressure. Accessory muscles may be used in breathing as they struggle to maintain adequate ventilation. This increased work of breathing, along with the anxiety, can cause marked fatigue.

Obstruction of the expiratory airflow is reflected in pulmonary function studies, which show an increase in residual volume, an increase in the functional residual capacity (FRC), and a decrease in the vital capacity (VC). Chest x-rays may reveal hyperinflation and atelectasis of the lungs. Rales and rhonchi may be heard throughout the lungs, along with inspiratory and expiratory wheezes.

Both the severity and the length of asthma attacks vary greatly. Treatment may bring the asthmatic attack under control rapidly, or the symptoms can become increasingly severe and prolonged. A severe and prolonged asthma attack that resists treatment is referred to as *status asthmaticus*. In this instance, more and more alveoli become either hyperinflated or collapsed; the arterial oxygen level decreases, causing hypoxemia; and the arterial carbon dioxide level rises. This rise in carbon dioxide can lead to respiratory acidosis. Unless treatment reverses the condition, the client will go into respiratory failure and die.

Medical Measures

Medications to dilate the bronchioles are used in both the prevention and treatment of asthmatic attacks. Examples include aminophylline-theophylline compounds and beta-adrenergic stimulators, which relax smooth muscle, and oral and parenteral corticosteroids, which moderate the inflammatory response. Cromolyn sodium, an inhaled medication that is not a bronchodilator but prevents the release of chemical mediators of anaphylaxis, is also used to prevent attacks.

In an acute asthma attack, the beta-adrenergic drugs (epinephrine, isoproterenol, metaproterenol, and terbutaline) and the theophyllines are used. Epinephrine may be given initially subcutaneously (0.3 to 0.5 mL of a 1:1000 solution) and repeated in 15 to 30 minutes if bronchospasm is not relieved. If the condition continues to worsen, intravenous aminophylline is started. The beta-adrenergic drugs are given either subcutaneously or by inhalation, along with aminophylline.

Status asthmaticus is refractory to the theophyllines and beta-adrenergic medications. Administration of intravenous corticosteroids is required (Mitchell & Petty, 1982).

In individuals with chronic persistent asthma or frequent attacks, continuous therapy is required. Theophylline administered orally is often accompanied by an oral or inhaled beta-adrenergic such as terbutaline and metaproterenol. If this is not effective, oral steroids such as prednisone may have to be given (Mitchell & Petty, 1982).

Sedatives or tranquilizers may be administered to calm the anxious client who is not threatened with ventilatory failure. Antibiotics may be prescribed if an infection is present. Clients whose asthma is triggered by common allergens may undergo treatment to reduce their sensitivity to the substances.

Since the client ill enough to visit the physician or emergency room is almost always suffering from hypoxemia, the administration of humidified oxygen is required and is guided by the monitoring of arterial blood gas values. The administration of fluids is also important; asthmatics are frequently dehydrated by diaphoresis, hyperventilation, and the inability to drink.

Breathing exercises along with bronchial drainage are ordered to assist in removing retained secretions. Because of the reported risk of sudden death, the use of IPPB is not advocated for acute asthma attacks (Mitchell & Petty, 1982). Aerosol therapy to loosen secretions may be ordered.

Careful monitoring of chest x-rays, arterial blood gas reports, pulmonary function studies, and sputum cultures is a necessary part of medical management, since these tests will reflect the client's response to treatment. If the client's condition worsens to the point of impending respiratory failure, the client will be intubated and placed on a mechanical ventilator.

Specific Nursing Measures

During an acute asthmatic attack, clients are frequently frightened, anxious, and exhausted because of labored breathing. It is important from the start to give clients all needed emotional support and assurance that the nurse will remain with them. Nothing is as terrifying as not being able to breathe and, even though the client and family may have been through the experience many times, each attack generates the fear of dying. To be effective, the nurse must overcome personal anxieties about acute asthmatic attacks by gaining a good understanding of asthma and its treatment.

Interact with the client and family in a calm and caring manner. Clients frequently prefer to sit up, bending forward. They can be made more comfortable if the bedside table is set so they rest their arms on it. To help allay the feeling of suffocation, clients may prefer not to be closed in (eg, by bedside curtains). A quiet environment with as few interruptions as possible should be maintained. Protect clients from drafts and chills; change wet linen from diaphoresis quickly.

Because shortness of breath interferes with ability to talk, do not tire the client further by trying to take an admission history or asking nonessential questions. Needed information can be obtained more easily from family members.

Any instructions given to asthmatics during an acute attack, such as instructions for breathing exercises, should be given slowly and repeated as necessary, since anxiety may interfere with the ability to comprehend what is being said (Traver, 1982). Clients should avoid any unnecessary exertion since they will need all their energy to breathe. As the condition warrants, activity levels can be increased, but initially, asthmatic clients require assistance in carrying out activities of daily living.

Monitor fluid intake and output; unless contraindicated, clients should receive 3000 to 4000 mL per day. The nutritional intake of asthmatics can be severely hampered if shortness of breath makes them unable to eat. Monitor their intake of food as well as fluids. High-nutrient liquid supplemental feedings are sometimes needed.

Attention to good bronchopulmonary toilet is essential. Breathing exercises along with bronchial drainage are important aspects of care. Suctioning may be required if secretions cannot be expectorated. Observe and chart the sputum expectorated for amount, consistency, and color.

Respiratory and cardiac assessment is an ongoing responsibility of the nurse, as is careful monitoring of blood gas values and pulmonary function studies. Cardiac dysrhythmias, tachycardia, tremors, nervousness, nausea, and headache are possible adverse effects from the beta-adrenergic stimulators as well as from aminophylline or theophylline. As the health professional with continuous client contact, the nurse is in the best position to synthesize the client's subjective reports and objective findings to evaluate client response to treatment.

Home Health Care

Since asthma is a chronic condition, clients, their families, and significant others require instruction in its cause, care, and treatment. If possible, help clients to identify precipitating factors in the development of their attacks and take measures to avoid them. This is especially important if specific allergens such as pollen, animal dander, or dust are involved. Other environmental irritants should be avoided, such as cigarette smoke, aerosol sprays, overly dry air, and extremes in temperatures. Since these irritants may precipitate an attack, encourage clients to seek medical care at the first sign of a respiratory tract infection, tonsillitis, or sinusitis. Clients should also avoid people with respiratory tract infections.

If emotional stress seems to be a precipitating factor, encourage the client to identify stressful factors and how they might manage stress more effectively. Stress management intervention should be aimed at identifying ways to prevent a stressor from disrupting the client's life or to lessen the degree of reaction. Stress management techniques such as relaxation training can be beneficial in assisting individuals to deal with stressful situations more positively.

Encourage asthmatics to maintain as active and as normal a life as possible, avoiding only activities that may precipitate an attack. An individualized medication program may help to control exercise-induced asthma. Sufficient rest is important, since fatigue may make it more difficult for asthmatic clients to handle daily stresses. Breathing exercises will help reduce the amount of residual volume of air in the lungs during an attack, and bronchial drainage will help to prevent the buildup of secretions.

Clients must be aware of the nature, proper administration, and side effects of the medications they are taking. Clients need to understand why they should not discontinue, start, or increase medication without consulting with the physician or care provider. For example, abrupt discontinuation of corticosteroids such as prednisone is likely to cause a serious "steroid rebound" effect (withdrawal syndrome). Propranolol (Inderal) should not be given to clients with asthma because of its potential to cause bronchoconstriction. Antihistamines and decongestants should be avoided because of their tendency to dry airway secretions, making expectoration difficult.

Chronic Bronchitis

The American Thoracic Society defines chronic bronchitis as a clinical disorder characterized by excessive mucus secretion in the bronchi, manifested by chronic or recurrent productive cough. The cough is present for a minimum of 3 months per year for at least 2 successive years, and other causes of productive cough, such as specific pulmonary infections, have been excluded.

There is conclusive evidence that cigarette smoking is the most consistently important factor in the development of chronic bronchitis. Atmospheric pollution from industry and automotive pollutants, such as sulfur oxides, nitrogen oxides, carbon monoxide, and many hydrocarbons, also irritates the respiratory structures, causing nonspecific inflammatory reactions in the lungs. Air pollution raises both the morbidity and mortality of chronic bronchitis sufferers. Occupational pollutants are also important predisposing factors in this disease. Some high-risk occupations are sandstone workers, copper miners, cotton strippers, and grinders.

Respiratory tract infections are associated with chronic bronchitis because recurrent infections damage the structures of the respiratory system. Conversely, the increased secretions of chronic bronchitis make individuals more susceptible to recurrent respiratory tract infections.

Nursing Research Note

Kneeshaw MF: Smoking cessation in nurses: A report on a self-selected population at the Presbyterian Hospital in New York City. *Occup Health Nurs* 1985; 33:338–342.

The number of nurses who smoke is greater than the average in the female population and greater than the number of physicians smoking. Cigarette breaks at this hospital were considered a good reason for a rest period, contributing to increased tobacco use among nurses.

A survey of nursing employees assessed the prevalence of smoking among nurses and determined the number of nurses who would be interested in a program that encouraged smoking cessation. Of the 32 nurses who stated they would be interested in a cessation program, only 3 actually attended.

As health care professionals, nurses should be role models for the general population and encourage cessation of tobacco use. Lung cancer has markedly increased in women. More research should be conducted to find ways to assist nurses with smoking cessation.

Genetic factors are believed to play a part in the development of the chronic obstructive pulmonary diseases, including chronic bronchitis. Relatives of bronchitic subjects have a higher prevalence of bronchitis than do relatives of controls. Chronic bronchitis is more common in men than women, occurs more frequently in whites than nonwhites, and is more common in city dwellers than those who live in the country.

The peripheral conducting airways are the primary site of pathologic changes. The chronic inflammatory response stimulates the bronchial mucous glands, causing hypertrophy and hyperplasia. This is accompanied by chronic inflammatory cell infiltration and edema of the bronchial mucosa. These factors combine with the hypersecretion of mucus to cause a narrowing of the bronchial airways, with increasing resistance to airflow. The narrowing increases the effort needed for breathing.

Cilia activity is either diminished or destroyed by the inflammation, which results in retained secretions. This mucus becomes an excellent medium for the growth of bacteria, subjecting individuals to recurrent respiratory tract infections, which in turn contribute to an increase in inflammation and mucus production (Traver, 1982). The inflammatory responses and retained secretions do not occur uniformly throughout the lungs, which results in ventilation–perfusion mismatching. Repeated infections along with inflammation and persistent obstruction can lead to necrotizing, scarring, and sometimes destruction of the small bronchioles.

Clinical Manifestations

In simple chronic bronchitis, the client experiences only a cough with intermittent wheezing. In the more severe forms, there are constant wheezing, sputum production, dyspnea, and episodes of acute respiratory failure. The changes in the airways usually occur gradually, over 25 to 40 years.

Individuals with chronic bronchitis tend to be overweight and dusky. The disease usually affects individuals between 40 and 55 years of age and has a gradual onset. The first symptom is an early morning cough, frequently described as a "cigarette cough." As the condition progresses, the cough, which is productive of copious secretions, becomes continual. The client experiences acute exacerbations from respiratory tract infections. Dyspnea becomes more and more severe, and the client becomes more inactive and debilitated. Table 16–4 compares characteristics of clients with predominant chronic bronchitis to those with predominant emphysema.

Those with chronic bronchitis are frequently referred to as "blue bloaters" because of their bloated, cyanotic appearance. The cyanosis is from the hypoxemia of chronic bronchitis, which is caused by alveolar hypoventilation. Why individuals with chronic bronchitis tend to hypoventilate is

Table 16–4
Characteristics of Clients With Predominant Chronic Bronchitis or Predominant Emphysema

Characteristic	Predominant Bronchitis	Predominant Emphysema
History	Recurrent pulmonary infections	Insidious dyspnea
Smoking history	Usual	Usual
General appearance	"Blue bloater," cyanotic	"Pink puffer," pursed lip breathing, use of accessory muscles
Weight loss	Absent or slight	Often marked
Dyspnea	Moderate	Severe, often disabling
Cough	Before onset of dyspnea	After onset of dyspnea
Sputum	Copious, purulent	Scanty, mucoid
Chest x-ray	Normal diaphragm position; cardiomegaly; increased bronchovascular markings at bases	Bilateral low, flat diaphragm; long, narrow cardiac silhouette; bullae; absence of bronchovascular markings in lung periphery
Cor pulmonale	Common	Uncommon, except terminally

not clearly understood, but it appears to be a type of compensatory mechanism (Wade, 1982). The hypoventilation results not only in a low arterial oxygen level (hypoxemia) but also in an elevation of carbon dioxide (hypercapnia). The combination of hypoxemia, hypercapnia, and possible respiratory acidosis can lead to vasoconstriction, resulting in increased vascular resistance. This causes an increase in pulmonary artery pressure and an increase in the work required by the right ventricle of the heart. This, in turn, can lead to right-sided heart failure, or cor pulmonale. Compensatory polycythemia may occur as a result of the chronic hypoxemia. Clubbing of the fingers because of the development of secondary polycythemia may also be present (Figure 16–5).

Medical and Specific Nursing Measures

The medical management of chronic bronchitis and specific nursing measures in the care of clients with chronic bronchitis are covered under pulmonary emphysema because they are so closely related.

Pulmonary Emphysema

Pulmonary emphysema is a chronically progressive pulmonary disease in which there is an enlargement of the air spaces distal to the terminal nonrespiratory bronchioles with destruction of the alveolar walls. Emphysema has been estimated to be three times more prevalent in men than in women. Although chronic bronchitis and emphysema can occur separately, they frequently coexist.

The etiology of emphysema is essentially unknown. The predisposing factors discussed under chronic bronchitis are applicable to emphysema. Cigarette smoking is again the major culprit.

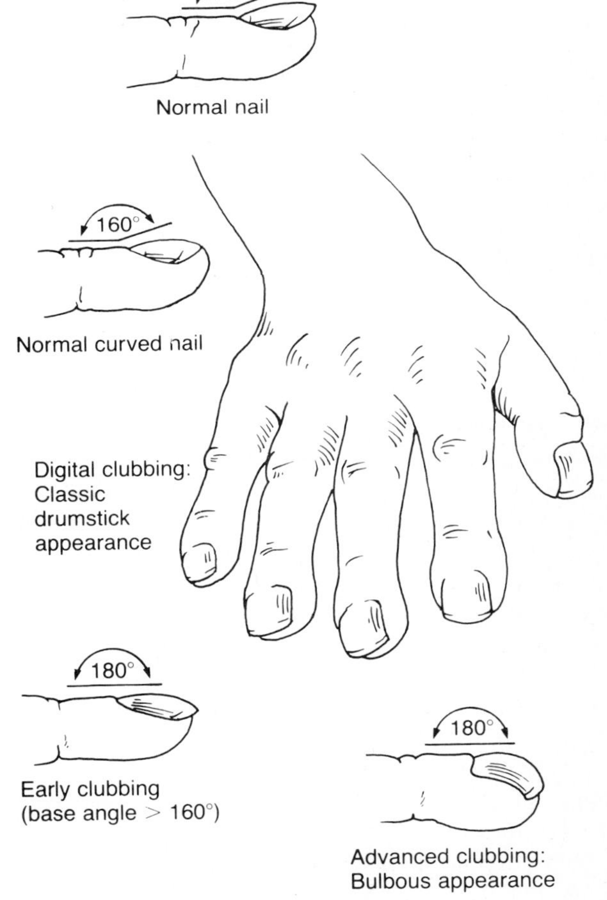

Figure 16–5

Clubbing of the fingers in chronic bronchitis.

Theories attempt to explain why certain people are more likely to develop emphysema. Research has shown an apparent failure of the connective tissue of the lungs to protect against protein digestion from enzymes released from the alveolar macrophages and leukocytes (Mitchell & Petty, 1982). Human serum, lung tissue, peripheral airways, and bronchial mucus have been shown to contain inhibitors of these enzymes. It is postulated that tissue damage to the lungs occurs when there is not enough of these enzyme inhibitors to control the enzymes released from the macrophages and the leukocytes.

The development of emphysema is insidious and progressive. The obstruction in emphysema typically begins in the small, peripheral bronchioles, due to inflammation, infection, retained secretions, and edema. The narrowing of the airways traps air in the alveoli. As the disease progresses, alveolar walls become disrupted by hyperinflation, and some alveolar tissue septa are destroyed. The alveolar walls degenerate into a lacy pattern made up of thin strands of collagen fibers. There is an accompanying destruction of the pulmonary capillaries of the involved alveoli and the development of air spaces. Because of the loss of elasticity of the lung tissue, the minute respiratory and terminal bronchioles tend to collapse prematurely during exhalation. This causes increased airway resistance and a slowing of expiratory airflow, making exhalation of air from the lungs more difficult. Ventilation–perfusion abnormalities occur, since the alveolar and vascular changes are not uniform throughout the lungs. Some alveoli will be ventilated and not perfused, and others will be perfused but underventilated.

Clinical Manifestations

Because emphysema has an insidious onset, symptoms may not appear until 20% to 30% of the lung tissue is destroyed unless an individual is active (Wade, 1982). Dyspnea on exertion is the first recognized symptom. As the disease progresses, the client must work harder and harder at breathing, especially exhalation. Individuals will often exhale through pursed lips to prolong expiration and reduce the tendency of airways to collapse, thus removing more air from the lungs. Clients use all their accessory muscles to breathe and usually sit with their hands firmly supported. The anterior–posterior diameter of the chest increases due to expansion of the chest wall and loss of lung elasticity, giving the chest a barrel-shaped appearance. Anorexia and weight loss are common, causing an emaciated appearance and concomitant muscle wasting (Figure 16–6). Cough and sputum production are not common, unless the client develops a respiratory tract infection—a frequent occurrence during the winter months.

Auscultation of the chest may reveal rhonchi, prolonged expiration, and diminished breath sounds. Hyperresonance is noted on percussion. Tactile and auditory fremitus is reduced. Chest x-ray may show a low, flattened diaphragm and hyperaeration of the lungs (Figure 16–7). Bullae—bubblelike structures containing air that project from the lung surface—can occur from progressive trapping of air and may be seen on chest x-ray. The cardiac silhouette is often lengthened and narrowed, although hypertrophy of the right ventricle can occur if cor pulmonale is developing (Mitchell & Petty, 1982). Pulmonary function tests usually show decrease in vital capacity and an increased resistance to expiratory airflow, with a decrease in forced expiratory volume and in maximal voluntary ventilation.

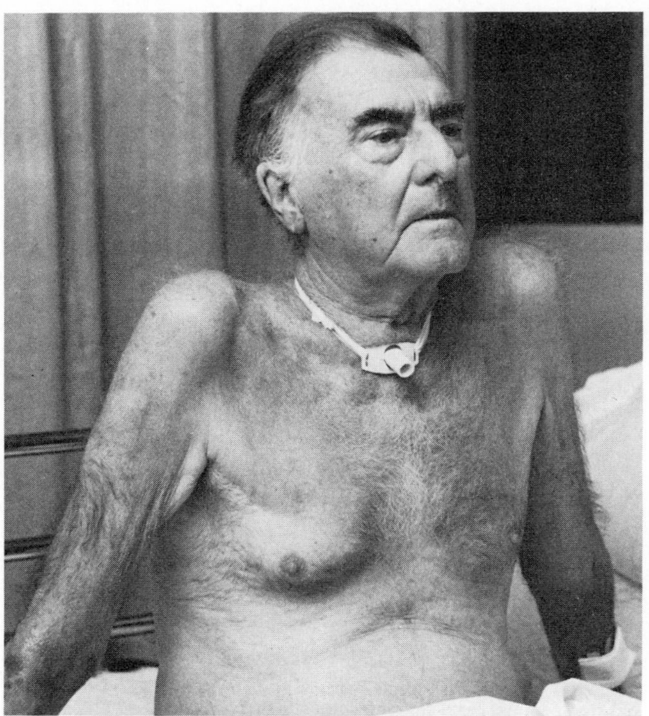

Figure 16–6

Typical appearance of a client with advanced pulmonary emphysema. *Photograph by Carol Payne-Zagon.*

Arterial blood gas values may show normal or slightly reduced arterial oxygen at rest. Even in the presence of severe disease, clients can maintain relatively normal blood gas levels. This happens because alveolar destruction is accompanied by pulmonary capillary destruction and, although this is not always uniform, the ventilation-to-perfusion ratio is close enough to maintain relatively normal blood gas values. In contrast, those with chronic bronchitis have a ventilation–perfusion mismatch that is more abnormal.

Those with COPD, especially emphysema, may show elevated arterial carbon dioxide levels. If elevation has developed gradually, the kidneys will have attempted to compensate for rising CO_2 levels by conserving bicarbonate, maintaining a normal pH. Therefore, clients whose

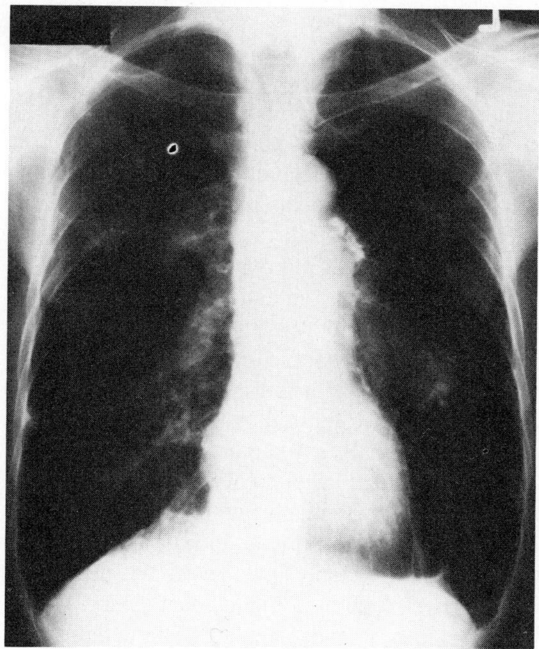

Figure 16–7

Chest x-ray of a male client with advanced pulmonary emphysema. Note the bilateral lowering and flattening of the diaphragm, the lengthened and narrowed cardiac silhouette, and the absence of bronchovascular patterns in the lung periphery. *Courtesy of Health Care Plan, Buffalo, NY.*

arterial blood gas values show an elevated CO_2 and a normal pH are considered to have compensated for respiratory acidosis.

The hematocrit is frequently elevated because of the development of polycythemia, giving clients a "pink puffer" appearance. With progression or exacerbation of the disease because of a superimposed respiratory tract infection, alveolar ventilation may be inadequate to maintain normal blood gas values. A low oxygen and an elevated carbon dioxide level with a low pH indicate respiratory acidosis that may lead to respiratory failure.

As with chronic bronchitis, finger clubbing may occur. Distended neck veins may be present along with cor pulmonale because of the loss of pulmonary vasculature, with a resulting increase in pulmonary vascular resistance.

Clients with emphysema can become totally disabled, unable to do anything for themselves except fight for every breath of air. They are frequently drained emotionally by anxiety, fear, and depression over their disease state.

Medical Measures

Since bronchitis and emphysema are chronic conditions that will last a lifetime, treatment centers around controlling the symptoms, retarding further deterioration of function, rehabilitation, and client education. Bronchodilators are used in the treatment of reversible bronchospasm, if present. Pulmonary function studies may be done before and after the administration of the medication to see if the medication has any effect on reducing the bronchospasm. Frequently used bronchodilators include theophylline and epinephrine or terbutaline.

Antibiotics are used to treat bacterial infections. They are given at the first sign of an upper or lower respiratory infection to prevent an exacerbation of chronic bronchitis that could lead to acute respiratory failure. Broad-spectrum antibiotics such as tetracycline or erythromycin are commonly prescribed.

Digitalis and diuretics are used in the treatment of right-sided heart failure. Digoxin is the most commonly used digitalis preparation, and the thiazide diuretics are most often used to treat the edema. Clients should be carefully monitored for hypokalemia and hypoxemia.

Yearly influenza vaccine is recommended for individuals with COPD to prevent added respiratory problems. The pneumonia vaccine should be given every 3 to 4 years, and the new antiviral agent amantadine, which affords protection against many A-strain viruses, is recommended for prophylaxis during epidemics (Mitchell & Petty, 1982).

Phlebotomy may be performed for clients experiencing symptoms of headache or mental clouding from very high hematocrits (over 60). The hematocrit is elevated because of the increased production of red blood cells (polycythemia), which is an adaptive response to hypoxemia.

In the treatment of chronic bronchitis and emphysema, surgery is limited to treatment of a spontaneous pneumothorax caused by rupture of an emphysematous bleb, which requires the insertion of chest tubes.

Specific Nursing Measures

The nurse must work with health team members in the care of clients with COPD. Frequently, physical and respiratory therapists are involved in client rehabilitation.

Clients with chronic lung conditions frequently feel angry, depressed, and anxious over their condition. It is important to know this, acknowledge their feelings, and answer their questions honestly. It is even more important that clients learn which aspects of their condition are reversible, such as accumulation of secretions and bronchospasm, and which are not. The potential for reversibility is greatest in treating chronic bronchitis and least in treating emphysema. Clients should understand that if they conscientiously carry out the treatment plan, they can expect improvement. By understanding their condition and how to manage their symptoms, they will be better able to cope with chronic respiratory disease.

Since infection is a threat, clients should be instructed to avoid persons who have colds or other respiratory tract infections. At the first sign of a cold, or of any change in the color, amount, or consistency of sputum, they should notify the physician. Sometimes clients have antibiotics on hand, which the physician has instructed them to take at the first sign of a cold. Stress that if the antibiotics do not begin to relieve the symptoms within 24 to 48 hours, clients should consult the physician.

Avoiding exposure to irritants is also important. Encourage clients who are still smoking to stop. It may help if clients understand that stopping smoking will result in some improvement of symptoms and will markedly retard further deterioration. Direct smokers to a smoking cessation clinic, to the American Lung Association, or the American Cancer Society for help on how to stop smoking. Nicorette gum, available by prescription, has been effective in aiding some smokers to give up their smoking habit.

Home Health Care

If clients are exposed to irritants on the job and there is no way of avoiding exposure, they may need to change jobs to avoid becoming completely disabled. Having to change jobs or stop working can be upsetting and result in financial problems. Nurses need to be aware of these feelings and help clients and their families work through them. Social workers can offer useful advice on how to manage finances.

Air pollution can aggravate respiratory disorders; clients should avoid high pollution levels by staying indoors. Daily pollution levels are often reported on television, especially when levels are high. Dusts, powders, and aerosol sprays may be a source of irritation and should be avoided or kept to a minimum. Home air conditioning may be helpful to decrease pollutants and maintain temperature control.

Bronchial hygiene is an important aspect of client instruction. Topics should include how to cough effectively, do breathing exercises, and aid bronchial drainage. To facilitate the expectoration of secretions and reduce bronchospasm, an IPPB machine may be ordered for use at home. Medications such as isoetharine (Bronkosol) and saline can be added to the nebulizer of the machine to loosen secretions and reduce bronchospasm. Steam inhalation may also loosen secretions. The nurse may have to teach clients and families how to procure and use the equipment.

Continuous home oxygen therapy may be required if the client's arterial oxygen level is low. Reservoir tanks can be placed in the home, and portable oxygen units can be filled from the reservoir. Because those with chronic bronchitis and emphysema may have a hypoxic drive to breathe, continuous low flow oxygen therapy must be carefully monitored with regular arterial blood gas levels. Clients and their families must know why it is essential to use only the flow of oxygen ordered by the physician and not to increase the flow. As with the IPPB machines, clients may require assistance in how to procure, use, and pay for oxygen equipment.

Review the most frequent symptoms of hypoxia and hypercapnia with the client and family since these symptoms may signify impending respiratory failure. Symptoms include increased shortness of breath, restlessness, lethargy, headache, and confusion.

Teach clients to weigh themselves daily, because a weight gain of 2½ kg (5½ lb) could indicate fluid retention from right-sided heart failure. Hydration is an important aspect of care because water helps to liquefy secretions in the lung. Unless contraindicated, instruct clients to drink 8 to 10 glasses of fluid a day. Coffee and tea have a diuretic effect and should not be counted as fluid intake.

Nutrition is another important aspect of care. High-calorie meals are necessary for clients with emphysema who are underweight and undernourished. Small, frequent meals may be more easily tolerated by those who are short of breath; eating large meals may require more energy than the client can afford. Also, large meals can interfere with the downward descent of the diaphragm during inspiration, adding to the breathing difficulty. (Gas-forming foods should be avoided for the same reason.) Salt-restricted diets may be necessary for those with right-sided heart failure. Foods high in potassium are important for clients taking diuretics.

The positive effects of physical reconditioning exercises have been well established in the literature. Those with chronic bronchitis and emphysema frequently fear exercise because of the dyspnea that may result. Exercise training and instruction are usually begun in the hospital and continued at home. Once breathing exercises are mastered, the client's tolerance to exercise is gradually increased by walking on a treadmill and/or riding a stationary bicycle. Stair climbing is also included. Clients continue to increase exercise until they reach their tolerance level. Blood gases, pulmonary function tests, and cardiac status are monitored.

Since walking and controlled breathing are the main components of the program, encourage clients to carry out these activities daily at home. If the weather is cold and rainy, clients can do their walking in a shopping mall. Pulmonary rehabilitation programs have helped clients return to more active and productive lives.

Acute Respiratory Failure

Acute respiratory failure is the sudden inability of the respiratory system and the heart to maintain adequate arterial oxygenation and adequate carbon dioxide elimination. The arterial blood gas level arbitrarily used to define acute respiratory failure is an arterial oxygen tension of less than 55 mm Hg, with or without carbon dioxide retention. An acute elevation of carbon dioxide to more than 50 mm Hg is referred to as acute ventilatory failure. Acute ventilatory failure can result in acute respiratory failure if the level of ventilation decreases enough that hypoxemia occurs. Acute respiratory failure is encountered frequently; it can be caused by a variety of conditions.

Arterial oxygen and carbon dioxide levels are maintained by the normal dynamics of ventilation, diffusion, and circulation. Should problems arise that alter any of these mechanisms, gas exchange can be impaired, resulting in respiratory failure. Of the diseases of the lungs, the chronic obstructive pulmonary diseases such as emphysema and chronic bronchitis are the most frequent causes of respiratory failure (Mitchell & Petty, 1982). Disturbances of the chest wall, such as kyphoscoliosis or neuromuscular diseases such as Guillain-Barré syndrome, can impair ventilation, leading to respiratory failure. Overdoses of certain drugs, such as narcotics, barbiturates, and tranquilizers, can depress or damage the respiratory center. Cerebral infarction or brain trauma can suppress the respiratory drive leading to respiratory failure (Mitchell & Petty, 1982).

Clinical Manifestations

The symptoms and signs of acute respiratory failure combine those of the underlying disease with the signs of hypoxemia, hypercapnia, or both. The onset of respiratory failure may be gradual and subtle, or it may be dramatic.

Clinical manifestations of hypoxemia affect the nervous system first because the brain is the organ most sensitive to oxygen deprivation. Neurologic symptoms include headache, mental confusion, anxiety and agitation, restlessness, impaired judgment, euphoria or depression, double vision, weakness, drowsiness, and coma. Effects on the cardiovascular system include tachycardia, hypertension, and dysrhythmias. Respiratory effects include tachypnea and dyspnea. But the hemoglobin saturation must be as low as 78% before cyanosis becomes apparent (Wade, 1982).

The marked increases in carbon dioxide levels depress the central nervous system, leading to symptoms of drowsiness or lethargy, inability to concentrate, headache, dizziness, muscle twitching, a gradual loss of consciousness, and coma. A rise in arterial carbon dioxide will decrease arterial oxygen because of hypoventilation. If the carbon dioxide level increases rapidly, the kidney will not have enough time to compensate by conserving bicarbonate, and respiratory acidosis will result. The four most common signs of acute respiratory failure are restlessness, headache, confusion, and tachycardia (Mitchell & Petty, 1982).

Medical Measures

Bronchodilators may be used to decrease edema of the airways and bronchospasm. Aminophylline may be administered as a bolus followed by intravenous drip. Corticosteroids may be administered to reduce bronchial inflammation and bronchospasm. Antibiotics may be necessary if an underlying infection is present. Cardiac drugs are given if cardiac failure or dysrhythmias occur. Sodium bicarbonate is administered in respiratory acidosis.

Acute respiratory failure is a medical emergency. It may require such life-saving measures as intubation and a mechanical ventilator. When the client's breathing is not as severely compromised as in COPD, respiratory failure can be treated by more conservative measures. These clients may be treated judiciously with the medications mentioned previously, closely monitored oxygen therapy, and chest physiotherapy.

Whether endotracheal intubation and mechanical ventilation will be required depends on the clinical evaluation of the client and on arterial blood gas abnormalities. If the client's arterial oxygen level cannot be maintained at 60 to 70 mm Hg, or if the rise in arterial carbon dioxide level results in respiratory acidosis, intubation and mechanical ventilation are required. Three general indications for endotracheal intubation and mechanical ventilation are unconsciousness, copious secretions that cannot be cleared by coughing, and severe hypoxemia or respiratory acidosis that does not respond promptly to lesser measures (Mitchell & Petty, 1982). Along with maintaining adequate ventilation, the underlying cause of the acute respiratory failure must be identified and treated.

Specific Nursing Measures

If the conservative approach to management is used in the treatment of respiratory failure, monitor the client carefully for symptoms and signs of hypoxia and hypercapnia. The COPD client who is difficult to arouse from sleep or is irritable may be exhibiting the symptoms of hypercapnia (Wade, 1982). Close monitoring of arterial blood gas values can also indicate any deterioration in the client's condition.

Besides monitoring the respiratory status, assess the client's cardiac status. Hypoxia, hypercapnia, and acidosis can lead to cardiac dysrhythmias and depressed myocardial contractility. Serum electrolyte values also require close monitoring.

Be alert to the possibility of carbon dioxide narcosis, especially in those with COPD. CO_2 narcosis occurs when the level of carbon dioxide in the arterial blood becomes so high that it no longer is a stimulus to breathe. The stimulus to breathe then comes from low arterial levels of oxygen. Oxygen should be administered continuously, since any interruption in the flow can result in a drastic drop in the arterial oxygen level. On the other hand, administering a high flow of oxygen raises the arterial oxygen levels, so the client no longer has any hypoxemic stimulus to breathe. Respiratory arrest can occur.

Some clients may find it difficult to keep an oxygen mask on or may be aggravated by a nasal cannula. They may find the oxygen irritating to the mucous membranes of the nose or mouth, experience a feeling of suffocation, or simply be confused. It is important to use the proper comfort measures when these oxygen delivery devices are used. Explaining to the client why the mask or cannula must be worn may help elicit more cooperation.

Provide bronchial hygiene instruction. If clients cannot raise secretions effectively, tracheobronchial suctioning may be necessary. Psychologic support for both clients and their families is important. Clients with acute respiratory failure are very ill, and many of the life-saving measures used in their treatment are frightening.

SECTION IV

Neoplastic Disorders

Bronchogenic Carcinoma

Lung cancer is the leading cause of cancer death in men and women. The average age at onset is around 60 years. The incidence of lung cancer has increased in women because of increased smoking rates in women. Among cancers, the survival rate for lung cancer is one of the poorest because this disease is seldom detected early and tends to metastasize quickly. More than 90% of lung cancers belong to the group called bronchogenic carcinoma, meaning that the cancer originates in the bronchi or bronchioles.

Since lung cancer is among the most preventable of all diseases, nurses can do much to alert the public to avoid the primary cause of lung cancer, which is cigarette smoking. Occupational factors, such as exposure to coal tars and asbestos; mining of radioactive ores; and exposure to arsenic, nickel, iron-oxide, or chromium, have also been documented as contributing to the development of lung cancer (Greco & Hande, 1982). Since everyone exposed to respiratory carcinogens does not develop lung cancer, certain host factors are believed to play a part in susceptibility. Lung cancer is more common in scarred and chronically diseased lungs.

Clinical Manifestations

Lung cancers are usually far along in their development before physical manifestations appear. The tumors have usually been present for a long time and may have metastasized. In general, symptoms and signs depend on the location and size of the primary tumor and whether metastasis is present (Greco & Hande, 1982). Localized symptoms of bronchogenic carcinoma can include cough or a change in a smoker's cough, dyspnea, hemoptysis, stridor or wheeze, and signs of obstructive pneumonitis. Figure 16–8 shows a chest x-ray of a male client with bronchogenic carcinoma of the right middle lobe.

The effects of spread to adjacent thoracic structures may cause the client's initial symptoms. Clients may experience pain in the chest where the tumor impinges on nerves or where it is invading the chest wall or mediastinum. Left vocal-cord paralysis can result from involvement of the left recurrent laryngeal nerve. The spread of the tumor to the outside surface of the lung may cause accumulation of fluid, resulting in a pleural effusion (Figure 16–9), which can cause chest pain and difficulty in breathing. Invasion of the mediastinum may cause obstruction of the superior vena cava or the esophagus. Pericardial effusion with tamponade may also result from invasion of the cancer to the mediastinum or chest wall. Sometimes the initial symptoms are associated with organs that are the primary sites of metastasis: the liver, brain, bones, kidneys, and adrenals.

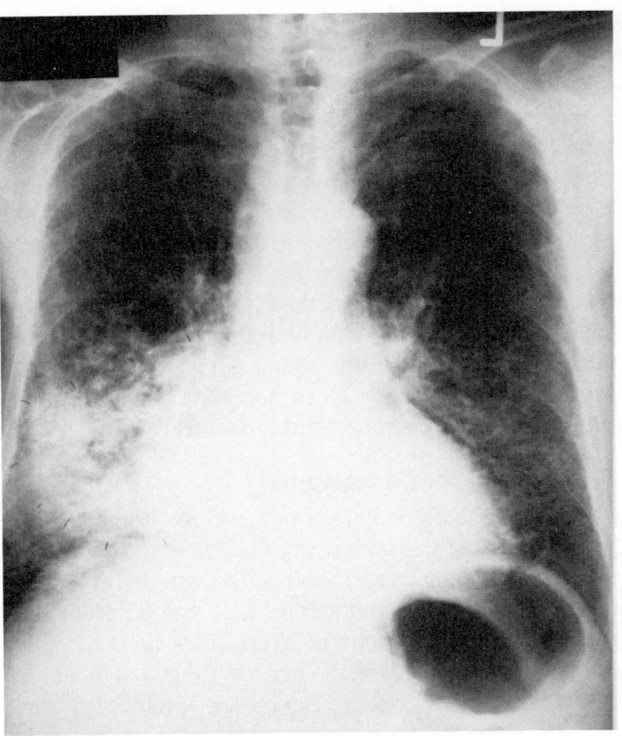

Figure 16–8

Chest x-ray of a male client with bronchogenic carcinoma of the right middle lobe. A normal gastric air bubble is evident on the client's lower left. *Courtesy of Health Care Plan, Buffalo, NY.*

Medical Measures

A careful history and physical examination are important in establishing the diagnosis of lung cancer. The history and physical are followed by a chest x-ray. When necessary, fluoroscopy, tomography, bronchoscopy, and angiography may be required to further define the nature and extent of involvement. The diagnosis of lung cancer requires histologic confirmation. Bronchoscopy may be carried out to locate the tumor, to obtain bronchial washings for sputum examination, or to take a biopsy specimen. Sputum cytology studies are done to test for the presence of cancer cells and identify the type. Bronchial brush biop-

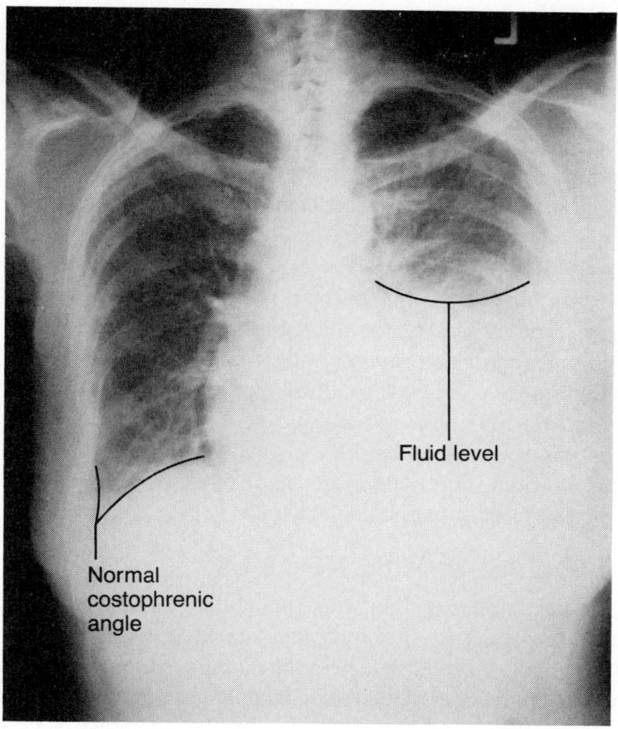

Figure 16–9

Chest x-ray of a female client with a left pleural effusion. Note the normal costophrenic angle (angle between the diaphragm and rib cage) on the right and the obliteration of the angle on the left. Also note the upward concavity of the fluid (effusion) level on the left. *Courtesy of Health Care Plan, Buffalo, NY.*

sies, percutaneous needle biopsies, scalene lymph node biopsy, and mediastinoscopy may be carried out to diagnose or rule out metastasis. Bone marrow biopsy may also be performed to check for metastasis. An exploratory thoracotomy may be performed as a diagnostic test when the previous measures have failed to locate a suspected tumor or show the extent of a known one. Usually sputum cytology, bronchoscopy, mediastinoscopy, and percutaneous biopsy are effective in the histologic confirmation of lung cancer. Complete blood counts and routine blood chemistries should also be performed (Greco & Hande, 1982).

The treatment of lung cancer depends on the cell type, the stage of the cancer, and the client's general condition. Basically, lung cancer can be treated in three ways: surgery, radiation therapy, and chemotherapy. One or a combination of these methods may be used.

Surgery is used primarily to treat individuals for whom all diagnostic evidence suggests that the entire tumor can be removed surgically. The presence of distant or extrathoracic metastasis is a contraindication for surgery. Palliative resections are not advocated since symptoms can usually be alleviated by other treatment. A thoracentesis may be performed to relieve pain or shortness of breath caused by a collection of fluid in the pleural space due to metastasis of the tumor.

Many clients receive radiotherapy at some time during their illness. It may be used as definitive treatment for localized intrathoracic lung cancers, in combination with chemotherapy, postoperatively in combination with surgery, or as a palliative treatment.

Chemotherapy is frequently used in treating lung cancer either because metastasis is present on diagnosis or because it is expected. (Metastasis occurs in 90% of clients with lung cancer.) The small-cell cancers have been shown to be the most responsive to chemotherapy, and partial and complete remissions have been reported. The chemotherapeutic regimen usually involves administration of cyclophosphamide, methotrexate, vincristine, doxorubicin, and procarbazine in varying three or four drug combinations concurrently (Petersdorf, 1983).

Specific Nursing Measures

Clients and their families may react in many ways to the diagnosis of lung cancer. There may be feelings of shock and disbelief, anger, depression, and anxiety. The nurse can assist clients and their significant others to work out their feelings, giving support and guidance as needed. Clients and their families need to be educated about lung cancer. They need to understand the various diagnostic procedures and therapeutic interventions. The side effects associated with radiation and chemotherapy need to be explained.

Many of these clients will not survive. Clients need to know the reality of their situation so they can organize their affairs and plan for the time they have remaining. Nurses often need to encourage physicians to be honest and direct with clients and families about the prognosis, because false hope may prevent them from coping realistically with the situation. There is a fine line between hope and realism; health care professionals do not want to destroy the client's desire to live or motivation to fight.

Pain is a great concern of both clients and families. Whether the client is hospitalized or cared for in the home, pain management approaches need to be planned so clients are comfortable but not overly sedated when they prefer to be alert. At other times, heavy sedation will be a great relief. The nurse may have to take the initiative in developing the pain management approaches, based on observations of the client.

Good nutrition is important to help clients maintain their strength and prevent tissue breakdown. Adequate vitamins, minerals, protein, and calories are necessary, even though clients undergoing treatment often do not feel like eating. Families can help clients by learning new food selection and preparation ideas.

Medications may need to be ordered to relieve nausea. Good oral hygiene can help to improve the taste of food.

Small and more frequent feedings are more readily tolerated. Supplemental vitamins and feedings may be necessary if the client's food intake is poor.

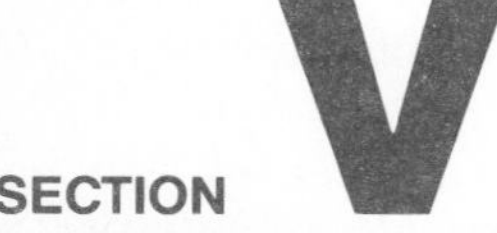

SECTION V

Traumatic Disorders

Chest trauma is an injury resulting from penetrating or blunt trauma to the chest. Penetrating chest injuries, also referred to as "open chest" trauma, result from penetration through the chest wall. Open chest trauma is caused by gunshot wounds, stab wounds, and wounds from other penetrating objects. Blunt chest trauma—nonpenetrating injury to the chest—is primarily caused by traffic accidents. Other causes include falls, blasts, explosions, and airplane crashes. Blunt chest trauma is by far the most common type of injury to the chest. Chest injuries may involve the bony framework of the chest, the heart, the great vessels, the lungs, or a combination of these. Damage to the liver and spleen are frequently associated with chest trauma. Chest injuries are particularly hazardous because damage to the many vital structures contained in this area can be life threatening.

If the client has a penetrating chest wound and the instrument (eg, knife) is still in place, it should not be removed. In most situations, the instrument serves as a mechanical tampon for the lacerated vessels, and removing the instrument may result in hemorrhage.

Rib or Sternal Fractures

Fractured ribs may pose few or many problems, depending on how many ribs are affected and whether there has been damage to the underlying tissue. A fractured sternum is usually not considered hazardous but, because of the amount of bone marrow in the sternum, there is some danger that the client may develop a fat embolism (Burrell & Burrell, 1982). Fractured ribs puncturing the wall of the trachea or bronchi, the aorta or other major blood vessels, or the heart can be a life-threatening emergency.

Fractured ribs and sternum are almost always caused by blunt chest injuries. Because the first and second ribs are relatively well protected, fractures of these ribs are usually associated with severe crushing injuries (Traver, 1982). Fractures of the fourth through eighth ribs are the most common.

Clinical Manifestations

With simple uncomplicated rib fractures, there may be pain, tenderness at the site, and splinting of the chest on the affected side. Splinting of the chest because of pain can result in shallow breathing, leading to atelectasis, retained secretions, and pneumonia. In clients who minimize breathing, low ventilation-to-perfusion ratios can occur, leading to hypoxemia and hypercapnia as well. Fractured ribs may also lead to secondary complications such as pneumothorax and hemothorax. In later years clients may experience arthritic pain in the region of an old rib fracture.

Medical Measures

Fractured ribs and sternum are diagnosed by a chest x-ray. Treatment of uncomplicated rib and sternal fractures primarily centers around the relief of pain. Analgesics such as aspirin or codeine are administered. In severe cases, intercostal nerve blocks may be required. Taping of the chest or the use of binders is no longer recommended because these methods limit chest excursion, leading to atelectasis and pneumonia (Traver, 1982).

Specific Nursing Measures

Explain to the client the importance of coughing and deep breathing to prevent atelectasis and pneumonia. Splinting of the chest will help the client breathe and cough more effectively with less pain. Monitor the administration of analgesics and watch for side effects, particularly respiratory depression. Also be alert for the possible complications of rib and sternal fractures.

Flail Chest

A flail chest occurs when multiple adjacent rib fractures and/or costosternal separations result in "floating" of a segment of the rib cage. Flail chest is the result of blunt trauma in which there is a crushing injury to the chest. The flail segment may occur anteriorly, laterally, or posteriorly. Posterior injuries occur less frequently because of the musculature and the protection afforded by the scapula (Traver, 1982).

Clinical Manifestations

A primary symptom of flail chest is the paradoxical motion of the chest wall during inspiration and expiration (Figure 16–10). The flail segment is pulled into the chest on inspiration because of the effect of the negative pleural pressure on the unstable segment. As the person exhales, the pleural pressure becomes more positive, and the flail segment moves outward. This can impair ventilation and lead to hypoxia, hypercapnia, and respiratory failure. A sternal flail, in which the sternum itself becomes free floating, can result in myocardial injury leading to heart failure. The degree of dysfunction is now thought to depend more on underlying damage than the flail injury itself. Flail chest may also be accompanied by a pneumothorax, a hemothorax, or both.

Mediastinal structures may shift toward the uninjured lung, compressing it and reducing the amount of ventilation

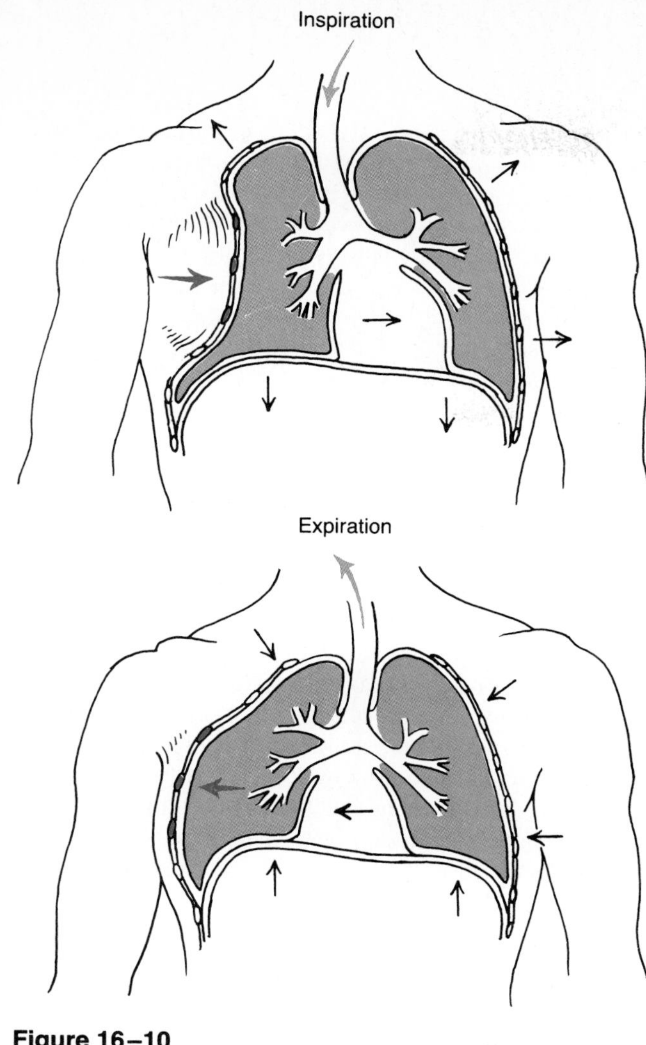

Figure 16–10

Flail chest. The blue arrows indicate movement of the flail segment on inspiration and expiration after multiple rib fracture.

the unaffected lung can provide. This mediastinal shift may also cause kinking and obstruction of major vessels.

Victims complain of pain, which tends to be severe, resulting in limited respiratory effort and an ineffective cough. Other manifestations include dyspnea, tachycardia, restlessness, and cyanosis (Burrell & Burrell, 1982).

Medical Measures

As a first-aid measure, the flail segment can initially be stabilized by exerting firm but gentle pressure on the segment with the palm of the hand. Sandbags, a pressure dressing, or positioning the client on the affected side may be used as temporary measures or to treat milder injuries. Supplemental oxygen and nerve blocks to decrease pain may also be needed.

If the client's ventilation becomes more severely compromised as reflected by hypoxemia and hypercapnia, the treatment of choice is intubation and mechanical ventilation. The positive pressure exerted by the ventilator causes internal stabilization of the flail segment and supports ventilation. Mechanical ventilation is usually continued only until the client can maintain adequate spontaneous ventilation and not until the flail segment has stabilized.

Surgical intervention to stabilize the flail through fixation of the broken rib fragments is seldom used. Closed chest drainage may be necessary if a pneumothorax or hemothorax is present.

Specific Nursing Measures

Coughing and deep breathing are imperative to prevent atelectasis and pneumonia. Suctioning may be required. Assess the client's level of pain and the effect of analgesics. Closely observe vital signs, level of consciousness, and respiratory and cardiac status. Nursing care of the client who is intubated is discussed in Chapter 14.

Pneumothorax

A pneumothorax occurs when there is a communication between the atmosphere and the pleural space, with resultant loss of the negative intrapleural pressure, causing partial or total collapse of the lung. A pneumothorax can be open or closed. In an open pneumothorax, the injury creates an opening in the chest wall, allowing air to flow into the pleural cavity (Figure 16–11). The increased intrapleural pressure causes a partial or total collapse of the lung.

In closed pneumothorax, also called spontaneous pneumothorax, the chest wall remains intact, and air enters the pleural space from the lung surface (Figure 16–12). A closed pneumothorax may be caused by blunt chest trauma,

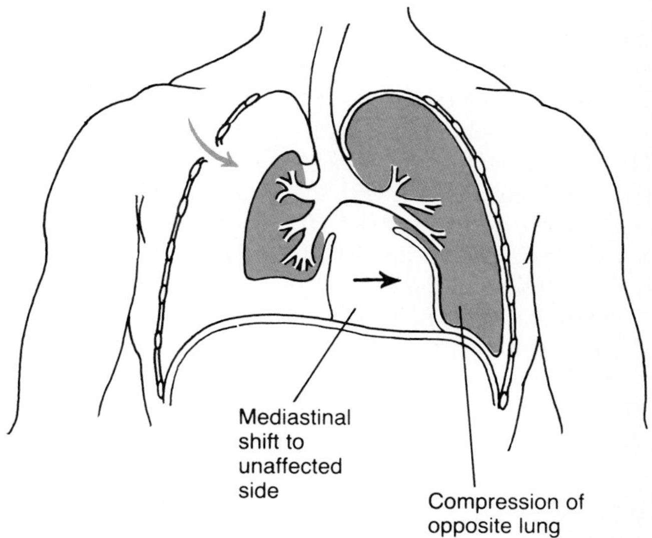

Figure 16–11

Open pneumothorax. An opening in the chest wall causes air to enter the pleural space, causing lung collapse and mediastinal shift to unaffected side.

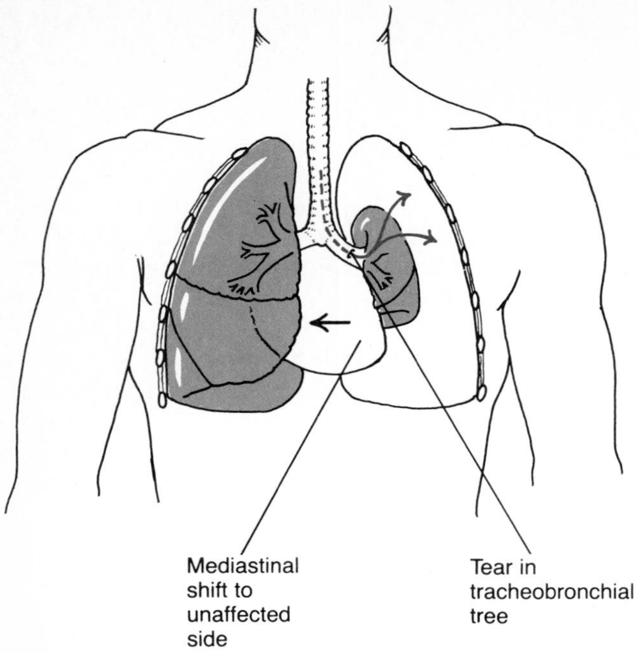

Figure 16–12

Closed pneumothorax. Tear in tracheobronchial tree allows air to enter pleural space, causing lung collapse and mediastinal shift to unaffected side.

in which a fractured rib pierces the lung, or from sudden compression of the thoracic cavity at the height of inspiration, with the glottis closed, causing rupture of the alveoli from excessive pressure (Hoyt, 1983). Pneumothorax can also be a complication of thoracentesis or CVP line insertion.

A spontaneous pneumothorax can also be caused by rupture of a bleb (a small vesicle) or a bulla (a large vesicle) on the lung surface, allowing air to leak from the lung into the pleural space. A bleb or a bulla may form from an infection or from congenital weakness in the lung tissue. Stress or strain, such as coughing or mechanical ventilation, can rupture the bleb or bulla (Woodin, 1982).

A tension pneumothorax is a complication of either a closed or open pneumothorax. Air enters the pleural cavity during inspiration but is unable to escape during expiration because the wound creates a one-way valve. With each inspiratory cycle, the amount of air increases, causing progressive compression of the lung. The high intrathoracic pressure on the affected side causes pressure on the mediastinum, resulting in a shift of the mediastinum (along with the heart, trachea, esophagus, and great vessels) to the unaffected side. This *mediastinal shift* compresses the unaffected lung, decreasing ventilation. Distortion of the vena cava impairs venous return to the heart with a resultant decrease in cardiac output. These abnormalities can lead to hypoxia, hypercapnia, and acidosis.

Clinical Manifestations

A client with a pneumothorax may have pain with breathing, dyspnea, tachypnea, and unilateral diminished breath sounds. The respiratory movement on the affected side may be diminished or absent. In an open pneumothorax, a sucking sound may be heard near the wound. There may be hyperresonance on the affected side. Tachycardia and hypoxemia can occur along with cyanosis. There may be subcutaneous emphysema in the neck and upper chest.

Symptoms of tension pneumothorax include marked dyspnea, severe chest pain, restlessness, agitation, cyanosis, intercostal retraction, nasal flaring, and tachycardia. Jugular vein distention and subcutaneous emphysema can occur (Traver, 1982). There may be asymmetric chest movement, with the affected side lagging behind the unaffected side during inspiration, or fixation of the chest can occur on the affected side.

Medical Measures

The diagnosis of a pneumothorax is confirmed by chest x-ray, which also shows the extent of lung collapse. The treatment of a pneumothorax involves the insertion of chest tubes to evacuate the air in the pleural space; a thoracentesis may be performed. In an open pneumothorax, the wound should be immediately covered with an occlusive petrolatum gauze dressing, followed by decompression and drainage of the pleural space with chest tubes. In a tension pneumothorax an emergency needle thoracostomy or insertion of a flutter valve or chest tube is done to relieve the life-threatening pressure in the pleural cavity (Hoyt, 1983).

Specific Nursing Measures

Careful assessment of the client's respiratory and cardiac status is imperative. Be on the alert for the symptoms and signs of a tension pneumothorax. When an occlusive dressing has been applied to an open pneumothorax, monitor the respiratory status of the client and remove the dressing if the client's breathing worsens, because the dressing may be creating a tension pneumothorax. Positioning the client in a semi-Fowler's position may facilitate breathing. Encourage deep breathing and coughing. In penetrating injuries, be alert to the possibility of infection introduced by the penetrating object. Be prepared to assist the physician in a thoracostomy and insertion of chest tubes. Nursing care of a client with chest tubes is discussed in Chapter 14.

Teach clients with a history of spontaneous pneumothorax to avoid scuba diving and flying in unpressurized aircraft at high altitudes.

Hemothorax

A hemothorax is the accumulation of blood in the pleural space. The usual sources of bleeding in a hemothorax are the pulmonary parenchyma and vessels, the intercostal and internal mammary arteries, the heart, the aorta and great vessels, and the liver and spleen.

A hemothorax may result from either blunt or penetrating trauma to the chest, but it is more common in penetrating trauma. A hemothorax should be considered in severe blunt or decelerating accidents (such as car crashes), which can result in ruptured intrathoracic vessels and cause aortic tears. Fractured ribs caused by blunt trauma are commonly responsible for lacerations leading to a hemothorax.

Clinical Manifestations

Symptoms and signs depend on the source and the amount of accumulated blood loss. A hemothorax may result not only in respiratory and cardiac impairments but also in hypovolemic shock if large amounts of blood are lost. The total accumulation of blood can range from less than 300 mL in a small hemothorax to over 1500 mL in a severe hemothorax. In a small hemothorax, the client may be asymptomatic. In more severe bleeding, partial or total lung collapse may occur as blood accumulates in the pleural cavity. There may be increasing dyspnea, asymmetrical chest movement, chest tightness, ecchymosis over the affected lung, and hemoptysis (Hoyt, 1983). Decreased breath sounds, tachycardia, restlessness, hypotension, and hypovolemic shock can occur. There may be a mediastinal shift to the unaffected side.

Medical and Specific Nursing Measures

A chest x-ray will confirm the diagnosis, showing accumulation of fluid in dependent areas and the amount of lung collapse. Clients with a small hemothorax may require no treatment because of the absorptive power of the pleura (Traver, 1982). In symptomatic clients, a thoracentesis may be performed initially. Chest tube drainage is the most effective means of treating a hemothorax. Replacement of lost blood volume is indicated. A thoracotomy may be necessary when there is a large amount of recurrent bleeding.

The nursing measures are comparable to those for pneumothorax. The emphasis is on monitoring for hypovolemic shock and carrying out fluid and blood replacement therapy.

SECTION 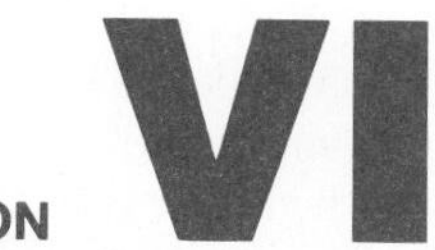

Surgery of the Thorax

Thoracic surgery refers to any surgical procedure of the chest wall or any organ between the diaphragm and clavicles. This section will deal specifically with surgery of pulmonary structures; Chapters 19 and 21 describe cardiovascular procedures.

A variety of incisions may be employed in thoracic surgery: the posterolateral and anterolateral approaches are used often in general thoracic surgery, whereas median sternotomy is employed for certain cardiothoracic procedures (Figure 16–13). Client and nursing implications are similar for each operation; they are discussed with pulmonary resections at the end of this chapter.

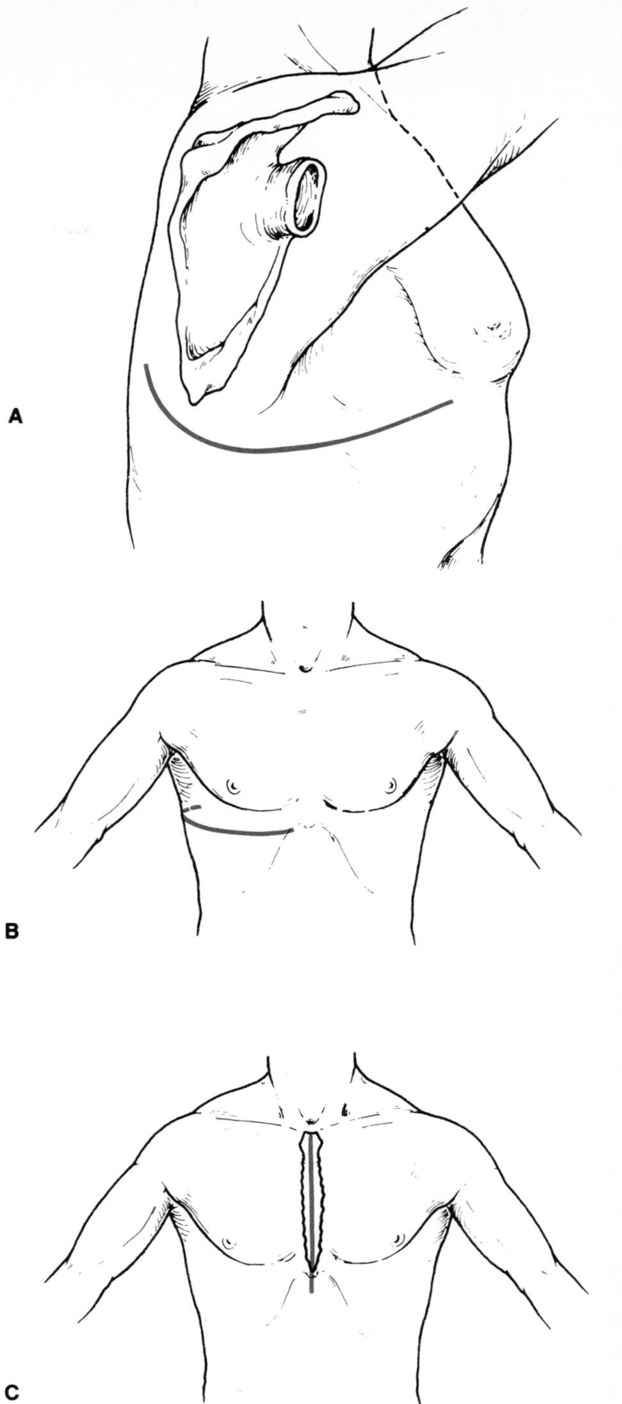

Figure 16–13

Incision sites for thoracic surgery. **A.** Incision site for posterolateral thoracotomy. **B.** Incision for anterolateral thoracotomy. **C.** Incision site for median sternotomy.

Thoracotomy

This procedure consists of opening the thorax for the purpose of inspecting, repairing, or removing tissue. If performed to inspect the area to diagnose suspected disease, the procedure is referred to as an *exploratory thoracotomy*. *Emergency thoracotomy* is sometimes performed in the emergency room for trauma victims. It is only appropriate when clients cannot be stabilized, and there is no time for transportation to the operating room. It has also been used when clients develop cardiac tamponade or other bleeding cardiopulmonary wounds. Emergency thoracotomy allows the physician to gain rapid access to perform open heart massage in an effort to maintain an adequate cardiac output.

Decortication

Decortication involves the removal of pleura that is pathologically thickened and restricts lung expansion. This is a formidable operation and may be associated with significant blood loss.

Thoracoplasty

Thoracoplasty involves the surgical alteration of the shape of the thoracic cage by removing sections of ribs. The purpose of the procedure is to collapse a diseased portion of a lung. It is rarely performed but may be indicated in the following situations (Glenn, 1983): (1) a client with tubercle bacilli consistently present in sputum cultures who is resistant to drugs but is not a candidate for pulmonary resection; (2) to obliterate an empyema cavity; or (3) to obliterate a noninfected residual pleural space.

Lung Transplantation

Lung transplantation is the removal of diseased lung tissue and replacement with lung tissue from a donor. Techniques have been developed to transplant one lung, both lungs, and the heart with both of the lungs.

Pulmonary Resections

The nature and extent of the disease and the condition of the client determine the type of pulmonary resection to be done. As little tissue as possible is removed to retain maximal pulmonary function.

The surgeon makes an incision (see Figure 16–13), spreads the ribs apart with a retractor, and removes or repairs lung tissue as appropriate.

Opening the thorax obliterates the normal negative pressure in the intrapleural space, allowing the lung to collapse. During surgery, the loss of negative intrapleural pressure is compensated for; the client is intubated and mechanically ventilated. Chest tubes must be placed prior to closure of the thorax, however, to restore the negative intrapleural pressure and assist in reexpansion of the lungs. After most pulmonary resections, a tube (sometimes more than one) is placed to allow for drainage of blood and fluid from the intrapleural space, and another for the removal of air. After placement of the chest tubes, the chest is closed.

The physiologic and psychosocial/lifestyle implications are summarized in Table 16–5.

Types of Pulmonary Resection

Pneumonectomy refers to the removal of a lung. A radical pneumonectomy also includes the removal of anterior and posterior mediastinal lymph nodes and excision of the tracheobronchial nodes on the involved side. Removal of an entire lung may be indicated to treat carcinoma of the lung or destruction of lung tissue as a result of extensive pleural disease (ie, tuberculosis). The phrenic nerve on the affected side is crushed or severed to paralyze the diaphragm in an elevated position. This reduces the size of the thoracic cavity on the operative side.

Lobectomy is the term used to describe the removal of one lobe of either lung. A lobectomy may be indicated for removal of diseased tissue as a result of bronchiectasis, an emphysematous bleb, carcinoma of the lung, or cysts.

A *segmental resection* may be employed to remove tissue if bronchiectasis, tuberculosis, well-localized primary or metastatic malignant neoplasm, or an emphysematous bleb has affected only a small portion of the lung.

A *wedge resection* consists of removing a small section or "wedge" of the lung. A wedge resection is used to remove small lesions on or near the surface of the lung. Indications include: to remove benign or inflammatory lesions, to obtain a biopsy from a client with diffuse lung disease, to remove metastatic growths, or to obtain tissue when lung cancer is suspected.

Nursing Implications

PREOPERATIVE CARE Many of those who undergo thoracic surgery have impaired pulmonary or cardiac function. Most are cigarette smokers and are at least in middle age. Those being treated for cancer may be debilitated by the disease process. Clients are usually admitted for extensive evaluation to determine if they can withstand the stress of thoracic surgery. In addition to routine preoperative tests, clients undergo an evaluation of nutritional status and of cardiac, pulmonary, and renal function. The results of pulmonary function tests and arterial blood gas analyses allow evaluation of respiratory status.

If evaluation indicates they will help, aggressive measures may be employed in an attempt to improve the client's nutritional or pulmonary status. This may involve the administration of hyperalimentation or enteral (tube) feedings. Respiratory therapy treatments containing bronchodilators may be prescribed to improve respiratory status. Ideally, the client should not smoke. The administration of antibiotics may be necessary in the preoperative period.

Table 16–5
Thoracic Surgery: Implications for the Client 

Physiologic Implications	Psychosocial/Lifestyle Implications
Significant discomfort varying with the type of incision Possible presence of chest tubes and other invasive tubes and drains Decrease in pulmonary function; extent depends on amount of functional lung tissue removed Pulmonary status may improve especially if tissue removed had significant perfusion without ventilation Altered sensation around surgical incision can last for months Potential complications include atelectasis, bronchopleural fistula, cardiac dysrhythmia, empyema, hemorrhage, hypotension, infection, persistent air leak, pulmonary edema, residual pleural space, respiratory failure, subcutaneous emphysema	Some clients must cope with the fear of recurring cancer and death Lung transplant clients face death if surgery is unsuccessful Need to learn and carry out arm and shoulder exercises Need to contact health care provider at earliest sign of respiratory infection Need to undergo follow-up care for evaluation of respiratory status Lifestyle changes (job change, stopping smoking, and so on, depending on pulmonary status)

Preoperative teaching is of extreme importance since client compliance will greatly affect progress following thoracic surgery. Family members should be included in preoperative preparation. Thoracic surgery is painful because of the incision and presence of chest tubes. Tell the client that medication for pain relief will be available and not to hesitate to ask for it. Clients will be asked to breathe deeply, to ambulate, and to perform shoulder exercises after surgery. Thoracic surgery affects several muscles that act on the shoulder—the trapezius, the rhomboideus major, the serratus anterior, and the latissimus dorsi. These muscles abduct, adduct, rotate, extend, elevate, and lower the shoulder.

Arm and shoulder exercises prevent stiffening of the shoulder and loss of muscle strength. For abduction and external rotation of the affected arm, ask clients to reach behind their heads and try to touch the opposite scapula. For internal rotation and adduction, ask clients to reach across their chests and touch the opposite acromion and also to reach behind their backs and touch the lower edge of the opposite scapula (Figure 16–14). The client should be taught (and should demonstrate) the shoulder exercises and the proper technique for coughing and deep breathing.

Psychologic preparation of the client and family may include a preoperative visit to the intensive care unit. Such a visit may decrease anxiety. The client must be prepared for the presence and function of the tubes (including chest tubes) that will be inserted during surgery. For chest tubes, it should be sufficient to say that they allow drainage of fluid or air so the lungs can function as they should.

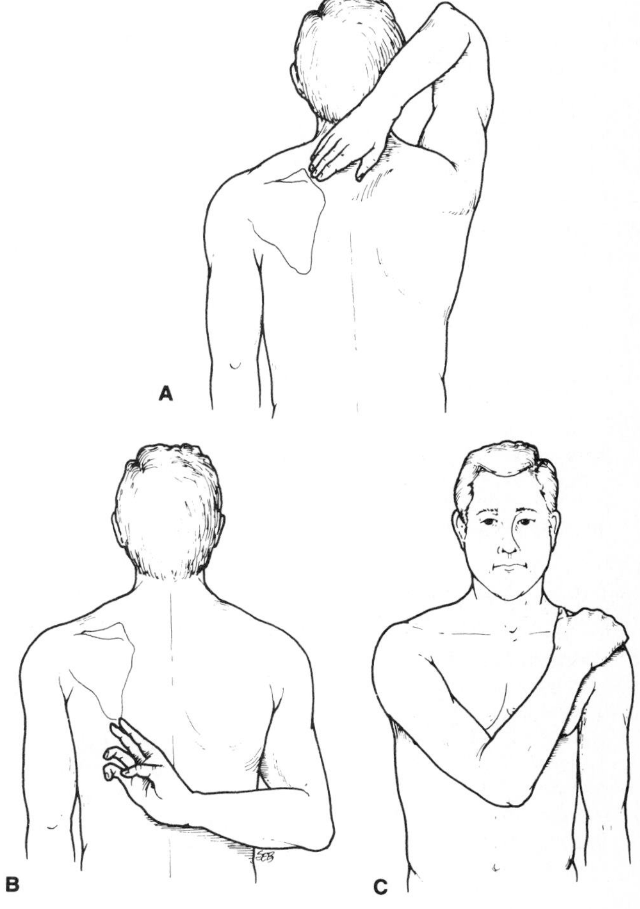

Figure 16–14

Arm and shoulder exercises for the postoperative thoracotomy client. **A.** External rotation and abduction. **B,C.** Internal rotation and adduction.

POSTOPERATIVE CARE Clients who have thoracic surgery are initially transported to a recovery room or intensive care unit for continuous observation. They should remain in the unit until they are stabilized. The client may

Table 16–6
Nursing Interventions for Complications of Thoracic Surgery

Complication	Nursing Intervention
Atelectasis The most common cause of atelectasis is retained bronchial secretions from ineffective coughing or guarding or hypoventilation because of pain. This results in collapse of a portion of the lung distal to the obstruction; infection may develop in the collapsed area.	Refer to nursing measures in the section on promoting optimum pulmonary ventilation.
Bronchopleural fistula A bronchopleural fistula, or opening between the bronchus and the pleural space, may occur during the first week after surgery. Thoracotomy is usually performed to reclose the bronchial stump; a pneumonectomy is occasionally required.	Assess for and report symptoms and signs that may indicate the presence of a bronchopleural fistula: hemoptysis, fever, subcutaneous emphysema, extensive air leak.
Cardiac dysrhythmia This is a common complication of thoracic surgery, especially sinus tachycardia, premature atrial contractions, premature ventricular contractions, atrial fibrillation, and atrial flutter.	Monitor the client's status continuously via ECG for a prescribed period. Note the presence of cardiac dysrhythmias. Take appropriate measures to alleviate side effects from the particular dysrhythmia.
Empyema Empyema is a fairly common complication of pulmonary resection, where the body cavity involved is the intrapleural space. Empyema is more likely to develop if the pleural space is not obliterated, and serosanguineous fluid collects in it. Most clients who develop empyema can be successfully treated with pleural drainage (chest tubes) and systemic antibiotics.	Assess and report symptoms and signs that could indicate the presence of an empyema: • Fever • Pleuritic pain • Dullness on percussion of the area Perform dressing change as needed. If the client is discharged with the wound still open, either the client or a family member or friend should be taught to change the dressing.
Hemorrhage Abnormal bleeding may be caused by a variety of factors. These include inadequate hemostasis at the time of surgery or inadequate coagulation mechanisms.	Monitor vital signs and report significant changes: • Increased pulse • Decreased blood pressure Observe for presence of blood on dressing. Monitor drainage from chest tubes and record hourly.
Hypotension Clients may become hypotensive after thoracic surgery because of a decreased cardiac output. This may result from fluid or blood loss, a myocardial infarction, or cardiac tamponade.	Refer to nursing intervention in the section on maintaining adequate cardiac output.
Infection Wound infections at the site of a lateral thoracotomy occur but are fairly uncommon.	Assess and report symptoms and signs of infection: inflammation, redness, tenderness, purulent drainage, tachycardia, persistent temperature elevation.
Persistent air leak Most of the openings in the lung parenchyma through which air can leak close spontaneously by the second or third day after surgery. An air leak that persists may be treated by injecting a sclerosing agent such as tetracycline into the pleural space and, if that is ineffective, by surgery (Glenn, 1983).	Assess the client's respiratory status. Monitor chest tube drainage; bubbling in the underwater seal chamber from the chest tube signals an air leak.
Pulmonary edema Pulmonary edema is a grave complication that results when fluid from the pulmonary capillaries effuses into the interstitial spaces and into the alveoli. A common cause of pulmonary edema after thoracic surgery is hypervolemia from overinfusion of fluids. Contributing factors may include myocardial infarction, decreased serum protein, and injury to pulmonary capillaries from sepsis or oxygen toxicity.	Assess for symptoms and signs of acute respiratory failure: • Tachypnea • Restlessness • Cyanosis Assess for symptoms and signs of pulmonary edema: • Rales on auscultation of the lungs • Productive cough • Diastolic gallop Observe for cardiac dysrhythmias that may accompany impaired blood gas exchange.

Complication	Nursing Intervention
The goal of treatment is to remove fluid from the pulmonary interstitial spaces and improve blood gas exchange. This may entail administration of diuretics and agents to improve cardiac output. Morphine sulfate may be prescribed to reduce the client's anxiety and peripheral vascular resistance. Oxygen is administered. Other therapeutic measures include rotating tourniquets and phlebotomy. Mechanical ventilation assistance may be needed (Glenn, 1983).	Administer oxygen and medication as prescribed. Provide for safety of client requiring rotating tourniquets (see Chapter 19).
Residual pleural space Residual pleural space is a complication that can affect respiratory status. When a portion of a lung is removed, the pleural space should be obliterated by further inflation of the remaining lung tissue, shifting of the mediastinum, and elevation of the diaphragm. If these do not occur, treatment may involve thoracoplasty using muscle tissue to fill the pleural space.	Monitor the client's respiratory status.
Respiratory failure Respiratory failure is a potential complication whose etiology is not always clear. An inability to get rid of bronchial secretions and pulmonary edema seem to be contributing factors.	Refer to Chapter 15 for nursing interventions.
Subcutaneous emphysema Subcutaneous emphysema is the presence of air under the skin; it occurs because of disruption of the respiratory tract. An occluded chest tube, for example, prevents the escape of air through the tube; the air travels under the skin instead. An air leak may also cause subcutaneous emphysema.	Assess for signs of subcutaneous emphysema: • Swelling or puffiness of the skin • Presence of crepitation Assess progression or resolution of subcutaneous emphysema: • Note and record daily the anatomic areas involved • Note the degree of swelling of the areas Provide comfort for the client by avoiding physical irritation of affected areas by sheets or equipment.

arrive from surgery with an endotracheal tube, pulmonary artery catheter (Swan–Ganz catheter), central venous pressure line (CVP), arterial line, peripheral intravenous lines, chest tubes connected to a closed water-seal drainage system, and a urinary catheter.

Nursing goals for the thoracic surgical client in the postoperative period include: maintenance of adequate cardiac output, promotion of optimal pulmonary ventilation, maintenance of normal fluid and electrolyte balance, relief from pain, promotion of optimal wound healing, promotion of recovery without residual dysfunction, and emotional support and encouragement. The nursing interventions relative to these goals are discussed below. Nursing interventions relative to complications of thoracic surgery are discussed in Table 16–6.

MAINTAINING ADEQUATE CARDIAC OUTPUT Once the client's condition has stabilized the client will be transferred to a postoperative unit. Monitor the client's blood pressure, respiratory rate, heart rate, and temperature until stable, and then as the client's condition requires. Report deviations to the physician immediately.

A change in body temperature alters the metabolic requirement and, thus, affects the cardiac output. If the client's temperature is greater than 102°F (39°C), an antipyretic is prescribed. If the temperature rises above 104°F (40°C), the client is placed on a cooling pad. A hypothermic client, conversely, is placed on a heating mattress and covered with blankets.

Drainage from the chest tubes must be monitored hourly. In the immediate postoperative period, it is wise to note the amount every 15 minutes. Persistent drainage of more than 200 mL per hour may require reexploration to achieve hemostasis. Clients should be encouraged to move their legs frequently while in bed to promote venous return to the heart and prevent the formation of clots.

PROMOTING OPTIMAL PULMONARY VENTILATION Most thoracic surgery clients can have the endotracheal tube removed immediately after surgery. Some, however, require assisted mechanical ventilation because of complications. Humidified oxygen is administered either by endotracheal tube or by mask to prevent hypoxia and liquefy secretions. Assess the client's color, respiration, and other vital signs. Auscultate the chest. Frequent analysis of arterial blood gas samples may be necessary.

The nurse must ensure that chest tubes remain in the intrapleural space, are patent, and connected to a closed water-seal collection receptacle. Carefully observe the amount and character of the chest tube drainage. The client who undergoes a pneumonectomy, however, may not have chest tubes; a majority of surgeons now elect *not* to place them after this surgery. The residual space gradually fills with fluid the first few days after surgery, but this fluid eventually solidifies. Some surgeons place a chest tube for the first 2 or 3 postoperative days, but keep it clamped, ordering it opened periodically to evacuate residual air. The nurse caring for a client who has a pneumonectomy must observe for symptoms and signs of a mediastinal shift.

As soon as the client regains consciousness, encourage coughing and deep breathing every hour for the first 24 hours. Coughing is more effective if the client is assisted to a sitting position with the feet resting on a chair. The incision should be supported anteriorly and posteriorly to minimize pain (Figure 16–15). Diaphragmatic breathing and postural drainage may be prescribed, depending on the amount of pulmonary secretions. If other measures are unsuccessful in the removal of pulmonary secretions, nasotracheal suctioning may be required.

The client should change position every 1 to 2 hours. Special precautions are usually ordered for clients after a pneumonectomy. Opinions differ among surgeons. In general, however, it is recommended that the client *not* be turned to the unoperative side. This is to allow maximum ventilation of the remaining lung. Many physicians specify that clients who undergo lobectomy or a segmental resection be positioned so their operated side is up, to facilitate expansion of the remaining tissue in the lung. After 1 or 2 days, these clients can usually be turned to either side. Clients who undergo other types of thoracic surgery can usually be turned from their back to each side.

The client may dangle the legs at the bedside the evening of surgery and should ambulate with assistance the first day after surgery, unless contraindicated for medical reasons.

MAINTAINING NORMAL FLUID AND ELECTROLYTE BALANCE Several measures can assist in determining the client's fluid status. Daily weights are obtained. The urine output is closely monitored and should amount to at least 30 mL per hour. Some clients will require a urinary catheter, but others will not. Elevated CVP readings can indicate that the client is hypervolemic and a reading below normal suggests hypovolemia. The normal reading is 5 to 12 cm of water. Intravenous fluid replacement is prescribed at specific rates by the physician. Administering fluids too rapidly, however, can lead to complications such as pulmonary edema.

If the abdominal cavity was not entered during surgery, clients can take fluids by mouth as soon as they are alert. Clients should be encouraged to drink a minimum of 1500 to 2000 mL of fluid each day unless contraindicated for medical reasons. The client can usually be advanced to the prescribed diet by the third postoperative day.

RELIEF FROM PAIN A narcotic analgesic such as meperidine or morphine is usually prescribed to be given every 2 to 3 hours as needed. Caution should be used when administering narcotic analgesics since they can lead to respiratory depression. Later, oral medication such as codeine, aspirin, or acetaminophen should be sufficient.

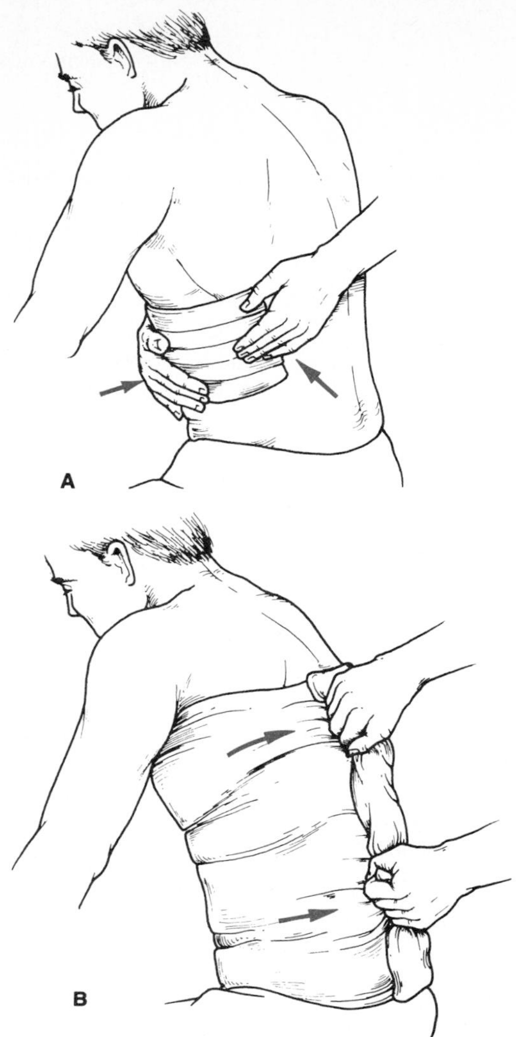

Figure 16–15

Support of a thoracotomy incision during coughing.

Pain medication should be administered 30 to 40 minutes before the client is asked to perform exercises that cause discomfort. This may increase client cooperation. Intercostal nerve blocks have been effective in reducing the pain in some clients.

PROMOTING OPTIMAL WOUND HEALING In the operating room, a light dressing is usually applied to the wound and secured with elastic adhesive tape. It may be taken off the first postoperative day to expose the wound to air. Bloody drainage on the chest dressing is unusual and should be reported to the surgeon. Cleansing of the wound may be necessary at regular intervals. The specific technique varies among surgeons and institutions. Sutures may be removed approximately 1 week after surgery.

PROMOTING RECOVERY WITHOUT RESIDUAL DYSFUNCTION As a result of anterolateral and posterolateral approaches in which nerve and muscle tissues are transected, the client may experience atrophy of the distal end of the transected muscle. In addition, altered sensation around the wound can last for months. The client will tend not to move the arm on the affected side because of the discomfort it causes. To combat these factors, the client is taught arm and shoulder exercises. Passive ROM exercises should be performed a few hours after surgery. The client should progress to active ROM exercises despite the discomfort they cause. Clients often need a great deal of encouragement to carry out these exercises.

EMOTIONAL SUPPORT AND ENCOURAGEMENT The environment, the presence of numerous tubes, and the pain can drain the client emotionally. The client and family members (and significant others) will require explanations and reassurance.

DISCHARGE TEACHING Prior to discharge from the hospital, clients should be able to care for themselves. They should know to report any symptoms and signs of a respiratory tract infection such as persistent fever, increased sputum production, and shortness of breath. They should understand why it is important to continue exercising the affected arm. Encourage clients to return for follow-up evaluation; this consists of assessment of the degree of wound healing and respiratory status. If the client was diagnosed as having cancer, an assessment will be made for recurrence or progression of the disease.

Chapter Highlights

Occupational lung diseases are preventable; nevertheless, they continue to affect a great many people, causing physical disability, lost earnings, suffering, and death.

Adult respiratory distress syndrome is associated with increased fluid in the lung. It can be caused by acute pulmonary infections, aspiration, inhalation of toxins and irritants, overdoses of drugs, and trauma.

Pneumonias, which can be community or hospital acquired, are the fifth leading cause of death in the United States.

Nurses play a significant part in the prevention of nosocomial or hospital-acquired pneumonias.

Client teaching regarding tuberculosis should stress that strict adherence to a prolonged treatment with antituberculosis drugs is necessary to cure the disease.

The prevalence of and death rate from chronic obstructive pulmonary disease (COPD) have increased markedly in recent years.

The most common diseases associated with COPD are chronic bronchitis and emphysema. Asthma, bronchiectasis, and cystic fibrosis are also included under this category.

Pulmonary rehabilitation programs, which encompass client teaching, respiratory hygiene measures, and conditioning exercises, form the cornerstone of intervention for COPD clients.

Lung cancer in this country is increasing at a greater rate in women.

Nursing interventions for clients with lung cancer center around helping them to cope with their diagnosis and treatment and to live as productive and fulfilling lives as their condition allows.

Acute respiratory failure is a life-threatening condition that occurs because of the lungs' inability to maintain adequate oxygenation of the blood.

Nursing intervention for victims of chest trauma centers around assessment of the airway, breathing, circulation, cervical spine, and level of consciousness.

Clients with elevated arterial carbon dioxide levels and low arterial oxygen levels are stimulated to breathe by the hypoxemia. Administration of high liter flows of oxygen can eliminate this hypoxemic drive to breathe, resulting in respiratory arrest.

In penetrating chest wounds when the instrument is still in place, it should remain in place until surgery; hemorrhage may result if it is removed.

During thoracic surgery, the loss of negative intrapleural pressure is compensated for by

intubating and mechanically ventilating the client.

Chest tubes are placed after most thoracic surgical procedures to restore the negative intrapleural pressure by allowing exit of air and fluid.

Vigorous pulmonary care is necessary in the postoperative period after thoracic surgery to prevent complications.

Thorough preoperative teaching of the client undergoing thoracic surgery is essential to ensure client and family cooperation in the postoperative period.

Bibliography

American Cancer Society: *Cancer Facts and Figures.* New York: American Cancer Society, 1987.

American Lung Association: *Occupational Disease: An Introduction.* New York: American Lung Association, 1983.

Anderson SJ: Sarcoidosis: A multisystem disease. *Am J Nurs* (Oct) 1982; 82:1566–1569.

Burrell LO, Burrell Z Jr: *Critical Care.* St. Louis: Mosby, 1982.

Cancer facts and figures. *Occup Health Nurs* (July) 1982; 30:42–43.

Cline B, Fisher M: A.R.D.S. means emergency. *Nurs 82* (Feb) 1982; 12:62–67.

D'Agostino J: Teaching tips for living with COPD at home. *Nurs 84* (Feb) 1984; 14:57.

D'Agostino J: You can breathe new life into your COPD patients. *Nurs 83* (Sept) 1983; 13:72–77.

Daniele R: Sarcoidosis: Diagnosis and management. *Hosp Pract* (June) 1983; 18:113–122.

Diethorn M: Prevention of sensory deprivation for the COPD victim's spouse. *Top Clin Nurs* 1985; 6(4):64–71.

Domigan-Wentz J: The CPAP mask: A comfortable approach to ARDS. *Am J Nurs* 1985; 85(7):813–815.

George R, Light R, Matthay R (editors): *Chest Medicine.* New York: Churchill Livingstone, 1983.

Gibbs CJ et al: Premenstrual exacerbation of asthma. *Thorax* (Nov) 1984; 39(11): 833–836.

Glenn W (editor): *Thoracic and Cardiovascular Surgery.* 4th ed. Norwalk, CT: Appleton-Century-Crofts, 1983.

Greco FA, Hande K: *Lung Cancer Management: Progress and Prospects.* Wayne, NJ: Lederle Laboratories, 1982.

Greifzu S, Crebase C, Winnick B: Lung cancer: By the time it's detected, it may be too late. *RN* (March) 1987; 52–58.

Hoyt S: Chest trauma: When the patient looks bad, act fast. When he looks good, act fast. *Nurs 83* (May) 1983; 13:34–41.

Hudak C, Lohr T, Gallo B (editors): *Critical Care Nursing.* Philadelphia: Lippincott, 1982.

Jett J, Cortese D, Fontana R: Lung cancer: Current concepts and prospects. *CA* 1983; 33:74–85.

Kane KK: Carotid artery rupture in advanced head and neck cancer patients. *Oncol Nurs Forum* (Winter) 1983; 10(1):14–18.

Katz LE: Postoperative complications of thoracic surgery: Their recognition and treatment. *AANA J* (June) 1980; 48(3):222–228.

Keller C, Solomon J, Reyes V: *Respiratory Nursing Care.* Englewood Cliffs, NJ: Prentice-Hall, 1984.

Kroksky NJ: Black lung and silicosis. *Am J Nurs* 1985; 85(8):883–886.

Mitchell R, Petty T (editors): *Synopsis of Clinical Pulmonary Disease.* St. Louis: Mosby, 1982.

Petersdorf RG et al: *Harrison's Principles of Internal Medicine,* 19th ed. New York: McGraw-Hill, 1983.

Petty TL: *Intensive and Rehabilitative Respiratory Care.* Philadelphia: Lea & Febiger, 1982.

Petty TL: Drug strategies for airflow obstruction. *Am J Nurs*; 87(2):180–184.

Raffin T, Roberts P: The prevention and treatment of status asthmaticus. *Hosp Pract* (Feb) 1982; 17:80A–80Z-6.

Ryan MA: Pneumonia: Aggressive treatment is the key. *RN* (Aug) 1982; 45:44–50.

Sexton DL, Munro BH: Impact of a husband's chronic illness (COPD) on the spouse's life. *Res Nurs Health* (March) 1985; 8(1):83–90.

Stockdale–Wooley R: Sexual dysfunction and COPD: Problems and management. *Nurse Pract* (Feb) 1983; 8:16–18.

Traver G: *Respiratory Nursing: The Science and the Art.* New York: Wiley, 1982.

Veith FJ et al: Lung transplantation–1983. *Transplantation* (April) 1983; 35(4):271–278.

Wade J: *Comprehensive Respiratory Care: Physiology and Technique.* St. Louis: Mosby, 1982.

Woodin L: Your patient with a pneumothorax: A patient in distress. *Nurs 82* (Nov) 1982; 12:50–56.

UNIT

4

The Client With Cardiovascular or Hematologic Dysfunction

CHAPTER 17

The Cardiovascular and Hematologic Systems in Health and Illness

> Other topics relevant to this content are: Electrocardiography and nursing implications, **Chapter 18;** Dietary management of hyperlipidemia, **Chapter 19.**

Objectives

When you have finished studying this chapter, you should be able to:

Identify the major structural and functional components of the cardiovascular system.

Describe the functions of the lymphatic system.

Delineate the formed elements of the blood and their purposes.

Explain the physiologic mechanisms that regulate the activity of the cardiovascular system.

Describe the pathologic conditions that lead to inadequate blood supply to the myocardium and to the peripheral tissues.

Give examples of internal and external factors that can influence bone marrow function.

Discuss alterations in other body systems that result from dysfunction in the cardiovascular system.

Identify and discuss the psychosocial/lifestyle effects of dysfunction in the cardiovascular system on the client and significant others.

This chapter reviews the anatomy and physiology of the heart, blood vessels, lymphatic system, and blood components in relation to aspects of nursing care most significant for adult clients. Pathologic changes are discussed in relation to their interference with cardiovascular function. The psychosocial aspects are discussed in relation to the effects of pathologic cardiovascular changes on the client's lifestyle.

SECTION 

Structural and Functional Interrelationships

The heart, which actually functions as two pumps, contracts and generates pressures to push the blood through the entire vascular system and back. The right side of the heart generates the pressures required to pump blood through the capillaries of the lungs (where exchange of gases, primarily oxygen and carbon dioxide, occurs) and to the left side of the heart. The left side of the heart generates pressure to push the blood throughout the systemic circulation.

In studying cardiovascular dynamics, the nurse should understand and be able to apply some laws of physics. Probably the most important is **Poiseuille's law,** which holds that the flow rate of a fluid through a tube is proportional to pressure differences and the diameter of the tube in relation to the length of the tube and the viscosity of the fluid. In the cardiovascular system, the heart generates the pressure, the diameter and length of the tubes are determined by the blood vessels, and the blood has a certain viscosity. To visualize the application of this law, imagine giving an injection. The more pressure applied to the plunger, the faster the fluid flows; the smaller the diameter and the longer the needle, the greater the pressure needed to make the fluid flow; and the more viscous the fluid, the greater the pressure needed to make the fluid flow. Factors that hinder flow involve *resistance,* which in this case is determined by the diameter and length of the tube as well as the viscosity of the fluid. In addition, the pressure depends on the amount of fluid in the container.

The Heart

The **cardiac output,** or the amount of blood the heart pumps per minute, is determined by the amount of blood the heart pumps with each stroke **(stroke volume)** and the number of strokes per minute **(heart rate).** The heart pumps about 70 mL of blood with each stroke at an average rate of 72 beats per minute; this accounts for an average of over 5000 mL of blood per minute. The heart can increase this quantity of blood by about four times by increasing its rate, the amount of blood it pumps with each stroke, or both. The heart's ability to do this depends on its ability to time contractions, its ability to contract, and the amount of blood available to pump.

Contractility of the Heart

Within its physiologic limits, the heart is able to pump all the blood returning to it without allowing it to back up into the veins. Because the body tissues regulate their own blood flow according to their needs, the amount of blood returning to the heart varies from moment to moment, and the heart is able to accommodate these changes. The muscle fibers of the heart act similarly to skeletal muscle fibers when stretched. The more they are stretched within physiologic limits, the greater the force of contraction. The myocardial fibers stretch with increased amounts of returning blood during diastole and contract with greater force during systole (called the Frank Starling law of the heart). **Preload** is the term that refers to the degree of stretch of myocardial fibers before contraction. **Afterload** is the term that refers to the tension the ventricles must develop in systole to pump against pressure in the aortic valve, aorta, and to resistance in the systemic and pulmonary arterioles.

Electrical Conduction in the Heart

When cardiac muscle cells are at rest, the inside of the cardiac cell membrane is electrically negative in relation to the outside. This electrical situation is referred to as the *resting membrane potential.* During *depolarization,* the first stage of the *action potential* (the change in electrical potential across the cell membrane when it becomes active), sodium ions rush into the cell and the cell membrane loses its electronegativity. Following this stage of the action potential, cardiac muscle contracts. *Repolarization,* the second stage of the action potential, is initiated by an outward flow of potassium ions which promotes return to the resting membrane potential. This electrical activity of the heart is visualized by placing electrical sensors on the surface of the skin and recording the electrical activity with an electrocardiograph (see Chapter 18).

Coronary Circulation

Like the other cells of the body, the heart needs blood flow to maintain cellular life and perform its work. It receives its blood supply from the left and right coronary arteries, which originate in the root of the aorta just above the left posterior and anterior cusps of the aortic valve. Blood flows into these arteries during ventricular diastole, when the aortic valve is closed by blood pushed backward by the recoil of the aorta at the beginning of ventricular diastole. The duration of ventricular diastole is important to ensure that the heart cells get sufficient blood supply. Note that when the heart cells contract, the contraction exerts pressure against the coronary vessels and inhibits blood flow.

The left coronary artery primarily supplies the left atrium and the majority of the left ventricle. This artery branches into the left anterior descending artery and the circumflex artery (Figure 17–1). In most persons, the left anterior descending artery and its branches supply the interventricular septum and surrounding myocardium. The circumflex artery and its branches supply the lateral wall and some of the posterior wall of the left ventricle. The right coronary artery supplies the right atrium; the right ventricle; and, in most persons, the A-V node and the inferior and posterior portions of the left ventricle (Figure 17–1).

Most cardiac veins empty into the coronary sinus, which drains directly into the right atrium. Some of the veins empty directly into all chambers of the heart.

Blood Vessels

The blood vessels carry the blood from the heart, provide an area for exchange of substances between the blood and interstitial spaces, and carry the blood back to the heart to be recirculated. Generally, the arteries and arterioles carry the blood to the capillaries (or sinusoids, which are larger and more irregular small tubes such as those found in the endocrine glands, liver, bone marrow, and spleen). There exchange takes place, and the venules and veins carry the blood back to the heart for recirculation. (Some exchange takes place in the capillary ends of the venules.)

The arteries are sometimes referred to as distribution or conduction vessels because they provide continuous blood flow to the periphery. Their walls are thick and elastic, enabling them to stretch to accommodate greater amounts of blood under high pressure during ventricular systole. Because of their elasticity, the arteries recoil during ventricular diastole and maintain sufficient blood pressure to promote blood flow through the system. They branch like a tree, and the branches get smaller as they extend away from the heart. The arteries are also called the *high-pressure blood vessels.*

Not all arteries end in arterioles. Some anastomose (unite) with other arteries. There are more anastomoses as the arteries decrease in size and move away from the heart. Anastomoses are especially prominent around joints, where external pressure during movement momentarily interrupts circulation. The anastomosed artery provides

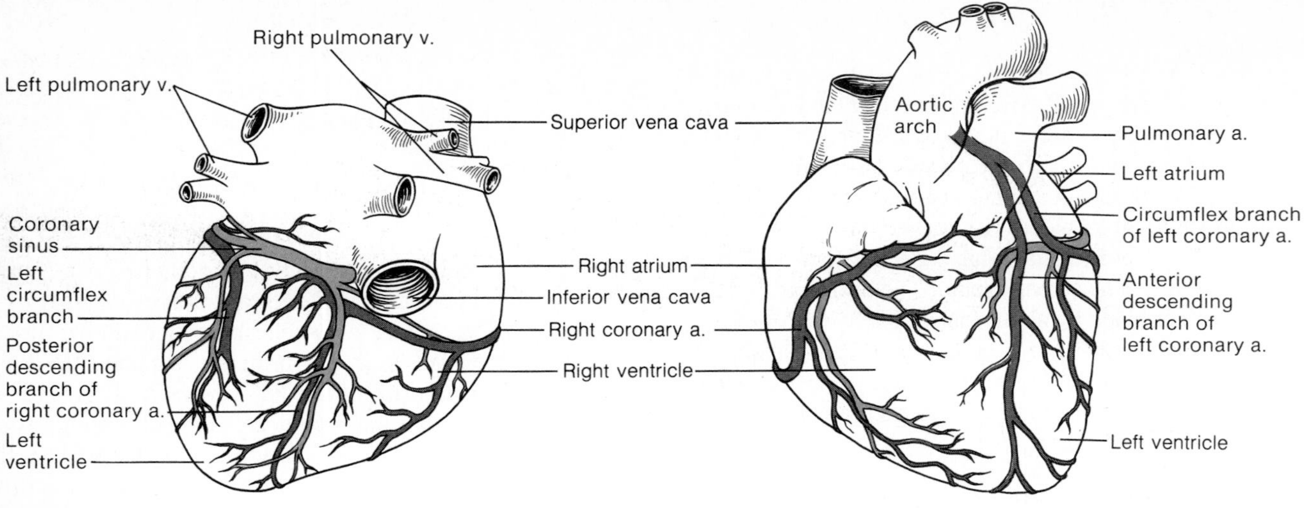

Figure 17–1

The coronary circulation.

the intermittent blood supply. When blood supply is compromised for a time from disease or injury, the anastomosed artery enlarges to provide collateral circulation. Sudden occlusion, however, may not permit sufficient time for the collateralization, and the involved tissue may die.

Some arteries develop connecting vessels that join veins, developing arteriovenous shunts, which divert the blood into the venous system rather than on to the capillary. These shunts are especially common in the skin of the hands, feet, nose, and ears and function in temperature regulation. When the body temperature is low, the shunts open and promote heat loss. Arteriovenous shunts are also common in the gastrointestinal tract. The connecting vessels close when absorption is taking place and open when it is not, shunting the blood to other areas.

The arterioles are short vessels a few millimeters long that branch into terminal arterioles, which feed the capillaries. The arterioles, referred to as the resistance vessels, have small diameters. The blood pressure drops from about 85 mm Hg when blood enters the arteriole to about 30 mm Hg at the beginning of the capillary.

In most tissue areas, each capillary is joined by an arteriole (sometimes called a *metarteriole*), which branches to serve other capillaries and ultimately joins a venule to form a capillary network. At the junction of each capillary and arteriole is a sphincter muscle, which opens to allow blood into the capillary and closes to divert blood to the venule or other capillaries in the network. The periodic opening and closing (about five to ten times per minute) of different spincters ensures irrigation of various parts of the capillary network. The most important factor in the regulation of the opening and closing of these spincters is the oxygen content in the tissues. Other substances that promote vasodilation are found in the area as well and may have some effect. When the oxygen concentration is low, the spincters open more often and permit more blood flow, resulting in more oxygen and nutrients to the area (autoregulation of blood supply).

Exchange take splace in the capillaries. The movement of substances both ways across the capillary membrane primarily occurs by diffusion, filtration, and osmosis. Primary factors that control the movement of fluid into the interstitial space include hydrostatic pressure (blood pressure), which tends to push fluid into the interstitial space, and colloidal osmotic (oncotic) pressure (primarily related to albumin and proteins), which tends to pull fluid in. The net effect is that fluid moves into the interstitial space at the arterial end, where hydrostatic pressure is about 30 mm Hg, and fluid moves back in at the venous side, where hydrostatic pressure is about 10 mm Hg (providing colloidal osmotic pressure is normal). Not all the fluid that leaves the capillaries returns to them. Some returns to the venous circulation by way of the lymphatics. Some protein substances and other larger particles leak out and are also returned by the lymphatics.

The venules collect the blood from the capillaries and small arterioles. There may be some fluid exchange in the venules. They also serve as one of the routes for the white blood cells' migration into and out of the tissues.

The veins are low-pressure vessels with thin walls and less muscle in the tunica media than arteries. They serve as conduits to return blood to the heart. Veins are referred to as *capacitance* or *reservoir blood vessels* because they hold over 60% of the blood. With the exception of the largest and smallest veins, most have valves that prevent blood from moving backward. As the body muscles contract, they exert external pressure against the veins, which promotes the forward flow of blood. When the venous pressure falls and the blood tends to run backward, the valves catch it until the muscles help move it forward again.

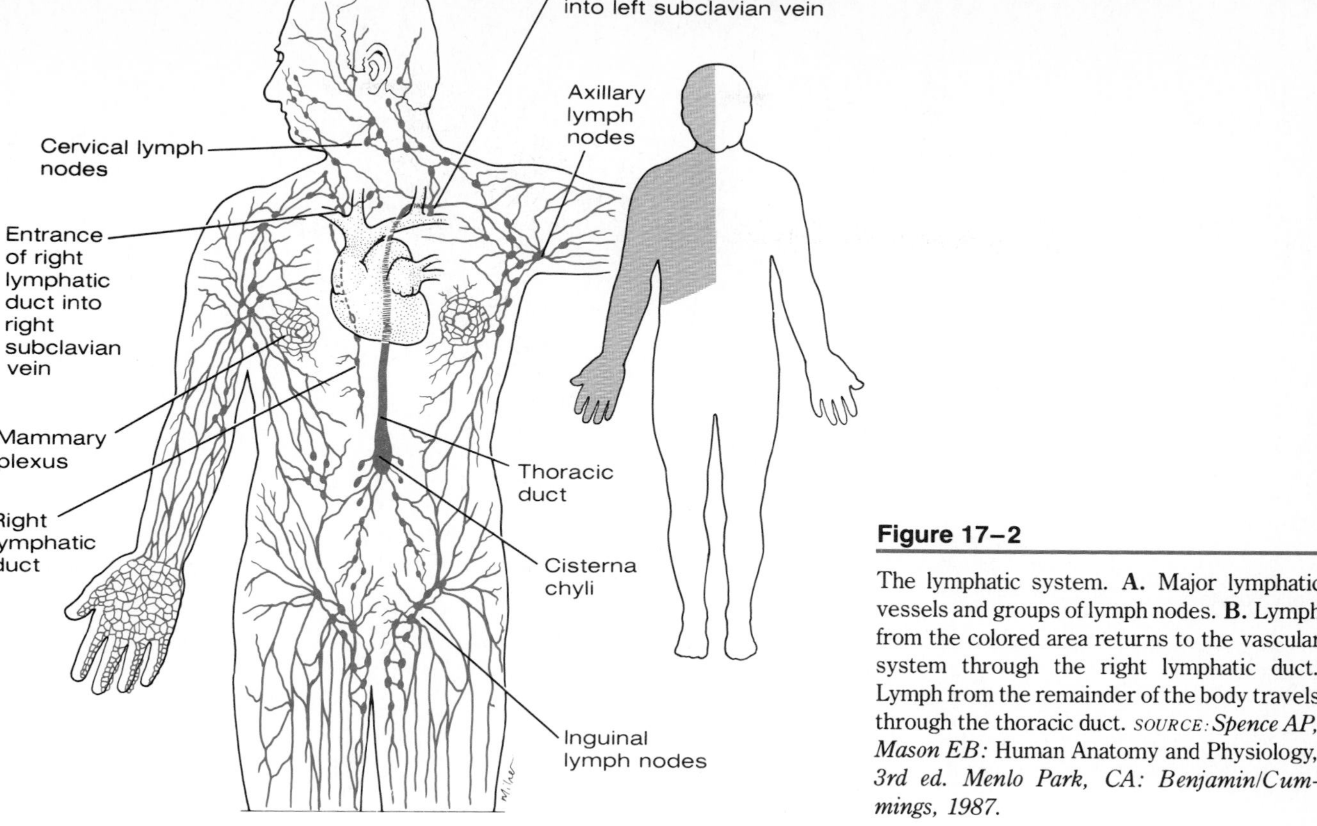

Figure 17–2

The lymphatic system. **A.** Major lymphatic vessels and groups of lymph nodes. **B.** Lymph from the colored area returns to the vascular system through the right lymphatic duct. Lymph from the remainder of the body travels through the thoracic duct. SOURCE: *Spence AP, Mason EB:* Human Anatomy and Physiology, *3rd ed. Menlo Park, CA: Benjamin/Cummings, 1987.*

The Lymphatic System

The lymphatics begin blindly in the tissue spaces as tiny vessels a little larger than capillaries, empty into progressively larger branches of lymphatic vessels, pass through the lymph nodes, and ultimately empty their fluid (lymph) into the venous system. The lymph from the legs and left side of the body empties into the thoracic duct and left subclavian vein. Lymph from the right side of the head, the right arm, and the right thorax empties into the right lymphatic duct and right subclavian vein (Figure 17–2). The lymphatics are similar to veins in structure but have many more valves. They are found almost everywhere there are blood vessels except in the central nervous system. Lymphatics have a great capacity for repair and the formation of new vessels.

The lymphatics serve an important function in preventing edema. The tiny vessels collect fluid and proteins from the interstitial spaces and promote their return to the circulation. The lymphatics drain about 120 mL fluid per hour and can drain about 20 times that much if necessary. They also collect the larger digested fat particles (chylomicrons) from the digestive system and empty them into the circulation.

In addition, the lymphatics play a key role in the body's defense against microorganisms. They collect microorganisms in the interstitial spaces and carry them along with the fluid into the lymph nodes (small masses of lymphoid tissue), where the lymphocytes and macrophages remove bacteria and other foreign substances from the lymph before sending it into the venous system.

The Spleen

The spleen is the largest lymphatic organ and is highly vascular. It is located in the left upper abdomen directly below the diaphragm, posterior and lateral to the fundus of the stomach. The spleen functions as a blood filtration system, trapping foreign particles and destroying bacteria and viruses. It also serves as a blood reservoir.

The spleen contains two types of pulp, red and white. The red pulp, which contains lymphocytes, macrophages, and erythrocytes, is the most abundant. Old erythrocytes are destroyed in the red pulp. Masses of white pulp, which surround the arterioles, are scattered throughout the red pulp. White pulp produces lymphocytes and sequesters lymphocytes, macrophages, and antigens.

The Bone Marrow

Bone marrow, contained inside all bones, collectively is one of the largest organs of the body. Hematopoiesis, or the formation of blood cells, is its primary function. There are two kinds of bone marrow: red and yellow bone marrow. Hematopoiesis is carried out by red (functioning) marrow. By adulthood, red marrow is confined to the pelvis, sternum, ribs, cranium, ends of the long bones, and the

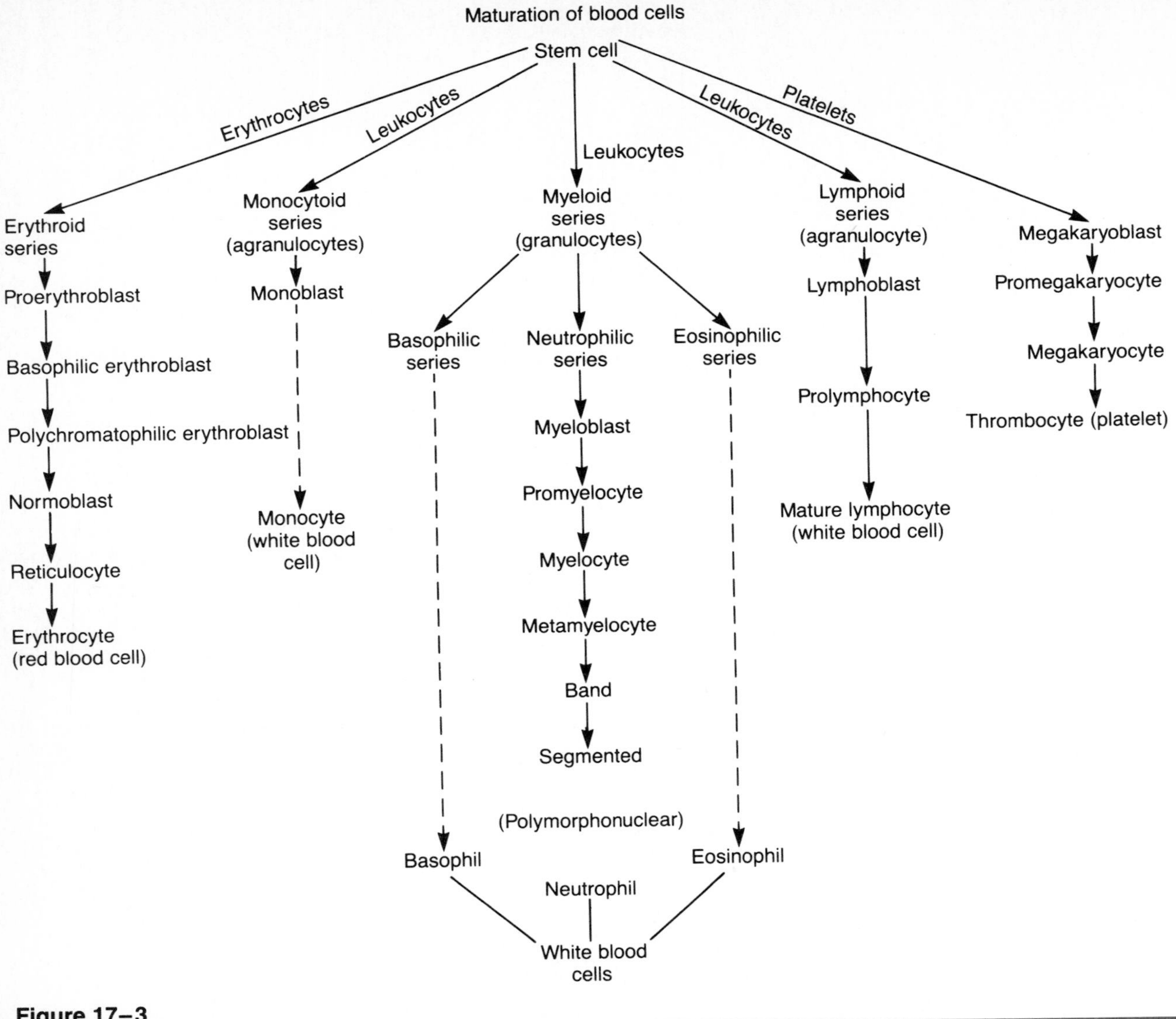

Figure 17–3

Maturation of blood cells. Dotted lines indicate that the maturation sequence is similar to that of the neutrophilic series.

vertebral spine. Yellow (fatty) bone marrow is red marrow that has changed to fat. It is found in the remaining bones and does not contribute to hematopoiesis.

All the blood components start as stem cells. These differentiate and become committed to one cell line—erythrocytes, leukocytes, or thrombocytes. They mature through orderly stages and are normally released into the bloodstream when they reach maturity (Figure 17–3). On occasion, when the demand for a particular blood cell is high, the bone marrow may respond by releasing the needed blood component too early. The nurse needs to know the functions of the blood components to interpret the clinical significance of the blood count.

The Blood

The purpose of the cardiovascular system is to circulate the blood to bring it into proximity with the body cells. Blood is the substance of life because it carries materials necessary to provide the correct environment in which the body cells can do their work.

When blood is centrifuged in a test tube, the erythrocytes form the bottom layer, the leukocytes and thrombocytes form the middle layer, and a clear fluid called *plasma* is on the top. The erythrocytes constitute about 45% of the volume and the plasma, about 55%; the volume of the leukocytes and the thrombocytes is negligible. The blood cells just mentioned are often referred to as the *formed elements of the blood*, or the *blood components*.

Erythrocytes

The erythrocytes (red blood cells) number about 5 million mL, carry about 14 g of hemoglobin per deciliter, and occupy about 45% of the blood volume. They are formed in the bone marrow and released in an immature form called *reticulocytes*. Because the life span of the erythrocyte is about 120 days, and the usual production of erythrocytes approximately equals the loss, the normal number of reticulocytes in the blood can be used to measure overall bone marrow activity. The reticulocyte count is expressed as a percentage with a range of approximately 0.5% to 1.5%. Values less than 0.5% may signal bone marrow suppression or failure, depending on the disease process involved. Conversely, values greater than the normal range can signal bone marrow recovery or increased activity. The stimulus prompting reticulocytosis varies from one client to another, depending on the underlying disease process.

The erythrocytes are vital to survival. They contain hemoglobin, which transports oxygen picked up in the lungs to the capillaries near the cells, where it is diffused for use by the cells. The erythrocytes also contain a large amount of carbonic anhydrase, which catalyzes the chemical reaction between carbon dioxide and water. This makes it possible for the blood to carry large amounts of carbon dioxide in solution; thus, the carbon dioxide can be picked up in the capillaries near the cells and carried to the lungs to be converted back to the gas form and exhaled. The erythrocytes also are important in maintaining an acid–base balance in the blood and are responsible for about 70% of the blood-buffering power.

The normal erythrocyte has a biconcave shape, like a doughnut without the hole. The biconcavity of the erythrocyte allows flexibility, pliability, and distortion without destruction. Flexibility and pliability are necessary to traverse the microcirculation. For the erythrocyte to survive, it must be able to squeeze through the smallest capillary, release its oxygen to adjacent cells, and reenter the venous circulation. Alterations in the normal biconcave shape (poikilocytosis) can cause increased erythrocyte fragility, increased splenic sequestration of erythrocytes, and anemia.

The mean corpuscular volume (MCV) of the erythrocyte ranges from 82 to 92 μm^3. Clients with anisocytosis (variations in erythrocyte size) may have erythrocytes larger than normal (macrocytic), smaller than normal (microcytic), or both. The anemias in particular are characterized by abnormal sizes of the erythrocyte.

As already mentioned, the erythrocyte contains the hemoglobin molecule. The adult hemoglobin molecule is composed of a heme (iron) portion and a globin (protein) portion. The protein portion is composed of two alpha and two beta polypeptide chains. Variations of the structure of these protein chains alter the hemoglobin molecule and create problems in oxygen transport. Sickle cell anemia and thalassemia are two such disorders in hemoglobin synthesis.

The erythrocytes contribute significantly to the viscosity of the blood and therefore influence the heart's ability to perform its function. When the quantity of erythrocytes is high, as in polycythemia, the heart must work harder to overcome the increased viscosity that impedes blood flow. The viscosity of the blood is measured by the packed cell volume (PCV), or hematocrit. The hematocrit is expressed as a percentage of the total blood volume and should be three times the hemoglobin concentration.

The erythrocytes carry antigens, of which over 50 have been identified. These antigen types are inherited (see Table 17–1). The most important to nursing are the ABO and Rh blood types because individuals produce antibodies against antigens other than the antigens they carry on their own erythrocytes. For instance, persons with type O erythrocytes have neither the type A nor B antigen and develop antibodies against them. If they receive a blood transfusion from persons with type A, B, or AB, their antibodies will attach to the donor's erythrocytes and cause agglutination (clumping). Because type O blood lacks antigens, it can be transfused into clients without causing reactions and is known as the **universal donor.** Persons with type A erythrocytes develop antibodies against type B

Table 17–1
ABO Genetics and Blood Types

Blood Type (Phenotype)	Genotype	Antigens on RBCs	Antibodies in Serum	% of Humans Who Have Blood Type	Compatible Donor Blood Types
A	AA	A	B	41	A, O
A	AO	A	B		
B	BB	B	A	9	B, O
B	BO	B	A		
AB	AB	AB	None	3	A, B, AB, O (universal recipient)
O	OO	None	A, B	47	O (universal donor)

SOURCE: Reprinted with permission from Vick RL: *Contemporary Medical Physiology*. Menlo Park, CA: Addison–Wesley, 1984, p. 367.

blood and therefore cannot receive type B or AB blood; persons with type B erythrocytes develop antibodies against type A blood, which results in agglutination with type A and AB erythrocytes. Persons with type AB erythrocytes have both A and B antigens and therefore can receive erythrocytes from any of the other three types. Type AB blood is known as the **universal recipient.**

Erythrocytes are also Rh positive or Rh negative, meaning that they either have the Rh antigen or they do not, respectively. The Rh system is different from the ABO system. Individuals who are Rh negative do not have antibodies against Rh-positive erythrocytes but develop them if Rh positive blood comes in contact with their blood.

Thrombocytes

The thrombocytes (platelets) are fragments of the megakaryocytes formed in the bone marrow and released into the bloodstream, where they are completely replaced over a 10-day period. They are important to the blood-clotting mechanism and clot retraction. Thrombocytes are especially important to the vascular system because they plug the many small ruptures that occur in small vessels daily. Without thrombocytes to plug the ruptures, blood leaks out and causes small hemorrhagic areas (petechiae) in the skin.

The thrombocytes swell, become sticky, and begin to adhere to one another when they come in contact with rough surfaces or are in areas of blood stasis. This characteristic is known as *platelet adhesion. Platelet aggregation* refers to the ability of thrombocytes to be mobilized to a site of injury and plug the leak. Adequate platelet numbers are necessary to promote the release of serotonin, which causes local vasoconstriction at the injury site and reduces the amount of bleeding following injury.

The thrombocytes are also important in clot retraction. A few minutes after a clot is formed, it retracts into the vessel and expresses fluid called *serum* over the next hour. This causes the ends of the damaged vessel to come together and promotes hemostasis.

Clotting Cascade

In addition to thrombocytes, a number of coagulation factors have been identified in the blood that contribute to hemostasis. The majority of these factors are produced in the liver. Table 17–2 lists the clotting factors and their site of production. Collectively, these clotting factors are referred to as the *clotting cascade.*

The term clotting cascade denotes an interdependent and orderly relation among these clotting factors, resembling a cascade or waterfall. A deficiency or defect of any one factor may contribute to a tendency to bleed in a particular client. Clot formation is not a random and haphazard event. The sequence of events leading to the formation of a fibrin clot is progressive and orderly. Clotting occurs in four stages.

Coagulation is initiated with injury to the wall of a blood vessel. Two pathways are activated. The *intrinsic pathway* describes events inside the injured blood vessel. The clotting events that occur on the outside of the blood vessel are called the *extrinsic pathway*. Roman numerals are used more often today than the factor names to represent the clotting factors. The clotting factors II, V, VII, IX, X, XI, and XII are continuously present in an inactive form in the circulation. When a vessel is injured, the clotting factors are transformed to their activated states, promoting clot formation. Stage I includes both the intrinsic and extrinsic pathways. The mechanism for activation of these pathways is injury. The *intrinsic pathway* is a sequence of events in which the next reaction is stimulated by the preceding one. In other words, injury initiates factor XII to stimulate factor XI, which converts factor IX to its activated form and so on. For successful progression of events, calcium and platelets must also be present.

The *extrinsic pathway* occurs simultaneously with the intrinsic pathway. With tissue injury, tissue thromboplastin is released. In the presence of factor VII, platelets, and calcium, tissue thromboplastin activates factors X and V, and the coagulation process continues.

Stage II of the clotting cascade consists of the conversion of prothrombin to thrombin by the plasma and tissue thromboplastin generated in stage I. Factors X, V, calcium, and platelets are vital to the successful completion of stage II.

Stage III begins with the action of thrombin on fibrinogen. Thrombin acts like an enzyme and splits fibrinogen into fibrin strands. The fibrin strands have the ability to mesh together side by side and end to end to form a clot. Factor XII (fibrin stabilizing factor) acts upon the fibrin clot, making it stronger, "more stable," and insoluble.

Stage IV is fibrinolysis, or the breakdown of the fibrin clot. This occurs once the blood vessel has been repaired. Fibrinolysis begins with the activation of plasminogen to plasmin. Plasminogen is normally found within the insoluble clot. Plasmin is an enzyme that breaks down the fibrin in the clot. Fibrin breakdown or digestion results in the release of fibrin degradation products (FDP) which inhibit clot formation by their anticoagulant activity and prevent unnecessary clot formation. An increase in FDP may be one of the factors responsible for the bleeding in disseminated intravascular coagulation (DIC).

Leukocytes

The leukocytes, or white blood cells (WBCs), are formed in the bone marrow and released into the blood, which they use for transit. Their primary purpose is to protect the body against invasion by foreign substances such as microorganisms. They also play a vital role in the normal inflammatory response. Leukocytes are classified as either granulocytes or agranular leukocytes (see Figure 17–3). Granulocytes consist of the neutrophils, basophils,

Table 17–2
The Coagulation System

Factor Number	Name(s)	Function	Site of Production
I	Fibrinogen	Protein acted on by thrombin to produce fibrin polymer, which forms structure of clot	Liver
II	Prothrombin	Precursor of thrombin	Liver (vitamin-K dependent)
III	Thromboplastin	Lipoprotein derived from tissue. In extrinsic coagulation cascade, interacts with other factors to produce prothrombinase	Thromboplastic activity present in most tissues
IV	Calcium	Necessary for function of extrinsic cascade, intrinsic cascade, and common pathway	
V	Proaccelerin (labile factor)	Accelerates plasma thromboplastin generation in stage I; speeds conversion of prothrombin in stage II	Liver
VII	Proconvertin	Interacts with thromboplastin and Ca^{2+} to activate factor X in *extrinsic* cascade	Liver (vitamin-K dependent)
VIII	Antihemophilic factor	Interacts with other factors to activate factor X in *intrinsic* cascade	Uncertain
IX	Plasma thromboplastin component, Christmas factor	Interacts with other factors to activate factor X in *intrinsic* cascade	Liver (vitamin-K dependent)
X	Stuart–Prower factor	Accelerates and amplifies prothrombin activation; point of *convergence* of *extrinsic* and *intrinsic* systems	Liver (vitamin-K dependent)
XI	Plasma thromboplastin antecedent	Activated by factor XII; accelerates thrombin formation in *intrinsic* cascade	Uncertain
XII	Hageman factor	Plasma factor activated by contact with negatively charged surfaces (collagen, glass, kaolin, fatty acids); activates factor XI to initiate *intrinsic cascade*	Uncertain
XIII	Fibrin stabilizing factor	Cross-links fibrin to make it stronger and less soluble	Liver

SOURCE: Adapted from Byrne CJ et al: *Laboratory Tests: Implications for Nursing Care*, 2nd ed. Menlo Park, CA: Addison–Wesley, 1986, p. 537–542; Vick RL: *Contemporary Medical Physiology*. Menlo Park, CA: Addison–Wesley, 1984, p. 392.

and eosinophils. These have similar stem-cell origins and contain granules that cause different staining reactions, which give them their names. Neutrophils stain a purplish hue; basophils, a bluish hue; and eosinophils, an orange color.

The neutrophils make up the largest number of the leukocytes and are most important to the body in defense against bacteria. Neutrophils include both a mature variety (segmented neutrophils, or segs) and an immature variety (bands). If not used by the body, bands mature to become segs. Neutrophils have the ability to phagocytize (engulf and digest) up to 25 bacteria before they die and are than phagocytized by larger macrophages. The number of neutrophils in the blood rises rapidly with the onset of bacterial infection, as does the WBC count. The differential count (a count of the number of each type of leukocyte in the blood) then demonstrates an increased percentage of segs and bands. An elevation of the percentage of bands above the normal level, referred to as a *shift to the left*, indicates the likelihood of a bacterial infection.

Neutrophils play an important role in the inflammatory response. Injured tissues and other leukocytes (basophils) are believed to secrete chemotactic substances that signal the bone marrow to release increased numbers of neutrophils, which squeeze out of the pores of capillaries (diapedesis) and move to the area where they are needed for phagocytosis.

Basophils are thought to prevent clotting in the microcirculation. They may also release histamine and inflammatory substances in infected tissue that are toxic to many microorganisms. The basophils also play a part in the allergic response because they secrete chemotactic substances that attract eosinophils.

The eosinophils also are involved in phagocytosis because they ingest antigen–antibody complexes. They also may be involved in allergic disorders, because their numbers increase during allergic reactions.

The agranular leukocytes consist of the monocytes and the lymphocytes. The monocytes have the ability to move into the tissues, where they become macrophages capable of phagocytosis. They also secrete a variety of substances involved in the body's defense and may play a role in the immune response.

The lymphocytes are agranular leukocytes that have attracted great interest since the advent of organ transplantation. They are formed in the hematopoietic organs, including the bone marrow, before birth, and migrate to a variety of body tissues before the birthing process begins. Lymphocytes continuously proliferate and travel throughout the body. Their cell division proceeds at much higher rates during invasion by viruses and foreign cells.

There are two kinds of lymphocytes: T-lymphocytes and B-lymphocytes. The T-lymphocytes travel from the bone marrow to the thymus before birth for storage, where they develop the ability to distinguish normal body tissue from foreign substances. T-lymphocytes are responsible for cellular immunity. They adhere to cells identified as foreign and secrete cytotoxic substances, killing the cells. The B-lymphocytes also migrate from the bone marrow before birth. The exact storage and processing place for B-lymphocytes in human beings is unknown. The B-lymphocytes are involved in humoral immunity; in the presence of an antigenic response, they produce antibodies. B-lymphocytes are also responsible for immunoglobulin production.

Both T-lymphocytes and B-lymphocytes can divide on stimulation by antigens, producing different types of cells such as memory cells, regulatory cells, and effector cells. Memory cells contain all the information from the lymphocyte that divided. Regulatory cells consist of the suppressor and helper cells, which either suppress or help the immune process and assist in the protection of the body. Effector cells are the T-lymphocyte killer cells and the B-lymphocyte plasma cells.

Regulatory Functions of the Cardiovascular System

The cardiovascular system needs a communications system to let it know how well it is performing its function. The vasomotor center located in the pons and medulla oblongata receives messages from the periphery and sends signals through the autonomic nervous system to the cardiovascular structures indicating what they are to do. These immediate adjustments are referred to as *autonomic reflexes.* To understand how these reflexes work, knowledge of the chemical mediators and the cardiovascular structural responses to them is necessary.

The postganglionic parasympathetic nerve fibers primarily secrete acetylcholine and are referred to as *cholinergic*. The postganglionic sympathetic nerve fibers, which secrete norepinephrine, are referred to as *adrenergic*. The sympathetic chemical transmitters to the sweat glands and a few blood vessels are cholinergic. (This helps explain why sweating is increased with strong sympathetic discharge.)

The heart is innervated by both parasympathetic and sympathetic nerve fibers. The parasympathetic fibers are primarily found in the atria, especially the S-A and A-V nodes. They are sparse in the ventricles. Parasympathetic stimulation to the heart results in a decreased heart rate (a negative chronotropic response) and decreased force of contraction (a negative inotropic response). The sympathetic fibers innervate the same areas as the parasympathetic fibers, but there is a greater number of sympathetic fibers in the ventricles. The heart responds to sympathetic stimulation by increasing its rate (a positive chronotropic response) and increasing its force of contraction (a positive inotropic response). Sympathetic stimulation increases metabolism in the heart and therefore creates the need for a greater blood supply.

The blood and blood vessels essentially respond to autonomic nervous system stimulation of the sympathetic nervous system. The blood responds to sympathetic stimulation by increasing coagulation. The blood vessels respond by either constricting or dilating. The capillaries neither constrict nor dilate in response to sympathetic stimulation.

The heart and blood vessels have two types of adrenergic receptors, alpha and beta. Blood vessels with alpha receptors constrict when stimulated by adrenergic chemicals, and those with beta receptors dilate when stimulated by adrenergic chemicals. This helps explain why some vessels (such as those in the abdomen and skin) constrict during strong sympathetic stimulation, whereas those in other areas (such as muscles) dilate.

The sympathetic nervous system affects the amount of blood circulating by influencing the heart rate and the force of cardiac contraction, as well as by changing the diameter of the blood vessels. These factors influence blood pressure and peripheral vascular resistance, which in turn affects blood flow. Several peripheral receptors send messages to the vasomotor center, which in turn promotes autonomic nervous system responses to regulate blood flow by influencing blood pressure. Some of these receptors are the baroreceptors, chemoreceptors, and atrial stretch receptors.

Baroreceptors are nerve receptors that respond to changes in blood pressure. This response is important to adjustments needed when changing positions, such as from lying to standing. The baroreceptors are stimulated by increases in blood pressure and send signals to the vasomotor center, which inhibits vasoconstriction and stimulates a parasympathetic response. This results in less vasoconstriction, a slower heart rate, less force of cardiac contraction, and lower blood pressure. When the blood pressure decreases, these receptors send fewer signals to the vasomotor center, which results in more vasoconstriction, increased heart rate, and a greater force of contraction, which raises blood pressure.

The baroreceptors are found in most of the large arteries in the chest and neck. Of greatest clinical importance are the baroreceptors in the bifurcation of the carotid artery. When the heart rate is very fast, this area may be massaged, stimulating the baroreceptors to send more signals to the vasomotor center, indicating that they sense the blood pressure to be very high. The vasomotor center responds by decreasing the heart rate.

Chemoreceptors sensitive to arterial oxygen, carbon dioxide, and hydrogen ion concentration are located in the carotid bifurcation (*carotid bodies*), and at the aortic arch (*aortic bodies*). When the hydrogen ion content is high, carbon dioxide content is high, and oxygen content is low, they send messages that excite the vasomotor center, resulting in sympathetic discharge in an effort to increase blood flow.

Stretch receptors in the atria send signals to the vasomotor center when the atrial pressure is high, indicating that blood is damming up in the heart. The vasomotor center responds by causing dilation of the peripheral arterioles, which results in less peripheral resistance and increases the ability of the heart to pump blood. When the arterioles to the kidney dilate, not only is renal filtration increased, but signals are sent to the hypothalamus, which results in a decreased secretion of antidiuretic hormone and a subsequent increase in urine production. This effectively decreases the circulating blood volume and subsequently decreases the blood pressure.

The vasomotor center responds with a powerful sympathetic response when it does not have enough blood supply (when the systolic blood pressure falls below 50 mm Hg); the response becomes stronger as the blood pressure is lowered below this point. This response is called the central nervous system ischemic response.

The activated sympathetic nervous system stimulates the adrenal medulla to secrete norepinephrine and epinephrine. These catecholamines have an effect on the blood vessels and heart that activates the sympathetic nervous system responses. Other organs, such as the kidneys and hypothalamus, also contribute their secretions to influence vasomotor activity.

This discussion has described responses to short-term changes in blood pressure. The receptors adapt as the blood pressure remains relatively stable over time (hours to days). The kidneys regulate longer term blood pressure and blood flow by regulating the body fluids.

Proper bone marrow function and hence integrity of the hematopoietic system are vital to the client's survival. Many factors have been identified that contribute to the regulation of hematopoiesis.

Erythropoiesis is influenced by the client's nutritional status, activity, age, chemical or radiation exposure, and drug therapy. Nutritional deficiencies in iron, vitamin B_{12}, and folic acid tend to decrease erythrocyte production and interfere with red cell maturation. Overall, the sedentary client has relatively less erythrocyte production. In the adult client, the sites of bone marrow activity are confined to the pelvis, sternum, ribs, cranium, and ends of the long bones and vertebral spine. This decrease in functional bone marrow mass may account in part for some of the anemias in the elderly population. Chemical and radiation overexposure may cause bone marrow damage and interfere with production of red cells, white cells, and platelets.

Tissue anoxia has been identified as causing an increase in erythropoiesis. Tissue anoxia stimulates the production of erythropoietin, a hormone made in the kidneys and liver. Erythropoietin stimulates the bone marrow to increase red cell production. Increases in altitude tend to increase erythrocyte production. At high altitudes, the amount of oxygen in the inspired air is diminished. This decrease in the amount of oxygen increases red cell production.

Drug therapy and chemical and radiation overexposure can influence the production of all blood cell components. Leukopenia may result in these situations. Leukocyte production is also influenced by chemotactic substances during an inflammatory response. These substances signal the bone marrow to increase the release of white cells necessary for a normal inflammatory response. Lymphocytes continuously travel throughout the body. Their proliferation is stimulated during the invasion of viruses and foreign substances (antigens).

SECTION 

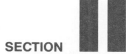

Pathophysiologic Influences and Effects

Any problem that interferes with an adequate blood supply (ischemia) may have serious consequences. Temporary ischemia may do no damage; however, the cells may not be able to perform their functions as well as usual. Continued ischemia injures the cells. The injury may be reversible if blood flow increases sufficiently to meet the tissue demands. If ischemia continues and irreversible damage occurs, the cells of the involved tissues or organs die. Tissue death is often referred to as *infarction, necrosis*, or *gangrene*.

The Heart

Within physiologic limits, the heart pumps all the blood that returns to it. The difference between the cardiac output at rest and the cardiac output when the physiologic limit is reached (which may be more than four times the resting state) is called the **cardiac reserve** and varies according to the condition of the heart and factors that may interfere with the heart's ability to pump effectively. When the physiologic limits are exceeded, heart failure results. When the cardiac reserve is used up, the body tissues become ischemic. The heart itself also becomes ischemic, which may result in injury or death to some of its tissues and a further reduction in its ability to pump blood.

Cardiac reserve is essential for adjustment to the normal changes in body activity and stresses that increase tissue demands, as well as for adjustment to changes in the environment. During increased activity, the tissue demands increase as the cells need more oxygen and nutrients to do their work. When the environmental temperature is low, the cells increase their metabolic rate to maintain body temperature and therefore need a greater blood supply. When the environmental temperature is high (especially when the humidity is high, reducing the effectiveness of sweating), blood is shunted to the skin to promote loss of body heat; this requires a greater cardiac output. Pregnancy, a normal physiologic process, requires a much greater cardiac output than the nonpregnant state.

Cardiac reserve is reduced by factors that increase the work load of the heart or decrease the heart's ability to pump blood. The work load of the heart increases when cardiac output increases and when the heart has to pump against increased resistance. Factors that decrease the heart's ability to pump blood include those that decrease blood return to the heart and the heart's ability to work.

Some disease conditions increase the tissue demands for oxygen and nutrients, resulting in increased cardiac output. Abnormal shunting of blood from arteries to veins requires an increase in cardiac output because the shunted blood does not meet tissue demands for nutrients. Another cause of increased cardiac output related to increased blood returning to the heart is *volume overload.* The increased blood volume may relate to increased fluid retention by the kidneys or overload of IV fluids.

The overall condition of the blood also affects cardiac output. Anemic states create a situation in which the blood is unable to carry enough oxygen and nutrients to meet cellular demands. Consequently, the cardiovascular system circulates the blood more often, increasing cardiac output. Increased output also may result from lack of availability of enough oxygen or nutrients for the blood to carry, as occurs in pulmonary disease, nutritional deficiencies, and liver disease.

Under some conditions, the heart pumps enough blood with each stroke, but some of it goes in the wrong direction. This happens with a ventricular septal defect after myocardial infarction, when blood is pumped from the left ventricle into both the aorta and right ventricle. The same situation exists with incompetent valves that do not close tightly, causing tricuspid, mitral, pulmonic, or aortic regurgitation. The heart has to pump the regurgitated blood again, increasing its work load.

When resistance to blood flow increases, the heart must create more pressure, increasing its work load and, subsequently, its need for more nutrients and a greater blood supply. When the resistance increases, the total amount the heart is capable of pumping diminishes, affecting the amount of cardiac reserve. A common condition that places additional strain on the left ventricle is diastolic hypertension. Other factors that increase the resistance against which the left ventricle has to pump include stenosis (narrowing) of the aortic valve or the narrowing of the blood vessels from conditions such as coarctation of the aorta and atherosclerosis. Increased pulmonary resistance, which is observed with some lung diseases and pulmonic stenosis, increases resistance for the right ventricle. Other conditions that cause resistance to blood flow through the pulmonary vessels include pulmonary emboli that block some of the vessels and increased viscosity of the blood.

Decreased blood return to the heart means the heart is unable to pump enough blood to meet the body's needs and possibly its own. Inadequate blood volume occurs with dehydration and massive hemorrhage. Mitral and tricuspid valvular stenosis inhibit ventricular filling during diastole and subsequently affect cardiac output. Disturbances in the heart's rhythm (**dysrhythmias** or arrhythmias) also may prevent the heart from having enough time to fill the ventricles completely. Inadequate blood supply to the myocardium as occurs in coronary artery disease decreases the heart's ability to pump blood and therefore reduces the cardiac reserve.

The Blood Vessels

Blood flow through the vessels depends on the vascular integrity and the ability of the blood vessels to perform their functions. To meet changing tissue demands for blood flow, the blood vessels must be able to change their diameters in response to normal local regulatory substances, temperature, vasoactive substances in the blood (eg, vasopressin, angiotensin, epinephrine), and the sympathetic nervous system. The arteries need to stretch during systole to accommodate the blood pumped from the heart and to recoil during diastole to move it on. The veins depend on muscular movement and the action of their valves to move the blood on. Disturbances in these functions result in the inability of the blood vessels to supply blood to the tissues properly, which results in ischemia.

Arterial Disorders

The blood vessels may lose integrity from trauma or disease processes that destroy their walls. The ultimate result is bleeding. If the vessel cannot contain the blood, it cannot fulfill its function to move the blood forward.

A common problem that inhibits the arteries' ability to stretch and recoil properly is atherosclerosis. In this disease process, atheromatous plaques, usually of lipid origin, develop in the tunica intima. Atheromatous plaques may become larger, progressively narrowing the arteries, causing atherosclerotic occlusive disease. As an artery narrows, it is unable to carry sufficient blood to the tissues it feeds, resulting in ischemia that may lead to tissue death. Sometimes an artery is able to handle enough blood during relative inactivity when tissue demands are low. When activity increases or tissue demands are higher, however, the narrowed artery is unable to accommodate enough blood flow, and the tissues become ischemic.

Some arterial obstruction results from inflammatory processes such as thromboangiitis obliterans, commonly called *Buerger's disease.* Diseases such as Raynaud's disease cause arterial spasms that decrease blood flow and may result in ischemia.

External pressures in excess of the arterial diastolic pressure inhibit arterial blood flow, and pressures that surpass the arterial systolic blood pressure stop blood flow through the artery. Common causes of obstruction to blood flow include tumors and swelling from injuries, such as burns. Clothing, bandages, or casts may tighten with swelling from bleeding or edema and obstruct blood flow. The constant weight of the body tissues on a vessel without intermittent relief of pressure may also obstruct blood flow.

Venous Disorders

The inability of the veins to move the blood on is called *venous insufficiency.* The most common cause is valves that do not function properly and promote damming up of blood in the veins. The hydrostatic pressure in the veins increases and causes edema in the tissues from which the blood empties into the involved vein. Complications of chronic venous insufficiency include thrombophlebitis, hemorrhage, stasis dermatitis, stasis cellulitis, and stasis ulcers.

Other factors that may inhibit venous flow, contribute to venous insufficiency, and result in edema include any event that causes enough pressure against the veins to inhibit blood flow. External pressure is commonly caused by garters or elastic used to hold stockings or socks up. Tumors or hematomas within the tissues may exert pressure against veins. Lack of the use of muscles that assist venous flow promotes venous stasis. Pressure on the veins from maintaining a constant position (eg, crossing the legs at the knees) also inhibits venous flow.

Embolus Formation

An *embolism* is the obstruction of a blood vessel by a blood clot or foreign substance such as air or fat. Emboli can occur in both the arteries and the veins. The most common type of embolus is a blood clot (thrombus) that forms in the heart or a blood vessel. The thrombus or a piece of it becomes dislodged and travels (then called a *thromboembolus*) until it gets to a vessel so small that it cannot move any farther; it then blocks any flow ahead of it. If the embolus is in a vein, it travels through larger and larger vessels until it arrives in the heart, where it moves through the right atrium and ventricle and into vessels in the lungs, which get smaller and smaller. When the embolus reaches a pulmonary vessel too small for it to pass through, it stops. It is then called a *pulmonary embolus.* When a blood clot breaks off in the left side of the heart or an artery, the thromboembolus travels through smaller and smaller arteries. When it comes to one smaller than itself, it stops and obstructs the blood flow ahead of it. The artery in which it stops may be anywhere in the systemic circulation (the brain, the legs, the arms, or the internal organs). The ultimate result may be death to the tissues ahead of it. Other types of emboli include fat, air, cholesterol, and pieces of tumors.

The Lymphatic System

The lymphatics remove fluid and particulate matter such as proteins and organisms from the interstitial spaces; carry these substances, which form the lymph, through the lymphatic vessels and into the lymph nodes for digestion by phagocytic cells; and return the processed lymph to the circulatory system. When the net amount of fluid remaining in the interstitial spaces exceeds the capability of the lymphatic vessels to remove it, edema results. Edema also may result from increased venous pressure when lymphatic drainage is normal. It also occurs with normal venous pressure if the lymphatics are diseased. Edema that results from improper function of the lymphatics is called **lymphedema.**

The lymphatics may function improperly because of primary or secondary problems. Primary lymphedema results from lack of formation of lymphatic vessels or distortion of the vessels. Secondary lymphedema is caused by the obstruction or surgical removal of the lymphatic vessels. Obstruction most commonly results from the pressure of tumors or from infections. Inflamed lymphatic vessels occur in **lymphangitis.** When the lymph nodes are involved and become swollen, the condition is called **lymphadenopathy.** In **lymphadenitis** the involved lymph nodes are inflamed.

The Bone Marrow

The bone marrow is a delicate organ and must be healthy to function properly. Bone marrow function is influenced by many internal and external factors. Internal factors include the client's age and nutritional status. External factors influencing normal hematopoiesis are chemical exposure, radiation exposure, and drug therapy. Overexposure can cause bone marrow suppression or failure, depending on the kind of agent the client is exposed to, the dose of the agent delivered during exposure, and the length of exposure. Any of these factors can disrupt the normal production of leukocytes, erythrocytes, and thrombocytes, making the client prone to infection, alteration in the oxygen-carrying capacity of the blood, and bleeding.

The Blood

The major purpose of the erythrocytes is to carry hemoglobin and subsequently oxygen to the capillaries for diffusion into the cells. Any condition that decreases the amount of hemoglobin, the number of erythrocytes, or the ability of the erythrocytes to flow through the capillaries decreases the oxygen supply to the tissues and may result in ischemia. In polycythemia the blood becomes viscous and cannot flow easily. This condition is caused by the bone marrow's high output of erythrocytes in response to tissue hypoxia. Anemia, a decrease in the number of erythrocytes or their ability to carry oxygen, may result from the inability of the bone marrow to produce enough erythrocytes, conditions that promote the rapid destruction of erythrocytes, or loss of blood through hemorrhage. Abnormalities of the erythrocytes that reduce their ability to carry oxygen include insufficient nutrients (such as vitamins and iron) or abnormal genetic material resulting in the production of defective erythrocytes or synthesis of abnormal hemoglobin.

The thrombocytes are necessary for blood to clot properly. Increased thrombocyte production is called *thrombocytosis*, and decreased or defective thrombocyte production is called *thrombocytopenia*. When thrombocytes are insufficient or defective, the client has an increased potential for bleeding.

The leukocytes protect the body from invasion by pathogenic organisms through phagocytosis and the immune response. The number of leukocytes normally increases (leukocytosis) in response to infection or tissue destruction. When a particular type of leukocyte increases in number, the condition is named according to cell type (eg, granulocytosis, neutrophilia). A decrease in the number of leukocytes (leukopenia) results in the inability of the body to defend itself against invasion of pathogenic organisms. This condition also is named by cell type (eg, agranulocytosis, lymphopenia). Disorders in leukocyte production and maturation make the client prone to overwhelming infection by invading microorganisms.

SECTION 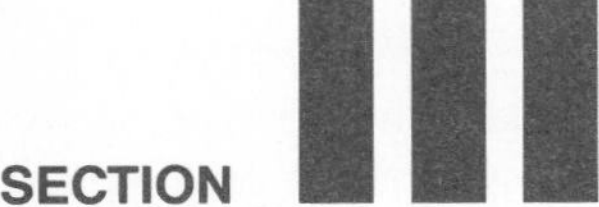

Related System Influences and Effects

All systems of the body rely on the cardiovascular system and blood-forming organs to supply them with the blood needed to perform their functions. Thus, a problem with the cardiovascular or blood-forming system may result in devastating consequences for the other systems. The other body systems also influence the ability of the cardiovascular and blood-forming systems to perform their functions.

Without a healthy nervous system, the blood vessels would not be able to respond to changes in a person's activity and position. The baroreceptors, as well as the other reflexes discussed earlier in the chapter, would not transmit messages to meet the moment-to-moment need for changes in blood flow. The temperature regulatory function of the cardiovascular system depends on communication between the vasomotor center and the hypothalamus, as well as the integrity of the skin.

The cardiovascular system depends on the respiratory system to make the necessary oxygen available to be picked up and to remove carbon dioxide from the blood. Without the necessary oxygen, the cardiovascular system would not be able to meet tissue needs. Lung-related problems may also increase the work of the heart, because they may promote increased resistance to blood flow as the heart responds to tissue hypoxia.

The cardiovascular system would not be able to pick up and deliver nutrients necessary for cellular function without proper intake of food and water and proper function of the gastrointestinal tract or the liver in metabolism (in processing and storing nutrients, as well as secreting substances necessary for digestion). Without the liver's role in the formation of blood-clotting factors, the integrity of the cardiovascular system would not be sustained.

The blood must be relatively free of waste products to provide the proper environment for the cells. Cellular health depends on the ability of the liver and kidneys to excrete waste products. In addition, the failure of the kidneys to excrete excess water—whether due to a problem with the kidneys, hypothalamus, or pituitary gland—would result in circulatory overload.

The musculoskeletal system must function properly to maintain the muscular activity that returns blood to the heart for recirculation. Healthy bones are essential to the ability of the bone marrow to produce blood cells.

The endocrine system, through its hormones, affects metabolism. The pituitary gland which secretes antidiuretic hormone and the adrenal glands which secrete aldosterone affect the cardiovascular system by regulating water and sodium balance. The adrenal glands are important in the secretion of epinephrine and norepinephrine in times of need to assist the sympathetic nervous system in promoting vasoconstriction.

SECTION 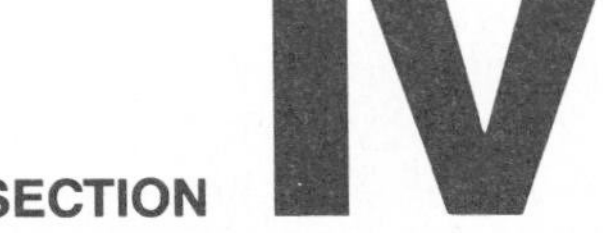

Psychosocial/Lifestyle Influences and Effects

A major physiologic problem caused by a disorder of the cardiovascular system, the blood, or the blood-forming organs is the inability to provide adequate nutrients to the cells. This disorder generally results in the client's need to reduce the metabolic demands of the body by decreasing activity levels. The adjustment to decreased activity may be temporary until the disease process is resolved, or it may involve a permanent change in lifestyle. A decrease in activity may not be compatible with the client's responsibilities for home or career. For some persons, a planned exercise program as part of rehabilitation also may be difficult.

Clients encounter other major physiologic problems with leukopenia and thrombocytopenia. The client with leukopenia must take special precautions to prevent infection. Once established, infection can be fatal; therefore, client education should be geared toward prevention. Clients may need to change their usual routine, especially during periodic leukopenic episodes. The client may need to avoid crowds or people with upper respiratory tract infections. Even a simple trip to the grocery store may be contraindicated during leukopenic episodes. The client and family or significant others may find this difficult to cope with.

Thrombocytopenia has its own set of restrictions to which the client must adjust. The client must be knowledgeable about measures to prevent serious bleeding episodes during thrombocytopenic periods. Lack of knowledge about the prevention of infection or bleeding episodes may make the client more prone to developing these complications. Decreasing the likelihood of these complications necessitates that clients take responsibility for learning about their disease processes and treatments. Taking responsibility for their own health care may be too stressful for some clients, however.

Adjustments may be needed in nutritional needs. Taking medications also may create an adjustment problem for some. Together, the changes in activity level, the changes in nutritional habits, the need to take medications, and the added responsibility of learning about a disease process and its treatment require adjustments in developmental and cultural aspects of living.

The nurse as counselor should assist clients by discussing their lifestyles in relation to the effects on the cardiovascular and blood-forming organs. Studies have shown that the level of compliance in both preventive and curative situations is low. A review of the literature by Dracup and Meleis (1982) found that about one-third to one-half of all clients studied did not follow suggested positive health practices. Even though not all clients will respond to recommendations, they all have the right to information so they can make informed decisions about lifestyle changes.

Developmental Influences

Developmental tasks that adults must perform include those related to their vocational, family, home, social, and leisure time responsibilities. Depending on the capabilities of the cardiovascular system and blood-forming organs, clients may need to make some changes in these responsibilities. Discuss the possibility of the client's returning to work. The need for alterations in activities of daily living to accomplish the responsibilities in the home also should be explored.

Activities such as family outings, sporting activities, and shopping trips may be physiologically too stressful or may put the client at an increased risk for developing serious infections if there is bone marrow dysfunction. Some changes may also be needed in living arrangements (eg, too many stairs to climb).

Discuss community activities in relation to the need for energy expenditure and the possible risk of infection. Some activities, such as being a volunteer fire fighter or participating in preparing dinners and bake sales, may be stressful to the cardiovascular and blood-forming systems and may need to be eliminated. Others, such as making telephone calls or stuffing envelopes for an organization, may be acceptable.

Leisure time activities also should be considered. Some persons use their leisure time in sedentary activities and may need to make no adjustments during the recovery period. Others who participate in activities requiring a high energy expenditure (eg, skiing and camping) may have difficulty adjusting. Some persons who have no hobbies or leisure time activities find having time on their hands stressful.

Sometimes eliminating an activity may be more stressful to the client than establishing a new leisure regimen. Probably the most important issue in counseling the client about a change in activity level is the importance the activity has for the client. Counseling may help clients decide what is most important for them. Some activities may need to be eliminated, some may be continued if they are spaced, and some may need no adjustment at all.

Cultural Influences

What a person believes is important plays a significant role in the development of cardiovascular disease as well as in his or her compliance with rehabilitation and treatment for both cardiovascular and blood disorders. Emotional stress has a physiologic effect on heart rate, blood pressure, and respiration. The extent to which a person is stressed and the effect of the stressor is related to its significance to the individual. The culture in which a person lives greatly determines the significance of emotional and physiologic stressors. The importance a person places on family, work, eating, social activities, and health care is related to cultural values.

Dietary Factors

Diet is important in all diseases. Without the proper nutrients, the cells cannot function properly. Certain dietary habits are associated with cardiovascular disease. A high blood cholesterol level has been determined to be a major risk factor in the development of atherosclerosis. Clients can control high cholesterol levels by changing to a diet low in saturated fat and cholesterol. Being overweight is a problem for many. Changing the dietary habits of one member of the family usually effects changes in the diets of others as well, which may place stress on the entire family. Dietary changes also have the potential for improving the entire family's health.

Economic and Occupational Factors

Changes in diet, occupation, activity level, and living arrangements, as well as the need for medication and the cost of health care may cause a severe economic burden for the client and family. In addition, persons with cardiovascular or blood disorders may have difficulty obtaining insurance because they pose a greater economic risk for health and life insurance companies than the general population. Consequently, insurance costs may be prohibitive, but the lack of insurance reduces economic security and brings more stress.

The client with a cardiovascular or blood disease may or may not be able to return to work. Job requirements may need to be adjusted, which can produce stress between the client and peers over work load. Workmen's compensation insurance may be available if the cardiovascular problem is related to the job. In cases of complete disability, the client may be eligible for Social Security compensation.

Environmental Factors

Environmental threats to the person with cardiovascular and blood problems include terrain and climate. Walking up an incline requires much more energy expenditure than walking on level ground. Environmental temperature extremes place an additional burden on the cardiovascular and blood systems. Cold temperature promotes vasoconstriction and shivering to generate body heat, and a person with an already diminished blood flow may experience ischemia. Shivering increases the metabolic needs and cardiac output. Hot temperature promotes dilation of the vessels near the skin, which also requires an increased cardiac output.

Sexual Expression

Clients with angina and those recovering from myocardial infarction or coronary artery bypass surgery often have fears about the resumption of sexual activity. The spouse may also be anxious, which can interfere with a satisfying intimate relationship. Males with hypertension may be taking antihypertensive medications that cause impotence, failure to ejaculate, or decreased libido.

Nursing Research Note

Sloan R: Achieving compliance to a reduced sodium diet. *Nurse Pract* (Feb) 1985; 10:25–26.

This research describes use of urinary chloride titrator sticks to evaluate client compliance to low-sodium diets, often prescribed in the treatment of hypertension. Test subjects were taught to use the chloride sticks on first morning urine specimens. Readings greater than +2 indicated noncompliance to sodium restrictions. Readings less than +2 demonstrated adherence to a dietary sodium intake of less than 85 mEq/day or a 2-g sodium restriction. Results suggest that with dietary instruction and use of chloride sticks, clients were able to adjust daily salt intake and monitor their own dietary restrictions with greater accuracy.

Chloride sticks may be an effective tool for nursing intervention. Results of daily chloride stick use can provide feedback to both the nurse and the client.

The nurse can be instrumental in identifying clients who have been unable to resume a satisfying sexual relationship because of fear of worsening their cardiac status or those with sexual dysfunction resulting from drug therapy. Careful history taking and a sensitive approach can pave the way for identifying sexual problems for which nursing interventions may be applied.

Chapter Highlights

The purpose of the cardiovascular system is to supply the body tissues with the nutrients and other substances they need, remove the waste products from the cellular environment, and circulate body defense substances.

Because of their elasticity and recoil, the arteries are able to continue blood flow during ventricular diastole.

The exchange of substances between the blood vessels and the interstitial spaces occurs in the capillaries.

The veins are capacitance vessels that serve as a reservoir for blood.

The erythrocytes carry oxygen to the cells.

The thrombocytes (platelets) are essential to the blood-clotting mechanism and clot retraction.

The granulocytes (neutrophils, basophils, and eosinophils) are primarily involved in phagocytosis.

The agranular leukocytes (monocytes and lymphocytes) are primarily involved in the immune response.

The autonomic nervous system influences heart rate and contraction. Parasympathetic activity speeds it up.

The sympathetic nervous system controls the diameter of the blood vessels. Some vessels dilate and some constrict in response to sympathetic activity.

The baroreceptors, chemoreceptors, and atrial stretch receptors monitor moment-to-moment changes in blood pressure and communicate with the vasomotor center.

Inadequate blood supply or decreased quality of the blood may produce ischemia of the cells, which in turn may lead to cellular death.

All the body systems depend on the cardiovascular system and blood-forming organs to supply their needs.

A problem with another body system will ultimately affect the cardiovascular and blood-forming systems.

An individual's lifestyle may contribute to the development of cardiovascular disease, and persons with cardiovascular problems may need to make changes in their lifestyles.

After a major cardiac event, both the client and sexual partner may be fearful about resuming sexual activity.

Bibliography

Byrne CJ et al: *Laboratory Tests: Implications for Nursing Care*, 2nd ed. Menlo Park, CA: Addison–Wesley, 1986.

Chesnewy MA, Rosenman RH: Type A behavior: Observation on the past decade. *Heart Lung* 1982; 11:12–19.

Conroy KM: Anergy: The hidden danger. *Heart Lung* 1982; 11:85–92.

Dracup KA, Meleis AI: Compliance: An interactionist approach. *Nurs Res* 1982; 31:31–36.

Erickson R: Tube talk: Principles of fluid flow in tubes. *Nurs 82* (July) 1982; 12:54–61.

Glenn WL et al: *Thoracic and Cardiovascular Surgery*, 2nd ed. Norwalk, CT: Appleton–Century–Crofts, 1983.

Heart Facts 1983. Dallas: American Heart Association, 1982.

Hurst JW et al: *The Heart*, 5th ed. New York: McGraw–Hill, 1982.

King NH: Controlling bleeding when the platelet count drops. *RN* (Aug) 1984; 47(8):25–27.

Mansen TJ: Does that CBC spell trouble? *RN* (July) 1984; 47(7):48–51.

Saxton DF et al: *The Addison–Wesley Manual of Nursing Practice*. Menlo Park, CA: Addison–Wesley, 1983.

Spittell JA (editor): *Clinical Vascular Disease*. Philadelphia: Davis, 1983.

Stites DP et al: *Clinical Immunology*, 4th ed. Los Altos, CA: Lange, 1982.

Williams WJ et al: *Hematology*, 3rd ed. New York: McGraw–Hill, 1983.

CHAPTER **18**

The Nursing Process for Clients With Cardiac Dysfunction

> Other topics relevant to this content are: The health history and physical assessment, **Chapter 5;** Nursing care of clients with cardiac disorders, **Chapter 19;** Nursing care of clients undergoing cardiac surgery, **Chapter 19.**

Objectives

When you have finished studying this chapter, you should be able to:

Specify the major components of the health history to be obtained from clients with cardiovascular disease.

Identify risk factors for cardiovascular disease.

Explain specific assessment approaches in evaluating clients with dysfunction of the cardiovascular system.

Identify the nursing implications of diagnostic studies commonly used to evaluate clients with cardiovascular dysfunction.

Determine appropriate nursing diagnoses for clients with disorders of the cardiovascular system.

Develop, with the client, realistic goals of care.

Anticipate the psychosocial/lifestyle implications of cardiovascular dysfunction on clients and their significant others.

Develop a nursing care plan for a client with cardiovascular dysfunction.

Implement nursing interventions specific to clients with cardiovascular disease.

Evaluate the effectiveness of the nursing care plan and modify it as necessary to meet client needs.

This chapter discusses the information to be obtained in a cardiovascular history, physical assessment of the cardiovascular system, and the common diagnostic tests used. The nursing diagnoses specific to clients with cardiovascular dysfunction, related nursing care, and the evaluation of care are discussed in Section II. A sample nursing care plan is included.

SECTION 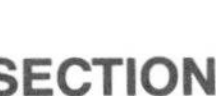

Nursing Assessment: Establishing the Data Base

Subjective Data

Obtaining a cardiovascular health history from the client is the first and most important step in cardiovascular assessment. Selection of diagnostic tests, interpretation of test results, and prescription of therapy all depend on the client's history. Most clients fear heart disease and often understate their symptoms. By carefully observing their nonverbal gestures, their reactions to questions, the words they use to describe symptoms, and their overall attitudes, the nurse can evaluate clients' emotional responses. Assessment of clients' emotional support systems is also beneficial, especially if invasive procedures must be performed or long-term disability is a possible outcome. Taking the time to get to know both clients and their families or significant others helps the nurse to correlate behavioral and emotional factors with the onset of cardiac symptoms.

The principal symptoms of heart disease are dyspnea, chest pain, palpitation, and syncope. Other common symptoms are fatigue and cough. The nurse should attempt to gain information about these symptoms, evaluating them according to the level of activity that precipitates the symptom. Clients may not experience any problems with minimal activity, but the symptoms may appear with exertion. This is the classic situation with cardiovascular dysfunction.

Dyspnea

Dyspnea, the most common symptom of both cardiac and pulmonary disease, is the condition of difficult or labored breathing. Clients report that it is difficult to breathe, that there is not enough air, or that they become short of breath with any activity. In heart disease, the dyspnea usually occurs with exertion: Clients cannot seem to get enough air into their lungs. In pulmonary disease, the dyspnea occurs both at rest and with exertion, and clients feel more difficulty during exhalation. The differentiation between cardiac and pulmonary dyspnea is difficult; the two diseases often coexist.

Dyspnea should be evaluated in relation to the extent of activity it takes to bring on the symptom. Ask clients if they can perform their normal daily activities without difficulty in breathing. If they have no problems with these activities, ascertain the highest level of activity they can attain without dyspnea (eg, the ability to climb two but not three flights of stairs without difficulty). Dyspnea associated with exertion is known as dyspnea on exertion (DOE). DOE is an early symptom of congestive heart failure (CHF).

PAROXYSMAL NOCTURNAL DYSPNEA **Paroxysmal nocturnal dyspnea** (PND) comes on during sleep. The client awakens suddenly, breathing with difficulty and having a sensation of suffocation. This usually occurs 2 to 5 hours after the onset of sleep and happens only once during the night.

PND occurs in clients with CHF and is due to pump failure of the left ventricle, which leads to fluid accumulation in the lungs. PND is relieved by sitting upright with legs over the side of the bed or by walking around the room. It usually subsides within 20 minutes without aftereffects, and the client can sleep the remainder of the night.

ORTHOPNEA **Orthopnea** is the form of dyspnea that develops when the client lies down. It is relieved within minutes by sitting up or standing. The client uses several pillows at night to elevate the head and prevent nocturnal breathlessness. In fact, the severity of the condition is often measured by the number of pillows the client needs. As heart disease advances and CHF progresses, the number of pillows required to provide relief increases. In severe heart failure, the client is unable to lie down and usually sleeps in a chair. To obtain information about this symptom, ask the client, "How well do you sleep?" Find out how many pillows the client normally uses and whether the number of pillows has increased to provide breathing comfort during the night.

Chest Pain

By far the most frightening cardiovascular symptom is chest pain. Because chest pain may have a variety of causes, the main objective in evaluating chest pain is to determine the origin. The most common origins are cardiac, pleuropulmonary, musculoskeletal, gastric, or psychosomatic. Pain originating from the heart is due to **ischemia** (deficiency of blood due to a constricted or obstructed blood vessel). Ischemic pain is referred to as either angina or myocardial infarction (MI) pain. The diagnosis depends on the client's history and subsequent physical examination.

The most serious cause of chest pain is pain from an MI. This cause should be considered first and, when the diagnosis of MI is ruled out, then questioning can be directed to other causes. When obtaining information about chest pain, assess the following aspects: the onset, location, radiation, duration, quality, alleviating and aggravating factors, and associated symptoms (see Chapter 5).

Chest pain due to MI is often described as a crushing substernal pain. The client may say, "It felt as if a ton of bricks was on my chest." A common gesture clients use is a tight fist over the center of the chest. The pain is usually associated with dyspnea, diaphoresis, and (less frequently) nausea and vomiting. The onset is acute and not associated with a precipitating event. The pain lasts longer than 5 minutes; nothing relieves it. Often, the pain radiates to the left arm, into the neck, or to the jaw and teeth. Occasionally, the client may have pain radiating into the right arm.

Like MI pain, angina is a constricting, pressure type of pain. Angina differs from the pain of an MI in that it is episodic and temporary, usually lasting less than 5 minutes. Also, the onset is associated with exertion, emotion, eating, or exposure to cold. Acute episodes are relieved by nitroglycerin and/or rest. For long-term management, angina is controlled by other cardiac medications, usually a beta-adrenergic inhibitor. If angina is uncontrollable and the client is unable to maintain an adequate lifestyle, coronary bypass surgery may be required.

Other serious causes of chest pain are pulmonary embolus and dissecting aortic aneurysm. Pain from a pulmonary embolus is described as knifelike shooting pain. The pain increases with inspiration and is often associated with a sudden onset of dyspnea, tachycardia, hypotension, diaphoresis, rales, and hemoptysis.

Pain from a dissecting aortic aneurysm is characterized as a sudden, tearing, intense chest pain with radiation to the back, flanks, and legs. Usually, the client has a history of hypertension.

Chest pain well localized to a specific area of the chest wall is usually due to a musculoskeletal problem. Tenderness in response to palpation is often present. An example is chest pain due to inflammation of the costochondral junctions of the ribs and sternum.

Stress and anxiety may also cause chest pain. This type of pain is usually localized in the left chest wall and does not radiate. The history assists in determining whether the chest pain is related to stress and anxiety.

Palpitation

Palpitation is an unpleasant awareness of the heartbeat. The client often describes a fluttering feeling in the chest or says that the heart seems to jump, race, pound, stop, or skip beats. Palpitations are most often due to rhythm disturbances such as premature contractions, atrial fibrillation, or sinus tachycardia. A variety of causes produces rhythm disturbances, however. Anxiety, stress, fatigue, or cardiac stimulants such as caffeine and nicotine are factors that precipitate palpitations. Detailed questions about the onset, relation to exercise, presence of associated symptoms such as shortness of breath or syncope, relieving factors such as stooping or breathholding assist in determining the significance of the palpitation. Drug toxicity may also cause palpitations. Therefore, a medication history, which includes asking *how* the client takes the medication, is necessary.

Syncope

Syncope, a transient loss of consciousness, is associated with muscle weakness and an inability to stand. It is due to inadequate blood flow to the brain, which may be a result of a cardiac rhythm disturbance or decreased cardiac output from valvular disease. Dizziness with an inability to maintain an upright posture is referred to as *near syncope.* The client should describe the circumstances that lead to dizziness or fainting. Syncope that occurs with exercise may be related to aortic or subaortic valve stenosis. This condition is serious and requires further documentation, usually through noninvasive testing.

A sudden loss of consciousness due to a heart block is known as a Stokes–Adams attack. This type of syncope commonly occurs in elderly clients and is followed by breathlessness and absence of pulse, usually lasting only seconds. Cardiac arrest may occur if respiration and circulation are not restored.

The elderly client may also develop another type of syncope caused by hypersensitivity of the carotid sinus bodies. The carotid sinus bodies are located in the carotid artery below the jawline. Pressure applied to the carotid artery may stimulate a vagal response that decreases the blood pressure and heart rate; exaggerated vagal response may produce syncope. The client may report episodes of fainting while shaving or buttoning a tight collar. Digitalis appears to increase carotid sinus sensitivity, making the client susceptible to syncope. Bilateral palpation of the carotids should never be performed.

Fatigue

Fatigue is a frequent concern of clients suffering from cardiovascular dysfunction. Clients describe muscle weakness and an inability to complete normal daily activities. They often need one to two naps a day to function. The fatigue is probably related to a combination of physical and emotional factors. Physically, the fatigue is thought to be related to insufficient blood flow to the tissues, the result of inadequate cardiac output. Depression may also cause fatigue. Fatigue is assessed by the level of activity tolerance.

Cough

Cough associated with cardiovascular disease is due to fluid accumulation in the lungs. The cough is described as dry, irritating, spasmodic, and nocturnal. Clients may cough after episodes of dyspnea. A productive cough with colored sputum may indicate a pulmonary problem.

Psychosocial Response

The heart's functioning is associated with life itself. A serious disruption of cardiovascular function can be a significant emotional and physical threat. The onset of heart disease is often considered a major life crisis. The life of a client who has a cardiac event (eg, an MI or cardiac surgery) may be either immediately threatened or altered. Survival cannot be guaranteed; former support systems may be diminished; roles as spouse, parent, and worker may be interrupted; and future plans often need revision. Central to this crisis is the fear of death, pain, disability, and physical dependence. Most clients respond to these fears by developing anxiety.

Anxiety can be manifested through a variety of physical, emotional, and behavioral responses. In cardiovascular assessment, it is important to appreciate that the physical responses to anxiety are similar to those of cardiovascular dysfunction: tachycardia, increased blood pressure and respiratory rate, fatigue, diaphoresis, or palpitations. Emotional and behavioral responses may include fear, apprehension, nervousness, crying, irritability, or withdrawal.

Anxiety may also be a result of the client's assessment of personal body image. An acute event poses a great threat to body integrity and function. The personal meaning of the heart to the client and the impact of the event on body image will greatly influence the client's convalescence. Client role responsibilities, knowledge of the severity of the disease, and the reaction of significant others are important components to assess.

To cope with anxiety and fear, the client may use denial. In the acute care setting, denial is used for defensive coping and serves to protect the client from perceived threats. As an effective coping mechanism decreasing the physical and emotional outcomes of anxiety, denial is beneficial in the acute phase of illness. Sustained denial, however, is maladaptive. The nurse must assist the client in identifying effective coping mechanisms.

Past Health History

After obtaining information about the client's symptoms, review the client's past health history, paying particular attention to information about previous hospitalization for cardiac problems. Ask the client whether any episodes of chest pain resulted in hospitalization. If cardiac surgery was performed, document the date, the type of surgery, number of bypasses, and any complications. If valvular surgery was performed, include the type of valve used (eg, porcine, ball and cage, or tilting disk). If a cardiac pacemaker was implanted, the client should know the type and have the model number available. Previous diagnostic procedures performed, such as ECGs, exercise stress testing, or cardiac catheterizations, add to the client's history.

Certain childhood diseases predispose the client to cardiovascular dysfunction. Childhood rheumatic fever can cause valvular disease that becomes evident in adulthood. Untreated streptococcal throat infections may also cause valvular disease. Maternal exposure to rubella in the first 2 months of pregnancy is associated with congenital heart defects. Many children who have had corrective surgery for congenital heart defects are now living through adulthood; therefore, information regarding the childhood cardiac problem should be obtained.

Medication and Dietary History

A medication history including prescribed and over-the-counter (OTC) medications should be obtained. OTC drugs may precipitate cardiac symptoms. Many antihistamines, decongestants, and antitussives contain sympathomimetic amines, which may cause palpitations or transient hypertension. Some antacid preparations contain large amounts of sodium, which may cause fluid retention and subsequent increase in blood pressure. If the client is taking a prescribed medicine, ask how the client is taking it, specifying the time of day and the amount.

A dietary history assists the nurse in evaluating the client's understanding of the relation between food and heart disease. Assess the eating of red meat, salt, dairy products, and sugar and estimate caloric intake. Evaluate the client's weight compared with the recommended ideal weight.

Risk Factors

An important component in cardiovascular assessment is evaluating the client's cardiovascular risk factor profile. Risk factors are personal characteristics and habits that increase the client's chances of developing coronary artery disease (CAD). The risk factors are divided into unalterable and alterable factors. The unalterable risk factors are sex (male) and a family history of heart disease or hypertension. Alterable risk factors include hypercholesterolemia, smoking, diabetes mellitus, obesity, physical inactivity, and oral contraceptive use. Personality may also contribute to CAD. A behavior pattern called type A behavior, characterized as competitive, compulsive, hard driving, and time oriented has been associated with twice the normal risk of developing CAD. The most prominent risk factors are hypertension, a high blood cholesterol level, and cigarette smoking.

Table 18–1
Classification for Diastolic and Systolic Hypertension

Diastolic Blood Pressure (mm Hg)	Category
<85	Normal blood pressure
85 to 89	High normal blood pressure
90 to 104	Mild hypertension
105 to 114	Moderate hypertension
≥115	Severe hypertension
Systolic blood pressure (mm Hg); when DBP <90 mm Hg	
<140	Normal blood pressure
140 to 159	Borderline isolated systolic hypertension
≥160	Isolated systolic hypertension

SOURCE: Reprinted from *1984 Report of the Joint National Committee on Detection, Evaluation, and Treatment of High Blood Pressure*. US Department of Health and Human Services. NIH Publication No 84-1088, June 1984.

HYPERTENSION Unequivocally, hypertension, either systolic or diastolic, increases the risk of developing CAD; the higher the blood pressure, the greater the risk. Hypertension causes coronary, cerebral, and renal vascular disease. It is the leading cause of death and disability among adults. The standard most often used to establish a diagnosis of diastolic or systolic hypertension is given in Table 18–1.

Symptoms often attributed to hypertension include headache, epistaxis, tinnitus, dizziness, and fainting. Unfortunately, uncomplicated hypertension is usually asymptomatic until significant organ damage occurs. Therefore, frequent screening is required.

CHOLESTEROL In evaluating cholesterol, ask about the client's previous history of elevated cholesterol levels and the therapeutic and preventive regimens the client is following. Ascertain how much the client knows about the role of cholesterol in developing CAD and whether the client understands the role of diet, exercise, and weight in controlling cholesterol levels. A diet low in saturated fats, high in polyunsaturated fats, and low in cholesterol is beneficial. A reduction in calories is usually recommended, especially if the client is overweight. Aerobic exercise appears to increase the high-density lipoprotein (HDL) levels, which appear to retard the development of CAD (see Diagnostic Studies). The optimal goal of client management is to achieve a serum cholesterol level below 200 mg/dL with a level of HDL higher than low-density lipoprotein

Table 18–2
Cholesterol Values for Adults at Moderate or High Risk of Heart Disease

Age	Moderate Risk	High Risk
20–29	⩾ 200 mg/dL	⩾ 220 mg/dL
30–39	⩾ 220 mg/dL	⩾ 240 mg/dL
40 and over	⩾ 240 mg/dL	⩾ 260 mg/dL

SOURCE: Reprinted from National Institutes of Health: *Lipid Research Clinics Population Study Data*. Vol. I, NIH Publication No. 80–1527, July 1980.

(LDL). Values for adults at moderate or high risk of heart disease according to age and cholesterol level are shown in Table 18–2. The client should limit the daily intake of cholesterol to less than 300 mg/day.

SMOKING The principal cause of death in cigarette smokers is CAD, not lung cancer. The risk is directly related to the number of cigarettes smoked per day. Smoking a pack or more a day increases the risk of heart disease at least threefold. How long smokers have been smoking and whether they inhale smoke do not appear to be significant. The risk can be reduced by discontinuing smoking. Within a year, the former smoker has the same risk as the non-smoker. The client should understand this encouraging fact.

When cigarette smoking is combined with oral contraceptives, the risk of CAD and MI is extremely high. Smokers who have hypertension and/or diabetes mellitus are also at greater risk.

After explaining the effect of cigarette smoking, offer the client assistance in smoking cessation. Group classes are effective, but if the client prefers individual help, the American Lung Association provides a written program. The health care provider should carefully review this program with the client. Informing the client of other community resources increases the client's chances of smoking cessation.

PHYSICAL INACTIVITY Exercise appears to be effective in preventing CAD by reducing other risk factors such as stress, obesity, and elevated cholesterol levels. Physically fit individuals are more likely to survive a cardiac event than sedentary individuals.

Clients should be encouraged to incorporate exercise into their lifestyle as a routine. Walking is usually recommended as an easy type of exercise that can be done anywhere. The amount and duration of exercise are prescribed *after* clients undergo a complete history and physical examination.

ALCOHOL AND CAFFEINE USE Excessive alcohol consumption causes an increase in serum lipid levels and caloric intake. Both effects contribute to CAD. A moderate consumption of alcohol (one glass of wine per day) has been associated with increased HDL levels, which may be positive. Documentation of the alcohol intake should include the client's pattern of drinking as well as the amount and type of alcohol consumed.

Caffeine is a cardiovascular stimulant causing tachycardia and dysrhythmias. It may contribute to other risk factors such as hypertension. Determine the client's intake of caffeine including coffee, tea, chocolate, and carbonated soft drinks. More than 16 oz per day is often considered excessive. Some clients who are especially sensitive to caffeine may experience symptoms with lesser amounts.

Objective Data

Physical Assessment

The physical assessment of the cardiovascular system begins with a general examination of the client. Whereas cardiac dysfunction may directly affect other body systems, systemic illnesses often have cardiac manifestations. For these reasons, a thorough examination of the client is necessary.

First, observe the general appearance of the client—physical build, skin color, pallor or cyanosis—and the client's emotional status. Assess whether the client appears to be in pain. The client experiencing pain may have overt signs. Typically, the client with angina sits quietly, whereas the client with acute MI pain is uncomfortable and moves continuously. With pericarditis, the client assumes a sitting position, leaning forward.

Tall clients with long extremities and arm spans exceeding their height may have Marfan's syndrome, which is associated with a variety of cardiac disorders. Note chest contour: Some thoracic deformities, such as kyphoscoliosis, pectus carinatum, and pectus excavatum, can affect the position of the heart and possibly cardiac function.

The general description is followed by detailed inspection. Note abnormal facial appearance, particularly facial edema, color, and skin texture. Rheumatic heart disease with severe mitral stenosis may cause cyanotic lips and jaundice. Constrictive pericarditis causes fluid retention, which can result in swelling of the face.

Skin color and temperature are important indicators of circulation. Pallor and cyanosis are key signs in assessing skin color. *Pallor* is the absence of the normal pink skin color. One cause of pallor is vasoconstriction, which decreases blood flow to the skin. In clients with deeply pigmented or dark skin, the conjunctivae and oral mucosa are examined for skin color changes.

Cyanosis is a blue tinge to the skin that appears when hemoglobin oxygen saturation is reduced. Cyanosis can take the form of central cyanosis or peripheral cyanosis. Central cyanosis is assessed in the lips, mucous membranes, and nail beds; peripheral cyanosis is found in the extremities. With prolonged central cyanosis, clubbing of fingers and toes can occur.

The nails are a good source of information regarding cardiovascular status. Circulation can be evaluated in the nail beds by applying pressure to the distal part of the fingernail and noting the pallor as the capillary blood flow is temporarily halted. When the fingernail is released, the color returns by capillary refill. The original color should be restored within 1 to 2 seconds or by the time the words *capillary refill* are said. The nail beds are also inspected for hemorrhagic areas resembling splinters, which can be seen in clients with bacterial endocarditis.

Temperature of the skin and extremities also reflects circulation. Cool, pale, wet, blue-tinged skin often indicates a decrease in circulation. This condition is seen in clients with an acute MI when the cardiac output is suddenly reduced. Warm and flushed skin appears in clients with a high cardiac output, as in hyperthyroidism.

Some skin lesions have also been associated with cardiac dysfunction. **Petechiae,** small red macules on the skin or mucous membranes, are observed in clients with infective endocarditis. **Xanthomas,** cholesterol-filled papules, are found on the eyelids or within the orbit of the eyes. These skin lesions are associated with hyperlipoproteinemia.

EDEMA **Edema** is a local or general accumulation of excess fluid in the body tissues. Edema in any dependent area such as the extremities, the sacrum, or the abdomen is important to recognize. Edema is distinguished as pitting or nonpitting. Pitting edema is considered more serious than nonpitting edema, but the presence of either type is significant. The depth of pitting and the extent and location of edema indicate the severity of the condition. Bilateral edema is associated with heart disease. Some cardiovascular causes of edema include CHF and constrictive pericarditis. Ask the client if shoes, rings, or clothes are getting uncomfortably tight. Tightness may reflect fluid retention in those areas. Changes in body weight also reflect fluid status. A weight gain in a short period may be due to fluid retention. Sudden increases in weight may indicate cardiac failure.

PULSES Arterial pulses provide significant information regarding cardiac output. Cardiac output, which depends on stroke volume and heart rate, can be assessed by the pulse rate and the quality of the pulse. Pulses should be examined bilaterally and include the carotid, brachial, radial, ulnar, femoral, popliteal, dorsalis pedis, and posterior tibial pulses. The rate, rhythm, and force are assessed. A pulse rate greater than 100 beats per minute **(tachycardia)** is considered abnormal for healthy adults. Although a variety of factors may cause tachycardia, the long-term effect is usually decreased cardiac output. A pulse rate below 60 beats per minute **(bradycardia)** is considered abnormal except in clients with well conditioned hearts (eg, marathon runners). In the diseased heart, bradycardia causes a decrease in cardiac output, possibly indicating heart block. An irregular pulse is associated with cardiac dysrhythmias. The quality of the pulse or force is assessed on a scale of 4 with 0 equal to unpalpable or absent and 4+ equal to full and bounding. A normal pulse is designated as 4+.

The absence of a pulse may be a normal variation, particularly the popliteal, ulnar, or posterior tibial pulses. A diminished or absent carotid pulse, however, usually indicates arterial disease. When a pulse is not palpable, a more distal pulse is assessed; for example, the dorsalis pedis pulse is assessed when the popliteal pulse is not palpable, and the radial pulse is assessed when the brachial pulse is not palpable. If distal pulses are felt, adequate circulation is present. If absent, other assessment parameters are noted such as skin temperature, skin color, and sensation.

Pulses are assessed bilaterally (for example, right radial and left radial). Asymmetric or unequal bilateral pulses are abnormal and may indicate a serious circulatory problem. An exception: the carotid arteries should never be palpated bilaterally. Palpation can overstimulate the pressure sensors (carotid sinus bodies), which will decrease heart rate and may result in syncope. As mentioned previously, the elderly client is especially susceptible.

BLOOD PRESSURE Blood pressure is routinely assessed in all clients. The indirect method is used, employing a sphygmomanometer, aneroid or mercury gauge, cuff, and stethoscope. The blood pressure is a good indicator of cardiovascular health. It reflects not only the physical state of the client but also the psychologic effect on the physical state.

Blood pressure is initially obtained in both arms with the client in supine, seated, and standing positions. The blood pressure in both arms should be comparable: A difference of more than 10 mm Hg is abnormal. The readings are recorded as shown in Table 18–3.

The cuff size is an important factor in obtaining accurate blood pressure. The cuff should be 20% wider than the diameter of the arm and cover two-thirds of the upper arm. If the cuff is too small, the reading will be elevated. Conversely, a cuff too large will artificially lower the read-

Table 18–3
Recording Blood Pressures

Client Position	Right Arm*	Left Arm*
Supine	120/80	122/84
Seated	126/80	130/84
Standing	130/80	136/86

*Use legs and arms when taking initial blood pressures of clients with a history of hypertension or vascular disease; use prone position for leg pressures.

ing. Positioning of the cuff and the level of the brachial artery are also important. The bladder of the cuff should be centered over the brachial artery with the lower edge 1 to 2 in above the antecubital space. The arm should be positioned so that the brachial artery is at the level of the heart; if below that level, the blood pressure will be artificially increased; if above that level, the blood pressure will be artificially decreased. These factors apply to any artery used.

Clients with a history of vascular disease or hypertension should also have initial blood pressure readings performed on both legs. Blood pressure in the legs is normally higher than in the arms. Lower blood pressure in the legs may indicate an abdominal aortic obstruction or coarctation of the aorta.

A large cuff is usually needed for leg blood pressures. The cuff is placed around the thigh, and the popliteal artery is auscultated. Leg pressures are best obtained with the client in the prone position.

Body position may have a significant effect on blood pressure in clients who take diuretics or who may have a fluid volume deficit. Standing up quickly from a supine position causes a drop in blood pressure. A slight drop in systolic pressure (less than 10 mm Hg) is normal. A drop in the diastolic pressure is abnormal.

Korotkoff sounds (ie, arterial vibrations) are indicators of blood pressure (Figure 18–1). As the blood pressure cuff is deflated, note (1) the onset of the first sound, (2) the muffling point of the sound, and (3) the disappearance of the sound. The onset of the first sound is the systolic pressure; the muffling point and the disappearance of sound have both been used as the diastolic pressure reading. In normal adults, the cessation of sound may best approximate the diastolic pressure. In hypertensive clients, there may be a silent interval between the systolic and diastolic pressure, known as the **auscultatory gap.** Noting the muffled sound may be more appropriate in these clients.

The systolic blood pressure is considered elevated when the reading is greater than 140 mm Hg; diastolic blood pressure is elevated when the reading is greater than 90 mm Hg. Systolic hypertension is seen often in elderly clients, usually due to atherosclerosis. Increased cardiac output from conditions such as thyrotoxicosis, anemia, anxiety, and aortic regurgitation can also cause systolic hypertension. Diastolic hypertension is associated with essential hypertension, arteriosclerosis, and renal disease. Low blood pressure or hypotension may be seen in clients with MI, shock, or hypovolemia.

Pulse pressure, the difference between the systolic and diastolic pressures, is also an indicator of cardiovascular status. The normal pulse pressure is between 30 and 40 mm Hg. A value greater than this is referred to as a widened pulse pressure. A widened pulse pressure can occur in conditions such as hypertension, aortic regurgitation, and thyrotoxicosis. A pulse pressure less than 30 mm Hg is called a narrowed pulse pressure and may occur in shock, pericardial effusion, severe aortic stenosis, and constrictive pericarditis.

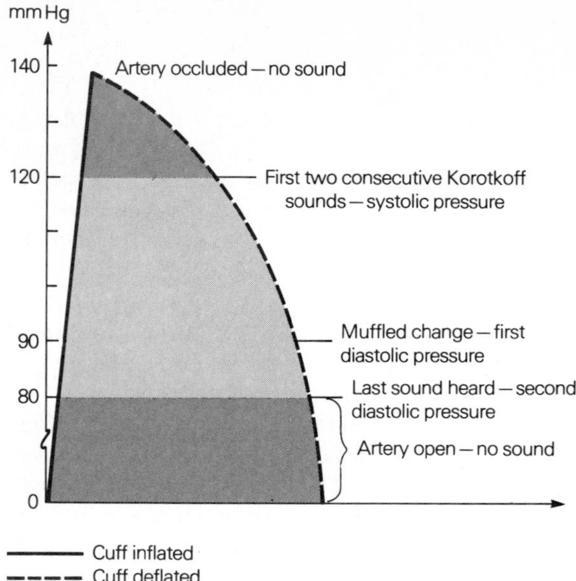

From above graph blood pressure may be recorded as 120/80 or 120/90/80.

Figure 18–1

Korotkoff sounds heard on auscultation of the blood pressure. SOURCE: *Saxton DF, et al.:* The Addison-Wesley Manual of Nursing Practice. *Menlo Park, CA: Addison-Wesley, 1983, p. 158.*

Diagnostic Studies

The assessment of the client with suspected cardiovascular dysfunction requires the examination of the blood and urine for abnormalities. Tests are performed to establish a diagnosis (eg, MI), to obtain general screening information, to assess risk factors, or to detect concurrent disease. The most common tests are serum lipids, serum cardiac enzymes, serum glucose, coagulation studies, complete blood count, electrolytes, urinalysis, and arterial blood gases.

SERUM LIPIDS The association between serum lipid levels (cholesterol, triglycerides, and lipoproteins) and CAD has been studied extensively. An elevated serum cholesterol level is directly related to the development of CAD: The higher the cholesterol level, the greater the risk. The inverse (ie, the lower the level, the lower the risk) is not true, however. Whether an elevated serum triglyceride level is a coronary risk factor is unclear. Some studies have documented an association between CAD and elevated triglyceride levels, but this association appears to be less predicative than the association of an elevated cholesterol level and CAD.

Cholesterol and triglyceride are bound to plasma proteins and transported in the blood as lipoproteins. The major lipoproteins are classified as chylomicrons, very low-density lipoproteins (VLDL), low-density lipoproteins (LDL), and high-density lipoproteins (HDL). The densities of lipoproteins vary according to the proportion of protein to fat and correspond to the protein portion of the lipoprotein (eg, HDL contains more protein than fat).

Each of the lipoproteins contains varying proportions of cholesterol, triglyceride, protein, and phospholipid. Chylomicrons and VLDL are composed primarily of triglyceride; LDL is predominantly cholesterol; an intermediate between VLDL and LDL called intermediate-density lipoprotein (IDL) contains a combination of triglycerides and cholesterol. HDL contains mostly protein but also has 20% cholesterol.

Elevated LDL levels are positively correlated with atherosclerosis. Therefore, clients with increased LDL are at risk for developing vascular disease. Elevated HDL is negatively correlated with atherosclerosis, however. In fact, studies demonstrate that elevated HDL levels appear to prevent plaque formation by converting cholesterol to a less active form. Elevated HDL levels may be a protective factor.

A total serum cholesterol level does not distinguish between LDL and HDL. Clients' health care management depends on this differential. A lipoprotein electrophoresis provides the information.

CARDIAC ENZYMES Cardiac enzyme studies are performed primarily to document acute myocardial damage. The enzyme levels most commonly obtained are creatine kinase (CK), CK isoenzymes, lactic dehydrogenase (LDH), LDH isoenzymes, and (less commonly) serum glutamic-oxaloacetic transaminase (SGOT).

Enzymes are catalytic proteins that accelerate biochemical reactions within cells. Each organ or tissue of the body contains specific enzymes, often similar enzymes, but in varying concentrations. Under normal conditions, the intracellular concentration of enzymes is high, and the extracellular or serum concentration is low. Serum enzyme concentrations increase when cell damage occurs and the enzyme leaks into the blood. Thus, cardiac muscle damage can be detected by measuring serum levels of enzymes specific to the heart. The severity of the damage can be assessed by the amount and duration of the elevation.

Found in high concentrations in both skeletal and heart muscle, CK is the most useful enzyme in the early diagnosis of MI. When the myocardium is injured, the serum CK level rises 3 to 6 hours after the event, peaks at 24 hours, and usually returns to normal within 72 to 96 hours. The specificity of CK activity is increased with the identification of the three CK isoenzymes: CK-MM, CK-MB, and CK-BB. CK-MM predominates in skeletal muscle, with small amounts in cardiac muscle. CK-BB is found primarily in brain and nervous tissue. The CK-MB has the highest concentration in the cardiac muscle, making this isoenzyme specific to the heart. Elevation in CK-MB level is diagnostic of MI and appears within 4 to 6 hours after the onset of chest pain, peaks within 24 hours, and returns to normal within 48 to 72 hours. If the client is not hospitalized within 24 hours from the onset of chest pain, the rise and peak of CK-MB may not be detected. CK-MM also increases and persists for approximately 5 days. Serial documentation of CK and CK isoenzymes provides a continuous assessment of myocardial necrosis.

LDH is found in most tissues of the body. The highest concentrations are in the heart, liver, brain, skeletal muscle, kidneys, and red blood cells. The specificity of LDH is improved when the LDH isoenzymes (LDH_1 through LDH_5) are measured. LDH_1 and LDH_2 are found primarily in the heart, red blood cells, and brain. Normally, LDH_2 is proportionately higher than LDH_1 in the serum ($LDH_2 > LDH_1$), but after a myocardial infarction, the ratio is reversed, and LDH_1 is higher ($LDH_1 > LDH_2$). This "flipped ratio" increases specificity in diagnosing MIs.

The LDH level is usually elevated within 8 to 12 hours after myocardial infarction, peaks within 24 to 48 hours, and remains elevated for 10 to 14 days. Because the LDH level remains elevated much longer than CK, it provides a significant diagnostic benefit in documenting MIs more than 35 hours old.

SGOT, now called aspartate aminotransferase (AST), was one of the original enzymes used in documenting cardiac muscle, liver, pancreas, kidneys, brain, testes, and spleen. SGOT isoenzymes have not been identified, so SGOT activity remains relatively nonspecific for myocardial damage. It is rarely used.

BLOOD COAGULATION STUDIES The major purposes of blood coagulation studies are to monitor the effectiveness of anticoagulant therapy and to detect deficiencies in serum clotting factors. Anticoagulant therapy with heparin is evaluated by obtaining the partial thromboplastin time (PTT). The therapeutic range is 1.5 to 2.5 times the normal value of PTT. The prothrombin time (PT) is used to monitor the effectiveness of therapy with an oral anticoagulant such as warfarin sodium. The therapeutic PT range is 2 to 2.5 times the normal value. Oral anticoagulants take 3 to 5 days to reach therapeutic levels; therefore, heparin and warfarin sodium are given in combination until the PT is prolonged.

Anticoagulant therapy may be used in clients with acute MI complicated by CHF to prevent clot formation. Clients who receive prosthetic valves often require chronic warfarin therapy to prevent clot formation on the valve. Certain medications may interact with the anticoagulants and potentiate or lessen the effect. For example, quinidine, salicylates, and adrenocorticosteroids increase PT; antihistamines, barbiturates, and chloral hydrate decrease PT. Pharmacologic resources should be consulted, and a complete medication history should be obtained and reviewed when anticoagulant therapy is used.

ELECTROLYTES Cardiac function depends in part on the body's electrolyte balance. Myocardial muscle requires adequate stores of calcium to maintain the force of contraction; potassium is needed to facilitate the myocardial cell's response to stimuli. Cardiovascular clients' most common electrolyte abnormality is potassium imbalance. Depletion of potassium can result from vomiting, diarrhea, diuretics, cardiac bypass surgery, and renal disease. Hypokalemia predisposes the client to dysrhythmias, particularly premature ventricular contractions and ventricular fibrillation, and contributes to digitalis toxicity. A high serum potassium level is usually a result of renal failure but may be caused by excessive potassium intake. Hyperkalemia slows the heart rate and may result in asystole or ventricular fibrillation.

Clients with CHF or an acute MI are most susceptible to electrolyte imbalance. Depletion of sodium, potassium, magnesium, calcium, and phosphorus may occur. Clients often complain of weakness, fatigue, and occasionally, muscle cramps. Serum electrolyte levels and ECG changes should be routinely monitored.

ARTERIAL BLOOD GASES Arterial blood gas (ABG) values are usually monitored when the client is acutely ill. The acid–base balance (pH) and oxygenation (PO_2) are the parameters observed. Although ABGs are not performed routinely in cardiovascular assessment, they are useful for detecting the acid–base imbalances and hypoxemia often found in unstable cardiac clients. Uncompensated CHF may result in hypoxemia and either respiratory alkalosis or respiratory acidosis. Cardiogenic shock may cause hypoxemia and metabolic acidosis. Clients with acute MI tend to hyperventilate; hyperventilation can lead to respiratory alkalosis and hypoxemia. Large doses of morphine for MI pain may depress respirations and cause respiratory acidosis.

CHEST X-RAY Significant information in the diagnosis of cardiac disease can be obtained through examination of the routine chest x-ray. The silhouette of the heart, cardiac chambers, and great vessels is observed, and the size and contour of the heart can be measured. Assessments are made by comparing the radiographic densities of the heart to those of surrounding structures such as the lungs. In addition to cardiac enlargement, calcifications in the coronary arteries and great vessels can be seen. Pulmonary involvement from CHF and other cardiac dysfunctions may be detected from x-ray examination. Pulmonary venous congestion and dilation of the pulmonary veins and artery may be observed.

A specific procedure called a cardiac series enhances the routine chest x-ray. The contrast in the x-ray film is increased by administering barium to the client. The esophagus is filled with barium, which makes it more opaque. Chamber enlargement or aortic dilation can be detected by noting the displacement of the esophagus.

ELECTROCARDIOGRAM The ECG graphically represents the electrical activity of the heart. Cellular activity of the cardiac muscle generates electrical impulses that flow through the heart, causing cardiac contraction and relaxation. The flow of electrical impulses that leads to contraction is called *depolarization*. Electrical recovery of the heart muscle is referred to as *repolarization*. This electrical activity of the heart muscle can be measured by a system of electrodes placed at specific points on the body surface. Only electrical activity generated by the atria and ventricles can be recorded by the body-surface ECG. The specialized conducting tissues within the heart do not provide enough voltage to be detected by the body-surface electrodes.

Figure 18–2 shows details of the normal ECG. The S-A node initiates the impulse, which is spread throughout the atria and into the A-V node, where the impulse is delayed while the atria contract to fill the ventricles completely. This produces a P wave on the ECG, signifying transmission of the depolarization wave through the atria. (The wave is written upright, because the sensor is near the apex of the heart.) There is a period of no electrical activity (signified by a straight line on the ECG) while the ventricles are filling (called the PR interval). Suddenly, the wave spreads through the bundle of His and into the ventricular septum (from left to right), which causes the inscription of the Q wave (the first negative deflection). The depolarization wave spreads rapidly through the right and left ventricles. Because the left ventricle has many more cells, the electrical sensor draws an upward R wave. The last part of the ventricle to depolarize is the left upper wall of the left ventrical, which causes the sensor to draw a small downward deflection, called the S wave. Atrial repolarization cannot be seen on the normal ECG because it occurs during ventricular depolarization and is hidden in the QRS complex. Another straight line signifies no electrical activity. Shortly thereafter, a T wave forms, which the sensor records when the ventricular muscle cells repolarize. Because ventricular repolarization occurs in a different sequence than depolarization, the T wave is upright.

There are normal time limits for these events to occur. During the ECG recording, the paper marked with light and dark horizontal lines moves under the writing instrument at a standard rate. The distance of five dark lines (counting the origin would make six) equals 1 second. The distance between two dark lines equals 0.2 seconds. The time necessary for the depolarization wave to be conducted through the various parts of the heart is significant in evaluating abnormalities of the heartbeat.

NURSING IMPLICATIONS The ECG is a noninvasive test that can be performed by a trained individual in any clinical setting. The nurse should prepare clients for the test by informing them about the purpose, procedure to be used, and the risks involved. Explain to clients that the ECG provides a graphic description of the heart rhythm, which yields information about their cardiac status and such matters as the effectiveness of their heart medicine.

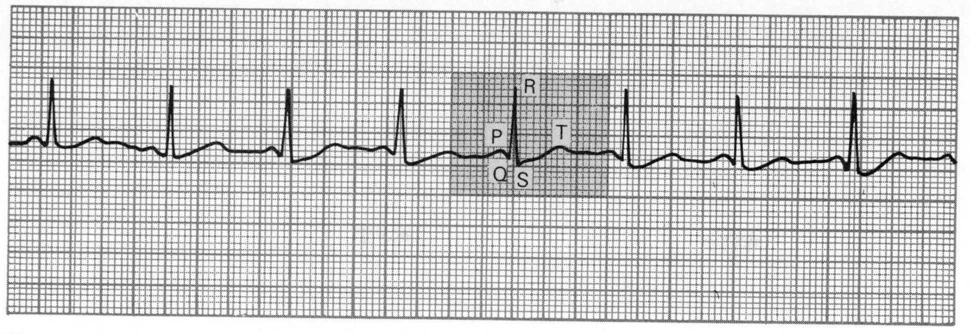

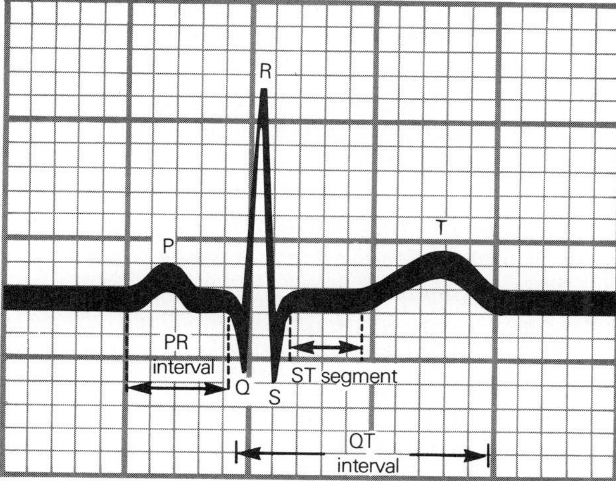

Figure 18–2

The normal electrocardiogram. A. Regular sinus rhythm. B. Details of ECG. SOURCE: *Saxton DF, et al.:* The Addison-Wesley Manual of Nursing Practice. *Menlo Park, CA: Addison-Wesley, 1983, p. 164.*

The ECG is performed with the client in a supine position; the client's chest is exposed for placement of electrodes. If hair is present, the electrode sites may need to be shaved. A conducting medium (creme, gel, or saline pads) is applied to the electrode sites if suction cups or metal plates are used. Adhesive electrodes are prepackaged with conducting gel. The client does not need to follow prior dietary restrictions, but occasionally certain medications are discontinued before testing. The client's watch may need to be removed if electrical interference is noted.

The risks are minimal: possible ecchymoses from the suction cups and a rare electrical hazard if proper electrical safety precautions are not followed. A written consent is not necessary, but the client should give verbal consent.

AMBULATORY ELECTROCARDIOGRAPHY (HOLTER MONITORING) A client's heart rhythm during daily activities can be evaluated by applying a portable ECG recorder that the client wears for a specific length of time, usually 24 hours. The ECG is recorded onto a tape, and the client documents in a diary daily activities as well as any symptoms occurring with the activity. After completion of the test period, the tape is translated into a standard graphic ECG reading by an electrocardioscanner. The ECG is reviewed, and the client's documentation is correlated with the interpretation. This technique of ambulatory ECG recording is often referred to as Holter monitoring.

Ambulatory ECG monitoring is used most often with clients whose symptoms may include episodes of dizziness, chest pain, fainting, or palpitations. This long-term monitoring permits a better correlation between the client's subjective information and objective findings. Clients who have had open heart surgery or an MI can be monitored for 24 hours prior to discharge to detect latent dysrhythmias or abnormal hemodynamic responses. The effects of therapy (drug, exercise, or diet) can also be evaluated with this test.

NURSING IMPLICATIONS Ambulatory monitoring is a noninvasive test similar to the standard ECG. The nurse should provide instructions to the client regarding the client's involvement in the procedure: The Holter monitor provides a recording of the heart rhythm for 24 hours, which, along with the client's diary, offers information about whether the heart rhythm is related to the symptoms the client has been feeling.

Three to five electrodes are applied to the chest. Not applying electrodes to the extremities provides the client freedom to move. The electrodes are connected to lead wires of a portable ECG tape recorder, and the tape is started.

The diary forms provided to clients should include headings for time, type of activity, and symptoms. The client is instructed to note the time and to record activities such as eating, walking, watching television, and sleeping and to note any associated symptoms such as dizziness, chest pain, fainting, or palpitations. The client may perform the usual activities but should avoid operating heavy machinery, microwave ovens, or electric shavers as well as bathing or showering. These activities may interfere with the electrical signals of the ECG recorder. The client may also be shown how to replace the electrodes if they are accidentally removed.

There are no inherent risks in ambulatory ECG monitoring. However, the client may suffer skin irritation from the long-term use of electrodes. A written consent may not be necessary, but a verbal consent should be obtained.

ECHOCARDIOGRAPHY The motion and dimensions of the cardiac structures can be measured by using high-frequency sound waves (ultrasound) and graphically recording the reflected sound (echo). This technique is called echocardiography. A sound-emitting transducer is applied to the client's chest and focused at the heart. As the sound transects the various structures, echoes are produced and recorded. Echocardiography is helpful in documenting valvular and congenital heart disease. In addition, the recording of cardiac movement permits objective assessment of cardiomyopathy, pericardial effusion, and ventricular aneurysm.

NURSING IMPLICATIONS Echocardiography is a noninvasive test that can be performed in any clinical setting that has an ultrasound machine. The nurse should explain to the client that the echocardiogram will provide a recording of the movement of the heart valves and ventricular walls, which can be used to measure the functional ability of the heart valves and the heart as a pump.

The client is placed in the recumbent position. A transducer, lubricated with a gel to facilitate movement and conduction, is applied to the client's anterior chest. As the transducer moves over the chest, images of the cardiac structures in motion are viewed. The images and the ECG are recorded. The client can expect the procedure to take about an hour.

Ultrasonography is a relatively new technology and, at this time, there are no proven risks. A verbal consent should be obtained; a written consent is not necessary. Echocardiography has some limitations: The procedure for obtaining good images is difficult, and clients who have a large, thick chest and those with a small heart are especially problematic. The procedure is also time-consuming.

EXERCISE TESTING (STRESS TEST) In the exercise test, the ECG is recorded during prescribed exercise. A motorized treadmill or a bicycle ergometer provides the method of exercise, and the work load is gradually increased to a prescribed level of stress. The objective of the test is to document the level of stress necessary to produce symptoms or signs. During the exercise, the ECG is monitored for changes: ST-segment depression, ventricular dysrhythmias, conduction defects, or severe heart-rate changes. Alterations in blood pressure are also monitored. The client is observed for symptoms of fatigue, chest pain, or shortness of breath.

The exercise test is noninvasive and is used primarily in the diagnosis and prognosis of CAD. The results of the test are best used in documentation of risk factors rather than as a statement of whether disease is present. There are some limitations in exercise testing. The correlations between positive (abnormal) exercise tests and the presence of CAD have been poor. There is a high degree of false-positive and false-negative results in the diagnosis of ischemic heart disease. Clients with significant CAD may have a negative test, but clients with no CAD may have a positive test. When the exercise test is performed in conjunction with myocardial perfusion studies, the correlation with CAD increases.

NURSING IMPLICATIONS Exercise testing is noninvasive, but because risks are associated with exercising until cardiovascular symptoms appear, the client should be thoroughly informed and a written consent obtained. The exercise test is performed with a cardiologist or physician present. Safety of the procedure depends primarily on adherence to the contraindications, termination of the exercise when the client exhibits untoward symptoms and signs, and availability of personnel and equipment to manage complications.

The client's understanding of the procedure and the importance of cooperation during the test are essential to successful exercise testing. To be adequately prepared, the client should know that the purpose of the test is to evaluate the effect of activity on the heart during exercise on a moving treadmill. The client's heart rhythm, blood pressure, and symptoms and signs will be continuously monitored. The client should either fast overnight or have only a light meal no later than 2 hours before testing. Some cardiac medications may be discontinued before testing. The client should wear loose-fitting clothes and supportive shoes. A cardiovascular history and physical exam are obtained along with a resting 12-lead ECG which is examined by the physician for any abnormalities that would preclude exercise testing. Several protocols for exercise testing have been developed and, depending on client characteristics and physician preference, one protocol is chosen.

The client is instructed to report any untoward symptoms and shown how to walk on the treadmill. The client exercises until one of the following occurs: A predetermined heart rate is reached and maintained; symptoms such as fatigue, chest pain, or dysrhythmias appear; or significant ST-segment depression occurs. In the post-exercise period, the ECG and blood pressure continue to be monitored until the client is completely recovered. The test is usually completed in approximately 20 minutes. The risk of an exercise test is small if contraindications and safety precautions are understood. A client with preexisting cardiovascular disease has the highest risk.

PHONOCARDIOGRAPHY Phonocardiography, the graphic recording of heart sounds heard during auscultation, is an extension of the physical exam. The heart sounds are translated into electrical impulses, amplified, and recorded by a microphone. Each component of the heart sounds and murmurs can be documented. External pulse recordings of either the carotid artery, jugular vein, or apical pulse are taken at the same time as the ECG, which provides a timing reference for the heart sound.

The client is placed in the normal auscultatory positions. A pressure-sensitive transducer is applied to the selected pulse, and the ECG reading is usually obtained through the standard limb leads. A special microphone, used in the same manner as a stethoscope, is applied to the various auscultatory points. A phonocardiography machine connects the three extensions and graphically records simultaneously the pulse wave, ECG, and heart sounds. The phonocardiogram is most useful in documenting heart sounds and murmurs that are almost inaudible with the ordinary stethoscope.

CARDIAC FLUOROSCOPY The movements of cardiac structures, the lungs, and coronary vessels may be viewed by fluoroscopy, permitting assessment of the degree of dysfunction of calcified heart valves and coronary vessels. In the past, the radiation exposure from this procedure was high, but now, with the use of image intensifiers and computers, the hazard is greatly reduced. The quality of the images has also improved. Fluoroscopy is also used for guiding the placement and positioning of temporary pacemakers and intracardiac catheters.

NURSING IMPLICATIONS Although the roentgenographic procedures are essentially noninvasive, the client should be informed about the radiation exposure. Roentgenographic procedures should be avoided during pregnancy.

NUCLEAR CARDIOLOGY Using radioactive tracer substances, cardiovascular abnormalities can be viewed, recorded, and evaluated. The use of radionuclide techniques in cardiovascular assessment is called nuclear cardiology. Radionuclides are unstable isotopes which, as they decay to a stable form, emit energy as gamma rays. The gamma rays are detected by a scintillation camera and converted to electrical impulses, which are then displayed and recorded.

The radionuclide techniques facilitate the evaluation of CAD, MI, ventricular wall function, valvular disease, and intracardiac shunts. The most commonly used radionuclides in nuclear cardiology are thallium (^{201}Tl), technetium pyrophosphate (^{99m}Tc-PYP), and ^{99m}Tc-labelled red blood cells. Each of the radionuclides has different individual properties that contribute to the cardiovascular assessment. In general, two kinds of studies are performed in nuclear cardiology: the myocardial perfusion/imaging study and the cardiac function/performance study.

A myocardial perfusion study assesses the blood supply in the various regions of the myocardium. Thus, this study shows the effect of CAD on myocardial perfusion. The most commonly used radionuclide in perfusion studies is ^{201}Tl, a potassium analogue. Like potassium, thallium readily diffuses across the cell membrane and accumulates in myocardial cells. Thallium uptake depends on coronary blood flow and ability of the myocardial cell membrane to extract the thallium from the blood. In CAD or coronary spasm where the coronary blood flow is decreased, the quantity of thallium reaching the myocardium is reduced, and the uptake of thallium within the cells is low. If myocardial cell membranes are destroyed or nonfunctional, as in an MI, the thallium is not extracted from the blood into the cell; hence, there is no thallium uptake.

The assessment of CAD has been greatly enhanced by combining exercise stress testing and thallium scintigraphy. Thallium is given intravenously during peak exercise, and the scan is performed immediately after the exercise test. This method permits detection of regions that may be perfused normally at rest but have reduced blood flow during exercise. A follow-up scan, about 2 hours after the first scan, is performed to assess the redistribution of blood into the regions that were previously underperfused. Redistribution indicates that the myocardium is viable.

Thallium scintigraphy is also used to evaluate the effect of pharmacologic agents on coronary blood flow. Perfusion studies performed before or after coronary artery bypass assess the ability of the grafts to increase coronary blood flow.

Technetium pyrophosphate (^{99m}Tc-PYP), which concentrates in zones of necrosis, is used in imaging MIs. The mechanism of the uptake, although not yet clear, appears to be related to the calcium deposits in the infarct zones. Any heart condition that results in myocardial cell damage may be assessed with ^{99m}Tc-PYP.

Ventricular function measurements including ejection fraction and cardiac output can be obtained through radionuclide angiography. The radionuclide used is sodium pertechnetate ^{99m}Tc, which attaches to red blood cells. Red blood cells labeled with ^{99m}Tc are large bodies that remain within the vascular system and thus provide for visualization of the vessels and cardiac chambers. Information from these studies is essentially the same as from contrast studies. However, radionuclide angiography is less invasive, requires less time, permits repeated studies, and has fewer inherent risks. Also, both right and left ventricular performance can be assessed at the same time.

NURSING IMPLICATIONS Radioisotope cardiovascular assessment is relatively noninvasive; the radiation exposure and risks are minimal. Because a radioisotope is used, there is no chemical toxicity. The studies do not require hospitalization or prior preparation. Nevertheless, the client should be given information regarding the purpose of the study, and the procedure should be fully explained. The radioisotope is injected intravenously and the client is asked to lie still during the test. A written consent is obtained.

CARDIAC CATHETERIZATION The most invasive but the most definitive test in the diagnosis of cardiac disease is cardiac catheterization. A catheter is passed into the right or left side of the heart to obtain information on cardiac pressures, cardiac output, oxygenation, and competency of intracardiac structures. When contrast dye is used to view the cardiac structures, the procedure is referred to as angiography. Most cardiac catheterizations are combined with angiography.

Right-heart catheterization is performed by inserting a catheter through either the basilic vein, superior vena cava, femoral vein, or inferior vena cava. With continuous cardiac pressure monitoring and fluoroscopy, the catheter is advanced into the right side of the heart. Intracardiac pressures (right atrial, right ventricular, pulmonary artery, and pulmonary wedge pressures) are obtained. Blood samples are also withdrawn. Contrast dye is usually injected to detect any regurgitation from the pulmonic or tricuspid valves or to detect cardiac shunts.

The left-heart catheterization procedure is more invasive. The heart is approached either by passing the catheter from the right heart through the atrial septum, using a special needle to puncture the septum, or by retrograde insertion, which is performed by advancing the catheter from the brachial or femoral artery up the aorta, across the aortic valve, and into the left ventricle. This approach is used when coronary artery angiography will be performed during the study. As with right-heart catheterization, pressure readings and blood samples are obtained. Pressures in the left atrium, left ventricle, and aorta and mitral and aortic valve status are evaluated. In addition, a ventriculogram (contrast dye injected into the ventricle) is performed, and calculations are made of end-systolic volume, end-diastolic volume, stroke volume, and ejection fraction.

For coronary arteriography, the catheter is advanced into the aortic arch and positioned selectively into the right and left coronary arteries. Contrast dye is injected, and films are taken. Observing the flow of the dye through the coronaries provides information about the site and severity of coronary lesions.

With the more sophisticated noninvasive tests available, the need for cardiac catheterization has decreased slightly. Nevertheless, when either valvular or vascular cardiac surgery is indicated, a cardiac catheterization is performed to confirm the diagnosis and to evaluate the surgical approach.

There are no absolute contraindications to cardiac catheterization. However, the client must be physically able to tolerate the procedure and subsequent cardiac surgery if necessary. Evidence of acute MI, uncompensated CHF, or severe dysrhythmias may be contraindications. The risks and the benefits are evaluated before the procedure is performed. Written informed consent is necessary.

NURSING IMPLICATIONS Because cardiac catheterization is an invasive test, it is often frightening to the client. The client's psychosocial readiness should be assessed. The purpose of the procedure should be explained. Tell the client that the information obtained will facilitate treatment, and only a cardiac catheterization can provide this information. The client is admitted to the hospital for the procedure, and the length of hospitalization varies depending on the outcome. Standard preoperative tests are usually performed: chest x-ray, ECG, CBC, and urinalysis. The client receives nothing by mouth after midnight or has only a liquid breakfast if the cardiac catheterization is scheduled for the afternoon. A mild sedative is usually given before the test. Nursing assessment includes the client's vital signs, evaluation of peripheral pulses, and auscultation of heart and lung sounds. The site of catheter insertion is prepared, the area is shaved if necessary, and usually a hexachlorophene scrub is done.

The client should be told how long the procedure usually takes, who will be present while it is going on, and what kind of physical environment it is done in. The client will be kept in a supine position, which may become uncomfortable. The injection of the dye often causes a warm feeling throughout the body—often compared to "hot flashes"—that the client may find disagreeable.

Postcatheterization care involves monitoring vital signs q. 15 min. ×4; then q. 30 min. ×2 or until stable; then q. 4 h. Peripheral pulses and possible bleeding at catheter insertion sites should be assessed with the vital signs. An intravenous line for medication and fluid replacement is usually required. The client is kept on bed rest 8 to 12 hours following the procedure.

DIGITAL SUBTRACTION ANGIOGRAPHY Digital subtraction angiography (DSA) is a new approach to the traditional angiogram. Instead of injecting contrast dye directly into an artery, dye is injected into the venous system via the superior vena cava so it circulates through the heart and into the arterial system. A fluoroscopic image-intensifier displays the vessels and focuses (intensifies) the image. A computer then converts images into numbers. The first image obtained before the injection of the contrast dye is subtracted from the postinjection images. The image obtained from the computer subtraction is an enhanced image of the arterial system. Several vessels rather than one vessel can be evaluated with one injection of contrast dye.

This technique has many advantages. It is less invasive than the conventional angiograms and requires less contrast dye, less time, and less radiation exposure, yet it provides better images. It requires no hospitalization and can be performed on high-risk clients.

HEMODYNAMIC MONITORING Intracardiac pressures can be measured and monitored continuously at the bedside in many critical care units. A balloon-tipped, flow-directed catheter is inserted percutaneously or by a venous cutdown into a large vein such as the internal jugular, subclavian, femoral, or brachial veins. The catheter (the Swan–Ganz catheter is the most common) is slowly advanced toward the right atrium; when it enters the right atrium, the balloon is inflated. Then the flow of blood carries the catheter through the tricuspid valve, the right ventricle, and the pulmonary valve into the pulmonary artery. The balloon finally wedges into a branch of the pulmonary artery. A pressure reading, the *pulmonary artery wedge pressure* (PAWP), is obtained, and the balloon is quickly deflated. The catheter floats back into the pulmonary artery and remains in this position for continuous monitoring. The pressures routinely monitored are the pulmonary artery systolic pressure (PASP) and diastolic pressure (PADP), PAWP, and the cardiac output. The PASP represents the pressure generated by the contraction of the right ventricle, whereas the PADP represents the filling pressure of the right ventricle. These pressures are monitored to assess right-sided heart function and pulmonary resistance. In the absence of lung dysfunction and mitral valve stenosis, the PAWP reflects left atrial pressure and left ventricular end-diastolic filling pressure. Thus, the function of the left heart can be assessed.

Catheters with a special temperature-sensing device, a thermistor, can be used to measure cardiac output by the thermodilution technique. A bolus of a solution with a known temperature is injected into the proximal port of the catheter, and the thermistor at the distal end measures the temperature change of the diluted solution. A bedside cardiac output computer connected to the catheter records the data, calculates the temperature curve, and displays the cardiac output.

These intracardiac pressure readings are valuable aids in the assessment of the critically ill client. Serial readings assist in evaluating the effectiveness of the therapeutic plan.

NURSING IMPLICATIONS As an invasive procedure, hemodynamic monitoring carries several risks. The catheter site, and subsequently the blood, may become infected. Endocarditis may occur but can be prevented by using sterile technique and observing the client for early signs of infection. Other serious complications include thromboembolism from blood clotting to the catheter; air embolism from balloon rupture, faulty line connections, or improper procedure; ventricular dysrhythmias due to ventricular irritation from the tip of the catheter floating back into the right ventricle; and pulmonary artery rupture from overdistention of the balloon or from the tip of the catheter piercing through the artery.

The client needs to be prepared for the procedure and the continuous presence of the catheter, intravenous line, and monitors. A written consent is necessary, but often, because the situation is critical and the client barely conscious, obtaining a written consent from the client may not be feasible. In this situation, the family may give written consent.

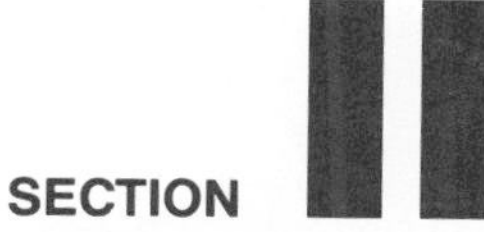

SECTION II

Nursing Diagnosis/Planning and Implementation/Evaluation

Information gathered from the client's health history, physical examination, and diagnostic studies is used to determine nursing diagnoses and the plan of care. Not every client will have the same needs. The Nursing Diagnosis box lists diagnoses **directly related** to cardiac dysfunction along with **potential** diagnoses for clients with cardiac problems. The most common nursing diagnoses for clients with cardiovascular dysfunction include fear; anxiety; disturbance in self-concept: body image; altered role performance; altered comfort: pain; altered sexuality patterns; and altered cardiac output: decreased. All of these diagnoses are discussed in the content that follows. The sample nursing care plan in Table 18–4 focuses on altered role performance; altered sexuality patterns; and altered cardiac output: decreased.

If the goals of care have not been met, reevaluation is required. The nurse and client should jointly review the nursing care plan. New objectives may need to be formulated; other nursing interventions may be added or modified; or the evaluation may show that more time is required to meet the objectives.

Fear and Anxiety

Clients who undergo a major cardiac event are under the stress of a life-threatening illness and are often consumed by the fear of death, pain, disability, physical dependency, and inactivity. Lack of knowledge may be fundamental to this fear. The client may use the call light frequently, ask many questions, and appear restless. If fear is unrelieved, the client will be at risk for developing anxiety that can lead to physical complications.

Anxiety is the most common emotional response of clients who are hospitalized for a coronary event. The physical responses to anxiety, which result from stimulation of the central nervous system, are likely to manifest themselves clinically as increases in pulse rate, blood pressure, and respiration, perhaps accompanied by heart rhythm irregularities or recurrent chest pain. This anxiety-induced

DIRECTLY RELATED DIAGNOSES

- Anxiety
- Activity intolerance
- Cardiac output, altered: decreased
- Comfort, altered: pain
- Fear
- Knowledge deficit
- Role performance, altered
- Self-concept, disturbance in: body image

OTHER POTENTIAL DIAGNOSES

- Adjustment, impaired
- Coping, ineffective: individual
- Tissue perfusion, altered: cerebral, cardiopulmonary, renal, gastrointestinal, peripheral

physical stimulation may be detrimental to the client's already compromised cardiac status. On the other hand, the client may not exhibit overt signs of anxiety and may camouflage true feelings by false cheerfulness. Denial of the seriousness of the cardiac event is a coping mechanism often used to diminish fear and anxiety.

Planning and Implementation

To reduce fear, offer the client information and reassurance. Knowledge and reassurance diminish anxiety and fear by enhancing the client's coping skills. The client is able to rehearse information mentally and formulate expectations. The following items should be thoroughly explained: room arrangements, use of equipment, monitoring procedures, routine hospital activities, visiting practices, purpose of diagnostic tests, and progression of self-care activities. Liberal visiting for family and significant others should be allowed.

In the acute setting, a mild sedative may be prescribed to relax the client. Diazepam (Valium) is often given. As the client's condition stabilizes, the nurse assists the client in recognizing the anxiety and the conditions that precipitate it. Reassurance and comfort are offered by conveying understanding, supporting the client's present coping mechanisms (which may include denial), and providing a calm environment. As anxiety diminishes, the client is assisted in identifying the threats and more effective coping mechanisms. The client's support systems are identified and included in providing emotional comfort to the client. Both the client and family are encouraged to attend cardiac rehabilitation classes.

Evaluation

As fear subsides, clients rest more comfortably, use the call light less frequently, and cope more effectively. As the client and significant others become more knowledgeable about the cardiac event, the situations that previously precipitated anxiety diminish. Significant others are able to provide effective emotional support because they have become more secure themselves.

Self-Concept, Disturbance in: Body Image

Clients who have had a cardiac event (MI, cardiac surgery, or heart transplant) may feel betrayed by their bodies because they can no longer do what they used to do. Most clients also subscribe to the culturally accepted view that the heart is not simply a mechanical pump but is also a person's vital center. Because of this, the impact of cardiac dysfunction on clients' lives depends to a large extent on clients' own ideas about what is happening to them.

Clinical manifestations of disturbances in self-concept are varied and often subtle. Each client reacts differently to the situation. In addition, there is often a time lag between the actual body change and the client's acceptance of this change. Often, this is displayed as denial, which is protective in the early phase of illness but a problem in convalescence.

To assess clients' self-concepts, find out how they feel about health problems in general, how they perceive the significance of this illness, and how well they are able to cope with their normal responsibilities. Some objective clues that may indicate a disturbance in self-concept include a lessening of the client's ability or willingness to make appropriate decisions, passive response to limitations, retrogression from well-role to sick-role behavior, and unwillingness to discuss problems or participate in cardiac rehabilitation classes. The client's assessment of the reaction of significant others to the cardiac event and their ability to be supportive is also important.

Planning and Implementation

To encourage the client's development of a positive self-concept, the nurse needs to develop a trusting relationship with the client. In the acute care setting, primary nursing works effectively. Ongoing efforts to provide information to the client and significant others clarify misconceptions and promote understanding of the plan of care.

As soon as possible, the client and significant others should be included in classes and encouraged to socialize with other cardiac clients and families. Whether the client will be able to return to work needs to be evaluated. If clients are unable to return to their former occupations, counseling should be provided. Career alternatives may be possible. Guidance regarding the disability is offered. Community resources are extremely helpful in the convalescent phase.

Evaluation

As self-concept improves, clients openly discuss the personal adjustments to be made and offer realistic goals for resuming career and family responsibilities. They read-

Table 18–4
Sample Nursing Care Plan for Clients With Heart and Major Blood Vessel Dysfunction, by Nursing Diagnosis

Client Care Goal	Plan/Nursing Implementation	Expected Outcome
Role performance, altered		
Improve body image; assume role responsibilities	Assign a primary nurse who can establish a trusting relationship with client and family; encourage client and family to express feelings and concerns; clarify misconceptions; encourage participation in group cardiac rehab classes; discuss physical progression and return to work; provide or obtain guidance in career alternatives if client unable to return to work	Client will show increased self-confidence and exhibit well behavior
Sexuality patterns, altered		
Resume normal sexual function; achieve satisfaction in sexual relationship	Provide information about normal recovery process from a cardiac event and the resumption of sexual activity; discuss use of exercise stress test in determining a safe activity level; clarify misconceptions; ascertain whether impotence is caused by medications; obtain a sexual history from the client and partner; discuss methods to minimize adverse cardiovascular responses to sexual intercourse; include use of prophylactic medications, eg, nitroglycerin	Client is able to discuss fears and problems; client achieves satisfying sexual relationship
Altered cardiac output: decreased		
Achieve cardiac tolerance of increased activity	Organize client care and provide undisturbed rest periods; establish gradual increases in activity; monitor client's response to increased activity; teach client to monitor pulse rate; assess the client's ability to provide self-care, especially in taking medications; identify the client's risk factors and suggest modifications: smoking cessation, weight reduction, stress reduction, etc; provide activity guidelines	Client is able to perform ADL; client will modify risk factors; client is able to identify factors that increase cardiac work load; adverse CV responses are reduced

ily participate in classes and maintain the prescribed level of activity.

Comfort, Altered: Pain

The client with cardiac dysfunction may develop acute chest pain from inadequate myocardial perfusion. Decrease in perfusion is most commonly a result of CAD. Myocardial ischemia or infarction may develop if inadequate perfusion persists. With acute myocardial pain, cardiac function is usually diminished, and a reduction in cardiac output may be noted. The client may experience shortness of breath; dizziness; weakness; nausea; vomiting; and changes in heart rate, rhythm, and blood pressure.

Some clients, who may not be surgical candidates or who may have decided against surgery, may have long-term chest discomfort called stable angina. Angina pain is usually infrequent and associated with precipitating factors such as exertion or stress. Stable angina usually lasts no longer than 30 minutes and is most often relieved with rest.

Planning and Implementation

The client's history is the most important factor in the assessment of cardiac pain. With MI pain, the client is hospitalized. Intravenous morphine sulfate and nasal oxygen are usually given. If the pain is not relieved, other medications such as intravenous nitroglycerin, propranolol, or a calcium antagonist may be used. Activities are restricted until pain is controlled. As perfusion of the myocardium improves, the pain subsides.

Stable angina is usually controlled by medication such as propranolol. Proper use of medication, identification of precipitating factors, and an evaluation of risk factors are important components in the client's management of pain. The following recommendations are usually offered: smoking cessation, weight reduction to ideal body weight, stress reduction, exercise for cardiac fitness, and proper diet. Blood pressure and serum lipids are monitored periodically. Teaching the client to recognize potential precipitating factors and to use prophylactic measures will assist in reducing recurrent pain.

Evaluation

Pain is relieved when the client can rest comfortably and physiologic responses to pain have resolved. For clients who have chronic angina, the incidence of acute pain is reduced. The client follows precautions to avoid chest pain. Planned activity is the key component. Through planned activity and prophylaxis, the client shows the ability to perform the activities of daily living.

Sexuality Patterns, Altered

Most clients who have cardiovascular disease experience a change in their sexual function. The most common cause of sexual dysfunction in these clients is lack of knowledge that results in fear. Clients may believe that sexual intercourse will cause another heart attack or that the stitches of new coronary blood vessels might rip apart. Their sexual partners may also fear inducing a cardiac event. Both clients and partners should be given guidelines regarding sexual activity. Previous marital or sexual problems may be exacerbated by the stress of the cardiac event.

Fatigue, pain, and shortness of breath due to cardiovascular disease also may cause sexual dysfunction. Because sexual intercourse induces elevated heart rate and blood pressure, clients must be physically ready to tolerate this stress. The energy expended during sexual activity, including orgasm, is equivalent to the energy required in moderate activity such as climbing stairs or walking 4 to 5 miles per hour. A stair-climbing test may be given to the client to determine physical readiness. Many antihypertensive agents can alter sexual function. Reserpine, clonidine, propranolol, and methyldopa are commonly reported to cause impotence, decrease libido, and decrease vaginal lubrication. Chronic use of potent diuretics such as furosemide and ethacrynic acid may also cause impotence.

Planning and Implementation

Sexual counseling of the client and partner begins before the client is released from the hospital and becomes part of the routine assessment in the long-term care of the client with cardiovascular dysfunction. An exercise stress test using a treadmill or stairs assesses the level of activity the client can safely achieve. Usually, the client who has had an uncomplicated MI may resume sexual activity in 5 to 8 weeks. Clients recovering from coronary artery bypass surgery may resume sexual activity in 3 to 6 weeks.

The first step in sexual counseling is the clarification of misconceptions regarding cardiovascular physiology and sex. A sexual history from the client and partner provides information on previous patterns and desires. The history taking may be the first opportunity the client and partner have had to express their sexual needs. Provide instruction and discussion about the physiologic and psychologic stress of sexual intercourse and interventions to minimize the physical impact of this stress.

Sexual intercourse should be planned to reduce its adverse effects. The client should wait at least 2 hours postprandial and should avoid excessive alcohol intake before intercourse. Prophylactic nitroglycerin or additional doses of propranolol may be used to prevent angina. The client is given written guidelines and instructed to report the following symptoms: chest pain during or after intercourse, persistent rapid heart rate, or persistent fatigue (Sadler, 1984).

Changes in sexual function in clients who take antihypertensive agents should be routinely assessed. If the client has developed side effects, the physician may alter the dosage or prescribe another medication. Clients rarely volunteer information about their sexual function; therefore, direct questions are required.

Evaluation

The majority of clients with cardiovascular dysfunction are able to resume sexual activity. Clients who maintain sexual relations often have improved self-confidence and a more positive outlook.

Cardiac Output, Altered: Decreased

Numerous systemic and cardiac factors affect the ability of the heart to pump blood adequately throughout the body. Only the direct cardiac factors will be discussed here.

The most common cause of inadequate cardiac output is a reduction in myocardial contractility, usually a result of myocardial ischemia secondary to CAD. Myocardial contractility may also be influenced by certain medications (eg, beta-adrenergics). Electrolyte imbalance such as calcium depletion can also decrease the cardiac output.

Any condition causing a decrease in ventricular filling (eg, mitral and tricuspid valvular stenoses) can cause a decrease in cardiac output. In these conditions, impeded blood flow through the valves causes ventricular pulmonary congestion, shortness of breath, edema, distended neck veins, tachycardia, dizziness, and fatigue.

Chronic ventricular overload also causes a decrease in cardiac output by decreasing the strength of myocardial contraction. Respiratory symptoms of heart failure are pronounced. The client often has severe shortness of breath, PND, orthopnea, and cough.

Abnormal cardiac rhythm and conduction disturbances can affect the cardiac output. In atrial fibrillation, atrial

Box 18–1
Symptoms of Inadequate Cardiac Output

Dyspnea	Fatigue
Paroxysmal nocturnal dyspnea	Dizziness
Orthopnea	Low urine output
Cough	Cool, clammy skin
Edema	Weak pulse

contraction is absent. This subsequently reduces ventricular filling, decreasing cardiac output. A very slow or fast heart rate may also be a precipitating factor. Box 18–1 summarizes the cardiovascular symptoms associated with an inadequate cardiac output.

Planning and Implementation

Factors that increase cardiac work load (ie, activities that increase heart rate and blood pressure) need to be identified. Stress, smoking, obesity, excessive activity, and fluid retention may be contributing factors. Nursing strategies are focused on reducing or eliminating precipitating factors. The management of underlying cardiac dysfunction is achieved with medical management.

The level of activity is increased as cardiac performance improves. An exercise stress test before the client's discharge will determine a safe level of activity. Planned activity with gradual increases and frequent rest periods is prescribed. Clients are instructed in monitoring their pulse rate to evaluate the cardiac response to activity: decreases in pulse rate during activity, resting pulse rate greater than 110, an irregular pulse, or pulse rate failing to return to normal within 3 minutes following the cessation of activity should be reported. Clients should report any symptoms such as shortness of breath, dizziness, or excessive fatigue. Clients are instructed to stop activity immediately and notify their health care provider if unrelieved chest pain and/or severe dyspnea occurs.

Psychologic stress may also contribute to a decrease in cardiac output. The client's understanding of the effects of stress on the heart's performance should be evaluated. Stress reduction techniques should be taught to clients and families.

Evaluation

With an adequate cardiac output, the client can increase activity without cardiovascular side effects, and the physical examination will not reveal signs of inadequate myocardial perfusion. After recovery from the cardiac event, the client can maintain the lifestyle of a healthy person. The client understands risk factors, is able to identify personal risk factors, and can make necessary modifications to alter the risk.

Nursing Research Note

Mills G, Barnes R, Rodell D, Terry L: An evaluation of an inpatient cardiac patient/family education program. *Heart Lung* 1985; 14(4):400–406.

Client knowledge, general intelligence and problem-solving abilities, dysfunctional behavior parameters (motivation), and demographic information were examined as potential predictors of compliance behavior in clients with ischemic heart disease who had been involved in a cardiac education program. An extensive statistical analysis revealed that a documented increase in knowledge can be attributed to client education programs. The clients themselves and how they are taught were found to be as important as the content. Although not definitive, some findings suggested that client education programs may motivate clients to be more compliant.

Because motivation correlates with compliance, nurses must identify techniques that enhance client motivation and incorporate these into client education programs. Programs for cardiac clients are highly desirable and useful for the knowledge gained by clients. Therefore, all nurses should encourage clients to attend these programs and should help reinforce the knowledge presented.

Chapter Highlights

The client's health history is the most important source of information in cardiovascular assessment.

The principal symptoms of heart disease are dyspnea, chest pain, palpitation, and syncope. Other symptoms often associated with heart disease include fatigue and cough.

An important component in cardiovascular assessment is evaluating the client's risk factor profile. Risk factors are personal characteristics and habits that increase the client's chance of developing CAD.

Clients who experience a major cardiac event are under the stress of a life-threatening illness and are often consumed by fear and anxiety.

Elevated serum cholesterol levels are directly related to the development of CAD: the higher the cholesterol level, the greater the risk. The inverse is not true. The relation of an elevated serum triglyceride level and CAD is unclear. An elevated HDL level appears to protect against the development of atherosclerosis. Conversely, an elevated LDL level is associated with increased risk of developing CAD.

Cardiac enzymes—CK and its isoenzymes and LDH and its isoenzymes—are elevated when the client has had a myocardial infarction.

Diagnostic studies commonly used in cardiovascular assessment include the ECG, the

ambulatory ECG (Holter) monitor, echocardiography, exercise stress test, phonocardiography, cardiac fluoroscopy, radionuclide studies, cardiac catheterization, and digital subtraction angiography.

Nursing diagnoses common to clients with cardiovascular dysfunction include fear; anxiety; disturbance in self-concept: body image; altered comfort: pain; altered sexual patterns; and altered cardiac output: decreased. The nurse's primary role in the care of clients with cardiovascular dysfunction is to facilitate physical and emotional adjustment. Modification of alterable risk factors is the major goal in the client's management.

Bibliography

Burgess AW, Hartman CR: Patient's perceptions of the cardiac crises—Key to recovery. *Am J Nurs* 1986; 86(5):568–571.

Cantwell J: Exercise and coronary heart disease: Role in primary prevention. *Heart Lung* 1984; 13:6–13.

Carpenito L: *Nursing Diagnosis.* Philadelphia: Lippincott, 1983.

Chobanian A, Loviglio L: *Heart Risk Book.* Toronto: Bantam, 1982.

Criss E: Digital subtraction angiography. *Am J Nurs* 1982; 82:1706–1707.

Dunckle J: Protocol: Congestive heart failure. *Nurse Pract* 1984; 9(9):15–24.

Goldberg L, Elliot DL: The effect of physical activity on lipid and lipoprotein levels. *Med Clin North Am* 1985; 69(1):41–55.

Goldschlager N: Use of the treadmill test in the diagnosis of coronary artery disease in patients with chest pain. *Ann Intern Med* 1982; 97:383–388.

Hallal JC: Caffeine: Is it hazardous to your health? *Am J Nurs* 1986; 86(4):422–425.

Kuller L: Risk factor reduction in coronary heart disease. *Mod Concepts Cardiov Dis* 1984; 53:7–11.

Morra L: Troubleshooting pulmonary catheters. *RN* (Feb) 1987; 46–47.

Pantaleo N et al: Thallium myocardial scintigraphy and its use in the assessment of coronary artery disease. *Heart Lung* 1981; 10:61–71.

Papadopoulos C: Sexuality of women after myocardial infarction. *Med Aspects Human Sexual* 1985; 19:215–223.

Rogers RR: Your patient is scheduled for electrophysiology studies. *Am J Nurs* 1986; 86(5):573–575.

Sadler D: *Nursing for Cardiovascular Health.* Norwalk, CT: Appleton–Century–Crofts, 1984.

Saul L: Heart sounds and common murmurs. *Am J Nurs* 1983; 83:1680–1689.

Scheidt S: Basic electrocardiography: Abnormalities of electrocardiographic patterns. *Ciba Clin Symp* 1984; 36(6):2–32.

Spangler RA: Update on pulmonary artery catheterization. *Nurs 85* 1985; 15(8):42–45.

Thomas S et al: Denial in coronary care patients: An objective reassessment. *Heart Lung* 1983; 12:71–80.

Tilkian S, Conover M, Tilkian A: *Clinical Implications of Laboratory Tests.* St. Louis: Mosby, 1983.

Tobis J, Nalcioglu O, Henry W: Cardiovascular applications of digital subtraction angiography. *Mod Concepts Cardiov Dis* 1984; 53:31–36.

US Department of Health and Human Services. National Institutes of Health: *1984 Report of the Joint National Committee on Detection, Evaluation and Treatment of High Blood Pressure.* NIH Publication No 84-1088, June 1984.

US Department of Health and Human Services. National Institutes of Health: *Lipid Research Clinics Population Study Data.* Vol. I. NIH Publication No. 80–1527, July 1980.

Willerson J et al: Recent advances in nuclear cardiology. (Part I & Part II) *Postgrad Med* 1981; 70(3):55–64, 69–72.

Winslow EH, Lane LD, Gaffney FA: Oxygen uptake and cardiovascular response in control adults and acute myocardial infarction patients during bathing. *Nurs Res* 1985; 34(3):164–169.

Resources

SELF-HELP GROUPS AND OTHER ORGANIZATIONS

American Heart Association
7320 Greenville Ave.
Dallas, TX 75231
Phone: (214) 750–5300

This association offers information, support groups, financial counseling, and classes related to heart disease, hypertension, and stroke, and sponsors hypertension screening clinics in many communities. Members are private citizens and professionals. Produces books, pamphlets, and audiovisual aids on heart disease for the public and for health professionals; a catalog is available. Local chapters exist nationwide.

Heartlife/AHP (Association of Heart Patients), Inc.
PO Box 54305
Atlanta, GA 30308
Phone: (404) 523–0826

This organization provides health education information on heart disease and offers its members a discount drug program, a life insurance program, and a quarterly magazine. It also supports the emotional needs of clients with pacemakers and their families, provides information about pacemaker technology, and publishes a newsletter ("Pulse"). It also provides a nationwide directory of pacemaker clinics, ID bracelets for clients, and a low cost telephone service that allows the client to check whether the pacemaker is functioning properly without leaving home.

Mended Hearts, Inc.
721 Huntington Ave.
Boston, MA 02115
Phone: (617) 732–5609

This nonprofit organization maintains chapters throughout the US and in some foreign countries. Members are persons who have undergone heart surgery. Volunteers share their personal experiences with others who will have or have had heart surgery. A volunteer will visit in the hospital or the home (with the physician's permission) and bring educational materials.

US Government High Blood Pressure Information Center
120/80 National Institutes of Health
Bethesda, MD 20892

This federal program serves as a clearinghouse for information on hypertension.

In Canada

Canadian Heart Foundation
1 Nicholas St., Suite 1200
Ottawa, Ontario, Canada K1N 7B7
Phone: (613) 237-4361

Hundreds of chapters are available throughout Canada which further prevention and treatment of cardiovascular diseases through research and professional and public education.

HOT LINES

Heartlife/AHP
Phone: (800) 241–6993
in Georgia (404) 523–0826, collect

Sponsored by Heartlife/AHP (Association of Heart Patients), Inc., this hot line provides up-to-date information on heart disease and pacemakers.

HEALTH EDUCATION MATERIAL

From: American Heart Association

"After a Heart Attack," a booklet that answers commonly asked questions about returning to normal activity after a heart attack.

"Inside the Cardiac Care Unit: A Guide for the Patient and His Family," a booklet describing the monitoring equipment and health personnel found in a cardiac care unit.

"Recipes for Fat-Controlled, Low Cholesterol Meals," a recipe book.

"Varicose Veins," a booklet describing the signs, symptoms, potential complications, and treatment of varicose veins.

From: Consumer Information Center
Pueblo, CO 81009

"What Every Woman Should Know About High Blood Pressure," a booklet on the relation between hypertension and being a woman who is black, pregnant, past menopause, or on birth control pills.

From: National Heart, Lung, and Blood Institute
Public Inquiries and Reports Section
9000 Rockville Pike
Bethesda, MD 20014
Phone: (301) 496-4000

Publishes pamphlets on cardiovascular health and disease.

CHAPTER **19**

Specific Disorders of the Heart

Other topics relevant to this content are: Common nursing diagnoses and planning and implementation of nursing care for cardiac clients, **Chapter 18**; Accurate assessment of blood pressure, **Chapter 18**; Diagnostic studies for clients with coronary artery disease, **Chapter 18**.

Objectives

When you have finished studying this chapter, you should be able to:

Identify risk factors that promote the development of heart disease.

Describe the subjective and objective findings in clients with hypertension, dysrhythmias, coronary artery disease, myocardial infarction, valvular disease, and heart failure.

Apply specific nursing measures to decrease the oxygen demands of the heart.

Discuss common medical and surgical interventions for clients with heart disease.

Anticipate the psychosocial/lifestyle implications of disorders of the heart on clients and significant others.

Specify appropriate nursing interventions for clients with cardiac dysfunction.

Explain the complications of cardiovascular surgery and the related nursing interventions.

Over 42 million Americans have one or more forms of heart or blood vessel disease, according to 1980 statistics from the American Heart Association. One out of every four adults is estimated to have high blood pressure. Cardiovascular disease is responsible for over 50% of all deaths, with myocardial infarction being the leading cause of death.

As these statistics indicate, a large proportion of a nurse's clients have heart or blood vessel disease or the potential for it. In all clients the nurse cares for, the probability of death from cardiovascular disease is at least one out of two. Nurses who have a good understanding of the cardiovascular system and associated problems are in a position to help prevent premature death from cardiovascular disease by providing nursing care and education. This chapter provides basic information about common heart problems and their nursing implications.

The care of the client requiring cardiovascular surgery is a fascinating and challenging area of nursing. Often the client's condition has reached life-threatening limits, and immediate surgery is required. In other cases, the disease process has slowly developed into a phase in which symptoms limit the client's activities and affect lifestyle.

Many of these are serious operations in which the risk is high for major complications. Because of this, the nursing needs of these clients are complex and demanding. Astute nursing care is essential to prevent, detect, and minimize these complications as well as to enhance the client's recovery and adaptation to long-term lifestyle changes.

SECTION **I**

Congenital Disorders (Clients Over Age 16)

Significant congenital disorders of the heart are usually identified and corrected early in life. Some persons reach adulthood without having had their congenital abnormality diagnosed or treated, perhaps because of inadequate medical care as a child or a lack of symptoms.

The two most common congenital heart problems in the adult are atrial septal defect, which may not produce symptoms until the fourth or fifth decade, and bicuspid aortic valve, which may never produce symptoms. Other congenital heart abnormalities found in adults, which may or may not have been diagnosed in childhood, include ventricular septal defect, pulmonic stenosis, coronary artery anomalies, and congenital heart block. For further information on congenital heart problems treated early in life, refer to a pediatric textbook. Congenital disorders diagnosed later in life are treated much the same as acquired defects discussed in this chapter.

A significant problem for adults who have had congenital problems diagnosed and treated early in life is obtaining health insurance. Because of the high cost of care that these persons may need, insurance rates are prohibitive. In addition, employers may be reluctant to hire individuals with a history of congenital heart disease because of the possible impact on an employer's group health insurance plan. Lack of adequate health insurance may discourage some clients from seeking needed care.

SECTION 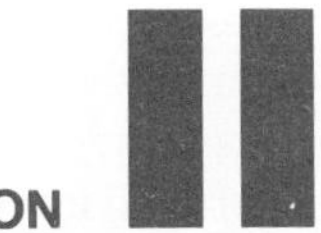

Disorders of Multifactorial Origin

Disorders of multifactorial origin that involve the heart may result from physiologic changes in the body, environmental influences, genetic characteristics, or psychosocial/lifestyle factors. Symptoms range from minor discomfort that is easily tolerated to life-threatening emergencies. Because these disorders are influenced by environmental and psychosocial/lifestyle factors, they are often preventable to some extent by changes in lifestyle.

Nurses can play a crucial role in the prevention of some of these cardiac disorders by educating the public. A person who understands the disease process and its effect on quality and length of life can make informed decisions regarding changes in lifestyle that will promote health. Education about the effects of diet, exercise, and smoking may promote healthier living. Educating the public about warning signs of heart attack may save lives. Detection and treatment of high blood pressure may prevent serious consequences of heart disease.

In the clinic and on the medical–surgical unit, nurses who are knowledgeable about abnormal assessment findings can refer clients for prompt medical evaluation. Astute detection of heart problems can mean the difference between life and death for clients who have been hospitalized for other reasons. For clients who are recovering from a heart problem, nurses can provide psychologic support to help them adjust to their new health status, to follow a rehabilitation program, and to make the changes in lifestyle that may minimize the effects of the disease.

Nursing assessment for stable clients with suspected heart disease involves a thorough history to identify risk factors including:

- Age and sex (Incidence of coronary artery disease increases with age and is higher in men than in women.)
- Family history of cardiovascular disease
- Cigarette smoking
- Elevated blood pressure
- Elevated blood lipid levels
- Obesity
- Diabetes mellitus
- Abnormal glucose tolerance
- Gout
- Use of oral contraceptives
- Sedentary lifestyle
- Emotional factors

Assessment and care planning for the cardiac client are described in Chapter 18. This chapter focuses on care of the ambulatory client or the client on a medical unit. For care given in the coronary care unit, refer to a cardiovascular nursing text.

Hypertension

High blood pressure, or hypertension, is a widespread chronic disease and a major health problem in North America. The incidence in blacks is twice that of whites. It is a significant cardiovascular risk factor and is the leading cause of cerebral vascular accident (CVA, or stroke). The mortality associated with hypertension is directly proportional to the diastolic and systolic blood pressures. As these pressures rise, mortality increases. Hypertension is usually detected between the ages of 20 and 40 years. Complications of hypertension are most prevalent after the age of 40.

According to most authorities, hypertension exists when the diastolic blood pressure is greater than 90 mm Hg. The systolic pressure may be normal or elevated. Isolated systolic hypertension is common in adults over 65 years of age and is most often due to atherosclerosis.

Hypertension is classified as either essential or secondary hypertension. Essential hypertension is the most common and affects aproximately 90% to 95% of clients. The cause of the elevated blood pressure is unknown, although there are often many contributing factors (eg, high-salt diet, obesity). Secondary hypertension, affecting approximately 5% of clients, is caused by a disease entity such as pheochromocytoma, renovascular disease, primary aldosteronism, or coarctation of the aorta. Oral con-

NURSING DIAGNOSES IN
Cardiac Dysfunction

DIRECTLY RELATED DIAGNOSES

- Anxiety
- Activity intolerance
- Cardiac output, altered: decreased
- Comfort, altered: pain
- Fear
- Knowledge deficit
- Role performance, altered
- Self-concept, disturbance in: body image
- Sexuality patterns, altered

OTHER POTENTIAL DIAGNOSES

- Adjustment, impaired
- Coping, ineffective: individual
- Tissue perfusion, altered: cerebral, cardiopulmonary, renal, gastrointestinal, peripheral

traceptives may also cause hypertension. Although the probability of secondary hypertension is low, the client's initial examination should always consider the possibility.

Clinical Manifestations

Hypertension has been called the silent disease or silent killer because clients are often asymptomatic until a CVA, myocardial infarction (MI), renal failure, or sudden death occurs. Persistent uncontrolled hypertension whether mild, moderate, or severe causes some degree of target organ damage to the heart, brain, or kidneys.

Cardiac manifestations of hypertension include angina, acute MI, left ventricular hypertrophy, acute pulmonary edema, congestive heart failure (CHF), and sudden coronary death. Renal involvement may begin as nocturia or proteinuria. More advanced renal damage leads to azotemia and renal failure. Cerebral strokes and transient ischemic attacks are often directly related to systolic hypertension. In fact, hypertension is a more potent risk factor for developing a CVA than coronary or renal disease.

Symptoms reported by clients that may be due to hypertension include dizziness, palpitations, chest pain, weakness, epistaxis, hematuria, and brief episodes of memory loss (transient ischemic attacks). Less frequently, severe hypertension may cause occipital headaches that are present when the client awakens in the morning and subside spontaneously within hours. Most often, clients are asymptomatic.

Essential hypertension is often described as mild diastolic elevation (90 to 104 mm Hg), moderate diastolic elevation (105 to 114 mm Hg), or severe diastolic elevation (>115 mm Hg). Because of increased morbidity in clients with diastolic pressures of 85 to 89 mm Hg, a high-normal category has recently been added to the classification.

When the average of two or more blood pressure readings shows a diastlic pressure greater than 90 mm Hg or systolic pressure greater than 160 mm Hg in three visits, the diagnosis of essential hypertension is confirmed. To ensure accurate measurements, the equipment (cuff and sphygmomanometer), environment, and the client's physical and psychologic state must be optimal.

Medical Measures

To reduce the morbidity and mortality associated with hypertension, nonpharmacologic and pharmacologic therapies are used. The client's condition is evaluated, and therapy is prescribed according to the severity of the blood pressure elevation, the client's symptoms, and the risk-factor profile. High-normal and mild hypertension are initially treated with a nonpharmacologic approach that includes weight reduction, dietary sodium restriction, moderation of alcohol intake, regular exercise, smoking cessation, stress reduction, and serum cholesterol reduction if needed.

WEIGHT REDUCTION Clients who are overweight (ie, 20% over their ideal body weight) are often hypertensive. Although the actual relation between obesity and hypertension is unclear, many studies have demonstrated that weight reduction can result in blood pressure reduction. In general, a 1 kg (2.2 lb) weight loss is associated with a 1.5 mm Hg decrease in diastolic pressure (McMahon, 1984).

SODIUM RESTRICTION In some clients, excessive salt/sodium intake correlates with the development of hypertension. Moderate restriction of sodium intake (2 g Na or 5 g NaCl) has lowered blood pressure in some, but not all, hypertensive clients. A combination of weight reduction and sodium restriction may provide the most benefit. Many OTC medications also contain sodium. Clients should be encouraged to read drug and food labels carefully.

ALCOHOL MODERATION Moderate alcohol intake may offer a protective effect in the development of cardiovascular disease. However, heavy alcohol consumption (ie, more than three or four hard-liquor drinks per day) is associated with increased blood pressure.

SMOKING CESSATION Cigarette smoking is a major risk factor in the development of cardiovascular disease. Nicotine causes constriction of both small and large blood vessels. When smoking is combined with hypertension, the risks are significantly increased. Although a cause-and-effect relation between cigarette smoking and the development of hypertension has not been documented, short-term nicotine use is known to increase both systolic and diastolic blood pressure.

EXERCISE Regular isotonic exercise such as walking, jogging, or swimming promotes cardiovascular fitness. Exercise facilitates weight reduction and promotes relaxation, which may result in lowering of the blood pressure. Clients who exercise regularly appear to have a lower incidence of cardiovascular disease than clients who remain sedentary or exercise irregularly.

If nonpharmacologic therapy is ineffective in lowering the blood pressure, or if faster results are desired, pharmacologic intervention is also prescribed. Clients with moderate or severe hypertension are usually treated immediately with both interventions.

PHARMACOLOGIC THERAPY Most health care providers use the *stepped-care* program in prescribing pharmacologic therapy. This approach has four steps (see Table 19–1).

Clients with mild hypertension who fail to respond to nonpharmacologic methods are routinely started at *step 1*, diuretic therapy. The diuretic works on the renal tubules, causing a sodium diuresis and subsequent volume depletion. A thiazide diuretic is usually selected, using the lowest effective dose.

Common side effects of diuretic therapy include hypokalemia, hyperuricemia, and carbohydrate intolerance. Cardiac dysrhythmias may develop if hypokalemia is present. Clients with a serum potassium level below 3.5 mEq/L may require a potassium supplement. Clients with gout often require treatment with probenecid or allopurinol.

If the diastolic blood pressure remains above normal (ie, >90 mm Hg), treatment is advanced to *step 2*. An antiadrenergic agent is added to the diuretic. The drugs in this group act on a variety of sites—centrally on the vasomotor center, peripherally by modifying catecholamine release, or on target tissue by blocking adrenergic receptor sites. Beta-adrenergic blocking agents (eg, propranolol) are the most commonly used agents in step 2. Recently, drugs that block the movement of calcium within smooth and cardiac muscle and drugs that inhibit the enzyme that converts angiotensin I to angiotensin II have been added to step 2.

Side effects of the drugs are often dose related. The therapeutic goal is to achieve hypertension control with the lowest dose and the fewest side effects. Therefore, a second drug is often substituted rather than using the maximum dose of a drug that may precipitate side effects. Sexual dysfunction is frequently reported by clients who are taking antihypertensive medication, especially adrenergic blocking agents. The mechanism of dysfunction is unclear, however. Psychologic factors, age, or other illnesses may contribute to the problem.

Step 3 is used when a variety of step 2 drugs combined with a diuretic have not achieved blood pressure control. The medications in step 3 are vasodilators that cause relaxation of smooth muscle, lowering peripheral resistance and blood pressure. The most common medication prescribed is hydralazine. Vasodilator therapy may cause a sympathetic reflex response (increased heart rate and cardiac output); therefore, an adrenergic blocking agent and a diuretic are often used in conjunction with the step 3 medication.

In severe hypertension or uncontrolled moderate hypertension, *step 4* is used. The approach in step 4 is substituting a step 2 agent for a peripheral adrenergic blocking agent. Guanethidine is frequently used. Side effects are common, however, and often contribute to poor client compliance. Some of the side effects include impotence, retrograde ejaculation, diarrhea, fatique, weight gain, and edema.

The stepped-care program appears to be effective for most clients, but the client's history and clinical condition should be evaluated. A flexible, individualized plan is the most effective approach.

Table 19–1
Stepped-Care Program: Antihypertensive Agents*

Antihypertensive Drug	Daily Dose Range
Step 1: Diuretic therapy	
Thiazides	
Chlorothiazide (Diuril)	250–500 mg
Hydrochlorothiazide (Oretic, HydroDIURIL, Esidrix)	25–50 mg
Sulfonamide diuretics	
Chlorthalidone (Hygroton)	25–50 mg
Loop diuretics	
Furosemide (Lasix)	40–120 mg
Ethacrynic acid (Edecrin)	50–200 mg
Potassium-sparing agents	
Spironolactone (Aldactone)	25–100 mg
Triamterene (Dyrenium)	50–100 mg
Step 2: Adrenergic inhibitors	
Beta-adrenergic blockers	
Atenolol (Tenormin)	25–100 mg
Metoprolol (Lopressor)	50–300 mg
Nadolol (Corgard)	20–120 mg
Propranolol (Inderal)	40–480 mg
Timolol (Timoptic)	20–60 mg
Central adrenergic inhibitors	
Clonidine (Catapres)	0.2–1.2 mg
Methyldopa (Aldomet)	500–2000 mg
Peripheral adrenergic inhibitor	
Reserpine (Serpasil)	0.05–0.25 mg
Alpha-1 adrenergic blocker	
Prazosin (Minipress)	1.0–20.0 mg
Angiotensin-converting enzyme inhibitors	
Captopril (Capoten)	37.5–150.0 mg
Slow-channel calcium-entry blocking agents	
Nifedipine (Procardia)	30–180 mg
Verapamil (Isoptin, Calan)	240–480 mg
Step 3: Vasodilators	
Hydralazine (Apresoline)	50–300 mg
Minoxidil (Loniten)	5–100 mg
Step 4: Peripheral adrenergic antagonist	
Guanethidine (Ismelin)	10–300 mg

*Most commonly used drugs

Specific Nursing Measures

Early detection, education, and promoting adherence to therapy are key factors in controlling blood pressure. The nurse's role is instrumental in each.

EARLY DETECTION The nurse is often the health care provider who takes the initial blood pressure on the client. Accurate measurement depends on the technique used (see Chapter 18). The client should be calm, quiet, and relaxed before obtaining the blood pressure. Restrictive clothing should be removed. If the initial reading is elevated, two more measurements 1 to 5 minutes apart should be obtained with the client in the supine position. The mean of the three readings is reported as the blood pressure.

Screening for hypertension may be performed at a variety of public events such as community programs, club meetings, company activities, fairs, or church functions. When nurses obtain elevated readings at these screening programs, they should urge affected clients to see their health care providers for a follow-up blood pressure check.

Client/Family Teaching

Perhaps the most significant factor in controlling blood pressure is the client's understanding of the disease and the treatment plan. Client education usually begins with the definition and cause of hypertension and the complications and risks associated with uncontrolled hypertension. The nonpharmacologic approach to hypertension management is initially emphasized.

After reviewing the client's health history and cardiovascular risk appraisal, an individualized nonpharmacologic approach is planned. Weight reduction and proper nutrition are the primary interventions. Give the client written guidelines such as a list of foods to avoid (ie, those high in sodium and cholesterol) and a calorie reduction diet. Assisting the client in menu planning is effective. Both the client and family may need additional nutritional counseling. A referral to a nutritionist may be helpful.

Clients who use antihypertensive medications need additional education. The purpose, dosage, and possible side effects of the medication should be explained. If more than one medication is used, the client must understand that each drug acts differently; therefore, substitution is inappropriate and dangerous. Skipping doses and discontinuing medication may cause rebound hypertension and possibly provoke a CVA or MI. Unpleasant side effects often result in poor drug compliance. Therefore, nurses need to investigate carefully any side effects the client experiences. Hypokalemia is a common side effect of diuretic therapy. The symptoms and signs include muscle weakness, apathy, hypotension, cardiac dysrhythmias, and prolonged Q-T interval on the ECG. Clients should be given a list of foods containing potassium to counterbalance the potassium loss (see Box 19–1). Occasionally, clients need a potassium supplement. Inform clients that if side effects occur, the drug dose can be altered by the physician to minimize the problem, or an alternative drug can be prescribed.

ADHERENCE TO THERAPY The predominant problem in controlling high blood pressure is the client's adherence to therapy. The nonpharmacologic approach requires personal lifestyle changes, and the pharmacologic approach may cause unacceptable side effects. Also contributing to poor compliance is the chronicity of hypertension, the asymptomatic nature of the disease, and the long-term management.

Involving the client in establishing the short-term and long-term goals of therapy is important in obtaining client cooperation. Clients are more likely to adhere to the hypertension regimen if they are active participants. Both nonpharmacologic and pharmacologic interventions should be instituted gradually, and a nonauthoritarian approach should be used. Management decisions may include negotiation between the client and health care provider. The client may decide on a weight reduction goal and select the foods to be sacrificed. For example, the client may negotiate for a daily beer but offer to give up salty pretzels. The nurse may also influence the client to consume "light" beer which is lower in calories and sodium.

Lack of adherence to antihypertensive medications may be from side effects, a dosage schedule of more than once

Box 19–1
Foods High in Potassium

Almonds	Grapefruit juice	Potato chips
Apricots	Honeydew melon	Potatoes (baked or boiled)
Artichokes	Meat (especially veal)	Poultry
Avocados	Milk	Prune juice
Bananas	Molasses (dark or light)	Prunes
Beans (lima, navy, pinto)	Nectarines	Pumpkin
Bran cereal	Nuts (brazil, cashew, chestnuts, peanuts, pecans, pistachio, walnuts)	Raisins
Bread (whole and grain)	Orange juice	Rhubarb
Broccoli	Oranges	Rhutabaga
Brussel sprouts	Papaya	Scallops
Cantaloupe	Parsnips	Shrimp
Chocolate	Peaches	Soybeans
Cocoa	Pears	Squash (winter)
Coffee (instant or percolated)	Pineapple	Tangerines
Dates	Pineapple juice	Tomato juice
Figs	Pomegranate	Tomatoes
Fish		Vegetable juice
Grapefruit		Wheat germ
		Yams

a day, or expense. The client's satisfaction with the medication as well as blood pressure response should be assessed at every visit.

Dysrhythmias

Disturbances in heart rate or rhythm are commonly referred to as cardiac dysrhythmias (arrhythmias). Dysrhythmias range from the common insignificant dysrhythmias found in persons with normal hearts to life-threatening dysrhythmias. The disturbance may be either in the automaticity of the cardiac cells or in the conduction of the impulses. Examples of disturbances in automaticity include an abnormal pacemaker site and **ectopic beats** (cardiac impulses originating outside the SA node). With a disturbance in conduction, a conducting heart cell may not depolarize when it is stimulated and completely "block" the conduction of the impulse ahead of it. The conducting cells to the sides of it conduct normally, but the conducting cell waits until the impulse is transmitted through abnormal pathways and propagated backwards. The cell then depolarizes, permitting the impulse to reenter the same abnormal pathway and set up an abnormal tachydysrhythmia. This is referred to as "reentry phenomenon."

Cardiac dysrhythmias are usually assessed by coronary care or critical care nurses using electronic monitoring equipment and ECG rhythm strips. However, all nurses routinely assess clients for the presence or absence of dysrhythmias by taking the pulse. A basic understanding of common disturbances in cardiac rate and rhythm as diagnosed from rhythm strips is helpful to nurses in the care of clients who may be susceptible to dysrhythmias or those who are being medically treated for prevention of cardiac dysrhythmias.

Ischemia or injury to cardiac cells is a frequent cause of dysrhythmias. Enlargement of the chambers of the heart sometimes affects normal conduction, resulting in dysrhythmias. Many drugs, including caffeine, nicotine, and alcohol, can be responsible for dysrhythmias. Disturbances in electrolyte balance or the normal physiologic environment of the cardiac cells may sometimes cause disturbances in rhythm. Some dysrhythmias are not abnormal but a normal physiologic response. Some common examples of normal physiologic response include sinus tachycardia associated with increased activity level and sinus bradycardia, which is quite often seen in athletes at rest.

Clinical Manifestations and Medical Measures

Because the clinical manifestations and treatment of dysrhythmias depend on the type of rhythm disturbance, common cardiac dysrhythmias will be discussed individually. Because dysrhythmias are named for their site of origin (sinus, atrial, atrioventricular [A-V], junctional, ventricular, etc) they will be presented in that order. Keep in mind that the rhythm strip alone does not provide sufficient information to make an unequivocal diagnosis of dysrhythmia. Often, several experts make different diagnoses from the same rhythm strip.

Drugs used to treat dysrhythmias reduce automaticity of ectopic foci, alter conduction velocity or cardiac membrane responsiveness (eg, quinidine), inhibit the effects of circulating catecholamines (eg, beta-adrenergic blockers), prolong action potential (eg, bretylium), or inhibit the influx of calcium ions (eg, calcium channel blockers).

NORMAL SINUS RHYTHM Under normal circumstances, the heart beats at a rate of between 60 and 100 beats per minute. The atria are electrically stimulated; these recorded electrical signals produce a P wave on the ECG (Figure 19–1; refer also to Figure 18–2). The impulse is slowed in the A-V node before being conducted through the ventricles and forming the QRS complex. The slowing permits the atria to contract and fill the ventricles with more blood before they contract. The amount of time from the beginning of the P wave to the beginning of the QRS complex is between 0.12 and 0.20 seconds, or 3 to 5 small

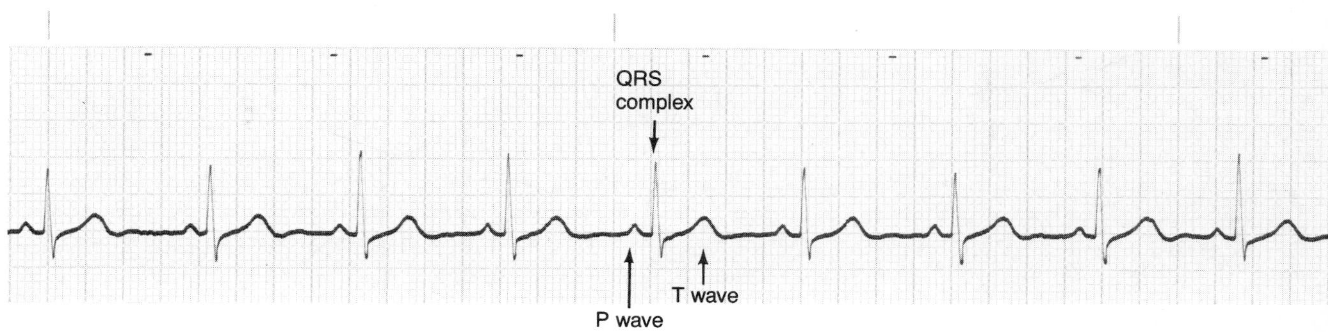

Figure 19–1

Normal sinus rhythm.

squares (0.04 seconds each) on the paper. Every P wave is followed by a QRS in normal sinus rhythm. Normal sinus rhythm has the following characteristics:

- P waves occur regularly. The distance between P waves is the same (ie, the distance between the first and second P waves is the same as the distance between the second and third P waves).
- P waves occur at a rate of between 60 (25 small squares between P waves) and 100 (15 small squares between P waves)
- Every P wave is followed by a QRS complex.
- The PR interval is the same for all cycles and is between 0.12 and 0.20 seconds. (It takes at least 0.12 seconds for an impulse to travel from the atria to the ventricles; therefore, what may appear to be a normal sinus rhythm may be an atrial rhythm.)
- The duration of the QRS complex is between 0.06 and 0.12 seconds (unless conduction is abnormally slow through the ventricles, as occurs with a bundle-branch block, which may produce a longer QRS complex).

SINUS DYSRHYTHMIA Sinus dysrhythmia is different from normal sinus rhythm only in the variation in the distance between the P waves (Figure 19–2). Most frequently, sinus dysrhythmia is seen in normal persons with slower heart rates that vary with respiration. The rate increases during inspiration and decreases with expiration. The P waves (and associated QRS complexes) are closer together during inspiration and further apart during expiration. Sinus dysrhythmia causes the pulse rate to vary slightly with breathing. There is no treatment for sinus dysrhythmia.

SINUS TACHYCARDIA The electrocardiographic difference between sinus tachycardia (Figure 19–3) and normal sinus rhythm is in the rate. The distance between P waves (and associated QRS complexes) is less than 15 small squares, which produces a heart rate of over 100.

Normally, the most common cause of sinus tachycardia is physical exercise. Depending on age and physical condition, an individual may increase the heart rate as high as 160 to nearly 200 beats per minute without problems. In the diseased heart, as the heart rate is increased past the physiologic limit, the ventricles do not have sufficient time to fill with blood, and cardiac output decreases. Decreased output may result in myocardial ischemia and lead to more serious dysrhythmias. Other causes of sinus tachycardia include removal of parasympathetic stimulation (such as with atropine and other vagolytic drugs); increase in sympathetic nervous system stimulation such as with fear or with administration of adrenergic drugs; use of stimulants such as nicotine, caffeine, and alcohol; and pathologic conditions such as fever, anemia, hypovolemia, and heart failure.

Sinus tachycardia causes the pulse rate to increase. In the diseased heart as the rate increases to the point that cardiac output is diminished, a weak pulse will reflect the decreased stroke volume.

Treatment is usually to remove the cause. When the client is symptomatic, drugs may be used (eg, propranolol, which blocks the effects of beta-adrenergic activity, or verapamil, a calcium channel blocker that decreases automaticity in the S-A node).

SINUS BRADYCARDIA The difference between normal sinus rhythm and sinus bradycardia is in the rate. The distance between the P waves in sinus bradycardia is greater than 25 small blocks, which produces a heart rate of less than 60.

Sinus bradycardia normally occurs in well-trained athletes, who may have heart rates as low as 35 or 40 during sleep. Sinus bradycardia occurs with stimulation of the vagus nerve, such as during vomiting or straining at defecation, as well as with the administration of parasympathetic drugs, beta-adrenergic blocking drugs, and calcium channel blocking drugs. It also occurs with increased intracranial or intraocular pressure as well as in some disease states.

Sinus bradycardia causes the pulse rate to decrease. The rate may be slow enough to cause symptoms of decreased cardiac output.

Treatment is not usually necessary unless the client has symptoms of insufficient cardiac output. Atropine may be used to inhibit the effects of parasympathetic stimulation, which slows the heart. Isoproterenol or another sympathomimetic drug may be used. When the sinus brady-

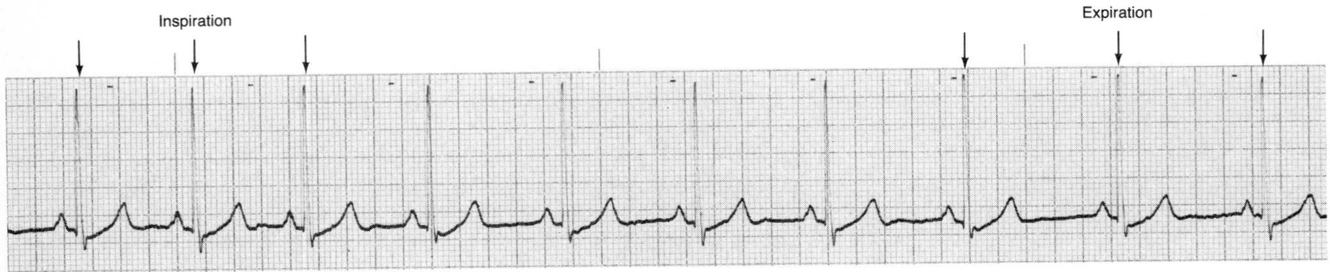

Figure 19–2

Sinus dysrhythmia. The heart rate varies with respiration, increasing during inspiration and slowing during expiration. Check the distance between the first three arrows and the last three arrows.

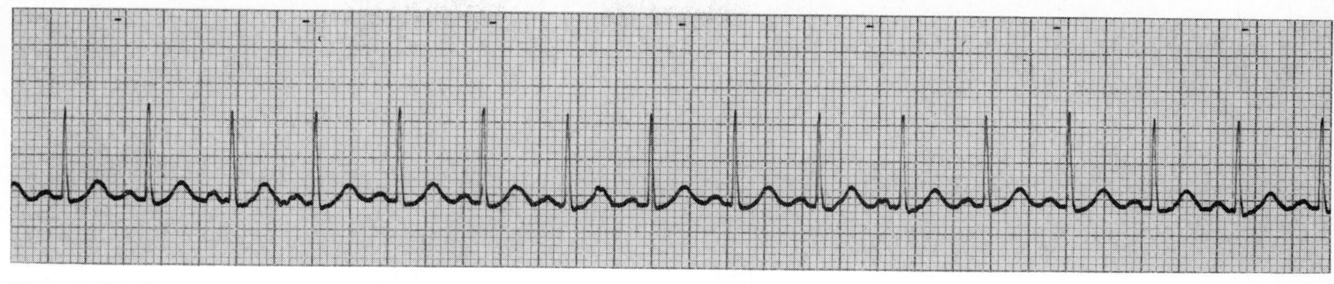

Figure 19–3

Sinus tachycardia. The heart rate is 130 beats per minute. Each complex has a P wave and QRS indicating a sinus tachycardia.

cardia is chronic and the client has symptoms, a pacemaker may be indicated.

PREMATURE ATRIAL COMPLEXES Premature atrial complex (PAC) (Figure 19–4) occurs when an area in the atrium promotes a premature depolarization of the atria, which results in a P wave of a different configuration than P waves of the dominant rhythm. If the impulse is conducted through the A-V junctional area, resulting in a QRS complex to follow, the PR interval is greater than 0.12 seconds. Because PACs usually result in depolarization of the sinus node, the sinus node has to reset its rhythm, and the subsequent normal sinus impulse comes later than expected. There is a pause after the premature P wave. Because the pause is usually not long enough for the normal P wave to occur where it originally would have, the pause is called *noncompensatory*. Sometimes, PACs are not conducted through the A-V junctional tissue and are called blocked PACs.

The etiology of PACs is the same as those of many dysrhythmias, including ischemia, drug effects, stimulants, and stretching of the atrial tissue. Persons with normal hearts may have PACs and note palpitations from them. With PACs, the major concern is that they sometimes promote the development of more severe dysrhythmias, including supraventricular tachycardia and atrial fibrillation. Treatment is not usually neccessary. If prone to supraventricular tachycardia, the client may be given digitalis, which slows conduction through the A-V node; propranolol, which inhibits the effects of sympathetic stimulation; or verapamil, which slows conduction through the A-V node. Other drugs used to decrease conduction and automaticity in atrial tissue include quinidine, procainamide, or disopyramide.

ATRIAL FLUTTER Atrial flutter (Figure 19–5) is characterized by sawtooth or flutter P waves. The atrial rate (P wave rate) is usually between 250 and 350 beats per minute. Because the A-V node has a physiologic limit that will not usually conduct more than 200 impulses per minute, atrial flutter causes a physiologic block, resulting in every other flutter wave being conducted through the A-V node. If the problem is untreated, the rate of the QRS complex is one-half that of the atrial rate. If treated, the flutter rate may be less than 250. The rate of impulses conducted will usually be an even number such as 2:1 or 4:1.

Persons with normal hearts experience occasional atrial flutter, but persistent atrial flutter is usually indicative of heart disease. Causes of atrial flutter include conditions that cause the atria to stretch, such as mitral or tricuspid stenosis or regurgitation, pulmonary emboli, MI, or ventricular failure. Other conditions such as thyrotoxicosis, alcoholism, and pericarditis may cause atrial flutter.

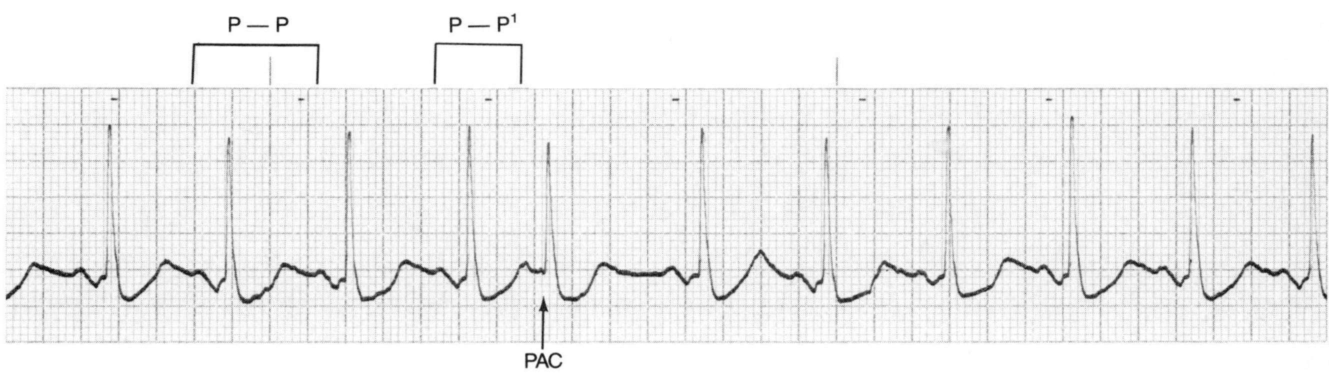

Figure 19–4

Premature atrial complexes fifth beat is a premature atrial contraction. Note that the P–P′ interval is shorter than the P–P interval. The P′ wave is partially buried in the preceding T wave. The QRS is normal.

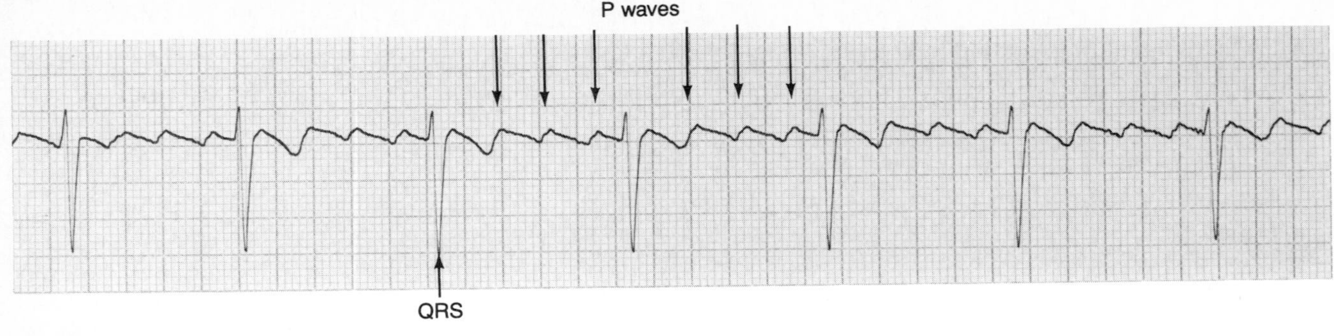

Figure 19–5

Atrial flutter. In atrial flutter the ECG forms a sawtooth pattern of P waves on the baseline.

The goals of therapy include terminating the rhythm or controlling the ventricular response as well as determining and treating the cause of the dysrhythmia. Direct current (DC) synchronous cardioversion is often effective in terminating the rhythm or converting it to atrial fibrillation, which is less dangerous because of a slower ventricular response. Drugs that block conduction through the A-V node (eg, digitalis, verapamil, and propranolol) may be used to control the ventricular response. Long-term management of atrial flutter includes the use of antidysrhythmic drugs, such as quinidine, procainamide, or disopyramide in combination with digitalis.

ATRIAL FIBRILLATION Atrial fibrillation (Figure 19–6) is characterized by an irregularly irregular QRS rhythm with QRS complexes occurring at a rate of between 100 and 150 in the untreated client. P waves are indistinguishable and may be represented by an undulating baseline or fine fibrillatory waves. The atrial rate is between 350 and 600, is chaotic, and does not support complete atrial contraction.

Atrial fibrillation may be experienced by persons with normal hearts, but chronic atrial fibrillation is usually indicative of heart disease. The causes of atrial fibrillation are the same as those of atrial flutter. Atrial fibrillation is considered less dangerous because it will not support as rapid a ventricular rate as atrial flutter. The stimulation of the A-V node is chaotic, and most stimulations are not capable of propagating an impulse because of the physiologic limits of the A-V node. Atrial fibrillation does not support atrial contraction. Therefore, because of the nature of the blood flow through the atria, clot formation and subsequent release of emboli when the rhythm is corrected are potential problems. The treatment of atrial fibrillation is much the same as for atrial flutter.

SUPRAVENTRICULAR TACHYCARDIA Supraventricular tachycardia includes any tachycardia in which the tissue responsible for pacing the heart is above the ventricles (above the bifurcation of the bundle of His). Supraventricular tachycardia promotes a ventricular rate between 150 and 250. The classification of supraventricular tachycardia includes sinus, atrial, and junctional tachycardia as well as tachycardia resulting from atrial flutter or atrial fibrillation. A tachycardia originating in the S-A node or atria should have a P wave before every QRS complex and a PR interval greater than 0.12 seconds. Junctional tachycardia may produce a P wave before the QRS complex with a PR interval less than 0.12 seconds. Or the P wave might be buried in the QRS complex or come after the QRS complex. This classification is useful because extremely fast rates may cause the P wave to be buried in the T wave or QRS complex in atrial tachycardia, and a P wave that comes after the QRS in a tachycardia originating in the junctional tissue may look like an atrial P wave. Other maneuvers or specific ECG studies may be done to determine the origin of the tachycardia. The differentiation of supraventricular tachycardia from ventricular tachycardia becomes a problem when the conduction through the ventricles is slowed and the QRS complex becomes longer than 0.12 seconds.

Although persons with normal hearts may experience supraventricular tachycardia, most supraventricular tachy-

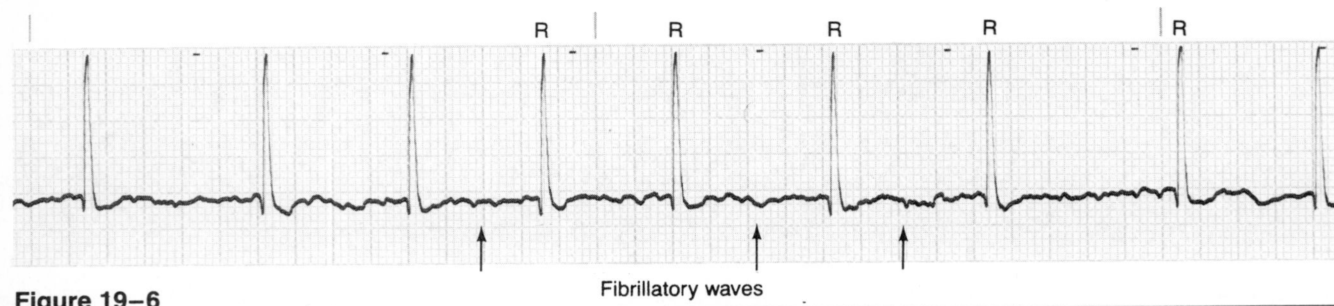

Figure 19–6

Atrial fibrillation. Atrial activity is manifested as fibrillatory waves—rapid, small, irregular waves. Note the varying R–R intervals. The ventricular rhythm is irregular.

cardia is associated with heart disease. The causes of supraventricular tachycardia are the same as those described under atrial flutter and sinus tachycardia.

The goals of therapy are to terminate the rhythm if possible or to slow down the ventricular response. The physician might massage the carotid sinus or apply pressure to the eyeballs to increase parasympathetic activity to terminate the rhythm, or decrease the ventricular response. The client might be encouraged to promote vagal nerve stimulation by gagging or simulating a diving reflex by dipping the head into cold water. Other treatment includes all the modalities discussed under atrial flutter: DC synchronous cardioversion to terminate the rhythm and administration of digitalis, verapamil, propranolol, quinidine, procainamide, or disopyramide. Sometimes a pacemaker is inserted, and in some cases, surgery is performed to remove accessory pathways.

PREMATURE VENTRICULAR COMPLEXES When an area in the ventricle promotes a premature depolarization of the ventricles, it is called a premature ventricular complex (PVC) (Figure 19–7). PVCs, like PACs, cause an irregularity in the pulse. The PVC may also produce a pulse wave that is less full and earlier than expected. The PVC may also occur early enough in the cardiac cycle so the heart does not have sufficient time to fill and the heart contraction does not eject sufficient blood to produce a pulse wave. The pulse wave that follows the PVC may be much fuller because of sufficient time to fill the heart between the premature contraction and the contraction that follows.

The major ECG feature distinguishing PVCs from PACs is a wide, bizarre-looking QRS complex (greater than 0.12 seconds), not preceded by a P wave, with a T wave that usually is inscribed in the opposite direction of the major deflection of the QRS. PVCs recorded on a rhythm strip cannot be distinguished with certainty from PACs. Generally, the PVC does not travel retrograde through the atria. As a result, the pause following the PVC is usually compensatory because the normal sinus node is not interrupted and maintains its rhythmicity. Sometimes the PVC does stimulate retrograde (backward) conduction through the atria and produces a retrograde P wave on the rhythm strip, interrupts the sinus mechanism, and produces a noncompensatory pause as the sinus mechanism is reset. If the PVC produces retrograde conduction, the P wave may precede, be buried in, or come after the QRS complex. If the P wave comes before the QRS complex, the PR interval will be less than 0.12 seconds.

PVCs are the most common type of rhythm disturbance and occur both in health and disease. They may cause discomfort in the neck or chest or palpitations. The frequency of PVCs increases with age. The causes of PVCs include ischemia, injury, drugs, caffeine, nicotine, alcohol, electrolyte imbalance, and extemes in heart rate. PVCs are of most concern in clients in the coronary care unit because they often presage more dangerous ventricular dysrhythmias.

Treatment may be to increase or decrease the heart rate if the PVCs are associated with extremes in heart rate. The initial therapy for PVCs in hospitalized clients is intravenous lidocaine. Other antidysrhythmic agents include procainamide, quinidine, disopyramide, propranolol, and phenytoin.

VENTRICULAR TACHYCARDIA When three or more PVCs occur in a row at a fairly regular rate of 110 to 250, the dysrhythmia is called ventricular tachycardia (Figure 19–8). Ventricular tachycardia may occur in people with healthy hearts and produce no symptoms. Ventricular tachycardia may be a life-threatening dysrhythmia in people with heart disease, especially if the dysrhythmia is sustained.

Persons who have ventricular tachycardia that is not sustained and produces no symptoms are not treated phar-

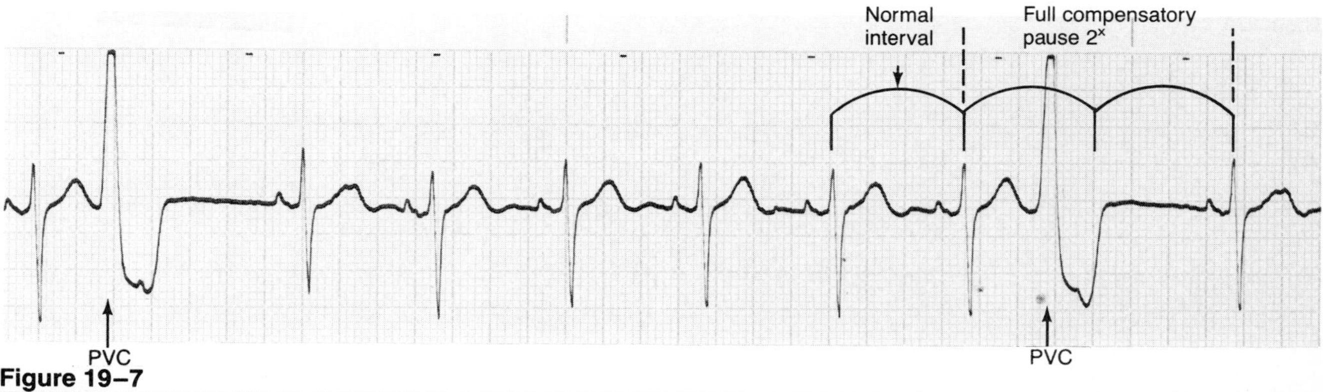

Figure 19–7

Premature ventricular complexes. The second and ninth beats are PVCs. Note that the QRS is greater than 0.12 sec, the R–R interval is shorter than the following beats, atrial depolarization follows the wide QRS, and a complete compensatory pause is present. A complete compensatory pause exists when the R–R interval containing the PVC is two times the R–R interval of the basic rhythm.

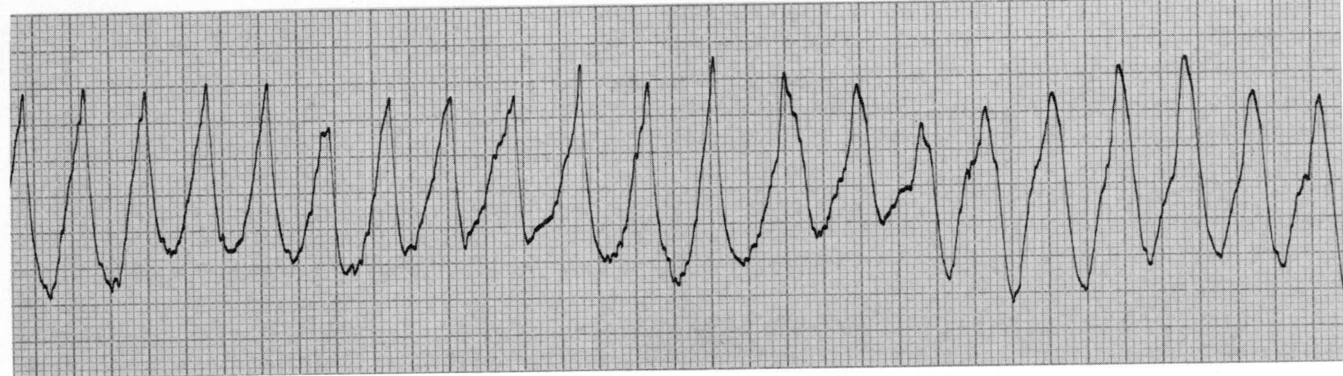

Figure 19–8

Ventricular tachycardia. With ventricular tachycardia a rapid succession of ventricular ectopic beats is seen on the ECG. The QRS complexes are wide and bizarre.

macologically but are followed closely by their physician. The usual first line of therapy for persons with ventricular tachycardia who have heart disease or are symptomatic is intravenous lidocaine. An artificial pacemaker is inserted if pharmacologic therapy is unsuccessful (see below). DC countershock may be used if the client is hemodynamically unstable.

VENTRICULAR FIBRILLATION Ventricular fibrillation (Figure 19–9) is a chaotic rhythm in which the ventricles produce completely disorganized depolarization and repolarization waves. Ventricular fibrillation is usually a terminal event associated with coronary artery disease. It may also be caused by ischemia, pharmacologic agents, electrical shock, and other dysrhythmias. The ECG features of ventricular fibrillation include irregular waveforms that vary in size. There are no distinguishable P waves, QRS complexes, ST segments, or T waves.

Because of the electrical disorganization, the ventricles do not contract as a unit, and there is no cardiac output. Ventricular fibrillation is a life-threatening dysrhythmia and usually will result in death if it is not treated within 3 to 5 minutes. DC countershock should be instituted as soon as possible. Cardiopulmonary resuscitation should be performed until the equipment is ready and continued as long as there is no effective rhythm.

FIRST-DEGREE A-V BLOCK First-degree A-V block is a delay in the transmission of impulses from the atria to the ventricles. All of the impulses reach the ventricles, which distinguishes first-degree block from the other forms of A-V heart block. The delay may be in the A-V node or the tissues beneath the A-V node. First-degree A-V block may be observed in healthy persons. Causes of first-degree heart block include pharmacologic agents, heart disease, hypoxia, congenital heart disease, lesions or calcifications of the conducting system, and other diseases affecting the heart. There is usually no treatment for first-degree A-V block, but attention is given to determining the cause and observing for progression to second- or third-degree heart block.

SECOND-DEGREE A-V BLOCK In second-degree A-V block some impulses are conducted from the atria to the ventricles and some impulses are not. The client may notice skipped heart beats. The causes of second-degree A-V block are the same as those of first-degree block. Second-degree A-V block is divided into type I and type II. The treatment for type I second-degree A-V block is the same as that of first-degree A-V block. If the heart rate is too slow and the client has symptoms of inadequate cardiac output, atropine may be used to increase the heart rate. If atropine is ineffective or contraindicated, an artificial

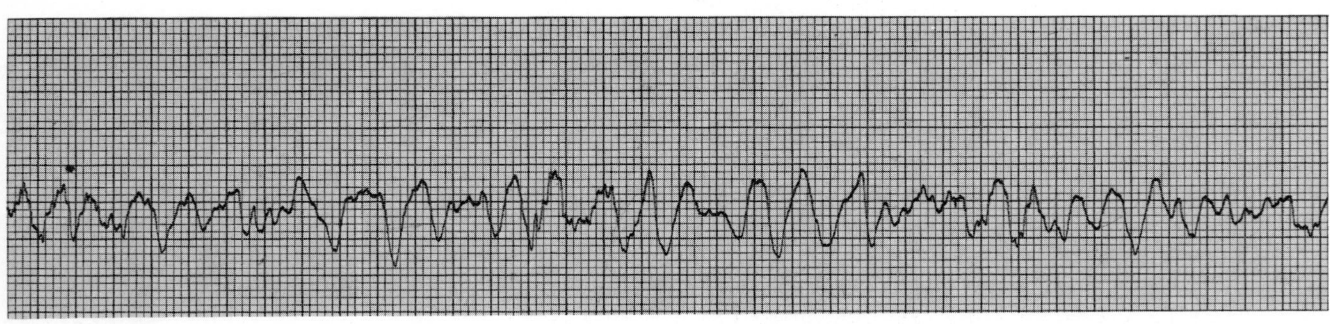

Figure 19–9

Ventricular fibrillation. Irregular wave forms occur that vary in size. There are no distinguishable P waves, QRS complexes, ST segments, or T waves. The rhythm is chaotic.

pacemaker may be used. Type II A-V block is considered more serious because the block is usually lower in the conductive system and more frequently progresses to complete A-V block. An artificial pacemaker is the usual treatment for type II A-V block.

COMPLETE A-V BLOCK Complete A-V block, sometimes referred to as third-degree A-V block, occurs when none of the impulses conducted through the atria reaches the ventricles. The causes of complete A-V block may be the same as first-degree A-V block. Emergency treatment of complete heart block may include administration of atropine or isoproterenol to increase the heart rate until an artificial pacemaker can be inserted.

Specific Nursing Measures

When assessing the client for a dysrhythmia, the nurse's major concern is whether the client has a sufficient heart rate to maintain cardiac output. The nurse determines this by the pulse rate; the critical care nurse gathers additional information by assessing on the ECG monitor the QRS complex that immediately precedes the pulse wave. Too fast a rate, or a tachycardia, may be dangerous because the heart may not have enough time to fill. Too slow a rate may be dangerous because cardiac output is determined by stroke volume and heart rate. Any time cardiac output is insufficient, the heart may not be able to supply its own muscle with sufficient nutrients, which may result in more severe dysrhythmias and heart failure.

If the rate is sufficient and the client is relatively stable, further assessment can take place. The nurse determines the regularity of the rhythm and the volume of the pulse. Is the volume of the pulse sufficient? An apical and radial pulse taken simultaneously might show a pulse deficit. An assessment of the radial pulse alone might reveal that some pulse waves are fuller than others. A perceptive nurse might associate these pulse findings with the probability of a rhythm disturbance.

Ask the client how he or she feels. Evaluate level of consciousness and mentation to determine adequacy of cerebral perfusion. Assess capillary refill, skin color and temperature, and pedal pulses to determine adequacy of peripheral circulation.

Several questions may be helpful in assessing the cardiac rhythm from a rhythm strip. Is the rate sufficient for adequate cardiac output? This is determined by the number of QRS complexes per minute, assuming that a pulse wave probably follows each QRS. If not, check the client before proceeding with further assessment because action may be required. If the rate is sufficient and the client is relatively stable, continue with the assessment. To determine origin of the heart rhythm and the atrial contribution to ventricular filling, ask:

- Are there P waves?
- What is their rate?
- What is their rhythm?
- Are the P waves related to the QRS complexes?
- What is the PR interval?
- Is the rhythm one that may decrease cardiac output or lead to serious dysrhythmias?

Pacemaker Implantation

For the client with a bradydysrhythmia, the treatment with lasting results is the implantation of a permanent **pacemaker,** a device that supplies electrical impulses to the heart muscle to stimulate the heartbeat. The pacemaker is powered by batteries that last from 8 to 10 years.

The pacemaker system has two components: (1) a pulse generator, which contains the electrical circuitry and batteries and is implanted in the chest or abdomen, and (2) the pacemaker electrodes, which are connected to the heart. Many different types of pacemakers are produced and can be programmed to stimulate the heart in a variety of pacing modes. For example, a pacemaker can pace only the atria, only the ventricles, or both. The pacemaker can pace continuously (fixed-rate pacing), or it can be programmed to pace the heart when needed (demand pacing). Newer self-adjusting units alter pulse rates slowly and smoothly like the natural heart does. Pacemakers also can be used temporarily with an external generator or can be permanently implanted. Temporary pacemakers are usually indicated for life-threatening situations in which the heartbeat cannot be stimulated by drugs or cardiopulmonary resuscitation.

Automatic implantable defibrillators for clients known to be at risk for fibrillation are also available in some medical centers. The defibrillator device, about the size of a deck of cards and weighing 1½ lb, was given Food and Drug Administration approval in late 1985.

Types of Pacemakers

TRANSVENOUS ENDOCARDIAL PACING Vein routes for either permanent or temporary transvenous endocardial pacing include cephalic, internal jugular, and external jugular routes. The cephalic vein is the most common site, because only one incision is required over the deltopectoral area for transvenous electrode and pacing generator box insertion under the skin (Figure 19–10). For temporary pacing, no incision is needed. An introduction sheath is placed into the vein, and the pacing electrode is passed through this sheath into the heart. The electrode is then connected to an external pulse generator.

EPICARDIAL PACING In epicardial pacing, the heart is stimulated to beat by an electrode sutured or screwed onto the epicardium. This method of insertion is used for permanent pacing. The most commonly used epicardial electrode is the flat lead, which is sutured to the surface of the heart, usually over the apex. A thoracotomy approach is

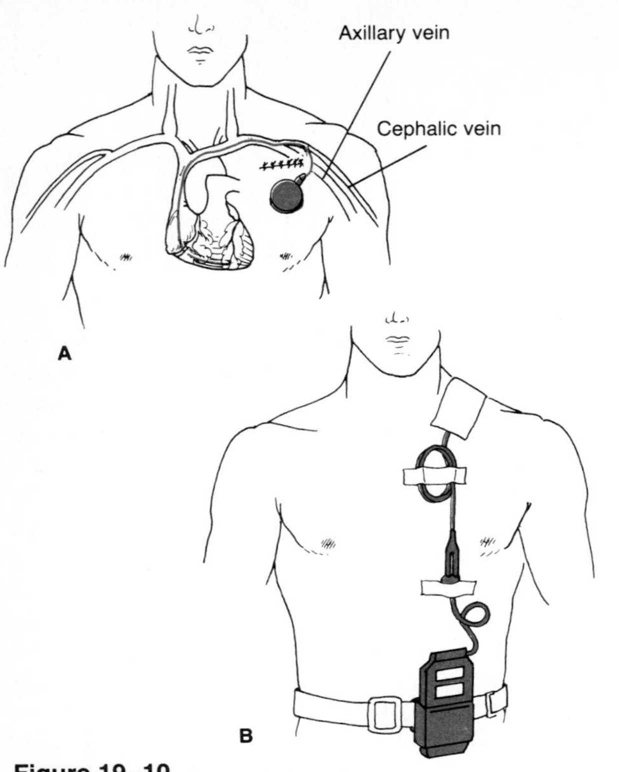

Figure 19–10

Transvenous endocardial pacing. **A.** Transvenous endocardial pacing using the cephalic vein with a pulse generator pocket on the anterior chest wall. **B.** External pulse generator for temporary pacing.

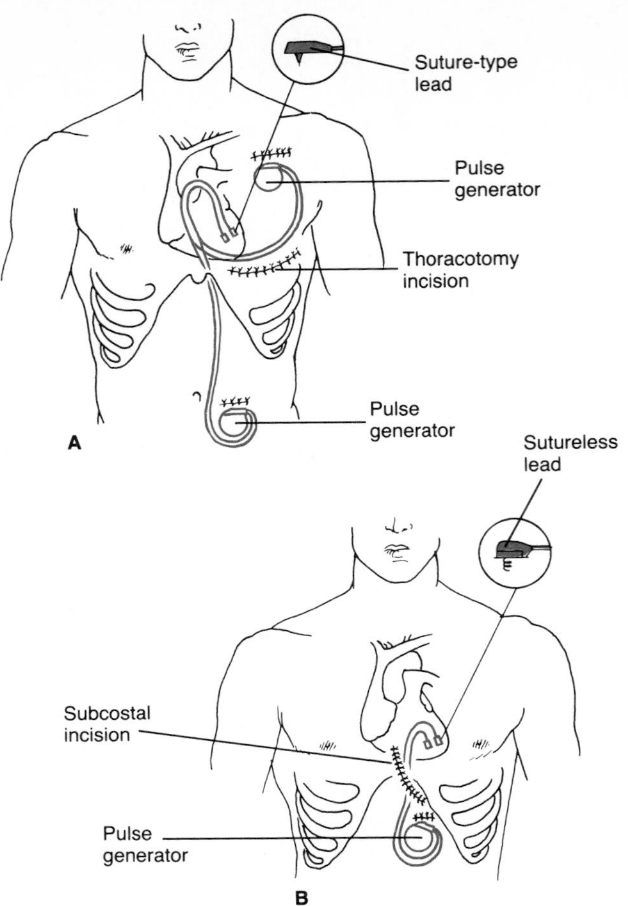

Figure 19–11

Epicardial pacing. **A.** The electrode is sutured to the surface of the heart. The pulse generator pocket can be on the anterior chest wall or on the abdomen. **B.** The electrode is screwed into the myocardium. The pulse generator pocket is on the upper abdomen.

required so the heart is in view for the suturing (Figure 19–11A).

The second type of myocardial electrode is a screw-in lead inserted into the myocardium by three clockwise turns. The advantage is that a thoracotomy approach is not required for insertion. An incision can be made in the subcostal area; the electrodes are slipped under the ribs and screwed into the myocardium (Figure 19–11B). Another advantage is that this lead is easily repositioned during implantation. The physiologic and psychosocial/lifestyle implications are in Table 19–2.

Nursing Implications

PREOPERATIVE CARE Because clients often fear pacemaker insertion, focus on reassuring clients and explaining the need for the pacemaker. Explain to clients in simple terms how the heart is stimulated to beat and how the heart's conduction system works. Clients must also understand where the incision is to be made; how the pacemaker will appear under the skin; and the fact that there will be a large, bulky dressing.

The procedure will take 30 minutes to 2 hours, depending on the approach. Warn clients that fluoroscopy will be used during the procedure. Also, blood pressure, heart rate, and heart rhythm will be continuously monitored. Restraints may also be necessary during the procedure. The client is kept NPO before pacemaker insertion. The upper chest is also shaved.

POSTOPERATIVE CARE After insertion, pacemaker function is closely monitored on the ECG, and vital signs are assessed frequently. The client remains in bed for 12 to 24 hours to allow for pacemaker electrode stabilization. Check the wound every 30 minutes for signs of bleeding. Record fluid intake and output to ensure that the client is well hydrated. Give medication for pain relief as needed.

Be especially alert for signs of pacemaker failure: hypertension, dizziness, light-headedness, chest pain, and ECG changes. Nurses who are monitoring the ECG need to have a thorough understanding of the types of pacemakers and the location of pacing spikes. A *pacing spike,* or *pacing artifact,* is a vertical line on the ECG that appears each time the pulse generator fires an impulse. This artifact is useful in identifying the type of pacemaker and any malfunctions related to pacing. Nurses must also be able to recognize pacemaker malfunction, such as lack of capture and competition.

Table 19–2
Pacemaker Implantation: Implications for the Client 

Physiologic Implications	Psychosocial/Lifestyle Implications
Bradydysrhythmia no longer present Possible pacemaker malfunction Pain, bleeding, or infection at insertion site Diaphragm twitching if electrode perforates myocardium or client has a thin-walled ventricle	Need to recognize signs of pacemaker failure (decreased heart rate, chest pain, dizziness, fainting, hiccups, undue fatigue, and shortness of breath) Need to carry an identification card and to alert airport security personnel to presence of pacemaker Avoidance of excessive arm movements and reaching 5 weeks postoperatively to prevent dislodging pacing electrode Need to take antibiotics before and after dental work to avoid bacterial endocarditis

In *lack of capture,* there is failure to pace the heart related to one of several possible problems such as a misplaced electrode, perforation of the ventricle, scar tissue at the site of the electrode with an inability to stimulate the myocardium, or an inadequate electrical output by the pulse generator from a weakened battery or mechanical dysfunction. *Competition* is said to exist when the pacemaker continues to fire despite the client's own underlying rhythm, which is at a heart rate similar to the pacemaker or higher.

Postoperative client teaching should include the factors discussed in Table 19–2.

Coronary Artery Disease

The coronary arteries that supply blood to the heart muscle may become diseased and fail to supply sufficient blood to enable the heart to perform its work. Disease of the coronary arteries usually results in obstruction to blood flow. The proximal sections of the major coronary arteries with as much as 80% blockage may continue to supply adequate blood to the heart when a person is at rest (Hurst el al., 1982). Further narrowing or increased activity usually results in ischemia to the heart muscle, however.

Coronary artery disease (CAD) resulting from atherosclerosis is the most commonly recognized cause of myocardial ischemia (Hurst et al., 1982). Lipoproteins (substances consisting of both fat and protein) have an important role in the development of atherosclerosis. There are five types of lipoproteins: the chylomicron, very low-density lipoprotein (VLDL), intermediate-density lipoprotein (IDL), low-density lipoprotein (LDL), and high-density lipoprotein (HDL). Chylomicrons and VLDL are composed mainly of triglycerides. LDL is predominantly cholesterol, and IDL is a combination of triglycerides and cholesterol. HDL is composed mainly of protein and is thought to serve a protective function against the development of CAD.

Although the complete cause of atherosclerosis is not known, empirical study has identified risk factors associated with the development of atherosclerosis. Factors that cannot be changed include heredity, sex (males are more prone), and increasing age. Other risk factors include cigarette smoking, elevated blood pressure, hyperlipidemia, obesity, diabetes mellitus, abnormal glucose tolerance, gout, use of oral contraceptives, and a sedentary lifestyle. Other causes of CAD include coronary artery spasms, congenital anomalies, thrombosis, embolism, trauma, inflammation, and external compression, such as that from tumors.

Clinical Manifestations

The person with CAD may never have symptoms of the disease until having a fatal MI. Some persons experience symptoms of heart failure and decrease their activity level. The most common symptom of CAD is **angina,** or chest pain that results from myocardial ischemia.

The pain of angina may last from 30 seconds to 30 minutes. The description of angina differs among individuals. It may be described as a heaviness; a squeezing, viselike pain; or crushing pain over or near the sternum. The pain may radiate into the arms, neck, or jaws. Most commonly, it radiates down the left arm on the side of the little finger (Figure 19–12). Difficulty in breathing may accompany the pain. Angina usually occurs with increased activity or exposure to a cold environment when myocardial oxygen need increases.

Angina is classified into three types: stable (chronic), unstable, and variant (Prinzmetal's) angina. The terms *chronic* or *stable angina* describe angina following increased activity, and the symptoms are relatively the same with each occurrence. *Unstable angina* refers to new or worsening angina. Variant or **Prinzmetal's angina** differs from stable angina in that it occurs at rest. Prinzmetal's angina differs from the other forms in that spasms of the coronary arteries occur at the time of the angina. Persons with Prinzmetal's angina may or may not have atherosclerosis of the coronary arteries. Persons with stable and unstable angina usually have atherosclerosis of the coronary arteries.

Persons with severe atherosclerosis or other forms of CAD may have normal resting ECGs. Those with angina usually have changes in the ST segment and the T wave

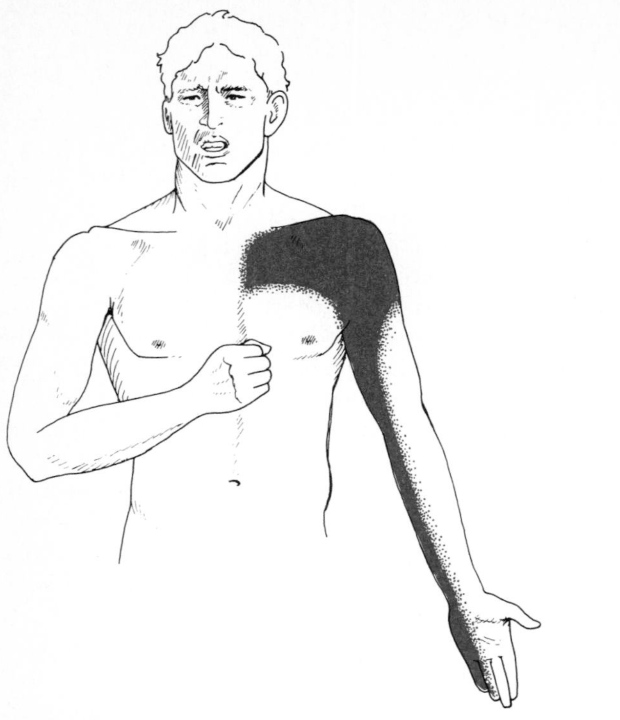

Figure 19–12

Typical pattern of anginal pain, radiating down the left arm on the side of the little finger.

of the ECG either during anginal attacks, as in the case of Prinzmetal's angina, or during stress electrocardiograms in the other forms. Stress ECGs are not usually performed when the client has pain.

After electrocardiographic diagnostic studies, other diagnostic tests may be performed to determine the cause of the angina and the extent of the CAD (see Chapter 18). The ECG may be followed by chest x-ray, cardiac enzyme laboratory studies, thallium perfusion scan, echocardiography, and cardiac catheterization with coronary arteriography and ventriculogram.

Medical Measures

There are six types of hyperlipidemia, also called hyperlipoproteinemia. Dietary management is directed to the specific elevated blood lipid. Table 19–3 summarizes the six hyperlipidemias and the suggested dietary management for each type.

Persons with new angina or worsening angina are admitted to the hospital for treatment of their symptoms and diagnosis of their problems. Because CAD may progress to MI and/or heart failure, the plan of care is directed at relieving symptoms and preventing progression of the disease as well as complications. Management may be medical, surgical, or a combination. Whether the client is treated with medication or surgery, lifestyle modification to diminish risk is of major importance.

Pharmacologic management includes the use of nitrates, beta-adrenergic blocking agents, and calcium channel blockers. The drugs may be used separately or in combination.

Nitrates relax the smooth muscle walls of the blood vessels, reducing venous return, which reduces preload. These agents also cause peripheral arteriolar dilation, reducing afterload. The nitrates also dilate healthy coronary vessels, which helps to redistribute blood to ischemic areas of the myocardium.

Beta-adrenergic blocking agents decrease oxygen requirements of the heart by inhibiting effects of circulating catecholamines on the beta-adrenergic receptors. Propranolol is the best known beta-blocking agent. Blocking effects vary depending on the type of beta receptor affected—beta 1 receptors (cardiac) or beta 2 receptors (bronchial and vascular smooth muscles). The effects of propranolol on the heart include decreased contractility, conduction velocity, and automaticity.

Calcium channel blockers inhibit the influx of calcium ions during depolarization of the membranes of cardiac and vascular smooth muscles. Although the exact mechanism is not known, the drugs have certain actions related to the relief of angina. Among these are dilation of main coronary arteries and arterioles and dilation of peripheral arterioles, which reduces peripheral resistance and decreases myocardial work and oxygen requirements. Calcium channel blocking agents also slow A-V conduction and can interfere with the sinus node impulse.

Surgical treatment depends on several factors including the age, psychologic status, and general health of the client. Also considered are diagnostic findings indicating the extent of the disease, the number of coronary arteries involved, the amount of tissue they supply, the placement of the lesions within the coronary artery, and the prognosis for the client with or without surgery.

When only one or two of the coronary arteries are involved and the lesions are easily accessible, percutaneous transluminal coronary angioplasty (PTCA) may be performed. The procedure involves the insertion of a balloon dilation catheter under fluoroscopic guidance into the coronary artery to the site of the lesion. The balloon is then inflated and compresses the plaque. PTCA is discussed in detail below. Sometimes the procedure is not successful, and emergency coronary bypass surgery must be done. The client is prepared for this possibility before the procedure. Coronary bypass surgery is also discussed below.

Specific Nursing Measures

Assessing the client's cardiovascular status to determine the effectiveness of medical management and any changes indicating deterioration is essential. Major nursing responsibilities include providing physical and psychologic comfort and security; keeping the client and family informed of all treatment approaches, diagnostic studies, and client progress; and providing health teaching and counseling

Table 19–3
Dietary Management of Hyperlipidemia

Type of Hyperlipidemia	Lipoprotein Involved	Lipid Component	Dietary Restriction
I	Chylomicrons	Triglyceride	Reduce total fat intake to less then 20% of total calories; avoid alcohol
IIa	LDL	Cholesterol	Reduce saturated fats, keep cholesterol intake below 300 mg/day
IIb	LDL, VLDL	Cholesterol, triglyceride	Reduce carbohydrate intake to 40% of total calories, avoid sweets; reduce fat intake to 40% of total calories; reduce saturated fats; keep cholesterol intake below 300 mg/day
III	IDL	Triglyceride, cholesterol	Same as for IIb
IV	VLDL	Triglyceride, cholesterol	Reduce carbohydrate intake to 45% of total calories; avoid sweets; reduce saturated fats; keep cholesterol intake between 300 and 500 mg/day
V	Chylomicrons, VLDL	Triglyceride, cholesterol	Reduce carbohydrate intake to 50% of total calories; avoid sweets; reduce saturated fats; reduce total fat intake to less than 30% of total calories; keep cholesterol intake between 300 and 500 mg/day; avoid alcohol

to assist the client and family to adjust to changes in lifestyle that may be necessary for reducing risk factors. Teaching should include information about cigarette smoking, elevated blood pressure, hyperlipidemia, obesity, diabetes mellitus, abnormal glucose tolerance, gout, use of oral contraceptives, sedentary lifestyle, and emotional factors.

Client/Family Teaching

The client should be well informed regarding the purpose of medications, side effects, and when to seek medical help. Clients should be taught to take their nitroglycerin before strenuous activity and before sexual intercourse. Over-the-counter drugs such as diet pills and decongestants must be avoided because they often will increase the heart rate. No drugs other than those specifically prescribed should be taken without consulting with the physician or pharmacist.

Encouraging the client to follow dietary guidelines requires careful instruction and follow-up. Clients will be instructed to avoid overeating and to eliminate or reduce salt and fat consumption; they may also be advised to lose weight. For clients who feel they cannot eat food without salt, advise them to avoid highly salted foods such as potato chips and ham. Suggest that they remove the salt shaker from the table. Caffeine should also be avoided because it may increase the heart rate.

Encourage obese clients to lose weight slowly according to a reasonable food plan. Advise them to avoid crash diets and to strive for nutritional balance. Help them to set a weight goal and to monitor their progress.

Teach clients to avoid any activity that precipitates angina. Moderate mild exercise is encouraged as long as pain is not induced and the exercise periods are balanced with periods of rest. Clients should avoid exercise after meals.

Because nicotine causes vasoconstriction, cigarette smoking is contraindicated and should be discontinued. Extreme cold should also be avoided because of vasoconstriction.

Provide emotional support for these changes in lifestyle. Empathize with the client and indicate that feelings of depression and discouragement are common reactions to changes in health status. Enlist the support of family and significant others in helping the client understand and cope with the condition.

Coronary Artery Bypass Surgery

In coronary artery bypass surgery, a graft consisting of the saphenous vein, internal mammary artery, or both brings a new blood supply to the distal portion of the stenotic coronary artery (Figure 19–13).

During heart surgery, the client requires constant hemodynamic and laboratory monitoring and cardiopulmonary bypass using the *heart–lung machine*. Most clients have a Swan–Ganz catheter or other thermodilution catheter inserted. A radial artery catheter measures arterial pressure. Urine output is monitored closely, as are blood electrolyte and blood oxygen levels.

The coronary artery bypass graft procedure begins with removal of the saphenous vein from the leg. The

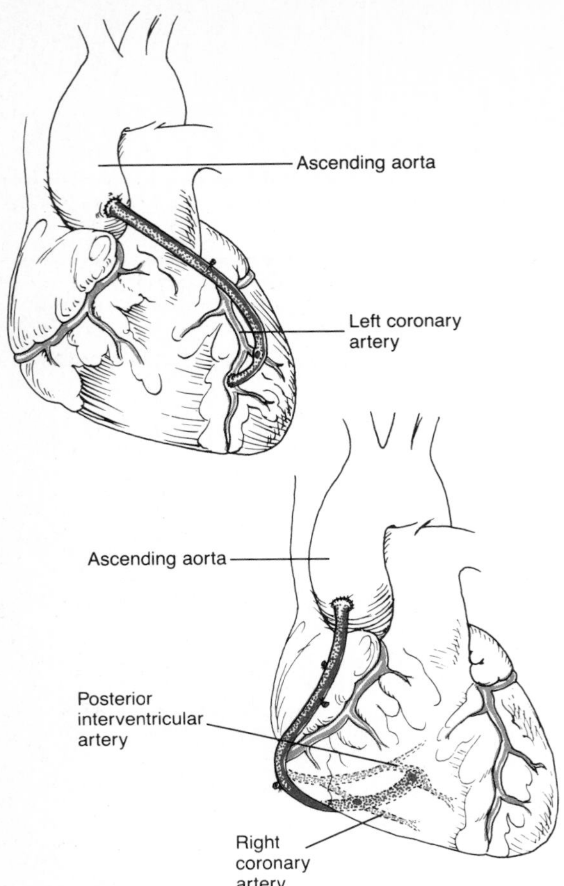

Figure 19–13

Coronary artery bypass grafts using the saphenous vein. **Top.** A single graft from the ascending aorta to the left coronary artery on the anterior surface of the heart. **Bottom.** A sequential graft (one vein graft that supplies two or more vessels) from the ascending aorta to the right coronary artery and the posterior interventricular artery on the posterior surface of the heart.

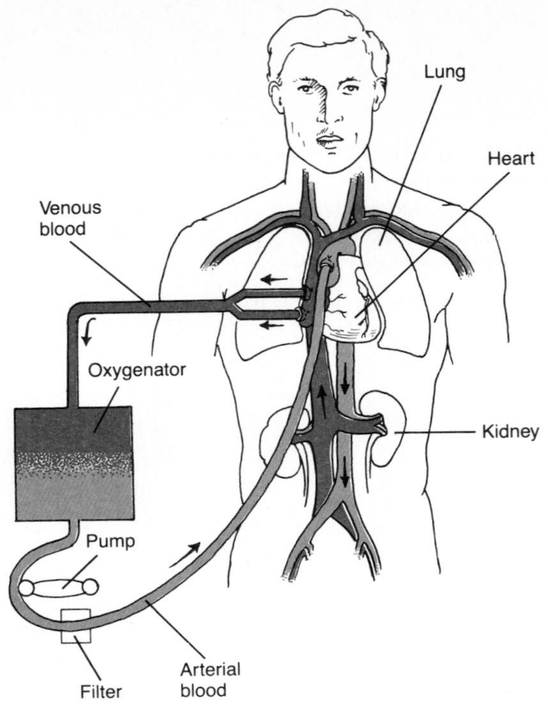

Figure 19–14

The heart–lung machine. Blood is diverted to the heart–lung machine through the cannulas in the superior and inferior venae cavae. Oxygen is bubbled through the blood in the oxygenator, and blood is then returned to the body through the arterial cannula in the ascending aorta.

incision is made on the medial aspect of the leg along the saphenous vein. While one surgeon prepares the vein graft, a second makes a medial sternotomy incision in preparation for placing the client on the heart–lung machine.

Cardiopulmonary bypass using the heart–lung machine (Figure 19–14) allows the heart to be stopped during the surgery and helps maintain a bloodless field. The procedure maintains minimal circulation and tissue perfusion, and the body is in a shocklike state. In addition, the body is cooled to reduce the metabolic tissue needs. As a result of this abnormal state, intravascular volume and electrolytes fluctuate during and after the surgery. Moreover, the mechanical components of the heart–lung machine injure red blood cells and platelets, causing hemolysis and abnormal platelet function.

The surgeon connects the saphenous vein graft to the aorta proximally and to the coronary artery distally. Blood flowing into the aorta then passes through the new graft to the coronary artery, restoring the blood supply to the ischemic myocardium. The internal mammary artery graft is based on the same principle; the difference is that the artery remains connected at its point of origin and is simply brought down to the stenotic coronary artery. The advantage is a greater longevity than the vein graft.

When the grafts are in place and tested for patency, the client is gradually removed from the heart–lung machine. This is a critical time in the surgery, because the heart must begin beating on its own.

After the bypass cannulas are removed, pacing wires are placed in the atria and ventricles and brought out through the skin. These wires are connected to an external pacing generator and placed in a demand mode. If the heart rate slows below the preset rate, the pacer automatically begins pacing the heart.

Anterior and posterior chest tubes are placed in the mediastinum and connected to a closed drainage system so drainage can be measured hourly. Free drainage through these tubes prevents the accumulation of blood around the heart and the development of life-threatening cardiac tamponade. The client is then taken to the recovery room or intensive care unit (ICU). The physiologic and psychosocial/lifestyle implications for the client are discussed in Table 19–4.

Nursing Implications

PREOPERATIVE CARE The nurse's most important role in the preoperative period is to prepare the client physically and psychologically for coronary artery bypass surgery. Physical preparations include ensuring that the client's nutritional state is optimal, preparing the skin by shaving and showering, cleansing the bowel with an enema, assessing preoperative laboratory values to ensure normal ranges (especially blood-clotting values), and assessing the client for any risk factors that would interfere with a smooth operation.

Client/Family Teaching

The value of preoperative teaching in psychologic preparation has been well documented and is included in the standard care of the heart surgery client. The client should thoroughly understand the normal heart anatomy and the heart problem. A heart model is helpful in giving these explanations. Clients often have misconceptions about the exact nature of their heart problems. They are often relieved to learn that their heart surgery is not as complicated as they envisioned.

Prepare clients for the possibility of transient postcardiotomy psychosis (confusion, delirium, and hallucinations). This condition usually resolves by the time the client leaves intensive care. When describing the tubes that will be present after surgery, also explain the sensations the client will experience. For example, the endotracheal tube is uncomfortable, and clients may feel they are not getting enough air. Some clients also experience a gagging sensation with this tube. Explain that this is a temporary discomfort and that the client will be getting sufficient air from the mechanical ventilator. A nurse will be with the client at all times while the tube is in place. The client also should know that the pain after heart surgery is an achiness and soreness that is especially felt with deep breathing. The pain is not sharp and unbearable, as some may think, and analgesics will be available.

Deep-breathing and coughing exercises are extremely important for the first 5 days following heart surgery. Before surgery, the client should practice these exercises and the use of the incentive spirometer.

POSTOPERATIVE CARE In the early postoperative period, the nurse must constantly assess the client because of the many physiologic changes with cardiopulmonary bypass surgery. Arterial pressure, pulmonary artery pressures, heart rate, and heart rhythm are evaluated every 15 minutes until the valves have stabilized. Chest drainage and urinary flow are measured hourly. Blood counts, clotting studies, and arterial blood gas measurements are performed regularly. The nurse carefully assesses the client's neurovascular, abdominal, and pulmonary functions and the circulatory function of the operated leg.

Table 19–4
Coronary Artery Bypass Surgery: Implications for the Client

Physiologic Implications	Psychosocial/Lifestyle Implications
Possible early complications of low-cardiac output syndrome, hypertension, hemorrhage, dysrhythmias, atelectasis, neurologic dysfunction, paralytic ileus, GI bleeding, infection or sepsis, renal failure, and hypokalemia	Postcardiotomy psychosis (confusion, delirium, and hallucinations)
Postpericardiotomy syndrome or possible late cardiac tamponade	Postoperative depression lasting up to 3 weeks
Improved heart pumping action	Changed self-image due to sternotomy and leg incisions
Relief of anginal pain	Risk-factor modification (change in diet, possible medications, elimination of smoking)
Relief of the symptoms and signs of heart failure	Improved quality of life
Temporary leg edema for about 6 weeks until deeper veins take over for saphenous vein	Avoid lifting heavy objects for 6 weeks and driving a car for 3 weeks
Need for antiplatelet therapy to prevent graft closure	Requires a 4- to 8-week convalescence
Stainless steel wire, used to close the sternum, remains permanently and is always visible on x-ray examination.	

The goal of nursing care in the immediate postoperative period is the prevention or early identification of the complications of cardiac surgery. In addition to a comprehensive nursing assessment, the nurse checks daily weights and chest x-rays to help monitor the client's fluid and pulmonary statuses. A weight gain of 1 kg in 24 hours is considered significant and may indicate the need for diuretic therapy. The nurse can identify atelectasis in the early postoperative period by decreased breath sounds and fever. When clients have been extubated, they should perform deep-breathing and coughing exercises every 2 hours. In many institutions, clients use an incentive spirometer hourly.

Clients on bed rest should perform range-of-motion (ROM) exercises and mild calisthenics. They gradually increase their activity until they are able to bathe and dress themselves and ambulate 400 ft unassisted and with minimal symptoms. A progressive exercise program is recommended; as clients are advanced to the next level, evaluate them for activity tolerance using heart rate, blood pressure, and heart rhythm as indicators (LaForge et al., 1984). Ambulation is often begun within the first 48 hours.

Adequate nutrition is important for any surgical client, particularly the heart surgery client. These clients are often nauseated and anorexic the first few days following surgery. Taste-bud function diminishes because the endotracheal tube rubs on the tongue surface. Fluid retention may necessitate a sodium-limited diet. Offer tasty high-protein foods in frequent small feedings. Custards, puddings, and milk shakes provide calories as well as protein. The dietitian should assist in planning individualized, attractive meals.

Client/Family Teaching

Discharge teaching begins the fifth or sixth postoperative day. Make sure the client and family or significant other clearly understand what normal recovery includes, what physical activity restrictions are appropriate, and what symptoms and signs to report. Clients must learn the dosages and side effects of medications. They must understand that they should not discontinue any medications without the physician's approval. If there is any wound drainage or separation, give clients dressing supplies, and instruct them in how to change dressings. All clients should know the signs of wound infection.

Diet instructions depend on special needs, but all cardiac surgery clients should follow a diet of no added salt for the first month because the body is undergoing changes in its fluid balance. Adequate intake of nutrients is also essential for proper wound healing, so the client should eat a diet high in protein, vitamins, and minerals. Eventually, a diet low in cholesterol and saturated fat can be followed.

The surgical leg tends to be edematous, so instruct the client to wear antiembolism support stockings during the day and to remove them at night. The operated leg should be elevated on a footstool when the client sits until the swelling has subsided.

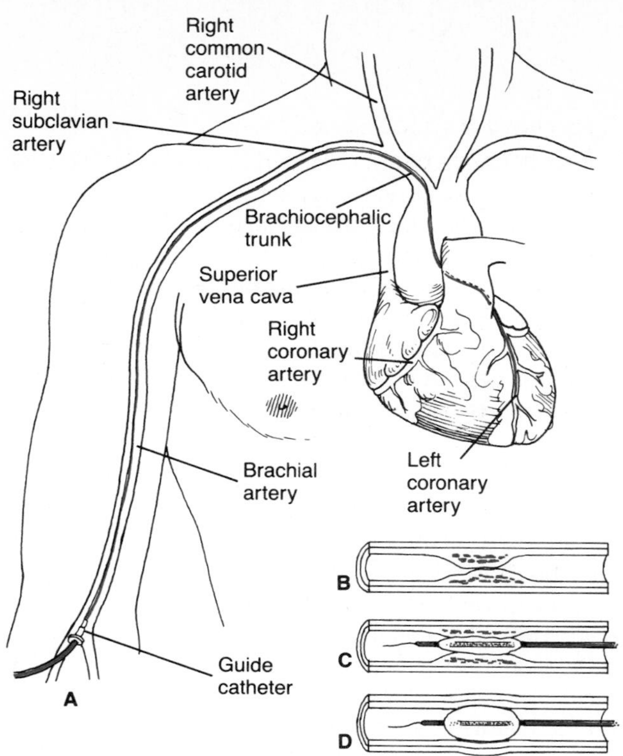

Figure 19–15

Percutaneous transluminal coronary angioplasty procedure. **A.** The guide catheter is threaded through the brachial artery to the blocked left coronary artery. **B.** An inside view of the blocked artery. **C.** The balloon dilation catheter is positioned in the artery so the balloon is within the obstruction. **D.** The inflated balloon flattens the obstruction against the vessel wall.

Percutaneous Transluminal Coronary Angioplasty

Percutaneous transluminal coronary angioplasty (PTCA) is an invasive but nonsurgical technique used in the treatment of CAD. PTCA is done in a cardiac catheterization laboratory using fluoroscopy. This procedure is only a few years old but is being performed worldwide.

A guide catheter is first inserted into the femoral or brachial arteries and advanced to the coronary arteries (Figure 19–15). A balloon dilatation catheter is advanced through the guide catheter and positioned within the stenosis. The balloon is then inflated under pressure, using a solution of saline and contrast material, and inflation is maintained for 3 to 5 seconds to compress the plaque and reestablish blood flow to the ischemic myocardium. The angiography is repeated to observe for lumen patency. The client is then transferred to the coronary care unit to be continuously monitored for complications. Physiologic and psychosocial/lifestyle implications for the client are summarized in Table 19–5.

Nursing Implications

PREOPERATIVE CARE The client is usually admitted the day before angioplasty. Preangioplasty diagnostic tests include: coronary angiogram, treadmill stress test, chest x-ray, ECG, blood chemistries, complete blood count, and glucose levels. Each client is blood typed and screened in preparation for possible heart surgery. Medications are started, including aspirin, dipyrimadole, nifedipine (Procardia), and nitroglycerin. A complete heart surgery preparation is done, and the client is placed on NPO status after midnight.

The nursing assessment is an important activity in the preoperative period. The client's cardiovascular assessment is documented in the nursing notes for reference in the early postoperative period.

Client education for this procedure is just as important as it is for heart surgery. Explain the coronary anatomy, the atherosclerotic process, the angioplasty procedure, and complications that can occur, particularly the potential need for heart surgery.

POSTOPERATIVE CARE The most important aspect of postangioplasty nursing care is observing the client for signs of coronary artery occlusion, including chest pain, ECG changes, dysrhythmias, and hypotension. These episodes may be treated with morphine sulfate for pain, IV or sublingual nitroglycerin, or a calcium antagonist such as nifedipine. If symptoms continue, coronary artery bypass surgery may be indicated.

Postangioplasty nursing assessment also includes monitoring vital signs every 15 minutes for an hour and then every 30 minutes until stable. A 12-lead ECG every 8 hours (three times in all) and continuous ECG monitoring are required. Assess the client's peripheral circulation (color, warmth, pulses, sensation, and mobility) every hour (four times), then every 2 hours (four times), and finally every 4 hours. Assess the catheter insertion site for bleeding, hematoma, or infection every hour (four times), then every 2 hours (four times), and finally every 4 hours. Monitor the client's urinary output every hour and breath sounds every 2 hours.

Maintain 5 to 10 lb of pressure on the catheter insertion site until all bleeding has ceased, and keep the head of the bed below 30°. Push fluids to assist in the elimination of contrast material.

On discharge, clients must understand the need for antiplatelet drugs and the necessity that they not be discontinued without the physician's consent. Clients also need instruction on symptoms and signs to report; these include new chest pressure or heaviness, recurrence of angina pectoris, dizziness, or light-headedness.

Myocardial Infarction

When blood supply to a portion of the myocardium is inadequate, the cells become ischemic and are injured. If blood supply remains low, the cells die. The death of myocardial cells is the condition called myocardial infarction (MI), or heart attack. The American Heart Association estimates that over one-third of Americans who have heart attacks will die, and most of them will die before they reach the hospital. The average victim does not seek help for about 3 hours after symptoms develop. Many deaths are from disturbances in heart rhythm, or dysrhythmias, that commonly occur within the first few hours after MI. The vast majority of clients with MI that nurses see will have their MI in the left ventricle.

MIs usually result from atherosclerotic CAD. Only about 4% of persons who have an acute MI have no evidence of atherosclerosis of the coronary arteries. In most clients with MI resulting from atherosclerosis, blood clots form on or adjacent to the atherosclerotic lesion. These clots cause MI by contributing to the occlusion of the coronary arteries (Braunwald, 1984).

Table 19–5
Percutaneous Transluminal Coronary Angioplasty: Implications for the Client

Physiologic Implications	Psychosocial/Lifestyle Implications
Fewer complications than with bypass surgery Possible complications of cardiac tamponade, myocardial infarction, dysrhythmias, hemorrhage, heart failure, hematoma formation, and thrombus formation at the insertion site Indefinite use of antiplatelet drugs Recurrence possible	Requires 2–3 day hospitalization Relief of anginal pain without the trauma of major surgery Elimination of the threat of immediate myocardial infarction Risk-factor modification (change in diet, elimination of smoking, need for exercise)

Clinical Manifestations

The symptoms and signs of MI include those described for CAD (newly developed chest pain, which may occur with rest or activity; chest pain lasting longer than 5 minutes or not relieved by three tablets of nitroglycerine taken 5 minutes apart; or chest pain accompanied by sweating, shortness of breath, nausea or vomiting, or a feeling of weakness). Some persons have an MI without ever having symptoms (a silent MI).

The diagnosis of an acute MI is made from at least two of the three usual findings: chest pain, ECG changes indicative of MI (newly developed abnormal Q waves), and enzymatic changes in creatine kinase (CK) and lactic dehydrogenase (LDH), discussed in Chapter 18. The location of the Q waves are diagnostic for the location of the infarction.

Medical Measures

Because elevated serum cholesterol and triglyceride levels are important risk factors for atherosclerosis, and atherosclerosis is the main cause of CAD and MI, careful attention to diet is essential. If dietary restriction does not reduce serum cholesterol and/or triglyceride levels, a 2-month trial of a hypolipidemic drug may be prescribed.

When the client has an MI, therapeutic management is aimed at relieving client discomfort, preventing and treating complications, promoting healing of the damaged myocardium, and promoting rehabilitation. More recently, for some who seek help early enough, early therapeutic management is directed to opening the blocked coronary artery or bypassing the blocked artery to enable enough blood to get to the ischemic area before extensive amounts of myocardial tissue die.

Of about every 150 persons admitted to coronary care units for suspected MI, only 100 have an MI (Marriott, 1982). The initial goal of promoting comfort is started when the client is first seen, which may be in the ambulance, clinic, or emergency room. Oxygen is provided by nasal cannula at about 2 to 4 L/min, the client is positioned for comfort, and nitroglycerin and morphine or another analgesic are ordered for pain control. Management is then directed to making the diagnosis while preventing complications, monitoring the client for indications of complications, and treating complications early when they occur.

Before the establishment of coronary care units, almost half (47%) of the 30% to 40% of hospital deaths for MI were from dysrhythmias; 43% were from circulatory failure; and the others were from embolism and ruptured ventricle. With coronary care units and ability to control dysrhythmias, the number of inhospital deaths has been reduced by about one-half. The majority of deaths are due to heart failure, cardiogenic shock, cardiac rupture, and papillary muscle dysfunction (Trevino & Massey, 1983). Therapeutic management continues to be directed at the early detection and treatment of dysrhythmias as well as early detection and treatment of the other complications.

Because in many instances, thrombosis is responsible for the complete occlusion of the coronary artery that produces the symptoms, newer therapies attempt to remove the clot as soon as possible after symptoms develop and before ischemia is prolonged enough to cause extensive infarction. Clients who have recently developed symptoms (less than 6 hours), may be candidates for parenteral or intracoronary streptokinase infusion if they have not had recent surgery, are not pregnant, have not had a recent cerebrovascular accident, have no bleeding disorders, and do not have severe hypertension. Streptokinase promotes fibrinolysis and essentially dissolves blood clots.

The client may be taken to the cardiac catheterization laboratory for this procedure. A cardiac catheterization is performed including a left ventriculogram and angiography of the coronary artery not involved. Then nitroglycerin is infused into the involved artery to ensure that the complete occlusion is not the result of coronary artery spasm rather than a blood clot. Streptokinase is then infused into the involved coronary artery first by a bolus and then by continuous infusion. The effects are observed through coronary arteriography about every 10 to 15 minutes. The therapy is completed in about 1 hour and is effective if the coronary artery is opened and left ventricular performance is improved. The atherosclerotic lesion remains at the site. When indicated by coronary anatomy and evaluation of the extent of the CAD, angioplasty may be carried out before transferring the client to the coronary care unit (angioplasty is discussed earlier and in Chapter 21). In the coronary care unit, bleeding is a major concern in addition to the usual complications of MI.

In some institutions, the streptokinase is given intravenously, and the client is closely monitored. Later, cardiac catheterization is performed for further diagnosis and treatment.

Coronary artery bypass surgery may be indicated for some clients. They may be taken to the operating room after the effects of the streptokinase have worn off (several hours) so there is minimal danger of bleeding.

Immediate use of streptokinase with or without angioplasty or coronary artery bypass surgery is not always indicated. These procedures must be done early to prevent extensions of the infarction. The possible benefits must be weighed against the risks for the individual client. When these procedures are not done, the extent of the CAD is either diagnosed just before discharge or about 6 weeks after the MI, depending on the attending physician's determination. Sometimes the CAD involves only one area, and there is no further myocardial tissue to preserve, so further treatment is not indicated. If the disease involves other areas of the coronary arteries, coronary artery bypass surgery may be indicated to prevent further damage. In all clients, measures to prevent progression of CAD are essential.

The usual course of treatment for clients with uncomplicated MI who do not have surgery involves admission to the coronary care unit, bed rest, liquid diet, and continuous monitoring for dysrhythmias and complications. The client and significant others are kept fully informed of the plan of care. During the first day, blood pressure is recorded every hour, and a cardiac assessment for evidence of complications such as heart failure is performed every 2 hours. By the second day, the client is given a soft diet and permitted to use the bedside commode and sit in a chair. Clients are closely observed during increases in activity for any signs of complications.

On the third or fourth day, when the threat of complications is significantly decreased, clients are transferred to a stepdown unit where they may continue to be monitored for dysrhythmias or to a regular medical surgical unit. By this time, a rehabilitation program has usually been started, and clients continue to increase activity while their tolerance to the activity is carefully assessed. Usually, clients are discharged within 10 to 14 days and are allowed to continue a gradual increase in their activity. Clients are usually permitted to return to work part time about 8 to 12 weeks after the MI.

Specific Nursing Measures

The goals of nursing care for a client with MI include relieving discomfort; preventing, detecting, and treating complications; promoting healing; and assisting in the rehabilitation program. The nursing care described under CAD is also applicable to the client with an MI.

The most common complications of MI include dysrhythmias, congestive heart failure, extension of the MI, rupture of a papillary muscle, ventricular septal defect, ventricular aneurysm, pericarditis, and thromboembolism. Thromboembolism can be prevented by having clients move their legs and feet while in bed and push their feet against a footboard. The nurse should be aware of the clinical manifestations of all potential complications and report significant findings to the physician so the medical treatment plan can be adjusted.

By the time clients have reached the general medical unit, their condition is usually stable, and a rehabilitation program has been started. Be especially observant of the client's response to increased activity. Spacing of activities and preventing physical stress are important.

Clients find the move to the unmonitored unit encouraging but also frightening because they are used to constant monitoring. Take extra care to provide an environment in which the client feels safe.

Straining at bowel movements should be avoided by providing bulk in the diet and use of stool softeners. Foods high in potassium are important because most clients are on diuretics. A diet low in carbohydrates and low in saturated fats may also be necessary, depending on the client's type of hyperlipidemia. Sodium should be restricted for clients with symptoms of heart failure. These dietary modifications are instituted during the client's hospitalization. Most of them will be continued throughout the client's life.

Client/Family Teaching

Clients should be given specific exercise instructions for home use based on predischarge exercise testing, clinical status, and activity level prior to the MI and during hospitalization. A progressive, individualized program is both physiologically and psychologically beneficial.

Walking is the major component of the early convalescent program. Teach clients to take their own pulses so they can monitor their own heart rate response to exercise. If the client has not had exercise testing prior to discharge, the pulse rate should not exceed 110 to 120 beats per minute with exercise.

In preparing clients for walking activities, tell them to walk on level ground and to avoid hills and steps, walking against the wind, and walking during periods of extreme heat, cold, or high humidity. They should wait at least 2 hours after eating before exercise.

Readiness to resume sexual activity following an MI is often gauged by the client's ability to climb two flights of stairs or walk vigorously around the block without symptoms such as chest pain or tachycardia. Sexual relations must be planned so that sexual activity after alcohol ingestion or after meals is avoided. Nitroglycerin can be used sublingually 5 to 10 minutes before sexual intercourse to prevent angina.

Teaching the client the importance of smoking cessation is another major nursing responsibility. Clients are usually anxious to do all they can to prevent another MI and are willing to embark on any program to improve their health. Nurses should use this opportunity and work to help both client and significant others understand the important lifestyle modifications to prevent future cardiac events. A case study for the client with MI is presented at the end of this chapter.

Valvular Disease

Diseases of the heart valve result in either stenosis of the involved valve, incompetency of the valve, or a combination. A stenotic valve impedes blood flow forward. An incompetent valve does not close after blood has entered the chamber ahead of it, permitting blood to flow back into the chamber when it should be moving forward. Both stenotic and incompetent valves may lead to heart failure.

Clinical Manifestations and Medical Measures

Most valvular problems require surgical treatment eventually, depending on the client's problems. The American Heart Association recommends secondary prophylaxis for prevention of streptococcal infections for persons who have had rheumatic fever, a common cause of valvular abnormalities. When rheumatic fever is a cause of the valvular problem, the client should take antibiotics continuously. Persons with valvular disease are also given antibiotic therapy for prophylaxis against infective endocarditis before and after dental procedures associated with bleeding, surgery, or procedures involving instrumentation of the genitourinary or gastrointestinal tracts. Specific treatment depends on the valvular abnormality.

Nursing Research Note

Hilbert G: Spouse support and myocardial infarction patient compliance. *Nurs Res* 1985; 34(4):217–220.

This researcher tested the hypothesis that a positive relation exists between spouse support and compliance for post-myocardial infarction (MI) clients. Using a sample of 60 postMI men and their spouses, the investigator measured support and compliance.

The results demonstrated no positive relation between spouse support and compliance. Compliance was not affected by client age, length of time since the MI, number of MIs, work status, number of marriages, social class, complications, ethnic background, religion, or education. There was a significant relation between compliance and enrollment in a cardiac rehabilitation program.

Because rehabilitation programs enhance compliance, clients should be encouraged to enroll in these programs. Although the findings did not link support and compliance, nurses still need to encourage spouse support and assistance in compliance.

TRICUSPID STENOSIS Although tricuspid stenosis is usually caused by rheumatic fever, other causes include systemic lupus erythematosus, right atrial tumors, metastatic carcinoid lesions of the tricuspid valve, and congenital malformations. The most common symptoms of tricuspid stenosis include dyspnea and fatigue. Because blood is hindered from flowing from the right atrium into the right ventricle during diastole, a diastolic murmur is heard best at the left sternal border or tricuspid area. Atrial fibrillation may also be present. Medical management includes sodium restriction and diuretics. Eventually, surgical repair or replacement of the valve is indicated.

TRICUSPID INSUFFICIENCY The most common cause of tricuspid insufficiency is a dilated right ventricle from right ventricular failure. Congenital malformations may also cause tricuspid insufficiency. The clinical manifestations are those of right ventricular failure and include distention of the jugular veins, hepatomegaly, jaundice, and peripheral edema. Because blood flows through the incompetent tricuspid valve into the right atrium during systole, a systolic murmur is heard at the left sternal border. Atrial fibrillation is usually present. Medical management centers on treating the cause of the tricuspid insufficiency.

PULMONIC STENOSIS The most common cause of pulmonic stenosis is congenital malformation. Other causes include rheumatic fever and metastatic carcinoid lesions of the pulmonic valve. Pulmonic stenosis is usually tolerated well and does not cause symptoms. When the problem is severe, the clinical manifestations are those of right heart failure. Because blood is hindered from flowing from the right ventricle into the pulmonary artery, a systolic murmur is heard at the pulmonic area or upper left sternal border. Persons with pulmonic stenosis usually require no therapy. Surgical repair may be necessary if the lesion is severe.

PULMONIC INSUFFICIENCY Pulmonic insufficiency is usually caused by pulmonary hypertension, infective endocarditis, or congenital malformations. Pulmonic insufficiency rarely causes symptoms unless severe enough to cause right heart failure. Because blood that is pumped into the pulmonary artery during systole regurgitates into the right ventricle during diastole, a diastolic murmur is heard in the pulmonic area (upper left sternal border). If the client develops problems related to pulmonic insufficiency, the treatment is aimed at the cause. Sometimes valve replacement is necessary.

MITRAL STENOSIS Mitral stenosis in the adult is usually the result of previous rheumatic fever. Other causes of mitral stenosis in the adult are rare. Mitral stenosis impedes blood flow from the left atrium into the left ventricle during diastole and produces a diastolic murmur, which is best heard at the apex (Figure 19–16A). The client usually does not develop a murmur or symptoms until several years after having had rheumatic fever. The most common symptoms are dyspnea and fatigue. As the stenosis increases, the symptoms become more severe and are related to pulmonary hypertension and right ventricular heart failure. Atrial fibrillation frequently accompanies mitral stenosis.

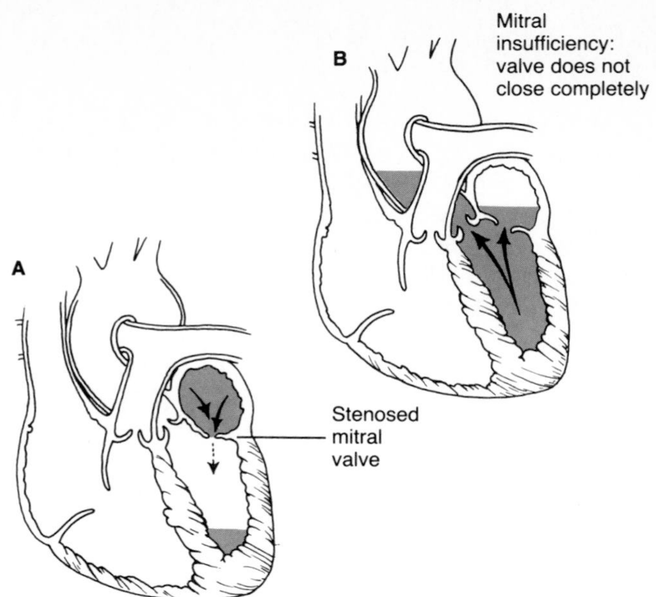

Figure 19–16

Mitral stenosis and mitral insufficiency. **A.** Mitral stenosis: during diastole blood flow from the left atrium to the left ventricle is impaired because the valve leaflets are diseased and do not open completely. **B.** Mitral insufficiency: normally during systole, all blood from the left ventricle is ejected through the aortic valve into the aorta. With mitral insufficiency some of the blood flows backward through the incompetent mitral valve.

Medical management includes treatment of atrial fibrillation with digitalis or antidysrhythmic drugs and anticoagulant therapy for prevention of blood clots and systemic emboli. Surgical therapy includes reconstruction or valve replacement.

MITRAL INSUFFICIENCY The most common causes of mitral insufficiency in the adult are rheumatic heart disease and mitral leaflet prolapse. Other causes include dilatation of the left ventricle, CAD, papillary muscle dysfunction, and congenital problems. Because mitral insufficiency results in blood flowing through the incompetent mitral valve into the left atrium during systole, a systolic murmur may be heard at the apex (Figure 19–16B). The clinical manifestations of mitral insufficiency vary depending upon the cause. Mitral insufficiency from rheumatic heart disease may cause no difficulties for many years and then produce manifestations associated with heart failure.

The medical management depends on the clinical manifestation and the cause. Management of the client with heart failure is discussed later in this chapter. The management of dysrhythmias has been previously discussed. Surgical treatment involves valve replacement.

MITRAL VALVE PROLAPSE Mitral valve prolapse, also called mitral leaflet prolapse, and Barlow's syndrome, deserves special mention because it is a common and usually benign clinical syndrome. It occurs more frequently in women and has a familial tendency. On auscultation at the apex, a mid- or late systolic click may be heard, sometimes accompanied by a late systolic murmur with a whooping sound.

Most clients with mitral valve prolapse never have clinical symptoms. Dysrhythmias, palpitations, syncope, and vague chest pain can occur, however. Treatment generally involves reassurance and propranolol for troublesome chest pains.

AORTIC STENOSIS The most frequent causes of aortic stenosis in the adult are congenital malformations; degenerative calcifications in the valve; and less frequently, the sequelae of rheumatic fever. The clinical manifestations of aortic stenosis depend upon the severity of the stenosis. Because blood flow is hindered from flowing into the aorta from the left ventricle during systole, a systolic murmur can be heard in the aortic area or right upper sternal border (Figure 19–17A). Left ventricular hypertrophy develops and can be diagnosed by an ECG. The pulse wave may be noted to rise slowly and have a small volume. The systolic blood pressure can be decreased and the pulse pressure also decreased. The client may notice no symptoms until late in the disease. Syncope, angina pectoris, or congestive heart failure can develop. After the onset of symptoms, incidence of sudden death increases.

Medical management centers around the observation of the progression of the stenosis and treatment of angina pectoris if it develops. Surgical replacement of the valve is recommended when the stenotic lesion becomes severe or when symptoms develop.

AORTIC INSUFFICIENCY The most common causes of aortic insufficiency in the adult include connective tissue diseases, rheumatic fever, endocarditis, syphilis, and diseases causing dilation of the aorta. Because blood pumped out of the left ventricle into the aorta during systole falls back into the ventricle during diastole, a diastolic murmur will be heard in the aortic area (Figure 19–17B). The pulse quickly increases in amplitude and then collapses. The systolic blood pressure is increased and the diastolic blood pressure decreased.

The client often has no symptoms for many years after the murmur is first heard. Later, as the regurgitation progresses, clients may notice a gradual increase in heart palpitations, palpitations in the neck, flushing, sweating, and chest pain. After development of symptoms, the person's condition usually rapidly deteriorates.

Medical management aims at following the client and observing for progression of valvular disease. Surgical replacement of the valve is recommended when the early

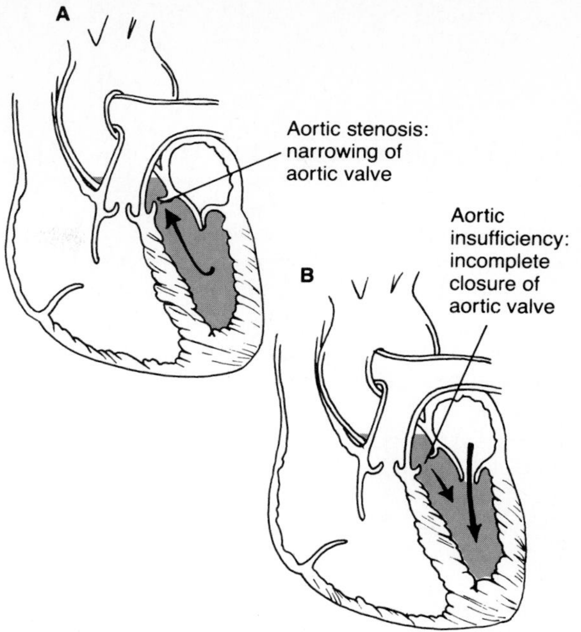

Figure 19–17

Aortic stenosis and aortic insufficiency. **A.** Aortic stenosis: during systole blood flow from the left ventricle through the aortic valve is impaired because of the stenotic aortic valve. **B.** Aortic insufficiency: during diastole some of the blood ejected through the aortic valve during systole flows backward through the incompetent aortic valve.

symptoms develop, before the valvular problem becomes severe.

Specific Nursing Measures

Nursing management centers on teaching the client about the need for prophylactic antibiotics while the condition is being managed medically. Clients who have had rheumatic fever are encouraged to take their antibiotics daily. Clients who have any type of valvular disease should be reminded to inform dentists and physicians planning invasive procedures about the valvular problem.

Heart Valve Surgery

Valvular heart disease is surgically treated by annuloplasty, mitral valve commissurotomy, or valve replacement. *Annuloplasty* involves the surgical repair of a native valve. The valve annulus is gathered with silk sutures, much like a skirt. This procedure is usually performed on the insufficient or regurgitant valve instead of valve replacement. Some believe it is better to maintain the client's original valve than to replace it, because artificial and tissue valves carry inherent risks and require significant lifestyle changes.

In *mitral valve commissurotomy,* an alternative to valve replacement, the valve leaflets are cut free from one another. A drawback of commissurotomy is that symptoms may recur, necessitating valve replacement. For this reason, commissurotomies are not performed as often as in the past.

Table 19–6
Heart Valve Surgery: Implications for the Client

Physiologic Implications	Psychosocial/Lifestyle Implications
Annuloplasty	
Complications and improvements similar to those of bypass surgery (see Table 19–4)	Postcardiotomy psychosis possible or depression
Abnormally high preload until ventricle adjusts to smaller volume	Temporary need for antidysrhythmic drugs
Susceptibility to pulmonary congestion	
Mitral valve commissurotomy	
Pulmonary complications and fluid overload in immeidate postoperative period	Postcardiotomy psychosis possible
Continuation of preoperative atrial dysrhythmias	Postoperative depression
Possible recurrence of symptoms and need for valve replacement	Changed self-image
Need for antiplatelet therapy	Risk-factor modification (change in diet, antidysrhythmic drugs, elimination of smoking)
	Improved quality of life
Valve replacement	
Same possible postoperative complications as bypass surgery (see Table 19–4)	Need for precautions related to increased clotting time caused by sodium warfarin
Thromboembolism is a risk	Need for endocarditis prophylaxis
Hemorrhage is a risk with sodium warfarin (Coumadin)	Need for reduction of sodium intake as a lifelong change
Possible hemolysis of red blood cells from turbulent blood flow through the valve	Annoying clicking of artificial valve
Risk of bacterial endocarditis	Improved quality of life
Diminished ventricular and atrial hypertrophy	
Reversal of vascular changes of pulmonary hypertension	
Improved exercise tolerance	
Diminished shortness of breath	

Valve replacement involves the removal of the native valve and the insertion of a prosthesis. Tissue valve prostheses originate from a pig (porcine valve) or cow (bovine valve) and are specially prepared for human use. The tissue valve has little risk of clot formation on the leaflets—a major advantage, because artificial valves are prone to clot formation and require that clients take sodium warfarin the rest of their lives. Tissue valves lack longevity, however. They begin to deteriorate after 5 to 10 years and too often require replacement.

Artificial valves are generally used in the young client, where valve longevity is important. Other factors are also considered when choosing a valve, such as bleeding history and plans for pregnancy. For example, if a client has a history of peptic ulcers or other bleeding problems, a tissue valve is preferred so sodium warfarin will not be needed. For a young female client who wishes to become pregnant, a tissue valve is also preferable because of the bleeding risk with sodium warfarin.

Clients having heart valve surgery are placed on the heart–lung machine during surgery. The physiologic and psychosocial/lifestyle implications for clients having annuloplasty, mitral commissurotomy, or valve replacement are discussed in Table 19–6.

Nursing Implications

PREOPERATIVE CARE The preoperative instructions for clients having heart valve surgery are similar to those given before bypass surgery, except no leg incision need be discussed. It is often helpful to show clients a heart model and discuss the location of the heart valves, the type of surgery to be performed, and the prosthesis to be used, if any. The physical preparations of the client are identical to those for bypass surgery.

POSTOPERATIVE CARE The postoperative nursing care of the heart valve surgery client is the same as for any client who has undergone heart surgery (see the discussion of bypass surgery for a summary of this care). Valve surgery always carries a higher risk for the development of pulmonary complications. Carefully monitor daily weights and 24-hour intake and output. Diuretic therapy is initiated for any signs of fluid retention. The client's fluid intake is limited to as little as 1200 mL per day, and sodium is restricted.

Atrial dysrhythmias are common. Occlusion or damage to the coronary arteries during valve replacement may result in ventricular dysrhythmias or acute MI. Continuous ECG monitoring provides early detection of these dysrhythmias.

The client's activity should progress according to how he or she is feeling. Discharge instructions on wound care, activity limitations, medications, and diet are similar to those for bypass surgery. See Table 19–6 for specifics.

Heart Failure

Heart failure indicates that the heart has failed to perform adequately its function of pumping blood throughout the circulatory system. Perhaps the best definition of heart failure is that of Hurst et al. (1982), who define heart failure as a condition in which the heart is no longer able to pump an adequate supply of blood to meet the metabolic needs of the body when there is an adequate venous return. The tems *forward* and *backward* heart failure have been used to indicate the symptoms the person exhibits as a result of heart failure. Forward failure produces symptoms related to low cardiac output, and backward failure produces symptoms related to increased venous pressure.

Left heart failure and *right heart failure* are terms describing the side of the heart that has the primary impairment. It is sometimes helpful to think of heart failure as left or right sided because the symptoms and signs may provide clues to the location of the primary problem. Keep in mind, however, that failure of one side of the heart usually leads to failure of the other side.

Heart failure may be acute or chronic. A person may not have any indication of heart disease and develop heart failure suddenly. A good example is the asymptomatic person with CAD who has an MI and develops acute heart failure with pulmonary edema. Chronic heart failure may also develop as a result of CAD as well as other forms of heart disease. The affected person may progressively reduce activity as the failure increases but attribute the decrease in activity to other causes such as normal aging.

Heart failure may be described as latent, compensated, and intractable. Latent heart failure implies that the heart is able to handle the circulatory needs at rest but fails with increased stress. Compensated heart failure is heart failure that was previously present, but cardiac output has been maintained at a normal level by therapy or by compensatory mechanisms. Intractable heart failure implies that heart failure persists when all therapies have been used.

Congestive heart failure is a state in which abnormal circulatory congestion occurs as the result of heart failure, and compensatory mechanisms are brought into play (Hurst et al., 1982). CHF may be classified as mild, moderate, or severe, based on the development of dyspnea in relation to activity. With mild CHF, dyspnea occurs with moderate activity; with moderate CHF, dyspnea occurs with mild activity; and with severe CHF, dyspnea occurs at rest (Hurst et al., 1982).

The causes of heart failure include conditions that overload the heart, affect cardiac rhythm or conduction, or decrease the ability of the heart to contract. The heart may become overloaded by decreased or increased preload and increased afterload. Examples of conditions that *increase preload* include increased venous return, incompetent valves that cause blood to be regurgitated back into the heart

Nursing Research Note

Quinless FW, Cassese M, Atherton N: The effect of selected preoperative, intraoperative and postoperative variables on the development of postcardiotomy psychosis in patients undergoing open heart surgery. *Heart Lung* 1985; 14(4): 334–340.

These researchers examined the relations between physiologic, environmental, and psychologic factors and the development of postcardiotomy psychosis. The most significant results occurred with the factors observed during the intraoperative period. They found that systolic blood pressure, perfusion time, and anesthesia time were all significantly correlated with the development of postcardiotomy psychosis. Of these, a low systolic blood pressure was most significant. It was interesting however, that all study participants developed some degree of postcardiotomy psychosis.

Nurses should be aware that postcardiotomy psychosis is common. They should educate their cardiac clients about the transient effect common to this type of surgery. The authors suggest that some type of checklist be developed so nurses can readily identify clients at risk for postcardiotomy psychosis—those having prolonged anesthesia and perfusion times along with hypotensive reactions.

chamber to be pumped again, and shunts or openings between chambers that promote the flow of blood from one side of the heart to the other. Conditions that *decrease preload* include insufficient blood return to the heart from bleeding or dehydration. When venous return is adequate, preload may be decreased by reduced ability of the ventricles to fill because of stenosis of the mitral or tricuspid valves or constriction of the pericardium, as in pericardial tamponade. Conditions that *increase afterload* include increased pulmonary or systemic blood pressure and stenosis of the valves through which the heart has to pump the blood, as in aortic or pulmonic stenosis.

Examples of disturbances in heart rhythm and electrical conduction include extremely fast or slow heart rate, fibrillation, and cardiac arrest. Conditions that decrease the ability of the heart to pump blood include diseases of the heart, toxic substances in the heart, and conditions that deprive the heart of oxygen. Examples of diseases of the heart muscle include MI and infections of the heart. Toxic substances include drugs and alcohol. Conditions that deprive the heart of oxygen include inadequate blood supply to the heart, as in CAD, or inadequate quality of the blood from anemia and other systemic diseases.

Left-sided heart failure occurs with pressure or volume overload of the left ventricle. Pressure overload can result from systemic hypertension, aortic stenosis, or coarctation of the aorta. Volume overload occurs with aortic or mitral regurgitation.

Left-sided heart failure can progress to pulmonary edema. In left heart failure, the left ventricle cannot pump out all of its blood, increasing the residual volume in the ventricle. Accumulating blood backs up into the left atrium, pulmonary veins, and the pulmonary capillary bed. *Pulmonary edema,* engorgement of the pulmonary vasculature with subsequent excessive accumulation of fluid in the interstitial spaces and alveoli of the lung, results.

Right-sided heart failure occurs with pressure or volume overload of the right ventricle. Pressure overload can result from pulmonary hypertension or stenosis of the pulmonic valve. Volume overload can result from an atrial septal defect.

Clinical Manifestations

The clinical manifestations of heart failure depend on the severity of the failure and the side of the heart that is predominantly affected. Depending on the severity, the client may notice difficulty in breathing; coughing of blood-tinged frothy sputum; fatigue; edema; nocturia; oliguria; weight gain; cerebral symptoms such as dizziness and syncope; or gastrointestinal symptoms such as anorexia, bloating, and abdominal pain. Table 19–7 lists common subjective and objective findings in left-sided and right-sided heart failure.

A chest x-ray may reveal an enlarged heart and pleural effusion. Although there are no ECG findings diagnostic of heart failure, the ECG probably will be abnormal because persons with heart failure generally have some form of heart disease.

Table 19–7
Subjective and Objective Findings in Left and Right Heart Failure

	Subjective	Objective
Left heart	Dyspnea Orthopnea Paroxysmal nocturnal dyspnea Cough Fatigue	Rales S_3 gallop Pleural effusion Peripheral cyanosis ↑ Respirations; Cheyne–Stokes respirations
Right heart	Abdominal pain Anorexia, nausea Bloating Fatigue	Distended neck veins Hepatojugular reflux Hepatomegaly Ascites ↑ CVP S_4 gallop ↓ urine output Peripheral edema

Medical Measures

The medical plan of therapy for heart failure is generally based on goals that include:

- Determining and eliminating or controlling the cause.
- Determining and treating the condition(s) that precipitated the heart failure.
- Improving the ability of the heart to contract and reducing the work load of the heart by:
  1. Decreasing the body demands.
  2. Decreasing preload.
  3. Decreasing afterload.

Eliminating the cause of heart failure depends on the disease process and the available treatment modalities. Keep in mind that all forms of heart disease have the potential to lead to heart failure.

The condition that precipitated the heart failure may be readily apparent and immediately treatable, such as inadvertent rapid administration of fluids, stresses of emergency surgery for another condition, or in the case of mild failure, the increase of sodium in the diet. Other stressors, such as other systemic diseases, may be less amenable to control. Decreasing the body demands to decrease the work load of the heart and subsequently improve its ability to pump blood may be accomplished by helping the client to decrease activity and, in some cases, by promoting improvement of the quality of the blood being pumped.

The person with chronic heart failure may need only to regulate the amount of physical activity to be free of symptoms. Sometimes discontinuing an activity is distressing to the individual, and spacing activity that cause symptoms may be appropriate. If the client is overweight, measures should be encouraged to reduce weight to decrease body demands for blood flow.

Clients with acute and severe heart failure may be confined to bed. They may be positioned in a sitting position to help them decrease the work of breathing. Oxygen may be administered by nasal prongs at 4 to 6 L/min if arterial oxygen saturation is low. Morphine sulfate may be given intravenously over a period of time to help decrease the work of breathing, decrease psychologic distress, and decrease the effects of sympathetic stimulation of the arteries and veins causing pooling of blood in the extremities so less blood is returned to the heart.

Control of the heart rate and rhythm to improve the ability of the heart to pump blood is managed by the use of antidysrhythmic agents. Sometimes the use of an artificial pacemaker is indicated.

In most cases, heart failure is related to increased preload, and measures to decrease preload will improve the heart's ability to contract. The severity of the heart failure will determine the measures necessary to decrease preload. When clients have a mild form of failure, preload can be decreased by reducing sodium intake. The physician will probably precribe a mild diuretic such as one of the thiazides. Antianginal drugs such as nitroglycerin and isosorbide dinitrate may also be prescribed to reduce preload through their vasodilating effects.

With severe heart failure, the use of the more potent diuretics such as ethacrynic acid or furosemide is necessary. In addition to antianginal drugs, antihypertensive agents such as nitroprusside, prazosin, or captopril may be used to promote pooling of blood in the veins. Nitroprusside and agents with properties that promote arterial dilation also decrease afterload. Additional measures such as rotating tourniquets or phlebotomy may also be necessary.

If the cause of heart failure is decreased preload, the treatment may be the administration of blood or fluids, depending on the cause. Use of this therapy may seem confusing because rapid fluid administration is contraindicated in most types of heart failure. To understand the rationale, consider that, if there is not enough blood to pump, the heart will pump it faster to meet body demands and subsequently become overloaded and fail. In these relatively infrequent instances, fluid administration is proper.

Measures to decrease afterload in a person with mild heart failure include therapies for control of high blood pressure. Antianginal drugs also decrease afterload by causing peripheral arteriolar dilation. As heart failure progresses, more potent drugs are used to promote arterial dilation. Hydralazine, minoxidil, phenoxybenzamine, and phentolamine are specific drugs for arterial dilation. Drugs such as nitroprusside, prazosin, and captopril that promote arterial dilation and venous dilation may also be used and will also decrease preload.

Digitalis glycosides are inotropic agents used for many years to improve the contractility of the heart. Digitalis preparations are usually prescribed for persons who have mild heart failure to promote better contraction of the heart and increase cardiac output. As heart failure progresses, the dosage of digitalis may be adjusted. In acute, severe heart failure, other inotropic drugs are used temporarily. These include catecholamines such as epinephrine, norepinephrine, isoproterenol, dopamine, dobutamine, and amrinone.

When these therapies are ineffective in relieving the symptoms of heart failure, mechanical assistive devices such as the intra-aortic balloon pump may be instituted. Cardiac transplantation or mechanical hearts may be a possible treatment.

Specific Nursing Measures

Nursing care involves continuous assessment of the client's cardiac status and the effects produced by drug therapies. Changes in the client's status indicating further deterioration should always be reported to the physician immediately so the medical plan of care can be adjusted.

When CHF progresses to pulmonary edema, the client should be assisted to a high Fowler's position with the legs dependent to decrease venous return. Support the lower arms on pillows to reduce strain and fatigue. Oxygen and IV morphine sulfate and IV diuretics may be ordered. Sometimes rotating tourniquets, by sphygmomanometer cuffs or automatic rotating-tourniquet machine, are applied to further reduce the volume of venous blood returning to the heart. Important nursing responsibilities in applying rotating tourniquets are:

- Measure and record a baseline blood pressure and take pulses in each extremity, marking their location.
- Apply stockinette to all extremities to protect the skin.
- Apply sphygmomanometer cuffs as high as possible on three extremities pumping them to 40 mm Hg of pressure. (Make every effort to find cuffs of the appropriate size to the client's extremities.)
- Use a flow sheet; rotate the tourniquets every 15 minutes in a fixed sequence (eg, clockwise), leaving one extremity unobstructed.
- Check arterial pulses frequently to be sure arterial flow is not impeded; check blood pressure in the unobstructed limb.
- If an IV is in place, a tourniquet should not be used on that extremity.
- When the treatment is discontinued, the sphygmomanometer cuffs should be removed gradually, one every 15 minutes, so as not to suddenly overload the venous system.

Client/Family Teaching

Explain the treatment in detail to the client and significant others. Prepare them for the discoloration of the peripheral skin while the tourniquets are in use, and assure them that arterial blood flow to the hands and feet will continue. Monitor urinary output. An increase in urine output is one measure of a decrease in blood volume.

Independent nursing action should be compatible with the goals of the medical plan of care. A major nursing measure is to provide an environment where clients feel safe and are assured of receiving proper care, whether in an acute care or outpatient facility. Clients may be frightened, and attention to their needs may increase or decrease the anxiety. Letting clients know that nurses will be assessing them frequently to determine the effects of the medical plan of care may be reassuring if they are told that this is routine and does not mean their condition is worsening.

Adjusting activity level may be a problem for many persons. In the acute care situation, the nurse should observe for untoward symptoms and signs as daily activities increase. Spacing activities to allow time for the heart to rest will promote a pattern of behavior that can be carried through to discharge. Involving clients by instructing them to be aware of symptoms with increased activity and planning for rest periods and activity periods should help them to be more aware of activity tolerance after discharge. Clients should be attentive to activities that bring on symptoms and avoid them if possible. If it is impossible to avoid some activities such as climbing steps, the activity should be spaced to allow for rest periods. If activity is severely compromised, nursing measures associated with care of clients with immobility are appropriate.

Correctly taking the prescribed medications is sometimes a problem. The client should be taught the reasons for each medication, the possible side effects, and the possible consequences if the medications are not taken.

Compliance with dietary advice is also difficult for clients. A low-salt diet is unpalatable to some, and a low-calorie diet is distressing to those who enjoy eating rich food. Knowledge of the long-term effects of noncompliance sometimes helps clients to comply. The nurse may be most effective in counseling the client to avoid very salty foods such as potato chips, ham, pretzels, and condiments. Clients will be more likely to follow this approach than a strict no salt diet. Removing the salt shaker from the table also helps because salting food is sometimes more of a habit than a real need.

Losing weight is a problem for most persons who need to lose it. Clients should be encouraged to lose weight slowly. They should be reminded that rapid weight loss or gain is usually related to fluid balance. Weighing themselves daily or weekly will help them to assess the effectiveness of the plan of therapy.

Depression may be a problem, as it is with most persons who lose their health or are forced to change their lifestyles. Acknowledging that these feelings are common may help. The family or significant others may also be helpful in providing the encouragement necessary for clients to be able to live with a disability.

Cardiac Arrest

Cardiac arrest implies that the heart has stopped beating. The term is used more loosely, however, for the practical purposes of determining the necessity for cardiopulmonary resuscitation (CPR). Braunwald's criteria (1984)—deepening cyanosis of rapid onset, absence of heart sounds, and a lack of detectable pulses in the major vessels—are sufficient findings to diagnose cardiac arrest. Most cardiac arrests occur before the victim reaches the hospital. Because so many deaths occur before hospitalization, the American Heart Association and the American Red Cross have developed a community effort for education and training in CPR for the public as well as professionals.

Cardiovascular disease is the most common cause of sudden death or death within 24 hours of onset of symptoms. The most common causes of sudden cardiac death are ventricular fibrillation, ventricular tachycardia, severe bradycardia, and asystole.

Medical Measures

The initial approach to cardiac arrest depends on whether the client is monitored. Hospitals and other health agencies have trained teams of personnel and guidelines to follow in the event of a cardiac arrest. When cardiac arrest occurs, basic cardiac life support is initiated, and the emergency plan developed by the agency is activated.

If the client is monitored and the cause of the arrest is ventricular fibrillation, a precordial thump is attempted to terminate the dysrhythmia. The client is thumped sharply on the midportion of the sternum to provide an electrical stimulus to restore a heart beat. If successful, lidocaine therapy is initiated. If unsuccessful, electrical countershock is performed. (Countershock involves application of an electrical current to the heart through the chest wall with a defibrillator.) If countershock is unsuccessful, CPR is started as would be done for any victim in any setting who is unresponsive.

CARDIOPULMONARY RESUSCITATION Cardiopulmonary resuscitation (CPR) must begin as soon as unresponsiveness and the absence of breathing and carotid pulses are noted. CPR provides for oxygenation of vital tissues (ie, brain and myocardium) until cardiac function can be restored, preventing irreversible cerebral or cardiac damage. The rescuer should call for help and then open the individual's airway using a head-tilt maneuver (Figure 19–18) and listen and feel for the victim's breath on the rescuer's cheek. For the victim with suspected neck injury, a jaw-thrust technique without head-tilt is a safer approach to open the airway. **The elapsed time should be no more than 3 to 5 seconds.** If the victim is not breathing, the rescuer should:

- Pinch the victim's nostrils to prevent an air leak.
- Take a deep breath.
- Seal the victim's mouth with his or her mouth and breathe forcefully two times with breaths of 1 to 1½ seconds each while watching for the victim's chest to rise.

If the victim's pulses are absent, cardiac compression must be instituted, using the following steps:

- Move the victim to a firm surface, such as the floor or a resuscitation board.
- Kneel on one side of the victim, keeping elbows straight and shoulders parallel, directly over the victim's sternum.
- Locate the correct anatomic landmark: 2 to 3 fingers above the xiphoid process.
- Place the heel of the working hand on the landmark with the heel of the second hand directly on top, interlacing the fingers. Only the heel of the working hand should be in contact with the victim's chest.
- Apply sufficient downward pressure to depress the

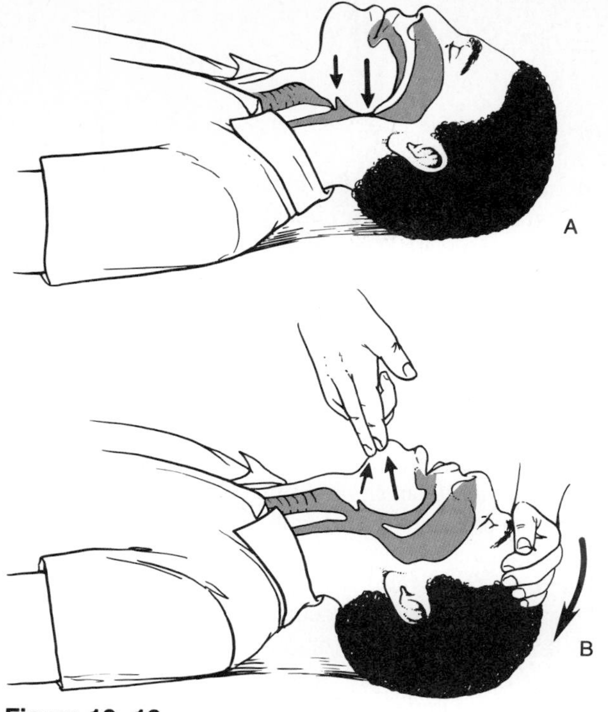

Figure 19–18

Opening the airway. **A.** Aortic obstruction produced by the tongue and the epiglottis. **B.** Relief by head-tilt and chin-lift.

sternum 3.8 to 5.0 cm (1.5 to 2 in). Release pressure to allow the heart to refill.

- Deliver 15 compressions at a rate of 80 per minute (and to 100 per minute, if possible), pacing the compressions by counting, "one-and, two-and, three-and, four-and, five-and, etc."
- Continue this cycle at a rate of *two breaths to 15 cardiac compressions at a rate of 80 to 100 compressions per minute (one breath to 5 cardiac compressions at a rate of 80 to 100 compressions per minute when two people are performing the procedure)* (*JAMA*, 1986).
- Pause after 1 minute to check the victim's carotid pulse and breathing. Thereafter, pause to check every 4 to 5 minutes.

If the victim is wearing secure-fitting dentures, they can be left in place to help the rescuer maintain an airtight seal. If dentures are loose, they should be removed. If the victim has a laryngectomy or tracheostomy, direct mouth-to-stoma ventilation should be used. If gastic distention occurs during CPR, reposition the airway to be sure it is patent.

Once CPR is initiated, it should be continued until the client's breathing and heartbeat are restored, the client can be turned over to an experienced resuscitation team, or the client is pronounced dead by a physician or coroner.

HEIMLICH MANEUVER Intervention for sudden airway obstruction is included as a part of basic life support instruction. Sudden occlusion of the airway is most common when a large or whole piece of food, such as a chunk of meat, a peanut, an ice cube, or a marshmallow, becomes lodged in the trachea. The passage of air is obstructed, and respiration ceases. Symptoms mimic those of an MI. This condition has been called the "café coronary" because it frequently occurs while dining in a restaurant. If the obstruction is not attended to immediately, death from a blocked airway will ensue in 4 to 6 minutes from cardiopulmonary arrest.

If the victim is conscious, the rescuer should:

- Validate with the victim that the airway is obstructed. (Ask the victim, "Can you breathe?")
- With the victim standing, rescuer behind, using an abdominal thrust (Heimlich maneuver) to clear the airway. (Make a fist with one hand. Place the thumb side of the fist in the midline of the client's abdomen, well below the tip of the xiphoid process. Grasp the fist with the other hand and press into the client's abdomen with a quick upward thrust.)
- Continue using separate abdominal thrusts until the airway is cleared or the victim becomes unconscious.
- Then place the unconscious victim in the supine, face-up position, turn the victim's head to the side and "sweep" the mouth using a cross-finger technique to remove any loosened material. Then attempt to ventilate.
- If unable to ventilate, place the heel of one hand in the abdominal midline, slightly above the navel and well below the tip of the xiphoid. The second hand is directly on top of the first. Press into the abdomen 6–10 times with quick upward thrusts.
- Use the finger sweep and attempt to ventilate again. Keep up these efforts as long as necessary (*JAMA*, 1986).

Specific Nursing Measures

Every nurse has a professional and ethical obligation to be certified in basic life support. Certification is available through the American Heart Association and the American Red Cross. Review the emergency plan in the agency, and be prepared for emergency action. In case of cardiac arrest in any setting, perform CPR according to the standards of the American Red Cross or the American Heart Association.

The nurse has a responsibility to educate the public concerning prevention of sudden airway obstruction, using the following guidelines:

- Avoid laughing or talking with food in the mouth.
- Take small bites.
- Have dentures fitted properly and use them when eating.
- Be familiar with the universal choking signal (Figure 19–19).
- If alone when the obstruction occurs, use a table edge, countertop, or chair to thrust against just below the rib cage in the middle of the upper abdomen.

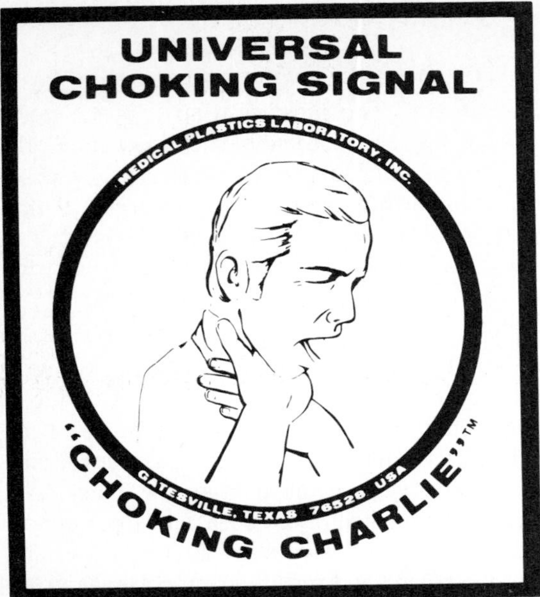

Figure 19–19

Universal choking signal. SOURCE: *Medical Plastics Laboratory, Inc., PO Box 38, Gatesville, Texas 76528.*

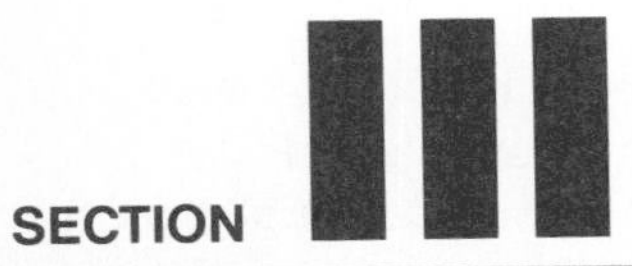

SECTION III

Infectious Disorders

Infections of the heart can follow systemic infections. These may be serious and if undiagnosed, can result in death. Clients with infections of the heart sometimes have prolonged recovery periods and may be prone to future heart problems. Infections can involve the endocardium (endocarditis), the myocardium (myocarditis), the pericardium (pericarditis), or a combination of these three layers. Involvement of all three layers, as frequently occurs with rheumatic fever, is called pancarditis.

Endocarditis

Endocarditis may result from invasion of the lining of the heart by organisms or from injury to the lining of the heart, a noninfective cause. Infective endocarditis involves the endocardium of the heart valves more frequently than the endocardium of the heart chambers. Infectious endocarditis may be acute, developing over a period of less than 2 weeks, or subacute, developing over several months. Although infectious endocarditis occurs in persons with no previous heart disease, it is most frequent in those with previous heart disease. In persons with no previous heart disease, infectious endocarditis is seen in drug abusers and in children under 2 years of age. In those with heart disease, it is associated with rheumatic heart disease, congential heart disease, previous cardiac surgery, and previous endocarditis (Hurst et al., 1982).

Microorganisms enter the bloodstream and lodge on the endocardial surface. They multiply and produce thrombosis, which stimulates the deposit of fibrin around the bacteria. This results in the formation of vegetations. On healing, the vegetations are covered by endothelium and calcium deposits. The endocardium becomes scarred, and the surface is susceptible to reinfection.

Although infectious endocarditis usually involves the left side of the heart, it also may involve the right side, especially in drug abusers. The most common complications include heart failure and embolization. If the right side of the heart is involved, emboli travel to the pulmonary circulation. If the left side is involved, emboli travel to the arterial circulation.

The organisms usually responsible for infective endocarditis are streptococci and staphylococci, although other organisms are sometimes responsible. The most common procedures providing portals of entry for the organisms include dental procedures that cause gingival bleeding, such as occurs with brushing of teeth; oral surgery; upper respiratory tract surgery; genitourinary and gastrointestinal surgery; and cardiac surgery. Intra-arterial and intravenous catheters are excellent avenues of entry for organisms, which may cause nosocomial infective endocarditis. Drug abusers are at risk because of contamination during drug use.

Clinical Manifestations

In the subacute form, the clinical manifestations persist over several weeks before the diagnosis is made. In the acute form, the clinical manifestations usually lead to hospitalization within a few days. The symptoms are described as flulike and include fever, chills, sweats, anorexia, fatigue, weakness, headache, and musculoskeletal aches and pains. Most persons develop cardiac murmurs during the course of the disease, and the pulse rate may be rapid. Heart failure may develop. If vegetations dislodge from the endocardium, there may be clinical manifestations of embolization. The client may have symptoms of microembolization originating in the left side of the heart, such as petechiae in the skin or mucous membranes or splinter hemorrhages under the nails. Other manifestations of larger arterial emboli might include decreased or absent arterial pulses in an extremity, cerebrovascular symptoms related to a stroke, abdominal pain related to infarctions of the spleen or bowel, back pain related to infarction of the kidney, or chest pain related to infarction of the myocardium. There may be clinical manifestations of pulmonary embolism, including increased respiratory and pulse rates, fever, pleuritic pain, or cough, if embolization originates in the right side of the heart.

Because the clinical manifestations are common to many types of illnesses, laboratory studies are important to medical diagnosis. Findings can include anemia, an elevated erythrocyte sedimentation rate, hematuria, isolation of the organism from blood culture, ECG changes, detection of valvular lesions by echocardiography, and evidence of CHF by chest x-ray.

Medical Measures

Medical management is critical because infective endorcarditis is usually fatal if untreated. The primary goal is to kill the infecting organisms as quickly as possible. If the organism is known, the antibiotic is chosen based on the sensitivity of the organism. When the organism is not known, nafcillin, ampicillin, and gentamicin are often used in combination therapy. Prolonged antibiotic therapy may be indicated for at least 4 weeks but may be extended for 8 weeks or longer to achieve a cure. Treatment for complications may also be necessary. Surgery to correct structural lesions may be indicated if heart failure becomes severe enough or if the client develops significant arterial emboli. Anticoagulant warfarin therapy for embolization is sometimes cautiously undertaken. The use of heparin is avoided.

Specific Nursing Measures

Nursing measures during the acute phase center around care related to infections and close assessment and reporting of subjective and objective findings that may indicate complications described previously. Because the client and family may be anxious, nursing approaches to decrease anxiety through careful explanation are important. Implement measures to preserve energy while promoting sufficient activity to prevent complications, as the client's condition indicates. Spacing of activities as well as other measures described for heart failure are appropriate.

The nurse can assist the client to prevent further episodes of endocarditis through health teaching about prophylactic antibiotic therapy. Explain that the client is prone to future episodes of endocarditis because scars that sometimes remain on the heart lining can trap bacteria and promote bacterial growth. With this information, the client may be more likely to comply with prescribed prophylactic antibacterial therapy when undergoing invasive procedures such as dental surgery.

Myocarditis

Myocarditis is an inflammatory process involving the myocardium caused by infectious agents, radiation, chemicals, pharmacologic agents, or metabolic disorders. Infectious myocarditis, which may be acute or chronic, frequently goes unrecognized. Most persons recover completely, although acute myocarditis is a common cause of acute dilated cardiomyopathy (previously called acute congestive cardiomyopathy). Several months or years after the initial myocarditis, an individual may develop clinical manifestations of CHF with ventricular enlargement and dysfunction. Progressive deterioration is usually followed by death within 4 years (Braunwald, 1984).

Any infectious agent may cause myocarditis. In North America, viruses are the most common cause, especially coxsackievirus B. Some common viral infections that have been identified as causing myocarditis are mumps, influenza, viral hepatitis, and infectious mononucleosis. Rickettsial, bacterial, spirochetal, fungal, protozoal, and metazoal infections can also cause myocarditis.

Clinical Manifestations

The clinical manifestations of myocarditis vary from no symptoms to symptoms of severe CHF. The manifestations are indistinguishable from those of systemic infection. The pulse rate may be higher than expected with the degree of temperature elevation. Transient ECG abnormalities may occur, including ST segment changes, T wave changes, and dysrhythmias, although these are also observed in clients with infections without myocardial involvement. Diagnosis is based on identification of the systemic infection and is suspected when ECG changes are present. When the client has CHF without an identifiable cause, a biopsy of the right ventricle may be diagnostic.

Medical Measures

Medical management centers around treating the client for the clinical manifestations. Antibiotic therapy may also be instituted against some organisms. The client should be observed closely for ECG changes and appropriately treated for dysrhythmias. Drugs, such as beta-blockers, which cause a negative inotropic effect are usually avoided in the treatment of dysrhythmias. If the client develops CHF, the treatment is similar to that previously described. Because persons with myocarditis are especially sensitive to the effects of digitalis, they should be observed closely for the development of digitalis toxicity. Adequate rest and oxygenation are also indicated.

Specific Nursing Measures

Nursing measures during the acute phase involve care of the client with an infection and assessment and reporting of cardiac dysrhythmias and signs of CHF. Because systemic infections may result in myocarditis, stress the importance of rest and provide supportive care of the client who has a systemic infection. The nursing care of clients with dysrhythmias and CHF was discussed earlier in this chapter.

Pericarditis

Pericarditis is an inflammation of the pericardium, the sac surrounding the heart. The infection, which may be acute or chronic, is frequently not properly diagnosed and sometimes results in death. Pericarditis may be caused by trauma, tumors, anticoagulants, bleeding disorders, systemic diseases, MI, as well as infectious agents. Pericarditis is frequently observed in clients who have had open heart surgery. Acute pericarditis is often misdiagnosed as pleurisy, MI, bronchopneumonia, or pulmonary embolism. Pericarditis may cause the life-treatening emergency of **cardiac tamponade,** an accumulation of a large amount of fluid in the pericardial sac, which prevents the heart from filling and consequently reduces cardiac output dramatically. Cardiac tamponade usually requires pericardiocentesis, an immediate surgical procedure to empty the pericardial sac. Pericarditis may also result in constrictive pericarditis, which may develop over months or years with the development of fibrosis of the pericardial sac. Constrictive pericarditis requires surgical removal of the pericardium, and recovery may require months.

Infectious pericarditis is most commonly caused by viral, bacterial, tuberculous, fungal, or parasitic organisms. Coxsackievirus B is a common viral cause, although mumps, influenza, poliomyelitis, varicella, hepatitis B, and viruses causing infectious mononucleosis are sometimes implicated. Bacterial pericarditis most commonly occurs by spread of intrathoracic infections. Common organisms include staphylococci, streptococci, gram-negative bacilli, *Neisseria, Salmonella,* and others. Fungal pericarditis usually develops from extension of infections of the lungs from inhalation of *Histoplasma* or *Coccidioides* organisms. *Aspergillus, Blastomyces,* and *Candida* may also be responsible organisms. Unusual infectious causes of pericarditis include the parasites *Entamoeba histolytica* and *Echinococcus granulosus.*

Clinical Manifestations

Chest pain, a pericardial friction rub, and serial ECG abnormalities are characteristic findings in the client with acute pericarditis. The chest pain is variable among clients and is sometimes indistinguishable from an MI. The chest pain can also be unlike MI pain, however. The pain is aggravated by lying supine, respiratory movements, and swallowing. It may be relieved somewhat by sitting up and leaning forward. A pericardial friction rub may be heard intermittently or may last as long as a week or more with some types of pericarditis. The sound is usually heard best at the left lower sternal border with the client sitting up and leaning forward upon inspiration and full expiration. The grating sound is similar to that of rubbing hairs together near the ear or squeaking leather. The ECG changes are ST and T wave changes. The client may also have dyspnea and manifestations of systemic infection including fever, chills, and sweating.

Constrictive pericarditis caused by fibrosis and calcification of the pericardium restricts filling of the heart and produces manifestations of systemic venous congestion including increased jugular venous pressure, edema, and abdominal swelling and discomfort related to liver congestion. Manifestations of pulmonary venous congestion including dyspnea, cough, and orthopnea may be present.

When pericarditis results in a **pericardial effusion** or accumulation of fluid in the pericardial sac, the clinical manifestations of cardiac tamponade occur. Pulsus paradoxus, diminished pulse pressure, distant heart sounds, and jugular venous distention may be present. *Pulsus paradoxus* is an exaggeration of the normal decrease in amplitude of the pulse and decrease in arterial blood pressure during inspiration. With severe tamponade, the palpated pulse may completely disappear during inspiration. The manifestations of tamponade may occur in the acute stage or after constrictive pericarditis has developed. The diagnosis of constrictive pericarditis is made after pericardiocentesis. Pericardiocentesis will not restore normal hemodynamics in constrictive pericarditis, and surgical removal of the pericardium is eventually necessary. The cause of the pericarditis is sometimes identified through laboratory examination of the pericardial fluid.

The client with acute pericarditis caused by a viral infection will usually report a recent cold or the flu and suggen development of precordial pain. A pericardial friction rub is usually present and may last up to a week. The client with pericarditis caused by a bacterial infection will usually have a history of fever, chills, night sweats, and dyspnea of a few days duration before seeking medical assistance. The client may have a pericardial friction rub but usually does not have the typical chest pain. Because bacterial pericarditis usually results in a pericardial effusion, the manifestion of cardiac tamponade from the development of purulent fluid in the pericardium will be apparent. Clients with fungal infections may develop a pericardial effusion rapidly or over a period of several months. Usually, they seek medical help for manifestations related to systemic infection. Those with pericarditis resulting from tuberculosis are usually not diagnosed as having pericarditis until the constrictive state, when the major symptoms are dyspnea and heaviness in the chest. A pericardial friction rub may or may not be heard in clients with all types of pericarditis.

Medical Measures

Medical management of the client with acute pericarditis includes hospitalization, rest, and close observation for the development of cardiac tamponande as well as treatment for the underlying problem. Nonsteroidal anti-inflammatory agents such as aspirin or indomethacin are used to control the pain. Sometimes they are not effective, however, and steroids may be necessary to control the pain. Specific antibiotic therapy is used when indicated, against the causative organism. When the client has constrictive pericarditis, surgical resection of the pericardium is usually performed.

Specific Nursing Measures

Nursing management includes providing an environment conducive to rest and the control of pain. The client is assessed for the development of cardiac tamponade as described previously.

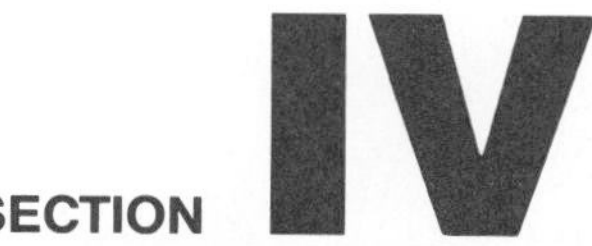

SECTION IV Obstructive Disorders

Many disorders can obstruct blood flow within the heart. Lack of blood flow to any tissue, including the heart, results in ischemia, injury, and infarction. With advances in cardiac surgery and better diagnostic studies, the obstructive problems of hypertrophic cardiomyopathy are diagnosed and treated with increasing frequency. Nurses are beginning to see persons with these problems more often in the clinical setting.

Hypertrophic Cardiomyopathy

Hypertrophic cardiomyopathy has more than 50 names. In the United States, it has most frequently been called idiopathic hypertrophic subaortic stenosis (IHSS). In Canada, it has been known as muscular subaortic stenosis. As these terms imply, the disease was once thought to involve hypertrophy of the ventricular septum, causing a stenotic obstruction to blood flow in the left ventricle during systole at an area beneath the aortic valve opposite the anterior leaflet of the mitral valve. More recently, the term has been changed because it has been found that not all persons have systolic obstruction to blood flow in the subaortic region.

The term *hypertrophic cardiomyopathy* is more appropriate because it indicates that the entire heart is enlarged even though the septum is more enlarged. Although the heart is enlarged, the ventricular chambers are small. Because of the hypertrophy, the ventricles are resistant to filling during diastole. The atria compensate for this by expanding. Hypertrophic cardiomyopathy is important to nurses because many of the therapies for heart problems are contraindicated in its treatment; in addition, the condition is frequently observed in young adulthood, and sudden death is common, especially during strenuous exercise and most commonly from dysrhythmias. Some persons have a long life with few or no symptoms, but many die within 10 years after symptoms begin. The cause of hypertrophic cardiomyopathy is not known, but it is thought to be genetically transmitted, because many persons have relatives with the problem or a familial history of sudden death.

Clinical Manifestations

Although many persons experience no symptoms of the disease and die suddenly, dyspnea is the most common symptom that prompts the client to seek medical assistance. Because there is resistance to diastolic filling, the left ventricular end diastolic pressure rises, and the client becomes dyspneic. Because of inadequate cardiac output, especially during strenuous exercise, angina, fatigue, and syncope may also occur. Exertion tends to bring on the symptoms. The ECG is usually abnormal with ST and T wave abnormalities and ventricular hypertrophy evidenced by large QRS complexes. Dysrhythmias are common. The chest x-ray may be abnormal or show left atrial enlargement or general cardiac enlargement. Echocardiography, radionuclide imaging, and phonocardiography are performed to assist in the diagnosis. Angiocardiography is often definitive.

Medical Measures

The goals of medical management center on attempts to minimize the consequences of hypertrophic cardiomyopathy. Because sudden death is the major problem, the client should avoid strenuous exercise, tachycardia, and hypotension, which increase likelihood of sudden death. Inotropic drugs such as digitalis and the sympathomimetics as well as hypotensive agents such as nitroglycerin should be avoided. Major therapeutic agents for the control of dysrhythmias include beta blockers or calcium channel blockers. Pacemaker therapy is sometimes indicated.

Atrial fibrillation is considered an emergency, and therapy is directed at prevention of the formation and embolization of blood clots through heparinization and cardioversion. If the client develops CHF, the usual therapy is digitalis and diuretics for those clients who do not have the obstructive component associated with hypertrophic cardiomyopathy. Use of the drugs may promote problems if the client has obstruction to blood flow, however. Antibiotic prophylaxis is prescribed for invasive procedures, because clients with hypertrophic cardiomyopathy can develop infective endocarditis of the aortic valve, mitral valve, or septum. Surgery is sometimes performed, replacing the mitral valve or removing a wedge of the hypertrophied myocardium from the left ventricular septum.

Specific Nursing Measures

The most important aspects of nursing care are client teaching and counseling. Clients are often hospitalized for the diagnostic procedures, and the nurse can provide support by preparing the client for changes in lifestyle that might be needed. Many persons with hypertrophic cardiomyopathy are young adults who have been active but must now avoid strenuous activity. Concerns regarding having children must be discussed. Although women with the condition seem to do remarkably well throughout pregnancy and delivery, the familial tendencies regarding the disease should be considered, especially if there is a strong history on both sides. Because there is a possibility of sudden death, families and significant others should be encouraged to learn basic life support.

Clients should be counseled regarding the drug regimen and the necessity to avoid inotropic and hypotensive agents. Any physician, dentist, or anesthesiologist treating the client for other problems should be alerted to avoid these drugs. Antibiotic prophylaxis is indicated during invasive procedures, because of the tendency to develop infective endocarditis.

Heart Transplantation

Heart transplantation is reserved for the client with intractable cardiac disease, extensive loss of ventricular function, severe CAD not amenable to bypass surgery, cardiomyopathy, and congenital heart disease when all forms of medical treatment have been exhausted. Recently, heart transplantation clients have had a 60% to 80% 1-year survival rate and a 30% to 50% 5-year survival rate (Copeland, 1984).

The first successful human transplant was performed by Christian Barnard in 1967. In this *heterotopic transplant,* the original heart was left in place, and the donor heart was transplanted on top of it. *Orthotopic transplant,* the removal of the recipient's heart and insertion of the donor heart, is the primary type of transplant performed in North America today.

The donor heart is usually from a brain-dead person of body size similar to the recipient's. The donor must be less than 35 years old and without any history of cardiac disease, cardiac trauma, serious infection, or malignancy. There must be histocompatibility between donor and recipient to minimize the possibility of rejection. The donor heart must be harvested, transported, and preserved for no more than 4 hours.

The client is placed on the heart–lung machine, most of the recipient's heart is resected, and the donor heart is transplanted (Figure 19–20). Temporary pacing wires ar mediastinal drainage tubes are placed. A direct pulmonary artery or direct left atrial pressure line may also be placed and passed through the chest wall. The physiologic and psychosocial/lifestyle implications for clients undergoing heart transplantations are discussed in Table 19–8.

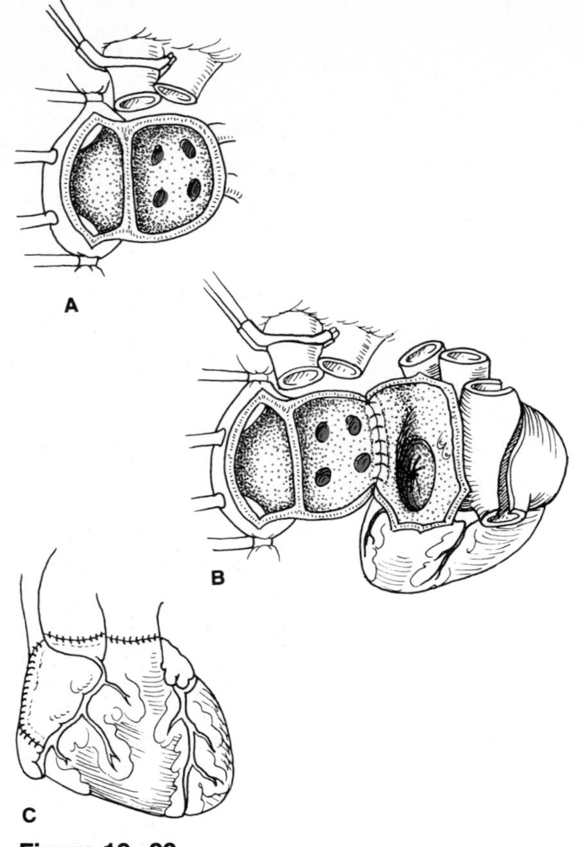

Figure 19–20

Orthotopic heart transplant. **A.** The posterior wall of the right and left atria and a ridge of atrial septum remain after the recipient's heart has been removed. **B.** The transplantation is begun by anastomosing the left atrium of the donor heart to the residual left atrial wall of the recipient. **C.** Transplantation is complete when the atrial walls, atrial septum, and great vessels have been joined.

Nursing Implications

PREOPERATIVE CARE Cyclosporine is administered to the client before surgery. The usual heart surgery preparations apply (see the discussion of coronary artery bypass surgery).

POSTOPERATIVE CARE The heart transplantation recipient requires the intensive nursing care necessary after any heart operation. One major difference with this operation is that the heart is denervated and therefore does not respond to vagal or sympathetic stimulation. Thus, atropine cannot be administered if the client has a bradydysrhythmia because the drug affects the heart rate via the vagus nerve (cranial nerve X). The client with myocardial ischemia also does not experience angina pectoris. Therefore, ischemic changes must be detected by ECG or myocardial enzyme studies.

Immunosuppressive drug therapy begins immediately after surgery. Conventional therapy uses azathioprine (Imuran), prednisone, and antithrombocytic globulin to prevent rejection. Cyclosporine can curb tissue rejection without inhibiting the body's infection-fighting mechanisms. This drug has been found to be highly effective and has facilitated early client rehabilitation.

Monitor the client for the side effects of immunosuppressive drugs and report them to the physician. Oral hygiene also becomes extremely important to prevent dental and gum disease that could be an infection source. The diet should be as high in protein as the drug regimen allows to encourage normal healing.

Protective isolation is maintained the first few weeks after surgery. Special precautions to prevent infection include inserting a suprapubic urinary catheter, using strict sterile technique with suctioning and dressing changes, washing all equipment with a bactericidal solution, observing wounds for early signs of infection, and auscultating the lungs for early signs of pulmonary congestion.

Monitor the client for signs of rejection. With conventional therapy, the signs include heart failure and diminishing QRS voltage. With cyclosporine therapy, clinical changes are not observed, and only myocardial biopsy is diagnostic. If rejection occurs after discharge, the client must be rehospitalized. Treatment usually consists of higher doses of corticosteroids or antithrombocytic globulin.

Discharge instructions are essential to successful rehabilitation. The client must have knowledge of:

- The purpose, dosages, and side effects to report of all medications and the need not to discontinue taking them without the physician's orders
- Situations to avoid that increase the risk of infection
- Good health care habits for teeth, skin, and so on
- Early signs of infection
- Treatment of injuries
- A diet low in saturated fat and cholesterol
- Activities allowed
- Clinic follow-up appointments
- Need for carrying a medical information tag or card

Table 19–8
Heart Transplantation: Implications for the Client

Physiologic Implications	Psychosocial/Lifestyle Implications
Denervation (no anginal pain or response to atropine)	Need to take precautions against infection
Two P waves in ECG	Lifelone need for immunosuppressive drugs
Higher resting heart rate	Drug side effects
Slowing of heart's response to exercise	Need for frequent physician visits
High risk of infection, especially the first 3 months after surgery	Low-fat, low-cholesterol diet
Possible rejection	Change in body image
Risk of coronary artery disease	Need to live close to hospital before, and a few months after, surgery
Risk of malignancy from cyclosporine	Guilt or depersonalization at having someone else's heart
Need to take aspirin and dipyramidole	Improved quality of life
	New roles for client and family members or significant others

Artificial Heart Implantation

The artificial heart (Figure 19–21) is an experimental device that is indicated for the client with intractable heart failure resistant to all known therapeutic measures. This type of heart failure occurs in individuals with severe CAD or cardiomyopathy. The procedure is done in only a few centers.

The surgical implantation of the artificial heart is technically simple compared with other heart surgeries. The client is placed on cardiopulmonary bypass, and the client's ventricles are excised, leaving the atria intact. The cuffs from the artificial heart are sutured onto the client's atria

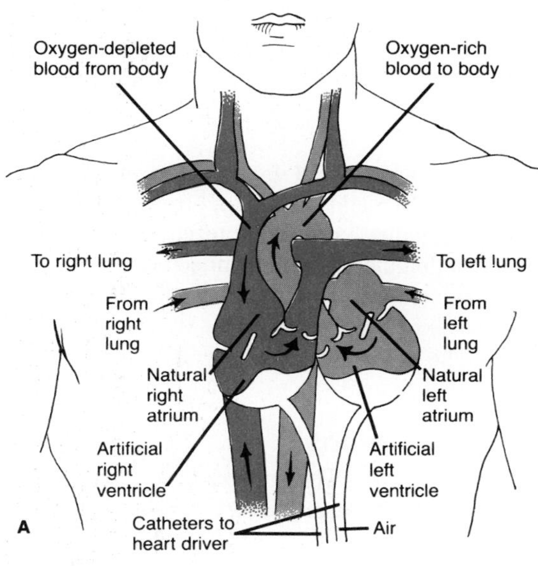

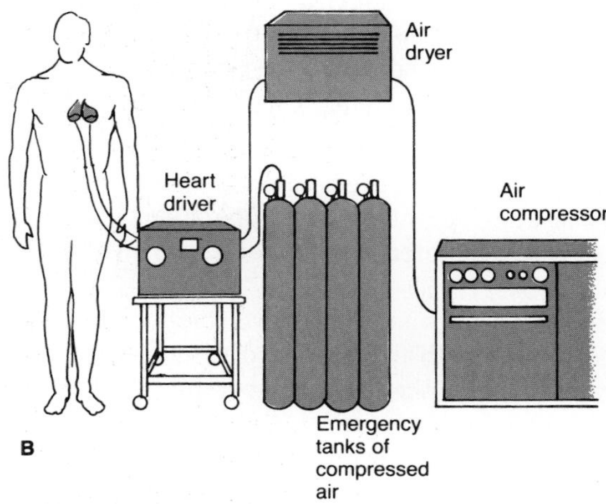

Figure 19–21

The artificial heart. **A.** The implant. **B.** The support system.

Table 19–9
Artificial Heart Implantation Implications for the Client

Physiologic Implications	Psychosocial/Lifestyle Implications
Implications not yet fully understood	Lifelong dependence on a mechanical device
Major complications are stroke, bleeding, emboli, hemolysis of red blood cells, and infection	Drive unit must be transported with client at all times
	Body image change
	Emotional responses such as anxiety and depression during the uncertainty of the postoperative period
	Regular ongoing health care requires client and family to move near the medical center
	Role changes for client and family

and great vessels. The artificial ventricles are then separately snapped into place and jointed together by a strip of Velcro. Special connecting lines, called tethers, are brought out through the abdominal wall and connected to the drive unit, which sends compressed air in and out of the heart. Researchers are exploring alternatives to the air-driven artificial heart. The physiologic and psychosocial/lifestyle implications are in Table 19–9.

Nursing Implications

PREOPERATIVE CARE The preoperative preparations are similar to those for coronary artery bypass surgery. A team of physicians, nurses, and social workers evaluates the client for a stable psychologic profile and ability to comply with the medical regimen and postoperative follow-up care. The client is also evaluated to be sure there is a stable home environment because living alone is not possible.

POSTOPERATIVE CARE The care of postoperative artificial heart recipients is a new challenge for critical care nurses. Not only does the client have the many tubes and lines present after any major heart operation, but he or she must also be monitored for any problems of mechanical failure.

The hemodynamics and fluid management of the client are also different from that of other cardiac surgery patients. If cardiac output falls, the drive pressure or heart rate is increased. Inotropic drugs cannot be used.

After the client is discharged from the ICU, the problem of mobility arises. The nurse must be creative in developing ways for the client to move while maintaining the integrity of the tethers. Rehabilitation must be individualized according to the client's reponse to surgery.

Ventricular Assist Implantation

Ventricular assist devices (VADs) are mechanical pumps that can be used temporarily or over the long term to provide assistance to an overburdened or poorly functioning ventricle. Temporary assist is indicated for ventricular dysfunction where recovery of the myocardium is anticipated. Temporary devices have also been used for support of the collapsed circulation prior to cardiac transplantation. Long-term assist is indicated for permanent damage to the myocardium.

There are many types of VADs available. Some devices are extracorporeal with the pump located outside the body and some are intracorporeal and implanted into the thoracic or abdominal cavity. VADs have the capability of supporting the left ventricle, right ventricle, or both ventricles simultaneously.

No matter what type of device is used, the principles remain the same. Blood is diverted away from the ventricle being assisted, passes through the pump and is returned to the corresponding major vessel (ie, pulmonary artery or aorta). Although the client's natural ventricle still contracts while the VAD device is in place, its load is much lighter since the blood is routed through the VAD. Permanent VADs are being developed. Powered by an electric motor about the size of a coffee mug, they do not require outside tubing nor tethers to an air-driven machine.

Chapter Highlights

Any disease affecting the heart may promote the development of heart failure.

Heart problems can result from congenital problems, multifactorial causes, degenerative changes, infections, and systemic diseases.

Heart disease may develop as a result of physiologic changes within the body, environmental factors, genetic characteristics, or psychosocial/lifestyle factors.

Avoidance of risk factors may retard the development of some forms of heart disease.

Avoidance of risk factors usually means that clients will need to change their lifestyles.

Cardiac dysfunction can result in long-term problems requiring surgery and/or lengthy medical treatment and major lifestyle changes.

The mental health of a client with heart problems may be affected because of loss of independence and self-esteem, changes in body image, and altered sexuality patterns.

Bradydysrhythmias are successfully treated by cardiac pacemakers, devices that supply electrical impulses to the heart muscle to stimulate

the heartbeat. Surgical implantation procedures depend on the type of pacemaker.

Many surgical procedures of the heart and major blood vessels use the heart–lung machine, and close client monitoring is needed by the nurse in the early postoperative period.

Heart surgery clients often experience postcardiotomy psychosis, confusion, and depression; a changed self-image; and the need to modify risk factors by dietary changes, medication, and the elimination of smoking.

A relatively new nonsurgical approach to coronary artery disease in worldwide use is percutaneous transluminal coronary angioplasty. It is used in preference to coronary artery bypass surgery whenever possible.

Transplantation and artificial heart implantation entail significant psysiologic and psychosocial adjustment.

Bibliography

Bohachick P, Rongaus AM: Hypertrophic cardiomyopathy. *Am J Nurs* 1984; 84:320–326.

Braunwald E: *Heart Disease,* 2nd ed. Philadelphia: Saunders, 1984.

Burgess AW, Hartman CR: Patient's perceptions of the cardiac crisis: Key to recovery. *Am J Nurs* 1986; 86(5): 568–571.

Burgess AW, Lerner DJ, Hartman CR: Policy issues for cardiac rehabilitation programs. *Image* 1983; 15(3):75–79.

Case RB et al: Type A behavior and survival after actue myocardial infarction. *N Engl J Med* 1985; 312:737–741.

Cisar NS, Morphew SF: Preoperative teaching: Aortocoronary bypass patients. *Focus* 1983; 10(1):21–25.

Cooley DA: *Techniques in Cardiac Surgery,* 2nd ed. Philadelphia: Saunders, 1984.

Copeland JG: Cardiac transplantation today. *J Cardiovasc Med* 1984; 30:528–536.

Craig H: Accuracy of indirect measures of medication compliance in hypertension. *Res Nurs Health* 1985; 8:61–66.

Dawson C: Hypertension, perceived clinician empathy, and patient self-disclosure. *Res Nurs Health* 1985; 8:191–198.

DeVon HA, Powers MJ: Health beliefs, adjustment to illness, and control of hypertension. *Res Nurs Health* 1984; 7:10–16.

Glenn WWL et al: *Thoracic and Cardiovascular Surgery,* 4th ed. Norwalk, CT: Appleton–Century–Crofts, 1983.

Gruendemann BJ, Meeker MH: *Alexander's Care of the Patient in Surgery,* 7th ed. St. Louis: Mosby, 1983.

Guzzetta CE, Dossey BM: *Cardiovascular Nursing: Bodymind Tapestry.* St. Louis: Mosby, 1984.

Haun AB, Barkin RL, Oestreich SJK: *Pharmacology in Nursing.* St. Louis: Mosby, 1982.

Heart Facts 1983. Dallas: American Heart Association, 1982.

Hurst JW et al: *The Heart,* 5th ed. New York: McGraw–Hill, 1982.

Hypertension in the elderly. *JAMA* July 4, 1986; 256 (1):70–74.

Jasinkowski NL: Aortic bypass: Trimming the postop risks. *RN* (June) 1983; 46:41–45.

Jasinkowski NL: The unique needs of a distal bypass patient. *RN* (March) 1982; 45:44–47, 122.

Jenkins CD et al: Coronary artery bypass surgery: Physical, psychosocial, social and economic outcomes six months later. *JAMA* 1983; 250:782–788.

Kern LS: Mechanical support of the failing heart. In: *Congestive Heart Failure.* Michaelson CR (editor). St. Louis: Mosby, 1983.

Kern LS: Surgical treatment of underlying heart disease: Coronary artery bypass, heart valve replacement, heart transplant. In: *Congestive Heart Failure.* Michaelson CR (editor). St. Louis: Mosby, 1983.

Kern LS, Gawlinski A: Stage-managing coronary artery disease. *Nurs 83* 1983; 13:34–40.

LaForge R et al: Cardiac rehabilitation programs: The Sharp Memorial Hospital Cardiac Rehabilitation Program. *J Cardiac Rehabil* 1984; 4(1):6–9.

Lamb LS, Di Giancomo BM: What to expect when your patient's scheduled for mitral valve replacement. *Nurs 85* 1985; 15(1):58–63.

Leon AS: Physical activity and coronary heart disease: Analysis of epidemiologic and supporting studies. *Med Clin North Am* 1985; 69(1):3–20.

Marriott HJ, Gozensky C: Arrhythmias in coronary care: A renewed plea. *Heart Lung* 1982; 11:33–39.

McMahon F: *Management of Essential Hypertension. The New Low-Dose Era,* 2nd ed. Mount Kisco, NY: Futura, 1984.

McMahon M, Palmer R: Exercise and hypertension. *Med Clin North Am* 1985; 69(1):57–70.

Mickus D, Monahan KJ, Brown C: Exciting external pacemakers. *Am J Nurs* 1986; 86(4):403–405.

New guidelines for hypertension management. *Am J Nurs* 1984; 84:976–978.

Nissen MB: Streptokinase therapy in acute myocardial infarction. *Heart Lung* 1984; 13:230–233.

Ornato JP: The resuscitation of near-drowning victims. *JAMA* July 4, 1986; 256(1):75–77.

Owen P: Defibrillating pacemaker patients. *Am J Nurs* 1984; 84(9):1129–1130.

Pender N: Effects of progressive muscle relaxation training on anxiety and health locus of control among hypertensive adults. *Res Nurs Health* 1985; 8:67–72.

Porterfield L, Posterfield JG: What you need to know about today's pacemakers. *RN* (March) 1987; 44–49.

Powers MJ, Jalowiec A: Profile of the well-controlled, well-adjusted hypertensive patient. *Nurs Research* 1987; 36(2):106–110.

Purcell JA: Shock drugs: Standardized guidelines. *Am J Nurs* 1982; 82:965–973.

Purcell JA, Burrows SG: A pacemaker primer: For CE credit. *Am J Nurs* 1985; 85:553–568.

Purcell JA, Holder CK: Intravenous nitroglycerine. *Am J Nurs* 1982; 82:254–259.

Quaal SJ: *Comprehensive Intra-Aortic Balloon Pumping.* St. Louis: Mosby, 1984.

Rodriguez SW, Reed RL: Thrombolytic therapy for MI. *Am J Nurs* 1987; 87(5):632–640.

Runions J: A program for psychological and social enhancement during rehabilitation after myocardial infarction. *Heart Lung* 1985; 14:117–125.

Ryan AM: Stopping CHF while there's still time. *RN* (August) 1986; 28–36.

Scherer P: ACLS guidelines: What nurses are saying about the drug changes. *Am J Nurs* 1986; 86(12):1352–1358.

Shank J: Postperiocardiotomy syndrome. *Cardiovasc Nurs* 1983; 19(3):11–14.

Sloan R: Achieving compliance to a reduced sodium diet. *Nurse Pract* (Feb) 1985; 10:24–26.

"Standards and guidelines for cardiopulmonary resuscitation and emergency cardiac care." *JAMA* June 6, 1986; 255(21):2841–3044.

The 1984 report of the Joint National Committee on detection, evaluation, and treatment of high blood pressure. *Nurse Pract* (July) 1985; 10:9–14, 19–26, 31–34.

Trevino S, Massey J: Risk factors for arrhythmias after myocardial infarction. *Heart Lung* 1983; 12:240–247.

Wessman JP: Preventing ventricular dysrhythmia following myocardial infarction. *Dimensions Crit Care Nurs* (Jan–Feb) 1985; 4:24–32.

Winslow EH, Lane LD, Gaffney FA: Oxygen uptake and cardiovascular responses in control adults and acute myocardial infarction patients during bathing. *Nurs Res* 1985; 34:164–169.

CASE STUDY

The Client With a Myocardial Infarction

I. Descriptive Data

Mr Gary Holzerland, a 42-year-old white male, arrived by ambulance at the medical center emergency department with acute substernal chest pain radiating to the left arm. He was admitted to the CCU with the diagnosis of possible myocardial infarction (MI). His wife was notified immediately.

II. Personal Data

Date and Time: December 22, 1987; 3 PM
Full Name: Gary Holzerland
Address: 143 Victoria Pl, Buffalo, NY
Sex: Male
Age: 42
Birthdate: 4-30-45
Race/Culture: Caucasian
Occupation: Computer systems analyst
Usual Health Care Providers: Dana Hanavan, NP; Matthew Sigman, MD
Social Security Number: 000-00-0000
Telephone: Home: 000-0000
Work: 000-0000
Marital Status: Married
Religion: Protestant

III. Health History

Source of Information: Client and wife
Reliability of Information: Mr Holzerland and his wife appear reliable
Chief Concern: Unrelieved substernal chest pain

History of Present Illness: During a business meeting, Mr Holzerland developed substernal chest pain, radiating to the left arm, associated with shortness of breath and diaphoresis, lasting longer than 5 minutes. He describes the pain as crushing, "like someone was sitting on my chest." Severity decreased with rest, but heaviness was constant. He denies palpitations, snycope, dizziness, or nausea and vomiting. Coworkers called an ambulance.

Mr Holzerland states that during the last 6 months he has experienced intermittent chest pain 1–2 times/wk, usually following a stressful encounter. The pain subsided with rest. He describes the pain as heavy, dull, nonradiating, and lasting less than 1 minute. Occasionally, he experiences "chest tightness" while playing racquetball, which is relieved if he stops playing. He feels the accompanying shortness of breath and tachycardia are related to the exercise. He denies DOE, orthopnea, PND, cough, wheezing, and hemoptysis; has 2–3 URIs every winter, of brief duration.

Mr Holzerland experiences burning epigastric pain following stressful situations, relieved with antacid; appetite and bowel pattern normal; no diarrhea, constipation, melena, or hematemesis; no history of peptic ulcer disease; has gained 15 lb in last 2 years; has a sedentary job.

Mr. Holzerland has a history of mild hypertension × 8 yr. He received no pharmacologic therapy for his blood pressure but was told to stop smoking, lose weight, reduce salt intake, and exercise regularly. He exercises 1–2 times/wk, watches his salt intake, has not lost weight, and smokes 1 pack of cigarettes per day × 20 yr. Last health evaluation was 2 years ago; his ECG, chest x-ray, and blood work were normal, and his blood

(continued)

CASE STUDY (continued)

The Client With a Myocardial Infarction

pressure was "slightly" elevated at that time. He did not consult his physician about his chest pain because he believed it to be related to stress at work and his sedentary lifestyle.

Past Health History:

Childhood: Has usual childhood diseases—chickenpox, mumps, rubella; no history of strep throat, scarlet fever, or rheumatic fever

Immunizations: Has routine childhood immunizations; tetanus booster (1980); received flu vaccine last winter

Medical Problems: Mild hypertension × 8 yr, no medications

Surgeries: Vasectomy, 1980

Transfusions: None

Special Diagnostic Procedures: None

Trauma: None

Allergies: No known allergies to medications, food, or environmental elements

Medications: No prescribed medications. Takes aspirin 600 mg q.d. for headache as needed; antacid 30 mL t.i.d p.r.n for "acid stomach"

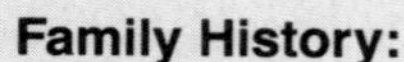

Family History:

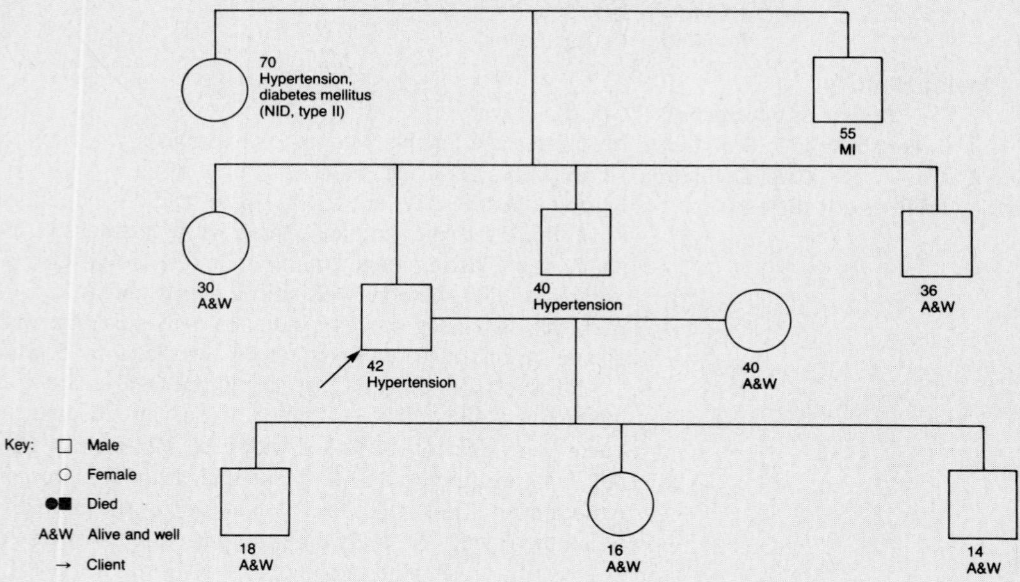

Personal/Social History: The client is married (20 years) and lives with his wife and three children in their home, which they own; is a college graduate with an MBA and works as a computer systems analyst with a well-known firm; usually works 10 hours a day, 5 days a week; states he has no time for hobbies. His wife works at home and participates in community volunteer programs. Mr Holzerland states his children are "good kids" with normal adolescent problems; his eldest child will be attending a private university next year; he expresses concern over their financial status if he is unable to work.

Habits: Mr Holzerland sleeps 6 hr/night without difficulty; he tries to follow a low-salt diet; eats two meals a day—lunch and dinner; admits to a heavy caffeine intake—6–10 cups of coffee/day; has an occasional martini at lunch and usually two martinis before dinner.

III. Health History, *Continued*

Review of Systems:

General: Feels "out of shape"; increased fatigue the last 6 months

HEENT: Experiences daily occipital headaches and stiff neck, relieved with aspirin, 600 mg; denies syncope, vertigo, blurred, or double vision

Respiratory: See HPI

Cardiovascular: See HPI

Genitourinary: No dysuria, incontinence, penile discharge, lesions, or impotence; no history of UTIs or kidney stones; no sexual problems

Musculoskeletal: No muscle weakness, joint swelling, or limitations in movement

Neurologic: No fainting, dizziness, loss of balance, weakness, or paresthesia

Endocrine: No heat or cold intolerance, history of goiter, excessive sweating, polydipsia, polyphasia, or polyuria; no difficulty in concentration

Psychologic: Often feels anxious and tense; states work is stressful but wife and family are supportive; expresses concern about missing work because "this is a busy time of year."

IV. Physical Assessment

Height: 5 ft 11 in

Weight: 200 lb

Vital Signs: Temperature 100°F (37.7°C); P. 100 apical, irregular; R. 24; BP RA 150/100, LA 145/98 (both supine); RA 154/100, LA 150/100 (both seated) Client is a 42-year-old white male in acute distress with unrelieved chest pain; appears anxious and restless

Relevant Organ Systems:

Thorax and Lungs: Thorax symmetrical, lungs resonant; breath sounds normal, no adventitious sounds

Cardiovascular: PMI @ 5th LICS, 8 cm from sternal border, 2 cm in diameter; no thrills, lifts, or heaves; apical HR 100 irregular, S_1 nl, S_2 split, S_4 present @ apex, no S_3 or ⓜ; carotid pulses = bilat, no bruit; JVP flat @ 30° angle; extremities: pale, cool, no edema; peripheral pulses 2+ = bilat

Abdomen: Bowel sounds active, no bruit: palpable abdominal aortic pulse; no organomegaly

Neurologic: DTRs 2+ = bilat

Mental Status: Alert but restless and apprehensive; responds appropriately

V. Diagostic Data

12-Lead ECG: Sinus tachycardia, elevated ST segment in leads V_1—V_4 and incomplete right bundle branch block (RBBB)

Serum Enzymes: Elevated CK and CK-MB isoenzyme; LDH and LDH_1 slightly elevated

Arterial Blood Gases: Shows a respiratory alkalosis and slight hypoxemia

Technetium 99M Pyrophosphate Scan: Increased uptake in the anterior surface of the heart

Echocardiogram: Indicates decreased contractility in the anterior surface including the septum; heart valves normal; delayed closure of the aortic and pulmonic valves; no ventricular aneurysm seen

Chest X-ray: wnl

CBC: WBC slightly elevated

Urinalysis: Specific gravity elevated

VI. Summary

The history, physical assessment, and diagnostic studies indicate that Mr Holzerland suffered an anterior-septal MI. The plan is to keep Mr Holzerland in the CCU until his condition is stable and then transfer him to an intermediate acute care unit.

(continued)

VII. Nursing Care Plan, by Nursing Diagnosis

Client Care Goals	Plan/Nursing implementation	Expected Outcome
Comfort, altered: Pain related to cardiac ischemia		
Reduce or eliminate chest pain	Bed rest until pain is relieved; continuous bedside monitoring; use morphine sulfate or other pain medication as prescribed; administer 2–4 L of O_2 by nasal cannula; monitor vital signs at onset, before and after medication, and after pain is relieved; notify MD if pain is unrelieved by prescribed medication; provide a quiet, calm environment; offer reassurance to client and family; refrain from nonessential procedures; obtain ECG as ordered	Client will be pain free; postinfarction angina is controlled; client will be able to perform activities without pain
Fear related to environmental stressor/hospitalization		
Achieve psychologic comfort and rest quietly	Facilitate client's coping mechanisms: provide relevant information and orientation to CCU routines, equipment, and procedures; offer reassurance to client and family; encourage expression of feelings regarding hospitalization, diagnosis, and sequelae; clarify misconceptions; identify a primary nurse for client and family; offer spiritual support; use diazepam as ordered; allow liberal visiting by family within client's tolerance	Diminished anxiety and fear within 48 hr; client and family will demonstrate effective coping mechanisms
Coping, ineffective individual related to denial		
Accept diagnosis of MI; use effective coping mechanisms	Assess denial: specific etiology, ie, fear of death, disabiltiy, loss of control, altered body image; do not reinforce denial or force client acceptance; for active denial (ie, disregards activity restrictions), assess consequences—are they detrimental? Convey concern and allow the client more control; assist client in identifying coping mechanisms that worked effectively in previous stressful events; utilize supportive resources: family, social services, or spiritual advisor	Client's use of denial decreases; client exhibits interest in learning about the heart attack and the rehabilitation process Client will perform activities within prescribed limits
Self-concept, disturbance in: self-esteem related to situational crisis of diagnosis of MI		
Accept alteration in body image over time; assume role responsibilities	Assign a primary nurse who can establish a trusting relationship with client and family; encourage client to express feelings; provide atmosphere of acceptance; clarify misconceptions; emphasize client's progress; encourage socialization with other cardiac clients and families; encourage participation in cardiac rehabilitation classes	Client expresses feelings about altered self-concept
Gas exchange, impaired related to decreased cardiac output		
Breathe comfortably at normal rate	Administer O_2 at 2–4 L as ordered; monitor ABGs; gradually increase client's activity	Vital signs will remain wnl with absence of dyspnea

Client Care Goals	Plan/Nursing implementation	Expected Outcome
Cardiac output, altered: decreased related to increased cardiac workload		
Perform ADL without risk; identify factors that increase cardiac work load	Organize client's care and provide undisburbed rest; monitor client's response to activity: vital sign changes, pain, shortness of breath, pallor, cyanosis, disequilibrium, confusion, development of dysrhythmias; establish gradual increases in activity; prophylactic medication prior to activity (eg, nitroglycerin); use of O_2 during periods of increased activity	Cardiac tolerance to increased activity will gradually improve
Bowel elimination, altered: constipation related to decreased activity		
Maintain normal bowel elimination pattern	Administer stool softener as prescribed; assist client to commode daily after breakfast; explain why straining should be avoided; encourage activity within prescribed limits; within dietary restrictions, encourage client to consume bran, fruit, and fluids; arrange environment, food, and client comfort to maintain the client's appetite	Bowel movement every 1–2 days without straining; client states why straining should be avoided
Knowledge deficit related to MI		
Acute phase: demonstrate understanding of CCU equipment and routines	Explain CCU routines and procedures client will encounter; assist client in feeling safe; prepare client and family for procedures, advancement of activities, and transfer from CCU	Client will be able to relax and experience less anxiety
Convalescent: identify personal cardiovascular risk factors	Discuss risk factors for CAD with client and emphasize the risk factors client can control; encourage client and family to participate in rehabilitation classes; offer nutritional counseling services; teach relaxation techniques to client and family; document teaching and evaluate client's learning	Client participates in learning and can identify own risk factors; client verbalizes plan to modify risk factors
Distinguish between angina and MI pain	Teach client and family how to differentiate angina from MI pain; offer written information and instruction	Client will state differences between angina and MI pain and give recommended treatment for each
State the names of prescribed medications, dosage, and administration	Discuss medications the client will be taking at home	Client and family will be able to identify each drug and state dosage and administration
Maintain supply of medications	Discuss importance of refilling drugs and to avoid "running out"; discuss resources available to client to cover expenses	Client and family will know how to obtain medication refills; client will be helped with sources to defray the cost of medications, if necessary
Explain prescribed activity levels	Discuss activity levels and why levels are progressed in steps; teach client to monitor the CV response by obtaining pulse rate and observing signs of fatigue, palpitations, or DOE; discuss the importance of adequate rest periods between activities	Client will state what activities are allowed within a given level; client progresses in activities within the cardiac rehabilitation guidelines; client will be able to monitor his own CV response

CHAPTER **20**

The Nursing Process for Clients With Vascular Dysfunction

Other topics relevant to this content are: The health history and physical assessment, **Chapter 5;** Dietary management of hyperlipidemia, **Chapter 19;** Nursing care of clients undergoing vascular surgery, **Chapter 21.**

Objectives

When you have finished studying this chapter, you should be able to:

Specify the major components of the health history to be obtained from clients with peripheral vascular disorders.

Explain specific assessment approaches in evaluating clients with peripheral vascular disease.

Compare and contrast arterial insufficiency and venous insufficiency.

Identify the nursing implications of diagnostic studies commonly used to evaluate clients with peripheral vascular dysfunction.

Determine appropriate nursing diagnoses for clients with peripheral vascular disease.

Develop, with the client, realistic goals of care.

Anticipate the psychosocial/lifestyle implications of peripheral vascular dysfunction for clients and their significant others.

Develop a nursing care plan for a client with peripheral vascular dysfunction.

Implement nursing interventions specific to clients with peripheral vascular problems.

Evaluate the effectiveness of the nursing care plan and modify it as necessary to meet client needs.

Nurses can play an instrumental role in the care of clients with peripheral vascular disease. A thorough nursing assessment aids in determining the extent of the circulation problem. Nursing interventions are effective in ameliorating the disease and may contribute to saving a client's limb. This chapter deals primarily with nursing care for arterial and venous insufficiency. For nursing implications of surgical treatment of vascular system dysfunction, refer to Chapter 21.

SECTION 

Nursing Assessment: Establishing the Data Base

Peripheral vascular disease can be readily detected through a precise, logical nursing assessment. The client's reports of particular kinds of pain, for example, may indicate vascular symptoms that can be confirmed through physical assessment and diagnostic studies.

Subjective Data

Begin the nursing assessment by taking a complete history that elicits the client's chief concern, current symptoms, past health history, habits, occupation, and lifestyle. Explore factors that can lead to peripheral vascular disease (eg, cigarette smoking, oral contraceptive use, hyperlipidemia, hypertension, diabetes mellitus, and genetic predisposition).

History of Present Illness

INTERMITTENT CLAUDICATION **Intermittent claudication,** the most common symptom of arterial insufficiency, is a cramping pain in a muscle brought on by exercise and relieved by rest. The pain usually develops in the legs after the client has walked a specific distance (eg, two blocks) and is relieved after leg rest of a few minutes. The client then can walk two more blocks and must rest again. Although the client experiences cramping pain in the muscle, the muscle is flaccid when palpated.

The cause of intermittent claudication is unknown but is thought to be due to the accumulation of toxic metabolites (lactic acid) in the tissues or to the release of histamine or other chemicals into the tissues near the nerve endings. It is probably not due to ischemia of the contracting muscle. The client who has calf pain usually has a blockage of the superficial femoral artery. Thigh pain may indicate a blockage in the iliac artery.

REST PAIN Rest pain occurs in clients who have advanced chronic arterial occlusive disease. This pain, which often occurs when the client is resting in bed at night, is usually experienced as a constant burning in the distal portion of the leg. Awakened from sleep, the client obtains relief by sitting up in a chair or allowing the legs to be dependent. The dependent position allows the arterial pressure in the legs to increase.

Blockage of a vessel by a thrombus or embolus, or severe arterial disease, may cause rest pain. These pathologic problems decrease the supply of blood to the surrounding tissues, resulting in ischemic pain. Ischemia, in turn, allows metabolites (lactic acid) to build up in the tissue and causes more pain.

Rest pain should not be confused with night leg cramps, which do not necessarily indicate a pathologic condition. Leg cramps can be brought on by just stretching the leg or foot quickly while asleep. Clients who are hypocalcemic may also experience cramping leg pain.

ADDITIONAL SYMPTOMS The functional ability or appearance of an extremity may change in conjunction with a gradual decrease in arterial circulation to the legs, which leads to atrophy of the muscles of the extremities. The male client with an occlusion of the aortic or femoral trunks may become impotent (Leriche's syndrome).

The client may have delayed healing after cuts or abrasions or a cold and pale extremity. When the blood flow is insufficient so the supply of nutrients is deficient, the extremities look pale, feel cool, and heal poorly. When a client says a limb is cold in a warm environment, suspect arterial insufficiency. The client may also report aching, tiredness, and a feeling of fullness in the legs following long periods of standing or sitting. These symptoms are associated with venous insufficiency and are relieved when legs are elevated for a short time.

Medication History

Obtain a history of current and past use of medications, both prescription and over-the-counter. Ask the client specifically about the use of ergotamine and oral contraceptives.

Ergotamine preparations, used to treat migraine headache, are vasoconstrictors. Although ergotamine is an excellent drug for migraine, it must be used carefully in limited amounts to avoid causing vasoconstrictive complications. Ergotamine preparations are contraindicated in peripheral vascular disease.

Oral contraceptives have been associated with thromboembolic complications, including thrombophlebitis in an extremity, pulmonary embolism, and myocardial infarction (MI). The cause of these complications is not known, although some abnormalities in clotting are suspected. Cigarette smoking with oral contraceptive use markedly increases the risk of cardiovascular side effects.

Habit History

CIGARETTE SMOKING Obtain a detailed history of the client's smoking habits. Cigarette smoking is absolutely contraindicated in clients with vascular disease. Smoking causes constriction of both small and large blood vessels and damages intimal cells. Nicotine also increases the aggregation of platelets (Miller & Roon, 1982).

DIET PATTERNS Nutritional assessment should include complete information on the daily diet of the client. Because elevated cholesterol and triglyceride levels are major risk factors for atherosclerosis, a diet high in calories, saturated fat, and cholesterol increases the client's risk for vascular disease. In a client with hypertension or a strong family history of hypertension, it is important to assess salt intake as well as ingestion of saturated fats and cholesterol.

Obese clients with peripheral vascular disease often have less claudication pain after they lose weight. A careful history that explores symptoms related to weight gain, which leads to a sedentary lifestyle and still greater weight gain, often helps the client make the association between increased weight and increased pain.

A complete dietary history should also be obtained from clients with diabetes mellitus or a strong family history of diabetes mellitus. A diabetic client with poor dietary control is at greater risk for vascular disease. Diabetics are more prone to leg and foot injuries because of peripheral neuropathy, are at greater risk for infection with resulting tissue destruction, and have amputation rates four times greater than nondiabetic clients with peripheral vascular disease (Miller & Roon, 1982).

Objective Data

Physical Assessment

INSPECTION Observe the color of the extremities in a comfortably warm environment because skin responds to changes in external temperature. Begin the examination of skin color by having the client walk barefoot. Foot pallor indicates vasodilation of the arteries in the muscles. With ambulation, the muscles of the legs and hips receive increased blood flow, and blood flow to the feet and skin is compromised.

Trophic changes in peripheral vascular disease occur because of ischemia and malnutrition of tissues. In looking for trophic changes, begin by looking at the symmetry and size of each limb and normal or decreased muscle mass. Inspect the groin, buttocks, and feet. Look for decreased muscle mass in the gluteal muscles, which is commonly seen in Leriche's syndrome. Inspect for loss of hair, especially on the toes and feet. Check for smooth, thin, shiny skin and thickened, blackish brown nails.

To check for arterial deficiency in the lower extremities, ask the client to elevate both legs to 45°. With arterial insufficiency, the legs are markedly pale, especially in the soles of the feet, toes, and heels. Called *pallor on elevation,* this occurs because the circulatory system cannot pump enough blood into the capillary system against gravity. In a client with a healthy vascular system, blood continues to perfuse the elevated extremities, although mild pallor does occur.

Another indication of arterial insufficiency is *dependent rubor.* Have the client elevate the legs for 60 seconds, then sit with the legs in a dependent position. Normally, color returns to the extremity within 10 seconds or less. When there is a delay in color return, arterial insufficiency is suspected. The appearance of a reddish blue color after a few minutes may indicate peripheral vessel damage. Rubor develops because of ischemia to the tissue. The dependent rubor sign usually indicates a 90% loss of blood flow.

While examining arterial status, also note venous filling. Venous filling is assessed with the feet in the dependent position. After 15 or 20 seconds of dependency, the veins of the dorsum of the leg should fill. With ischemia, there may be a delay of 40 to 60 seconds before the vein fills. With varicose veins, there is rapid venous filling as blood flows backward unchecked by the incompetent valves.

Test *capillary refill* for assessment of the circulation to the foot. Normally, compressing the nail beds or the sole of a foot causes blanching, which is followed by rapid return of normal color. In the ischemic foot, the return to normal color after blanching takes much longer, signifying a delay in capillary filling.

Leg ulcers or cellulitis may be present. Arterial ischemic leg ulcers are caused by chronic occlusion of small arterioles and arteries, resulting in skin breakdown and ulceration. In venous stasis ulcers, the venous blood pools in the tissues of the extremities. This pooling of venous blood provides an excellent medium for bacterial growth, causing skin lesions and infections.

Arterial ulcers have a pale base, are very painful, and usually occur on the lateral lower leg above the lateral malleolus. Venous ulcers are usually moderately painful and usually involve the medial aspect of the ankle.

Pregangrene and frank gangrene are present in the client with chronic arterial insufficiency. Gangrene develops first in the most distal part of the legs. Gangrene results from severe and prolonged ischemia to an area, usually caused by a complete or almost complete blockage of blood flow. In pregangrene, which is reversible, the skin has a purple-black color that does not change when pressure is applied. Frank gangrene, characterized by skin that is black, shriveled, hard, and dry, is irreversible. Table 20–1 compares the common findings in arterial and venous insufficiency.

PALPATION Assessment of all peripheral pulses is essential in clients with possible peripheral vascular disease. Pulses are evaluated according to their:

- Absence or presence
- Rate and rhythm
- Quality and strength
- Symmetry

Pulses are described according to a numerical classification from 0 (absent pulse) to 4+ (a normal full, bounding pulse).

Palpate the *carotid pulse* in the neck just below the mandible and anterior to the sternocleidomastoid muscle. Take care not to palpate the carotid sinus, which is located in the upper portion of the carotid artery just above the bifurcation between the internal and external carotid arteries at the angle of the mandible. Palpating the carotid sinus area sends impulses from the carotid sinus stretch receptors that increase parasympathetic nervous activity and decrease sympathetic nervous activity. Within 3 to 4 seconds, a parasympathetic effect of decreased heart rate and vasodilation will occur and can lead to significant cerebral hypotension, with resulting syncope (Fetzer–Fowler, 1983).

Palpation of the *ulnar* and *radial* pulses provides information about circulation to the hands and fingers. Allen's test (Figure 20–1) can also be used to evaluate the patency of the radial and ulnar arteries. The *brachial* pulse is assessed in conjunction with the radial and ulnar pulses to evaluate arterial blood flow to the arms and hands.

Palpation of the *aorta* in the upper abdomen may detect a prominent pulsation with lateral expansion, which may indicate an abdominal aortic aneurysm. Diminished, unequal, or absent *femoral* pulses suggest aortoiliac occlusive disease.

Palpate the *popliteal* pulse deep in the popliteal fossa, posterior to the knee. The client should be supine with the knee slightly bent. Use the fingertips of both hands to locate the popliteal artery. This pulse is usually more difficult to find than other pulses. If it is absent, the superficial femoral artery may be occluded.

Palpate the *posterior tibial* pulse in the groove between the medial malleolus and the Achilles tendon and the *dorsalis pedis* pulse on the dorsum of the foot. Although the congenital absence of one of these pedal pulses is considered normal, both pulses should not be absent on the same foot. If both are impalpable, the branches of the popliteal artery or the anterior tibial artery may be occluded.

During palpation of the peripheral pulses, assess the skin temperature. The areas to be checked should be exposed and at rest for several minutes. Compare the temperature of each limb with the other in similar surroundings. To detect differences in temperature, use the dry, cool dorsum of the fingers rather than the warm, moist palmar surface of the fingers.

Diminished motor sensory ability may result from poor blood supply to distal nerve fibers. Assess motor function by having the client flex and extend the toes, and evaluate sensory function by asking the client to identify the part of the foot the nurse is touching.

Palpate each calf for signs of deep phlebitis. Tenderness and increased firmness and tension suggest thrombophlebitis. If phlebitis is suspected, palpate for tenderness or palpable cords and feel for warmth accompanied by redness or discoloration, which indicate superficial thrombophlebitis. Palpate for varicose veins by checking for thickened walls and tortuous veins.

The client with thrombophlebitis may have a positive *Homans' sign,* which is elicited by forcefully dorsiflexing the client's foot with the knee bent. Pain in the calf may indicate deep-vein thrombophlebitis (DVT). Homans' sign is a common clinical assessment for DVT but is not a sensitive or specific test. More specific approaches to evaluation include assessing the client for pain, aching, or a full sensation in the leg; inspecting and palpating the leg for

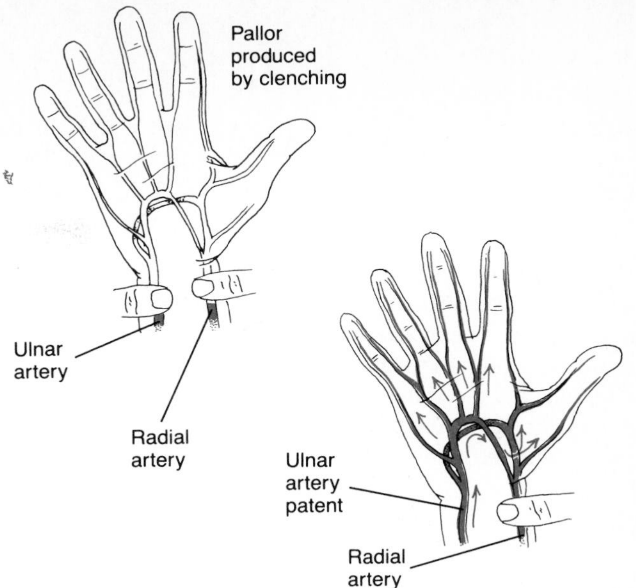

Figure 20–1

Allen's test. Position the client's arm on a flat surface. Compress both the radial and ulnar arteries while the client clenches the fist tightly. After 1 minute, the client extends the fingers quickly while the examiner releases pressure on the ulnar artery but continues compression of the radial artery. If there is adequate ulnar circulation, color will return promptly. Persistent pallor indicates occlusion of the ulnar artery (Bates, 1983). This maneuver is repeated, maintaining compression of the ulnar artery while releasing pressure on the radial artery. In this instance, persistent pallor indicates radial artery disease.

Table 20–1
Comparison of Findings in Arterial and Venous Insufficiency

Assessment	Arterial Insufficiency	Venous Insufficiency
Skin changes	Smooth, shiny, thin; loss of hair over the toes and foot; thickened blackish brown nails	Rough, thickened, brown pigmentation around ankles; stasis dermatitis
Skin color	Pallor on elevation and dependent rubor	Feet normal or slightly cyanotic in a dependent position
Skin temperature	Cool	Warm
Pulses	Absent or decreased; a bruit may be heard over an arterial plaque or aneurysm	Normal; no bruits
Pain	Sharp pain that increases with walking; resting helps relieve pain	Heavy aching, tiredness, and feeling of fullness; elevation of legs helps
Edema	Absent	Present; worse at end of day
Ulcers of ankles and feet	Very painful pale base; occur on lateral lower leg above the lateral malleolus and on the toes; also occur in areas of trauma	Moderately painful, pink base; occur on medial aspect of ankle
Gangrene	May develop Pregangrene: skin purple-black (reversible) Frank gangrene: skin black, shriveled, hard, and dry (irreversible)	Does not develop

swelling, tenderness, discoloration, increased heat, and dilated superficial veins; and unexplained tachycardia and fever (Miller & Roon, 1982).

Diagnostic Studies

SKIN TEMPERATURE STUDIES Skin temperature of the extremities can be evaluated in a variety of ways. Immersing one extremity in warm water while observing the other extremity gives a gross evaluation of arterial disease. In the healthy client, the temperature in an unimmersed arm will rise with the temperature in the immersed arm because of reflex vasodilation. In clients with arterial disease, no reflex vasodilation is detected.

In a cold pressure test, the client's normal blood pressure and pulse pressure are compared to pressures taken after immersion of the hand in ice water. The healthy client has a slight increase in blood pressure and no increase in pulse pressure, whereas the client with occlusive arterial disease has a significant increase in both blood and pulse pressures.

Excessive variations in skin-surface temperatures may indicate arterial disease. Skin temperatures are normally in the range of 14 to 16°F (−10 to −9°C) below normal body temperatures. Lower temperatures in the extremities than in the trunk may indicate impeded arterial flow. Direct skin thermometers (thermistors) are used to measure skin surface temperature.

In the cold stimulation test, normal finger temperature is recorded by skin thermometers. The hands are then immersed in ice water for 20 seconds. Digital temperature should return to normal within 15 minutes. If the return to normal temperature takes 20 to 40 minutes, the client is exhibiting Raynaud's phenomenon, attacks of severe pallor in the fingers or toes (sometimes also the ears and nose) brought on by cold or sometimes by emotion. Raynaud's phenomenon is usually linked to arterial insufficiency but sometimes appears by itself without causal disease. In that case, it is called Raynaud's disease. Thus, the cold stimulation test does not conclusively indicate arterial insufficiency.

DOPPLER ULTRASONOGRAPHY The Doppler ultrasonography test is so named because it makes use of the Doppler effect—the alteration of sound by contact with a moving body. The transducer of the test instrument placed on the skin sends out bursts of ultra-high-frequency (UHF) sound; between bursts, it picks up echoes of the UHF sound that have been changed by bouncing off red blood cells flowing in a vein or artery. The difference between the transmitted and received UHF signals is an audible signal, the nature of which indicates the condition of the vein or artery. The sound also indicates blood pressure in areas of low blood flow. The ankle-arm pressure index (API), the ratio of ankle to brachial systolic pressure, provides information about vascular sufficiency, as do pressure gradients at adjacent sites. Because the test is noninvasive, involving only the moving about of the transducer on the skin, the nurse usually needs only to explain the procedure to allay clients' fears.

TREADMILL TEST FOR INTERMITTENT CLAUDICATION The treadmill test aids in discriminating between clients with true intermittent claudication and those with conditions that mimic claudication. ECG monitoring is often done concomitantly.

The Doppler probe is used to measure the systolic pressure at the dorsalis pedis and posterior tibial arteries. The client then walks on the treadmill until claudication develops. Foot and ankle pressures are again obtained. In peripheral vascular disease, these pressures fall with exercise.

IMPEDANCE PLETHYSMOGRAPHY Impedance plethysmography is a noninvasive test to measure the venous flow in the extremities. It is helpful in detecting DVT in the popliteal and iliofemoral systems.

The impedance plethysmograph works on the principle that electrical resistance in a vein is proportional to blood volume. The plethysmograph is used in conjunction with a blood pressure cuff to discover whether a blockage in a vein prevents the normal buildup and release of venous blood in response to temporary vascular occlusion by the cuff.

LUMBAR SYMPATHETIC BLOCK With the client in a prone position, procaine hydrochloride is injected into the sympathetic ganglia that innervate the lumbar spine at the level of the second or third lumbar vertebra. Successful blocking of the sympathetic tracts results in increased circulation with drying and warming of the skin of the extremity on the side of the block.

NURSING IMPLICATIONS Clients experience initial discomfort with needle insertion and tingling and warmth in the extremity for several hours after the procedure. Postprocedure nursing care includes careful assessment for shock, which can result from sudden fluid shift into the peripheral circulation.

LOWER LIMB VENOGRAPHY Lower limb venography (also called phlebography) assists in determining patency of the tibial–popliteal, superficial femoral–common femoral, and the saphenous veins. A contrast medium is injected into the superficial and/or deep veins of the extremity. X-rays are taken while the legs are placed in a variety of positions. Venography is the definitive test for DVT and also is used to locate a vein for possible arterial bypass grafting. The test is expensive and may cause localized clotting.

RADIONUCLIDE VENOGRAPHY Radionuclide venography using ^{125}I fibrinogen is used to detect thrombi in the leg veins; it is not a good test for thrombi in the pelvis and groin. It is less expensive and less hazardous than venography with a contrast medium and may be used for clients who are too ill to undergo contrast venography or are sensitive to the dye. The ^{125}I fibrinogen is incorporated into thrombi when present. The initial scan is done 12 hours after injection and repeated in 24 hours to verify the findings.

ANGIOGRAPHY Angiography (arteriography) is the radiographic examination of one or more arteries after injection of a contrast medium (such as Hypaque) into an artery. For visualization of the arteries in the lower extremities, the contrast medium is injected into the femoral artery. Several x-rays are taken during the last few seconds of the injection, and another series is taken immediately after the injection. Concentrations of radioactivity, or "hot spots," indicate arterial blockage.

NURSING IMPLICATIONS Angiography is an invasive diagnostic procedure. A consent form is required. Ask the client about iodine allergy because the contrast medium contains iodine. Tell clients undergoing angiography that they will experience a burning sensation at the injection site and a flushing warm feeling in the extremity (and sometimes in the whole body) that lasts a few seconds.

Following the procedure, the client is on bed rest, and vital signs are monitored every 15 minutes until stable. Check the injection site for local inflammation and internal and external bleeding. Ecchymosis is an indication of internal bleeding. Assess the peripheral pulses each time vital signs are taken and evaluate the affected extremity for skin color, warmth, numbness, and pain. Encourage the client to drink plenty of fluids to assist the kidneys in excretion of the contrast medium.

SECTION 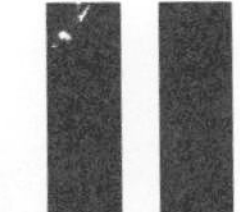

Nursing Diagnosis/Planning and Implementation/Evaluation

Information gathered from the client's health history, physical examination, and diagnostic studies is used to determine nursing diagnoses and the plan of care. Not every client will have the same needs. The Nursing Diagnosis box lists diagnoses **directly related** to vascular dysfunction along with **potential** diagnoses for clients with vascular problems.

The most common nursing diagnoses for clients with peripheral vascular disease include altered tissue perfusion: peripheral; skin integrity, impaired; altered comfort: pain; disturbance in self-concept: body image. All of these diagnoses are discussed in the content that follows. The sample nursing care plan in Table 20–2 focuses on impairment of skin integrity and alteration in comfort, pain.

If the goals of care have not been met, reevaluation is required. The nurse and client should jointly review the nursing care plan. New objectives may need to be formulated; other nursing interventions may be added or modified; or the evaluation may show that more time is required to meet the objectives.

Tissue Perfusion, Altered: Peripheral

Inadequate tissue perfusion may be related to arterial or venous thrombus formation and obstruction, vasoconstriction, or inflammatory effects. The major goal of care is to maximize tissue perfusion by reducing risk factors, maintaining a proper environment, wearing nonconstrictive clothing, balancing rest and exercise, and doing specialized exercises.

Planning and Implementation

SMOKING CESSATION Smoking is one of the major contributing factors in the development of peripheral vascular disease. The importance of decreasing, or preferably eliminating, smoking cannot be overemphasized. Nicotine causes vasospasm and constriction of the arteries and also increases the heart rate, which increases the work load of the heart and circulatory system. The carbon monoxide that is inhaled by the smoker decreases the oxygen-carrying capacity of the hemoglobin so less oxygen is delivered to the tissues.

Smoking is extremely difficult for many clients to give up. Provide the client with information about smoking cessation programs, self-help groups in the community, and nicotine chewing gum as a temporary aid for clients with a high nicotine dependence who are also attempting behavior modification. Clients with peripheral vascular disease who do not quit smoking face serious sequelae including gangrene and amputation.

DIETARY MANAGEMENT Dietary instruction is essential for clients with peripheral vascular disease. Obesity increases stress on the heart and increases venous congestion, impeding proper nutrition to body cells. A properly balanced weight-reduction diet should be prescribed and carefully monitored by the nurse or physician.

When serum lipid levels are elevated, dietary management is directed to the specific elevated serum lipid. Clients with an elevated cholesterol level are given a low-cholesterol diet. Clients with an increase in the triglyceride level are given a diet low in saturated fats and low in carbohydrates. More specific diets for the six types of hyperlipidemia are described in Chapter 19. Clients with hypertension are placed on a diet low in sodium.

NURSING DIAGNOSES IN
Vascular Dysfunction

DIRECTLY RELATED DIAGNOSES

- Comfort, altered: pain
- Self-concept, disturbance in: body image
- Skin integrity, impaired: potential
- Tissue perfusion, altered: peripheral

OTHER POTENTIAL DIAGNOSES

- Adjustment, impaired
- Hypothermia
- Knowledge deficit
- Nutrition, altered: less than body requirements
- Nutrition, altered: more than body requirements

ENVIRONMENTAL TEMPERATURE AND WEARING APPAREL A warm environment is important for a client with peripheral vascular disease because it causes vasodilation, which in turn increases blood supply to the extremities. Warm clothing such as bed socks or long underwear achieve the required warmth. Direct heat applied to the extremities is not advisable: most clients with peripheral vascular disease suffer from peripheral neuropathy, which diminishes the ability to sense heat accurately, predisposing the client to burns. Clients should understand the importance of checking bathwater temperature with the arm rather than the foot because of peripheral neuropathy.

Clients should avoid constrictive clothing such as elastics, garters, girdles, knee-high nylon socks, and tight waistbands. Such items compromise circulation to the already deficient areas. Shoelaces should not be tied too tightly.

Clients should wear thermal underwear, heavy socks, and gloves in cold weather. Chilling of the feet and/or body causes vasoconstriction, which leads to inadequate circulation to the extremities.

EXERCISE AND POSITION CHANGE The client with peripheral vascular disease must understand the importance of daily exercise. Exercise provides necessary muscle contraction for movement of arterial blood to the peripheral areas of the body, for return of venous blood to the heart, and for the development of collateral circulation. The exercise regimen must begin gradually, and a mod-

Table 20–2
Sample Nursing Care Plan for the Client With Vascular System Dysfunction, by Nursing Diagnosis

Client Care Goals	Plan/Nursing Implementation	Expected Outcome
Skin integrity, impaired: actual related to impaired circulation		
Describe hazards of skin breakdown and injury to extremities; remain protected from injury and infection; monitor skin changes correctly	Assess skin for signs of breakdown; instruct client and family about skin changes such as thickening, drying, cracking, and areas of ulceration; monitor skin color, temperature, and peripheral pulses; keep skin clean and dry; instruct client and family about the importance of protecting extremities from exposure to extremes in temperature and from trauma; instruct client and family about the importance of physical exercise	Skin integrity is normal; shows no signs of breakdown or infection
Comfort, altered: pain related to vascular insufficiency		
Experience a decreased level of pain	Determine the source of pain and eliminate, if possible (eg, by administration of analgesics as ordered); provide distraction (eg, reading, television, visitors); position extremities to relieve pressure; instruct client not to sit or stand for long periods, not to sit with legs crossed, to elevate feet (venous insufficiency), or provide a flat position for feet (arterial insufficiency); provide for balanced exercise and rest periods; provide warmth to extremities by controlling environmental temperature; instruct client on the importance of nonconstrictive clothing; administer analgesics as ordered	Client comfortable and free of pain

erate daily exercise program must be continued. Excessive exercise increases the metabolic demands of the body, increasing the work load of the circulatory system.

Clients should rest after exercise periods. Elevating the feet above heart level is helpful to the client with venous insufficiency. Clients with arterial insufficiency should rest lying flat; raising the legs increases the work of the arterial system and impedes perfusion to the legs.

Clients should not maintain one position for too long. Sitting for long periods with knees bent or crossed causes undue pressure on the popliteal vessels, which decreases circulation to and from the area and results in leg swelling and pain. Standing for long periods also causes venous congestion because the veins have to work against gravity to return blood to the heart.

The best form of moderate exercise to increase blood flow to the legs is walking. Rest periods are important during the walking regimen. If pain develops with walking short distances, rest at regular intervals should become part of the exercise program. Clients should be aware of their level of pain tolerance; those with a high tolerance need to be careful not to walk too much at one time; clients with low tolerance may have to push themselves to get enough exercise.

Evaluation

The following expected outcomes demonstrate the client's understanding of measures to promote tissue perfusion. The client:

- Demonstrates an active interest in smoking cessation programs
- Shows a decrease in the number of cigarettes smoked in a cigarette count
- Discusses the importance of maintaining the prescribed diet and proper weight
- States reasons for avoiding direct application of heat
- Explains importance of preventing exposure to extremes in temperature and use of warm clothing in winter
- Describes proper wearing apparel for avoiding vasoconstriction
- Lists ambulation requirements
- Explains balance of rest and activity throughout the day
- States rationale for avoiding prolonged standing, sitting in one position, crossing legs, and elevating legs

Skin Integrity, Impaired: Actual

Clients with peripheral vascular disease suffer from decreased blood supply to the extremities, particularly the feet. Therefore, clients must learn to protect skin integrity through generalized foot care and to promote skin integrity by stimulating increased blood flow to the skin.

Planning and Implementation

Clients should take meticulous care of their feet. They should wash their feet daily with mild soap and warm water and rinse them thoroughly. They must dry the feet completely, using a patting motion. Rough drying of the feet can cause tissue trauma. The feet should be kept soft by use of lanolin lotions to prevent drying and cracking between the toes, which leads to infection. If drying and itching occur on the feet or legs (especially in the elderly), clients should take fewer baths and use lanolin or superfat soaps. Hard, scaly areas; discoloration; or swelling of the legs must be reported to the physician.

Corn and callous removers or other chemicals should not be used. Toenails should be cut straight across after a bath has softened them. If there is a problem with hard, overgrown nails, a podiatrist should cut the nails routinely.

Fungal infections of the feet can be prevented by keeping the feet dry. The client who perspires may use foot powder judiciously. Clients should change their socks daily (or more often, if indicated). Leather-soled shoes are preferable to rubber soles because rubber impedes evaporation of moisture and provides a dark, moist area in which fungi can breed.

The feet should always be protected by socks and slippers or shoes. The client should not walk barefoot. Shoes should not be constricting, and new shoes should be broken in slowly. All these measures diminish the potential for trauma to the feet. Trauma, no matter how minor, requires physician consultation.

Clients should not scratch itchy spots on the feet or legs because scratching can break down the skin, and broken skin can progress to leg ulcers. Calamine lotion may be used on itchy areas.

Even with meticulous care of the legs and feet, some clients will develop leg ulcers. Preventing infection in the ulcerated area is essential. Whether the client remains at home or is hospitalized, strict aseptic technique is required with ulcer care because the impaired circulation to the extremity decreases the availability of nutrients to promote fast healing. Wet dressings are applied with sterile gloves and allowed to dry before removal to facilitate removal of the necrotic tissue. Protective agents such as zinc oxide or petrolatum are used in dressings.

Dressing or soaking the ulcer can be painful. Pain medication should be administered 30 minutes before ulcer care.

Clients with chronic ulcers learn to be meticulous in their care when they understand that infection is potentially limb threatening. Severe leg ulcers may need skin grafting. A visiting community health nurse can assist the client and family with proper ulcer care.

Evaluation

The following expected outcomes demonstrate the client's understanding of measures to maintain skin integrity. The client:

- Explains reasons for washing feet and changing socks daily and for keeping feet dry
- Demonstrates foot care including patting rather than rubbing feet dry
- Discusses approaches to avoiding trauma to legs and feet
- Demonstrates the proper care of leg ulcers
- Lists symptoms and signs of infection
- Specifies symptoms and signs that require medical attention

Comfort, Altered: Pain

In peripheral vascular disorders, pain may result from the inflammatory response that produces tissue edema and pressure on nerve endings and/or from tissue hypoxia. Analgesics may be ordered for symptomatic relief. Tranquilizers may help reduce anxiety, which can increase pain perception. Vasodilators may be used to increase blood supply to the ischemic area.

Planning and Implementation

Nursing measures to alleviate pain include isolating the source of the pain and taking measures to diminish it, providing distraction for the client, and promoting relaxation and comfort. Teach clients about the action, expected therapeutic effect, dosage, frequency of administration, and potential side effects of any medication prescribed.

Evaluation

The following expected outcomes demonstrate the client's understanding of measures to promote comfort. The client:

- Explains the balance of rest and activity
- Specifies pain-relief approaches following exercise
- States dosage, action, side effects, and frequency of administration of prescribed pain medication

Self-Concept, Disturbance in: Body Image

Depending on its severity, peripheral vascular disease causes a number of body changes. Any of these changes can affect a client's self-concept and relationships with significant others. Skin-color changes, muscle atrophy, swelling, leg ulcers, and amputation all have the potential to affect the client's body image negatively. An unsightly extremity, pain, or fear of injury to the affected limb may cause the client or the sexual partner to avoid sexual intercourse. This change in an intimate relationship will add to the client's poor self-image and may increase anxiety and fear.

Planning and Implementation

Peripheral vascular disease is usually a chronic, lifelong problem. Treatment is often slow with frequent setbacks, which add to the discouragement and frustration of clients and significant others. Fears of chronic disease and becoming a burden to the family are not unrealistic. Clients feel a loss of control over their disease and their lives. The nurse should assist both clients and families to express these fears.

Teach the client about the disease process and the symptoms and signs that should be reported to the physician. Realistically and honestly encourage the client when progress is made. Involve the client and significant others in the plan of care, so that a realistic plan for living with peripheral vascular disease can be made. Involve the client in all decision making, which is essential for maintaining feelings of self-worth. Encourage the client and sexual partner to discuss any fears they have about resumption of sexual intercourse. Suggest positions they can try that will be sexually satisfying and yet avoid trauma to the extremity.

Evaluation

The following expected outcomes demonstrate the client's improved body image. The client:

- Makes decisions about her or his life based on a sound knowledge base
- Verbalizes feelings about body changes
- Resumes satisfactory intimate relations

Nursing Research Note

Ventura M et al: Effectiveness of health promotion interventions. *Nurs Res* 1984; 33(3):162–167.

The purpose of this research was to determine whether participation in a health promotion program for clients with peripheral vascular disease would improve their level of exercise, reduce smoking, and enhance foot care. The sample size was 84 with a study group of 44 subjects, and a control group of 40 subjects. The study group received three booklets about exercise, living with peripheral vascular disease, and foot care and a pamphlet about smoking reduction. The control group received no special intervention.

There was no significant difference between the control group and experimental group in smoking and foot care, although there was a trend toward reducing smoking and improving foot care. Members of the experimental group who chose to increase their activity showed greater increases over the control group in frequency, distance, and length of exercise. Overall, there was no difference between groups in blood pressure indices after intervention, nor was there a change in symptoms.

This study demonstrates that health promotion activities have some benefit. Client education, support, and encouragement may facilitate behavior modification with improved health outcomes.

Chapter Highlights

Nursing assessment to determine the adequacy of peripheral circulation includes evaluation for color, temperature of extremities, the presence of pulses, and trophic changes.

Tissue perfusion may be altered by degenerative changes, trauma, infection, and inflammation.

A diet with large amounts of cholesterol or saturated fats, a family predisposition to atherosclerosis or diabetes mellitus, and high stress levels can cause alterations in circulation.

Clients with peripheral vascular disorders often have edema, symptoms of intermittent claudication, and/or pain in the extremity.

Peripheral vascular disease can result in long-term degenerative changes requiring extended medical treatment and adaptation to changes.

Quality of ambulation, perfusion to the extremities, and venous and arterial competency are important criteria in the assessment of peripheral vascular disorders.

Smoking is absolutely contraindicated in clients with peripheral vascular disease. Clients cannot hope to achieve improvement in symptoms unless they abandon their cigarette habit.

Oral contraceptives and drugs containing ergotamine (often used for clients with migraine headaches) are also contraindicated in vascular disease.

The most important goals of a nursing care plan for a client with peripheral vascular disease are to increase perfusion of tissues, to maintain skin integrity, and to keep the client comfortable.

Bibliography

Bastarache MM et al: Assessing peripheral vascular disease: Noninvasive testing. *Am J Nurs* 1983; 83:1552–1556.

Bates B: *A Guide to Physical Examination,* 3rd ed. Philadelphia: Lippincott, 1983.

Baum PL: Heed the early warning signs of PVD. *Nurs 85* (March) 1985: 15:50–57.

Durbin N: The application of Doppler techniques in critical care. *Focus Critical Care* (June) 1983; 10:44–46.

Fetzer-Fowler S: Carotid sinus massage. *Critical Care Nurse* (July–Aug) 1983; 3:26–30.

Hudson B: Sharpen your vascular assessment skills with the Doppler ultrasound stethoscope. *Nurs 83* (May) 1983; 13:55–57.

Kim MJ, Moritz DA: Classification of nursing diagnosis. In: *Proceedings of the Third and Fourth National Conferences.* New York: McGraw–Hill, 1982.

Miller DC, Roon AJ: *Diagnosis and Management of Peripheral Vascular Disease.* Menlo Park, CA: Addison–Wesley, 1982.

Petersdorf RG et al: *Harrison's Principles of Internal Medicine,* 10th ed. New York: McGraw–Hill, 1983.

Peterson FY: Assessing peripheral vascular disease at the bedside. *Am J Nurs* 1983; 83:1549–1551.

Raab D: Peripheral vascular disease: How to recognize it, how to treat it. *Can Nurse* (Sept) 1982; 78:30–33.

CHAPTER **21**

Specific Disorders of the Peripheral Circulation

Objectives

When you have finished studying this chapter, you should be able to:

Identify the clinical manifestations and nursing care of clients with Raynaud's disease, Raynaud's phenomenon, and Buerger's disease.

Discuss the pathophysiology, clinical manifestations, and nursing care of clients with abdominal, thoracic, peripheral, and dissecting aortic aneurysms.

Specify nursing approaches in the care of clients with varicose veins and venous leg ulcers.

Discuss the pathophysiology, clinical manifestations, and the medical and surgical management of arterial and venous occlusive disease and lymphedema.

Explain the major types of traumatic injuries to the peripheral circulation and discuss the nursing implications related to the care of these clients.

Educate clients and their significant others about the surgical procedures presented in this chapter.

Specific disorders of the peripheral circulation may involve any condition of the vascular system that alters circulation through the aorta, arteries, veins, and lymphatic vessels. The alteration in circulation may be due to a multifactorial, degenerative, infectious, obstructive, or traumatic disorder.

There are a wide variety of surgical procedures associated with these disorders. Some procedures involve the direct removal, replacement, or manipulation of a blood vessel; others require diversion of blood flow; and still others, such as lumbar sympathectomy, indirectly affect blood flow.

Many clients having these surgeries have a long history of peripheral vascular disease. In addition to the specific preoperative and postoperative nursing measures described, remember to implement the recommended nursing measures, health teaching, and lifestyle changes. In some instances, clients with advanced peripheral vascular disease may require amputation of an extremity. Amputation is discussed in Chapter 46.

SECTION 

Disorders of Multifactorial Origin

Disorders of multifactorial origin involving the peripheral vascular circulation can cause symptoms ranging from mild discomfort to severe pain and loss of sensation. Alteration in circulation to the extremities can lead to poor nutrition and oxygenation of tissues; ulceration and subsequent loss of digits or an entire extremity may result. Conditions discussed in this section include Raynaud's disease, Raynaud's phenomenon, and Buerger's disease.

Raynaud's Disease and Raynaud's Phenomenon

Raynaud's disease is an idiopathic benign disorder characterized by vasospasm of the peripheral small arteries and arterioles of the upper extremities, especially the hands; the feet are rarely affected. The disease is more common in women than in men and often begins in the late teens.

The cause of Raynaud's disease is unknown, but the following theories have been suggested: (1) excessive adrenergic stimulation, selective to the arms, resulting in the constrition of small arteries and arterioles, which causes the characteristic changes in color, temperature, and sensation of the fingers; (2) intrinsic vascular-wall hyperactivity to cold and emotional stresses; or (3) an antigen–antibody immune response. The latter is the most likely theory because abnormal immunologic test results usually accompany the disease.

Raynaud's phenomenon is also characterized by vasospasm of the arteries, but the vasospasm is secondary to another underlying condition. Raynaud's phenomenon is seen with connective-tissue disease (especially scleroderma); thoracic outlet syndrome; exposure to polyvinyl chloride, lead, arsenic, or ergot; continuous trauma such as that with typing, piano playing, or jackhammer use; and drug therapy (mainly ergotamine, methysergide, and propranolol).

Clinical Manifestations

When the client is exposed to cold or a stressor, the fingers first blanch and turn completely white (the *pallor* phase); the fingers next become blue (the *cyanotic* phase); finally, the fingers turn red (the *rubor* phase). In the pallor phase, the fingers become cold. They begin to warm in the rubor phase. Numbness and tingling may occur during these phases. The thumbs are often not involved. If the disease is severe or long-standing, trophic changes, skin ulcerations, and gangrene may develop.

Medical Measures

Drugs that interfere with the action of sympathetic nerves by blocking vasoconstriction are often used in Raynaud's disease. These drugs include reserpine, guanethidine (Ismelin), methyldopa (Aldomet), phenoxybenzamine (Dibenzyline), or prazosin (Minipress). Nifedipine (Procardia), a calcium channel blocking agent with a peripheral vasodilating effect, has been used experimentally in Raynaud's disease.

Temporary cervicothoracic sympathetic block may be done to assess the amount of vasodilation that could be gained by a cervicothoracic sympathectomy. Cervicothoracic sympathectomy is performed in severe cases of Raynaud's disease to reduce vasospasm and pain. In some instances, gangrenous fingers are amputated to remove necrotic tissue. Medical treatment of Raynaud's phenomenon is directed toward the underlying disease process.

Specific Nursing Measures

Teaching clients to abstain from smoking and to avoid exposure to cold are the major nursing responsibilities for clients with both Raynaud's disease and Raynaud's phenomenon. Urge the client to stop smoking, explaining that nicotine, a vasoconstrictor, aggravates the disease process. Encourage and support the client in these efforts and involve significant others. Teach approaches that have been helpful to others in giving up cigarettes—smoking clinics, self-help groups, behavior modification, biofeedback, hypnosis, and nicotine gum. Some persons can quit "cold turkey," but many cannot. Clients may have to experiment with several approaches before they find the one that works for them. Many of these methods are costly; however, continuing to smoke costs more in the long run, not only in health and health-related expenses but also in the actual cost of cigarettes. Significant others who live with the client should also give up cigarettes to help the client become and remain a nonsmoker. Health-care providers who do not smoke are also good role models.

Warn clients against exposing hands to cold. Measures to prevent chilling, such as wearing adequate clothing for total body warmth and use of warm gloves and socks in cold weather, are essential. Also urge clients to use gloves when handling frozen foods or when cleaning the freezer or refrigerator. Clients with Raynaud's disease or Raynaud's phenomenon should avoid jobs that expose them to constant cold. Teach clients to avoid applying heat directly to cold extremities; burns can result.

Teach clients to avoid secondary causes of vasospasm, such as occupational use of pneumatic tools or exposure to toxins and vasoconstricting drugs. Explain the need to avoid constrictive clothing such as tight cuffs and elastic wristbands.

Clients on vasodilating drugs should be taught the action, expected therapeutic effect, dosage, frequency of administration, and any side effects of the drug. Women with Raynaud's disease or Raynaud's phenomenon should not use oral contraceptives because of the danger of thromboembolism.

Buerger's Disease

Buerger's disease (thromboangiitis obliterans) is an inflammatory, obstructive, nonatheromatous disease that affects small and medium arteries and veins (unlike atherosclerosis, which involves only arteries). Diminished blood flow to the legs and feet from thrombus development and vessel spasm results in leg ulceration and gangrene. Arteries of the upper limbs may also be involved.

Buerger's disease is an idiopathic disease, occurring mainly in men from 20 to 40 years of age. There is a high incidence of the disease among smokers.

Clinical Manifestations

The chief symptom in Buerger's disease is pain. Intermittent claudication of the arch of the foot is common. There may also be rest pain, which signifies that ischemia is increasing in severity. When the feet are exposed to cold, there is a cold feeling of the extremity, followed by cyanosis and numbness, and later by reddening and hot, tingly sensations. There may be ulceration and gangrene of fingers and toes. There may also be migratory superficial thrombophlebitis manifested as painful, red, swollen lumps under the skin. In the later stages of the disease, the limbs may become red and/or cyanotic in a dependent

DIRECTLY RELATED DIAGNOSES

- Comfort, altered: pain
- Self-concept, disturbance in: body image
- Skin integrity, impaired: actual
- Skin integrity, impaired: potential
- Tissue perfusion, altered: peripheral

OTHER POTENTIAL DIAGNOSES

- Adjustment, impaired
- Hypothermia
- Knowledge deficit
- Nutrition, altered: less than body requirements
- Nutrition, altered: more than body requirements

position. Muscle atrophy, ulceration, and gangrene around the nails and toes can occur.

Findings on physical examination are (Petersdorf et al., 1983):

- Intense rubor of the feet
- Absent foot pulses in the presence of normal femoral and popliteal pulses
- Absent or reduced radial and/or ulnar pulses

Medical Measures

Vasodilating drugs such as tolazoline (Priscoline) or papaverine (Pavabid) may be used with some clients. The only effective treatment approach is complete abstinence from tobacco, however.

Temporary lumbar sympathetic block may be done to assess the amount of vasodilation that might be gained by a lumbar sympathectomy. Lumbar sympathectomy (see Obstructive Disorders section later in this chapter) is performed to reduce vasospasm and pain and to increase collateral circulation. Gangrenous digits may have to be amputated to remove necrotic tissue.

Specific Nursing Measures

Encourage the client to stop smoking. This is the single most important aspect of care. Refer to the discussion of smoking under Raynaud's disease.

Client/Family Teaching

Educate the client about the importance of keeping the extremities warm, wearing adequate clothing for total body warmth, and avoiding constricting clothing. Keeping room temperature at 71°F (21°C) aids in maintaining a stable body temperature. Clients should avoid all situations that exacerbate vasoconstriction, such as exposure to cold water, refrigerators, freezers, cold weather, vibrating tools, oral contraceptives, beta-adrenergic blocking agents, and ergotamine preparations.

Educate the client about the importance of not remaining in one position, either standing or sitting, for too long. Explain the necessity for leg movement, ankle rotation, and knee bending on long trips to stimulate circulation. Reinforce the importance of not crossing the legs and not sitting too close to the chair edge, which can compromise popliteal circulation. Elevating the head of the client's bed a few inches (eg, by putting blocks under it) may enhance circulation to the extremities.

Encourage the client to drink fluids to increase vascular volume and decrease blood viscosity. Reinforce the exercise regimen prescribed by the physician. Walking is recommended unless pain is severe. Trauma to the extremities must be avoided because of the danger of lesions that will not heal, infection, and gangrene.

Educate the client and significant others about foot care, including the use of warm water, mild soaps, rinsing well, and patting rather than rubbing dry. Also reinforce the importance of applying lotions to keep skin moist, preventing drying and cracking. Encourage the client to wear supportive slippers and properly fitted shoes to minimize trauma to feet. Demonstrate how to check the extremities for symptoms and signs of decreased blood flow, such as a change in color or temperature of the limb, cuts that do not heal, cracking skin, and thickening of the nails.

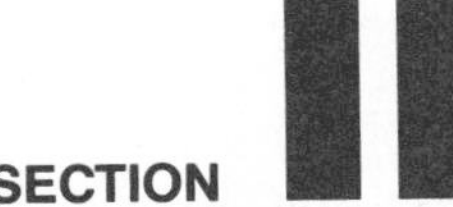

SECTION II

Degenerative Disorders

The degenerative disorders of the peripheral circulation affect both the arterial and the venous systems. This section discusses aneurysms of the aorta, peripheral arterial aneurysms, and venous insufficiency with resultant varicose veins and venous leg ulcers.

Arterial Aneurysms

An aneurysm is a sac or dilatation of the arterial vessel wall that develops because of a weakness in the arterial wall. It can be localized or diffuse. Aneurysms occur most often in the aorta and the cerebral arteries, but they may develop in any artery.

There are many types and shapes of aneurysms (Figure 21–1). A true aneurysm is the outpouching or dilatation of all three layers of an artery. Involvement of the entire circumference of the artery is called a *fusiform aneurysm,* the most common type. A *saccular aneurysm,* an outpouching involving one side of the artery, looks like a sac or pouch and is attached by a small neck. A *false aneurysm*

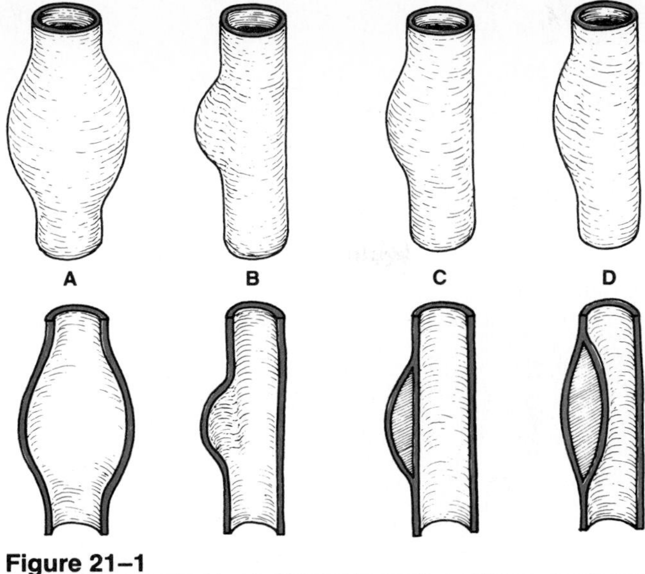

Figure 21–1

Types of aortic aneurysms. **A.** Fusiform: a spindle-shaped expansion of the entire circumference of the artery. **B.** Saccular: an outpouching involving one side of the artery. **C.** False: a pulsating hematoma, often mistaken for an abdominal aneurysm. **D.** Dissecting: a hemorrhagic separation between the medial and internal arterial layers.

is actually a pulsating hematoma. A disruption in the arterial wall allows an accumulation of blood to be held in place by the surrounding tissue.

A *dissecting aneurysm* occurs when blood between the medial and intimal layers of the arterial wall begins to split the arterial layers. This can lead to rupture of the artery and death from internal hemorrhage and shock.

Aneurysms are also classified according to the specific blood vessel and the area of that vessel they involve (eg, a femoral aneurysm, an aneurysm of the aortic arch, and an abdominal aortic aneurysm). Very small aneurysms resulting from infection are called mycotic aneurysms.

The most common cause of an aneurysm is atherosclerosis, which weakens the arterial wall and gradually distends the arterial lumen at the weakened area. Infections, congenital defects, syphilitic aortitis, and cystic medial necrosis associated with Marfan's syndrome or hypertension are other causative factors (Petersdorf et al., 1983).

Clinical Manifestations

The specific manifestations are associated with the location of the aneurysm. The symptoms may not develop until the aneurysm has enlarged and exerts pressure on surrounding organs.

ABDOMINAL AORTIC ANEURYSM The abdominal aorta just below the renal arteries is the most common site for aneurysms. The aneurysms are usually caused by atherosclerosis but may also occur secondary to trauma, syphilis, or infection. Men over age 60 are the most frequently affected. Smoking cigarettes increases the risk.

Abdominal aortic aneurysms develop slowly; the client may remain asymptomatic for years. Clients may gradually become aware of a prominent abdominal pulsation and dull abdominal or low-back pain. Low-back pain radiating to the groin from compression of the lumbar nerves may signal aneurysm enlargement.

Physical findings include an expansile pulsating mass in the midabdomen, usually slightly to the left of midline. Bimanual palpation can aid in identifying the lateral borders of the aneurysm. A systolic bruit is heard with auscultation. Peripheral pulses may be decreased.

Often, abdominal aortic aneurysms are detected on an abdominal x-ray, which demonstrates a curvilinear calcification in the wall of the aneurysm. Ultrasonography can confirm the diagnosis. The size and shape of the aneurysm and presence of thrombi can be detected on ultrasonography. Aortography also demonstrates the size and shape of the aneurysm as well as the condition of blood vessels proximal and distal to the aneurysm.

When an abdominal aortic aneurysm ruptures, the client experiences persistent severe abdominal and back pain; the pain is sometimes not unlike renal colic. Because the retroperitoneal space contains the rupture, a tamponade effect sometimes occurs, temporarily preventing further hemorrhage. Clients may remain stable for several hours before developing signs of shock such as weakness, tachycardia, and hypotension. Without immediate surgical intervention, clients will die of exsanguination.

THORACIC AORTIC ANEURYSM The thoracic aorta (the section of the descending aorta within the thoracic cavity distal to the origin of the left subclavian artery) is the second most likely location for aortic aneurysms (Zimmerman & Ruplinger, 1983). Thoracic aneurysm (Figure 21–2) is usually caused by atherosclerosis or trauma.

Thoracic aneurysms may cause dysphagia as a result of esophageal compression or hoarseness from pressure on the recurrent laryngeal nerve. The client may also experience dyspnea. A deep aching pain that increases in the supine position is a common symptom.

Physical assessment of the client may reveal dilated superficial veins on the chest, neck, and arms; edema of the chest wall; cyanosis; aortic murmur; discrepancy in radial pulses; and an abnormal pulsation on the chest wall over the region of the aneurysm. Blood pressure may vary between arms.

A comparison of a current chest x-ray with a previous one can demonstrate widening of the aorta. Aortography can show the location and the size of the aneurysm. An ECG can help distinguish the chest discomfort of thoracic aneurysm from that of myocardial infarction.

DISSECTING AORTIC ANEURYSM Dissecting aortic aneurysm, which is caused by degenerative disease of the aortic tunica media and intima, is not a true aneurysm. The more appropriate term is *dissecting hematoma* because

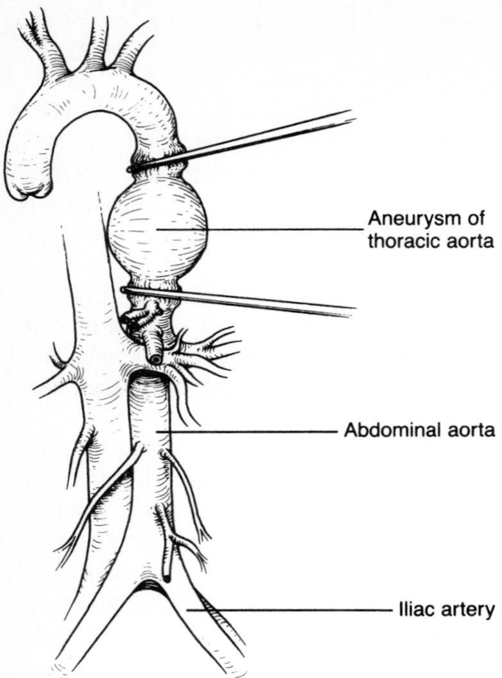

Figure 21–2

Thoracic aortic aneurysm.

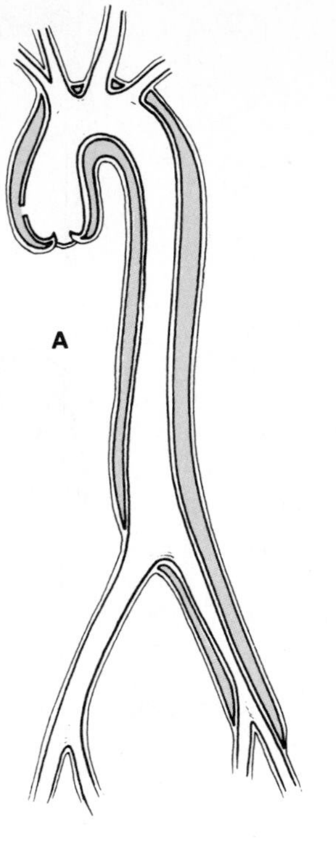

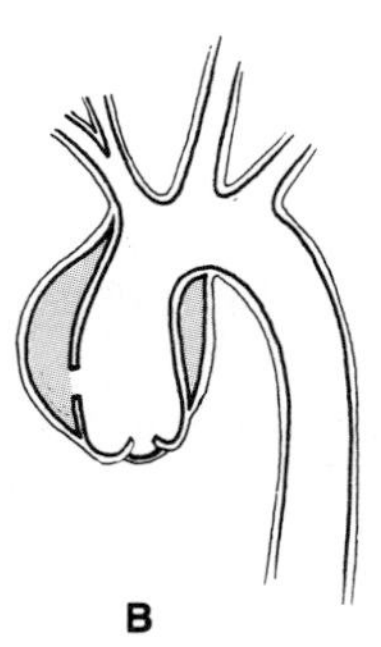

Figure 21–3

Dissecting aortic aneurysm. **A.** Dissecting aneurysm that begins in the ascending aorta near the aortic valve and extends to the external iliac arteries. **B.** Dissecting aneurysm limited to the ascending aorta.

of the hemorrhagic separation of the arterial layers (Figure 21–3).

Causes include hypertension and Marfan's syndrome. Dissecting aneurysms can also be iatrogenic (eg, from arterial lines or intra-aortic balloon insertion) (Zimmerman & Ruplinger, 1983).

Clients with dissecting aortic aneurysm experience an abrupt onset of excruciating pain that almost immediately reaches a peak of intensity—very different from the gradually increasing intensity of an MI. Pain can be felt in both the anterior and posterior chest. The pain has a tendency to migrate as the dissection progresses.

The client is pale, diaphoretic, and in acute distress. Syncope may occur. There may be associated neurologic defects (ie, weakness, paraplegia). Diagnostic tests include an ECG to distinguish between MI and dissecting aneurysm of the aorta. A chest x-ray may show a widening mediastinum or left pleural effusion from extravasation of blood. An aortogram is the most definitive diagnostic test; it can show the aneurysm's size and location.

PERIPHERAL ARTERIAL ANEURYSM Aneurysms of the femoral and popliteal arteries are usually fusiform or saccular. Fusiform lesions can affect one leg or both legs (25% of clients), and may accompany aneurysms of the abdominal aorta. They affect mostly males aged 50 to 70. Hypertension is present in 40% to 50% of clients. Peripheral aneurysms usually occur secondary to atherosclerosis but also may be caused by trauma, infection, or previous vascular surgery. These aneurysms tend to progress rapidly to embolization and gangrene because of the intermittent compression of the aneurysm by flexion of the knee.

Some clients are asymptomatic. Others notice a vigorous pulse in the popliteal region or upper thigh. The aneurysm rarely enlarges sufficiently to cause local pain and tenderness. Rupture seldom occurs. Venous distention may be seen secondary to compression of adjacent veins. There may be symptoms of ischemia in the leg or foot due to acute thrombosis in the aneurysmal sac or embolization of a thrombus fragment. After arterial occlusion, there is severe pain, loss of pulse and color, coldness, and eventually, gangrene.

Bilateral palpation reveals a pulsating mass in the region of the inguinal ligament. A firm, nonpulsating mass can be palpated when pooling of blood in the aneurysmal sac causes thrombosis. Ultrasonography and arteriography are helpful in diagnosis.

Medical Measures

The usual treatment of choice for aneurysms is surgery to prevent rupture and thrombosis. Aneurysm surgery is covered below.

Specific Nursing Measures

Nursing management is aimed at providing emotional support and health teaching if surgery is not immediately indicated. Teach the client and family to watch for early symptoms and signs of changes in vascular function, such as alteration or discrepancy in pulses and color changes in the extremities. Also warn the client to avoid Valsalva's maneuver—bearing down during a bowel movement or holding the breath while moving up in bed. The nurse also assists clients to prepare emotionally for surgery.

Make sure that the client and significant others understand the potential complications of an untreated aneurysm. Periodic physical examination and abdominal x-ray or ultrasonography can demonstrate expansion of the aneurysm. Electing to have an expanding aneurysm surgically repaired while the client is in relatively good health is better than having emergency surgery when the aneurysm is leaking or has ruptured. Although the surgery is major and not without risk, morbidity and mortality are considerably lower when aneurysms are surgically repaired under elective rather than emergency conditions.

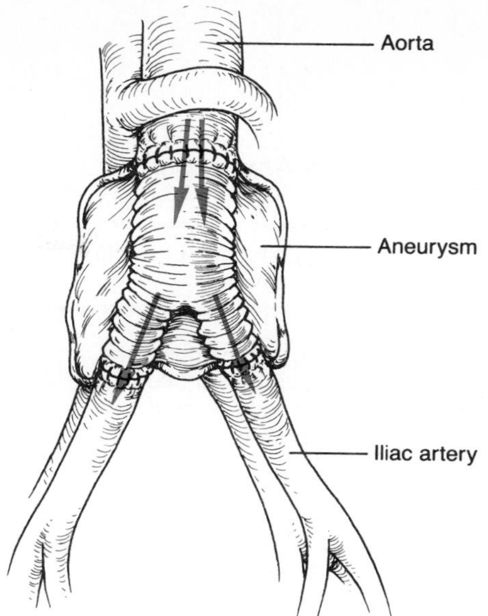

Figure 21–4

Abdominal aortic aneurysm repair. The aneurysm is resected. The synthetic graft is anastomosed to the aorta and the iliac arteries. The aneurysm is then sutured over the graft itself to provide added support to the graft.

Repair of Aortic and Peripheral Aneurysms

An aneurysm repair is a resection of the aneurysm and restoration of normal blood flow through replacement of the damaged section with a Dacron or Teflon graft. Hypothermia is induced during aortic surgery to decrease the need for oxygen at the tissue level and to decrease the production of metabolic waste products. The repair of thoracic aorta aneurysms requires opening the chest and usually the use of the heart–lung machine. Abdominal aneurysm resection involves ligation of the inferior mesenteric artery, clamping of the iliac arteries, and cross-clamping of the aorta at the neck of the aneurysm. Aneurysms may also occur in the peripheral arteries and may be repaired by synthetic grafts or natural grafts using a portion of a vein.

Repair of an abdominal aortic aneurysm is illustrated in Figure 21–4. The physiologic and psychosocial/lifestyle implications of aneurysm repairs are in Table 21–1.

Nursing Implications

PREOPERATIVE CARE Prepare the client having thoracic aneurysm repair preoperatively as described in the discussion of coronary artery bypass surgery. Surgical preparations are usually rushed. The client is often anxious, because the symptoms appeared suddenly, and the decision to have surgery was made quickly. The goal of nursing care at this time is to stabilize the client's blood pressure with nitroprusside and offer emotional support to the client and family or significant other.

The preoperative care of the client having abdominal aortic or peripheral repair is similar to that of the bypass surgeries discussed earlier. Baseline measurements of vital signs and vascular status are important and serve as a basis for evaluating postoperative progress.

POSTOPERATIVE CARE The client with thoracic aortic aneurysm repair is usually unstable in the immediate postoperative period and requires constant monitoring of arterial pressure. The goal of nursing care is to maintain a pressure high enough for tissue perfusion but not so high that stress is placed on suture lines. Because of the constant monitoring required, the client is usually kept in an intensive care unit for 2–3 days before being sent to a cardiovascular floor.

Nursing assessment includes evaluating circulation to the extremities, assessing for stroke, monitoring hourly urine output for decreased kidney perfusion, monitoring clotting studies to prevent coagulopathy, monitoring the ECG for signs of complete heart block and MI, assessing breath and heart sounds, and monitoring pulmonary and right atrial pressures for signs of hypovolemia or heart failure. Vasodilating agents are given intravenously to control arterial pressure. Give analgesics liberally, especially if a thoracotomy incision was used. Finally, emphasize breathing exercises with any thoracic or cardiac surgery client. Follow guidelines in the earlier cardiac surgery section.

The client with an abdominal aortic aneurysm repair will be taken to the intensive care unit for 1 to 2 days for

Table 21–1
Repair of Aortic and Peripheral Aneurysms: Implications for the Client

Physiologic Implications	Psychosocial/Lifestyle Implications
Possible thrombi or emboli	Regular exercise and avoidance of situations that could produce trauma or infection
Possible prosthetic endocarditis	Lifestyle modifications to reduce risk of atherosclerosis (see Chapter 20)
Clamping of aorta and tributary arteries may cause malfunction of the organs supplied by them	Regular health care supervision
Possibility of future aneurysms	Prophylaxis against bacterial endocarditis or graft infection
With repair of thoracic aortic aneurysms and dissections, possible complications of complete heart block; conduction disturbances; myocardial ischemia with risk of myocardial infarction, lethal dysrhythmias, or both; congestive heart failure; renal failure; respiratory insufficiency	Postcardiotomy psychosis if heart–lung machine used
	Possible need for antihypertensive and anticoagulation medications

continuous assessment or to a vascular surgery floor. Here, pulse (radial and apical) and blood pressure are monitored every 15 minutes until stable, then every hour for 24 hours. Peripheral perfusion should be monitored by evaluating the peripheral pulses as well as evaluating the color and temperature of the skin and determining the presence or absence of diaphoresis, pain, or numbness. Assess the client for any signs of bleeding, which can occur anywhere along the graft site and at the anastomoses. Abdominal girth should be measured and dressings checked for excessive bleeding or drainage every hour, and then every 4 to 8 hours. Dressings are either changed or reinforced according to the surgeon's preference.

While the client remains on bed rest for the first 48 hours postoperatively, keep the bed flat initially, then assist the client to turn gently from side to side at regular intervals. Encourage the client to dorsiflex and extend the feet to prevent congestion of venous blood in the lower extremities. Administration of analgesics at this stage allows the client to move with less distress and helps to make coughing and deep breathing easier. Determine the location and the severity of any pain. Back pain may indicate retroperitoneal hemorrhage or thrombus at the graft site.

Assist the client with initial ambulation and guard the client against any injury. The client must remain erect when ambulating to prevent kinking and tension of grafts. Monitor the client for any signs of infection, such as elevated temperature or redness at the incision line, so appropriate treatment measures can be taken early.

The client with an abdominal aortic aneurysm repair will have a nasogastric tube. Note the quality and amount of the nasogastric tube losses and monitor electrolyte levels daily.

The client is likely to have a number of fears and anxieties about the surgery itself, restrictions on activity, the change in self-image, possible loss of a limb, and death. Create an environment that facilitates discussion of these fears and concerns. Encourage the family to become involved in the client's postoperative care and provide them with opportunities to ask questions and discuss their concerns. The general nursing care of the client having abdominal aortic or peripheral aneurysm repair is similar to that discussed for bypass surgery.

Varicose Veins

Varicose veins are dilated, tortuous, elongated branches of the greater and lesser saphenous veins. Resulting from incompetent valves (Figure 21–5), they are a major cause of venous insufficiency. Varicose veins are common in persons whose occupations require long periods of standing (eg, waitresses, nurses). Heredity is also a factor.

It is not known whether the valvular incompetence of varicose veins is caused by dilation of the veins or whether the dilation of the valvular ring occurs first and then causes secondary valvular incompetence. During pregnancy, varicosities may appear because of hormonal changes, increased pelvic venous blood flow, or increased intra-abdominal pressure of the enlarged uterus, which prevents good venous return.

Infections and trauma to the veins with accompanying thrombophlebitis may also lead to varicose veins. Poor posture with sagging abdominal organs, obesity, systemic disease (ie, portal hypertension), and chronic constipation with straining at stool all contribute to venous engorgement in the legs and eventually to varicose vein formation.

Clinical Manifestations

Clients with superficial varicosities are often asymptomatic. Their varicosities are dark, tortuous, raised veins that become more prominent when they stand or cross their legs. Over time, dilation of the veins produces venous stasis with edema and fibrotic changes in fatty tissue and changes in the skin pigmentation.

Symptoms vary from minimal to incapacitating, depending on the location and severity of the varicosities. Nodular protrusions occurring along the veins as a result of sclerosed valves may result in disfigurement of the leg. Clients may report dull aching, heaviness, pain, and muscle cramping as well as a generalized tiredness and discomfort in the legs that tends to increase in hot weather and with prolonged standing.

Medical Measures

Treatment approaches range from conservative medical treatment to surgical intervention for severe varicosities. Medical management is aimed at decreasing the amount of blood pooling in the veins of the lower extremities and decreasing the venous pressure in the superficial veins. Compression of the superficial veins by support hose or elastic bandages decreases the volume of venous pooling.

A client with mild symptomatic varicosities may gain relief of symptoms and edema with support hose and leg elevation. A client with severe venous insufficiency requires regular periods of foot elevation and use of elastic bandages.

Surgical ligation and stripping of the greater or lesser saphenous veins is indicated for clients with recurrent leg ulcers. This surgical procedure and related nursing care are discussed below.

Specific Nursing Measures

Nursing intervention is directed toward client education to decrease intra-abdominal pressure, promote venous return, and maintain skin integrity. Teach the client to avoid sitting or standing for long periods, to keep the legs uncrossed, and to use low chairs that are not too deep so the feet can touch the floor to avoid putting pressure on the popliteal fossae. Tight, restrictive clothing, such as girdles, binders, garters, and elastics, must be avoided. Constipation can be managed with bran, fresh fruits and vegetables, psyllium seed, and exercise. When obesity is a contributing factor, the client should be on a weight-reduction diet.

Support stockings or elastic bandages should be donned before getting out of bed. If this is inconvenient (eg, if the client always showers in the morning), the client should resume the supine position and elevate the legs before applying the stockings. Support stockings and elastic bandages are applied from the toes upward, providing greater support to the lower leg, with a gradual decrease in pressure in the knee, thigh, and groin areas. Venous pooling is increased with constriction at the knee or groin. The ankle should be flexed several times to promote venous return before stockings or elastic bandages are applied. Clients should walk at least once each hour and elevate the legs above heart level four to six times a day or more, depending on symptoms.

Teach the client the importance of preserving skin integrity. The feet should be carefully cleaned with mild soaps, rinsed well, and patted (not rubbed) dry. Moisturizing creams or lotions should be applied to the dry skin of the lower legs and feet. The client should maintain a well-balanced diet that includes vitamins, proteins, and minerals.

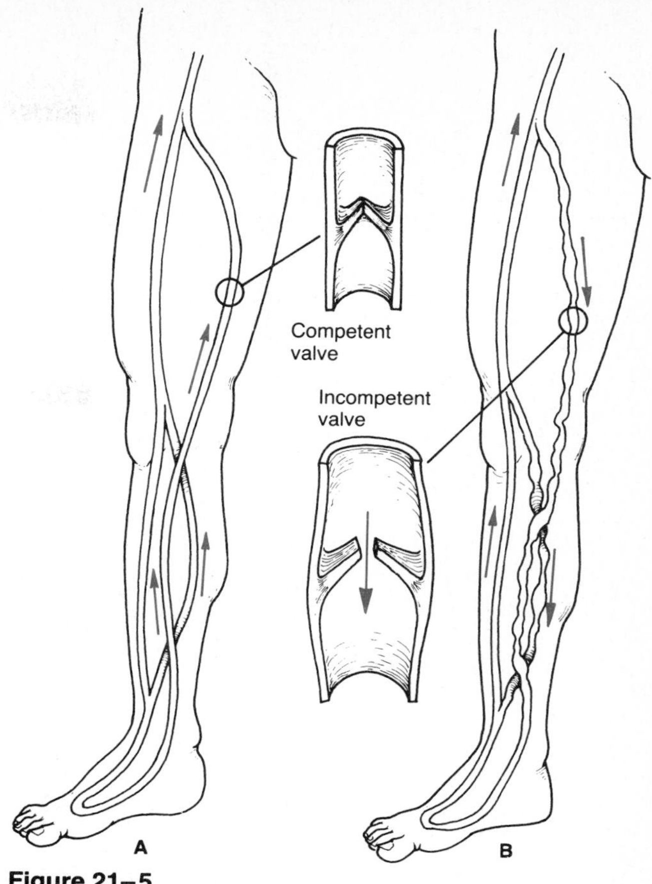

Figure 21–5

A. Competent valves with normal blood flow patterns. No backflow of blood occurs. **B.** Incompetent valves with backflow of venous blood.

Vein Ligation and Stripping

Ligation and diversion of a vein above the varicosity and removal of varicosed veins are carried out on enlarged tortuous veins that cause great discomfort. This procedure prevents secondary edema, ulceration, pain, and fatigue in the affected extremity.

The great saphenous vein is ligated close to the femoral vein through an inguinal incision. A second incision is made in the medial aspect of the ankle. The vein is stripped (pulled) by a plastic or metal vein stripper which is threaded through the lumen of the vein from the ankle to the groin and then pulled upward through the inguinal incision bringing the vein with it (Figure 21–6A). The bleeding that occurs as these tributaries are broken off can usually be controlled in surgery by pressure, elevation of the extremity, and electrocautery.

The procedure is more complex when the saphenous vein is extremely tortuous or when incompetent perforating veins are also involved. In these cases, other smaller incisions have traditionally been used to resect the veins involved.

After the groin is sutured, sterile dressings are applied along the incisions, and compression bandages are applied

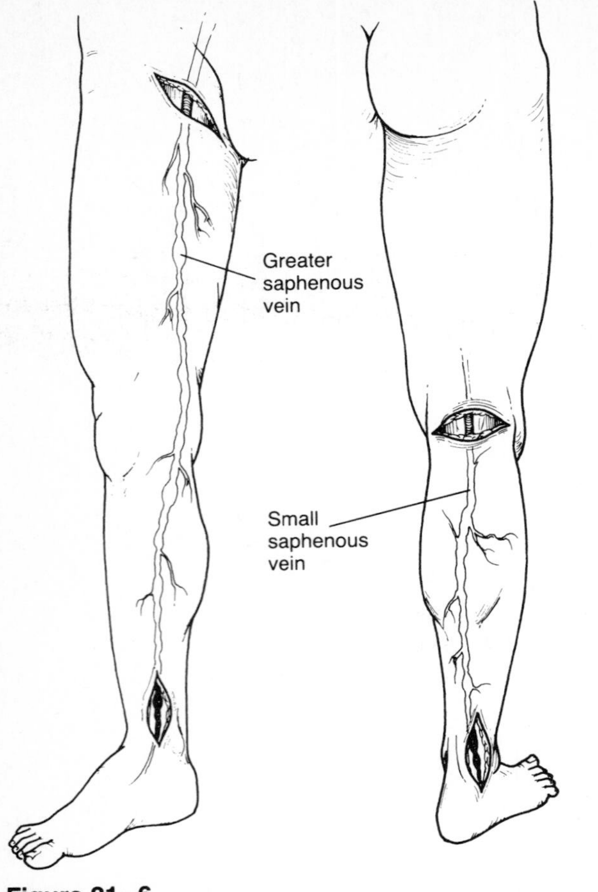

Figure 21–6

Incisions for vein ligation and stripping for varicosities of the great (**A**) and small (**B**) saphenous veins.

from the foot to the groin. See Figure 21–6B for an illustration of incision sites for the small saphenous vein. The physiologic and psychosocial/lifestyle implications are in Table 21–2.

Nursing Implications

PREOPERATIVE CARE In addition to routine preoperative preparation, instruct the client in the importance of early ambulation, frequent walking, avoiding sitting for long periods, and elevation of the limbs to prevent venous stasis. Sometime during the evening before surgery, the surgeon will mark the client's veins with a felt-tip pen while the client is in a standing position. Inform the client that the purpose is to aid the surgeon to identify the veins to be operated on. Since the client will be lying on the operating table, the varicosities may appear less prominent and more difficult to locate without markings.

POSTOPERATIVE CARE In addition to the usual postoperative care, the client who has had a vein ligation and stripping should be assessed for bleeding every 2 hours. If hemorrhage occurs, apply pressure over the area, elevate the foot, and notify the vascular surgeon immediately. For the first 4 hours after surgery, the client should be kept recumbent with the foot of the bed elevated to promote venous return to the heart.

Ambulation is encouraged the day of surgery and short, frequent walks the following days. Early ambulation is important in preventing thrombus formation in the remaining veins of the extremities. Ambulating after vein ligation and stripping is painful, so administering analgesics approximately 30 minutes before ambulation will increase the client's comfort and willingness to ambulate. Assist the client with ambulating and guard against trauma to the legs. Check the compression bandages after each ambulation to make sure they remain snug and in place.

Clients are usually discharged from the hospital after 2 or 3 days. Instruct clients to elevate the extremities routinely for 10 to 18 hours each day during the first week at home and not to stand or sit for long periods. By the third and fourth week, the client may slowly resume normal activities modified by the necessary lifestyle changes.

Venous Leg Ulcers

Venous leg ulcers result from incompetent valves in the perforating veins. Venous ulcers are found in the lower third of the lower leg and are common posterior and superior to the medial and lateral malleoli. These ulcerations are shallow and have a rim of bluish discoloration and erythema. They can penetrate to the level of the deep fascia or tendons but not through them. They may also erode through veins or arteries. Occasionally, the ulcers encircle the leg. Before ulceration, a firm edema is present that decreases slowly and minimally when the client's legs are elevated. A brown pigmentation of the lower leg is observed in a client with long-standing venous insufficiency. It can frequently be found around healed ulcers.

Table 21–2
Vein Ligation and Stripping: Implications for the Client

Physiologic Implications	Psychosocial/Lifestyle Implications
Hemorrhage and thrombus formation possible complications	Weight-loss program if necessary
Varicosities may occur in superficial collateral vessels	Avoid restrictive clothing
Elimination of option of using saphenous veins for future coronary artery bypass surgery if needed	Elevate extremities at regular intervals throughout day
	Prevent constipation and straining at stool
	Regular exercises and walking to decrease stasis

Venous leg ulcers may appear spontaneously or following trauma. The underlying problem is venous insufficiency. Postphlebotic syndrome (discussed later in this chapter) and stasis account for most leg ulcers. Ulcerations are more common in clients with deep vein abnormalities and incompetent perforating veins than in clients with varicose veins alone. In venous insufficiency, the tissue of the lower legs has a decreased resistance to infection. Thus, trauma and abrasions may result in ulcer formation.

Clinical Manifestations

Because of high venous pressure, localized varicosities and edema occur, with an increase in deposition of fibrous tissue. With long-standing venous insufficiency, the edema, initially soft and pitting, becomes firmer and may decrease only slowly and minimally upon elevation. The edema then acquires a "woody" feeling, termed **brawny induration** because of increased connective tissue in the subcutaneous tissue. Ulcer formation is preceded by a localized area of redness, tenderness, and brawny induration.

The diabetic client is prone to ulcer formation because of vascular changes that occur in diabetes mellitus. The diabetic's leg ulcers heal slowly, and skin grafting is often required.

Medical Measures

To stimulate ulcer repair and maintain skin integrity around the ulcer, a semirigid boot of paste (eg, Unna's paste) may be applied to the client's ulcerated leg. These boots are used for the ambulatory client to provide stability, support, and protection to the ulcerated area as well as to promote healing. The Unna's paste boot is somewhat inconvenient to apply; an elastic bandage over a layer of foam rubber and a medicated dry gauze may be applied instead. These protective ulcer dressings are left in place for several days but may be changed as necessary, depending on the drainage from the ulcer.

There are different approaches to the pharmacologic management of leg ulcers. Some physicians avoid application of local medications and debriding agents. Others use enzymatic debriding agents such as fibrinolysin or collagenase to clear away necrotic tissue. Debridement provides a clean layer of granulation tissue to serve as a base for optimal healing. Dextranomer (Debrisan), a nonenzymatic agent, is effective for draining wounds. Dextranomer is available as small spherical beads that absorb secretions by exerting a suctionlike force on exudates and tissue particles. The bead layer changes color according to the infecting organism. A grayish yellow color indicates the beads have become saturated and should be completely removed. Irrigation or whirlpool treatments may be necessary to remove residual patches of saturated dextranomer. Beads can be reapplied every 12 hours or more often if necessary.

Topical antibiotics are rarely used. Systemic antibiotics are prescribed according to wound culture and sensitivity results.

Specific Nursing Measures

Nursing intervention is directed toward promoting healing of ulcers, preventing infection, and educating clients to maintain optimal health of the extremities. While engaged in client care, continually reinforce proper ulcer-care technique and make clear the rationale for the care regimen.

Cleanse the extremities with mild soap and warm water and apply moisturizing lotion to the unaffected skin. Using aseptic technique, debride the ulcer as prescribed (ie, irrigate the ulcer with sterile normal saline and/or dilute hydrogen peroxide and use enzymatic debriding agents or dextranomer). Another approach is to use wet-to-dry dressings for debridement of the ulcer. First, apply wet sterile saline dressings. When they are dry, gently remove the dressings, which bring with them devitalized tissue.

Instruct the client and significant others to elevate the client's extremities above heart level for 30 minutes at least every 2 hours. Teach proper application of supportive stockings or bandages. Encourage as much regular exercise as the client can tolerate to stimulate venous return. Encourage a high-protein diet with adequate vitamin C and E to aid in healing and connective tissue repair. If the client is obese, a weight-loss diet is indicated. The dietitian can help plan a diet to meet the client's particular needs. As in all disorders of the peripheral circulation, clients should eliminate constrictive clothing from their wardrobes, be attentive to proper foot care, avoid trauma, and abstain from smoking.

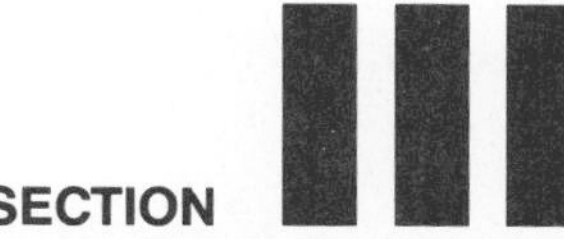

SECTION III

Infectious Disorders

Lymphangitis and Lymphadenopathy

Lymphangitis is an acute or chronic inflammation of the lymphatic vessels generally caused by a streptococcal infection of an extremity. Lymphadenopathy or lymph node enlargement can be generalized or regional. Table 21–3 lists the suspected causes of lymph node enlargement by region and conditions associated with generalized lymphadenopathy.

Clinical Manifestations

Lymphangitis is characterized by red, warm, tender streaks spreading up an arm or leg toward the regional lymph nodes from a focal point of infection. Chills, fever,

Table 21–3
Causes of Lymph Node Enlargement

Region of Lymphadenopathy*	Suspected Cause
Occipital nodes	Ringworm of scalp, seborrheic dermatitis, pediculosis capitis
Posterior auricular nodes	Rubella, infections of the auricle
Anterior auricular nodes	Lesions of the conjunctivae and eyelids, keratoconjunctivitis, ophthalmic herpes zoster
Cervical lymph nodes	Upper respiratory infections, oral or dental infections, mononucleosis, tuberculosis, coccidioidomycosis, lymphoma, leukemia
Supraclavicular lymph nodes**	
Right side	Malignancy of the lungs or esophagus
Left side	Malignancy of the stomach, kidney, ovary, or testis
Axillary lymph nodes	Local infections, metastatic breast cancer
Epitrochlear nodes	Local infections in the area of drainage
Inguinal nodes	Vaginitis, urethritis, urinary tract infections, herpes, syphilis, chancroid, malignancy

*Generalized lymphadenopathy involving three or more lymph node groups often occurs in rubella, rubeola, mononucleosis, scabies, leukemia, Hodgkin's disease, lymphosarcoma, systemic lupus erythematosus, sarcoidosis, dermatomyositis, and amyloidosis.

**Enlargement of the supraclavicular nodes is always considered abnormal.

and generalized malaise usually occur. The regional lymph nodes become enlarged and tender.

Lymph node characteristics in lymphadenopathy, whether regional or general, provide important clues to diagnosis. Nodes may be tender or painless, firm or rock hard, movable or fixed, discrete or matted together. The location, size, and characteristics of the enlarged nodes should be carefully documented.

Although lymph node enlargement is often clinically significant, some people have a chronically enlarged node that remains palpable after an infection resolves. Such nodes are not usually problematic. Change in the node should be checked by the client's health care provider, however.

Medical Measures

Therapeutic approaches are aimed at treating the cause. Antibiotics, fluids, rest, warm soaks, and drainage of infected areas are all possible approaches, depending on the cause of the inflamed lymph vessels and lymph nodes.

Specific Nursing Measures

Nursing care for clients with lymphangitis is aimed at promoting drainage of the lymph nodes by elevating the extremity and applying warm moist packs to the inflamed area. Nurses often have opportunities to advise clients with lymph node enlargement in normal daily contact with family, friends, and neighbors. Those with cervical lymph node involvement accompanying a viral upper respiratory infection (URI) do not need to be referred to a care provider unless the URI persists for several weeks. Those currently under treatment for an infection (eg, vaginal) in the region of lymph node enlargement (eg, inguinal) need an explanation of the function of lymph nodes and why they enlarge. All others should be referred to a care provider, because the node enlargement may signal an infection that requires treatment, or the lymphadenopathy could herald a more serious health problem.

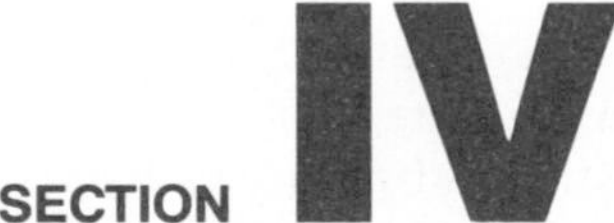

Obstructive Disorders

Obstructive disorders of the peripheral circulation develop as a result of changes that occlude the normal pathway of circulation. Circulatory occlusion may cause gradual or sudden changes in tissues, resulting in ischemic ulcerations, gangrene, and/or edema. Acute and chronic arterial occlusive disease, thrombophlebitis, chronic venous insufficiency, and lymphedema are discussed in this section.

Acute Arterial Occlusion

Acute arterial occlusion is a sudden interruption of the blood supply to all or a part of an extremity. The clinical manifestations depend on the location and extent of the occlusion as well as on the availability of collateral circulation. The major causes of acute arterial occlusion are embolism, thrombosis, and injury.

Embolization of a thrombus from the heart is the most frequent cause of an acute arterial occlusion in the upper extremities. These emboli develop as a result of a pros-

Table 21–4
Sites of Occlusion in the Arterial System

Site of Occlusion	Clinical Manifestations
Carotid arterial system (including the external and internal carotids)	Neurologic dysfunction (ie, transient ischemic attacks, or TIAs) that occurs because of reduced cerebral circulation, which also produces sensory or motor dysfunction; transient monocular blindness; transient hemiparesis, aphasia, dysarthria; decreased mental ability; confusion and headache; possible bruit over the carotids; manifestations may last for a few seconds or 5 to 10 min and may be present for up to 12 h; 20% of clients with TIAs suffer a stroke (Petersdorf et al., 1983)
Innominate (brachiocephalic) artery	TIAs of brain stem and cerebellum (visual disturbances, vertigo, falling down without loss of consciousness, and dysarthria); claudication of the right arm and a bruit over the right neck
Subclavian artery	TIAs with visual disturbances, vertigo, falling down without loss of consciousness, and dysarthria; arm claudication after exercise, with potential gangrene of the fingers
Mesenteric artery (including the superior mesenteric artery, which is most often affected, the celiac axis, and inferior mesenteric)	Sudden acute abdominal pain, nausea, and vomiting; bowel ischemia, necrosis, and gangrene because of a possible infarct; leukocytosis and shock
Aortic bifurcation (saddle occlusion), considered a medical emergency	Muscle weakness, numbness, paresthesia and paralysis; ischemic signs of sudden pain, cool pale legs, and absent or diminished pulses
Iliac artery (Leriche's syndrome)	Claudication of buttocks and legs (relieved by rest), diminished or absent leg pulses, bruit over the femoral arteries, and impotence; atrophy of the lower extremities is a late manifestation
Femoral and popliteal artery	Intermittent claudication of the legs, ischemic pain, leg coolness and pallor; potential gangrene

thetic heart valve, atrial fibrillation, or MI. Emboli are carried from the left side of the heart through the circulatory system until they reach an artery too small to allow passage. Arterial thrombus formation also occurs in an atherosclerotic vessel where there is a rough surface. Emboli break off from the thrombus formation and lodge in the arterial system. In the lower extremities, over half of the emboli lodge in the superficial femoral or popliteal artery.

Clinical Manifestations

Severe pain and loss of both motor and sensory function are the symptoms of acute arterial embolism. If acute arterial occlusion involves a critical segment of the arterial tree where there is poor collateral circulation, the initial symptom is pain in the most distal part of the limb, which is then quickly followed by pallor, coldness, and a sensation of numbness. In the first hour, cutaneous sensation is lost. After 6 hours, ischemic muscular contractures, focal gangrene, and subcutaneous hemorrhage develop. Table 21–4 lists clinical manifestations for obstructions in different arterial systems.

When the artery is not completely blocked and allows sufficient blood flow to prevent tissue death, there may be only loss of pulses distal to the occlusion, decreased skin temperature, decreased systolic pressure in the distal portion of the limb, and ischemic pain at rest. Active or passive ROM of the limb increases the pain. If there is adequate collateral circulation, the client may experience only numbness or weakness of the limb.

Medical Measures

Remember that acute arterial occlusion is a life-threatening medical emergency. If the embolus or thrombus blocks off a major artery, immediate embolectomy is performed under local anesthesia (see below). Intravenous heparin therapy is instituted immediately to reduce emboli formation and expansion. Analgesics are administered for relief of pain. Morphine sulfate may be used not only for its analgesic effect but also for decreasing the clients anxiety level.

Thrombolytic agents such as streptokinase or urokinase may be given IV for lysis of intravascular deposits of fibrin. The danger of hemorrhage is increased when thrombolytic agents are given concurrently with an anticoagulant. Aspirin and indomethacin therapy should also be avoided during thrombolytic treatment because of the potential for bleeding.

Specific Nursing Measures

Nursing care of clients with an acute arterial occlusion involves monitoring vital signs and frequently assessing the extremities. The client should be on bed rest in a warm room. Protect the involved extremity from injury (eg, from hard surfaces and tight or heavy bed covers) by a bed cradle. Keep the extremity level or just slightly dependent. Give analgesics as necessary (as ordered) to improve client comfort.

On admission the client may be prepared for emergency surgery. The client should understand that immediate surgery is necessary to preserve viability of the extremity. Both client and significant others will be anxious and fearful. Pain can alter the client's ability to think clearly and respond calmly to the situation. Be sensitive to the fears and frustrations of both client and significant others, explaining all treatments and medications clearly, while completing surgical preparations in a timely and sensitive manner. Continuous assessment for bleeding is important when anticoagulants or thrombolytic agents are used.

Arteriosclerosis Obliterans

Arteriosclerosis obliterans is a chronic arterial occlusive disease of the extremities. It can involve the aorta, the common iliac artery, the superficial femoral artery, the posterior tibial artery at the ankle, and the anterior tibial artery at its origin. The lesions are segmental and localized, often obstructing one section of the artery and leaving other sections uninvolved.

Arteriosclerosis obliterans is most often seen in older men. Clients with diabetes mellitus develop the disease at an earlier age and have greater involvement of the lower leg.

Clinical Manifestations

Clinical manifestations occur because progressive arterial obstruction prevents oxygen and nutrients from being supplied to the tissues. Pain is the most common symptom—both intermittent claudication and rest pain. There may be numbness and tingling of the digits and coldness in the digits or feet on exposure to cold. Tissue necrosis and/or gangrene in the terminal digit can occur.

Other manifestations include thin, pale, shiny, taut skin with loss of hair on the lower part of the legs. In severe disease cyanosis, dependent rubor, and edema of the feet and legs can occur.

Leriche's syndrome (caused by slowly progressive atherosclerotic occlusion of the terminal aorta and the iliac vessels) has a characteristic cluster of manifestations, which depend on the location and extent of the plaque formation. Intermittent claudication in the lower back, buttocks, thigh, calf, or foot occurs with exercise and is relieved by rest. Impotence, muscle atrophy, and leg weakness also occur.

Medical Measures

Medical approaches include control of hypertension, hyperlipidemia or diabetes mellitus when present. Analgesics are used for pain. Vasodilator drugs are not usually effective.

Surgical approaches include bypass grafting of the affected segment, endarterectomy, and balloon catheter dilation. Lumbar sympathectomy may be done to increase blood flow, which may relieve pain and promote healing of small ulcers. Amputation is sometimes necessary.

Specific Nursing Measures

Nursing intervention is directed toward client education regarding stopping smoking, modifying the diet, avoiding constrictive clothing, providing warmth and avoiding trauma to the extremity, foot care, and an exercise program to stimulate peripheral circulation. Refer to Section I earlier in this chapter and Chapter 20 for a complete discussion of these nursing interventions.

Phlebothrombosis and Thrombophlebitis

Thrombus formation in a vein is called **phlebothrombosis.** Inflammation of a vein with thrombus formation is called **thrombophlebitis.** Venous stasis, trauma, and increased coagulability of blood lead to thrombus formation. Because there are no inflammatory symptoms and signs with phlebothrombosis and because the thrombus does not adhere to the wall of the vein as in thrombophlebitis, there is greater danger of pulmonary embolism with phlebothrombosis. This discussion refers mainly to thrombophlebitis, which has definite subjective and objective findings. Remember, however, that the possibility of phlebothrombosis exists in clients who are immobilized, postsurgical, postpartum, in a leg cast or traction, or on oral contraceptives, particularly if they smoke cigarettes.

Thrombophlebitis can occur in the deep or superficial veins of the legs. The saphenous vein is the most common site of superficial thrombophlebitis. In deep vein thrombophlebitis (DVT), the iliofemoral vein, popliteal segments, or small veins of the calf are most often involved. DVT can also cause distention of the superficial veins because of the backflow of blood through communicating veins.

Clinical Manifestations

In both deep vein and superficial vein thrombophlebitis, clinical manifestations vary with the site and length of the disease process. With inflammation of the endothelial lining of the vein, redness, swelling, and increased warmth occur along the path of the vein. Temperature may also be elevated.

As the thrombus enlarges causing greater reduction in blood flow, there is pain, dependent cyanosis, a positive Homans' sign, and an increase in the circumference of the extremity. The client may experience muscle cramping.

Inflamed superficial veins feel like firm cords when palpated. Palpation may elicit tenderness over the involved segment. Frequent, deep palpation must be avoided because of the possibility of dislodging a thrombus. Pulmonary embolism is not a danger with superficial thrombophlebitis but is a definite concern with DVT.

Diagnosis of thrombophlebitis is aided by noninvasive tests such as Doppler ultrasonography and impedance plethysmography. The ^{125}I-labeled fibrinogen test may help in detecting the thrombus. Contrast venography may also be done. See Chapter 20 for a description of these tests.

Medical Measures

Anti-inflammatory agents such as ibuprofen or indomethacin are usually prescribed for superficial thrombophlebitis. Anticoagulants are seldom used. Anticoagulants are indicated if the thrombosis progresses proximally or if the involved segment of the superficial thrombosis is near the deep venous system at the groin.

For DVT, intravenous heparin is the treatment of choice. The partial thromboplastin time (PTT) should be maintained at about two times the control time. Oral anticoagulation with warfarin sodium is prescribed for 4 to 6 weeks after the acute stage of DVT in uncomplicated clients. Oral anticoagulation may be extended when the popliteal, femoral, or iliac vessels are involved. The prothrombin time (PT) of clients on warfarin sodium must be carefully monitored and kept at about twice the control time.

Intravenous thrombolytic (fibrinolytic) therapy with streptokinase may be helpful in dissolving the clot, preventing damage to the valves of the vein, and preventing development of chronic venous insufficiency and postphlebitic syndrome. Bleeding is a danger with streptokinase treatment, especially if the client is also on anticoagulants.

Specific Nursing Measures

Clients with superficial thrombophlebitis are usually cared for at home. They or their significant others must be taught to elevate the affected limb for 15 minutes every 3 to 4 hours, to apply moist heat, and to use anti-inflammatory agents. Clients should wear support stockings during ambulation.

The client with DVT should be on complete bed rest for at least 7 days, with the affected limb elevated above heart level. Apply elastic bandages or stockings from the toes up with even support along the entire leg. Remove them daily for inspection and gentle cleansing of the skin. When pillows are used for leg elevation, they should support the entire length of the leg to prevent compression of the popliteal space. Continuous applications of moist heat will reduce the inflammation and decrease pain. The client should do exercises in bed by pressing the foot against a footboard. The unaffected leg should be exercised more actively.

Measure and record the circumference of the extremity daily and compare with the initial measurement. Make an identifying mark on the extremity to ensure that each nurse measures in the same place. Monitor the PTT in clients on heparin therapy and the PT in clients on warfarin sodium.

Observe the client for any signs of bleeding—hematuria; bleeding gums; dark, tarry stools; coffee ground emesis. Be alert to symptoms and signs of pulmonary embolism—restlessness, sudden pleuritic pain and dyspnea, hypotension, tachycardia, and hemoptysis.

Home care of clients with DVT involves instructing them about periodic leg elevation, use of support hose at all times when ambulatory, and frequent walking, which aids in emptying the leg veins. Clients should not sit or stand for long periods. Instruct clients who return home on warfarin sodium to have a weekly PT to monitor the level of anticoagulation. Clients on anticoagulants should not take any other medication without first checking with their physician or pharmacist. Aspirin and nonsteroidal anti-inflammatory drugs such as indomethacin must be avoided because they increase anticoagulant activity that could lead to bleeding.

Assisting clients to prevent future episodes of thrombophlebitis is a major nursing responsibility. Periodic leg elevation above heart level, elastic stockings, walking, not crossing the legs, and avoiding periods of prolonged sitting or standing are beneficial approaches. Obesity and constipation, which increase intra-abdominal pressure and promote venous stasis, should be avoided. Instruct clients about weight loss and high-fiber diets as appropriate. Ade-

Nursing Research Note

Vanbree N, Hollerbach A, Brook G: Clinical evaluation of three techniques for administering low-dose heparin. *Nurs Res* 1984; 3(1):15–19.

The effect of methods of administering low-dose heparin on the incidence of postinjection abdominal bruising was investigated. Three techniques were compared. All three methods were the same in site, preinjection skin preparation, skin holding, drug dose and packaging, angle of needle insertion, needle withdrawal, and postinjection skin preparation. Differences in techniques were: (1) during technique 1, the roll of tissue was released after needle insertion, and the plunger was aspirated; (2) in technique 2, the roll of tissue was not released, and the plunger was not aspirated; (3) in technique 3, the tissue roll also was not released, and the plunger was not aspirated, but 0.2 mL of air was injected after injection.

There was no significant reduction in incidence of abdominal bruising regardless of the technique used. Women 60 years and older had the most numerous and largest bruises compared with other subjects.

Nurses must continue to investigate different approaches to low-dose heparin therapy that may reduce bruising. Care must be taken with current technique to minimize tissue trauma. Because older women are at highest risk for bruises, nurses must take extra care in technique.

quate hydration will prevent concentration of blood. Clients should never take ergotamine preparations or oral contraceptives. They also should not smoke.

Embolectomy, Thrombectomy, and Endarterectomy

An *embolectomy* is the removal of an occluding embolus from an artery by means of a surgical incision into a blood vessel with the aim of restoring normal blood flow. Embolectomy is the procedure of choice when a major vessel to an extremity is occluded. This procedure is most effective in acute arterial occlusion if it is performed within 6 hours of the occlusion, because tissue damage is progressive and often reaches an irreversible stage by the sixth hour. After this time, saving the extremity may be impossible, and amputation may become necessary.

A *thrombectomy* is the removal of a thrombus from a vessel. The objectives of a thrombectomy are to reduce venous insufficiency and to minimize postphlebotic disability. Clients with iliofemoral involvement or recent onset of thrombosis are candidates for this procedure.

For both surgeries a balloon catheter such as a Fogarty catheter is passed beyond the point of clot attachment. The balloon is then inflated, and the catheter is withdrawn along with the clot (Figure 21–7). This may have to be repeated, to ensure removal. After the operative area is closed, pressure dressings to prevent bleeding are usually applied.

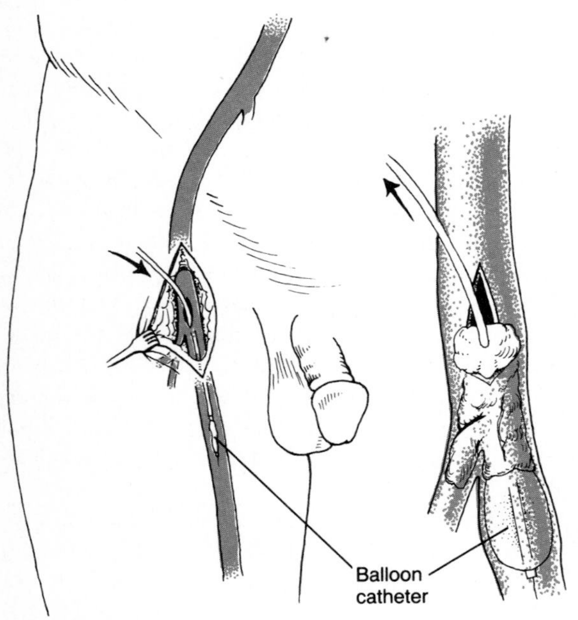

Figure 21–7

Embolectomy. **A.** The balloon catheter is inserted into the common femoral artery. **B.** The catheter is withdrawn along the embolus.

Table 21–5
Embolectomy, Thrombectomy, and Endarterectomy: Implications for the Client

Physiologic Implications	Psychosocial/Lifestyle Implications
Alleviates pain from vasospasm and ischemia; maintains viability of affected extremity	Alleviates fear of losing extremity to amputation
Potential complications of bleeding, thrombus, or embolus	Anxiety over possibility of thrombus or embolus
Long-term anticoagulant therapy	Regular daily exercise; avoidance of long periods of sitting or pressure on peripheral vessels to prevent stasis

An *endarterectomy* involves surgically incising an artery to remove an obstruction such as a progressive atheroma. This procedure is most often indicated for lesions of the femoral artery, the aortic bifurcation, or the carotid artery. The physiologic and psychosocial/lifestyle implications are similar for all three surgeries, and are discussed in Table 21–5.

Nursing Implications

PREOPERATIVE CARE Before surgery, measures are essential to prevent fragmentation of the embolus or thrombus that would result in occlusion of distal vessels. These measures include keeping the client on bed rest and protecting the extremity from trauma. A bed cradle keeps linens off the extremities, avoiding pressure and providing protection. A soft pillow between the legs helps to prevent the client from accidentally bumping the affected extremity. Family and nursing personnel should also be reminded to avoid bumping or jarring the extremity or the client's bed. Do not elevate the affected extremity; it should be kept level or in a slightly dependent position.

Obtain baseline vital sign measurements for comparison in the postoperative period. Preoperative vascular assessment will help to determine postoperative changes. Obtain peripheral pulses distal to the occlusion, noting their presence or absence and pulse strength. Measurements should be obtained for both extremities. It may be necessary to use a Doppler flow-meter (see Chapter 20). Note and record the color, temperature, and sensations in both extremities. Administer anticoagulants, thrombolytics, analgesics, and antispasmodics as necessary.

POSTOPERATIVE CARE The client is maintained on bed rest for 8 to 10 hours postoperatively. Monitor vital signs and compare them to their preoperative baselines. The blood pressure should not vary significantly from preoperative levels; variations predispose the client to thrombus formation.

Assess vascular status, paying particular attention to the pulses palpable distal to the site of the occlusion and to the color, temperature, and sensation in the affected extremity. Be alert to any changes. Observe the pressure dressings for evidence of bleeding and be aware of potential signs of hemorrhage such as increased pulse, decreased blood pressure, restlessness, and pallor. Renal function is an excellent indicator of vascular perfusion: if hemorrhage occurs, oliguria follows shortly. If an endarterectomy involves the aortic bifurcation, also monitor the client for abdominal distention or rigidity and assess the client's bowel sounds.

As with any postoperative client, encourage coughing and deep breathing every hour and observe for indications of cardiac, renal, and pulmonary complications as well as infection. Range-of-motion (ROM) exercises are especially important in preventing stasis. Encourage the client to turn and move in bed to stimulate circulation to the affected extremity. Other activities and ambulation are determined mutually with the surgeon.

In addition to administering analgesics, attempt to create a comfortable environment for the client when performing ROM exercises and while deep breathing and coughing. Administer anticoagulants or thrombolytics as ordered.

Before discharge from the hospital, clients will need information on the daily exercise routine and the anticoagulant therapy regimen they are to follow. Health teaching for clients undergoing anticoagulant therapy is discussed in Chapter 19.

Percutaneous Transluminal Angioplasty

Percutaneous transluminal angioplasty (PTA) of a peripheral artery is preferred to bypass surgery for reperfusion of an area. The most common peripheral vascular angioplasties are the aortoiliac and femeropopliteal. Iliac artery dilations are generally the easiest and most likely to be successful in the long term. A complete discussion and illustration of this surgical approach is in the cardiac surgery section on PTCA. The physiologic and psychosocial/lifestyle implications are similar to those for PTCA. These implications are discussed in Table 19–5.

Nursing Implications

PREOPERATIVE CARE Obtain and record vascular assessments of the extremity—color, warmth, presence and strength of pulses, sensation, and mobility. Use of a Doppler flow-meter to assess circulation may be vital. These preoperative baseline measurements are important indicators of postoperative progress. Prepare the client to expect frequent assessments of vital signs and vascular status and restriction of activity and mobility in the early postprocedure period.

POSTOPERATIVE CARE Care of the client after a PTA includes assessing the vital signs and vascular status. Color, temperature, and pulses distal to the operative site are monitored for presence and strength every 15 minutes the first hour, then hourly for the next 4 hours. The client should be kept flat in bed for 8 hours and instructed to keep the catheterized extremity in an extended position to minimize bleeding potential. Inspect the operative area for evidence of hematoma formation or bleeding.

After the first 8 hours on bed rest, the client can have the head of the bed elevated to a semi-Fowler's position. An increase in the client's activity level is usually permitted within 24 hours, beginning with sitting at the side of the bed or sitting up in a chair on the evening following the procedure.

An anticoagulation regimen is instituted postoperatively and continued indefinitely. Explain to the client the importance of taking this medication as directed upon discharge as well as the need for follow-up visits.

Peripheral Arterial Bypass

Today every effort is made to salvage an ischemic limb by arterial bypass surgery, provided the client has a lesion that can be bypassed and is not considered a poor surgical risk. The decision for surgery is made after angiographic and tomographic studies to determine the extent of the occlusion.

A *femoropopliteal bypass* is one in which a graft extends from the femoral to the popliteal arteries. The autogenous saphenous vein graft is used as the bypass material. The types of femoropopliteal bypass routes are illustrated in Figure 21–8.

A graft extending from the aorta down to the femoral arteries (Figure 21–9) is an *aortofemoral bypass*. A synthetic graft is used as the bypass material.

An **extra-anatomic bypass** (EAB) is one in which a synthetic graft extends from one artery to the other. In a *femorofemoral EAB*, a subcutaneous suprapubic tunnel is created. The graft is anastomosed to the femoral artery that has good vascular flow, passed through the suprapubic tunnel, and then anastomosed to the inadequately perfused femoral artery.

In an *axillofemoral EAB*, a graft placed subcutaneously on the side of the chest extends from the axillary artery to the femoral artery through a tunnel between the two sites, and anastomosed to the poorly perfused femoral artery. The physiologic and phychosocial/lifestyle implications are summarized in Table 21–6.

Nursing Implications

PREOPERATIVE CARE Nursing implications for the client having arterial bypass are similar to those for the vascular surgeries discussed earlier. Baseline measurements are necessary for postoperative comparison. Inform

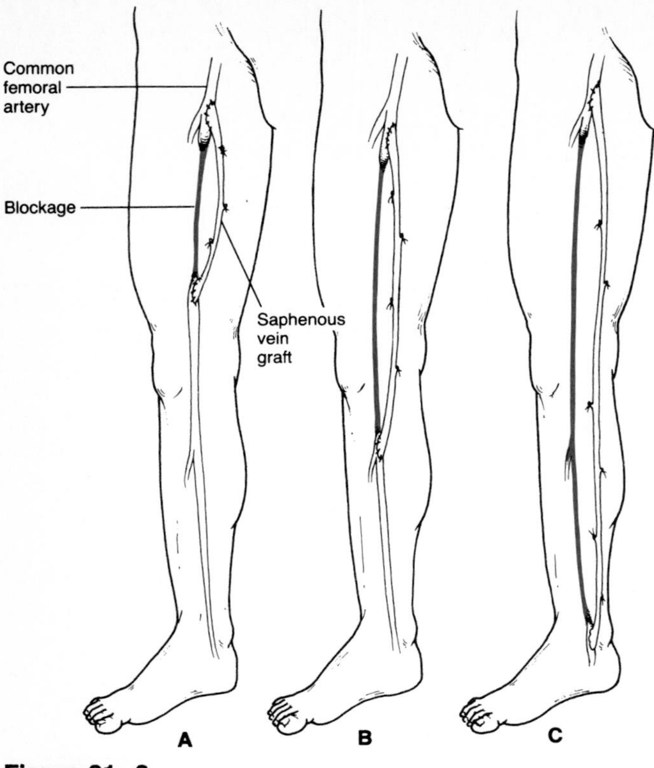

Figure 21–8

Femoropopliteal bypass. **A.** Bypass to proximal popliteal artery. **B.** Bypass to tibioperoneal trunk. **C.** Bypass to ankle.

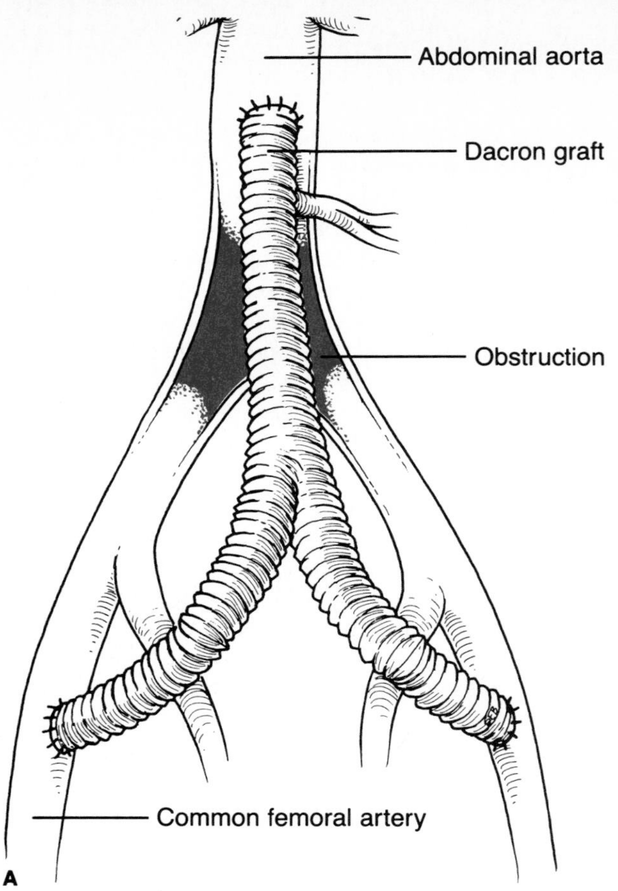

Figure 21–9

Aortofemoral bypass.

the client that postoperative discomfort in the operative area is due to manipulation of tissue necessary in order to perform the bypass, and that analgesics will be available for pain relief.

POSTOPERATIVE CARE Careful vascular assessments hourly for the first 12 hours (refer to the earlier discussion in the section on embolectomy) and at least once per shift thereafter, are crucial for the client having had arterial bypass surgery. Thrombi broken off by an increase in blood pressure or blood velocity can become emboli, a major complication of this surgery. Signs of embolization of a major arterial supply to an extremity could include rapid, severe pain; pallor; cyanosis; coolness; and the absence of pulses distal to the site of the obstruction. If the embolus has lodged in a small vessel, warmth and function may return to the extremity.

Vital signs must also be carefully monitored because hypotension increases the potential of thrombus formation and clotting of the graft. Also, leakage of blood around the anastomosis of the graft may be minimal or can occur as a steady leak, both of which can lead to hemorrhage.

When checking pulses of the client with an EAB, check the arterial pulses in the donor arm, in the axillofemoral graft itself, or the femorofemoral graft as it passes above the prominence of the symphysis pubis, and in the revascularized legs. Teach the client how to check the graft pulses so that the client will be prepared to carry out this procedure independently after discharge from the hospital.

Monitor the color and clarity of the urine as well as the urine output postoperatively because perfusion to the kidneys may have been decreased during surgery. Assess the incision lines for healing and the presence of infection; signs of infection should be reported to the surgeon immediately.

Clients who have had bypass surgery are restricted to bed for usually the first 48 hours. Assisting the client to change positions at regular intervals and using supportive devices will increase the client's comfort. After the first 48 hours of bed rest, the client is assisted to ambulate slowly. Although ambulation is encouraged, actual knee or hip flexion for longer than 30 to 45 minutes is discouraged. Joint flexion may cause kinking of the graft and thrombus formation. If there have been no complications, the client may sit up in the chair on the third postoperative day. Because the client should not flex the hip to 90°, a reclining chair is preferable. On the fourth postoperative day, the client may be assisted to the bathroom and may increase mobility as tolerated on the fifth day. Liberal administration of analgesics during these first few days after surgery will help the client to ambulate and decrease discomfort.

Carry out abdominal assessments on the client who has had an aortofemoral bypass. These include measurement of the abdominal girth each shift, assessment of bowel sounds, and monitoring nasogastric tube losses so fluid replacement needs can be determined.

The client who undergoes a femoropopliteal bypass—whether to the proximal popliteal artery, the tibioperoneal trunk, or to the ankle—develops edema within the first few days postoperatively. Edema can last for weeks or months, resolving gradually. Elevating the leg and using elastic compression stockings (if ordered by the surgeon) help to reduce edema. Monitor the edema by measuring and recording ankle, calf, and thigh circumference daily before the client gets out of bed in the morning. Instruct the client not to sit with the legs in a dependent position for more than 30 to 45 minutes; doing so will only increase the edema.

The client with an EAB should not have femoral arterial blood gases drawn because of the potential for damaging the donor artery. All laboratory slips should be marked with this precaution, and a sign should be placed over the client's bed or on the client's door. Mark the chart as well.

Offer the client the opportunity to discuss feelings about the prognosis and any concerns about the surgery, its effects, or the change in self-image. Clients may understandably be worried about graft rejection. Graft rejection, although rare, can occur with synthetic grafts. Carefully assess perfusion to the grafted area. Sometimes, however, a body rash and elevated temperature may be the only cues to graft rejection. Encourage the involvement of significant others in the client's care, providing them the opportunity to express their concerns and anxieties as well.

Table 21–6
Peripheral Arterial Bypass: Implications for the Client

Physiologic Implications	Psychosocial/Lifestyle Implications
Thrombosis and emboli possible early complications	Avoid body positions that could cause kinking of graft
Complication of postoperative myocardial infarction, bleeding from anastomosis site, intestinal ischemia	Avoid restrictive clothing
Rejection or failure of graft possible	Monitor graft pulses daily if EAB performed
Possible impotence from clamping arteries that supply pelvis during surgery	Increased use of limb on grafted side while avoiding sudden, forceful use of limb
Subcutaneous tunnel in EAB susceptible to injury	Daily exercise to prevent stasis
Indefinite anticoagulant therapy	Visible subcutaneous tunnel or leg edema may alter body image and restrict choice of clothing, exercise, and recreation
	Sexual dysfunction and lack of ability to reproduce if impotent

Insertion of Intracaval Filter/ Plication of Inferior Vena Cava

The intracaval (umbrella) filter is a tiny device that partially occludes the inferior vena cava. An intracaval filter is used when a client has deep vein thrombophlebitis (DVT) or pulmonary emboli and is unable to withstand anticoagulants because of blood dyscrasias, hemorrhage, hepatic dysfunction with alteration in the clotting mechanism, major visceral injury, or a history of cerebrovascular accident or other neurologic conditions. The procedure is also indicated if the client cannot withstand major surgery.

The umbrella filter is inserted under local anesthesia in a cardiac catheterization laboratory. The filter is attached to a stylet and folded inside a capsule, passed through a small incision into the right internal jugular vein, into the right atrium, and out through the inferior vena cava to the level of the third or fourth lumbar vertebra, distal to the renal veins. When correctly situated, the stylet is pushed forward to eject the umbrella from the capsule. The capsule then springs open, and the spokes fix to the wall of the vein (Figure 21–10).

Plication (partial occlusion) of the inferior vena cava is also performed to prevent movement of pulmonary emboli through the inferior vena cava. It is a major surgical procedure and is used less often than insertion of the intracaval filter. Plication of the inferior vena cava is carried out in an operating room under a general anesthetic. The vena cava is not cut; suture ligaments or Teflon clips are used to strain the blood or partition the inferior vena cava.

Because the intracaval filter is used more often than plication, the following discussion focuses on intracaval filter insertion. The principles can be applied to the care of the client who has had a plication. The physiologic and

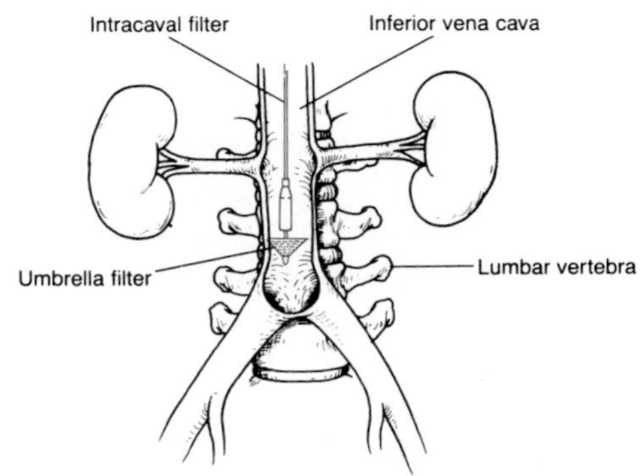

Figure 21–10

The intracaval filter in place.

psychosocial/lifestyle implications are similar and are discussed in Table 21–7.

Nursing Implications

PREOPERATIVE CARE Because this procedure is carried out while the client is awake, the client's anxiety level is likely to escalate. Thorough preparation of the client before the procedure will aid in decreasing anxiety levels and increasing cooperation during the procedure. The client should be told why this procedure is being done, what the filter looks like and what it does, and what sensations to expect during the procedure.

POSTOPERATIVE CARE Vital signs should be monitored every half hour until they return to a stable level, usually after 3 hours. Assessment of the insertion site is important: Hematoma development may indicate jugular bleeding, which requires immediate notification of the physician. Daily dressing changes with a bactericidal ointment are often recommended until the sutures are removed.

The client remains on bed rest for 24 hours after the procedure. Leg exercises during this period promote venous return to the heart. It is best to keep the foot of the bed elevated 15° when the client is in bed. Encourage the client to ambulate and not to sit except during meals and when going to the bathroom.

Instruct the client in preventing peripheral venous stasis and edema in the lower extremities. Ambulating, avoiding sitting for long periods, performing isometric calf exercises, elevating the legs, and wearing elastic support hose indefinitely help prevent these problems.

If plication of the inferior vena cava has been performed, it will be necessary to follow general postoperative nursing assessments and interventions as well as the nursing implications described in this section.

Table 21–7
Insertion of Intracaval Filter/Plication of Inferior Vena Cava: Implications for the Client

Physiologic Implications	Psychosocial/Lifestyle Implications
Trapped clots may cause stasis of blood and edema in lower extremities	Regular and frequent walking to prevent stasis
Possible formation of thrombi or emboli	Long-term anticoagulant therapy
Air embolism or filter migration into vascular system possible	Indefinite wearing of support hose
	Surgical correction if filter clots or migrates

Lumbar Sympathectomy

A lumbar sympathectomy is the severing of the sympathetic nerve fibers supplying the peripheral vessels. This severing causes relaxation of the small vessels and collateral channels of the legs, resulting in peripheral vasodilation and improved blood flow. A lumbar sympathectomy may be used in clients who are at high risk for corrective vascular surgery. This procedure is indicated only in clients whose vessels are elastic and only mildly or moderately occluded. A lumbar sympathectomy may also be done before vascular surgery to reduce the risk of postoperative thrombosis because it results in peripheral vasodilation and improved blood flow.

A lumbar sympathectomy is performed through an incision in the midflank area or the lower abdomen. The sympathetic ganglia that innervate the lumbar spine are removed, and the fibers are cut. This operation may be done unilaterally or bilaterally. The physiologic and psychosocial/lifestyle implications for the client are discussed in Table 21–8.

Nursing Implications

PREOPERATIVE CARE Prepare the client for what to expect in the postoperative period and provide the usual preoperative care. Because the client will be prone to postoperative orthostatic hypotension, instruct the client to request assistance for ambulation, especially in the early postoperative period.

POSTOPERATIVE CARE After this procedure, the client is positioned on one side, and vital signs are taken every

Table 21–8
Lumbar Sympathectomy: Implications for the Client

Physiologic Implications	Psychosocial/Lifestyle Implications
Mild discomfort from constant warmth and heaviness in extremities from pooling of blood	Need to wear elastic support hose during walking hours for discomfort
Chance of inability to ejaculate after bilateral sympathectomy that includes the first or second lumbar ganglion	Sexual dysfunction and sterility possible after bilateral sympathectomy.
Excessive perspiration in area above where nerve fibers have been severed; no perspiration in areas below	Lifestyle modifications related to peripheral vascular disease
	Avoidance of hot baths

15 minutes until they have stabilized. A complication to be especially alert for is shock: The dilated vessels of the extremities and lower abdomen will provide for pooling of blood.

As with any surgical procedure, the client must be carefully assessed for urinary retention and abdominal distention; because of the nature of this surgery, these problems are more likely. An in-dwelling urinary catheter and a rectal tube may be necessary to relieve these symptoms.

Reposition the client every hour and encourage coughing and deep-breathing exercises. Assist the client to ambulate with assistance the day after surgery. Be alert for orthostatic hypotension and take measures to ensure the client's safety. Apply elastic support hose before the client gets out of bed to sit. This will decrease pooling of blood in the legs.

Clients are usually discharged in 5 days. Instruct the client to balance exercise with rest at home and to elevate the extremities frequently during the day. Support hose worn during the first few weeks or months at home may increase comfort. Also instruct the client not to take hot baths; they may cause further vessel dilatation leading to hypotension.

Chronic Venous Insufficiency

Destruction of the venous valves, which leaves the deep veins of the legs functionally inadequate, is the cause of chronic venous insufficiency. The most common factor in the development of chronic venous insufficiency is single or multiple episodes of DVT. For this reason, chronic venous insufficiency is often called postphlebitic syndrome.

Clinical Manifestations

Chronic dependent edema of the ankles occurs, which is worse at the end of the day. The skin around the malleoli develops a brownish pigmentation and subcutaneous fibrosis occurs, manifested as induration. There is also lymphatic obstruction. The skin is thin, shiny, atrophic, and cyanotic. An acute weeping dermatitis is sometimes seen. Varicosities may appear due to incompetence of the perforating veins. These chronic changes eventually lead to stasis ulcer formation. Any trauma to the region of the lower leg and foot can result in ulcers that will not heal.

Medical Measures

Medical approaches are directed toward reducing the venous pressure in the legs. This is accomplished by leg elevation and the use of heavy elastic support stockings or pneumatic compression boots. Leg ulcers are treated with saline compresses, an Unna's paste boot, or a gauze dressing impregnated with a nonallergenic, self-adhering compound. Skin grafting is necessary for some ulcers. See the discussion of venous leg ulcers in Section II of this chapter.

Specific Nursing Measures

Instruct the client to keep the legs elevated above heart level at night. The legs should also be elevated intermittently during the day. Close-fitting, heavy-duty elastic support stockings are essential. Clients must understand that failure to wear the stockings will contribute to increasing edema and ulceration, which markedly interfere with ambulation and quality of life. Also refer to nursing responsibilities discussed under preventing future episodes of thrombophlebitis.

Lymphedema

Lymphedema is swelling of a part of the body as a result of insufficient lymph drainage. There is stasis of lymph with resultant chronic swelling, which can vary from mild to severe. The severity of the edema is directly related to the degree of obstruction and protein concentration in the interstitial spaces.

Lymphedema is caused by interference with the flow of lymph from an extremity. It can result from trauma, infection, allergy, malignancy, or the congenital absence of a developed lymphatic system.

When the normal outflow of lymphatic fluid is obstructed, the pressure in the lymphatic vessels builds up as the lymph begins to flow backward. Valves become incompetent, and protein accumulates in the interstitial spaces. This protein begins to draw or retain fluid that would normally be reabsorbed by the bloodstream.

Clinical Manifestations

The swelling in lymphedema is initially manifested as a soft edema, which then progresses and becomes harder, due to fibrosis. In later stages, skin becomes thick and brown.

Medical Measures

There is no cure for lymphedema. Measures used to control the manifestations of the disease include application of a pneumatic cufflike apparatus and regular light massage to the affected limb to enhance lymph drainage. Elastic support stockings are prescribed to help drain the legs and for cosmetic reasons.

Thiazide diuretics are sometimes prescribed to prevent fluid retention. Antibiotics may be used if there is any evidence of infection.

Specific Nursing Measures

Weigh the client twice a week and measure the circumference of the extremity. Seeing whether fluid retention is increasing, decreasing, or stabilizing allows for evaluation of therapy. Examine the involved extremity (ie, pulses, skin color, and temperature) daily. Teach the client to observe for changes in the extremity and to notify the physician if there is an increase in limb size; an absence in pulse; or a change in skin color, temperature, or texture.

Another nursing objective is to increase client comfort and promote lymph return. Emphasize elevation of the affected limb or limbs during sleep and several times during the day. The foot of the bed can be raised on a chair or blocks. Teach the client the hazards of a prolonged dependent limb position.

Client/Family Teaching

Demonstrate the correct method of massaging the extremity to client and significant others. The extremity should be massaged gently, using lotions, from the most distal point to the lymph nodes that drain the area (ie, from toes upward to the inguinal nodes).

The client should be correctly measured for elastic support hose and taught the proper way to don these stockings. Also, the correct procedure for application and use of the pneumatic cuffs should be taught. A number of pneumatic pumping devices is available for intermittent compression of the extremity. The pressure used is 30 mm Hg for the deeper lymphatic vessels and 20 mm Hg for the more peripheral lymphatic vessels. Pneumatic pumping therapy is evaluated by measuring the extremity before and after therapy.

Nutritional management includes instruction about sodium restriction to decrease fluid retention. The client may also be on diuretic therapy and should maintain an adequate potassium intake to counterbalance the potassium loss caused by diuretics. A well-balanced weight-reduction diet is appropriate for clients who are obese because elevated intra-abdominal pressure interferes with lymph return.

Emphasize meticulous hygiene to the skin and nails of the involved extremities and avoidance of trauma (eg, cuts and burns) that can lead to infection. The client should also understand the importance of regular medical examinations.

The physician should order a regular exercise program that can be implemented by the nurse. If an exercise program is not suggested, the nurse should ask the physician about the possibility of instituting one.

The nurse must be able to provide emotional support to the client who feels disfigured or who feels rejected because of an unshapely extremity. The client needs to be able to express feelings of exasperation and anger because of the body change and its effect on relationships and lifestyle. Withdrawal and depression can occur. The client's active involvement in making decisions about care can foster greater independence and control over the disease process and its management. The nurse must listen, encourage, and aid both the client and significant others in learning to cope effectively with this chronic disease.

SECTION V

Traumatic Disorders

The aorta and peripheral arteries can suffer penetrating and nonpenetrating traumatic injuries. A penetrating injury is the sort produced by a knife or bullet. Nonpenetrating injuries result from physical force delivered to the external body, as in a hammer blow to a thumb or a sudden slam against the dashboard or windshield in an automobile accident.

Traumatic injuries to blood vessels are frequently complicated by fractures that can obstruct or compress the vessel. Blunt injuries to extremities can cause contusions of vessels with resultant thrombosis.

Penetrating and Nonpenetrating Wounds of the Aorta

Penetrating wounds of the aorta and/or vena cava are a common cause of death from hemorrhage with chest injuries. These penetrating injuries usually result from stabbing or missile penetration. Nonpenetrating injury of the aorta, which occurs following blunt trauma, is important to recognize because surgery can most often save these clients. The great majority usually die quickly from exsanguination, but 15% to 20% survive the initial insult. Rupture can be delayed, with some clients forming aneurysms several months or years after the traumatic injury.

Rupture from blunt trauma is usually an indirect result of acceleration–deceleration forces generated in automobile accidents, vehicle–pedestrian accidents, aircraft accidents, and falls from great heights, but it occasionally results directly from a hard blow to the chest. The tear can involve one or all layers of the aorta and part or all of the circumference of the aortic wall. Immediate fatal hemorrhage is prevented in some clients because the tunica adventitia is not torn.

Clients who survive longer than 2 months after injury usually develop a false aneurysm of the aorta and then proceed through an uneventful course. They may remain asymptomatic for many years until massive enlargement occurs. Calcification develops at different times during development of the aneurysm, and the first clue of aneurysm formation is often seen on x-rays of the chest.

Clinical Manifestations

Clients who survive a penetrating injury are first seen with symptoms and signs of massive intrathoracic bleeding and severe shock. Later, however, an aneurysm may be discovered when a chest x-ray is done. If the aneurysm begins to expand, the symptoms and signs are those of the organs it compresses.

Medical Measures

With penetrating injuries, the treatment is immediate thoracotomy and reanastomosis of the aorta. An arterial prosthesis may be necessary.

Therapeutic approaches to nonpenetrating wounds of the aorta include resection and graft replacement of the traumatized area. Many physicians advocate resection of all trauma-induced aneurysms. If the aneurysm is leaking, a chest x-ray shows widening of the mediastinal area.

Specific Nursing Measures

Nursing care of the client with a penetrating wound or suspected blunt wound of the aorta includes assessment of the client's circulatory status and the body's response to the insult. Observe the client for signs of hypotension, cardiac, and respiratory arrest. Cardiopulmonary resuscitation may be needed.

Prepare the client for emergency surgery. Keep the client warm and continuously monitor vital signs, urine output, and level of consciousness. Give medications as ordered. Support of the client and significant others, who will probably be frightened and anxious, is important. Explain all procedures and give them as much feedback as possible in this emergency situation.

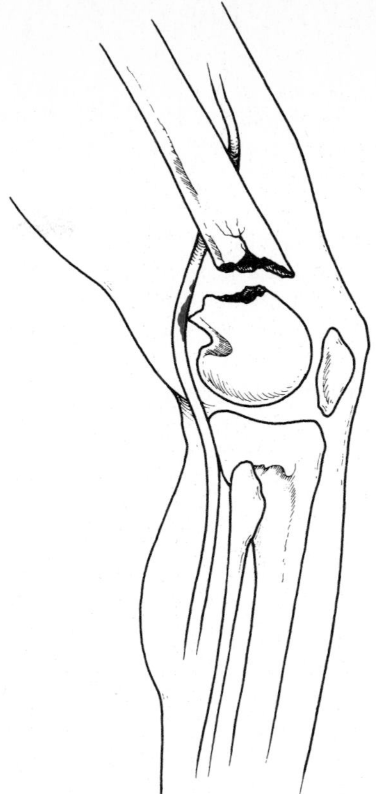

Figure 21–11

Arterial contusion accompanying a fracture.

Peripheral Arterial Trauma

Most injuries of the peripheral arterial system are either lacerations or transections of the arterial wall. Some uncommon injuries include arterial spasm, arterial contusion, and arteriovenous fistula.

Lacerations or transections made by a knife or ice pick are clean, incised wounds, and injury to the arterial wall is usually minimal. If the trauma is from a high-velocity missile such as a bullet, the tunica intima and tunica media will be disrupted some distance from the actual arterial wall laceration. This necessitates a greater area of debridement during surgery.

Arterial contusion or spasm often occurs when there are fractures and extensive soft tissue injuries from blunt trauma (Figure 21–11). Multiple injuries often obscure the arterial injury. Arterial spasm occurs most frequently in response to a brachial artery injury accompanying a fractured humerus.

Arterial contusion from a blunt injury is characterized by multiple areas of breakage in the arterial wall with intramural hemorrhage. The tunica intima becomes separated and prolapses into the lumen, obstructing arterial flow. The typical bumper injury produces contusion of the popliteal artery.

Most arterial injuries result from penetrating wounds that partially or completely disrupt the arterial wall. Nonpenetrating injuries are not as common but carry a serious prognosis, partially because of possible crushing injury to the arterial wall and because of the potential delay in diagnosis.

Clinical Manifestations

Loss of blood predisposes 50% of clients to shock. Hemorrhaging results from the arterial injury itself or from associated body injuries. With profound shock, severe peripheral vasoconstriction may conceal the arterial injury.

In blunt trauma, there is usually multiple organ injury. If an extremity suffers either blunt injury or penetrating wounds, fractures and nerve trauma often occur. When femoral artery injury is associated with a fractured femur, the incidence of gangrene is high.

In the extremity, arterial injury often produces four abnormal findings. They are best remembered as the "4 Ps"—paralysis, paresthesia, loss of pulses, and pallor. Of these, paralysis and paresthesia are the most important clinical manifestations because loss of neurologic function indicates tissue ischemia, which slowly progresses to gangrene unless the arterial blood flow is improved. Absence of pulse in one extremity and a normal pulse in the opposite extremity indicate arterial injury. (Keep in mind that there could also be a congenital absence of a pedal pulse. This possibility reinforces the importance of documenting pulses on a routine physical exam.) The presence of a peripheral pulse does not exclude the possibility of arterial injury. A lacerated arterial wall could be sealed with a blood clot, and arterial blood could still flow.

Bright red pulsatile bleeding, even in small quantities, is highly suggestive of arterial injury. On the other hand, bleeding may be totally absent, but a tense hematoma (from extravasation of blood into the fascia) may be palpated around the wound. A systolic bruit may also be audible over the traumatized artery.

Remember that arterial injury may be present if there is a penetrating wound near a major artery. Unrecognized secondary hemorrhage, a false aneurysm, or an arteriovenous fistula may develop.

Medical Measures

The most urgent problem is control of bleeding, which is accomplished by tightly packing the wound with gauze and then applying a pressure dressing. Tourniquets increase the risk of permanent injury to a peripheral nerve and should be avoided. Because of shock, rapid infusion of fluid is instituted until the systolic blood pressure rises to 80 mm Hg. After this, additional fluids may be given gradually. A total of 1000 to 2000 mL of fluid is necessary. Whole blood or volume expansion with Ringer's lactate solution, dextran, or plasma is also used. Tetanous toxoid is given prophylactically, and antibiotics are often started.

Specific Nursing Measures

Nursing care of the client with peripheral arterial trauma is aimed at evaluation of the extremity according to the "4 Ps." Assess the extremity for paralysis and paresthesia. Pulse assessment must be continuous because a pulse may be present even though there is arterial injury. Palpate the extremity for a hematoma formation, which may be a manifestation of extravasation of blood into the fascia. Be alert for bright red bleeding and aid in controlling the bleeding by applying a pressure dressing.

Assessment of all vital signs is important in detecting any changes in systemic status. The client may be ashen or pale and shiver due to peripheral vasoconstriction. If there is marked blood loss, the client's level of consciousness may be altered. The client may be anxious, irritable, confused, or comatose. As shock progresses, heart rate and rhythm vary. Initially, tachycardia occurs, followed by bradycardia as shock progresses.

Hypotension will be seen if 25% of the blood volume has been lost from the vascular tree. A reflex hypertensive state may be noted in shock. This is due to sympathetic and adrenal stimulation.

Preparation of the client for surgery involves insertion of an intravenous infusion and, in hypotensive states, volume expansion. A pulmonary artery catheter or central venous pressure line may be inserted before surgery.

Chapter Highlights

Blood flow may be disrupted by tumors, infection, obstruction, trauma, or rupture of the vessel.

Embolectomy, thrombectomy, and endarterectomy are surgical procedures that clear obstructed blood vessels.

Obstructed arteries may be bypassed surgically. Percutaneous transluminal angioplasty is an option for removing blood vessel obstructions in clients who are poor surgical risks.

Emotional stress, inactivity, degenerative changes, infection, and trauma may lead to ischemic changes in the periphery.

The emotional status of a client with peripheral vascular disease may be affected because of loss of independence and self-esteem, changes in body image, and altered sexuality patterns.

The nurse must assess the client for the principal complications of vascular surgery: bleeding and thrombus formation. Clients need long-term anticoagulant therapy and regular exercise to prevent thrombus formation.

Aortic aneurysms are repaired with a Dacron or Teflon graft. Peripheral aneurysms are bypassed with a synthetic or vein graft.

Blood flow to and from the extremities can be aided by client education regarding diet, exercise, wearing apparel, care of the feet, avoidance of cold, and smoking cessation.

Obstructive disorders of the peripheral circulation require astute nursing assessment, which involves inspection for temperature and trophic changes, palpation for hard masses or absent or diminished pulses, and auscultation for bruits.

The presence of a pulse does not necessarily mean a vessel is supplying adequate circulation to an area, and absence of a pulse could be congenital.

Although peripheral arterial disease seldom causes death, it may eventually result in limb loss and devastating physical and psychologic disability.

Irreparable damage can occur to arterial or venous tissue and surrounding organs when there is interference with normal blood flow and nerve supply.

Bibliography

A single syndrome for Raynaud's disease: *Emerg Med* (May) 1982; 14:175–176.

Baum L: Abdominal aortic aneurysm? *Nurs 82* 1982; 12:34–41.

Doyle JE: Treatment modalities in peripheral vascular disease. *Nurs Clin North Am* 1986; 21:241–253.

Ekers MA, Satiani B: EAB: A new route for vascular rehabilitation. *Nurs 82* (Nov) 1982; 12:34–41.

Fahey VA, Finkelmeier BA: Iatrogenic arterial injuries. *Am J Nurs* 1984; 84:448–451.

Foley WT et al: *Advances in the Management of Cardiovascular Diseases.* Chicago: Yearbook Medical Publishers, 1982.

Ginsberg R, et al.: Percutaneous transluminal laser angioplasty for treatment of peripheral vascular disease. *Radiol* 1985; 156:619–624.

Goldberger E: *Textbook of Clinical Cardiology.* St. Louis: Mosby, 1982.

Hinnant JR, Stallworth JM: Simplified surgery for varicose veins. *AORN J* 1981; 34:135–150.

Logan J, Ziebell E: Axillofemoral artery bypass for lower limb ischemia. *Can Nurse* (Sept) 1982; 78:25–29.

Malseed R: *Pharmacology: Drug Therapy and Nursing Considerations.* Philadelphia: Lippincott, 1982.

McMahan BE: Why deep vein thrombosis is so dangerous. *RN* 1987; (Jan):20–23.

Miller DC, Roon AJ: *Diagnosis and Management of Peripheral Vascular Disease.* Menlo Park, CA: Addison–Wesley, 1982.

Petersdorf RG et al: *Harrison's Principles of Internal Medicine,* 10th ed. New York: McGraw–Hill, 1983.

Price SA, Wilson LM: *Pathophysiology: Clinical Concepts of Disease Processes,* 2nd ed. New York: McGraw–Hill, 1982.

Raab D: Peripheral vascular disease: How to recognize it, how to treat it. *Can Nurse* 1982; 78:30–33.

Rutherford RB: Lumbar sympathectomy: Indications and technique in vascular surgery. In: *Vascular Surgery,* 2nd ed. Rutherford RB (editor). Philadelphia: Saunders, 1984.

Taylor DL: Thrombophlebitis: Physiology, signs, and symptoms. *Nurs 83* (July) 1983; 13:52–53.

Thompson DA: Teaching the client about anticoagulants. *Am J Nurs* 1982; 82:278–281.

Wyngaarden JB, Smith L: *Cecil Textbook of Medicine,* 16th ed. Philadelphia: Saunders, 1982.

Zimmerman TA, Ruplinger J: Thoraco-abdominal aortic aneurysms: Treatment and nursing interventions. *Crit Care Nurse* (Nov–Dec) 1983; 3:54–63.

CHAPTER **22**

The Nursing Process for Clients With Disorders of the Blood and Blood-Forming Organs

Other topics relevant to this content are: The health history and physical assessment, **Chapter 5;** Care of the client with nutritional deficits, **Chapter 6;** Self-help groups and other organizations related to leukemia, lymphoma, Hodgkin's disease, and multiple myeloma, **Chapter 10;** Pulmonary edema, **Chapter 19;** Risk factors for AIDS, **Chapter 23;** Care of clients with iron deficiency anemia and polycythemia vera, **Chapter 23.**

Objectives

When you have finished studying this chapter, you should be able to:

Specify the major components of the health history to be obtained from clients with disorders of the blood and blood-forming organs.

Explain specific assessment approaches in evaluating clients with disorders affecting the blood and blood-forming organs.

Identify the nursing implications of diagnostic studies commonly used to evaluate clients with disorders of the blood and blood-forming organs.

Determine appropriate nursing diagnoses for clients with disorders of the blood and blood-forming organs.

Develop, with the client, realistic goals of care.

Anticipate the psychosocial/lifestyle implications of disease of the blood and blood-forming organs on clients and their significant others.

Develop a nursing care plan for a client with a disorder of the blood and blood-forming organs.

Implement nursing interventions specific to clients with disease of the blood and blood-forming organs.

Implement nursing interventions specific to clients having a transfusion of blood or blood components.

Evaluate the effectiveness of the nursing care plan and modify it as necessary to meet client needs.

Clients with disorders of the blood and blood-forming organs have special needs, partly because a disturbance in blood production or bone marrow functioning can affect every organ system. These disorders can produce symptoms that become life threatening. Many clients' lives become uncertain in a number of ways—bleeding is often a constant threat; discomfort can evolve into severe pain; recurrent infections that are resistant to treatment can be life threatening; and weakness can become incapacitating fatigue. There may be little energy to devote to family, friends, job, school, or recreation. Therefore, both physiologic and psychosocial support are essential nursing measures.

SECTION 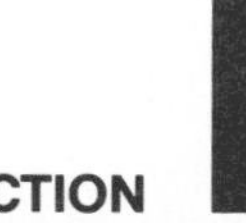

Nursing Assessment: Establishing the Data Base

Dysfunction of the blood or blood-forming organs can affect every organ system. For this reason, presenting symptoms can be varied and widespread.

Subjective Data

Initially, clients may report nonspecific symptoms such as weakness, fatigue, or malaise. Encourage clients to describe these and other symptoms in their own words and to explain how the symptoms affect their daily activities.

History of the Present Illness

BRUISING AND BLEEDING Ask clients if they have bruised easily lately or had larger bruises than normal; this fact may signal problems either with platelet production or consumption or with a clotting factor. Ask about the nature of the bruises: What causes them? Do they appear without injury? Also obtain information about when the client first noticed the bruising.

Petechiae, red to brownish pinpoint hemorrhages in the skin, may go undetected; clients may or may not spontaneously report them. Ask the client "Have you noticed any pinhead-sized reddish discolorations on your skin, especially where clothes fit snugly, such as at your belt line?"

Thrombocytopenia is the most frequent cause of bleeding and can accompany the leukemias, the lymphomas, or idiopathic thrombocytopenic purpura. Thrombocytopenia can also be a side effect of the chemotherapeutic treatment of any malignancy. Bleeding commonly occurs in a number of body systems. For example, clients may experience epistaxis and/or bleeding from the gums. Epistaxis may cause significant blood loss. Bleeding from the gums can interfere with the client's sense of taste; clients may report that nothing tastes good.

Gastrointestinal bleeding, appearing as hematemesis and melena, may occur with thrombocytopenia or gastrointestinal tumors. Frequently, the blood loss in the gastrointestinal tract is occult and can only be detected through chemical testing.

Female clients with thrombocytopenia may have menorrhagia, resulting in severe blood loss. When interviewing the female client about blood loss during menses, be specific and thorough in the questioning. Ask about color and amount of menstrual flow. Amount of menstrual flow can be documented by the number and size of the sanitary pads or tampons the client uses per day.

Ask about bleeding in other organ systems the client may have observed. Has the client noticed any hematuria? If so, what is the extent of the bleeding? Is the urine pink tinged, or is it grossly bloody? Determine also whether the client has noticed any bleeding into the sclera or any pulmonary bleeding.

LYMPHADENOPATHY Clients sometimes report a painless mass in the area of the cervical lymphatic chain. Enlargement of the lymph nodes of the neck is most common in Hodgkin's disease but may also accompany non-Hodgkin's lymphoma or the leukemias. Clients may also report swelling in the groin or edema of the lower extremities. This may occur in clients with lymphoma (Hodgkin's and non-Hodgkin's) who have inguinal lymph node involvement that impedes the normal flow of lymphatic fluid.

PAIN Clients with hematopoietic dysfunction are also subject to pain. Hemarthroses (bleeding into the joints) may accompany bleeding disorders and result in joint pain. Other hematologic dysfunctions—the leukemias, the lymphomas, and multiple myeloma—may be accompanied by bone pain. High uric acid levels sometimes found in the hematologic malignancies may initiate a painful gouty arthritis.

Abdominal tenderness may be due to splenomegaly, though splenomegaly is not always accompanied by abdominal tenderness. Abdominal pain may be due to intestinal obstruction caused by invasion of lymphoma into the gastrointestinal tract. Determine whether the client has a sore tongue. Severe iron deficiency anemia, pernicious anemia, and vitamin deficiencies commonly cause this symptom.

INTEGUMENTARY CHANGES Frequently, clients having disorders of the blood and blood-forming organs have abnormalities in skin texture, appearance, or color. As the largest organ of the body, the skin provides valuable information about clients' bone marrow function.

Clients should be asked about changes in skin color. Have they or their significant others noticed pallor or flushing? Pallor, especially if it occurs over weeks or months, may not be noticed. Jaundice is a color change clients usually easily recognize as abnormal. Jaundice may represent a hemolytic process involving erythrocytes, with or without accompanying hepatic dysfunction. Determine when change in color was first noticed. Approximations may have to suffice (eg, "Did you notice you were first becoming jaundiced around Christmas or Thanksgiving?"). Correlate changes in skin color with the onset of fatigue or decreased activity tolerance. Ask clients whether they noticed a change in skin color at about the same time their tolerance to activity changed.

Pruritus may or may not be present, depending on the disorder; it frequently accompanies Hodgkin's disease and non-Hodgkin's lymphoma, although the exact cause of the pruritus is unknown. Clients tend to regard pruritus as a nuisance and not to associate it with the blood disorder. Questions about pruritus should focus on the approximate time the client first noticed pruritus, what aggravates it, and what home remedies seem to relieve the itching. Ask also about the condition of the skin of the lower extremities because they seem to be especially vulnerable to blood abnormalities.

NEUROLOGIC CHANGES Headache is a common problem for clients with hematologic disease. Its causes are varied. Headache may accompany anemia or polycythemia vera. It may be present with central nervous system (CNS) involvement in leukemia or lymphoma, as a result of CNS infection, or with CNS hemorrhage secondary to thrombocytopenia.

Alterations in vision may accompany the blood disorders and be related to neurologic changes. The client can experience diplopia or blurred vision with CNS involvement of the leukemias or from retinal hemorrhage.

Numbness and tingling of the extremities may be present in pernicious anemia. With modern therapeutic measures, however, neurologic complications of pernicious anemia are rare.

Loss of deep tendon reflexes frequently accompanies the use of vincristine and vinblastine. Loss of the reflex in itself causes no problem for the client. However, gait abnormalities, gross or fine motor uncoordination, footdrop, or slurred speech while clients are taking plant alkaloids may indicate neurologic toxicity of the drug. If neurologic toxicity is suspected, use of the drug is discontinued.

Dizziness or light-headedness may be experienced with any of the anemias. If the blood loss has been gradual, extending over weeks or months, the client's body may have adapted to the decreased oxygen-carrying capacity of the blood. Gradual blood loss does not cause the fluid volume deficits that occur in sudden major hemorrhage. Clients who have idiopathic thrombocytopenic purpura or leukemia with profound thrombocytopenia may have an altered consciousness level because of a cerebral hemorrhage.

CARDIOVASCULAR AND RESPIRATORY CHANGES Clients with anemia can have tachycardia, palpitations, or chest pain. They may even seek medical treatment because of congestive heart failure. The degree of effect of the anemia on the cardiovascular system is related to the amount and the rapidity of blood loss. With the chronic anemias, the client may have no cardiovascular symptoms because of the body's ability to adapt to small blood losses over a long time.

Clients with anemia sometimes have shortness of breath or dyspnea, usually with exertion. Sometimes, however, clients have difficulty breathing even at rest. The effect of anemia on the respiratory system is similar to its effects on the cardiovascular system: the client's symptoms depend on the amount and the rapidity of blood loss.

GASTROINTESTINAL CHANGES Clients with disorders of the blood and blood-forming organs frequently have gastrointestinal symptoms. Some symptoms such as anorexia, nausea, and vomiting are relatively nonspecific to the disease process, whereas other symptoms pinpoint the hematologic deficit. For example, clients with chronic iron deficiency may report difficulty swallowing due to atrophy of the oral mucous membrane. The sore tongue of clients with certain anemias or vitamin deficiencies was discussed earlier, as was the anorexia of clients with gingival oozing or epistaxis.

Ulcerations of the oral mucosa or the mucosa elsewhere in the gastrointestinal tract can result from the side effects of chemotherapeutic agents used in the treatment of the leukemias and the lymphomas, placing clients at risk for bleeding, infection, and changes in elimination. Clients who are immunosuppressed are more likely to have infections of the oral mucosa such as candidiasis. Clients taking Vinca alkaloids may also be constipated.

DRUG USE AND CHEMICAL AND RADIATION EXPOSURE Because many drugs interfere with normal hematologic function, the history should make note of any prescribed or over-the-counter (OTC) medications the client takes. Antineoplastic drugs as well as some antibiotics such as chloramphenicol cause bone marrow suppression. Sedatives, hypnotics, analgesics, laxatives, and aspirin may cause or worsen hematologic abnormalities.

The use of aspirin is so common that both the client and the nurse can overlook or disregard its significance. Aspirin reduces platelet aggregation (the ability of platelets to be called to an injury site), increasing the potential for bleeding, especially in clients with compromised hematologic function. Thus, determining the client's use of aspirin and noting when the client last used aspirin are especially important.

Alcohol consumption must also be assessed. Alcohol abuse damages the liver; liver damage alters the production of clotting factors.

Exposure to chemicals increases the incidence of hematologic disorders. Clients may come into contact with chemicals through their jobs or avocations, by living in a contaminated area, or by using certain cosmetics. At increased risk for developing hematologic disorders are clients who are continuously exposed to asbestos, asphalt, industrial dyes, lead, and dry-cleaning fluid. Dyes used in fabrics and even on the client's own hair may cause hematologic injury. Clients living close to industrial plants are also at increased risk.

Exposure to radiation also increases the incidence of hematologic disorders. Clients who live close to nuclear power plants or work with radioactive materials may be at increased risk, as are clients who have been accidentally exposed to high amounts of radiation or purposely exposed for therapeutic purposes.

Past Health History

Allergies and preexisting medical conditions such as liver disease should be documented. Note previous diagnoses of blood disorders such as anemia or mononucleosis or gastrointestinal malabsorption problems. Determine how many and what kinds of infections the client has had. What part of the body has been affected? Do the infections recur? Do they respond to treatment? What symptoms are evident (ie, Is the temperature elevated? Is there a pattern? Does the client have night sweats?)?

Ask about the client's bleeding tendencies after injury, surgery, or dental extraction: Has the client had any problems with abnormal bleeding or bruising? The client's history of receiving blood transfusions—the number of transfusions, why they were administered, and whether there were any complications during or following the transfusion—should be documented.

Ask about the client's surgical history. Has the client had a splenectomy or surgical resection of the duodenum? Removal of the stomach and duodenum interferes with the client's ability to properly absorb vitamin B and sets the stage for a surgically induced pernicious anemia. Information about the client's postoperative healing may give clues to the client's bone marrow integrity and competence of immune response.

Diet History

The diet history may provide important clues about the causes of some hematologic disorders. Information about intake of iron, vitamin B_{12}, and folic acid may be revealed in clients' listings of the kinds of foods they eat regularly. High alcohol intake may suggest why a client has a diminished appetite or vitamin deficiencies. A diet low in foods high in iron may indicate the cause of the client's anemia; knowing that a client takes vitamin B injections suggests the possibility of pernicious anemia. Although diet history alone cannot diagnose hematologic abnormalities, it can aid in both the diagnosis and management of disorders of the blood and the blood-forming organs.

Family Health History

Certain hematologic disorders and other hematologic dysfunctions tend to run in families. The family history should include any history of anemias, jaundice, liver dysfunctions, red blood cell disorders, sickle cell disease, clotting disorders, and malignancies.

Objective Data

Physical Assessment

The collection of objective data begins with a complete physical examination, which requires the skills of inspection, palpation and, to a lesser extent, auscultation and percussion. The physical assessment is organized according to areas of the body from head to toe.

SKIN Inspection and palpation of the skin can give valuable information about the status of the client's hematologic system. Clients with hepatic or biliary disease with elevated bilirubin levels may have a hemolytic anemia (destruction of erythrocytes), which manifests itself as jaundice. Clients having reduced hemoglobin levels may be cyanotic. Clients with polycythemia vera frequently have ruddy complexions.

Color of the client's skin depends not only on the level of the client's hemoglobin but also on the amount of pigmentation in the skin. If clients have darkly pigmented skin, disorder-induced color changes may be obscured by the client's natural skin tones or hues. Hence, skin color cannot be used as the sole indicator of overall oxygenation of body tissues. To assess skin color properly in these situations, closely inspect the client's oral mucosa, conjunctivae, and the fingernail beds. Another good way to assess oxygenation to tissues without interference from skin pigmentation or hemoglobin level is to inspect the color of palmar creases. Have the client open the hand with fingers fully extended. If oxygenation to the body tissues is adequate, the palmar creases should be pink.

Clients having problems with platelets—production, life span, or function—and those with clotting-mechanism dysfunction have alterations in skin integrity that can be observed on physical examination. Frequently, the nurse observes purpura (redness), ecchymoses, or petechiae. **Ecchymoses** (hemorrhagic spots larger than petechiae) may be dark purplish, brown, yellow, or greenish, depending on the age of the lesion, and they may or may not be precipitated by a bump or injury. Lesions can be flat or elevated and may be painful or tender to palpation. Petechiae are most common when clients have disorders of platelet function, life span, or decreased platelet numbers. Petechiae can occur over any part of the skin but are most common where pressure has been applied to a body part (eg, after application of a tourniquet or blood pressure cuff). Petechiae are usually flat, nontender lesions that do not blanche with pressure.

Pruritus in clients with Hodgkin's disease or non-Hodgkin's lymphoma may be so severe that the skin is excoriated from scratching. Leg ulcers in clients with sickle cell anemia are most frequent over the medial and lateral malleoli. Ulcerations may be present at the time of the physical examination, or the nurse may observe healed scars over the lower extremities.

EYES Jaundice of the sclera may accompany jaundice of the skin. Retinal or scleral hemorrhages may be observed with thrombocytopenia. Conjunctival pallor can be seen in many of the anemias.

MOUTH Tissue oxygenation also may be assessed using the gingivae of the mouth as the guide. With optimal tissue oxygenation, the gingivae appear pink, but pallor indicates inadequate oxygenation. The tongues of clients with pernicious anemia and iron deficiency anemia may be smooth. Nutritional deficits, in general, may cause the tongue to become red and smooth (see Chapter 6).

Bleeding or oozing from the gums or teeth may occur in any client having a bleeding disorder, whether due to platelet abnormalities or clotting-factor deficiencies. Infections and lesions of the oral mucosa frequently develop in clients with leukopenia. Inspect the client's mouth daily, noting any of these alterations in skin integrity.

LYMPH NODES The lymph nodes make up part of the lymphoreticular system, which is responsible for the body's defense against invading pathogens. Lymph node enlargement is frequent among clients with hematologic and lymphoreticular disorders, particularly malignant ones. During palpation it is important to note whether the lymph nodes are enlarged, mobile or fixed, tender or painless.

THORAX Sternal tenderness or pain upon palpation may accompany the leukemias and the lymphomas in the presence of a mediastinal mass. Auscultation of heart sounds may reveal tachycardia and cardiac murmurs if the client is severely anemic. The tachycardia and murmur usually resolve following the administration of packed red blood cells.

Auscultation of the lungs may reveal diminished or absent breath sounds that may be related to a malignant pleural effusion or tumor obstruction. The presence of adventitious sounds (described in Chapter 5) may indicate pulmonary bleeding, pulmonary edema, or pneumonia. Decreased diaphragmatic excursion (movement) may be due to splenomegaly or hepatomegaly.

ABDOMEN Clients with disorders of the blood and blood-forming organs frequently have hepatomegaly, splenomegaly, or both. An increase in liver size, with or without tenderness, is a significant finding in the blood disorders. The spleen normally is not palpable in the adult. The finding of splenomegaly in an adult is significant because splenomegaly is present in many hematologic disorders.

NERVOUS SYSTEM Clients with vitamin B_{12} deficiency, such as those with pernicious anemia, can have neurologic dysfunction manifested as cerebral, spinal cord, or peripheral nerve involvement. Leukemic clients with meningeal involvement may have headache, visual impairment, or cranial nerve involvement. Clients who have neutropenia or thrombocytopenia may have neurologic dysfunction due to CNS infection or bleeding.

Diagnostic Studies

COMPLETE BLOOD COUNT WITH DIFFERENTIAL The complete blood count (CBC) with white blood cell (WBC) differential (Diff) is one of the most important tests for evaluating the status of the client's hematologic system; the CBC with Diff provides a measure of the blood's ability to carry and transport oxygen (erythrocyte measurements) and to resist invading infectious organisms (leukocyte measurements).

The CBC erythrocyte measurements consist of a red blood cell count, hemoglobin, hematocrit, various erythrocyte indices (such as mean corpuscular volume, mean corpuscular hemoglobin, and mean corpuscular hemoglobin concentration), and a stained red cell examination (film or peripheral blood smear). The CBC leukocyte measurement includes a WBC count. In addition to the total WBC count, the CBC with Diff determines the various types of leukocyte cells (neutrophils, basophils, eosinophils, lymphocytes, and monocytes).

RED BLOOD CELL COUNT The red blood cell count (RBC), or erythrocyte count, is the measurement of the number of erythrocytes circulating in 1 μL of whole blood. Factors or disease states that result in an elevation of the erythrocyte count are high altitude; hemoconcentration resulting from shock, trauma, or hemorrhage; anoxia; and polycythemia vera. The erythrocyte count may be decreased in anemia, Hodgkin's disease, or the leukemias.

HEMOGLOBIN Hemoglobin (Hb) is the main component of the erythrocyte or RBC. Disease states or pathologic conditions that contribute to an elevation in the hemoglobin level include polycythemia or erythrocytosis, hemoconcentration in shock or immediately after hemorrhage, and high altitude. Hemoglobin levels are decreased in anemia resulting from increased blood destruction or decreased RBC production.

HEMATOCRIT The hematocrit (Hct) or packed cell volume (PCV) measures the percentage of a given volume of whole blood occupied by erythrocytes. Disorders that result in an elevated hematocrit are polycythemia vera and hemoconcentration from shock, surgery, or hemorrhage. A decrease in hematocrit can be caused by anemia resulting from diminished blood production or increased red blood cell destruction, the leukemias, and the lymphomas. If hematocrit is done separately from the CBC, a sample of blood may be obtained by a finger prick.

ERYTHROCYTE INDICES The erythrocyte indices are three different values that examine the size, weight, and hemoglobin content of the average erythrocyte. These three values—mean corpuscular volume (MCV), mean corpuscular hemoglobin (MCH), and mean corpuscular hemoglobin concentration (MCHC)—reflect red cell morphology. Abnormalities in the erythrocyte indices in conjunction with the stained red cell examination provide a way of classifying anemias and suggesting their possible causes.

STAINED RED CELL EXAMINATION The stained blood smear is examined to determine abnormalities in the size, shape, or structure of erythrocytes as well as the staining properties. This microscopic examination helps in the diagnosis of anemia, leukemia, and thalassemia and in determining harmful effects of chemotherapy and radiation.

WHITE BLOOD CELL COUNT AND DIFFERENTIAL The total WBC count, or leukocyte count, determines the number of circulating white blood cells in 1 μL of whole blood. An elevated WBC (or leukocytosis) can accompany anoxia, anemia, infections, mononucleosis, the leukemias, polycythemia vera, and transfusion reactions and may also occur immediately following trauma or hemorrhage. Leukopenia, or a decreased WBC, may accompany agranulocytosis, anemia, hypersplenism, and the leukemias.

The differential WBC count (Diff) determines the distribution of the kinds of WBCs. The Diff count is usually reported in percentages, which should add up to 100. The Diff classifies leukocytes as monocytes, lymphocytes, or granulocytes. Granulocytes are further classified as neutrophils, eosinophils, or basophils. Neutrophils are divided into and reported as either banded (a juvenile form) or segmented (the mature neutrophil). The Diff not only reports leukocyte morphology but also identifies and reports immature or atypical leukocytes. An increase in the number of immature leukocytes is often called "a shift to the left."

ERYTHROCYTE SEDIMENTATION RATE The erythrocyte sedimentation rate (ESR) is the rate at which erythrocytes in anticoagulated whole blood settle to the bottom of a tube. The ESR's great value is to indicate the presence of an active inflammatory disease process. The ESR is elevated in leukemia, malignant lymphoma, Hodgkin's disease, severe anemia, and agranulocytosis but may be within the normal range in polycythemia.

RETICULOCYTE COUNT The reticulocyte count is considered the most useful test in the evaluation of anemia and is a good index of effective erythropoiesis and bone marrow response to anemia. Reticulocytes are nonnucleated, immature RBCs capable of oxygen transport. They remain in the blood for 24 to 48 hours, after which they are mature. An elevated reticulocyte count, or reticulocytosis, occurs in disease states or conditions that cause a relative anoxic or hypoxic state in the client. A decreased reticulocyte count, or reticulocytopenia, occurs in disease states or conditions in which the bone marrow's ability to respond to hypoxic or anoxic states by an outpouring of reticulocytes has been impaired.

PLATELET COUNT The platelet count measures the number of circulating platelets, or thrombocytes, per μL of whole blood. Platelet values may be altered by many of the disorders of the blood and blood-forming organs. Thrombocytosis is an elevation in the number of platelets. Decreased platelets is called thrombocytopenia. Platelets are usually reported as adequate, low adequate, or high adequate.

BLEEDING TIME The bleeding time, a test that records the duration of active bleeding, provides information on vascular response to injury and helps to evaluate platelet function. The two principal methods of performing the bleeding time are Duke's and Ivy's methods. In Duke's method, bleeding time is measured by observing active bleeding after a puncture on one of the client's ear lobes. Ivy's method, preferred because it is less liable to variation among testers, measures the bleeding time after two small punctures on the client's forearm. Pressure is applied by inflating a blood pressure cuff up to 40 mm Hg. The client's bleeding time may be prolonged in any of the leukemias, asplastic anemia, disseminated intravascular coagulation (DIC), idiopathic thrombocytopenic purpura, infectious mononucleosis, multiple myeloma, and pernicious anemia.

TOURNIQUET TEST The tourniquet test, or Rumpel–Leede capillary fragility test, measures capillary strength and may be used to identify platelet defects or deficiencies. It is, however, one of the least scientific of the coagulation studies. This test utilizes a blood pressure cuff inflated to midway between the systolic and diastolic pressures (to a maximum of 100 mm Hg) and sustained for 5 minutes. The number of petechiae on the forearm within a 5 cm circle at least 1 in from the cuff are then counted.

CLOT RETRACTION TEST Clot retraction estimates the quantity and quality of platelets and fibrinogen. A clot normally retracts or pulls away partially from the sides of a test tube in 1 to 2 hours, and completely retracts in 12 to 24 hours, expressing serum as it shrinks. When platelet numbers are low, platelet quality is poor, or fibrinogen level low or poorly functioning, clot retraction is slowed. This test can be useful in the diagnosis of disorders of platelet dysfunction or deficiency and in diseases involving low fibrinogen levels or increased destruction of fibrinogen. Examples of these disorders are the acute leukemias, the thrombocytopenias, hypofibrinogenemia, and aplastic anemia.

PROTHROMBIN TIME Prothrombin time (PT) evaluates stages II and III in the coagulation cascade. An increased PT may be present in the acute leukemias, DIC, factor VII or X deficiency, polycythemia vera, and multiple myeloma. This test is also used to regulate warfarin therapy.

PARTIAL THROMBOPLASTIN TIME The partial thromboplastin time (PTT) is a general evaluation of the entire coagulation system except for factors VII, XIII, and platelets and can also be used to regulate heparin therapy. A prolonged PTT can occur in DIC and in deficiencies of factors V, VIII, IX, X, XI, or XII.

SERUM FERRITIN LEVEL Serum ferritin determinations evaluate the amount of iron stored in body tissues. Depleted iron supplies depress the synthesis of ferritin. Clients with iron deficiency anemia, have decreased serum ferritin levels. The test helps to distinguish between iron deficiency anemia and anemias associated with chronic disease.

TOTAL IRON-BINDING CAPACITY Total iron-binding capacity (TIBC) measures the amount of available transferrin (a protein that binds with iron and transports it throughout the body) in the blood. TIBC increases as iron levels and iron stores decrease. Elevated TIBC is found in iron deficiency states, infancy, pregnancy, and blood loss. Decreased TIBC is found in iron overload states such as hemochromatosis, pernicious anemia, and blood transfusion overload.

BONE MARROW EXAMINATION Examination of the client's bone marrow, one of the most common hematologic diagnostic tests, provides information about the character, integrity, and production of the client's erythrocytes, leukocytes, and thrombocytes. Bone marrow examination can be done either by aspiration or biopsy.

Bone marrow aspiration is usually performed when only a small amount (less than 5 mL) of marrow is needed for diagnosis. Bone marrow aspiration is used to diagnose and evaluate clients having any of the anemias, the acute leukemias, neutropenia, or thrombocytopenia and as part of the staging process for some of the solid tumor malignancies such as Hodgkin's disease, multiple myeloma, and non-Hodgkin's lymphoma. *Bone marrow biopsy,* a surgical procedure usually performed under local anesthesia, is done when a larger amount of bone marrow is required to aid diagnosis or evaluation. The most common sites for bone marrow examination in the adult are the sternum and the iliac crest (especially the posterior iliac crest).

NURSING IMPLICATIONS Bone marrow aspiration is routinely performed in clients' rooms or in a treatment room on the nursing unit. Teach clients and their families about the reasons for the aspiration and describe what to expect. In particular, prepare the client for a sharp but brief pain (suction pain) when bone marrow is aspirated into the syringe.

For a *bone marrow aspiration* using the iliac crest, the client should be lying on either side with hips and knees flexed at 90° angles if the anterior iliac crest is used, or prone if the posterior iliac crest is used. When the sternum is used for sampling, the client can be supine. The skin site for puncture is prepared in a circular fashion using an iodine cleansing agent, and the overlying skin, subcutaneous tissue, and periosteum are anesthetized. When anesthesia is obtained, an aspiration needle with stylet is advanced through the skin and tissue until it meets bone. Penetration of the periosteum requires a twisting motion. As the aspirate is withdrawn into a syringe, clients may experience the suction pain and hear a crunching or grinding sound. To avoid mechanical injury, clients must hold completely still during the aspiration. This may be difficult for some. Be prepared to support them emotionally and gently restrain them when necessary. Once the bone marrow sample is obtained, the needle is removed, and immediate pressure is applied using a sterile gauze sponge. When hemostasis is assured, an adhesive bandage or small sterile dressing should be applied. A pressure dressing may be used if the client is prone to bleeding or is thrombocytopenic. Encourage clients to resume the same kinds of activities they were performing before aspiration. Analgesic medication is usually not indicated following the procedure. Assess the aspiration site for signs of hemorrhage and for symptoms and signs of infection.

For *bone marrow biopsy,* a small incision (3 mm to 4 mm) is made through the skin overlying the bone to be used, and a wedge specimen or a large needle specimen of bone marrow is obtained. Clients undergoing an open biopsy may require analgesic medication. Care of the incision includes keeping it clean and dry and assessing the wound for symptoms and signs of hemorrhage or infection. Clients are usually able to resume their normal activities following the biopsy but are asked to leave the dressing in place and avoid getting it wet for 48 hours.

LYMPHANGIOGRAPHY Lymphangiography is the radiographic examination of the lymphatic system. Radiopaque dye is injected into the lymphatic chains in the client's feet. First, a blue dye to stain the lymphatic vessels is injected intradermally between each of the first three toes of each foot. The dorsum of each foot is then anesthetized. An incision is made into the dorsum of the foot between the second and third toes, and the lymph nodes are identified and isolated. The lymphatic chain is then cannulated, and the radiopaque dye is injected. X-ray films (lymphangiograms) are taken immediately and as the contrast dye moves up the lymphatic chain to the level of the third and fourth lumbar vertebrae. A second set of films is taken 24 hours later when the contrast medium has filled the lymph nodes. The dye remains in the lymphatic chains up to 6 months following its initial injection, so subsequent x-rays and follow-up can determine disease status without the need to repeat dye injection. Lymphangiography is performed for clients with edema due to an obstruction in lymphatic drainage and for clients suspected of having Hodgkin's disease or non-Hodgkin's lymphoma.

Normally, the lymphatic system shows complete filling with the dye on the initial set of films. Twenty-four hours later, the lymph nodes are shown as opaque, well-defined nodes. With a metastatic process, filling defects and lack of opacification are demonstrated. Primary lymphedema shows fewer shortened lymphatic vessels on x-ray films. Secondary lymphedema appears as abruptly terminating vessels.

NURSING IMPLICATIONS Client and family education is the primary responsibility of the nurse. The procedure is lengthy, ranging from as little as 2 hours to as long as 8 hours, depending on the skill of the radiologist and the ease with which the lymphatic chain is identified and isolated. Clients must lie supine and hold completely still.

When clients are returned to the nursing unit after the procedure, the incisions on the dorsum of the feet should be observed for symptoms and signs of bleeding, infection, and inflammation. Clients may resume normal activities but must keep their feet dry. Clients should not get their feet wet when bathing until after the sutures are removed—usually about 5 days after the procedure. Pain or discomfort at the incision sites ordinarily does not require analgesic medication nor interfere with ambulation. To minimize discomfort that could result from shoes rubbing against the incisions, clients should wear soft shoes, such as moccasins or slippers.

Although expected, one of the most alarming side effects of the lymphangiogram is a bluish green discoloration on the dorsal skin of the feet, in the urine, and in the veins of the lower extremities. Some clients have even reported that their feces turn bluish green. This color change may last from 2 to 5 days, depending on the individual client's rate of excretion of the dye. The bluish green discolorations are expected and predictable; they indicate that the client is adequately excreting the dye. Tell clients about the color change to allay their anxiety.

SECTION 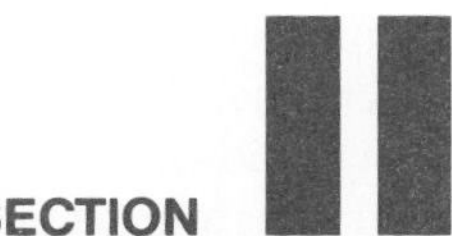

Nursing Diagnosis/Planning and Implementation/Evaluation

Information gathered from the client's health history, physical examination, and diagnostic studies is used to determine nursing diagnoses and the plan of care. Not every client will have the same needs. The Nursing Diagnosis box lists diagnoses **directly related** to disorders of the blood and blood-forming organs along with **potential** diagnoses for clients with problems of the blood and blood-forming organs. The most common nursing diagnoses for clients with disorders of the blood and blood-forming organs include altered comfort: pain; impaired gas exchange; impaired physical mobility; impaired skin integrity; potential for infection; altered nutrition: less than body requirements; knowledge deficit; and ineffective individual and family coping. All of these diagnoses are discussed in the content that follows. The sample nursing care plan in Table 22–1 focuses on altered comfort: pain; altered nutrition; and ineffective coping.

If the goals of care have not been met, reevaluation is required. The nurse and client should jointly review the nursing care plan. New objectives may need to be formulated; other nursing interventions may be added or modified; or the evaluation may show that more time is required to meet the objectives.

Comfort, Altered: Pain

In Hodgkin's disease, pain results from pressure by the enlarged lymph nodes on normal tissue. In the leukemias, chloromas (localized congregations of leukemic cells within organs and tissues) may cause pressure and pain. In clotting disorders, bleeding into a joint or body cavity may cause pain. Hyperuricemia, which frequently accompanies malignant disorders, may precipitate a goutlike joint pain.

Planning and Implementation

Touch denotes acceptance and caring to most clients. Back rubs should be given, keeping this principle in mind. Back rubs also improve circulation and promote relaxation. The amount and quality of the time the nurse spends with the client daily assist in fostering a trusting nurse–client relationship. Trust creates a bond that promotes comfort.

Clients with blood disorders may be so anxious that their perception of pain is heightened. Antianxiety drugs may aid in the overall plan to promote client comfort.

Nonpharmacologic measures that may promote comfort should be used as much as possible. Clients should be encouraged to keep up interests they pursue when not hospitalized. Some clients have sedentary vocations or avocations (eg, paperwork, sketching, knitting) that can be done while hospitalized. These interests and activities may serve as distractions from pain.

Clients undergoing chemotherapy or radiation may have ulcerations in the mouth and along the GI tract to the rectum. Provide good mouth care by using nonalcoholic-based mouth rinses and gentle teeth cleansing by using soft-bristled brushes or sponge or gauze tooth cleaners. A soft diet may relieve the discomfort of oral ulcerations. Topical anesthetics may be used as needed and before meals to decrease the discomfort associated with mastication when ulcers are present. Rectal discomfort of ulceration can be relieved by providing meticulous perineal care and sitz baths and relieving diarrhea or preventing constipation.

Evaluation

Clients will remain as pain free as possible and be able to perform their own activities of daily living independently, when appropriate. Elicit clients' subjective statements about their pain and examine clients' vital signs, noting especially any tachycardia, tachypnea, or rise in systolic blood pressure above baseline measurements. Clients having pain frequently demonstrate nonverbal clues in response to painful stimuli (eg, facial grimacing, diaphoresis, and muscle tension). The response the nurse sees depends largely on the client's attitudes toward pain.

Gas Exchange, Impaired

Any interference with normal erythrocyte production, function, or activity may impair oxygen transport and exchange to body tissues. In any anemic client, the oxygen-carrying capacity of the blood is reduced by a low hemoglobin concentration or a decreased number of circulating erythrocytes or both. Gas exchange may be impaired in disease processes disrupting coagulation. Whether the bleeding is caused by a coagulation abnormality, or by thrombocytopenia, blood loss may be severe enough that the oxygen-carrying capacity of the blood is diminished or impaired.

NURSING DIAGNOSES IN
Disorders of Blood and Blood-Forming Organs

DIRECTLY RELATED DIAGNOSES

- Comfort, altered: pain
- Coping, ineffective family: disabling
- Coping, ineffective individual
- Gas exchange, impaired
- Infection, potential for
- Knowledge deficit
- Mobility, impaired physical
- Nutrition, altered: less than body requirements
- Skin integrity, impaired: potential

OTHER POTENTIAL DIAGNOSES

- Activity intolerance
- Adjustment, impaired
- Grieving, anticipatory
- Powerlessness
- Self-concept, disturbance in: body image
- Sexuality patterns, altered
- Social interaction, impaired
- Tissue integrity, impaired: oral mucous membranes

Planning and Implementation

The interventions for both anemia and bleeding problems are geared toward increasing the total oxygen-carrying capacity of the client's blood. Nursing intervention begins with a review of the results of the most recent blood work. This information provides a basis for planning care and developing observational criteria.

The nurse's assessments of clients' responses to decreases in oxygen-carrying capacity are important. Assess clients' skin color, temperature, and moisture. For example, one client will have pallor and shortness of breath with an Hb value of 9.0 g/dL, but another client with a similar Hb may be asymptomatic. It is essential to listen to clients' statements about shortness of breath or difficulty in breathing, headache, and dizziness. Monitor the client's vital signs, especially noting changes reflecting decreased oxygen-carrying capacity such as tachycardia and tachypnea and orthostatic hypotension. Note the client's tolerance to activity and adjust the client's activity level appropriately. With impaired gas exchange, the client needs to have balanced periods of rest and activity and may need assistance to complete activities of daily living.

When the client is receiving a transfusion, be alert for possible allergic reactions and administer antihistamines before transfusion, if necessary. Clients receiving transfusion therapy need to be educated about the use of blood products (see Section III in this chapter).

Besides transfusion therapy, clients may also require iron supplements and an iron-rich diet to enhance the formation of hemoglobin. Client education must accompany the use of iron supplements and food sources rich in iron (see Chapter 23). In general, self-medication with OTC iron supplements should be discouraged.

Oxygen therapy may be administered to further promote gas exchange. Elevating the head of the client's bed facilitates downward movement of the diaphragm, allows greater lung expansion, and increases the volume of air taken into the lungs, promoting better gas exchange.

Evaluation

Clients who are exchanging gas optimally are not fatigued or weak; have vital signs within the normal limits established for them; remain oriented to time, place, and person; and have skin that is pink, warm, and dry. Determine whether other factors influence this goal. For example, sleep deprivation or nutritional deficiencies may cause fatigue; infection may elevate the body temperature; hypovolemia may decrease the blood pressure; and orientation to time, place, and person may be affected by drugs.

Physical Mobility, Impaired

Fatigue, weakness, or dyspnea on exertion (DOE) may accompany the anemias; the client may limit physical movement to avoid these symptoms. In bleeding disorders, such as idiopathic thrombocytopenic purpura, actual bleeding into the joints may destroy joints, with loss of joint motion and function. Pain may also limit the client's mobility.

Planning and Implementation

Problems of immobility must be counteracted by range-of-motion (ROM) exercises and frequent position changes. If clients cannot perform active ROM, the nurse should initiate and perform passive ROM. A physical therapist may help clients maintain mobility. Ambulation of the client as soon as possible, within limits, is important to prevent the hazards of immobility. To prevent pulmonary involvement caused by immobility, encourage the client to turn, cough, and deep-breathe.

Because pain severely alters clients' tolerance to movement, plan a course of action to minimize pain and maximize mobility. For instance, activity in a client with multiple myeloma reverses the negative calcium balance caused by skeletal degeneration and can prevent spinal cord compression. An effective analgesia regimen will facilitate mobility.

Evaluation

The plan of care is effective when the client is able to tolerate increases in activity without undue fatigue and gradually resume self-care.

Table 22–1
Sample Nursing Care Plan for Clients With Disorders of the Blood and Blood-Forming Organs, by Nursing Diagnosis

Client Care Goals	Plan/Nursing Implementation	Expected Outcome
Comfort, altered: pain related to disease process		
Remain comfortable throughout the therapy and the disease process	Administer analgesics for pain p.r.n. as ordered (nonaspirin products); aid pain relief by comfortable positioning of client; aid client in position changes; use pillows for support and change position q. 2h; provide good mouth care: mouthwashes, gentle teeth care, and soft diet to relieve discomfort of oral ulcerations; use topical anesthetics p.r.n. and a.c.; relieve rectal and anal discomfort from ulceration by providing meticulous perineal care, sitz bath, and preventing constipation and relieving diarrhea; use distraction and diversional activities; offer antianxiety agents; gently rub back; spend unhurried time with client every day	Clients will remain pain free, will independently perform own ADLs when appropriate, will state they are comfortable; skin warm and dry; relaxed body posture; vital signs within normal limits
Nutrition, altered: less than body requirements related to inadequate intake		
Maintain optimum nutritional status	Initiate dietary consult; inquire about client's food preferences, remembering that neutropenic clients are not allowed fresh fruits and vegetables because of potential infection; offer small, frequent feedings; avoid temperature extremes in foods served if oral ulcers present; serve meals attractively and remove unpleasant stimuli from surroundings at mealtime; assist client in selecting easily chewed foods that meet requirements from the basic four food groups; maintain daily calorie count; weigh client q.d; administer antiemetics when client is receiving chemotherapy—do not wait until client becomes nauseated or vomits before giving the antiemetic; perform oral hygiene daily using soft toothbrush/gauze/sponges for oral care; note condition and integrity of ginginvae, buccal mucosa, tongue; observe characteristics of saliva (ie, thin, abundant or stringy, scant); encouarge frequent rinsing of mouth with cool water to keep mucous membranes moist; apply lubricant to lips as needed	Eat ¾ of meals, snacks served; maintain stable weight; feel energetic
Coping, ineffective individual related to disease process		
Individual regains sense of control	Establish therapeutic relationship between client and nurse; spend "quality" time with client every day; answer questions honestly but do not destroy client's defense mechanisms—allow client to express denial; assess client's coping ability, note any clues to ineffective coping (eg, giddiness/inappropriate joking about diagnosis, reluctance to begin learning about home	Make decisions about health care and ask questions about disease process; open lines of communication between nurse and client, and client and family

(continued)

Table 22–1
Sample Nursing Care Plan for Clients With Disorders of the Blood and Blood-Forming Organs, by Nursing Diagnosis, continued

Client Care Goals	Plan/Nursing Implementation	Expected Outcome
	care needs) and effective coping (eg, asking questions regarding illness, alterations in lifestyle from illness, denial, crying, asking questions about death/dying)	
Coping, ineffective family: disabling related to conflicting coping styles		
Expresses unresolved feelings	Establish therapeutic relationship between significant others and nurse; spend "quality" time with family every day; answer questions honestly but do not destroy family's defense mechanisms; assess family's coping ability, note any clues to ineffective coping (eg, giddiness/inappropriate joking about diagnosis, reluctance to begin learning about home care needs) and effective coping (eg, asking questions regarding illness, alterations in lifestyle from illness, denial, crying, asking questions about death/dying	Assist in decision making about client's health care; ask questions about disease process; open lines of communication between client and family

Skin Integrity, Impaired and Infection, Potential for

Whenever leukocyte production, function, or activity is interfered with or interrupted, the client has an increased risk for developing infection. Clients with leukemia, lymphoma, Hodgkin's disease, and multiple myeloma are likely to undergo chemotherapy or radiation therapy at some point during their illnesses. These treatments leave the client leukopenic. The oral and gastric mucosa are sites of irritation and ulceration from chemotherapy. These sites may be portals of entry for potentially harmful microorganisms.

Planning and Implementation

Clients with blood disorders are predisposed to pressure ulcer formation and poor wound healing. When clients are on prolonged bed rest, frequent turning and positioning are essential. Continued assessment of the skin for redness on body prominences and pressure areas is required along with good skin care techniques and ambulation, when possible. Evaluate the oral mucosa each day and every 8 hours in clients who are neutropenic or thrombocytopenic. The use of soft-bristled toothbrushes or cotton swabs, as well as the use of soothing nonalcohol mouthwashes every 2 to 4 hours, should be recommended for mouth care. Tell these clients not to use toothpicks or dental floss.

Manage predisposition to infection by monitoring the client's vital signs, especially the temperature, every 4 hours. At the first sign of infection, obtain blood, urine, throat, and stool cultures for the identification of the organism. Because these clients may lack the ability to form pus or may have an altered ability to produce an inflammatory response, the typical symptoms and signs of infection may be absent. Therefore, it is important always to listen to the client's concerns. Antibiotic therapy will be administered whenever infection is suspected; the dosage may be high. Toxic reactions to antibiotic therapy need to be assessed. Look for electrolyte abnormalities such as hypokalemia, hypomagnesemia, and hypocalcemia; oliguria; hearing loss, and the more common symptoms of nausea, vomiting, and diarrhea. Granulocytes may be ordered as supportive therapy when the client's total WBC is exceedingly low.

It is important that both nurse and client practice good hand-washing. Isolation of the client is controversial. The client should be educated to avoid contact with individuals with known infections, with recently immunized individuals, and with large crowds.

Evaluation

The plan of care is effective when the client's skin is intact. The client with a normal temperature is probably free of infection.

Nutrition, Altered: Less Than Body Requirements

Anorexia, nausea, vomiting, and weight loss may accompany antineoplastic drug treatment of the blood disorder, further compromising and altering the client's nutritional status. Stomatitis, mucositis, or other oral lesions may limit the client's ability to chew and swallow food in adequate amounts. Alterations in the client's sense of taste may make mealtime and eating unpleasant.

Whereas clients with malignant disorders have general nutritional deficits, clients with anemia have nutrient deficiencies specific to the anemia. For example, clients having iron deficiency anemia have different nutritional needs than those with pernicious anemia. Nutritional support for each of these clients must take into account the individual's deficiency.

Planning and Implementation

Nursing interventions should promote optimal nutritional intake. Seek the advice and suggestions of a nutritionist. Subtle weight losses may go undetected, so it is advisable to weigh the client daily. Inquire about the client's food preferences, recalling that fresh fruits and vegetables may not be allowed for severely neutropenic clients because these food items are a potential source of infection. Clients should be offered small, frequent feedings to avoid expending unnecessary energy while eating and digesting meals. Meals should be served attractively; unpleasant stimuli, such as bedpans and emesis basins, should be removed in an attempt to entice the client to eat.

For clients with oral ulcerations, avoid temperature extremes in foods served. Warm or cool foods are better than hot or cold ones. Choose foods that are easily chewed and meet the requirements of the basic four food groups. Performing oral hygiene before meals stimulates the secretion of the salivary glands, the first step in digestion.

Clients receiving chemotherapy frequently experience nausea and vomiting which can be effectively controlled, in most clients, with antiemetic medication. The antiemetic should be administered before chemotherapy and subsequently on a regular schedule until the client is nausea free. An as-necessary regimen usually does not curb nausea effectively. In any case, try to anticipate the client's needs and do not wait until the client becomes nauseated or vomits before giving the ordered antiemetic.

Evaluation

Expected outcomes indicating clients are getting adequate nutrition include subjective statements about the way they feel, the amount of food they eat daily, and their weight. Clients who are improving or maintaining an optimum nutritional status should feel energetic, eat at least three-fourths of the food offered, and maintain a stable weight or, in the case of improving nutritional status, gain weight.

Knowledge Deficit

Clients with disorders of the blood and blood-forming organs often do not know much about the disease process and treatment programs. This group of disorders is complex and may seem overwhelming to clients and their significant others. Clients must understand the disease process, the function of the blood-cell components, medications, and symptoms and signs indicating a need for medical and nursing interventions in order to be able to knowledgeably participate in their own care.

Planning and Implementation

Encourage both the client and significant others to become involved in all health teaching sessions. Listen to the client and significant others discuss fears and anxieties, and support them when they ask questions. Assess their ability and readiness to learn. Remember to teach at the client's level of understanding when the client is ready. General content may include the disease process, functions of the blood cells, and the treatment regimen. It is always helpful to list symptoms and signs that indicate a need for medical or nursing intervention.

Remember that all clients need review and reinforcement of content taught. Once diagnosed, clients with blood disorders are taught about the disease process, pharmacologic and dietary management, home care management, alterations in lifestyle, and the symptoms and signs that warrant immediate intervention. The amount of information given to the client in a relatively short period is enormous and often overwhelming. It is unrealistic to expect the client to comprehend and manage this large amount of information and the associated instructions during one hospitalization period or clinic visit. Continual reassessment of the client's knowledge level and reteaching when indicated are essential nursing functions. Consider providing phone numbers for the client to call when questions arise after discharge and including outpatient caregivers in the client's care before discharge. A well thought out teaching program also promotes effective coping.

Evaluation

After implementing the teaching plan, evaluate how much clients and their families have learned. Ask clients to repeat or recall the content in their own words. Observing clients making decisions about their health care based upon principles of content taught suggests that they have learned. Clients' stating that they feel comfortable about the prospect of going home, or at least look forward to going home, indicates that self-care and home management of the disorder are not troublesome to them because they have learned how to manage their health problem.

Coping, Ineffective Individual and Coping, Ineffective Family: Disabling

Clients with blood disorders may have to alter their lifestyles temporarily or permanently. These alterations may require that the client learn new coping methods.

For the adult client with leukemia, the poor long-term

prognosis is the issue facing the client and family. Grieving may accompany the diagnosis, and the client and family may begin to cope ineffectively. The client may try to be strong for the family's sake, and the family may be overly solicitous toward the client. Clients with disorders like Hodgkin's disease, which primarily affects young individuals, may be anxious and fearful about whether they can attain career and personal goals and about the effect of antineoplastic agents on future fertility. Clients may be anxious about diagnostic procedures because they lack knowledge or have misconceptions about what will happen to them.

Planning and Implementation

Initially, the nurse needs to establish a therapeutic relationship with the client and significant others. Spend "quality" time with the client each day. This may involve planning a 15-minute period of each day with the client, doing whatever the client wishes.

Assess the client's and family's coping ability. Note any clues to ineffective coping, such as giddiness or inappropriate joking about the diagnosis. Effective coping may be demonstrated when the client asks questions about the illness or alterations in lifestyle imposed by the disorder.

Honesty promotes trust and aids the establishment and maintenance of a therapeutic nurse–client relationship. Temper this principle with knowledge about the protective qualities of defense mechanisms. Answer the client's questions honestly but without destroying the client's defense mechanisms. This balance is difficult to achieve, because defense mechanisms may be the client's or family's only method of coping with the disease process. Demonstrate acceptance of the defense mechanisms and support the client's attempts to cope positively with the illness. An example is the client with a diagnosis of leukemia who uses denial to cope with the diagnosis. Denial may serve to protect the client from a reality too difficult to face. In this situation, support the client's attempts to deal with the reality of the diagnosis, but do not destroy or take away the client's use of denial before the client has given evidence of being ready to give it up.

Evaluation

Outcomes to evaluate indicating that the client and the client's family have achieved a sense of control are the kinds of communication techniques used by the client and family, the questions they ask, and their ability to make decisions about health care. Open communication between the nurse and client, between the nurse and family, and especially between the client and family demonstrate positive coping behaviors. The fact that the client and family ask questions pertinent to the disease process and treatments prescribed indicates an attempt to deal with the altered health patterns. Clients who carefully think through decisions they make affecting their health are demonstrating effective coping mechanisms.

SECTION 

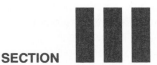

Blood and Blood Component Administration

Blood and blood components are administered primarily to provide adequate tissue oxygenation. The other purposes are to restore circulatory blood volume or to restore coagulation factors. With current methods, clients need only receive the missing components, avoiding unneeded blood products that may cause a transfusion reaction or circulatory overload. Nurses may be involved in providing care to donors as well as to recipients.

Blood Donation

Prospective blood donors are carefully screened before donating blood to protect the health and safety of both donor and recipient. Nurses often have responsibility for screening donors according to criteria established by the American Association of Blood Banks and the Centers for Disease Control.

Blood donors should be in good health, and suspicion of disease should disqualify a potential donor. Other aspects of a client's health history that will disqualify a potential donor include a history of AIDS, hepatitis, syphilis, or malaria.

A potential donor's temperature, pulse, respirations, and blood pressure should be within normal limits. Donors should be between 17 and 65 years of age and weigh at least 110 lb (50 kg) for a standard 450 mL donation. Less than the standard 450 mL is taken from donors who do not meet the weight minimum. A hemoglobin screening test should identify that the donor's hemoglobin level is within normal limits for sex.

A phlebotomy, or venesection, the rapid withdrawal of blood from a peripheral vein, is the method used to obtain blood from donors. A phlebotomy may also be a therapeutic measure for clients with polycythemia vera because it reduces the circulating blood volume and the red blood cell mass. (Polycythemia vera is discussed in Chapter 23). Phlebotomy is also sometimes used in the treatment of clients with acute pulmonary edema to reduce the venous return to the heart, decreasing congestion of the pulmonary vessels and lung capillaries. (Pulmonary edema is discussed in Chapter 19.)

All donated blood is typed and tested for the hepatitis B antigen, for specific antibodies to confirm the ABO grouping, for syphilis, and recently, for acquired immune deficiency syndrome (AIDS). Testing for exposure to AIDS in blood donors began in response to situations in which persons have contracted AIDS after blood transfusions. Detection of this antibody does not indicate that the donor has or will develop AIDS. It does mean that the donor has, at some point in time, been exposed to the AIDS virus. Blood containing this antibody is not used for donation. It is speculated that tests for exposure to the AIDS virus are not yet sophisticated enough to be able to detect its presence early. Potential donors are also screened to determine if they are at increased risk for AIDS (see Chapter 23 for a description of risk categories). Individuals found to be at risk are not considered for donation and are discouraged from donating blood in the future. Research into the development of more specific determinations of AIDS exposure is ongoing. Although the number of blood donors has decreased because donors fear contracting the disease during blood donation, this has not been proven to occur. Fear of contracting AIDS from blood transfusion has led to an increased use of autologous blood transfusion.

Administration of Blood or Blood Components

Before a transfusion, the nurse verifies the type of blood or blood component the client is to receive, the number of units to be given, the date of infusion, and the rate of infusion. Be sure also to check with the client and the client's chart for previous transfusion reactions. Clients with a history of transfusion reactions may need diphenhydramine (Benadryl) and prednisone before receiving blood.

The nurse then follows hospital policy to obtain the blood from the blood bank. The blood bank may send only one unit at a time, especially if the product requires refrigeration to prevent any breakdown of blood components. Refrigeration also decreases the risk for growth of bacteria.

Determine that the intravenous infusion was started using an 18- or 19-gauge needle. In pediatric clients or elderly clients, a 21-gauge needle can be used. Assure that the priming solution is 0.9% NaCl and that this setup remains until the transfusion is completed. The IV 0.9% NaCl provides a continuous route for flushing purposes, does not result in clotting of citrated blood, and also is necessary as a maintenance route in case of a transfusion reaction.

After obtaining the blood component, check the label on the blood bag with another nurse against the requisition form for:

- The client's name and hospital number
- The physician's name
- The client's blood group and Rh factor
- The donor's blood group and Rh factor
- VDRL (Venereal Disease Research Laboratories) results
- The expiration date

Ask the client to identify herself or himself by name and check the blood bag label against the client's identification band. Also check the bag for air bubbles or discoloration. If these conditions are present, do not use the blood and send the unit back to the blood bank.

A baseline set of vital signs should be obtained before the unit of blood is piggybacked into the 0.9% NaCl solution already hung. Figure 22–1 illustrates the equipment used. The blood should infuse slowly at first (20 to 30 drops/minute). Remain with the client for the first 15 minutes of the infusion to evaluate the client's response to the blood infusion; the symptoms of an adverse reaction usually occur during this first 15-minute period. After the first 15 minutes, the flow rate is adjusted to allow for infusion in 1 to 2 hours; if the client cannot tolerate this rate of infusion, the flow may be slowed still further. Elderly clients and clients with heart disease may need slower infusions. The rate of infusion of whole blood and red cell components should not exceed 4 hours because of the potential for bacterial growth.

To discontinue the infusion, flush the tubing with 50 mL of 0.9% NaCl and remove the IV device. Return a completed blood form with the empty blood bag wrapped in a plastic bag to the blood bank. Documentation in the client's chart should include the blood component delivered and the blood unit number, the starting and completion time, and the client's response to the transfusion.

When transfusing a client with a blood product, keep several important points in mind. No medications of any kind should be infused with the blood because of possible incompatibility and the potential for contamination. In addition, a filter is required for blood or blood-component administration to prevent infiltration of fibrin clots and other blood debris. A cryoprecipitate-platelet infusion set is used to provide for complete component infusion. If longer tubing is used for small-volume products, some of the components may be lost to the client because they are trapped in the longer tubing.

Transfusion Reactions

Whenever administering any blood or blood component, be aware that, because blood is a protein substance, it has the potential for initiating an antigen–antibody reaction (a transfusion reaction). A reaction to the delivered blood can occur even with the best type-and-crossmatch results. Be on guard whenever administering a blood product.

The types of transfusion reactions are outlined in Table 22–2. These reactions may be mild enough to go unnoticed, or they may be severe enough to result in anaphylaxis. In general, the greater the number of transfusions the client receives, the greater the risk for developing antibodies against blood or blood products. Because of the large number of transfusions received by sickle cell anemia

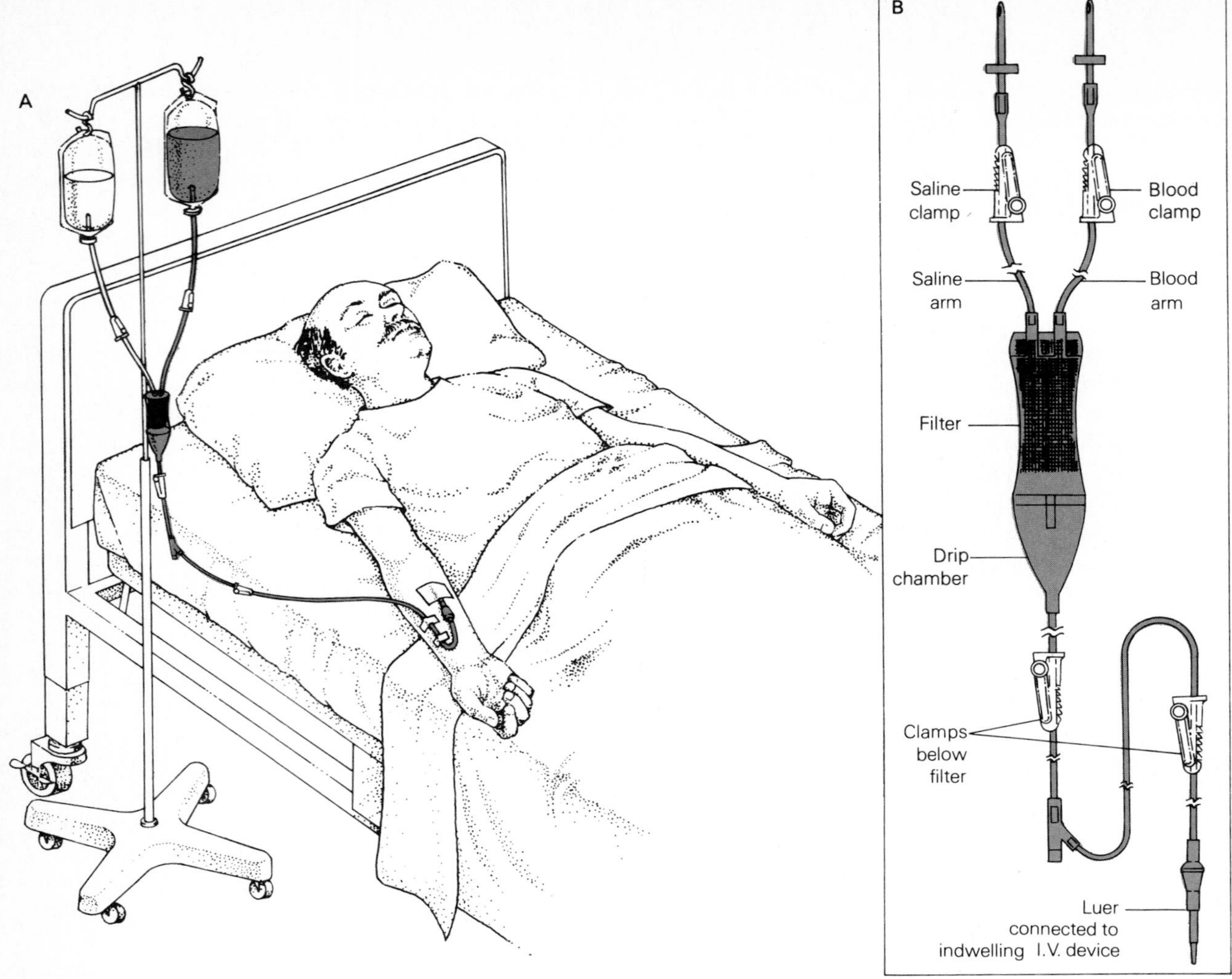

Figure 22–1

Blood or blood component administration. **A.** Client with standard Y-type blood administration set. **B.** Detail of standard Y-type blood administration set. *SOURCE: Saxton DF, et al.:* Addison-Wesley Manual of Nursing Practice. *Menlo Park, CA: Addison-Wesley, 1983.*

or oncology clients, be especially attuned to their increased risk for developing a reaction. With any reaction during a transfusion:

- Stop the infusion of blood.
- Switch the infusion to the 0.9% NaCl solution.
- Take vital signs every 5 minutes.
- Notify the physician.
- Notify the blood bank of a possible transfusion reaction.
- Obtain urine specimens for examination.
- Send the remaining blood in the blood bag back to the blood bank with the transfusion reaction form attached.

Institutions may vary in the steps to follow in a suspected transfusion reaction. This information is only a basic guideline. Become familiar with the institution's specific protocol.

Autologous Blood Transfusion (Autotransfusion)

Autotransfusion is the process for removing whole blood from a client, storing it, and then reinfusing it into the same client at a later date. Autologous transfusion has several advantages for the client who has had or will have a 1000 mL or greater blood loss. Such blood loss can occur in trauma (with massive hemorrhage) or before, during, or after cardiothoracic surgery. Autotransfusion can also be used in clients who have rare blood that is difficult to crossmatch.

The methods for collecting and reinfusing a client's own blood are: elective phlebotomy, perioperative phlebotomy, intraoperative salvage and reinfusion, postoperative mediastinal collection, and collection and reinfusion from a client with a traumatic hemothorax. The advantages, disadvantages, and contraindications for autotransfusions are outlined in Table 22–3.

Elective phlebotomy is the withdrawal of the client's own blood for use at a later date. Blood may be collected from a client scheduled for surgery up to 8 weeks before the operation, so that autologous blood is available at the time of surgery. Elective phlebotomy is also used for clients with rare blood types. Clients with rare blood types or

Table 22–2
Transfusion Reactions

Type of Reaction	Clinical Observation	Imediate Nursing Actions
Hemolytic	Immediate onset (may be delayed when Rh incompatibility involved); facial flush, burning sensation along vien, fever, chills (temperature elevation to 40.6°C [105°F] or higher); chest pain, labored respirations; headache; low-back pain; shock	Stop transfusion; noticy physician; administer oxygen, epinephrine; fluids as ordered
Allergic	Urticaria, rash, pruritus; in rare instances, asthma, pulmonary edema, facial or glottal edema; anaphylactic shock	Stop transfusion; notify physician; administer antihistamine
Febrile	Fever and chills about 1 h after start of infusion; headache, flushing, tachycardia, genreal malaise; symptoms persist for 8–10 h	Stop transfusion; notify physician; keep client covered; administer antipyretic
Bacterial	Chills and fever; hypotension; dry, flushed skin; abdominal and extremity pain; vomiting and bloody diarrhea	Stop transfusion; notify physician; administer broad-spectrum antibiotic, as ordered
Circulatory overload	Chest constriction, dyspnea, dry cough, rales at base of lung, pulmonary edema	Stop or slow transfusion; place client in sitting position; notify physician; apply rotating tourniquets, if ordered
Air embolism	Cyanosis, dyspnea, shock, cardiac arrest	Stop transfusion; lower client's head and turn client on left side (air collects in right atrium where it can be gradually released to the lungs); notify physician

SOURCE: Adapted with permission from Saxton et al: *Addison–Wesley Manual of Nursing Practice.* Menlo Park, CA: Addison–Wesley, 1983.

Table 22–3
Advantages, Disadvantages, and Contraindications to Autotransfusion

Advantages	Disadvantages	Constraindications
Reduced usage of blood from blood bank	Potential contamination with gastrointestinal secretions if abdominal wound blood used	In contamination with gastrointestinal secretions occurs
Decreased cost to client	Potential for air embolus if air not aspirated from donating system	If abdominal wound is more than 4 h old
Eliminate transfusion reaction		If there is cancerous lesion in cavity from which blood is taken
Eliminate transmission of hepatitis, syphillis, and AIDS through blood transfusion		
Avoid religious conflicts		

clients with rare antigens or antibodies who are difficult to crossmatch may have their blood frozen in case a transfusion is needed at a later date. A process of deglycerolization decreases the possibility of allergic and febrile reactions and preserves the red blood cells.

A second type of autotransfusion is perioperative phlebotomy with concomitant hemodilution. This technique is usually carried out just after the client has been anesthetized but before the surgery is performed. One or two units of blood are withdrawn while 500 to 1000 mL of crystalloid or colloid is infused.

Intraoperative salvage or reinfusion of shed blood is the third type. The blood is collected and filtered during surgery in a commercially available autotransfusion system. Anticoagulants are then added, and the blood is reinfused into the client.

Postoperative collection of blood from mediastinal tubes from cardiac surgical clients is another type of autotransfusion. An autotransfusion collection system is attached to the client's mediastinal tubes at the completion of surgery, and the blood is collected by gravitational flow. The blood from the mediastinum does not require anticoagulation because of defibrination. Defibrination occurs as a result of the mechanical action of the heart and lungs as well as contact with the pericardial surface.

Collection and reinfusion of blood in the emergency department from a client with a traumatic hemothorax can also be used as an autotransfusion. Because there is no need to anticoagulate blood collected from the chest, an autotransfusion unit that works with chest tubes is attached, and the blood is rapidly reinfused.

Apheresis

Apheresis is the process of separating whole blood into its major components—plasma, thrombocytes, erythrocytes, and leukocytes—and removing one of these components for use. Apheresis is used to replace cell components that are defective or insufficient.

Four types of apheresis may be performed. *Plasmapheresis* (plasma exchange) removes multiple liters of plasma that contain abnormal substances (ie, antigen–antibody complexes) and replaces this amount with a similar plasma solution. *Lymphapheresis* (leukapheresis), removes abnormal or excessive WBCs. *Platelet pheresis* removes abnormal or excessive platelets. *Red cell pheresis* removes abnormal or excessive erythrocytes.

Although not a cure for blood diseases, apheresis is a way of interfering with the disease process or preventing further pathophysiologic changes. Apheresis is used in conjunction with routine therapy and is a last resort to control the disease process.

Blood Substitutes

The search for a blood substitute has focused on the replacement of the oxygen-carrying capacity of erythrocytes. The experimental replacement for erythrocytes has fallen into three categories: perfluorochemicals, stroma-free hemoglobin, and oxygen-binding chelates.

Perfluorochemicals

Perfluorochemicals are synthetic compounds related to Teflon and Freon. Perfluorochemicals dissolve 40% to 60% oxygen per unit volume, approximately three times the capacity of blood, and also have a carbon-dioxide-carrying capacity three times greater than their ability to carry oxygen.

Perfluorochemical therapy requires the concomitant administration of 70% to 100% oxygen because perfluorochemicals do not extract oxygen from the air as hemoglobin does. This high oxygen administration exposes the client to oxygen toxicity (Leser, 1982). Another limitation of perfluorochemicals is the potential for thrombus formation, especially in the lungs, caused by alteration of platelet membranes. The lungs are a prime target because perfluorochemicals are excreted mainly by respiration. A third limitation is the lack of clotting factors, which are not replaced by perfluorochemicals. Infection could be a serious limitation because leukocytes are not replaced by perfluorochemical therapy. Thus, prophylactic antibiotics may need to be added to the perfluorochemicals. There is no need to crossmatch or type perfluorochemicals; because there are no antigens, they can be transfused immediately. Although frozen, refrozen, and autoclaved, perfluorochemicals will last indefinitely. There is also a decreased risk of hepatitis.

Be aware of potential spleen and liver damage by assessing for organ enlargement and enzyme change. Oxygen toxicity and lung damage, which can occur from platelet aggregation, must be assessed if the client develops a cough, nasal congestion, a sore throat, and substernal discomfort. Careful monitoring of vital signs, lab values, and wound sites aids in the detection of bleeding and infection.

Stroma-Free Hemoglobin

Stroma-free hemoglobin uses human hemoglobin stripped of the elements that clog capillaries. The substance has several advantages over other synthetic blood products: It functions well at low levels of oxygen, it has a colloidal osmotic effect and thus works as a plasma expander, it has a universal compatibility, and it can be stored indefinitely. However, it can only be obtained from human donors; when it is metabolized, iron accumulates and iron toxicity develops; it will not solve problems related to agents that are toxic to hemoglobin (ie, carbon monoxide) because it will most likely be affected as well; and because it is a volume expander, the client with anemia who has an adequate circulating blood volume but a poor hemoglobin value must be monitored carefully for fluid overload (Leser, 1982).

Oxygen-Binding Chelates

Oxygen-binding chelates are erythrocyte substitutes that contain elements that act like hemoglobin (ie, they bind oxygen to themselves). Because these products use iron, they are subject to the same difficulties as stroma-free hemoglobin, particularly the development of iron toxicity. Also, this chelate requires storage temperatures of −45°C to −40°C and is therefore impractical to use (Leser, 1982).

Chapter Highlights

Disorders of the blood and blood-forming organs have the potential for causing widespread bodily changes, placing every other body system at risk for dysfunction.

Tissue changes make clients with disorders of the blood and blood-forming organs especially prone to alterations in comfort level.

Information regarding the client's tendency for bleeding episodes is an important part of establishing a thorough data base.

A detailed account of the client's exposure to drugs and chemicals is an important part of the nursing assessment because many drugs and chemicals may interfere with normal hematologic functioning.

Nursing assessment to determine abnormalities in blood-forming organs includes evaluation of color changes in the skin and mucous membranes and assessment of organ enlargement and tenderness.

Changes in skin pigmentation and integrity, eyes, oral mucosa, range of motion, condition of the joints, and neurologic function may provide clues about the progress of the disorder.

The CBC and WBC differential are the most important laboratory tests in diagnosing disorders of the blood and blood-forming organs. In bleeding disorders, coagulation studies are also important.

Common nursing diagnoses for clients with disorders of the blood and blood-forming organs include altered comfort: pain, impaired gas exchange, impaired physical mobility, impaired skin integrity, potential for infection, altered nutrition: less than body requirements, knowledge deficit, and ineffective client and family coping.

Blood or blood-component transfusions are indicated for provision of adequate tissue oxygenation, restoration of circulatory blood volume, and restoration of coagulation factors.

The nurse administering blood or blood components must ensure that the correct protocol is followed. This includes assessment of the client before the transfusion and close monitoring of the client during and after transfusion therapy.

Autotransfusion eliminates the possibility of a transfusion reaction and the transmission of hepatitis, syphilis, and AIDS.

Apheresis is not a cure for diseases such as hemolytic anemia, systemic lupus erythematosus, and leukemias but a way of interfering with pathophysiologic changes of the disease process.

Bibliography

Bahu GAB: Administering blood safely. *AORN J* 1983; 37:1073–1077+.

Bates B: *A Guide to Physical Examination,* 3rd ed. Philadelphia: Lippincott, 1983.

Benson ML, Benson DM: Autotransfusion is here—Are you ready? *Nurs 85* (March) 1985; 15:46–49.

Byrne JC et al: *Laboratory Tests: Implications for Nursing Care,* 2nd ed. Menlo Park, CA: Addison–Wesley, 1986.

Centers for Disease Control: Possible transfusion-associated acquired immune deficiency syndrome (AIDS). *MMWR* 1982; 31:652–654.

Centers for Disease Control: Prevention of acquired immune deficiency syndrome (AIDS): Report of interagency recommendations, *MMWR* 1983; 32:101–103.

Dyer KE: Lymphangiography. In: *Diagnostics.* Springhouse, PA: Intermed, 1982.

Freedman ML: New thoughts on old blood. *Emerg Med* (July 15) 1982; 14:148–150+.

King C: Exploring the neck and lymphatics. *RN* (June) 1982; 45:48–55.

King NH: Controlling bleeding when the platelet count drops. *RN* (Aug) 1984; 47:25–27.

Kirsch CM: Reticulocyte count. In: *Diagnostics.* Springhouse, PA: Intermed, 1982.

Leser DR: Synthetic blood: A future alternative. *Am J Nurs* 1982; 82:452–455.

Lopez JA, Hausz M: Therapeutic apheresis. *Am J Nurs* 1982; 82:1572–1578.

Masoorli ST, Piercy S: A step-by-step guide to trouble-free transfusions. *RN* (May) 1984; 47:34–42.

Rutman R, Miller W (editors): *Transfusion Therapy: Practices and Procedures,* 2nd ed. Rockville, MD: Aspen, 1985.

Smith LG: Reactions to blood transfusions. *Am J Nurs* 1984; 84:1096–1101.

Resources

Leukemia Society of America, Inc.
733 3rd Ave.
New York, NY 10017
Phone: (212) 573–8484

Supports research, client assistance, and public and professional education about leukemia and allied disorders including the lymphomas and Hodgkin's disease. Maintains a list of state and local agencies that offer financial assistance to leukemia clients as well as to those with Hodgkin's disease or non-Hodgkin's lymphoma.

National Foundation–March of Dimes
303 S. Broadway
Tarrytown, NY 10591
Phone: (914) 428–7100

This organization is concerned with preventing birth defects and genetic diseases. It disseminates information, sponsors research, and provides referrals for genetic counseling and treatment centers.

National Leukemia Association
585 Stewart Ave.
Suite 536
Garden City, NY 11530
Phone: (516) 222–1944

This organization raises funds to sponsor research and to help clients and their families with the costs of laboratory tests, radiation therapy and chemotherapy, blood transfusions, and related expenses not covered by the client's health insurance plan.

National Rare Blood Club
164 Fifth Ave.
New York, NY 10010
Phone: (212) 243–8037

This organization maintains a list of individuals who donate their rare blood without charge whenever needed. Membership information is in their brochure entitled *National Rare Blood Club of the Associated Health Foundation.*

HOT LINES

AIDS Hot line
Phone: (800) 342–AIDS (Mon-Fri, 8:30 AM to 5:30 PM EST)

Sponsored by the US Public Health Service, this hot line gives a recorded informational message on AIDS. If the caller stays on the line, someone will be available to answer questions or respond to concerns.

National Gay and Lesbian Task Force Crisis Line
Phone: (800) 221–7044 or (212) 529-1604;
5 PM to 10, Sat 1 PM to 5 PM
Provides up-to-date information on AIDS.

HEALTH EDUCATION MATERIAL

From: AIDS Project
3670 Wilshire Blvd., Suite 300
Los Angeles, CA 90010
Phone: (213) 738-8200

From: National Library of Medicine
Literature Search Program
Reference Section
8600 Rockville Pike
Bethesda, MD 20209
Phone: (301) 496-4000

A bibliography on AIDS is available. Include name and address typed on a gummed label (no return postage is necessary).

CHAPTER 23

Specific Disorders of the Blood and Blood-Forming Organs

Other topics related to the content in this chapter are: Nursing care of clients receiving chemotherapy or radiation therapy, **Chapter 10;** Health teaching for clients on anticoagulants, **Chapter 19.**

Objectives

When you have finished studying this chapter, you should be able to:

Describe the clinical manifestations and medical and surgical measures for disorders of the blood and blood-forming organs.

Apply appropriate nursing interventions in the care of clients with disorders that affect blood cells, bone marrow, and coagulation.

Explain the importance of psychosocial support in the nursing care of clients with disorders of the blood and blood-forming organs.

Instruct clients in measures to avoid or eliminate situations that may adversely affect hematopoeisis or the coagulation mechanism.

Describe the nursing care of the bone marrow donor and the bone marrow recipient.

Discuss the role of prevention in nursing interventions related to clients with acquired immune deficiency syndrome (AIDS).

Specify the nursing interventions common to the care of clients with neoplastic disorders of the blood and blood-forming organs.

Disorders of the blood and blood-forming organs pose complex problems for clients, their families, and nurses. Many of these disorders disrupt the immune system, reduce the ability to fight infection, and interfere with the ability to maintain vascular integrity and transport oxygen to the tissues. Thus, these conditions not only compromise health, they also threaten life. In addition to these physiologic problems, clients must cope with interrupted career plans, altered family roles, changes in lifestyle, and possibly the uncertainty of their future. Congenital disorders such as sickle cell anemia, thalassemia, spherocytosis, G-6-PD, hemophilia, and von Willebrand's disease are discussed in pediatric nursing textbooks and will not be repeated here.

SECTION 

Disorders of Multifactorial Origin

Multifactorial disorders of the blood and blood-forming organs may be precipitated by (1) a nutritional deficiency, (2) environmental or chemical toxins, (3) other disease processes, or (4) no known cause. Any of the bone marrow elements may be involved, resulting in an inability of the body to resist infectious organisms, a deficiency in the blood's ability to coagulate, or an alteration in the body's ability to transport oxygen to tissues. Some acquired hematologic diseases interfere in only one of these functions; in others, the entire bone marrow may fail.

Aplastic Anemia

Aplastic anemia is characterized by a decrease in the hematopoietic tissue, its replacement by fatty bone marrow, and marked pancytopenia. The three hallmarks of aplastic anemia are *leukopenia, anemia,* and *thrombocytopenia.*

NURSING DIAGNOSES IN
Disorders of Blood and Blood-Forming Organs

DIRECTLY RELATED DIAGNOSES

- Comfort, altered: pain
- Coping, ineffective family: disabled
- Coping, ineffective individual
- Gas exchange, impaired
- Infection, potential for
- Knowledge deficit
- Mobility, impaired physical
- Nutrition, altered: less than body requirements
- Skin integrity, impaired: potential

OTHER POTENTIAL DIAGNOSES

- Activity intolerance
- Adjustment, impaired
- Grieving, anticipatory
- Powerlessness
- Self-concept, disturbance in: body image
- Sexuality patterns, altered
- Social interaction, impaired
- Tissue integrity, impaired: oral mucous membranes

The etiology of aplastic anemia can be classified as idiopathic or secondary. Idiopathic aplastic anemia has no known cause and can be further classified as either congenital (Fanconi's anemia) or acquired. Secondary aplastic anemia involves the client's prior exposure to stimuli such as chemical (eg, benzene or dichlorodiphenyltrichloroethane [DDT]), radiation, environmental toxins, drugs (eg, chloramphenicol or cytotoxic drugs), or immunologic injury. Aplastic anemia may also be related to a defect in the regulation of blood cell production by the bone marrow, a defect of the bone marrow tissue, or both. Regardless of the etiology, the overall result is a decrease in the amount of functional bone marrow.

Clinical Manifestations

Clinical manifestations of aplastic anemia are related to the pancytopenia. Clients have symptoms of severe bone marrow depression: pallor, fatigue, repeated infections, malaise, and bleeding tendencies. Bleeding tendencies may be occult or conspicuous, major or minor, such as gastrointestinal bleeding versus gingival oozing; or in the form of purpura or petechiae.

Diagnosis is made by bone marrow aspiration, bone marrow biopsy, or both. The bone marrow is found to contain primarily hypocellular fatty deposits.

Medical Measures

Supportive therapy is prescribed to help the client maintain as normal a life as possible. Therapy includes blood and platelet transfusions. Infections are treated aggressively, especially when the client is symptomatic. Reverse isolation may be used, possibly including a laminar air flow unit to purify the air. A high-fiber diet allows easy defecation, because straining at stool can precipitate a bleeding episode. Bone marrow transplantation (see below) is effective for clients with aplastic anemia. Both steroids and androgens hold promise for the treatment of children but not adults.

Specific Nursing Measures

Pay particular attention to the client's safety; avoid infection and prevent bleeding episodes. This means not using intramuscular injections or straight-edged razors. Special soft toothbrushes and stool softeners may be needed. Blood component therapy in the form of packed RBCs, platelets, and granulocytes may be administered.

The client with aplastic anemia may be prohibited from engaging in sexual intercourse because severe leukopenia and thrombocytopenia increase the possibility of infection or bleeding. Suggest sexual counseling or refer the client to a sex counselor when indicated.

Maintaining existing relationships between the client and family members and significant others should be a primary goal guiding nursing care. Include family members and significant others in the client's care and education whenever possible. Securing close contact and involvement with family members and significant others can provide the client needed affection and a feeling of belonging.

Pernicious Anemia

Pernicious anemia is characterized by a metabolic defect involving the absence of intrinsic factor (IF), a protein (possibly a globulin) secreted by the gastric mucosa. (Intrinsic factor is discussed in Chapter 40.) Its chief purpose is to combine with extrinsic factor (vitamin B_{12}) for transport to the ileum. Once deposited in the ileum, vitamin B_{12} can be absorbed. In the absence of IF, vitamin B_{12} deficiency develops.

Vitamin B_{12} is necessary for proper growth and maturation of all body cells; but cells of the bone marrow, the gastrointestinal tract, and the central nervous system (CNS) are especially vulnerable to deficiencies in this vitamin. Vitamin B_{12} deficiency affects normal erythropoiesis and granulocytopoiesis, but the major impact of vitamin B_{12} deficiency is on the erythrocyte. The erythrocyte demonstrates both anisocytosis (abnormal size)—in this case, it is abnormally large—and poikilocytosis (abnormal shape). The membrane of the vitamin B_{12}-deficient erythrocyte is also extremely fragile and ruptures easily. The effect on the erythrocyte is so profound that anemia develops.

Vitamin B_{12} also plays a major role in the proper formation of myelinated nerves. Vitamin B_{12} deficiency causes widespread demyelination of nerves and degeneration of white matter. Untreated pernicious anemia has a progressive and usually terminal course. Spontaneous remissions have been known to occur but are rare.

Pernicious anemia is thought to be caused by a single autosomal dominant defect. It occurs predominantly in light-skinned, blue-eyed people of northwest European, Scandinavian, or British descent. The disorder seems to involve a predisposition for atrophy of the secreting glands of the gastric mucosa (found on postmortem examination). Along with this atrophy, IF, pepsin, and hydrochloric acid are absent in the gastric juices. Other causes of pernicious anemia include gastrectomy, gastric cancer, infestation by fish tapeworms, and malabsorption problems involving the ileum.

Clinical Manifestations

The onset of pernicious anemia occurs in late middle adult life. The first clinical manifestations are usually those of anemia. Clients demonstrate pallor with slight icterus, as well as lassitude and weakness disproportionate to the degree of existing anemia.

The loss of vibratory sense may be the first clue in the diagnosis of pernicious anemia. Numbness and tingling of the extremities can follow. As demyelination and degeneration continue, paralysis and psychosis may develop. Once neurologic damage has occurred, neurologic function may not be regained.

The stomach atrophies and loses its acid- and enzyme-secreting abilities, developing achlorhydria and achylia. The remainder of the intestinal tract enlarges, and digestion becomes difficult as the disease progresses.

Pernicious anemia is diagnosed by the Schilling test. Gastric analysis may also be used. In addition, multiple laboratory studies are performed on the peripheral blood both before and after the initiation of vitamin B_{12} therapy. Quantitative erythrocyte counts may be as low as 2 million μL; the hemoglobin level is approximately 8 g/dL; and mean corpuscular volume (MCV) is elevated. Only the mean corpuscular hemoglobin count (MCHC) is normal. As already stated, the peripheral blood smear demonstrates anisocytosis and poikilocytosis.

Medical Measures

Current treatment of pernicious anemia includes regular injections of vitamin B_{12}. After the diagnosis of pernicious anemia and the initiation of vitamin B_{12} therapy, the client's hemogram quickly returns to normal. Improvement may begin as early as 4 days after the initiation of vitamin therapy. In addition, a dramatically increased sense of well-being accompanies the hematologic improvement. Vitamin B_{12} therapy administered before the onset of neurologic symptoms and signs is ideal. When these symptoms and signs have already appeared, prompt and accurate diagnosis and treatment are imperative. Physical therapy may help restore some use and function, but residual neurologic damage may persist for life.

Specific Nursing Measures

Nursing management of pernicious anemia includes client support and education during the diagnostic phase, client education about the disease process and the importance of compliance with lifelong vitamin B_{12} therapy, and assessment and rehabilitation of clients with neurologic changes. The client with pernicious anemia will need assistance to complete activities of daily living until the lassitude and weakness are resolved. Encourage these clients to rest frequently and make every effort not to tire them by long and vigorous days of testing.

The client with pernicious anemia is committed to a lifetime of vitamin B_{12} therapy. Noncompliance causes the return of symptoms and possibly more dramatic consequences, such as neurologic involvement. Thus, these clients must understand the rationale for vitamin B_{12} therapy and comply completely with the chemotherapeutic regimen.

Iron Deficiency Anemia

Iron deficiency anemia is a microcytic, hypochromic disorder of the erythrocyte; in other words, the erythrocyte is small and pale because of a reduction in hemoglobin concentration. The causative factor is usually inadequate dietary intake of foods containing iron. Clients at high risk for iron deficiency anemia are the elderly, and menstruating, pregnant, and lactating females. Blacks have a higher incidence of iron deficiency anemia than whites.

Clinical Manifestations

Clinical symptoms and signs of iron deficiency anemia depend on the condition's severity. The client feels chronically tired and may be pale. Laboratory studies indicate a hemoglobin level of less than 12 g/dL, decreased serum ferritin levels, increased total iron-binding capacity, and decreased iron stores in the bone marrow. Clients with severe anemia may have malaise, tachycardia, and shortness of breath on exertion.

Medical Measures

Iron supplementation may be given by a parenteral or oral route. The injectable iron preparation is often painful and may lead to necrosis if misplaced into fatty tissue, so the oral route is preferred. Clinical improvement is seen in 2 to 4 weeks. The client should eat a diet high in iron.

Specific Nursing Measures

The focus of nursing measures is client education regarding the importance of adequate iron for optimum body function. Education is important in gaining client compliance with iron therapy. Initiate a dietary referral and give the client a list of foods high in dietary iron for home use. Explain the side effects of iron therapy. The most common are gastrointestinal and include constipation or diarrhea, abdominal cramping, and gastric distress. Stool color will change from normal brownish to either a dark green or black. Warn the client to keep all iron preparations out of the reach of children.

Administer oral iron preparations with citrus juice to enhance absorption. If parenteral iron therapy is prescribed, use the Z-track method with a 20-gauge, 2- to 3-in needle injected in the dorsogluteal site only (see a nursing fundamentals text).

Disseminated Intravascular Coagulation

Disseminated intravascular coagulation (DIC) is an acute abnormal stimulation of the normal hemostatic mechanism. In DIC, balance in the clotting cascade is disrupted. The abnormal stimulation of coagulation is explosive, resulting in widespread thrombi formation that eventually exhausts clotting factors and platelets. The existing degree of clotting activates the fibrinolytic process. These two events can result in major bleeding episodes.

DIC does not exist alone; it coexists with a variety of other acute disease processes that damage cells in some way and thus potentiate stimulation of the normal hemostatic mechanism. Disorders or situations associated with DIC include malignancies, sepsis, shock, abruptio placentae, postextracorporeal bypass, respiratory distress syndrome, malaria, and venomous bites. Mismatched blood and fat emboli can initiate DIC by releasing excessive factor XII.

Clinical Manifestations

The client with DIC may have bleeding tendencies, tissue damage from ischemia, erythrocyte damage, and hemolysis with a potential for shock. These problems have either occult or overt symptoms and signs. Symptoms and signs of bleeding include epistaxis; petechiae; ecchymosis; bleeding from surgical sites, placental detachment areas, or old sites of injury; positive findings of blood in the stool or emesis; fall in blood pressure; postural hypotension; tachycardia; decreased packed red cell volume; and restlessness.

Manifestations of thrombosis depend on the specific organ or body system affected. The kidneys are a prime target organ, and hematuria is the most common clinical evidence that the renal system is affected. Thrombosis also can affect the CNS; changes in the level of consciousness may signal interruption in cerebral blood flow. Characteristic skin changes such as acrocyanosis, in which the client experiences generalized sweating with cold, mottled toes and fingers, also occur.

A battery of laboratory analyses is used in the diagnosis of DIC in conjunction with the client's symptoms and signs. These tests measure the client's coagulation. Platelet counts are decreased; PT and PTT are prolonged. Fibrinogen levels are decreased, and levels of fibrin degradation products (fibrin split products) are elevated. A protamine sulfate test is strongly positive, and coagulation factor assay demonstrates a reduction in factors II, V, and VII.

Medical Measures

The pharmacologic management of DIC is controversial. Currently, heparin, or blood components such as packed RBCs, platelets, plasma, and factor replacements, or both are used. Some think that DIC is best managed by no treatment at all, because treating the client's symptoms and signs may worsen the clotting–bleeding phenomenon. The overall goal of therapy is removing the stimulus that initiated the DIC process.

Specific Nursing Measures

The nursing care of DIC clients is complex. The overall nursing goal is to protect them from bleeding by applying pressure to bleeding sites, avoiding intramuscular injections, keeping the client's nails trimmed, and having both male and female clients shave with an electric razor instead of a straight-edged razor.

The client undergoing heparin sodium or blood component therapy needs additional support and explanations. Heparin may be given either continuously or intermittently by IV drip, and the nurse must closely monitor the prescribed flow rate. The client receiving heparin must be assessed continuously for bleeding. Blood component therapy, although prescribed to replace depleted coagulation factors consumed by the systemic clotting phenomenon, may stimulate additional clotting. Changes in the client's level of consciousness, pallor or cyanosis of body parts, or oliguria or anuria may indicate additional clotting. Notify the physician immediately if these changes occur so the medical management of the client can be adjusted.

Because clients with DIC have other disorders simultaneously, the stress levels of the DIC client and significant others are high. The client and family or friends require thorough teaching and psychosocial support to cope effectively with this complex, confusing disease.

SECTION 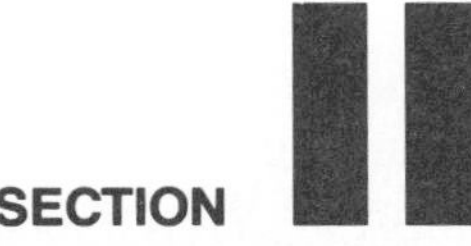

Immunologic Disorders

Immunologic disorders of the blood and blood-forming organs affect the body's ability to resist infectious agents. Without an adequate immune system or a competent bone marrow, the client is prone to life-threatening infections.

Aquired immune deficiency syndrome is discussed here. Congenital immunologic disorders are in pediatric nursing texts.

Acquired Immune Deficiency Syndrome

Acquired immune deficiency syndrome (AIDS) is a specific defect in immunity against disease. Clients with this immune system defect are unable to defend against disease and are prone to debilitating, often fatal opportunistic infections.

The causative agent of AIDS is a retrovirus known as the human immunodeficiency virus (HIV-1). This virus tends to seek out and reproduce in T-lymphocytes and, in so doing, injures and kills the lymphocytes.

Mode of Transmission

The presence of the AIDS virus has thus far been demonstrated in blood, semen, saliva, and tears. Whether it can be transmitted through saliva and tears is not yet known.

Sexual transmission, especially homosexual transmission among men through receptive anal intercourse, is the most common. Semen can carry infected lymphocytes that are transferred through minute breaks in the rectal mucosa that occur during anal intercourse. The question of transmission by oral–genital contact remains unanswered.

The AIDS virus can also be transmitted parenterally by using contaminated needles or through contaminated blood and blood products such as whole blood, cellular components, plasma, and clotting factor concentrates that have not been heat treated. Thus far, other blood products such as immune globulin, albumin, plasma protein fraction, and hepatitis B vaccine have not been implicated (Bennett, 1985). AIDS can also be transmitted by an infected mother to a fetus or newborn infant.

Incidence and Risk Factors

The first cases of AIDS appeared simultaneously in New York City and Port-au-Prince, Haiti, in 1978 (Bennett, 1985). The Centers for Disease Control (CDC) first began publishing incidence reports in June 1981 related to these first cases of AIDS as well as others diagnosed in San Francisco and Los Angeles. Since then the number of AIDS cases has escalated in geometric proportions—reported cases have doubled about every 10 months. More than half of these persons have died, most within 2 years of diagnosis. The rapid progress of the disease is thought to be related to the tremendous speed with which the HIV virus reproduces. The number of AIDS cases reported by the CDC through April 1987 are illustrated by state in Figure 23–1. The CDC has predicted a continuing alarming rise in the incidence of AIDS, estimating that there will be

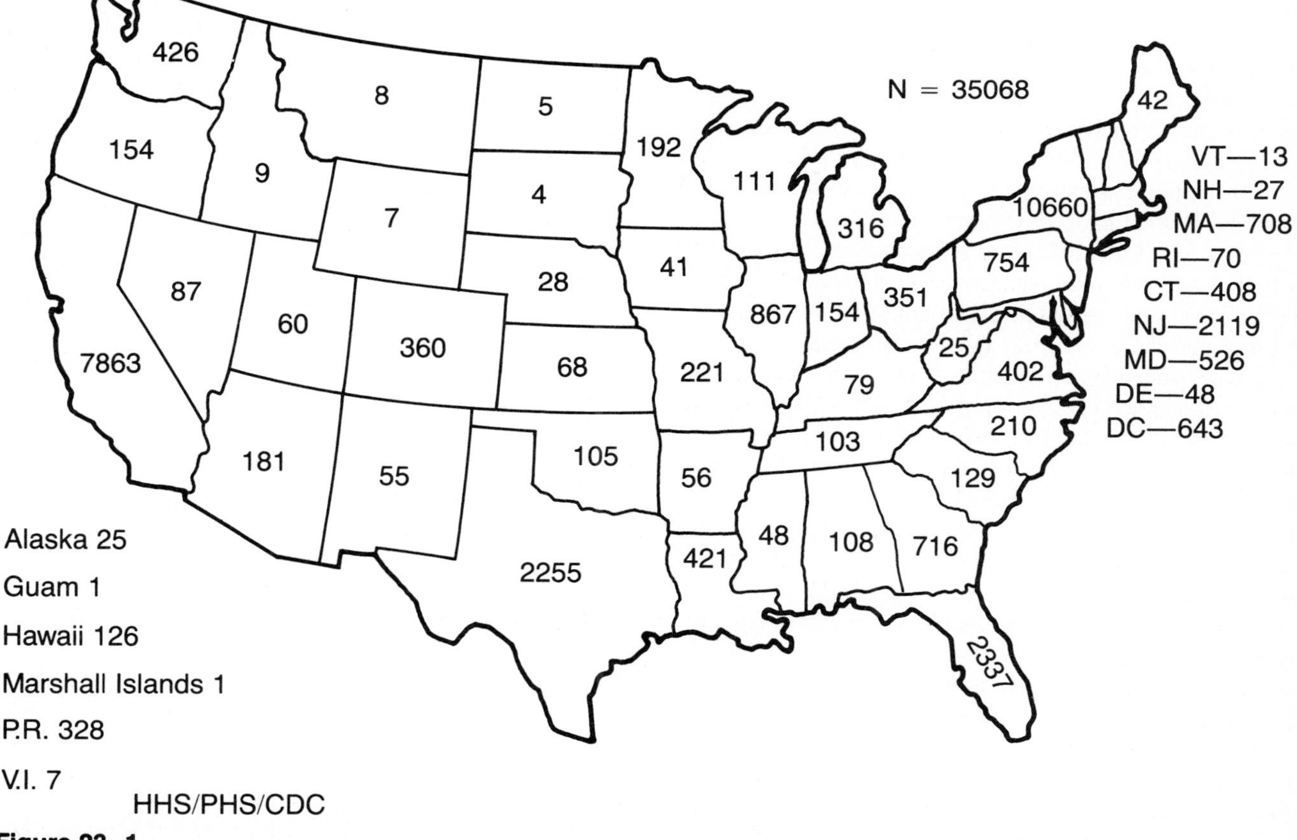

Figure 23–1

AIDS cases reported to the CDC, by state, through April 27, 1987. *SOURCE: Centers for Disease Control, Atlanta, GA.*

approximately 200,000 cases on record by 1988. According to the World Health Organization, in the Americas, the countries other than the United States with the highest number of reported cases were Brazil, Canada, and Haiti in that order.

Several groups have been identified in the United States as being at high risk of developing AIDS: Homosexual/bisexual men represent approximately three-quarters of all AIDS cases; parenteral drug users are the category with the second highest incidence. Female sexual partners of bisexual men and children of AIDS clients are also at high risk. Only 9% of cases have occurred outside the two highest risk groups. Of this number, 3% are categorized as unknown.

The incidence among heterosexuals in the US has increased to approximately 4%. In Africa, however, AIDS occurs about equally among men and women. This has led to speculation that AIDS, which has been largely confined to homosexual and bisexual men, will spread to and among the general population. Figure 23–2 illustrates the risk factors for specific populations in the United States.

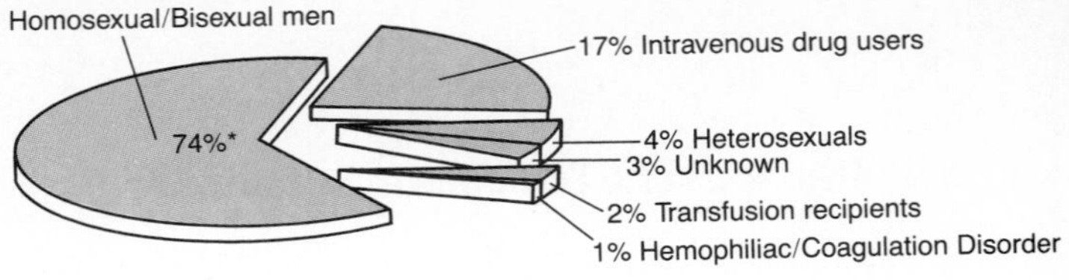

Figure 23–2

AIDS in the United States. Populations at risk as of April 27, 1987. SOURCE: *Centers for Disease Control, Atlanta, GA.*

Clinical Manifestations

The incubation period for AIDS is unknown. The time between exposure to the virus to onset of symptoms ranges from about 6 months to more than 5 years. In transfusion-associated cases, the mean is 2 years (Benenson, 1985). The onset of AIDS is usually insidious. Early in the disease, clients have nonspecific symptoms such as fatigue and weakness, lymphadenopathy, anorexia and weight loss, recurrent diarrhea, pallor, fever, and night sweats. This group of symptoms has been termed AIDS-related complex (ARC) when it occurs in persons who have had the symptoms for at least three months and test positive for the virus. Not everyone who has ARC develops full-blown AIDS. The symptoms gradually increase in severity, usually until the client becomes ill with an opportunistic disease. The unusual occurrence of *Pneumocystis carinii* pneumonia or Kaposi's sarcoma in clients who have not had a past diagnosis of an immune disorder and have not received immunosuppressive therapy is the single most important piece of data suggesting AIDS. Although the line that separates AIDS from ARC is unclear, a person is usually considered to have AIDS once the client develops a life-threatening infection.

Pneumocystis carinii pneumonia is a rare parasitic protozoan lung infection otherwise almost always seen in cancer clients or transplant recipients who have received immunosuppressive agents. This serious, often fatal lung infection is characterized by shortness of breath and fever. The shortness of breath may be so profound that the client may experience air hunger. The infection begins insidiously; possibly the only symptoms are fever, sore throat, chills, and a nonproductive cough. Within months, the infectious process becomes so extensive that dyspnea, cyanosis, painful respiration, and air hunger become pronounced. High fever with night sweats may also be present. By this time, the protozoa have invaded lung tissue and created cystic pockets that impede the oxygen-carbon dioxide exchange across the alveolar membrane. Clients may require oxygen administration via an artificial ventilation device. (For a discussion of pneumonia, see Chapter 16.)

Kaposi's sarcoma is a rare, usually mild skin cancer that typically occurs in males over 60 years of age with a Mediterranean ancestry. Skin changes include dark purplish, sometimes ulcerating lesions that usually appear over the lower extremities (Figure 23–3). Kaposi's sarcoma is rarely fatal in clients without AIDS. In the AIDS client, who is often younger than the usual Kaposi's sarcoma client, the disease is virulent and invasive, often involving internal organs; mucous membranes; and the face, arms, and chest. Median years of survival following diagnosis of Kaposi's sarcoma for the client without AIDS ranges from 8 to 13 years, compared to as little as 15 months for the AIDS client.

Although there is no one laboratory or diagnostic test to determine whether a client has AIDS, a blood test to screen for the HIV-1 virus was approved for use in March 1985 by the US Food and Drug Administration. Having antibodies to the virus does not indicate that the person has AIDS or even that the person will, with any certainty, develop AIDS in the future. Demonstrating antibody formation to the virus simply means that the person has been exposed to the virus and has developed antibodies in response to it. This finding allows blood donation centers to screen out potential donors who might possibly be incubating the disease. There is some concern that a 3- to 6-week "window" (and perhaps as long as 6 months) exists in which persons infected with the AIDS virus may not test positive. Other laboratory findings are lymphopenia, hypergammaglobulinemia, and diminished reactivity to antigens.

Once the diagnosis is made, the course of AIDS is predictable. Repeated, life-threatening opportunistic infections (eg, *Pneumocystis carinii* pneumonia and overwhelming candidiasis, cytomegalovirus infection, or disseminated herpes simplex infection, among others) requiring hospitalization are the rule. The nonspecific early symptoms described earlier increase in severity along with the progression of the disease. Central nervous system

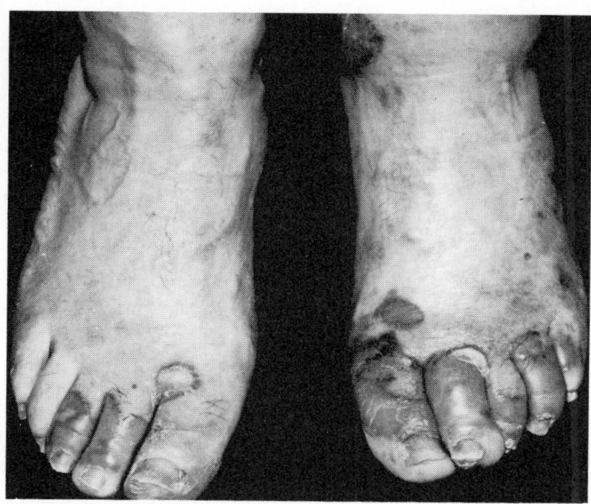

Figure 23–3

Typical skin changes in Kaposi's sarcoma. SOURCE: *Binnick SA:* Skin Diseases: Diagnosis and Management in Clinical Practice. *Baltimore, MD: Williams & Wilkins, 1982.*

changes including dementia have been observed in later stages of the disease.

Medical Measures

AIDS has no known cure. Of those diagnosed with the disease in 1981, 92% have died. Immunotherapy with interferon has been used for clients with Kaposi's sarcoma. Although interferon treatment has had some success, it does not correct the immune defect in AIDS. Interleukon-2 may help fight the severe immunodeficiency by increasing the ability of the impaired lymphocytes of AIDS clients to fight infection. The substance has been shown to improve infection-fighting activity in the test tube; it is not yet shown to work in vivo. Clinical trials now test interleukon-2 activity in AIDS clients.

Experimentation is also under way to develop drug therapy for AIDS. A drug developed in France that interferes with the virus's multiplication, HPA-23, was approved for experimental use in the United States in late 1985. Another experimental agent that appears to prevent viral multiplication and is less toxic than HPA-23 is azidothymidine (AZT). A third drug, available in Europe, Mexico, and Canada but not in the United States, is isoprinosine. This drug reportedly stimulates the immune system and has also been used for herpes genitalis, hepatitis B, and genital warts. Another drug that seems to stimulate the immune system and also increases the body's production of interferon and interleukon-2 (natural antiviral agents) is ABPP, an experimental drug for cancer clients, soon to be tested in AIDS clients. Researchers are also investigating the potential uses of other drugs such as suramin sodium (Antrypol, Germanin), used to treat African sleeping sickness caused by a protozoal parasite spread by the tsetse fly; and ribavirin (Virazole), an antiviral agent said to be effective in certain forms of influenza and in herpesvirus infections. Complicating drug treatment is the fact that the HIV-1 virus also attacks the brain, which is difficult for drugs to reach.

Antibiotic therapy is used for clients with infection. For example, *Pneumocystis carinii* infections are treated with either a combination of trimethoprim and sulfamethoxazole or with pentamidine isethionate (Lomidine). Refer to the other specific disorders chapters for treatment of other infections.

Research into the development of a vaccine is ongoing. Vaccine development could, however, be a slow process. For example, although the hepatitis B virus was identified as early as 1968, an effective vaccine did not become available until 1983. The development of a vaccine is likely to be a difficult task. The virus behaves much like the influenza virus, changing its structure frequently. It would be difficult to develop a vaccine that would be effective against all forms of the virus.

Specific Nursing Measures

Prevention is the focus of AIDS nursing measures today. Prevention strategies for AIDS are given in Box 23–1. Nurses can play an important role in educating clients, their significant others, and the public in risk-reduction strategies and in identifying individuals at risk.

In caring for clients with AIDS, the CDC recommends that blood–body fluid precautions be instituted. Equipment

Box 23–1
Prevention Strategies for AIDS

- Avoiding sexual contact with persons *known* to have AIDS
- Avoiding sexual contact with persons *suspected* to have AIDS
- Practicing "healthy sex" (no exchanges of body fluids including semen, urine, saliva, feces, or blood; no contact of body fluids with mucous membranes)
- Avoiding unnecessary transfusions of blood or blood products
- Encouraging autologous transfusions for elective surgery whenever possible
- Administering only heat-treated coagulation factor to hemophiliacs
- Screening all potential blood donors carefully
- Encouraging AIDS clients and persons at high risk not to donate blood, plasma, organs for transplantation, or semen for artificial insemination
- Advising parenteral drug users to use only clean, disposable needles and syringes and not to share drug equipment
- Recommending that seropositive women delay pregnancy
- Providing educational programs on AIDS for the public and school children
- Using appropriate blood/body fluid precautions with known or suspected AIDS clients

contaminated with blood, excretions, or secretions should be disinfected concurrently. Body fluids and body tissues should be handled with caution. In addition, if the client has an opportunistic infection, other isolation precautions specific to the infectious disease should be observed. The likelihood of transmission to health care personnel if precautions are observed is small.

Clients with AIDS have many emotional needs. They often are rejected by significant others, leading to increasing isolation. Families or friends of homosexual AIDS clients may have abandoned the clients before they became ill because of the stigma still associated with homosexuality. When they confront a diagnosis of AIDS, these clients may truly be isolated and alone.

Fear surrounds AIDS clients because of the increasing incidence of AIDS and the yet-unknown factors that influence its transmission. Health care personnel may be fearful of caring for AIDS clients and reject clients because of the diagnosis or because the clients may be homosexual. Giving holistic care to AIDS clients requires a nonjudgmental and accepting approach that promotes open communication. These clients can be very ill and require skilled physiologic and psychosocial nursing care.

Because AIDS is universally fatal, AIDS clients may demonstrate signs of depression, grief, and mourning, along with other adaptations to death and dying. Assess these clients for these psychosocial alterations and intervene appropriately. Inform clients as more support groups for AIDS clients form (see the resources list at the end of Chapter 22).

Because anorexia and weight loss accompany AIDS, it is important to promote optimal nutritional intake while monitoring the client's nutritional status. A palatable diet that is high in calories and proteins, served attractively, and easily digestible is ideal for AIDS clients. Flexibility in menu planning and meal time is advised. Small frequent meals may be easier for the client to eat.

Other nursing care measures depend on the specific opportunistic diseases affecting the client. These are discussed in the appropriate chapters in this text. Nursing care for clients with brain involvement is similar to that for clients with organic mental disorder. (Consult a psychiatric nursing text.)

SECTION 

Neoplastic Disorders

Neoplastic disorders of the blood and blood-forming organs include the leukemias, lymphomas, and multiple myeloma. These disease processes can involve infiltration and disruption of normal bone marrow function and alteration of the usual protective mechanism of the immune system.

Leukemia

Leukemia is characterized by an accumulation and proliferation of abnormal cells in the bone marrow. The leukemic cells are initially confined to the bone marrow but subsequently invade other organs and tissues as well as the peripheral blood. The accumulation of the leukemic cells in the bone marrow prevents normal hematopoiesis. The result is functionally incompetent bone marrow. The client's peripheral WBC count is generally greater than 50000/μL. It is possible, however, to have a WBC count near or below normal limits and still have leukemia.

The literature reveals possible chemical, viral, radiation, and genetic stimuli preceding the development of leukemia. It is nearly impossible, however, to identify the causative factor or factors for individual clients diagnosed as having leukemia.

Types of Leukemia

Leukemia occurs in acute forms (involving proliferation of immature cells) and chronic forms (involving proliferation of mature cells) and can affect the erythrocyte or any of the white cell precursors. This discussion focuses on the four common types of leukemia.

ACUTE LYMPHOCYTIC LEUKEMIA Acute lymphocytic leukemia is a malignant disorder involving the lymphoid series. The abnormal leukemic cell does not mature. Instead, leukemic lymphoblasts accumulate in the bone marrow, crowding out precursors for normal myelopoiesis, erythropoiesis, and megakaryocytopoiesis.

Acute lymphocytic leukemia is predominantly a disorder of children. It is the most common malignancy in childhood and ranks as the second leading cause of death in that age group. The peak incidence is between the ages of 2 and 10 years. A second rise in incidence occurs during middle and older adulthood.

CHRONIC LYMPHOCYTIC LEUKEMIA Chronic lymphocytic leukemia is a proliferative disorder of lymphoid tissues. Abnormal and incompetent lymphocytes initially are found in the lymph nodes; the disease progresses to involve the reticuloendothelial system (liver and spleen) and invade the bone marrow. The abnormal and incompetent lymphocytes accumulate in the blood. Eventually, the lining of the respiratory and gastrointestinal tracts, as well as the skin, are infiltrated by leukemic cells. As the disease process continues, abnormal lymphocytes eventually replace normal bone marrow elements. This process interferes with normal myelopoiesis, erythropoiesis, and megakaryocytopoiesis.

Chronic lymphocytic leukemia has an insidious onset and is usually found by accident upon routine blood count examination. It is the most common leukemia of the Western hemisphere and primarily affects the elderly population.

ACUTE MYELOGENOUS LEUKEMIA Acute myelogenous leukemia is a malignant disorder involving the myeloid cell line of the bone marrow. Other marrow elements can be affected as well. The terminology for the varieties of AML is confusing, but remember that the descriptors identify cell line precursor affected. Examples of varieties or types of AML include acute granulocytic leukemia (AGL), acute promyelocytic leukemia (AProL), acute myelomonocytic leukemia, and erythroleukemia.

Acute granulocytic leukemia is the most common variety of the AMLs. Often the terms AML and AGL are used interchangeably. Acute granulocytic leukemia involves abnormal proliferation and accumulation of immature granulocytes in the bone marrow. The immature granulocytes may proliferate slower or faster than normal granulocytes. Regardless of the speed of cell division, however, the abnormal leukemic cells eventually crowd out normal myelopoiesis or granulopoiesis, erythropoiesis, and megakaryocytopoiesis. Normal hematopoiesis is impaired.

The incidence of AGL peaks at several ages. The majority of acute leukemias diagnosed during the neonatal period and early infancy are AGL, and a second peak incidence occurs in the eighth and ninth decades of life. Approximately one-third of all clients are over 60 years old.

CHRONIC GRANULOCYTIC LEUKEMIA Chronic granulocytic leukemia is a malignant disorder characterized by an abnormal and excessive accumulation and overgrowth of mature granulocytes in the bone marrow, blood, and spleen. These abnormalities are associated with a unique chromosomal abnormality, the Ph^1 (Philadelphia) chromosome. The granulocytes also seem to have lengthened life spans and may or may not retain their ability to fight infection through phagocytosis.

The onset and progression of CGL are insidious. Remission may last for as long as 4 years, but almost 70% of clients undergo an acute transformation, or "blast crisis." In this stage, the leukemia resembles AGL but is not amenable to chemotherapy; death usually occurs within months.

Approximately 20% of all leukemias in the Western hemisphere are CGL. The disease occurs in adolescence but it is more likely to occur between the ages of 25 and 60 years with the peak incidence in the fourth decade of life. In the neonate, CGL tends to have a rapid progression of infiltration and invasion.

Clinical Manifestations

The clinical manifestations of leukemia are related to the varying degrees of anemia, thrombocytopenia, and leukopenia. Anemia can appear as pallor, fatigue, malaise, shortness of breath, dyspnea, or decreased activity tolerance. Thrombocytopenia frequently has symptoms of petechiae, easy bruising, bleeding gums, occult hematuria, or retinal hemorrhages. When present, leukopenia leaves the client at risk for infection from bacterial, viral, fungal, or protozoal organisms.

Other manifestations of leukemia include lymphadenopathy, joint swelling and pain, weight loss, anorexia, and varying degrees of hepatosplenomegaly. Sternal tenderness is frequent in CGL, and gingival hyperplasia frequently accompanies AGL.

CNS involvement is possible in any of the leukemias. Meningeal involvement causes increased intracranial pressure. Its symptoms and signs include irritability, nausea and vomiting, headache, personality changes, blurred vision, cranial nerve dysfunction involving CN III and CN IV, and changes in the level of consciousness.

Medical Measures

Antineoplastic drug therapy varies with the type of leukemia. Combinations of drugs may be used initially to destroy actively dividing cells, and to reduce the quiescent leukemic cell population for 2 to 3 years after diagnosis.

Remission is never completely established with the chronic leukemias; instead, the chronic leukemias are more or less controlled with antineoplastic drugs for as long as possible. CLL is also treated with apheresis and interferon. In CGL, treatment is aggressive in an attempt to eradicate the Philadelphia chromosome to try to delay the onset of "blast crisis." The usefulness of autologous bone marrow transplantation is being investigated. Blood counts, especially WBC determinations, are carefully monitored, and dosages of medications are adjusted accordingly. Drug therapy for the chronic leukemias may be administered intermittently or continuously.

In both children and adults, the CNS acts as a sanctuary for leukemic cells. Once CNS invasion by abnormal cells occurs, conventional routes of chemotherapy are not successful because systemic treatment does not adequately penetrate the blood-brain barrier. Therefore, the intrathecal route is used in CNS treatment. Some treatment protocols combine intrathecal medication with cranial irradiation. Regardless of the protocol, the purpose remains the same: to eradicate leukemic cells from the sanctuary of the CNS.

Specific Nursing Measures

Nursing care of all leukemic clients centers around potential or actual neutropenia, anemia, and thrombocytopenia caused by replacement of the normal bone marrow cellular elements by leukemic cells or destruction by antineoplastic chemotherapy. Chemotherapeutic treatment also can lead to bone marrow suppression. The nurse must help the leukemic client deal with pain, develop coping skills, and accept body image changes. Clients receiving chemotherapy need special nursing attention.

INFECTION Infections can be fatal for the leukemic client who is immunosuppressed because of the chemotherapeutic regimen. Infection is related to the degree of granulocytopenia.

It is the nurse's responsibility to prevent infection. Clients should be isolated when leukopenic. Several different techniques may be used. Some institutions have laminar airflow units; some use protective isolation or reverse isolation techniques. Regardless of the isolation technique, the purpose is to protect the client against infection. In addition, screen all visitors, and staff members who are even mildly ill should avoid caring for these clients. Once remission has been established and the client is discharged, teach the client to avoid large crowds and contact with contagious persons.

Avoid taking rectal temperatures and administering enemas and suppositories whenever possible to avoid damage to the rectal mucosa and consequent contamination by the gastrointestinal flora. Also avoid intramuscular injections, which compromise the skin integrity and create a portal for bacterial invasion and abscess formation.

Clients may have an altered inflammatory response and may not exhibit the usual signs of inflammation and infection, such as purulent discharge. For this reason, frequently assess the leukemic client for indicators of infection such as an elevated temperature. Client complaints should be taken seriously and investigated quickly. Whenever infection is suggested in a leukopenic client, cultures of the blood, urine, throat, and other sites may be taken in an attempt to identify the location of infection and the causative organism. Granulocytes and broad-spectrum antibiotics are given.

Clients should not receive immunization of any kind during this time. It is the nurse's responsibility to be aware of immunosuppressed clients and to refrain from administering immunizations to them.

ANEMIA Leukemic clients frequently need replacement transfusion therapy in the form of packed RBCs. Facilitate breathing by elevating the head of the client's bed. To decrease the client's energy requirements, help the client perform activities of daily living as needed. Offer frequent rest periods throughout the waking hours to prevent exhaustion.

HEMORRHAGE Thrombocytopenia resulting in hemorrhage can be life threatening to the leukemic client. Nursing care centers around preventing major hemorrhagic episodes. Leukemic clients with thrombocytopenia need safe, gentle nursing care with continuous assessment of symptoms or signs of hemorrhage. Changes in level of consciousness (intracranial bleeding), hematemesis, and epistaxis may occur with or without injury.

Not all bleeding is apparent or life threatening. Nursing assessment includes observing for signs of occult bleeding and testing stools, emesis, and urine for occult blood. Carefully assess clients who have had an invasive procedure such as arterial blood gas determinations, oral suctioning, NG tube insertion, or bone marrow aspiration or biopsy.

Nursing management is also directed toward preventing injury. Rectal temperatures, enemas, rectal suppositories, and intramuscular injections are avoided because they can cause severe hemorrhagic episodes. Encourage clients to wear protective foot coverings whenever ambulating. They should use soft toothbrushes and electric razors instead of blades. Platelet concentrates may be given.

Anticoagulants, aspirin or aspirin-containing products, and medications containing guaifenesin should not be administered to the client with leukemia because they interfere with adequate platelet function. Aspirin is found in many OTC cold and influenza medications, and guaifenesin is in OTC cough suppressants. Febrile episodes are controlled with acetaminophen (rather than aspirin) and antibiotics, if needed. Remind clients that anticoagulants, aspirin, and guaifenesin should be avoided and discourage self-medication with OTC drugs.

PAIN The leukemia client may have pain, most commonly in the bones and joints, because of pressure caused by the infiltration and accumulation of leukemic cells in the bone marrow. Hemarthrosis may also occur and can be painful. The nurse may administer narcotics to control the pain, or chemotherapy may be administered when the pain is thought to be caused by leukemic infiltration.

COPING SKILLS The client with leukemia requires the support of family members, friends, and national or local support groups. Continuously assess the client's coping ability and offer support when needed by initially establishing a one-to-one relationship with the client and significant others. Spending time with the client regularly demonstrates concern about the client's welfare.

Assess the client's knowledge of the disease process and treatment, and begin teaching about the disorder and therapy to offer the client some sense of control. Answer the client's questions honestly, but do not destroy defense mechanisms that protect the client from an intolerable reality. For example, the nurse who notices that the client occasionally demonstrates denial but complies with the medical and nursing prescriptions should allow the client to express the denial, because it may be the client's only way to cope with the disease process.

BODY IMAGE CHANGES Body image changes caused by chemotherapy or radiation therapy interfere with the client's ability to cope positively with the disease process. Emphasize that alopecia is only a temporary consequence of treatment. Until the client's hair does grow back, wigs, toupees, decorative scarfs, or caps can promote a positive self-concept.

Client/Family Teaching

The leukemic client and family or significant others need extensive teaching with information on the leukemic disease process, procedures during the diagnostic and maintenance phases of treatment, radiation therapy, antineoplastic drug therapy, symptoms and signs warranting medical intervention, precautions needed for home care, restrictions on activities of daily living and employment, community resources, and OTC medications to be avoided. Teaching must be planned carefully to avoid overwhelming the client. Coordination of the teaching between the acute care and ambulatory care settings is most important.

DIET With weight loss, a diet high in proteins and calories is needed. Supplemental high-protein, high-calorie feedings may need to be added to the client's 24-hour regimen. Fluid retention caused by corticosteroids can be decreased by a reduced-sodium diet. Because these clients frequently may continue corticosteroid therapy after discharge from the hospital, they may need instruction not only about a sodium-restricted diet but also about the preparation of foods without salt.

Hodgkin's Disease

Hodgkin's disease is a malignant disorder of the lymph nodes characterized by the presence of Reed–Sternberg cells (giant binucleated malignant reticulum cells having prominent nucleoli) on histopathologic examination. Hodgkin's disease metastasizes predominantly via the lymphatics along predictable, connecting pathways. This disease represents 40% of all malignant lymphomas. Hodgkin's disease occurs in persons of all ages, but one-half of all clients are between the ages of 20 and 40. Less than 10% of all cases occur before 10 years of age. The overall incidence of Hodgkin's disease is higher in the male population, and males have a poorer prognosis (Bakemeier et al., 1983).

The exact etiology of Hodgkin's disease is unknown. Both genetic and environmental factors seem to be predispositions. Family members are at increased risk, but the disease does not seem to be contagious.

Clinical Manifestations

The usual clinical presentation of Hodgkin's disease is painless lymph node enlargement that may be accompanied by fever, night sweats, pruritus, weight loss, and malaise. Usually, enlarged nodes are above the diaphragm; the cervical nodes are most commonly involved (Figure 23–4). Other supradiaphragmatic nodes that can be involved are the axillary and mediastinal nodes. Symptoms and signs associated with axillary and mediastinal lymphadenopathy include cough, dyspnea, and superior vena cava obstruction. Less commonly, subdiaphragmatic lymphadenopathy is present, most likely in the inguinal nodes. Mesenteric nodes are rarely involved.

Other clinical manifestations may include retroperitoneal lymph node enlargement, hepatosplenomegaly, and bone involvement. These usually occur later, as the disease becomes more generalized. However, a small number of clients may have generalized disease at the time of diagnosis.

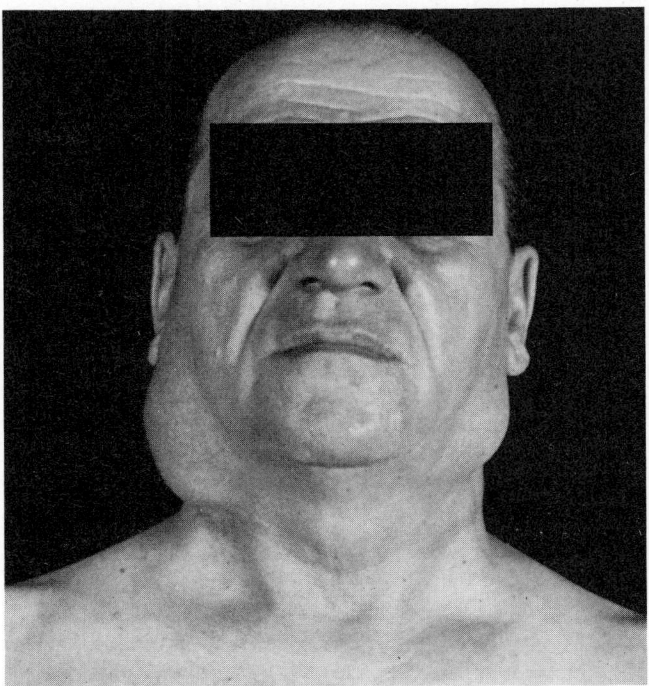

Figure 23–4

Enlargement of cervical lymph nodes due to malignant lymphoma. *SOURCE:* Introduction to Human Disease, *by Leonard V Crowley. Copyright 1983 by Wadsworth, Inc. Reprinted by permission of Wadsworth Health Sciences Division, Monterey, CA and the author. Photo provided by Dr. Crowley.*

Extensive testing is required to diagnose and stage Hodgkin's disease properly. The performance of laparotomy and splenectomy is controversial. Splenectomy carries a risk in itself, and the splenectomized client has an increased risk for infection. Although laparotomy can identify unsuspected nodal and splenic metastasis not found on radiologic examination, it is currently recommended only when the results may influence the choice of therapeutic approach. Another important diagnostic procedure is lymph node biopsy, which establishes the diagnosis of Hodgkin's disease by the presence of Reed–Sternberg cells.

Medical Measures

Even clients with disseminated disease have a chance for long-term disease-free periods, and those with localized disease have an excellent chance for cure. Radiation therapy is the primary treatment for Hodgkin's disease stages. Chemotherapy has its place in the management of more disseminated disease. Even clients with widespread disease at the time of diagnosis and those with evidence of cross-resistance to one chemotherapeutic protocol still have a chance for long-term survival. Today the major chemotherapeutic protocols involve combinations of antineoplastic drugs. Radiation therapy and chemotherapy also can be combined to give the client the greatest chance for long-term sustained remission.

Clients who have had a weight loss of greater than 10% of body weight before diagnosis need special nutritional considerations and testing. Serum protein studies may be indicated; if total serum protein and albumin levels are low, a diet high in protein and carbohydrates is needed. Nutritional supplements also may be administered. These clients should consider food part of the medical prescription.

Specific Nursing Measures

Nursing management of the client with Hodgkin's disease is complex. Emotional support and client education are important in all phases of care.

During the diagnostic phase, the client may seem overwhelmed by the number and invasiveness of the diagnostic procedures. Explain all procedures thoroughly to the client and family or significant others. Be alert to the need to have questions clarified and to ventilate feelings.

These clients are prone to the same problems as anyone receiving radiation therapy or chemotherapy. Because the majority of Hodgkin's disease clients are between 20 and 40 years of age and are receiving radiation therapy, chemotherapy, or both, reproduction may be impaired. These therapies are also teratogenic; they cause an increased rate of spontaneous abortion or genetically defective offspring. Sperm banking offers the male client the possibility of fathering normal offspring at a later time.

Especially troublesome are problems caused by nausea and vomiting, bone marrow suppression, and alopecia. The client with nausea and vomiting is prone to developing disturbances in electrolyte balance. Thus, antiemetics should be given routinely, and IV fluids must be regulated to maintain homeostasis.

Bone marrow suppression can lead to leukopenia, anemia, and thrombocytopenia. These conditions make the client prone to the problems of infection, deficits of oxygen transport, and major and minor bleeding episodes. Monitor the client's complete blood count and note when the values are low.

During leukopenic episodes, the major nursing goal is prevention of infection. Clients should avoid crowds and frequently assess themselves for symptoms and signs of infection. This self-assessment necessitates detailed instruction by the nurse.

Oxygen transport problems may be caused by anemia or a large mediastinal mass. Clients with these problems should be encouraged to alternate activity with rest periods. Use of a Fowler's or semi-Fowler's position for resting or sleeping may relieve dyspnea. Monitoring the client's heart and respiratory rates before and after activity may provide clues to the client's ability to tolerate activity. When anemia is severe, administer blood component therapy in the form of packed RBCs.

Overt or occult bleeding episodes are another client problem caused by bone marrow suppression. Special oral hygiene using soft toothbrushes may be needed to prevent gingival oozing. Straight-edged razors and drugs interfering with platelet function are contraindicated.

Body image changes may be difficult for the client to endure and may damage self-esteem. Clients 20 to 40 years old—the age group most commonly affected by Hodgkin's disease—undergo many changes. They are establishing intimate relationships, planning families, and attaining career goals. This is one of the most productive periods of life. The diagnosis of Hodgkin's disease, even with its good chance for cure, still brings the fears associated with cancer. Feelings of loss of control, rejection, and isolation may overwhelm the client.

The nurse is in a prime position to offer these clients emotional support, restored feelings of control, and relief from some of the feelings of rejection and isolation. Use a calm, unhurried, reassuring approach whenever interacting with these clients. Provide accurate information about Hodgkin's disease, radiation therapy, and chemotherapy, and correct misconceptions about the disease process. Allow clients to make decisions about their schedules whenever possible. Attempt to meet any physical and emotional needs they may have.

Non-Hodgkin's Lymphoma

Included in the classification non-Hodgkin's lymphoma (NHL) are all malignant lymphomas that cannot be classified as Hodgkin's disease. The exact etiology is unknown. Theories of causality center around viruses and immunosuppression. Most likely to develop the condition are clients 50 to 70 years old, but NHL is not limited to the adult population. Males carry a slightly higher risk for NHL than females.

Clinical Manifestations

The clinical manifestations of NHL are similar to those of Hodgkin's disease: painless lymph node enlargement with or without fever, sweating, weight loss, malaise, and pruritus. There are also differences between NHL and Hodgkin's disease. Extranodal involvement with unpredictable and widespread metastasis occurs early in the course of NHL and is frequently present upon diagnosis. Manifestations may include involvement of the skin, gastrointestinal tract, bone, and bone marrow. Transformation to leukemia occurs in approximately 13% of NHL cases with high peripheral lymphocyte counts (Bakemeier et al., 1983).

Medical Measures

The primary purpose of surgery in the treatment of NHL is the diagnosis and clinical staging of the disorder.

Radiation therapy is the primary treatment modality in localized disease. In advanced disseminated disease, radiation therapy is combined with adjuvant chemotherapy. For advanced lymphoma, chemotherapy is prescribed. Multiagent regimens carry the best chances for long-term disease-free survival. Nutritional management of clients with NHL is similar to that in Hodgkin's disease.

The prognosis for the client with NHL is variable. Favorable outcomes are increasingly frequent for localized disease, and long periods free of disease are becoming more common for clients with disseminated disease. The development of less toxic, more effective chemotherapeutic treatment protocols holds great promise for NHL clients.

Specific Nursing Measures

Nursing management of NHL clients is similar to the nursing management for Hodgkin's disease and multiple myeloma. Oncologic emergencies occur more frequently in NHL than in Hodgkin's disease, however (see Chapter 10). Superior vena cava obstruction and spinal cord compression are two of the most common. Other complications of NHL include CNS involvement, infections, the development of other primary malignancies, bone involvement, and joint effusions.

Multiple Myeloma

Multiple myeloma, also called plasma cell myeloma (PCM), is a malignant disorder characterized by the proliferation of abnormal plasma cells in the bone marrow. Single or multiple tumors containing abnormal plasma cells are found throughout the marrow, and immunoglobulin synthesis is disturbed. Multiple myeloma is disseminated throughout the body, ultimately involving the lymph nodes, liver, spleen, and kidneys.

Multiple myeloma occurs exclusively in people over 40 years old. The peak incidence is in the sixth decade of life, and the male-to-female ratio is 2:1. The exact etiology is unknown, but research data suggest a genetic stimulus.

Clinical Manifestations

The onset of multiple myeloma is insidious. A presymptomatic phase may last from 5 to 20 years. During this time, the client's only complaint may be frequent infections, particularly pneumonia. The earliest initial and most frequent complaint is bone pain. Spontaneous pathologic fractures may also occur. Skeletal changes are caused by loss of calcium from bone tissue resulting in hypercalcemia, as well as by invasion of the bone marrow by abnormal plasma cells.

Anemia, fatigue, repeated infection, and bleeding tendencies (such as purpura and epistaxis) represent dysfunction or impairment of bone marrow function. Anorexia, nausea, vomiting, weight loss, and confusion also may be presenting symptoms and signs.

About half of clients have renal insufficiency. Renal function is impaired by hypercalcemia, hyperviscosity of the blood caused by proteinemia, and hyperuricemia. Most commonly, the disease affects the renal tubules, resulting in proteinuria. Characteristic of multiple myeloma is the loss in the urine of a light-chain protein, the Bence–Jones protein.

Diagnosis involves multiple tests. Complete blood counts with quantitative platelet determinations may demonstrate granulocytopenia, anemia, and thrombocytopenia. Serum studies show hypercalcemia, hyperuricemia, and proteinuria. Prothrombin time and partial thromboplastin times may be altered. The erythrocyte sedimentation rate is elevated. Quantitative immunoglobulin assays indicate a monoclonal immunoglobulin abnormality. Radiologic studies of the ribs, spine, skull, and pelvis show a characteristic "punched-out" or "honeycombed" appearance. A 24-hour urinalysis may demonstrate Bence–Jones protein.

The diagnosis of multiple myeloma is confirmed by bone marrow biopsy. Normally, the plasma cell concentration in the bone marrow is approximately 5%; in multiple myeloma, abnormal plasma cell proliferation may range between 30% and 95%.

Medical Measures

Antineoplastic agents are used to induce and maintain a remission in multiple myeloma. Prednisone may be added to the client's chemotherapeutic program. Remission-induced rates currently approach 60%, and survival is approximately 2 to 5 years.

Supportive pharmacologic management may enhance renal function and promote an optimal level of comfort. Diuretics, particularly furosemide (Lasix), may prevent complications such as congestive heart failure secondary to impaired renal function. This drug also enhances the excretion of calcium ions and therefore is useful in controlling or reducing hypercalcemia. Oral phosphate drugs also promote calcium ion excretion but must be used with caution in clients already having renal impairment. Allopurinol (Zyloprim) reduces uric acid formation, preventing uric acid nephropathy caused by hyperuricemia prevalent in multiple myeloma. Narcotic analgesics used in conjunction with muscle relaxants control the pain associated with malignant invasion of the bone marrow by plasma cells.

Dehydration can become a life-threatening complication because of renal shutdown. Acute renal failure can be precipitated by the accompanying hyperuricemia, proteinemia, hypercalcemia, and increased viscosity of the blood. At no time should these clients have a sustained period without fluid intake. If an NPO status is necessary for diagnostic procedures, an IV route with an appropriate flow rate is warranted. Renal disease is easier to prevent than treat. If renal shutdown occurs, hemodialysis may be necessary.

Specific Nursing Measures

The two foremost goals of nursing management for clients with multiple myeloma are maintaining optimal hydration and promoting optimal physical activity. Clients with multiple myeloma have a fluid need requirement above the maintenance need, and 1½ to 2 times the normal fluid requirements (approximately 4 to 5 L/day) should be forced. Urine output should show the appropriate increase. Ambulation must be maintained because the activity increases circulation, decreases demineralization of bones by slowing the loss of calcium, and can reduce the occurrence of spontaneous fractures. Use assistive devices such as splints, canes, or walkers to reduce the discomfort and fear associated with full weight bearing. Before expecting cooperation with ambulation, make sure the client is relatively comfortable by administering non-narcotic analgesics and muscle relaxants. Accompany clients taking these drugs whenever they are ambulating.

Monitor the client's blood counts for values indicating leukopenia, anemia, or thrombocytopenia. Administer blood component therapy (packed RBCs, or platelets) as ordered. Use safe, gentle nursing techniques when thrombocytopenia and anemia are present. (Refer to the discussion of care of the leukemic client with thrombocytopenia and anemia.)

Clients with multiple myeloma can experience severe anorexia, weight loss, nausea, vomiting, diarrhea, or constipation related to the disease process itself, the effects of chemotherapy and radiation therapy, or immobility. The nurse should attempt to make meals enjoyable. Antiemetics should be used as a forethought, not an afterthought. Offer a diet high in proteins, vitamins, minerals, and carbohydrates. The client may more easily tolerate small, frequent meals (perhaps six a day).

The client with multiple myeloma has complex psychosocial needs. Because the peak incidence is middle adulthood, the client is likely to be facing financial responsibilities of a mortgage and college tuition for children, other family monetary responsibilities, unemployment, divorce, or death of a spouse. Middle adulthood also can be a time of career success. Complications of disease progression and the side effects of treatment may alter the client's self-esteem and feeling of control. Provide an environment that promotes self-esteem and gives the client a sense of control over the body. Establish a trusting relationship, maintain open and honest communication, encourage the client and family or significant others to participate in care as much as possible, and provide a sense of control through client education.

A teaching plan for the client with multiple myeloma includes education about the disease process, the significance of antineoplastic drug and radiation therapy, the importance of ambulation and adequate hydration, and pain management.

Polycythemia Vera

Polycythemia vera is a myeloproliferative disorder characterized by panmyelosis (marked erythrocytosis, leukocytosis, and thrombocytosis). Splenomegaly is also present. The erythrocytosis is so massive that hypervolemia and hyperviscosity of the blood result. The red blood cell mass may be two to three times normal without a concurrent rise in plasma volume.

Eventually, the bone marrow undergoes myelofibrotic and osteosclerotic changes, anemia occurs, and immature granulocytes appear in the bloodstream. Extension and infiltration of erythrocytes primarily, and to a lesser extent, leukocytes and platelets, into the spleen, liver, and lymph nodes can develop. Transformation of polycythemia vera into leukemia and other myeloproliferative disorders has been reported.

This disorder is primarily a disease of the middle-aged and older adult. Incidence is slightly higher in males, but there is no known geographic or regional distribution. The exact etiology is unknown. A viral agent has been implicated in mice, but polycythemia vera is not transmitted by contact with clients or their blood.

Clinical Manifestations

Polycythemia vera has an insidious onset and a lengthy, progressive course. Because this disorder is systemic, clinical manifestations are varied and may not suggest the underlying disease process. Any organ system may be involved.

Clients have alterations in their peripheral blood counts. The hemogram shows elevated levels of hemoglobin, circulating erythrocytes, hematocrit, and reticulocytes. Leukocytosis and thrombocytosis are also present.

As in many myeloproliferative disorders, the basal metabolic rate is elevated without any evidence of alteration in thyroid function. Hyperuricemia and hyperuricosuria are also evident in the presence of leukocytosis. Symptoms of gouty arthritis may become apparent if uric acid levels are left untreated.

The skin takes on a characteristic ruddy appearance, especially over the face and hands. Pruritus and eczema-like dermatologic changes may also be present. In addition, these clients may be sensitive to extremes of hot and cold.

Clients may have an elevated systolic and diastolic blood pressure, left ventricular hypertrophy, palpitations, and angina in response to the increased work load on the heart. Other cardiovascular symptoms and signs include dizziness, exertional dyspnea, and peripheral edema. Sluggish circulation with resultant thrombi formation may precipitate infarctions of the spleen, heart, and brain.

CNS symptoms are common. Disturbances in cerebral blood flow may cause headaches, vertigo, tinnitus, and visual problems such as diplopia and blurred vision.

Hypervolemia and consequent venous distention can cause hemorrhage when vessels are weakened and rupture. Some hemorrhages, such as bleeding esophageal varices, may be life threatening. Other bleeding may be covert, or may be minute, such as petechiae and ecchymoses. Epistaxis is common. Hemorrhoids may also occur.

Peptic ulcer disease is 10 times more common in polycythemia vera clients than in the general population. The exact reason for this increased incidence is unknown.

Medical Measures

Repeated phlebotomies may be necessary to reduce the viscosity of the blood adequately, and iron deficiency anemia can result. Supplemental iron can correct this deficiency. Phlebotomy does not correct the panmyelosis of this disease; it only reduces hypervolemia and hyperviscosity. Phlebotomy is further discussed in Chapter 22.

Once the peripheral blood count is normalized, radiation therapy or chemotherapy is begun. Radioactive phosphorus (^{32}P) is a safe, easy, and effective mode of inducing myelosuppression in the client with polycythemia vera. Recently, alkylating agents have been shown to effect myelosuppression as well. The introduction of ^{32}P and antineoplastic agents to the treatment program of polycythemia vera has lengthened the average survival time to approximately 13 years (Williams et al., 1983).

The client with polycythemia vera who has an increased basal metabolic rate may have lost weight before diagnosis. Small, frequent, high-calorie, high-protein meals should be served. Dietary supplements high in calories and proteins may need to be added to the client's nutritional regimen.

Specific Nursing Measures

Phlebotomy is not without risk. Volume loss may precipitate symptoms and signs of shock, so the assessment of vital signs and the symptoms and signs of hypovolemia during phlebotomy is crucial.

When chemotherapeutic agents are administered, assess their adverse or toxic effects. Hyperuricemia can result from a dramatic and rapid reduction in leukocytes. A decreasing urinary output seen while accurately measuring the client's intake and output may be the first indication of uric acid nephropathy.

Make mealtime pleasant and productive and monitor the client's weight carefully. Regardless of whether there is an elevated basal metabolic rate or peptic ulcer disease, maintaining adequate hydration is essential for these clients. Dehydration compounds the hyperviscosity of polycythemia vera and may precipitate thrombotic episodes.

Stress the need for adequate activity to promote vascular integrity, prevent stasis, and promote a sense of control over life. Because these clients have a life expectancy of approximately 13 years after diagnosis, it is essential for them to return to their usual patterns of everyday life.

Client education is another important aspect of nursing management to improve compliance with the medical and nutritional regimens. In addition, client education may foster autonomy and a sense of control over the disease process. Instruction should include explanations of the disease process, the rationale for phlebotomy and radiation therapy or chemotherapy, the importance of compliance with the dietary prescription and fluid needs, and the effectiveness of maintaining optimum activity levels. Encourage clients who smoke to stop smoking. Over a long time, smoking increases the hematocrit level, increasing the viscosity of the blood.

Bone Marrow Transplantation

A bone marrow transplantation (BMT) is the replacement of diseased or deficient bone marrow with healthy marrow from a suitably matched donor. It is done primarily to reconstitute hematologic and immunologic function in clients with leukemia, severe combined immunodeficiency, or aplastic anemia. BMT is also being used on a trial basis for clients with thalassemia.

The donor is given either spinal or general anesthesia, and multiple bone marrow aspirations are taken from the anterior and posterior iliac crests over 30 to 40 minutes. Altogether, about 100 needle aspirations consisting of about 700 mL of bone marrow are obtained. The bone marrow is infused in the recipient through a central vein over a 4-hour period.

Although the procedure is brief, the preparations for bone marrow transplantation are complicated and lengthy. The recipient receives both chemotherapy and radiation therapy. These procedures are discussed in the section on nursing implications.

In BMT, there are a number of clients to consider—the donor, the recipient, and the donor's significant others. The physiologic and psychosocial/lifestyle implications for all these persons are discussed in Table 23–1.

Graft-versus-host disease (GVHD), a tissue incompatibility syndrome in which competent T-lymphocytes from the donor circulate and attack host tissue primarily in the skin, liver, and gastrointestinal tract, is a common complication. GVHD threatens graft success. The disorder usually develops within 1 to 2 weeks after BMT, the most critical period, but may develop as late as 2 to 12 months after the transplant. Transplant failure leads to eventual relapse.

Veno-occlusive disease, another complication of BMT, usually occurs in the first 3 weeks after transplantation and is fatal in about one-third of these clients. This condition, which occurs in up to 25% of clients, affects the liver

Table 23–1
Bone Marrow Transplantation: Implications for Donor and Recipient

Physiologic Implications	Psychosocial/Lifestyle Implications
Donor:	
No known long-term effects; bone marrow replaced naturally within a few weeks	Satisfaction in providing gift of bone marrow
Possible need for blood transfusion or iron replacement	Period of high stress while success of transplant is uncertain
Soreness at aspiration sites for first week	Sadness, anger, sense of failure, and need to grieve if graft is not successful
Infection possible	
Recipient:	
Sterility from total body irradiation	Lengthy hospitalization and posttransplantation care
Infection is common complication for 12 to 18 months; bleeding and veno-occlusive disease possible	Isolation and restriction of visitors and mobility
Graft may fail	Lifestyle modifications to avoid infection
Hematologic and immune functioning restored	Loss of control with dependence on family and health care providers
Extreme discomfort from side effects of chemotherapy and total body irradiation	Alteration of family roles
No known long-term effects; bone marrow replaced naturally within a few weeks	Anxiety and stress until graft is known to be successful
	Body image changes from chemotherapy and total body irradiation

(Nuscher et al., 1984). Symptoms of veno-occlusive disease include:

- Ascites
- Hepatomegaly
- Heart failure
- Encephalopathy
- Elevated serum bilirubin

This complication is most common in clients who have undergone intensive radiochemotherapy before BMT. In some instances, the syndrome resolves without major aftereffects.

Nursing Implications

PREOPERATIVE CARE OF THE DONOR The donor will probably be admitted to the hospital the day before the transplant so any preoperative preparation, including an anesthesia assessment, can be completed. It is likely that a complete history and physical, chest x-ray, electrocardiogram, and blood studies will have been done on an outpatient basis before this time.

The donor should also be offered the opportunity to discuss concerns about the BMT. The nurse's role is supportive during this time but also includes reinforcing or clarifying the information the donor has previously received.

POSTOPERATIVE CARE OF THE DONOR Check the donor's pressure dressings for bleeding on the first day. Use aseptic technique when removing the pressure dressings and replacing them with bandages on the following day.

Instruct the donor to observe for and report any signs of infection—tenderness, swelling, redness, purulent drainage, or acute pain—and to take showers rather than baths until the bone marrow aspiration sites have healed. The donor will probably be discharged from the hospital on the second or third postoperative day to wait out the results of the BMT. Remind the persons who constitute the donor's support system that the donor may be anxious during the postoperative period and worried about whether the donated bone marrow is "good enough" to act as a lifesaver for the recipient. The donor will need their understanding support during this period.

PREOPERATIVE CARE OF THE RECIPIENT Before admission to a transplant unit, the client has a central venous catheter inserted into either the cephalic vein or the subclavian vein to facilitate the administration of parenteral drugs, blood products, TPN, and the bone marrow infusion.

The BMT recipient may be cared for in a number of environments—reverse isolation in a single room, a clean environment in a laminar airflow unit, or a germ-free environment in a laminar airflow unit—depending on the protocol in the institution. The client is in this environment for 5 to 7 days before the BMT takes place while efforts focus on suppressing the recipient's tissue-rejection potential by destroying bone marrow function and destroying all malignant cells.

Once the client has been immunosuppressed, the client is at risk of infection from normal body flora, so steps are taken to protect the client from this source of infection before immunosuppression. These steps may include baths and showers with an antimicrobial skin cleanser such as chlorhexidine gluconate (Hibiclens), antibiotics to sterilize the gastrointestinal tract, antimicrobial creams for instillation in the vagina, and often includes the administration of trimethoprin-sulfamethoxazole (Bactrim, Septra) to inhibit the growth of *P. carinii,* the organism that most often causes posttransplantation interstitial pneumonia. Some protocols also include the oral administration of antifungal agents and the topical application of antifungal powders to the axilla, groin, and other **intertriginous areas** (apposed surfaces of the skin), such as the creases of the neck and beneath pendulous breasts, to prevent fungal infection.

The two components of the immunosuppressive regimen are chemotherapy and total body irradiation. Clients who wish to father children may arrange for sperm banking before total body irradiation. In some centers, the chemotherapy is done first; in others, it follows total body irradiation. The most common agent used for chemotherapy is cyclophosphamide (Cytoxan). The variations in dosage for both chemotherapy and total body irradiation depend on the reason for the bone marrow transplantation (clients with leukemia and Hodgkin's disease receive the higher doses) and the protocol of the institution. Once the immunosuppressive regimen has been completed, the bone marrow transplant is performed, usually after a day of rest for the client.

Restrictions are begun in the pretransplant period and continued throughout the client's hospitalization. Personnel and family members dress in sterile garb, and visitors other than the family are discouraged. Food and liquids are sterilized before being served if the client is able to tolerate an oral diet. Again, the extent of these restrictions depends on the protocol in the transplant unit.

Both the pretransplant and the posttransplant periods are times of great discomfort and stress for the client. There are numerous uncomfortable and discouraging effects of both chemotherapy and total body irradiation, including nausea, vomiting, diarrhea, stomatitis, weakness, anorexia, and alopecia. Refer to Chapter 10 for the nursing care for clients undergoing chemotherapy and radiation therapy.

POSTOPERATIVE CARE OF THE RECIPIENT Engraftment (the appearance of normal erythrocytes, leukocytes, and thrombocytes in the bone marrow) takes from 2 to 4 weeks after BMT. While without a functioning bone marrow, the client is subject to infection and bleeding. Chemotherapy and total body irradiation cause the client to feel worse rather than better, and the nurse is constantly challenged to find ways to reduce the client's discomfort. During hospitalization, bone marrow aspirations are usually done weekly to assess bone marrow function. The uncertainty of whether the transplant will be successful remains a concern of clients, family, and the transplant team.

INFECTION The suppression of the client's bone marrow makes the client granulocytopenic. Protecting the client from infection is essential to the client's survival. Change IV tubing, central venous catheter dressings, and the client's bed linen and clothing daily. Daily baths with antimicrobial soaps should remain a part of the routine. Monitoring pulmonary hygiene; protecting skin integrity; and avoiding urinary drainage catheters, IM injections, and rectal medication help to prevent infection. Weekly cultures monitor the client's germ-free status and detect colonization before it becomes infection.

Assess the client's skin, mouth, throat, axilla, perineum, and rectum for signs of infection; check all body fluids and excreta for color and consistency; and obtain cultures if infection is suspected. Monitor vital signs and assess the lungs every 4 hours. The possibility of interstitial pneumonia, a frequent complication in immunosuppressed clients, warrants these continuous 4-hour assessments. A temperature of 38°C (100.4°F) or greater should be investigated by cultures with sensitivity determinations, chest x-ray, and urinalysis. IV wide-spectrum antibiotic therapy is instituted until the results of the cultures and sensitivities are obtained, after which specific antimicrobial therapy can be given.

Daily infusions of granulocytes are often given to the client with a granulocyte count below 500 μL and with a fever that fails to respond to antimicrobial therapy. In some institutions, granulocytes are administered routinely as a prophylactic measure. Granulocytes and all blood products are irradiated before infusion to eliminate any T-lymphocytes that could contribute to GVHD. Side effects and nursing measures with blood and blood product infusion are discussed in Chapter 22.

STOMATITIS The management of stomatitis is always aimed toward increasing the client's comfort and oral intake. Additional goals with the BMT client are to decrease bacterial and fungal superinfections and to decrease mucosal ulcerations that may cause bleeding in this client whose platelet count is low. The frequency of mouth care will need to increase as mucosal deterioration increases.

BLEEDING Assessing for petechiae, gastrointestinal bleeding, and conjunctival and cerebral hemorrhage is essential because the BMT client's low platelet counts may lead to these conditions necessitating infusions of platelets or packed red blood cells. Encourage family members to donate their blood for this purpose. Avoid IM and SC injections and rectal temperatures. Clients should not shave to avoid bleeding from cuts and nicks as well as impairment of skin integrity.

NUTRITION Clients are usually started on TPN 24 hours after the last dose of chemotherapy to prevent or reverse the catabolic state of malnutrition. The amounts to be infused are determined weekly by a nutritional support team and based on monitoring electrolytes, minerals, liver function, kidney function, and hematologic tests. Optimal nutritional status is essential during BMT. Anorexia, gastrointestinal and metabolic changes, and increased need for nutrients during periods of infection and fever combined with malnutrition increase the incidence of morbidity and mortality in BMT clients. Encourage as much oral intake as possible.

GRAFT-VERSUS-HOST DISEASE Because GVHD can occur despite the measures to prevent it discussed earlier, low-dose methotrexate or cyclosporine may be administered for 4 to 6 months after BMT. The onset of GVHD is serious because it signals the possibility that grafting has not been successful. At present, there is no known cure for GVHD, although the administration of high doses of corticosteroids has sometimes proven helpful. Clients who do not respond to steroid therapy may receive antithymocyte globulin (Nuscher et al., 1984).

Be alert for the development of both early onset and late onset GVHD. An early sign is impairment of skin integrity characterized by a rubellalike rash that begins on the face, palms of the hands, and the soles of the feet, eventually progressing to the trunk and the rest of the limbs. The skin may become dry and scaly, progressing to blistering and eventual desquamation (peeling). In some clients, the condition progresses to a chronic form in which inelasticity of the skin leads to contractures, scarring, impaired physical mobility, possible skin ulceration, and muscle wasting. Some clients do not have the early signs but rather begin with the chronic form up to 1 year after the transplant.

GVHD may also involve the gastrointestinal tract, causing nausea and vomiting, abdominal cramping, malabsorption, and bleeding. Clients can lose from 500 mL to 6 L of fluid per day in severe diarrhea that is a dark green-brown (Nuscher et al., 1984). Hepatic involvement causes pruritus, jaundice, ascites, and fatigue. The liver is enlarged and the serum bilirubin, alkaline phosphatase, and serum glutamic-oxaloacetic transaminase (SGOT) levels are elevated.

Assess the extent, nature, and location of the client's discomfort and administer analgesics accordingly. Topical creams and soothing oatmeal baths may help relieve the discomfort of pruritus. Petrolatum gauze may be used to cover blistered or desquamated areas. Keep the client's perianal area clean after each bowel movement. Soothing ointments may help irritated skin and also help to promote skin integrity.

Not only does GVHD cause physical discomfort, it also causes emotional distress. Clients who develop GVHD and their families may experience depression, anger, and fear of death. As clients lose hope, they may become reluctant to participate in self-care or refuse medical treatment. Sometimes clients withdraw from interaction by sleeping or refusing visitors. Explaining this behavior to family members will help them to understand it, tolerate it, and be supportive of the client. It is important to serve as an anchor for clients as well as their families by encouraging self-care, joining with them in the hope that symptoms will subside, pointing out any subtle signs of improvement, and sustaining them through despair and discouragement.

Client/Family Teaching

Discharge planning begins approximately 2 weeks after BMT. At least 2 weeks before discharge, the client and family should begin to perform the required care under nursing supervision. Instruct the family in skills such as caring for the central venous catheter, administering TPN, and administering medications.

Advise them to prevent infection by proper handwashing, avoiding contact with the client if they are ill, and remaining healthy. The client should avoid contacts with crowds and animals for at least the first 100 days after the transplant. Teach the client and family about the early signs of infection and GVHD.

Emphasize the importance of continued health care and assessments by dentists and dietitians because late-developing GVHD is a possibility. Until the immune system has regained normal function, the client is susceptible to infection, especially viral infection. Referral to a visiting nurse service is a resource for both client and family. Encourage clients and their families to identify the support systems available to them—other family members, friends, neighbors, community services, self-help groups, mental health counselors—and to plan to use them after discharge.

Splenectomy

Splenectomy, the surgical removal of the spleen, is usually performed for a spleen ruptured by trauma (eg, automobile accidents, knife or bullet penetration, or blows to the spleen) or because of severe hypersplenism. Because of recent evidence that the immune system may be compromised by spleen removal, splenectomy is usually reserved for life-threatening circumstances. The physiologic and psychosocial/lifestyle implications are discussed in Table 23–2.

Nursing Implications

PREOPERATIVE CARE The client about to undergo a splenectomy because of trauma may be in shock from blood loss. A major responsibility is to monitor the client's vital

Table 23–2
Splenectomy: Implications for the Client 

Physiologic Implications	Psychosocial/Lifestyle Implications
Compromised immune system with greater risk of infections (particularly pneumococcal infections) and adverse effect on antibody development	Temporary anticoagulant therapy
Thrombosis is early complication	Adequate rest and nutrition
Abdominal distention possible because of organ manipulation or thromboses in portal system	Stop smoking
Subphrenic abscess and atelectasis of the left lower lobe with pneumonia are possible complications	Contact with health care provider necessary for infection or exposure to infectious disease; may require prophylactic antimicrobial therapy and periodic pneumococcal vaccine (Pneumovax)

signs and undertake preparations for surgery as soon as possible. Anxiety may accompany the urgent nature of the client's condition as well as result from tissue hypoxia related to blood loss. Support and reassurance of the client and family are important in the preoperative period.

POSTOPERATIVE CARE Routine postoperative care for abdominal surgery is performed along with monitoring for hemorrhage and potential shock. The client with idiopathic thrombocytopenic purpura has an increased tendency for hemorrhage because the platelet level is decreased from its preoperative level. Platelet transfusion may aid in reducing this threat. The traumatized client is also a potential candidate for hemorrhage from trauma to other body sites.

Because the platelet count automatically rises after surgery up to five times the normal level before subsiding within about 7 days after surgery, the client is at risk for thrombosis and thromboembolic phenomena. Take measures to reduce the risk of postoperative thrombosis and assess the client regularly to detect possible thrombophlebitis. Insertion of an intracaval filter or plication of the inferior vena cava may be necessary in some clients.

Assess for abdominal distention and apply abdominal binders snugly to decrease distention and increase the client's comfort. Monitoring for abdominal distention is important in determining the possibility of thrombi being lodged in the portal system.

Monitor the client's temperature carefully. Temperature elevation (38.3°C or 101°F) for 7 to 10 days postoperatively may be related to thrombosis of the splenic vein. Temperature elevation may also occur in conjunction with the development of a left subphrenic abscess. Assessment of respiratory status and respiratory distress are also indicated and give clues to the possibility of subphrenic abscess.

Before discharge, instruct the client on avoiding situations with high infection risk and explain the lifestyle modifications necessitated by removal of the spleen. Remind the client of the need for regular health care follow-up.

Chapter Highlights

Multifactorial hematologic disorders may interfere with one or more of the following functions of the bone marrow elements: resistance to infectious organisms, coagulation, or the transportation of oxygen to tissues.

These multifactorial disorders include aplastic, pernicious, and iron deficiency anemia and disseminated intravascular coagulation (DIC).

Acquired immune deficiency syndrome (AIDS) is an immunologic disorder involving the T-lymphocytes. Prevention is crucial because AIDS has no known cure.

Neoplastic hematologic disorders—the leukemias, lymphomas, and multiple myeloma—involve infiltration and disruption of normal bone marrow function and an alteration in the usual protective mechanism of the immune system.

Nursing care of the client with leukemia centers around leukopenia, anemia, and thrombocytopenia. In addition, the client may need help in dealing with pain, ineffective coping skills, body-image changes, and the side effects of chemotherapy.

The nursing care of clients with multiple myeloma includes promoting comfort and preventing spontaneous fractures and renal shutdown.

Nursing management of polycythemia vera clients centers around reducing hypervolemia and hyperviscosity, providing client education, promoting vascular integrity, and preventing stasis.

Bone marrow transplant is a life-saving measure used when other treatments for aplastic anemia, severe immunodeficiency, leukemia, and Hodgkin's disease have failed.

Splenectomy is almost always an emergency procedure performed to control bleeding from a ruptured spleen, although it is sometimes done in hypersplenism.

Bibliography

American Cancer Society: *Facts and Figures*. New York: American Cancer Society, 1987.

Bakemeier RF et al: The malignant lymphomas: Hodgkin's disease and non-Hodgkin's lymphoma, multiple myeloma, and macroglobulinemia. In: *Clinical Oncology for Medical Students and Physicians*. Bakemeier RF (editor). Rochester, NY: American Cancer Society, 1983.

Benenson AS: *Control of Communicable Disease in Man,* 14th ed. Washington, DC: American Public Health Association, 1985.

Bennett JA: AIDS epidemiology update. *Am J Nurs* 1985; 85:968–972.

Brown MH, Kiss ME: Standards of care for the patient with "graft-versus-host disease" post bone marrow transplant. *Canc Nurs* 1981; 4:191–198.

Caza B, Ross CA: Living with leukemia. *Can Nurse* (Sept) 1981; 77:32–36.

CDC: Update: Prospective evaluation of health-care workers exposed via parenteral or mucous-membrane route to blood or body fluids from patients with acquired immunodeficiency syndrome. *MMWR* 1985: 34:101–103.

Consalvo D, Gallagher M: Winning the battle against Hodgkin's disease. *RN* 1986; 49 (Dec) 20–25.

Curran JW et al: The epidemiology of AIDS: Current status and future prospects. *Science* 1985; 229:1352–1357.

Ersek MT: The adult leukemia patient in the intensive care unit. *Heart Lung* 1984; 13:183–193.

Farrant C: Multiple myeloma: Controlling pain, prolonging survival. *RN* 1987; 50 (Jan):38–42.

Ford R et al: Veno-occlusive disease following marrow transplantation. *Nurs Clin North Am* 1983; 18(9):563–568.

Hutchinson MM, Itoh K: Nursing care for the patient undergoing bone marrow transplantation for acute leukemia. *Nurs Clin North Am* 1982; 17(12):697–711.

Kayser SR: Thrombosis. In: *Applied Therapeutics: The Clinical Use of Drugs,* 3rd ed. Katcher BS, Young LY, Koda–Kimble, MA (editors). San Francisco: Applied Therapeutics, 1983; 333–360.

Levitt DE: Multiple myeloma. *Am J Nurs* 1981; 81:1345–1347.

Maxwell MB: When the cancer patient becomes anemic. *Cancer Nurs* 1984; 7:499–503.

Nuscher R et al: Bone marrow transplantation. *Am J Nurs* 1984; 84:764–772.

Reich P: *Hematology: Physiopathologic Basis for Clinical Practice,* 2nd ed. Boston: Little, Brown, 1984.

Rodman MJ, Smith DW: *Clinical Pharmacology in Nursing,* 2nd ed. Philadelphia: Lippincott, 1984.

Spivak J (editor): *Fundamentals of Clinical Hematology,* 2nd ed. Philadelphia: Harper & Row, 1984.

Stewart FM et al.: Bone marrow transplantation: Three treatments for disease. *AORN J* 1985; 42:196–205.

Thomas ED: Bone marrow failure and bone marrow transplantation. In: *Harrison's Principles of Internal Medicine,* 10th ed. Petersdorf RG et al (editors). New York: McGraw–Hill, 1983.

Turner JG, Pryor E: AIDS: Risk containment for home health care providers. *Fam Community Health* 8(3):25, 1985.

Turner JG, Williamson KM: AIDS: A challenge for contemporary nursing. *Foc Crit Care* Part I, 13(3):53, 1986; Part II, 13(4):41, 1986.

Williams WJ et al: *Hematology,* 3rd ed. New York: McGraw–Hill, 1983.

Yasko JM: *Guidelines for Cancer Care: Symptom Management.* Reston, VA: Reston, 1983.

UNIT 5

The Client With Urinary Dysfunction

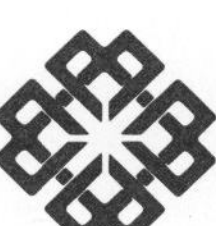

CHAPTER **24**

The Kidneys and Urinary System in Health and Illness

Other topics relevant to this content are: Electrolytes and acid–base balance, **Chapter 3;** Renin-angiotensin-aldosterone system, **Chapter 35.**

Objectives

When you have finished studying this chapter, you should be able to:

Describe the structural components of the urinary tract and their major anatomic relationships.

Identify the functions of the nephron.

Explain the major circulatory variables that contribute to renal function.

Describe renal–hormonal mechanisms for maintaining fluid balance and regulating blood pressure.

Trace the pathway for the formation and excretion of urine.

Identify the primary electrolyte and acid–base abnormalities associated with failure of renal regulation.

Describe the general effects of uremia.

Discuss general psychosocial and cultural considerations relevant to the kidneys and urinary system.

The urinary system includes the kidneys, ureters, urinary bladder, and urethra. Although this system has as a major function the removal of waste products from the body, it actually accomplishes much more than that. The urinary system is also essential to the maintenance of homeostasis. The kidneys rid the body of a variety of metabolic waste products as well as conserve or excrete fluid and electrolytes as needed to maintain the internal balance of these substances. To do so, the kidneys filter a volume equivalent to all of the blood plasma in the body every 5 minutes. A person can live with only one kidney. If both kidneys fail, however, many of these waste products cannot be removed from the body. To prevent death in these cases, a kidney transplant or dialysis is necessary. The importance of the ureters, bladder, and urethra must not be overlooked. They transport urine, and the bladder also stores it. All structures function together to accomplish these important tasks.

SECTION 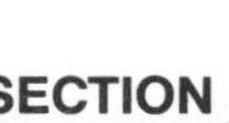

Structural and Functional Interrelationships

Structure of the Kidneys

The kidneys lie in the retroperitoneal space of the posterior abdominal cavity on either side of the vertebral column. Thus, a surgeon can expose them without opening the peritoneal cavity. Layers of muscle surround the posterior surfaces of the kidneys, and abdominal organs surround their anterior surfaces.

The position of the kidneys is not fixed but varies somewhat with a person's position. When the client is in the supine position, the kidneys lie between the 12th thoracic and 3rd lumbar vertebrae. When the client is standing, the kidneys may descend to the top of the iliac crest. For a client in Trendelenburg's position, the kidneys ascend to the 10th intercostal space.

The right kidney is lower in the abdomen than the left because of the presence of the liver in the right upper quadrant. The lower portion of each kidney descends beneath the lower portion of the rib cage. The angle formed between the lower rim of the rib cage and the vertebral column is referred to as the costovertebral angle (CVA).

Each kidney is surrounded by three layers of tissue. The fibrous renal capsule, the innermost layer, covers the surface of the kidney. The adipose capsule, a mass of perirenal fat, surrounds the renal capsule. The third layer, the renal fascia, surrounds and encloses the kidney and adipose capsule and anchors the kidney to the posterior abdominal wall. The perirenal fat, renal fascia, and surrounding muscles protect and support the kidneys.

The cross-sectional view in Figure 24–1A shows three general regions of each kidney: the cortex, the medulla, and the pelvis. These structures are located inside the renal capsule; two of them, the cortex and the medulla, are often referred to as the *renal parenchyma.* The cortex is a highly vascularized area of tissue very sensitive to changes in blood flow. The medulla, located deep in the cortex, consists of 8 to 18 triangular renal pyramids. The renal pyramids are composed of collecting ducts that drain urine into the calyces. The cortex covers the bases of the pyramids, and the tips (or papillae) project toward the renal pelvis. Cortical tissue known as *renal columns* dips into the medulla to separate the pyramids, and blood vessels that supply the cortex and medulla pass through these columns. Urine flows from the papillae into a minor calyx, and several of the funnel-shaped minor calyces emerge to form a major calyx. The major calyces join to form the renal pelvis, which is the expanded upper end of the ureter.

Blood is supplied to the kidneys by the renal artery of the abdominal aorta. Each renal artery branches into increasingly smaller arteries, which supply progressively smaller areas of the kidney. Blood returns to the general circulation through a series of renal venules and veins; the renal vein of each kidney returns blood into the inferior vena cava.

The *nephron,* the functional unit of the kidney, is primarily responsible for most of the mechanisms that provide internal homeostasis. Each kidney contains approximately 1.25 million nephrons, and each nephron in turn is composed of a vascular and tubular system that allows for the formation of urine (Figure 24–1B). The nephrons are located in the renal parenchyma. Most nephrons are in the cortex (cortical nephrons), but juxtamedullary nephrons begin in the cortex and extend deep into the medulla.

The vascular system of the nephron consists of the glomerulus and Bowman's capsule, both located in the cortex of the kidney. The glomerulus is composed of a knot of capillaries. Bowman's capsule, or the glomerular capsule, surrounds the glomerulus.

The tubular system of the nephron begins with Bow-

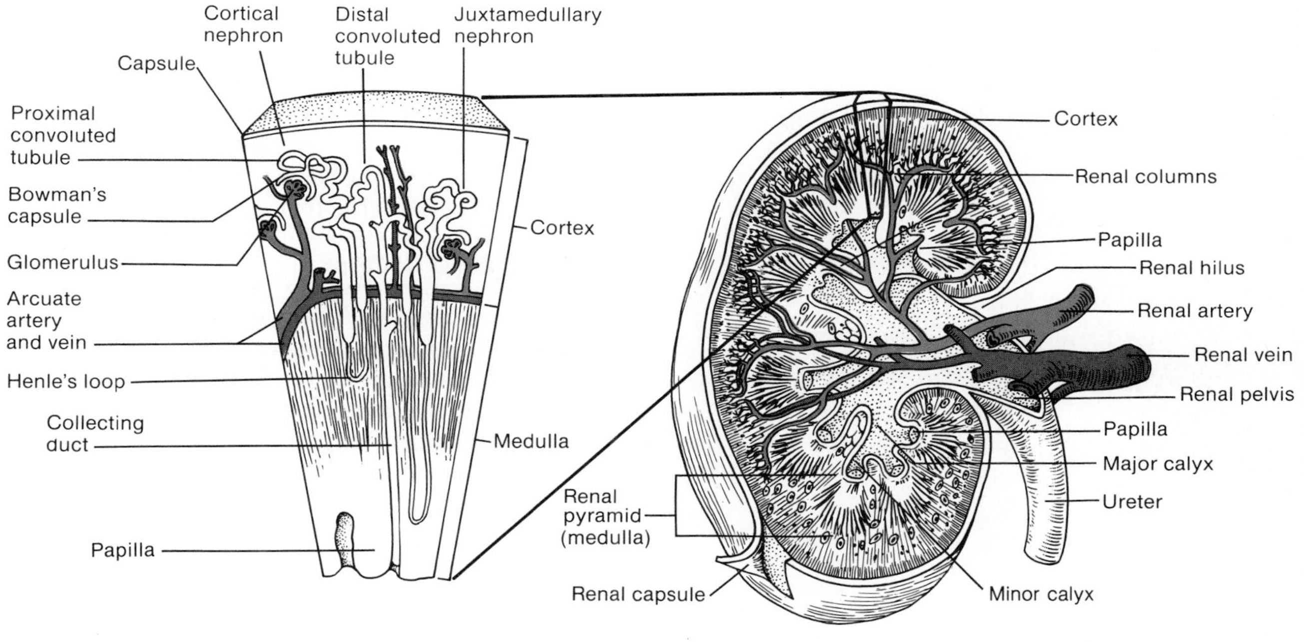

Figure 24–1

A. Longitudinal section of kidney showing internal structure. **B.** Longitudinal section of kidney showing location of cortical and juxtamedullary nephrons.

man's capsule, which is invaginated around each glomerular tuft to form a sac. Bowman's capsule narrows into the proximal convoluted tubule, which changes direction many times until it straightens into the descending limb of Henle's loop and angles downward toward the pelvis of the kidney. The hairpin loops of tubular tissue are much longer in juxtamedullary nephrons than in cortical nephrons and are contained within the pyramids of the medulla. The ascending limb of Henle's loop then becomes the distal convoluted tubule. The distal convoluted tubules of several nephrons enter a collecting duct within a pyramid of the medulla from which they drain into the calyceal system of the renal pelvis through the tips of the papillae.

Structure of the Ureters

From the renal pelvis, ureters transport urine to the urinary bladder. Each kidney normally has a single ureter, which is responsible for emptying the urine formed by that kidney. Although the ureter's length varies with the size of the individual, an average ureter is around 30 cm (almost a foot) long. The ureter's diameter ranges from 2 to 8 mm at various points in its structure.

The ureters descend between the parietal peritoneum and the body wall to the pelvic cavity, where they enter the bladder on its posterior inferior surface (refer to Figure 24–2). Before opening into the bladder, the ureters travel obliquely through the bladder wall. As a result, pressure in the bladder can compress the ureters and help prevent urine from flowing back into the ureters, especially during bladder emptying.

Each ureter is composed of both longitudinal and circular muscular fibers responsible for the peristalsis of urine into the urinary bladder. The narrow points of the ureter are at the junction of the ureter and the renal pelvis, the ureteropelvic (U-P) junction; the point at which the ureters cross over the iliac vessels; and the point of ureteral entry into the bladder, the ureterovesical (U-V) junction. The importance of these locations is described in the section on nephrolithiasis and urolithiasis in Chapter 26.

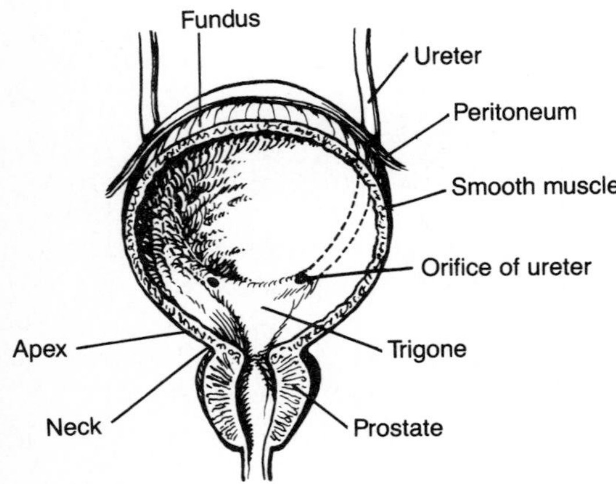

Figure 24–2

Opened male urinary bladder showing trigone. SOURCE: *Vick RL: Contemporary Medical Physiology. Menlo Park, CA: Addison-Wesley, 1984.*

Structure of the Urinary Bladder

The urinary bladder, a muscular sac capable of tremendous distention, is used to store formed urine. The bladder rests on the floor of the pelvic cavity and is retroperitoneal. Its anterior surface lies just behind the pubic symphysis. In males, the bladder is in front of the rectum, whereas in females it lies just anterior to the uterus and the superior portion of the vagina.

The major anatomic areas of the bladder are the fundus, the apex, the neck, and the trigone (Figure 24–2). The fundus is the upper portion of the bladder, and the apex is the bottom portion of the bladder closest to the pelvic floor. The bladder neck is the most inferior portion of the bladder and contains the internal sphincter. It is actually a group of thickened fibers of the detrusor muscle, which evolves into the smooth muscle of the urethra. The trigone is an area of the posterior wall of the bladder defined by the urethra and the two ureteral slits, where the ureters enter the bladder. Special characteristics of this area of muscle are responsible for separating the upper urinary tract from the lower urinary tract during normal micturition.

The nerve supply to the bladder is both sensory and motor. Sympathetic fibers arise from T-9 through L-2, and parasympathetic and somatic nerves arise from S-2 through S-4. The motor nerve supply to the bladder involves parasympathetic supply to the detrusor muscle and sympathetic supply to the trigone. The pudendal nerves, which are under voluntary control, supply the external sphincter and the muscles of the pelvic floor.

Structure of the Urethra

The urethra is a muscular tube lined with mucous membranes that exits from the inferior surface of the urinary bladder and carries urine to the exterior of the body. The urethra of the male is about 21 cm long and about 8 to 9 mm in diameter. In the female, the urethra is about 4 cm long and about 8 mm in diameter. Because of the proximity of the anus and vagina to the urethra, normal microorganisms found in those regions may more easily migrate into the bladder. This accounts for why women are more likely than men to have bladder infections.

Regulatory Functions of the Kidneys

The kidneys and urinary system maintain internal homeostasis of body fluids and their composition. A variety of mechanisms maintain this fluid and electrolyte balance, and the end result is the production of urine. This final product represents the work of the kidneys and results in the removal of nitrogenous waste products, as well as the regulation of fluid, electrolyte, and acid–base balances. In addition, the kidneys produce hormones and additional substances that influence other metabolic and chemical processes (see Unit 7).

Formation of Urine

The basic function of the nephron is to cleanse the blood of unwanted substances as it passes through the kidney. This results in the formation of urine and is accomplished through three specific processes that occur in the nephron: glomerular filtration, tubular reabsorption, and tubular secretion.

GLOMERULAR FILTRATION Glomerular filtration is the ultrafiltration of blood across a semipermeable membrane in which fluid, electrolytes, and certain nonelectrolytes are filtered but plasma proteins remain. Glomerular filtration occurs within the glomerulus, across the glomerular capillary membrane. Small pores within the lining of the capillary loops of the glomerulus (called the *basement membrane*) allow the passage of fluid and certain particles.

Certain conditions must exist for glomerular filtration to occur. There must be adequate fluid volume (blood volume or plasma) in the intravascular space, as well as adequate hydrostatic pressure to overcome the forces that oppose glomerular filtration. The pumping of the heart and vascular resistance provide the hydrostatic pressure. The vascular tone, or blood flow, within the kidney is under two types of control: (1) extrinsic factors such as sympathetic nerve fibers from the celiac and renal nerve plexuses and (2) intrinsic control, called *autoregulation of renal blood flow.* Each has a definite purpose (Guyton, 1985).

The sympathetic nervous system provides extrinsic control of renal blood flow when an emergency situation exists. Normal renal blood flow is 1200 mL/min, but this flow may be decreased to 200 mL/min when blood is needed to supply the heart, brain, or skeletal muscle. This is a strong vasoconstrictor response to the release of epinephrine and norepinephrine by the sympathetic nervous system.

Autoregulation of blood flow maintains a constancy of glomerular filtration through the kidney's unique ability to regulate the resistance of the afferent and efferent arterioles to the flow of blood. Because of this autoregulation, arterial blood pressure can vary widely—between 80 and 180 mm Hg—while renal blood flow and glomerular filtration remain basically unchanged.

The product of glomerular filtration is glomerular filtrate. The normal glomerular filtration rate is 130 mL/min. Thus, roughly 187,000 mL of glomerular filtrate is formed in 24 hours. Glomerular filtrate is composed of water, sodium, potassium, calcium, magnesium, chloride, bicarbonate, phosphate, and other anions; glucose; urea; creatinine; uric acid; and amino acids. The filtrate does not contain protein, because the glomerular membrane is almost completely impermeable to all plasma proteins. For all practical purposes, glomerular filtrate is the same as plasma except it has no significant amount of plasma proteins. If all these substances were excreted as urine, death would occur immediately. Therefore, much of the filtrate is returned to the blood via tubular reabsorption.

TUBULAR REABSORPTION In tubular reabsorption, the initial refinement process, water and specific electrolytes and nonelectrolytes from the tubular filtrate are reabsorbed into the plasma of the peritubular capillaries or vasa recta. Tubular reabsorption occurs throughout the tubular system of the nephron, but much of it occurs within the proximal convoluted tubule.

The tubules have a limited capacity for reabsorption of some substances. For example, the threshold for reabsorption of glucose may be limited when the blood level of glucose is exceedingly high or when renal tubular surfaces are altered through injury. Reabsorption is primarily accomplished through diffusion and active transport. In *diffusion,* molecules move from an area of greater to lesser concentration or greater to lesser pressure. With some substances, however, expenditure of energy may be necessary to move the molecules. *Active transport* occurs through this expenditure of energy—basically, the release of adenosine triphosphate (ATP).

Normally, reabsorption from the tubular filtrate into the blood is sufficient to maintain normal serum levels of the various electrolytes. However, reabsorption of some nonelectrolytes (eg, urea, creatinine, and uric acid) is not readily accomplished. The organism benefits from this because these substances are removed or cleared from the body.

Reabsorption of water is by osmosis. Water is reabsorbed primarily in the proximal convoluted tubule. If greater water reabsorption is needed to maintain balance, however, the permeability of the distal tubule and collecting duct may be increased.

This reabsorption of water reflects the kidneys' ability to concentrate or dilute the urine as necessary. Sensitive osmoreceptors in the hypothalamus sense the plasma osmolality. Only slight alterations in the osmolality of the blood are required to trigger appropriate regulatory mechanisms. A combined response by the neuroendocrine system and the kidneys will ensure that the serum osmolality is returned to the normal range by the release of antidiuretic hormone (ADH) from its storage area in the posterior pituitary. The ADH alters the permeability of the distal convoluted tubules and collecting ducts so more or less water can be reabsorbed as needed. When ADH secretion increases, so does the reabsorption of the water in the tubules; when ADH secretion decreases, more water is excreted by the kidneys. Maintenance of intravascular volume is always the primary goal of the homeostatic mechanism. Thus, normally functioning kidneys concentrate or dilute urine to maintain normal serum osmolality.

TUBULAR SECRETION The third major process in urine formation is tubular secretion, the process by which ions in the tubular cells are secreted into the lumen of the tubule to be excreted in the end product, urine. Tubular secretion of potassium and hydrogen regulates the serum potassium level and serves as the kidney's acid–base balancing mechanism.

The kidneys regulate acids and bases in conjunction with other body regulatory mechanisms (ie, the blood buffers and the lungs). The kidneys are responsible for the secretion of the fixed acids of normal metabolism, whereas the lungs excrete the volatile acids. The blood buffers provide moment-to-moment regulation. The fixed acids derive primarily from the metabolism of protein. The kidneys regulate their excretion by conserving bicarbonate, excreting sodium in exchange for the secretion of hydrogen, and secreting ammonia.

Thus, the processes of filtration, reabsorption, and secretion create the end product, urine. Urine is composed primarily of water, sodium, potassium, chloride, urea, creatinine, and uric acid. The volume of urine is normally about 1500 mL per 24 hours, but it depends on the amount of solute that must be excreted.

Blood Pressure Control

The kidneys regulate blood pressure through the maintenance of fluid volume and the release of the hormone renin, which stimulates powerful vasoconstrictive responses. Fluid volume in the extracellular compartment, and specifically the plasma, is controlled by the kidneys' ability to concentrate or dilute urine in response to the serum osmolality. Thus, hypertonic plasma stimulates the release of ADH, the reabsorption of water, the expansion of intravascular volume, the decrease of urine output, and the elevation of blood pressure. This primary mechanism of volume expansion is partially responsible for the regulation of blood pressure.

Renin release influences blood pressure. When renin is liberated from the juxtaglomerular cells it acts on angiotensinogen, a glycoprotein made in the liver and normally found in plasma, converting it to angiotensin I. Another converting enzyme in the pulmonary capillary bed acts on angiotensin I to change it to angiotensin II, a powerful vasoconstrictor that elevates blood pressure through peripheral vasoconstriction. Angiotensin II also triggers the release by the adrenal cortex of aldosterone, a mineralocorticoid that helps control sodium utilization. With the release of aldosterone, the distal convoluted tubule of the nephron reabsorbs sodium, and water reabsorption follows the sodium reabsorption increasing plasma volume. Thus, angiotensin II has two main effects that help to elevate blood pressure: peripheral vasoconstriction and plasma volume expansion. When ADH production increases, aldosterone production usually does as well.

When cardiac output is severely decreased because of loss of circulating blood volume, vasoconstriction within the kidneys will severely limit intrarenal blood flow and maintain flow to more vital organs, the heart and brain. This is an excellent example of the kidneys' role in the preservation of the whole organism because if renal vasoconstriction is not abated, death of the renal parenchyma results.

Process of Micturition

Micturition, also called *urination* or *voiding,* is a complex physical process under a variety of neural controls. For the toilet-trained person, urination is voluntary and can be interrupted or initiated upon cerebral command, as long as motor and sensory nerve pathways are intact. Micturition normally is a painless function that occurs five to six times a day and possibly once at night (2–3 times at night in the elderly because of decreased bladder capacity and weakened sphincter and detrusor muscles). The average person voids a total of about 1500 mL of urine per 24 hours. This amount is affected by fluid intake, the ingestion of diuretics, sweating, temperature, vomiting, and diarrhea.

The adult usually perceives an initial desire to empty the urinary bladder when about 150 mL of urine has accumulated there. However, the bladder can distend to a much larger capacity, and it often does before there is a feeling of bladder fullness. Since urine accumulates gradually in the bladder, the slow distention of the muscular sac accommodates larger and larger quantities of urine.

Micturition involves a number of responses that occur almost simultaneously. Initially, there is the felt need to void. After the person has determined that environmental conditions are satisfactory, a series of nerve impulses are activated to allow the release of urine. First, the muscles of the pelvic floor are relaxed, which relaxes the urethral opening and allows the descent of the urinary bladder. Next, the trigone contracts, which ensures closure of the U-V junction and prevents the reflux of urine into the ureters. Trigonal contraction also causes contraction of the bladder neck, which makes the bladder more funnel shaped. Finally, the detrusor muscle of the bladder, which is continuous with the urethral lining, contracts. Detrusor contraction increases the pressure within the bladder and results in bladder emptying.

The cerebral control mechanism can interrupt the voiding process at any point identified as appropriate. When the bladder is empty, the detrusor muscle relaxes, the bladder neck closes, the trigone assumes its normal tone, and the perineal muscles resume their normal tone.

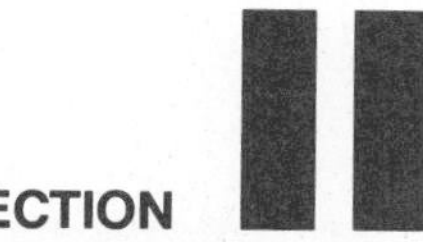

Pathophysiologic Influences and Effects

Alterations in urine formation and excretion have profound effects on homeostasis. Failure to maintain the chemical balance of the fluids of the various fluid compartments will result in death unless the balance is restored. Manifestations of alterations in urine formation and excretion may include changes in the clearance rates of substances, changes in the amount and composition of the urine and the pattern of its excretion, elevated blood pressure, decreased maturation of red blood cells, and changes in the excretion of metabolic waste products.

Alterations in Fluid Volume

With renal dysfunction, the inability to control fluid volume may have a variety of sequelae. For example, a loss of the ability of the kidneys to concentrate urine may be the earliest observation of renal pathology. Continuous loss of dilute urine in turn may result in volume depletion and thus low blood pressure. *Hypovolemia* will eventually alter renal function, because adequate blood volume is required to establish a pressure gradient so that glomerular filtration can occur.

Although the kidneys have the capacity for some autoregulation of blood flow, they also will deprive the renal parenchyma of necessary blood volume if the organism demands are greater elsewhere. Fluid deficits can also occur with abnormal decreases in the ingestion of water or excessive water losses from diarrhea, vomiting, or rapid dehydration.

Failure of the kidneys to excrete water and thus maintain normal fluid volume also has serious consequences for the overall functioning of the body. *Hypervolemia* puts severe strain on the cardiovascular system. Hypertension will cause long-term problems related to ventricular hypertrophy and increased peripheral vascular resistance. More immediate changes that are due to fluid shifts, particularly into the lungs, will impair adequate diffusion of gases and can cause severe hypoxia.

The response to ischemia of any renal tissue is the liberation of renin and the stimulation of the renin–angiotensin–aldosterone system. The release of renin is triggered to increase renal blood flow in response to hormonal mechanisms, but it is also associated with increased volume retention and volume expansion. Particularly, this can happen in kidney tissue damage that affects the normal formation of urine, but aldosterone and ADH are being produced normally. Therefore, overhydration is more common as the client reaches end-stage renal disease.

Electrolyte Imbalances

Hyperkalemia is the most frequently encountered imbalance in chronic renal failure. The kidney tubules also may fail to conserve potassium correctly and thus excrete large amounts. *Hypokalemia* can alter the medullary interstitium of the kidney and impair renal function.

Hypernatremia can occur in clients with end-stage renal disease when urine volume drops to very low levels. In these cases, even a restricted salt intake results in sodium and water retention with edema and pump failure. Since sodium conservation occurs primarily in the renal medulla, deterioration of this area produces *hyponatremia* which leads to decreased extracellular fluid. As the circulating blood volume decreases, the glomerular filtration rate decreases, and renal function is further compromised.

When the glomerular filtration rate decreases to around 30 mL/min, the renal excretion of phosphate also decreases. The body's response to *hyperphosphatemia* causes the calcium level (nonprotein-bound or ionized) to decrease. In renal insufficiency, the kidney is unable to produce 1,25-dihydroxycholecalciferol. Without it, calcium cannot be utilized. This further contributes to the development of hypocalcemia.

The ongoing process of hyperphosphatemia and hypocalcemia with subsequent production of parathormone results in secondary hyperparathyroidism. Untreated, this leads to serious bone pathology known as *renal osteodystrophy* (discussed later in this chapter).

When urine output is low and a normal magnesium intake continues, *hypermagnesemia* can occur. It may also be aggravated by the administration of magnesium-containing laxatives and antacids.

Accumulation of Uremic Toxins

Azotemia is the accumulation of uremic toxins (urea, uric acid, and creatinine) in the blood. **Uremia** refers to azotemia with clinical symptoms. The accumulation of uremic toxins in renal failure can result in neurologic complications, gastrointestinal bleeding, and skin changes resulting from urochrome pigments deposited in the skin. This pigmentation, combined with anemia, results in the pale yellow–gray color characteristic of clients with renal failure. Pruritus, also common, is thought to be the result of a buildup of the urochrome pigments in the skin as well as the crust of urate crystals that accumulates on the skin (called **uremic frost** because it is similar in appearance to frost on a window on a cold morning).

The accumulation of uremic toxins also causes neurologic changes that range from fatigue, decreased ability to concentrate, irritability, and insomnia to depression, peripheral neuropathy, and retinopathy. Coma, convulsions, and death can occur if the toxins are not removed.

Uremic toxins and gastrointestinal bleeding cause nutrition-related problems. The gastrointestinal tract becomes inflamed and irritated because of the uremic toxins. This results in loss of appetite, nausea, vomiting, and diarrhea—problems that further complicate fluid and electrolyte imbalances. The irritability of the gastrointestinal tract, compounded by altered platelet function, causes the gastrointestinal bleeding so common in clients with impaired kidney function. The buildup of ammonia in the body results in a characteristic **uremic fetor**—a urinelike odor of the client's breath accompanied by a bad taste in the mouth (described by some as metallic)—which greatly alters the appeal of food. Associated pancreatitis may also impair digestion.

Alterations in Urine Output

Urine output may greatly increase in certain situations, such as in the diuretic phase of acute renal failure. However, a decreased urine output is the more common alteration. This may be temporary, as with the oliguric phase of acute renal failure, benign prostatic hyperplasia, or kidney stone obstruction of the urethra, or it may be a long-term sequela common with acute tubular necrosis and chronic renal failure.

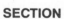

SECTION III

Related System Influences and Effects

Since the kidneys and urinary system perform multiple functions related to the performance of many body systems, impairment of renal function can affect other body systems to varying extents, and other body systems can influence renal function.

Integumentary System

Dry, pale, yellow–gray skin is characteristic of renal failure. Nails and hair are also brittle and dry. Pruritus may become so severe that clients scratch until they bleed. This break in skin integrity increases the client's susceptibility to infection. Edema from sodium and water retention, as well as poor nutritional status, can also make the skin highly susceptible to breakdown. Pressure ulcers may form within hours if clients are not frequently repositioned. (See Unit 13.)

Cardiovascular System

Uremic pericarditis is fairly common for clients with end-stage renal disease. The cause of this inflammatory response is believed to be related to nitrogenous waste products not removed by dialysis. Massive pericardial effusions (greater than 2000 mL) may accumulate over a period of days to weeks, seriously altering cardiovascular hemodynamics, possibly leading to cardiac tamponade.

Accelerated atherosclerotic processes have been observed in clients with chronic renal failure. An increased incidence of death from coronary artery disease seems to be associated with the effects of chronic essential hypertension, ventricular hypertrophy, and possible alterations in lipid metabolism associated with uremia. In addition, diffuse atherosclerotic processes that include cerebral, aortic, and peripheral vessels are not uncommon. Clients with these conditions frequently develop renal failure as a result of chronic glomerulonephritis, nephrosclerosis, renal artery stenotic lesions, or atheromatous embolization.

Uncontrolled hypertension, either from volume or hormonal response, greatly increases peripheral vascular resistance in small blood vessels throughout the body. The loss of elasticity of the arterioles in the kidneys as well as other organs, such as the retina of the eye and the small vessel circulation of the brain, will seriously affect the long-term functioning of those organs.

Cardiac dysrhythmias may result from the kidneys' inability to regulate potassium. The problems of fluid overload have been discussed earlier.

Respiratory System

The interrelation of the renal and respiratory systems is important in maintaining an acid–base balance. Although this balance is partially restored in the client with renal failure by medication and control of diet, these conservative measures can accomplish only so much. Dialysis may assist, but the lungs must help to control this narrow range of imbalance minute to minute. Clients with obstructive lung disease have carbon dioxide retention with respiratory acidosis. Thus, when renal and respiratory diseases exist simultaneously, the ability to combat metabolic acidosis is severely impaired because of the already present respiratory acidosis. Gas exchange is further hampered by pulmonary edema and anemia states.

Nervous System

Uremic encephalopathy (the development of altered mentation and intellectual processes, speech manifestations, and the presence of tremors and myoclonus) is characteristically associated with the onset of uremic manifestations. Grand mal seizures may develop if the encephalopathic process is not corrected.

Peripheral neuropathies are common in the client with end-stage renal disease who requires chronic dialysis. These neuropathies are neither clearly understood nor easily treated.

Musculoskeletal System

Musculoskeletal manifestations of renal failure are collectively referred to as **renal osteodystrophy.** A variety of problems, including osteomalacia, osteoporosis, and osteitis fibrosa cystica, may result from the chronic stimulation for release of parathormone because of elevated phosphorus levels and decreased calcium levels in the serum. Bone pain, increased tendencies for fractures, and metastatic calcifications throughout the body result from this chronic imbalance.

Hematopoietic System

Clients with renal failure have a chronic normochromic, normocytic anemia. Hematocrit values fall to 20% to 30%, and hemoglobin values drop to 7 to 8 g/dL. For clients with coronary artery disease, decreased circulating red blood cell mass may exacerbate anginal attacks or increase tendencies to develop arrhythmias, particularly if hypoxia occurs.

Although the platelet count is normal, and there is no alteration in the ability to produce platelets, in the uremic environment the platelets do not promote the clotting mechanism as well and bleeding time may be prolonged. Impaired platelet function in the uremic environment is believed to be responsible for the frequent and easily induced bleeding into the skin and mucous membranes of the client with either acute or chronic renal failure.

Gastrointestinal System

Uremia profoundly affects the gastrointestinal system. The inability to eat or retain food results in loss of weight and a breakdown of muscle and fat. Uncorrected, profound debilitation results, because the client is less able to combat infections and make appropriate immune responses.

The effects of uremia may be observed throughout the gastrointestinal system. As has been described, the client will notice a bad taste in the mouth (described by some as metallic) and a urinelike odor to the breath. Alteration in taste sensation, known as *hypogeusia,* involves both loss of acuity and loss of ability to discriminate tastes. These significant changes in the ability to taste foods, along with uremic fetor, make eating less pleasurable.

Parotitis, gastritis, pancreatitis, and colitis may occur at varying stages in the development of uremia. Irritation of the gastric and intestinal mucosa often is accompanied by vague discomfort, nausea, vomiting, eructation, and diarrhea. Bleeding from the mucous membrane lining the gastrointestinal tract is common because platelet abnormalities alter the clotting mechanism. The bleeding generally is occult, but gross bleeding with severe gastritis is also common.

Reproductive System

The loss of renal function and the development of uremia also affect the reproductive systems of both men and women. Both experience a loss of libido, and men frequently become impotent. Fertility is affected as well: Men have lower testosterone levels and a decrease in sperm formation, whereas women ovulate and menstruate less often, if at all. Successfully carrying a pregnancy to term is rare.

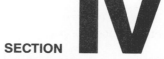

SECTION

Psychosocial/Lifestyle Influences and Effects

Sex

Sex influences the structure of the urinary system in an important way. As has been discussed, because the urethra is shorter in women, they are more prone to cystitis (bladder infection) than men. Stress urinary incontinence is not uncommon in women who have experienced relaxation of the pelvic muscles as a result of pregnancy.

Developmental and Cultural Influences

Urination is important in our daily routines. In fact, people who have stopped urinating almost completely because of renal failure frequently describe the absence of this physical act from the habits of a usual day as odd, unusual, and difficult to get used to.

Our society has specific values and attitudes toward the organs associated with the urinary tract, as well as toward urination itself. Most young children learn that control is probably the most important aspect related to urination. Urine should also be delivered into appropriate

Nursing Research Note

Hilbert G: An investigation of the relationship between social support and compliance of hemodialysis patients. *AANNTJ* (April) 1985; 12:133–136.

This study tested the hypothesis that higher levels of social support would be associated with higher levels of compliance in hemodialysis clients. The results indicated that age, income, educational level, and time hospitalized did not significantly affect compliance. Compliance was greatest when support was given by a significant other and consisted of information and feedback and telling the client what to do.

Compliance was found to be greatest for the medication regimen, followed by fluid restriction, and diet. In addition, length of time on dialysis and compliance were inversely related; as the length of time on dialysis increased, compliance decreased.

Nurses should assess client support systems when planning care and evaluating compliance. Including supportive individuals in teaching and client care may enhance overall compliance. Actions such as offering information, giving positive feedback, and reminding the client to follow prescribed regimens can be beneficial. Because this research found that compliance declines as time on hemodialysis increases, nurses may need to reassess more frequently and more closely for compliance. Re-education may be helpful.

receptacles, not bedding or clothing. Urinary disorders that cause loss of control over urination are particularly distressing.

The proximity of the urethral orifices to the genitalia contributes to the difficulties some people encounter in talking about these areas of the body. Cultural and societal attitudes toward these "private parts" create a challenge in nursing interventions with clients who have problems associated with the genitourinary system.

Other aspects of sociocultural background and lifestyle also greatly influence people's health care practices. A concern for and awareness of preventive measures during the early years can help people avoid lifelong problems related to kidney and urinary tract function (eg, females should be taught to wipe from front to back).

Dietary Habits and Medications

A high-salt diet can contribute to the development of hypertension, which can lead to renal disease. For people with diagnosed renal problems, salt and protein restrictions may limit the pleasure of eating. They can avoid certain foods and beverages in their own homes with some discipline, but visiting friends or dining in restaurants presents difficulties that may not be controlled so easily. Many social functions involve sharing food and drink. People who must strictly limit fluid intake may feel pressure to explain why they must avoid fluids. Thus, the altered health state is always a part of life. Participation and sharing are social expectations, and some people prefer to avoid these situations rather than not do what is expected.

Among medications that may have a toxic effect on the kidneys are a number of antibiotics including penicillin, neomycin, kanamycin, and amphotericin. Probably the most nephrotoxic category of antibiotics, however, is the aminoglycosides (gentamicin, tobramycin). Other nephrotoxic drugs include the sulfonamides, salicylates, thiazides, and furosemide.

Economic Factors

The costs of renal dialysis and transplantation are high. Although the government pays for most of the costs, minor expenses add up to thousands of dollars. Moreover, a loss of income may result if the client is a wage earner.

Occupation and Avocation

Exposure to nephrotoxic chemicals may be related to occupation or hobbies. Carbon tetrachloride, used in dry cleaning and various industrial processes, is nephrotoxic, as are methyl alcohol, phenols, and ethylene glycol. Several metals used in the fabrication of jewelry and some electronic components are nephrotoxic, including gold, lead, copper, uranium, arsenic, mercury, and cadmium.

Jobs that require travel, flexible hours, or physical energy may prove difficult to maintain. The need to change careers or develop new skills, in addition to coping with physical illness, may be an enormous challenge or too much to cope with for the client with kidney disease.

Roles and Relationships

For the client with serious kidney dysfunction, as in end-stage renal disease, the psychosocial effects are numerous. Lifestyle, family life, and work commitments usually are interrupted, often in substantial ways. The client usually must make major adjustments in various roles. Stress accompanies the effort to maintain the existing lifestyle in the face of vast uncertainty about the future, and both clients and all those near them are affected (especially spouses and children). Powerlessness, helplessness, and hopelessness are all components of the newly experienced dependency created by renal failure.

Sexual Expression and Reproduction

Surgical procedures such as urinary diversion may require the client to wear an appliance on the abdomen to collect urine, and clients with such appliances may be reluctant to participate in sexual activity. They and their partners may find it necessary to alter their sexual behaviors to accommodate the appliance, a catheter, or a dialysis fistula. Clients and their sexual partners may have to discuss and experiment with alternate positions for sexual intercourse, and intercourse may be somewhat unpleasant or even uncomfortable or painful.

The client's reproductive ability may also be altered. For example, certain surgical procedures (such as radical cystectomy in men) may cause impotence. Because hormone levels are not regulated in the presence of chronic renal failure, many female clients have amenorrhea and are unlikely to become pregnant. In men, low testosterone levels and decreased sperm formation significantly reduce the ability to fertilize an ovum. Active prevention of pregnancy in women receiving dialysis is indicated for a number of reasons. For one, pregnancy increases the circulating blood volume. In addition, the low hemoglobin values of most chronic renal failure clients are inadequate to support a healthy fetus. Attempting to have a baby while on dialysis can be harmful to both mother and fetus.

If the renal problem is genetically transmitted, as in polycystic kidney disease, reproduction may be discouraged.

Body Image and Self-Concept

Because where and how we urinate is essentially culturally prescribed, it is intimately linked to our view of ourselves and to our self-concept. A person faced with the problem of disposing of a plastic bag full of urine, or who finds that passing flatus means that urine is likely to leak over the body or clothing, may feel dirty and out of control of basic body functions. The person may also worry about being offensive to others because of odor.

To conceal urinary diversion appliances or drainage tubes, a client may find the choice of clothing limited to nonrestrictive and comfortable styles. Not being able to wear a preferred style of clothing—in other words, sacrificing fashion for comfort—may provoke anxiety in people who highly value being fashionable. Being unclothed and seen in the nude may also create great discomfort to the client concerned about body changes.

The client with a transplanted kidney may have to deal with concerns about having another person's organ within his or her own body. The knowledge that a related donor has sacrificed a healthy kidney for the client's benefit may become a burden of guilt. The guilt may be increased if the donor kidney is rejected by the client's body.

Chapter Highlights

The nephron is the functional unit of the renal parenchyma, and each kidney has over 1 million nephrons.

Glomerular filtration, tubular reabsorption, and tubular secretion are the processes that remove nitrogenous waste and maintain electrolyte and acid–base balances.

The glomerular filtration rate requires adequate intravascular volume and hydrostatic pressure to effect the clearance of creatinine and urea nitrogen.

Tubular reabsorption moves water and electrolytes from tubular filtrate into the plasma.

Tubular secretion regulates potassium and hydrogen ion levels.

Control of micturition is voluntary as long as motor and sensory nerve pathways are intact.

The failure to excrete nitrogenous waste products and middle molecules creates the uremic environment.

The major uremic symptoms affect the gastrointestinal system (anorexia, nausea, and vomiting), the nervous system (muscle cramps, lethargy, and inability to concentrate), and the integumentary system (severe pruritus).

Hypervolemia in renal failure may result in hypertension and peripheral or pulmonary edema.

Developmental and psychosocial forces are influential in the formation of attitudes and values about urination.

The proximity of urinary system organs to the organs of reproduction and sexuality influences the adult client's attitude toward urinary system dysfunction.

Dysfunction in the urinary system may affect the client's modes of sexual expression, limit reproductive ability, and alter the client's body image and self-concept.

Bibliography

Artinian BM: Role identities of the dialysis patient. *Nephrology Nurse,* 1983, pp 10–14.

Felsenfeld AJ: Dialysis osteomalacia and aluminum toxicity: A form of renal osteodystrophy. *ANNA J* 1985; 12(3):189–191.

Guyton AC: *Textbook of Medical Physiology,* 7th ed. Philadelphia: Saunders, 1985.

Lancaster LE: Selected endocrine problems related to end-stage renal disease. *J Neph Nurs* 1985; (Nov–Dec):277–285.

O'Brien ME: *The Courage to Survive.* New York: Grune and Stratton, 1983.

Orr ML: Cost containment and patient choice in the end-stage renal disease program. *AANNT J* 1982; 9(Dec):11–15.

Pickering L, Robbins D: Fluid, electrolyte, and acid–base balance in the renal patient. *Nurs Clin North Am* 1980; 15(3):577–592.

Rose BR: *Pathophysiology of Renal Disease.* New York: McGraw–Hill, 1981.

Schrier RW: *Renal and Electrolyte Disorders.* Boston: Little, Brown, 1980.

Smith DR: *General Urology,* 10th ed. Los Altos, CA: Lange, 1981.

Spence AP, Mason EB: *Human Anatomy and Physiology,* 3rd ed. Menlo Park, CA: Addison–Wesley, 1987.

Taylor DL: Renal hypertension: Physiology, signs and symptoms. *Nurs 83* 1983; 13(10)44–45.

CHAPTER **25**

The Nursing Process for Clients With Kidney and Urinary Dysfunction

Other topics relevant to this content are: The health history and physical assessment, **Chapter 5;** Care of the client with a cardiac dysrhythmia, **Chapter 19;** Care of the client with a blood transfusion reaction, **Chapter 22;** Care of the client with renal failure, **Chapter 26;** Care of the client following urinary diversion procedures and surgical procedures to correct incontinence and urinary retention, **Chapter 26.**

Objectives

When you have finished studying this chapter you should be able to:

Specify the major components of the health history to be obtained from clients with urinary system dysfunction.

Explain specific assessment approaches in evaluating clients with dysfunction of the urinary system.

Identify the nursing implications of diagnostic studies commonly used to evaluate clients with kidney and urinary dysfunction.

Determine appropriate nursing diagnoses for clients with disorders of the urinary system.

Develop, with the client, realistic goals of care.

Anticipate the psychosocial/lifestyle implications of kidney and urinary dysfunction for clients and their significant others.

Develop a nursing care plan for a client with urinary system dysfunction.

Implement nursing interventions specific to clients with urinary system disease.

Evaluate the effectiveness of the nursing care plan and modify it as necessary to meet client needs.

Describe nursing interventions for hemodialysis and peritoneal dialysis.

The nursing process with problems of the kidneys and urinary tract encompasses a wide range of assessments and interventions. This chapter discusses nursing responsibilities generally applicable to kidney and urinary system dysfunction.

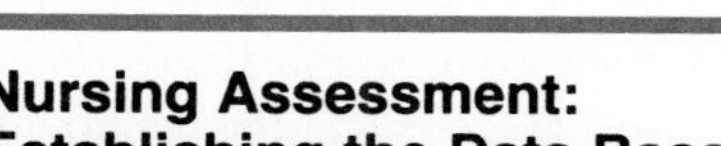

Nursing Assessment: Establishing the Data Base

Subjective Data

Consideration of the client's normal pattern of urination and the discussion of changes in this pattern involve questioning the client about the urinary volume, timing characteristics, micturition control, and appearance of urine. Clients often experience anxiety in discussing this aspect of their daily activities. Urination is a culturally established act performed in privacy. Language referring to the process frequently involves colloquial expressions or terminology unique to a particular family or group, and medical or biologic terms may not be familiar to the client. Thus, communication about the exact nature of the problem may be difficult. In addition, the proximity of the urinary tract to the sexual organs may cause further embarrassment or anxiety during the assessment process. The nurse's calm, confident approach to the interview and examination may make the client more comfortable.

The nurse should question the client about any changes in micturition. What color is the urine? How many times a day does the client void? Is there trouble initiating the stream or difficulty holding the urine? Does the client get up at night to void? How many times? When did this begin? Is there pain with urination? Does the client have urgency or hesitancy with voiding? Are there problems with incontinence? Does the client void excessive amounts?

Are there changes in the color of urine? Changes in the urine's appearance may have caused the client to seek medical advice. Hematuria may be a serious sign because it may indicate cancer of the urinary system. It also may be related to anticoagulant therapy, excessive exercise, infection, or trauma. If the urine is alkaline, clients may describe their urine as being bright red or coffee colored. If the urine is acidic, blood gives the urine a cloudy or smoky appearance. Cloudy urine, however, is usually related to pus in the urine (pyuria). In severe pyuria, the urine may be malodorous. Almost colorless urine usually results from excessive fluid intake, chronic renal disease, diabetes insipidus, or diabetes mellitus. Dark yellow-orange urine suggests dehydration or ingestion of medications or foods that discolor the urine. It is important to know when a change in urine color began and if it is related to other events, is constant, or is intermittent.

Pain is not always present with disorders of the kidneys and urinary tract; it is more common in acute conditions. The client's history must include descriptions of the character, location, distribution, onset, duration, and frequency of the discomfort. Is it related to voiding? What brings it on? What relieves it?

Pain from within the kidney is described as a dull ache. Usually the pain is always present and not interrupted with position change. The client will point to the **flank** region (the part of the body between the ribs and the ileum) and say the pain also extends into the lower abdomen or the umbilical area. Renal colic and ureteral colic cause severe, excruciating pain of sudden onset. The pain, located in the flank area and radiating to the groin, is accompanied by nausea, vomiting, and paralytic ileus.

Bladder pain in the suprapubic area is usually the result of bladder spasms, which can be contractions of the detrusor muscle responsible for normal micturition. Urgency and burning on urination are also common in clients with cystitis or urethritis (irritation of the urethra). Cystitis may produce burning both during and after urination, whereas urethritis usually causes burning during urination only. Strangury (slow and painful voiding of small amounts of urine) often accompanies severe bladder infection.

Some women with symptoms of burning on urination may actually have a vaginal infection. Ask the client about any signs of vaginal discharge. Has she noted any vaginal or perineal itching or dyspareunia (pain with sexual intercourse)?

In men, scrotal pain can be due to inflammation and swelling of the testicle or epididymis. Rectal and perineal fullness and pain suggest prostatitis. A weak urinary stream, dribbling, or inability to initiate the stream can be caused by benign prostatic hyperplasia. Metastasis of prostatic cancer to the pelvis can cause leg and back pain.

Stress incontinence is a common problem for women. A weakness can develop in the bladder–urethral sphincter mechanism through the stretching of pelvic muscles during childbirth or the pressure of the uterus on the bladder during pregnancy.

In the elderly (especially those who have had pregnancies), relaxation of pelvic musculature also contributes to the incontinence. Frequent catheterizations and the use of forceps during delivery increase the chances for development of stress incontinence. When questioned, many women state that they have to wear sanitary pads, adult diapers, or even plastic pants at all times to prevent embarrassment.

Does the client maintain an adequate fluid intake (1500 to 2000 mL a day) to help prevent urinary tract infections (UTIs) and renal calculi? Does the client have an excessive intake of milk and vitamin D, which could lead to hypercalciuria? What are the client's exercise habits? Proteinuria, hematuria, or both can be a normal finding in people who exercise excessively. Immobility because of a fracture, thrombophlebitis, or surgery can predispose the client to the development of renal calculi.

A medication history is essential, because many drugs can damage the kidney. Has the client taken any prescription drugs recently? What OTC (over-the-counter) medications does the client routinely take? The client also may be exposed to nephrotoxins on the job or with certain hobbies. See Box 25–1 for a list of nephrotoxic substances.

The client's health history may be significant. Has the client ever had problems that could lead to nephropathy, such as frequent streptococcal infections, recurrent UTIs, renal calculi, hyperuricemia (as occurs in gout), or hyper-

Box 25–1
Nephrotoxic Substances

Phenacetin* (usually combined with aspirin)

Some antibiotics (especially the aminoglycosides)

Nonsteroidal anti-inflammatory agents (ibuprofen and fenoprofen)

Anesthetics (methoxyflurane)

Radiographic contrast media

Carbon tetrachloride

Lead

Cadmium

*Although this product is no longer available, clients may experience problems related to past use.

calcemia (as occurs in hyperparathyroidism, sarcoidosis, or metastatic bone disease)? Has the client ever had an indwelling catheter, cystoscopy, or x-rays of the renal system? Is there a history of trauma?

Is there a family history of any congenital disorders such as polycystic kidney or congenital malformations of the urinary tract? A strong family history of diseases such as diabetes mellitus or hypertension is also significant because these diseases tend to run in families and can cause renal problems.

Objective Data

Physical Assessment

Objective data are obtained in the physical assessment of the client through inspection, auscultation, percussion, and palpation. Objective data are also obtained through a variety of diagnostic studies. The physical assessment skills and diagnostic studies specific to the kidneys and the urinary system are discussed below; general information is discussed in Chapter 5.

INSPECTION The first stage of data collection is inspection of the client. Examination of the skin is important; uremic clients have a characteristic ashen, yellow skin coloring, and uremic frost may be visible. The eyes of uremic clients are often sunken and give the client a wasted appearance that is exaggerated with muscle wasting and edema. The edema associated with renal failure is generalized rather than dependent. Bruises are common.

The integument also provides clues to renal involvement in clients not yet diagnosed as having urinary system problems. In a hypernatremic state, the skin is dry and flushed, and the body temperature is elevated. Examination of the mucous membranes of the nose and mouth is important. With hypernatremia, the mucous membranes are dry and sticky, and the tongue is rough and dry. Tetany including carpopedal spasms occurs with hypocalcemia. Skin turgor provides an important assessment of the client's hydration status.

Respirations should be observed. Rapid respirations suggest metabolic acidosis, infection, or fluid overload. Kussmaul's respirations are common with metabolic acidosis. Shallow respirations and shortness of breath may be signs of hypokalemia. Shortness of breath may also suggest pulmonary edema, congestive heart failure, or both.

Inspection of the abdomen will reveal some important findings with many clients. Scars may represent surgical procedures or trauma. There may be urinary or fecal diversions or cutaneous fistulas. The abdominal contour may be altered if the bladder is distended or the kidneys are enlarged, as with polycystic kidney disease. With significant bladder distention, the umbilicus may be displaced toward the client's head. In the male, the penis should be inspected for lesions, scars, or discharge.

The urine should be inspected for blood, color, cloudiness, and precipitates. If any discharge is present at the urinary meatus, a specimen should be obtained before the client gives a urine sample.

AUSCULTATION Auscultation of the lungs may provide evidence of crackles or rhonchi related to fluid overload. Cardiac irregularities and faint heart sounds may be heard with potassium imbalances. Auscultate the abdomen before palpating it. Listen for renal bruits. Listen also over each costovertebral angle (CVA). A bruit over one or both renal arteries suggests the possibility of renal artery stenosis.

PERCUSSION Percussion of the urinary bladder will elicit a dull sound in the suprapubic region if the bladder is distended. Bladder distention may extend to the level of the umbilicus or higher. A variation of the normal percussion technique can detect discomfort or pain over the kidney. Tenderness over the CVA suggests infection in the kidney or perinephric area. The client should assume a sitting position, and the nurse should gently strike each CVA with the heel of the hand.

PALPATION Palpation can define the borders, and thus the size and contour, of internal organs. Palpation of normal-sized kidneys is difficult except in individuals who are thin or have poorly developed muscles. The right kidney is more readily palpable because it is normally lower in the abdomen and slightly more anterior than the left kidney.

Figure 25–1 illustrates the technique for kidney palpation. Deep palpation is necessary to identify the kidney. In this method, the lower pole of the right kidney may be palpated when the client takes a deep breath. In another method of kidney palpation, called *capturing,* hand placement is the same, but the right hand exerts greater pressure. The client is asked to exhale and then to stop breathing. If the kidney has been captured, it will be felt as the

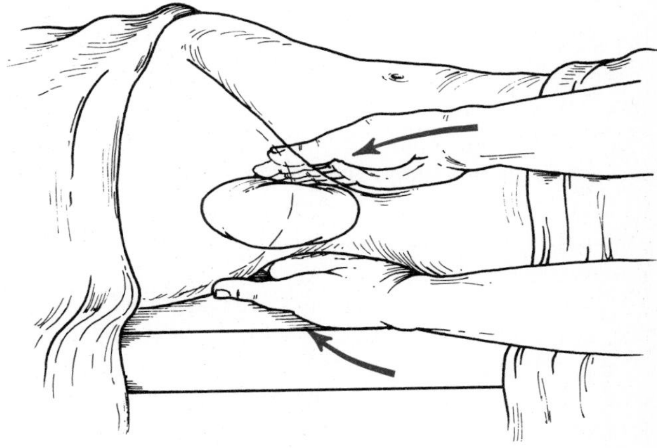

Figure 25–1

Technique for kidney palpation.

pressure of the fingers is released. The client may feel this procedure, but it is not painful.

If abdominal masses are present and are thought to be enlarged kidneys, do not attempt kidney palpation, because tumor cells may be liberated with manipulation if the masses are hypernephromas. Furthermore, if the masses are polycystic kidneys, palpation may aggravate bleeding.

The male prostate gland should be palpated during the rectal examination. In women, pathologic conditions in the reproductive organs may affect the urinary tract. The pelvic and rectal examinations are important when assessing clients with kidney and urinary system dysfunction.

Diagnostic Studies

A wide variety of diagnostic studies are used to assess kidney and urinary system dysfunction. The tests most often used to assess kidney function are the serum creatinine, the blood urea nitrogen (BUN), and the creatinine clearance. These tests are referred to as *renal function studies*.

SERUM CREATININE Serum creatinine measurements primarily reflect the ability of the kidneys to excrete creatinine, the waste product of skeletal muscle metabolism derived from the breakdown of phosphocreatine. The normal serum creatinine level is 0.6 to 1.5 mg/dL (Byrne et al., 1986), but it varies with sex and individual muscle mass characteristics (women generally having less muscle mass). Serial changes in serum creatinine levels are significant in evaluating and interpreting renal function, because this substance is excreted entirely by the kidney and is therefore directly proportional to excretory function. Unlike the BUN level, the serum creatinine level normally remains constant and is not influenced by other variables such as dehydration, malnutrition, or hepatic function. Only renal disorders will cause an abnormal elevation in creatinine.

BLOOD UREA NITROGEN (BUN) The BUN is a general indicator of renal ability to excrete urea nitrogen. The normal BUN level is 6 to 20 mg/dL (Byrne et al., 1986). Urea nitrogen is synthesized by the liver using protein sources for the conversion, so a functioning liver is required for this test. Because dietary proteins form the primary source of urea nitrogen, a diet high in proteins will increase BUN levels, especially in the presence of renal disease. The metabolism of hemoglobin also results in the production of urea nitrogen.

Nearly all primary renal diseases cause BUN levels to rise, as do certain medications such as steroids, tetracyclines, tobramycin, gentamicin, and chemotherapeutic drugs. Hydration changes such as hemoconcentration or hemodilution also alter the BUN level. In dehydration, a decreased renal blood flow leads to decreased excretion of urea nitrogen and increased serum BUN levels. Since urea synthesis depends on the liver, the BUN level may be normal in hepatorenal syndrome or any time there is combined liver and kidney disease. The BUN level is normal not because the renal excretory function is good, but because hepatic function is poor, and BUN formation is therefore decreased.

CREATININE CLEARANCE The best test to measure overall renal function is the creatinine clearance, a mathematical calculation that compares the amount of creatinine filtered in a 24-hour urine collection with the amount of creatinine that remains in the serum. Because almost all creatinine is excreted, and other variables do not influence muscle metabolism and renal excretion, creatinine clearance is regarded as the best indicator of renal function. Although a 24-hour collection is preferred, a 12-hour or shorter collection may be acceptable in some situations.

The normal creatinine clearance value for men is 107 to 141 mL/min; for women it is 87 to 132 mL/min. For practical purposes, a rate of 100 mL/min may be considered normal to allow a comparison of the clearance to a percentage value. For example, a creatinine clearance value of 100 mL/min is 100%, or normal. A creatinine clearance value of 50 mL/min suggests that 50% of renal function is lost and 50% remains. After the initial calculation, subsequent increases of the serum creatinine level imply that renal function is deteriorating; in other words, the kidneys are clearing less creatinine, and the serum level is increasing. If a creatinine clearance were calculated, it would be decreasing, because less creatinine would be measured in the urine as more accumulated in the serum. The trend is what is significant. The serum level will not increase until at least 50% of renal function has been lost.

Dialysis or transplantation generally is not required until the creatinine clearance values drop below 5 mL/min. Occasionally, however, symptoms may dictate that dialysis be started before the levels get that low.

ROUTINE URINALYSIS A routine urinalysis is a urologic screening test to assess the nature of urine produced. It includes:

- Measurement of color, pH, and specific gravity
- Determination of the presence of glucose, protein, blood, and ketones
- A microscopic examination of the urine sediment for cells, casts, bacteria, and crystals

The pH and the presence of protein, glucose, ketones, or blood in the urine can be detected easily using reagent strips. A plastic stick to which several separate reagent strips are affixed for testing various substances is most common. Completely immerse the reagent strip in well-mixed urine and remove it immediately to avoid dissolving the reagents. Hold the strip in a horizontal position to prevent possible mixing of the chemical reagents, and compare it with the test chart at the specified time.

URINARY pH Urine is normally slightly acidic, because the kidneys excrete hydrogen ions. The first voided morning specimen is generally most acidic because of alterations in ventilation during sleep. Food usually results in the production of a more alkaline urine. The range of urinary pH is 4.6 to 8, averaging around 6.

COLOR The color of urine ranges from pale yellow to amber because of the pigment urochrome. The color indicates the urine's concentration and varies with the specific gravity. Dilute urine is straw colored, and concentrated urine is a deep amber. Abnormally colored urine can result from the ingestion of certain foods or medicines or from a pathologic condition.

SPECIFIC GRAVITY Specific gravity, a measure of the concentration of particles in the urine, reflects the ability of the kidney tubules to concentrate or dilute urine. The normal specific gravity is 1.016 to 1.022, but it can range from 1.001 to 1.040. The specific gravity increases in clients with:

- Dehydration, because the kidneys absorb all available free water, which makes the excreted urine very concentrated
- Pituitary tumor that causes the release of excessive amounts of antidiuretic hormone (ADH), resulting in excessive water absorption
- Decrease in renal blood flow, as in hypotension, heart failure, or renal artery stenosis
- Glucosuria and proteinuria, because of the increased number of particles in the urine

In contrast, the specific gravity decreases in clients with:

- Overhydration
- Diabetes insipidus, in which there is inadequate secretion of ADH, which decreases water reabsorption
- Chronic renal failure, because the kidney has lost its ability to concentrate urine through water reabsorption

In clients with chronic renal failure, the specific gravity is usually stable at about 1.010 despite changes in intake because the kidney can no longer respond to changes.

Specific gravity can easily be measured with a hydrometer (refer to a nursing fundamentals text).

PROTEIN (ALBUMIN) The normal protein content of urine is less than 8 mg/dL. The first voided morning specimen is preferred to detect the presence of protein in the urine. Since the client has not been up and exercising, orthostatic and transient proteinuria generally can be ruled out. Stress and cold weather exposure over time also can contribute to transient proteinuria. Higher-than-average protein levels found on routine analysis should be evaluated further for total protein by a 24-hour collection. Most protein excreted in the urine is albumin and may be referred to as *albuminuria.* Other abnormal proteins may be identified, however, and require investigation by other methods, such as urine electrophoresis.

KETONES Normally, there are no ketones in the urine. *Ketonuria,* or ketones in the urine, occurs when there is incomplete metabolism of fats. This condition may be observed in diabetic ketoacidosis. However, nondiabetic clients who follow a diet high in protein and low in carbohydrates in an effort to lose weight quickly will form ketones. Ketonuria also may be seen in the presence of dehydration, starvation, or excessive aspirin consumption.

GLUCOSE Normal urine contains only small amounts of glucose—usually less than 15 mg/dL. *Glucosuria,* or glucose in the urine, occurs when the renal threshold for reabsorption of glucose is exceeded. The ability of the renal tubule cells to reabsorb glucose is exceeded when the blood glucose level is about 180 mg/dL, but this varies with individuals. When the renal tubules are impaired, glucosuria will occur at lower blood glucose levels. Aging, pregnancy, and diabetes mellitus of several years duration will increase the renal threshold for glucose.

BLOOD Any disruption in the blood–urine barrier, whether at the glomerular or tubular level, will cause blood cells to enter the urine. *Hematuria* occurs when more than two to three red blood cells are found in the sediment of urine on microscopic examination. Hemoglobinuria, or free hemoglobin in the urine, is an abnormal finding. Hemolysis of red blood cells that results in hemoglobinuria may occur in various hemolytic anemias and following some blood transfusion reactions.

BILIRUBIN *Bilirubinuria,* or bilirubin in the urine, should be suspected when the color of the urine is dark gold or brown. Normally, there is no detectable bilirubin in the urine. Its presence indicates liver dysfunction or an obstruction to the flow of bile in the biliary tract.

WHITE BLOOD CELLS White blood cells, or pus cells, in the urine are referred to as *pyuria.* This condition indicates that an infection exists somewhere in the urinary tract. However, 4 to 5 white blood cells per high power field is not significant.

EPITHELIAL CELLS Epithelial cells line the urethra and vagina and are commonly found in the urine. Their presence indicates the expected turnover of cells. Cells from within the kidney (renal cells), however, suggest a pathologic condition in the kidney.

CASTS Casts are abnormal elements formed in the renal tubules and molded to the lumen of the tubules. A mucoprotein material along with various cells, such as red blood cells, white blood cells, or epithelial cells, form the cast. Casts are named for the predominant cellular element they contain. For example, white blood cell casts suggest kidney infection, whereas red blood cell casts suggest damage to glomerular capillaries or ruptured tubular walls. Hyaline casts, composed of various types of protein, are the most common. In fact, they may be found in people with fever or those who exercise strenuously. They may indicate the mildest form of tubular damage. As casts degenerate, they may become granular or waxy, but these forms are not usually found in normal urine.

CRYSTALS Crystals found in the urine sediment indicate that the client may either have a renal calculus or be at risk for forming one. Urate crystals occur in the urine of clients with gout, whereas phosphate and calcium oxalate crystals occur in the urine of clients with hyperparathyroidism of malabsorptive states. The type of crystal found varies with urine pH. Urate crystals are in acidic urine, and calcium oxalate crystals are in alkaline urine.

BACTERIA Few if any bacteria are normally present in urine, and large numbers of bacteria suggest infection in the urinary tract. Normal urine contains less than 1000 bacteria per mL of urine. A count greater than 100,000 colonies per mL of urine indicates a urinary tract infection. Some debate exists about the minimal colony count at which there is evidence of infection and not contamination.

URINARY ELECTROLYTES AND OSMOLALITY Urinary electrolytes and osmolality can be measured using a random sample of urine or 24-hour collection. The random sample yields a quick analysis of the urine content, especially when the client is oliguric or anuric. The 24-hour collection for analysis of total urinary excretion of certain electrolytes will provide more information regarding the specific nature of the renal problem. Sodium, potassium, chloride, and calcium are electrolytes commonly measured in 24-hour collections. The amount present in the urine reflects how well the kidney is excreting or conserving these electrolytes.

Urinary osmolality reflects the ability of the kidneys to concentrate or dilute urine to maintain the osmotic balance between cells, tissues, and plasma. Urine osmolality is interpreted in comparison with the plasma osmolality. For example, if the plasma osmolality is elevated, the kidneys should reabsorb water and excrete a more concentrated and smaller volume of urine. In contrast, if the plasma osmolality is low, the kidneys should excrete a less concentrated and larger volume of urine. This maintains the proper osmotic balance among cells, tissue, and plasma. The ratio of urine osmolality to plasma osmolality should be greater than 1:1. Urine osmolality may range from 300 to 1090 mOsm/kg, depending upon sex and activity (Byrne et al., 1986). Variations in urinary osmolality also depend on the amount of solute to be excreted.

ULTRASONOGRAPHY Ultrasonography of the kidney can locate renal cysts, differentiate renal cysts from solid renal tumors, demonstrate renal or pelvic calculi, and guide a percutaneously inserted needle for cyst aspiration or removal of a biopsy specimen (Pagana & Pagana, 1982).

NURSING IMPLICATIONS The test is best performed prior to any barium contrast studies, or all barium must be removed first with cathartics. No preparation for the client is required other than to advise the client to not empty the bladder prior to ultrasonography. A full bladder enhances organ and tissue delineation. Instruct the client to lie quietly in the prone position for about 15 minutes. If a biopsy is done at the same time, 30 minutes may be necessary (refer to the section on renal biopsy). Warn the client about the copious amounts of lubricant that will be applied to the skin to enhance transmission of the sound waves. Nonhealing open wounds may be a deterrent to the placement of the lubricant but do not necessarily make the test impossible to perform. After the procedure, remove the lubricant from the client's back.

X-RAY OF THE KIDNEYS, URETERS, BLADDER An abdominal flat-plate x-ray of the abdomen is called a KUB or plain film. This simple x-ray does not involve any client preparation or injection of contrast media; the client is in the supine position. The KUB will generally determine the presence of two kidneys, as well as provide a general outline of the kidneys, from which their size may be grossly determined. The left kidney is normally about 0.5 cm longer than the right. Thus, if the left kidney is not slightly larger, it may represent a pathologic condition on that side. The KUB may also identify tumors, malformations, and calculi. The study is contraindicated in the pregnant client.

NURSING IMPLICATIONS Explain the KUB x-ray to clients and reassure them that it will not hurt. It should be scheduled before any barium studies to ensure adequate visualization.

INTRAVENOUS PYELOGRAPHY An intravenous pyelogram (IVP) is a fluoroscopic examination that involves the IV injection of a contrast medium, which is carried through the blood into the kidneys and then filtered and excreted into the ureters and bladder. The IVP will give some information on function of the kidneys, as reflected by the uptake and excretion of dye. Well-functioning kidneys take up and excrete the dye rapidly, whereas delayed uptake and excretion indicate a decrease in function. The IVP also provides information about the presence or absence of kidneys; the pole-to-pole size of the kidneys; the depth of the renal cortex; the integrity or contour of the calyces; the size of the renal pelvis; the presence of stones in the pelvis, the ureters, and the bladder; and the size of the ureters and their patency (Figure 25–2). Complications of IVP include allergic reaction, infiltration of the contrast agent, and renal shut-down and failure.

The IVP films yield the best information when the bowel has been cleansed of stool, air, and fluid. Therefore, clients are usually given a laxative the evening before the

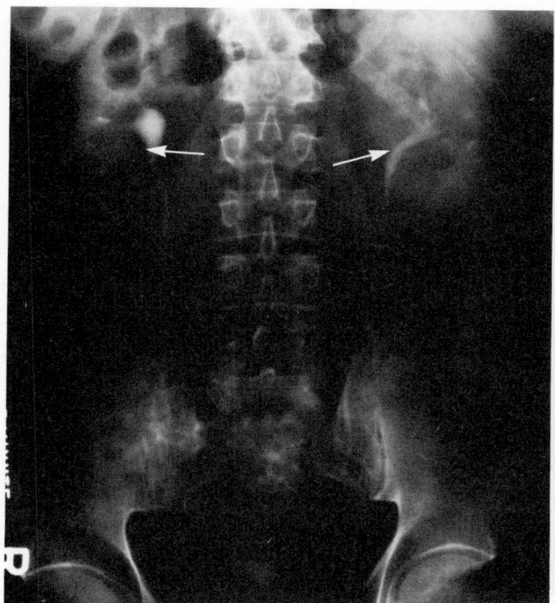

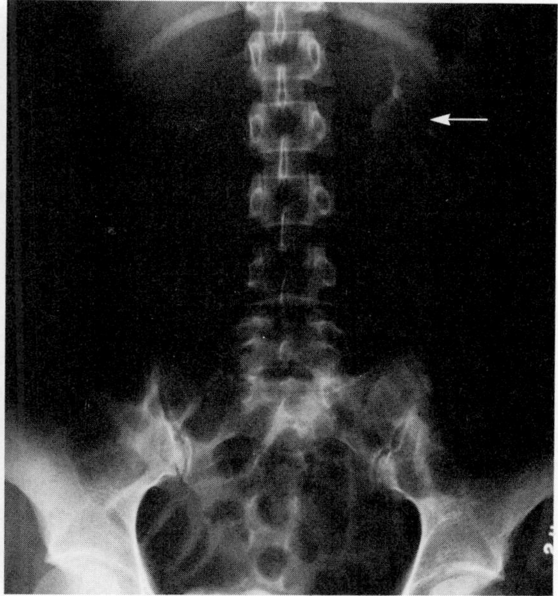

Figure 25–2

Intravenous pyelogram. **A.** The renal pelves and calyces fill normally on both sides, and both ureters are visualized. **B.** After 2 hours, the ureter and kidney on the right are not visualized; they are functioning normally and the dye has cleared. A calculus in the left ureter causes dilation of the calyx shown here.

procedure, and preparatory enemas or suppositories are generally administered. In addition, the client is usually NPO. After the dye has been administered intravenously, x-ray films are taken at 1-, 5-, 10-, 15-, 20-, and 30-minute intervals (and sometimes longer). The client is then asked to void, and another film is taken to assess bladder emptying.

NURSING IMPLICATIONS Explain the purpose and procedure of the test and that it takes about 45 minutes. Emphasize that it will not hurt except for the placement of the IV needle. Give cathartics as ordered the evening preceding the examination, and keep the client NPO after midnight. Ask the client about allergy to iodine. Explain that the dye can cause flushing of the face, a feeling of warmth, and a salty taste in the mouth. Assess the IV site for infiltration. Encourage fluids after the test has been completed.

In elderly clients or clients with known renal insufficiency (ie, elevation of the serum creatinine level above 1.5 mg/dL), diabetes mellitus, or multiple myeloma, tests using contrast media are contraindicated. Other renal diagnostic tests are recommended, if possible.

CYSTOSCOPY A cystoscopy is a procedure in which a cystoscope is inserted into the bladder via the urethra to visualize directly the internal bladder wall and the contents of the bladder. A cystoscopy is indicated to identify the origin of hematuria as well as to diagnose and remove tumors, stones, or any other foreign material. The application of electrical current to the lesion (fulguration) to remove bladder tumors may be carried out during the cystoscopic examination. A cystoscope also can be used to implant radium seeds into a tumor, place catheters in the ureters to drain the renal pelvis, and coagulate bleeding areas.

A cystoscopy is performed under general or local anesthesia. During the procedure, the client is supine, with the legs and feet supported in a lithotomy position. Strict aseptic technique is essential during the procedure. The cystoscope is available in a variety of sizes from 12 to 26 F. Its wide-angle lens allows viewing of the interior bladder surfaces. A panendoscope will be used to examine the urethra visually, because its lens is more directly in line with the instrument. Retrograde pyelography, which involves the direct injection of dye into each ureter through the cystoscope, also may be performed during cystoscopy. It is indicated if obstruction is suspected in the ureters or the renal pelvis. Because the dye is not directly injected into the bloodstream, this procedure avoids the risk of an allergic reaction to the contrast media.

NURSING IMPLICATIONS In explaining the procedure to clients, tell them the cystoscope is inserted into the bladder in the same manner as a catheter (Figure 25–3). Because it is rigid and not flexible as a catheter would be, the procedure may cause mild to moderate discomfort. Give enemas as ordered to clear the bowel. Keep the client NPO if general anesthesia is to be used. A liquid breakfast may

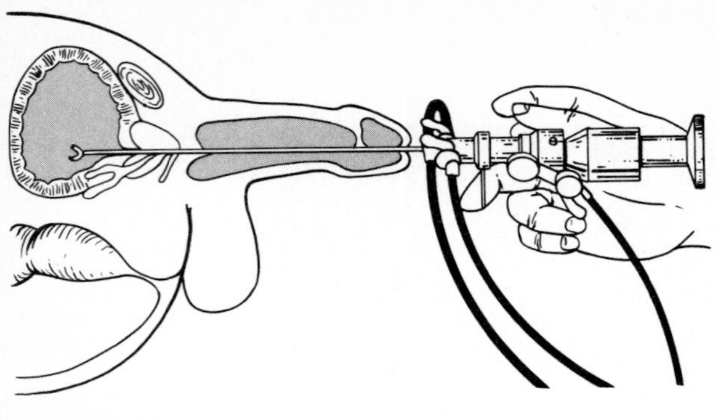

Figure 25–3

Cystoscope insertion.

be given if local anesthesia is to be used. Administer preprocedure sedatives as ordered to help reduce anxiety as well as bladder spasms.

Postoperatively, record careful measurement of urinary output. Measure vital signs at least every 4 hours and report any elevation in temperature immediately. Urinary instrumentation is a major cause of nosocomial urinary tract infections, but prompt detection and treatment may prevent complications such as sepsis and acute renal failure. A small amount of pink-tinged urine is a common postprocedure finding, but it will gradually decrease over 24 to 48 hours.

The client may experience back pain, bladder spasms, urinary frequency, and burning on urination. Warm sitz baths and mild analgesics may be ordered. Sometimes belladonna and opium (B & O) suppositories are given to relieve bladder spasms. Encourage fluids. Occasionally, antibiotics are ordered 1 day before and 3 days after the procedure to reduce the incidence of bacteremia. Perforation of the bladder is a rare but possible complication of cystoscopy, and should be considered if the client experiences severe abdominal pain.

CYSTOGRAM AND VOIDING CYSTOURETHROGRAM The cystogram outlines the contour of the bladder and identifies any reflux or urine from the bladder into the ureters toward the kidney (ureterovesical or U-V reflux). For this test, a catheter is inserted into the urinary bladder, and dye is injected through the catheter into the bladder. No reflux should occur, but if it does, it will be detected when the dye is injected. The voiding cystourethrogram (VCU or VCUG) is performed in a similar manner. It provides additional information about strictures or urethral disorders as the client is observed voiding. This test is particularly embarrassing to the client so it requires some psychologic preparation. It is important that the client have the opportunity to discuss and understand thoroughly why the test is necessary and how it will help in the diagnostic process. Assurance that there will be as much privacy as possible may help diminish concerns.

URODYNAMIC STUDIES Urodynamics involve the physiology of micturition. A variety of tests is available to study known or suspected problems related to nerve innervation of the bladder, incontinence, or variations in the urinary pattern. The uroflometer measures the rate of urine flow during voiding. The normal flow rate, expressed in volume (milliliters) per second, for a man is 20 to 25 mL/s; for a woman it is 25 to 30 mL/s. A decreased flow rate may be observed with obstruction or decreased innervation.

CYSTOMETROGRAPHY In cystometrography, a cystometrogram measures changes in pressure within the bladder. A catheter is inserted into the urinary bladder, water is instilled into the bladder via the catheter, and measurements of the internal pressure are recorded. Since part of the test is to determine how the client feels as bladder pressure increases, the client is asked to note when bladder fullness is detected and when the urge to void is felt. The normal bladder capacity is 400 to 500 mL, and the urge to void is felt at around 50 to 100 mL below the capacity. Bladder pressure increases when the client is told to urinate and decreases when urination is completed. This increase in pressure is related to the contraction of bladder musculature during the voiding process.

URETHRAL PRESSURE PROFILE Pressures within the urethra can be measured and calculated in a variety of combinations. The primary measurements determine the peak pressure in the urethra and the pressure on closure of the urethra. Variations in pressure and pressure distribution help identify the type of incontinence present.

ELECTROMYOGRAPHY A component of urodynamic studies, electromyography (EMG) determines alterations in the voluntary control of urination as maintained by the external sphincter. Normally, when the bladder is filling and the external sphincter is relaxed, there is electrical activity in the muscles; EMG records this. With voiding, the pelvic muscles relax, the external sphincter (detrusor muscle) contracts, and there is an absence of electrical activity. Various methods may be used to measure this muscle activity. Cutaneous electrodes, needle electrodes, an anal catheter, or an anal plug (sometimes called a *rectal plug*) may be used.

Determine which method has been selected before initiating client instruction. A great deal of explanation is needed for the client, because needle electrodes are quite uncomfortable. The needle electrode is placed near the urethra in the female client and through the perineum in the male client. Needle placement is difficult, and information may be hard to obtain. The anal plug is generally preferred for overall perineal muscle evaluation and produces only a slight sensation of pressure.

NEPHROTOMOGRAPHY Nephrotomography provides radiographic visualization of the kidney using the tomographic technique, usually following the IV injection of radiopaque dye. Tomographic techniques involve x-ray films of various planes and varying depths of kidney tissue which permits detailed study of alterations in structure. Refer to the discussion on IVP earlier in the chapter for nursing implications associated with nephrotomography.

COMPUTERIZED TOMOGRAPHY A computerized tomography (CT) scan of the abdomen is often done to identify kidney size and structural alterations within the urinary system. It may be done with or without contrast media. The scan picks up images at varying levels—from 3 to 13 mm apart—so small lesions, tumors, or defects can be pinpointed precisely. In addition to the kidneys, the retroperitoneal space, adrenals, bladder, and prostate can be visualized well. The IV injection of contrast media may be contraindicated for the same reasons as the IVP. A CT scan without contrast media may provide detail adequate for the diagnostic process, however.

NURSING IMPLICATIONS Clients must lie motionless throughout the CT scan. Explain the procedure, show the client a picture of the machine if possible, and encourage the client to verbalize fears. Keep the client NPO for 4 hours before the test to prevent food in the stomach or duodenum from confusing the final picture.

RENAL SCAN The renal scan, a nuclear medicine procedure, demonstrates blood flow to each kidney following the IV administration of a small amount of radioisotope. A variety of isotopes may be used for imaging. Pictures are taken immediately following injection of the isotope and at various intervals thereafter.

The renal scan is used to:

- Show the size, shape, and location of the kidneys
- Detect localized infections
- Detect renal infarctions
- Detect renal arterial atherosclerosis or trauma (uptake of the isotope is delayed on the affected side)
- Monitor rejection of a transplanted kidney (in chronic rejection, uptake is delayed)
- Detect primary renal disease (uptake is delayed)
- Detect pathologic renal conditions in clients who cannot have an IVP because of dye allergies

Some examiners request that Lugol's solution be administered before the isotope injection and for several days following the scan to block the uptake of the isotope by the thyroid gland. The client is unsedated and nonfasting when the radionucleotide (^{131}I or ^{125}I) is given. It takes only minutes for the isotope to be concentrated in the kidneys. A gamma-ray detecting device then is passed over the kidney area, and the uptake is recorded on either x-ray or Polaroid film. The test is contraindicated in pregnant women.

NURSING IMPLICATIONS Explain the procedure to the client, and encourage verbalization of concerns. Assure clients that they will not be exposed to large amounts of radioactivity, and tell them there will be no pain during the procedure except the discomfort of starting an IV. Also explain that the procedure usually takes about 1 hour.

Nurses should take precautions with the urine of a client who has had a renal scan. The ambulating client may use the toilet without concern for disposal of the isotope. Wear gloves when caring for an incontinent client, and bag linens for special handling. Pregnant health care providers should avoid contact with the client for at least 24 hours.

RENAL ANGIOGRAPHY Renal angiography is a test that allows further study of kidney structure. It specifically delineates the vascular supply. Intravenous injection of radiopaque contrast media is followed by a series of films as the dye is taken up by the kidneys. Delays in uptake, alterations in contour of the kidney, and vessel abnormalities provide useful information about renal function. Stenosis (narrowing) of the renal artery is best demonstrated with this study.

During the procedure, a local anesthetic is injected into the femoral area, and a catheter is threaded through the femoral artery into the aorta. From there, it is directed into each renal artery, and dye is subsequently injected. The client may experience an intense burning feeling throughout the body that dissipates in seconds. This test can identify stenosis of the renal artery, localize aneurysms, and can also show vascular tumor masses or infarcted areas of renal parenchyma in detail. Renal arteriography may be contraindicated in clients with dye allergies, atherosclerosis, and physiologic instability. Concerns during the procedure include sensitivity to dye, dislodgment of thrombi, and excessive bleeding at the catheterization site.

NURSING IMPLICATIONS Explain the procedure, being sure to show where the catheter will be inserted, and prepare the client for the burning feeling that occurs when the dye is injected. Encourage the client to verbalize concerns regarding the angiography. Question the client about iodine allergies. Ensure that a written informed consent form is on the chart as this is an invasive procedure and carries some risk. Bowel cleansing with enemas and/or cathartics prior to the procedure helps to ensure adequate visualization of the kidneys. Keep the client NPO after midnight on the day of the study, and administer preprocedure medication as ordered. Have the client void immediately before the procedure.

Postprocedure care includes the frequent assessment of vital signs and inspection of the catheter insertion site for bleeding or hematoma formation. In addition, the color, temperature, and nature of pulses in the extremity involved should be assessed along with a basic check of neurologic function. Apply cold compresses to the puncture site as needed, to reduce swelling and discomfort. Force fluids after the procedure to prevent dehydration from the osmotic diuretic effects of the dye.

Symptoms of abdominal or flank pain may indicate that

significant bleeding is occurring. Because bleeding is the major complication, changes in vital signs, abdominal pain, or flank pain should be reported immediately to the physician. The client is kept in bed for 12 to 24 hours, and the IV infusion normally in place following the procedure is maintained for the duration of bed rest. Since dehydration increases the risk of renal damage, the IV line may be kept open for a longer period. Urine output and serum creatinine levels should be monitored for at least 5 to 7 days after the procedure, particularly in the high-risk client.

RENAL BIOPSY A biopsy of kidney tissue may be necessary to determine the exact nature of renal pathology. Direct tissue examination allows assessment of the glomeruli—particularly the cellular elements of the glomeruli, the glomerular basement membrane, and the supporting tissue for the glomerular tuft. In addition, biopsy permits examination of the tubules and interstitium for evidence of inflammatory responses, fibrosis, or scarring. Renal biopsy is almost always indicated when unexplained proteinuria or hematuria are evident. Biopsy can identify the cause of the proteinuria or hematuria and thus allow the prescription of appropriate treatment.

A renal biopsy may use either open or closed technique. An open renal biopsy is a surgical procedure in which a flank incision is made and a piece of kidney tissue obtained by direct visualization of the kidney. A closed biopsy is usually performed with the kidney visualized under fluoroscopy or by ultrasonography.

In any kind of closed renal biopsy, the client assumes the prone position. A rolled blanket is placed under the lower abdomen to angle the kidney closer to the surface and to straighten the spine. Clients with lung disease or difficulty breathing may not be able to tolerate this position for the time required, which varies from 30 to 45 minutes. The client must be reasonably alert and cooperative as well as able to respond to requests to alter the breathing pattern; this is essential because changes in the level of the diaphragm will alter the position of the kidney. The client must be able to take a deep breath and hold it while the needle is introduced into the renal cortex. The left kidney is chosen for renal biopsy, since the right kidney is so near the liver.

The procedure involves thorough cleansing of the skin with povidone–iodine and draping the area around the site where the needle will be introduced. A local anesthetic is injected cutaneously and then into progressively deeper layers of tissue. A spinal needle determines the depth of the kidney beneath the surface of the skin. The biopsy needle then is inserted as close as possible into the spinal needle's path. After the biopsy needle has been placed into the kidney, just beneath the capsule, the client's breathing pattern is observed. When the needle is properly positioned to obtain kidney tissue, the needle's angle with the skin will go back and forth with respiration. When tissue is obtained, the client is asked to take a deep breath and hold it to minimize kidney movement. Usually three pieces of tissue are needed for the stains and tests that will be used to identify the exact pathologic conditions.

NURSING IMPLICATIONS The nurse must prepare clients for a kidney biopsy both intellectually and emotionally. Most clients immediately fear cancer when they hear the word *biopsy.* They should be assured that cancer is rarely a consideration when a renal biopsy is performed; usually its purpose is to evaluate conditions leading to renal failure.

Prebiopsy physical preparation involves ensuring that clotting studies (prothrombin time, partial thromboplastin time, and platelet count) are normal. It is also important that hypertension be controlled, because uncontrolled high blood pressure increases the bleeding potential. Depending on when the biopsy is scheduled, clear liquids may be allowed. The client is usually kept NPO for 5 to 6 hours prebiopsy. Assess vital signs prior to the procedure for baseline comparison.

After the biopsy, apply pressure over the site for about 5 minutes, and apply a bandage. Measure the client's vital signs immediately and then every 15 minutes for an hour, every half hour times 2, and hourly for 6 hours. The client should lie flat in bed with a sandbag or blanket roll under the flank to provide direct pressure. The head of the bed may be raised slightly. Bed rest is maintained for 24 hours. The client may take foods and fluids immediately. Hemoglobin and hematocrit are usually checked about 6 to 24 hours after the procedure.

Serious bleeding after a renal biopsy is extremely rare when the biopsy is performed by experienced and well-trained nephrologists. However, changes in vital signs or flank pain that radiates into the front of the abdomen may signify bleeding, so notify the physician immediately if this develops. Expect to start an IV infusion to restore intravascular volume; normal saline and possibly blood transfusions will be administered. Bleeding that cannot be controlled with volume or blood replacement may necessitate surgical intervention for control. The most serious consequence of uncontrolled bleeding would be the loss of the kidney. Pink-tinged urine or small amounts of frank blood are not uncommon for 24 hours after the biopsy. Tell the client to expect this to prevent undue alarm. Large amounts of blood in the urine are not expected, however. Advise the client to avoid heavy exercise, activity, or athletic endeavors for 1 to 2 weeks after the biopsy.

The time required to process the tissue specimens varies, depending on laboratory facilities. Almost all processing requires at least 48 to 72 hours; however, the results of some stains may not be available for a week or longer. Since the results of the tissue examination may determine treatment or provide evidence of disease progression or remission, waiting for the results of the biopsy is an anxious time for the client. Nursing support during this waiting period can assist the concerned client and family.

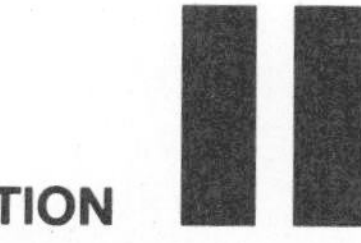

SECTION II

Nursing Diagnosis/Planning and Implementation/Evaluation

Information gathered from the client's health history, physical examination, and diagnostic studies is used to determine nursing diagnoses and the plan of care. Not every client will have the same needs. The Nursing Diagnosis box lists diagnoses **directly related** to kidney and urinary dysfunction along with **potential** nursing diagnoses for clients with kidney and urinary problems. The most common nursing diagnoses for clients with kidney and urinary disease include altered comfort; potential for impaired skin integrity; potential for infection; fluid volume deficit; fluid volume excess; altered thought processes; altered nutrition: less than body requirements; impaired gas exchange; self-concept disturbance: body image; altered sexuality patterns; altered tissue perfusion: renal; and altered patterns of urinary elimination. The sample nursing care plan in Table 25–1 focuses on six of these diagnoses: altered sexuality patterns; altered tissue perfusion: renal, cardiopulmonary; incontinence, total; incontinence, functional: stress, urge, reflex; urinary retention; and altered patterns of urinary elimination. The others are discussed in the narrative.

If the goals of care have not been met, reevaluation is required. The nurse and client should jointly review the nursing care plan. New objectives may need to be formu-

Table 25–1
Sample Nursing Care Plan, by Nursing Diagnosis

Client Care Goals	Plan/Nursing Implementation	Expected Outcomes
Sexuality, altered patterns related to loss of libido		
Accept altered sexual patterns; identify alternatives for sexual pleasure	Explore factors contributing to impotence or loss of libido; suggest alternatives for sexual expression; recommend sex counselor	Client will begin to verbalize fears about sexual patterns and discuss problems/alternatives with sexual partner
Tissue perfusion, altered: renal, cardiopulmonary related to decreased kidney function		
Maintain adequate tissue perfusion	Monitor vital signs and urinary output; assist with dialysis for fluid overload; administer packed red blood cells and 0_2 as ordered; be alert for electrolyte imbalances that may result in dysrhythmias	Blood pressure of no more than 140/80; hemoglobin values around 7–8 g/dL, absence of dysrhythmias or fluid excess
Incontinence, total related to urinary diversion		
Care for and accept urinary appliance or alternate means of voiding	Instruct client in self-care of various urinary diversions (Chapter 26); discuss implications of urinary diversion	Client demonstrates self-care of urinary appliance or urinary diversion
Incontinence, functional; reflex, stress, urge related to disease process		
Maintain urinary continence	Instruct client in care following procedures to correct incontinence problems (Chapter 26)	Client will have improvement in urinary incontinence
Urinary retention related to chronically overdistended bladder		
Reduce urinary retention	Instruct client in care following procedures to correct urinary retention (Chapter 26)	Client will void in a normal manner; bladder is not distended
Urinary elimination, altered patterns related to polyuria, oliguria		
Accept altered urinary elimination patterns	Explain reasons for altered elimination patterns (such as anuria with end-stage renal disease, or polyuria when concentrating ability of kidneys ceases)	Client will manage alteration in urinary elimination without difficulty

NURSING DIAGNOSES IN Kidney and Urinary Dysfunction

DIRECTLY RELATED DIAGNOSES

- Comfort, altered: pain
- Fluid volume deficit
- Fluid volume excess
- Gas exchange, impaired
- Incontinence, functional
- Incontinence, reflex
- Incontinence, stress
- Incontinence, total
- Incontinence, urge
- Infection, potential for
- Nutrition, altered: less than body requirements
- Self-concept, disturbance in: body image
- Sexuality, altered patterns
- Skin integrity, impaired: potential
- Thought processes, altered
- Tissue perfusion, altered: renal, cardiopulmonary
- Urinary elimination, altered patterns
- Urinary retention

OTHER POTENTIAL DIAGNOSES

- Home maintenance management, impaired
- Knowledge deficit
- Powerlessness
- Self-concept, disturbance in: self-esteem
- Social interaction, impaired

lated, other nursing interventions may be added or modified, or the evaluation may show that more time is required to meet the objectives.

Comfort, Altered: Pain

Clients with renal or ureteral calculi experience excruciating pain when passing a stone. Renal abscesses and infections of the urinary tract, including cystitis and urethritis, produce moderate pain. Tumors, enlarged polycystic kidneys, and a distended urinary bladder also result in discomfort for the client. Mild or severe generalized itching accompanies end-stage renal failure and the development of uremia. Dry skin or perspiration and other moisture will worsen the pruritus.

Planning and Implementation

The pain of renal colic experienced by clients with renal or ureteral calculi will require narcotic analgesics for relief. Morphine sulfate is generally given intravenously to provide immediate pain relief, and subsequent doses may be given subcutaneously until the stone is passed or removed. Non-narcotic analgesics, urinary antiseptics, antibiotics, and increased fluid intake may be prescribed to control the discomfort associated with infectious processes. Analgesia may also be needed to relieve the bone pain associated with the hypocalcemia of renal failure. Clients with polycystic kidney disease should avoid aspirin and aspirin-containing compounds because of the potential for bleeding within the cysts.

Pain associated with renal surgery will require narcotic analgesia during the initial 24 to 48 hours, and extensive surgery may cause discomfort for a longer period. Belladonna and opium suppositories may relieve the pain of bladder spasms following prostate surgery, bladder surgery, and kidney transplant surgery (because the new ureter is surgically placed through the bladder wall).

Pruritus in uremic clients with end-stage renal disease is often not relieved by starting dialytic treatments. Interventions that may provide comfort include keeping the client's fingernails short and avoiding agents known to dry the skin (eg, soaps and lotions that contain alcohol). Bathing without soap will remove the uremic frost that compounds itching. (The bath water will be yellow because of the urochrome pigments.) Oil-based lotions and soaps containing lanolin or high fat content should be encouraged. In addition, encourage clients to take phosphate-binding agents as prescribed. Control of the phosphorus–calcium balance will moderate the production of parathormone, which is believed responsible for pruritus in uremic clients.

The aluminum hydroxide antacids (Nutrajel, ALternaGel, Alu-Cap, Amphojel, Basaljel) promote phosphate excretion. They should not be taken with iron because they combine with iron, preventing its absorption. Vitamin D and calcium supplements should also be given to correct the calcium deficit once the hyperphosphatemia has been normalized. Observations that may indicate the presence of hypocalcemia are sore feet, muscle weakness, joint pain, generalized bone aching, and spontaneous fractures. Medications such as trimeprazine tartrate (Temaril) and diphenhydramine (Benadryl) may provide relief from the itching. Diphenhydramine sometimes causes drowsiness and is excreted by the kidney so the dosage should be low to avoid toxicity.

Evaluation

Nursing interventions related to comfort are successful if the client is resting, moving, or sleeping comfortably. Facial expressions and body movements should be relaxed and without tension. Relief from pruritus is successful if the client does not constantly scratch or ask to be scratched or if skin is free of excoriation from frequent scratching.

Skin Integrity, Impaired: Potential

A number of factors contribute to the potential for alterations in skin integrity in renal clients. Poor nutrition, chronic anemia, and pruritus with associated scratching are present in uremic clients with end-stage renal failure. In addition, edema, immobility, alteration in skin sensation, and decreased mental alertness and responsiveness can contribute to problems of skin breakdown. Slowed wound healing has been observed in uremic clients, further contributing to the potential for impairment of skin integrity.

Planning and Implementation

The alleviation of pruritus will promote the maintenance of skin integrity through decreasing the scratching that is difficult to control. Uremic clients who become immobilized for any reason are prone to the development of decubitus ulcers, so they should be turned every 1 to 2 hours and positioned to relieve pressure on edematous areas. A low-sodium diet, fluid restriction, and diuretic therapy or perhaps dialysis may be prescribed to lessen edema. The regulation of parathormone secretion will also decrease pruritus. Other fundamental nursing measures should be implemented to prevent skin breakdown. Nutritional support may promote healing and improve skin integrity.

Evaluation

Data supporting the maintenance of skin integrity include healed surgical incisions without redness or drainage, absence of excoriation from scratching, absence of decubitus ulcers from pressure, and evidence that the client is eating the prescribed diet.

Infection: Potential For

Urinary tract instrumentation is the most common cause of nosocomial UTIs. Clients with stones in the kidneys, ureters, or bladder may develop infections. In-dwelling urinary catheters, stents, ureteral tubes, and nephrostomy tubes also may contribute to the client's potential for infection. Urinary stasis associated with a neurogenic bladder is an excellent medium for ascending UTIs, which can become systemic.

Planning and Implementation

Maintain sterile technique during dressing changes and at sites where catheters have been inserted into the blood or urinary system. No client should be catheterized unless absolutely necessary. Intermittent catheterization is preferable to the placement of a continuous in-dwelling urinary catheter. Vascular access routes for hemodialysis and catheters for peritoneal dialysis should all be cared for meticulously. For shunt care, some medical centers use clean technique, whereas others use aseptic technique. All institutions use sterile technique for insertion or cannulation of access sites to prevent the development of bacteremic infection.

For the client with an in-dwelling catheter, a closed drainage system (one that is closed to outside air) including the catheter connecting tube and collection bag must be maintained. The catheter must be secured to prevent movement and injury to the urethra. For female clients, the drainage tubing should be taped horizontally to the thigh. For male clients, the catheter should be secured by taping it horizontally to the thigh or the abdomen. The client should be assessed for symptoms and signs of urinary tract infection such as fever, chills, and bloody or cloudy urine. The urethral meatus should also be observed for drainage or irritation.

The following principles apply to the care of a client with a closed urinary drainage system.

- Use strict aseptic technique when inserting in-dwelling catheters or when obtaining specimens.
- Keep the entire collection system closed.
- Avoid obtaining specimens from connecting tubing (which may not be self-sealing) if the system does not have an inline port; use a sterile needle and syringe to aspirate through the catheter.
- Prevent reflux of urine by keeping the drainage bag below the bladder at all times; do not allow the drainage bag to rest on the floor.
- Prevent kinking or twisting of the drainage tubing.
- Drain the collection bag at least every 8 hours.
- Remove catheters as soon as possible.
- Change catheters whenever crusting develops at the catheter-meatal junction or in the catheter itself, or if it becomes necessary to manipulate the catheter to maintain the flow of urine.
- Irrigate catheters only when necessary; if irrigations are necessary to maintain patency, use a closed three-way system.
- Maintain a liberal fluid intake (if not contraindicated) to keep the urine dilute and to retard crusting and infection.

Home Health Care

When clients with urinary drainage catheters are cared for at home, the client or caregiver should be taught the proper care and maintenance of the catheter. The perineal area or penis should be washed daily with soap and water, and rinsed and dried thoroughly. The rectal area should be cleansed the same way after each bowel movement.

Instruct the client and caregivers regarding the symptoms and signs of infection (characteristics of urine, redness at the urethral meatus, odor, discharge, or pain). They should understand the importance of notifying the physician or nurse if any of these occur.

Teach the client and caregivers to assess for malfunction of the catheter (decreased urine flow, bladder distention, discomfort and/or leaking around the catheter). They should be taught how to remove the catheter safely at home, if a major problem occurs with the client's urinary drainage.

Evaluation

Evaluation of the absence of infection includes a normal body temperature, a normal white blood cell count, and the absence of chills. In addition, the client should not have foul-smelling urine or wound drainage, and catheter and vascular sites should be free of erythema, drainage, and tenderness.

Fluid Volume Deficit
Fluid Volume Excess

Loss of fluid or blood volume through the use of diuretics, infection processes, hemorrhage, or fluid shift to the interstitial space (which occurs in the nephrotic syndrome) may result in a fluid volume deficit. For clients with normal renal function, this may contribute to decreased renal perfusion and the development of prerenal azotemia. Clients who undergo hemodialysis or peritoneal dialysis also may have too much fluid removed during the treatment and experience a fluid volume deficit (hypovolemia).

Excess circulating fluid volume, or hypervolemia, occurs when the client is oliguric because of renal failure. This problem may occur acutely with sudden loss of renal function or develop as end-stage renal failure progresses. Excesses in fluid volume contribute to cardiopulmonary decompensation and must be corrected.

Planning and Implementation

Oral or IV fluid replacement will be necessary if the client becomes fluid-depleted from diuretic therapy, surgical drainage, or dialysis. Blood or plasma expanders also may be given to restore intravascular volume. Careful measurement of the client's intake and output, weight, and vital signs is essential to assess fluid volume status. In addition, the client's dry weight may need to be reevaluated. Dry weight is weight after dialysis without evidence of edema and with the client's blood pressure in the normal range.

Fluid volume excess may be avoided in dialysis clients if they understand the need to control fluid intake. Instruct clients to restrict fluid intake to the amount of urinary output in 24 hours plus 600 mL. If there is no urine output, fluid should be limited to no more than 1000 mL and perhaps to no more than 500 mL per day. Intravenous infusions should be administered with microdrip tubing to avoid excessive fluid administration. Medications administered piggyback should be dissolved in the smallest possible volume of fluid.

A plastic glass with lines marking the amount of fluid will help the client control fluid intake. Also helpful is a list of the amount of fluid in common containers used in the hospital. Fluid restriction may be prescribed as a guideline; however, the client eventually will need to assume responsibility for control of thirst and fluid intake and thus may impose his or her own fluid restriction. Staff members can assist the client to control fluid intake by not placing the water pitcher at the bedside. Intake and output, weight, and blood pressure should be monitored to assess the client's fluid status. Clinical manifestations of fluid excess can include edema, hypertension, and shortness of breath.

Evaluation

Normal blood pressure generally indicates stabilization of fluid volume. Body weight should be stable, reflective of the client's dry weight. The client should demonstrate knowledge of the fluid allowance, how to calculate fluid intake and loss, and how to compare weight changes with feelings of physical well-being. For example, the client who suddenly becomes short of breath should suspect that dry weight has been exceeded and the blood pressure is elevated. Other manifestations of normal fluid volume include absence of syncope or light-headedness with changes in posture. The client should not feel nauseated or thirsty; peripheral edema should be minimal, and there should be no rales or congestion in the lung fields.

Thought Processes, Altered

Changes in the sensorium, inability to concentrate, and impaired memory of recent events are common manifestations of uremia. Nitrogenous waste products accumulate because of impaired renal excretion, metabolic acidosis occurs because of inadequate acid excretion and a bicarbonate deficit, and electrolyte disturbances arise with renal failure. These biochemical alterations cause a progressive deterioration in mental functioning. Clients become increasingly lethargic and drowsy until dialysis can correct the metabolic alterations. Dietary alterations may temporarily slow the development of these altered mental functions. The use of potent diuretics also can contribute to electrolyte imbalances and altered thought processes.

Planning and Implementation

For the uremic client, removal of nitrogenous waste products and control of metabolic acidosis usually improves thought processes. Hemodialysis or peritoneal dialysis is usually necessary when thought processes are impaired. In addition, modifying the diet to restrict protein intake may decrease cognitive impairment. If the client has impaired mental functioning, explanations should be short and concise. Because of impaired memory of recent events, the client will need frequent reinforcement of previous explanations. The nurse should assure clients and family members that the loss of clear thought processes is temporary and will be normalized with adequate dialysis.

In addition to assessing the client's level of orientation to person, place, and time, observe the client for slurred speech, tremors, myoclonus, and asterixis. The client with uremic encephalopathy is vulnerable to seizures, so safety precautions should be initiated. Pad the siderails and assist the client when ambulating or out of bed. Monitor the client for drug toxicity that can occur because of limited renal excretion of drugs.

Evaluation

Successful correction of altered mental functioning can be determined through orientation to person, place, and time; clarity of the client's speech; improved alertness and ability to remember explanations; and the absence of asterixis. No tremors or myoclonus should occur.

Nutrition, Altered: Less Than Body Requirements

The client with acute or chronic renal failure always has altered nutritional status. Nausea, vomiting, and anorexia are common manifestations of each of these processes in which there is azotemia. In addition, clients commonly experience a metallic taste in the mouth, and some foods may no longer taste good to them. Hypogeusia is a common problem for clients with end-stage renal failure. Dietary modifications (low-salt, low-potassium diets) prescribed for clients with renal failure complicate efforts to maintain good nutrition. The loss of proteins via peritoneal dialysis and loss of water-soluble vitamins via either peritoneal or hemodialysis further complicate nutritional status. Clients with altered renal function who are acutely or critically ill from sepsis or other problems will also experience nutritional deficits.

Planning and Implementation

The diets of clients with altered renal function generally require modification or restriction. Clients with hypertension should be on a no added salt diet, which is restricted to 4 g of sodium. If severe hypertension or heart failure is also present, the dietary sodium content may be restricted to 2 g/day.

Protein allowances also may be adjusted. Clients who are losing excessive protein, such as clients with nephrotic syndrome who have proteinuria or peritoneal dialysis clients who may lose up to 70 g/wk of protein in the dialysate, need a high-protein diet of 100 g/day or more. In contrast, clients with end-stage renal failure who are becoming uremic or are undergoing chronic hemodialysis generally are prescribed a diet restricted in protein (around 40 to 60 g/day for clients who have not yet started dialytic therapy; 50 to 70 g/day for dialysis clients). Protein in foods should be of high biologic value (ie, contain a high proportion of essential amino acids) to ensure that essential amino acids are provided (Table 25–2). Adequate protein and calories must be provided so the client's own muscle mass is not catabolized as a source of energy.

When clients stop excreting urine, potassium intake also must be restricted, because fatal cardiac dysrhythmias will occur with excessively high serum potassium levels. The nurse should observe for signs of hyperkalemia which

Table 25–2
Protein Foods of High and Low Biologic Value

High Biologic Value	Low Biologic Value
Meat	Potatoes
Fish	Rice
Poultry	Spaghetti
Eggs	Bread
Cheese	Other vegetable products

include muscle weakness, which can result in a flaccid paralysis of the extremities, and cardiac dysrhythmias. The potassium allowance is generally equivalent in milliequivalents to the grams of protein. For example, a 60-g protein diet and a 60-mEq potassium diet would be compatible. Each gram of protein provides a milliequivalent of potassium; therefore, potassium may not be more restricted than protein. Foods with a high potassium content are listed in Box 19–1 in Chapter 19.

Often, the dietary restriction of potassium is not enough to prevent hyperkalemia. To lower dangerously high potassium levels, sodium polystyrene sulfonate (Kayexalate) may be administered in addition to dialysis. Kayexalate is a cation-exchange resin in which sodium is exchanged for potassium, and the potassium is excreted in the stool. One gram of Kayexalate will decrease the serum potassium level by 1.0 mEq/L. It may be administered orally, by nasogastric tube, or rectally, and its effectiveness is enhanced by retention in the bowel for at least 6 hours. Because it causes constipation, Kayexalate often is administered with sorbitol and water. A 30-mL Foley catheter with the balloon inflated distal to the anal sphincter has proven helpful in enhancing rectal retention. This procedure can, however, be extremely uncomfortable for the client.

The general caloric recommendation for clients maintained on chronic dialysis is about 35 kcal/kg of ideal body weight. Chronic dialysis clients who become ill with other problems or require surgery usually have dietary limitations temporarily removed so that nutritional needs may be met through a more liberal choice of foods. This is to ensure healing and prevent further debilitation from infection or stress. Nutritional supplements may be offered, such as milk shakes made with a high-carbohydrate and high-fat additive. Potassium restrictions, however, are not removed.

Severely debilitated or critically ill clients in severe need of adequate nutrition will be fed via parenteral or enteral alimentation. In general, protein intake is not restricted when these methods of feeding are required. If necessary, more frequent dialysis can control fluid and BUN levels. With parenteral or enteral alimentation and concurrent dialysis, serum electrolyte levels should be monitored. Rapid imbalances of electrolytes may produce critical situations if careful monitoring is not part of the routine.

Promoting a well-balanced diet for a client who often has no appetite or a metallic taste in the mouth is a challenge for the nurse, especially if the previously mentioned restrictions must be followed. Appetite may be improved by providing oral hygiene and fresh air, minimizing movement, and administering prescribed antiemetics. A mouthwash of sodium acid phosphate will relieve the uremic fetor (ammonialike breath). Sucking on hard candy can also relieve the bad taste. Work with the dietitian to provide appetizing meals, perhaps in small, frequent feedings supplemented by nourishing snacks. The mealtime environment should be pleasant and free of odors. The client's food preferences should be considered.

Evaluation

Improvement of nutritional status may be assumed if the client is eating the prescribed diet without nausea and vomiting. Over a period of several weeks to months, laboratory values for albumin, total protein, and electrolytes should become normal. Other evidence of adequate nutrition includes healing of wounds and maintenance of skin integrity.

Gas Exchange, Impaired

The impairment of oxygen–carbon dioxide exchange leading to inadequate oxygenation may be caused by renal disorders or surgical intervention. If the kidneys fail to excrete hydrogen ions and regenerate adequate bicarbonate, the lungs must compensate for the increased load of metabolic acids by increasing the rate and depth of breathing, also known as Kussmaul's respirations. Respiratory fatigue from continued compensation may lead to decreased oxygenation, especially if infection or cardiac problems are present. Flank incisions or thoracoabdominal approaches for renal or urologic surgery may limit respiratory movements. Chronic anemia impairs gas exchange and results in increased cardiac workload.

Planning and Implementation

For clients with metabolic acidosis from acute or chronic renal failure, oxygen–carbon dioxide exchange may be improved with the administration of sodium bicarbonate or with the institution of dialysis. Sodium bicarbonate may also be administered to treat hyperkalemia, because correcting metabolic acidosis helps to correct hyperkalemia. Correction of metabolic acidosis and the lowering of serum potassium levels are an important part of stabilizing the client with acute renal failure. Sodium bicarbonate may be administered orally in tablet form or intravenously. The major risk associated with IV administration of sodium bicarbonate is that it may further expand extracellular fluid volume and worsen problems of hypervolemia, if they are present. Since the correction of acidosis can lead to calcium deficits, it is important to observe for signs of tetany. The dialysate used for either peritoneal dialysis or hemodialysis contains acetate, which converts to bicarbonate when absorbed. Thus, dialysis will provide for the replacement of depleted bicarbonate stores.

Decreased oxygenation due to fluid accumulation in the lungs may impair gas exchange; thus ventilation should improve when dialysis removes fluid from the lungs. Respiratory rate, pulse rate, and arterial blood gases should be monitored to prevent cardiopulmonary arrest.

In addition to sodium bicarbonate and dialysis, oxygen will usually be prescribed via a cannula. Ensure that the airway is patent and help the client into a semi-Fowler's position to ease respiratory effort. Moderately or completely unresponsive clients should be positioned on their sides to prevent aspiration of secretions or stomach contents. Clients who hypoventilate because their surgical incision makes breathing painful should receive analgesics before coughing and deep-breathing exercises.

Evaluation

Indications that oxygenation is adequate include arterial blood gases that give evidence of a pH between 7.35 and 7.45, a carbon dioxide content of 38 to 42 mg/dL, and an oxygen level greater than 60%. In addition, the client should have no subjective feelings of respiratory distress and should perform normal exercise without undue respiratory embarrassment. Slight tachypnea is common in clients who use respiratory compensation for metabolic acidosis, but the client usually is not aware of the increased respiratory rate.

Self-Concept, Disturbance in: Body Image

Altered kidney and urinary tract function cause a variety of body image changes. Urinary diversions may result in cutaneous stomata and necessitate the client's wearing an external pouch. In-dwelling urinary catheters or a suprapubic tube may also be used to provide permanent or temporary urinary drainage. If chronic renal failure develops, dialysis requiring vascular access or permanent peritoneal catheter placement will alter the client's body image. In addition, chronic dialysis clients often produce minimal urine. Not urinating, after a lifetime of this habit, commonly causes a significant change in body image. Furthermore, dependence on a machine for the preservation of life causes major alterations in lifestyle and often precipitates crises in role relationships and sexuality. Finally, the amount of time required for dialysis per week (12 to 15 h/wk for hemodialysis and 32 to 48 h/wk for peritoneal dialysis) may necessitate job changes or reliance on disability insurance.

Body image changes also accompany renal transplantation. Having a part of someone else's body can create emotional turmoil. Also, the use of steroids following transplantation results in many changes such as softening of skin, thinning of hair, osteoporosis, moon face, buffalo hump, and weight gain.

Planning and Implementation

Listen to the client's concerns and anxieties. Encourage clients to express their feelings about urinary diversion procedures or the need for vascular or catheter access for dialysis. After the initial period of shock passes, opportunities to talk with other clients who have successfully managed these adjustments may be helpful. Nurses who patiently support clients learning new self-care practices will promote feelings of confidence and ease the burdens associated with changed body image.

Suggest that changes in skin color—the ashen-yellow appearance—may be partially masked by colors such as bright red or blue that tone down the yellow. Orange, green, yellow, and white should be avoided. Severe edema may be hidden by loose-fitting clothing. Gain the client's confidence, however, before discussing these sensitive subjects. Explaining the physiologic changes that contribute to body changes will help the client cope.

The client having a kidney transplant also has special needs. Professional counseling and ventilation of feelings with the nurse will help the client learn to live with the fact that his or her kidney once was in someone else. The client also will need guidance in adjusting to the long-term effects of immunosuppressive therapy.

The development of renal failure may necessitate major lifestyle changes. The client may have to quit working entirely, change jobs, or work part-time. Feelings of not being worthwhile are common. Someone may need to be hired to carry out household tasks, or other family members will have to take on additional responsibilities. All these changes require crisis intervention by the health care team, because they may seem insurmountable at first. Government aid for the care of renal failure clients may ease the financial burden.

Evaluation

Successful nursing interventions result in the client's ability to verbalize freely feelings related to self-concept, self-esteem, changes in body image, altered performance of roles, and altered sexuality. If the client fails to discuss feelings in all areas, however, nursing interventions have not necessarily failed. Respect for appropriate timing and sensitivity to the client's need for delay or denial of feelings to cope with other stressors is another successful nursing intervention. The transplant recipient should demonstrate increasing ability to cope with having a donor kidney and with the effects of immunosuppressants.

SECTION 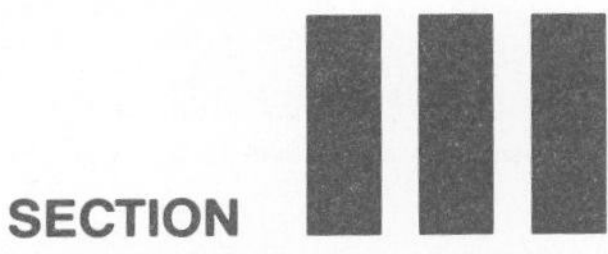

Dialysis

When conservative treatment of renal failure is no longer effective, and renal function has deteriorated to the point where death will ensue, dialysis therapy must be started. Kidney transplantation, another alternative for clients with chronic or end-stage renal disease, is discussed in Chapter 26.

Principles and Types of Dialysis

The combination of three principles—diffusion, osmosis, and filtration—permits the removal of metabolic wastes and excess electrolytes and fluids from the client with renal failure by artificial means. Dialysis involves the differential *diffusion* of substances (solute) across a semipermeable membrane that separates two fluid compartments containing substances of different concentrations. The pressure gradient produced results in the flow, or diffusion, of substances to the less concentrated area. This process continues until the concentrations are equal on each side. *Osmosis,* the movement of fluid or solvent from a lower concentration to a higher one, also occurs during dialysis. *Filtration,* the movement of both solvent and solute across a semipermeable membrane under force, also occurs. An increase in hydrostatic pressure on one side of the membrane used for dialysis drives fluid and dissolved substances into the opposite side.

Dialysis affects only fluid, electrolyte, and acid–base imbalances (and only during the time it is performed), so it cannot completely substitute for renal functions such as the production of erythropoietin and renin; detoxification of drugs; and intermediary metabolism of glucose, insulin, and vitamin D.

There are two types of dialysis: **peritoneal dialysis** and **hemodialysis.** In peritoneal dialysis, the client's own peritoneal lining serves as the semipermeable membrane, whereas in hemodialysis, an artificial kidney contains the semipermeable membrane. Refer to Table 25–3 for a comparison of the advantages of the two types of dialysis.

Indications for Dialysis

In acute renal failure, dialysis is usually begun when acidosis, hyperkalemia, and other uremic symptoms no longer can be controlled. In chronic renal failure, dialysis should be started before the appearance of symptoms of uncontrolled hypertension and acidosis, bone disease, peripheral neuropathy, uremic encephalopathy, and severe anemia. This is generally when creatinine clearance values fall below 5 mL/min and serum creatinine levels are greater

Table 25–3
Advantages of Hemodialysis and Peritoneal Dialysis

Hemodialysis	Peritoneal Dialysis
• Requires 12–15 h/wk compared to up to 48 h with peritoneal dialysis • Can be used when peritoneal dialysis is contraindicated because of abdominal lesions • Causes rapid reversal of fluid and electrolyte imbalances • Does not result in protein loss	• Can be started in 1 h (this includes time for catheter placement) • Is a simple procedure • Because it is slow, there are fewer distressing symptoms • Anticoagulants are not necessary • Does not cause blood loss • Can be done on an ambulatory basis which is less expensive and allows client flexibility

than 10 mEq/L (Saxton et al., 1983). Clients who begin dialysis before these problems arise are more likely to remain complication-free and sustain normal life activities than clients who begin dialysis after these symptoms arise.

Client Implications in Dialysis

The client usually decides the mode of dialysis to be used, and the health care team gives support and recommendations. Factors that influence this decision include answers to the following questions: What aspects of the client's lifestyle, work goals, or travel considerations may influence the method of dialysis selected? Is the client capable of self-care? Continuous ambulatory peritoneal dialysis (CAPD) may be the best alternative for a motivated, active person. What social support system does the client have? Family members often can be taught to carry out dialysis at home, although the training program is extensive and usually requires 8 to 12 weeks. Do physical complications or limitations make one mode of dialysis less than ideal or contraindicated? The client should participate actively in the selection of the method for chronic dialysis or the client may choose to have no dialysis at all. Some clients may prefer to die rather than to face chronic dialysis or renal transplantation.

Hemodialysis

Hemodialysis removes nitrogenous waste products, excess electrolytes, and excess fluid from the blood via a specially processed, cellophanelike dialyzing membrane. The membrane, housed in a dialyzer in the artificial kidney machine, maintains sterility and integrity. A vascular access provides a route for blood to exit the body and then return to the vascular system.

While outside the body, the blood is pumped through the artificial kidney machine, composed of a pump, a semipermeable membrane, and a source of dialysate solution for the removal of waste products from the blood. In addition to these basic components, a variety of devices monitor and ensure the safety of the system. Regulation of the pump adjusts the rate of blood flow; the goal for blood flow is usually 200 to 300 mL/min.

The client is heparinized before dialysis is initiated, the machine is loaded with a heparinized solution before blood is sent through the dialyzer, or both. Blood flows from the client's body through plastic tubing into the artificial kidney and returns to the client's vascular system through plastic tubing. The blood is warmed after dialysis before it returns to the client.

Dialysate is a solution composed of water, glucose, sodium, chloride, potassium, calcium, and acetate or bicarbonate. It contains varying amounts of substances to help remove as much or as little water, electrolytes, and waste products from the blood as are indicated by the client's laboratory values. While blood is pumped through the semipermeable membrane, dialysate is delivered into the plastic cylinder containing the membrane. The flow of dialysate thus continuously surrounds the membrane, but the dialysate does not come in direct contact with the blood inside. While the dialysate is in contact with the membrane, waste products and excess electrolytes diffuse into it from the blood. The dialysate exit is at the end of the plastic cylinder opposite the blood entry point, which minimizes the possibility of the waste products being reabsorbed.

Removal of water is by osmosis and filtration. Because the glucose concentration in the dialysate is greater than the glucose concentration in the blood, water moves from the blood into the dialysate by osmosis. The higher the glucose concentration of the dialysate, the more water is removed by osmosis. If water were removed only by this method, however, the time required for the process would be very long. Therefore, more water may be removed by increasing the hydrostatic pressure applied to the blood as it flows through the dialyzer, resulting in the ultrafiltration of the blood. Another method of pressure application to increase removal of water is the use of negative pressure, or suction. Negative pressure is applied to the membrane, and water is pulled from the blood as it passes through the dialyzer.

Indications/Contraindications

Hemodialysis can treat acute or chronic renal failure. Because it corrects hyperkalemia, metabolic acidosis, or hypervolemia in 1 to 2 hours, it is the dialysis of choice in emergency situations. Hemodialysis is preferred over peritoneal dialysis whenever there is a hypercatabolic state, a diaphragmatic leak, severe respiratory insufficiency, a large abdominal wound, intra-abdominal cancer, abdominal adhesions or scar tissue, peritonitis, or critical volume excesses such as pulmonary edema. Hemodialysis is contraindicated when there are clotting disorders, circulatory instability, or cardiovascular disease. Some treatment centers consider diabetes a contraindication to hemodialysis because of the possibility that large amounts of heparin may result in blindness for the diabetic client.

Procedure

Hemodialysis requires a vascular access. A variety of vascular accesses are available. For clients with chronic renal failure, the **arteriovenous** (AV) **fistula** is the preferred access. An AV fistula is the internal anastomosis of an artery to a vein, and for hemodialysis the nondominant forearm usually is chosen (Figure 25–4). After 8 to 12 weeks, the vein wall becomes thickened and more muscular, resembling an artery. The fistula also distends and becomes prominent. At this point, the fistula is considered mature and is expected to be able to withstand frequent venipunctures and to provide adequate blood flow for the hemodialysis procedure. The average lifetime of a fistula is about 3 to 4 years.

A bovine graft is a section of a blood vessel from a cow that has been treated to avoid contamination. It is implanted with one end in an artery and the other in a vein. Like the fistula, it is internal. If possible, at least 1 week should elapse between the bovine graft surgery and use of the graft. This type of access is used in the same way as the AV fistula.

A Gore-Tex graft is a synthetic tube used in place of a bovine graft or fistula. It is placed in the same manner as the bovine graft: One end of the tube is attached to an artery and the other to a vein. Two weeks should elapse from the time of surgery to the time of dialysis. This access also is used in the same way as the fistula.

A cannula, or **arteriovenous shunt,** is another form of vascular access used for hemodialysis. It is an external connection of an artery to a vein in which two pieces of synthetic tubing form a loop (Figure 25–5). One limb of tubing is sutured into an artery, and the other is sutured into a vein. The two limbs of shunt tubing are joined by either a t-connector or a straight connector. The t-connector has the advantage of allowing blood to be withdrawn, or fluids or medication to be administered intravenously via the cannula, thus avoiding venipuncture. In some centers, a straight connector is used, especially when a cannula has a tendency toward clotting. It is thought that a disadvantage of the t-connector is increased resistance to blood flow through the slightly narrowed diameter of its lumen. A straight connector is generally preferred for outpatients with a cannula. Their external junction may be disconnected and attached to tubing to accomplish extracorporeal blood flow through the artificial kidney machine. Cannulas are considered temporary forms of vascular access. Because they can be used immediately, they may be appropriate for clients with acute renal failure or those with chronic renal failure while a fistula develops. The lifetime of a cannula is usually less than 1 year. The cannula is typically placed in the dominant forearm, although the other arm, a thigh, or an ankle may be selected. The dominant forearm is preferred as a temporary site so that when a permanent access is developed, the client will have the more usable hand and arm for activities during the dialysis treatment.

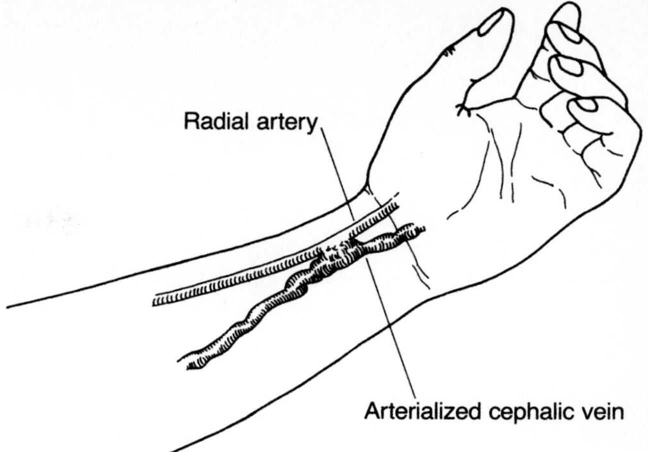

Figure 25–4

Arteriovenous (AV) fistula for hemodialysis. SOURCE: *Holloway N:* Nursing the Critically Ill Adult: Applying Nursing Diagnosis, *3rd ed. Menlo Park, CA: Addison–Wesley, 1988.*

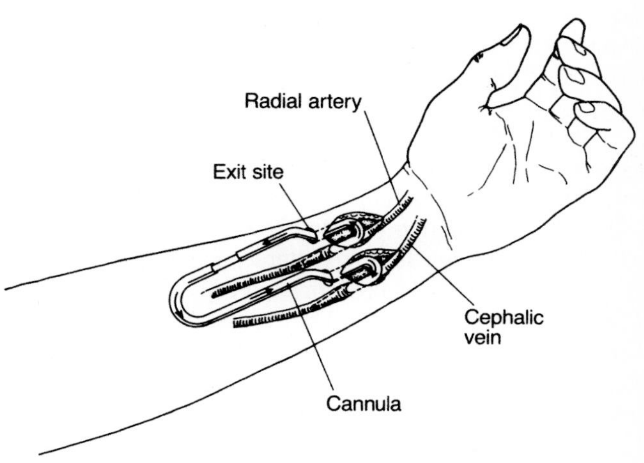

Figure 25–5

Standard AV shunt (cannula) for hemodialysis. SOURCE: *Holloway N:* Nursing the Critically Ill Adult: Applying Nursing Diagnosis, *3rd ed. Menlo Park, CA: Addison–Wesley, 1988.*

Nursing Implications

Because the artificial kidney machine or its monitoring system can malfunction and cause death, it is necessary to obtain informed consent from the client or guardian prior to initiating the treatment. The physician explains the benefits and risks of the procedure, and the nurse frequently obtains the signature and, if there is lack of client understanding, initiates further teaching.

Check the blood pressure at the beginning of the treatment and at least every 30 minutes throughout. Hemodialysis treatments for the client with end-stage renal failure commonly last 4 hours three times a week. However, the client with acute renal failure who is extremely catabolic or requires parenteral nutrition may need hemodialysis more frequently to maintain fluid and electrolyte balance and remove nitrogenous wastes.

Monitor the vascular access for patency, absence of infection, and absence of bleeding. The cannula and fistula should be checked for patency every hour for the first 24 hours after insertion and then at least every 4 hours by palpation of the thrill and auscultation of the bruit. A thrill is a rippling sensation palpable on the venous side of the cannula or fistula. It is usually more readily palpable in a fistula than a cannula. The bruit, heard through the stethoscope, is a rushing or roaring noise or "swoosh" timed with each heartbeat. Failure to detect a thrill or bruit when either was previously present suggests loss of patency, usually because of clotting of the access. A properly trained nurse should declot a cannula immediately, as time is critical. Clotted fistulas may require surgical intervention. In either case, once patency has been established, measures to prevent reclotting—continuous heparin infusions, administrations of Low Molecular-Weight Dextran (LMD), and antiplatelet agents such as dipyridamole (Persantine)—should be considered.

The client and significant others should be instructed in checking patency of the access at least every 4 hours. Some medical centers suggest checking every 1 to 2 hours, especially following dialysis. The client with a fistula should be taught to:

- Keep the arm elevated and extended at first.
- Avoid lying on the access (such as having the arm curled under the head while sleeping).
- Avoid wearing constricting clothing or jewelry on the affected extremity.
- Allow no venipunctures or blood pressure cuffs or tourniquets to be placed around the extremity.
- Watch for symptoms and signs of infection.

The nurse should also follow these rules when caring for a client who has had surgery for a fistula, as well as check for capillary refill in the extremity. In some centers, clients receive specific instructions on exercises or activities to increase the strength of the vessel walls until the fistula is mature and ready to be used (ie, for approximately 8 to 12 weeks). Emphasize to the client that the vascular access is a lifeline and should be protected as such. A fistula does not require a dressing, since it is internal.

The client with a cannula requires slightly different care. Because the cannula can be used immediately, no exercises are needed. Also teach the client with a cannula to check for patency, as previously discussed. In addition, advise the client that the blood should be bright red. If the blood is dark or if clots can be seen in the tubing, the cannula must be declotted immediately. Although the cannula is wrapped in gauze to prevent separation or infection, a small loop of tubing should be made easily accessible by lifting up a piece of the gauze. This permits visualization of the blood in the tubing and assessment of the warmth characteristic of the tubing of a patent cannula. The same restrictions apply to the cannula as to the fistula, for example, no blood pressure cuffs or tourniquets, no restrictive clothing or jewelry, and no lying on the access.

The subclavian and femoral catheters do not have an arterial-to-venous flow so there is no thrill or bruit. Patency of these catheters is maintained through intermittent irrigations with a dilute heparin-saline solution or by the intermittent instillation of a heparinized saline solution.

Infection at the insertion site and, subsequently, of the bloodstream is a common problem and source of concern for the client with vascular access. Frequent manipulations and the presence of foreign materials in the blood make the cannula, the subclavian catheter, and the femoral catheter all likely sites for infection. Use aseptic technique whenever the tubings are disconnected and blood exposed, such as when attaching or disconnecting bloodlines or placing a t-connector or straight connector. The skin over the fistula puncture sites should be prepared carefully with a bactericidal solution.

Since the cannula is external, preventing infection is particularly important. Thoroughly cleanse the cannula site after washing the hands. Wear sterile gloves when opening the cannula. Do not pull or tug on the tubing. Some health care centers suggest scrubbing the client's skin with bactericidal soap and rinsing the area with sterile saline, whereas others recommend swabbing exit sites with hydrogen peroxide. Next, apply a bactericidal ointment at the exit sites, and put dry, sterile gauze under the tubing. It is important to keep the tubing from touching the skin, so wrap the area with gauze, and cover the tubing lightly with gauze. Leave some tubing accessible to check patency, however.

Bleeding is another complication of the vascular access. If a cannula pulls apart, the client can bleed to death in minutes; for this reason, bulldog or alligator clamps should be attached to the plastic wrap or elastic bandage that covers the gauze around the cannula. This way, the cannula tubings can be clamped off immediately should they become disconnected. The fistula, bovine graft, or Gore-Tex graft require direct pressure over the two venipuncture sites to control hemorrhage. Blood clots at each site will form in about 10 minutes. If new bleeding develops, direct pressure over the site for about 10 minutes will usually result in hemostasis. If bleeding occurs around the subclavian or femoral catheter insertion site, direct pressure, topical hemostatic agents (such as thrombin), or a pressure dressing may be required to stop it.

The client receiving hemodialysis treatments needs extensive physical care. The client's emotional needs are just as great. Because peritoneal dialysis and hemodialysis create essentially the same psychologic stresses, the psychologic implications of both types will be described after the following discussion of peritoneal dialysis.

Peritoneal Dialysis

During peritoneal dialysis the peritoneal membrane serves as the semipermeable membrane for dialysis. The peritoneal membrane allows the diffusion of small molecules such as electrolytes, urea, creatinine, uric acid, and glucose, all of which have molecular weights below 200. It is impermeable to large molecules such as blood cells and proteins, which have molecular weights greater than 50,000.

During peritoneal dialysis, a catheter (a common one is the Tenckhoff catheter) is placed into the abdominal cavity (Figure 25–6). A temporary or permanent catheter may be inserted at the client's bedside, but the permanent catheter generally is inserted in surgery. Dialysate is then instilled through the catheter into the abdominal cavity. Through diffusion and osmosis, excess electrolytes, nitrogenous waste products, and fluid are transported from the blood into the dialysate. The dialysate is then drained, and new, pure dialysate is instilled.

A complete cycle involves new fluid running in (inflow phase), sitting for diffusion and osmosis (dwell time), and being drained out (outflow phase). The length of each cycle affects the efficiency of dialysis. During the inflow phase, which usually lasts about 5 to 10 minutes, about 2 L of dialysate are allowed to flow into the abdominal cavity after it has been warmed to enhance diffusion and minimize discomfort. During the dwell phase of about 30 minutes, dialysis takes place. Initially, the exchange rate is rapid, but it slows down in later cycles, when dialysate and blood composition are similar. The outflow phase, which lasts about 20 minutes, begins when the dialysate flows out of the abdomen. These cycles may be accomplished manually, with the aid of an automatic peritoneal dialysis machine, or through continuous ambulatory peritoneal dialysis (CAPD).

With manual peritoneal dialysis, the fluid is exchanged every 60 minutes for 30 to 40 hours. This method is slow and inefficient, but it effectively clears waste products and removes fluid when rapid decreases are not required.

With an automatic peritoneal dialysis machine, the

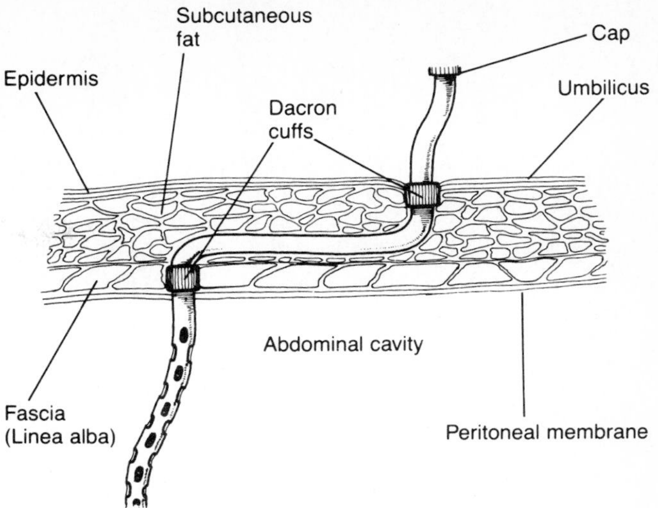

Figure 25–6

Catheter placement for peritoneal dialysis. The permanently implanted catheter exits from a point different than the insertion site through a subcutaneous tunnel.

cycling and the amount of dialysate to be infused are preset. Pressure alarms inform the nurse of any problems with inflow or outflow. About 10 to 16 hours of treatment are necessary two or three times a week. Intermittent peritoneal dialysis (IPD) by machine is relatively easy to learn, and many clients do this form of therapy at home. Clients who select IPD for use at home usually require the assistance of a second person. Midway through the procedure, eight new 2-L bottles of dialysate must be added to the system. The bottles are cumbersome, and the tubing that connects the machine to the peritoneal catheter is not long. Therefore, the client generally has limited freedom to move about. Furthermore, reaching up to place the bottles on the hangers above the machine requires more strength and mobility than many home IPD clients have.

The client using CAPD enjoys greater freedom and independence. The same permanent peritoneal catheter is used, but dialysate is always present in the abdominal cavity. The dialysate is drained into a bag attached by tubing to the peritoneal catheter four times a day, every day of the week (Figure 25–7). Exchanges are timed to occur about every 4 to 5 hours and at bedtime. This lack of machine dependency is appealing to many people who want to maintain as normal a lifestyle as possible. With CAPD, the client assumes responsibility for all aspects of the dialysis procedure. For those unable to assume responsibility for the procedure, the significant other can receive training to help provide this treatment. Many clients who have experienced other modes of therapy report that they feel better more consistently with this form of continuous dialysis.

Indications/Contraindications

Peritoneal dialysis, a relatively simple procedure, may be used when hemodialysis is not available. It is often cho-

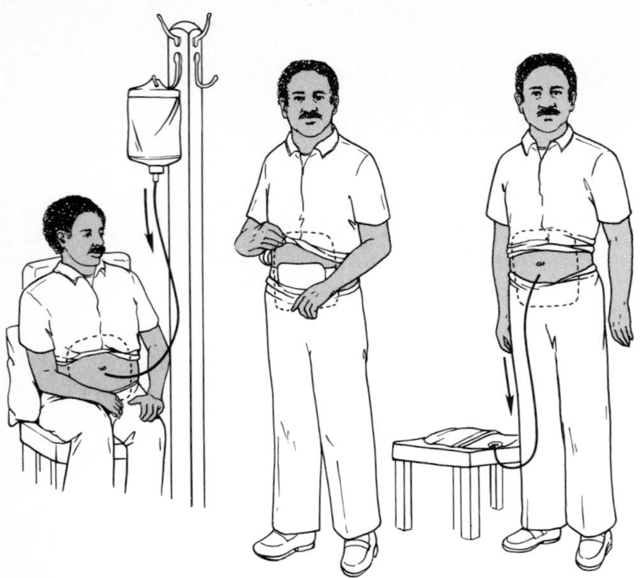

Figure 25–7

Client performing COPD at home.

sen over hemodialysis for clients with acute renal failure when immediate results are not critical. Some advantages of peritoneal dialysis are that it can be used for clients with clotting disorders, cardiovascular disease, exhausted vascular access sites, inadequate veins (the very young and very old), and diabetes, as well as for clients who refuse blood transfusions.

Peritoneal dialysis is contraindicated in clients with active pathologic conditions in the abdomen, including diaphragmatic leaks, abdominal wounds, abdominal cancer, abdominal adhesions, or infected abdominal wall, as well as for respiratory insufficiency or a hypercatabolic state.

Complications

The primary complication of peritoneal dialysis is peritonitis. Instruct the client to report any abdominal discomfort or change in the appearance of the peritoneal fluid. Normally, the peritoneal fluid returned is clear and uncolored. Cloudy, discolored, or bloody fluid suggests that infection is present, and appropriate treatment is required without delay. Other symptoms of infection include fever and abdominal tenderness. Instillation of antibiotics into the peritoneal cavity accompanied by several peritoneal flushings may effectively treat infection. If the peritonitis persists, catheter removal may be necessary to eradicate the infection. Multiple episodes of peritonitis are believed to result in the development of scar tissue in the peritoneal membrane, which decreases the surface area available for clearance of waste products.

Hyperglycemic and hyperosmolar syndromes may occur during the procedure, especially when the dialysate contains high glucose levels. The blood absorbs solute at the same time that water flows out of the blood by osmosis, which causes an increased solute concentration in the blood. These changes can lead to hyperosmolar coma with hypovolemia that can lead to shock. Treatment involves monitoring serum glucose levels and administering insulin to reverse the high serum glucose levels. Occasionally, salt-poor albumin may be required to increase the amount of interstitial fluid movement into the plasma.

Protein loss is unavoidable during peritoneal dialysis; this necessitates an increased dietary intake of high-quality protein such as eggs, meat, fish, and poultry, which contain all the essential amino acids. Other complications include perforation of the bowel, bladder, or major blood vessel during catheter insertion; respiratory distress, especially at the onset of dialysis; and outflow obstruction by either a change in the client's position, peritonitis, or formation of a fibrin clot.

Nursing Implications

Nursing care of the client during peritoneal dialysis procedures includes monitoring blood pressure, pulse rate, temperature, and body weight. The specific method of peritoneal dialysis and the stability of the client determine the frequency of monitoring. Obtain all measurements prior to beginning the dialysis treatment and at its conclusion.

After the peritoneal catheter has been placed, the catheter site and the dressing should be kept clean and dry. The dressing should be occlusive. Temporary catheters are usually removed after the completion of the treatment and replaced if necessary. If more than one or two peritoneal dialysis treatments are anticipated, a permanent peritoneal catheter is generally placed. The Dacron Teflon cuffs on the permanent catheter stabilize the catheter in the subcutaneous tissue and form a partial barrier to the entrance of bacteria (Figure 25–6).

The IPD catheter is capped at the end of the dialysis treatment. After capping, gauze is placed under the catheter to protect the skin. A dressing placed over the catheter protects the catheter insertion site from the environment. No dressing is usually necessary over the CAPD catheter. After the site has healed, the client may shower or swim in chlorinated pools, although the client should avoid sitting in bath water.

Dietary protein allowances are liberalized for the client who selects peritoneal dialysis because of the protein loss that occurs in the dialysate. Maintaining a good appetite and consuming adequate protein may be difficult for some clients. Foods high in potassium should be avoided. However, for clients performing CAPD, potassium restriction may be unnecessary because the CAPD process is so efficient. Each client should be individually assessed according to blood work and dietary patterns.

Dialysate often affects the gastrointestinal system during dialysis, and clients can experience diarrhea while undergoing IPD. A bedside commode is needed because the client's catheter is hooked to the machine and limits movement.

Although peritoneal dialysis generally offers some increased independence (particularly CAPD), many clients experience significant changes in body image. The permanent peritoneal catheter and/or the presence of 1 to 3 L of dialysate in the peritoneal cavity both alter body contour. Although the tube and drainage bag can be concealed reasonably well, a slim waist and flat abdomen are not possible. Thus, the client may need to alter clothing selection. If possible, the client should discuss clothing style preferences with the surgeon prior to placement of the catheter, since the identification of the normal waistline or belt line can enhance comfort after surgery.

Psychosocial/Lifestyle Implications of Dialysis

Clients with chronic renal failure must adjust to the fact that they have a chronic and terminal illness. Life can be prolonged with dialysis or transplantation, but death may occur any time complications arise. For instance, if the peritoneal lining becomes infected, peritoneal dialysis is no longer possible. If all four limbs have exhausted vascular accesses, hemodialysis is not possible. Therefore, clotting or infection is a serious threat to these clients.

Client/Family Teaching

Adjusting to a chronic illness involves phases similar to the changes that occur with the death of loved ones. First, people are shocked to hear the news. Then they become angry and depressed or deny the existence of death. Acceptance finally occurs, it is hoped. Thus, certain psychologic reactions are normal and expected, and the nurse should help the client work through these feelings and offer support. The client's family also must adjust to the diagnosis of a chronic illness. They must go through the same changes as the client, as well as endure the lifestyle changes that result from such events as the client's loss of employment.

Some clients never accept their diagnosis or dependence on a machine and become suicidal. A client with a cannula can pull it apart and die from hemorrhage within minutes. Clients suspected of being suicidal should not be left unattended. Failure to follow dietary (potassium) and fluid restrictions may be an indirect way of committing suicide. Death may occur from hyperkalemia-induced cardiac arrest, or from fluid overload which results in pulmonary edema and subsequent suffocation.

During the process of adjustment, regression, anxiety, hostility, or depression are not uncommon responses. Regression occurs because of increasing dependency on others. Anxiety results from fears of death, dialysis, uremia, physical and socioeconomic changes, and altered family relationships. This reaction is intensified if impotence becomes a problem. Hostility, which is directed toward family and health care providers, is related to all the restrictions on the client. Depression occurs with the realization that major lifestyle changes must take place to allow for diet modifications and the hours needed for dialysis.

The client's family may experience similar reactions. Roles and relationships must withstand severe strains. New marriages or marriages in trouble are usually more affected than stable, long-term ones. A family that was close before dialysis probably will become more supportive and helpful. A family that was not close, however, may dissolve. The family can greatly affect the client's attitude toward dialysis.

Since acceptance of the dialysis treatment and compliance with the dietary and medical regimen are important to the client's well-being, the nurse must help the client and significant others adjust to all the stresses. If this cannot be accomplished, the inability to cope can lead to a deterioration in physical status that may result in death.

Chapter Highlights

Subjective symptoms that prompt the client with kidney or urinary system problems to seek health care are usually related to a change in the amount or general appearance of urine or alterations in comfort.

Because of anxiety related to renal and urinary function and proximity to external genitalia, clients may have difficulty communicating their concerns.

Creatinine clearance and serum creatinine values are the best indicators of renal function.

A urinalysis will provide many clues to the cause of the client's symptoms.

For the client with altered comfort related to pain, promoting comfort includes administering analgesics appropriate to the source and severity of pain, avoiding nephrotoxic analgesics, and providing other nursing comfort measures.

Nursing measures to relieve pruritus for the client with urinary dysfunction include keeping the client's fingernails short, avoiding agents that dry the skin, removing urochrome pigments on the surface of the skin, using oil-based lotions, controlling the phosphorus–calcium balance, administering antipruritic medications, and using ultraviolet light.

Nursing measures to maintain skin integrity include providing a nutritious diet that follows the limitations placed on the client, relieving pruritus, repositioning and turning the client with edema every 1 to 2 hours, and providing good skin care.

Restoration of fluid volume involves fluid restrictions, diuretics, and dialysis for fluid volume excesses or the administration of fluids with appropriate electrolytes for fluid deficits.

Helping the client maintain satisfactory mentation involves assisting with dialysis to remove nitrogenous wastes and control metabolic acidosis, giving clear and concise instructions, and promoting safety.

Nursing measures to overcome nutritional imbalances include encouraging the intake of a well-balanced diet that is low in sodium and potassium for renal failure clients, high in protein for clients who have proteinuria or are undergoing peritoneal dialysis, or low in protein for clients undergoing hemodialysis.

Promoting adequate oxygen–carbon dioxide exchange in the client with urinary dysfunction involves correcting metabolic acidosis with dialysis and the administration of sodium bicarbonate, removing excess fluid with dialysis, encouraging surgical clients to cough every hour, and administering oxygen as needed.

Nursing measures to improve the client's self-concept and sexuality involve listening to the client and encouraging ventilation of feelings related to ostomies, dialysis, transplantation, and role changes.

Dialysis to cleanse the blood of uremic toxins, excess water, and electrolytes works on the principles of diffusion, osmosis, and filtration.

With hemodialysis, a vascular access is necessary, the time involved is about 12 to 15 hours a week, and an artificial kidney contains the semipermeable membrane across which waste products flow.

With peritoneal dialysis, the peritoneal membrane serves as the semipermeable membrane, there are fewer risks, and up to 48 hours a week are involved in treatment.

Bibliography

Binkley LS: Keeping up with peritoneal dialysis. *Am J Nurs* 1984; 84:729–733.

Byrne CJ et al: *Laboratory Tests: Implications for Nursing Care.* 2nd ed. Menlo Park, CA: Addison–Wesley, 1986.

Cairoli OM, Voyce PK: *Memory Bank for Hemodialysis.* Pacific Palisades, CA: Nurseco, Inc, 1982.

Chambers JK: Bowel management in dialysis patients. *Am J Nurs* (July) 1983; 83:1051–1052.

Chambers JK: Staff nurse perceptions of the nursing diagnoses most commonly experienced by hospitalized dialysis patients. *ANNA J* 1986; 13(3)26–31.

Eichel CJ: Stress and coping in patients on CAPD compared to hemodialysis patients. *ANNA J* 1986; 13(1):9–13.

Fleming LM, Kane J: Step-by-step guide to safe peritoneal dialysis. *RN* (Feb) 1984: 44–47.

Holloway NM: *Nursing the Critically Ill Adult: Applying Nursing Diagnosis,* 3rd ed. Menlo Park, CA: Addison–Wesley, 1988.

Lancaster LE: *The Patient with Renal Disease.* 2nd ed. New York: Wiley, 1984.

McConnell EA, Zimmerman MF: *Care of Patients With Urologic Problems.* Philadelphia: Lippincott, 1983.

Pagana KD, Pagana TJ: *Diagnostic Testing and Nursing Implications: A Case Study Approach.* St. Louis: Mosby, 1982.

Perras ST, Mattern ML, Zappacosta AR: Presentation of treatment modalities for the ESRD patient: Peritoneal dialysis. *AANNT J* 1984; 11:43–46.

Saxton DF et al: *Addison–Wesley Manual of Nursing Practice.* Menlo Park, CA: Addison–Wesley, 1983.

Sims TN, Ulrich B: Successful utilization of subclavian catheters for hemodialysis and apheresis access. *AANNT J* 1983; 10:41–44.

Voith AM: A conceptual framework for nursing diagnoses: Alterations in urinary elimination. *Rehab Nurs* 1986; (Jan–Feb): 18–20.

Wheeler D, Coleman S: Manual peritoneal dialysis multiple bag set-up for CAPD patients. *Nephrol Nurse* 1983; (March–April): 17–21.

Resources

SELF-HELP GROUPS AND OTHER ORGANIZATIONS

American Council on Transplantation (ACT)
700 N. Fairfax St.
Suite 505
Alexandria, VA 22314
Phone: (703) 836–4301

The American Council on Transplantation (ACT) was formed in 1984 to address concerns related to organ and tissue donation and transplantation. ACT is a federation of member organizations such as the ANA, NATCO, AHA, and AMA, as well as individual lay and professional members. The purposes of ACT are to promote public and professional education about the need for increased availability of donated organs and tissues and advances in successful transplantation of organs and tissues. A major focus is to work for coordinated voluntary efforts to assure equitable access and distribution of donated organs and tissues. A quarterly newsletter is published and a hot line is available.

Help For Incontinent People
PO Box 544
Union, SC 29379
Phone: (803) 585–8789

This newly organized nonprofit organization is designed to promote national interest in the problem of incontinence. The organization publishes a quarterly newsletter, "The HIP Report," and other resources of interest to the public and health professionals.

National Association of Patients on Hemodialysis
and Transplantation (NAPHT)
505 Northern Blvd.
Great Neck, NY 11021

This organization, made up largely of clients, promotes the well-being of clients with kidney dysfunction and provides education for lay persons and professionals on kidney disease and treatment. There are several local chapters. They publish a newsletter and several pamphlets and brochures. Kidney client ID card available.

National Kidney Foundation
2 Park Ave.
New York, NY 10016
Phone: (212) 889–2210

This voluntary agency is concerned with the prevention and treatment of kidney diseases. It sponsors a national program of organ donors, research, education, and client services through local chapters. Publications on the organ donor program, kidney function, and kidney disease are available. Persons interested in donating their kidneys should contact a local affiliate for information.

United Network for Organ Sharing (UNOS)
PO Box 28010
2024 Monument Ave.
Richmond, VA 23228
Phone: (800) 446–2726

A computer network that lists the names of persons waiting for a kidney transplant as well as their blood and tissue types. Has recently consolidated with the North American Transplant Coordinators (NATCO) to handle all organ matchups in the US.

United Ostomy Association, Inc.
1111 Wilshire Blvd.
Los Angeles, CA 90017

Persons who have had urostomies, colostomies, or ileostomies belong to this national organization through its almost 500 local chapters in the United States and Canada. It provides local support groups and also serves as an educational resource and publishes pamphlets and brochures.

In Canada:

Calgary Ostomy Society
210 86th Ave., SE, Apt. 91
Calgary, Alberta, Canada T2H 1N6
Phone: (408) 228–4487

A Canadian chapter of the United Ostomy Association. For information on other Canadian affiliates write to the US national headquarters listed above.

HOT LINES

American Council on Transplantation
Phone: (800) ACT–GIVE

This national phone number is maintained to answer questions about organ and tissue donation and transplantation.

HEALTH EDUCATION INFORMATION

American Cancer Society
(local chapters or national headquarters)
"Urinary Ostomies: A Guidebook for Patients," second edition
"Living With Your Urostomy"
These are available at no charge to clients or health professionals.

Jeanette K. Chambers, RN, MS
Renal Clinical Nurse Specialist
Riverside Methodist Hospital, Dialysis Unit
3535 Olentangy River Road
Columbus, OH 43214

"Living with Kidney Failure," 44 pages, illustrated. $8.00 each. (Discounts for multiple copies.) Books mailed postpaid. Send check or money order payable to Riverside Methodist Hospital.

SPECIALTY ORGANIZATIONS

American Association of Nephrology Nurses and Technicians
Suite 219
505 N. Tustin
Santa Ana, CA 92705

American Board of Urologic Allied Health Professionals
Suite 256
2222 N.W. Lovejoy
Portland, OR 97210

American Nephrology Nurses Association (ANNA)
Box 56
Pitman, NJ 08071
Phone: (609) 589–2187

The goal of this organization is to provide education and support for nurses involved in the care of clients with kidney disease. Sponsors regional meetings and a national conference and publishes the ANNA journal, a bimonthly publication.

American Urological Association, Allied
6845 Lake Shore Drive
Raytown, MO 64133
Phone: (816) 358–3317

Membership in this organization is composed of RNs, LPNs, and any allied care workers who have completed an approved course of instruction and are actively engaged in urology. Dues, $50 new members; $45 renewals.

Council of Nephrology Nurses and Technicians
National Kidney Foundation

Membership in the council is open to nurses interested in nephrology nursing. An annual educational program and business meeting coincides with the meeting of the National Kidney Foundation.

International Association for Enterostomal Therapy, Inc.
2081 Business Center Dr.
Suite 290
Irvine, CA 92715
Phone: (714) 476–0268

This organization provides care and rehabilitation to persons with abdominal stomas, and to those with incontinence. Members are enterostomal therapists and interested others who are licensed to practice medicine or nursing. Dues, $65.

North American Transplant Coordinators Organization (NATCO)
℅ Mark Reiner
J-286 Department of Surgery
J.H. Miller Health Center
Gainesville, FL 32610
Phone: (904) 375–0084

The major purposes of NATCO are to provide a forum for discussion of issues common to transplant coordinators and to educate new transplant coordinators. The organization also maintains a donor registry. Membership is open to all transplant coordinators, many of whom are RNs. An annual meeting and periodic training courses are conducted.

CHAPTER 26

Specific Disorders of the Kidneys and Urinary System

Other topics relevant to this content are: Dialysis, **Chapter 25.**

Objectives

When you have finished studying this chapter, you should be able to:

Discuss the clinical manifestations and nursing interventions for polycystic kidney disease.

Identify medical and surgical treatment measures and nursing implications for acute tubular necrosis, urinary incontinence, and neurogenic bladder.

Discuss the nursing implications of caring for these clients in the preoperative and postoperative periods.

Describe clinical manifestations, medical treatment, and nursing measures for clients with analgesic abuse nephropathy, nephrosclerosis, and renal artery stenosis.

Discuss the clinical manifestations and treatments for membranous nephropathy, nephrotic syndrome, and acute and chronic glomerulonephritis.

Explain the complications of kidney and urinary system surgery and the related nursing interventions.

Describe the clinical manifestations and nursing implications for the client with infectious processes in the urinary tract (urethritis, cystitis, acute and chronic pyelonephritis, and renal abscess).

Explain the circumstances associated with renal cell and bladder cancer and surgical interventions for clients with these disorders.

Discuss alterations in body image encountered by clients requiring urinary diversion and their relationship to self-image, sexuality, and role relationships.

Discuss risk factors, symptoms and signs, and nursing care of clients with urinary calculi.

Identify the symptoms and signs of the three types of kidney transplant rejection.

Identify types of trauma of the urinary system and the nursing care involved for the client with trauma to the kidneys, bladder, and ureters.

Specific disorders of the kidneys and urinary system include life-threatening illnesses with long-term implications. Disorders of the urinary system may be generally classified as congenital, multifactorial in origin, degenerative, immunologic, infectious, neoplastic and obstructive, and traumatic. Many of these disorders result in acute renal failure or chronic renal failure (end-stage renal disease; ESRD). Surgical interventions for dysfunction of the kidneys and the urinary system may be used for palliative effects or to achieve a cure. In many disorders, surgery is reserved for cases in which more conservative medical treatment has not proven effective.

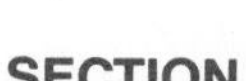

SECTION I

Congenital Disorders

Polycystic Kidney Disease

Polycystic kidney disease (PCKD or PKD) is an inherited disorder in which cysts form within the nephrons (Figure 26–1). These grapelike clusters of cysts are filled with fluid from tubular filtrate and thus are composed of water and electrolytes. The disease has two forms—one affecting adults and the other affecting children. The adult form

NURSING DIAGNOSES IN Kidney and Urinary Dysfunction

DIRECTLY RELATED DIAGNOSES

- Comfort, altered: pain
- Fluid volume deficit
- Fluid volume excess
- Gas exchange, impaired
- Incontinence, functional
- Incontinence, reflex
- Incontinence, stress
- Incontinence, total
- Incontinence, urge
- Infection, potential for
- Nutrition, altered: less than body requirements
- Self-concept, disturbance in: body image
- Sexuality, altered patterns
- Skin integrity, impaired: potential
- Thought processes, altered
- Tissue perfusion, altered: renal, cardiopulmonary
- Urinary elimination, altered patterns
- Urinary retention

OTHER POTENTIAL DIAGNOSES

- Home maintenance management, impaired
- Knowledge deficit
- Powerlessness
- Self-concept, disturbance in: self-esteem
- Social interaction, impaired

is a regular autosomal dominant hereditary disorder, whereas the childhood form is an autosomal recessive disorder. Both kidneys are involved in both disorders. Because the disorder may affect the renal medulla, salt wasting or sodium loss may be a problem that requires sodium replacement. Weakness of cerebral blood vessel walls with resultant intracranial bleeding is also associated with PCKD.

Clinical Manifestations

Symptoms in the adult form generally are not present until the client is at least 30 years of age, and more commonly 40 to 50. Initial symptoms often include flank pain and hematuria. Hypertension also is common, because polycystic kidneys lose their ability to regulate sodium balance. As the size of the kidneys increases over the years, the client may notice the abdomen enlarging and the polycystic kidneys become palpable. Palpation should be done *gently*, however, to prevent discomfort and possible bleeding. Accompanying urinary tract infections and hematuria are common. Uremia develops gradually.

Medical Measures

Treatment of the client with PCKD is supportive and determined by the problems that develop. Heat and analgesics may be useful in controlling the discomfort from the enlarged kidneys. If bleeding occurs, heat should not be used, however, and bed rest should be instituted in an attempt to control the hemorrhage. Because the cysts often rupture and bleed, blood transfusions may be needed to stabilize the hemodynamic status of the client if significant bleeding develops. Aminocaproic acid (Amicar) may control bleeding that does not stop spontaneously. In addition, the client with bleeding into the cysts should be observed carefully for the development of acute renal failure from obstruction by clots or sloughed tissue.

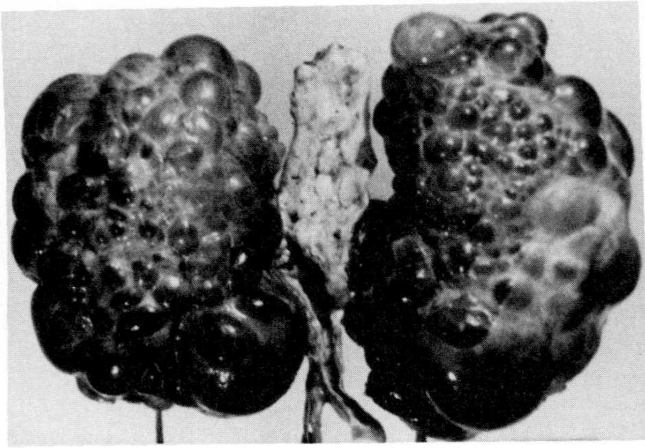

Figure 26–1

Polycystic kidneys. *Courtesy of Millard Fillmore Hospital, Buffalo, NY.*

If necessary, antibiotics will be prescribed to eradicate infection which develops in the cysts. Antihypertensives and diuretics will be prescribed as renal function deteriorates. A sodium supplement may be required if there is severe salt wasting from damage to the medulla. Because end-stage renal disease may develop, the client should avoid known nephrotoxic agents, which may compromise renal function prematurely.

A unilateral or bilateral nephrectomy may be required if conservative medical therapy cannot control bleeding or infection. Surgical intervention is delayed as long as possible, however, since erythropoietin production and water excretion still occur despite the formation of the cysts.

Specific Nursing Measures

If bleeding develops, the vital signs and blood count must be monitored closely. Observe and carefully measure urinary output, because acute renal failure may develop. Analgesics should be administered to control discomfort from the cysts. The monitoring of temperature and white blood cell counts also is important, because infection is a potential problem.

Client education to maximize understanding of the disease and self-care management is an important consideration. The client should understand the methods prescribed to help control hypertension. For example, sodium restriction may be recommended as part of the dietary modification if the client is retaining sodium. Careful assessment is important, because restricting sodium in a client who is losing sodium may result in the development of renal insufficiency from volume depletion and lack of renal perfusion. Furthermore, if the renal medulla is affected, clients will need to take in more sodium to correct for the salt wasting. As azotemia progresses, dietary restriction of protein and potassium may be prescribed to minimize or delay the onset of uremic symptoms.

With the progression of renal insufficiency, the client and significant others will need information about dialytic alternatives and transplantation. The age at which end-stage renal failure develops for the client with PCKD will vary, but it is usually after 50 years.

SECTION 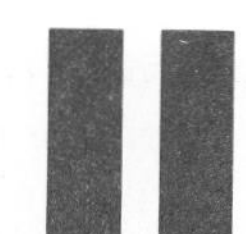

Disorders of Multifactorial Origin

A combination of alterations, because of exposure to toxins or altered vascular or neurologic function, may result in kidney or urinary tract dysfunction. Acute renal failure, chronic renal failure, acute tubular necrosis, urinary incontinence, and neurogenic bladder are disorders that are commonly of multifactorial origin. Renal failure is discussed separately at the end of this chapter.

Acute Tubular Necrosis

Acute tubular necrosis (ATN) represents about 75% of the cases of acute renal failure. In this condition, intrarenal problems result in an abrupt, sudden deterioration in renal function in which nitrogenous waste products accumulate in the blood. Acute renal failure and *acute tubular necrosis* are sometimes used interchangeably, but distinction may be made as follows: All ATN produces acute renal failure, but not all acute renal failure is from ATN.

The causes of ATN are generally grouped as postischemic, nephrotoxic, or pigment-related. Postischemic causes include all mechanisms that result in ATN. For example, hypotension due to hemorrhage or lack of cardiac pumping ability may alter renal blood blow and cause subsequent renal damage. Nephrotoxic causes of ATN include exposure to antibiotics, contrast media, organic solvents, or other drugs that result in inflammatory responses. These substances are listed in Box 25–1 in Chapter 25.

The heme pigments hemoglobin and myoglobin may also cause ATN. Hemoglobin injury to renal tubules is possible when there is hemolysis of red blood cells, as in a transfusion reaction. In rhabdomyolysis, the breakdown of skeletal muscle causes the release of myoglobin, a large molecule that cannot be removed adequately by the tubules. Rhabdomyolysis can develop in many situations, including in severe crushing injuries, with prolonged and extensive exercise, following seizure activity, with viral syndromes affecting the muscles, and when large muscles are deprived of adequate blood and oxygen for a time (Frank & Admire, 1982).

Clinical Manifestations

Clinical manifestations of ATN depend on several factors. One consideration is the cause of ATN. With contrast-induced and aminoglycoside ATN, the client is usually non-oliguric; he or she continues to excrete normal volumes of urine, but BUN and serum creatinine levels are elevated. Oliguric clients may have hypertension, peripheral edema, and pulmonary edema as a result of fluid retention. Hyperkalemia (with possible ECG manifestations), hyperphosphatemia, hypocalcemia, and metabolic acidosis are also common. With metabolic acidosis, hyperkalemia is intensified, and thus life-threatening arrhythmias are possible.

Characteristics of rhabdomyolysis include oliguria, rapid onset of azotemia, and hyperkalemia. Urine may be dark brown or black, although the color change is transient and may not be detected. Serum creatinine phosphokinase (CPK) levels are greatly elevated in clients who have rhabdomyolysis and may reach levels of 30,000 to 40,000 units. Serum aldolase also is elevated, and myoglobin is found in the urine.

Uremic manifestations also may be present in clients with ATN, particularly as azotemia and metabolic acidosis worsen. The BUN and serum creatinine levels increase daily. Uremic symptoms include nausea, vomiting, anorexia, muscle cramps, pruritus, and lethargy. Examination of the urine produced by a client with ATN reveals the presence of brown cellular casts and many cells of the tubular epithelium (Schrier, 1980). Clients with ATN pass through the same four phases as those with acute renal failure discussed later in this chapter: onset, oliguric, diuretic, and recovery phases.

Medical and Specific Nursing Measures

Both medical and specific nursing measures are similar to those for the client with acute renal failure.

Urinary Incontinence

The client with urinary incontinence is unable to control the flow of urine, and urine leaks spontaneously. Loss of urinary control may result from increased intra-abdominal pressure, relaxation of pelvic muscles, trauma to the external sphincter, cystitis, decompensation of the bladder, or impairment in cerebral blood flow.

Clinical Manifestations

In *true,* or *total, incontinence,* the client experiences a constant loss of urine via the urethra. In *stress incontinence,* the client loses urine in upright positions when

Nursing Research Note

Burns P et al.: Kegel's exercises with biofeedback therapy for treatment of stress incontinence. *Nurse Pract* 1985; 10(2):28–34.

Two case studies described the effectiveness of Kegel exercises when combined with biofeedback therapy in reducing symptoms of urinary stress incontinence. Kegel exercises were found to be effective in decreasing incontinence episodes. Biofeedback therapy was found to be beneficial in assisting clients to identify the pubococcygeal muscle as well as providing immediate feedback and reinforcement of muscle activity.

Kegel exercises have important implications for nurses working in the area of women's health. These exercises, which can be easily taught in the primary care setting and in the hospital, offer the client hope for relief of incontinence symptoms.

coughing, laughing, sneezing, or otherwise increasing the intra-abdominal pressure. *Urgency incontinence* is characterized by a strongly felt need to void followed by loss of urine; this can occur in any position. *Paradoxical incontinence,* also called overflow incontinence, is primarily manifested by constant dribbling.

Medical Measures

If cystitis is causing the symptoms of incontinence, appropriate antibiotics should be prescribed. Pharmacologic agents may be prescribed for the treatment of stress incontinence that is not corrected by perineal exercises before surgical intervention is attempted. Agents that increase contraction of urethral smooth muscle, such as phenylpropanolamine hydrochloride (Ornade), an alpha-adrenergic stimulant, also may be prescribed. If upper motor neuron disease has resulted in increased detrusor muscle irritability, parasympatholytic agents such as dicyclomine hydrochloride (Bentyl), propantheline bromide (Pro-Banthine), or methantheline bromide (Banthine) may decrease the irritability and promote continence (McConnell & Zimmerman, 1983).

Surgical interventions may repair a vesicovaginal fistula, suspend the bladder, remove bladder tumors, or insert an artificial sphincter device. In addition, urinary diversion may be necessary to preserve the function of the upper urinary tract.

Specific Nursing Measures

Nursing care of the client who has urinary incontinence requires patience, understanding, and concern for the preservation of the client's dignity. Because urinary incontinence is associated with infant and toddler behavior, it is disturbing to the adult's self-esteem, self-concept, and self-image. There may be concern about altered sexual functioning if surgical intervention is necessary. Nursing support with appropriate preparation for diagnostic procedures may be helpful to the adult client.

If perineal exercises (Kegel exercises) are prescribed, the nurse should explain the proper method (see Chapter 49). Obese clients with stress incontinence should be advised that weight loss may improve muscle compliance and promote continence. The client with incontinence should know that adequate fluid volume—2000 to 3000 mL/day—should be consumed, because inadequate fluid intake may further decrease the functional capacity of the bladder. Wearing incontinence pads or specially designed undergarments helps preserve the client's dignity.

Neurogenic Bladder

A neurogenic bladder occurs in clients whose normal neural innervation of bladder contraction is interrupted. The result may be sensory disruption, motor disruption, or both. A neurogenic bladder may have a variety of causes. Diabetes mellitus may result in autonomic neuropathy resulting in a sensory deficit. Neurologic disease such as multiple sclerosis or amyotrophic lateral sclerosis also may result in a neurogenic bladder. Another cause is spinal cord injuries or tumors that interrupt normal nerve transmission. One method of describing the neurogenic bladder is to consider the origin of the problem as either low motor neuron (sacral) or upper motor neuron (suprasacral).

Clinical Manifestations

The client with a lower motor neuron neurogenic bladder will have lost the perception of bladder fullness and not experience a desire to urinate. As a result, overflow incontinence occurs because of greatly extended bladder capacity. The distended bladder may be palpated and percussed. The client with an upper motor neuron neurogenic bladder will also experience spontaneous voiding when the bladder is stimulated. However, the bladder is hyperirritable, and voiding is not complete.

The client with a neurogenic bladder is more susceptible to the development of a UTI because of ineffective bladder emptying and also because catheterization carries increased risk. Repeated infections put the client at risk of developing chronic renal failure. In addition, the risk of urinary tract obstruction from struvite kidney stones increases in the client with a neurogenic bladder.

Medical Measures

Parasympathomimetic agents may be prescribed for the client with a lower motor neuron neurogenic bladder to improve the contraction of the detrusor muscle. Examples include bethanechol chloride (Urecholine) and neostigmine (Prostigmin). For clients with an upper motor neuron neurogenic bladder, other pharmacologic agents may be prescribed. Bladder spasms or contractions may be

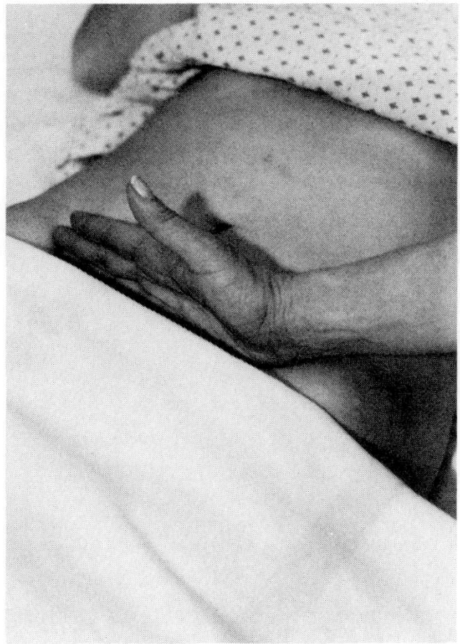

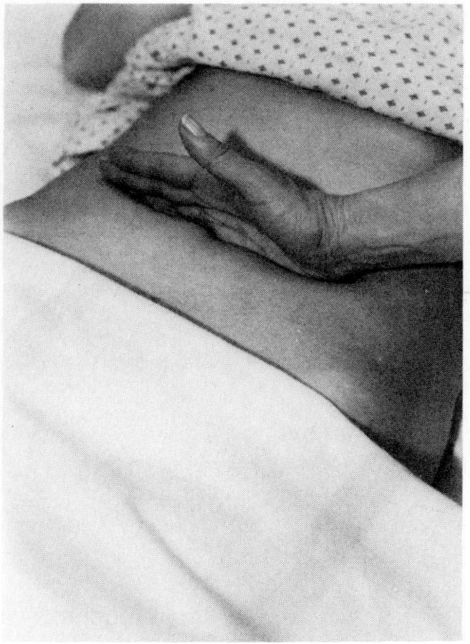

Figure 26–2

Credé's maneuver. **A.** Manual pressure applied to the bladder can be employed to facilitate the removal of urine for clients whose bladders are irreversibly flacid (eg, clients with neurogenic bladders). Usually the procedure is performed every 4 to 6 hours to prevent the bladder from becoming overly distended. **B.** When the client is in a comfortable position, place the ulnar surface of your hand at the umbilicus. Instruct the client to bear down with the abdominal muscles, if possible. Press downward and sweep your hand onto the suprapubic area, using a kneading motion to initiate urination. Continue the maneuver every 30 seconds until urination ceases. SOURCE: *Swearingen PL:* Addison–Wesley Photo-Atlas of Nursing Procedures. *Menlo Park, CA: Addison–Wesley, 1984, p. 474.*

inhibited with medications such as the parasympatholytics, which include propantheline bromide (Pro-Banthine) and methantheline bromide (Banthine). Sympathomimetic agents such as ephedrine sulfate, phenylpropanolamine hydrochloride (Ornade), or imipramine hydrochloride (Tofranil) also may be useful in contracting the bladder neck and improving continence (McConnell & Zimmerman, 1983). Muscle relaxants such as diazepam (Valium) may reduce skeletal muscle spasms.

In addition to pharmacologic agents, voiding or catheterization programs may be prescribed. For the client with lower motor neuron neurogenic bladder, bladder massage (Credé's maneuver) or intermittent catheterization may be used. Clients with upper motor neuron neurogenic bladders may be able to stimulate bladder contraction by reflex contraction of the spastic bladder, which may be precipitated by stroking the abdomen, genitalia, or thighs. Digital rectal stimulation also may result in reflex voiding. These methods are used in conjunction with intermittent catheterization.

Transurethral bladder neck resection with or without external sphincterotomy or continent vesicostomy may be performed for the client with lower motor neuron neurogenic bladder. Depending on the type of procedure required, it may not be possible to preserve continence. Surgery may convert the spastic bladder into a flaccid bladder. This procedure, bilateral anterior/posterior sacral rhizotomy, commonly results in impotence.

Specific Nursing Measures

Emotional support and educational interventions are extremely important nursing measures for the client with a neurogenic bladder. Concern for preservation of the client's dignity and privacy should accompany all diagnostic and therapeutic interventions.

Client/Family Teaching

Teach the client to perform Credé's maneuver on the bladder to promote emptying (Figure 26–2). The client should sit on the toilet while performing Credé's maneuver.

Many clients will also need to learn intermittent self-catheterization. A clean technique of intermittent self-catheterization is adequate and will not result in an increased incidence of urinary tract infection. The male client will be able to see his own urethra readily. Hold a mirror to assist the female client. A method may need to be created to allow the client to do this by herself at home. Reusable catheters generally are soaked in a solution of povidone–iodine (Betadine) and water when not being used. The client washes his or her hands before beginning the technique and then cleans the urinary meatus and surrounding area with a solution such as Betadine prior to the catheter insertion. At the beginning, the schedule for intermittent catheterization is every 2 hours. The time between catheterizations may increase gradually, usually by ½ to 1 hour increments. The final schedule usually requires catheterization every 4 hours. Maximizing fluid intake before 6 PM will minimize problems with nocturnal incontinence or the need for awakening at night for self-catheterization.

Continent Vesicostomy

A continent vesicostomy involves the formation of an internal pouch using existing bladder tissue and a stoma also formed from bladder tissue. Intermittent self-catheterization through a nipple valve that exits the skin provides for urinary drainage. The continent vesicostomy is indicated for the client with a neurogenic bladder. Physiologic and psychosocial/lifestyle implications are discussed in Table 26–1.

Nursing Implications

PREOPERATIVE CARE Any infections of the urinary tract should be eradicated preoperatively. Encourage and facilitate the client's clarification of postoperative expectations, including feelings and concerns related to changes in self-concept, body image, and sexuality. Antibiotics may be given preoperatively to sterilize the urinary tract.

POSTOPERATIVE CARE Postoperative considerations include careful monitoring of renal function and the prevention of infection. Closed urinary drainage systems for the suprapubic and stomal catheters should be ensured to prevent the introduction of infectious microorganisms. Intravenous fluid and electrolyte replacement will be required until normal intestinal motility returns. Careful measurement of fluid intake and output is important. Meticulous skin care should be done daily or as needed to keep the skin dry and free from irritation.

Catheter irrigation will be required by the client at home for about a month after surgery, until each catheter is removed. Intermittent self-catheterization may be done with clean technique at home. The client should be instructed to drink a normal amount of fluids and carry or wear identification indicating the presence of the vesicostomy. Clients may avoid embarrassing leakage of urine during sexual intercourse if they empty the bladder in advance.

Table 26–1
Continent Vesicostomy: Implications for the Client

Physiologic Implications	Psychosocial/Lifestyle Implications
Careful monitoring of renal function	Improved quality of life with urinary continence
High fluid intake to decrease chances of infection	Altered body image
	Altered sexual identity, self-esteem, and self-concept
	Need to learn self-catheterization of nipple and stoma care

SECTION 

Degenerative Disorders

Degenerative changes may occur in the glomeruli, the tubules, or in the blood vessels that supply the kidney. Glomerular disorders will be discussed in the next section, because much of the recent research links glomerular pathology to immunologic processes.

Degenerative processes occur over a long time—often 20 to 30 years or longer—and the client is usually unaware that these changes are taking place. Over a period of years, degeneration of renal function generally results in end-stage renal failure.

Analgesic Abuse Nephropathy

Analgesic abuse nephropathy, a tubular interstitial disorder, is caused by the chronic ingestion of phenacetin-containing compounds or agents that combine aspirin or acetaminophen with phenacetin. Phenacetin-containing compounds have been removed from the US market in both prescription and nonprescription medications. However, because the effects may not be seen for a number of years, nurses still see clients with this condition. There are many cases of analgesic abuse nephropathy in the southern states where many people took "headache powders" (containing phenacetin) regularly. Although the long-term effects of aspirin continue to be controversial, many physicians and scientists do not believe aspirin alone results in nephropathy. Aspirin–acetaminophen combinations, however, have been demonstrated to cause renal tubular damage similar to that caused by phenacetin-containing compounds.

Clinical Manifestations

A client with a history of a chronic pain disorder is the most likely to develop analgesic abuse nephropathy. Headaches, back pain, and chronic problems with arthritis are common in these clients' histories.

Necrosis of the papillae may result in the sloughing of papillary tissue into the ureters. There may be flank pain and hematuria. Other manifestations may include symptoms of uremia—anorexia, nausea, vomiting, muscle cramps, and pruritus—if there is a significant decrease in the creatinine clearance.

Medical Measures

Agents to control hypertension and infections are often administered, but the client must stop taking analgesic agents that cause deterioration of renal function to prevent further deterioration. Alternative therapies for the control of pain must be identified, or the client must be assisted to learn new methods for coping with the discomfort or the stress. Dialysis or transplantation will be necessary when end-stage renal failure with uremia develops.

Specific Nursing Measures

Nursing management for the client with analgesic abuse nephropathy should focus largely on educational efforts to help the client alter practices harmful to his or her long-term health status. The client must thoroughly understand the implications of continued abuse of analgesics that are harming residual renal function. Alternative methods for coping with and controlling pain, such as relaxation or biofeedback, must be explored. If end-stage renal disease has developed, the client and family or significant others will need emotions and educational support about the dialytic alternatives and possibilities for renal transplantation.

Nephrosclerosis

Nephrosclerosis results from untreated or uncontrolled systemic hypertension acting on the vascular supply of the kidney. It may be classified as benign or malignant according to the severity of the rise in diastolic blood pressure. With *benign nephrosclerosis,* the diastolic reading is less than 115 mm Hg, whereas *malignant nephrosclerosis* is found with diastolic readings greater than 130 mm Hg. The renal tissue deterioration is caused by a combination of the thickening of the walls of the blood vessels and the resulting ischemia to the interstitium. The tubules are particularly sensitive to the decreased blood supply. Fibrosis also occurs.

Clinical Manifestations

Benign nephrosclerosis is associated with aging and usually affects clients over 60. It is less often fatal than the malignant form because it progresses more slowly. In this condition, the urine has a low specific gravity that is fixed, as well as a small amount of protein. Renal insufficiency and end-stage renal disease arise late in the disease process as more glomeruli are damaged. The client with well-controlled hypertension is much less likely to develop end-stage renal disease from nephrosclerosis.

The client with malignant nephrosclerosis is usually from 30 to 50 years of age. This form progresses rapidly. The client will first identify problems related more to the severely elevated blood pressure than the kidneys. They include visual disturbances, severe headaches, or altered neurologic functioning. The urine will contain blood and protein. As renal function falls, BUN and serum creatinine values will rise. Death may occur in a few months and, if the blood pressure cannot be lowered, usually results from a stroke or heart attack rather than renal failure.

Medical Measures

Pharmacologic agents are used to treat nephrosclerosis and hypertension. If the diastolic pressure is severely elevated, potent antihypertensive agents are given to lower the blood pressure rapidly. This is usually done in an intensive care unit to allow close monitoring. First, fast-acting powerful vasodilators such as sodium nitroprusside (Nipride) and diazoxide (Hyperstat) are administered. Then agents for long-term management are administered to control the hypertension and prevent cardiovascular, cerebral, and renal complications. Unfortunately, the control of blood pressure may result in a decreased blood supply to the kidney and, subsequently, decreased renal function. However, uncontrolled hypertension places a tremendous burden on cardiac function and stresses cerebral blood vessels. Dialysis or transplantation will be necessary for the client with end-stage renal failure.

For clients with severe malignant hypertension and malignant nephrosclerosis, bilateral nephrectomy may be necessary to control the hypertension. This surgical intervention is used rarely, only when all known methods for blood pressure control have been tried without success. Dialysis or transplantation would then be necessary to prevent death from uremia.

Specific Nursing Measures

Administering the agents necessary to control hypertension in the acute phase and monitoring the client to prevent or detect complications are major nursing objectives. Thromboembolic phenomena may cause deterioration of cardiac or cerebral functioning as a result of severe hypertension, so frequent measurement of blood pressure through conventional cuff measurements or by arterial line monitoring in the intensive care unit (if indicated) will be necessary.

With uremia, the client will require monitoring and preparation for eventual dialysis. Health teaching for self-care should address the appropriate methods of taking the antihypertensive agents prescribed, as well as other drugs such as diuretics, and include blood pressure assessment. If dialysis is necessary, provide educational and emotional support of the client and family or significant others.

Renal Artery Stenosis

In renal artery stenosis, the narrowing of the lumen of the renal artery results in diminished blood flow to the kidney, the release of renin, and the stimulation of the renin–angiotensin system. It may occur unilaterally or bilaterally. Severe high blood pressure, as well as ischemia to the renal interstitium and tubules, results. The cause of renal artery stenosis is diffuse atherosclerosis that includes the renal vasculature.

Clinical Manifestations

The onset of mild, moderate, or severe hypertension before the age of 30 or after the age of 50 is characteristic of renal artery stenosis. An abdominal bruit over one or both renal arteries may also be heard, but this does not occur consistently.

Medical Measures

If hypertension is severe as a result of renal artery stenosis, a hypertensive crisis may result. Pharmacologic measures and bed rest are essential to prevent a cerebral vascular accident. Since these clients characteristically have an increased production of renin, an agent such as captopril (Capoten) that blocks the normal renin–angiotensin–aldosterone system is ideal. Without angiotensin formation and release, there usually is a profound decrease in blood pressure. An acceptable pharmacologic regimen for lifetime control of the high blood pressure is essential for the long-term health of the client.

Percutaneous transluminal renal angioplasty (see Chapter 21) is an option that may be increasingly available to clients with renal artery stenosis. A balloon-tipped catheter is used to dilate the renal artery at the point of narrowing to increase renal blood flow, improve renal function, and decrease blood pressure.

Renal artery bypass surgery may be performed to restore blood flow to the renal parenchyma. A severely atrophic kidney (less than 9 to 10 cm) is not generally considered for revascularization. However, this atrophic kidney may be a major source of renin production, so nephrectomy may be indicated.

Specific Nursing Measures

Regardless of the treatment method selected, nursing interventions will be directed toward physical and emotional support of the client. Since a variety of risks and benefits are associated with any method, the client will be anxious during decision making. The nurse must understand the rationale for the various alternatives that will be explained to the client, because supportive discussion that clarifies and validates the client's understanding is important.

Renal Revascularization

Revascularization procedures are commonly used to restore renal function, or at least to prevent further deterioration, or to regain control of high blood pressure. In situ revascularization procedures include endarterectomy, resection and end-to-end anastomosis, and renal artery bypass graft. The endarterectomy and resection with anastomosis are less common and have less chance of long-term patency than the renal artery bypass graft. The graft is sutured into the aorta and then into the renal artery distal to the site of stenosis. The graft material may be a portion of saphenous vein or made of a synthetic material.

Renal bench surgery (ex vivo surgery) and autotransplantation are indicated when there are complicated disorders of the renal artery and one or more of its branches that would require a lengthy period of surgery and anesthesia. Renal bench surgery involves removing the kidney, placing it on the table, repairing the renal vasculature, and reimplanting the kidney into the right iliac fossa after adequate blood flow is ensured. The physiologic and psychosocial/lifestyle implications are discussed in Table 26–2.

Nursing Implications

PREOPERATIVE CARE The avoidance of contrast media or nephrotoxic antibiotics is essential whenever possible before surgery to avoid further compromising renal function. Intravenous fluids may be required to correct fluid volume deficit, and electrolyte imbalances also should be corrected. The management of hypertensive crises is described in Chapter 19. General preoperative preparation should be instituted.

POSTOPERATIVE CARE Monitor the client's postoperative urine output and vital signs at least hourly. Daily weights provide information regarding overall hydration. Hemodynamic monitoring with a flow-directed, balloon-tipped catheter such as a Swan–Ganz catheter may be needed temporarily to determine the intravascular volume. An arterial line may also be placed intraoperatively and continued postoperatively to facilitate the control of blood pressure. The physician should clearly delineate the desired blood pressure parameters for the nurse, who should report deviations immediately to the physician. The physician also should clearly specify fluid replacement and urine flow parameters, and exceptions to these should also be reported promptly. The client's hydration balance and adequate renal perfusion should result in an acceptable flow of urine (at least 30 to 50 mL/h).

Institute turning, coughing, and deep breathing immediately after surgery. Ambulation, or at least sitting at the bedside and standing, should occur within the first 24 to 48 hours. In the interim, institute leg exercises, elastic support stockings, and positioning that avoids circulatory stasis.

Meticulous aseptic treatment of all invasive lines and catheters is essential to prevent the development of local infections that could become systematic and place the kidneys under greater stress. Good nutrition also is important to the healing process, so encourage the client to eat well.

Daily monitoring of serum creatinine levels and electrolytes should continue during the postoperative period. Other blood tests that should be performed regularly are hemoglobin, hematocrit, and white blood cell (WBC) counts. Leukocytosis and temperature elevation should be promptly assessed.

During this time, the client needs to be encouraged about progress being made, because the healing process is seemingly slow. The client should receive instructions related to lifestyle implications.

Table 26–2
Renal Revascularization: Implications for the Client 

Physiologic Implications	Psychosocial/Lifestyle Implications
Possible improvement in the quality of life by restoring blood supply and renal function, preventing further deterioration in renal function, or helping control hypertension Potential complications are: hemorrhage, acute renal failure, thromboembolic phenomena, infection Severe postoperative hypotension causing graft closure Severe postoperative hypertension causing bleeding at the sites of anastomoses Temporary dialysis may be required	Limit activity 4 to 8 weeks Possible need for assistance at home Possible lifestyle alterations for temporary dialysis (see also Chapter 25) Anxiety and uncertainty over whether sufficient renal function will be regained

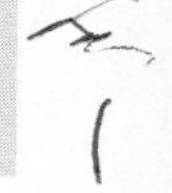

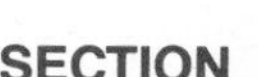
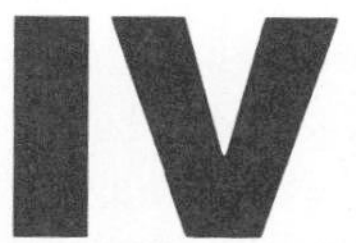

SECTION IV

Immunologic Disorders

Advances in electron microscopy and techniques of analyzing tissue obtained from renal biopsy have enabled increasingly accurate diagnosis of the pathologic processes resulting in glomerulonephritis (the term referring to all glomerular disorders). For this reason, the term *glomerulonephritis* has only limited application to specific diseases; most glomerular disorders are identified by the immunologic processes that cause them.

Current classification describes glomerulonephritis, or all glomerular disorders, as glomerulopathies or glomerulonephridities (interchangeable terms). The effects on the client are variable, depending on the etiology and whether there is response to treatment. There may be spontaneous reversal, progression to total deterioration requiring dialysis or transplantation to sustain life, or stabilization of the current situation.

Nephrotic Syndrome

Nephrotic syndrome, or nephrosis, occurs in any condition that seriously damages the glomerular capillary membrane, thus allowing increased permeability of the membrane to plasma proteins. A variety of glomerular diseases, such as chronic glomerulonephritis, lupus nephritis, poststreptococcal nephritis, Kimmelstiel–Wilson syndrome, toxic nephropathy, and membranous nephropathy, can result in the nephrotic syndrome. The primary cause of nephrotic syndrome, however, is membranous nephropathy.

Membranous nephropathy may develop from malignancies or endogenous antigens such as DNA; DNA antigens and antibodies to DNA occur in systemic lupus erythematosus and may result in lupus nephritis. Exogenous antigens that may result in membranous nephropathy include hepatitis B virus, gold, and penicillamine.

Clinical Manifestations

Nephrotic syndrome is characterized by renal losses of protein that exceed 3.5 g/24 hours, hypoalbuminemia, edema, hyperlipidemia, and a hypercoagulable state. The client will notice the development of edema, primarily in dependent areas. The client may notice periorbital or facial edema upon awakening, and edema in the legs and feet will be apparent as the day progresses. Urinalysis will reveal the presence of protein. Although the mechanisms are unclear, increased incidences of arterial and venous thrombosis have been noted in clients with nephrotic syndrome.

Medical Measures

If renal biopsy has identified an immunologic basis, corticosteroids, cytotoxic agents, or both are prescribed. These substances decrease the large amounts of protein lost by decreasing the immunologic response. Corticosteroids may be given as bolus therapy (eg, 1 g intravenously every day for 3 to 5 days). Then, during the active stages of immunologic activity, the client may receive 1.0 to 1.5 mg/kg/day of prednisone. With stabilization, the dosage of prednisone is converted to alternate-day therapy in an attempt to decrease the incidence and severity of side effects. Cytotoxic agents such as azathioprine (Imuran) and cyclophosphamide (Cytoxan) may also be prescribed for some forms of immunologic processes that have led to the nephrotic syndrome.

If renal deterioration is not responsive to pharmacologic management, plasmapheresis may be attempted. For some immunologically based disorders, this effectively removes the circulating immune complexes or the antigens and antibodies. If renal deterioration continues, however, dialysis or transplantation is necessary.

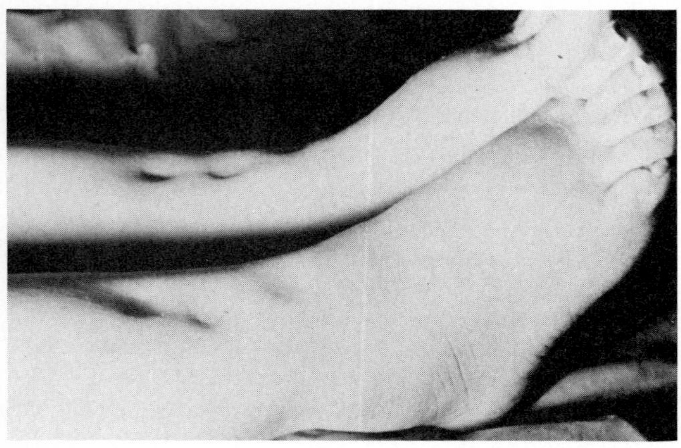

Figure 26–3

Severe pitting edema in a client with nephrotic syndrome. *Courtesy of Millard Fillmore Hospital, Buffalo, NY.*

Specific Nursing Measures

Many clients with nephrotic syndrome require considerable nursing care. Profound edema is common in these clients (Figure 26–3) so meticulous skin care is essential. Difficulties with skin breakdown and immobility are also common; thus, devices to prevent skin breakdown, such as mattresses that provide pressure relief, should be used. Routinely inspect dependent parts for evidence of erythema and the need for pressure relief. Immobility from edema, as well as the hypercoagulable state associated with nephrotic syndrome, make the client susceptible to the development of thromboembolic phenomena.

Instruct the client to do hourly leg and toe exercises to increase circulation, as well as institute range-of-motion (ROM) activities unless contraindicated by the known presence of thrombotic processes. Hourly position changes for the client confined to bed, chair activity, and ambulation (if allowed) should be encouraged, and the client should be supported in attaining alterations in activity. The eyes of clients with periorbital edema may swell shut and need to be irrigated with sterile normal saline.

Nutritional management may include a diet high in protein foods because renal losses of protein are extensive (see Table 25–2 in Chapter 25). When massive edema is present, fluid restriction may be prescribed. Since edema occurs in the lining of the gastrointestinal tract as well as the periphery, clients frequently experience anorexia and feelings of abdominal fullness. Smaller and more frequent servings may be more appealing. Monitoring daily weights and measuring fluid intake and urinary output will help determine the effectiveness of diuretics prescribed.

Many opportunities will arise in which the nurse can help the client understand the rationale for medications and other interventions. This is important, because many clients will continue with these pharmacologic and dietary interventions for some time. Clarify the purpose and methods of self-care procedures to facilitate the client's assuming responsibility for this facet of care.

Acute Glomerulonephritis

Acute glomerulonephritis (postinfectious glomerulonephritis or acute nephritic syndrome) generally has a sudden onset and causes changes in the urine such as proteinuria and hematuria. It is commonly associated with a recent infectious process, and the etiology is exposure to an exogenous antigen to which antibodies are formed and subsequently deposited in the glomerulus. For example, the group A beta-hemolytic streptococcus organism has certain strains that are associated with the ability to evoke a glomerulonephritis. Not all group A beta-hemolytic streptococcal infections will cause glomerulonephritis, however.

Clinical Manifestations

The client usually reports having had a recent upper respiratory tract infection, often with a sore throat. The urine may be the color of cola. There may be evidence of decreased urinary output, peripheral and periorbital edema, and hypertension. The urine contains protein and red blood cell casts.

Medical Measures

Hypertension related to decreased glomerular filtration and the hypervolemic state may need to be controlled. The administration of diuretics and antihypertensive agents is often required during the acute phase of illness as well as for a while into the recovery phase or if permanent renal insufficiency results.

Short-term hemodialysis or peritoneal dialysis may also be necessary if acute renal failure develops. There is evidence that this syndrome is progressive in a number of adult clients. Continued follow-up for the treatment of hypertension and careful management to prevent further renal insufficiency from developing are indicated.

Specific Nursing Measures

During the period of acute illness, the client should be kept in bed if there are several symptoms of volume overload, heart failure, or severe hypertension. Otherwise, encourage modest activity that includes ambulation. Supportive measures to increase comfort and allow the time needed for healing are important. The nursing care plan should include careful monitoring of fluid status during the period of oliguria, daily weighing, and measurement of intake and output.

Fluid restrictions will be prescribed to correlate with the amount of urine produced, plus about 600 mL to account for insensible losses. If blood chemistry measurements indicate an elevated BUN level, dietary protein may be restricted. Sodium intake may be limited if hypertension is present. In any case, a nutritious diet is important during the acute phase of this syndrome. The client and family or significant others must understand the need for consistent follow-up after the acute illness is past; it is estimated that progressive renal deterioration occurs in 50% or fewer of clients, often depending on other factors involved in their overall health status.

Chronic Glomerulonephritis

In chronic glomerulonephritis, glomerular disorders have resulted in chronic renal failure or end-stage renal disease. Renal deterioration has usually been a long, slow process, and the client generally is unaware of this loss of function. The cause of chronic glomerulonephritis is usually not known although it is thought to be the result of repeated antigen–antibody reaction or autoimmune response. Because the kidneys are atrophic, little is gained from biopsy; the amount of kidney tissue that could be obtained would only demonstrate scarring. The client is past the time when the disease might have been reversed; loss of renal function is permanent.

Clinical Manifestations

Protein, red blood cells, leukocytes, and waxy casts are often present in the urine of clients with chronic glomerulonephritis. Urine specific gravity fixates at about 1.010 because the nephrons lose their urine-concentrating ability. Hypertension and the nephrotic syndrome also may be present. Significant renal deterioration commonly occurs before the client is aware of it. Eye changes, sudden nose bleeds, elevated blood pressure, or uremic manifestations of chronic renal failure (anorexia, nausea, vomiting, muscle cramps, pruritus, fatigue, and lethargy) may be initial symptoms.

Once the condition is diagnosed, the client may have good health for 10 to 30 years or may develop end-stage renal disease in 1 to 2 years. The client's state of health is determined by the extent of glomerular necrosis, the extent of renal vasculature sclerosis, and the extent of the autoimmune activity. As the disease progresses, the client will develop severe headaches, shortness of breath, angina, edema, dry skin, nocturia, and polyuria. Eye changes from retinal artery thickening include seeing black spots or flashes of light, as well as dimness of vision.

Medical and Specific Nursing Measures

Specific medications prescribed for the client with chronic glomerulonephritis include diuretics and antihypertensives. These agents control the fluid retention and elevated blood pressure that result from renal deterioration. When renal function deteriorates to a level at which diuretics are no longer effective, dialysis or transplantation are necessary to prevent death from uremia. Dietary modifications, fluid restriction, prevention of skin breakdown, control of electrolyte and acid–base balances, and removal of waste products are also required.

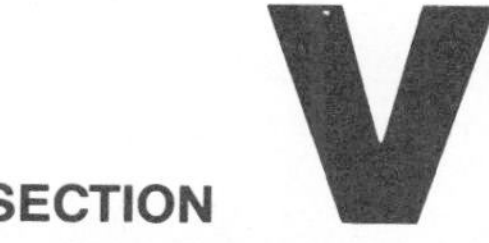

SECTION V

Infectious Disorders

Infections within the urinary tract are a common clinical problem. They may be localized to a specific anatomical structure or become a systematic process through infection of the blood.

The routes of infection in the urinary tract include the blood (hematogenous route), the lymphatic system (lymphatogenous route), or ascending or descending routes (eg, traveling up the urinary tract from urethra to bladder, or traveling down the urinary tract from kidney to bladder).

In-dwelling or suprapubic catheters placed for the control or facilitation of urinary drainage are often associated with the development of infections. Urinary tract infections are the most significant of hospital-acquired infections: 41% of the nosocomial infections are within the urinary tract (the highest of any category), and invasion of the urinary tract by either a catheter or other instrument precedes 75% to 100% of the hospital-acquired infections. Urinary tract infections produce significant discomfort. When there is a continuous site of infection, end-stage renal failure may develop from the infection and associated scarring.

Urethritis

Urethritis, or inflammation of the urethra, may result from bacterial infection, traumatic irritation, or hypersensitivity to detergents or bubble bath. Bacterial causes of urethritis include *Chlamydia trachomatis* and *Neisseria gonorrhoeae*. The herpes simplex virus type 2 also may cause urethritis.

Clinical Manifestations

The client usually complains of discomfort with urination. Female clients also may experience generalized discomfort in the labial tissues. The urethra may be red, but there is generally no drainage. Examination of urine will show pus in the first morning specimen and the absence of pus or white blood cells in the specimen collected immediately following.

Medical Measures

Bacterial urethritis is treated with antibiotics appropriate to the eradication of the pathogens. Urethritis may result in the inability to expel urine from the bladder. In such cases, the flow of urine must be reestablished to prevent deterioration of renal parenchyma. If strictures develop, gradual dilatation with progressively larger instruments or direct internal repair of the stricture will be required.

Postmenopausal women may experience symptoms similar to bacterial urethritis; these respond to the topical application of estrogen preparations.

Specific Nursing Measures

Instruct clients about taking the prescribed antibiotics, the proper application of topical ointments or creams, the need for women to wipe from front to back after urination or defecation and the need to void before and after intercourse, and the need for the uncircumcised man to clean beneath the foreskin routinely. Urethritis may occur from sexual activities resulting in transmission of bacteria between partners. Reinfection frequently results when one partner is not adequately treated, so treatment of both is necessary.

Cystitis

Cystitis, or inflammation of the urinary bladder, usually is the result of bacterial contamination. It also can be caused by a fungal infection or fibrosis of the bladder wall. Bladder calculi, urinary diverticuli, or an in-dwelling urethral or suprapublic catheter will increase the likelihood of cystitis developing. Because of the relatively short female urethra and its proximity to the rectum and vagina, women are much more susceptible than men to cystitis. Recent literature suggests that sexual intercourse, as a single variable, does not cause urinary tract infection. In healthy subjects, bacteriuria increases following sexual intercourse; however, this increase is transient and does not produce the symptoms commonly referred to as "honeymoon cystitis" (from frequent intercourse).

Clinical Manifestations

The client with cystitis generally experiences a burning discomfort upon urination. There may also be a frequency, urgency, nocturia, bladder spasms, or incontinence. The urine may be cloudy or cola colored from the presence of red blood cells, white blood cells, or both. Other symptoms may include fever, general feelings of fatigue, and pelvic and abdominal discomfort. When cystitis is associated with urinary tract obstruction at the bladder neck, the client may have symptoms of urinary obstruction and/or acute renal failure resulting in uremia.

Medical Measures

If cystitis has resulted in obstruction or acute renal failure, the obstruction must be removed immediately and the infection treated and eradicated. Failure to remove the obstruction and treat the infection may result in permanent renal damage. Antibiotics effective in eradicating the bacteria causing the cystitis will be prescribed. Any infected foreign bodies such as calculi must be removed to eradicate the source of the infection.

Specific Nursing Measures

Nursing interventions for the care of clients with cystitis are supportive and educational. Methods to promote comfort may include sitz baths for local comfort and the administration of mild analgesics as prescribed; phenazophridine hydrochloride (Pyridium) is often given for the first 2 to 3 days to lessen the pain and bladder spasms. Warn the client that this drug colors the urine red or orange and may stain fabrics. Warm compresses or sitz baths as well as opium and belladonna suppositories may assist the client in achieving adequate relaxation for natural micturition. Oil of peppermint held near the urethra also has been useful. Avoid urethral catheterization whenever possible, since additional contamination may result from the procedure. The administration of antibiotics is essential to the supportive management. The continued monitoring of renal function involves measurement and recording of fluid intake and output. Clients with cystitis should have a liberal fluid intake of at least 3 L/day. Encourage the client to void frequently, even if it is uncomfortable, to help wash out contaminating microorganisms.

Include several specific points in the client's education. An important point is that moisture around the urethral meatus provides a medium that enhances bacterial growth and puts the client at risk for an ascending urinary tract infection. Cotton briefs are more absorbent than nylon and do not trap moisture. The client should avoid nylon panty hose or other tight clothing, if possible. If the client's urine is routinely alkaline, the goal should be to acidify the urine to inhibit bacterial growth; drinking cranberry or prune juice will help. Urine may become alkaline through the ingestion of juices such as tomato, orange, grapefruit, or apple. Irritants such as coffee, tea, or soft drinks containing caffeine, should be avoided.

Pyelonephritis

Pyelonephritis, or inflammation of the renal pelvis, may occur bilaterally or unilaterally. *Acute pyelonephritis* is the result of bacterial invasion of the renal pelvis and medulla—usually an infection that has ascended from the lower urinary tract. In *chronic pyelonephritis,* infectious processes tend to persist or recur, resulting in renal parenchymal deterioration from scarring. A major cause of chronic pyelonephritis is believed to be ureterovesical reflux, in which infected urine ascends into the ureters and, consequently, the renal pelvises due to inadequate closure of the U-V valves during voiding. Most authorities believe that bacteriuria alone does not cause renal failure, but that structural alterations along with the infection produce serious renal deterioration.

Progressive kidney changes begin with parenchymal scarring in the periphery of the kidney. As the scarring progresses, it causes calyceal dilation and narrowing of the necks of the calyces. Kidney atrophy is the end stage.

Clinical Manifestations

ACUTE PYELONEPHRITIS The client with acute pyelonephritis is usually quite ill with fever, chills, nausea, and vomiting. Severe pain or constant dull aching over the kidney in the flank area may be present unilaterally or bilaterally.

CHRONIC PYELONEPHRITIS Unless there is an acute episode of a new infectious process, the client generally is unaware of chronic pyelonephritis. If the client notices anything, it may be only bladder irritability, chronic fatigue, or a slight aching over one or both kidneys. Eventually, the client develops hypertension, and the kidneys atrophy. Salt wasting occurs when the medulla is damaged.

Medical Measures

ACUTE PYELONEPHRITIS Antibiotics are administered to eradicate the infectious process. Follow-up cultures must be obtained to ensure that the urine is sterile. Recurrence of the infection necessitates reculturing to ensure that another organism has not invaded the urinary tract or that a resistant strain has not developed. Antispasmodics may be prescribed to alleviate bladder spasms. Any obstruction must be surgically removed.

CHRONIC PYELONEPHRITIS The major goal of medical management of chronic pyelonephritis is to prevent further damage to the renal parenchyma. In addition to appropriate antibiotics for the treatment of bacterial infections, agents that suppress the formation of new bacteria are generally prescribed. Urinary antiseptics such as the sulfonamides or nitrofurantoin may be administered. Antihypertensive agents also may be necessary. Surgical correction of structural abnormalities should be considered when possible. If end-stage renal failure develops, dialysis or transplantation will be necessary.

Specific Nursing Measures

ACUTE PYELONEPHRITIS Nursing measures for the client with acute pyelonephritis are directed toward support during the period of illness and education about the self-care measures necessary to attain or maintain health. Assist the client with such basic care needs as hygiene, nutrition, elimination, rest, and sleep—important components in the healing process. Fluid balance should be monitored and recorded accurately. Antibiotics should be administered to ensure that appropriate 24-hour blood levels are achieved.

Education about self-care in the convalescent phase of acute pyelonephritis should include discussion about how to take the prescribed medications. Appropriate follow-up to evaluate the effectiveness of therapy is essential. Likewise, it is extremely important that the client seek assistance if a new infection is suspected.

CHRONIC PYELONEPHRITIS Nursing interventions for the client with chronic pyelonephritis should include educational efforts to maximize understanding about self-care needs. The appropriate administration of prescribed medications, adequate fluid intake to ensure removal of metabolic wastes, and adequate nutrition for continued health are all components of the nursing care plan. If significant renal deterioration has occurred, the client and family or significant others will need support in understanding the dialytic or transplantation options available.

Renal Abscess

The client with a renal abscess is acutely and possibly critically ill. Single or multiple sites of bacterial abscess may be present. Renal abscesses are most common in clients with a history of pyelonephritis, chronic obstruction, or calculous disease. Staphylococcal skin infections may also spread to kidney parenchyma and result in an abscess.

Clinical Manifestations

The client usually has pain in the costovertebral angle, fever, and chills. Physical examination may reveal edema and a palpable mass.

Medical Measures

Penicillin-type antibiotics must be given immediately. If the infection is associated with chronic pyelonephritis, other broad-spectrum antibiotics may be necessary. Medical treatment aims at supporting the client while the antibiotics eradicate the infection. For example, IV fluid administration may be required. If severe bacteremia develops, septic shock may follow and cardiopulmonary support may be required. Surgical drainage of the abscess may be necessary. Partial or complete nephrectomy may be required if significant renal deterioration has occurred.

Specific Nursing Measures

Administration of the prescribed antibiotics is a priority nursing action. Anticipate IV administration of the antibiotics to ensure adequate absorption of the drug. In addition, parenteral fluid replacement may be necessary if the client is not able to tolerate fluids and food. Nursing interventions also include careful monitoring of vital signs, including temperature. Changes in level of consciousness, along with hypotension, may signify that the infection is becoming systemic. Measurement of intake, output, and daily weights should be part of the nursing care plan. The client will often be weak from the infection and require temporary assistance with hygienic measures. In addition, the client may be susceptible to problems of immobility, such as atelectasis, skin breakdown, and thrombophlebitis. Initiate appropriate interventions to prevent the sequelae of these problems.

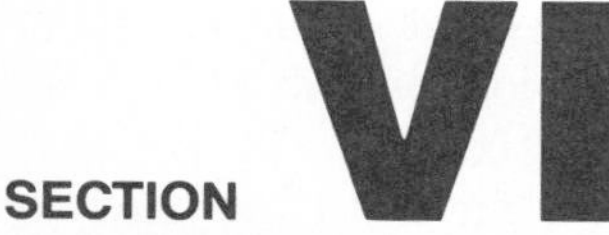

Neoplastic and Obstructive Disorders

Neoplastic and obstructive disorders of the kidneys and urinary tract are fairly common in the adult client. The most common nonmalignant obstructive disorders of the kidneys and the urinary system result from the formation or calculi or the effects of their obstruction, or from hyperplasia of prostatic tissue (prostatic disorders are discussed in Chapter 49). The most common malignant disorder of the urinary system is bladder cancer.

Approximately 67,300 new cases of cancer in the urinary system were estimated for 1987, while deaths were estimated at 20,000. Of these new cases, over 45,000 would be bladder cancers with over 10,000 deaths and over 21,000 cancers of the kidneys or other urinary organs with 9400 deaths (American Cancer Society, 1987). Because these tumors tend to develop in later life (the fifth, sixth, and seventh decades and beyond), clients with neoplastic disorders of the kidneys and urinary tract may already have other health alterations that require management. Consequently, the individual client must be carefully assessed so that the therapeutic interventions selected will maximize the quality of life.

Renal Cancer

Renal adenocarcinoma, sometimes called hypernephroma, accounts for about 80% of renal tumors and occurs about 66% more often in men than in women. Adenocarcinomas occur in the renal parenchyma and may secrete various hormones such as ACTH, gonadotropins, erythropoietin, and hormones that resemble parathormone and insulin. About 15% of kidney cancers are transitional or squamous cell carcinomas of the renal pelvis. This form of kidney cancer has an equal incidence in men and in women.

There may be hemorrhage or necrosis within the kidney, and enlargement of the kidney from the tumor. Because the tumor frequently grows for months before detection, the tumor may be quite large before the client seeks medical assistance. The tumor typically spreads to other structures by blood or lymph. The liver, lungs, long bones, ureter, and other kidney are the most common sites of metastasis.

Clinical Manifestations

Gross hematuria is the most common manifestation of a renal cell carcinoma. The client may identify dull flank pain, but this is generally a late symptom that develops as the tumor enlarges and presses upon adjacent structures. Occasionally, the client identifies a mass in the flank region, but this is rare. Other manifestations of a renal carcinoma may include nausea or vomiting, which result from the direct involvement or displacement of abdominal contents. Metastatic symptoms include weakness, loss of weight, and bone pain.

Medical Measures

In general, the renal cell carcinoma is not responsive to available chemotherapeutic agents or radiation therapy. Recent research indicates that interferon may be useful. Hormonal therapies may be useful for hormone-producing tumors.

The intentional embolization of the involved kidney by purposefully occluding the renal artery may be performed prior to surgical intervention. This procedure, sometimes referred to as a *medical nephrectomy,* decreases the blood supply to the kidney with the tumor and facilitates the technical aspects of surgery. In addition, renal artery embolization may be performed to control hemorrhage.

Surgery is the primary intervention and the procedure of choice is a radical nephrectomy. Because spontaneous remission of renal carcinomas has occurred, surgical debulking of the tumor mass is indicated even if obvious metastases are present.

Specific Nursing Measures

In general, nursing interventions for the client with cancer of the kidneys or urinary tract include providing comfort; providing emotional support during the diagnostic, therapeutic, and convalescent period; and educating the client in self-care and optimal decision making. In addition, the nurse must continually assess the client to prevent complications associated with the therapeutic interventions or the disease process. The prevention of problems such as infection, urinary tract obstruction, and acute renal failure depends on constant assessment for their potential development. The client and family or significant others should be involved throughout. Emotional support and educational counseling of the family or significant others should facilitate the posthospitalization convalescence and rehabilitation. Specific nursing care revolves around the surgical intervention as discussed below.

Nephrectomy

A *nephrectomy* is a surgical procedure in which a kidney is removed. It may be indicated in instances of chronic infection, trauma, hemorrhage, tumor, hypertension resistant to treatment, an infected calculus, or a desire to donate a kidney to a relative. A *radical nephrectomy* includes the removal of a kidney, adjacent perinephric fasciae and fat, the superior adrenal gland, and nearby lymph nodes. This procedure is indicated when there is renal cell carcinoma. A *partial nephrectomy* may be performed in clients with significant renal deterioration as evidenced by an elevated serum creatinine level or decreased 24-hour creatinine clearance rate, or in clients who have only one kidney. If a tumor is present, however, removal of the entire kidney may be necessary, and a partial nephrectomy may not be possible.

For a healthy client requiring a simple nephrectomy, a lumbar–flank incision may be selected. (This position is illustrated in Figure 11–5.) The thoracoabdominal or the transabdominal approach is preferred for wide visualization for removal of tissue. The physiologic and psychosocial/lifestyle implications for the client are discussed in Table 26–3.

Table 26–3
Nephrectomy: Implications for the Client

Physiologic Implications	Psychosocial/Lifestyle Implications
Dialysis or transplantation if inadequate kidney function remains	Need for emotional support
Decreased perfusion	Need for assurance of possibility to live with one healthy kidney
Avoidance of nephrotoxins	Potential need for dialysis or transplantation may be anxiety-provoking
Possible complications are: infection and bacteremia, hemorrhage, electrolyte imbalance, pneumonia	Avoidance of contact sports
Adrenal insufficiency possible after radical nephrectomy	Return to activities in 8 weeks
	Avoidance of heavy lifting for at least 8 weeks

Nursing Implications

PREOPERATIVE CARE Adequately hydrate the client to promote the excretion of waste products before surgery. Teach clients how to splint an incision to ensure that coughing and deep breathing will be done postoperatively.

A complete blood count (CBC) and coagulation profile (prothrombin time, partial thromboplastin time, and platelet count) should be obtained, and any problems should be corrected prior to surgery. Electrolyte values should also be monitored and corrected as necessary. The measurement of BUN and serum creatinine levels preoperatively will allow comparison with postoperative values.

POSTOPERATIVE CARE A major objective of postoperative nursing care is to ensure adequate oxygenation and the prevention of postoperative pulmonary complications. Atelectasis and pneumonia are significant possibilities; because lumbar–flank incisions involve the accessory muscles of respiration, postoperative discomfort is a major deterrent to deep breathing and coughing exercises. Medications administered liberally will facilitate relief of pain and maximum relaxation. In turn, the client who is relaxed and reasonably comfortable (but not oversedated) can more easily perform breathing exercises. Incentive spirometry or other respiratory therapy techniques may also promote maximum respiratory excursion. Splinting of the incision will decrease pain upon coughing. Finally, ambulation on the first postoperative day improves pulmonary function. (If the pleural cavity has been entered, a chest tube will be in place. Refer to Chapter 14 for discussion of client care when a chest tube is present.)

Alterations in gastrointestinal function, including paralytic ileus, intestinal obstruction, or hemorrhage, are common following renal surgery. Fluids and foods should not be taken orally until active peristalsis, identified by the return of bowel sounds and the passage of flatus, is present. Paralytic ileus is the most common complication. To treat it, a nasogastric tube generally is placed, and the client is kept NPO. Encourage ambulation if the client is able. Intestinal obstruction may develop if there was significant manipulation of the bowel during surgery. Hemorrhage in the gastrointestinal tract may result from generalized stress. A more detailed discussion of these complications is presented in Unit 8.

Wound care is another important postoperative nursing objective. The type of incision and the nature of the surgery determine whether drains will be placed. For example, a lumbar–flank incision does not usually require drain placement. In any case, the use of aseptic or clean technique (protocol differs among institutions) is essential when caring for the incision or drains. Keep the dressing and incisional site clean and dry.

Postoperative renal function is assessed through the careful measurement of intake and output; monitoring of serum creatinine, BUN, and electrolyte levels; and the measurement of urine specific gravity. The nurse also may take central venous line measurements, especially if large amounts of fluids are infused. Hourly outputs often are recorded, and IV infusions of an amount equal to the output may promote perfusion of the remaining kidney. In this case, hourly CVP readings are often recorded as well to avoid overhydration. Recording daily weights also is useful in assessing the client's hydration status.

Intraoperative hemorrhage, dehydration, and altered hemodynamics (associated with the hyperextended position) may alter renal perfusion. Consequently, the detection of the prerenal azotemia that may develop is important.

Home Health Care

Discharge planning includes the provision of emotional support and education about activities related to self-care. The client should avoid lifting and other major activities for at least 8 weeks, depending on the specific surgical procedure and the client. Thus, the involvement of the family and significant others in posthospital plans is valuable. The client should receive information regarding the injuries that may be sustained in contact sports. If radiation, chemotherapy, or chronic dialysis are needed, the nurse should provide referrals to appropriate clinical nurse specialists, social workers, and nutritionists.

Bladder Cancer

Bladder malignancies are most commonly found in men over 50. The bladder tumor commonly involves transitional cells of the ureteral orifices or bladder neck. Bladder neoplasms commonly metastasize to the organs supplied by the lymph nodes of the bladder and to the hypogastric, common iliac, and lumbar vessels.

A variety of substances have been described as potentially carcinogenic to the bladder, and suspected carcinogens have been identified in the urine of clients with bladder cancer. For example, there is a well-established link between prolonged exposure to industrial compounds such as the aniline dyes and development of bladder cancer. Tryptophan and the tars of smoking have been strongly linked with bladder cancer, but the evidence is not unequivocal.

Clinical Manifestations

Painless hematuria is the primary clinical manifestation of bladder cancer. The hematuria is intermittent, so the client may ignore the earliest manifestation of the pathologic process. Obstruction of the urinary tract by the tumor may alter the outflow of urine, causing intermittent anuria and polyuria; there also may be bladder distention. Infection may cause symptoms of dysuria, such as burning, frequency, or urgency. Other urinary flow alterations may include a decrease of the force or volume of the urinary stream.

Medical Measures

Considerable research continues in the administration of various chemotherapeutic agents for the treatment of bladder cancers. Methods of administration include direct bladder instillations, intra-arterial infusions, IV infusion, and oral ingestion. Many chemotherapeutic agents (including 5-fluorouracil, methotrexate, bleomycin, mitomycin-C, and hydroxyurea) have been used in an attempt to demonstrate a significant clinical response. More recently, doxorubicin and cyclophosphamide or cisplatin have been tried; reports of effectiveness are variable, and results are not conclusive. Because of the high association of tryptophan metabolites with bladder cancer, Smith (1981) recommends the administration of pyridoxine to those with a confirmed diagnosis, because pyridoxine neutralizes tryptophan metabolities.

Bladder malignancies may be treated by transurethral removal, partial cystectomy, or radical cystectomy. Urinary diversion procedures also may be necessary.

Specific Nursing Measures

Nursing care for the client with bladder cancer is the same as for anyone diagnosed as having cancer. A discussion of postoperative nursing care for these clients follows.

Cystectomy

A *partial cystectomy* involves the surgical excision of a portion of the urinary bladder. This procedure generally is indicated only when there is a single, primary tumor too large for transurethral resection via cystoscopy. The tumor and adjacent bladder muscle are resected and the size of the urinary bladder decreased.

A *radical cystectomy* involves the removal of the urinary bladder and adjacent structures; it necessitates permanent urinary diversion. Indications for a radical cystectomy include malignancies not treatable with less conservative measures. In the man, a radical cystectomy involves the removal of the urinary bladder, pelvic peritoneum, prostate, seminal vesicles, and pelvic lymph nodes; removal of the urethra remains controversial. In the woman, a radical cystectomy includes removal of the urinary bladder, pelvic peritoneum, urethra, uterus and broad ligaments, part of the anterior vaginal wall, and pelvic lymph nodes. The physiologic and psychosocial/lifestyle implications for both partial and radical cystectomy are discussed in Table 26–4.

Nursing Implications

PREOPERATIVE CARE Prior to surgery, the goal is to have the client in the best possible state of health. The client who has had radiation therapy or chemotherapy has had some time to adjust to the diagnosis of cancer. However, all clients and family need a good deal of support and time to ask questions or ventilate feelings.

POSTOPERATIVE CARE Postoperatively, the client with a partial cystectomy will generally have in-dwelling and suprapubic catheters. Accurate measurements and record-

Table 26–4
Cystectomy: Implications for the Client 

Physiologic Implications	Psychosocial/Lifestyle Implications
Partial cystectomy	
Decreased bladder size postoperatively	Diminished capacity of bladder that requires frequent voidings to avoid embarrassing accidents
Bladder's gradual return to normal size in about 6 months	Cystoscopy every 3 months for 2 years to evaluate effectiveness of surgery
Potential complications are: thromboembolic phenomena and infection	
Radical cystectomy	
Urinary diversion procedures necessary (see Tables 26–5 and 26–6)	Dependence on urinary diversion selected
Pelvic congestion and peripheral edema from removal of lymph nodes	Fear and anxiety associated with cancer
Potential complications are: thromboembolic phenomena and infection	Altered body image
	Loss of reproductive ability
	Impotence

ing of intake and urinary output from each catheter are important. Catheter drainage will be continued until all identifiable urinary leakage has ceased.

Fluid intake after surgery should be at least 2000 mL per day, but advise the client to limit fluid intake prior to sleeping or when toilet facilities are not readily available. Until bladder capacity is normal, instruct the client to void frequently. He or she should identify the location of toilet facilities in advance of the need to urinate to prevent embarrassment from urinary incontinence. The nurse should offer support to the client, family, and significant others during any further cancer treatment.

Postoperatively, leg exercises and early ambulation are particularly important for the client with a radical cystectomy because of the lymph node removal and the tendency to develop congestion and edema. Thrombosis with embolization is another potential complication following this surgical procedure. Bowel sounds and gastrointestinal motility should return in 3 to 5 days after surgery. The client will be NPO and receiving IV fluids until peristalsis returns. Carefully measure intake, output, and vital signs during the postoperative period. Other postoperative care depends on the type of urinary diversion selected.

Ileal and Sigmoid Urinary Conduits

Ileal conduit, ureteroileal urinary conduit, ileal bladder, ileal loop, Bricker's procedure, or ureteroileostomy are terms describing the same basic urinary diversion procedure. A portion of the ileum is resected and used as a new passage for urine. The open end of the resected segment is brought to the surface of the skin in the form of a stoma (Figure 26–4A).

In the *sigmoid conduit,* or colon conduit, a portion of the sigmoid colon is resected and used to move urine (Figure 26–4B). The physiologic and psychosocial/lifestyle implications of these forms of urinary diversion are discussed in Table 26–5.

Nursing Implications

PREOPERATIVE CARE Preoperatively, the client should receive thorough explanations about the need for evaluation of the intestinal tract. The client should assist in selecting a comfortable site for stoma placement (generally in the upper right lower quadrant of the abdomen). The surface of the skin at the site should be free of scars and deep tissue folds. In addition, the site should be readily

Nursing Research Note

Williamson M: Reducing post-catheterization bladder dysfunction. *Nurs Res* 1982; 31:28–30.

This study determined the effect of bladder reconditioning before removal of an in-dwelling catheter on bladder dysfunction postcatheterization. One group of women had their in-dwelling catheters clamped for 3 hours with a 5-minute drain period for a total of 9 hours. The control group had no conditioning, and the indwelling catheter was just removed.

Those clients who underwent reconditioning resumed normal bladder elimination significantly sooner than the control group. Residual urine volumes for both groups did not differ significantly. However, for the control group, residual urine volumes after the first normal micturition following catheter removal were 10 times the mean baseline residual volume. The group with reconditioning had residual volumes 1.3 times the mean baseline.

This study suggests an intervention to assist clients to return to normal urinary elimination sooner after catheterization. Reconditioning was found to shorten the amount of time needed to resume normal micturition. It also reduced residual urine volumes after the first normal voiding and therefore may help to reduce bladder infection.

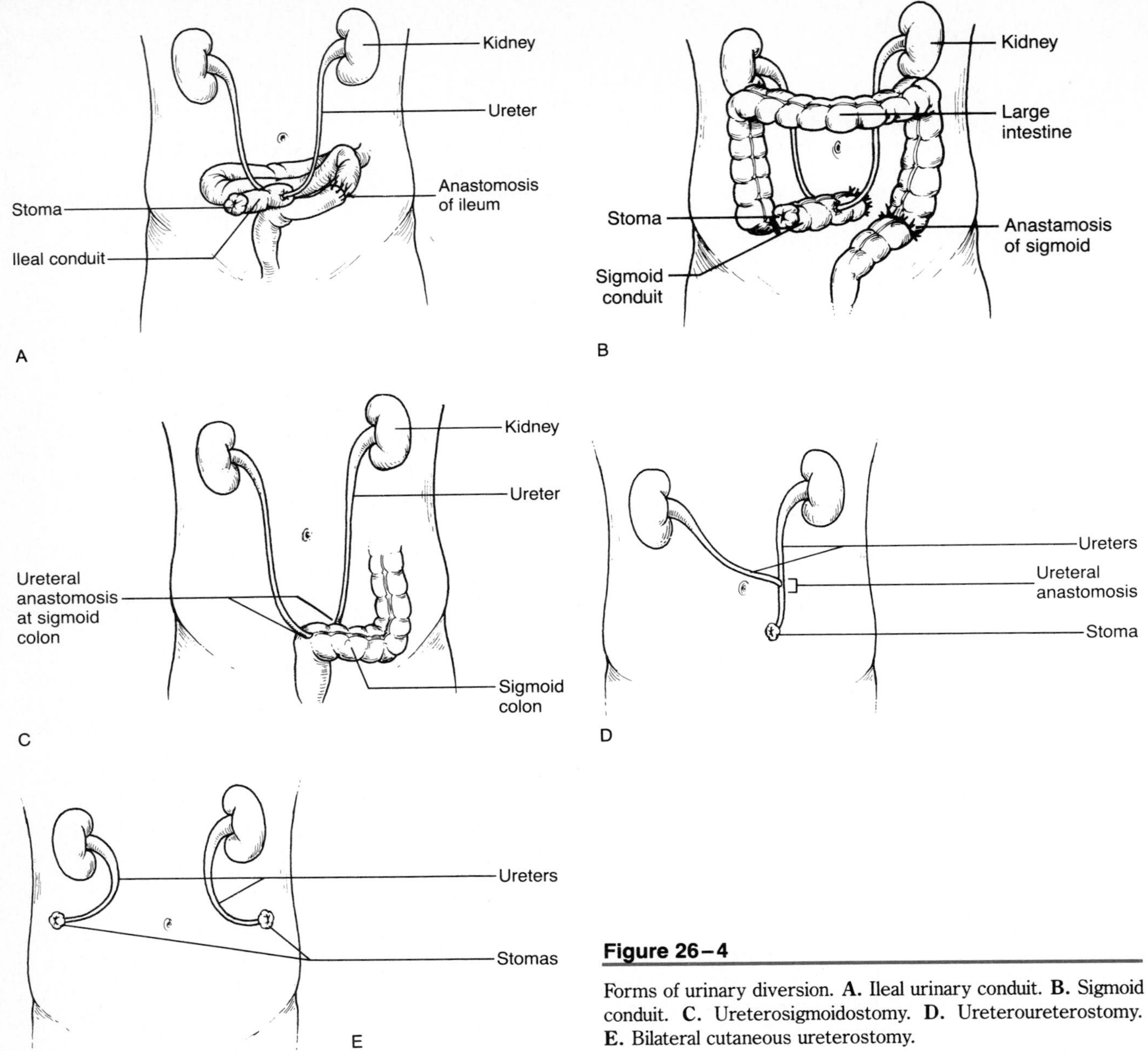

Figure 26–4

Forms of urinary diversion. **A.** Ileal urinary conduit. **B.** Sigmoid conduit. **C.** Ureterosigmoidostomy. **D.** Ureteroureterostomy. **E.** Bilateral cutaneous ureterostomy.

Table 26–5
Ileal and Sigmoid Urinary Conduits: Implications for the Client

Physiologic Implications	Psychosocial/Lifestyle Implications
Reabsorption of water and electrolytes from conduit leading to imbalances	Altered body image and sexual identity related to stoma and appliance
Deep vein thrombosis and embolization	Embarrassment from drainage and odor from stoma leading to social isolation
Skin irritation around stoma	Potential alterations in self-concept and self-esteem
Potential complications are: wound infection and dehiscence, obstruction of ureter and small bowel, stomal gangrene	Need to care for stoma and appliance
Renal calculi and pyelonephritis are potential long-term complications	

accessible to the client. Having the client wear a pouch filled with water for several days during the preoperative period may help ensure that the site selected is optimally functional and comfortable, as well as help with the post-operative adjustment by helping the client know what to expect. Several different pouches may be tried to ensure comfort and compatibility with normal clothing. An enterostomal therapist is invaluable for all preoperative teaching.

Preoperative bowel preparation is achieved through a low-residue diet, a laxative or enemas, or oral neomycin to reduce the risk of infection. Three days is generally needed for bowel preparation procedures. Cardiovascular evaluation is also important in determining whether the client can withstand the lengthy surgery.

POSTOPERATIVE CARE The goals of postoperative nursing management are to preserve renal function and assist the client in adapting to an altered body image. The client will have a nasogastric tube inserted until bowel motility returns (usually in 3 to 5 days). Urine will flow into a pouch placed over the stoma at the time of surgery. Lack of urine flow during the first 12 to 18 hours may be the result of edema at the site of ureteral implantation and should be reported immediately to the surgeon. Carefully measure and record intake and output, as well as monitor serum creatinine and BUN values. Electrolyte balance should also be assessed by daily laboratory data.

Early ambulation will prevent venous stasis and the development of atelectasis, as well as promote the return of peristalsis. The lengthy time required for this procedure, particularly when performed with a radical cystectomy, increases the client's risk for postoperative deep vein thrombosis and embolization. The administration of narcotic analgesics in the early postoperative period will achieve pain control.

Preserving renal function depends upon proper stoma care and the absence of infection. If the area is kept clean, infection probably will not develop. Stoma care involves several factors. Assess the stoma for adequate vascular supply; it should be red or pink. If the stoma becomes purple, surgical intervention may be required to correct the blood supply to the stoma.

The choice of the correct appliance promotes proper stoma care and functioning. Clients may choose disposable or reusable appliances. The appliance should be ¹⁄₁₆ inch larger than the diameter of the stoma. After about 1 month, the stoma size should stabilize.

Home Health Care

The collecting appliance should be changed every 4 to 5 days or whenever it is leaking. Instruct the client to remove the face plate and then bend over quickly and remain that way for a minute to allow the conduit to empty completely. The client then washes and rinses the skin, taking care to dry the skin before reapplying the appliance. The skin around the stoma is highly sensitive to urine, so skin care and the correct application of an appliance for urine collection are important in preventing skin breakdown. Another problem is the congealing of mucus in the stoma; a high fluid intake will help prevent this. A gauze wick or tampon inserted at the stoma will absorb urine and keep the skin dry during appliance application. The client should apply a skin barrier or protectant if needed. Next, gentle pressure applied around the appliance removes air bubbles and secures the adhesive or cement and the appliance to the skin. Taping around the appliance will give extra security.

Clients often wear leg bags to be sure the collecting bag at the stoma does not get too full and empty itself. An adapter attaches the drainage apparatus to the leg bag and tubing. At night the client may prefer to snap a tubing with dependent drainage to a collection bottle to have uninterrupted sleep.

Odor control may be a challenge for the client with a urinary conduit. Foods that give urine a strong odor, such as tomatoes and asparagus, should be avoided. Wearing an appliance too long without cleaning it will also create an odor. Ascorbic acid intake will help suppress odors, as will white vinegar introduced into the drain spout at the bottom of the pouch. After rinsing the bag in warm water, soak it in a vinegar-and-water solution for 30 to 60 minutes. After the bag is rinsed, dried (avoiding sunlight), and powdered with cornstarch, it can be stored until the next use. Other tips on caring for the appliance and managing odor control may be obtained from the local ostomy association (see the Resources list in Chapter 25).

The urinary conduit or other forms of urinary diversion force the client to make major emotional adjustments. The external stoma creates a change in body image, along with potential alterations in self-concept, self-esteem, and sexual identity. Learning to adjust to pouch drainage, odor control, and skin irritation prevention and management requires considerable effort and perseverance. Close personal contact, including sexual intimacy, may be difficult for the client to resume. The lack of privacy in health clubs or other locker facilities may cause the client to avoid previous recreational activities; clients often prefer to isolate themselves socially rather than risk embarrassment. Assisting the client in learning self-care and adjusting to changes in body image requires time, patience, and continuous support from the family or significant others and the health care team.

Ureterosigmoidostomy and Ureteroileosigmoidostomy

Ureterosigmoidostomy and ureteroileosigmoidostomy are urinary diversions in which the flow of urine is directed into the rectum. A *ureterosigmoidostomy,* which is usually done for the client with small bowel disease, involves the implantation of the ureters into the sigmoid colon (Figure 26–4C). A *ureteroileosigmoidostomy* is done for the client who is not a candidate for other urinary diversions, but who, because the small bowel is healthy, is able to have a portion of it used to form a pouch that attaches to the colon. This procedure minimizes the spread of bacteria and reflux of urine back to the kidneys because the ureters are attached to a section of the ileum rather than directly to the sigmoid colon. These procedures do not require an external pouch because urine is passed via the rectum. Table 26–6 summarizes physiologic and psychosocial/lifestyle implications for the client with ureterosigmoidostomy or ureteroileosigmoidostomy

Nursing Implications

PREOPERATIVE CARE The client having ureterosigmoidostomy or ureteroileosigmoidostomy needs a thorough understanding of the procedure and potential postoperative problems.

Physical preparation for the surgical procedure involves a liquid or low-residue diet, enemas, and antibiotics to sterilize the bowel. Preoperative assessment of the client's ability to retain urine in the rectum may be made by administering a small-volume enema (200 to 300 mL) and measuring the time the client can hold the fluid.

Emotional preparation for surgery includes offering the client opportunities to discuss what is expected in the postoperative period. The client should verbalize and explore feelings about body image changes associated with a new procedure for voiding. Men should consider and explore their feelings associated with urinating in a sitting position.

POSTOPERATIVE CARE A rectal tube is inserted when the client is in the operating room for the collection and measurement of urinary output. Gentle irrigations with small amounts of normal saline may be required to prevent obstruction from stool or mucus. In addition to the rectal tube, two ureteral catheters, which serve as stents to keep the ureters patent at the site of anastomosis, will also exit the rectum and drain into one collection bag. The rectal tube will empty into another bag. Provide regular skin care to the anal area and keep the area as dry as possible.

Careful measurement of fluid intake and output is important. Intravenous fluids and electrolytes will be necessary until intestinal motility returns. The client will be NPO and may have a nasogastric tube in place initially.

Infection in the urinary tract is always a potential problem. The development of fever and flank pain indicates infection in the urinary tract. Sudden decreases in urinary output may occur with infection or obstruction of the catheters or rectal tube.

Home Health Care

Following the acute postoperative period, nursing care will revolve around educating the client for maximum self-care in the future. The client should understand that dietary modifications will be necessary to provide a high-potassium, low-chloride, and low-calcium intake. Chloride intake may be reduced if salt intake is limited. High-potassium and low-salt foods are listed in Chapter 19. Calcium, which occurs in milk and dairy products, should be consumed in limited quantities. In addition, medications may be prescribed to supplement potassium and bicarbonate consumption.

Foods that readily produce gas should be avoided (eg, beans, cabbage, cauliflower, brussels sprouts, prunes, and raisins). Gum chewing, using straws, and smoking, which cause air to be swallowed and thus increase flatus production, also should be avoided.

Table 26–6
Ureterosigmoidostomy and Ureteroileosigmoidostomy: Implications for the Client

Physiologic Implications	Psychosocial/Lifestyle Implications
Urinary continence except with expulsion of flatus or fecal incontinence	No external pouch
Anal irritation from urine	Altered body image
Reabsorption of electrolytes and fluid leading to hyperchloremia, metabolic acidosis, hypokalemia, and possibly hypomagnesemia	Male's need to adjust to sitting to urinate
Hypercalcemia predisposing client to calculi	Embarrassment if incontinent
Increased serum ammonia levels may cause encephalopathy	Frequent emptying of colon necessary to minimize problems of electrolyte reabsorption
Pyelonephritis, ureteral obstruction, and increased risk of colon adenocarcinoma are potential long-term complications	Need to make diet adjustments to prevent complications (high potassium, low chloride, low calcium)
Usually not considered for long-term diversion	

The client should avoid enemas, laxatives, diagnostic enemas, and activities that would increase intrarectal pressure; an increase in intrarectal pressure will result in reflux and possible infection of the urinary tract. The client should get up once or twice at night to empty the rectum of urine.

Because the urine flows into the stool, constipation is generally not a problem. A liberal fluid intake of 2 to 3 L per day should be consumed.

Cutaneous Ureterostomy

In the cutaneous ureterostomy, another form of urinary diversion, the ureters are brought to the surface of the skin for drainage. Several types of cutaneous ureterostomies may be performed, and they may be considered temporary or permanent urinary diversions. The procedure is not recommended for long-term diversion, however, because of infection and progressive narrowing of the stomas. The *unilateral cutaneous ureterostomy* involves a single ureteral stoma. A *ureteroureterostomy* involves the anastomosis of one ureter into the side of the other; one ureter is brought to the surface (Figure 26–4D). The *bilateral (or double-barreled) cutaneous ureterostomy* involves each ureter's surfacing onto the skin with a stoma for urine drainage. Typically, the bilateral ureteral stomas are placed at the midline, or sometimes on the lateral aspects of each side of the abdomen (Figure 26–4E). The physiologic and psychosocial/lifestyle implications are discussed in Table 26–7.

Nursing Implications

PREOPERATIVE CARE Offer the client opportunities to express concerns and clarify expectations about the proposed urinary diversion. Encouraging the client to reflect upon the effect of the diversion of urine on his or her lifestyle may facilitate the recovery period.

POSTOPERATIVE CARE Plan for the prevention of the complications of immobility to which the elderly and debilitated are prone. Early ambulation, turning, coughing, and deep breathing exercises should be instituted. Routine postoperative measurement of intake and output, daily weights, and vital signs is essential. Early detection of infection also is imperative, because the direct opening into the urinary tract may result in pyelonephritis or sepsis. A high fluid intake will minimize the development of pyelonephritis. Other care and management of the stoma is similar to that for the client with a urinary conduit.

Urinary Calculi

Calculi (stones) in the urinary tract are a relatively common problem, especially for men, but rare in black men. They usually occur within the same family. There is a high incidence of recurrence; the incidence of a second calculus within 2 years is reported to be as high at 40%.

Table 26–7
Cutaneous Ureterostomy: Implications for the Client

Physiologic Implications	Psychosocial/Lifestyle Implications
Little surgical time; good for debilitated clients	Altered body image, self-concept, and self-esteem
Infection is potential complication	Possible social isolation because of pouch leakage and odor
Skin irritation	Need for self-care assistance

Most calculi are composed of calcium salts (calcium oxalate or calcium phosphate), uric acid, or struvite (magnesium ammonium phosphate, a triple salt). The majority of calculi originate in the renal parenchyma (nephrolithiasis) and are passed out into the ureters or bladder (urolithiasis). When associated with infection or obstruction, renal calculi may be life threatening.

A number of factors contribute to the formation of calculi. The primary factors influencing calculi formation are the degree to which the urine is supersaturated with an element normally excreted, the pH of the urine, the presence of substances that inhibit the formation of crystals, the stasis of urine, and a special preexisting environment.

Clients with pathologic conditions in which large amounts of calcium phosphate or uric acid are excreted may develop calculi. A dietary excess of foods containing calcium or purine, immobilization, primary hyperparathyroidism, hypervitaminosis D, and renal tubular acidosis may result in hypercalciuria. Medications taken in excess, such as the antacids or vitamin C, may also result in hypercalciuria or excess calcium oxalate.

The pH of the urine may also influence calculus formation. Normally, urine is slightly acidic with a pH of 5 to 6. With infection, the urine is slightly alkaline (pH above 7). Uric acid and cystine calculi will form in acidic urine; calcium phosphate calculi will dissolve in acidic urine; and calcium oxalate calculi are not influenced by the pH of the urine. Struvite calculi are associated with infection from urea-splitting bacteria. Bacteria such as the *Proteus* strains convert ureas to ammonia, and the alkaline urine contributes to the formation of struvite calculi.

Exactly how calculi form is not clearly understood. However, certain substances that the kidney excretes (pyrophosphate, magnesium, and citrate) are believed to inhibit the formation of calculi, and decreases in the levels of these substances have been associated with calculus formation. Calculus formation is enhanced when there are

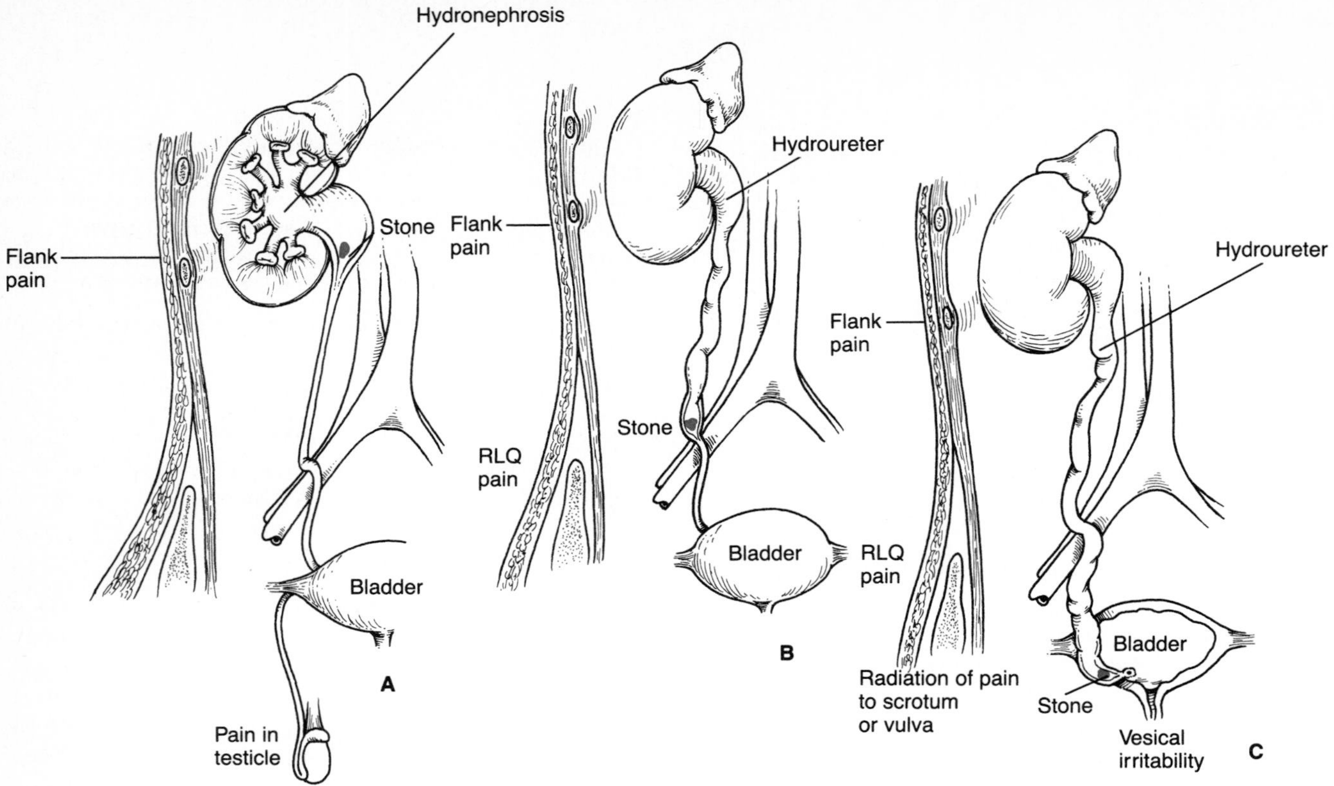

Figure 26–5

Radiation of pain and location of lodged calculi. **A.** Calculus lodged at the ureteropelvic junction. Distention of the renal pelvis and renal capsule causes severe costovertebral angle pain. Hyperperistalsis of smooth muscle of the ureter causes pain to radiate along the course of the ureter and into the testicle, which is hypersensitive. **B.** Calculus lodged at the iliac bend (the point at which the ureter crosses over the iliac vessels). Pain symptoms are like those in A with the addition of pain in the lower quadrant of the abdomen. **C.** Calculus lodged at the ureterovesical junction. Pain symptoms are like those in A and B with the addition of pain radiating into the bladder, scrotum, or vulva. Urgency, frequency, and burning on urination may result from inflammation of the bladder wall around the ureteral orifice.

old scars (either from infection or surgical procedures in the urinary tract) or when urinary stasis or urinary crystallization is already present.

Clinical Manifestations

The primary clinical manifestation of nephrolithiasis or urolithiasis is pain, and its location may suggest the location of the calculus (eg, the client may describe a calculus in the kidney pelvis as dull, intermittent flank pain). In some situations there may be no discomfort at all. However, if the calculus moves down into the ureter and becomes lodged at a narrow point in the ureter, the client may describe the pain as excruciatingly severe, an 11 on a scale of 10. Severe intermittent pain results as the musculature of the ureter goes into spasm (**colic**) in an attempt to move the calculus out of the ureter by peristalsis. The characteristics of the radiating pain indicate the location of the lodged calculus (Figure 26–5). The client commonly experiences nausea and perhaps vomiting. He or she may also report the presence of blood in the urine and, if infection is present, chills and fever.

Medical Measures

Narcotics are generally necessary for relief of the pain associated with renal or urinary calculi. Antispasmodics may also be prescribed to relax the ureteral musculature. If infection is present or if instrumentation is necessary to remove the calculus, antibiotics will be prescribed.

Clients with calculi too large to pass spontaneously may be able to avoid urologic surgery for calculus removal through a technique called *lithotripsy*. In this treatment, the client is supported and suspended in a large tank of water (Figure 26–6). An extracorporeal shock wave lithotripter sends shock waves through the water to the calculus, which shatters and is excreted within several days. Clients liken the feeling of the shock waves to having a rubber band snapping their backs. Lithotripsy is expected to be used in the near future in 60% to 80% of all cases where large calculi cannot be voided without assistance.

Kidney stones can also be broken down with ultrasound vibrations and flushed out of the kidney with water. Ultrasound treatment requires a small incision, about ⅓ inch long. It shares the major advantage of lithotripsy—

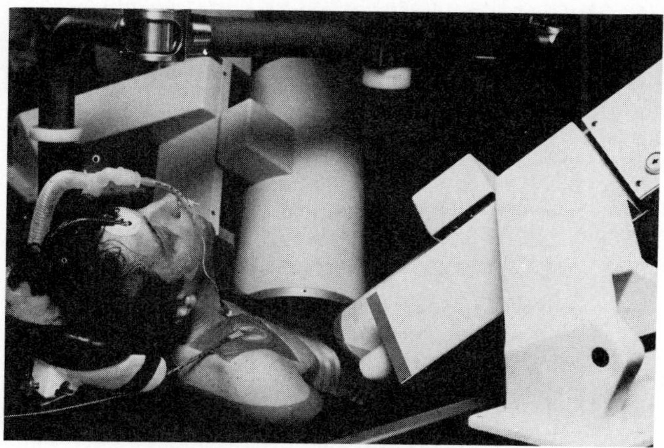

Figure 26–6

Client receiving lithotripsy treatment. The client is anesthetized and immersed in water where he will receive up to 1000 shock waves over a period of 30 to 45 minutes.

making major surgery a thing of the past for clients with kidney stones. However, if the calculus does not pass spontaneously or if there is intractable pain, persistent infection, or obstruction, surgical removal of the calculus will be necessary.

The long-term management of the client identified as a calculus-former should emphasize obtaining a high-volume, dilute urine. Dietary modifications depend on the chemical content of the calculus. Medications that alter urine composition, or alter the urinary pH to create the desired environment, are given to prevent calculus development and are more effective than dietary modifications. Table 26–8 summarizes the dietary modifications and pharmacologic treatment.

Specific Nursing Measures

Care of the client with renal or urinary calculi presents challenges to the maintenance of comfort and the prevention of infection. The prescribed medications should be administered to afford the client relief from pain. Initially, the client may require IV administration of morphine sulfate to obtain relief. Antibiotics should be administered as prescribed to ensure that bacterial growth ceases.

The client may achieve the goal of obtaining a high-volume, dilute urine to inhibit stone formation and to flush out small stones by consuming 4 L fluid per day; water is the ideal liquid. It is important to void before bedtime and to consume fluids so the client will awaken in the middle of the night to empty the bladder. When awakened, the client should drink more water to ensure a constant dilution of urine. Intravenous fluids may be required if the client cannot take them orally. A high fluid intake of 3 to 4 L/day is usually recommended for the remainder of the client's lifetime.

In addition to measuring intake and output carefully, an essential nursing intervention is the straining of all urine through a fine mesh gauze contained in a funnel-shaped container. The goal of the straining procedure is to obtain a calculus or calculus fragments that may be analyzed by the laboratory for chemical characteristics.

The goal for client education is the prevention of recurrence, if possible. If surgery is necessary, nursing care will depend on the method chosen. Potential complications of lithotripsy are bruising and hemorrhage.

Lithotomy

A *nephrolithotomy* is any surgical procedure in which the parenchyma of the kidney is incised for the removal of a calculus or small tumor or the correction of altered anatomic structure and vascular abnormalities. Although *lith* literally means "stone," this procedure may be performed to correct any intrarenal abnormality. In a *pyelolithotomy,* an incision is made into the renal pelvis, generally to remove a calculus from it. This procedure is indicated when a calculus is infected and the infection cannot be eradicated, or when an obstruction to the outflow of urine results in hydronephrosis. A *ureterolithotomy* involves incising the ureter to remove a calculus that is not passing spontaneously. The site of the incision depends on the location of the calculus. Postoperatively, one or two wound drains and a ureteral catheter are placed. The physiologic and psychosocial/lifestyle implications of surgery to remove a urinary calculus are discussed in Table 26–9.

Nursing Implications

PREOPERATIVE CARE Preoperative care is the same as is described for the nephrectomy client.

POSTOPERATIVE CARE Postoperative nursing implications are similar to those indicated for the client requiring a nephrectomy. Although the lithotomy client will not have lost a portion of renal parenchyma, maximizing renal reserve is still important. Use meticulous aseptic techniques for the proper care of the ureteral catheter or the ureteral stent that will be in place along with a Foley catheter. The ureteral catheter ensures that local edema in the ureter will not result in hydronephrosis after the calculus is removed, and it must not be dislodged.

If a ureterolithotomy was performed, a stent is used to ensure patency of the ureter during the period of ureteral tissue healing and to allow the ureter to heal without stricture or fistula formation. Without the catheter, edema of local tissue in the ureter could result in ureteral obstruction.

A ureteral **stent** is a hollow tubelike device made of soft, flexible silicone that is placed within a ureter. The double-J ureteral stent (Figure 26–7) prevents movement of the stent without restricting the client's activities. Nurs-

Table 26–8
Urinary Calculi: Nonsurgical Treatment

Type	Conditions Promoting Formation	Dietary Modifications	Medications	Goal of Urinary pH
Calcium phosphate	Hypercalciuria	Decrease dietary calcium if normally a high calcium intake; increase fluid intake	Cellulose phosphate; thiazide diuretics (eg, Diuril, Hydrodiuril); avoid antacids that contain calcium; use aluminum hydroxide antacids that bind with phosphorus	Less than 6
Calcium oxalate	Hyperoxaluria	Increase fluid intake; decrease calcium oxalate intake (avoid tea, cocoa, colas, instant coffee, and beer); avoid citrus fruits, grapes, cranberries, beans, spinach, apples, mushrooms, beets, turnips, and most nuts	Cholestyramine, pyridoxine, and methylene blue; avoid antacids that contain calcium	Less than 6
Uric acid	Hyperuricemia and uricosuria	Low purine diet may help; increase fluid intake; limit intake of ham, beef, halibut, trout, and salmon	Allopurinol; avoid uricosuric agents such as the thiazide diuretics and aspirin; give sodium bicarbonate to increase urine pH	Greater than 6.5
Struvite (triple phosphate or magnesium ammonium phosphate)	Presence of *Proteus* bacteria strains in the urinary tract: bacterial splitting of urea results in high-ammonia, highly alkaline urine	Encourage eggs, meat, poultry, fish, and cereals; increase fluid intake; limit phosphate intake	Antibiotics (long term); methionine; ascorbic acid	Between 5.5 and 6.2

Table 26–9
Lithotomy: Implications for the Client

Physiologic Implications	Psychosocial/Lifestyle Implications
Renal function is preserved Potential complications are: infection, pneumonia, electrolyte imbalance, hemorrhage Avoidance of nephrotoxins	Education on diet, fluid intake, testing of urinary pH, and medication administration in attempt to prevent further calculi development (see Chapter 25) Restricted activity and avoidance of heavy lifting for 6–8 weeks

ing care involves monitoring for bleeding and purulent drainage from the stent, measuring output, and observing for stent dislodgement (colicky pain and decreased urine output).

The dressing will need to be changed frequently during the first 24 hours after surgery. Drainage via the wound drain is frequently copious and sanguineous in the early postoperative period. The amount will diminish and the color will return to clear amber, usually within 48 hours. Infection is a potential postoperative problem. Elevated temperature or an abnormal odor of the drainage may indicate an infection in the urinary tract. The nursing care plan should include careful measurement and recording of intake and output and daily weights to detect changes in urinary output and fluid imbalances, as well as prompt collection

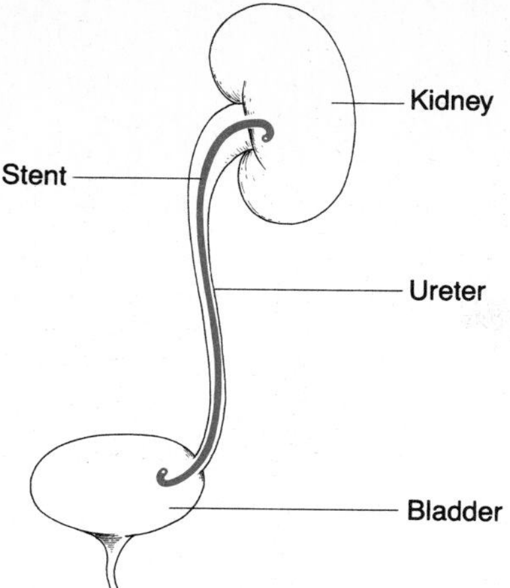

Figure 26–7

Double-J ureteral stent.

of specimens. Monitor laboratory work for changes in the serum creatinine level and any evidence of leukocytosis. In addition, the client should be monitored for the development of hemorrhage, wound infection, atelectasis, and sepsis.

Postoperative respiratory complications such as atelectasis or pneumonia are a major consideration for the client who has had a lumbar–flank incision. The client who guards against the use of respiratory muscles may limit deep breathing and adequate postoperative coughing to clear secretions. Sufficient pain relief will facilitate the necessary coughing and deep breathing exercises. Direct external support also may assist the client with these exercises. In addition, liberal fluid intake will loosen and thin secretions and facilitate expectoration. Acute renal failure from obstruction or sepsis is another possible complication.

A nephrostomy tube may be placed if fragments of a renal calculus remain. This U-shaped or circular tube inserted directly into the kidney is attached to closed gravity drainage or to a urostomy appliance. Its purpose is to divert urine temporarily or permanently or to instill irrigating fluid.

Care of the nephrostomy tube includes evaluating for bleeding at the site, ensuring that the catheter drains freely, and never clamping the tube (any blockage of the tube will result in acute hydronephrosis). Encourage a large fluid intake to dilute both urine and elements that form calculi. An acidic urine also will prevent calculus formation. The tube can be irrigated (usually by the physician) to flush out fragments using small amounts (10 mL or less) of a solution with an acid pH, such as renacidin or hemiacidrin. Irrigations are controversial because they are potential causes of renal damage or infection. If there is a nephrostomy tube from each kidney, maintain separate output records for each. Leg bags permit the ambulatory client to move about. Teach clients how to avoid further calculi development.

Hydroureter and Hydronephrosis

A *hydroureter* is an enlargement of the lumen of the ureter as the result of obstruction distal to the point of the enlargement (see Figures 26–5B and C). Unilateral hydroureter might occur as a result of an obstruction within the ureter from a calculus at the U-V junction, whereas bilateral hydroureter might occur from an obstruction at the bladder neck or within the urethra. When obstruction to the urinary outflow causes the accumulation of fluid under pressure in the renal pelvis, it results in distention of the renal pelvis and calyces. This condition, known as *hydronephrosis,* is accompanied by severe atrophy of the renal parenchyma (see Figure 26–5A).

Clinical Manifestations

Pain is a common manifestation as the ureteral musculature enters a spasm. In bilateral hydroureter, symptoms will include a decrease in or absence of urinary output. Bladder distention may also be present if the obstruction is distal to the bladder neck. With hydronephrosis there may be dull flank pain, local tenderness, and vomiting or gastrointestinal upset as the distended kidney presses on the stomach. Infection or renal failure develops if the problem is not corrected quickly.

Medical Measures

Medical treatment includes diagnostic testing to identify the cause of the obstruction and pharmacologic treatment to manage the symptoms:

- Narcotics for relief of pain
- Antispasmodics to relieve ureteral spasm
- Antibiotics and urinary antiseptics to prevent or treat infection
- Antiemetics to control nausea and vomiting

Urinary catheterization will be necessary if there is urinary retention with bladder distention. An in-dwelling catheter may be required to continue urinary drainage and prevent recurrence of the obstruction. A nephrostomy tube may be used to drain urine from the renal pelvis. Antibiotics may be prescribed if infection is present. Surgical interventions may be required, such as ureterolithotomy, cystoscopy with prostatic resection (see Unit 11) or fulguration of bladder tumors, or nephrectomy if irreparable kidney damage has occurred.

Specific Nursing Measures

Take careful measurements of the client's intake, output, and weight. Providing adequate pain relief is essential. Educational preparation for diagnostic tests and emotional support for proposed procedures will be necessary. The client is likely to have concerns about permanent alteration in kidney function and thus may be quite anxious. Other measures depend on the type of pharmacologic management or surgical intervention selected.

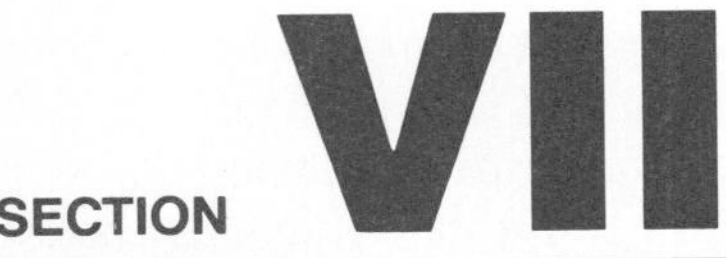

Traumatic Disorders

Injuries to the kidneys, ureters, or bladder may significantly affect the client's overall health. Preservation of renal function is the primary goal. Loss of a single kidney from trauma may not be life threatening assuming the other kidney is functioning adequately, but it can have serious consequences (see client implications for nephrectomy above). In addition, clients who experience renal trauma are often victims of other abdominal trauma that may be life threatening.

The history of the client with a traumatic disorder is often the most significant part of the diagnosis. Gunshot or stab wounds are quite obvious, but only the history may disclose less obvious traumatic events. Physical sports involving heavy direct contact, such as football or ice hockey, may result in injuries that did not seem significant at the time. Other sports generally not labeled as contact sports, such as baseball, basketball, snow skiing, tobogganing, and horseback riding, all may involve heavy blows to the back or ribs. A history of rib fractures, chest injuries, or abdominal injuries should always suggest the potential for renal trauma.

Renal Trauma

The kidneys are well protected from injury because of their structural placement partially within the rib cage and under the strong muscles of the back and spine. However, about 50% of all injuries involving the urinary system are reported to involve the kidneys. Minor injuries include contusions, hematomas, and simple lacerations of the cortex. Major injuries involve significant laceration of the renal parenchyma, loss of renal parenchyma, or injury to a major branch of the renal artery. Critical injuries involve lacerations of the renal artery, renal vein, or renal pelvis. A transplanted kidney is not as well protected from injury, so abdominal injuries to the transplant recipient may result in significant renal trauma.

Abdominal gunshot or stab wounds may affect either or both kidneys. Automobile accidents, automobile–pedestrian accidents, motorcycle accidents, or sports injuries may result in blunt trauma. All levels of involvement—minor, major, or critical—may occur.

Clinical Manifestations

Gross or microscopic hematuria, flank pain, abdominal pain, or a combination are the most common manifestations of renal trauma. Flank pain may be related to the direct force of the injury or to bleeding in the parenchyma or under the capsule. A significant hematoma may develop in the retroperitoneal spaces, and blood clots that form and descend into the ureter may result in pain that mimics renal colic and obstruction.

Medical Measures

Emergency measures include appropriate radiologic testing to evaluate the extent of traumatic injury; abdominal ultrasonography, CT scan, and renal arteriography are among the most useful tests. Significant hemorrhage occurs with renal pedicle injuries; therefore, blood, volume expanders, and fluids are administered parenterally to support blood pressure and perfusion of vital organs. Surgical intervention is required to control hemorrhage, preserve renal functions, and prevent death.

For nonpenetrating and minor renal injuries, a conservative approach is generally accepted, including bed rest; monitoring of laboratory data such as hemoglobin, hematocrit, serum creatinine, and BUN levels; and careful evaluation of fluid balance. Minor bleeding ceases from the tamponade effect within the kidney capsule. Recall that the kidney is contained in a capsule that expands or stretches only minimally. As bleeding occurs, blood fills the renal capsule, exerting pressure on the source of bleeding and thus stopping the hemorrhage (the tamponade effect).

Penetrating injuries, in contrast, necessitate surgical exploration to ensure that bleeding is controlled and other tissue tears, especially intraperitoneal lacerations, are repaired. Nephrectomy, partial nephrectomy, and renal bench surgery with autotransplantation are potential surgical interventions for renal trauma.

Antibiotics are generally prescribed for clients with penetrating renal trauma. Antibiotic dosages must be adjusted approximately when compromise of renal function is present or the development of toxicity is evident. Gunshot and stab wounds often perforate the peritoneum and abdominal organs such as the intestine, so analgesics are required to control the pain.

Specific Nursing Measures

Monitor urine output and vital signs hourly, laboratory values (eg, hemoglobin, hematocrit, BUN, and electrolytes), and fluid balance. Observe the client for hypovolemic shock that may occur because of hemorrhage or peritonitis from urine leaking into the peritoneum. The administration of blood, fluids, volume expanders, antibiotics, and medications for pain relief is a primary nursing responsibility.

Ureteral Trauma

Ureteral injuries are relatively rare, because the ureters are deep and well protected. When it occurs, however, injury to the ureter or ureters is significant because of the resulting loss of continuity for urinary drainage. The majority of ureteral injuries result from penetrating trauma such as gunshot or stab wounds or from accidental ligation or unintentional incision during another surgical procedure.

Clinical Manifestations

Alteration in urinary output is the most common manifestation of ureteral trauma. Anuria is common, and abdominal pain, fever, and chills may be present if peritonitis develops from the leakage of urine into the peritoneum. In addition, if there is an abdominal incision, urine may leak to the surface or exit via a drain.

Medical Measures

Recognition of ureteral injury should be followed by surgical measures to reconstruct the continuity of the urinary tract. Peritonitis, if present, should be treated without delay by antibiotics. In addition, analgesics will promote comfort. Renal function and fluid replacement must be monitored carefully until the integrity of the ureter has been reestablished.

Specific Nursing Measures

Assess urine output and observe the client for symptoms of peritonitis (elevated temperature, abdominal discomfort, and tenderness).

Bladder Trauma

Nonpenetrating injuries to the bladder are usually contusions, whereas penetrating injuries result in rupture with leakage of urine. Although the bladder is somewhat protected by its position in the lower pelvis, bladder injury is common with pelvic fractures. A full bladder is an increased risk to injury from perforation during a traumatic or compression injury. Gunshot and stab wounds may penetrate the urinary bladder. Automobile injuries, especially from seat belt placement over a distended bladder, and automobile–pedestrian accidents are common causes of bladder trauma. The risk of bladder injury from seat belt use is minimized by keeping the bladder nondistended.

Clinical Manifestations

Manifestations of bladder injury include hematuria, difficulty with voiding, or absence of urine output. Suprapubic pain or tenderness is common, as is scrotal or perineal swelling from the extravasation of urine into these issues.

Medical Measures

The immediate recognition and treatment of bladder rupture are important in saving the client's life. Conservative treatment—rest and constant drainage via a Foley catheter—is used for bladder contusions. A suspected bladder tear or laceration, however, requires surgical exploration. Surgical intervention also is needed to repair penetrating bladder trauma. Antibiotics are usually required to treat the infection that occurs with leakage of urine into the peritoneum or other tissues.

Specific Nursing Measures

Major nursing implications include recognizing symptoms that may identify a previously undetected bladder rupture; for example, persistent, unidentified fever may result from leakage of urine.

Monitor intake and output to ensure that fluid balance is achieved. Alterations in urinary output should be detected as soon as possible so corrective measures may be initiated.

Appropriate health teaching and emotional support should be provided, because the client and family or significant others will be concerned about normalization of urinary function. In addition, they may have concerns about sexuality or sexual function.

SECTION 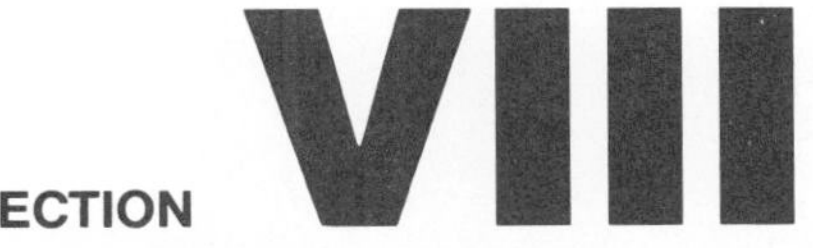

Renal Failure

Acute renal failure that is reversible occurs rapidly over a period of hours or days. Causes of acute renal failure are divided into three categories: prerenal, renal, and postrenal. *Prerenal causes* diminish renal perfusion but do not cause tubular damage unless prolonged. Examples are shock, severe hemorrhage, severely diminished cardiac output, and renal artery stenosis or thrombosis. Damage to the renal parenchyma characterizes *renal causes,* which result from acute glomerulonephritis or ATN. *Postrenal causes* include any cause of urinary tract obstruction, such as bilateral ureteral stones, benign prostatic hypertrophy, or carcinoma. Therefore, in prerenal and postrenal causes the kidney is normal, but with renal causes the kidney is damaged. About 75% of all acute renal failure is caused by ATN (Holloway, 1988). Despite the cause, clients with acute renal failure cannot excrete waste products or regulate fluid, electrolyte, and acid–base balances.

The four phases of acute renal failure are: onset, oliguric, diuretic, and recovery. The *onset phase* can be as short as 24 hours or as long as one week. Detection of acute renal failure and prevention of further renal damage are the priorities during this period. In the *oliguric phase,* urine output falls below 400 mL/day. This phase usually begins within 48 hours of the renal insult and may last up to 2 weeks. During this phase serum creatinine and BUN levels rise steadily. The *diuretic phase* begins when urine output rises above 400 mL/day, but BUN and creatinine levels continue to increase. Regeneration of kidney tubules occurs during this phase, which generally lasts about 2 weeks. During the *recovery phase,* which lasts about 4 to 12 months, laboratory values begin to stabilize and return to normal. Hyperkalemia is the most common and serious problem. Dialysis will most likely be required if uremia develops, and it should continue until the client stabilizes in the recovery phase. A description of the stages of acute renal failure, fluid allowance, and dietary modification is in Table 26–10.

Chronic renal failure, which is irreversible, is a slow, gradual loss of renal function that develops over a period of months or years. Chronic renal failure is characterized by three stages: diminished renal reserve, renal insufficiency, and uremia. Renal damage occurs in the *diminished renal reserve stage.* Nitrogenous wastes do not accumulate, however, because 50% of renal function still exists. With *renal insufficiency,* nitrogenous wastes in the blood increase slightly, but the kidneys function well enough to sustain life. Metabolic or physiologic stresses may be difficult for the kidneys to handle, however. During the *uremic stage,* the creatinine clearance value falls below 10 mL/min. Nitrogenous wastes and fluid, electrolyte, and acid–base imbalances may necessitate dialysis or renal transplanta-

Table 26–10
Stages of Acute Renal Failure

Stage	Duration	Laboratory Data	Urine Output	Fluid Allowance	Dietary Modification
Onset	24 h–1 wk	↑ Creatinine ↑ BUN	Normal or decreasing	No restriction	None
Oliguric/anuric	8–15 days (average)	↑ Creatinine ↑ BUN ↑ Potassium ↑ Phosphorus ↓ Calcium ↓ Bicarbonate	Oliguria: $<$400 mL/24 h Anuria: $<$100 mL/24 h	600 mL + urine output for previous 24 h	Restricted potassium; low protein to control BUN; high-calorie, high-carbohydrate diet and fat to meet nutritional needs; parenteral or enteral nutrition may be needed; no added salt if hypertensive
Diuretic					
Early	Variable	↑ Creatinine ↑ BUN ↑ Potassium ↑ Phosphorus ↓ Calcium ↓ Bicarbonate	Greater than 400 or 100 mL/24 h; may reach 2 or 3 L per day	At least equal to urinary output plus 600 mL/24 h	Continue as above; monitor lab data
Late	Variable	↑ ↓ Creatinine ↑ ↓ BUN ↑ ↓ Potassium ↑ ↓ Phosphorus ↓ ↑ Calcium ↓ ↑ Bicarbonate	Usually stabilizes between 2 and 3 L/24 h	As above	Protein and potassium no longer restricted; high caloric needs remain
Recovery	Up to 12 m	Creatinine and BUN levels stabilize near preinsult normal	Around 1500 mL/24 h	Normal	Normal diet; sodium not restricted unless high blood pressure remains

tion to sustain life. A case study for the client with chronic renal failure is presented at the end of this chapter.

Renal Transplantation

Renal transplantation is a surgical procedure in which the kidney of one person (the donor) is placed into the body of another person (the recipient). The donor may be a relative from the immediate family (a living-related donor or LRD), or a cadaver (CAD). For clients with end-stage renal disease (chronic renal failure), a renal transplantation is necessary to maintain life without the need for chronic dialysis.

The left kidney of the donor is preferred, because the left renal vein is longer. In addition, the ureter of the donor is also removed and included in the transplantation procedure. The kidney transplant recipient's own kidneys are not removed unless chronic infection is present. However, the kidneys may have been removed previously because of problems with hypertension or infection.

The renal transplant is placed in the right lower quadrant, generally in the anterior iliac fossa (Figure 26–8). The peritoneal cavity is not incised, so the kidney is placed retroperitoneally. Three anastomoses are necessary to ensure that the transplanted kidney will be able to function normally: The renal artery is usually anastomosed to the hypogastric artery or internal iliac artery; the renal vein is anastomosed to the iliac vein; and the ureter must be anastomosed to a ureter or the bladder.

Recipient Selection

Renal transplantation should be considered for the client who has systemic effects of uremia, or whose renal function has deteriorated to a creatinine clearance rate of 5 mL/min. Clients with severe cardiovascular problems, connective tissue disorders, or immune problems are not the best transplant candidates. These disorders can cause the same kidney destruction in a transplanted kidney.

Staff evaluate each client individually for the potential benefit from transplant surgery. After a complete physical examination, a psychiatric evaluation also is conducted to be sure the client is mentally able to withstand the procedure and the idea of having someone else's kidney in his or her body.

Donor Selection

The LRD makes a conscious, voluntary decision to donate a kidney to a family member. To help a loved one, he or she takes on the restrictions associated with living with one kidney, such as avoiding all contact sports. This individual and family decision is different from the circumstances that surround the gift of an organ from a CAD, who voluntarily indicated the desire to have his or her organs used in the event of death or whose next of kin made the decision to donate. Difficult decisions in a time of crisis—accepting the unexpected death of a loved one and agreeing to the organ donation—may be facilitated through nursing counseling and education. The dignity and level of care provided for the CAD donor client should be of the highest level throughout the entire period. The donor client's family, while coping with the grief of the loss of a loved one, may feel a sense of satisfaction and some happiness that the organ donation will help another person to live without the restriction of chronic dialysis.

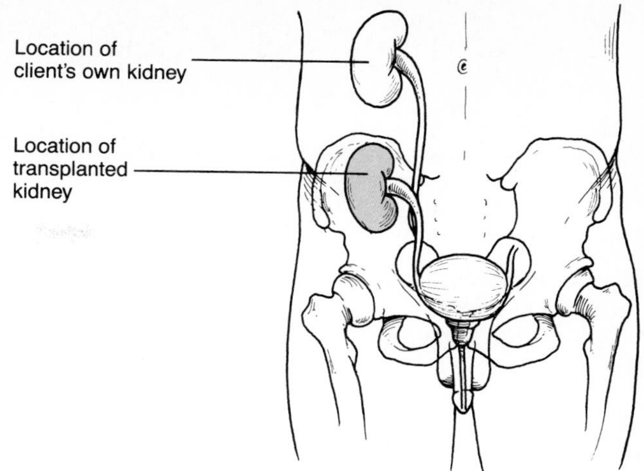

Figure 26–8

Location of transplanted kidney in the anterior iliac fossa.

Potential LRDs include full-blooded mothers, fathers, sisters, brothers, sons, or daughters over the age of 18. An identical twin provides the best possible match. First, the donor relative's ABO blood compatibility with the recipient must be established. Following the determination of ABO blood compatibility, histocompatibility testing is done.

Before surgery, the donor client is given an in-depth physical examination, and a health history is taken to ensure excellent health. Renal function, blood chemistries, and electrolytes are evaluated, and a glucose tolerance test is performed. The donor's ability to live without one kidney must be established.

The names of clients without potential LRDs are placed on a national computer network, the United Network for Organ Sharing (UNOS), that lists all clients and describes their blood types and HLA requirements. This network enables transplant centers to communicate a client's transplant needs and the availability of CAD kidneys and is described in the resources listing at the end of Chapter 25.

The CAD must have met established criteria for brain death, be free of systemic diseases, and have normal kidney perfusion and renal function. Once brain death and other criteria for donation have been established, renal perfusion must be maintained to keep the kidney viable.

The physiologic and psychosocial/lifestyle implications for an LRD are discussed in Table 26–3 on nephrectomy. The implications for the renal transplant recipient are discussed in Table 26–11.

Table 26–11
Renal Transplant: Implications for the Recipient Client 

Physiologic Implications	Psychosocial/Lifestyle Implications
Potential complications are: pneumonia, GI bleeding, rejection of kidney	Improved quality of life
Postoperative anuria in transplanted kidney may require temporary dialysis	Altered mental states from steroids; mainly euphoria, but sometimes depression
Systemic effects of lifetime steroid therapy	Immunosuppressive drugs taken for life of kidney
Increased risk of infection from immunosuppressant therapy	Need to avoid crowds to prevent infection
	Body image changes associated with immunosuppressants
	Adjustment to someone else's kidney
	Constant fear of rejection of kidney
	Financial concerns
	Changes in family roles are often required

Nursing Implications

PREOPERATIVE CARE Transplant recipients need a great deal of emotional care before and after surgery. Answer their questions honestly but avoid terrifying them with possible difficulties. Good preoperative teaching can help the client understand the preparation necessary for surgery, as well as what to expect during and after surgery. The client is usually dialyzed the day before surgery to correct the fluid, acid–base, and electrolyte imbalances, as well as to remove urea and other dialyzable body wastes. For the CAD transplant recipient, dialysis is done a few hours before surgery if the client has not been dialyzed that day.

Blood is drawn to determine leukocyte counts and prothrombin time, as well as hemoglobin, hematocrit, serum bilirubin, creatinine, and electrolyte values. Typing and crossmatching of leukocyte-poor blood is also done. A sample is sent for final tissue type crossmatch. A physical examination, chest x-ray, and ECG are completed, along with other usual preoperative measures. Weigh the client before surgery.

The client will receive IM or PO antibiotics and IV push methylprednisolone sodium succinate (Solu-Medrol) in the afternoon preceding surgery. Azathioprine (Imuran) is given 2 days before surgery when possible, and heparin is given 1 hour before surgery. Usually IV antibiotics, Solu-Medrol, and azathioprine are sent to the operating room with the client in the appropriate dosage. A 0.5% solution of neomycin also may be sent with the client for bladder irrigation before surgery.

POSTOPERATIVE CARE On the client's arrival from the operating room, weigh the client on the bed scale before assisting the client into bed. Any bedclothes must be weighed separately once the client is in bed and their weight subtracted. The daily weight is compared to the baseline weight to determine whether the client is retaining fluid or diuresing following the transplant surgery.

The usual postanesthetic checks are carried out, and blood pressure, pulse, respiration, and CVP are monitored at least hourly. Temperature is recorded every 4 hours. Urine output is recorded (a Foley catheter is placed during surgery), and urine specific gravity and sugar are checked hourly. The urine should be clear or light pink, indicating that clots are not developing. Take extreme caution to maintain catheter patency: no clots, no kinking or twisting, no pressure, and direct gravitational flow. Obstruction and bladder distention can result in excessive tension upon the sutures of the ureteral anastomosis and can seriously jeopardize the success of the surgical procedure. A backup of urine may also cause an infection to develop.

Monitor the results of urine and blood studies and chest x-rays. Urinalysis and cultures for bacteria and fungus are performed when the urinary catheter is removed, when the temperature is 101° F (38° C) or above, and weekly.

If oliguria or anuria develops, the cause must be identified and corrected as soon as possible. Postoperative anuria suggests an acute rejection process or a blockage of the catheter. Oliguria may result from hypovolemia or ischemic injury that causes acute tubular necrosis (ATN).

At least two IV lines are used for IV and fluid therapy: a central venous line and a peripheral line. Some institutions prefer a flow-directed, balloon-tipped catheter. Replacement of urine output with D5/0.5NS and administration of supplemental potassium is regulated according to urine and serum values. The protocols for fluid replacement may vary from center to center.

Analgesics are prescribed on a p.r.n. basis. Transplant recipients may not have pain as great as other abdominal surgical clients because the transplanted kidney is in the retroperitoneal space. Nevertheless, they do have pain. Assess the client's need for analgesics and offer them. The bladder spasms that are quite severe and common following surgery can be relieved by belladonna and opium suppositories. Keeping the client comfortable will make coughing, ambulating, and sleeping easier. Do not gatch the bed at the knee or elevate the foot of the bed. Both of these actions may increase the potential for thrombosis. Initiate ambulation as soon as possible, preferably the first postoperative day.

Pneumonia is a major concern in the renal transplant client. Thus, the nurse must maintain pulmonary function through rigorous attention to postoperative turning, coughing, and deep breathing exercises. Adequate hydration will assist in the mobilization of secretions. Incentive spirometry is commonly prescribed to decrease alveolar hypoventilation. Other measures, such as intermittent positive-pressure breathing treatments or the administration of medications through nebulization may be needed to ensure adequate clearance of pulmonary secretions.

Immunosuppressive agents increase the possibility of infection, particularly from cytomegalovirus (CMV) or from *Pneumocystis carinii.* In the past, reverse isolation was used to reduce this threat, but the cause of most infections was the client's own flora. Reverse isolation is now used only if the WBC count falls below 800. Prevention and early detection of infection are major nursing goals. Aseptic technique for appropriate procedures, handwashing before and after each client contact, and use of common sense to avoid unnecessary exposure to persons with upper respiratory tract infections are essential. Persons with upper respiratory tract infections who must be in contact with the transplant recipient should wear a mask and follow strict handwashing techniques.

The client may have a nasogastric tube attached to low suction until peristalsis of the gastrointestinal tract returns. Often the client is merely kept NPO and started on liquids as peristalsis returns. Routinely check nasogastric drainage and stool for blood, because gastrointestinal bleeding is a major risk in the transplant client given high doses of immunosuppressants after surgery to avoid or treat rejection. Other factors that contribute to gastrointestinal bleeding include the stress of surgery and the alteration in platelet aggregation associated with uremia. Consequently, antacids are commonly prescribed as often as hourly; low-magnesium, low-sodium, phosphate-binding antacids are the most common. Laxatives may be needed if antacids are taken every 2 hours or more.

After removing the client's urinary catheter, instruct the client to void hourly while awake and awaken the client every 4 hours at night to void. This prevents pressure in the bladder, which could disrupt the anastomosis of the ureter to the bladder.

TRANSPLANTATION REJECTION Rejection cannot be prevented completely, but with proper management rejection can usually be reversed and renal function returned. If rejection is irreversible, the donor kidney is removed.

Early diagnosis of kidney rejection is mandatory. Maintain a close, constant observation of the client to detect symptoms such as a swollen and tender kidney, weight gain, elevated temperature and blood pressure, decreased urine output, anorexia, drowsiness, and elevated serum creatinine values.

Hyperacute rejection (anuria with failure of the kidney to function) occurs immediately after the kidney is implanted. There is no treatment for hyperacute rejection, and a transplant nephrectomy is performed immediately. *Acute rejection* may develop within 1 week or as long as 2 years after the transplant surgery. The symptoms are similar to those of acute renal failure with oliguria. Steroid medications are increased, and the client is supported until the rejection passes. An episode or two of acute rejection occurs for almost all clients. Most episodes reverse, but some do not. *Chronic rejection* occurs gradually, generally over months to years. Its onset is detected by gradually worsening renal function as determined by elevation of the serum creatinine and BUN levels. Other electrolyte abnormalities may also be present, such as elevated phosphorus and decreased bicarbonate. Edema and hypertension may be increasing. No treatment for chronic rejection exists, and the graft eventually is lost.

In an attempt to increase graft survival, a number of centers now use donor-specific transfusions (DSTs). This procedure involves the administration of 200 mL of fresh blood from an LRD donor to the proposed LRD recipient every 2 weeks for three transfusion administrations.

Treatment of rejection includes the administration of large doses of steroids; doses of 1000 to 2000 mg are common. Methylprednisolone sodium succinate (Solu-Medrol) should never be given quickly; it is given over 20 to 30 minutes for 6 to 7 days, depending on the duration of the rejection and the age of the client. Such high doses require antacids to prevent gastrointestinal bleeding; 30 mL of an antacid is given every 2 hours if the client is receiving 1 g of Solu-Medrol, and 30 mL every hour if the client is bleeding or receiving 2 g of Solu-Medrol. Furosemide (Lasix) IV should not be given within 2 hours of Solu-Medrol infusions to prevent cardiac arrhythmias. Ambulation helps to prevent the muscle atrophy that accompanies high-dose steroid therapy.

Client/Family Teaching

Client education about the pharmacologic regimen that will be prescribed to prevent the rejection of the graft is extensive. Advise the client to wear identification jewelry that clearly notes that the client is a transplant recipient and requires immunosuppressive agents. Inform the client that therapy normally taken may not be adequate if excessive physiologic or emotional stress occurs. The stress of trauma, surgery, or infection may precipitate an adrenal crisis if it precipitates adrenal insufficiency.

Commonly prescribed immunosuppressants include prednisone, azathioprine (Imuran) and cyclophosphamide (Cytoxan), usually in combination. Prednisone is administered with either azathioprine or cyclophosphamide. Cyclosporine is also administered in combination with corticosteroids. Complications with long-term steroid use are discussed in Chapter 31. Cyclosporine is administered to clients at high risk for the development of rejection or in whom rejection has been detected. Prior to the availability of cyclosporine, transplantation might not have even been tried in these high-risk clients, or the amount of immunosuppressive drugs required to save the graft would have resulted in death to the client from infection. Side effects of cyclosporine are discussed in Chapter 19 in the section on heart transplantation.

Immune suppression also may be achieved by the use of antilymphocyte and antithymocyte preparations to provoke the formation of antibodies to the antigens administered in the agent. These agents are largely experimental and may be in the form of a serum or a globulin. Problems include hypersensitivity reactions, the possibility of anaphylaxis, and the development of opportunistic infections.

The need for the client to understand the importance of taking the prescribed medications cannot be overemphasized. Clients must understand that doses cannot be missed. If they have the flu and cannot take the medication by mouth, the client should seek medical care and receive it intravenously. Emergency IM administration of prednisone should be taught to the client, family, or significant others. Instruct clients about any other medications they may take, such as anticoagulants or antihypertensives.

Help the client learn the symptoms and signs of rejection. Many transplant centers ask the client to keep a log of daily weights, blood pressure, and temperature measurements to help the physician monitor the client's progress. Regular creatinine values, WBC counts, and prothrombin times are often recorded in the log as well. Compliance increases when the client understands the rationale for treatments. In some transplant centers, selected clients, under nursing supervision, give themselves their own medications and record weight, vital signs, and laboratory values.

The client should understand the need to avoid crowds and any risk of infection. Follow-up visits for the evaluation of renal function and overall health status are equally important.

The client must also receive psychologic and emotional support from the nurse to adjust to psychosocial and lifestyle changes. Renal transplant clients always live in fear of rejection. If hyperacute or acute rejection occurs, the joy of receiving the new kidney quickly becomes sorrow. If irreversible rejection occurs later, the loss of the kidney means returning to dialysis, awaiting retransplantation, or both.

Chapter Highlights

Acute tubular necrosis (ATN) is the most common cause of acute renal failure, the sudden deterioration in renal function. It may present a life-threatening situation that requires prompt intervention and management.

A kidney transplant is an alternative to dialysis for clients with chronic renal failure.

Clients with urinary incontinence have physical discomfort, as well as social and emotional embarrassment.

A neurogenic bladder may increase the client's potential for the development of infection, obstruction of the urinary tract, or chronic renal failure.

A continent vesicostomy, which involves the formation of an internal pouch and stoma from existing bladder tissue that can be catheterized via a nipple, is indicated for clients with a neurogenic bladder.

Urinary tract infections account for more than 40% of all nosocomial infections. Treatment of these infections involves the correct administration of antibiotics, ingestion of about 3 L/day of fluid, and client education about hygiene measures to help prevent the development of future infections.

A nephrectomy is the surgical removal of a kidney that is indicated when there is chronic infection, trauma, hemorrhage, tumor, uncontrolled hypertension, an infected calculus, or a desire to donate a kidney to a relative.

A cystectomy involves the surgical excision of all or part of the bladder and is indicated when a large tumor is present.

A urinary diversion procedure is required after a radical cystectomy and may include an ileal conduit, sigmoid conduit, ureterosigmoidostomy, ureteroileosigmoidostomy, or cutaneous ureterostomy.

Clients with a tendency toward formation of urinary calculi should avoid dehydration and maintain a liberal fluid intake. Dietary changes or medications may be prescribed for treatment.

Most common traumatic occurrences interrupt the structural integrity of the kidney or kidneys,

ureter or ureters, or bladder, as well as the vascular supply to these structures.

Symptoms and signs of kidney transplant rejection include elevated blood pressure, temperature, and serum creatinine value; decreased urine output; a swollen and tender kidney; drowsiness; anorexia; and weight gain.

Bibliography

American Cancer Society: *Cancer Facts and Figures.* New York: American Cancer Society, 1987.

Barrett N: Continent vesicostomy: The dry urinary diversion. *Am J Nurs* 1979; 79(3):462–464.

Brown, RO: Nutritional support in acute renal failure. *AANNT J* 1983; 10:25–29.

Buszta C et al: Pregnancy and the renal transplant patient. *ANNA J* 1985; 12(3):183–186.

Cain L, Bigongiari L: The percutaneous nephrostomy tube. *Am J Nurs* 1982; 82:296–298.

Chambers JK: Save your diabetic patient from early kidney damage. *Nurs 83* 1983; 13(5):58–64.

Cockett ATK, Koshiba K: *Manual of Urologic Surgery.* New York: Springer–Verlag, 1980.

Corbet D, Russin M, Hunter P: Extracorporeal shock wave lithotripsy: The nurse's role. *ANNA J* 1985; 12(5):289–293.

Fairman JA: Sexual concerns of the renal transplant patient in the ambulatory care setting: A format for nursing intervention. *AANNT J* 1982; 9(Dec):45–48.

Frank LI, Admire RC: Rhabdomyolysis. *Urol Clin North Am* 1982; 9(2):267–273.

Freed SZ: Urinary incontinence in the elderly. *Hospital Practice* 1982; 10(March):81+.

Glenn JF (editor): *Urologic Surgery,* 3rd ed. Philadelphia: Lippincott, 1983.

Harcum P: Renal nutrition for the renal nurse. *ANNA J* 1984; 11:38–44.

Hart M, Adamek C: Do increased fluids decrease urinary stone formation? *Geriat Nurs* 1984; 5:245–248.

Henrich WL: Nephrotoxicity of non-steroidal anti-inflammatory agents. *Am J Kidney Dis* 1983; 2(4):278–284.

Hinkle MT, Bowditch RW: The great stent mystery: Can you solve it? *Nurs 81* 1981; 11(April):94+.

Holloway NM: *Nursing the Critically Ill Adult: Applying Nursing Diagnosis.* 2nd ed. Menlo Park, CA: Addison–Wesley, 1988.

Irwin BC: Renal transplantation: Advances in immunology. A nursing perspective. *AANNT J* 1983; 10(4):11–15, 22.

Lancaster LE: *The Patient With Renal Disease.* 2nd ed. New York: Wiley, 1984.

McConnell EA, Zimmerman MF: *Care of Patients With Urologic Problems.* Philadelphia: Lippincott, 1983.

McConnell J: Preventing urinary tract infections. *Geriat Nurs* 1984; 5:361–362.

Porter GA, Bennett WM: Nephrotoxin-induced acute renal failure. In: *Contemporary Issues in Nephrology, Vol 6, Acute Renal Failure.* Brenner BM, Stein JH (editors). New York: Churchill Livingstone, 1980.

Price S, Wilson L: *Pathophysiology: Clinical Concepts of Disease Processes,* 2nd ed. New York: McGraw–Hill, 1982.

Richard C: Management of patients with renal and genitourinary disorders. In: *ACCN's Clinical Reference for Critical Care Nursing.* Kinney M, et al (editors). New York: Mc-Graw–Hill, 1981.

Robbins KC et al: Donor-specific transfusions as pretreatment for living related donor transplants and implications for nursing. *Nephrol Nurse* 1983; 5(May/June):4+.

Rose BD: *Pathophysiology of Renal Disease.* New York: McGraw–Hill, 1981.

Rubin P (editor): *Clinical Oncology for Medical Students and Physicians: A Multidisciplinary Approach.* New York: American Cancer Society, 1983.

Ruge CA: Shock (wave) treatment for kidney stones. *Am J Nurs* 1986; 86(4); 400–401.

Schrier RW: *Renal and Electrolyte Disorders,* 2nd ed. Boston: Little, Brown, 1980.

Smith DR: *General Urology,* 10th ed. Los Altos, CA: Lange, 1981.

Solomon J: Does renal failure mean sexual failure? *RN* 1986; (August):41–43.

Sos FA et al: Percutaneous transluminal renal angioplasty in renovascular hypertension due to atheroma or fibromuscular dysplasia. *New Engl J Med* 1983; 309:274–279.

Woods JE: *Clinical Organ Transplantation in Surgical Immunology,* Munster A (editor). New York: Grune & Stratton, 1976.

CASE STUDY

The Client With Chronic Renal Failure

I. Descriptive Data

Mrs Ethel Redding, a 73-year-old black woman, is currently undergoing outpatient peritoneal dialysis 3 days a week for end-stage renal disease secondary to hypertensive nephrosclerosis. She is hypertensive, weak, and anorexic.

II. Personal Data

Date and Time: Sept 5, 1987, 11 AM
Full Name: Ethel Joy Redding
Social Security Number: 000-00-000
Address: 700 Third Ave., Waverly, KS
Telephone: Home: 000-0000
Sex: Female
Age: 73
Birthdate: 4-5-14
Marital Status: Widowed
Race: Black
Religion: Lutheran
Occupation: Retired post office employee
Usual Health Care Provider: Dr John Hoak

III. Health History

Source of Information: Client
Reliability of Informant: Reliable
Chief Complaint: Extreme tiredness and inability to eat

History of Present Illness:

Mrs Redding has had severe hypertension for 12 years. A low-sodium diet and antihypertensive drugs failed to control her blood pressure adequately. In November 1983, she went into renal failure secondary to hypertensive nephrosclerosis. She was placed on hemodialysis. She had several fistula failures and revisions in both arms and the left leg. Following the clotting of the last fistula in her right arm, a Tenckhoff peritoneal catheter was inserted (October 1985). She has been on peritoneal dialysis since that time. During peritoneal dialysis, she has episodes of cramping, nausea, and diarrhea. She associates her decrease in appetite with the peritoneal dialysis procedure.

In October 1984, Mrs Redding had a pacemaker inserted because of a dysrhythmia and was placed on disopyramide (Norpace) 100 mg q.d. and digoxin 0.125 mg Mon, Wed, and Fri. She also takes a stool softener, iron, folate, thiamine, and a multivitamin. Mrs Redding is on a 2 g Na, 50–60 g protein, 50 mEq K^+ diet. However, she lives alone, cooks for herself, and finds it difficult to follow the dietary restrictions.

Past Health History:

Childhood: Measles, mumps, chickenpox
Immunizations: Td, 1982
Surgeries: Pacemaker, Oct 1984; various access (fistula) procedures from 1983–1985
Transfusions: Approximately 5 during hemodialysis
Pregnancies: None
Trauma: None
Allergies: None

Current Medications:

Multivitamin, ī q.d.
Thiamine tablet, ī q.d.
Folate, mg ī q.d.
Disopyramide, 100 mg q.d.
Digoxin, 0.125 mg M,W,F
Ferrous gluconate, 325 mg t.i.d.
Surfak, q.d.

Family History:

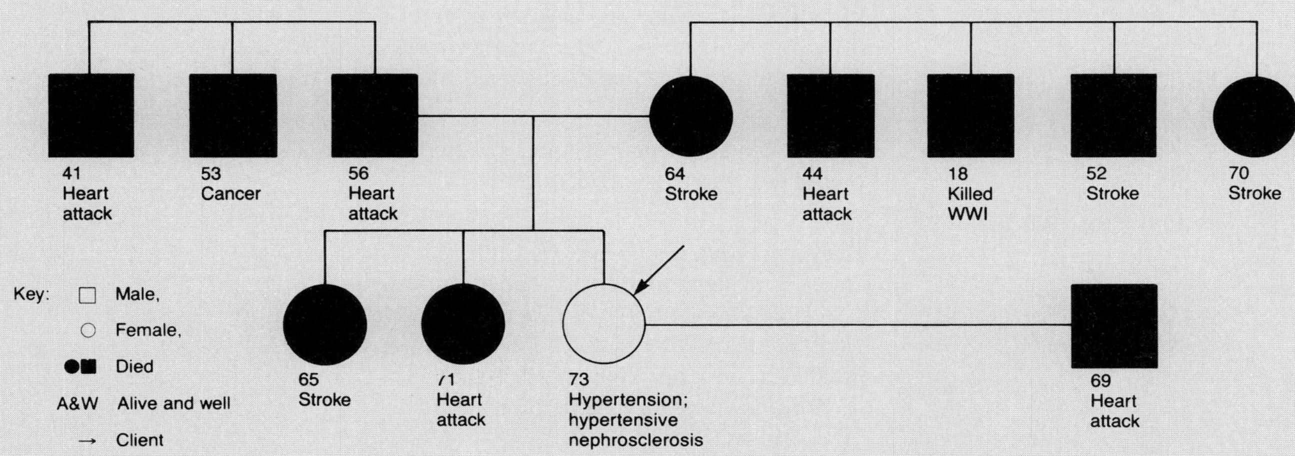

Personal/Social History: The client lives alone in a house she owns. She has several friends who visit her often and transport her to and from dialysis. She is supported by Social Security, and Medicare covers the medical expenses. Her family and husband are deceased. She has no children. A low-salt, low-protein, low-potassium diet is prescribed, which she does not follow carefully because she enjoys ham, tomatoes, beans, and bacon. She attends church regularly. Overall health has been deteriorating for past 3½ years because of renal failure.

Review of Systems:

Skin: Some episodes of itching

Cardiovascular: History of dysrhythmia; pacemaker since 1984; hypertension; arteriovenous fistula failures in extremities

Urinary: Has passed no urine in 3 years

Hematopoietic: History of low hemoglobin values; chronic fatigue

IV. Physical Assessment

Height: 5 ft 3 in

Weight: 128 lb (dry weight)

Vital Signs: BP 160/96; pulse 96; respirations 20; temperature 36°C or 96.8°F

Relevant Organ Systems:

Skin: Pale yellow skin; several healed scars on extremities from previous fistulas, pacemaker site; Tenckhoff catheter present; generalized edema

Chest: Shortness of breath on exertion and during fill stage of dialysis; rales in lower lobes bilaterally

Cardiovascular: Pacemaker set for 72 beats to fire as necessary; generalized edema predialysis; predialysis weight of 134 lb (dry weight is 128)

(Continued)

CASE STUDY (continued)

The Client With Chronic Renal Failure

Gastrointestinal:	Eats 1/8 of food on tray; severe abdominal cramping and diarrhea during dialysis; Tenckhoff catheter with abdominal placement
Urinary:	Anuric
Musculoskeletal:	Some neuromuscular irritability; fatigue
Psychologic:	Sometimes she feels life isn't worth living; feels she is a burden to her friends who take her and pick her up from dialysis 3 days a week; dietary restrictions eliminate all her favorite foods, although often she goes off her diet because food is one of her main enjoyments in life

V. Diagnostic Data

Present predialysis abnormal laboratory results showed decreased hemoglobin and hematocrit and elevated blood urea nitrogen, creatinine, potassium, and triglyceride values

VI. Medical Regimen

Diet, 2 g Na, 50–60 g protein, 50–60 mEq K^+
Dialysis: 15 h/week, Mon, Wed, Fri
Use a 30% solution if 0–3 lb above dry weight
Use a 50% solution if 4–5 lb above dry weight
Add 250 mL of D50 in water if more than 6 lb above dry weight
4000 U heparin per 2000 mL dialysate
40 mEq KCI to every bottle of dialysate

VII. Nursing Care Plan, by Nursing Diagnosis

Client Care Goals	Plan/Nursing Implementation	Expected Outcomes
Noncompliance (with fluid and dietary restrictions) related to negative consequences of treatment regimen		
Will discuss feelings about her illness and the dietary and fluid restrictions; compliance with dietary and fluid restrictions will improve	Nonjudgmental, supportive approach to client; attempt to understand how disease and necessary restrictions affect her life; work with client regarding foods; methods of food preparation; seasonings that limit sodium, protein, and potassium. Consider more frequent meals. Involve nutritionist; help client understand process of fluid retention and its relation to diet, energy levels, and breathing; since depression is an additional cause of fatigue, consider referral to a mental health nurse clinician	Has improved understanding of reasons for fatigue, shortness of breath; feels comfortable verbalizing her feelings of frustration; improved compliance with diet restrictions, absence of cramping and diarrhea during dialysis
Fluid volume excess related to kidney failure		
Maintains target weight	Assess predialysis weight and lung sounds; change full time and dialysate amounts as needed to minimize diarrhea and cramping; encourage and praise client appropriately; inform client of target weight to maintain between dialysis treatments	Weight gain of no more than 8 lbs. between dialysis treatments; improved breathing pattern

Client Care Goals	Plan/Nursing Implementation	Expected Outcome
Bowel elimination, altered: constipation related to medication side-effects		
Normal bowel function	Administer ferrous gluconate after dialysis and not with antacid; explain that iron turns stools black and also causes constipation; encourage continuing use of stool softener; monitor of bowel function	Will take iron and stool softener as prescribed; will not become constipated
Activity intolerance related to fatigue secondary to low hemoglobin		
Decreased fatigue	Instruct client to perform activities with frequent rest periods; pace activities	
Skin integrity, impairment of: potential for, related to itching and edema		
Client will be more comfortable; decrease in or absence of itching	Dialysis to remove excess fluid; explain causes of itching to client	Increase in client comfort; maintenance of skin integrity
Skin integrity, impairment of: potential for infection related to peritoneal catheter		
Will recognize symptoms and signs of infection; understands and is comfortable with home care of peritoneal catheter	Use sterile technique when hooking up catheter to dialysis machine; teach client symptoms and signs of infection; teach correct home care of abdominal skin and peritoneal catheter	Client will recognize symptoms and signs of infection; will care for abdominal skin and catheter without problems

UNIT 6

The Client With Neurologic Dysfunction

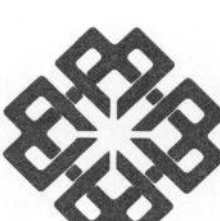

CHAPTER 27

The Nervous System in Health and Illness

Other topics relevant to this content are: Assessment of mental status, **Chapter 5;** Electrocardiography and nursing implications, **Chapter 18.**

Objectives

When you have finished studying this chapter, you should be able to:

Identify the major structural and functional components of the nervous system.

Explain the physiologic mechanisms that regulate the activity of the nervous system.

Specify the role of neurons in message transmission throughout the body.

Describe some pathologic conditions that lead to nervous system dysfunction.

Discuss alterations in other body systems that result from neurologic dysfunction.

Identify and discuss the psychosocial/lifestyle effects of neurologic dysfunction on the client and significant others.

Every physical, mental, and emotional aspect of a person's existence is influenced by continually changing internal and external environments. To deal with these changes effectively, the nervous system must perceive and interpret the changes and then quickly initiate, coordinate, and modulate body responses. The nervous system is always "on alert." Its job is endless because the environment is never static.

SECTION I

Structural and Functional Interrelationships

An understanding of neurologic structure and function and the interdependence of body systems is an essential part of the nurse's knowledge base. With this knowledge, the nurse can effectively assess and plan care for the client with nervous system dysfunction.

Structure of the Neuron

Neurons (nerve cells) are primary components of the nervous system. Working alone or as units, they detect environmental changes and initiate body responses to maintain homeostasis. Each neuron is composed of a cell body, an axon, and a varying number of dendrites. Both axons and dendrites vary in size and shape. The *axons*, ranging in length from miniscule to over a meter, transmit messages throughout the central and peripheral nervous systems. Each cell has only one axon, but axonal branching is common and allows for broader dissemination of neuronal transmissions. *Dendrites*, the processes of neurons that conduct electrical impulses to the cell body, also have varying branching patterns. These characteristics allow for efficient transmission and reception of impulses throughout the body.

Many central and peripheral axons are wrapped in

insulating sheaths of a white fatty substance called *myelin*. The myelin is encased in special cells lying end to end along the axons. Junctures, known as nodes of Ranvier, occur where these cells abut, allowing for more rapid transmission of electrical impulses. Axons often branch at these nodes.

Two distinct types of cells cover axons of the central nervous system (CNS) and peripheral nervous system (PNS). Those located in the CNS are known as oligodendrocytes. These cells and the neurons they protect cannot be replaced or repaired if damaged. On the other hand, Schwann's cells, which surround PNS myelinated and unmyelinated axons, form the neurilemma, the outer membrane that supports and protects PNS axons and sometimes facilitates the healing of damaged axons.

Groups of neurons called nuclei provide routes for the transmission of complex afferent and efferent impulses. Clusters of neurons in the PNS are referred to as ganglia. *Fasciculi* are bundles of neurons encased in a covering called perineurium, whereas groups of fasciculi, encased in a covering called epineurium, are referred to as *nerves*. Most nerves are mixed nerves that contain afferent (toward the CNS) and efferent (from the CNS) fibers.

CNS and PNS neurons cannot function independently. Their nutritional and physical support and protection are provided by other cells commonly referred to as glial cells. Glial cells, unlike neurons, are able to undergo mitosis. *Astrocytes*, star-shaped cells with many projections, are the largest and most numerous glial cells. They provide structural support and nutrition to neurons and maintain a biochemical environment supportive of nerve impulse transmission and synaptic activity. If nervous tissue is destroyed, astrocytes multiply in a process called gliosis to fill in the area or line a cavity.

Central Nervous System Structures

The brain is structurally divided into components according to its embryologic development. These components, known as the forebrain, midbrain, hindbrain, and spinal cord, are further divided according to their location within the adult brain.

The Cerebral Cortex

The outer area of the cerebral cortex is composed of gray matter in complex folds called *gyri* or convolutions separated by deep depressions called *fissures* and shallow depressions called *sulci*. These folds make the surface area much greater. The patterning of gyri and sulci is similar in all individuals. Each hemisphere of the cerebral cortex is divided into lobes. The names of the bones of the skull correspond to the lobes of the brain that they protect.

Nerve fiber tracts establish connections between areas within the brain. The *corpus callosum* consists of fibers extending between the right and left hemispheres. The internal capsule also allows networking between areas within the brain. The internal capsule comprises two distinct sections referred to as anterior and posterior limbs. Here afferent and efferent fibers extend from an extensive fan-like radiation of fibers in the cerebrum to link it with the brain stem and spinal cord.

The *basal ganglia*, bodies of gray matter, are located within the white matter of the cerebral hemispheres. This area contains the caudate nucleus, putamen, globus pallidus, thalamus, subthalamus, substantia nigra, and the red nucleus. These structures have many and varied functions including sensory and motor activities and transmission of afferent and efferent signals to appropriate parts of the nervous system. The *hypothalamus*, a small but extremely important area of the brain, is situated just below the thalamus. It receives input from all parts of the body both by neuronal transmission and its blood supply. The hypothalamus, in turn, influences body functions via these same routes.

The *limbic system* comprises a group of structures that influence behavior and responses to stimuli. For example, the sensory system, cerebral cortex, and limbic system are involved in the stimulation of visceral and somatic effectors, which result in psychologic expressions of behavior and emotions (Carpenter & Sutin, 1983).

The *brain stem*, which lies between the diencephalon and the spinal cord, has three sections—the midbrain (superior portion), pons (center portion), and the medulla oblongata. The medulla oblongata joins the spinal cord at the foramen magnum located at the base of the skull. The brain stem contains many fiber tracts that transmit messages to and from the brain. It also serves as a relay station between the cerebellum and brain. Ten of the twelve cranial nerves (CN) located here function much like peripheral nerves (spinal nerves). With the exception of CN IV, the trochlear nerve, they are unlike peripheral nerves in that they innervate tissues ipsilaterally—that is, on the same side of the body.

The Cerebellum

The cerebellum lies in the posterior inferior portion of the cranial vault. It is made up of two hemispheres connected in the center by a structure called the vermis. The superficial area of the cerebellum is composed of gray matter, which lies in even, horizontal folds forming fissures and sulci. White fiber tracts lying below the gray matter provide extensive afferent and efferent connections with the brain stem, cortex, thalamus, and basal ganglia. The cerebellum receives afferent signals via the spinal cord and brain stem. Cerebellar efferent signals travel to the brain stem, thalamus, and motor cortex.

The Spinal Cord

The spinal cord is continuous with the brain stem. It begins at the foramen magnum and descends through the vertebral canal to the level of the first or second lumbar vertebra. Nerve roots known collectively as the *cauda equina* extend off the base of the spinal cord and travel for some distance before exiting at the appropriate intervertebral foramina.

The spinal cord contains neuronal cell bodies, ascending sensory tracts, and descending motor tracts. A cross section of the cord shows a gray center shaped like a capital H surrounded by white fibers. The gray area is made up of neuronal cell bodies, internuncial neurons, neuroglial cells and synapses. Within the center of the gray matter lies the central canal, which is continuous with the fourth ventricle. It may contain CSF but is often filled with cellular debris.

The white fiber area of the cord contains myelinated and unmyelinated fiber tracts, which transmit the many messages essential for maintenance of the body's complex functions. Both sensory and motor tracts are located on each side of the cord.

There are 31 pairs of spinal nerves, each numbered according to the level of the cord section from which it originates. There are 8 pairs of cervical nerves, 12 pairs of thoracic nerves, 5 pairs of lumbar nerves, 5 pairs of sacral nerves, and 1 pair of coccygeal nerves. The first pair of cervical nerves exits between the occipital bone and the first cervical vertebra. Because there are 8 cervical nerves and only 7 cervical vertebrae, spinal lesions are identified according to the cord level rather than the vertebral level. Generally, each cord segment is named for the vertebral body below its exit point.

Peripheral nerve trunks extend from anterior and posterior roots, which unite in the intervertebral foramina. On emerging from the vertebral foramina, they form mixed nerves, which divide into anterior and posterior branches and extend into the periphery to skeletal muscles and skin. Also present are white rami containing autonomic nervous system fibers. The posterior rami divide into smaller nerves connected to the muscles and skin of the posterior surface of the head, neck, and trunk. Anterior rami (except for the thoracic nerves) divide to supply fibers to the skeletal muscles, skin of the extremities, and the anterior and lateral surfaces. Subdivisions of the anterior rami form three complex networks or plexuses, which contain fibers from many nerves. These plexuses are the *cervical plexus, brachial plexus,* and *lumbosacral plexus.* Smaller nerves emerge from these plexuses and continue to subdivide to innervate distal regions of the extremities.

The Autonomic Nervous System

The autonomic nervous system (ANS) comprises two efferent subsystems—the sympathetic and parasympathetic subsystems. Organs influenced by the ANS are controlled by one of the two subsystems (Figure 27–1).

THE SYMPATHETIC NERVOUS SYSTEM Sympathetic nervous system impulses are transmitted to the periphery by tracts of sympathetic fibers containing cell bodies and dendrites that extend within the intermediolateral gray horns of the spinal cord from thoracic spinal nerve 1 to lumbar spinal nerve 2. Because of its location, the sympathetic nervous system is often referred to as the *thoracolumbar division.* Axons leave the cord with the anterior roots of the thoracic and first four lumbar spinal nerves. After exiting, they quickly join the sympathetic trunk via white rami. The sympathetic trunks located on both sides of the cord extend from the second cervical vertebra to the coccyx. The axons, on entering the trunks, extend branches up and down the chain. The sympathetic nervous system preganglionic axons terminate on many postsynaptic ganglia present in organs.

THE PARASYMPATHETIC NERVOUS SYSTEM Cell bodies of the preganglionic neurons of the parasympathetic nervous system are located in two areas. The nuclei of CN III, VII, IX, and X are located in the brain stem and the lateral gray columns of the sacral cord. In the sacral region, parasympathetic axons are present in spinal nerves. Because of these anatomic locations, the parasympathetic nervous system is often referred to as the *craniosacral division* of the ANS.

Speech Centers

About 95% of the population have their speech centers in the left hemisphere of the cerebral cortex. Speech centers in the remaining 5% are in the right hemisphere or (rarely) in both. There is a relation between the preferred hand and the hemisphere controlling speech: most *right-handed* persons' speech centers are in the *left hemisphere; left-handed* persons' speech centers tend to be in the *right hemisphere.* The term *cerebral dominance* refers to the hemisphere containing the speech centers. Two areas within the brain concerned with speech and language are Broca's motor speech area located in the frontal lobe and Wernicke's area located in the superior posterior aspect of the temporal lobe (Figure 27–2).

Cerebral Hemisphere Specialization

Research has demonstrated that both hemispheres have many types of specialization in addition to speech. The dominant hemisphere appears to excel in mathematic calculation and logical analysis of problems, whereas the other hemisphere appears better able to understand complex visual patterns and spatial relations and to appreciate music. Development and effective use of these special skills require that the fibers connecting the hemispheres be intact.

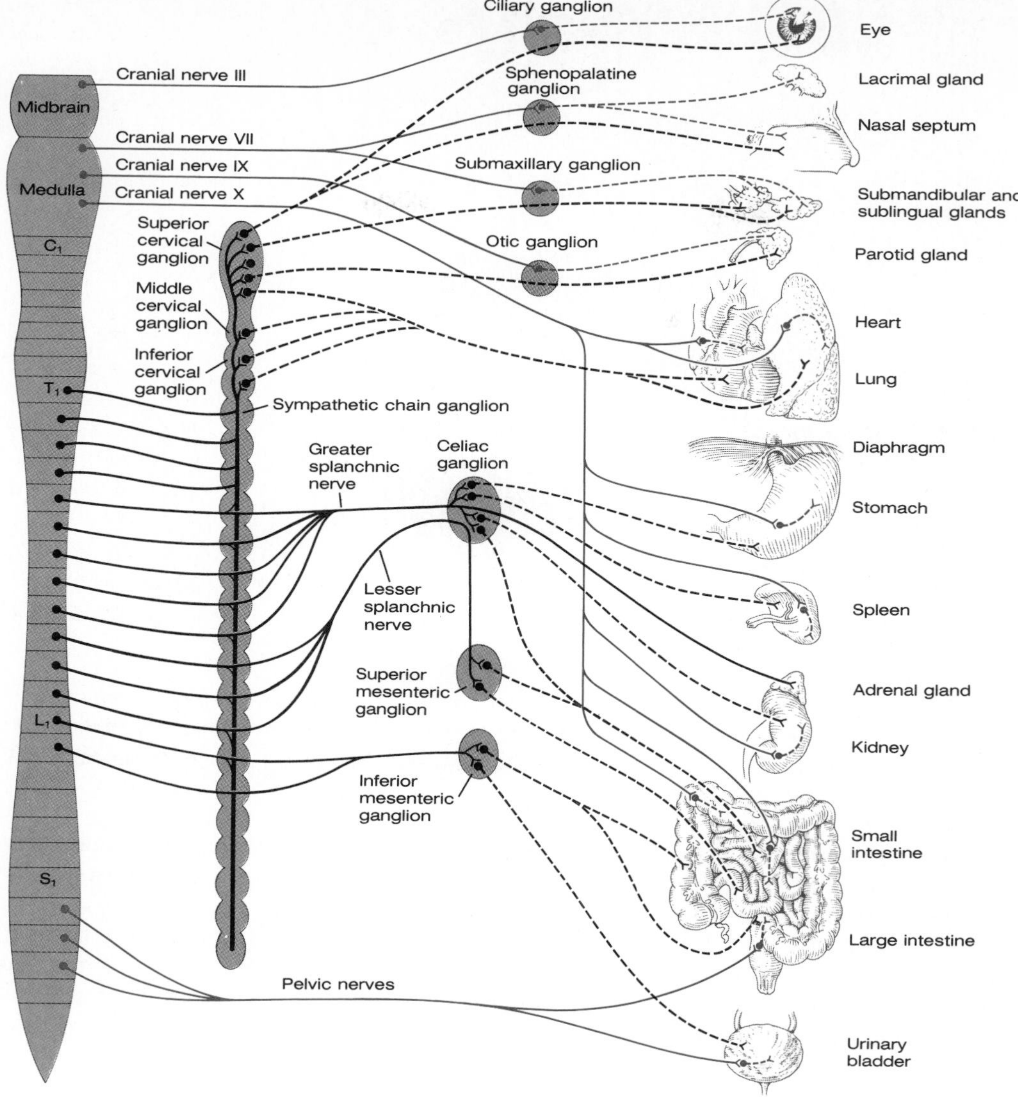

Figure 27–1

Components of the autonomic nervous system. The parasympathetic division is shown in color; the sympathetic division is shown in black. The solid lines indicate preganglionic nerve fibers; the dotted lines indicate postganglionic nerve fibers. SOURCE: *Spence AP, Mason EB:* Human Anatomy and Physiology, *3rd ed. Menlo Park, CA: Benjamin/Cummings, 1987.*

The Blood–Brain Barrier

The blood–brain barrier theory stems from observations that only water, oxygen, carbon dioxide, and alcohol can readily enter or leave the capillaries of the CNS. Large molecules penetrate slowly through special systems or not at all. This protective barrier is believed to prevent sudden, extreme fluctuations in the composition of CNS tissue fluid while allowing nutrients to pass. The blood–brain barrier is thought to be formed within the capillaries by a continous layer of endothelial cells connected by tight junctions. The basement membrane surrounds the endothelium. Astrocytes that lie in close opposition are no longer considered part of this barrier (Carpenter & Sutin, 1983).

The blood–brain barrier protects most of the brain and cord tissue. Exceptions are the pineal body and the posterior lobe of the hypophysis, among others, which are believed to be nourished by vessels with fenestrated endothelia that provide specific sites for the transfer of proteins and solutes irrespective of molecular size and lipid solubility. Tight junctions at the intracellular clefts of the choroid epithelium serve as the blood–brain barrier in the vascular choroid plexuses of the CSF system (Carpenter & Sutin, 1983).

Function of the Nervous System

Neuronal Function

Functionally, neurons are recognized as being *motor* (efferent) neurons, *sensory* (afferent) neurons, or *inter-*

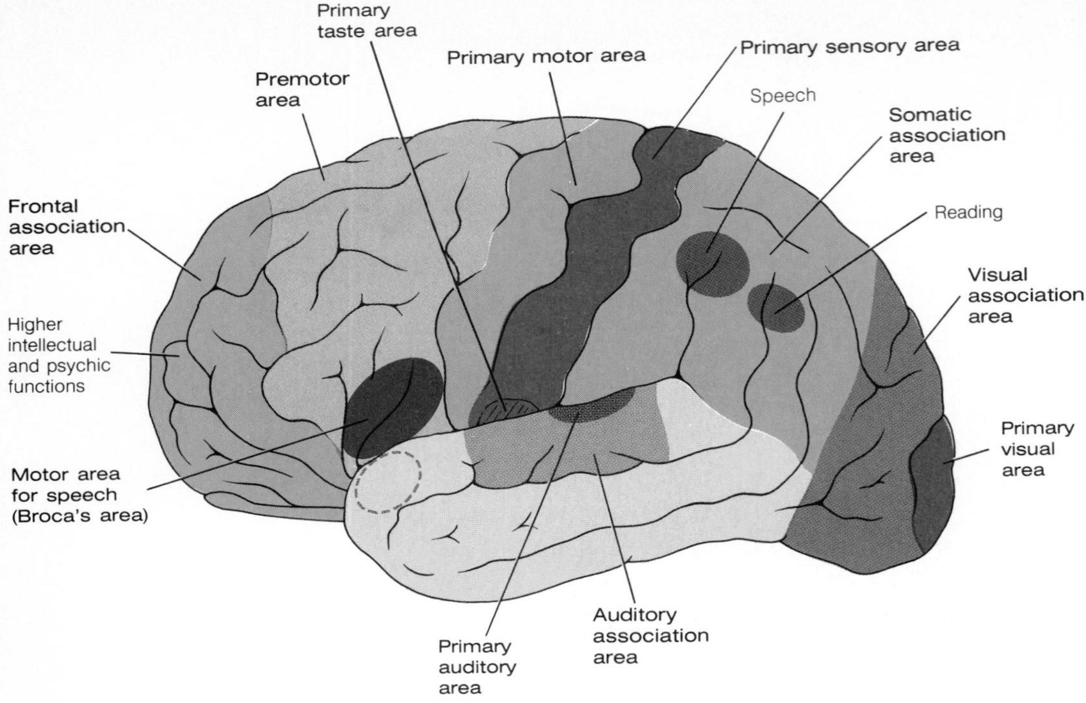

Figure 27–2

Major functional areas of the cortex. SOURCE: *Spence AP, Mason EB:* Human Anatomy and Physiology, *3rd ed. Menlo Park, CA: Benjamin/Cummings, 1987.*

nuncial neurons (transmitters of messages from neuron to neuron). Neuronal messages are transmitted through electrical impulses. The necessary voltages are created by positive and negative forces produced when ions line up inside and outside the cell's plasma membrane. When a nerve is in a resting state (known as a resting membrane potential), the electrical charge outside the wall is positive; inside, the charge is negative.

The principal extracellular cation is sodium; the main intracellular anion is potassium. With adequate stimulation of the cell, the charge is reversed as sodium moves into the cell and potassium moves out. This reversal results in a flow of electric current. With sufficient stimulation, the reversal of polarity travels along the entire axon. This process, known as an *action potential*, requires only a few milliseconds. Quickly, electrical forces and ion concentration forces re-establish the resting membrane potential. If a stimulus is not sufficient to produce an action potential, and another stimulus occurs before the membrane has completely stabilized, depolarization will be facilitated. (See Chapter 18 for a comparable discussion related to the ECG.)

Information is transmitted from one neuron to another at *synapses* following the initiation of an action potential. In humans, chemical synapses initiate almost all action potentials. These synapses, located where axons and dendrites meet, use various neurotransmitters, which are stored in and released from the axon terminal following an action potential. Action potentials are believed to increase the permeability of the axon terminal to calcium, allowing it to move into the axon terminal to stimulate the release of neurotransmitters into the synaptic cleft. The neurotransmitter diffuses across the cleft and attaches to postsynaptic receptors.

The influence of neurotransmitters on the postsynaptic receptor depends on the combination of impulses received. This combination is derived from the total number and frequency of impulses received over a period of time from one or multiple synapses. Strong stimuli activate a greater number of neurons. Myelinated fibers speed the transmission of impulses. Inhibitory impulses also influence the postsynaptic receptors' response. Through these combinations, the nervous system "fine tunes" synaptic activity needed to manage the body's complex functions. Nerve impulses are binary (ie, either "on" or "off"), so the CNS must discriminate among stimuli by interpreting variations in strength, frequency, and number of stimuli received.

There are many other neurotransmitters. About 30 are known or suspected to play a role in nerve-impulse transmission. Some have multiple actions. For example, norepinephrine is involved in the maintenance of arousal and dreaming sleep and regulation of moods; dopamine has roles in the regulation of emotional responses and control of complex movements; and endorphins and enkephalins are believed to be involved in the perception and integration of pain and emotional experiences.

Cerebral Function

THE FRONTAL LOBES The frontal lobes are involved in mental, emotional, and physical functions. Anterior por-

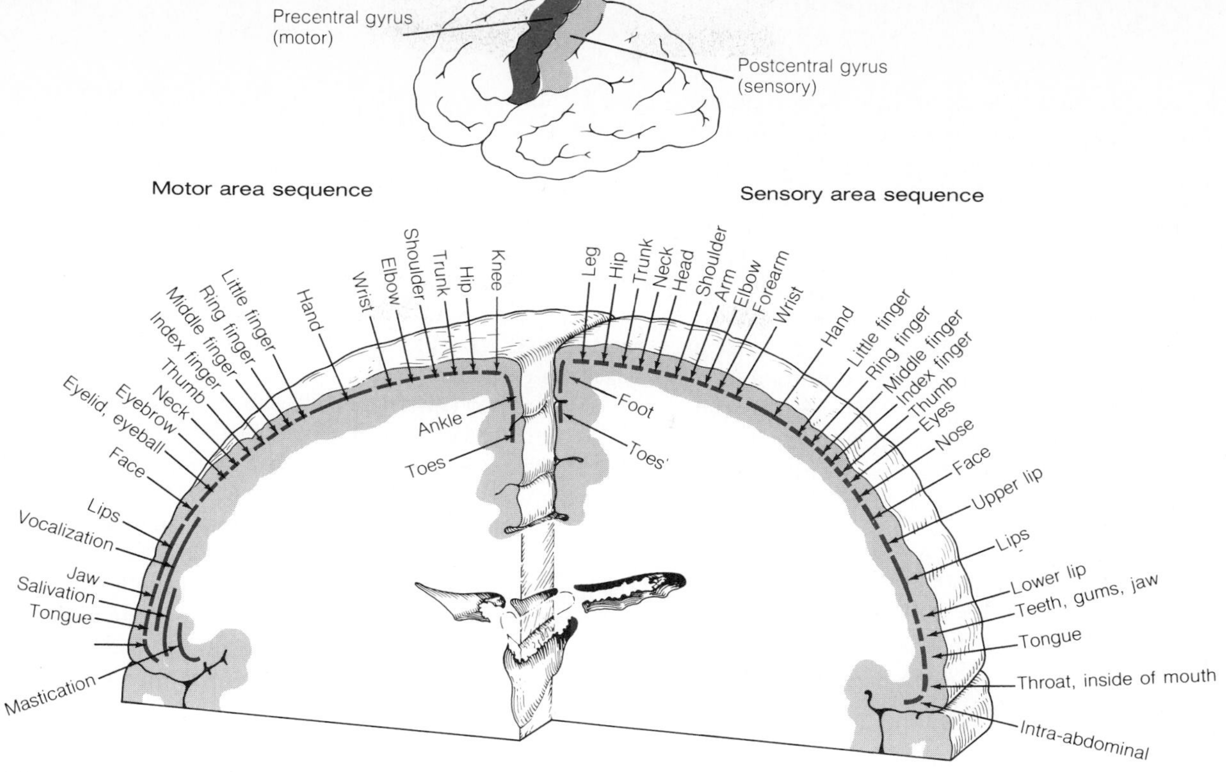

Figure 27–3

Frontal section of the cerebrum. **Left.** Through the precentral gyrus, showing the locations of neurons within the cerebral cortex that control voluntary motor movement of specific structures. **Right.** Through the postcentral gyrus, showing the locations of regions of the cerebral cortex that receive sensory nerve impulses from specific body structures. SOURCE: *Spence AP, Mason EB:* Human Anatomy and Physiology, *3rd ed. Menlo Park, CA: Benjamin/Cummings, 1987.*

tions have major roles in the control of conscious and unconscious behaviors such as personality, social behavior, judgment, and complex intellectual activity. The central and posterior portions of the frontal lobes control motor function. The primary motor areas control voluntary movement via the pyramidal tracts. The premotor areas control and coordinate complex, learned movements such as typing, writing, scanning eye movements, conjugate deviation of the eyes, and movement of the head. These activities are effected via the extrapyramidal tracts and described in the following section on function of the CNS. Pyramidal and extrapyramidal centers control movements on the opposite side of the body. The dominant frontal lobe also contains Broca's motor speech area (see Figure 27–2).

THE PARIETAL LOBES The parietal lobes interpret sensory input. The postcentral convolutions, organized similarly to the major motor strip (Figure 27–3), receive conscious sensory input. Sensations perceived on one side of the body are interpreted by the contralateral parietal lobe. Somatic sensations perceived are pain, temperature, touch, pressure, and proprioception (awareness of position in space and muscle activity). The parietal lobes contain the somatesthetic association areas, which lie in the superior portion of the lobes and extend to the medial surface of the hemisphere. Many other connections within the parietal lobe allow for interpretation of sensory input such as stereognosis (perceiving and understanding an object by touch and relating the sensations to experience and knowledge). Awareness of body parts and the establishment of body image also take place here. The angular gyrus located in the parietal lobe of the dominant hemisphere is responsible for interpretation of written language (Price & Wilson, 1982).

THE INSULA The insula, thought by some to be a fifth lobe of the brain, lies deep within the lateral fissure where it is covered by portions of the frontal, temporal, and parietal lobes (Spence & Mason, 1987). It is believed to be involved in visceral activities related to intra-abdominal sensations and visceral motility. Little information is available regarding function.

THE TEMPORAL LOBES The temporal lobes receive input from three senses—hearing, taste, and smell—and have a role in memory processes. Association fibers, especially in the dominant lobe, allow the comparison of sensory input with past experiences. Association fibers, particularly those of the dominant lobe, interrelate somatesthetic visual and auditory stimuli to give them meaning (Conway–Rutkowski, 1982). Wernicke's area, also located on the dominant side, is involved in the hearing component in speech and in the formulation of language.

THE OCCIPITAL LOBES The occipital lobes contain the primary visual areas and visual association areas (refer to Figure 27–2). The primary visual areas receive information and perceive color. The visual association areas give visual input meaning and have a role in visual reflexes for fixing the eyes on a stationary or moving object. To appreciate the function of the association areas, consider the problems that arise when the areas are damaged. Injury to the medial surface on the dominant side can result in loss of the ability to recognize objects and know their function, although recognition of faces still is possible. A consequence of damage to the nondominant side may be the inability to recognize faces and differentiate various forms of life such as horses and elephants (Price & Wilson, 1982).

THE THALAMUS The thalamus, a large ovoid gray mass, surrounds the third ventricle. Specific areas within the thalamus receive axons from the cord, brain stem, cerebellum, basal ganglia, and various parts of the cerebellum. These connections allow it to influence motor function and have a role in arousal, alerting mechanisms, and reflex movements.

The thalamus influences the motor cortex through its connections with the pyramidal tract neurons. It is involved with the initiation of movement, control of muscle tone, and regulation of cortical reflexes through connections with the cerebellum, globus pallidus, and substantia nigra (Carpenter & Sutin, 1983). The thalamus interprets and relays sensory impulses from all parts of the body except the olfactory nerve. Recognition of crude sensations such as pain, temperature, and touch also takes place here. Sensory impulses that the thalamus is unable to interpret are relayed by it to appropriate primary sensory and association nuclei in the cerebral cortex. The thalamus is even involved in emotional responses, interpreting sensations as pleasant or unpleasant.

THE HYPOTHALAMUS The hypothalamus, a small but extremely important area of brain tissue situated just below the thalamus, plays a major role in the maintenance of many homeostatic functions. Numerous regulatory activities initiated here are effected through the pituitary gland and the ANS.

The pituitary gland, also known as the hypophysis, lies below the hypothalamus in the sella turcica. Hypothalamic nuclei influence pituitary gland function through neural and endocrine activity.

The hypothalamus receives input from all parts of the body. ANS activity is initiated in response to input received from areas within the thalamus, medulla oblongata, spinal cord, and limbic system. The influence of the hypothalamus on ANS activity includes the regulation of heart rate, blood pressure, and body temperature. In temperature regulation, the ANS lowers body temperature through the activation of vasodilation and sweating. It raises temperature by initiating (through shivering, vasoconstriction, and piloerection) increases in heart rate, basal metabolic rate, and mobilization of carbohydrate reserves.

The limbic system, important in emotions and behavior, surrounds the hypothalamus and has connections with it. Hypothalamic connections with the thalamus, which interprets feelings of pleasantness and unpleasantness, and with the reticular activating system, which influences wakefulness, provide additional input to which the hypothalamus responds.

Many hypothalamic activities are initiated by changes in the perceived composition of its blood supply. For example, specific areas within the hypothalamus are sensitive to changes in water balance, glucose, and insulin levels. The hypothalamic response to an increase in osmotic pressure illustrates this sensitivity: With a loss of body fluid, the hypothalamus detects an increase in osmotic pressure. In response, it initiates the release of antidiuretic hormone by the posterior pituitary gland to concentrate the urine and stimulate the thirst center to increase the oral intake of fluid.

Other centers within the hypothalamus regulate appetite. Specific nuclei credited with the initiation of feeding behavior and satiety have been identified. These centers are reciprocal in their inhibition of one another. The hypothalamus also influences gastrointestinal function and sexual activity.

THE LIMBIC SYSTEM The limbic system influences memory, drives, motivation, visceral functions, and interactions with the environment. Emotional expressions believed to evolve from this complex group of structures include rage, placidity, fear, and attack reactions.

Research with animals has demonstrated that the limbic system contains centers of reward and punishment with both serving as important motivators of behavior and affecting memory (Guyton, 1982). The *hippocampus* is thought to be involved in the transfer of short-term memory into long-term memory, especially with events related to elements perceived in the environment.

The *amygdala* is thought to have major responsibilities for the control of behavior in social and environmental circumstances. It is also believed to influence visceral responses to emotions and various movements related to posturing and eating (Guyton, 1982).

The Brain Stem

The brain stem comprises the midbrain, pons, and medulla oblongata. Each of these structures has unique responsibilities, but the three function as a unit to serve as a conduit for impulses passing to and from the cerebral cortex and the spinal column. The midbrain, the uppermost portion of the brain stem, contains afferent and efferent nerve tracts that travel to and from the cerebral hemispheres. It also houses the red nucleus, which serves as a relay station for coordination of impulses traveling between the cerebellum and cerebral hemispheres, and the corpora quadrigemina, which are involved in reflex responses to visual stimuli and the relay of auditory impulses.

The *pons* sits between the midbrain and the medulla oblongata and anterior to the cerebellum. It contains nerve fiber tracts that provide communication between upper and lower levels of the CNS and the cerebellum. The lower third of the pons contains respiratory reflex centers influenced by the carbon dioxide levels of the blood and spinal fluid. The pons also influences vasomotor activity.

The *medulla oblongata* forms the inferior portion of the brain stem. The pyramids for the motor tracts are located on its ventral surface. Sensory tracts ascend through the medulla to the thalamus. Major reflex centers in the medulla influence respiratory and cardiovascular function.

The Reticular Activating System

The reticular activating system regulates spinal motor activity as well as voluntary and reflex muscle activity. Projections to the diencephalon and cortex effect and maintain arousal and alerting states. In addition to maintaining wakefulness, this system also participates in the regulation of sensory input from the periphery, regulation of respirations, and vasomotor activity.

The Cranial Nerves

The functions of cranial nerves vary; some are motor, some sensory, and others mixed. Motor nerves are innervated with proprioceptive (sensory) branches. The parasympathetic branch of the ANS provides a visceral component for some cranial nerves. The 12 pairs of cranial nerves, identified by Roman numerals, are ordered by their position within the skull.

The two cranial nerves I, the *olfactory nerves*, are sensory nerves responsible for the perception of odors. Nerve impulses originating in the olfactory nerves are transmitted to the temporal lobes for interpretation.

The *optic nerves*, cranial nerves II, are sensory nerves that originate in the retina of the eye. Nerve impulses are transmitted to the occipital lobe, where vision is perceived. Optic nerves projecting back from the orbits meet at the optic chiasm. Here each tract divides, the inner halves joining with fibers from the opposite orbit. From this point, each tract carries fibers from both eyes.

Cranial nerves III, the *oculomotor nerves*, emerge from the midbrain and enter the orbits through the superior orbital fissures. They are responsible for movement of four of the six extrinsic eye muscles as well as opening the eyelid.

The *trochlear nerves*, cranial nerves IV, are motor nerves that are responsible for voluntary movement of the eyeball through innervation of the superior oblique muscles.

Cranial nerves V, the *trigeminal nerves*, have both sensory and motor fibers. Deep and superficial sensory fibers innervate the face and anterior portion of the head through the ophthalmic, maxillary, and mandibular branches. Sensory fibers for pain, light touch, and proprioception can be readily identified. The motor components of this nerve are responsible for mastication.

Cranial nerves VI, the *abducens nerves*, enter the orbits with cranial nerves III and IV. Their function is to roll the eyes outward.

The *facial nerves*, cranial nerves VII, supply motor neurons for the facial and scalp muscles. Sensory fibers supply the taste buds for sweet, sour, and salt on the anterior two-thirds of the tongue. Parasympathetic fibers supply the lacrimal glands and the submandibular and sublingual salivary glands.

The *vestibulocochlear nerves*, cranial nerves VIII, have two sensory divisions, the auditory and the vestibular. Both originate at inner-ear receptors located in the petrous portion of the temporal bones. The two divisions, enclosed in a single sheath, pass to the brain stem just below the pons. Some of the vestibular fibers travel directly to the cerebellum. Auditory impulses are transmitted to the temporal lobes for interpretation.

Cranial nerves IX, the *glossopharyngeal nerves*, innervate the tongue and the pharynx. The motor component is important in swallowing. Sensory responsibilities include perception of bitter taste on the posterior one-third of the tongue; sensory awareness for the mucous membranes of the pharynx, tonsils, and middle-ear cavity; carotid body receptor sensitivity to serum oxygen and carbon dioxide levels; and baroreceptor information regarding blood pressure.

Cranial nerve X, the *vagus nerve*, carries motor impulses to the pharynx and larynx, and sensory impulses from them. Extensive parasympathetic nerve fibers innervate the pharynx, larynx, and trachea and extend into the thorax and abdomen. Thoracic and abdominal vagal branches influence the function of the esophagus, lungs, aorta, stomach, gallbladder, spleen, small intestine, kidneys, and upper two-thirds of the large intestine.

Sensory fibers from the vagus nerve related to visceral functions generally operate at an unconscious level. An exception is nausea which is perceived via the vagus nerve.

Cranial nerves XI, the *accessory nerves*, are actually formed by two nerves. One projects from the medulla; the other, projecting from the fifth or sixth cervical segment of the spinal cord, is actually a spinal nerve. Fibers from the cranial portion join with the vagus nerve to supply muscles of the larynx and pharynx. Fibers from the spinal component innervate the trapezius and sternocleidomastoid muscles.

The *hypoglossal nerves*, cranial nerves XII, are motor

nerves that exit from the medulla oblongata and pass through the hypoglossal canals located beneath the tongue. These nerves are responsible for tongue movement.

The Cerebellum

The cerebellum modulates and coordinates skeletal muscle activity and maintains body posture and muscle tone. It controls movement with both excitatory and inhibitory signals, which fine tune movements in ways the cerebral cortex is incapable of carrying out. Each hemisphere influences the movement on the ipsilateral side of the body. It modifies activity initiated elsewhere in the body. There is no conscious input.

Activities of the cerebellum derive from the multiple inputs from the CNS and PNS. Afferent fibers travel to the cerebellum from the cerebral cortex by way of the corticocerebellar tracts and the pons. Peripheral afferent impulses from muscle spindles, Golgi tendon organs, skin, and joint receptors travel to the cerebellum via the ventral and dorsal spinocerebellar tracts. (See Table 27–1 and Figure 27–4 for more information on these tracts.) The reticular substance of the brain stem and vestibular tracts also provide the cerebellum with information.

Cerebellar efferent impulses are sent to the motor cortex via the thalamus. Additional efferent signals are transmitted to the basal ganglia, red nucleus, reticular formation of the brain stem, and vestibular nuclei. The connections with the vestibular nuclei integrate changes in the direction of body movement and posture. The semicircular canals of the inner ear perceive these changes and

Table 27–1
Major Ascending and Descending Tracts of the Spinal Cord

Spinal Cord Tract	Responsibilities	Crossover Point
Sensory Tract—Ascending		
Fasciculus gracilis	Carry information to parietal lobe regarding lower limb movement and position; sensations of fine touch from receptors located in the muscle, joint, and skin.	Cross in medulla
Fasciculus cuneatus	Carry information about upper extremities, trunk, and neck. Proprioception—conscious stereognosis (being able to perceive and understand objects by touch) from receptors located on muscle, joint, and skin. Synapse in thalamus—ascend to sensory cortex in parietal lobe.	Cross in medulla
Spinothalamic:		
• Lateral	Convey impulses of pain and temperature from surface and viscera.	Cross in spinal cord
• Ventral	Convey impulses of crude touch and pressure, itch, and tickle. Synapse in thalamus—ascend to sensory cortex in parietal lobe.	Cross in spinal cord
Spinocerebellar:		
• Dorsal	Unconscious proprioception from neuromuscular receptors.	Uncrossed—directly to cerebellum
• Ventral	Sensory information originates in muscle spindles and Golgi tendon apparatus; coordination of posture and limb movement.	Uncrossed—directly to cerebellum
Motor Tract—Descending		
Corticospinal:		
• Lateral	Volitional movements, especially in distal parts of extremities.	Cross in medulla
• Ventral	Innervate muscles of upper extremities and neck.	Cross where they synapse with lower motor neurons
Tectospinal (includes reticulospinal tracts)	Optic relay centers—mediate reflex postural movements in response to visual and perhaps auditory stimuli.	Cross in the brain stem
Rubrospinal (includes reticulospinal tracts)	Control muscle tone in flexor muscle groups. Require an intact cerebellum.	Some cross in brain stem; some uncrossed
Vestibulospinal	Influence derived from vestibular nuclei and cerebellum. Exert facilitory influence on reflex activity in the spinal cord and spinal mechanisms that control muscle tone.	Uncrossed
Olivospinal	Role unclear; may serve as relay centers from basal ganglia to spinal motor nerves.	Cross in the brain stem

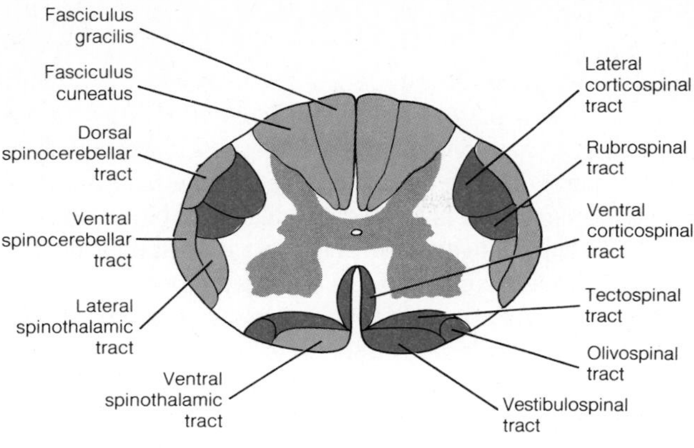

Figure 27–4

Main fasciculi of the spinal cord. The ascending (sensory) tracts are labeled only on the left side. The descending (motor) tracts are labeled only on the right side. *SOURCE: Spence AP, Mason EB:* Human Anatomy and Physiology, *3rd ed. Menlo Park, CA: Benjamin/Cummings, 1987.*

transmit this information to the cerebellum via the vestibular nerve and the brain stem. Balance is maintained through the modification of muscle tone. The cerebellum has no direct influence on lower motor neurons. The cerebellum is also involved with predictively coordinating visual clues with bodily motion. For example, the cerebellum provides persons with input on how rapidly they are approaching an object.

The Spinal Cord

The spinal cord is a conduit for messages to and from the higher levels within the CNS and participates in reflex motor activities. Descending pathways within the cord carry motor instructions to the anterior horn (ventral roots) from the cerebral cortex, brain stem, and cerebellum. Impulses synapse in the anterior horn (motor gray area) just before leaving the cord. This synaptic activity involves upper motor neurons, located within the cord, and lower motor neurons, which extend beyond the cord. Ascending (dorsal) roots transmit sensory impulses from the skin and viscera to the cord and CNS. Synaptic activity necessary for transmission of signals occurs at various levels within the cord. Dermatome charts provide a "map" of the area of skin supplied by the dorsal root of each spinal nerve.

Specific sensory and motor tracts have been identified within the spinal cord. These tracts, located within the white matter, are identified as anterior, lateral, and posterior funiculi. These funiculi, further divided into tracts called fasciculi, carry similar types of nerve impulses to specific destinations (Figure 27–4).

Motor Function

Effective skeletal muscle function involves many components of the CNS and PNS. Muscle function requires the perception and interpretation of sensory stimuli for movements and an intact motor system to initiate and carry out muscle contraction. Areas of the nervous system involved in motor function include the premotor cortex, the primary motor area, pyramidal and extrapyramidal tracts, basal ganglia, thalamus, brain stem, spinal cord, and cerebellum.

The premotor cortex (associative cortex), positioned just anterior to the major motor strip, is involved in muscle activities that produce hand skills, voluntary eye movements, eyelid blinking, and vocalization. Function of the premotor area requires intact connections with the sensory association areas of the parietal lobe, the temporal lobe, frontal lobe, occipital lobe, components of the basal ganglia, primary motor cortex, thalamus, brain stem, and spinal cord.

The primary motor area is believed responsible for the initiation of movement by individual groups of muscles such as those involved in the movement of fingers, toes, and mouth. The cross section of the precentral gyrus (see Figure 27–3) illustrates specific areas of the primary motor area identified as initiating willed movement by various muscles. Note the large amount of gray matter (nerve cells) allocated to muscle groups involved in complex movements of the hands and mouth.

Nerve cells of the major motor strip and their conducting fibers make up the *pyramidal* (corticospinal) motor system. Nerve fibers descend from the motor strip through the internal capsule, midbrain, and pons to the medulla oblongata where the pyramidal fibers cross. After crossing, the fibers descend in the spinal cord to appropriate levels. Most pyramidal fibers descend via the lateral corticospinal tracts to ventral horns of gray matter in the cord. Some motor fibers travel via ventral corticospinal tracts.

Extrapyramidal motor tracts (those that exclude the pyramidal tract) are more complex in their arrangement and synaptic activity in the cerebrum and brain stem. A functional, rather than an anatomic unit, the extrapyramidal tracts are involved in maintaining balance and posture by facilitating some muscle movements and inhibiting others. Movements initiated in one hemisphere influence movements on the opposite side of the body. The basal ganglia, bodies of gray matter deep within the white matter of the cerebral hemispheres, are part of the extrapyramidal tract. Specifically, they are the caudate nucleus, putamen, and the globus pallidus. In addition, the thalamus, subthalamus, substantia nigra, and red nucleus have roles in motor function. Multiple connections exist among all of these areas. A second pathway allows for feedback control of extrapyramidal motor activity.

The basal ganglia have three motor functions. A major responsibility of the basal ganglia as a whole is believed to be the inhibition of postural muscle tone. The caudate nucleus and putamen, collectively referred to as the *striate body*, are thought to initiate and regulate gross intention movements such as body posture and major arm movements. This regulation involves pyramidal and extrapyramidal pathways. The globus pallidus is believed to provide background muscle tone for intended movements initiated by the striate body or the cerebral cortex (eg, the muscle contractions needed to support the arm and trunk while using a typewriter or a tennis racket).

Final pathways for extrapyramidal signals into the cord are the reticulospinal tracts that lie in both the ventral and lateral tracts of the cord. Also involved in transmission to a lesser degree are the rubrospinal, tectospinal, vestibulospinal, and possibly the olivospinal tracts.

Reflex Movements

Reflexes differ from voluntary muscle activity in that they are automatic, stereotypic movements that do not require cortical processing. Reflex actions may involve skeletal, smooth, and cardiac muscles and glands. *Monosynaptic* and *polysynaptic* reflexes are carried out through neural pathways known as spinal reflex arcs. They are initiated by various noxious stimuli such as pain, rapid stretch, and fear.

Monosynaptic reflexes involve a sensory receptor, an afferent neuron to carry impulses to the cord, and a synapse within the spinal cord between the afferent neuron and the efferent neuron, which transmits the impulse to the effector. A common example of a monosynaptic impulse is the knee jerk, elicited by tapping a tendon with a reflex hammer. In this example, the stretching of the patellar tendon causes a reflex contraction of the quadriceps muscle.

A polysynaptic reflex response involves an additional activity, a synapse with an internuncial neuron within the cord. With this reflex, muscle (or other sensitive tissue) subjected to a noxious stimulus produces a polysynaptic reflex. This activity can be complex, with signals sent to neurons above, below, and on to the opposite side of the spinal cord. These additional synapses are part of the automatic actions designed to initiate actions to protect the body.

The Autonomic Nervous System

Autonomic nervous system activity is initiated by centers in the spinal cord, brain stem, hypothalamus, and limbic system. This system helps to regulate visceral functions, maintain homeostasis, and combat stress. Afferent messages reach these centers via sensory nerve transmission. The ANS usually operates at an unconscious level.

Sympathetic and parasympathetic activities are effected by preganglionic and postganglionic fibers that stimulate target organs. Two neurotransmitters, acetylcholine and norepinephrine, are required for impulse transmission. Acetylcholine is the transmitter for parasympathetic preganglionic and postganglionic synapses and preganglionic sympathetic synapses. Norepinephrine is the transmitter required for almost all sympathetic postganglionic synapses.

The sympathetic nervous system helps the body to respond quickly to emergencies. Its network of branching axons provides for extensive and rapid stimulation of the sympathetic chain when quick responses are needed. Fear or rage can stimulate the sympathetic nervous system to produce an increase in heart rate, dilation of blood vessels, a rise in blood sugar, and secretion of epinephrine and norepinephrine to reinforce and prolong the body's response to the stress. Parasympathetic nervous system activity primarily maintains body functions under normal conditions. For example, it decreases the heart rate and promotes digestive activity.

Some activities initiated by the sympathetic nervous system oppose parasympathetic impulses (eg, countering the parasympathetic nervous system's slowing effect on the heart by increasing the rate and force of contraction). It also slows peristalsis and increases the tone in sphincters, thereby slowing digestion and absorption of nutrients.

The sympathetic nervous system, the major regulator of blood pressure, always maintains some tone within the vessel walls. Blood pressure is decreased when sympathetic nervous system activity is reduced. Parasympathetic fibers do not innervate the smooth muscles of blood vessels. The only way the system can decrease the blood pressure is by slowing the heart rate and decreasing the force of cardiac contraction.

Protection and Maintenance of the Nervous System

Understanding the complex and wonderful capabilities of the nervous system helps in appreciating the system's means of protection and maintenance. Recognizing the safeguards of the bony cranial vault and vertebral column is easy. Less obvious but also valuable is the protection provided by the hair, skin, scalp, fascia, muscle, meninges, fluid cushioning, and complex vascular supply. The superficial structures help to limit injuries from external trauma, and the ventricular and vascular systems provide an environment for optimal neuronal function.

The *meninges* within the cranial vault and vertebral column protect the CNS from physical harm and support the cerebrospinal fluid system and the circulation. The *dura mater*, the outermost layer of meninges, forms a double layer over the brain tissue. Its outer layer forms an inner periosteal lining for the skull and vertebral canal. In the cranium, the inner layer of dura, for the most part fused with the outer layer, helps to secure the brain to the cranial vault. To provide extra support and protection, the inner layer of dura separates in areas, dipping down between the longitudinal fissure, between the cerebellar hemispheres, and between the cerebrum and cerebullum and passing over the pituitary gland nestled in the sella turcica. In other areas, dura layers separate to form venous sinuses that collect and carry venous blood away from the brain. Arachnoid processes (villi) project into the dural sinuses.

In the spinal cord, the inner layer of dura is continuous with the spinal dura mater. The spinal dura extends to the second sacral vertebra where it joins with the external filum terminale and attaches to the back of the first segment of the coccyx. The middle layer of the meninges, the *arachnoid,* is a thin, fibrous membrane that adheres closely to the inner surface of the dura allowing only a narrow space between the two. The inner layer of the meninges, the *pia mater,* adheres so closely to the brain that it follows the contour of the fissures and sulci. The space between the pia mater and arachnoid is bridged with weblike strands of arachnoid called trabeculae. A rich network of pial blood vessels extends into the brain. The area between the arachnoid and pia mater is called the *subarachnoid space.* Located here are arteries, veins, arachnoid trabeculae, and CSF. Within the spinal cord, fibrous bridges join the pia mater with the arachnoid and dura mater. These bridges, known as denticulate ligaments, help to stabilize the cord within the spinal canal.

The Cerebrospinal Fluid System

The CSF protects the brain and spinal cord by supporting the tissues, acting as a shock absorber, and serving as a medium in the transfer of elements from the bloodstream to nervous system tissues. CSF flows through an elaborate ventricular system located within the brain and through the subarachnoid space surrounding the brain and spinal cord (Figure 27–5). Two large ventricles are positioned within each cerebral hemisphere. Their central portions extend into the parietal lobes. The anterior horns project into the frontal lobes, the inferior horns extend into the temporal lobes, and the posterior horns project into the occipital lobes. A small third ventricle lies below and communicates with each lateral ventricle via a small channel known as the foramen of Monro. The thalamus forms the lateral walls of the third ventricle. The third

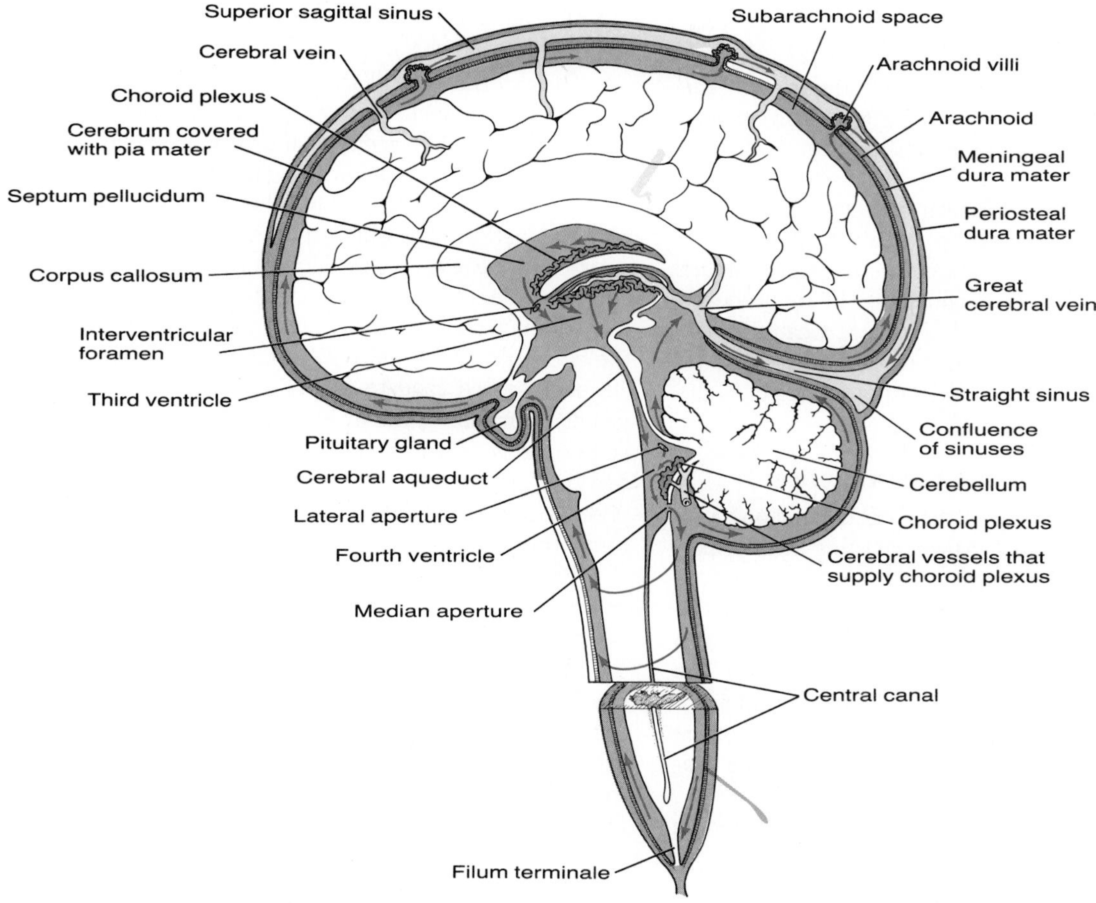

Figure 27–5

The location of the cerebrospinal fluid (red) surrounding the brain and spinal cord. The arrows indicate the direction of the fluid's flow. Blood is shown in light red. *SOURCE: Spence AP, Mason EB:* Human Anatomy and Physiology, *3rd ed. Menlo Park, CA: Benjamin/ Cummings, 1987.*

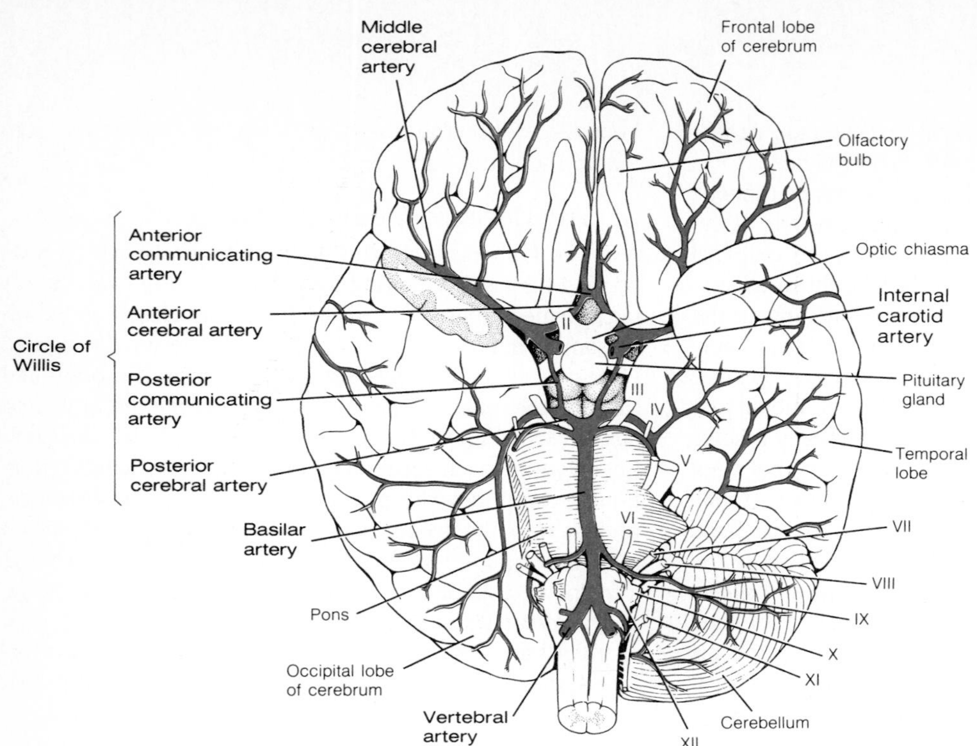

Figure 27–6

Arteries of the base of the brain, forming the circle of Willis around the pituitary gland. To provide an unobstructed view, part of the right temporal lobe and the right cerebellar hemisphere have been removed. Roman numerals indicate cranial nerves. SOURCE: *Spence AP, Mason EB:* Human Anatomy and Physiology, *3rd ed. Menlo Park, CA: Benjamin/ Cummings, 1987.*

ventricle is connected via the cerebral aqueduct to the fourth ventricle, which lies below. The pons and medulla are positioned below the fourth ventricle. The cerebellum lies above.

CSF flows from the ventricular system to the arachnoid space of the brain and spinal cord by way of the lateral apertures (foramina of Luschka) and the median aperture (foramen of Magendie). CSF is constantly being produced by capillary tufts, called choroid plexuses, located in the ventricles. Arachnoid villi, projecting into the dural sinuses, provide routes for the reabsorption of CSF into the venous circulation.

Central Nervous System Circulation

The viability and function of the CNS depend on a rich and continuous blood supply. Major arteries supply oxygenated blood to the arterioles, which branch into capillaries where actual uptake of oxygen and nutrients occurs. The brain utilizes approximately 20% of the body's oxygen supply and requires about 400 kcal of glucose per day. The average cerebral blood flow is about 750 mL per minute.

Two major arteries branch directly off the arch of the aorta to establish the blood supply to the head—the brachiocephalic artery and the left common carotid artery. The brachiocephalic artery divides into the right common carotid artery and the right subclavian artery. The two common carotid arteries move up the neck along the trachea where they separate into the internal and external carotid arteries. *Carotid sinus baroreceptors,* sensitive to changes in blood pressure, are located at this point of separation. *Carotid bodies,* also located here, monitor changes in the blood's oxygen, carbon dioxide, and pH levels.

The external carotid arteries supply the scalp and parts of the head and neck. Secondary branches of the external carotids, the middle meningeal arteries, supply blood to the meninges of the brain. The right and left internal carotid arteries, after passing through the carotid canals, branch into the anterior cerebral arteries and middle cerebral arteries at the level of the optic chiasm. The right and left anterior cerebral arteries are connected by the small anterior communicating artery to form the anterior portion of the circle of Willis (Figure 27–6). Anterior cerebral arteries perfuse the caudate and putamen nuclei of the basal ganglia, portions of the internal capsule, corpus callosum, and portions of the frontal and parietal lobes. The middle cerebral arteries are the major suppliers of blood to the precentral and postcentral gyri and feed portions of the temporal, parietal, and frontal lobes.

The vertebral arteries, whose source is the subclavian artery, travel to the brain via the foramina of the cervical vertebrae and the foramen magnum. At the level where the medulla and pons meet, the vertebral arteries join to form the basilar artery. The basilar artery separates at the rostral border of the pons, forming the posterior cerebral arteries. Posterior communicating arteries extending back from the internal carotid arteries complete the anastomosis with the posterior cerebral arteries to form the circle of Willis. This anastomosis, intended to maintain circulation to the brain tissue if one of the vessels closes, is not always functional. Other vessels providing collateral circulation are vessels at the base of the brain; small pial anastomotic branches on the surface; external carotids to the eyes; and anterior, middle, and posterior cerebral anastomoses on the surface of the brain.

Passage of venous blood from surface and deep brain tissue takes place via thick veins lacking valves. The blood flows into the dural sinuses and then drains into the internal jugular veins. Three dural sinuses are of particular importance. The *superior sagittal sinus* serves as a major route for the removal of the constantly forming CSF. The *cavernous sinus* drains blood from the eye, orbit, and face. The *transverse sinus* lies close to the ear.

REGULATION OF CEREBRAL BLOOD FLOW Control of blood flow in the CNS is essential for viability and optimal function. The body can use several built-in mechanisms to maintain effective circulation.

Three major factors that have a direct and potent effect on cerebral blood flow by producing vasodilation are elevations in carbon dioxide concentration, hydrogen ion concentration, and oxygen concentration. (Elevated carbon dioxide levels lead to an increase in hydrogen ion concentration.) The increase in hydrogen ion concentration causes vasodilation of the cerebral vessels. Vasomotor reflex responses that affect the body's general vascular perfusion also affect the perfusion of blood in the CNS. Vasomotor centers in the pons and medulla maintain vascular tone through impulses transmitted via the spinal cord to all blood vessels in the body. The reticular areas of the brain stem and hypothalamus have both excitatory and inhibitory effects on vasomotor activity. The hypothalamus also influences vasoconstriction activity through excitatory or inhibitory action on the vasomotor centers. It also helps to regulate total body water and therefore blood pressure by increasing or decreasing the release of antidiuretic hormone.

A severe drop in blood pressure to 50 mm Hg or less will result in ischemia in the vasomotor center. The resulting local increase in concentration of carbon dioxide causes a profound stimulation of blood vessels—some to the point of occlusion. This response, meant to shunt the blood to the CNS, is known as the ischemic response.

Cushing's phenomenon occurs when an increase in pressure in the CSF system equals the pressure in the cerebral vascular bed, hampering the flow of blood to the brain. At this point, the CNS ischemic response is initiated to raise the CNS blood pressure above the CSF pressure to facilitate blood flow to the brain (Guyton, 1982).

SPINAL CORD CIRCULATION Multiple arteries feed the spinal cord. The vessels join, forming a complex network that supplies the vertebrae, periosteum, and dura. Branches supply the ventral and dorsal roots and penetrate deeply into the cord. Anterior and posterior spinal arteries extending the length of the cord originate from the carotid and vertebral arteries.

The venous system of the spinal cord is a rich network. The internal vertebral venous plexus, located between the dura mater and vertebral periosteum, is made up of anterior and posterior venous channels that extend from the skull to the sacral region. Thoracic, abdominal, and intercostal veins as well as the external vertebral venous plexus have connections with the internal vertebral plexus at each intervertebral space. There are no valves in this venous network. As a result, blood flow varies depending on pressure. With elevation of intra-abdominal pressure, venous blood from the pelvic plexus passes into the vertebral venous channels. If the jugular vein is occluded, blood from the skull can drain via the vertebral channels. On the other hand, this venous plexus is believed to provide potential routes for metastasis of neoplasms (Carpenter & Sutin, 1983)

SECTION 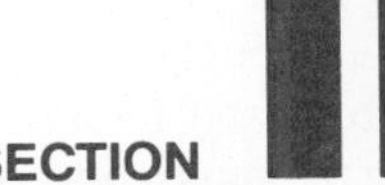

Pathophysiologic Influences and Effects

The nervous system's complex structure and diverse functions predispose it to a multitude of pathologies, each capable of causing varying types and degrees of dysfunction. The protective structures and mechanisms discussed in the preceding section are obviously not fail proof. In fact, these protective structures often produce or contribute to nervous system trauma. The rigid skull and vertebral column allow little room for neuronal swelling, tumor growth, or circulatory congestion. Trauma may also occur when external forces drive the nervous tissue against the inside of the bony structures. Fractures and bony degenerative processes can perforate or crush neurons or supportive tissues.

The elaborate CSF system, designed to support and cushion the CNS, is subject to risks from a localized or generalized buildup of CSF if reabsorption is impeded. This extensive fluid system also provides routes for the spread of infection. Foramina of the skull and vertebral column, serving as avenues for the passage of blood vessels and nerves traveling to and from the periphery, also provide routes for microorganisms into the CNS.

Meningeal tissues, too, present hazards as well as protection. With increases in intracranial pressure (ICP), herniation of brain tissue through the tentorial notch formed by the tough dura can seriously injure the brain stem and surrounding tissues. The dura mater, pia mater, and arachnoid tissues also provide extensive, uninterrupted routes for the spread of infection.

The CNS's circulatory bed, so important in providing nourishment, presents risks to the same structures it serves. The circulation provides routes for migrating microorganisms and even tumors from all parts of the body. Additional risks include an increase in ICP from hemorrhage and abnormal vascular structures.

The neurons, nerves, and nerve tracts, with their long communication chains and multiple connections needed for effective afferent and efferent activity, form the most complex part of the nervous system. Because of their presence throughout the body, these neurologic structures are vulnerable to many pathologic elements including alterations in the biochemical environment, structural damage from disease, degeneration of the myelin sheath, trauma, and neurotransmitter abnormality.

Inflammation and Infectious Processes

Inflammatory processes affecting nervous tissue alter the metabolism and thus the tissue's nutritional and immune processes. Infectious processes destroy tissue through the toxins released by the organisms. The CNS can become inflamed with trauma, lumbar punctures, and infectious processes such as meningitis. Meningitis illustrates well the response of the CNS to inflammation. This infection of the pia mater and arachnoid membranes can be caused by a variety of microorganisms. Its symptoms—headache, fever, stiffness in the back and neck, as well as pain when the neck is forcefully moved—reflect the inflammatory response of the meninges. The infectious process may cause alterations in the level of consciousness, behavior, and motor and sensory function as well as convulsions.

Inflammatory processes are known to attack the spinal cord's gray matter. Inflammation can occur in response to acute infections such as measles or pneumonia or can be part of a primary infectious process such as poliomyelitis. The inflammatory processes can cause necrosis, emboli, or thrombotic complications. Sensory and motor deficits may result.

Trauma, Tumors, and Compression

Trauma to the nervous system may result from external forces or elements within the nervous system. The skull and vertebral bodies make it difficult to discover, locate, and assess trauma or physical changes. Symptoms indicating progressing damage are sometimes subtle or lacking until the condition is too advanced to treat effectively.

At times, the system's response to the trauma causes more damage than the insult itself. This secondary damage occurs when edema, bleeding, and increased ICP destroy nervous tissue by compression or restriction of circulation. Edema results from trauma associated with contusions and laceration, trauma to capillary walls, or from hematomas or tumors that obstruct venous blood outflow. The obstruction causes the blood to back up and fluid to move out of the capillaries. Expanding tumors not only cause an increase in ICP and edema; they may also cause bleeding by damaging vessels. All these elements, which cause an increase in ICP, carry the hazard of herniation through the tentorial notch or foramen magnum.

Spinal injuries may cause many of the same problems as cranial injuries, but the complexity of the vertebral column's structure and the concentration of neural tracts at all levels of the cord present special concerns. Injuries to the spinal cord are more common in areas of greater mobility such as the lower cervical spine and the lumbar juncture (T-12, L-1, L-2). Vertebral injuries can cause compression of nerve roots by bone, ligaments, extruded disk material, hematomas, and disruption or overstretching of the neural tissue. Edema caused by trauma can compromise cord function.

Peripheral nerves are responsible for all input for somatic sensations and somatic reflex activity and for all output for the control of striated muscle and other peripheral effector structures. Damage to peripheral nerves will result in loss of sensory or motor functions below the site of the lesion. Some severed peripheral nerves may heal and function may be restored if the integrity of the tissue can be maintained and the nerve ends surgically aligned. Peripheral nerve damage may result from compression of nerves by ruptured disks or by compression from anatomic structures.

Nursing Research Note

Power DJ, Craven RF: ALS and aging: A case study in autonomy and control. *Image* (Winter) 1983; 15:22–25.

The clinical case study is one approach in qualitative research. This case study of a client with amyotrophic lateral sclerosis (ALS) in a long-term care setting assessed the client's balance between ADL and coping resources and support systems. The authors discuss the physiology of aging and the pathophysiology of ALS. Proposed nursing interventions, their rationale, and their expected and actual outcomes are presented.

The authors learned that the demands of daily living stimulated collaboration between the client and the nurse to develop an individualized plan of care. The case study suggests that the maintenance of autonomy and control is basic to attaining a high quality of life.

Degenerative Processes

Many nervous system diseases can be categorized as degenerative. Their causes vary, as do their severity and influence on lifestyle. Upper and lower motor neuron diseases are examples of degenerative processes manifested in the nervous system. Progressive muscular atrophy follows degeneration of lower motor neurons in the spinal cord because the muscles are no longer stimulated to contract. The disease amyotrophic lateral sclerosis (ALS) is manifested by degeneration of the upper motor neurons in the medulla oblongata and lower motor neurons in the spinal cord.

Hereditary and Congenital Diseases

Hereditary diseases result from inborn errors that affect development, maturation, or aging. These illnesses present varying degrees of risk to offspring both in the threat of developing the disease and carrying it on to another generation. For example, Huntington's chorea, a hereditary disease that causes mental and physical deterioration, is transmitted through an autosomal dominant gene. Each child born of an affected parent has a 50% chance of developing the disease.

Congenital defects causing CNS abnormalities or malfunctions may occur alone or in combination. Causes include a hereditary tendency, intrinsic factors such as inadequate circulation for the embryo, and in-utero exposure to infectious diseases such as rubella.

SECTION 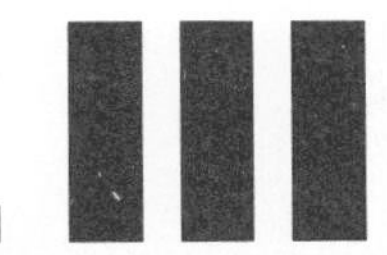

Related System Influences and Effects

The nervous system orchestrates activities to maintain body functions and homeostasis. The central nervous system's control over other major bodily systems has already been discussed. A brief discussion of other system activities that support CNS function will help complete the picture.

Each major system has a role in maintaining homeostatic activity through the regulation of the body's biochemical environment. Alteration in system functions by disease or trauma can result in abnormal neuronal activity or tissue destruction within the CNS. For example, effective pumping by the heart is essential to nourish the CNS and remove waste. Along with the respiratory system, the heart provides the oxygen necessary for function. Failure of these systems quickly results in neuronal death.

The kidneys serve several functions to support the nervous system. They participate in the maintenance of water balance and thus blood pressure. The kidneys also are important in maintaining electrolyte and acid–base balance. They even have a role in ensuring an adequate oxygen supply through the manufacture of erythropoietin, the hormone that stimulates the production of oxygen-carrying red blood cells.

Gastrointestinal absorption maintains an adequate nutritional level of food elements, vitamins, and minerals. The liver also helps by maintaining an effective level of blood glucose and other nutrients. Detoxification of drugs and other foreign substances are other ways in which the liver helps to maintain homeostasis.

An example of the influence of abnormal liver function on CNS function is hepatic coma. With this condition, the liver is unable to convert ammonia, the end product of amino-acid metabolism, into urea. As a result, the ammonia concentration becomes elevated and may reach toxic levels. Alterations in mental function and coma can occur.

The endocrine system, which has multiple roles in the regulation of body function, influences metabolism, heart rate, water balance, and mental function. Pathology within this system can cause a variety of neurologic abnormalities or deficits.

SECTION 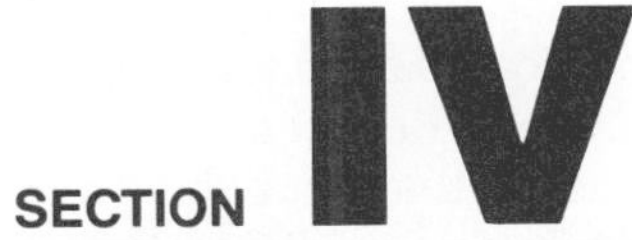

Psychosocial/Lifestyle Influences and Effects

Developmental Factors

Changes with aging are the result of alterations in effector tissues, receptor systems, and impairment of the body's homeostatic regulatory system.

Implications for Elderly Clients

Athletic ability gradually declines with age, along with skills requiring rapid sensory and motor coordination. Isometric muscle strength is maintained through the fifth decade, after which there is a gradual decline related to a decrease in the number of muscle fibers and muscle atrophy. Loss of muscle mass, especially in the thigh, calf, and intrinsic hand muscles occurs even in the active elderly (Katzman & Terry, 1983). Gait changes, such as slowing of step, are believed to be related to a decrease in muscle mass, loss of large motor nerve fibers regulating motor function, stiffening of joints, and proprioceptive impairment.

Epidemiologic studies indicate that physical exercise contributes to longevity by decreasing the incidence of heart disease. Studies suggest that exercise may reverse or retard age-related changes in synaptic function and nerve-conduction velocity. Physical training in the elderly has been found to improve heart rate, cardiac output, blood pressure, and joint mobility and to decrease stiffness, although it has not improved pulmonary function. Research has also shown that those who are active physically can outperform younger sedentary individuals.

Intellectual performance as measured by vocabulary and information comprehension peaks between 20 and 30 year of age and is maintained through life or until the mid-70s, in the absence of disease. Mental dexterity, especially learning and memory, shows some deficit, especially after age 70. As with physical activity, individuals who continue to be active mentally can perform better than some 20-year-olds. However, the speed of central processing for mental functioning is impaired with age (Katzman & Terry, 1983).

The loss of vibratory perception in the lower extremities usually begins at about age 50. Touch becomes significantly diminished due to skin changes and a decrease in the number of sensory receptors. Corneal sensitivity, an accurate measurement of sensory perception, shows a decrease in sensitivity in the aged. Visual, auditory, gustatory, and olfactory senses are also diminished.

Cortical size and blood flow decrease over time. The weight of the brain peaks in the early 20s and then undergoes a slow decline. Cerebral blood flow in the adult is about 50 to 60 mL per minute per 100 g of tissue. (The base requirement for normal cortical function is a little less than 40 mL per minute per 100 g.) Between 30 and 70 years of age, the rate of flow decreases about 20% (Kenney, 1982). Alterations in blood flow from atherosclerosis, structural changes such as the positioning of vessels in the vertebral column, and heart disease can easily decrease the oxygen supply, compromising neuronal function.

Changes in autonomic nervous system function in the elderly can be seen in the deterioration of pupillary, cardiovascular, thermal, and secretory functions. It is not clear whether these changes are the result of peripheral or CNS changes.

The elderly face the threat of altered homeostasis due to health problems unrelated to neurologic pathology such as cardiac, respiratory, kidney, and gastrointestinal disturbances. If an imbalance occurs, the nervous system can be affected. Psychologic reactions to stress can also alter neurologic function.

Sociocultural and Lifestyle Influences

Neurologic disease processes frequently force clients and their significant others to deal with devastating and wide-ranging alterations in lifestyles. These alterations may include the shattering of hopes and dreams for themselves and perhaps for their offspring. Neurologic disease may cause tremendous financial strain and perhaps even the need to seek public assistance. Clients may suddenly be forced to become receivers rather than contributors to life, family, and community.

Depending on the time of onset of the disease, educational or professional aspirations may be interrupted. Many neurologic diseases strike early, leaving deficits or a slowly progressing loss of function. Alterations in function from neurologic diseases may be accompanied by changes in physical appearance that can seriously affect self-concept and body image. Examples include awkward gait, drooling, distorted facial expression, tremors, and being wheelchair-bound.

Mental function may also be altered, affecting interaction with others. Common problems include confusion and changes in intellect. Mental function may be further compromised by alteration in sensory perceptions such as vision, hearing, touch, and smell. These changes in function as well as the experience of the disease contribute to a negative change in the individual's body image. Many characteristics valued by society may be lost.

Even though society has become more accepting toward persons who are different from others or from the images created by advertisers, interactions with the disabled may still be strained. Perhaps part of this discomfort is the result of conscious or unconscious concern about one's own susceptibility to illness. The physical, mental, and emotional deficits often experienced by persons with neurologic diseases, along with society's difficulty in relating to them, can cause clients and their loved ones to become isolated from others. The alteration in physical function and body image, as well as self-consciousness and possibly depression, can result in self-imposed isolation. Clients may have limited opportunities for environmental or social interaction. This physical and mental isolation affects how clients feel, live, work, and play.

Chapter Highlights

Neurons, the cells that regulate intricate and gross body functions, require a homeostatic biochemical environment and an extensive system of support and protection to function effectively.

Central nervous system neurons cannot be repaired or replaced. Some peripheral neurons may be repaired.

Complex intercommunication among individual neurons and neurons within functional units and hemispheres of the brain is required for nervous system function and body function.

Specialized areas of function have been identified within the nervous system. Effective function is based on the presence of neurotransmitters and effective intercommunication among parts of the nervous system.

The limbic system, on receiving multiple input from the internal and external environments, influences physical and emotional responses.

The autonomic nervous system, composed of the sympathetic and parasympathetic nervous systems, regulates visceral functions, maintains homeostasis, and combats stress.

Nervous tissue requires constant nourishment and removal of waste products.

Cerebrospinal fluid is constantly being produced and must be reabsorbed to prevent excessive pressure within the central nervous system.

Many of the nervous system's structural components protect vital brain tissue but are subject to pathology, which may harm brain tissue.

Blood vessels and peripheral nerves provide routes for foreign elements to enter the central nervous system.

The effects of pathology on nervous system function depend on the size of the lesion, its location, and the reaction of the system to the insult.

The nervous system is subject to harm when other body systems fail.

For many, keeping active mentally and physically can slow the aging process.

Deficits caused by neurologic disease can alter all aspects of life.

Planning care for clients with neurologic problems requires assessment for psychosocial and lifestyle problems as well as for physical deficits.

Bibliography

Angevine JB, Cotman CW: *Principles of Neuroanatomy*. New York: Oxford, 1981.

Anthony CP, Thibodeau GA: *Textbook of Anatomy and Physiology*. St Louis: Mosby, 1983.

Carpenter MB, Sutin J: *Human Neuroanatomy*. Baltimore: Williams & Wilkins, 1983.

Chusid JG: *Correlative Neuroanatomy and Functional Neuroanatomy*, 19th ed. Los Altos, CA: Lange, 1985.

Conway–Rutkowski BL: *Carini and Owens' Neurological and Neurosurgical Nursing*, 8th ed. St. Louis: Mosby, 1982.

De Young S: *The Neurologic Patient: A Nursing Perspective*. Englewood Cliffs, NJ: Prentice–Hall, 1983.

Diseases. Springhouse, PA: Intermed, 1983.

Eliasson SG, Prensky AL, Hardin WB: *Neurological Pathophysiology*. New York: Oxford, 1979.

Groër ME, Shekleton ME: *Basic Pathophysiology: A Conceptual Approach*, 2nd ed. St Louis: Mosby, 1983.

Guyton AC: *Human Physiology and Mechanisms of Disease*. Philadelphia: Saunders, 1982.

Katzman R, Terry R: *The Neurology of Aging*. Philadelphia: Davis, 1983.

Kenney RA: *Physiology of Aging: A Synopsis*. Chicago: Year Book Medical Publishers, 1982.

Pallett P, O'Brien M: *Textbook of Neurological Nursing*. Boston: Little, Brown, 1985.

Price SA, Wilson LM: *Pathophysiology: Clinical Concepts of Disease Processes*, 2nd ed. New York: McGraw–Hill, 1982.

Spence AP, Mason ER: *Human Anatomy and Physiology*, 3rd ed. Menlo Park, CA: Benjamin/Cummings, 1987.

CHAPTER 28

The Nursing Process for Clients With Neurologic Dysfunction

Other topics relevant to this content are: Assessment of mental status and sensory and motor function, **Chapter 5;** The Heimlich maneuver, **Chapter 19;** Care of the client undergoing cystometrography, **Chapter 25;** Care of the client with spinal cord injury, **Chapter 29;** Care of the client with carpal tunnel syndrome, **Chapter 46.**

Objectives

When you have finished studying this chapter you should be able to:

Specify the major components of the health history to be obtained from clients with neurologic dysfunction.

Explain specific assessment approaches in evaluating clients with dysfunction of the nervous system.

Identify the nursing implications of diagnostic studies commonly used to evaluate clients with neurologic dysfunction.

Determine appropriate nursing diagnoses for clients with disorders of the nervous system.

Develop, with the client, realistic goals of care.

Anticipate the psychosocial/lifestyle implications of neurologic dysfunction for clients and their significant others.

Develop a nursing care plan for a client with neurologic dysfunction.

Implement nursing interventions specific to clients with dysfunction of the nervous system.

Evaluate the effectiveness of the nursing care plan and modify it as necessary to meet client needs.

The pervasive influence of the central nervous system (CNS) on mental and physical functions often complicates the analysis of neurologic symptoms. Identification of nervous system pathology can be difficult because symptoms are often far removed from the source. For example, a cerebrovascular accident (CVA) can result in weakness in a lower extremity. Furthermore, because of similar symptoms and signs some diseases of the CNS can confound the diagnosis; for example, subarachnoid hemorrhage, stroke, and hydrocephalus all create symptoms of increased intracranial pressure (ICP).

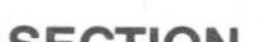

SECTION I

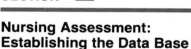

Nursing Assessment: Establishing the Data Base

The rewards from neurologic assessment are many. Symptoms and signs may be identified in time to prevent serious or extensive neurologic damage. A neurologic assessment also provides an opportunity to teach the client about body function and health and adds to the nursing knowledge needed to develop a comprehensive care plan.

Subjective Data

Collection of subjective data from clients with CNS diseases can be especially difficult because the disease often compromises the client's ability to provide reliable information. In some instances, the client will be unresponsive, unconscious, or unreliable as a historian. At these times, family members, friends, or persons who were present when the problem arose should be consulted.

The fear or apprehension that often accompanies possible diagnosis of neurologic disease can limit client disclosure. The nurse's expressed interest in the client's problems along with appropriate teaching and support while collecting the data can comfort the client and family, build confidence in the nurse, and increase willingness to share symptoms and concerns.

Essential to a neurologic assessment is a review of the client's long-term and recent health history because neurologic problems can result from diseases affecting other systems. Neurologic problems are also sometimes misdiagnosed as psychiatric problems. Other health problems must also be considered in planning treatments or care. For example, plans for diet, medications, and intravenous therapy will be more complex if the client with neurologic dysfunction also has diabetes, cirrhosis, or renal disease.

Communication with the client during the assessment must be well planned. Keep in mind that terminology describing neurologic problems can be foreign to individuals without a health care background. Therefore, when seeking information from the client, use lay terminology or descriptive terms to avoid miscommunication or intimidation. For example, when describing sensations, use the words *numbness* and *tingling* rather than *paresthesia.* Encourage more thorough disclosure by giving examples of symptoms. Consider this approach: "Mrs Smith, do you have any difficulty in seeing, such as blurred vision or spots or lines in your vision?" This approach helps clients understand what kind of information is sought.

Skin, Nails, and Hair

Integumentary changes are important symptoms in many neurologic disorders. Ask about changes in the skin, hair, and nails. Hair loss can signal nutritional deficiencies related to the inability to eat because of dysphagia, depression, or altered level of consciousness. Question the client about skin changes or overgrowths of skin, port-wine stains, or nevi. **Café au lait spots** (spots of light brown patchy skin pigmentation) and disfiguring overgrowths of skin resembling polyps are seen in neurofibromatosis. Because these growths can also occur in the CNS, it is important to inquire about other symptoms of an enlarging CNS mass such as headache, sensory changes, alteration in level of consciousness, mood changes, and alteration in motor function.

Head and Neck

Client symptoms related to the head and neck should be carefully reviewed during the history of the present illness (HPI). Headaches are common in a variety of health problems, including stress, tumors, meningitis, or one of the many diseases causing increased ICP.

The history or presence of earache accompanied by diminished hearing and possibly ear drainage often suggests otitis. Ear infections can spread into the brain via adjacent blood vessels and the mastoid bone of the skull. Infections of the scalp, paranasal sinuses, and the nasopharynx also present the risk of meningitis or encephalitis because of their proximity to venous sinuses, blood vessels, and foramina. These channels facilitate the spread of infection into the CNS.

Reported hearing loss may be the result of a conduction problem or of damage to CN VIII or to cortical tissue. Question the client about **tinnitus** (ringing or buzzing in the ears). If emotional or behavioral changes are reported, ask whether the client has been having auditory hallucinations, which can result from temporal lobe lesions. Keep in mind that damage to the auditory receptive area in the temporal lobe of the dominant hemisphere can also cause difficulty in understanding the communication of others. Dizziness and vertigo are significant symptoms of tumors or degenerative changes in the vestibular branch of CN VIII, the brain stem, or the cerebellum.

Uncontrolled head movements are significant for Parkinson's disease, other extrapyramidal disease processes, and multiple sclerosis. A partial loss of motor function of the face can be the result of Bell's palsy, CVAs, or pathology affecting the nuclei of the brain stem. Loss of smell from insult to the olfactory bulbs or tracts can be related to shearing trauma, orbital fractures, or tumors.

A loss of taste, perceived by CN V and CN IX, can suggest local or CNS pathology. On the other hand, many older clients comment on loss of taste or decreased taste without the presence of pathology.

Visual changes can result from many elements affecting CN II, its optic radiations, the occipital lobe, CN III, CN IV, CN VI, and their related nuclei in the brain stem. Diseases causing visual changes include multiple sclerosis, myasthenia gravis, stroke, tumors, and trauma.

CN IX, X, and XII direct muscle activity related to talking, chewing, and swallowing. A deficit may be evident during the history. Many disease processes affect these cranial nerves including stroke, tumor, myasthenia gravis, amyotrophic lateral sclerosis (ALS), and multiple sclerosis. Help the client to identify problems by inquiring about difficulty in chewing, swallowing, a need for conscious effort to chew or swallow, choking, excessive accumulation of saliva or food in the mouth, and fatigue from chewing, which may even limit intake and result in weight loss. Speech problems stemming from pathology in these areas may include difficulty in formulating words and in articulation.

Bowel and Bladder

Bowel and bladder function is controlled by various components of the autonomic nervous system. Thoroughly review symptoms such as constipation, urinary retention, and fecal and urinary incontinence.

The client may be unable to expel stool if thoracic spinal cord segments T-1 through T-12 are injured. This problem occurs because voluntary control of abdominal contraction, important in the contraction of the rectal wall, can be lost. In addition, spinal cord injury or disease above or involving sacral nerves S-3, S-4, and S-5 can result in incontinence because of the loss of sphincter tone and reflex activity. Diseases of the cerebral cortex that interfere with mental function can also cause fecal incontinence.

Urinary bladder dysfunction can occur with diseases affecting the cerebral cortex; parasympathetic fibers of S-2, S-3, and S-4; sympathetic fibers from T-11 and T-12 and L-1 and L-2; and peripheral nerve fibers. Examples of CNS diseases are tumors, ruptured disks, and tabes dorsalis. Incontinence or urinary retention can also stem from peripheral nerve damage from diabetes and herpes zoster (Samuels, 1982). Transient urinary retention can follow lumbar puncture or lumbar myelography.

Sexual Function

Occasionally, clients mention concern about sexual dysfunction. Careful and sensitive questioning is needed to establish that problems exist. Sexual dysfunction can occur in men and women who have had insults to the parasympathetic fibers from spinal cord segments S-2, S-3, and S-4; sympathetic fibers from the lumbar spine; or peripheral nerves from these segments. For clients who report sexual dysfunction, take a careful and thorough medication history because many medications have been implicated in impotence. These include anticholinergic agents; drugs with significant anticholinergic side effects such as tricyclic antidepressants, phenothiazines, and antivertigo drugs; narcotic stimulants or psychedelic drugs; drugs that induce depression such as reserpine, methyldopa, propranolol, and other antihypertensive drugs; and ethyl alcohol.

Motor Function

Changes in motor function are often unique to a disease process. Inquiry into changes in motor function should include thorough questioning about localized or generalized weakness. Asking specifically about difficulty arising from or turning in bed; flopping of ankles during walking; and difficulty in moving legs to go up and down steps or in lifting objects, brushing teeth, or keeping eyes open will help clients explain their symptoms better.

Attend to reports of widely separated areas of motor deficit as well as isolated or continuous areas, because disseminated patches of deficit often occur in multiple sclerosis. Symptoms of **ataxia** (lack of muscle coordination) should raise concern about degeneration of the posterior tracts of the spinal cord or cerebellar dysfunction. Uncontrolled movements stemming from faulty basal ganglion function may herald the development of Parkinson's disease, Huntington's chorea, or other diseases affecting the basal ganglia. Reports of uncontrolled movement can also be related to seizure activity.

Spasticity of muscles (increased resistance to passive stretch with rapid extension or flexion of a joint) occurs with CVAs or multiple sclerosis, which release muscles from upper motor neuron control. In contrast, **flaccidity** (decreased or absent muscle tone) can result from isolation of muscles from neuronal impulses. This pathology occurs when anterior horn motor neurons are destroyed, as in poliomyelitis or ALS. Flaccidity may also be seen with peripheral nerve damage from trauma or peripheral nerve inflammation as in Guillain–Barré syndrome. Reports of weakness can be attributed to a variety of disease processes such as entrapment of nerves, as seen in carpal tunnel syndrome (see Chapter 47), or as a weakness that increases with exertion, as with myasthenia gravis.

Twitching (localized, spasmodic contraction of a single muscle group) of the trapezius muscle may occur with lesions in the nucleus of CN XI. Twitching may also occur in other muscles affected by poliomyelitis, spinal cord disease, motor root and peripheral nerve disease, ALS, and muscular dystrophy (Chusid, 1985). Diseases affecting sternocleidomastoid functions are muscular dystrophy, polyneuritis, and poliomyelitis. **Fasciculations** are fine, rapid, twitching movements originating in small groups of muscle fibers. Fasciculations in muscles that are becoming atrophied indicate lower motor neuron disease.

Other abnormal movements include spasm of a muscle or muscle groups (**myoclonus**), tremors, paucity of movement, and rigidity of movement. **Dyskinesias** (defects in voluntary movement) including facial and limb **chorea** (involuntary twitching of the limbs or facial muscles), **athetosis** (slow, twisting, snakelike movements in the upper extremities), and **dystonia** (intense, irregular torsion muscle spasms) can result from antipsychotic medications or from Huntington's chorea.

Sensory Function

Diseases of the spinal cord's sensory tract can alter or even prevent transmission of stimuli to the brain for interpretation. Symptoms of pathology causing alteration in transmission include numbness, tingling, pain, increased or decreased sensitivity to touch, and alteration in perception of cold and heat. The loss of these sensations may be partial or complete. In addition, clients often show evidence of trauma and burns, incurred because of the absence of a sensory warning of impending injury. Many sensory deficits result from peripheral neuropathy and follow peripheral nerve distribution patterns.

Common sensory disturbances include neuritis, neuralgia, root pain, and herpes zoster. **Neuritis,** characterized by pain and tenderness along the course of the nerve, results from inflammation, trauma, or infection. It can progress to complete loss of sensory and motor function. **Neuralgia,** an uncomfortable, painful, burning sensation, may occur spontaneously or from unintentional stimulation of "trigger zones." Trigeminal neuralgia is typical of this process. **Root pain** occurs with lesions of the dorsal roots of the spinal nerves. The pain is sharp and lightninglike. Coughing and sneezing increase the pain. The pain may result from ruptured disks, cord tumors, fractures, inflammatory diseases of the vertebrae, or meninges. Herpes zoster, a viral inflammatory process, is characterized by painful blisters that follow the cutaneous nerve roots. Transient motor paralysis may accompany the condition.

Clients may also report sensory changes following peripheral nerve damage from trauma, metabolic diseases such as pernicious anemia and diabetes, and entrapment of nerves as in carpal tunnel syndrome. Reports of enlarging joints or loose joints may be given by clients with diabetic neuropathy, syringomyelia, spinal cord disorders, and peripheral nerve injuries. Joint deterioration results when the joints, lacking sensation, are repeatedly injured (Chusid, 1985).

Objective Data

A thorough neurologic assessment of clients with probable nervous system disease is important initially and throughout the nurse–client interaction. Comprehensive baseline data assist in effective evaluation of the client's changing status. In addition to the formal assessment, frequent contact with the hospitalized client during treatments and activities of daily living will allow close observation of client actions.

Physical Assessment

MENTAL STATUS Keep in mind when assessing mental function that many clients and family members view the brain with awe. Their concern over the diagnosis of a disease affecting the brain can cause fear. In addition, some tests may seem to be a test of intelligence and may cause misunderstanding and apprehension. Therefore, the purpose of the exam should be explained and the testing carried out in a nonthreatening and supportive manner in a quiet and private environment.

The client's mental status is an important component of the neurologic assessment, providing valuable insights into the cause of disease and its effect on the body. Determination of level of consciousness is often used to evaluate improvement or decline of health status in clients with brain trauma or tumors. See Chapter 5 for a sequential approach to the mental status exam.

Assessment of level of consciousness begins with noting the degree of alertness. Is the client awake and alert? If sleeping, is the client aroused by verbal stimuli or tactile stimulation such as touch or gentle shaking, or does the client respond only to a noxious stimulus? After arousal, is alertness maintained once the stimulus is removed? Does the client appear drowsy, restless, irritable, or combative? Question the client regarding time, place, person, and self. If the client is becoming disoriented, awareness of time will usually be lost first, then place, then person, and last self. Inappropriate responses to such questioning may not necessarily indicate mental dysfunction. The client may fail to respond appropriately because of a language barrier, impaired hearing or vision, or some degree of expressive or receptive dysphasia. The trauma client may be confused about time or place because of a period of unconsciousness or the rapidity of events. The client transferred from another hospital or even from another unit may have trouble keeping up with the changes. This is especially true of the elderly.

Long periods of hospitalization can easily cause a client, even without a neurologic problem, to lose track of the date. An extended stay in an intensive care unit, where there is round-the-clock activity, can readily lead to confusion about time of day. Ask the client to follow simple commands, such as "squeeze my hand," "hold up your arm," "wiggle your toes." The response permits assessment of motor function as well as mental function. If the client does not respond to verbal or tactile stimulation, a noxious or painful stimulus may be needed. As a general rule, the stimulus should be the least that will elicit a response and yet not inflict damage. Even in the unconscious client, noxious stimuli may cause a precipitous rise in blood pressure.

Charting should include the stimulus used as well as a description of the client's response to it. Responses are usually classified as appropriate, inappropriate, or absent. In an appropriate response the client localizes the unpleasant stimulus and attempts to withdraw from it or push it away. An inappropriate response involves random or purposeless movements and decerebrate or decorticate posturing. In extreme situations no response can be elicited and the client remains flaccid. Because subtle changes in level of consciousness can be significant, precise documentation and clear communication are essential. Avoid words like confused, stuporous, and comatose. Instead describe the clients behavior, what is said, and what can or cannot be done. At change of shift, it may be especially beneficial for the nurse coming on duty and the nurse reporting off duty to do an assessment together. In this way, the nurse about to assume responsibility for the client has a clearer picture of the client's condition. Subtle or minor changes that may be significant are less likely to be missed or misinterpreted.

The Glasgow Coma Scale is an objective measure of level of consciousness that can also be somewhat predictive of recovery (Table 28–1). Coma is defined as a score of 7 or less. With a score of 3 or 4, there is an 85% chance of dying or remaining vegetative. A score above 11 is associated with an 85% chance of moderate disability or good recovery.

STATION AND GAIT Observation of the client's **station** (manner of standing) and gait will give many clues. Postures can be influenced by mental and physical problems. The degree of decrease in the level of consciousness

Table 28–1
Levels of Consciousness: Glasgow Coma Scale

Faculty Measured	Response	Score
Eye opening	Spontaneous	4
	To verbal command	3
	To pain	2
	No response	1
Motor response	To verbal command	6
	To painful stimuli:	
	• Localizes pain	5
	• Flexes and withdraws	4
	• Assumes decorticate posture	3
	• Assumes decerebrate posture	2
	• No response	1
Verbal response (arouse client with painful stimuli, if necessary)	Oriented, converses	5
	Disoriented, converses	4
	Uses inappropriate words	3
	Makes incomprehensible sounds	2
	No response	1

SOURCE: Adapted from Teasdale G, Bennet B: Assessment of coma and impaired consciousness: A practical scale. *Lancet* 1974; 2(7872):81.

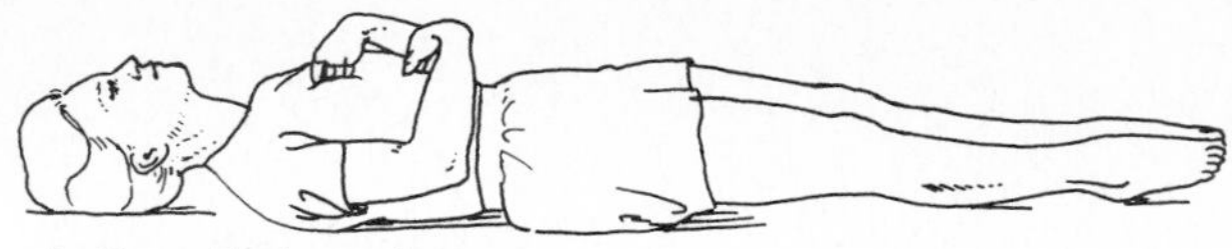

A. Decorticate posture

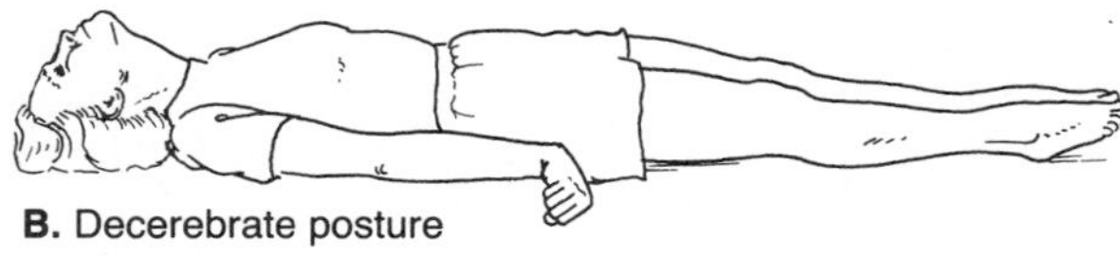

B. Decerebrate posture

Figure 28–1

Decorticate and decerebrate posturing. **A.** Decorticate posture: the client's arms are adducted with elbows and wrists in rigid flexion, the hands rotated internally and fingers flexed; the lower extremities are hyperextended. **B.** Decerebrate posture: the client has hyperextended upper and lower extremities; **opisthotonos** (head extended, body arched) is an exaggerated decerebrate posture seen in tetanus, when the body may be supported on the back of the head and the feet during a convulsion.

affects posture, which can vary from slouching to flaccid with no response to stimuli. Two types of posture in unresponsive clients can be significant in identifying the level of CNS involvement, giving evidence of decortication or decerebration. The postures can occur spontaneously or in response to a stimulus such as testing for reflexes.

With **decorticate posturing** (Figure 28–1A), the client demonstrates hyperflexion of the upper extremities and hyperextension of the lower extremities. Lesions on the cerebral hemisphere or internal capsule are believed to cause decorticate postures by interrupting the corticospinal pathways. With **decerebrate posturing** (Figure 28–1B), both the upper and lower extremities are hyperextended. Decerebrate posture can occur when a diencephalic lesion of the hemisphere extends, causing midbrain and upper pontine damage.

Unusual gait, stance, or sitting posture can result from motor or sensory deficits as in stroke or tabes dorsalis. Clients with Parkinson's disease have a typical shuffling and propulsive (**festination**) gait. The normal arm swing is also lost.

SKIN AND HAIR Trophic changes on the face and extremities are often noticeable at the beginning of the exam. Café au lait spots, frequently accompanied by subcutaneous nodules, are seen on any part of the body in neurofibromatosis. Autonomic nervous system (ANS) abnormalities are suspected with abnormal colorations ranging from erythema to cyanosis; temperature changes, either coolness or increased warmth; and variations in skin moisture, either dryness or sweating. Melanomas—malignant skin tumors—metastasize to the CNS. Burns and bruises of the extremities suggest decreased sensation.

Decreased sensory awareness can result in decubitus ulcers. In the spinal and posterior fossa areas, look for tufts of hair and abnormal pigmentation, suggesting underlying neural tube deformity.

Baldness can result from nutritional disorders, anxiety, or chemotherapy. Pluckable or shedding hair and brittle hair are signs of nutritional deficiency. Chemotherapy may temporarily affect the hair follicle, causing hair loss. A client with nervous dysfunction may show signs of patchy baldness from pulling out hair without being aware of doing so; thus, the baldness may suggest sensory dysfunction. Baldness may also suggest nutritional deficiency, which can result from neurologically based dysphagia, depression, or dulled consciousness.

HEAD AND NECK A major portion of the neurologic exam focuses on the head and neck because of the concentration of nervous tissue in this area. Keep in mind that, although the skull protects the brain, foramina are portals for organisms and can be obstructed by tumors and calcifications. Palpation can reveal trauma, tender areas, and bony elevations. If the history includes a report of severe and often unpredictable facial pain, like that of tic douloureux (trigeminal neuralgia), avoid palpating or stimulating an identified trigger zone. Asymmetry in facial muscles can indicate a deficit in motor function.

Auscultation over the closed eyes may reveal bruits stemming from a variety of vascular changes such as arteriovenous malformation, stenosis of the carotid arteries or aorta, dilation of vessels to meet the increased nutritional needs of a vascular meningioma, or distortion of blood vessels by a space-occupying lesion (Conway–Rutkowski,

1982). With arteriovenous malformations or aneurysms of the temporal lobe, bruits may be heard directly over the site.

CRANIAL NERVES Assessment of the individual cranial nerves is essential when pathology is suspected in the head, neck, and shoulders. The widespread influence of CN X must be considered with the general assessment.

Assessment of an individual's ability to smell is a test of CN I. Loss of smell (**anosmia**) can result from a shearing force with a blow to the head or pressure from a tumor on the olfactory bulb or tract.

Visual changes provide a vast array of information about the function of CN II, III, IV, and VI. The extension of CN II from its exit site on the retina (optic disk) to the occipital lobe makes it vulnerable to a variety of lesions. Identifying problems of visual acuity and loss of peripheral vision can help to establish the location of the pathology. For example, partial loss of a visual field suggests injury to the optic tracts. Loss of vision can occur with occipital lobe trauma; the inability to interpret visual input can occur with parietal lobe trauma. **Papilledema** (edema and inflammation of the optic nerve at its point of entrance into the eye ball—also called choked disk) results from increased ICP.

Cranial nerves III, IV, and VI are responsible for eye movements needed for focusing. CN III controls eye movement medially, upward, and downward. Diseases affecting CN IV will result in loss of the ability to look down and laterally in the involved eye. Deficits in CN VI function will be evidenced by the loss of ability of the affected eye to look laterally. With any of these deficits, the client might have double vision (**diplopia**) or dizziness. Observe also for nystagmus, which can be physiologic or due to central or labyrinthine lesions. It can also occur with certain drugs, for example, phenytoin (Dilantin), bromides, barbiturates, and alcohol (Chusid, 1982). Squinting or tilting the head to facilitate focusing are additional signs of pathology.

Cranial nerve III also controls elevation of the eyelid. Ineffective closure of the lid is a common problem in myasthenia gravis and in pathology in the brain stem as in stroke or head injury. Parasympathetic fibers traveling with CN III are responsible for constriction of the pupil. Pupillary size and reaction (or lack of reaction) to a light stimulus are significant in various neurologic diseases. Pupillary change is of special concern when increased ICP or brain stem pathology is suspected. Using an assessment guide similar to that in Figure 28–2 will aid in measuring pupil size.

Tumors, injury, and disease processes can alter function in CN V causing pain, loss of sensation, or paresthesia. Motor and sensory abnormalities of the face can also be seen with CN VII pathology. The motor component of this nerve innervates all facial muscles. Its sensory component perceives taste on the anterior two-thirds of the tongue.

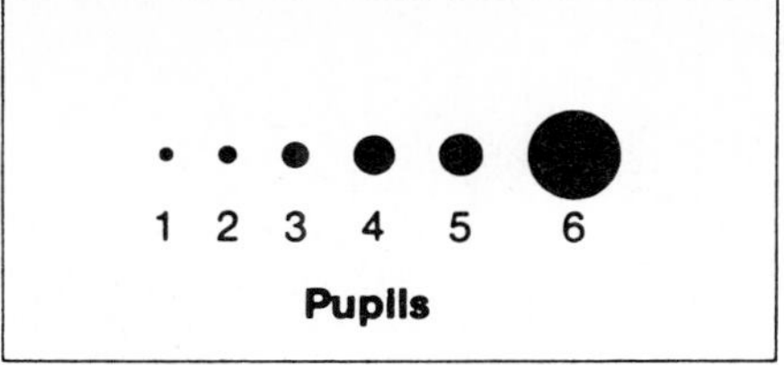

Figure 28–2

Pupil gauge. SOURCE: *Swearingen PL:* The Addison-Wesley Photo-Atlas of Nursing Procedure. *Menlo Park, CA: Addison-Wesley, 1984.*

With Bell's palsy, which affects CN VII, the client experiences unilateral drooping of the mouth, collection of food between cheek and gum, tearing of the eye, loss of deep sensation (position and vibratory sense), and inability to close the eye. Pathology involving CN VIII causes hearing loss (cochlear branch) or disturbances in balance (vestibular branch).

Cranial nerves IX and XII can be affected by tumors, trauma, hemorrhage, ALS, and bulbar diseases. Aspiration of food or saliva is a serious threat to clients when these cranial nerves are affected. Other signs of involvement include the collection of food or saliva in the mouth, choking, loss of weight, and a poor nutritional state. The client's gag reflex and ability to chew, to form a bolus of food, and to swallow must be carefully assessed.

Cranial nerves IX and X also have a major role in perception of pain, touch, and temperature. All are important for safe chewing and swallowing. Loss of sensitivity in the pharynx, together with the loss of taste on the posterior one-third of the tongue, occur with CN IX pathology.

Cranial nerve XII controls motor function of the tongue. Lesions affecting its movement can result from unilateral or bilateral upper or lower motor neuron lesions. Signs of CN XII pathology include deviation of the tongue on protrusion, flaccid or spastic paralysis, atrophy, and fasciculations. If the lesion is bilateral, dysphagia (difficulty in swallowing), **dysarthria** (poorly articulated speech), and difficulty in chewing will be present. CN XII is also harmed in poisoning by lead, alcohol, arsenic, and carbon monoxide (Chusid, 1985).

Cranial nerve XI is affected by a number of diseases that can limit contraction of the sternocleidomastoid and trapezius muscles. These diseases include multiple sclerosis, syphilis, meningitis, poliomyelitis, and muscular dystrophy. Alteration of muscle function can result from pathology in the medulla, in the cervical cord and its peripheral nerves, and from cortical lesions. Signs of CN XI pathology include atrophy of muscle, inability to rotate the head to the healthy side, unequal strength in pushing against resistance, inability to shrug the involved shoulder, or dropping of this shoulder. Look for the involved scapula to be displaced downward. Bilateral nuclear or peripheral lesions cause difficulty in rotating the head or raising the chin. The head droops forward. Atrophied trapezius mus-

Nursing Research Note

Feroli–Lord K, McGinty–Maquire M: Toward a more objective approach to pupil assessment. *J Neurosurg Nurs* 1985; 7(5):309–312.

This descriptive study examined the differences between a hand-held tongue depressor pupil gauge and a printed millimeter scale sheet to assess pupillary size. The tongue depressor was held next to the client's eye and moved up and down until it best correlated with pupil size. The printed millimeter tool was on a sheet of paper, and size was compared to scaled drawings and diagrams of millimeter circles. Forty-two pairs of nurses were randomly assigned to either the tongue depressor pupil tool or the printed millimeter sheet tool. An investigator watched as each pair of nurses individually assessed pupil size with the tools. Twenty-eight pairs were in the tongue depressor group, and 14 pairs were in the standard pupil measurement group. There was no significant difference between measurements in either group. However, the tongue depressor group had higher interrater reliability, indicating that different nurses using the tool measured pupil size the same.

This research indicates that millimeter pupil gauges that can be held near the client's eye provide a more consistent and reliable measure of pupil size for nursing practice; using such a tool decreases subjective pupil measurement. The tool must be placed near the eye for best measurement. Developing such a tool on a tongue blade is inexpensive, convenient, and disposable.

cles give the shoulder a square appearance. Central paralysis causes similar limitations in movement but no atrophy. Muscles are spastic. Unilateral central involvement can result in **torticollis** (tilting of the head to one side in response to muscle contraction) (Chusid, 1985). Fasciculation in involved muscles may be observed, felt, or heard on auscultation. Pain with rotation of the head suggests cervical arthritis.

MOTOR FUNCTION Alteration in motor function can result from cortical, cerebellar, spinal cord, or peripheral nerve pathology as well as psychiatric disturbances. Observed changes in motor function provide valuable information about the disease process and nursing care needed.

Assessment of motor function includes examination of the physical structure of muscles and their ability to function normally. The structure of muscles gives information about their innervation, strength, and nutritional status as well as about the type of physical activity usually undertaken. Muscle mass and bulk are influenced by age, sex, and heredity. Poliomyelitis is an example of a disease that wastes muscle. Muscular dystrophy also results in muscle wasting, but the enlargement of muscle with connective and fatty tissue can be deceiving. Clients with myasthenia gravis, a disease of the neuromuscular junction, demonstrate a greater degree of weakness during exercise.

Muscle tone, the response of a limb to movement, can be increased or decreased by disease. Increased tone can be seen in extrapyramidal tract disorders such as Parkinson's disease or in upper motor neuron damage as in stroke. A pronounced increase in tone is referred to as **rigidity**. Rigidity can be increased when the individual concentrates on movement and when another limb is moved (Snyder, 1983). In **cogwheel rigidity**, seen in Parkinson's disease, the examiner feels predictable fluctuations in the intensity of muscle tone. Spasticity is seen in pyramidal tract disease. Joint contractures are often seen in clients with a history of spasticity. Flaccidity of muscle (**hypotonia**) is observed with lesions of the sensory and motor components of the reflex arc (Conway–Rutkowski, 1982). Fasciculation can be seen with denervation of muscle, with drug therapy, dietary deficiencies, fever, and uremia.

Other abnormal movements such as chorea, athetosis, dystonia, and tremor can be seen in extrapyramidal tract dysfunction. Choreic movements are rapid, jerky, and semipurposeful. In athetosis, less purposeful movements are slower, sinuous, and continuous. They are exaggerated with voluntary movements or emotional stimuli. These movements do not occur during sleep but can interfere with speech, eating, smooth respiration, and other activities (Conway–Rutkowski, 1982).

Cerebellar control of coordination, balance, and the judgment of distance can be limited or destroyed by a number of pathologies such as trauma, congenital deficits, disease, and medications. Signs, which may be subtle or obvious, include tremor, ataxia, exaggerated arm swing, hypotonia, and impaired posture without loss of motor power (Conway–Rutkowski, 1982).

Useful in diagnosing lumbar disease is *Lasègue's sign,* which assesses pain and limitation in motor function. For this test the client lies supine and is asked to do straight leg raises. With lumbar disk disease, leg raising on the affected side will be limited. Root pain can occur on the affected side when the opposite leg is raised. If a lesion is present in the upper lumbar area, pain is increased when the hip is hyperextended (Conway–Rutkowski, 1982).

SENSORY FUNCTION Sensory changes, significant in all disease processes, are especially important in neurologic problems; they are often the first or only symptom of a disease or disease progression. Neurologic sensory changes call for careful planning to ensure client safety and maintenance of optimal function because lack of attention to symptoms of pain or paresthesia (eg, with clients who have spinal cord or root injuries) could lead to a permanent loss of motor and sensory function. Sensory changes can result from disease or trauma of the parietal lobe, thalamus, brain stem, spinal cord, and peripheral nerves. They include alteration or loss of touch, pain, or temperature sensitivity and the loss of vibratory and position sense.

Assessment of sensory function is covered in Chapter 5. Assessment includes testing of superficial sensation (light touch, pain, and temperature) and deep sensation (position and vibratory senses). The absence of sensory changes when motor deficits are present can help to confirm a diagnosis. In both Guillain–Barré syndrome and ALS, profound motor deficits occur while sensation remains unchanged.

SUPERFICIAL AND DEEP TENDON REFLEXES Reflex changes provide valuable information about diminished sensations or paralysis in the conscious and unconscious client. These changes can provide early warning of pathology involving the corticospinal pathways, anterior horn cells, their axonal projections, and the afferent sensory component of muscles. Reflex responses also help to localize the level of a spinal cord injury.

When assessing deep tendon reflexes (DTRs), view asymmetry and diminished, increased, or absent reflexes in light of other neurologic findings. Superficial reflexes such as the abdominal and cremasteric responses are of limited value because of the superimposed cortical pathway. Therefore, lesions of either the cortical tract or the lower motor neuron can result in abnormal reflexes (Conway–Rutkowski, 1982). Furthermore, when checking these reflexes, keep in mind that lesions above the decussations (crossings) of the corticospinal tract result in loss or diminished reflexes on the opposite side of the body. Lesions below this level result in a loss of reflexes on the same side as the lesion.

A superficial reflex frequently used for discovering an upper motor neuron lesion is **clonus**, a continued rapid flexion and extension of the foot. This reflex is elicited by quickly dorsiflexing the foot. The wrist and patella can also be tested. Note that if the clonus stops quickly, it may be a normal response (Chusid, 1985).

MENINGEAL IRRITATION Assessment for nuchal (neck) rigidity, Kernig's sign, and Brudzinski's sign aid in diagnosing meningeal irritation as in meningitis or subarachnoid hemorrhage. In nuchal rigidity, the client is unable to place the chin on the chest because neck flexion is limited by involuntary muscle spasm.

To test for Kernig's and Brudzinski's signs, the client is in the supine position. For Kernig's sign, one hip is flexed to 90° with the knee also flexed to 90° (Figure 28–3A). If meningeal irritation is present, the client in this position will be unable to extend the knee past 90° without pain. To test for Brudzinski's sign, the client is supine with the legs extended. When the examiner flexes the client's neck, if meningeal irritability is present, the hips and knees will spontaneously flex to avoid the accompanying pain (Figure 28–3B).

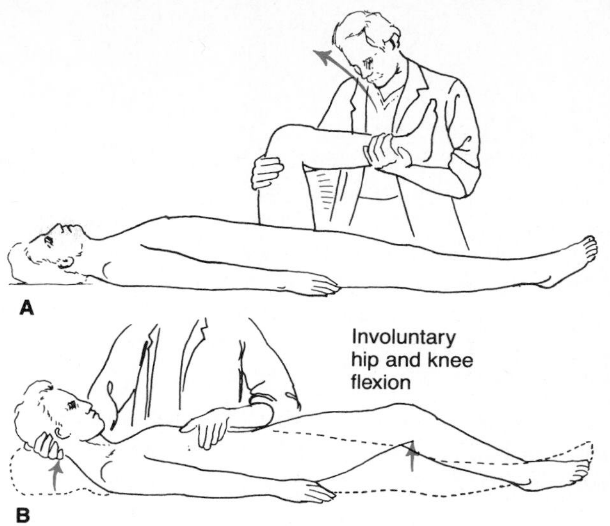

Figure 28–3

Kernig's sign and Brudzinski's sign—two signs of meningeal irritation. **A.** Kernig's sign: with client supine, flex hip and knee to about 90°; then attempt to extend the knee. **B.** Brudzinski's sign: with client supine and legs extended, passively flex the client's neck.

Diagnostic Studies

SKULL FILMS These x-rays are used as a basic noninvasive screening for trauma and neoplasms. They can reveal pathologic changes such as pituitary gland tumors. They can detect calcified abnormalities, such as aneurysms, or abnormal position of the calcified pineal gland (calcification is normal in the adult).

NURSING IMPLICATIONS Explain the purpose for the procedure and steps involved. Comb tangled or braided hair, and remove pins and wigs. Glass eyes can produce confusing shadows in a radiograph, so their presence should be noted (Snyder, 1983).

SPINAL FILMS Radiography may reveal changes in spinal bones resulting from fractures, tumors, or infections. It may also show the bony ridges and spur formations characteristic of osteoarthritis and help to identify congenital defects.

ELECTROENCEPHALOGRAPHY Electroencephalography (EEG) is essentially a noninvasive test that records a portion of the brain's electrical activity. The EEG is valued for its ability to reveal abnormal brain-wave patterns that help in diagnosing seizure disorders, brain tumors, abscesses, and psychologic disorders. The analysis of brain waves is possible because specific types of normal and abnormal brain waves have been identified. Diagnosis is made by evaluating patterns and characteristics of brain waves recorded, along with the client's clinical state. An absence of brain waves establishes brain death. Note, however, that acute drug intoxication or severe hypothermia resulting in a loss of consciousness can also cause a flat EEG.

The client is placed in a bed or on a lounge chair in a quiet secluded area. Surface electrodes, or occasionally needle electrodes, are positioned on or in the scalp. The client is instructed to close the eyes, relax, and rest quietly. Various stimuli are introduced to determine whether seizure activity can be produced. The client may be asked to hyperventilate for 3 minutes, to watch a flashing light, to endure a sensory stimulus such as a minor electrical shock, to observe a black-and-white checkerboard, and to listen to sounds through earphones. The client must be observed carefully and protected if seizure activity occurs. If a sleep EEG is requested, the client will be instructed to stay awake the night before the test. A sleeping medication may be given to promote sleep.

NURSING IMPLICATIONS Instruct the client to eat meals as usual with the exception of coffee, tea, cocoa, and cola, which the physician may want withheld because of their stimulant effect. Medications that may influence the test are often withheld. These include anticonvulsants, tranquilizers, barbiturates, or sedatives. Be sure the hair is clean and free from oils, sprays, or pins.

An explanation of the procedure and its purpose, the function of the electrodes, and the length of the test will help the client relax. The test usually takes 40 to 60 minutes with pretest and posttest care taking another hour.

Following test completion, assist clients in removing the electrode paste from the hair. At the same time, observe them for seizures and recovery from any sedation given during the test. The physician's order for resumption of medications is reviewed with the client. Check vital signs and neurologic signs as appropriate.

COMPUTERIZED TOMOGRAPHY Computerized tomography (CT) scanning is used to diagnose intracranial and spinal cord lesions. Scans are also used to monitor the effects of surgery, radiotherapy, or chemotherapy on tumors and to reveal vascular displacement, hematomas, cerebral atrophy, infarction, edema, and hydrocephalus. An iodinated contrast dye is sometimes administered to make large blood vessels visible or to define lesions. Administered intravenously, the dye increases the blood density and delineates intracranial masses.

NURSING IMPLICATIONS Explain the purpose of the exam. If no contrast medium is to be used, restriction of food and drink is not necessary. With use of dye, the client fasts for 4 to 6 hours to prevent emesis if nausea occurs. Before administering a contrast dye, identify any allergies to shellfish, iodine, or contrast media because use of the dye may be contraindicated. Skin testing to determine allergy is sometimes done.

Explain details about the procedure including special positioning, noise emitted by the machine, and length of the test. Some machines require the client to be strapped to the table, which moves into a gantry during the test. Loud clacking noises are normally emitted during this time. The test takes 15 to 30 minutes if no dye is used; with dye, the time is doubled. Clients receiving the dye should know that it is normal to feel flushed and warm and that sometimes a headache or salty taste or nausea occurs.

POSITRON EMISSION TOMOGRAPHY Positron emissions tomography (PET) is a noninvasive nuclear-imaging technique available in large medical centers. It is used to study oxygen uptake, blood flow, and glucose utilization in clients with cerebrovascular disease, seizure disorders, cardiovascular disease, and some degenerative disorders. With PET, viable tissue can be discriminated from nonviable tissue and the amount of nutritional blood flow to an area can be identified. PET is combined with computerized tomography. See nursing implications for CT scanning.

MAGNETIC RESONANCE IMAGING Magnetic resonance imaging (MRI) is based on the fact that the hydrogen nuclei in abnormal tissues behave differently in a magnetic field. A computer can manipulate these differences into a detailed picture of the organ under study. This noninvasive study does not require contrast media or exposure to radiation.

The client lies supine in a huge doughnut-shaped magnet. Bone tissue is not visualized with MRI but soft tissue close to bone is easily viewed. This enhances the use of MRI for problems of the skull and spine.

RADIONUCLIDE SCAN OF THE BRAIN The radionuclide scan detects intracranial masses; vascular lesions; and areas of ischemia, infarction, and hemorrhage. A radionuclide, usually administered intravenously, accumulates in affected areas if the blood–brain barrier has been compromised. Oral or intra-arterial administration can also be used. Some scans also include oscilloscope scanning of the carotid and cerebral blood flow. After the radioactive isotope has circulated for at least 1 hour, a scanner records the accumulation of isotopes. Another scan can be done 3 to 4 hours after injection.

NURSING IMPLICATIONS Ask about allergies to the isotope. No dietary or fluid restrictions are required. Potassium perchlorate is sometimes given to block uptake of the isotope by the thyroid, choroid plexus, and salivary glands (Conway–Rutkowski, 1982). Discuss the steps of the procedure and its time requirements, and inform the client that the injection will be the only discomfort. Have the client remove all jewelry and metal objects from the head and neck. To prevent client apprehension, explain that the radioisotope is harmless to self and others and is quickly excreted from the body. This test is often combined with CT scanning and angiography to help confirm the diagnosis.

CEREBRAL ANGIOGRAM The cerebral angiogram is used to diagnose intracranial lesions. A radiopaque contrast medium is injected into blood vessels of the head and neck to allow visualization of intracranial and extracranial vessels (Figure 28–4). The cerebral angiogram can reveal aneurysms; arteriovenous malformations; and displacement of vessels by masses, edema, or herniation. The test

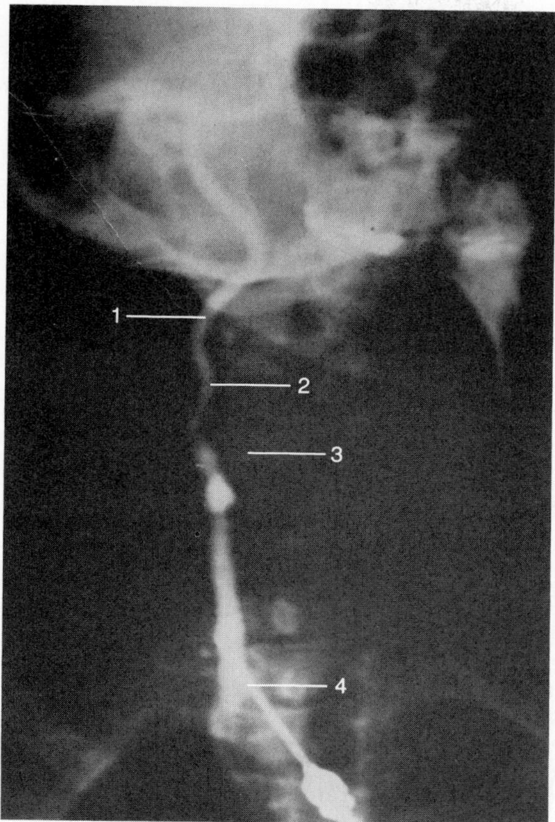

Figure 28–4

Cerebral angiogram performed through the carotid artery. **1**, External carotid artery; **2**, region of carotid bifurcation; internal carotid artery cannot be seen because of atheromatous plaques occluding the lumen; **3**, superior thyroid artery; **4**, needle in the common carotid. *Courtesy of Millard Fillmore Hospital, Buffalo, NY.*

is also used during surgery to check the position and integrity of aneurysm clippings.

The contrast material can be injected into a variety of sites. The most common are the carotid, brachial, and femoral arteries. Catheters are used in the more distal sites. Injection is done under local or general anesthesia in a special procedures area where resuscitation equipment is available or in the operating room. This test is contraindicated in clients with renal, hepatic, thyroid, or clotting disorders as well as in those who are hypersensitive to iodine or contrast materials.

NURSING IMPLICATIONS Client education includes review of the procedure's purpose. The physician explains the risks, which include CVA, thrombus, allergic reactions, seizures, pulmonary emboli, and visual disturbances. A consent must be signed. To reduce apprehension, inform the client that a supine position, with the head secured to prevent movement, will be required throughout the test, which lasts approximately 2 hours. In addition, tell the client that periodic assessment of heart function and blood pressure are routine.

Careful explanation of sensations expected when the dye is injected is essential to reduce fear, because having the contrast medium injected into the blood vessels of the head can be painful. The sensations vary from warmth to severe burning behind the eyes and in the jaw, teeth, tongue, and lips. Even fillings in the teeth can feel warm. The sensation of heat lasts 4 to 6 seconds after the dye is injected. More than one injection may be needed.

Nursing care also includes collection of baseline data and preparation of the client. Record vital signs and neurologic status. Mark pulses distal to the puncture site to facilitate assessment after the procedure. If the carotid site is used, document the neck measurement to allow comparison after the test (Snyder, 1983). Hairpins, nets, and dentures must be removed. The client should also void.

Preprocedure medications can include phenobarbital, to help the client relax, and atropine sulfate, to protect against a reflex response (hypotension, syncope, and bradycardia) by the carotid artery. The client should be well hydrated to promote clearance of the dye by the kidneys but should fast for 6 to 8 hours before the test. Shave the injection site and prepare it with an antiseptic solution. Local anesthetic is usually given before insertion of the catheter or needle.

Immediately following the removal of the needle or catheter from the artery, apply pressure to the puncture site for 15 minutes to prevent hemorrhage and development of a hematoma. Record vital signs and neurologic checks every hour for 4 hours, then every 4 hours for 24 hours. Also record intake and output.

Carefully monitor the puncture site, surrounding areas, and the distal extremity. Examine the puncture site for redness, swelling, and superficial or deep hematoma. A pressure dressing and ice bag may decrease the risk of bleeding and discomfort. When the carotid artery is used, monitor the client for respiratory distress and swallowing difficulty, which may indicate excessive edema or an expanding hematoma. For femoral or brachial sites, monitor pulses in the distal limb for 12 hours. Maintain the limb in an extended position and observe it for normal temperature, color, and sensation. Do not monitor blood pressures in the involved arm. Notify the physician immediately of any untoward effects. The client should rest quietly in bed for 12 to 24 hours, with diet and medications given as tolerated.

ELECTROMYOGRAPHY AND NERVE CONDUCTION STUDIES Electromyography (EMG) records electrical activity in muscle at rest and during contraction. Findings allow differentiation of muscle disease from lower motor neuron dysfunction. Recorded electrical patterns can be specific to various diseases such as myositis, dystrophy, and myasthenia gravis. EMG can be used to assess function in the spinal cord, nerve root, nerve plexus, peripheral nerves, or myoneural junction. The test can detect and measure regeneration of nerve and muscle before clinical signs appear. This information can be used to predict recovery (Snyder, 1983).

A nerve conduction test is often administered along with an EMG. This test measures the strength and speed of conduction in the sensory and motor fibers of peripheral nerves. Motor conduction studies are valued for assessing nerve damage when minor symptoms of motor weakness or atrophy exist. Sensory fiber conduction rates are especially useful for diagnosing neuropathies in clients with diabetes, alcoholism, metabolic and nutritional disorders, and trauma. Sensory nerve fiber conduction is assessed with a single electrical stimulus. The action potential is recorded by an electrode placed on the skin where the nerve is close to the surface. The recorded conduction time is compared with established norms for healthy nerves.

NURSING IMPLICATIONS Fluid or food intake is not restricted for this test. The physician may, however, request that cigarettes, coffee, tea, cola, or medications be restricted before the test. A written consent is obtained. Educate clients about the time EMG takes (1 hour or more), steps of the procedure, the need to insert a needle into the muscle, and the changing of needle position that will probably cause discomfort. In addition, stress the need for client cooperation in flexing and relaxing muscles during the test. To prepare a client for a nerve conduction test, outline the steps of the procedure and warn the client to expect mild electrical shocks.

Treat residual pain after the test with warm compresses and prescribed analgesics. Consult with the physician to determine whether medications withheld for the test should be resume.

LUMBAR PUNCTURE Lumbar puncture is an invasive procedure to obtain samples of CSF, to measure fluid pressure, and to reduce pressure in conditions such as subarachnoid hemorrhage. Lumbar puncture is also done to instill antibiotics; steroids; and dye, air, or oxygen for diagnostic studies and to evaluate CSF flow.

Lumbar puncture can be done at the bedside or in the diagnostic lab. The procedure is done with the client positioned to one side with head and knees flexed toward the abdomen. The client is assisted in maintaining this position, which separates the vertebrae, allowing the needle to enter the subarachnoid space at the level of L-3 and L-4 (Figure 28–5). Aseptic technique is required.

Contraindications for LP include skin lesions in the lumbar area, epidural infection or abscess, or lumbar deformity near the puncture site. LP is also contraindicated with increased ICP because of the risk of brain compression or herniation through the tentorial hiatus when the spinal fluid pressure is lowered. In some circumstances, such as when meningitis is suspected, it is crucial to establish a diagnosis despite the danger of the procedure, and LP may be justified.

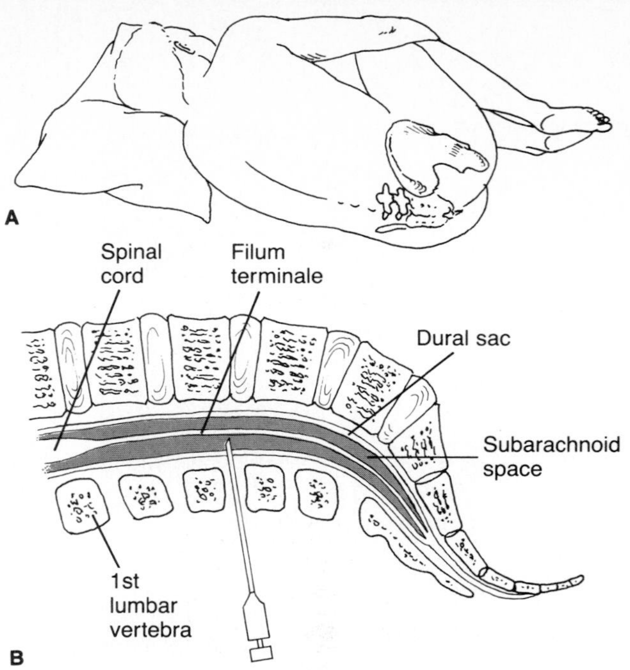

Figure 28–5

Lumbar puncture. **A.** Client position for lumbar puncture with neck and hips flexed to increase space between the vertebrae. **B.** Position of the spinal needle in the subarachnoid space, below the termination of the spinal cord.

Complications of LP include headache, transitory low back pain and root irritation, and meningitis or abscess. Headache is believed to result from the loss of CSF at the puncture site, which lowers the spinal fluid pressure and places tension on the intracranial structures.

NURSING IMPLICATIONS Carefully explain the purpose of the test and steps of the procedure because clients often fear this test. Emphasize the importance of lying still in the flexed position during the LP. Inform the client of the brief episodes of pain when the anesthetic and spinal needle are inserted. A discussion of postprocedure activity is also helpful. Have the client void before the LP.

After an LP, most physicians require the client to remain flat in bed for 4 to 24 hours, but turning should be encouraged. Forcing fluids will help to promote replacement of withdrawn spinal fluid. Headaches, experienced by many, can be treated with prescribed analgesics. Carefully monitor vital signs and neurologic status including signs of increased ICP and root pain radiating down the back of the leg. Observe for signs of meningitis and drainage or discharge at the puncture site. Report abnormal findings to the physician.

MYELOGRAM In a myelogram, fluoroscopy and radiography are combined to study the subarachnoid space, spinal cord, and vertebral bodies. The test reveals spinal cord tumors, herniated or ruptured intervertebral disks, and nerve root injury. In this study, a spinal tap is used to replace a small amount of CSF with a radiopaque dye or gas. The client is positioned on a movable table that tilts to various positions to allow the flow of dye through the subarachnoid space. Abnormalities in flow provide the diagnostic information.

NURSING IMPLICATIONS Explain the procedure and postprocedure routine. Determine any client allergies to iodine, shellfish, or radiographic dye, and obtain a written consent from the client. Maintain the client in a fasting state for 4 to 8 hours, and record baseline vital signs and neurologic status. Administer a cleansing enema to reduce x-ray shadows, a sedative to relax the client, and atropine to reduce secretions, as ordered.

Client education should cover information about the procedure including the length of time (1 hour or more); the purpose of the LP; the usual response to the dye, which includes flushing, a warm sensation, a salty taste, headache, nausea and vomiting; the positioning and strapping to the table with the head hyperextended to prevent the dye from entering the cranium; and the need to tilt the table during the study and to remove the dye.

After the procedure, position the client's head to keep the dye from entering the cranium. The physician should order a specific head position for a prescribed period of time depending on whether an iodized oil or a water-soluble iodine contrast was used. In addition, monitor vital signs and neurologic status including nuchal rigidity, nausea and vomiting, and reports of back pain and spasms for at least 24 hours or as indicated by the institution's policy. Headache can be treated by positioning and analgesics. Encourage plenty of fluids and monitor intake and output as well as the ability to void.

CEREBROSPINAL FLUID ANALYSIS Because CSF is in contact with the components of the CNS, CSF is valuable in the diagnosis and evaluation of disease progression or healing processes. CSF is colorless and consists of water and traces of protein, glucose, sodium, chloride, and potassium. The average volume in adults ranges from 100 to 150 mL. CSF pressure in the supine client ranges from 7 to 20 cm/H_2O.

The collection and handling of CSF should be carefully controlled to ensure proper analysis. The fluid must be collected in sterile tubes and delivered to the laboratory immediately. Some diagnostic evaluations require processing within 1 hour.

Certain analyses of CSF require special considerations. For example, the evaluation of the glucose level requires that a blood glucose level be obtained not more than 3 hours before the tap. The additional information is necessary because serum glucose levels are reflected in the CSF. The serum glucose level, rather than a neurologic disease process, may be the cause of the abnormal CSF levels. Similarly, CSF chloride levels can be affected by serum chloride levels. Because of this influence, CSF chloride levels will not be valid if the client has received IV therapy with electrolyte solutions close to the tap or at the time of the tap.

SECTION 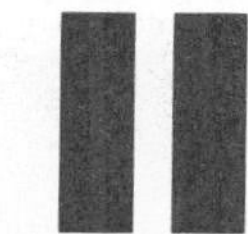

Nursing Diagnosis/Planning and Implementation/Evaluation

Information gathered from the client's health history, physical examination, and diagnostic studies is used to determine nursing diagnoses and the plan of care. Not every client will have the same needs. The Nursing Diagnoses box lists diagnoses **directly related** to neurologic dysfunction along with **potential** nursing diagnoses for clients with neurologic problems. The most common nursing diagnoses for clients with neurologic disease include ineffective airway clearance; ineffective breathing pattern; altered cardiac output: decreased; altered nutrition: less than body requirements; altered bowel elimination: constipation and/or incontinence; altered urinary elimination patterns; altered sexuality patterns; self-care deficit; altered communication: verbal; sensory/perceptual alterations; and impaired physical mobility. The sample nursing care plan in Table 28–2 focuses on three of these diagnoses: altered communication: verbal, sensory/perceptual alterations, and impaired physical mobility. The others are discussed in the narrative.

If the goals of care have not been met, reevaluation is required. The nurse and client should jointly review the nursing care plan. New objectives may need to be formulated; other nursing interventions may be added or modified; or the evaluation may show that more time is required to meet the objectives.

Airway Clearance, Ineffective

Patency of the respiratory tract depends on proper positioning, effective function of the muscles of respiration, and healthy respiratory tract mucosa. Neurologic diseases often cause dulled consciousness, confusion, and decreased motor function. Clients may not be able to assume positions independently that keep the tongue from obstructing the airway. Disease processes such as myasthenia gravis or ALS that affect cranial nerve function, as well as conditions affecting level of consciousness, can make it difficult to swallow or cough to clear the airway of sputum, foreign objects, or vomitus.

Ingestion of adequate fluids can be a problem for clients with various neurologic problems. Those with mental limitations may forget to drink. Those with communication problems may not be able to tell of their thirst or dry

NURSING DIAGNOSES IN
Neurologic Dysfunction

DIRECTLY RELATED DIAGNOSES

- Airway clearance, ineffective
- Breathing pattern, ineffective
- Bowel elimination, altered: constipation
- Bowel elimination, altered: incontinence
- Cardiac output, altered: decreased
- Communication, impaired: verbal
- Mobility, impaired physical
- Nutrition, altered: less than body requirements
- Self-care deficit
- Sensory/perceptual alterations: visual, auditory, kinesthetic, gustatory, tactile, olfactory
- Sexuality, altered patterns
- Urinary elimination, altered patterns

OTHER POTENTIAL DIAGNOSES

- Adjustment, impaired
- Comfort, altered: pain
- Coping, ineffective individual
- Injury, potential for
- Role performance, altered
- Skin integrity, impaired: actual, potential
- Self-concept, disturbance in: body image
- Self-concept, disturbance in: self-esteem
- Swallowing, impaired
- Thermoregulation, ineffective
- Thought processes, altered
- Tissue perfusion, altered: cerebral
- Unilateral neglect
- Urinary retention

mouth. Those who are limited physically may not be able to obtain or safely ingest liquids. These situations can result in dehydration with drying and crusting of the mucosal tissue in the oropharynx and respiratory tree with damage to mucous cells and cilia. This damage compromises the ability to expel organisms, increasing the risk of respiratory tract infections.

Planning and Implementation

For the physically impaired or **obtunded** (lethargic, drowsy) client, careful positioning with pillows and special devices promotes drainage of secretions, maintains a patent airway, and reduces the risk of aspiration. This includes careful positioning during meals, supplemental oral intake, nasogastric feedings, and oral care. A suction machine should be at hand if choking is a risk or secretions are unmanageable. Active or passive ROM exercises and frequent position changes help to promote mobilization of secretions. In an emergency, the nurse may need to initiate the Heimlich maneuver (see Chapter 19) or oxygen therapy if obstruction is suspected.

Steps to ensure adequate hydration promote healthy respiratory function both by promoting the elimination of secretions and the destruction of organisms. Careful, ongoing assessment of the oropharyngeal mucosa, breath sounds, and ability to manage secretions are necessary because the client's condition may change quickly, and the change may not be obvious.

Evaluation

Expected outcomes following effective nursing interventions for ineffective airway clearance include absence of adventitious breath sounds, absence of symptoms and signs of hypoxia, adequate fluid intake, absence of tenacious secretions, absence of inflammation and drainage in the oropharynx, and no episodes of choking or aspiration.

Breathing Pattern, Ineffective

Changes in body functions from neurologic diseases can cause ineffective breathing that interferes with the brain stem's regulation of respiratory function. Neurogically based changes in body function (eg, decreased level of consciousness, immobility, obstruction of airway, and aspiration) can result in decreased ventilation, decreased gas exchange, and hypoxia. Hypoxia presents two threats: anoxia in vital neurons and dilation of cerebral vessels leading to an increase in ICP.

Pathologic conditions producing an increase in intracranial pressure can lead to herniation, damaging respiratory centers in the brain stem. This trauma and other pathologies involving the brain stem, such as stroke or tumor, alter the rate, depth, and rhythm of respirations. Diseases, injuries, or infections affecting phrenic innervation of the diaphragm can result in loss of stimulus for breathing.

Hyperventilation can result from physical problems such as encephalitis, drug overdose, and hypoxia. It can also be initiated by psychologic stress or pain, both common in neurologic diseases.

Planning and Implementation

Many neurologic diseases and injuries of CNS predispose clients to ineffective respiratory function. Care for clients who are not breathing effectively may include oxygen therapy or ventilator assistance. In some instances, the equipment should be on standby in case it is needed suddenly. Notify the physician immediately if the breathing pattern becomes tachypneic, bradypneic, or markedly irregular suggesting a worsening of the client's condition.

Clients may be placed on a ventilator soon after the onset of the illness or trauma, or the ventilator may be used in the future if their disease progresses. In both instances, psychologic support and special planning for client communication are needed.

Nursing care for clients having trouble breathing because of apprehension or pain is focused on determining the cause and planning interventions. Analgesics should be given as

Table 28–2
Sample Nursing Care Plan for Clients With Nervous System Dysfunction

Client Care Goals	Plan/Nursing Implementation	Expected Outcome
Communication, altered: verbal related to expressive and/or receptive aphasia		
Interact safely with environment; express needs/feelings; improve communication through speech or alternative forms of communication; adapt to alteration in lifestyle and self-image	Assess client's ability to perceive and integrate sensations; work with speech pathologist to develop a program to be used by health care team and family to improve communication with client; record in care plan techniques for client to use and avoid; assess client's ability to understand communication of others; record results and incorporate them in care plan; provide a safe and supportive environment that prevents sensory overload, promotes independence, limits frustration, and promotes communication efforts and adaptation of body image and lifestyle; determine client and family expectations; initiate actions to prevent sensory deprivation and isolation; support client efforts with communication by: acknowledging attempts and positive results; attending to communication; refraining from interrupting client; making short, concise statements; and using facilitative techniques, gestures, and alternative communication systems when appropriate; plan for follow-up services after discharge	Communicates effectively regarding physical, intellectual, and emotional needs; attends to communications of self and others; functions effectively in the environment
Sensory/perceptual alterations related to altered sensory reception, transmission and/or integration		
Participate in activities to maintain safety and integrity of involved sensory systems and systems compensating for deficit; use compensatory methods to ensure safety and optimize interactions with the environment; make use of support from health care system and family; function at optimal safe level of independence	Assess client's ability to perceive and integrate by senses; determine effects of deficit on lifestyle (physical and psychosocial); seek therapies for control of pain; consult with health team to determine causes, extent of limitations, prognosis, and therapies; provide a safe and supportive environment that allows periods of activity and rest; determine and implement techniques to preserve and enhance use of remaining senses; promote independence by teaching the use of other senses and tools that can compensate for deficits; confer with OT and PT to coordinate client care goals and gain an understanding of their approaches that can be reinforced during nurse–client interactions; involve client and family in problem-solving activities to deal with deficits and crises	Alteration in sensory function is corrected or compensated for: no additional dysfunction occurs; pain is managed; psychologic issues are resolved; client perceives the environment in an enriching and realistic manner; client develops and maintains an optimal level of function after discharge
Mobility, impaired physical related to neuromuscular impairment		
Actively plan and participate in activities to maintain or improve ROM; express frustrations and adapt to necessary alterations in lifestyle; seek out	Assess and record ROM; evaluate potential for development of limitations in light of diagnosis, such as upper or lower motor neuron disease; plan therapies to improve or maintain current ROM through activities planned by PT, OT, and nursing and	No contractures or limitations in motor function will occur—exercises and adaptive equipment will be used to limit loss of motor function or compensate for limitations in mobility; client will maintain interaction with the environment to greatest

(continued)

Table 28–2, (Continued)
Sample Nursing Care Plan for Clients With Nervous System Dysfunction

Client Care Goals	Plan/Nursing Implementation	Expected Outcome
community groups to interact with others and gain new information regarding illness and assistance available	through use of splints and positioning techniques; periodically reevaluate ROM to determine effectiveness of program; confer with PT and OT regarding how spasticity may facilitate mobility or hamper positioning; assess limitations in movements resulting from tremors, rigidity, or other uncontrolled movements. Confer with OT regarding adaptive devices to optimize levels of independence; confer with physician regarding effectiveness of medications used to control spasticity, rigidity, or uncontrolled movements; optimize opportunities to interact with environment in spite of limitations through activities that promote independence and feelings of usefulness and improved self-esteem; assist client and significant others in problem solving and identifying strengths and support systems; plan for discharge; teach importance of follow-up care; provide information on self-help groups, common interest groups, and community organizations	possible extent; client will share feelings about loss of mobility and will adapt lifestyle; family and community will support client physically and emotionally; client will describe purpose and side effects of medications

ordered if positioning and other comfort measures are not effective and if vital signs are stable.

Evaluation

Expected outcomes following effective nursing interventions for ineffective breathing pattern include normal vital signs, symmetrical chest expansion, normal breath sounds, normal chest x-ray, normal blood gases, and absence of anxiety.

Cardiac Output, Altered: Decreased

Impairment of cardiac output can follow injury to the brain stem's vasomotor center, which influences cardiac function via the ANS. The brain stem's vasomotor center also controls blood pressure. With sharp elevations in blood pressure initiated to perfuse a severely edematous brain, the vasomotor center initiates reflex slowing of the heart, reduces contractility, and produces vasodilation (Price & Wilson, 1982). Cardiac output can also be compromised by anoxia stemming from alterations in respiratory function, as discussed earlier.

Decreases in vasomotor tone with various neurologic problems can affect cardiac function because of the decrease in blood returning to the heart. In addition, spinal cord injuries producing spinal shock severely decrease vasomotor tone. Orthostatic hypotension after long periods of bed rest is also the result of a loss of vasomotor tone.

Planning and Implementation

Nurses must be knowledgeable about disease processes that threaten cardiac output, such as brain stem trauma or ANS dysfunction, to provide comprehensive monitoring of clients at risk. Nursing actions must focus on the assessment of heart rate, rhythm, and effectiveness of beat to anticipate decreases in output that could threaten the integrity of both cardiovascular and CNS function. Because of the influence of high and low blood pressures on cardiac function, blood pressure must also be carefully monitored and treatments provided to maintain a safe range. To ensure oxygenation of the heart muscle, attend to neurologic deficits hindering respiratory function. Anticipate the need for resuscitation when spinal shock (discussed in the section on spinal cord injury in Chapter 29) or other events produce hypotension.

Evaluation

Adequate cardiac output is reflected by normal vital signs, lack of orthostatic hypotension, and clarity of mental status.

Nutrition, Altered: Less Than Body Requirements

The physical, psychologic, and social influences accompanying neurologic diseases can have a profound effect on an individual's nutritional status. Common physical problems that may limit intake include lact of exercise, which stimulates the appetite; inability or awkwardness in self-feeding; social isolation; difficulty in chewing and swallowing; fear of choking; and limited energy for eating.

For the individual at home, physical and mental deficits can make buying food and preparing meals challenging. A limited income (eg, because of illness-related unemployment) can also influence the amount and type of food available. As a result, the quality and quantity of food consumed may be reduced.

Sight, smell, taste, and touch—all important to an interest in eating—are altered by many neurologic diseases. In addition, mental changes from injury to the cerebral cortex or the psychologic response to disease can diminish interest in eating.

Planning and Implementation

Physical problems of neurologic origin (eg, weakness, limited ability to feed oneself, or a decreased level of consciousness) frequently mean clients have difficulty eating. Adaptive devices to facilitate cutting and eating food, supplemental feedings, arranging for someone to assist the client with food shopping and meal preparation, and contact with organizations like Meals-on-Wheels may help correct the nutritional problems.

Depression, isolation, and fear are common psychosocial problems that often contribute to a disinterest in food. Plans to correct such situations consider each client's needs. Plans might include encouraging involvement of the family at mealtime, arranging for the client to eat with others on the unit, or providing music and special positioning at mealtime.

Evaluation

Nutritional status is improved when there is evidence that the rehabilitation period includes an emphasis on meal planning. Efforts are made to involve the client in as much planning and preparation as she/he is capable of. Support systems and community resources are involved so that the full responsibility of planning, shopping, cooking, and clean-up are not the client's alone. Companionship at mealtime helps to assure adequate intake.

Bowel Elimination, Altered: Constipation

Many neurologic diseases can cause constipation. Neurologic alterations can result in decreased fluid intake, decreased physical activity, inability to monitor bowel patterns, inability to initiate changes in diet to correct constipation, limitations in using toilet facilities, and increased dependence resulting in a lack of privacy.

Diseases such as stroke, myasthenia gravis, and ALS often produce paralysis of the lips, tongue, mouth, pharynx, and larynx (**bulbar paralysis**). The resultant difficulty in swallowing frequently reduces fluid intake. Stools become hard and difficult to pass.

Immobility from motor neuron damage or decreased level of consciousness limits abdominal muscle contraction, and bowel activity slows. More water is absorbed from the stool, making its passage difficult. Positioning constraints, as with spasticity or contractures, are often outcomes of neurologic diseases. These limitations can prevent a client from assuming positions that facilitate defecation. For example, being confined to bed for treatment of a lumbar disk problem often causes constipation brought about by both immobility and positioning constraints.

Aphasia often accompanies neurologic disease that damages the cerebral cortex. Because communication is impaired, clients may be unable to make their needs known, so they become constipated.

The client's loss of toilet privacy frequently accompanies the physical disabilities of weakness, paralysis, and immobility. Embarrassment over exposure during toilet activities and related helplessness can hamper normal defecation.

Planning and Implementation

Nursing techniques for the client with limited motor function who needs to increase fluid intake to keep stools moist include proper positioning and the use of special cups, straws, and other adaptive devices. Recognizing the client's physical and mental deficits allows for effective planning and assistance. If the client's communication is limited, family or friends may be able to suggest favored fluids and foods that will increase fluid intake and bulk to relieve or prevent constipation.

Privacy can often be provided to reduce embarrassment and feelings of helplessness. A Posey vest might allow safe positioning so the client can be left alone to use the toilet. A padded toilet seat or bedpan may increase comfort and promote defecation, especially for the client who has mobility problems or who is very thin. For the immobile client who is hesitant to ask for the bedpan or assistance, offering help regularly demonstrates acceptance of the client's needs and a willingness to help. If the client is unable to report symptoms or signs of constipation because of confusion, forgetfulness, or communication problems, daily monitoring of bowel function allows early treatment and prevention of constipation and impactions.

Evaluation

Client evidence of efforts to decrease constipation include increased fluid intake and attempts to let others know of the need to defecate. Significant others demonstrate their understanding of the problem by providing privacy for the client during toileting activities; offering the bedpan, commode, or assistance to the bathroom in a helpful and kind manner; providing fluids and foods that will aid the client in having a daily bowel movement; and carefully monitoring the client's bowel function.

Bowel Elimination, Altered: Incontinence

Bowel incontinence may accompany a wide variety of disease processes. Sphincter control can be lost because of cortical, spinal cord, or peripheral nerve damage. Recovery of control may or may not be possible. Clients whose personalities change following brain trauma may have temporary or chronic loss of bowel continence. Aphasia predisposes some clients to incontinence because they cannot express their need to defecate. Tube feedings and medications may cause diarrhea, which the physically or mentally compromised client may not be able to control.

Planning and Implementation

Bowel incontinence presents profound psychosocial as well as physical problems. The client's frame of reference and responses must be considered. The client's unique problems determine what actions are needed.

Keep in mind that time is needed after CNS trauma for the edema to resolve and the intact neurons to resume normal activity. With time, communication can be established with aphasic clients. Precious moments are gained by having a clean bedpan in the bed and an over-the-bed trapeze available to help the client get onto the pan alone. A bedside commode is another possible solution for the client who has some warning of an impending bowel movement. The staff's strategies for prompt answering of the call light help to meet the client's physical and psychologic needs. Evaluation of dietary or medication regimens and consultation with the physician and dietitian can assist in locating and eliminating bowel irritants that hamper control. Education of the client, staff, and family on the potential for control and the purpose of bowel training programs promote commitment and effort by all. A consulting psychologist may assist in developing a behavior modification program for the client with mental dysfunction.

Throughout the process of regaining bowel control, or when efforts to regain control are exhausted, the nurse must use techniques (physical and psychologic) to maintain the client's dignity and self-esteem. Special underpants can keep moisture and other irritants away from the skin and control odor. These pants may allow a fairly normal lifestyle.

Evaluation

Incontinence is reduced when the client's diet is free of irritants and diarrhea-producing foods. Accidents are reduced when the client has easy access to the bedpan or commode. Bowel retraining programs are successful when the client, significant others, and staff are in accord about the procedure to be followed.

Urinary Elimination, Altered Patterns

Urinary retention or urinary incontinence can result from diseases affecting the cerebral cortex, spinal cord, and peripheral nervous system. With CNS dysfunction, the client often has both a diminished awareness of bladder fullness and a decreased ability to empty the bladder. Alterations in consciousness from trauma, electrolyte imbalance, anoxia, and disease processes can produce temporary or permanent urinary incontinence.

Planning and Implementation

Work closely with the physician to determine the cause of the incontinence and the client's potential for regaining control. Diagnostic procedures, such as cystometrography (see Chapter 25) may be needed.

Bladder training programs consisting of regularly scheduled attempts to void help many clients with cortical injury to relearn bladder control. Partial control of function may keep the client continent if steps are taken to provide frequent toileting or access to toilet equipment. Intermittent self-catheterization may be an option for some clients with urinary retention.

Special pants for incontinent clients that protect the skin and control odor may be helpful for the client who is unable to regain control. These pants reduce the need for dependence on an in-dwelling catheter.

There is a potential for urinary retention after surgery, myelogram, or LP, which increases the risk of urinary tract infections and reflux into the ureters. Carefully monitor client voiding patterns after any of these procedures and accurately record urine output.

Evaluation

The expected outcomes for a client with neurologic dysfunction and alteration in urinary elimination following effective nursing interventions are: no symptoms or signs of bladder distention, retention, or incontinence; and proper self-catheterization or in-dwelling catheter management for those who require it.

Sexuality, Altered Patterns

Sexual dysfunction can result from spinal cord trauma, peripheral nerve trauma, or diseases that damage the peripheral nerves necessary for sexual activities. Medication regimens can also produce sexual dysfunction. Mental changes stemming from brain damage may result in inappropriate sexual behaviors.

Planning and Implementation

Nursing care for the client with sexual dysfunction seeks to create an atmosphere in which clients feel comfortable in expressing their concerns. The nurse can facilitate discussion by maintaining a professional and matter-of-fact approach toward body functions. If inappropriate behaviors result because of mental changes, maintain a professional approach. Behavior modification or psychotherapy may be needed. Consultation with a mental health–psychiatric nursing clinical specialist can be helpful to clients, family members, and nursing staff.

Evaluation

Expected outcomes following effective nursing interventions for sexual dysfunction in clients with neurologic disease include client ability to discuss the problem with care providers and with the sexual partner and an interest in learning about alternative approaches for meeting sexual needs.

Self-Care Deficit

Neurologic diseases predispose clients to many types and degrees of self-care deficits. Planning effective care depends on determining how the following factors influence the treatments and activities planned for or by the client: cause of the illness, its current and expected degree of influence on self-care, the prognosis and expected outcomes for the treatments anticipated by health care providers, the client's personality and response to deficits, and the family's interest and ability to support the client mentally and physically.

Planning and Implementation

At times, the seriously ill or physically impaired client needs the nurse or family members to provide what are normally self-care activities. Meeting these needs in a supportive manner promotes feelings of safety and security that can foster recovery or adaptation to a change in lifestyle.

If and when a client is able to begin to participate in self-care, the nurse's role gradually changes to that of facilitator to encourage the client's effort and to reduce frustration in learning to overcome physical impairments. Nursing actions must be specific for each client's needs. When possible, work closely with the occupational therapist to encourage the client to apply skills learned during therapy and during nurse–client interactions.

Evaluation

Expected outcomes following effective nursing interventions for clients with self-care deficits include obvious client efforts to participate in his/her own care and a willingness to learn new skills to become more independent in self-care activities.

Chapter Highlights

A major focus of nursing care for the client with neurologic disease is to prevent the disease from progressing, because damaged neurons are irreparable.

The nervous system is predisposed to a wide variety of diseases and traumas because of its complex and widespread structures.

The nervous system is vulnerable to diseases affecting other body systems.

The nervous system's influence over other body systems may produce symptoms suggesting malfunction of other systems.

Physiologic and psychosocial/lifestyle influences affect the client's response to neurologic disease during all stages of the illness.

Although some deficits from neurologic disease processes do not cause obvious structural changes, they may produce severely limiting disabilities that last a lifetime.

Clients require support when diagnostic studies are ordered because most neurologic tests are invasive, lengthy, and frightening; they often produce considerable discomfort and involve some risk to the client.

Nursing assessment must be an ongoing process for clients with neurologic disease because improvement or decline in their condition will require prompt changes in the plan of care.

Nursing interventions for clients with neurologic diseases often involve supportive measures for other body systems the nervous system can no longer effectively control.

Family members and significant others of clients with neurologic disease are often presented with monumental physical, psychosocial, and lifestyle challenges.

Bibliography

Assessment. Springhouse, PA: Intermed, 1982.

Bates B: *A Guide to Physical Examination,* 3rd ed. Philadelphia: Lippincott, 1983.

Chusid JG: *Correlative Neuroanatomy & Functional Neurology,* 19th ed. Los Altos, CA: Lange, 1985.

Conway–Rutkowski BL: *Carini and Owens' Neurological and Neurosurgical Nursing,* 8th ed. St Louis: Mosby, 1982.

Diagnostics. Springhouse, PA: Intermed, 1982.

Fisher J: What you need to know about neurologic testing. *RN* (Jan) 1987: 47–53.

Goldberg B, Chiverton P: Assessing behavior: The nurse's mental status exam. *Geriatr Nurs* (March–April) 1984; 94–98.

Hackett C: Limbering up your neurovascular assessment technique. *Nurs 83* (March) 1983; 13:40–43.

Kallail KJ, Hemphill MK: Notes from a young aphasic patient in a nursing home. *Nurs Health Care* 1985; 6:379–381.

Konikow NS: Alterations in movement: Nursing assessment and implications. *J Neurosurg Nurs* (Feb) 1985; 17(1):61–65.

Mitchell PH et al: *Neurological Assessment for Nursing Practice.* Reston, VA: Reston, 1984.

Ozuna J: Alterations in mentation: Nursing assessment and intervention. *J Neurosurg Nurs* (Feb) 1985; 17(1):66–70.

Price SA, Wilson LM: *Pathophysiology: Clinical Concepts of Disease Processes,* 2nd ed. New York: McGraw–Hill, 1982.

Samuels MA: *Manual of Neurologic Therapeutics,* 2nd ed. Boston: Little, Brown, 1982.

Scherer P: Assessment: The logic of coma. *Am J Nurs* 1986; 86(5):551–556.

Snyder M (editor): *A Guide to Neurological and Neurosurgical Nursing.* New York: Wiley, 1983.

Vogt G, Miller M, Eslaur M: *Mosby's Manual of Neurologic Care.* St. Louis: Mosby, 1985.

Wahlquist GI: Evaluation and primary management of spasticity. *Nurse Pract* 1987; 12(3):27–32.

Whitney FW: Guidelines for neurological consultation. *Nurse Pract* (July–Aug) 1982; 7:13–18.

Resources

ORGANIZATIONS

Alzheimer's Disease and Related Disorders Association (ADRDA)
70 E Lake St
Chicago, IL 60601
Phone: (800) 621–0379; in Illinois (800) 572–6037

This organization provides information to the public and to health professionals, advocates and aids research, provides emotional support to family and friends, and makes referrals to other appropriate services.

American Parkinson's Disease Association
116 John St
New York, NY 10038

Thirteen satellite centers throughout the United States maintain extensive information for the public and health professionals, and offer diagnostic and treatment services.

Epilepsy Foundation of America
4351 Garden City Dr
Suite 406
Landover, MD 20785
Phone: (301) 459–3700

This voluntary organization provides information on seizure disorders, referrals, advocates the civil rights of persons with seizure disorders, monitors related legislative activity, and sponsors self-help groups for clients and their families. Members are eligible for discount prescription drugs.

Myasthenia Gravis Foundation, Inc
53 W Jackson Blvd
Suite 909
Chicago, IL 60604
Phone: (312) 427–6252

Chapters throughout the United States provide education, raise funds for research, and sponsor low-cost diagnostic and treatment clinics and discount drug plans.

ALS (Amyotrophic Lateral Sclerosis) Association
15300 Ventura Blvd
Suite 315
Sherman Oaks, CA 19403
Phone: (818) 990–2151

The ALS maintains an information bureau, recommends neurologists who specialize in the treatment of ALS, directs clients and families to manufacturers of aids and appliances, and raises funds for research. Volunteers with personal experience are available to answer letters and telephone calls. Maintains an information center for the medical profession, patients, and families.

National Ataxia Foundation
600 Twelve Oaks Center
15500 Wayzata Blvd
Wayzata, MN 55391
Phone: (612) 473–7666

This organization sponsors a network of clinics for persons with ataxia and offers referrals for medical, social, emotional, and financial support.

Huntington's Disease Society of America, Inc
140 W 22nd St, 6th Fl
New York, NY 10011
Phone: (800) 345–HDSA; in New York (212) 242–1968

This agency maintains a comprehensive listing of specialists and sponsors educational programs and raises funds for research.

National Headache Foundation
5252 N Western Ave
Chicago, IL 60625
Phone: (312) 878–7715; toll free (800) 843–2256 outside IL

This nonprofit organization makes information available and offers referrals to health professionals who are members of the American Association for the Study of Headache.

National Multiple Sclerosis Society
205 E 42nd St, 3rd Fl
New York, NY 10017
Phone: (212) 986–3240

Chapters throughout the United States sponsor diagnostic and treatment clinics, group recreation programs, personal counseling by trained volunteers, and free loan of equipment and appliances.

National Paraplegia Foundation
333 N Michigan Ave
Chicago, IL 60601
Phone: (312) 346–4779

This voluntary health agency encourages research and helps paraplegics through self-help, counseling, and information services. Volunteer counselors help clients adjust to wheelchair living. Offers referral to sources that provide special equipment.

Parkinson's Disease Foundation
William Black Medical Research Building
Columbia University Medical Center
640–650 W 168th St
New York, NY 10032
Phone: (212) 923–4700

Offering information and referral for persons with Parkinson's disease and other diseases of the basal ganglia, this organization serves as a clearinghouse for clients, families, and health professionals.

US Government
National Institute of Neurological and Communicative Disorders and Stroke
Office of Scientific and Health Reports
Bldg 31, Rm 8A06
Bethesda, MD 20892
Phone: (301) 496–5751

Provides information about research on stroke and stroke prevention.

In Canada

Canadian Paraplegic Association
520 Sutherland Dr
Toronto, Ontario M4G3V9
Phone: (416) 423–5690

Multiple Sclerosis Society of Canada
130 Bloor St W, Suite 700
Toronto, Ontario M5S1N5
Phone: (416) 924–4406

Migraine Foundation
390 Brunswick Ave
Toronto, Ontario M5R2Z4
Phone: (416) 920–4916

HOT LINES

Counseling for families and friends of those with Alzheimer's disease and related diseases (Alzheimer's Disease and Related Disorders Association)
Phone: (612) 830–1043

Counseling for psychologic support for clients with amyotrophic lateral sclerosis (National ALS Foundation)
Phone: (212) 679–4016

NURSING ORGANIZATIONS

American Association of Neuroscience Nurses
22 S Washington St, Suite 203
Park Ridge, IL 60068

Members include RNs actively engaged or primarily interested in neurologic or neurosurgical nursing. Dues, $53 a year.

Association of Rehabilitation Nurses
2506 Gross Point Rd
Evanston, IL 60201
Phone: (312) 475–7530

Members include RNs interested in rehabilitative nursing practice. Dues, $40 a year.

Canadian Association of Neurological and Neurosurgical Nurses
296 Palace Road
Kingston, Ontario K1N7B7

CHAPTER **29**

Specific Disorders of the Nervous System

Other topics relevant to this content are: Care of the client with cancer, **Chapter 10;** Credé's maneuver to assist in voiding, **Chapter 26;** The Glasgow coma scale, **Chapter 28;** Care of the client with a pituitary tumor, **Chapter 34;** Care of the client with Crutchfield tongs, **Chapter 45;** Care of the client with a penile implant, **Chapter 49.**

Objectives

When you have finished studying this chapter, you should be able to:

Enumerate the nursing precautions with clients having possible subarachnoid hemorrhage from a ruptured cerebral aneurysm.

Anticipate the nursing interventions for clients with seizures.

Compare and contrast the common types of headache and their management.

Identify the risk factors of cerebrovascular accident and discuss the role of the nurse in stroke prevention.

Distinguish among Alzheimer's disease, Parkinson's disease, and amyotrophic lateral sclerosis and describe nursing care priorities for each.

Compare and contrast myasthenia gravis and multiple sclerosis and describe nursing care priorities for each.

Describe the problems that occur from compression of cranial or spinal structures by tumors.

Discuss the principal types of head trauma and spinal injuries, their treatment, and specific nursing responsibilities.

Define the surgical procedures presented involving the brain and spinal cord.

Apply an understanding of the physiologic and psychosocial/lifestyle implications of each surgical procedure to the nursing care of the client.

Discuss nursing implications of caring for these clients in the preoperative and postoperative periods.

Explain the complications of neurosurgery and the related nursing interventions.

Diseases of the nervous system include those of congenital, multifactorial, degenerative, immunologic, infectious, neoplastic, and traumatic origin. Because of the complexity of the nervous system, symptoms and signs associated with malfunction are multiple and varied. Many of the disorders in this chapter (eg, Alzheimer's disease, cerebrovascular accident, and spinal cord injuries) cause severe physiologic and psychosocial/lifestyle problems for clients and their significant others and present a tremendous challenge to the health care team.

Surgical intervention for neurologic disorders is broad in scope and complex. The significance of a neurosurgical procedure is not necessarily indicated by the operation listed on the OR schedule. The schedule may state only the operative method for reaching the area of the pathology and not the definitive treatment. For example, craniotomy is only the means for exposing the intracranial contents. A laminectomy, though, may constitute a surgical remedy if the client's problem stems from bony compression of the spinal cord or its nerve roots. On the other hand, if the client has a spinal cord tumor, laminectomy is only the means for exposing that lesion. This distinction is important because, although general nursing considerations apply to each of the basic approaches, the specific nature, location, and extent of the pathology have considerable bearing on the plan of care and its implementation. As a general rule, the outcome and risks can be directly correlated with the size and location of the lesion and the client's preoperative condition.

SECTION I

Congenital Disorders

A congenital disorder of the nervous system can be defined as a developmental defect. A variety of these defects may be present at birth. Although the causes of maldevelopments are often unknown, a majority are considered to result from the hereditary transmission of a chromosomal abnormality or are secondary to embryonic damage from teratogenic agents.

Neurofibromatosis

Neurofibromatosis (NF) is a hereditary disorder with an autosomal dominant mode of inheritance. Neurofibromatosis is characterized by a variety of congenital abnormalities. The skin, PNS, CNS, bones, endocrine glands, and sometimes other organs are affected. Usually, some form of benign tumor is the typical finding. The disorder is most commonly classified according to what parts of the nervous system are affected: peripheral, central, or both. The first definitive account of its clinical and pathologic features is credited to von Recklinghausen in 1882, and NF is therefore also known as von Recklinghausens's disease. The poignant portrayal of John Merrick in the movie *The Elephant Man* brought this disorder into public awareness, although fibrous dysplasia accounted for more of Merrick's disfigurement than NF.

NF occurs in all races and nationalities. Although it can affect both sexes equally, the disease is slightly more common in males. Each child of an affected parent has a 50% chance of inheriting the gene and developing NF. NF can also result from a new or spontaneous mutation of a dominant gene.

Clincial Manifestations

The earliest signs of NF are usually light to dark brown patches of cutaneous pigmentation called café au lait spots. The spots vary in diameter from several millimeters to centimeters. The patches are an early diagnostic clue because they are rarely associated with other pathologic states. Any individual with six or more café au lait spots is considered at risk for NF. Diagnosis is based on the presence of six or more café au lait spots of 0.5 cm or more in conjunction with neurofibromas. Another clinical manifestation is diffuse axillary pigmentation (axillary freckling).

Café au lait spots commonly increase during childhood, and skin tumors typically increase in number and/or size during puberty and pregnancy. For some, the disorder stabilizes during adulthood, but in others, the symptoms progress usually between the late teens and early 20s and again in the 60s. The course of the disease is not easy to predict.

About a third of all NF clients are asymptomatic and diagnosed incidentally. That is, the clinical manifestations are observed during a routine physical examination when the individual is being evaluated for symptoms of another disorder. These clients have mild cutaneous abnormalities.

In the peripheral form of NF, multiple cutaneous and subcutaneous nodules occur. Cutaneous tumors are located in the dermis as discrete, soft, or firm papules. Their size varies from millimeters to centimeters. They also vary from flat to conical or lobular. If pressed, these soft nodules feel like a seedless grape, which aids in distinguishing lesions of NF from other tumors.

Clients with NF also have a high incidence of CNS tumors, including tumors of the meninges (meningiomas), tumors of the glial cells (astrocytomas, ependymomas, glioblastomas), and a high incidence of neurofibromas of cranial and spinal nerves. In many cases, clients have a variety of these tumors. A form of central NF involving bilateral acoustic neuromas (CN VIII) may be the only central finding. Clinical symptoms usually are progressive hearing loss accompanied by tinnitus.

Medical Measures

NF has no cure. The most promising approach is surgery for removal of symptomatic lesions. In cases of multiple CNS lesions, the decision to have surgery depends on the severity of symptoms, risk for survival, and the quality of life. Some have advocated aggressive plastic surgical treatment for cosmetic reasons or for removing lesions that might degenerate into sarcomas. Radiotherapy is not justified because of unsatisfactory results and the risk of x-ray exposure.

Treatment decisions involve ethical issues that frequently require a multidisciplinary approach including the client and significant others, neurosurgeons, nursing staff, a psychiatrist, a social worker, and a chaplain. After this group has thoroughly explored the issues, the client and family will be in a better position to decide on treatment.

Specific Nursing Measures

The client with NF is often unaware of the implications of the diagnosis. Initial reactions of shock and disbelief can be intensified by stereotypes like "the elephant man." Help the client recognize that there are many variants of the

NURSING DIAGNOSES IN
Neurologic Dysfunction

DIRECTLY RELATED DIAGNOSES

- Airway clearance, ineffective
- Breathing pattern, ineffective
- Bowel elimination, altered: constipation
- Bowel elimination, altered: incontinence
- Cardiac output, altered: decreased
- Communication, impaired: verbal
- Mobility, impaired: physical
- Nutrition, altered: less than body requirements
- Self-care deficit
- Sensory/perceptual alterations: visual, auditory, kinesthetic, gustatory, tactile, olfactory
- Sexuality, altered patterns
- Urinary elimination, altered patterns

OTHER POTENTIAL DIAGNOSES

- Adjustment, impaired
- Comfort, altered: pain
- Coping, ineffective individual
- Injury, potential for
- Role performance, altered
- Skin integrity, impaired: actual, potential
- Self-concept, disturbance in: body image
- Self-concept, disturbance in: self-esteem
- Swallowing, impaired
- Thermoregulation, ineffective
- Thought processes, altered
- Tissue perfusion, altered: cerebral
- Unilateral neglect
- Urinary retention

disease and that no two individuals have the same course and prognosis. Erroneous ideas should be dispelled. Explain the current extent of the illness and possible treatment strategies. Emphasize support for the client's right to make decisions regarding treatment choices.

A difficult task is helping the client recognize the uncertainty of the disease course and prognosis. Inform clients that lesions can change from asymptomatic to symptomatic at any time, that new ones can develop spontaneously without warning, and that others may remain dormant for long periods; in fact, clients may experience symptom-free periods. The nurse may play a key role in teaching the client and family to live one day at a time and to resume as normal a lifestyle as possible. Emphasize the importance of reporting new symptoms immediately and seeking medical attention early.

Cerebral Aneurysms

A cerebral aneurysm is an abnormality of the wall of a cerebral artery caused by a structural weakness in the vessel. Most common is a focal deficit in a vessel wall that results in a sacular dilation. As pressure in the artery increases, adjacent nervous tissue is compressed and/or arterial rupture and hemorrhage occurs. The majority of cerebral aneurysms are called *berry* aneurysms because of their saccular appearance. Others appear as a ballooning or puckering of a vessel without a distinct neck. Cerebral aneurysms vary from 2 mm to 3 cm with an average size of 8 to 10 mm.

Most cerebral aneurysms occur in the anterior circle of Willis. The circle of Willis is crucial to total brain circulation because it forms an anastomosis between the internal carotids and the vertebral–basilar system providing a means of collateral circulation. About 85% of cerebral aneurysms occur in the anterior cerebral and anterior communicating arteries, the internal carotid and posterior communicating arteries, and the middle cerebral artery at its trifurcation. The most frequent sites are the posterior communicating and internal carotid arteries. The incidence of aneurysms in the vertebral–basilar system is only about 15%. Most cerebral aneurysms occur at vessel bifurcations, where there is potential for weakness.

When an aneurysm ruptures, it can bleed into the subarachnoid space or into the cerebral tissue. In first incidents, blood usually escapes from the aneurysm dome into the subarachnoid space (the space between the arachnoid and pia layers of the meninges where CSF circulates). Bleeding into this area is a *subarachnoid hemorrhage* (SAH), whereas bleeding into cerebral tissue causes an intracerebral hematoma. More than 70% of spontaneous subarachnoid hemorrhages are caused by ruptured cerebral aneurysms. Ruptured cerebral aneurysms cause three major medical complications: rebleeding, cerebrovasospasm, and communicating hydrocephalus. The major cause of death in the unoperated client is rebleeding within the first 2 weeks following the initial bleed.

Although the exact etiology of cerebral aneurysms is unknown, several theories have been proposed. One well-known explanation suggests that aneurysms arise from congenital defects in the media of arterial walls. Another theory suggests that aneurysms develop from remnants of pre-existing fetal vessels. A third possibility is that aneurysms follow arteriosclerotic changes in blood vessels and hypertensive effects.

Clinical Manifestations

The majority of clients with cerebral aneurysms are asymptomatic until an aneurysm ruptures. Rupture is the most prevalent diagnosis among clients between ages 35 and 65 years. Although premonitory signs of subarachnoid hemorrhage are common, clients sometimes ignore them. The most common symptom of a ruptured cerebral aneurysm is the *sudden* onset of a severe headache, often described as "explosive." The headache may be associated with nausea and vomiting, visual disturbances, motor deficits, and a loss of consciousness. All of these signs can be related to an intense rise in ICP. In addition, meningeal irritation often occurs, causing nuchal rigidity, positive Kernig's and Brudzinski's signs, photophobia, blurred vision, irritability, restlessness, and low-grade fever. Meningeal signs diminish as the blood clears from the CSF.

Fewer than a third of clients with cerebral aneurysms seek health care before rupture. These clients usually show signs of oculomotor nerve pressure or compression from an aneurysm in a posterior communicating artery. Clinical signs include an eyelid ptosis; a dilated and sluggish nonreactive pupil; and a restriction of extraocular movement in upward, inward, and downward gaze.

Regardless of the symptoms and signs, the client's condition is grave and the prognosis guarded. To interpret clinical findings, a grading system is employed. The most widely adopted system is the Botterel scale (Table 29–1). The criteria provide baseline data for future comparison and a method for determining prognosis and suitability for neurosurgical intervention. On admission, clients are assigned to one of the categories and their status revised with changes in condition.

Lumbar puncture (LP) was a major diagnostic tool in confirming a subarachnoid hemorrhage before the CT scan. The classic lumbar puncture findings are a grossly bloody spinal tap from a recent bleed and a xanthochromic one from a bleed occurring 6 to 12 hours before the spinal tap. Xanthochromic or straw-colored CSF results from the release of bilirubin during the breakdown of red blood cells. An elevated CSF cell count and protein level are expected in these clients.

The CT scan has had a major impact on the diagnosis and management of clients with SAH. A CT scan without contrast enhancement can verify the presence of blood in the cisterns (enclosed spaces or CSF reservoir cavities), which indicates a SAH. The CT scan also rules out a subdural or intracerebral hematoma. Lumbar puncture is contraindicated in these conditions. With a hematoma, the elevated ICP and the negative pressure created by lumbar puncture could cause a brain shift, which could lead to brain compression and herniation through the tentorial hiatus. A CT scan can also demonstrate the presence of communicating hydrocephalus and, with contrast, may indicate the location of the aneurysm itself.

An LP is done when a CT scanner is unavailable or when a CT scan is not confirmatory. The spinal tap may demonstrate elevated ICP above 250 mm H_2O pressure or higher. Even with the increased pressure, the risk of herniation is markedly decreased because of the nature of the increased pressure. The initial increase in CSF pressure is not due to an absorption problem, but there is the potential for developing communicating hydrocephalus later.

The cerebral angiogram is most valuable in outlining the vasculature and identifying abnormality and displacement of vessel lumina. Because of the high incidence of multiple aneurysms (in 10% to 15% of clients), four-vessel angiography is the procedure of choice. This study examines complete anterior–posterior cerebral circulation by assessing both the carotid and vertebral arteries.

Table 29–1
The Botterel Scale for Grading Ruptured Cerebral Aneurysms

Category	Criteria	Survival Rate
Grade I (minimal hemorrhage)	Client alert, neurologically intact, with a minimal headache and slight nuchal rigidity	65%
Grade II (mild hemorrhage)	Client alert with minimal neurologic deficits, such as CN III palsy (eg, ptosis, diplopia), with a mild to severe headache and nuchal rigidity	55%
Grade III (moderate hemorrhage)	Client has definite change in level of consciousness, is drowsy or confused; nuchal rigidity is present with mild focal deficits	45%
Grade IV (moderate to severe hemorrhage)	Client stuporous or semicomatose with mild to severe hemiparesis, nuchal rigidity, and possible early decerebration	30%
Grade V (severe hemorrhage)	Client decerebrate, comatose, with a moribund appearance	5%

Angiography is also the primary diagnostic tool for identifying vasospasm, a major complication of aneurysm rupture. The procedure can identify clients with vasospasm who have no clinical signs. Vasospasm is a process in which the lumen of the parent and adjacent vessels to the aneurysm becomes narrowed. The narrowing decreases cerebral blood flow to brain tissue supplied by the affected arteries and their branches. Cerebrovasospasm is thought to be related to the vasoactive effects of the blood-bathing arteries in the subarachnoid space.

Symptoms of acute vasospasm occur 1 to 3 hours after the initial aneurysm rupture. Chronic vasospasm occurs 3 to 4 days later. Its onset is often slow and insidious. Symptoms vary depending on the severity of the vasospasm and its effects on cerebral blood flow. Other considerations include cerebral perfusion pressure and the degree of autoregulation maintained. Regional alterations may cause focal neurologic deficits such as aphasia or hemiparesis. Diffuse alterations result in level of consciousness changes. Neurologic deterioration in the absence of headache, raised systolic blood pressure, or increased meningeal signs usually suggests development of or increase in cerebrovasospasm.

On the other hand, a deterioration or change in neurologic status may be related to an aneurysm bleed. The major cause of death in the unoperated client is *rebleeding* for the 2 weeks following initial aneurysm rupture. The risk of rebleeding is greatest within 24 hours and again 7 to 10 days after the initial bleed. When the aneurysm first ruptures, a fibrin clot forms over the rupture, sealing the dome. Seven to 10 days later, the fibrin clot undergoes lysis, leaving the aneurysm vulnerable to rebleeding.

Medical Measures

Therapy is based on the clinical and neurodiagnostic findings. The primary focus of medical care after initial aneurysm rupture is to prevent rebleeding. Aminocaproic acid (Amicar) prevents destruction of the clot that has sealed the dome of the aneurysm following initial rupture; it also enables endothelial repair and fibrous tissue development to take place. Extended use (3 weeks or more) of aminocaproic acid has been associated with thrombophlebitis and pulmonary embolism.

Cerebrovasospasm is treated by a number of protocols:

- Calcium channel blockers such as verapamil (Calan) and nifedipine (Procardia) have been used in an attempt to prevent, reverse, or inhibit vasospasm. These drugs are thought to prevent calcium from entering vascular smooth muscle, reducing vasospasm.
- Kanamycin sulfate (Kantrex) and reserpine (Serpasil) have been used together to prevent cerebrovasospasm. Kanamycin sulfate inhibits serotonin levels in the gastrointestinal tract. Reserpine depletes brain norepinephrine and serotonin. There is no evidence that this protocol is effective once angiography diagnoses vasospasm.
- Isoproterenol (Isuprel) and aminophylline combined relax vascular smooth muscle. Dysrhythmias can develop with this regimen; therefore, cardiac monitoring is advised.
- Isoproterenol (Isuprel) and lidocaine (Xylocaine) are used in combination. Isoproterenol dilates vascular smooth muscle, and lidocaine prevents potential dysrhythmias.

Another common protocol is to expand blood volume and to assist cerebral perfusion by using colloids (albumin) and packed red blood cells to maintain a hematocrit of 35% to 45%. A central venous pressure catheter or ICP monitor can be used to modify fluid therapy. The ICP must be kept below 15 to 20 mm Hg; serum sodium and osmolality levels are carefully monitored to prevent water intoxication. Management of postoperative cerebrovasospasm with hypertensive therapy is less dangerous because the aneurysm is surgically repaired and in no danger of rebleeding.

Communicating hydrocephalus, the third most common complication of SAH, can occur with the bleed or weeks later. It is caused by a malabsorption or blockage of CSF from the arachnoid villi into the venous sinuses. The drainage of the arachnoid villi is blocked by the breakdown products of blood resulting from the initial subarachnoid hemorrhage. Hydrocephalus should be suspected if any of these signs appears:

- Mental status changes
- A decrease in level of consciousness
- Dementias
- Flat affect
- Urinary incontinence
- Disturbances in gait

Hydrocephalus is confirmed by a CT scan that shows an enlargement of the ventricles and a decrease in CSF space due to a decreased absorption of CSF. Surgery may be required if clients do not recover spontaneously. Ventricles can be drained by ventriculosubgaleal shunt to manage the problem for 2 to 3 weeks. Long-term management requires a ventriculoperitoneal shunt (see a pediatric textbook for specifics of care).

Surgical repair that includes clipping of the aneurysm neck is the best treatment of a ruptured intracranial aneurysm. This procedure is recommended for clients who are neurologically stable. The appropriate timing for surgery is controversial. Early operation is sometimes advocated, 24 to 48 hours after rupture, in clients who are asymptomatic. The rationale is to treat the client before the peak risk of rebleeding and before cerebrovasospasm increases and communicating hydrocephalus develops. This group of clients, however, constitutes only a small number. Those who demonstrate more extensive signs of meningeal initiation or neurologic deficit may be at greater risk if operated on during the first week following aneurysm rupture. Despite the continuing interest in early surgery, there is not enough statistical evidence to indicate that it has merit except in asymptomatic clients.

Specific Nursing Measures

Unfortunately, about 40% to 50% of clients with subarachnoid hemorrhage due to ruptured intracranial aneurysms die from catastrophic bleeds before receiving medical attention. For those who do have medical care, mortality and morbidity rates can be greatly reduced with careful nursing and medical management. The acute care of such clients presents the nurse with a formidable challenge. Nursing care is aimed at preventing rebleeding, the most life-threatening complication for these clients. Subarachnoid aneurysm precautions are instituted to manage actual or potential alterations in neurologic status from rebleeding (Box 29–1).

The majority of clients are in good health and inde-

Box 29–1
Nursing Precautions for Clients With Ruptured Cerebral Aneurysms

Provide a quiet, dark environment with complete bed rest.

Assess neurologic and vital signs every hour for 24 hours, then every 2 to 4 hours if client is stable. Report any changes in vital signs, especially elevations in systolic blood pressure above 120 mm Hg or a 20 mm Hg rise above baseline.

Report immediately to the physician any new or worsening neurologic deficits. Important signs to watch for are restlessness, confusion, and a decrease in level of consciousness. Cardinal symptoms and signs of rebleeding include increased or severe headache, significant increase in systolic blood pressure, and increased signs of meningeal irritation. Other neurologic signs to watch for are motor weakness, change in pupillary size and function, and dysphasia. Document all changes and nursing actions taken.

Administer complete hygiene and feed the client.

Restrict visiting privileges to significant others as designated by the client. Provide brief periods for visitation and instruct client and significant others about the importance of precautions to prevent rebleeding.

Avoid external stimuli that can increase stress (eg, telephone, television, smoking).

Caution client to avoid straining on defecation. Administer stool softeners and mild laxative as ordered.

Give no enemas.

Keep the head of the client's bed elevated at 30° to decrease intracranial pressure.

Administer sedatives and/or anticonvulsant medications as ordered and monitor serum drug levels.

Medicate clients with mild analgesics for headaches only as ordered.

Administer antifibrinolytic agent (aminocaproic acid) via continuous intravenous infusion pump or orally, as ordered. Observe clients for side effects such as thrombophlebitis, diarrhea, and rash.

Be aware that these protocols may have to be modified in some cases by the physician to decrease clients' anxiety and agitation.

pendent until the aneurysm rupture. The unexpected hospitalization and impending surgery may be difficult for clients to cope with, and their first reaction may be denial. Assist clients to acknowledge their concerns without forcing them into acceptance. During a period when the client's denial is beneficial, the nurse can respond by listening empathically and reflecting accurately the client's comments. Demonstrate an accepting attitude toward the client's concerns, establish a regular time for sharing feelings, and maintain consistency in nursing management.

Clients may feel a loss of self-control and independence because of the subarachnoid hemorrhage precautions. Offer clients whatever choices are available and assist them to identify alternatives. Give ongoing updates of their neurologic condition and prepare them in advance for any diagnostic tests.

Neurologic status can also be altered by cerebrovasospasm. Potential neurologic deficits to watch for are described in the earlier clinical manifestations section. Report and document all changes as well as nursing actions taken. Maintain adequate client hydration. The intravenous fluid rate is usually titrated according to serum osmolality, blood pressure, and/or CVP measurement. Keep a strick intake and output record during acute changes in neurologic status.

Clients' cardiovascular status may change because of hypothalamic dysfunction. A common cardiac change in a client with a subarachnoid hemorrhage is sinus bradycardia with ST-segment or T-wave changes. Monitor ECG pattern and vital signs with the neurologic assessment.

Seizure Disorders

Seizures are generally defined as sudden, involuntary abnormal discharges of electrical energy in the neurons of the brain. These discharges are usually rapid and excessive with the foci of disturbance in the cerebral cortex. Seizures may be a primary disorder or secondary to CNS disease. The term *epilepsy* is used to indicate that an individual experiences seizures. "Fit" and convulsion are other common synonyms. It has been estimated that approximately 1% of the population in the United States suffer from epilepsy (Conway–Rutkowski, 1982). Seizures can be classified according to etiology, clinical signs, and EEG patterns. The "International Classification of Epileptic Seizures" is a common classification (Box 29–2).

Some seizure disorders originate from antenatal, perinatal, or postnatal problems. Seizures can occur with conditions that cause vascular hemorrhage or hypoxia. Seizures can be a prominent feature of cerebral palsy and cerebral arteriovenous malformations. Febrile periods during infancy and childhood can lead to seizures. Seizures may also develop during the course of a degenerative disease. Sometimes the etiology of seizures is unknown.

The onset of a majority of seizure disorders occurs before the second decade. Those occurring later that are unrelated to trauma are usually caused by cerebrovascular or neoplastic disease. Less commonly they are caused by neuroinfective disorders such as meningitis or encephalitis. Seizures can develop during withdrawal from alcohol, sedatives, tranquilizers, and antidepressants. Toxic intoxication from heavy metals or carbon monoxide may induce seizures. Certain cardiac, liver, and kidney diseases may cause seizures.

Factors that can precipitate seizures in clients predisposed to them include nutritional deficiencies, emotional stress, alcohol abuse, and excessive fatigue. Noncompli-

Box 29–2
International Classification of Epileptic Seizures

I. Focal or partial seizures

Simple (general without an impairment of level of consciousness)
- Motor (eg, Jacksonian seizures)
- Sensory or somatosensory
- Autonomic

Complex (the spread of simple or partial to a generalized convulsive form such as temporal lobe or psychomotor)

II. Generalized seizures (without a local onset, bilaterally symmetric)

Absences (petit mal)

Tonic–clonic (grand mal)

Infantile spasms

Bilateral massive myoclonus

Clonic seizures

Tonic seizures

Atonic seizures

Akinetic seizures

III. Unilateral seizures

IV. Unclassified seizures (when complete data is not available)

V. Classification of paroxysmal forms

Benign febrile seizures

Convulsive equivalent syndrome

Breath-holding spells

ance with anticonvulsant drug therapy places a client at risk for seizures.

Clinical Manifestations

Partial or focal seizures usually affect a specific body part. The symptoms of an attack depend on where the cerebral focus is. For example, the Jacksonian or focal motor seizure occurs in the motor strip of the cerebral cortex. It is also known as the Jacksonian march because the seizure usually begins in an extremity or the facial muscles with tonic–clonic activity that spreads over the same side of the body. Seizure activity will occur on the opposite side of the body from the irritable cerebral foci. When the seizure activity spreads to involve the other side of the body, it is then considered generalized and may involve a loss of consciousness. Usually a tumor or irritant such as scar tissue causes the attack.

Partial seizures may involve only sensory symptoms like numbness or tingling of a body part. Clients may experience dizziness or visual, auditory, gustatory, or olfactory symptoms. More complex partial seizures involve cognitive signs including a feeling of "déja vu" (a feeling that things are all very familiar), fear, unreality, anxiety, or a dreamy state. Psychomotor seizures usually cause a sudden change in behavior. Motor automatisms can occur in which purposeful patterned activity is carried out by the client with no memory of the behavior. Clients may do something that is out of character or inappropriate to the situation. The behavior may be preceded by various hallucinations such as olfactory, visual, or gustatory. These episodes are not usually related to an environmental stimulus. A common phenomenon is the "uncinate" fit. These are olfactory seizures with unusual odors or tastes that are unpleasant experiences for the client. Seizures involving visual hallucinations are described as flashes of light or a formed image. Those involving auditory hallucinations may involve a nondescript noise or a well-developed sound. It is important to recognize that hallucinatory seizures may be the aura phase preceding a generalized seizure. Any partial seizure can become generalized if the seizure activity spreads from the original focus to other parts of the brain. However, most focal seizures do not become generalized nor do they involve a loss of consciousness.

Generalized seizures are most commonly described as convulsions, or grand mal seizures. This type usually consists of three phases: an aura, an ictal, and a postictal state. The aura is a warning sign of the convulsive, or ictal, phase of a seizure, and the postictal phase represents the period after a convulsion during which the client may be dazed, confused, or asleep. It is not uncommon for generalized seizures to have a marked focal component. This may be demonstrated during any phase of the seizure. Auras that involve very descriptive neurophysiologic phenomena can suggest a cortical focus. Some examples include paresthesias, auditory hallucinations, or a vivid remembrance of a former experience.

Petit mal attacks are a special type of minor epileptic seizures. They are idiopathic with an onset in childhood or adolescence. They rarely continue into adulthood. Petit mal is known as an absence attack. Attacks usually last from a few seconds to less than a minute. The frequency of the seizure can be as high as several hundred per day. The seizure usually consists of a short staring episode in which there is a pause in the child's conversation. Words may be skipped or repeated. Head nodding and eyelid fluttering may occur during an attack. These absence attacks can be accompanied by myoclonic jerks. Some clients have akinetic petit mal attacks that involve a brief duration of sudden falling to the floor or dropping of objects. They can last only a fraction of a second.

The diagnosis of a seizure disorder is based on a detailed client and family history, electroencephalograms (EEGs), and the accurate assessment of seizure activity as reported by the client and observed by the family and/or health team members. An EEG is often the most valuable diagnostic test.

Medical Measures

Seizure disorders caused by CNS disease are treated by removing the causative agent (eg, a craniotomy may be done to remove a brain tumor or a burr hole drilled to evacuate a subdural hematoma). Follow-up includes the use of anticonvulsants for about one year or longer dependent on whether or not the client remains seizure free.

The primary medical treatment for idiopathic seizure disorders includes various anticonvulsant drug regimens. The objective is to reduce the excitation threshold of the neurons to a level that requires a much higher stimuli than normal to initiate a seizure. Choice of drug therapy depends on an accurate diagnosis of the type and frequency of seizures. The goal is to achieve optimal seizure management using the lowest dose of anticonvulsants with the least side effects.

For grand mal, or generalized major motor, seizures, the hydantoins are especially useful. The most common is phenytoin (Dilantin). This is often combined with phenobarbital. If the major seizures have a focal onset, primidone (Mysoline) and carbamazepine (Tegretol) are used. This combination is also recommended in the treatment of partial complex (psychomotor) seizures. For generalized petit mal seizures, the drug choice is the succinimides. This is followed by the benzodiazepines of which diazepam (Valium) is one. Diazepam has a very short half-life and has limited use in the oral form. IV diazepam is the drug of choice for status epilepticus (rapid succession of seizures without regaining consciousness).

One of the newest anticonvulsant medications is valproic acid (Depakene). It is most effective in managing petit mal seizures. It is less effective for focal motor seizures. Sometimes phenobarbital is added to valproic acid to treat petit mal because many children will progress from petit to grand mal.

The treatment of epilepsy requires a precise regulation of drug dosage. Long-term management requires determination of therapeutic drug levels as well as actual or impending drug toxicity. Subtherapeutic drug levels can be caused by noncompliance or by problems with drug absorption. For example, drug absorption can be affected by gastrointestinal or liver dysfunction depending on where the drug is metabolized. Correcting specific organic problems can help. Sometimes drug doses may be increased or administered in a more soluble form. Serum drug levels must be used as reasonable guides for drug regulation, because clients may remain seizure-free with slightly higher or lower than therapeutic drug levels. With long-term use and high drug doses, various symptoms can occur. An acnelike rash can develop, especially with barbiturates (eg, phenobarbital). Drowsiness may occur with barbiturates or primidone.

The administration of high levels of the hydantoins can cause cerebellar signs such as an ataxic gait, slurred speech, and intention tremors. Nystagmus and blurred vision can also occur. A common side effect of phenytoin is a diffuse red patchy rash, especially over the trunk area. Phenytoin can also cause severe gingival hyperplasia (see Chapter 37). Valproic acid may cause gastrointestinal irritation. The drug can be given with meals. The most serious complications of anticonvulsant therapy are blood dyscrasias and liver dysfunction. The hydantoins are the most responsible for these complications. Clients must be well informed about action, dosage, side effects, and toxicity of the drugs.

Surgical interventions may be recommended for clients who are intractable to various anticonvulsant regimens. Candidates for surgery must be carefully evaluated. The goal is to remove part or all of the seizure focus. Surgery can be done to excise scar tissue in posttraumatic epilepsy or to remove part of the temporal lobe in temporal lobe epilepsy. Surgery may also create scar tissue that can become a potential future focus for seizure activity.

Specific Nursing Measures

Help the client and family to understand epilepsy by using an analogy. The brain may be referred to as the biologic equivalent of a computer. That is, brain cells connect and communicate through tiny electrical components that are similar to the interconnections found in a computer. When there is an abnormal burst of electrical energy, a computer may shut down whereas the brain may experience a physical reaction known as a seizure. A seizure may be described as a temporary period during which the brain is "overcome" by intense, rapid spurts of electrical energy.

The primary goal of nursing care during a seizure is to prevent client injury and to protect the client's airway. Place the client in a lying position on a flat surface (eg, bed or floor). The side-lying position will promote drainage of secretions and prevent the tongue from falling back and obstructing the airway. Breathing can be facilitated by loosening the client's clothing, especially anything tight around the neck. At the onset of a generalized major motor or grand mal seizure, place a firm soft object between the teeth to prevent biting the tongue. Wash cloths, handkerchiefs, or a padded tongue blade are recommended. Force should *never* be used in placing the object. Do not attempt to open a clenched jaw. Remove all potentially harmful objects around the client. Protect the client's head from injury by cradling the head or placing a soft object under it. *Never* restrain the client during a seizure. Call for help, report the seizure to the physician immediately, record all symptoms and signs of an attack, and administer anticonvulsant drugs as ordered. Place all clients with a history of seizures on seizure precautions, including the following:

- Keep an oral airway, padded tongue blade, and oropharyngeal suction equipment at the client's bedside.
- Maintain the client's bed in the lowest position and pad the siderails.
- Provide a protected environment free of potentially harmful objects in the event of a seizure.
- Indicate on the Kardex and nursing care plan that the client is on seizure precautions.

One of the most important nursing actions when caring for a client with an active seizure disorder is accurate observation of seizure symptoms and signs. General assessment guidelines are found in Box 29–3.

Teach clients and their significant others approaches to managing any future seizures. Provide written information. Assist them to react to the diagnosis and vent their feelings. The long-term management of epilepsy requires courage and acceptance by the client and family. Compliance with medication regimens is essential. Teach the client about drug side effects and the need for continuous monitoring of blood levels. Encourage clients to avoid factors that might precipitate seizures such as infections, stress, and trauma.

Box 29–3
Seizures—General Assessment Guidelines

A. Ictal (convulsive phase)

Note date, onset, time, duration, and cessation of seizure activity.

Describe the course of the seizure: site of focal onset (thumb, mouth, toe), progression, and sequence of spread.

Evaluate pupillary size and reaction to light.

Assess status of entire body:
- Did the client cry out, lose consciousness, fall to the ground?
- Did the eyes or head deviate to one side?
- Did tonic–clonic movements of the extremities occur?
- Did nystagmus occur?
- Did eyelids flicker or eyeballs roll, close, or open?
- Was there clenching of teeth or jaw?
- Did the client bite the tongue or cheek?
- Was there any drooling or frothing from the mouth?
- Were there any tremors or marked jerking of limbs?
- Was client incontinent of urine and/or feces?
- Were there changes in speech, color, or breathing pattern?
- Were there changes in body posture (stiffening, relaxation, twisting)?
- Was skin diaphoretic?

What was the level of consciousness? Was client confused, irritable, excited?

B. Postictal (after seizure ceases)

Assess the client for memory impairment; depression; headache; muscle aching; sleepiness; change in level of consciousness, respirations, or heart rate.

Evaluate the client for possible injury during the seizure (eg, bruises, lacerations).

Check for paresis or paralysis of extremities.

Question the client about activity at the onset of the seizure and whether an aura occurred.

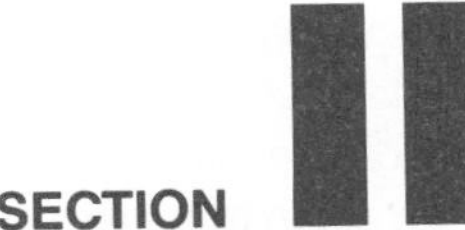

SECTION II

Disorders of Multifactorial Origin

Nervous system disorders of multifactorial origin can be associated with lifestyle factors, trauma, environmental toxins, and inherited defects, to name a few. Health problems in this section include headaches, trigeminal neuralgia, Bell's palsy, and cerebrovascular disease.

Headache

Headache symptoms account for a large proportion of phone calls and visits to physicians. A number of pain-sensitive structures and mechanisms can be involved in headache, including the skin and periosteum over the outer skull; the dura with its venous sinuses and tributaries; branches of CN V, CN IX, and CN X; and branches of large arteries at the brain's base. Headache can result from compression, traction, displacement, or inflammation of these structures. Pain can be referred from other cranial structures such as the scalp, neck, and extraocular muscles as well as the paranasal sinuses and air cells of the mastoid.

Tension headaches, characterized by a sustained constriction of scalp and neck muscles are the most common form. Tension headaches occur by themselves or as the residual effect of a migraine. These headaches are usually caused by tension or poor posture; they may or may not have a vascular component.

The classic *migraine headache* is a clinical condition recognized for centuries. Although the exact cause is unknown, attacks are thought to be precipitated by chemical changes in and around affected blood vessel walls. One common theory is that migraine results from spasm of intracranial blood vessels and a dilation of extracranial blood vessels. The spasm sometimes produces an aura, or warning of an attack, and the dilation leads to headache. Several biochemical agents have been considered in causality—norepinephrine, serotonin, and bradykinin. Migraines have a familial tendency, occurring in a 3:1 ratio on the maternal side. They have also been associated with a history of allergic disorders within the same family—asthma and eczema being common ones (Bickerstaff, 1980). Migraine attacks have been associated with stress, fatigue, overwork, the menstrual cycle, dietary intake (eg, chocolate, cheese, wine), and the letdown of weekends or vacations. They are more common in women, beginning in the teens, and often occur in clients with perfectionistic personalities.

Cluster headaches, also known as atypical migraines, are more common in men. The term *cluster* refers to the tendency for a rapid succession of attacks over days or weeks followed by a remission. They were previously considered to be caused by histamine sensitization but are now thought to have a vascular cause.

Temporal arteritis causes severe, unremitting headaches in the region of the temporal artery. An inflammation of this artery causes a tenderness and palpable thickness, and the site sometimes becomes nodular. Temporal arteritis affects men and women about equally but occurs most often among the elderly. It is not a common cause of headache but requires prompt diagnosis and treatment. If untreated, the condition can affect the ophthalmic artery and lead to blindness. Involvement of the intracranial arteries can lead to stroke syndromes.

The headache associated with mild hypertension is usually not characteristic and is similar to a tension headache. Frequent, intense headaches may be associated with severe hypertensive episodes and can be similar to those caused by intracranial lesions.

Ocular headaches can be caused by acquired or congenital conditions. Glaucoma is a common cause of intense headache from increased intraocular pressure. Sharp pain radiates over the ophthalmic branch of the trigeminal nerve. Contraction of scalp and neck muscles causes occipital headaches. Ocular headaches can also be caused by hyperopia, astigmatism, and an imbalance of ocular muscles. Myopia rarely causes severe ocular headaches.

A number of *ear, nose,* and *throat* diseases have been implicated in headache. Mucous membranes of the nasal and paranasal sinuses are more pain sensitive than the sinuses themselves. Inflammations of the superior sinuses can cause pain in the anterior head and between the eyes; an inflammation of the inferior sinuses generally leads to discomfort in the teeth, jaws, and temples.

Lumbar puncture headache is caused by a traction on the structures at the base of the brain after the removal of CSF via the lumbar subarachnoid space. The mechanism is similar to that in increased ICP.

Meningitis also can result in severe headache and nuchal rigidity. Meningeal irritation is caused by blood or pus mixing with CSF.

Headaches of intracranial origin are related to a distortion of pain-sensitive structures in early stages of organic disease. During later stages, increased ICP may displace pain-sensitive structures at a location distal from the specific site of the problem. Etiology may include space-occupying lesions, cerebral trauma, cerebral edema, hydrocephalus, or vascular anomaly.

Supratentorial headaches result from stimulation of pain receptors above the tentorium. Pain impulses travel via CN V, causing headaches in the front half of the head. On the other hand, infratentorial or posterior fossa headache problems cause "occipital" headaches, or pain in the back of the head. Pain receptors are stimulated by CN II in these clients.

Clinical Manifestations

Tension headaches are often mistaken for migraine. Involvement of the scalp muscles leads to more prolonged pain sensation. The pain is often described as a "pressure" or tightness around the head and neck. Tension headaches usually have no aura, cause no alterations in sleep patterns, and are not accompanied by vomiting.

The classic characteristics of migraine headache include throbbing and the tendency of attacks to alternate sides of the head and to be unilateral. Unilateral headaches always occurring on the same side may indicate a serious neurologic problem, especially a vascular anomaly. The initial symptoms of a migraine are caused by the specific blood vessels that go into spasm. Some attacks are preceded by an aura type of visual disturbance. One common aura includes **teichopsia** (flashing lights zigzagging across the visual fields) and **fortification** (colored patterns with a dark center and jagged edges). Clients may have visual field defects such as **homonymous hemianopia** (loss of half of the visual field) and **bitemporal hemianopia** (loss of the peripheral visual fields) (Figure 29–1). **Scotomas** (blind gaps in the visual fields) are patchy losses or complete loss of vision. Less common is unilateral numbness of the face or extremities. Some clients experience vertigo, tinnitus, extremity tingling, and dysarthria. The type of aura depends on which cerebral blood vessels are in spasm. Symptoms last from several minutes to an hour, followed by the headache. At this point, some clients briefly lose consciousness. Migraine headaches are associated with nausea and vomiting, accounting for the popular term "sick headache." A migraine headache can persist for as long as 2 days.

Common signs of cluster headache are nasal stuffiness, facial flushing, sweating, and sometimes edema of the affected side. Cluster headaches are sustained, occur in rapid succession, and may have an onset during sleep. Intense, unilateral pain in the orbital and temporal region is not uncommon. Attacks last from 30 to 90 minutes. Unlike other forms of migraine, they usually have no aura or warning preceding onset.

With temporal arteritis, the client has severe localized headache, anorexia, and fever. Visual disturbances can develop, such as visual field defects or sudden blindness. The disorder is diagnosed by clinical symptoms, artery palpation, an elevated erythrocyte sedimentation rate, and leukocytosis. In some clients, a temporal artery biopsy may be performed.

Hypertensive headaches can be pulsatile and are char-

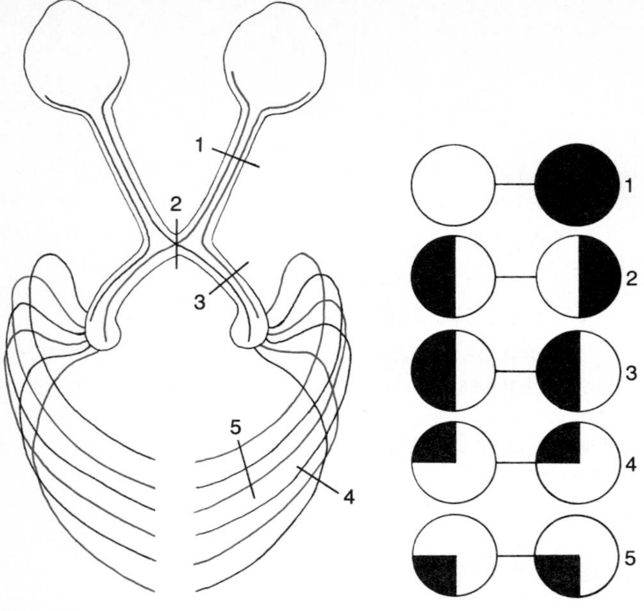

Figure 29–1

Visual field defects caused by lesions in the visual pathways. *1,* Right optic nerve lesion results in blindness of the right eye. *2,* Lesion at the optic chiasm causes bitemporal hemianopia. *3,* Lesion in the right optic tract causes left homonymous hemianopia. *4,* Partial lesion of optic radiation; homonymous left upper quadrant defect. *5,* Partial lesion of optic radiation; homonymous left lower quadrant defect.

acterized by pallor, nausea, vomiting, and tachycardia. They tend to occur on arising. When associated with vomiting, they are similar to headaches related to intracranial lesions. Hypertensive headaches can signify a pheochromocytoma (adrenal cortex tumor).

The symptoms and signs of ocular headaches vary according to their cause. A common symptom is orbital pain that radiates to the occiput. Occular headaches do not usually awaken a client, are more frequent with eye use, and may be alleviated by rest. Constant eye strain precipitates attacks.

Headaches related to increased ICP are usually worse when the client first awakens. These headaches are related to an irritation, traction, or compression on dural sinuses or cerebral blood vessels. If the client has slept on a flat bed, the headache may be intensified by a decrease in central venous drainage by gravity. These headaches vary from mild to excruciating and from generalized to localized, depending on tumor location, type, and growth rate. It may be associated with vomiting, papilledema, or visual disturbances.

Medical Measures

Muscle tension headaches may be treated by increasing circulation to the affected area, relaxing neck and shoulder muscles. Circulation can be stimulated by applying moist or dry heat, improving posture, performing stretching and ROM exercises, and using acupressure. Acupressure relieves pain through a technique of applying pressure to stimulate certain body points. Biofeedback has been used to help clients learn to control muscle contraction and relaxation. Muscle relaxation drugs may be helpful for clients who do not respond to other measures. In some cases, local anesthetic may be injected into muscle trigger points to relieve pain and spasm.

There is no panacea for migraine headaches, but a number of medications are more or less effective. Acute attacks are commonly treated with ergot preparations, (cranial vasoconstrictors), which if given during the aura stage, may prevent the headache. A physician sometimes uses dihydroergotamine mesylate (DHE 45) during a probable migraine attack to confirm the diagnosis.

At headache onset, ergotamine tartrate 2 mg orally may be given, followed by 1 mg every half hour to a maximum of six tablets per attack. If the client is vomiting, a rectal suppository or inhalation form of the drug can be given. Another alternative may be dihydroergotamine mesylate 0.5 mg to 1 mg IM with a repeat dosage 1 hour later as needed to a maximum of 3 mg. Some clients need an antiemetic such as dimenhydrinate (Dramamine) to prevent gastrointestinal side effects. Long-term overuse of ergot preparations can result in mild malaise and chronic headache, symptoms sometimes mistaken for an actual migraine. Ergot preparations are best reserved for severe attacks, cannot be used frequently, and are not recommended as preventive treatment. Ergot preparations should not be used by clients with peripheral vascular disease, coronary artery disease, hypertension, or impaired hepatic or renal function. Pregnant women should not take ergot.

Caffeine products are also cranial vasoconstrictors and are a household remedy for migraines. A compound of caffeine 100 mg and ergotamine tartrate 1 mg (Cafergot) is effective for some clients. Usually, two tablets are given at headache onset, followed by one tablet every half hour, not to exceed six tablets per attack or ten per week.

Methysergide maleate (Sansert), a serotonin antagonist, has been used to prevent attacks and treat intractable cases of migraine headache. Long-term use is not recommended because it may cause retroperitoneal fibrosis or peripheral vascular insufficiency. The drug should be given for no longer than several continuous months and be stopped slowly to prevent untoward effects. Short-term therapy with methysergide maleate may alter the pattern of migraine frequency enough to permit smooth drug reduction and discontinuation.

Propranolol (Inderal) has been effective for migraine prophylaxis but has no effect on a headache that has already started. The dosage is individualized. Amitriptyline (Elavil) has also been used in migraine prevention. Its ability to offset headache does not seem to be related to its antidepressant effect.

Some clients obtain a prophylactic effect by using minor

tranquilizers or barbiturates to decrease levels of stress and anxiety that tend to precipitate their migraines. Clients who understand their predisposition to headaches and take appropriate precautions (eg, avoiding a glass of wine at the time of the menses) can participate in their normal activities without much difficulty. The frequency of attacks tends to decrease with age and may subside for menopausal women. On the other hand, hypertension or use of oral contraceptives may induce, intensify, or prolong an attack.

Although cluster headaches differ from migraines, they also respond to the vasoconstrictive effects of ergot preparations. The previous restrictions and precautions also apply. Some clients with cluster headaches respond well to indomethacin (Indocin). This drug should be used for short-term therapy only and clients monitored closely for gastrointestinal side effects and blood dyscrasias. Indomethacin should be administered with meals or milk and the client's blood count periodically evaluated.

Temporal arteritis requires prompt diagnosis and early treatment. Steroid therapy with ACTH or cortisone acetate relieves pain and prevents involvement of other arteries, especially the ophthalmic artery. The condition often responds to drug therapy over time. Sometimes surgical division of the temporal artery is recommended.

Hypertensive headaches are treated with antihypertensive drug therapy. Persistent ocular headaches may require evaluation by an ophthalmologist to detect or treat astigmatism, hyperopia, or muscle imbalance. Avoiding continuous activities that cause eye strain may help to prevent attacks. For headaches of intracranial origin, refer to the sections on cerebral aneurysms, meningitis, and neoplasms.

Specific Nursing Measures

Obtaining a complete history and a description of headache characteristics is important to identify factors that precipitate the migraine headache. Nursing care is directed toward assisting the client to develop strategies to decrease the frequency and duration of migraine attacks. One strategy is to maintain a headache log to document duration of headaches, intervals between them, and probable precipitants. A log enables clients to recognize the patterns of their headaches. Some clients need to be assisted to identify and avoid dietary factors that induce headache. Decreasing intake of cheese, wine, and chocolate may be helpful. Eliminating salt for several days before menstruation is beneficial in some cases. Client education about drug regimens is crucial to avoid untoward side effects. Tell clients to notify their physician of any change in the severity, duration and frequency of migraines. Particularly important is having clients report any persistence of headaches on one side of the head consistently. Women with a history of migraine headaches should not take oral contraceptives.

The nursing care of clients with muscle contraction headaches is similar to that for clients with migraines. Emphasize proper diet, rest, and exercise. These clients often respond well to self-help groups that heighten their awareness of the relation between lifestyle patterns and headache onset. Courses in assertiveness training may teach individuals to set appropriate limits for themselves and others. Strategies to reduce stress and tension may be internalized and practiced after the client has worked in a group process problem-solving setting. Evaluate the techniques developed by clients to reduce their tension headaches and teach them how to manage medication use, physical exercise, and diet modifications effectively.

Trigeminal Neuralgia

Trigeminal neuralgia (tic douloureux) is the most common neurologic disorder to affect CN V and is also the most frequent of the neuralgias. The etiology can be associated with other neurologic disorders such as MS, tumors, or aneurysms. Often the cause is unknown. Paroxysms of recurrent excrucitating, sharp, stabbing pain of short duration along one or more branches of the trigeminal nerve characterize this disorder. The intensity of the pain often causes clients to wince; thus the word "tic" is used to describe the condition. Recurrent episodes of pain are not only disabling, but are anticipated with fear and anxiety. Although trigeminal neuralgia can occur at any age, the onset is most often between the fourth and sixth decades of life.

Clinical Manifestations

An attack of trigeminal neuralgia is often described as paroxysms of excruciating pain with a lightninglike stab that burns. The onset is usually abrupt and related to a precipitating event that irritates a "trigger" point. Dental caries, sinusitis, trauma, and hot or cold temperatures or fluids can stimulate a trigger point. The usual sites for these sensitive spots are the mouth, lips, cheek, tongue, face, or nose. Movements such as speaking, brushing the teeth, washing the face, shaving, laughing, and facial movements in the maxillary and mandibular divisions of CN V can precipitate an attack. An important diagnostic point is that during or following an attack there is no objective loss of cutaneous sensation. Diagnosis is usually made on the history of facial pain as well as the client's ability to identify any precipitants.

Medical Measures

A plethora of medication regimens have been used to treat trigeminal neuralgia over the years but most have been unsuccessful. Standard analgesics are ineffective. Morphine provides some relief but is contraindicated because of its addictive properties. Sometimes phenytoin (Dilantin) is given intravenously to prevent an acute attack although long-term use of oral phenytoin is not effective in treating paroxysms of trigeminal neuralgia. Carbamazepine (Tegretol), an anticonvulsant, has controlled the disorder in some clients. Clients on carbamazepine must carefully be monitored for blood dyscrasias.

Injections of absolute alcohol into the gasserian ganglion have been used with clients intractable to other medication therapies. When effective, it causes a loss of sensation in the affected divisions of the trigeminal nerve. The length of symptom remission is variable. Surgical interventions have also been attempted involving resection of the retrogasserian rootlets, causing a permanent facial anesthesia in the sectioned branch. Sometimes the rootlets are decompressed and manipulated to retain sensory function. Several microneurosurgical techniques to relieve pressure on CN V are currently being used in major neurosurgical centers with more promising results.

Specific Nursing Measures

Preventing attacks of trigeminal neuralgia is the priority of nursing care. Document a detailed history of precipitating factors and describe the client's trigger points on the nursing care plan. Place clients in an environment that avoids exposure to drafts or excessive heat or cold. Encourage ambulation between attacks to prevent hazards of immobility. Assist clients to anticipate their own needs and help them with hygiene and meals as needed to prevent precipitating an attack. Give prescribed medications on time to promote adequate blood levels. Document the client's response to all medications given.

Clients often lose weight because they fear that chewing movements will precipitate an attack. Encourage food choices that avoid excessive chewing. Teach clients to chew on the unaffected side and to avoid liquids and solids of extreme temperatures. Frequent, small feedings are often helpful. For some clients, temporary intravenous therapy, or hyperalimentation, may be necessary.

Fearing an attack of pain, clients may avoid washing their faces, performing mouth care, and shaving. Recommend tepid tub baths. Mild mouthwash can be used for oral hygiene. For clients with loss of corneal sensation, teach special eye care to avoid complications. Refer to nursing measures in Bell's palsy for specifics of eye care.

Clients may develop ineffective coping patterns due to the disabling and extremely painful nature of trigeminal neuralgia. Use a kind, understanding approach. Reassurance, support, and comfort measures to minimize attacks are essential. Review preventive measures with the client and significant others.

Bell's Palsy

Bell's palsy is the most common neurologic condition to affect the facial nerve, CN VII. An inflammatory, edematous reaction is thought to occur in or around CN VII resulting in nerve compression, which is characterized by an abrupt onset of a flaccid facial paralysis. There is a loss of facial expression on the affected side, an inability to close the eyelid on the ipsilateral side, and a deviation of the mouth toward the contralateral side. Bell's palsy occurs most often between the third to fifth decades of life with an equal distribution between sexes. Most clients with Bell's palsy recover without residual neurologic deficits. The period of recovery varies and can range from several weeks to as long as a year.

Previous infection, prolonged exposure to cold temperatures, and psychologic trauma have been suggested as possible causes of Bell's palsy. Concurrent herpetic vesicles in the external auditory meatus of some clients with Bell's palsy suggest a viral cause (Conway–Rutkowski, 1982). Bell's palsy usually has no identifiable precipitant, however. The facial nerve can be affected by many other conditions such as brain tumor, traumatic injury, meningitis, middle ear infection, intracranial hemorrhage, or demyelinating disease.

Clinical Manifestations

Bell's palsy often begins with pain behind the ear followed within several hours or 1 to 2 days by a flaccid facial paralysis. The client is unable to wrinkle the forehead, close the eyelid, whistle, blow out the cheek, or smile (Figure 29–2). The affected eye may tear excessively and saliva may drool from the affected side of the mouth. Impairment of taste in the anterior two-thirds of the tongue can occur. Bell's phenomenon refers to the upward and slightly inward positioning of the eyeball that occurs when the client attempts to close the eyelid. The corneal reflex is usually absent. **Hyperacusis** (abnormal sensitivity to sound) can result from nerve involvement to the stapedius muscle. There is usually a loss of deep facial sensation and hypesthesia occurs in some clients.

Medical Measures

Treatment is symptomatic, supportive, and aimed at preventing complications. Protection of the cornea is a priority when the client cannot voluntarily close the eyelid. Electrical stimulation with a weak galvanic current can be done to massage and stimulate facial muscle tone and prevent atrophy. Steroids may be given to reduce facial nerve inflammation. Less commonly vasodilating drugs are given to stimulate circulation and restore blood supply to the affected area. The application of moist heat several times a day for 15 to 30 minutes is a more conservative method of stimulating circulation and may also decrease facial pain. A facial sling is sometimes recommended to prevent muscle stretching and sagging, improve muscle tone, facilitate eating, and improve lip alignment. When spontaneous recovery does not occur over time, surgical procedures may be done. This involves either an end-to-end suturing

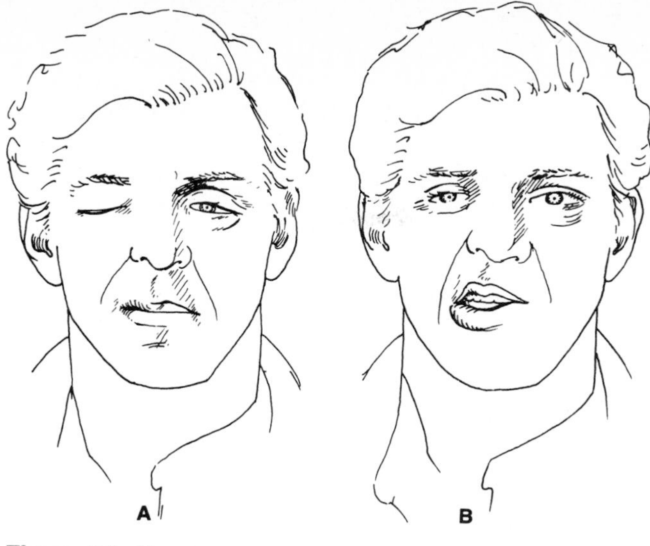

Figure 29–2

A client with left-sided Bell's palsy—paralysis of CN VII. **A.** Note the sagging of the left side of the face and inability to close the left eyelid. **B.** Note that when the client smiles only one side of the face moves.

of the affected nerve or an anastomosis of CN XI or CN XII to the facial nerve.

Specific Nursing Measures

The priority of nursing care is to prevent alterations in protective mechanisms related to loss of the corneal reflex. Cover the affected eyelid with a clear plastic eye bubble or a cloth patch. Avoid gauze patches that can cause corneal scratching. Taping of the eyelid is an effective alternative. Instill artificial tears every 2 to 4 hours and more often as necessary to clear mucus and debris from the eye. This prevents eyeball dryness when the client is unable to produce tears spontaneously. Teach client to manually close the affected eyelid during the period of recovery. As eyelid movement begins, teach client to practice progressive movement toward lid closure. Clients should wear protective glasses during the day and an eye patch or eyelid tape at night.

A second objective is to prevent alterations in protective mechanisms related to sensorimotor changes until paralysis subsides. Instruct the client to chew on the unaffected side to prevent food from collecting and lodging in the paralyzed side. This also prevents the client from biting the mucous membranes inadvertently where sensation is absent. Give frequent mouth care to prevent the development of parotitis. Instruct the client to avoid extreme temperatures of foods to prevent injuries to areas lacking sensation. Privacy for clients during meals avoids embarrassment because of drooling and awkward chewing.

Maintain facial muscle tone by applying a facial sling to prevent stretching of weakened muscles and improve lip alignment. This also facilitates eating and drinking. Stimulate circulation to affected muscles with warm, moist compresses. Teach clients to massage facial muscles three to four times a day from the chin upward on the affected side. When return of facial movement occurs, have the client practice various facial expressions in a mirror.

Clients may have alterations in body image related to changes in facial appearance and function. Assist the client and family to be realistic about the length of facial dysfunction. In 80% of clients with Bell's palsy, recovery is complete in several weeks to months. During the regenerative period, teach the client the rationale for protective measures and techniques in activities of daily living to support the natural course of recovery. Help the client to understand that there is not much that can be done to hasten nerve regeneration. Provide clients with opportunities to verbalize feelings about changes in appearance and give positive reinforcement as they progress.

Cerebrovascular Accident

Cerebrovascular accident (CVA), or stroke, is a syndrome in which cerebral circulation is interrupted. CVA causes sudden onset of neurologic deficits that vary according to the location and extent of vascular interruption. As a result, cerebral ischemia and infarction may occur. A CVA may or may not be preceded by warning signs.

CVAs account for more than 10% of all deaths in the United States each year, making them the third leading cause of death. An additional two million individuals are disabled, making CVAs the second most common cause of chronic disability.

Stroke tends to run in families. It is more frequent in men than in women and in blacks than in whites. (The higher incidence in blacks is considered related to their greater incidence of hypertension, a predisposing factor in stroke.) The highest incidence of stroke is among those between 75 and 85 years old. On the other hand, about one out of seven individuals under age 65 sustains a stroke.

CVA is divided into two major types: ischemic and hemorrhagic. In an *ischemic* episode, cerebral blood flow is suddenly impaired and no longer sufficient to enable affected brain cells to function adequately. In hemorrhagic stroke, the rupture of a cerebral blood vessel causes bleeding into the subarachnoid space or directly into brain tissue (intracerebral hemorrhage).

Cerebral thrombosis accounts for at least half of all CVAs. A cerebral thrombosis is caused by a shortage of cerebral blood supply, commonly because of an *atheroma,* a hard, fatty degenerative plaque that forms on the inner wall of an artery. Atherosclerosis is the most common cause of an ischemic CVA. Thrombotic stroke usually is a progression from partial to complete occusion of the vessel, with an initial transient ischemic attack (TIA) or warning sign, the reversible ischemic episode, stroke in evolution, and the completed stroke. Clients may experience one, several, or all syndrome stages.

In an embolic stroke, the clot usually forms outside

the brain in the heart, neck, or thorax. Usually, a segment of the original clot breaks off and travels via the bloodstream to the brain. The embolus eventually lodges in a vessel too small to permit passage. The process is known as cerebral embolism with causation. The neurologic deficits are similar to those with thrombotic stroke. Embolic stroke develops within a few seconds to minutes without warning signs. The risk factors for cerebrovascular occusive disease are listed in Box 29–4.

A cerebral thrombosis may be specifically attributed to a number of conditions, the most frequent being atherosclerosis and inflammatory disease processes that damage arterial walls. An intracranial mass can also mechanically constrict cerebral arteries. Hematologic disorders and diseases that increase coagulation can lead to thrombus formation. Conditions causing inadequate cerebral perfusion such as hypotension and dehydration may increase the risk of thrombosis, as may problems of prolonged vasoconstriction such as malignant hypertension. Trauma, on the other hand, only occasionally causes cerebral thrombosis.

Cerebral embolism also has specific risk factors. The most common causes are myocardial infarction, myocarditis and endocarditis, rheumatic heart disease, postcardiac surgical procedures, atrial–septal defects, and atrial dysrhythmias. (The risk of embolic stroke for clients with atrial dysrhythmias is five times greater than for those without.) Another major risk is a disorder of the aortic, carotid, or vertebral–basilar circulation. Less frequent contributors to embolic stroke are air, fat, tumors, and foreign objects. A major risk of posterior fossa surgery in the sitting position is an air embolism; fat emboli are usually associated with fractures of long bones. Finally, any condition that increases coagulation, such as taking oral contraceptives or diseases such as sickle cell anemia or polycythemia vera, potentiates the risk for embolic stroke.

Box 29–4
Risk Factors for Cerebrovascular Occlusive Disease

- Atherosclerosis
- Hypertension
- Diabetes mellitus
- Obesity
- Elevated serum cholesterol, lipoprotein, triglyceride, and uric acid levels
- Cigarette smoking
- Sedentary lifestyle
- Hypothyroidism
- Use of oral contraceptives
- Sickle cell anemia
- Coagulation disorders
- Polycythemia vera
- Dehydration, especially combined with any of above conditions

Clinical Manifestations

The clinical symptoms and signs of occlusive stroke vary according to which cerebral blood vessel and its branches are involved. Symptoms and signs also depend on the site, size, and degree of occlusion or infarction. Involvement of the middle cerebral artery is the most common form of all cerebral occlusions. A massive infarction of the affected hemisphere occurs with an occlusion of the main stem of this vessel.

An occlusion of the internal carotid artery may not be evident if collateral circulation is sufficient. When symptoms do occur, they are similar to those caused by middle cerebral artery occlusion. An internal carotid artery occlusion is considered when the client has repeated TIAs. Atheromas of the internal carotid artery in the neck may lead to embolic occlusions of the middle cerebral artery.

The diagnosis of the cause of a CVA can be difficult. The client's history should investigate risk factors and trace symptoms and signs. The physical exam focuses on neurovascular and neurologic status. Neurovascular assessment includes vital signs, cardiac rhythm, blood pressure, and pulses. The heart and great vessels are assessed for bruits. Funduscopic examination evaluates the vasculature of the retina. Some clinicians attempt to determine the effects of precipitant events such as body position changes on blood pressure; head turning; carotid sinus massage; and Valsalva's maneuver.

CSF analysis is important to distinguish cerebral thrombosis from hemorrhage. The CSF is normal in the majority of clients with cerebral thrombosis and bloody in a large proportion of clients with hemorrhagic stroke.

Angiography is valuable in the definitive diagnosis of arterial stenosis, occlusion, or hemorrhage. A femoral angiogram, which permits selective catheterization of the aortic arch, is the procedure of choice. This study visualizes extracranial and intracranial circulation. It also avoids directly puncturing an atheromatous vessel, eliminating risk of precipitating an occlusion. Digital venous angiography is another accepted method for differentiating between a stenosis and occlusion.

The CT scan is valuable for detecting signs of cerebral infarction as early as the first day of a CVA. The scan readily distinguishes thrombosis from hemorrhagic embolic infarction. In cases of TIA, the CT scan is generally normal. Doppler studies of the neck are done to evaluate extracranial circulation as well as to detect a possible carotid lesion in the neck.

Cerebral blood flow is sometimes evaluated for decreased regional perfusion by radionuclide studies. Serial isotope scanning examinations may be done. In cases of vascular lesions, uptake around the infarct will be increased. Repeated investigation demonstrates an improving condition, suggesting a vascular lesion rather than a tumor.

Ocular testing may include an ophthalmologic examination with the pupils dilated. The retinal vessels are checked for emboli, which could be fragments of an ulcerated plaque or of thrombotic origin. Laboratory tests usually include the complete blood count with platelets, electrolytes, glucose level, blood urea nitrogen and creatinine, uric acid, and cholesterol level.

Medical Measures

Treatment of cerebrovascular occlusive disease varies according to etiology. Routine treatment for TIAs with aspirin to prevent platelet aggregation has been more effective in men than women. Anticoagulants help to alleviate microembolism; however, an underlying atheromatous process may continue to progress. Complete occlusion of the affected vessel may result.

It is crucial for the physician to establish whether the source of cerebral ischemia is carotid disease of the neck or intracranial vessel disease. Clients undergoing surgery for carotid stenosis who have not had a CVA should have their diagnosis confirmed by angiography. Candidates for surgery include those who have had one or more temporary strokes, including TIAs. Surgery is usually more urgent for a client who has bilateral carotid artery disease and impairment in the vertebral or basilar system. However, the best surgical results are in clients with minimal or no permanent neurologic deficits and in those where cerebrovascular disease only affects one of the major vessels with an obstruction of approximately 80% of the lumen. The procedure of choice for clients with carotid disease of the neck is a carotid endarterectomy. The operation involves the surgical excision of the thickened, atheromatous tunica intima of the affected vessel.

Cerebrovascular occlusive disease caused by emboli is best treated by identifying and controlling the foci for the emboli. Varicosities in the lower extremities may require a high saphenous vein ligation. Cardiac problems such as atrial fibrillation, mitral stenosis, or atrial dysrhythmia are treated. Vasculitis related to collagen diseases can be managed with steroid therapy.

Clients who sustain completed strokes receive supportive therapy. Comatose clients require various life-sustaining interventions such as airway maintenance, fluids, electrolytes, and measures to prevent complications. Sometimes artificial airways are necessary. Although intermittent catherization is preferred, in-dwelling urinary catheters or condom catheters may be used. Continuous collection of urine helps prevent decubiti.

The acute onset of a completed stroke may be accompanied by marked cerebral edema that can lead to brain stem compression. The client is at risk for potential herniation. Signs of impending herniation include pupil dilation, deterioration in level of consciousness, irregular respiratory pattern, hiccoughs, and motor deficits. Aggressive therapy is required to reduce increased ICP. Bolus infusions of mannitol and dexamethasone (Decadron) are often used. Urea solutions may be given IV if no signs of hemorrhage accompany increased ICP.

Cerebral vasodilating agents may also be used in the acute phase. The most potent cerebral vasodilator in current use is an inhalation mixture of 5% CO_2 and 95% O_2. The mixture can be given via mask every hour for 15 minutes during the first 48 hours after a completed stroke. In some clients, however, vasodilators may increase cerebral blood flow by shunting blood away from an ischemic site.

Anticoagulant therapy is best used in clients with an evolving stroke caused by thrombi or emboli. Its use is contraindicated in clients with hypertensive states or blood dyscrasias. When indicated, heparin is the drug of choice during the acute phase and warfarin sodium (Coumadin) for long-term management. Heparin therapy is best monitored by checking the partial thromboplastin time or clotting time; warfarin anticoagulation is assessed by checking the prothrombin time.

During acute phases of a stroke, convulsive episodes can be managed with phenytoin (Dilantin), diazepam (Valium), and phenobarbital. Loading doses of intravenous phenytoin must be given slowly in divided doses to prevent cardiac dysrhythmias. Phenytoin is only compatible in solution with normal saline. Clients require careful cardiac monitoring during the loading time. Diazepam cannot be diluted in an intravenous Soluset solution. It should be given as prepared by the manufacturer. For clients who are hypertensive, antihypertensive medications should be used to decrease the systolic blood pressure to 150 to 160 mm Hg.

Specific Nursing Measures

The first nursing priority in acute stroke is to prevent ineffective airway clearance and to manage increased ICP. Clients are at risk for obstructed airways and hypoxia. A patent airway and adequate ventilation are essential to prevent atelectasis, pneumonia, respiratory arrest, and increased ICP. Assess the depth and rate of respirations frequently and auscultate the chest for adventitious sounds. For clients with marked deterioration in level of consciousness, an oral airway should be inserted and a side-lying position maintained. Respiratory treatments should not be instituted vigorously, or the ICP may elevate proportionately.

Standard measures for managing increased ICP are:

- Elevating the head of the bed at least 30° to promote central venous drainage.

- Maintaining a patent airway to help prevent an accumulation of CO_2. (An elevated partial pressure of carbon dioxide [Pco_2] causes vasodilation of cerebral blood vessels that can lead to increased ICP.)
- Providing gentle respiratory care and avoiding straining at defecation.
- Frequent monitoring of neurologic signs and reporting promptly changes from the baseline.
- Avoiding frequent head rotation. (Neck muscles can compress the jugular veins, impeding central venous drainage. Turn clients with head and shoulders as a unit to avoid this problem.)

Recognize the rationale for medication regimens used to treat stroke in evolution and their side effects. These regimens are discussed under medical measures.

Maintenance of skin integrity and the management of immobility are major nursing care objectives that influence future rehabilitation. Circulation can be impaired if the paretic or paralyzed side is not carefully positioned. Affected limbs should be supported with splints and elevated to prevent or treat dependent edema. Motor deficits are usually accompanied by sensory loss. The client will not be able to report circulatory impairments on the affected side. Check peripheral pulses in the hands and feet periodically.

Good skin care and maintaining clean, dry, and wrinkle-free linen decrease interruptions in skin integrity. Carefully schedule active and passive ROM exercises as well as repositioning in the side-lying and prone positions to decrease problems of immobility. Hip flexion contractures can be avoided with a prone position, and footdrop can be prevented with footboards for side-lying and supine positions.

After respiratory dysfunction, the second major complication of immobility is thrombophlebitis and pulmonary embolism. Thigh-high elastic stockings and ROM exercises are ordered as preventive measures. Be alert for client symptoms and signs of calf stiffness, aching, or pain and check for Homans' sign. Also check for local signs of calf or thigh redness, swelling, and increased temperature. Measure calf and thigh circumferences every shift and document the comparisons. Watch for respiratory distress such as shortness of breath or chest pain that could indicate a pulmonary embolism.

Alteration in communication patterns is one of the most distressing problems for a client with stroke. Receptive and/or expressive dysphasia may be present. Establish effective communication by written or visual cues and provide an appropriate type of call bell for the unaffected extremity. A trusting relationship can develop if the nurse treats the client with respect and demonstrates a knowledge of the deficit. Speak to the client directly in a slow, patient manner. Remember that hearing is intact. Listen carefully, allow the client time to answer, and offer appropriate cues. These measures conserve the client's energy and avoid frustration. Discuss the communication problem and plans for rehabilitation with the client and significant others. This is particularly helpful for those with expressive aphasia (the inability to formulate and use expressive language). Place objects within easy reach of the unaffected side. Clients with receptive aphasia (the inability to comprehend and integrate receptive language) need frequent reorientation and a safe environment.

Alterations in elimination patterns are a potential problem for the stroke client. Plan a regular voiding pattern for continent clients. Offering the bedpan every 2 or 3 hours and using Credé's maneuver can assist the client to void. (Credé's maneuver is discussed in Chapter 26.) Clients may develop constipation or fecal impaction. Administer psyllium, carthartics, or suppositories as ordered. Encourage adequate fluid intake including water and fruit juice. Auscultation of bowel sounds is important to detect any signs of a paralytic ileus. See specific nursing measures for clients with multiple sclerosis for additional guidelines for bladder and bowel management.

Alterations in visual function can accompany a CVA. Assess the client's visual acuity, approach clients on the side of best visual perception, and teach them to use the best field of vision. Be alert for diplopia or nystagmus. Alternate eye patching can correct diplopia.

REHABILITATION Maximum rehabilitation of the client with a CVA depends on an active rehabilitation program involving care providers, consultants, client, and significant others. The client may have cognitive, sensory-perceptual, motor, and/or communication deficits. A physical therapist, speech therapist, nutritionist, and occupational therapist may all need to contribute their expertise.

Depending on the status of the lower extremities, the client may initially be confined to a wheelchair or may begin balance training progressing to ambulation with assistance (eg, walker or cane). The affected upper extremity should be in a sling to prevent shoulder subluxation. Splints or soft rolls can be used to maintain functional hand positions. Special aids for eating (eg, wide-handled spoons) are often helpful. Other special equipment such as raised toilet seats, safety rails, or long-handled brushes can assist the client in various self-care activities. Physical and occupational therapists can be a tremendous source of assistance to the staff and to the client and significant others in these areas. For the client with **dysphasia,** long-term rehabilitation requires the assistance of a speech therapist.

Major emphasis should be placed on reduction of risk factors (Box 29–4). Clients may need to be on a weight loss diet, restricted in sodium if the client is hypertensive and/or in cholesterol and carbohydrates if the client has a form of hyperlipidemia or is diabetic. Clients should stop smoking because of the vasoconstrictive properties of nic-

Table 29–2
Nursing Interventions for the Client with CVA

Potential Client Problem	Nursing Interventions
Contractures; decreased muscle strength; thrombosis and pulmonary embolism	Change client position at least q. 2 hr; maintain correct body alignment; ROM — passive to affected extremities, active to unaffected extremities; quadriceps and gluteal setting exercises
Subluxation of affected shoulder; shoulder–hand syndrome	Sling for affected arm; arm supports; exercise of affected arm (interlace fingers, place palms together, lift affected arm over head frequently)
Orthostasis	Check supine BP; elevate client slowly from lying to sitting, sitting to standing—taking BP in each position; if BP drops significantly, do not attempt to ambulate client; BP will stabilize with daily efforts at gradual elevation
Sensory–perceptual alterations	Approach client from unaffected side; keep necessary objects within reach of unaffected side; encourage self-feeding for improving hand-to-mouth coordination
Dysphasia	Speak slowly and distinctly to client; minimize environmental distractions; encourage attempts to verbalize
Decreased self-concept	Actively involve client in decision making; encourage every effort to participate in own care; be supportive to significant others so they can remain strong and continue their support of the client during the frustrating times

otine and should use little to no alcohol. Encourage clients to be involved in all decision making regarding their health with the goal of total self-management. Teach clients returning home on anticoagulants the action of the drug and the dangers of taking any other medicine without permission of their physician. Emphasize the fact that no OTC drugs can be taken because many of them contain aspirin or aspirinlike products that can cause bleeding. Support groups can be a potential source of comfort, strength, and management strategies for both clients and their significant others. Table 29–2 lists some potential problems for clients with stroke and helpful nursing interventions.

SECTION 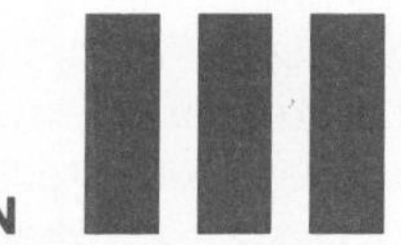

Degenerative Disorders

Degenerative disorders of the nervous system are those with an unknown etiology that have an insidious onset and involve atrophy of neurons and nerve fibers. It is not uncommon for degenerative diseases to occur after a long period of normal nervous system function. The disease course is gradual and progressive over many years.

Alzheimer's Disease

Alzheimer's disease (AD) is a progressive, degenerative disorder that causes cerebral atrophy. Affecting more than 2.5 million Americans, AD is the fifth leading cause of total disability in the United States and the fourth leading cause of death among the elderly. Each year it claims the lives of 120,000 Americans. Experts predict that in the next century AD will be the leading cause of death (Schneider and Emr, 1985).

The disorder develops insidiously, marked by progressive organic mental changes and language dysfunction. *Dementia,* the deterioration of intellectual capacity, is characteristic of AD. This disorder is thought to account for at least half of all cases of dementia in the elderly (McKinstry, 1982).

The cause of AD is unknown, although several theories have been proposed. One theory suggests that the disease is the result of the brain's generalized reaction to a number of harmful processes. Another suggests that a specific agent such as a toxin, slow virus, genetic deficit, metal deposit, or an immunologic dysfunction causes the disorder (McKinstry, 1982). Current research is aimed at identifying a genetic marker responsible for AD. Evidence of a familial pattern supports this area of investigation. Researchers expect to find a biologic marker unique to the disease such as a peripheral abnormality, a specific sensory organ change, or a diagnostic blood test.

In late 1986, researchers identified an abnormal protein, A-68, that appears in the brain of AD victims and also in the spinal fluid of living persons thought to have the disease. A-68 is unique to AD, although it is not known whether the protein is a causative factor. Depending on further studies, a routine laboratory test could be developed that would make possible early and accurate diagnosis. Until such a test is developed, definitive diagnosis can only be made at autopsy.

Another research focus has been on the role of neurotransmitters. The most substantial finding has been the deficiency of acetylcholine in the brain of affected clients.

This finding has encouraged further research into acetylcholine precursors as a potential treatment, similar to the use of L-dopa in Parkinson's disease. These studies involve the role of lecithin and choline in treating Alzheimer's disease. Findings have been inconclusive.

Clinical Manifestations

The clinical diagnosis of Alzheimer's disease is presumptive. A confirming diagnosis is best made by microscopic examination in a postmortem to identify the characteristic neuronal degeneration. Therefore, diagnosis is made by exclusion. First, the signs of dementia are established. Then identification of the pathology is attempted: Is it curable and reversible, or is it irreversible? Treatable causes of dementia may include general paresis, myxedema, normal pressure hydrocephalus, intracranial masses, avitaminosis, and depression. Other irreversible causes of dementia include alcoholism, Huntington's chorea, and multiple cerebrovascular infarction.

Box 29–5
Stages of Alzheimer's Disease and Associated Symptoms

Stage I

- Emotion/mood
  - depression
  - anxiety
  - fatigue
  - decreased activity
- Memory deficits
  - recent
  - delayed

Stage II

Language difficulties

Stage III

- Language/motor
  - aphasia
  - apraxia
  - agnosia
  - echolalia
- Psychiatric
  - hallucinations/delusions
- Sleep
  - altered sleep/awake cycles

Stage IV

- Decreased arousal
- Disruptive behavior
- Urinary/fecal incontinence

These manifestations may vary widely in time of onset, rate of progression, and severity, but they tend to follow the sequence outlined here.

Reprinted with permission from Cutler NR, Narang PK: Drug therapies. *Geriatric Nursing*, 1985; 6(3):162.

The diagnostic work-up for Alzheimer's disease should be exhaustive because the psychosocial/lifestyle implications of the diagnosis can be devastating for both client and family.

Symptoms have been divided into three stages: mild, moderate, severe, and terminal (see Box 29–5). During a period of from 2 to 15 years, the person with AD gradually slides into a childlike dependency. The average time from diagnosis to death is seven years (Jolles and Hijman, 1983).

The first stage is marked by memory loss caused by the patchy loss of neurons throughout the cerebral cortex. Judgment and logic compensate for memory deficits as long as enough frontal lobe neurons remain intact. Other aspects of first-stage Alzheimer's disease are irritability, mood swings, flattening of affect, and agitation.

As the disease progresses into the second stage, judgment and logic decline. Disorientation and language difficulties begin.

The third stage is marked by global aphasia. The aphasia includes motor and expressive speech deficits (Broca's aphasia) and sensory comprehension deficits (Wernicke's aphasia). Speech deficits are more difficult to assess because the pattern is different than in other neurologic problems such as cerebrovascular disease. The neuronal damage in Alzheimer's disease is symmetrical, preventing the opposite hemisphere compensation common in hemorrhagic stroke.

During this third phase, clients forget learned, socially acceptable behaviors. They neglect hygiene and develop inappropriate eating habits and poor elimination patterns. Clients lose portions of their ability to see, to hear, and to feel pain. A common sensory deficit is **agnosia,** the inability to recognize familiar objects in the environment through the senses of touch and vision. Clients may have seizures. Behavioral problems include **perseveration** (repetition of a motor or verbal action) and **hyperorality** (an insatiable need for oral stimulation by chewing or tasting objects). This second stage varies from 2 to 12 years; regression is more rapid in younger persons and men.

The fourth or terminal stage is the impaired confusional stage, marked by the progression of both generalized and focal deficits. The client eventually becomes mute and unresponsive and has anorexia and **apraxia** (the inability to carry out a learned, voluntary act when motor function is intact).

Medical and Specific Nursing Measures

No means of prevention or treatment is yet available for AD. In late 1986, however, early results of a study showed some success with the drug *tetrahydroaminoacridine* (THA) in helping to restore some cognitive function (Davis and Mohs, 1986). Further drug trials are underway.

Box 29–6
Adapting Environment to Client

- Individualize care
- Recognize strengths
- Provide environmental cues for orientation
- Maintain patient's home schedule
- Adapt schedule of diagnostic procedures to patient's needs
- Communicate clearly
- Maintain balance of ADL and DDL with patient's coping resources and social supports
- Learn who the patient was
- Foster sense of control
- Time the giving of information
- Maintain consistency in staff–patient interactions

Reprinted with permission from Schafer SC: Modifying the environment. *Geriatric Nursing*, 1985; 6(3) 159.

In planning care, consider that the adjustments and compensations the client develops at an early stage of the disease will not remain for future use. Clients need increased supervision and manipulation of the environment; see suggestions summarized in Box 29–6. In fact, a major part of the nurse's role is to teach and role model the following concepts for families (Gioella and Bevil, 1985): structured environment, safety, activity, respite, and support. In addition, the nurse can provide important counseling, teaching, and referral services.

The client is not well attuned to the present, but reminiscing can be supportive because long-term memory is more intact. Encourage the family to help the client reminisce about familiar persons and events. Reminiscing is comforting and increases the client's self-confidence. Communication strategies are important. Conversation should be clear and simple, using short words and sentences that are readily understood. Repetition is required. Keeping a log of effective techniques can be helpful. Clients frequently refuse treatment during this stage. Never pressure them. Reapproach a task when the client is more receptive.

During the final stage, comprehensive, supervised care is required. Maintaining a safe environment is a major priority. Suggestions for protective measures include:

- Providing an identification necklace or bracelet with the client's name, address, and telephone number for those with a tendency to wander
- Securing hazardous areas by installing safety locks that are difficult for clients to reach or use
- Keeping toxic fluids and firearms locked up and preventing access to lighters and burners
- Providing an uncluttered environment to prevent falls
- Keeping objects in the same place to decrease client confusion

Help families to recognize the need for skilled care and think about alternative placement for the client. Appropriate referrals to social service agencies assist families in investigating the chronic care facilities. Families need support in dealing with the anxiety and guilt of separation from the client as well as the change in their own roles and responsibilities.

Parkinson's Disease

Parkinson's disease is a degenerative process of nerve cells in the extrapyramidal system: basal ganglia, thalamus, substantia nigra, red nucleus, and reticular formation. The disease has a slow, gradual course. Parkinsonism is one of the most common neurologic disorders, affecting both men and women over age 50.

The causes of Parkinson's disease are not known. The condition may result from an accelerated aging process or from a virus causing gradual destruction of dopaminergic neurons, or it may be an inherited genetic defect. Several forms of the disease have been described according to etiology:

- Idiopathic (in which the cause is unknown)
- Arteriosclerotic (related to a defective blood supply to the basal ganglia)
- Postencephalitic (occurring after encephalitis)
- Posttraumatic (following an ischemic episode to the brain)
- Toxic (following inhalation of carbon monoxide, manganese, or mercury)
- Neurosyphilitic (as a complication of syphilis, now rare)
- Drug induced (pseudoparkinson's disease, related to high doses of antipsychotic drugs)

Clinical Manifestations

Diseases of the basal ganglia are clinically manifested as disturbances of movement: tremor, rigidity of muscles, and dyskinesias. Dyskinesias involve a problem in initiating or performing a movement quickly. Clients report feeling stiff and sore in the joints and are slow in performing activities of daily living.

Tremor is the most common initial symptom. Classic signs of tremor in clients with Parkinson's disease include pill rolling of the thumb and forefingers at rest, to-and-fro head tremors, and tremulous voice quality. The involuntary resting tremors differ from the intention tremors of clients with cerebellar disease. In parkinsonism, tremors vary from mild to severe to incapacitating. They are aggravated by fatigue and stress and dissipate when the client sleeps or performs a purposeful activity. After the hands, the larger joints and the lower extremities become involved. Eventually, tremors are so marked that it is impossible for a client to control or conceal them.

Rigidity occurs either at the same time as tremors, or long before, as the only sign of the syndrome. Muscular rigidity has been described in three ways: the rhythmical jerking interruption of passive ROM as "cogwheel" rigidity, mild resistance as "plastic" rigidity, and total resistance as "leadpipe" rigidity.

Hypokinetic features include paucity of movement and hypertonicity of antagonistic muscles despite client attempts to relax. These signs are caused from the irregular, asynchronous pattern of neuronal discharges. Bradykinesia is observed as difficulty initiating voluntary movement marked by episodes of "freezing" of movement. Facial expression becomes masklike (masklike facies) with a fixed stare and paucity of facial movement. Clients assume a bent-forward, stooped position, and adjustments are uncoordinated. The gait consists of small, short shuffling steps that are slowly initiated. Movements become propulsive with an acceleration in gait. Clients lose their armswing when walking and have difficulty ceasing motion. The feet fail to move before a change in position from sitting to standing and vice versa. Clients also lose finesse of movement. Their bodies tend to turn all at once (like a statue) rather than in the normal sequence.

Handwriting is cramped and small (**micrographia**) with signs of tremor; the voice tends to be a monotone with no range. Speech becomes rapid, unpunctuated, and incomprehensible. **Pallalia** (involuntary sentence repetition) and **echolalia** (parrotlike repetition of words spoken by others) may be heard.

Other symptoms include insomnia, dysphagia, weight loss, and drooling (sialorrhea); shiny, oily skin with scalp seborrhea; and involuntary rapid eyelid blinking (blepharospasm). Oculogyric crisis can occur—sudden, forceful spasms of the eye muscles in which the eyeballs deviate and jump up and down. There is also evidence that parkinsonism affects the sensory system. Tingling, numbness, and crawling sensations of the extremities have been reported. The client's intelligence is not affected. Other distressing symptoms include alterations in mood, paranoid ideations, and depression.

The diagnosis is based on the history, neurologic examination, electromyography, clinical signs, handwriting analysis, and an HVA analysis. HVA is diminished in urine and in the cerebrospinal fluid. The disease is best classified by the scale in Box 29–7.

Box 29–7
Stages in Parkinson's Disease

Stage I: Unilateral involvement

Stage II: Bilateral involvement

Stage III: Bilateral involvement with impaired posture and mild imbalance; disability is mild; client independent

Stage IV: Bilateral involvement with postural instability; client requires considerable assistance

Stage V: Fully developed, severe disease; client confined to wheelchair or bed

SOURCE: Hoehn M, Yahr, M: Parkinsonism: onset, progression and mortality, *Neurology* 1967; 17:433.

Medical Measures

During the past decade, the treatment of choice has been to increase available dopamine. A derivative of dopamine, such as levodopa (L-dopa), taken orally, is converted into dopamine in the brain. The drug compensates for the client's deficit and is most effective for those with an akinetic form of the disease. The masklike facies should disappear. The client can initiate, turn, stop, and accelerate movements better. Tremor is usually less responsive to the drug but may decrease on prolonged therapy. The rapid appearance and disappearance of symptom relief (the "on–off" phenomenon) can be avoided by prescribing smaller amounts of L-dopa in divided doses. In some cases, a drug "holiday" may be required.

Because most L-dopa taken by mouth is destroyed before reaching the brain, carbidopa (Sinemet) is also given. A smaller dose of L-dopa is needed, more levodopa is available to the basal ganglia, and peripheral side effects are reduced. Dyskinesia remains a major side effect, but some clients prefer this reaction to their original akinesia. Bromocriptine mesylate (Parlodel) is a dopamine agonist that decreases dopamine turnover. It allows a reduction of levodopa dosage for clients experiencing dyskinesias.

The antiviral drug amantadine (Symmetrel) was accidentally found to prevent neuronal reuptake of natural dopamine. Amantadine improves rigidity but has little effect on tremor and is best used for clients with minimal symptoms.

Anticholinergic drugs may be used early in the disease when tremor is a predominant problem. These drugs reduce cholinergic activity by decreasing the excitation effects of acetylcholine. Common drug choices include benztropine mesylate (Cogentin), ethopropazine (Parsidol), and trihexyphenidyl (Artane). These drugs indirectly control rigidity, tremor, and drooling.

Although antihistamines have only a minimal effect on Parkinson's symptoms, they can be combined with anticholinergic drugs for clients unable to tolerate other combinations. Diphenhydramine (Benadryl) is the most commonly used antihistamine. For sedation, diazepam is preferred over barbiturates or hypnotics that could cause an excitation of symptoms.

The major objective of physical therapy for parkinsonian clients is to prevent contractures and atrophy while reducing muscular rigidity. Physical therapy can maximize the level of function. A basic program for clients includes general ROM of all joints as well as walking, sitting, and stretching maneuvers. Exercises should be done to improve speech and facial expression.

Severe tremor may be resistant to medical treatment. Surgery for clients whose condition is intractable interrupts the extrapyramidal pathways. The most common procedure is thalamotomy. Criteria for this stereotaxic surgery are severe unilateral tremor that is a manifestation of nondominant hemispheric disease; no signs of lip, chin, and tongue involvement in clients under 65; good general health; and freedom from atherosclerotic disease. A bilateral thalamotomy can result in speech disturbances, memory deficits, and poor urinary control. L-dopa has greatly reduced the use of stereotaxic surgical procedures.

Specific Nursing Measures

The goal of nursing care is to assist the client to manage self-care deficits and to handle alterations in body image. Mobility must be maintained. Purposeful activity can reduce or eliminate tremors, whereas bed rest can lead to contractures and muscular atrophy. Gait training includes teaching the client to walk by placing each foot down as heel, ball, and toe instead of shuffling. Pivotal heel maneuvers can aid turning. Ambulation may require supervision.

Client/Family Teaching

Help clients to recognize that feelings of depression and frustration may result from alterations in body image and loss of independence. Nursing approaches should assist clients to share their feelings, recognize their reaction as a realistic coping mechanism, and encourage and support as much independence as possible.

Teach clients to perform activities of daily living with minimal assistance to foster self-confidence. Assistive devices may be required to maintain a safe environment. Guardrails in bathtubs and hallways may prevent falls because of client tremors and loss of protective reflexes. Showers can be taken with a special chair. Other self-help devices include clothing that is easier to wear (eg, with Velcro fasteners instead of zippers and slip-on instead of laced shoes).

Interruption in skin integrity is a potential problem because of drug therapy and autonomic dysfunction. Daily or as-necessary bathing can reduce excessive perspiration and seborrhea.

There is a potential for altered nutrition and elimination patterns. Weight loss may result from difficulty in eating related to tremors and the diuretic effect of drug therapy. Constipation is a common problem caused by immobility and anticholinergic drug effects. Recommendations include use of psyllium, stool softeners two or three times a day, a daily glycerin or bisacodyl (Dulcolax) suppository, and increased bulk in the diet. Monitor the client's weight pattern, maintain a high-calorie and controlled protein diet, and provide small frequent feedings and assistive eating devices.

Recognize the effects of diet on drug absorption. Ineffective drug absorption is a potential problem because of obesity, alcohol intake, and diet. Obesity increases vascular problems, decreases mobility, and affects levodopa regulation. (Fat cells absorb and release levodopa erratically.) Reducing diets are best planned with nutritional counseling. Teach clients to avoid or limit alcohol intake to no more than two glasses of wine or beer with dinner. Alcohol antagonizes the effects of L-dopa and can also increase the risk of depression. A high-protein intake may also block the effects of L-dopa, an amino acid, by competing for intestinal and blood–brain barrier absorption with other protein by-products. Protein intake should be decreased by 50%. Include limiting protein products such as milk, poultry, fish, meat, cheese, nuts, eggs, soybean products, sunflower seeds, and whole grain in client and family teaching. Also emphasize limitation of caffeine intake because caffeine promotes the development of abnormal body movements.

Document the client's baseline symptoms—especially tremor, rigidity, and dyskinesia—before medications are initiated. Therapeutic effects are measured against the baseline.

The common side effects of prescribed medications should be recognized. These include dryness of the mouth, nausea, postural hypotension, and dysrhythmias such as sinus tachycardia. Frequent mouth care alleviates dryness related to anticholinergic drug effects. For nausea, give antiemetics as ordered. For postural hypotension, assist the client to make gradual position changes, apply antiembolism stockings, and record standing and supine blood pressures at least twice a day. Monitor and report heart rate changes.

Drug therapy can also precipitate abnormal involuntary movement. Clients and significant others are taught what choreiform and athetoid movements look like. Abnormal movements to report are head nodding, tongue protrusion, facial grimacing, exaggerated gestures, and unusual breathing patterns. Drug dosages must be reduced to prevent the "on–off" phenomenon.

Medication may also have to be adjusted if clients exhibit behavioral problems. Observe and report the following symptoms: irritability, outbursts of anger, hostility, delirium, hallucinations, and paranoid ideation. A safe environment must be maintained.

Give the client and significant others a list of symptoms and signs to report to the physician when the client returns home. A discharge plan should include instructing the client and family in the factors decreasing medication absorption, potential side effects of medication, how to maintain a safe environment, and a plan for daily living.

Amyotrophic Lateral Sclerosis

Amyotrophic lateral sclerosis (ALS) is a progressive degenerative CNS disease with a relentless, fatal course. The term *amyotrophic* refers to the muscle atrophy from the degeneration of ventral horn cells. *Lateral sclerosis* pertains to the demyelination of the corticospinal tract.

The disease affects both upper and lower motor neurons of the pyramidal tracts of the CNS. The three major aspects of the motor neuron disease are progressive muscle atrophy, progressive bulbar palsy, and upper motor neuron deficits.

The course of ALS varies from 1 to 4 years. The survival rate is 5 years for 20% of clients and 10 years for another 10%. Men are more frequently affected than women in a ratio of about 2:1. Disease onset occurs between ages 40 and 70, most frequently in the fifth and sixth decades. The cause of ALS is unknown. Researchers are currently investigating viral, metabolic, infectious, toxic, immunologic, and specific life events as possible causes.

Clinical Manifestations

To make a differential diagnosis in ALS, a myelogram is often performed to rule out any other degenerative disease or treatable condition. Diagnosis in early stages of ALS can be difficult if no signs of lateral sclerosis are evident and when only one aspect of the spinal cord or brain stem is involved. A characteristic finding is absence of sensory signs.

A complete history, physical, and neurologic examination are done. Electromyography demonstrates muscle wasting, atrophy, fasciculations, and fibrillations. Nerve biopsy is normal, whereas a muscle biopsy may demonstrate degenerative fibers interspersed with normal ones. Laboratory tests find normal CSF and a continuous elevation of serum enzyme levels: aldolase, SGPT, and especially CK.

Clinical manifestations vary and are related to the anatomic areas of involvement. ALS usually includes a combination of the syndromes of progressive muscle atrophy, bulbar palsy, and primary lateral sclerosis. Initial symptoms include skeletal muscle weakness and atrophy that progresses from distal to proximal and unilateral to bilateral involvement in the upper extremities. These symptoms are accompanied by fasciculations and a decrease or absence of DTRs.

With total paralysis and lower cranial nerve involvement, the "locked-in syndrome" occurs. Clients are fully conscious of the environment and themselves, but "locked in" by a paralyzed body. All movement and ability to verbalize are absent. The client may only be able to communicate by eyelid movement and blinking. The immediate cause of death is often respiratory muscle weakness and bulbar palsy causing respiratory failure.

Medical Measures

There is no specific or effective treatment for this relentless, progressive disease. Supportive symptomatic therapy is recommended to improve and, in some cases, extend life. The quality of life should be a primary consideration when planning treatment.

Drug researchers have advocated the administration of guanidine HCl and small amounts of detoxified snake venom to arrest disease progression, although no conclusive evidence supports this regimen. Symptomatic drug therapy includes diazepam, baclofen (Lioresal), and dantrolene sodium (Dantrium) to control spasticity. Neostigmine methylsulfate (Prostigmin) is used temporarily to manage bulbar weakness. Analgesics are used to control pain. Short-term use of anticholinergic drugs is helpful in relieving sialorrhea. Alternative feeding methods are solutions to swallowing problems. Efforts are made to prevent infections, especially of the respiratory tract. In many cases, tracheostomy and mechanical ventilation are mandatory to maintain respiratory function. Regardless of treatment, the prognosis is poor, and survival is brief for most clients.

Specific Nursing Measures

Nursing priorities for the client with ALS vary depending on the stage of disease. A common problem is ineffective communication patterns related to muscular weakness, dysarthria, and respiratory complications. Provide adequate time to anticipate client needs, offer explanations of care, identify client problems, and encourage client participation in decisions about nursing care. Alternative communication methods may be necessary: the use of an alphabet and number board, writing, common object cards, and eye blinking. The client must be assisted to use whatever method is most feasible and least likely to cause fatigue.

Monitor any alteration in nutritional status due to swallowing and chewing impairments. Some management suggestions include small, frequent feedings to prevent fatigue and choking. Provide a soft diet high in calories, protein, and carbohydrates with an adequate daily fluid intake. When feeding clients with ALS, elevate the head of the bed, keep oropharyngeal suction equipment nearby, and allow adequate time for meals. To evaluate nutritional status of hospitalized clients, obtain weights three times a week, check calorie counts, and review serum albumin and protein levels. Tube feedings may be necessary for some clients.

Alterations in mobility accompany increased motor paresis. To keep clients independent as long as possible, active and passive ROM exercises and physical and occupational therapy are helpful. Assistive devices may be necessary for daily activities. Clients should remain out of bed and up in a chair as long as their condition permits. Treatments and rest periods should be coordinated to avoid excessive fatigue. Changing the client's position with supportive devices provides comfort and minimizes the hazards of immobility. These interventions and antispasmodic drugs should reduce spasticity. For management of bladder and bowel incontinence, refer to specific nursing measures for clients with multiple sclerosis.

Management of ineffective breathing patterns related to muscle weakness or aspiration often becomes a nursing priority. Aspiration may occur from dysphagia and excessive salivation. Preventive measures include monitoring the client during eating, suctioning if necessary, assessing respiratory patterns around meal times, and administering anticholinergic drugs as ordered. Good oral hygiene must be provided.

When respiratory involvement progresses, the maintenance of a patent airway and adequate ventilation become the nursing priorities. Assess respiratory function every 1 to 2 hours including observation of rate, depth, and rhythm of respirations and auscultation of breath sounds. Encourage frequent coughing and deep breathing. Monitoring of tidal volume, vital capacity, and arterial blood gases becomes crucial. Chest physical therapy including postural drainage may be required as well as nasotracheal and oropharyngeal suctioning every hour and as necessary. Keep intubation and ventilatory equipment on standby.

A major nursing concern should be the management of anticipatory grieving related to the terminal nature of this disease. The most difficult nursing task often becomes helping the client and significant others to accept the seriousness of the condition. The nursing objective should be to facilitate client–family communication of anxieties and fears to assist them in their grieving process, and to help identify support systems such as social services, mental health liaisons, and community agencies. Communicate to the client and family that nursing care is available to promote optimal client comfort and safety.

SECTION 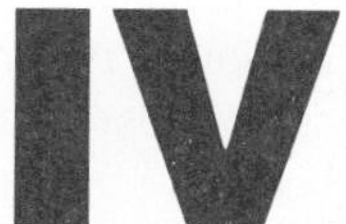

Immunologic Disorders

Myasthenia gravis, multiple sclerosis, and Guillain-Barré syndrome are thought to have an autoimmune component. They are covered in this section although the exact etiology of each disease remains unknown.

Myasthenia Gravis

Myasthenia gravis is a chronic neuromuscular disorder that affects voluntary (striated) muscles. The disease is characterized by fluctuating muscle weakness that becomes worse with use and shows some improvement with rest. The course of the disease is variable. Onset is usually gradual, marked by either a stable period or rapid progression of symptoms. Respiratory infections and emotional stress may greatly exacerbate symptoms. The highest mortality rate is seen in the first year of the disease.

The disease is common, with incidence estimated at 1 in 10,000. Peak incidence is between the second and third decades; onset is rare in the first decade of life or after age 70. Under age 40, females are affected approximately two to three times as often as males. In later life, the incidence is about equal.

This disorder usually persists for life, although there may be periods of spontaneous improvement for weeks or months followed by worsening. This disease is not hereditary, but 15% of the infants born to myasthenic mothers have a transient case of the disease. With treatment, infants recover fully in 2 to 3 months.

Despite numerous theories and a great deal of research, the cause of myasthenia gravis remains unknown. There is general agreement that the defect occurs at the neuromuscular junction, and myasthenia gravis is now considered an autoimmune disease. In the normal individual, there are approximately 38 million acetylcholine receptors at each neuromuscular junction. In the client with myasthenia gravis, acetylcholine receptors are reduced by about 20%. An autoimmune reaction is now known to cause the acetylcholine receptor deficiency.

The autoimmune attack is directed against acetylcholine receptors. Immunoglobulin G (IgG) antibodies, detected in the serum of 90% of myasthenic clients, react against the acetylcholine receptors. These autoantibodies cause two different types of adverse effects: they can prevent receptors from responding to acetylcholine, and they can cause receptor portions of a muscle cell to degenerate rapidly. Both conditions cause fewer receptors to be available at the neuromuscular junction.

The thymus gland is also considered to be involved in myasthenia gravis. The thymus gland, located beneath the sternum, plays an important role in normal immunity. Active from birth until puberty, the gland is thought to initiate the body's immune response and to cease functioning after puberty. In about 85% of myasthenic clients, however, the thymus gland is abnormal and remains active. An autoimmune reaction is probably triggered by the lymphocyte or musclelike cell abnormalities of the thymus gland.

Clinical Manifestations

The most characteristic finding in myasthenia gravis is an increasing weakness of certain voluntary muscles with activity, and some improvement with rest. The muscles of the eyes are often most affected. The eyelids droop (ptosis), the eyes squint, and there may be double vision (diplopia). The ptosis may be unilateral or bilateral and intensifies when the client attempts to gaze upward. Pupillary response to light and accommodation remain normal.

Other muscles affected are those of facial expression, chewing, swallowing, and speech. The mobility and expression of the face is altered so attempts to smile look like a snarl. The affect is flat, and the jaw muscles hang loosely. When chewing, clients with myasthenia gravis often become fatigued and must rest.

Clients with CN IX and CN X deficits experience problems with managing saliva, choking, and nasal regurgitation. Speech deficits include a weak voice that fades with conversation and diminishes to a whisper. Speech becomes nasal, monotonous, and dysarthric.

The shoulder and neck muscles are often affected. The head tends to fall forward, and clients have difficulty holding their arms above the head, so reaching for an object and fixing the hair are difficult. The muscles for fine hand movements can also be affected, resulting in difficulty in writing, serving, and moving the hands to the mouth. The most life-threatening situation occurs when the intercostal and/or diaphragm muscles are affected. An early sign of respiratory involvement is breathlessness. Respiratory weakness can develop rapidly.

The diagnosis of myasthenia gravis is based on the history of voluntary muscle weakness, a physical exam that identifies muscle fatigability on repetitive action, and the clinical signs previously described. The Tensilon test is the most discriminating diagnostic study. Tensilon is a short- and rapid-acting cholinergic drug that dramatically improves the muscle strength of a myasthenic client. This test can distinguish between myasthenic and cholinergic crises.

Radiologic studies include CT scans to reveal thymomas and thymus scans to reveal hyperplasia or a thymoma. Chest x-ray and mediastinal tomograms may also reveal a thymoma.

In myasthenia gravis, the EMG shows that the amplitude of the evoked muscle's action potentials decreases rapidly. This reaction can be diminished or prevented with a single 2-mg IV dose of Tensilon.

Medical Measures

Drug therapy is the first line of treatment. The drugs—pyridostigmine bromide (Mestinon), neostigmine bromide (Prostigmin), and occasionally ambenonium chloride (Mytelase)—act by inhibiting anticholinesterase, preventing the rapid destruction of the neurotransmitter acetylcholine. Although this effect does not change the basic abnormality, it increases the amount of acetylcholine available, partially compensating for symptoms of a defective neuromuscular transmission. There are no set rules for determining the amount of anticholinesterase medication a client may need. Drug dosage must be individualized to provide the greatest symptom relief and the fewest side effects. Pyridostigmine usually provides a smoother action with fewer gastrointestinal side effects.

Corticosteroids are sometimes prescribed for clients who do not respond well to anticholinesterase drugs. Current practice recommends giving prednisone 100 mg every other day for 10 days. Clients are hospitalized for close observation during the initial treatment period on full-dose therapy. Symptoms intensify at 7 to 10 days of treatment but improve after treatment ends. This treatment is given with anticholinesterase therapy. As improvement is shown, the steroid is reduced slowly to the lowest effective dose. The effectiveness of immunosuppressive drug therapy for these clients has not been conclusively established.

The surgical removal of the thymus gland (thymectomy) is indicated for clients with thymomas and hyperplasia of the gland. The procedure is most effective for young women within the first 2 years of diagnosis and least effective for older men with thymomas. The removal of the thymus gland without an associated tumor produces a high rate of improvement or remission of symptoms in clients with early onset.

Plasmapheresis is usually performed on clients whose disease is refractory to standard treatments. Potential complications such as loss of clotting factors, hemolysis, and fluid and electrolyte imbalances must be considered. Clients undergoing this procedure remain on their medication in adjusted lower doses.

Specific Nursing Measures

The care of clients with myasthenia gravis presents a formidable challenge. What was once a catastrophic disease with a high mortality and morbidity rate has become, in many cases, a treatable condition. Careful nursing assessment, management, and evaluation can make a major difference in treating clients in crisis. Nursing priorities for myasthenic clients depend on whether the client is stable or in crisis. For clients in crisis, ineffective breathing patterns can be a life-threatening problem.

In myasthenic crisis, the client experiences an abrupt exacerbation of motor weakness, usually from undermedication. The neuromuscular junction is no longer responsive to drug therapy. This crisis may also occur in a myasthenic client receiving no medication.

Cholinergic crisis is caused by overmedication with cholinergic (anticholinesterase) drugs. Excessive medication results in a depolarization block. An acute exacerbation of myasthenic muscle weakness also occurs in this crisis. Symptoms and signs of myasthenic and cholinergic crises are listed in Table 29–3.

Evaluate the client's ability to swallow. Check this by gently placing a hand over the anterior neck and instructing the client to attempt "dry" swallowing. This maneuver is preferable to giving the client liquids that might induce choking or aspiration. If the swallowing reflex is intact, test the gag reflex. Suction apparatus should be available during testing.

Test upper extremity strength by asking the client to do a repetitive act such as squeezing and releasing an object placed in the hand and flexing and extending the elbow. Assess lower extremity strength by having the client alternate dorsiflexion and plantar flexion of the feet repeatedly or flex and extend the knees. Baseline assessment of the various muscle groups of the client in crisis is essential for future comparisons, diagnosis of the problem, and intervention.

Table 29–3
Symptoms and Signs of Myasthenic and Cholinergic Crises

Myasthenic Crisis	Cholinergic Crisis
Sudden marked crisis in blood pressure and pulse	*Generalized weakness
*Extreme restlessness and apprehension	*Dysphagia
*Increased diaphoresis, secretions, and lacrimation	Dysarthria
*Severe cyanosis and dyspnea that may lead to respiratory arrest	*Dyspnea
*Dysphagia (difficulty swallowing)	Nausea and vomiting
Absent cough reflex	Abdominal cramps and diarrhea
Urinary and fecal incontinence; urinary output	Miosis, pallor
*Dysarthria (difficulty speaking)	*Increased copious secretions: salivation, lacrimation, phlegm, perspiration
*Generalized muscle weakness	Blurred vision
	Muscle twitching
	*Apprehension

*Indicates that dyspnea, dysphagia, dysarthria, generalized weakness, increased secretions, and apprehension are common to both myasthenic and cholinergic crises.

For clients who develop respiratory failure, endotracheal intubation creates an emergency airway. Long-term management includes a planned tracheostomy. A volume-cycled ventilator should be used during periods of acute respiratory insufficiency. During the acute phase, current practice recommends discontinuing all anticholinesterase medication to allow a "rest period" for the neuromuscular junction. Once the client's condition stabilizes, small doses of anticholinesterase medication can be restarted. During this period, the client is generally fed by nasogastric tube. To prevent aspiration, check for proper tube placement before each feeding, check the amount and type of stomach aspirant, and feed the client in the upright position with an inflated tracheal or endotracheal cuff. Aspiration of feedings can lead to major complications for myasthenic clients with bulbar paralysis.

Intensive chest physiotherapy should be carried out during crises to prevent respiratory complications. In addition, a bedside physical therapy program should be instituted to prevent muscle atrophy or contractures. Adequate hydration and antiembolism support stockings should be used to prevent thrombophlebitis.

The most difficult nursing challenge for a client in crisis is how to handle ineffective coping patterns that result from the client's complete dependency. The crisis may persist for a long time, placing a great emotional strain on the client. The nurse must be able to anticipate clients' needs while helping them to identify concerns and preferences for care. Clients with chronic illnesses often become well informed about their diseases and treatment approaches. They want to participate in decision making for their care as well as identify successful techniques they have developed.

To develop an accurate, detailed plan of care, an effective communication system must be provided. Ordinary communication devices are not usually effective for clients in crisis. Alternatives may include a bell tied to the client's ankle and wrist, a light touch bell under the client's shoulder, or a special communication device that requires head turning or forehead movement.

Myasthenic clients often experience fear and anxiety because of the disease sequelae. The client needs constant help to express fears and establish realistic goals. Ensure sufficient time for ventilation of the client's feelings and avoid frustration-producing conditions.

Clients with myasthenia gravis often have long-term muscle weakness that worsens with activity and fatigue. Anticholinesterase drugs should always be administered *exactly on time*. Assess the client's strength and motor ability with drug administration, and observe and report side effects. Give medications with milk or food to prevent gastrointestinal irritation. Give the medication at least 45 minutes before meals to ensure optimal muscle strength during meals. In addition, plan nursing care to provide rest periods and prevent excessive fatigue. Teach alternative methods of communication such as lip reading; writing; and use of erasable boards, pictures, and gestures. Be sure to provide adequate listening time.

Alterations in protective mechanisms can occur, such as incomplete eyelid closure. Corneal abrasion or ulceration is a potential problem. Provide routine eye care with normal saline every 4 to 6 hours and as necessary. Lubricate the cornea with artificial tears every 2 hours and as appropriate; provide a protective eye shield if necessary. Eye patching may be alternated every 2 to 4 hours and clients taught compensatory techniques. Clients may have diplopia and require assistance with daily activities.

Clients on long-term anticholinesterase drug therapy may have periods of altered gastrointestinal function. Common concerns include nausea, diarrhea, abdominal cramping, and constipation. The type and frequency of discomfort should be monitored. Gastrointestinal symptoms may indicate anticholinesterase toxicity. Anticholinergics (atropine sulfate) should be administered as ordered and small frequent feedings given. Antiemetics and antidiarrheal agents may also be necessary. For clients with constipation, enemas should be avoided to prevent a crisis. Mild cathartics and suppositories can be used. Alterations in diet and fluid regimen may be helpful. Educate clients about actions of drugs and specific factors that might precipitate an increase in muscle weakness.

Multiple Sclerosis

Multiple sclerosis (MS) is a degenerative disease with a chronic course, marked by variable periods of remission and exacerbation. The disorder is the most common neurologic condition causing demyelination of the CNS. Myelin sheaths and nerve conduction pathways are affected. Myelin can be destroyed anywhere in the CNS white matter, followed by the development of patches of plaques (scars), a recovery period, and subsequent degeneration. Plaques may develop in the cerebral hemispheres, brain stem, cerebellum, and in the spinal cord. The PNS is not involved per se. Eventually remyelination becomes less likely, and neurologic deficits result from permanent sclerosis. In early stages of the disease, it is more common to have periods of both remission and exacerbation. Later, exacerbations are more common, longer, and more severe.

Approximately 500,000 cases of multiple sclerosis occur in the United States per year. Although females are affected slightly more often than males, the difference is not significant. Because at least two-thirds of all cases occur between the ages of 20 and 40, MS is known as the "crippler" among young adults. MS tends to occur more frequently in cold, damp climates.

The cause of multiple sclerosis is unknown. Most theories involve a viral or immunologic cause. Many theories postulating a vascular, traumatic, nutritional, allergic, or infectious cause have been tested, but none has adequately explained the etiology. It had been thought that a slow virus identical to or similar to the measles virus might be responsible for MS. Now attention is focused on the age of onset of measles because MS incidence is higher in clients who had measles later than in infancy or early childhood. Those with MS have a high level of measles specific antibody in their serum. This finding lends support to an immunologic explanation for MS. An autoimmune reaction might occur in which a person develops antigens that act against normal antibodies.

Serologic studies have identified a much higher-than-normal incidence of certain antigens, the most significant of which is the HLA-Dw2. Also important is the B-lymphocyte alloantigen. The significance of these findings is not clear, but it suggests that these antigens might be markers for a "susceptibility" gene that is possibly an immune-response gene.

Clinical Manifestations

Symptoms differ among clients, depending on the areas of the CNS affected, duration of disease, and disease expression. Some clients have only mild exacerbations, long remission periods, and minimal disabilities, whereas others have frequent relapses with increasing residual deficits followed by deterioration. The symptoms are discussed according to the clients' subjective concerns and objective clinical findings. The most common initial symptoms are fatigue, visual disturbances, and motor weakness.

All symptoms tend to subside after white matter degenerates initially. Relapses increase as sclerosis becomes more extensive during subsequent exacerbation periods. The diagnosis of MS is presumptive based on report of the symptoms, with an emphasis on remission and exacerbation, the neurologic exam, and CSF analysis.

The examination of CSF is diagnostically significant. The CSF shows an elevation of gamma globulin in two-thirds of clients with MS. A major diagnostic finding is abnormal brain stem auditory-evoked, somatosensory-evoked, and visual-evoked response studies. Abnormalities occur in a high percentage of clients with MS.

Several factors can precipitate disease onset as well as cause an exacerbation. Infections, pregnancy, and trauma can precipitate the onset of MS or a relapse. Menstruation, extreme cold or heat, fatigue, and stress can cause an exacerbation of symptoms.

VISUAL SYMPTOMS AND SIGNS The client describes visual disturbances as double and blurred vision, decreased acuity, loss of peripheral vision, and blind spots. Clinical examination often reveals optic neuritis. This common early sign accounts for the blurring and loss of vision as well as orbital pain. Nystagmus occurs in almost three-fourths of all clients. Pupillary response is slowed in the affected eye. A sign strongly suggestive of MS is internuclear ophthalmoplegia (paralysis of ocular muscles) on lateral gaze.

MOTOR SYMPTOMS AND SIGNS The client usually reports stiffness, weakness, and clumsiness of the extremities, which are initially more frequent in the legs than arms. Limbs become heavy and spastic, causing a "jumping" of affected limbs, especially at night. Clients may also report a decrease in motor strength after a hot bath or shower; strenuous exercise can also decrease motor strength. The clinical exam finds muscular weakness, spasm, and spasticity.

REFLEX CHANGES On clinical exam, DTRs are found to be hyperactive. Clonus occurs as well as Babinski's sign. The abdominal reflex, a superficial reflex, is frequently absent in MS.

SENSORY ALTERATIONS Common client concerns include numbness and tingling (paresthesia) of the face and affected extremities. Disturbing symptoms are feelings of burning or crawling (formications) and shocklike sensations. Clients may report loss of position sense, which is often accompanied by feelings of extremity swelling and tightness. Clinical examination shows paresthesia, decrease or loss of position sense, and vibration. *Lhermitte's sign*, transient sensations of electriclike shock extending bilaterally down the arms, back, and trunk, is evoked on neck flexion.

CEREBRAL DEFICITS Frontal lobe involvement can lead to emotional lability and deterioration of intellectual function. Clients feel irritable and apathetic, have a short attention span, and have difficulty doing calculations and thinking abstractly. They report lapses in memory and inappropriate episodes of laughing or crying. They sometimes report seizures. Neurologic examination shows deficits of memory, affect, judgment, and reasoning. Later signs include confusion, disorientation, and depression. The CT scan demonstrates nonspecific ventricular enlargement and/or cortical atrophy in approximately 40% of clients with MS. An abnormal EEG and neuropsychologic deficits can be observed.

BRAIN STEM SIGNS Clients are often concerned about speech impairments, which are a result of spastic weakness in the muscles responsible for speech. Initially, speech is slurred; later, speech becomes garbled, staccatolike, and unintelligible. **Scanning speech**—speech that is slow and deliberate, punctuated with pauses between syllables—is a common characteristic of MS. Other brain stem signs include reports of dizziness, vertigo, nausea, diplopia, tinnitus, dysphagia, facial weakness, and loss of sensation.

CEREBELLAR DEFICITS Cerebellar involvement is more frequent in later stages of the disease. Clients note clumsiness, loss of balance and coordination, and tremors. Clinical exam reveals truncal ataxia, **dysmetria** (inability to measure distance properly in muscular acts), and intention tremors. The ability to perform alternating movements is impaired. Head tremors are observed in the final stage of the disease.

BLADDER AND BOWEL PROBLEMS Clients often have urinary hesitancy, urgency, frequency, dysuria, nocturia, retention, or reflex emptying. Constipation and incontinence are common problems.

SEXUAL PROBLEMS Men may be impotent or have difficulty sustaining erections. Women report absence of sexual desire and decreased vaginal secretions.

Medical Measures

Because numerous treatment protocols have been tried over the last several decades, clients are often confused about long-term treatment and prognosis. There is no curative treatment for MS. Intervention is supportive according to symptoms. The drugs of choice are corticosteroids, which reduce edema and inflammation at sites of demyelination. High doses of ACTH can shorten an acute exacerbation if given early enough and can produce clinical improvement in some cases. Steroids do not alter the course of the disease however; the drugs are considered ineffective in the long term and do not prevent relapses.

Recently, public attention has focused on diet in the treatment of MS. Previously, low-fat diets were encouraged because incidence of MS has been low during years when famine prevailed. Gluten-free diets and diets high in linoleic acid (sunflower seed oil) are still being investigated. The consensus among most neurologists is that no statistically valid controlled studies have demonstrated the value of any special diet.

Physical therapy is aimed at maintaining function and preventing complications of immobility. Muscle spasms can be treated with muscle relaxants such as diazepam and dantrolene sodium. These drugs must be carefully regulated to prevent increased muscle weakness.

Clients with severe symptoms that do not respond to drug therapy are sometimes considered for palliative surgical procedures. Thalamotomies can be done to eliminate intention tremors of cerebellar origin. It should be recognized, however, that this is a destructive procedure with variable results. Clients with severe swallowing problems might require a gastrostomy.

Plasmapheresis is a new treatment aimed at removing autoantibodies, similar to its use in myasthenia gravis. It is important to consider potential complications such as the loss of clotting factors, hemolysis, and fluid and electrolyte imbalances.

Specific Nursing Measures

Clients with multiple sclerosis must recognize that they may experience various stages of loss and acceptance as the disease progresses. Although the symptoms may be minimal at disease onset, there is a tendency for neurologic deficits to progress. Teach clients strategies to cope with periods of symptom exacerbation and progression. Symptoms and signs of relapse should be identified early. Instruct the client to avoid extreme fatigue, emotional stress, and infection. Clients should adjust daily schedules to include regular exercise, rest periods, and proper dietary habits. Also assist clients to reach realistic goals and potentials during periods of remission.

Client/Family Teaching

During periods of exacerbation, steroids may be used. Medication selection depends on the severity of the client's symptoms. The objectives of the medication regimen are to reduce the acute inflammatory response, expedite a remission, and promote the level of recovery. Clients may require bed rest at this time in a relaxed, quiet environment. It is crucial to prevent any secondary infections from steroids or restricted activity. Side effects of steroids to be alert for include fluid retention, hypertension, electrolyte imbalance, and gastric irritation. To prevent gastric irritation, antacids may be given with steroids or between meals if medication is given with meals. Hypokalemia is not uncommon. Therefore, potassium supplements are given or high-potassium foods increased. Although vitamins have not been proven effective, some clients feel better taking them. Linoleic acid may have an effect on myelin formation.

A common problem is alteration in elimination patterns. Urinary incontinence or urinary retention and constipation may occur. For bladder problems, in-dwelling catheters with a closed drainage system may be required. Catheter care should be done at least twice a day. Clients can be taught to clean their own catheters with warm water and soap using hydrogen peroxide for encrustations. If unusual or foul-smelling drainage is noted around the meatus or in the urine, notify the physician. Encourage fluid intake to about 3 L per day. Cranberry juice (200 mL) given four times a day can keep the urine pH acidic and possibly decrease the incidence of urinary tract infections. In-dwelling catheters are changed every 10 to 14 days or once a month, depending on the client's urinary status. Intermittent catheterization is recommended because of the lower incidence of bladder infections and the potential for increasing bladder tone between catheterizations. To prevent or manage constipation, administer a suppository daily or as necessary at the same time of day, give stool softeners as prescribed, and provide bulk in the diet. Establish a regular schedule for bowel movements.

Impairment in mobility is another common problem. Loss of motor strength and coordination are the most frequent concerns. The degree of deficit varies. Approaches to prevent disuse atrophy and increase muscle strength include resistive exercises and muscle stretching and active and passive ROM every 4 to 6 hours. Assistive devices (eg, braces, walkers) may be required to prevent injury. Encourage as much ambulation as the client can tolerate. Handrails may be needed in bathrooms and halls and on stairways. Hand controls may be necessary in the client's automobile. Encourage clients to maintain as normal an activity level as possible.

Clients may also experience a loss of protective mechanisms because of sensory deficits. Caution clients to avoid extreme temperatures and hazards because they may not feel the pain associated with such injuries. Compensatory mechanisms can include the use of eye-hand coordination when manipulating objects.

Alterations in sensory perception are common, especially visual disturbances such as decreased visual acuity and diplopia. To combat visual loss, organize objects for easy reach and orient the client to new settings. A magnifying glass and large-print reading material can be invaluable. For diplopia, alternate patching of the eye with a dark cloth eyepatch can correct this disturbing problem.

Self-care deficits can occur because of intention tremors and spasticity. To manage intention tremors, avoid fatigue and place objects within easy reach. Clients can be helped to learn how to anticipate their needs and reorganize their environments. Otherwise, they may experience unnecessary frustration. A number of interventions can diminish spasticity. In addition to exercises mentioned under impaired immobility, muscle relaxants, warm tub baths, and sleeping prone can help. Hot baths must be avoided because they can increase the metabolic rate, causing more weakness. Flexor spasms can diminish with position changes, such as sleeping in the prone position.

Alterations in body image and self-esteem can lead to depression and a sense of hopelessness. It is crucial for both clients and their families to have an accurate understanding of the disease and to use appropriate resources, especially the National Multiple Sclerosis Society. Clients need to function to the level of their ability and tolerance, to continue socialization, and to find diversional activities that decrease anxiety and fatigue.

Clients may have periods of emotional lability that do not appear appropriate to a given situation. Teach family members to be understanding when the client has changes in mood. Open communication in families is essential for optimal coping patterns to develop, especially in chronic illness. Foster a positive attitude to maintain as near a normal lifestyle for the client as possible.

Guillain–Barré Syndrome

Guillain–Barré syndrome, also known as acute infectious polyneuritis, causes a demyelination and degeneration of peripheral nerves and anterior and posterior spinal nerve roots. The disease is characterized by acute, rapid ascending symmetrical motor and sensory deficits. Cranial nerve involvement can occur. There is a potential for respiratory failure. Symptom progression occurs within about 2 weeks of the initial signs, and progression can cease at any time.

Guillain–Barré syndrome can affect any age group, race, or sex; however, it is more common in young adults and more severe in pregnant women and the very young or old. The pathophysiologic signs include an inflammation of peripheral nerves and infiltration of them by perivascular lymphocytes. The inflammatory process is marked by edema and exudate that leads to compression of nerve roots. Segmental demyelination causes an ascending bilateral pattern of paresthesias and paralysis along with cranial nerve dysfunction.

Guillain–Barré syndrome is a disease of unknown etiology. The major theories propose an immunologic, infective, or viral cause. About half of diagnosed clients have had a mild respiratory or gastrointestinal infection 1 to 3 weeks before the onset of polyneuritis. Additional preceding events are other viral illnesses, certain surgical procedures, lymphomatous diseases (particularly Hodgkin's disease), and the influenza vaccine. In 1976, national attention was focused on Guillain–Barré syndrome when swine flu immunizations were suspended. More than 100 individuals in different states developed symptoms of the disease after receiving swine flu immunization.

Current research efforts have focused on Guillain–Barré syndrome as an autoimmune disease. The syndrome may represent an autoimmune response to antibodies formed in reaction to damage of body tissue. Whether this is a response to a prodromal illness, an immunization, or unknown agent remains to be established. An alteration in cell-mediated immunity may be responsible for the hypersensitivity reaction of tissue in this disease.

Clinical Manifestations

Clinical signs and disease course help to distinguish Guillain–Barré syndrome from other forms of polyneuritis. An acute onset of symptoms with a rapid progression of motor weakness and paralysis are characteristic findings. The bilateral progression of symptoms from distal to proximal in an ascending pattern is common.

The disease is usually characterized by a history of a preceding respiratory or gastrointestinal infection, a latent period of about 2 weeks, and then symptom onset. Paresthesias and weakness of proximal, distal, and trunk muscles occur. The absence of atrophy is significant. There is an abrupt onset of flaccid motor paralysis from involvement of the anterior roots of lower motor neurons. Symptoms ascend symmetrically from lower extremities and can stop at any level of the CNS. Respiratory distress can result from diaphragm and intercostal muscular weakness. Cranial nerves may become involved. Bladder and bowel sphincter function usually remain intact.

The cardinal signs include paresthesias, paralysis, and CSF findings. Symptoms progress over several days to 2 months, with an average duration of intensive symptoms for about 10 days. Recovery usually takes several weeks to a year. Relapse is infrequent.

The major diagnostic tests are the examination of CSF and nerve conduction tests. The CSF findings include the unusual finding of a high protein level without cellular abnormality, the so-called albuminocytologic dissociation. Nerve conduction studies usually demonstrate a slowing of conduction time.

Medical Measures

The acute care of clients with Guillain–Barré syndrome involves maintaining a patent airway. Clients are best cared for in a hospital where potential respiratory and cardiac complications can be detected and monitored. Respiratory insufficiency is high because of dysfunction of the phrenic nerve (affecting diaphragm excursion) or the vagus nerve (affecting laryngeal function), or thoracic nerve root damage. Hypoxia is a common complication that requires endotracheal intubation or a tracheostomy with ventilatory support. Aggressive respiratory protocols should be instituted to prevent complications.

Controversy persists regarding steroid therapy. Prednisone or ACTH given during acute stages of the illness is thought to speed recovery. Steroids are considered to have little therapeutic value when given in later stages. When steroids are given, clients must be monitored for fluid retention, gastrointestinal irritation, and electrolyte imbalance. Potassium replacement is often indicated. Dosages are usually tapered to prevent an acute episode of adrenal insufficiency.

Throughout the illness, proper nutrition should be maintained by nasogastric or gastrostomy tube when the oral route cannot be used. Physical therapy programs can be instituted once the client's condition has stabilized. Motor strength should be frequently evaluated because return of function is not always symmetrical. It is important to prevent back problems from premature ambulation of clients with asymmetric muscle function. When respiratory muscle function begins to return as paralysis recedes, the client should be slowly weaned from the ventilator. The tracheostomy may be closed through the decannulation process.

Specific Nursing Measures

Clients with Guillain–Barré syndrome have a potential for alterations in cardiovascular status related to autonomic dysfunction. During the acute phase, frequently evaluate vital signs. Sometimes clients are placed on cardiac monitoring.

Measure clients for antiembolism stockings, change their position at least every 2 hours, and perform passive ROM exercises for 15 minutes four times a day. When repositioning the client, assess respiratory function and handle extremities gently because of change in pain sensation. Cranial nerve dysfunction can occur. Important assessments for CN VII include checking all facial movements, lacrimation, and the anterior two-thirds of the tongue for taste. In addition, some clients lose corneal sensation from CN V dysfunction. Care of eyes is essential to prevent drying and corneal abrasion. Normal saline eye care twice a day, administration of artificial tears every 2 to 4 hours, and the use of a plastic eye bubble will protect the eyes. CN IX and CN X must be assessed by checking the gag, cough, and swallowing reflexes. Oropharyngeal suction setups and alternative methods of feeding must be available. Other changes clients may manifest are inability to shrug their shoulders or turn their heads to the extreme lateral position from deficit of CN XI. Dysfunction of CN XII will manifest as paresis and deviation of the tongue.

A major concern of clients with Guillain–Barré syndrome is alteration in comfort. Clients require complete maintenance of hygiene needs not only during the acute phase of illness but also for varying periods during convalescence. Maintenance of basic hygiene and cleanliness fosters better self-esteem and a more positive body image. Provide good mouth care and prevent interruption in skin integrity.

Clients' knowledge deficits may cause them fear and anxiety. The fact that Guillain–Barré syndrome strikes swiftly and clears slowly largely accounts for the alterations in coping patterns. Be supportive, provide a safe environment, and acknowledge to the client any signs of neurologic improvement. Clients must be given sufficient opportunity to help plan their nursing care so they can begin to regain control and reduce their feelings of powerlessness. Psychosocial support systems can aid in optimal client rehabilitation, goals, and plans.

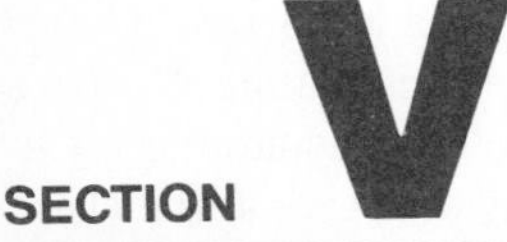

SECTION V

Infectious and Inflammatory Disorders

The nervous system's parenchyma, blood vessels, and protective coverings may be infected by many of the pathogenic microorganisms that affect other organs of the body. Nervous system infections including meningitis, encephalitis, myelitis, brain abscesses, and herpes zoster are covered in this section.

Meningitis

Meningitis is an inflammation of the meninges caused by a viral, bacterial, or fungal organism. It is classified according to the location of CNS involvement. Meningoencephalitis is an inflammation that is more extensive, involving not only the meninges but also cerebral tissue.

There are three major types of meningitis—aseptic, septic, and tuberculous. *Aseptic* meningitis is thought to occur from viral inflammation or meningeal irritation. *Septic* purulent meningitis is caused by infection of the pia and arachnoid from pus-forming bacteria. The third major type is *tuberculous* caused by the tubercle bacillus.

The pathophysiology of meningitis can best be described by tracing the route of the causative organism throughout the CNS. Once the pathogen enters the subarachnoid space, the infection spreads because of the open communication over the brain's convexity. Arachnoid cells become edematous from the inflammatory process. The infection extends along the blood vessels of the pia and then penetrates the sulci. It is not uncommon for affected blood vessels to become engorged, leading to thrombosis or rupture. The accumulation of exudate over the convexities, in the cisterns or the ventricles, can cause obstruction of CSF flow. The exudate may extend to involve the spinal cord. If the brain surface adjacent to the meninges becomes involved, secondary encephalitis and neuronal degeneration can occur.

Clinical Manifestations

The clinical course can be acute, subacute, chronic, or recurrent. Headache, fever, meningeal irritation, and mental status changes are the most common. Clients will complain of severe headaches, the worst they have ever experienced. Meningeal signs will include nuchal rigidity; opisthotonic positioning (extensor rigidity with legs hyperextended, forming an arc with the trunk); photophobia; and pain down the back and limbs. Generalized hyperirritability with hypersensitivity/hyperalgesia, alterations in mental status, decreased level of consciousness, restlessness, confusion, hallucinations, and delirium can occur. There may be generalized seizures and increased ICP due to cerebral edema and communicating hydrocephalus. There also may be medullary signs such as vomiting, respiratory difficulties, and a weak, rapid pulse. Cranial nerve involvement causes visual disturbances, ptosis, pupil abnormalities, strabismus, deafness, nystagmus, and vertigo.

In meningococcal meningitis there can be a skin rash, evidenced by petechiae in which skin stroking yields tache cerebrale (meningitis streak). The onset of tuberculous meningitis is less acute. The client may have vague symptoms with a progressive listlessness and headache. Eventually, similar symptoms and signs as in other types of meningitis occur. The onset of viral meningitis is less severe with symptoms comparable to the previous general description.

Diagnosis is based on history of prior infection or exposure, symptoms and signs of an existing infection, clinical neurologic signs, and diagnostic tests. Skull x-rays are ordered to look for fractures, and infected sinuses or mastoids. Chest x-rays are checked for pneumonia and lung abscesses. CSF studies reveal increased CSF pressure from 200 to 700 mm/water. The appearance of the CSF varies according to the organism. In bacterial infection, the CSF is turbid to purulent. In tubercular infection, the CSF is clear, xanthochromic, or like ground glass. In viral infection, the CSF is usually clear. An important differential diagnosis is the glucose level, which is low in bacterial and tubercular infections but normal in viral infections.

Medical Measures

The diagnosis of bacterial meningitis is confirmed by lumbar puncture. CSF pressure will be increased; the fluid will be milky or cloudy, with many polymorphonuclear leukocytes and a low glucose level. Culture confirms the type of bacteria, and results of sensitivity tests indicate appropriate drug therapy. Prognosis is good with antibiotic therapy.

In the acute phase of meningococcal meningitis, it is possible to infect others. It is spread by nasopharyngeal and droplet secretions from the respiratory tract. This organism is usually controlled within 24 hours of antibiotic therapy. Isolation procedures to protect others should be maintained until cultures are negative.

In tuberculous meningitis the CSF shows fewer cells and low glucose and chloride levels. Tuberculous meningitis was fatal in the past. Prognosis has improved with a prolonged course of drug therapy including streptomycin injections together with oral isoniazid (INH) and rifampin. Streptomycin is given intrathecally (via lumbar puncture) in some clients. Drug treatment should be continued for a minimum of 3 months.

Specific Nursing Measures

The major priority in the care of a client with meningitis is management of the acute phase of infection. Frequently assess level of consciousness and neurologic signs. Maintain appropriate infection control precautions according to institution and infection control guidelines. Clients with meningococcal meningitis or meningitis of unknown etiology are kept in isolation. Administer antibiotics on a strict schedule to maintain blood levels.

Clients will have a febrile period. Monitor the client's temperature every 1 to 2 hours if higher than 101°F (38°C). Give tepid sponge baths, axillary and groin compresses, and antipyretic drugs as ordered. Hypothermia blankets are used for temperatures above 102 to 103°F (39°C). A cooling blanket reduces fever by conduction and radiation. Provide frequent skin care with a lanolin lotion. If shivering develops during hypothermia treatments, the temperature could increase. Chlorpromazine (Thorazine) is sometimes used to counteract shivering.

Fluid volume deficits can occur due to fever and inadequate intake. During pyrexic states, potassium; sodium; vitamin A, B complex, and C are lost. Requirements for protein, carbohydrates, and fat increase. Fluid administration at a minimum of 3000 mL/24 hours is required to replace fluid lost by evaporation or urinary output. A balance must be achieved that will provide enough fluid to maintain hydration without increasing ICP. Monitor serum electrolytes daily during febrile periods and maintain strict intake and output. Give oral fluids, intravenous fluids, and/or tube feedings as needed. Intermittent or in-dwelling bladder catheterization may be necessary for clients with impaired levels of consciousness.

Sensory perceptual alterations can occur because of photophobia, hyperalgesia, and hyperirritability. Maintain a quiet, dark, nonstimulating environment to reduce photophobia. Hyperirritability may be caused by hypoxia or bladder distention, which should be ruled out before considering it a neurologic problem. Plan nursing care to minimize overstimulating the client. Restricted visiting hours may be necessary to promote rest.

For headache management, keep the head of the bed elevated unless contraindicated. Maintain good body alignment and position the client every 2 hours. Provide cold compresses and avoid overstimulation. Salicylates and codeine, the drugs of choice, are usually ordered.

Encephalitis

Encephalitis is an infection of brain tissue caused by viruses, pyogenic bacteria, fungi, or parasites. Viruses are the most common. Epidemic encephalitis begins in a reservoir and is transmitted to humans (eg, equine encephalitis begins in squirrels, horses, wild birds, chickens, or garter snakes; a mosquito or tick bites the reservoir animal and transmits the virus to a human host). Incubation periods vary according to the host's susceptibility, reaction to, and strength of the pathogen.

Encephalitis begins with the pathogen gaining access to the CNS. This occurs via the bloodstream or along peripheral and cranial nerves. The cortex, white matter, and meninges develop a nonsuppurative inflammation. There is a degeneration and destruction of cortical neurons with demyelination. Patches of hemorrhage, necrosis, and cavitation can occur, depending on the type of pathogen involved. Diffuse cerebral edema results.

Viruses are the most common pathogens. Type I herpes simplex virus has the potential to cause acute encephalitis in the adult and Type II can cause neonatal encephalitis from vaginal delivery of a mother with genital herpes. Other latent viruses that can cause encephalitis include herpes zoster, cytomegalovirus, Epstein–Barr virus, mumps, rabies, and measles. The severity of encephalitis depends on the pathogen.

Clinical Manifestations

A prodromal illness often precedes neurologic signs. Usual symptoms are headache, fever, malaise, sore throat, and vague aches and pains. This is often followed by marked alteration in level of consciousness from lethargy to coma. Confusion and disorientation with abrupt behavioral disturbances may occur. Objective signs include motor and sensory deficits, tremor, and ataxia. Hyperirritability, meningeal signs, seizures, and cranial nerve palsies are possible.

Diagnosis depends on a number of factors. The health history may reveal a preceding infection or related precipitating factor. The client may have symptoms and signs of an existing infection. Serum and urine laboratory studies may be of little value because they demonstrate findings consistent with a number of infectious diseases. Elevated CSF pressure with a xanthochromic appearance of CSF occurs with hemorrhage. CSF may also show elevated protein, decreased glucose, and an elevated WBC. A CT scan identifies edematous tissue areas and a brain shift.

It is essential to make a quick and accurate diagnosis. Isolation of the organism is not always possible. The only conclusive diagnostic method is by special fluorescent antibody studies and viral culture of cerebral tissue from a brain biopsy.

Medical Measures

Medical approaches are mainly symptomatic and supportive. There is no effective drug to treat encephalitis. The use of steroids such as dexamethasone (Decadron) combats cerebral edema. Potent antiviral drugs (eg, adenine arabinoside or Ara-A) have been used for the treatment of viral strains. Antiviral drugs in combination with steroids may prevent a fatal outcome. All clients do not recover completely, however. Those surviving an acute episode can have residual neurologic deficits including seizures, dysphasia, memory deficits, or personality changes.

Specific Nursing Measures

Nursing priorities for the client with encephalitis are similar to those outlined for meningitis with several major differences. Clients with acute encephalitis have more marked alterations in level of consciousness and behavioral manifestations. Restlessness, agitation, and dementia are more severe. There are also sleep pattern disturbances in which the sleep–wake cycle is less predictable. Minimal stress will increase agitation and hostility. Carefully control environmental stimuli; set limits; and provide a safe, supervised environment. Use a calm, soothing approach because the client's behavior may be unpredictable. Education of significant others is crucial to increase their awareness and guide them in their interactions with the client.

Neurologic deficits may increase rapidly due to cerebral edema and necrosis. Assess neurologic signs frequently during the acute stage, and report changes promptly. There is a potential for fluid volume overload related to intravenous antiviral drug administration. Administer these drugs on a strict time schedule as ordered. Maintain accurate intake and output. Observe for possible drug side effects, including nausea, vomiting, diarrhea, weight loss, and transient alterations in blood cell and liver function tests. Other nursing measures include elevating the head of the bed and monitoring electrolytes and respiratory and cardiac status. Explain all procedures and tests to the client and family; allow time for verbalization of anxieties; and encourage participation in care planning.

Myelitis

The term *myelitis* refers to an inflammation of the spinal cord. The most common viral diseases causing myelitis are poliomyelitis and herpes zoster. Myelitis may develop after an infection such as measles, varicella, or gonorrhea or may follow cowpox or antirabies vaccination. Myelitis associated with meningeal inflammation may be triggered by various organisms such as the tubercle bacillus, funguses, or parasites. Myelitis can also be related to epidural spinal abscesses and spinal arachnoiditis.

Clinical Manifestations

The viruses that cause myelitis usually have an affinity for motor and sensory neurons rather than spinal tracts. Neurons of the anterior horn are affected by poliomyelitis; those of the dorsal root ganglion are affected by herpes zoster. In most cases, inflammations involving motor and sensory tracts are not viral in origin. In postinfection or postvaccination myelitis, neurologic symptoms and signs develop over a few days and may involve both the brain and spinal cord or primarily the spinal cord. Following an isolated attack, the degree of recovery is variable over several weeks. Acute multiple sclerosis can be confused with myelitis because of manifestations similar to those that occur after a viral infection. Symptoms and signs develop more insidiously in acute MS, however.

Clinical findings in clients with spinal cord involvement include paresis, numbness of the feet and legs more than arms, dysuria, and sometimes headache and stiff neck. As the skin rash related to the initial infection fades, neurologic symptoms and signs develop, progress, stabilize, and then recede. CSF analysis demonstrates an elevated lymphocyte count with normal glucose and a normal or slightly elevated protein level. Neurologic involvement can extend to the brain stem, cerebellum, cerebrum, and optic nerves in some clients. In myelitis related to vaccines, the PNS may be more involved than the CNS.

Inflammatory conditions of the meninges can lead to a myelitis. This type of myelitis is often a sign of generalized disease. The disease can involve the epidural space, the dura, or the pia and arachnoid.

The diagnosis of myelitis includes evidence of an acute infection with a history of sudden motor paresis accompanied by other neurologic deficits. The CSF analysis may be within normal limits, and assessments such as Queckenstedt's test may demonstrate no blockage.

Medical Measures

Treatment is supportive but usually without therapeutic value. If an autoimmune disorder is responsible for the myelitis, steroids are recommended (ACTH or prednisone). Some clients make remarkable recoveries; some sustain severe and irreversible deficits. A certain proportion of clients who have relapses have multiple sclerosis as the underlying disease.

Specific Nursing Measures

Nursing care is aimed at preventing hazards of immobility and alterations in comfort. Bed rest is usually indicated during the acute phase of the illness. It is important that rehabilitation measures be instituted early. (Refer to nursing measures for clients with a CVA.)

Brain Abscesses

An abscess may form around or within the brain as a result of a local or systemic focus of infection. Brain abscesses are purulent collections that are usually encapsulated. Although abscesses can form anywhere in the brain, the most common sites are the temporal lobes, frontal lobes, and the cerebellum. Brain abscesses tend to become deeply situated within the hemispheres, because the infection has a tendency to spread into the white matter.

Most brain abscesses develop secondarily to a primary source of infection. Of these, at least 40% are caused by a mastoiditis, otitis media, or sinusitis. Approximately a third are hematogenous, resulting from a septic focus in the pulmonary system or, less often, from a cardiac or pelvic source. In about 20%, no source is identified. A smaller percentage results from direct invasion by traumatic injury, such as gunshot wounds, basilar skull fractures, and compound skull fractures with dural tears.

Clinical Manifestations

During the inital stage of organism invasion of the brain, the client experiences chills, fever, malaise, and appetite loss. The most common presenting symptom of an intracranial abscess is headache, which may be associated with vomiting and papilledema. Other common presenting symptoms are alterations in level of consciousness, especially drowsiness and confusion, and partial or generalized seizures. Focal neurologic deficits vary according to the anatomic location of the abscess. These include various motor, sensory, and speech disturbances.

In contrast, a subdural abscess tends to produce even more profound symptoms than brain abscesses. A subdural abscess affects the cortical blood vessels, causing thrombosis, arteritis, and eventually ischemia. The abscess usually arises from an acute sinusitis. A headache occurs with a rapid deterioration in neurologic status including seizures, hemiplegia, and dysphasia.

Brain abscesses in the early stages can have an insidious onset and progress through suppurative encephalitis accompanied by edema. Without treatment, brain compression or abscess rupture into the ventricle or subarachnoid space can be fatal.

Diagnosis is usually made by history of a previous infection, neurologic exam, and CT scan. A lumbar puncture is not recommended because a brain abscess acts as a mass lesion. The negative pressure created by the procedure can lead to a brain shift and herniation. When meningitis is the presumptive diagnosis, however, a lumbar puncture may be justified. The most important diagnostic test is the CT scan, which can demonstrate displacement of the lateral ventricles from a cerebral abscess or dilation from an abscess in the posterior fossa. The CT scan usually isolates an abscess, which is observed as an area of decreased density (Jennett & Galbraith, 1983). Cerebral angiography may be recommended in the absence of CT scanning in clients whose clinical picture is unclear.

Medical Measures

Intervention is aimed at diagnosing and managing the primary infection source, providing for abscess drainage, and administering an effective antibiotic regimen. The most crucial aspect of treatment is drainage and elimination of the abscess by neurosurgical intervention. Most cerebral abscesses can be drained via a burr hole aspiration. Some may require more than one aspiration. Traumatic and cerebellar abscesses cannot be eliminated by this method, however. Antibiotic therapy is given for at least 6 weeks to reduce virulence of the organism, eliminate the pathogen, and penetrate the cavity. Prognosis is usually good after an effective regimen of antibiotics and/or surgery.

Specific Nursing Measures

Management of the acute infection is a priority of nursing care. Administer antibiotics on a strict schedule to maintain therapeutic blood levels. Carefully inspect intravenous sites and rotate them every 48 to 72 hours to prevent thrombosis or phlebitis. During antibiotic therapy, watch for the development of opportunistic infections. The growth of other organisms results from imbalances in natural flora, especially in the mouth and gastrointestinal tract.

Monitor the client for alterations in level of consciousness. Sudden increases in ICP can result from cerebral edema that may surround an acute abscess. Frequent assessment of neurologic and vital signs, head of bed elevation to 30°, restricted fluid intake, and avoiding any stimulant that can raise intracranial pressure are necessary components of care.

Monitor clients for potential seizures. Administer anticonvulsants as ordered with periodic checking of serum blood levels. During actual seizures, protect the client from self-injury and maintain a patent airway. A careful description of seizure onset, course, and duration may assist the physician in localizing the abscess site. Interventions for headache include providing a quiet environment, changing position to promote comfort, and administering mild analgesics as ordered. Reduce knowledge deficits by preparing clients psychologically and physically for surgery for aspiration of the abscess and intrathecal medication. Discharge teaching should include methods of preventing future abscesses if caused by an infected tooth, ear infection, or sinus problem.

Herpes Zoster

Herpes zoster (shingles) is a viral disorder that affects the posterior root ganglia. The disease is characterized by cutaneous eruptions of vesicles along the distribution of involved spinal or cranial nerve roots. The highest percentage involves spinal ganglia. Herpes zoster occurs mainly in adults; the incidence is higher in women than men and during the spring and fall.

Herpes zoster develops from reactivation of the virus responsible for chickenpox, the varicella virus. In fact, children can develop chickenpox if exposed to an adult with shingles. Adults with shingles have all had chickenpox in the past. There also seems to be a relation between herpes zoster and certain systemic infections, spinal diseases, neoplasms, and immunosuppressive therapy. Probably, these conditions reactivate the virus.

Clinical Manifestations

Mild to severe neuralgic pain in the affected nerve root distribution is the most common presenting symptom. The pain may be burning, tingling, sharp, or dull. Pain may be concurrent with or followed by skin reddening and an eruption of vesicles. Over the next 1 or 2 weeks, these lesions become pustules and then develop a crust. After healing, a pigmented scar may appear. If an infection or ulceration accompanies the vesicles, the scarring may be permanent.

Less often, sensory and motor dysfunctions develop in the affected nerve root. With meningeal involvement, nuchal rigidity, headache and changes in level of consciousness can occur. The virus rarely causes an encephalopathy.

Diagnosis is usually based on the sudden onset of root pain followed by the characteristic distribution of shingles. The lesions are unilateral and do not cross the midline of the body. They follow a characteristic bandlike distribution that follows nerve root lines; therefore, they are transverse on the hemithorax and vertical on an extremity. If lesions are widespread, diagnosis may be difficult.

There are potential complications from an attack of herpes zoster. The main ones are scarring of the skin, facial palsies, and postherpetic neuralgia. In elderly or debilitated clients, the neuralgia can persist for months or years. The skin may also be hypersensitive to touch. Unfortunately, this variant does not respond well to treatment. Less commonly, some individuals develop Guillain–Barré syndrome following herpes zoster.

Medical Measures

No specific antiviral treatment is effective. Zoster immune globulin is not helpful during an attack but may be preventive. Most treatment is aimed at giving local care to the vesicles. Topical corticosteroids can alleviate local pain and itching and may shorten the stage of vesicle eruption. Antibiotics may be administered to prevent or treat secondary infections related to shingles. During the acute phase, bed rest and analgesics can be supportive.

Postherpetic neuralgia is a difficult condition to treat. Intractable cases may require neurosurgical sectioning of affected nerve roots or occasionally irradiation to the site. Treatment results are variable.

Specific Nursing Measures

The primary objective of nursing management is care of interruptions in skin integrity. Instruct clients to avoid scratching vesicles to prevent spreading the lesions and promoting infection. Skin eruptions can be treated with topical applications of corticosteroids. Open vesicles require wet–dry saline and povidone–iodine compresses. Systemic steroid therapy may be used. Be alert for side effects of steroids. Clients experience alterations in comfort due to localized pain and itching. Comfort measures include positioning techniques (especially during bed rest), skin treatments, and analgesics as ordered.

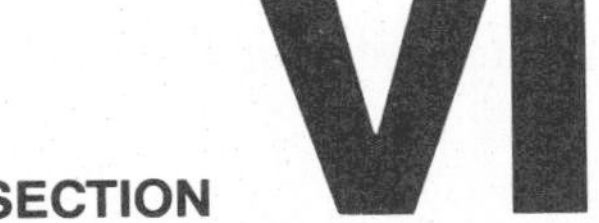

SECTION VI

Neoplastic and Obstructive Disorders

Tumors within the cranium can be either primary or metastatic. Primary tumors are classified as primary intracranial intracerebral tumors or primary intracranial extracerebral tumors. Primary intracerebral tumors arise from the supporting cellular elements of the brain, such as glial cells. Primary extracerebral tumors arise outside the substance of the brain. Metastatic tumors are found predominantly within the substance of the brain, which they reach through the systemic circulation. The histologic appearance of a metastatic tumor is identical to the organ of tumor origin.

Cranial Tumors

Glioblastoma multiforme accounts for approximately 55% of all glial tumors. The most malignant of the glioma group, this tumor has a propensity for rapid growth. Clients with a confirmed diagnosis of glioblastoma multiforme and surgical removal without any additional treatment have a median survival of 14 weeks. The addition of radiation and chemotherapy prolongs median survival to approximately 1 year. About 25% of cerebral gliomas are astrocytomas. These tumors may be slow growing and surgical resection can result in cure.

Meningiomas account for approximately 25% of the primary intracranial tumors. They arise from the arachnoid layer and are well circumscribed and encapsulated. Meningiomas are usually slow growing and occur frequently around the parasagittal area. They are considered benign because they do not invade the surrounding brain but produce symptoms by compression. Surgical removal of these tumors is curative. Any involved bone must be removed to prevent recurrence.

Neuromas arise from Schwann's cells of the cranial nerves. Neuromas are usually solitary lesions, but they can occur on multiple cranial nerves in neurofibromatosis. Their clinical presentation depends on the particular cranial nerve involved. An acoustic neuroma is a benign lesion arising from the vestibular portion of CN VIII.

Clinical Manifestations

Tumors produce symptoms by invasion or compression of surrounding neural structures. The neurologic symptoms and signs of any tumor affecting the brain depend on the location of the tumor and its rate of growth. Disruption of neural structures by the tumor can cause an insidious deterioration of neurologic function or an acute neurologic disturbance. In the latter instance, the client may have a seizure without any previous history of neurologic symptoms. In some cases, hemorrhage within the tumor results in an acute deterioration of neurologic status.

Besides directly disrupting neural structures, tumors may produce symptoms as a consequence of the resulting edema in the brain surrounding the tumor. The edema contributes to the mass effect of the tumor and can result in ICP elevations and concomitant cerebral herniation. In addition, tumor obstruction of the CSF pathway may result in symptoms usually attributed to hydrocephalus.

Preoperative evaluation of a client suspected of having a brain tumor relies principally on neuroradiologic studies. CT scanning and, more recently, magnetic resonance imaging (MRI) are the usual initial diagnostic studies. The size and anatomic location of the tumor can frequently be determined from these studies. In a CT scan, intravenous contrast agents aid in determining the extent of tumor vascularity. In some institutions, positron emission tomography (PET) enables the clinician to evaluate the metabolic activity of the tumor. Cerebral angiography defines the blood supply of the tumor and aids in preoperative diagnosis. In addition, angiography contributes valuable information in planning the neurosurgical removal or elimination of these lesions.

Medical and Specific Nursing Measures

Medical and nursing approaches to the care of clients with brain tumors, including those undergoing neurosurgical procedures, are covered below and in Chapter 34. General care of the client with a malignancy is found in Chapter 10.

Burr Hole

A burr hole, a hole drilled into the skull, has numerous diagnostic and therapeutic indications. It is often used to gain access to one of the lateral ventricles to introduce air into the ventricular system for diagnostic studies, to reduce intracranial pressure (ICP) by the removal of cerebrospinal fluid (CSF), as the initial step in a ventricular shunting operation, or to place a catheter in the ventricle (ventriculostomy) for intermittent or continuous drainage of CSF, for instillation of antibiotics or chemotherapeutic agents, or for monitoring of intracranial pressure.

A burr hole may be adequate for the drainage of some intracranial cysts, abscesses, hematomas, and hygromas, avoiding a major craniotomy. A burr hole may be used to obtain samples of brain tissue for histologic examination. In head trauma, rapid drilling of a burr hole in the temporal area may be life saving if the brain is severely compressed by a rapidly accumulating epidural hematoma. A burr hole is sometimes all that is required to elevate a section of bone in a depressed skull fracture, relieving pressure on the underlying brain.

A burr hole is often drilled under local anesthesia, although if the client is restless or unable to cooperate, general anesthesia may be preferred. Because the skin incision is small, little hair removal is necessary. (Some surgeons or clients may prefer to have the entire scalp shaved.) The physiologic and psychosocial/lifestyle implications are discussed in Table 29–4.

Table 29–4
Drilling of Burr Holes: Implications for the Client 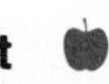

Physiologic Implications	Psychosocial Implications
Usually involves minimal manipulation of the intracranial contents Postoperative pain is usually minimal Intraoperative blood loss is usually minimal Because the cranial vault has been entered, possible complications are similar to those for craniotomy or craniectomy and include: hemorrhage, increased intracranial pressure, seizure activity, infection	Depends on the underlying pathologic condition; with head trauma, the most significant factor is the extent of brain damage inflicted at the time of the initial injury When done for diagnostic purposes, several days of anxiety and uncertainty follow before the diagnosis is confirmed Need to adjust to the diagnosis and/or the need for further treatment may significantly alter lifestyle

Nursing Implications

PREOPERATIVE CARE Although a burr hole is usually considered a minor surgical procedure, the preoperative preparation is generally the same as for any intracranial procedure. Nursing observations and interventions are discussed in detail in the following section on craniotomy and craniectomy.

Provide opportunities for the client and family to express their fears and to ask questions. If the procedure is to be done under local anesthesia, the client must be prepared for what to expect. If the client is comatose, disoriented, or confused, preparation may be impossible but should be attempted.

In some instances, a burr hole may not achieve the goal of surgery (eg, drainage of subdural hematoma or elevation of depressed skull fracture), and a craniotomy or craniectomy may be necessary. The client and significant others should be prepared for that possibility.

Many surgeons prefer and hospital policy may dictate the precaution of crossmatching a unit of blood. If a more involved operative procedure might be necessary, additional blood will be reserved, the preoperative scalp preparation will be more extensive, and additional intraoperative monitoring may be used.

POSTOPERATIVE CARE Mild analgesics are usually sufficient to relieve headache. Narcotics are avoided because of their depressant effect on the central nervous system (CNS) and respiratory system and because their effect may mask changes in neurologic status.

In the trauma client who exhibits signs of postoperative hypovolemia or shock, be alert to the possibility of blood loss from other sources (eg, intra-abdominal bleeding).

Take care to maintain the integrity of any tubes or drains. The type and quantity of drainage should be noted. Meticulous care must be taken to maintain the sterility of any external drainage or monitoring system because an intraventricular infection can be especially devastating.

Craniotomy and Craniectomy

A craniotomy and craniectomy are the means of exposing or gaining access to the brain and cranial nerves so intracranial disease (tumors, abscesses, hematomas, and vascular lesions) can be surgically treated. The cranium may also be opened to excise an area of cortex or disrupt various nerves and fiber tracts for the relief of pain, seizures, tremors, spasms, or severe mental disturbances that do not respond to pharmacologic therapy. Craniotomy or craniectomy is often indicated in the treatment of skull fractures and other traumatic head wounds, not only to repair the bony defect but to repair dural tears; decompress the underlying brain; inspect for bleeding or cortical damage; and, in some instances, to debride the brain of foreign material. CSF leaks, occurring spontaneously or as a result of trauma or surgery, may also require intracranial repair.

If a neoplasm is present, the goal of surgery is usually the total removal of the pathology while preserving the normal neural and vascular structures. When this is not possible, the surgeon must decide whether to risk possible neurologic impairment or to leave a tumor that will regrow. Many factors influence this decision. A few considerations are the age and preoperative condition of the client; histology of the lesion, its rate of growth, and its proximity to vital structures; the amount of disability that may be induced; and the client's ability to cope.

A *craniotomy* is an incision or opening into the cranial cavity. A flap of bone is cut in the skull and secured back in place after the intracranial portion of the procedure. On the other hand, *craniectomy* involves permanent removal of bone. This type of opening is used primarily for posterior fossa operations (suboccipital craniectomy; discussed later in this chapter) because the posterior neck muscles provide good protection. It may also be employed for the subtemporal approach to the middle fossa because the bone in this area is extremely thin, and temporalis musculature is heavy enough to provide safe coverage. Craniectomy may also be indicated in the presence of infection, when the bone is invaded by tumor, or when the ICP is elevated to an extent that replacement of the bone flap would compress the brain.

Because of the size and extreme delicacy of the structures that must be dissected and manipulated during many neurosurgical procedures, it is imperative that the operative site remains relatively immobile and that any chance of inadvertent movement is eliminated. Immobilization and proper alignment are usually accomplished by means of a pinned headrest device.

The location of the skin incision and bone flap depends on the location of the pathologic condition. The location and dimensions of the opening are carefully planned in advance so it can be kept small and placed accurately. The size of the opening may not correspond with the size of the lesion. The overall aim is to provide optimal exposure with as little brain retraction as possible. For a good cosmetic result, with few exceptions the skin flaps are placed in the area covered by the hair. Unfortunately, little can be done cosmetically for the bald client or when trauma dictates the area of the incision.

Whenever possible, the cortical incision is placed to avoid damage to the cortex (eg, through a sulcus). When nondestructive approaches are not possible, a corticotomy (incising an area of overlying cortex) may be necessary to reach the lesion.

Benign tumors are regularly removed piecemeal. The inner portion of the tumor is removed to achieve an internal decompression. As the tumor is shrunk, it tends to fall away from the surrounding brain and neural and vascular structures. This technique facilitates safer tumor removal. Carcinomas and abscesses are usually removed in one piece if possible to prevent the dissemination of tumor cells or infectious agents to the surrounding brain or into the subarachnoid space where disease can spread via the CSF circulation.

When the bone is to be replaced, small holes are drilled into the bone flap and in the surrounding cranium, and the bone flap is sewn or wired back into place. A drain is often left in the wound and may be placed in the tumor bed or the subdural, extradural, or subgaleal space (under the galea aponeurotica, the broad flat tendon that lies against the top of the skull). A closed drainage system is preferred to an open drain which can become a migratory pathway for microorganisms. The physiologic and psychosocial/lifestyle implications are discussed in Table 29–5.

Table 29–5
Craniotomy/Craniectomy: Implications for the Client

Physiologic Implications	Psychosocial/Lifestyle Implications
Postoperative cerebral edema, and periorbital edema and ecchymosis reach their peak between 48 to 72 hours and influence the neurologic status	Impact of surgery is influenced by: extent of the injury or underlying disease; degree and duration of the preoperative neurologic impairment; degree of neural damage resulting from the surgery; ultimate prognosis for the underlying disease
Postoperative pain (headache) is usually minimal	Common concerns are fear of death, paralysis, disfigurement, personality changes, loss of independence, survival in a vegetative state, becoming a burden to family, and financial worries
Mild hyperpyrexia and neck pain in the first 48 hours may be expected as a result of the introduction of blood into the subarachnoid space	Hospitalization requires possibly extensive, time-consuming, and costly preoperative diagnostic workup; 7–10 days postoperative hospitalization; and 4–6 weeks of rehabilitation
Potential complications include: intracranial hemorrhage/hematoma; increased intracranial pressure/herniation; seizures; infection; CSF leak; fluid/electrolyte and/or metabolic/hormonal imbalance such as diabetes insipidus or SIADH; hydrocephalus; complications related to the hazards of immobility and/or a depressed level of consciousness	Depression in the first postoperative week is common even with a favorable surgical outcome and good prognosis; it is thought to be physiologic rather than psychologic in origin
Mild headaches may persist after discharge but can usually be controlled with OTC pain relievers	Postoperative sequelae may be transient or permanent; client may require assistance with ADL, a period of rehabilitation therapy, and significant alteration in lifestyle
Need to protect incision line; hair can be shampooed 3–4 days after sutures are removed, avoid direct heat (hairdryer, hot curlers) until hair has regrown to a reasonable length; hat should be worn in full sunlight	Seizures may require limitation of activities, travel, driving a motor vehicle, or a change in occupation; prophylactic anticonvulsant therapy usual for one year following surgery
Risk of postoperative seizures, especially after surgery in the frontotemporal region or in clients with seizures preoperatively	Visible deficits can result in significant changes in body image and loss of self-esteem
Postoperative impairment will depend on the location and extent of neural damage and may be transient or permanent. Deficits may include: impaired level of consciousness; mental status changes; focal motor and/or sensory impairment; language disturbances; cranial nerve dysfunction (eg, anosmia, visual deficits, oculomotor palsies)	Personality changes, emotional disturbances, or conceptual disorders related to organic brain damage or disease can be very difficult for family to handle
Abscess formation in the operative site and osteomyelitis of the bone flap are potential late complications	Language disturbances can be extremely frustrating for the client and family and frequently cause depression
	Strenuous exercise such as jogging or tennis should be avoided for a few weeks

Nursing Implications

PREOPERATIVE CARE One of the most important nursing measures is the assessment and documentation of the baseline neurologic status to provide a standard by which postoperative progress or deterioration can be measured. Assessment should include:

- Mental status
- Level of consciousness
- Responsiveness
- Behavior
- Speech
- Motor, sensory, and cranial nerve function
- Pupillary size, position, response to light, and any abnormality of extraocular movements

The frequency of preoperative neurologic assessment

depends on the condition of the client and the physician's orders. If any decline in neurologic status is observed—no matter how slight or subtle—increase the frequency of neurologic and vital sign assessments and promptly report and record changes.

Preoperative recordings of vital signs are important in assessing postoperative cardiovascular and respiratory status. The documentation of the client's preoperative weight may be extremely important if the client develops postoperative diabetes insipidus or SIADH. It may also be valuable in assessing the nutritional status of a client with a depressed level of consciousness who is unable to take oral feedings.

Any significant existing health problems such as hypertensive, renal, cardiac, or respiratory disease should be documented. Such health problems may adversely affect the intraoperative and postoperative course by interfering with optimal cerebral perfusion, oxygenation, and metabolic processes, and should be corrected or controlled whenever possible. These system abnormalities and the current medication regimen (eg, insulin, antihypertensive medication) should be communicated to nurses in the OR, recovery room, and intensive care unit (ICU). Laboratory values should be checked and any abnormality promptly reported.

The client's blood should be typed and cross-matched. The number of units placed on reserve depends on the nature of the lesion. Preoperative hemoglobin and hematocrit values are useful in assessing blood loss and in determining the need for replacement. Because hemostasis within the brain is critical, the prothrombin time is often ordered. Clients, especially those with a history of headaches, should be questioned regarding the use of aspirin. In general, they should take acetaminophen (Tylenol) instead to avoid possible increased bleeding.

Be sensitive to the fears of the client and family regarding the impending surgery. Assigning one nurse consistently to the client so rapport can be established is extremely helpful. Provide the client and family with opportunities to express their fears and concerns and to ask questions. Whenever possible, accompany the physician during discussion of the surgery with the client and family to be able to clarify and reinforce the information given and to provide support. Learning about possible complications can be emotionally devastating for the client and family. Reinforce accurate perceptions and correct misconceptions. Realistic positive expectations should be emphasized.

Remember that as the day of surgery approaches, the stress level of the client and family is likely to increase, and their displaced anger, frustration, or inability to cope may be directed toward nursing staff. Involvement of the liaison mental health nurse or social worker early in the preoperative period may be beneficial. A visit by a priest, minister, rabbi, or other clergy can provide a great deal of comfort and support for many persons.

Because fear of the unknown is a significant stress factor, prepare the client for what to expect in the perioperative period. Explain the preoperative routines, such as the placement of a peripheral IV line, a central venous pressure (CVP) line, and an in-dwelling catheter. Familiarize the client with postoperative routines (eg, pupil checks, motor testing) and expected sensations (eg, headache, the sensation of having to void produced by the in-dwelling catheter). Provide routine preoperative teaching.

Also prepare the client for the hair removal procedure. The amount of hair removed depends on the area to be exposed, the extent of the incision, and the surgeon's preference. Some surgeons prefer that the entire head be shaved to facilitate the preparation and maintenance of the sterile field. Other advantages are that the head dressing is easier to apply and keep in place, regrowth is more even, and wigs may fit better. Encourage the client to discuss the extent of hair removal with the surgeon preoperatively. Allowing the client to participate in the decision provides some degree of control over the situation.

Because hair loss is often traumatic for client and significant others, it is preferable to shave the scalp after the client is anesthetized. This also spares the client discomfort. It is also preferable to do the shave as close to the time of incision as possible to reduce the time bacteria have to colonize in skin nicks or cuts. After the shave, the entire area is thoroughly washed with an antibacterial agent and painted with an antiseptic solution. Some surgeons may also prescribe a shampoo with povidone–iodine, hexachlorophene, or other antimicrobial soap the night before surgery to reduce the bacteria on the skin.

Clients' reactions to the loss of hair vary. Many clients, both male and female, are devastated by it, but others consider it relatively trivial. Often, if the hair is long enough, sections can be combed and secured away from the operative site. The remaining hair may be adequate to cover the shaved area. In the case of posterior fossa surgery, the hair loss often is not even apparent from the front.

Be sure the family understands that the surgery is long and explain how to get information about the client's condition and the progress of the surgery. They should also know when they can expect to talk with the surgeon and see the client following surgery. Because this is such a stressful time, a written form with the necessary information is helpful. The family should be alerted to the array of infusion lines and monitoring devices that will be in place as well as the presence of the head dressing and wound drain. Stress that these are normal measures and do not indicate a problem or complication. If there is any possibility that the client will remain intubated and on a ventilator, explain this in advance. The family should also be made aware of the significance and importance of assessing vital signs and neurologic status because these are often perceived as cruel or inconsiderate disturbances.

POSTOPERATIVE CARE The nurse on the postoperative unit should obtain a thorough report from the operating room nursing staff before receiving the client. In some instances, it may be supplemented by information from the surgeon or the anesthesiologist. Specific information regarding the surgical procedure itself, and untoward events that may have occurred intraoperatively, may influence postoperative care.

As soon as possible after the client is admitted to the postoperative unit, assess the client's neurologic status, including level of consciousness, pupillary reaction and eye signs, motor function, and vital signs. This initial baseline postoperative assessment will serve as a basis for determining subsequent progress or deterioration. Compare the findings with preoperative findings. Auscultate breath sounds bilaterally.

Observe the site and type of wound drain as well as the quantity and characteristics of the drainage. Check the head dressing to be sure it is dry and intact. A bloodstained area remote from the operative site is not unusual; it is usually the result of oozing from the site of a skull pin used for intraoperative fixation of the head. Note the size of the stain and reinforce the dressing. In most instances, this bleeding will stop on its own or respond to mild pressure applied to the site for a few minutes. Occasionally, a skin suture may be required.

During the critical 24 to 48 hours following intracranial surgery (in some cases this period may be extended), the nurse's main task is to recognize promptly any potential complications and to implement preventive measures. Changes in neurologic condition are often related to changes in ICP. Acute changes in ICP postoperatively are most likely to result from intracranial bleeding or severe edema. Regardless of the cause, markedly increased pressure can cause irreversible damage or death if not controlled. It is important to recognize the change early so appropriate therapy can be instituted.

LEVEL OF CONSCIOUSNESS Level of consciousness is the most sensitive indicator of ICP and, in most instances, provides the first clue to a deteriorating condition. Assessment of level of consciousness is described in Chapter 28.

EYE SIGNS Assessment of pupillary activity includes observation of their size, shape, equality, and reactivity to light. A pupil that previously reacted briskly and now reacts sluggishly could be an early sign of increasing ICP and should be reported promptly. A sudden dilated and nonreactive pupil is an ominous sign of impending uncal herniation and requires immediate attention.

Abnormality of eye movements or pupillary response may have causes other than neurologic ones. Check the client's history for previous eye surgery or trauma. Various drugs administered intraoperatively also affect pupil size and reactivity, but this reaction is bilateral. Atropine and scopolamine, which are frequently given preoperatively, dilate the pupil. Pupils may become bilaterally dilated and fixed following a seizure, but they usually recover within minutes. In the trauma client, recent ingestion of drugs or alcohol may be a factor. The surgical procedure or the underlying pathologic condition may have damaged the optic nerve or any of the cranial nerves responsible for eye movements. In these circumstances, deficits are to be expected.

MOTOR FUNCTION In testing motor function, check for the presence or absence of movement, assess the strength and symmetry of movement, and observe for abnormal or inappropriate movements. In the conscious client, motor strength of the upper extremities is best tested by assessing grip strength and presence of pronator drift. Proximal muscle strength can be tested by asking the client to close the eyes and hold both arms out forward with the palms up. If one arm gradually drifts down or turns inward (pronator drift), it may be an early indication of hemiparesis. In the lower extremities, subtle changes are best detected if the client is asked to dorsiflex, plantar flex, and leg raise against the resistance of the examiner's hand.

Focal motor deficits not present before the surgery may be the result of edema in the operative area. These deficits are often transient, and severity may vary in relation to the degree of swelling. In many instances, the deficit is a direct and predictable consequence of the surgical procedure. If the deficit, which can be sensory as well as motor, does not correlate anatomically with the operative site (eg, left-leg weakness should not occur following left-sided brain surgery), the possibility of vascular injury, peripheral nerve injury, or brain damage remote from the operative area should be considered and investigated.

In the comatose client or in one whose level of consciousness prevents active participation in the examination, begin the assessment by observing general posture and the presence of any spontaneous movements. Stimulate the client to elicit a response. Apply the stimulus, which should be the least that will elicit a response, to both sides of the body. Movements in response to a noxious stimulus are usually graded as either purposeful (or appropriate), inappropriate, or absent. Note that many unresponsive clients exhibit a grasp reflex that can be misinterpreted as a response to command. To distinguish a grasp reflex from a voluntary motor activity, ask the client to grip and release repeatedly. Inappropriate movements, which can occur spontaneously or in response to a stimulus, include decorticate and decerebrate posturing (see Figure 28–2 in Chapter 28). These responses are usually bilateral but can occur unilaterally or in combination. The total absence of response to a noxious stimulus is viewed as a grave sign (see the Glasgow Coma Scale in Table 28–1 in Chapter 28 for an objective measure). When assessing motor function, consider preoperative deficits as well as factors that may limit movement such as pain, armboards, or intravenous lines or monitoring equipment.

INTRACRANIAL PRESSURE Prevention of increased ICP is one of the most important aspects of nursing care of the postcraniotomy client. Untreated increased ICP can result in shifting of the intracranial contents and displacement of a portion of the brain through or around linings or openings within the intracranial cavity. This herniation can be life-threatening unless promptly recognized and treated. The process reaches its catastrophic irreversible conclusion when midbrain hemorrhage is produced by venous obstruction.

Early and frequently subtle signs of increasing ICP may include a change in the severity or pattern of headaches, visual disturbances, nausea with or without vomiting, restlessness, irritability, or the tendency to fall asleep under circumstances that previously had kept the client awake. If the client exhibits any signs of increased ICP, the surgeon should be promptly notified.

Increased ICP secondary to cerebral edema can often be prevented or at least limited by various medical and nursing interventions. Unless otherwise ordered, the head of the bed should be kept elevated to at least 30°. This position enhances venous drainage from the head. Make certain the client does not slide down in bed, lowering the degree of head elevation. Avoid any position that allows for neck flexion because this can impede venous outflow through the jugular veins. Assist clients in turning or changing position to avoid straining or Valsalva's maneuver. Stool softeners are often administered to prevent straining.

Steroids are almost routinely ordered. Because these drugs cause gastric irritation, they are usually administered with an antacid and/or cimetidine (Tagamet). Dehydration is another method frequently employed to minimize swelling. Oral fluid intake may be severely restricted, and intravenous infusions may be limited to the minimal rate required to keep the vein open or to administer medications. In the alert client, thirst can be the major discomfort. Frequent mouth care and moist, cold gauze applied to the lips and tongue provide some degree of comfort. Often the surgeon allows the client to suck on ice chips periodically. Lollipops provide relief without adding to fluid intake if the client is alert enough to suck on them safely. If the neurologic condition is stable and the client is alert and thirsty, more liberal fluid intake on the second postoperative day may be allowed.

Intracranial pressure and central venous pressure may be monitored. Measure urine output carefully to assure that renal perfusion is adequate. This monitoring is especially important when dehydration and hypotensive techniques are employed. Output should be at least 30 mL per hour.

Monitor respiratory status carefully because anoxia and hypercarbia result in cerebral vasodilation, increasing ICP. Encourage deep breathing as soon as the client is alert enough to cooperate. In the extubated client, oxygen via face mask or nasal cannula is usually administered for the first 12 to 24 hours. Humidification is often added to decrease the viscosity of secretions. Suction the intubated client every 2 hours or as necessary. Avoid vigorous suctioning because it increases ICP. As a general rule, limit suctioning to 15 seconds or less. In many institutions, the procedure for suctioning a neurosurgical client includes hyperventilation and hyperoxygenation with 100% oxygen via Ambu bag both before and after suctioning to reduce the risk of hypercarbia. In other facilities, the Ambu bag is avoided to prevent the venous pressure increase that its positive cycle induces. For the same reason, vigorous coughing, IPPB, and postural drainage are avoided. Arterial blood gases are periodically monitored.

Surgery in or around the hypothalamus can disturb temperature regulation mechanisms, and wide fluctuations in temperature may occur. In such cases, it might be advantageous to prepare the postoperative bed with a hyper/hypothermia mattress before the client arrives. Attempt to keep the client normothermic because shivering increases ICP as well as the metabolic needs and oxygen consumption of the brain. Chlorpromazine (Thorazine) may be administered to prevent shivering. Regardless of the cause, hyperthermia should be treated with antipyretic medications, cooling blanket or mattress, and/or alcohol or ice water sponge baths.

If medical interventions fail to reduce the ICP adequately, surgery is likely. The procedure may include placement of an intraventricular catheter or shunting system for the removal of CSF, removal of the bone flap, or possible lobectomy to relieve pressure. Headache following cranial surgery is expected and usually can be relieved by mild analgesics such as aspirin or acetaminophen. Occasionally, codeine is required for adequate comfort. More potent narcotics are contraindicated because their CNS depressant effect may mask changes in level of consciousness. In addition, they may depress respirations, contributing to increased ICP. Elevating the head of the bed and maintaining a quiet, dark environment is often helpful.

Anticipate the administration of furosemide (Lasix) or mannitol and hyperventilation with oxygen via Ambu bag or mechanical ventilator to reduce the intracranial volume. Hypothermia or barbiturate therapy (the administration of phenobarbital or pentobarbital in doses sufficient to produce complete unresponsiveness) may also be instituted in an attempt to reduce the metabolic demands. The therapy requires complete mechanical ventilation with an endotracheal or cuffed tracheostomy tube.

A postoperative hematoma results in a marked and often extremely rapid rise in the ICP that can be devastating to neurologic function and life threatening. Take care to maintain the blood pressure within the prescribed parameters. In some instances, this can be an extremely difficult task involving the manipulation of several drugs such as propranolol (Inderal), nitroprusside (Nipride), and nitroglycerin, alone or in combination. With pharmacologic manipulation of the blood pressure, continuous monitoring of the mean arterial pressure via arterial catheter is strongly recommended. Take great care to maintain the integrity of the monitoring lines as well as the wound drain. Check the amount and type of drainage hourly, and promptly report any sharp increase in amount. Restless or uncooperative clients may require mitts to prevent inadvertent disruption of monitoring or infusion lines. Restraints may occasionally be necessary but should be used only as a last resort.

If the client's condition is rapidly deteriorating because of a hematoma, be prepared for the surgeon to return the client directly to the operating room for re-exploration and evacuation of the hematoma. Examination of the wound may reveal elevation of the bone flap. In cases where there is no bone flap, the wound may appear tense and bulging. In rare instances, where minutes may make the difference between life and death, the surgeon may elect to open the wound in the recovery room or intensive care unit to decompress the brain stem. Occasionally, the situation progresses so rapidly that the surgeon does not have enough time to provide adequate explanation to the family or to even obtain consent for the surgery. Needless to say, this is a period of confusion and extreme anxiety for the family. It may be especially difficult for them to understand if the client was doing well initially before a sudden deterioration in condition. Offer support and provide as much explanation and information as possible.

Changes in vital signs from increased ICP are usually a late sign and most often signal impending herniation. With any decline in level of consciousness, motor function, or pupillary reactivity, pay careful attention to respiratory rate and pattern. The particular respiratory pattern may provide a clue to the area of the brain or brain stem being compressed. Some fluctuations in vital signs usually occur long before the appearance of the classic Cushing's reflex. *Cushing's reflex,* which includes a rising blood pressure, bradycardia, and respiratory irregularity, is a compensatory mechanism and an ominous sign of impending intracranial crisis. This stage is followed, often rapidly, by the late decompensatory stage in which blood pressure falls; the pulse becomes rapid, irregular, and thready; and the respiratory pattern becomes increasingly irregular and includes periods of apnea. If the rising ICP is not checked and the client is allowed to deteriorate to this point, intervention is likely to be ineffective.

Nursing Research Note

Watson C, Ross J, Ramsey M: Identification of neurosurgical patients susceptible to pulmonary infection. *J Neurosurg Nurs* 1984; 16(3):123–127.

This research tested the effectiveness of a tool to identify clients at high risk for development of pulmonary infection and investigated the efficacy of a pulmonary protocol in preventing infections in this group.

Using a quasi-experimental design, the researchers identified two groups of high-risk clients using a tool they had developed—the Pulmonary Infection Risk Assessment Tool. The first group identified during a pilot study served as the control. A second group received the pulmonary protocol: a pulmonary assessment every 4 hours; turning every hour or out of bed four times daily; incentive deep breathing every 2 hours; pulmonary physical therapy every 2 hours; suctioning of tracheostomy clients or those with altered levels of awareness; humidified oxygen or compressed air; forced fluids to 2500 mL daily; and, in alert clients, effective breathing technique training.

The results indicated that the tool overidentified clients at high risk for pulmonary infection, and the pulmonary protocol did not significantly reduce infection. The incidence of infection was 33% in the experimental group, and 35% in the control group. In both groups, clients who had diminished levels of consciousness, pre-existing chronic obstructive pulmonary disease, were receiving steroids, had undergone lengthy surgery, or had paralyzed palates, exhibited the greatest incidence of infection. The authors note that the pulmonary protocol was not consistently implemented unless the client showed clinical evidence of pulmonary compromise.

When providing nursing care to neurologically impaired clients, clients at risk for pulmonary complications must be identified. Consistent and aggressive nursing intervention should be planned and implemented to prevent such complications.

ENDOCRINE FUNCTION Diabetes insipidus and SIADH can complicate the postoperative course of any craniotomy/craniectomy client especially following head trauma or surgery in the area of the pituitary gland and hypothalamus. Although the symptoms for each of these syndromes appear to be opposite, both carry the danger of severe fluid and electrolyte imbalance. Therefore, the nursing measures are similar for both. Care of clients with diabetes insipidus and SIADH is discussed in Chapter 34.

INFECTION The head dressing should be kept clean, dry, and intact and should be reinforced as necessary if drainage is noted. Strict adherence to aseptic technique is essential when the dressing is changed, when the drain or sutures are removed, and when the wound-drainage reservoir is emptied. Care should be taken to maintain the integrity of any wound drain because blood collecting within the surgical wound provides an excellent culture medium for the growth of microorganisms. Restless or confused clients may attempt to remove their head dressings and, even if they fail, can introduce organisms into the incision line. Mitts or restraints may be necessary to protect the wound from contamination.

If infection at the operative site is suspected, a specimen of any drainage or exudate should be sent for culture and sensitivity testing. A slight elevation in temperature (to 100° F or 38° C), with or without some mild neck stiffness, is not uncommon about the second or third postoperative day and is the result of the introduction of blood into the subarachnoid space at the time of surgery. Persistent or spiking temperatures, especially accompanied by severe headaches or the tendency to keep the neck immobile and in an extended position, are the classic signs of meningitis and are cause for concern and prompt therapeutic measures. Anticipate a lumbar puncture will be done to confirm the diagnosis and to obtain a specimen for culture and sensitivity testing. The tap may also have a therapeutic effect by lowering the ICP.

Infection from extracranial sources also seriously threatens neurologic function and life. Comatose clients or those with limited mobility are especially prone to pneumonia and urinary tract infections. In addition, invasive monitoring and infusion lines predispose clients to bacteremia and septicemia.

If infection occurs, prompt, adequate, and appropriate antibiotic therapy is essential. Treat the temperature elevation and headache as previously described in the section on intracranial pressure. Carefully monitor input and output and serum electrolyte levels. Attempt to maintain an adequate fluid and caloric intake. To protect staff and other clients, observe appropriate infection control precautions.

SEIZURES Seizure precautions should be instituted on all clients following supratentorial craniotomy or craniectomy. In many clients, the risk is minimal but should always be anticipated if the client is known to have any history of seizure activity, if the surgery involves the frontotemporal area, or if there has been a large amount of cortical manipulation or resection. Trauma, especially if cortical damage was inflicted, and subarachnoid or intracerebral hemorrhage may also increase the likelihood of a postoperative seizure.

Anticonvulsant medications are almost routinely ordered postoperatively, and administration is often instituted preoperatively to ensure an adequate blood level during the period immediately following surgery.

A seizure in the early postoperative period may signal an intracranial complication such as meningitis or a hematoma. The seizure, which results in increased venous and arterial blood pressure and ICP, may precipitate an intracranial hemorrhage. Observations regarding the nature of the seizure activity should be documented and immediately reported to the surgeon. For more specific details on care of the client with seizures, see the section on seizure disorders earlier in this chapter.

CEREBROSPINAL FLUID LEAKAGE Leakage of CSF from the wound or from the nose or ear is a serious threat because microorganisms can enter the skull through whatever opening allows the escape of CSF. If fluid leaks from the ear or nose, attempt to obtain a sample of the fluid and do not place packs in the ear or nose. CSF is glucose positive and can easily be tested with a chemical reagent strip used to check the glucose content of urine. For the test to be valid, the fluid sample should be free of blood, because blood also tests glucose positive.

If fluid is leaking from the wound edges, reinforce or change the dressing as necessary to keep it dry and prevent contamination. If endotracheal suctioning is required, do it via the mouth rather than the nose. Because of significant risk of infection, be alert to any rise in temperature, neck stiffness, or increased headache.

Conservative management includes measures to decrease ICP (discussed previously) in the hope that the leak will seal spontaneously. Frequent or daily spinal taps may be done to drain CSF and keep the ICP low. Acetazolamide (Diamox) may be given to decrease CSF production.

Additional skin and/or galeal sutures may be required to stop leakage. Many leaks seal without the need for surgery. When leakage persists following an adequate trial of conservative therapy, re-exploration of the wound may be necessary to repair the dural defect.

LATER POSTOPERATIVE CARE The client without any serious neurologic sequelae usually progresses through the postoperative phase much as any client who has undergone a major general surgical procedure. Diet is usually increased as tolerated, and most clients are taking a regular diet by the second postoperative day. Ambulation is begun early, with many clients out of bed in a chair on the day after surgery. Monitoring devices and lines as well as intravenous infusions are usually discontinued after 48 hours. The urinary catheter is removed as soon as the client is able to use a bedpan, commode, or toilet. Because postoperative edema usually reaches its peak between 48 and 72 hours, reduction of the steroid dosage is begun on about the third or fourth day. Clients undergoing postoperative radiation therapy usually remain on steroids during treatment because the radiation often results in cerebral edema. While still hospitalized, the client's level of physical activity will gradually increase.

DISCHARGE TEACHING Discharge teaching should include a warning regarding too rapid an increase in activity. During the first week or so at home, the client will tire easily and need a nap or rest by late afternoon. Reassure the client that this is normal, that strength and endurance will increase daily, and that it may take a few weeks before a feeling of well-being returns. Involve the family and include both oral and written instructions in discharge teaching. (Refer to Table 29–5.)

Instruct the caregivers to assess the home carefully before bringing the neurologically impaired client home. Loose throw rugs and low furniture that could prove to be hazards to the client should be removed. Caution caregivers to avoid frequent environmental changes, however, to avoid further confusing a disoriented client.

In assessing a client's potential for future adjustment, remember adjustment largely depends on the extent of the impairment. Adaptation to disability does not really begin until after the person returns home and makes the necessary adjustments. Often the involvement of the social worker and other allied health professionals is necessary to make appropriate referrals and arrangements to ensure a smooth transition from hospital to home or other health care facility.

Suboccipital Craniectomy

A *suboccipital craniectomy* involves the removal of a portion of the posterior occipital bone. Because the muscles of the neck are thick enough to protect the underlying brain, the bone is usually removed and discarded.

This approach is indicated for lesions involving the infratentorial portion of the brain, those structures that lie beneath the tentorium. It allows access to the contents of the posterior fossa including the cerebellum, brain stem, fourth ventricle, and the lower cranial nerves. The approach is also used to expose and treat aneurysms and vascular malformations involving the vertebral arteries and the posterior branches of the circle of Willis. CN V through CN XII can be visualized, and tumors arising from or surrounding them can be excised. These nerves can be decompressed or interrupted for the relief of pain or spasm (eg, trigeminal or glossopharyngeal neuralgia or hemifacial spasm).

During the operative procedure, it is frequently necessary to manipulate the cerebellum, cranial nerves, and the structures adjacent to the brain stem. The specific implications and potential complications related to the anatomic structures within the posterior fossa will be discussed in this section and are summarized in Table 29–6.

Nursing Implications

PREOPERATIVE CARE Specific nursing measures for clients undergoing suboccipital craniectomy depend on the neurologic manifestations of the disease. The general nursing interventions outlined in the previous section on supratentorial craniotomy also apply.

Depending on the size, location, and nature of the posterior fossa lesion, clients require varying degrees of vigilance for respiratory status. Lesions that compress or distort the brain stem or produce hydrocephalus place the client at greater risk of sudden medullary compression. Vascular lesions also present a special danger because a sudden episode of bleeding can precipitate respiratory failure. Clients with cerebellar hemangioblastomas may also be at risk because the size of these cystic lesions tends to fluctuate. The preoperative unit should be equipped with equipment for emergency intubation and ventilatory support. The client at risk should be placed on an apnea monitor as a precaution. The client and family should be prepared for the possible need for intubation and mechanical ventilation in the immediate postoperative period.

Client/Family Teaching

Both client and family need to be prepared for what may be a complicated postoperative course. Try to determine the level of understanding. Accurate perceptions should be reinforced, misconceptions clarified, and realistic expectations stressed.

Some clients with benign lesions may be admitted for a diagnostic work-up and readmitted later for surgery. When elective posterior fossa surgery is planned, it can be suggested that the male client grow a beard (the beard will, to some extent, disguise or conceal a postoperative facial weakness or paralysis) and that the female client allow her hair to grow as long as possible before the surgery. Often, hair not directly in the operative field can be secured out of the way. Postoperatively, the hair will cover the operative scar and the shaved area. This improvement in appearance may be especially helpful to the client suffering a severely altered body image as a result of facial paralysis.

Document the preoperative body weight in case a tracheostomy and some alternative means of feeding (nasogastric tube, gastrostomy, or hyperalimentation) may be necessary to protect the tracheobronchial tree and to provide adequate nutrition.

The client with lost or impaired hearing on one side who is now at risk of losing hearing on the other side needs to be prepared for the possibility of total deafness. Alternative means of communication should be established and practiced during the preoperative period.

POSTOPERATIVE CARE Except for seizure precautions, all of the nursing measures outlined in the previous section on supratentorial craniotomy/craniectomy are generally applicable. An intraoperative ventricular tap constitutes a supratentorial operation, however. It may, therefore, carry a minimal risk of postoperative seizures and bleeding within the cerebral hemisphere.

HEMORRHAGE AND EDEMA Hemorrhage or edema within the posterior fossa is even more dangerous than in the cerebral hemisphere because of the vital local structures. Because rapid herniation can occur with little or no warning and without decline in the level of consciousness, vigilant monitoring of respiratory status is imperative. Carefully observe the respiratory rate and pattern and monitor blood gases regularly. Any irregularity, especially slowing of the rate with periods of apnea, may be evidence of impending respiratory arrest and should be reported immediately. An apnea monitor is advisable following operative manipulation of the brain stem or the anterior–inferior cerebellar artery or when posterior fossa sur-

Table 29–6
Suboccipital Craniectomy: Implications for the Client 

The implications are similar to those for a supratentorial intracranial procedure (see Table 33–2) except that in a suboccipital craniectomy, seizures are absent and normal intellectual function is preserved.

Physiologic Implications	Psychosocial/Lifestyle Implications
The high concentration of vital structures within a small area make posterior fossa surgery especially hazardous	Ataxia may impair mobility and necessitate rehabilitation, ambulatory aids, and assistance with ADL. Bilateral damage may prove incapacitating
Permanent or transient ipsilateral dysfunction can be caused by the lesion itself or operative manipulation of the cerebellum, brain stem, or specific cranial nerves	Clients with damage to CN V need to protect and care for the affected eye
Some degree of cranial nerve dysfunction is to be anticipated following surgical manipulation. It can be permanent or transient, depending on the condition of the nerve	The deformity from CN VII paralysis, whether transient or permanent, often has a profound effect on body image. Some degree of depression can be expected. Following anastomosis or nerve grafting, retraining exercises may be required
CN V dysfunction results in lost or decreased corneal sensation that predisposes the client to keratitis; manipulation of CN V or its ganglion can result in painless, noninfectious herpes simplex eruptions on the affected side of the face; damage to the motor branch of CN V results in weakness of the muscles of mastication	Loss of hearing from damage to CN VIII causes significant lifestyle changes; bilateral damage to the vestibular branches of CN VIII may be incapacitating
Dissection of CN VI results in diplopia that may last several months	Loss of CN IX and CN X function may lead to permanent dependence on tracheostomy and/or gastrostomy. This requires significant lifestyle alterations for client and family. It may also interfere with placement of the client in a rehabilitation center or nursing home
Damage to CN VII results in facial paralysis; if anatomically intact, function almost always returns: If not, plastic surgery may be required. Recovery rate is variable and may take up to 2 years	Changes in certain occupations and recreational activities may be necessary
CN VIII is especially sensitive and neural hearing loss is usually permanent; tinnitus, vertigo, or alteration of space perception are usually transient	Body image and self-esteem alterations depend on the type and extent of cranial nerve damage
Loss of CN IX, CN X, and CN XII function that occurs in younger clients or is gradual is usually compensated for well. Dysphagia and loss of the gag reflex predispose the client to aspiration	Psychosocial/lifestyle impact also depends on the prognosis for the underlying disease
Lateral exposures, which involve opening the mastoid cavity, carry a higher risk of CSF leak	Loss of function may cause anxiety
The risk of GI hemorrhage from stress or Cushing's ulcer is somewhat higher following posterior fossa surgery	Mental health counseling may be required for severe anxiety or prolonged depression
Damage during surgery to the anterior inferior cerebellar artery carries a significant risk of fatal brain stem infarction	Cranial defects difficult to conceal may alter body image and cause apprehension; may require wearing a football helmet or other protective headgear
Compression of the respiratory center in the brain stem (ie, by edema or hematoma) can result in respiratory arrest that occurs with little or no warning and without a decline in the level of consciousness	
Potential complications include: hemorrhage/hematoma; increased ICP; herniation resulting in respiratory arrest; infection; CSF leak; hydrocephalus; GI hemorrhage; ataxia	

gery is combined with any dissection of the upper cervical spinal cord.

Be alert to other warning signs, which may include neck pain or stiffness and tingling in the arms on neck extension as a result of pressure on the cervical cord. Some clients may faint if they move the head too far. This movement probably raises pressure by completing the block to CSF circulation in addition to causing pressure directly on the medulla (Jennett & Galbraith, 1983). Headache, especially with vomiting, may also be a warning sign. Hiccups may be an early sign of medullary irritation, especially if associated with respiratory irregularity, such as sighing. Equipment for emergency intubation and ventilatory support should be readily available. Because respiratory arrest is frequently rapidly followed by cardiac arrest, a defibrilator and the necessary drugs and solutions should also be accessible.

In the early postoperative period, if the wound appears tense and bulging, hematoma is usually suspected. The surgeon is likely to re-explore the wound to decompress the brain stem and achieve hemostasis. Edema is treated with the measures outlined in the previous section. Ventricular drainage may be instituted or a ventricular shunting system inserted to relieve hydrocephalus.

Unless otherwise ordered, the head of the bed should be elevated to at least 30°. Turn the client every 2 hours. Although the bone has been removed, the neck muscles provide sufficient protection for the underlying brain, and there are usually no special positioning precautions or restrictions.

PAIN These clients may have more postoperative pain than clients who have undergone a supratentorial operation because of the incision through the neck muscles. Head movement can be painful during the first few days. Take care to maintain the head in alignment when turning the body and to provide support for the neck area when the client is moving or turning. Mild analgesics usually provide sufficient relief, and the client is usually reasonably comfortable as long as movements of the head and neck are limited.

CRANIAL NERVE DYSFUNCTION Cardiac irregularity in the early postoperative period may be the result of manipulation of CN IX or CN X or may be secondary to a central venous catheter within the right atrium. The location of the tip of the catheter can usually be determined by chest x-ray. The irregularity can often be reversed almost immediately if the catheter is withdrawn a few inches.

To protect the tracheobronchial tree, no oral intake should be permitted until the gag reflex can be checked. Once the gag reflex, swallowing, and cough have been assessed, the initial intake should be supervised by the physician or an experienced nurse. Suction apparatus should be immediately available. Swallowing should first be tested by a small sip of water so that if aspiration occurs, it will cause little harm.

Because of the delicacy of neural tissues, some degree of paresis is always anticipated when the surgical procedure involves manipulation of cranial nerves. The degree and duration of the dysfunction greatly influence the nursing care plan.

Because of its anatomic location, damage to CN III is unusual but may be seen following dissection of lesions that extend high along the tentorial margin. Isolated dysfunction of CN IV is relatively rare but is difficult to recognize clinically. When dysfunction occurs, the diplopia is usually mild. The client can learn to compensate for it by tilting the head slightly so the visual images fuse. Damage to CN VI (the abducens nerve) interferes with outward movement of the eye. Diplopia is most severe with lateral gaze to the affected side. If the nerve is anatomically intact, recovery is usually complete but may take several months. Treatment consists of alternating eye patches to eliminate one visual image. If there is a CN III palsy, no cover will be necessary as long as ptosis is present. If diplopia is accompanied by damage of CN V or CN VII, the affected eye will be patched rather than using alternating patches.

Cotton ophthalmic eye patches are contraindicated for the client with damage to the ophthalmic division of CN V: the client without corneal sensation may be unable to detect a partially opened lid, and the cotton gauze irritates or abrades the cornea. Instead, the eye should be taped closed or covered with a cone of stiff paper or other material that covers the eye without actually touching it. A piece of exposed x-ray film is a suitable material. Transparent coverage for the eye that allows for binocular vision as well as assessment of pupillary function and extraocular movements is available. It also traps moisture, providing an additional degree of protection and comfort for the eye. These features can be especially beneficial when the client also has a facial nerve paresis or paralysis that markedly decreases lacrimation and the inability to raise the lower lid to close the eye adequately. For the client with diplopia, an opaque eye covering that eliminates one visual image may be preferable. In such cases, tape can be placed on the outside of the shield to render it opaque. If facial nerve function is intact and the client has adequate lid closure, the eye need only be shielded or taped closed during sleep or if the level of consciousness is depressed.

Lubricate the eye with artificial tears or some other ophthalmic lubricant every 4 hours, and inspect it for redness or signs of irritation or infection. If the condition is expected to be long term or permanent, teach the client to inspect the eye with a mirror every morning and evening and to seek medical attention if any redness is noted. The client will need to tape the eye closed or wear a shield for sleep. Eyeglasses that incorporate a side piece (moist chamber) should be worn outdoors to protect the eye from foreign bodies. Contact lenses are contraindicated.

Most clients soon learn to compensate for the chewing difficulty that results from damage to the motor portion of CN V by chewing on the opposite side. In the initial recovery period, foods that require extensive chewing should be avoided. Loss of sensation from the sensory portion of CN V can predispose the client to injury to the tongue, lips, and buccal mucosa. After the client eats, check the mouth for pockets of food retained on the anesthetized side. Frequent mouth care is essential, and the mouth should be inspected daily for any signs of ulceration or infection. Teach the client to continue these practices at home. Regular dental care is also imperative because tooth decay and periodontal disease can go undetected because of the lack of pain.

Following operations that involve manipulation of CN V or its ganglion, cutaneous lesions of herpes simplex can be expected about the fourth postoperative day. Reassure the client that they are painless, noninfectious, and will resolve in a week or so without scarring or any other sequelae and will not recur. Also reassure family members, other clients, and staff members that these lesions are not contagious and that there is no need to isolate or otherwise restrict the client.

Damage to CN VII affects a number of functions (Figure 29–3). Resulting facial paralysis causes the mouth to droop on the affected side and causes difficulty with eating and drinking. Liquids often present the greatest problem. Most clients learn to compensate by tilting the head slightly and using the unaffected side. The impaired taste sensation on the anterior two-thirds of the affected side of the tongue and decreased salivation are often not troublesome enough to disturb the client or interfere with adequate nutritional intake. Speech may be slightly slurred because of mouth droop, but the deficit is mild and compensated for quickly. Faint flickers of movement of the lower lid can sometimes be observed when the client forcibly attempts to close the eye. This usually signals the start of recovery of function. If the flickers are observed early in the postoperative period, recovery often occurs rapidly (within days or weeks) and provides encouragement for the client.

In the early postoperative period, it may be difficult to assess damage to CN VIII because of hemotympanum (blood behind the eardrum). The client with hemotympanum usually feels fullness or stuffiness in the ear and speech sounds are muffled. The process is self-limiting and requires no treatment. Caution the client against forceful nose blowing. Nasal decongestants may increase comfort by reducing the stuffiness. If hearing is present, it will usually improve as the fluid is absorbed. If blood or fluid drains from the external canal, allow it to drain freely. Packs or irrigation should never be used. Examination with an otoscope may predispose to infection. As a general rule, the ear should be left alone for at least 6 weeks, after which crusting or exudate can be gently cleansed and the eardrum adequately inspected.

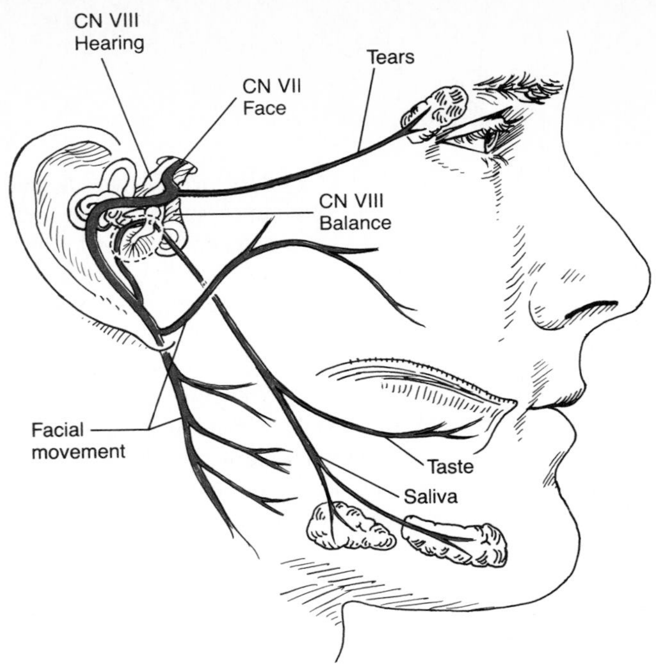

Figure 29–3

Areas affected by facial nerve injury.

Stressing realistic expectations for hearing is important. Neural hearing loss is almost always irreversible. Cochlear implants do not function if CN VIII is absent and offer no hope in this situation. When any amount of hearing is present preoperatively, testing is usually done to provide a baseline for postoperative comparison. Hearing loss secondary to neural damage is most often characterized by loss of speech discrimination rather than loss of volume. Often, the person may be unaware of gradual loss. These clients often find they have switched the ear with which they use the telephone without even realizing it. Strategies to use when talking with hearing-impaired clients are discussed in Chapter 51.

Clients with tinnitus can be referred to hearing specialists who can recommend devices designed to mask tinnitus. Occasionally, the problem is so distressing that the surgeon will re-explore the wound and intentionally section the nerve. Unfortunately, in some instances the tinnitus persists even after the nerve has been cut.

Encourage clients who have lost the vestibular portion of CN VIII to use touch and sight to compensate for the loss. Teach them to avoid quick head turns or sudden movements. The elderly client or one with any degree of visual impairment or cerebellar ataxia may need help with ambulation. Handrails may be helpful, and the home should be cleared of clutter to protect the client from injuries. Bilateral vestibular loss can usually be managed as long as the person is able to maintain visual orientation to the environment. To prevent injury, a night light should be left on or within easy reach at the bedside.

The degree of dysfunction resulting from impaired

function of CN IX, CN X, and CN XII may vary. The combination of functional impairment of the pharynx and vocal cords results in the loss of adequate airway protection and makes the client especially susceptible to spillage of pharyngeal contents into the trachea. A primary goal of nursing management is to prevent aspiration. Suction apparatus should be available at the bedside at all times. Once the client is able to participate in self-care, the suction should be kept within easy reach and the client encouraged to suction the mouth as often as necessary.

A client with swallowing difficulty should always be fed in the upright position and supervised closely the entire time. Fluids are generally more difficult to handle. Most clients are better able to manage soft or semisolid foods because these stimulate the swallowing reflex. Instruct the client to place the food on the unaffected side and to tilt the head in that direction. Provide a calm, comfortable, nondistracting environment and allow the client as much time as necessary. Care should be taken that the client does not become overtired because fatigue makes swallowing more difficult.

Monitor input and output and daily weight and evaluate the caloric and nutritional adequacy of oral intake. If caloric or nutritional intake is not adequate, nasogastric feedings or hyperalimentation may be necessary. If the swallowing deficit is expected to be long term or permanent, gastrostomy may be considered. Follow oral feedings with mouth care and inspect the mouth carefully because food tends to be trapped on the affected side.

Clients with severe or long-lasting deficits may require tracheostomy to facilitate adequate pulmonary toilet. The combination of tracheostomy and upper gastrointestinal feeding can be especially hazardous. To prevent soiling of the tracheobronchial tree, the cuff on the tracheostomy tube should be inflated. The client should be maintained in an erect position during feeding and for at least 30 minutes afterward to lessen the danger of gastric regurgitation and aspiration.

Because phonation depends on the action of the musculature of the tongue, lips, pharynx, larynx, and soft palate, many clients also experience varying degrees of dysarthria. Speech is often slurred and indistinct. Damage to the vagus nerve may result in vocal cord paralysis that results in a hoarse, raspy, and sometimes barely audible voice. The person with a long-standing deficit needs to be treated with genuine concern by the nursing staff as well as family and significant others. Recognize the client's frustration and be accepting of anger or depression. Maintain a calm, relaxed, and unhurried environment. Remember that comprehension is usually intact. Although communication should be kept brief and simple, treat the person as an adult and avoid using "baby talk." Encourage clients' efforts to speak and praise them for any success, regardless how small. Use alternative methods of communication as necessary. Speech therapy is often helpful but as a general rule should not be instituted until the person expresses readiness. The client and family can also be taught environmental management, support behavior, and behaviors to enhance communication (Boss, 1984).

Ataxia is frequently aggravated by surgery and may interfere with early ambulation. On the other hand, recovery, especially in younger clients, is often remarkable, and the condition is usually temporary. For other clients, some degree of disability may be permanent. For them, physical therapy is usually necessary. Rehabilitation is directed at the restoration of mobility and self-care.

Antacids and cimetidine should be administered with steroids because of the risk of Curling's stress ulcer and gastrointestinal hemorrhage. Carefully monitor blood pressure, hematocrit, and hemoglobin levels. Frequent or daily examination of stool for occult blood may detect gastrointestinal bleeding early.

CSF accumulation in the tissues of the operative area is easily recognizable: The wound appears to bulge and is soft and fluctuant to touch. The nursing measures are described in the previous section on craniotomy and craniectomy.

In the absence of complications, the usual postoperative course is similar to that of the client undergoing a craniotomy. Late complications may include infection, hydrocephalus, CSF leak, and tumor recurrence. Discharge teaching should include preparing the client and family to manage any postoperative deficits or complications.

Cranioplasty

Cranioplasty is the surgical correction of a defect in the cranial vault. This procedure usually involves insertion of a substitute material that has been prepared and shaped to fit into or over the defective area. It may be done as part of the closure of a craniectomy or as a separate procedure.

Cranioplasty is most often done to protect the intracranial contents or to improve the client's appearance. The procedure may also be performed to relieve headaches, vertigo, and the local tenderness and throbbing that sometimes occurs when the bone flap has been left out after craniectomy.

Repair of a bony defect may be indicated following extensive or comminuted skull fractures or when osteomyelitis, radiation necrosis, or erosion or invasion of a bone flap by a tumor necessitate removal of the bone flap. In fact, these complications may occur several years after the original surgical procedure or radiotherapy. When markedly increased ICP precludes replacement of the bone flap, a secondary cranioplasty is often required.

The client's own bone flap may be placed in a sterile container at the time of original surgery for later use. Or, an autogenous graft of other bone or cartilage may be used. In most instances, however, a foreign substance is used. Methyl methacrylate, a synthetic acrylic substance that is inert and causes no tissue reaction, has simplified cranioplasty procedures. It can be molded to the desired shape, contour, and thickness, placed over the defect, and allowed to harden.

A modification of this procedure uses a sheet of wire mesh (usually stainless steel) that is cut, molded, and secured to the prepared bone edge and then impregnated with methyl methacrylate.

In the past, metal plates of stainless steel, tantalum, or Vitallium were common. Incompatibility between the metal alloys in the plate and the metal alloys in the screws used to fix the plates to the surrounding skull can lead to a reaction that eventually erodes the bone. Metal plates are also radiopaque, which presents difficulties if the client requires radiologic studies or if the lesion necessitates follow-up with x-ray or CT scanning. Because of their magnetic properties, these plates preclude use of magnetic resonance imaging (MRI) as a diagnostic tool. If metal plates are used, they should be nonmagnetic, or the client should be warned never to have an MRI scan.

The physiologic and psychosocial/lifestyle implications are discussed in Table 29–7.

Nursing Implications

PREOPERATIVE CARE Preoperative preparation is basically the same as for a client undergoing a craniotomy or craniectomy although usually not as extensive. As with any intracranial procedure, a baseline neurologic assessment should be performed and well documented to assess the postoperative condition adequately. The client's blood should be typed and possibly cross-matched. Clients, especially those with a history of headaches, should be questioned regarding aspirin use. Report any recent use to the physician. Encourage the client to express fears and expectations. Reinforce realistic expectations about relief of symptoms and cosmetic results.

Unless there are existing medical problems (eg, heart, pulmonary, or renal disease), arterial and central venous lines are not often used. Because little or no brain retraction is usually required and because it is desirable to maintain the normal contour of the brain, osmotic diuretics are often withheld.

POSTOPERATIVE CARE Postoperatively, cranioplasty clients usually do not require intensive care management unless there are serious underlying medical problems. Because the cranial vault has been entered, however, the usual vital signs and neurologic status should be monitored for at least 24 hours. The urinary catheter can usually be removed as soon as the client is awake and alert. Steroids and anticonvulsants may be ordered. Seizure precautions should be observed if the client has a history of seizures of if the surgery involved the frontal or temporal area.

Clients with cranioplastic plates sometimes develop subgaleal fluid collections. Often the fluid collection is worse

Table 29–7
Cranioplasty: Implications for the Client

Physiologic Implications	Psychosocial/Lifestyle Implications
Because the cranial cavity is entered but there is usually little or no manipulation of the intracranial contents, edema and an accompanying decline in neurologic status should not be expected unless extensive dissection was required	Relief of apprehension, enhanced self-esteem, and improvement in physical appearance
Skin sutures left in place for about 2 weeks	Occasionally a client not at risk following craniectomy may require cranioplasty to relieve the apprehension associated with the cranial defect to be able to resume normal activities
The most frequent complication is infection, which is usually local but can lead to meningitis	Postoperative cranioplasty infection can prove very disruptive because of the need for prolonged antibiotic therapy, repeat hospitalization, and reoperation
Resection of dura and/or a foreign body reaction may lead to the development of a subgaleal fluid collection over the cranioplasty site	Hospitalization for approximately one week
Autogenous bone may undergo some degree of absorption	Need to wait 6–12 months following infection to replace the cranioplasty plate can severely disrupt lifestyle, exhaust financial reserves, and often results in some degree of depression
Clients with metal plates may experience headaches associated with extremes of heat or cold	Cosmetic results may not always live up to the client's expectations resulting in disappointment and depression
A blow of sufficient force to shatter bone will also shatter acrylic plates; reinforcement with wire adds strength to the acrylic plate and reduces the risk of breakage	Disappointment if preoperative symptoms such as headache, throbbing, or local tenderness do not subside following cranioplasty
Repeated operations in the same area may result in devascularization of the skin flap necessitating skin grafting or extensive plastic surgical repair	Concern over long-term effects of repeated operations

in the morning and lessens or disappears completely as the day goes on. This phenomenon probably is related to position, because pressure rises and fluid accumulates during sleep. The accumulation is unsightly and annoying but is usually painless and often subsides gradually without treatment. Treatment is required only if swelling threatens the integrity of the suture line.

Because infection is the main danger, attention to aseptic technique is imperative in any aspect of wound care such as suture removal and caring for the wound drain. The postoperative course progresses rapidly, and the client can usually be discharged within a week. Because the operation involves reopening a previous incision line, the skin sutures are left in place longer than usual—about 2 weeks.

Teach the client and family to care for the incision until sutures are removed in the physician's office or the outpatient department. Discharge teaching should include symptoms and signs of infection. Any inflammation, tenderness, or wound drainage should be reported to the physician.

Spinal Cord Tumors

Spinal cord tumors are classified not only by their histologic type but by their relation to the dura and spinal cord. They are of two principal kinds:

- Extradural tumors, which lie outside the dura; usually metastatic
- Intradural tumors, subdivided into extramedullary (within the dura but not within the spinal cord itself) and intramedullary (within the substance of the spinal cord)

Meningiomas and neurofibromas are the most common *intradural extramedullary* tumors. Meningiomas are most frequent in the thoracic region and much more prevalent in women. Neurofibromas can occur at any level. Because they arise from the nerve root, they can be intradural, extradural, or a combination. Both meningiomas and neurofibromas are benign, slow growing, and most prevalent in the fourth through sixth decades of life. They grow between the spinal cord and dura and slowly displace the cord.

Intramedullary cord tumors are relatively rare. The majority of these tumors arise from the connective tissue cells of the CNS, particularly the ependymal cells that line the central canal of the spinal cord and the astrocytes. Ependymomas may be totally intramedullary, usually forming an encapsulated, well-demarcated lesion that expands the cord, or they may involve the cauda equina. Astrocytomas vary in their degree of malignancy and resectability. Some are reasonably well demarcated whereas others infiltrate between all the viable fibers of the cord. Infiltrating tumors are unresectable because, unlike the brain where certain areas of nervous tissue can be sacrificed without causing significant damage, no such leeway exists within the spinal cord (Jennett & Galbraith, 1983).

Clinical Manifestations

Metastatic tumors of the spine cause epidural compression of the spinal cord. Metastases rarely occur to the cord itself or to the epidural tissue but generally occur in the vertebrae. They cause compression either by progressive growth with gradual cord compression or by destruction of the vertebrae with sudden collapse and sudden compression of the cord. With the sudden compression, paraplegia or quadriplegia occurs within hours, or even instantaneously depending on the level of the lesion. Pain at the site of the collapse is often agonizing. Sometimes the symptoms develop over hours or days but may have been preceded by a week or so of backache.

Total motor and sensory loss with sudden vertebral collapse is rarely recoverable, regardless of the treatment, and surgical intervention is not usually indicated. On the other hand, slowly progressive paralysis from continued tumor growth is usually diagnosed while some function remains, and appropriate treatment may lead to significant recovery. The most frequently affected site is the thoracic spine, and the most common lesions are from lung, breast, and prostate cancers. Some clients have no known primary malignant lesion. Even after histologic confirmation and extensive diagnostic investigation, evidence of the primary site may not become evident before their death.

The symptoms and signs of meningiomas and neurofibromas include root pain and progressive paresis, usually with a partial Brown–Séquard syndrome (ie, loss of vibration and position sense below the level of the lesion ipsilaterally and loss of the perception of pain and temperature contralaterally), when they occur in the cervical and thoracic regions.

Lumbar neuromas often present a clinical picture similar to that of a herniated disk. Because of slow growth, symptoms may develop over years before treatment is sought. The diagnosis is confirmed by CT scan, myelography, or both. In the client with neurofibromatosis, the possibility of multiple tumors, both meningiomas and neurofibromas as well as intramedullary lesions, should be considered. A full laminectomy is done and usually extends a level above and below the lesion.

Intramedullary cord tumors enlarge the cord and interfere with its function by destroying cord parenchyma from within or by pressure on surrounding normal cord. They usually first damage the sensory fibers of the spinothalamic tract, which crosses in the center of the cord, producing a band of sensory loss in the cutaneous distribution corresponding to the level of the lesion. The client loses the appreciation of pain and temperature, whereas the sensation of light touch, which travels in the uncrossed tracts of the dorsal columns, remains intact. As the lesion enlarges, it interferes with the vertically running fiber tracts within the cord and causes motor weakness, which is of an upper motor neuron type. The diagnosis is usually made by myelography, which demonstrates the widened cord.

Medical and Specific Nursing Measures

Care of the client undergoing spinal surgery is covered below. General care of the client with a malignancy is found in Chapter 10.

Spinal Surgery

Most neurosurgery of the spine is aimed at relieving *compression.* Although the most frequent spinal operation is the resection of a herniated lumbar disk, there are numerous other conditions for which a laminectomy is performed. These include the treatment of injuries such as fractures and dislocations; excision of tumors and vascular malformations; drainage of abscesses and hematomas; correction of deformity or disease of the vertebral bodies; repair of congenital malformations; and for bony compression of the cord or nerve roots due to narrow canal syndrome or arthritic bone-spur formation. Although less common, laminectomy may also be performed for the insertion of a subarachnoid shunt, for lysis of arachnoidal adhesions, and for the treatment of intractable pain by the sectioning of posterior nerve roots (rhizotomy) or the interruption of spinothalamic fiber tracts within the cord (cordotomy).

The traditional laminectomy for the treatment of herniated lumbar disk is discussed in Chapter 46. In recent years, the large laminectomies and fusions have given way to progressively smaller procedures and in many institutions, these procedures have been replaced by a microsurgical approach. The use of Crutchfield tongs to treat cervical fractures or dislocations is discussed later in the section on spinal cord injury and in Chapter 45.

Microlumbar Diskectomy

Surgery for the removal of a herniated lumbar disk is the most common spinal operation and the eighth most common operation in the United States. Approximately 200,000 operative disk procedures are done annually (Maroon & Abla, 1985).

Microlumbar diskectomy is the microsurgical technique used in the treatment of a lumbar disk. This procedure does not involve a laminectomy, the incision is much smaller, there is less soft tissue and muscle dissection, and there is minimal alteration of the lumbar spine.

Because the skin incision is small (1-inch), it must be placed precisely over the involved interspace. Most often, skin sutures are not used. Instead, the wound edges are approximated and held together with sterile wound tapes. Blood loss is ordinarily less than 50 mL. Physiologic and psychosocial/lifestyle implications are discussed in Table 29–8.

Nursing Implications

PREOPERATIVE CARE Preoperative preparation includes the standard measures and teaching appropriate for any surgical client. A thorough assessment of motor and sensory function as well as the characteristics and distribution of the pain should be documented for postoperative comparison. Analgesics and muscle relaxants are frequently prescribed, and steroids may also be administered to reduce the nerve root irritation. Because straining aggravates pain by increasing intrathecal pressure, stool softeners are often ordered. Because most clients have pain, they should be asked about prolonged or recent use of aspirin.

POSTOPERATIVE CARE Some surgeons prefer to have the client remain flat in bed for 2 hours postoperatively to promote hemostasis. Most allow the client to assume whatever position is most comfortable and to be out of bed as soon as completely recovered from the anesthesia. Immediate assessment includes motor and sensory testing and comparison of the findings with the preoperative status. Question the client about the relief or persistence of back and leg pain. Monitor vital signs as for any postsurgical client.

Although damage to the great vessels is rare and is usually discovered at surgery, it can cause retroperitoneal hematoma that may not be detected for several hours until the client develops a mass or exhibits signs of shock. Although impairment of blood supply to the lower extremities is also rare, assess vascular status of the legs. Check the dressing for any sign of bleeding or CSF leakage.

Assess the bladder for distention. Notify the physician if the client does not void within 6 hours following surgery. Allowing the male client to stand to void or encouraging the female client to get out of bed and use the toilet is often sufficient to stimulate voiding. If not present preoperatively, bladder dysfunction is rare following disk surgery but can occur as a result of manipulation of the cauda equina nerve roots and is usually transient. As with any neurosurgical client, any decline in function from the immediate postoperative status or any acute increase in pain should be promptly reported.

Most clients have less pain after the operation than before. Narcotics are rarely necessary unless the client has a psychologic or physiologic dependence on them. Because the stability of the spine has not been affected, logrolling (turning the client as a unit) is not necessary. Clients are often apprehensive about movement, fearing that they can do damage or that movement will precipitate pain. They need to be reassured and encouraged to ambulate as soon as possible.

Table 29–8
Microlumbar Diskectomy: Implications for the Client

Physiologic Implications	Psychosocial/Lifestyle Implications
Relief of pain and recovery of function vary depending on the degree and duration of preoperative compression; when sciatica has persisted for years, the nerve root may be so damaged that some degree of pain, sensory loss, or decreased DTRs may persist indefinitely	Lifestyle is usually enhanced by the relief of chronic or recurrent back and sciatic pain
Following cauda equina compression, motor recovery is gradual but often continues over a period of 18 months or more; control of bladder function is regained slowly and recovery may be incomplete	Most clients require no analgesics, can ambulate immediately, and are discharged on the second or third postoperative day
80%–90% of clients make a complete recovery	Sexual activities are not restricted; progressive athletic activities are encouraged
Inflammatory changes in the compressed nerve root may continue to cause postoperative pain before it resolves; persistence or recurrence of sciatic pain after initial postoperative relief may indicate recurrent herniation	Muscle-strengthening exercises may be required
Incisional pain is minimal and stability of the spine remains intact	Heavy manual labor and strenuous sports may be restricted for a month or so
Because of immediate ambulation, the risk of complications associated with immobility is low	Long-term follow-up is not necessary
Potential complications include hematoma, infection, CSF leak due to dural perforation, and recurrent disk herniation	Obese clients should be encouraged to begin a weight control program
	Clients with long-term preoperative restriction of activities may need physical therapy or a program of exercises to increase strength and develop supportive musculature

A full regular diet can be resumed as soon as bowel sounds have returned. Ambulation and activities are progressively increased, but some surgeons prefer that the client lie flat while in bed. This measure is taken because the semisitting position with the head of the bed elevated often precipitates muscle spasms in the lower back. Therefore, it is preferable to have clients dangle their legs at the side of the bed or sit in a straight-backed chair.

Most clients are discharged on the third postoperative day. When adhesive strips have been used for skin closure, the client is often instructed to shower after about a week, when the tapes can be removed.

Discharge teaching includes proper body mechanics. Encourage obese clients to begin a program for weight control. Some clients, especially those with long-term preoperative restriction of activity, may require physical therapy or an exercise program to increase strength and develop supportive musculature.

Anterior Cervical Diskectomy

Most often, herniated cervical disks are approached anteriorly through an incision made parallel to the clavicle. If a posterior approach is used, an incision is made much like that described for the microlumbar diskectomy. The physiologic and psychosocial/lifestyle implications are discussed in Table 29–9.

Nursing Implications

PREOPERATIVE CARE Preoperative medical management and nursing care are similar to those for the client with a lumbar herniated disk. The client should avoid excessive flexion, extension, and rotation of the head. Often a cervical collar is worn preoperatively to maintain the neck in alignment and to reduce pain by limiting movement. As with any neurosurgical client, document a baseline motor and sensory assessment. Record the history and description of the pain syndrome. In addition, evaluate the client for muscle wasting or atrophy and difficulty in performing activities of daily living.

POSTOPERATIVE CARE Postoperatively, following a baseline assessment of motor and sensory function, assess neurologic status and vital signs as ordered or as indicated by the client's condition. In most instances, these assessments decrease in frequency as the client's condition improves and are often discontinued or reduced to once per shift after the first 24 hours. Assess swallowing and speech. Inspect the dressing frequently for signs of bleeding, and monitor the neck area closely for swelling or shift in the position of the trachea. Because tracheal compres-

Table 29–9
Anterior Cervical Diskectomy: Implications for the Client 

Physiologic Implications	Psychosocial/Lifestyle Implications
Herniated cervical disk may cause spinal cord compression as well as nerve root pressure; recovery depends on the degree and duration of compression	Discharge from the hospital by the third day is likely
Pain is usually minimal	Activities that involve straining or stretching of the cervical spine (such as driving a car) may be restricted for a few weeks
Hoarseness may result from retraction of the trachea or stretching of the recurrent laryngeal nerve; usually resolves within a few days	Activities are usually unrestricted by the end of a month to 6 weeks
Transient dysphagia can occur because of prolonged retraction of the esophagus	Freedom from analgesics, muscle relaxants, and cervical collar
Bleeding and hematoma formation can cause tracheal compression and compromise respirations; esophageal perforation is a rare complication	Unless occupational or leisure activities impose severe strain on the cervical spine, no change in lifestyle is necessary
Since bone removal is minimal, the stability of the spine is not affected unless multiple levels are involved	Clients with long-term preoperative restriction of activities may need physical therapy or a program of exercises to increase strength and develop supportive musculature
Spontaneous fusion usually occurs within 6 months	
Early ambulation lessens the risk of complications related to immobility	

sion can be life threatening, have emergency respiratory support equipment available. Report any decline in function or sharp increase in pain to the physician.

Pain is usually minimal, but steroids, mild analgesics, and muscle relaxants may be necessary. Often, a cervical collar is prescribed for a few days to provide support and minimize muscle movements of the neck. Most often, the client is permitted to ambulate the evening of surgery or the following day. Activities are gradually increased, and the client often is discharged within 3 days.

Activities that involve excessive stretching or straining of the cervical spine (eg, driving, tennis) are restricted for a few weeks, but normal lifestyle can almost always be resumed without restrictions. As with lumbar diskectomy, the client who has had a long period of restricted activity preoperatively may require general muscle-strengthening exercises to achieve optimal function and well-being.

Multilevel Posterior Laminectomy

Multilevel posterior laminectomy is the removal of one or more of the vertebral laminae. Most indications for this procedure involve compression of the spinal cord on its nerve roots because of conditions such as stenosis of the cervical or lumbar canal, spinal cord tumors, or a metastatic lesion from elsewhere in the body.

When the laminectomy is performed for the treatment of spinal stenosis, bone removal is all that is required to treat the condition. Bone removal permits the dural sac to expand backward and eliminate compression of the cord. When underlying pathology is to be treated, the procedure varies from this point on, depending on the lesion and its resectability.

The exposed dura may be covered with a sheet of absorbable gelatin sponge (Gelfoam). Frequently, a wound drain is left in place. Subcutaneous and skin closure is done with separate suture layers. This closure is remarkably strong. After healing is complete, the scar provides adequate protection for the spinal cord, so the absence of the bony structure does not lead to damage or injury. Also remarkable is the fact that this extensive bone removal does not produce significant instability, providing either the anterior or lateral structures are intact. Accordingly, no fusion or stabilization is required. If adequate hemostasis has been maintained throughout the procedure, blood loss is often below the amount that requires replacement. The physiologic and psychosocial/lifestyle implications are discussed in Table 29–10.

Nursing Implications

PREOPERATIVE CARE Clients' needs for preoperative care vary with the degree of functional disability. If the client is able to ambulate, observe the posture and gait. Note impairment or difficulty in carrying out activities of daily living. Test all four extremities for motor strength and sensation, including the perception of pinprick, temperature, light touch, and joint position sense. Examine the skin for evidence of burns, bruises, or scars that might indicate an area of sensory impairment. Document any area of decreased sensation or hyperalgesia (excessive sensitivity) and communicate the findings to other staff members. Appropriate precautions can then be taken to

Table 29–10
Multilevel Posterior Laminectomy: Implications for the Client 

Physiologic Implications	Psychosocial/Lifestyle Implications
Recovery depends on: location, nature, and extent of underlying disease; degree and duration of neurologic impairment; ultimate prognosis for the underlying disease	Improvement in quality of life, especially with spinal stenosis and benign intradural tumors
For spinal stenosis and benign intradural tumors, surgery will halt the progress of neurologic deterioration; recovery of function may be partial or complete	Loss of bowel, bladder, and sexual function greatly affects body image and self-esteem; depression and despair are common
For the client with a metastatic lesion, decompression, if performed early enough, may allow for return of function and maintenance of bowel and bladder control	The need for and type of active rehabilitation varies with the location and degree of dysfunction
Recovery for the client with an intramedullary tumor varies with the malignancy of the tumor and the degree of resectability	Profound lifestyle changes may be required, especially when the onset of dysfunction is sudden and unexpected (ie, trauma, metastatic disease), or when the cervical cord is involved
The client with a slowly developing paralysis (even when complete) may recover a surprising degree of function; improvement may be slow but continues for many months	Grieving over loss of function, regardless of cause, or possibility of death from an as yet undetected malignancy elsewhere in the body
Postoperative pain is severe for about the first 3 days because of extensive muscle dissection	
Bladder and/or bowel function may be temporarily or permanently impaired; respiratory function may be impaired, depending on the level of the lesion	
Clients with foramen magnum or high cervical lesions may develop sleep apnea due to bilateral damage in the area of C-1, which interferes with the normal respiratory response	
Possible complications include: hemorrhage; infection; CSF leak; complications in clients with spinal cord lesions are related to the hazards of immobility or specific motor or sensory deficits	

avoid injury to an insensitive area and to protect the client from unnecessary pain or discomfort when a hyperalgesic area needs to be touched.

Care needs to be taken with the temperature of bath or shower water because decreased sensation can predispose the client to thermal injuries. For the client with a cervical or high thoracic lesion, pay special attention to the status of respiratory function. Question the client about any existing pulmonary problems that might complicate intraoperative or postoperative management. Also assess bowel and bladder function. Question the client about urinary frequency, urgency, dribbling, or retention; constipation or diarrhea; and fecal or urinary incontinence. Male clients may report impotence or difficulty in attaining or maintaining an erection.

The frequency of motor and sensory testing depends on the physician's orders and the client's condition. As with any neurologic condition, any deterioration should promptly be reported.

Although it is relatively rare, be aware that a spinal tap, performed for removal of CSF for diagnostic purposes or for the instillation of contrast material for myelography, can precipitate an acute deterioration in the client's neurologic condition. Deterioration occurs because of alterations in the CSF dynamics; the reduction of pressure below blocks the circulation of CSF within the thecal sac. Immediate surgical decompression is often necessary to prevent catastrophic loss of function.

Preoperative teaching should prepare the client and family for expected postoperative sensations, devices, and routines (eg, monitors, cervical collar, motor and sensory testing). Warn them that incisional pain will be severe, but adequate medication will be provided to maintain comfort. Help them to understand that pain is to be expected and is not an indication of any problem or complication. Also reassure them that the stability of the spine will not be affected and that turning and ambulation, although painful, will not be harmful.

POSTOPERATIVE CARE A baseline assessment of motor and sensory function is done as soon as the client is awake enough to cooperate and to answer questions. Even before this, observe the client's ability to move the extremities, either spontaneously or in response to a stimulus. Response to stimulus also gives some indication of sensory function.

Severe incisional pain is apparent almost immediately after the client's emergence from the anesthetic, and adequate analgesia is needed. If respiratory status is not compromised, intravenous or intramuscular meperidine (Demerol) or morphine may be administered every 3 to 4 hours. With adequate monitoring of blood pressure and respiratory status, a continuous intravenous infusion of morphine may be administered. Using this method, a surprising degree of relief can be achieved with significantly smaller doses than when the drugs are administered intermittently. The dosage is gradually reduced over 2 to 3 days, when oral analgesics are usually sufficient. Steroids are often prescribed to prevent or minimize the cord and nerve-root swelling that results from surgical manipulation.

After surgery in the cervical area, emphasize the assessment of respiratory status. Often, these clients are left intubated until adequate spontaneous respirations can be assured. Following extubation, remain vigilant because edema or bleeding at the operative site can lead to respiratory failure. After the excision of a tumor at the foramen magnum or C-1 to C-2 level, an apnea monitor is advisable because these clients may develop sleep apnea. They breathe adequately while awake, but when they fall asleep their respirations become irregular and they may fail to breathe. The exact mechanism for this phenomenon is unclear, but it is know that the syndrome results from bilateral damage in the C-1 area of the cord, which interferes with the normal respiratory response to a rising blood CO_2 level.

Often, an in-dwelling catheter is left in the bladder during the initial postoperative period. Following its removal, assess bladder function and notify the physician if the client fails to void within 6 hours or if distention occurs. Bladder dysfunction may be transient or permanent and may necessitate the continued use of an in-dwelling catheter, a schedule for intermittent catheterization, or use of Credé's maneuver. (Intermittent catheterization and Credé's maneuver are discussed in Chapter 26.) Bethanechol chloride (Urecholine) may be administered to stimulate the bladder.

When bowel sounds have returned, the client is usually allowed to begin oral intake. Diet is progressed as rapidly as tolerated, and a high-protein, high-vitamin, high-bulk diet is encouraged. Stool softeners or a daily bowel regimen may be necessary to facilitate elimination.

If mobility is impaired, position clients to prevent complications and turn them every 2 hours. Perform active or passive range-of-motion exercises regularly to stimulate circulation, maintain muscle tone, prevent contractures, and maintain joint mobility. Because the stability of the spine has not been impaired, many surgeons do not think that logrolling is necessary. Because movement is painful, however, spinal alignment should be maintained. Clients with extensive incisions may benefit from logrolling in the initial postoperative period. A turning sheet facilitates turning. Unless the client is receiving continuous intravenous pain medication, turning and other potentially painful activities should be scheduled, as much as possible, to coincide with the time when pain medication is at maximum effectiveness. During changes in position, examine the skin for any signs of breakdown and massage areas prone to pressure ulcers to stimulate circulation. Prevention of pressure ulcers is discussed in Chapter 55.

Often the client is ambulated with assistance, if only for a short time, on the first postoperative day. Ambulation, participation in self-care, and other activities progress according to the location and extent of the neurologic dysfunction. When neurologic damage is limited, the client can often be discharged within a week and may resume normal activities within a month to 6 weeks.

A decline in the neurologic condition may indicate a postoperative hemorrhage. A drop in the hemoglobin and hematocrit or changes in vital signs may help to differentiate bleeding from deterioration secondary to swelling or ischemia. Prompt detection is essential so the hematoma can be evacuated and the cord decompressed before permanent damage occurs. In the cervical area, the prompt detection of any decline in respiratory status can be life saving because a hematoma can result in sudden respiratory collapse.

Although the leakage of CSF through the wound is infrequent, the potential for this complication is increased when the dura has not been closed. A CSF leak may be evidenced by frank seepage of fluid through the suture line or by swelling at the operative site. Often, the fluid collection is only apparent when the client is up and about, and subsides or disappears completely when the client lies in bed.

Infection can occur early or late and can be superficial and localized, or the client may exhibit symptoms and signs of meningitis. Most other complications in clients with spinal cord tumors are related to the hazards of immobility or the client's specific motor or sensory deficit.

SECTION VII

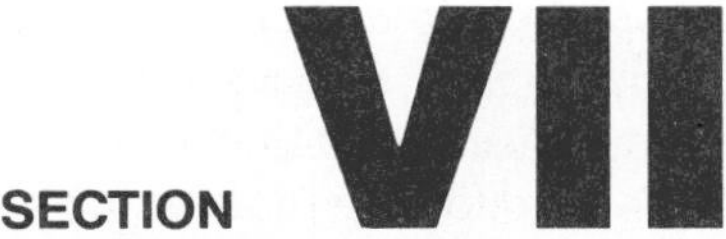

Traumatic Disorders

Craniocerebral trauma is the major cause of death in persons between the ages of 1 and 44 years and contributes to more deaths than strokes in persons aged 45 to 64.

Close to 6.5 million head injuries occur yearly in the United States (Friedman, 1983). There are approximately six to nine thousand new clients with spinal cord injury in the United States. The highest incidence occurs in young, previously healthy men. Serious injury leads to complete incapacitation and emotional devastation for the client and the cost of long-term rehabilitation and maintenance programs have a tremendous impact on the total health care system.

Head Trauma

Serious cerebral injury can result from a number of factors, including motor vehicle, sports, and industrial accidents as well as assaults and falls. Regardless of the nature of the injury, it is important to consider the Monro–Kellie hypothesis (closed-box theory), which states that the skull is a rigid sphere filled to capacity with contents that are basically noncompressible. These components include CSF, the vascular system, and brain tissue. All maintain a fairly constant volume. Therefore, any increase in the volume of one intracranial component occurs at the expense of the others; otherwise, ICP increases. (The theory does not apply to infants, because their skulls are not yet rigid.)

Among the methods for classifying head injuries are mechanism and severity of injury. Mechanisms include direct (acceleration or deceleration) and indirect causes. A direct acceleration injury occurs when the stationary head is struck by a moving object, such as a baseball. A direct deceleration injury occurs when the head in motion strikes an immovable object, such as when a person falls from a bicycle onto the pavement. In an indirect injury, the traumatic force is not directly applied to the head but is usually transmitted through an impact to the neck or buttocks.

Another major classification is closed and open head injury, referring to whether the skull and the dura mater are intact. A closed head injury is a nonpenetrating, blunt injury with no break in the integrity of the skull and dura mater. Severity ranges from slight to moderate to severe. Injuries include scalp bruises or lacerations, depressed fractures with no dural tears, and linear fractures that are undisplaced. Brain concussions (jarring), contusions (bruising), and lacerations (tearing) may occur. Closed head injuries can also result in hemorrhage, cranial nerve injury, and cerebral edema.

An important phenomenon in closed head injury is coup–contrecoup. The *coup injury* is bruising of the brain directly below the point of injury resulting from impact to the skull; there are visible signs of injury. *Contrecoup* refers to the rebound effect of injury, the mass movement of the brain opposite to the site of impact. For example, a blow to the frontal region (coup) causes damage to the occipital region (contrecoup) of the brain. Injuries include lacerations and hemorrhage causing sensory and motor dysfunctions.

In open head trauma, a penetrating injury breaks the integrity of the skull or dura. Cerebral contusions or lacerations occur. The most frequent fractures are linear, at the base of the skull. Depressed and comminuted fractures are less frequent but more serious because of dural tears and lacerations of brain tissue. Infection is a high risk in open head injuries.

Clinical Manifestations

SKULL FRACTURES Clinical findings are related to specific types of skull fractures and brain injuries. The location of a skull fracture is most crucial for determining damage to the underlying structures: the meninges, blood vessels, and the brain itself. Distinction is made between fractures of the cranial vault and the base of the skull. Fractures are classified as linear, comminuted, depressed, compound, and basilar.

Linear skull fractures are usually simple breaks in bone continuity anywhere in the skull. A simple crack or several straight lines appear. Both the outer and inner table of the skull can be affected. These fractures usually cause no problem, but those in the temporal bone can damage the middle meningeal artery and cause epidural bleeding. *Comminuted skull fractures* are multiple fragmentations of the bone. When these involve the inner table of the skull, bone fragments can be driven into the dura or brain. These structures may be compressed or torn. *Depressed skull fractures* are caused by trauma from sharper, penetrating injuries. Brain lacerations and infections are common. Less serious forms of these fractures are caused by blunter objects that do not fragment the inner table of the skull. A *compound skull fracture* is a scalp laceration along with a depressed skull fracture. Debris (hair, dirt, and foreign material) penetrates the wound. The dura may or may not be torn. A *basilar skull fracture* involves injury to the base of the skull. The middle and anterior fossa are more often affected than the posterior fossa. The most common type involves the extension of a linear fracture into the base of the skull. These fractures usually involve the petrous portion of the temporal bone. Basilar skull fractures can indicate severe trauma and should be suspected in any significant head injury.

CONCUSSIONS, CONTUSIONS, AND LACERATIONS Brain injury is classified as a concussion, contusion, or laceration that may or may not be associated with vascular rupture and cranial nerve damage. A cerebral *concussion* is considered the most benign form of brain injury. A concussion is characterized by a loss of consciousness for 5 minutes or less and memory loss of events preceding and following trauma. Other symptoms may include dizziness, spots before the eyes, and a dazed state. In the past, a concussion was believed to cause no structural brain damage. Current data indicate conclusively that there is microscopic damage in virtually all cases. Residual deficits are clinically observable if carefully sought and may be long lasting.

A cerebral *contusion* is a bruising of the brain. There may be petechial hemorrhage of cortical tissue and white matter with tearing of the pia mater. Contusions are commonly found beneath depressed skull fractures and around penetrating injuries of the frontal and temporal lobes. Contusions cause unconsciousness that persists for longer than 5 minutes. An initial period of shock is followed by signs of cerebral irritability.

A cerebral *laceration* is a tearing of the brain tissue followed by intracerebral bleeding. Prolonged unconsciousness, immediate neurologic deficits, and a deterioration in condition can be expected.

EPIDURAL, SUBDURAL, AND INTRACEREBRAL HEMATOMAS The major vascular hemorrhages from trauma include epidural, subdural, and intracerebral hematomas. An *epidural* hematoma is a life-threatening hemorrhage in the epidural space, which is between the inner table of the skull and the dura. Trauma to the temporal bone from a linear fracture constitutes the most common form. The fracture causes tearing of the middle meningeal artery and its branches. Most epidural hematomas are from arterial bleeds. Classically, the trauma causes an initial loss of consciousness, followed by a lucid interval. Unconsciousness follows that is both rapid and often unexpected. Epidural hematomas require prompt surgical intervention.

Subdural hematomas are collections of blood from clots in the subdural space between the arachnoid and dura that usually involve venous bleeding. The three types include acute, subacute, and chronic hematomas, referring to the time interval between initial injury and symptom development. Acute hematoma occurs within 48 hours; subacute, within 2 weeks; and chronic, more than 2 weeks after injury. Subdural hematomas can develop over an entire hemisphere. Chronic subdural hematomas can increase in size over time, probably due to rebleeding.

Acute subdural hematomas are often associated with massive cerebral or brain stem injury. Although bleeding is mostly venous, it develops quickly with rapid onset of symptoms. Common clinical symptoms and signs are headache, drowsiness and confusion, slow responses, and restlessness. These worsen over time. A critical sign of deterioration is an ipsilateral dilation of the pupil that becomes unreactive.

Subacute subdural hematomas usually develop 7 to 10 days after injury and are associated with less severe brain contusions. The course is slower with a much better survival rate. Persistent cerebral pressure causes prolonged alteration in level of consciousness.

Chronic subdural hematomas commonly occur from more trivial injuries. At first, a small hemorrhage fills the subdural space. Several weeks later, a vascular membrane forms around the collection, which slowly enlarges. Symptoms may not occur for several weeks or months. Because of this time lapse, the initial injury may not be recalled. Progressive headache, confusion and drowsiness, slow responses, and seizures occur. Pupillary changes and motor deficits result, similar to those in subacute subdural hematomas. Papilledema may develop as well.

An intracerebral hematoma, a collection of blood in brain tissue, is a complication in a small percentage of all head traumas. The hematoma may accompany the contrecoup phenomenon. Most are related to contusions and occur in frontal and temporal areas. Lesions can be single or multiple. They may occur deep within the hemispheres but are rare in the cerebellum. Symptom onset may be slowed because of gradual or delayed bleeding.

Medical Measures

The treatment of head trauma includes medical or surgical therapy or both. The initial management of head trauma clients not only includes diagnosis of head injury but also an awareness of potential respiratory problems or injury to other systems. These other problems are important, because anoxia or shock may complicate the initial head injury. The survival rate has improved with central head trauma units. Standards ensure that clients have immediate stabilization of vital signs, that further injury is prevented, and that intracranial edema is reduced. The primary focus is on maintenance of a patent airway. In these centers, the conditions requiring surgery, such as epidural hematomas, are diagnosed, and surgical intervention is prompt. In a large group of clients with closed head injury, no surgery is necessary. Client management depends on neurologic care that includes maintenance of airway and blood pressure, monitoring of ICP, and appropriate antibiotic therapy as necessary. Treatment of cerebral edema includes use of dehydrating agents such as mannitol, which withdraw water from intracranial tissue. High-dose steroid therapy is usually administered although studies show no benefit. Hyperventilation therapy is employed in clients with severe head trauma to decrease P_{CO_2}, reducing cerebral vasodilation and thereby decreasing ICP. Although controversial, current data indicate that these procedures are beneficial for the brain-injured client. Assessment approaches such as the Glasgow Coma Scale are beginning to permit institutions to compare data about modes of therapy and outcomes.

Specific Nursing Measures

The initial nursing priority for the care of the client with acute head injury must be maintenance of effective airway clearance and breathing pattern. Respiratory control may be interrupted by direct trauma to the cerebrum or brain stem. Compromised respiration leads to increased ICP, which causes ischemia to respiratory centers. An inadequate airway or ventilation may be caused by a number of factors. Mechanical complications include upper airway obstruction and poor pulmonary toilet. Gag reflex absence, phrenic nerve damage, or aspiration can compromise pulmonary status. Clients with alterations in level of consciousness are at greatest risk for hypoventilation because of shallow respiration and potential for respiratory failure or arrest. Check for airway patency and adequate pulmonary toilet, and assess, report, and document breathing patterns and breath sounds.

Be sure that the client's head and neck are immobilized and *not* manipulated until cervical injury is ruled out by cervical spine x-ray or CT scan. Avoid neck hyperextension, flexion, and rotation. Manipulation can cause an airway obstruction or can seriously complicate a cervical injury. If respiratory resuscitation is required, the jaw thrust maneuver can be used. Do *not* suction nasal passages until basal skull fractures and dural tears have been ruled out. Clear the mouth and oropharynx of foreign bodies. Gentle oropharyngeal suctioning can be done to maintain an effective airway. If the airway is not patent, endotracheal intubation or a tracheostomy will be indicated.

Clients with potential for respiratory complications may be repositioned after the cervical spine is stabilized. The semiprone lateral position facilitates drainage of secretions, or the clients can be turned from side to side. Position should be changed at least every 2 hours. Assess respiratory rate, rhythm, and pattern every 1 to 2 hours or as necessary. Evaluate chest excursions and breath sounds at the same interval. Arterial blood gases are monitored initially, after 4 hours, and subsequently as necessary. Neurologic dysfunction can cause specific changes in respiratory patterns. Teach conscious clients to do deep breathing exercises. Coughing should be avoided as it increases ICP.

Assess the neurologic status of the client with acute head trauma immediately after respiratory airway patency is established. The level of consciousness is the single most important aspect of the clinical nursing observation, because it is maintained by the normal functioning of the cerebral cortex and the ascending reticular activating system of the brain stem. Consciousness is assessed on a continuum from full reaction to no reaction to various kinds of stimuli. At present, no levels of consciousness terms are universally accepted. Therefore, it is best to describe the stimulus given and the response obtained (see Glasgow Coma Scale in Chapter 28).

Care of clients with basal skull fractures includes assessment for "raccoon" eyes or bilateral periorbital ecchymosis and hemorrhage; Battle's sign, an ecchymosis of the mastoid region; and hemotympanum, blood behind the eardrum. Cerebrospinal fluid leaks may occur as rhinorrhea or otorrhea. Never probe or irrigate the nose or ear when a CSF leak is suspected. If drainage occurs, collect the fluid in a test tube and test it with a Dextrostix for the presence of glucose. A glucose positive result can confirm a CSF leak, since glucose is present in CSF but not in mucus. If drainage cannot be collected for testing, carefully inspect the client's gown and linen. The halo sign, a combination of bloody or darker drainage encircled by a lighter yellowish stain, signifies a bloody leakage of CSF. Basal skull fractures are considered serious head injuries due to the proximity of the fracture site to vital brain stem areas. Brain stem edema can result in severe respiratory and cardiac dysfunction. Assess the client frequently for any alterations in neurologic, respiratory, or cardiac status.

Nursing Research Note

Parson LC, Peard–Smith AL, Page MC: The effects of hygiene interventions on the cerebrovascular status of severe closed-head injured persons. *Res Nurs Health* 1985; 8:173–181.

This study measured physiologic responses by the severe closed-head injured client to three nursing interventions: oral care, body hygiene, and in-dwelling catheter care. The physiologic responses measured were heart rate, mean arterial blood pressure, mean intracranial pressure, and cerebral perfusion pressure.

All three interventions produced increases in heart rate, mean arterial pressure, mean intracranial pressure, and cerebral perfusion pressure. Oral care and body hygiene produced a greater rise in all four measures than did catheter care. These elevations all returned to baseline within 1 minute following completion of the care. Although the nursing interventions raised physiologic measures, the cerebral perfusion pressure was never less than 50, the minimal pressure needed to perfuse the brain adequately.

The results indicate that these nursing measures can be performed safely on clients with severe closed-head injuries. The interventions help to reduce associated complications of immobility, oral decay, and urinary tract infection.

Spinal Cord Injury

The vast majority of spinal pathology results from traumatic injury. The highest incidence is in young men in the second and third decades of life. Spinal injury usually results from a sudden catastrophic event in a previously healthy individual. The leading causes in the United States are car and motorcycle accidents, sports accidents (football, diving), and penetrating injuries (gunshot or stab wounds).

Fracture-dislocations can occur anywhere along the spine. The mechanisms of injury vary according to the area of the spine involved. Cervical injuries, the most common, are usually related to flexion–extension maneuvers during a traumatic injury. Fracture-dislocations in the thoracic and lumbar areas usually arise from compression injuries, as in falls from high places. Spinal column fracture-dislocations may also result from pathologic bone processes: metastatic, infectious, or degenerative disease. This discussion focuses on traumatic injuries to the cervical spine because of its potential to cause the most extensive neurologic deficits.

Dislocation fractures of the high cervical vertebrae (C-1 to C-2) can occur as a result of fractures or congenital defects of the odontoid process or from arthritic changes that weaken the ligaments in this area. A forward movement of the skull and C-1 and C-2 vertebrae can compress the cervical cord. These fractures can occur in the body or posterior elements of the spine causing a forward or backward dislocation of cervical vertebrae and compromising the neural canal. Additional compression can result from bony fragments or disk material that impinges on the spinal cord.

Instability is often observed on cervical spine radiographs where a misalignment is seen. This situation is exemplified by "locked facets," in which an upper cervical vertebra is dislocated forward on the adjacent lower vertebra. The vertebra is held in position because of slippage of the upper facet on the lower facet. In some cases, however, the spine appears to be aligned although the spinal cord is actually or physiologically severed (transection). At the time of injury, damage to the support structures of the spine results in a vertebral subluxation that compresses neural elements and then returns to a normal position. The position of the vertebra is unstable, however, and any movement can result in dislocation or transection.

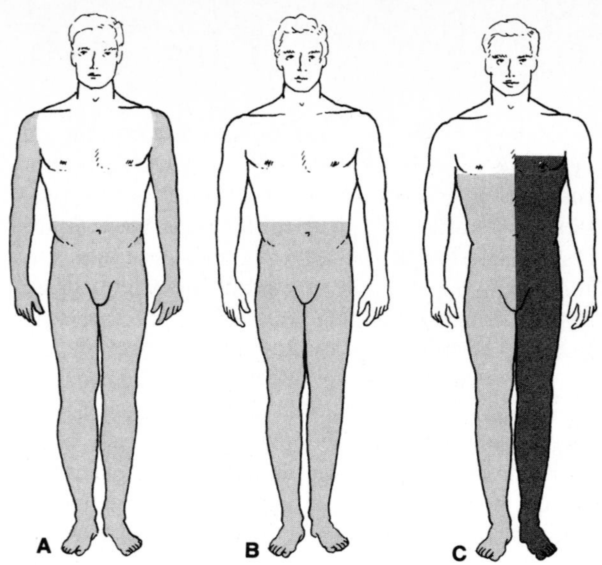

Figure 29–4

Spinal cord injury with paralysis. **A.** Quadriplegia—paralysis of all four extremities. **B.** Paraplegia—paralysis of both legs. **C.** Brown-Séquard syndrome—the client with an injury to the left cord has motor paresis and loss of vibration and proprioception on the left with loss of pain and temperature sensation on the right, one to two segments below the level of injury.

Clinical Manifestations

The extent of a client's functional loss depends on the degree of spinal cord injury. *Complete* spinal cord transection causes a total loss of motor and sensory function below the level of injury with irreversible spinal cord damage.

In the cervical area, millimeters can be crucial for spinal nerve-root function. With cervical cord transection, **quadriplegia** (paralysis of all four extremities) results, with varying degrees of respiratory and arm paralysis, depending on the injury level. Cord transection of the thoracic spine through L-1 and L-2 causes **paraplegia** (paralysis of both legs) (Figure 29–4). A common classification system relating neurologic deficits to anatomic level of injuries is outlined in Table 29–11.

The classification in Table 29–11 is more helpful in evaluating spinal-cord injury than one based on structural changes in the cord. For example, a complete cord transection can cause visible damage to cord tissue or only minimal gross structural change. In either, the individual sustains an immediate flaccid paralysis, loss of sensation, and usually loss of reflexes below the level of injury. Some reflexes may be intact initially, then disappear within a few days, indicating "spinal shock," or the loss of all reflex activity below the level of injury. The loss can last for days, for weeks, or several months. As paralysis subsides, reflexes usually return, and flaccidity changes to involuntary spastic movement. Recovery of any motor or sensory function is rare when there is complete paralysis of these functions for several days after injury.

With incomplete spinal cord injuries, degrees of sensory and motor deficit below the level of damage vary, resulting in one of several spinal cord syndromes. The most common is *anterior-cord syndrome,* caused by acute flexion injuries to the cervical spine. The anterior spinal artery and/or ventral part of the spinal cord is injured. Complete loss of motor function occurs with preservation of dorsal column sensation, known as "sacral sparing." Below the level of injury, there are hyperesthesia and hypalgesia with some preservation of position sense as well as vibration, pressure, and touch sensation.

The *central-cord syndrome* usually involves hyperextension injuries, primarily in the elderly with osteoarthritic spines. The central gray matter is the main site of injury. Central-cord syndrome is characterized by a greater loss of motor power in the arms than in the legs accompanied by varying degrees of sensory and bladder dysfunction. A flaccid paralysis at the site of injury and a spastic involvement below the level of injury occur.

The *Brown–Séquard syndrome,* also known as a hemisection of the spinal cord, usually follows penetrating injuries of a rotation–flexion nature. On the ipsilateral side of cord injury, motor paresis and loss of vibration and proprioception occur. On the contralateral side of the injury, one to two segments below, there is loss of pain and temperature sensation (Figure 29–4). Clients who sustain injuries to the lower spinal cord, conus medullaris, and cauda equina may experience signs of both upper and lower motor neuron dysfunction.

A number of factors are examined to assess the degree of spinal cord damage. The first consideration may be the mechanism of injury. A compression of the cord can occur from ligaments, bone, herniated disk material, or hema-

Table 29–11
Classification of Neurologic Deficits According to Level of Spinal Cord Injury

Level of Injury	Neurologic Deficit
Cervical C-1 to C-2	Quadriplegia: no respiratory function with an immediate respiratory arrest if untreated
C-3 to C-4	Quadriplegia: loss of phrenic nerve innervation to the diaphragm causing absence of respirations
C-4 to C-5	Quadriplegia: no motor power in the arms
C-5 to C-6	Quadriplegia: gross motor function in the arms only
C-6 to C-7	Quadriplegia: no triceps function; biceps spared
C-7 to C-8	Quadriplegia: no intrinsic muscle function in the hands; triceps spared
Thoracic T-1 to T-12 and Lumbar L-1 to L-2	Paraplegia; arm function preserved; some loss of intercostals; loss of bladder, bowel, and sexual function
L-2 and below	Cauda equina damage: a combination of loss of sensory, motor, bowel, bladder, and sexual function; degree of injury depends on which nerve roots are involved
Sacral	Loss of bowel, bladder, and sexual function

tomas. A contusion causes a bruising of the cord. In transection injuries, the spinal cord is actually or physiologically severed. A hemorrhage known as hematomyelia can occur within the cord substance.

Another important factor influencing the degree of spinal injury is the diameter of the spinal canal, the amount of space the spinal cord has to move within to avoid compression. This factor is especially crucial in the cervical area. This space tends to be wider in children and narrower in persons with various congenital anomalies, arthritic changes, and conditions such as spondylosis.

Neurons do not regenerate within the cord substance. Spinal cord necrosis can result from a number of factors such as disturbances in circulation causing poor cord perfusion, edema, and progressive hemorrhage of central gray matter.

Medical Measures

The first priority in initial treatment of an acute spinal cord injury is handling of the client's spine with extreme caution. Proper handling can prevent further dislocation of fractured or already dislocated bone. At the scene of injury, the client should be moved with the head and neck immobilized. There should be no movement of the cervical spine, especially flexion. The client should be placed supine on a rigid frame or stretcher with sandbags (or other firm objects) applied to both sides of the head and neck. Place a firm roll under the nape of the neck. Any life-threatening injury to another body system or signs of systemic shock should be treated immediately. For emergency life support, the neck should *not* be hyperextended. The jaw-thrust maneuver can be used for mouth-to-mouth resuscitation.

Formerly, clients with acute spinal trauma had prompt surgery to "decompress" their injured cord. Today the immediate goal of trauma care is to stabilize bony malalignments and ligamentous instability. Stabilization is usually achieved in cervical injuries with the application of skeletal traction by Crutchfield or Gardner–Wells tongs. (Crutchfield tongs are illustrated in Chapter 45.) Realignment may be achieved with skeletal traction or an open reduction later. In most trauma units, early fixation and spinal traction have replaced decompression laminectomies.

Another goal of therapy is to reverse the effects of vertebral body fractures. Neurosurgery replaces the injured vertebra with bone, acrylic, or a combination. The advantage of acrylic is early mobilization for the client, whereas bone fusion requires some internal fixation. For clients who remain unstable, a halo frame and body jacket vest are applied for several months until stabilization is achieved. In the lower thoracic and lumbar areas, internal fixation can be achieved using rods.

Spinal-cord-injured clients are at greatest risk in the first week to 10 days after trauma. During this time, shock, pulmonary dysfunction, infection, and paralytic ileus can be major problems. Clients who sustain quadriplegic injuries require intensive total medical and nursing management. The posttraumatic care of paraplegic clients mainly involves management of bladder and bowel dysfunctions, skin care, nutrition maintenance, and physical therapy.

Specific Nursing Measures

The most intensive nursing care is required for clients with acute, unstable cervical fractures resulting in quadriplegia. The first objective for the nurse admitting these clients to an ER, ICU, or trauma unit is absolute immobilization of the head and neck with sandbags and a firm roll under the nape of the neck. Once the client is placed in tongs and cervical traction, follow physician's orders for client positioning. Pin sites must be cared for once per shift. The tong sites are cleansed with hydrogen peroxide and saline to remove exudate. Culture unusual or foul-smelling drainage and report it to the physician. After cleansing the sites, apply povidone–iodine ointment as ordered around pin sites. Maintain the integrity of the tongs and skeletal traction. If the tongs come out, keep the client's head in a neutral position, remain with the client, and call for immediate help. Caution the client to avoid any head and neck movement.

The client with an acute cervical injury should not be turned until the fracture is reduced and stabilized. Turning the client requires an explicit order from the physician. When a turning order has been verified, a minimum of three staff members is required to logroll the client. One person is assigned to support the client's head. Carefully explain the turning or transferring procedure to the client and provide reassurance. In some institutions. Stryker frames or circle beds are used to care for clients. More recently, the Rota Rest bed has been recommended to provide safe stabilization and reduce the hazards of immobility.

Continuous monitoring of the client's neurologic status including respiratory, motor, and sensory function is essential. Assess the client's level of consciousness and evaluate pupillary response. Report the progression of any neurologic deficit immediately.

With high cervical lesions, there will be ineffective airway clearance and alterations in breathing patterns. Assess the adequacy of respiration and ventilation. Specific assessment includes the rate, depth, and rhythm of respirations. Periodically check tidal volumes and arterial blood gas values. Many clients require endotracheal or tracheostomy tubes with ventilatory support. Oxygen administration will be ordered by tracheostomy tube, tracheostomy collar, or ventilator.

High cervical injuries frequently cause respiratory arrest. During this emergency, the neck *must not* be hyperextended. Instead, the jaw thrust maneuver is used for mouth-to-mouth resuscitation. The client then requires careful nasotracheal intubation or an emergency tracheostomy. For clients admitted with respiratory function intact, observe respiration carefully. During spinal shock, it is not uncommon for the level of injury to ascend one or two levels above actual damage due to massive spinal cord edema. When this occurs, clients with high cervical injuries may develop respiratory dysfunction and/or arrest even if they did not have the problem initially. This group of clients is at high risk for pulmonary complications such as pneumonia and atelectasis.

To alleviate early spinal cord edema, large doses of intravenous or intramuscular dexamethasone (Decadron) may be given. Steroids may cause gastric distress as well as other side effects such as behavioral changes, elevated glucose levels, and an acnelike rash.

Clients are also at risk for abdominal distention and paralytic ileus. Keep the client NPO until bowel sounds return. Use a rectal tube if not contraindicated to relieve abdominal distention. Carefully monitor the client for gastrointestinal bleeding from stress ulcers related to steroid therapy. For clients with ulcer histories, cimetidine (Tagamet) may be ordered with the steroids. Remind the physician if the client has an ulcer history. If gastrointestinal bleeding is suspected, test gastric secretions and stool specimens for occult blood. A nasogastric tube may be passed if signs of a gastric ulcer are identified. Protocols for irrigation vary (eg, continuous iced saline, room temperature saline, or vasopressin drips for gastrointestinal bleeding). Obtain immediate complete blood counts and specimens for blood typing and crossmatching.

In developing a plan of care to prevent hazards of immobility, emboli, skin breakdown, and bowel and bladder dysfunction, refer to specific nursing measures for clients with stroke. In addition, it is helpful to begin a bowel management program by administering a cleansing enema. To establish a bowel reflex, provide a combination of bulk in the diet, stool softeners, prune juice, and daily suppositories. Abdominal massage and digital stimulation can help. Establish a schedule for defecating and administer the daily suppository at the same time each day.

Assess the client for symptoms and signs of thrombophlebitis and pulmonary embolism because the client cannot give subjective reports of calf pain. When managing skin care, consider the type of bed the client is in. A Rota Rest bed is preferred. If unavailable, a circle bed or Stryker frame can provide sufficient turning capability to assess and care for all skin areas. Changing clients to a prone position may evoke fear and anxiety about falling or suffocation. Assess vital signs, tidal volume, or vital capacity before turning. These clients have a potential for hypoxia, hypotensive episodes, and vagal reflexes.

The most sensitive area of nursing care is the client's psychologic reaction to paralysis. Body image and the client's entire future have been suddenly and irrevocably altered. Assess available support systems, prevent sleep deprivation and sensory overload, and provide time to talk with clients or just be with them.

Understand and prepare significant others for the client's angry outbursts or other behaviors that reflect attempts to cope. These behaviors are healthy and cathartic. Recognize the range of emotion the client experiences, with the goal of supporting the client in progressing toward eventual acceptance and resolution. Encourage clients to make as many decisions about their care as possible to help them regain a sense of control over self and environment.

The acceptance of permanent disability may take a long time. Acknowledge client concerns without forcing acceptance. Denial can be beneficial for a time. Be an empathic listener who can accurately reflect the client's comments and feelings. A consistent, supportive approach is essential.

Client/Family Teaching

Sometimes clients develop an extreme dependence on the acute care setting, the care providers, and ventilatory support. The client experiences varying degrees of anxiety about separating from a stable group of caregivers and support systems. A careful, well-planned approach is required for the task of separation. Provide simple explanations for ventilatory weaning. It is helpful to discuss the criteria for weaning from ventilation and the client's achievement of the appropriate goals. Remain with the client being weaned and check vital signs and respiratory status at intervals. Institute short periods of weaning initially and have all backup equipment available and functioning. Prepare clients for any setbacks and reinforce their progress. Clients' confidence levels can improve by encouraging them to assume responsibility for timing of certain treatments and reminding the staff of the schedule.

Once vertebral fractures fuse, clients can be transferred to stretcher chairs. Hypotension and dizziness may occur, so mobilization must be done progressively. Abdominal binders and antiembolism stockings can be used to decrease hypotensive episodes and periods of dizziness.

Sexual dysfunction is a major concern that clients may or may not verbalize during the acute stage of injury. Factors that determine future potential for sexual function are the anatomic level of injury, the client's personality and former sexual experiences, and the effectiveness of sexual counseling. The most important fact to convey is that a caring, loving relationship is possible with another individual. The majority of female clients can physically participate in intercourse. Assistive information about technique, positions, and catheter taping is helpful. Male clients have greater sexual potential when they have a high cervical or thoracic lesion because of reflexogenic ability. Lumbar and sacral injury can destroy the reflex arc, decreasing the potential for an erection. For these clients, prosthetic devices such as penile implants (see Chapter 49) can be used. Clients may give cues that signal appropriate timing for discussion of sexual issues. If they do not, the nurse should initiate the discussion.

Anticipate autonomic dysreflexia with quadriplegics and paraplegics who sustain high thoracic lesions. Autonomic dysreflexia results from exaggerated autonomic responses to stimuli. Bladder or bowel distention or skin stimulation can trigger the response. Autonomic dysreflexia is an emergency that may lead to increased ICP and severe hypertension. Assess the client for severe headache, flushing, bradycardia, elevated blood pressure, and diaphoresis. When symptoms occur, elevate the client's head to lower blood pressure, assess patency of the in-dwelling catheter, and check for a fecal impaction. Anesthetic ointment can be topically applied in the rectum before feces are removed to decrease the stimulation of manual removal. Antihypertensive drugs may be necessary [eg, hydralazine hydrochloride (Apresoline)]. The nurse can help prevent episodes of dysreflexia by preventing conditions that result in stimulus overload (eg, fecal impaction or bladder distention).

Chapter Highlights

An explosive headache is the most common symptom of a client with rupture of an intracranial aneurysm. Clients with ruptured intracranial aneurysms should not be given enemas or any form of stimulus that can increase ICP.

Never restrain a client having a major generalized motor (grand mal) seizure. Never use force to insert an oral airway into a client having a grand mal seizure.

Bell's palsy is characterized by a flaccid facial paralysis. The priority of nursing care for clients with Bell's palsy is protecting the cornea.

Occlusive cerebrovascular disease is caused by a thrombus or embolus. Hemorrhagic cerebrovascular disease is caused by an aneurysm rupture or AVM bleed.

The most common initial symptom of Parkinson's disease is tremor.

Medication for treating myasthenia gravis must be given at the exact time ordered.

Guillain–Barré syndrome can develop after a respiratory or gastrointestinal illness. The onset is characterized by ascending symmetrical sensory and motor deficits.

Clients with meningococcal (bacterial) meningitis must be isolated until therapeutic antibiotic levels are achieved. Diagnosis of viral encephalitis has greatly improved with electron microscopy.

Teach clients to seek medical treatment for dental caries, ear infections, and sinusitis to prevent development of a brain abscess.

There is a relationship between the chicken pox and herpes zoster virus.

A client's head and neck must be immobilized and not manipulated if cervical trauma is suspected. Use the jaw thrust maneuver to resuscitate a client with cervical injury.

Never suction the nasal passageways of a client with head trauma until basal skull fractures and/or dural tears have been ruled out.

Basal skull fracture is characterized by Battle's sign, ecchymosis of the mastoid region, and hemotympanum.

Spinal shock following an acute spinal cord injury can increase the functional level of injury for weeks after injury.

Postoperative neurosurgical clients must be carefully observed for any subtle or sudden decline in neurologic status.

The prognosis and recovery of many neurosurgical clients are based on the extent of damage to neural tissue inflicted by the lesion and/or the surgical manipulations.

Most neurosurgical clients and their families fear that death, disability, disfigurement, loss of intellectual function, and personality changes will result from the surgical procedure.

Cerebral edema and periorbital edema are expected reactions to manipulation and retraction of brain tissue.

A postoperative hematoma is the most devastating and dreaded complication of intracranial surgery.

One of the most important nursing measures is the assessment and documentation of the baseline neurologic status to provide a standard by which postoperative progress or deterioration can be measured.

Level of consciousness often provides the first clue to a client's deteriorating neurologic condition.

Seizure precautions should be instituted on all clients following supratentorial craniotomy or craniectomy.

Suboccipital craniectomy is especially hazardous because of the concentration of vital structures in this small area.

Most neurosurgery of the spine is aimed at relieving compression. Recovery of function and relief of pain depend on the degree and duration of spinal cord or nerve root compression and the nature of the underlying pathology.

Bibliography

Adams RD, Victor M: *Principles of Neurology,* 2nd ed. New York: McGraw–Hill, 1981.

American Association of Neuroscience Nurses: *Core Curriculum for Neuroscience Nursing.* Chicago: The American Association of Neuroscience Nurses, 1983.

Baggerly J: Rehabilitation of the adult with head trauma. *Nurs Clinic NA* 1986; 21(4):577–587.

Bickerstaff E: *Neurology,* 3rd ed. London: Hodder and Stroughton, 1980.

Boss BJ: Dysphasia, dyspraxia and dsysarthria: Distinguishing features, Part I. *J Neurosurg Nurs* 1984; 16(3):151–160.

Boss BJ: Dysphasia, dyspraxia and dysarthria: Distinguishing features, Part II. *J Neurosurg Nurs* 1984: 16(4):211–216.

Cohen S et al: Radioimmunoassay of myelin basic protein in spinal fluid. *New Engl J Med* 1976; 295:1455.

Conway–Rutkowski: *Carini and Owens' Neurological and Neurosurgical Nursing.* St. Louis: C. V. Mosby, 1982.

Cutler NR, Narang PK: Drug therapies (Alzheimer's disease). *Geriatric Nursing* 1985; 6:160–163.

Drayton-Hargrove S, Reddy MA: Rehabilitation and long-term management of the spinal cord injured adult. *Nurs Clinics NA* 1986; 21(4):599–610.

Eisendorf, Cohen: *J Fam Pract* 1980.

Eldridge R. Fahn S (editors): *Advances in Neurology,* Vol. 14. Dystonia, NY: Raven, 1976.

Forster FM: *Clinical Neurology,* 4th ed. St. Louis: C. V. Mosby, 1978.

Friedman W: Head injuries. *Clinical Symposia* 1983; 35(4):2–32.

Gioella EC, Bevil CW: *Nursing Care of the Aging Client: Promoting Healthy Adaptation.* Appleton-Century Crofts, 1985.

Hakim AM, Mathieson G: Basis of dementia in Parkinson's disease. *Lancet* 1978; 2:729.

Hayter J: Patients who have Alzheimer's disease. *Am J Nurs* 1974; 8:1460–1463.

Hayward R: *Essentials of Neurosurgery.* London: Blackwell, 1980.

Hickey J: *The Clinical Practice of Neurological and Neurosurgical Nursing.* Philadelphia: Lippincott, 1981.

Horwitz NH, Rizzoli HV: *Postoperative Complications of Intracranial Neurological Surgery.* Baltimore: Williams & Wilkins, 1982.

Jennett B, Galbraith S: *An Introduction to Neurosurgery,* 4th ed. Chicago: Year Book, 1983.

Jolles J, Hijman R: The neuropsychology of aging and dementia. In: *Aging of the Brain.* Gispen, WH, Trabers J (editors). Elsevier, 1983.

Kaminski, D: Air embolism during surgery in the sitting position: Prevention, detection and treatment. *Neurosurg Nurs* 1975; 7(2):65–71.

Kolata G: Alzheimer's research poses. *Science* (Jan) 1982; 215.

Malis LI: Arteriovenous malformations of the brain. In: *Neurological Surgery,* Vol. 3. Youmans JR (editor). Philadelphia: W. B. Saunders, 1982.

Maroon JC, Abla A: Microdiscectomy versus chemonucleolysis. *Neurosurg* 1985; 16(5):644–649.

Mathis M: Personal needs of family members of critically ill patients with and without acute brain injury. *J Neurosurg Nurs* 1984; 16(1):36–44.

McKinstry D: Diagnosis, cause and treatment of Alzheimer's disease. *Research Resources Reports* (June) 1982; VI(6).

Merritt HH: *A Textbook of Neurology,* 6th ed. Philadelphia: Lea & Febiger, 1979.

Michenfelder JD, Gronert GA, Rehder K: Anesthesia in Neurological Surgery. In: *Neurological Surgery.* Youmans, JR (editor). Philadelphia: Saunders, 1982.

Mulford E: Degenerative diseases or "slipped" disc? The clues are clear-cut. *RN* (Feb) 1981.

Panel of Neuromuscular Disorders. Washington, D.C.: Department of Health, Education, and Welfare, 1979.

Plum F, Posner JB: *The Diagnosis of Stupor and Coma.* Philadelphia: F.A. Davis, 1980.

Power DJ, Craven DF: ALS and aging: A case study in autonomy and control. *Image* (Winter) 1983; 15:22–25.

Rhodes M, Grosser B: Complications of posterior fossa craniotomy. *J Neurosurg Nurs* 1983; 15(9):51–56.

Rhodes PR (editor): *Core Curriculum for Neurosurgical Nursing in the Operating Room.* Chicago: American Assn Neurosurgical Nurses, 1980.

Ricci M: Neurologic assessment: Keeping it ongoing. In: *Coping With Neurological Problems Proficiently.* Robinson J (editor). Horsham, PA: Intermed Communications, 1979.

Ricci M (editor): *Core Curriculum for Neuroscience Nursing.* Park Ridge, IL: American Assn Neuroscience Nurses, 1984.

Rundy EB: *Advanced Neurological and Neurosurgical Nursing.* St. Louis: C.V. Mosby, 1984.

Schafer SC: Modifying the environment (Alzheimer's disease). *Geriatric Nursing* 1985; 6:157–159.

Schawlb D, Zahr L: Nursing care of patients with an altered body image due to multiple sclerosis. *Nursing Forum* 1985; 22(2):72–76.

Schneider EL, Emr M: Alzheimzer's disease: research highlights. *Geriatric Nursing* 1985; 6:135–138.

Smith J, Geist B: Evaluation and care of the acute craniotomy patient. *J Neurosurg Nurs* 1978; 10(3):102–111.

Stern WE: Preoperative evaluation: Complications, their prevention and treatment. In: *Neurological Surgery.* Youmans JR (editor). Philadelphia: Saunders, 1982.

Swift-Bandini, N: *Manual of Neurological Nursing,* 2nd ed. Boston: Little, Brown, 1982.

Tucker C: Safety assessment for the postictal confusional phase following complex partial seizure. *J Neurosurg Nurs* 1985; 17(1):201–207.

Wells P, Geden E: Paraplegic body support pressure on convoluted foam, waterbed, and standard mattresses. *Res Nurs Health* 1984; 7:127–133.

Wilkins RH, Odom GL: General operative technique. In: *Neurological Surgery.* Youmans JR (editor). Philadelphia: Saunders, 1982.

Youmans JR (editor): *Neurological Surgery,* (3 volumes). Philadelphia: Saunders, 1982.

CASE STUDY

The Client With Head Trauma

I. Brief Descriptive Data: Joseph Holmlund, a 32-year-old certified public accountant and father of two young daughters, was brought unconscious to the emergency department following a head injury. The injury resulted from being hit with a baseball during a ball game.

II. Personal Data

Date and Time: June 25, 1988; 6:15 P.M.
Full Name: Joseph Stephen Holmlund
Social Security Number: 000-00-0000
Address: 16 Juliet St., Warren, Ohio
Telephone: Home: 000-0000
Work: 000-0000
Sex: Male
Age: 32
Birthdate: 2/6/56
Marital Status: Widower
Race: Caucasian
Religion: Born-again Christian
Occupation: Certified Public Accountant
Usual Health Care Provider: Geraldine Kostusiak, M.D.

III. Health History

Source of Information: Two members of the baseball team, who were present when the injury occurred, and Mr. Holmlund's fiancee, Donna Shipman.
Reliability of Information: Reliable
Chief Concern: Unresponsive 32-year-old man who sustained a head injury 7 hours ago.

History of Present Illness: During a baseball game 7 hours ago, Joe was accidently hit on the right side of his head by a hardball traveling at high speed. He fell to the ground and lost consciousness for several minutes. He awakened somewhat dazed, with a headache, but felt well enough to remain at the game. Later, while lying on his couch at home watching TV, he fell asleep; his fiancee was unable to arouse him. She called the paramedics and Joe was rushed to the emergency room.

His fiancee states that his general health has been excellent. He has never had surgery or been treated for a medical problem. To her knowledge he has not had a previous head injury. He takes no medications; does not smoke or drink; no known allergies.

Past Health History: Unknown except for fiancee's report.

Family History: Daughters × 2—ages 4 and 7; both A&W.
Wife died, age 28—automobile accident.
Brother—age 39, A&W; lives in Nevada.
His parents are both dead, cause unknown.
Nothing known about other blood relatives.

Personal/Social History: Joe lives in a condominium with his 2 daughters; his youngest attends a day care center and the oldest is in second grade. They have had some difficulty adjusting to the tragic death of Mrs Holmlund 2 years ago. Joe recently joined the baseball team to get some exercise and recreation. Donna has known Joe for 8 months—they became engaged 6 weeks ago.

Review of Systems: Unknown

IV. Physical Assessment

Height: 6 ft 2 in

Vital Signs: BP 100/60; pulse 106; resp. 22; temperature 98°F (36.7°C)

Relevant Organ Systems:

Head: Boggy swelling, right occiput.

Neurologic: Cerebral function—no response to painful stimuli with absence of gag, cough, and corneal reflexes.

Cranial nerves:
I: Not tested
II: Fundi benign
III, IV, VI: Ptosis of right eyelid with fully dilated, fixed pupil unresponsive to light; left pupil reacting somewhat sluggishly to light
V: Corneal reflex absent; no response to painful stimuli
VII: Facial muscles appear symmetrical; lacrimation adequate
VIII: Caloric testing done confirming deep coma
IX, X: Gag reflex absent
XI: Not tested
XII: No atrophy or deviation of tongue noted
Motor system: No atrophy or tremors; spastic paralysis of the left extremities noted
Sensory system: No response to deep, painful stimuli
Reflexes: DTRs hyperactive

V. Diagnostic Data

A stat CT scan was done, revealing a right epidural hematoma; an emergency craniotomy was scheduled. The surgeon contacted Mr Holmlund's brother, Leon, in Nevada (his closest living relative), explaining the gravity of the situation. Leon agreed to wire permission for the procedure.

VI. Preoperative Regimen

Mr Holmlund was intubated and given hyperventilation therapy to maintain P_{CO_2} between 25–30 mm Hg (by decreasing P_{CO_2}, cerebrovasodilation is reduced causing a decrease in ICP)
Dexamethasone (10 mg) given IV bolus followed by 4 mg IV q. 6 hrs
Mannitol 1 Unit given IV stat
An in-dwelling catheter was inserted

VII. Surgery:

An emergency craniotomy was performed down to the base of the skull; the right middle meningeal artery was isolated at the foramen spinosum; a large right epidural hematoma was evacuated, arterial bleeders were coagulated, and a Hemovac was inserted
Mr. Holmlund was transferred from the OR to the Intensive Care Unit

VIII. Nursing Care Plan, by Nursing Diagnosis:

Client Care Goal	Plan/Nursing Implementation	Expected Outcome
Airway clearance, ineffective related to deep coma		
Effective air exchange through ET tube	Maintain patent airway by suctioning ET tube PRN; assess lung sounds bilaterally; monitor baseline and ongoing ABGs; maintain functional AMBU bag with O_2 source, suction machine, and ventilator; provide source of humidification for ET tube	No signs of respiratory distress or aspiration

(Continued)

CASE STUDY (Continued)

The Client With Head Trauma

VIII. Nursing Care Plan, by Nursing Diagnosis:

Client Care Goal	Plan/Nursing Implementation	Expected Outcome
Gas exchange, impaired related to cerebral edema		
Reduce cerebral edema	Administer hyperventilation therapy via ventilator as ordered; maintain P_{CO_2} between 25–30 mm Hg as ordered	Maintain state of respiratory alkalosis; cerebral edema will decrease
Sensory/perceptual alteration: visual, kinesthetic, tactile related to altered level of consciousness		
Reduce anxiety levels for comatose client by recognizing hearing is intact	Explain all procedures to the client and provide reassurance despite comatose state	Client will not experience anxiety or fear related to knowledge deficits
Tissue perfusion, altered: cerebral related to neurologic trauma		
Prevent further deterioration in client's neurologic status	Perform accurate baseline neurologic assessment for further comparison; continue to monitor all neurologic parameters q. 15 min until stable, then q. ½–1 hr	Comparison of neurologic assessment to a baseline aids in documenting client progress
Assess neurologic status according to which parameters may change first	Critical aspects of assessment are level of consciousness, pupil signs, and motor function; document neurologic findings on standard assessment sheet as designated by institution	Neurologic status will be assessed accurately and any changes recognized early
Prevent unrecognized deterioration in neurologic status	Report any new or worsening signs of neurologic deterioration to the physician immediately; anticipate emergency neurodiagnostic procedures, especially CT scan; prepare to accompany client to procedures; maintain ongoing rapport with significant others; provide psychologic support; give explanations and rationale for therapeutic measures; anticipate measures; anticipate emergency surgical interventions	All changes in the client's neurologic condition will be reported promptly Significant others will have decreased anxiety
Injury, potential for related to potential for infection secondary to CSF leak		
Prevent meningitis related to CSF leak	Never suction head trauma clients through nasal passageways until ordered by the physician	Meningitis will not develop
Fluid volume excess related to altered regulatory mechanisms		
Decrease ICP Promote central venous drainage	Administer steroids and osmotic diuretics as ordered; Maintain HOB at 30° elevation; avoid any unnecessary stimuli; keep ventricular tap set on standby; avoid positioning with any neck compression	Increased ICP will not develop
Ensure adequate urinary output	Maintain and monitor strict I&O and patency of Foley catheter; also check lab values for problems with function	Renal function will be maintained; urinary output wn1

Client Care Goal	Plan/Nursing Implementation	Expected Outcome
Family processes, altered related to illness of family member		
Assess significant others' needs; significant others to identify personal strengths	Keep significant others informed of client status; refer to social services for home support; encourage significant others to verbalize concerns and feelings; provide psychological support	Significant others will express concerns and seek social service support as needed; family unit will be maintained.

UNIT 7

The Client with Endocrine Dysfunction

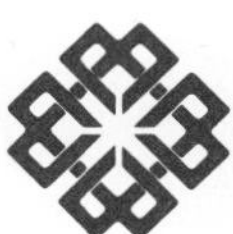

CHAPTER 30

The Endocrine System in Health and Illness

Other topics relevant to this content are: Exocrine functions of the pancreas, **Chapter 35;** Structure and function of the gonads, **Chapter 47.**

Objectives

When you have finished studying this chapter, you should be able to:

Identify the major structural and functional components of the endocrine system.

Explain the physiologic mechanisms that regulate the activity of the endocrine system.

Describe some pathologic conditions that lead to endocrine dysfunction.

Discuss alterations in other body systems that result from endocrine dysfunction.

Identify and discuss the psychosocial/lifestyle effects of endocrine dysfunction on the client and significant others.

The endocrine system can be thought of as a communications system that links all other body systems and affects nearly all physiologic aspects of life. The system functions as an interrelated unit with the nervous system to maintain homeostasis.

SECTION 

Structural and Functional Interrelationships

The endocrine system is a complex of glands that are not anatomically continuous but are interrelated so they function as an organ system. Traditionally, the endocrine system has been defined as a system of glands that secrete hormones directly into the bloodstream. In contrast, the exocrine glands secrete their hormones through ducts or directly into the intestinal lumen or onto the skin.

The principal functional units in the system are the endocrine glands: the pituitary, thyroid, parathyroid, adrenal, and pineal glands; the cells of the islets of Langerhans in the pancreas; the gonads (ovaries and testes); and the thymus (Figure 30–1). The kidneys also perform an endocrine function. Some of these glands are solely endocrine in function, whereas others form parts of larger organs that may have both endocrine and nonendocrine functions.

Structure of the Endocrine Glands

Pituitary Gland

The pituitary gland (hypophysis) is located in the sella turcica at the base of the skull. It lies just below the hypothalamus and is connected to it by a stalk containing blood vessels and nervous tissue. The pituitary gland is composed of an anterior and posterior lobe (**adenohypophysis** and **neurohypophysis,** respectively), each of which performs specific functions, and a rudimentary intermediate lobe.

Thyroid Gland

The thyroid gland lies in the anterior central portion of the neck below the larynx. It is composed of two lobes joined by a strip of tissue called the *isthmus.* The thyroid gland lies anterior to the trachea and receives an abundant blood supply. Knowing the proximity of the thyroid gland to the recurrent laryngeal nerve, which innervates the larynx, is critical for postoperative care. Damage to the recurrent laryngeal nerve during surgery can affect the client's breathing and voice production.

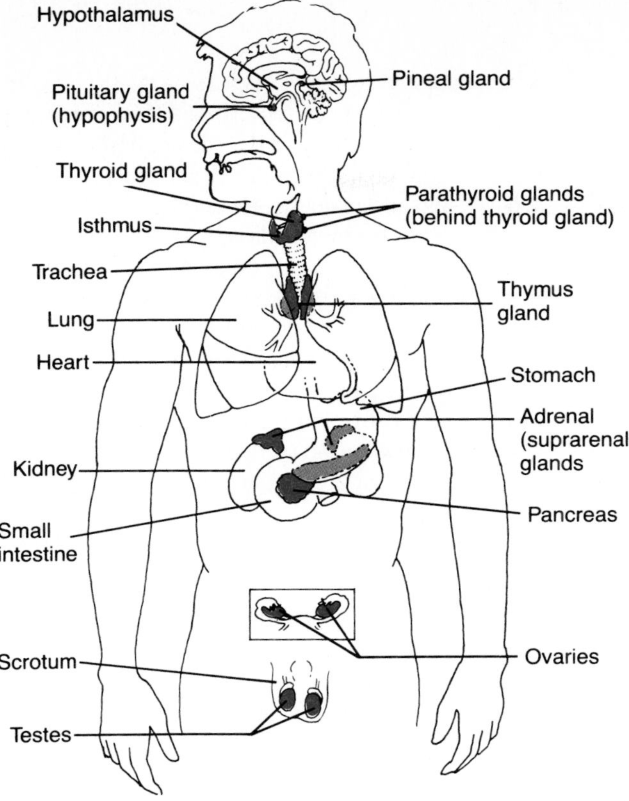

Figure 30–1

The endocrine glands and related structures.

Parathyroid Glands

The parathyroid glands are paired and usually total four, although the actual number may vary; some persons have two glands and others, as many as six. They are usually located on the posterior surface of the thyroid gland, beneath the capsular covering. The parathyroid glands may actually be embedded in the tissue of the thyroid; because of their minute size and variability in number and location, they are often hard to locate. This can result in their accidental excision during thyroid surgery, causing temporary hypoparathyroidism if more than three glands are affected. If this should occur, one gland can produce the necessary amount of hormone if it is able to increase in size sufficiently to meet the increased demand.

Adrenal Glands

The adrenal glands are paired and located in the retroperitoneal space at the upper pole of each kidney. Because of this position, they may be referred to as the *suprarenal glands*. Each adrenal gland consists of an outer portion (the cortex) and an inner portion (the medulla), which differ in both anatomic structure and function. The adrenal glands receive an abundant blood supply. The medulla of the adrenal gland functions as part of the sympathetic nervous system, whereas the cortex has only minimal nervous system innervation.

Pancreas

The pancreas lies transversely deep in the abdomen along the posterior aspect and can be found in the epigastric area and left upper quadrant. Both sympathetic and parasympathetic nerve fibers innervate it. The pancreas performs both endocrine and exocrine functions. The islets of Langerhans are involved in endocrine function and contain at least three types of hormone-secreting cells: alpha, beta, and delta. The alpha cells are thought to secrete glucagon; the beta cells, insulin; and the delta cells, somatostatin.

Gonads

The gonads—the testes and the ovaries—are the organs of reproduction. The gonads are discussed in Chapter 47.

Thymus

The thymus is a flat structure consisting of two symmetrical lobes located in the mediastinal cavity anterior and superior to the heart. The size of the thymus varies with age. Compared with body size, it is the largest at birth and for the first 2 years of life; it then grows slowly until puberty, when it begins to atrophy.

Pineal Gland

The pineal gland (epiphysis cerebri) has a characteristic pinecone shape and is attached to the posterior portion of the third ventricle of the brain. It is composed of an anterior and posterior lobe and secretes a substance that acts as a base for calcium deposits within the gland. Calcification of the pineal gland starts at age 19, and by age 60, most pineal glands are partially calcified. The relation of this process to the actual function of the pineal gland in adults has led to much discussion and research.

Function of the Endocrine System

Generalized functions of the endocrine system include:

- Maintaining the body's internal environment
- Responding to internal and external challenges (stress, infection, and trauma)
- Growth and development
- Reproductive and sexual functions

The endocrine glands perform these functions through the secretion of hormones.

Hormones

A **hormone** may be defined as a "chemical substance synthesized by an endocrine gland and secreted into the bloodstream, which carries it to other sites in the body where its actions are exerted" (Vander, Sherman, & Luciano, 1980). Hormones may function independently, in conjunction with other hormones, or as a step in a series of related actions. They may influence the action, metabolism, synthesis, and/or transport of another hormone—one of the integrative aspects of the endocrine system.

Hormones can be differentiated into two major categories: local hormones that have specific local effects and general hormones that are transported by the circulation to distant sites, where they have a physiologic effect. The endocrine hormones are summarized in Table 30–1.

MECHANISM OF HORMONAL ACTION Hormones travel throughout the body via the bloodstream, yet the body's response to them is highly specific. Only certain cells, known as **target cells,** have the capability to respond to a specific hormone in a characteristic way. Their response depends on the presence of specific receptors for a particular hormone. This response is called **hormone–target cell specificity,** and the process is known as **hormone–receptor binding.** The initial interaction between a hormone and its target cell receptor initiates a chain of biochemical events that eventually provokes a cellular response. This often involves a hormone-induced change in the activity of a specific enzyme found in the target cell that might change the rate of reactions within the cell, change the growth of the cell, or control the cell's secretion. Because cells are exposed to many hormones, complex hormone–hormone interactions can occur in target cells. These interactions may be inhibitory, synergistic, or permissive (ie, one hormone, by its presence, potentiates the effect of the second hormone).

CIRCULATION OF HORMONES Most hormones are not secreted at a constant rate. After secretion into the bloodstream, they circulate in a free form or are bound to proteins. Polypeptide hormones and the catecholamines are essentially unbound in the circulation. These free hormones are directly available to the target tissues, and only they can affect the target cells. The protein-bound forms are thought to represent a hormonal reserve, because the protein binding may prevent excretion of the hormone by the kidney. The amount of circulating free hormone is usually quite small and exists in equilibrium with the bound fraction.

REGULATION OF HORMONES There are five major influences on the secretion of hormones by the endocrine glands: the hypothalamus, hypothalamic releasing factors, anterior pituitary hormones, the autonomic nervous system, and nutrient and ion concentrations in the plasma. The hypothalamus affects hormones secretion by secreting a series of peptides called *releasing factors (RFs),* which stimulate or inhibit the release of hormones by the anterior pituitary gland. The hypothalamus also directly manufactures oxytocin and antidiurectic hormone (ADH), or vasopressin. This relationship is shown in Figure 30–2.

The hypothalamic releasing factors cause the anterior pituitary gland to secrete growth hormone (GH), prolactin, thyroid-stimulating hormone (TSH), the gonadotropic hormones follicle-stimulating hormone (FSH) and luteinizing hormone (LH), and adrenocorticotropic hormone (ACTH). The anterior pituitary hormones directly control the release of thyroid hormone (T_3 and T_4), cortisol, testosterone in the male, and estrogen and progesterone in the female.

The release of epinephrine and norepinephrine from the adrenal medulla, the gastrointestinal hormones, insulin and glucagon from the pancreas, and renin from the kidney are under the direct control of the autonomic nervous system. The adrenal medulla and posterior pituitary are under neural influence and function as part of the autonomic nervous system. The secretion of parathyroid hormone (PTH), insulin, glucagon, aldosterone, and thyrocalcitonin is directly controlled by the amount of these hormones in the serum.

FEEDBACK, AUTONOMY, AND DIURNAL VARIATION IN HORMONAL REGULATION **Feedback mechanisms** are also involved in the regulation of hormone secretion. For example, the anterior pituitary gland secretes TSH, which stimulates the thyroid to secrete thyroxine (T_4) and triidothyronine (T_3). As the serum levels of T_4 and T_3 rise, the secretion of TSH by the anterior pituitary gland is suppressed. If the serum levels of T_4 and T_3 fall, the anterior pituitary gland increases its secretion of TSH. Feedback loops can exist simply between a gland and an organ or in a more complex feedback system involving the hypothalamus, pituitary gland, and target glands.

In some clients with excessive hormone levels caused by a tumor of the involved endocrine gland, feedback inhibition does not suppress the overproduction of the hormone, and the tumor functions autonomously. An example is primary hyperparathyroidism secondary to parathyroid adenoma, a condition in which PTH secretion continues in spite of high serum calcium levels.

Diurnal variation is another of the control mechanisms affecting hormonal secretion. A 24-hour cyclical variation in the secretory rates of certain hormones can be seen. For example, GH levels are highest in the first 90 minutes after sleep begins. These **circadian rhythms** have been found to be different for each hormone.

Regulatory Functions of the Endocrine System

Hypothalamus

The hypothalamus functions as an integral part of both the endocrine and nervous systems. In its neural role, it receives and processes innervations from the thalamus, cerebral cortex, spinal cord, and brain stem. This results in the control of such bodily functions as temperature, respiration, arterial blood pressure and circulation, and metabolism. The hypothalamus also controls certain

Table 30–1
The Major Hormones: Their Sources and Effects

Endocrine Gland, Organ, or Organ System	Hormone	Target	Effect
Hypothalamus	Thyrotropin releasing factor (TRF)	Anterior pituitary	Secretion of TSH
	Corticotropin releasing factor (CRF)	Anterior pituitary	Secretion of ACTH
	Growth hormone releasing factor (GRF)	Anterior pituitary	Secretion of GH
	Somatostatin	Anterior pituitary	Inhibition of the secretion of GH, prolactin, and TSH
	Luteinizing hormone releasing factor (LRF)	Anterior pituitary	Secretion of LH and FSH
	Luteinizing hormone inhibiting factor (LIF)	Anterior pituitary	Inhibition of the secretion of LH and FSH
	Prolactin releasing factor (PRF)	Anterior pituitary	Secretion of prolactin
	Prolactin inhibiting factor (PIF)	Anterior pituitary	Inhibition of the secretion of prolactin
Anterior pituitary gland (adenohypophysis)	Thyroid-stimulating hormone (TSH)	Thyroid	Secretion of T_4, T_3, and calcitonin
	Adrenocorticotropic hormone (ACTH)	Adrenal cortex	Secretion of glucocorticoids (cortisol), mineralocorticoids (aldosterone), and sex hormones
	Growth hormone, or somatotropic hormone (GH, or STH)	Bones, muscles, organs	Promotion of growth and metabolism
	Luteinizing hormone (LH)	Ovarian follicle	Formation of corpus luteum; production of estrogen
	Interstitial cell-stimulating hormone (ICSH)	Testes	Production of testosterone
	Follicle-stimulating hormone (FSH)	Ovaries or seminiferous tubules	Development of ovarian follicle; secretion of estrogen; production of sperm
	Prolactin, or luteotropic hormone (LTH)	Corpus luteum, breasts	Maintenance of corpus luteum; secretion of progesterone; stimulation of milk secretion
Intermediate pituitary gland	Melanocyte-stimulating hormone (MSH)	Skin	Pigment deposition
Posterior pituitary gland (neurohypophysis)	Antidiuretic hormone (ADH), or vasopressin	Distal tubules of kidney	Reabsorption of water
	Oxytocin	Uterus, breasts	Stimulation of uterine contraction; secretion of milk; facilitation of movement of sperm in fallopian tubes
Thyroid gland	Thyroxine (T_4), triiodothyronine (T_3)	Widespread targets	Increase in metabolic rate; energy metabolism; regulation of growth; stimulation of gluconeogenesis; mobilization of fats; effect on protein metabolism

(continued)

Table 30–1
The Major Hormones: Their Sources and Effects (continued)

Endocrine Gland, Organ, or Organ System	Hormone	Target	Effect
Thyroid gland	Calcitonin	Skeleton	Decrease in plasma calcium levels
Parathyroid glands	Parathyroid hormone (PTH) or parathormone	Bones, kidneys, GI tract	Increase in plasma calcium levels; regulation of phosphorus excretion
Adrenal cortex	Glucocorticoids (eg, cortisol)	Widespread targets	Effect on carbohydrate, fat, and protein metabolism; promotion of gluconeogenesis; mobilization of amino acids; suppression of inflammation; response to stress; effect on plasma glucose levels; lipolysis
	Mineralocorticoids (eg, aldosterone)	Distal renal tubules	Maintenance of fluid balance; reabsorption of sodium; excretion of potassium
	Sex hormones (eg, androgens, estrogen, progesterone)	Gonads	Influence on development of secondary sex characteristics and growth
Adrenal medulla	Epinephrine, norepinephrine	Widespread targets	Vasoconstriction; increase in blood pressure; gluconeogenesis; sympathetic response to stress; stimulation of metabolism; secretion of ACTH
Pancreas	Insulin	Widespread targets	Decrease in plasma glucose aids glucose transport into cells; decrease in protein catabolism
	Glucagon	Liver, muscle, adipose cells	Increase in plasma glucose via glycogenolysis, gluconeogenesis, and lipolysis
	Somatostatin, or growth hormone inhibiting factor (GIF)	Pancreas, stomach	Inhibition of the secretion of insulin and glucagon
Gonads:			
Female ovaries	Estrogen	Reproductive tissues	Development of secondary sex characteristics; maturation of sexual organs; sexual functioning
	Progesterone	Uterus, breasts	Development of mammary tissue; maintenance of pregnancy; preparation of endometrium
Male testes	Testosterone	Widespread targets	Anabolism; development of secondary sex characteristics; maturation of sexual organs; sexual functioning
Kidneys	Renin	Renin substrate	Angiotensin I (regulation of blood pressure)
	Erythropoietic stimulating factor (ESF)	Bone marrow	Red blood cell production
	1,25-dihydroxycholecalciferol	Kidneys	Serum calcium levels

Endocrine Gland, Organ, or Organ System	Hormone	Target	Effect
Gastrointestinal tract	Gastrin	Stomach	Increase in gastric secretion and motility; production of pepsin and intrinsic factor
	Secretin	Stomach, pancreas	Decrease in gastric secretion
	Cholecystokinin–pancreozymin (CCK–PZ)	Pancreas	Decrease in gastric motility
	Gastric inhibitory peptide (GIP)	Gallbladder, stomach	Secretion of enzymes
	Somatostatin		
Thymus	Thymosin	Immune system	Lymphocyte development
	Thymopoietin	Immune system	Probable blocking of neuromuscular transmissions
Pineal gland	Melatonin	Hypothalamus, midbrain, gonads	Inhibition of GH secretion; decrease in plasma LH; increase in sleepiness; possible increase in well-being; sexual maturity

behavioral functions, including the emotional states of fear, anxiety, anger, rage, pleasure, and pain, as well as the states of sleep, wakefulness, and alertness. The hypothalamus, as it is influenced by the autonomic nervous system, affects all the unconscious activities of the body.

In its endocrine role, the hypothalamus has two functions:

- Regulating the anterior pituitary gland by producing and secreting releasing factors
- Producing and secreting two hormones, oxytocin and ADH, which are stored in the posterior pituitary gland

The hypothalamic releasing factors are proteins that act on the anterior pituitary gland to stimulate or inhibit the release of tropic hormones (THs). Both inhibiting factors (IFs) and releasing factors (RFs) have been identified; it is thought, although still unproven, that the hypothalamus may produce both an inhibiting and a releasing factor for each of the anterior pituitary hormones.

The release or inhibition of these hypothalamic hormones is controlled by various neurotransmitters such as serotonin, acetylcholine, norepinephrine, and dopamine (Ryan, 1980). The THs released from the anterior pituitary gland then act upon a target gland or tissue to produce a specific response (Figure 30–2). In regulating the secretion of these releasing factors, the hypothalamus processes input from both the circulatory and nervous systems. The releasing factors are secreted into the pituitary portal venous system and transported to the anterior pituitary gland.

The hypothalamus also secretes the hormones oxytocin and ADH. The storage and release of ADH are influenced by such factors as plasma osmolality, blood volume, physiologic and psychologic stress, and input from the central nervous system. ADH is produced in the hypothalamus and then transported to the posterior pituitary gland where it is stored.

Anterior Pituitary Gland

In response to the releasing factors from the hypothalamus, the anterior pituitary gland secretes several hormones, some of which control hormonal secretion by other glands. Some of the effects of the hypothalamic factors on the anterior pituitary gland are inhibitory, such as those of prolactin inhibiting factor (PIF), luteinizing hormone inhibiting factor (LIF), and growth hormone inhibiting factor (GIF), and some stimulate secretion.

The anterior pituitary hormones secreted include TSH, ACTH, GH, and LH—also called interstitial cell-stimulating hormone (ICSH) in men—FSH, and prolactin. In general, GH, ACTH, and TSH are concerned with metabolic activities, whereas LH, FSH, and prolactin are concerned with reproduction. ACTH, TSH, FSH, and LH exert their effects on target glands, either increasing their size or their secretions. Prolactin and GH directly affect the metabolism of specific target tissues. (See Table 30–1 for a summary of the major hormones.)

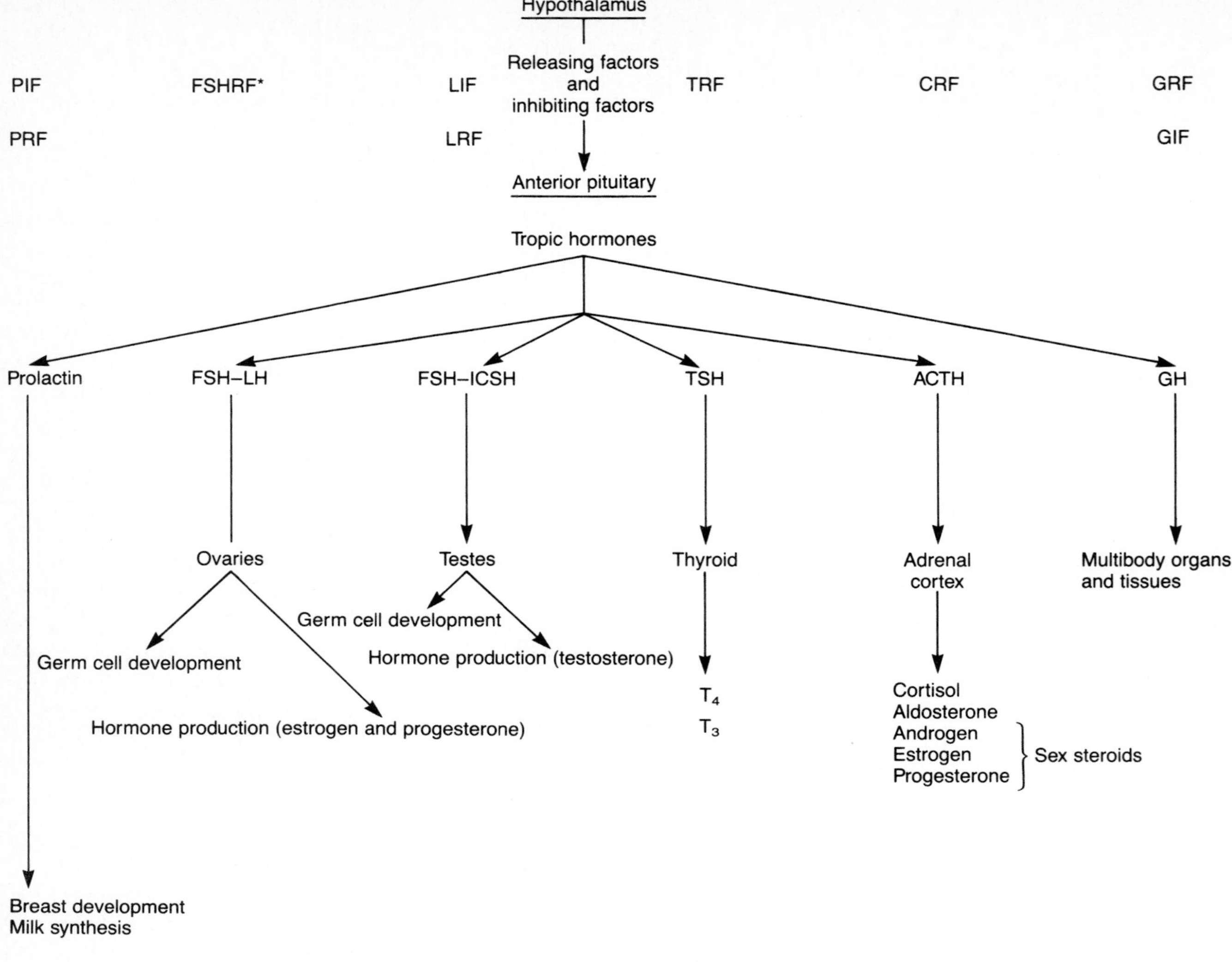

*Follicle-stimulating hormone releasing factor

Figure 30–2

The relationship of the hypothalamus, anterior pituitary gland, and target organs.

Posterior Pituitary Gland

The posterior pituitary gland does not produce any hormones; it stores and releases the two hypothalamic hormones, ADH and oxytocin. The hypothalamus mediates the release of these hormones from the posterior pituitary gland into the circulation when stimulated by the neurotransmitters acetylcholine or norepinephrine.

Adrenal Cortex

In response to stimulation by ACTH from the anterior pituitary gland, the adrenal cortex secretes three major types of hormones: glucocorticoids (eg, cortisol), mineralocorticoids (eg, aldosterone), and sex hormones (eg, androgens, estrogen, and progesterone). These hormones affect metabolism, fluid balance, and the development of secondary sex characteristics, respectively. All three types of hormones secreted by the adrenal cortex are structurally similar steroids, which results in some overlapping of their effects. However, each type of steroid produces a fairly distinct physiologic response.

GLUCOCORTICOIDS The glucocorticoids function in carbohydrate, fat, and protein metabolism and play an important role in the body's response to stress and emotional well-being. The principal glucocorticoid secreted by the adrenal cortex is cortisol, which constitutes 95% of cortical production. Corticosterone and cortisone are also produced. Cortisol has many physiologic actions and affects many tissues of the body (Table 30–1).

MINERALOCORTICOIDS The principal and most potent mineralocorticoid secreted by the adrenal cortex is aldosterone. Also secreted are desoxycorticosterone and corticosterone, but their actions are of minor importance. Aldosterone increases the reabsorption of sodium and the excretion of potassium. This is accomplished as an exchange of sodium ions for potassium or hydrogen ions, which results in the excretion of potassium and hydrogen into the urine and the retention of sodium. As sodium is reabsorbed into the blood, it brings with it water and chlorides, which mechanically increases the blood volume. This action of aldosterone is vital to the maintenance of the extracellular fluid volume. Aldosterone also promotes sodium reabsorption to a lesser degree from the sweat glands, salivary glands, and gastrointestinal tract.

Aldosterone is an important factor in the maintenance of circulatory homeostasis through its effect on electrolyte balance and its control of blood volume. It is the most potent hormonal regulator of electrolyte excretion.

The ratio of serum sodium levels to serum potassium levels is another important regulator of aldosterone secretion. If the serum potassium level rises or the serum sodium level decreases, changing the sodium–potassium ratio, the adrenal cortex will be stimulated to produce aldosterone. Prostaglandins are also thought to be involved in aldosterone secretion (Williams, 1981) through the regulation of sodium and water excretion and the release of renin.

SEX HORMONES The sex hormones produced by the adrenal cortex are the androgens and smaller amounts of estrogen and progesterone. This group of hormones has less physiologic impact than the other adrenal hormones but does affect reproductive function.

Adrenal Medulla

The adrenal medulla is considered a part of the sympathetic division of the autonomic nervous system, which controls the secretion of its hormones. Because the functions of the sympathetic nervous system and the functions of the hormones of the adrenal medulla are the same, they can compensate for each other. Thus, the medullary hormones are not essential to life but play an important role in the body's response to stress. About 15% of the hormonal secretion by the adrenal medulla is norepinephrine, and 75% is epinephrine. The nerve endings in the sympathetic nervous system also secrete norepinephrine.

Epinephrine is considered chiefly a hormone, whereas norepinephrine functions as both a hormone and a neurotransmitter. Although constant amounts of norepinephrine and epinephrine are secreted into the bloodstream, stress triggering the sympathetic nervous system can dramatically increase their output. The overall effect of the adrenal medullary hormones is to prepare the individual physiologically to function during an emergency. They have widespread effects in the body.

NOREPINEPHRINE Norepinephrine increases the contraction of the blood vessels, which increases peripheral resistance and causes the blood pressure to rise. This hormone also dilates the pupils of the eyes, increases the force and rate of myocardial contraction, and inhibits the activity of the gastrointestinal system. It causes peripheral vasoconstriction, which diverts blood away from less-needed areas (eg, the gastrointestinal tract) toward the heart and skeletal muscles, which are needed for the fight-or-flight response. Because of the length of time norepinephrine is retained in the circulation (two or three circulation times), it has an effect ten times larger than that of the sympathetic nervous system (Muthe, 1981).

EPINEPHRINE Epinephrine increases body metabolism and, in conjunction with glucagon, elevates the plasma glucose levels by **glycogenolysis** (the conversion of glycogen to glucose). Epinephrine also inhibits the secretion of insulin and elevates blood lipid levels by promoting **lipolysis** (the breakdown of fat). All these actions provide the body with a plasma glucose source for increased energy expenditure. Epinephrine is also able to constrict the arterioles of the skin selectively (causing pallor) while dilating the blood vessels of the heart and skeletal muscles. This effect increases the blood flow to these structures, which also is vital to the stress response.

REGULATION OF SECRETION Through innervation from the sympathetic nervous system, the secretion of the adrenal medullary hormones is influenced by emotional stresses (fear, anxiety), and physiologic stresses (childbirth, hypoxia, immobilization, physical exercise). The relation between the psychologic–emotional state and the endocrine system is one of the body's major homeostatic mechanisms for protecting the individual from harm and physiologic stresses in a way that preserves integrity.

Thyroid Gland

In response to stimulation by TSH, the thyroid gland secretes two types of hormones: iodinated (T_3 and T_4) and noniodinated (calcitonin). The ratio of T_4 to T_3 in the circulating blood is approximately 20:1. These hormones have similar functions but differ in the rapidity and degree of action. By far the more potent form of the hormone, T_3 is secreted in small quantities by the thyroid gland. Its increased potency (five times that of T_4) is thought to arise from the fact that it is not bound to proteins in the plasma and thus can work more readily. In peripheral tissues, T_4 is also converted to T_3. Because T_4 and T_3 have similar functions, they will be referred to collectively as *thyroid hormone* from here on.

In response to elevated plasma calcium levels, the thyroid gland releases calcitonin into the circulation. This acts on bones, where it inhibits the further release of calcium and thereby lowers serum calcium levels. It also inhibits osteoclastic activity, stimulates the transformation of osteoclasts (bone breakdown cells) and osteoblasts, and decreases the absorption of calcium from the gastrointestinal tract.

For thyroid hormones to be synthesized, iodine, pro-

Box 30–1
Major Functions of Thyroid Hormone

Metabolic effects. Thyroid hormone increases the rate of both protein synthesis and catabolism. The anabolic action of T_4 promotes growth; this hormone also enhances the synthesis of enzymes.

Carbohydrate metabolism. All processes of carbohydrate metabolism are affected by T_4. It stimulates gluconeogenesis and the utilization of glucose by the cells. It also potentiates the effect of insulin on glycogen synthesis and increases the absorption of glucose and galactose by the gut. Thyroid hormone also regulates the magnitude of the effect of epinephrine and norepinephrine on carbohydrate metabolism.

Fat metabolism. T_4 affects the synthesis, mobilization, and breakdown of fats, with its greatest effect being on fat degradation. It stimulates cholesterol synthesis and the mechanisms that remove cholesterol from the circulation. It regulates the conversion of carotene to vitamin A in the liver, stimulates lipid turnover, and stimulates the release of free fatty acids.

Metabolic rate. Thyroid hormone regulates the metabolic rate of all cells and increases the body's overall consumption of oxygen and depth of respiration. It increases heat production and regulates the heat-dissipating mechanism.

tein, and vitamins (especially A, B complex, B_{12}, and thiamine) must be present. Iodine is absorbed from the gastrointestinal tract and transported via the bloodstream in the form of inorganic iodine. Through a special mechanism known as the *iodine pump,* the thyroid gland is able to absorb and concentrate the iodine and convert it to form thyroid hormone. The thyroid gland is thought to need about 2 mg of ingested iodine each week. Normally, the thyroid stores enough thyroid hormone to maintain circulating plasma levels for several weeks. It is the only endocrine gland that is able to do this.

Thyroid hormone has widespread physiologic actions that involve all body systems and affect many tissues and organs. Its major effects are on metabolic activities and the activities of other body tissues (Box 30–1). Thyroid hormone has both extracellular and intracellular effects. The response to thyroid hormone is based on both the dosage and state of the recipient target cells.

Thyroid hormone also affects red cell production; milk production during lactation; regulation of fertility and the menstrual cycle; mental processes and development of the central nervous system; maintenance of cardiac rate, force, and output; maintenance of normal muscle and skin tone; maintenance of GH secretion, skeletal maturation, and tissue development; and maintenance of secretions from the gastrointestinal tract.

Parathyroid Glands

The parathyroid glands produce and secrete one hormone, parathyroid hormone (PTH). The basic function of PTH is the regulation of serum calcium and phosphorus, which is also regulated by vitamin D and calcitonin. Calcium is the chief cation of the body and is necessary for the integrity of the bony structures and many neuromuscular and metabolic activities.

The three target sites for PTH are the kidneys, the bones, and the gastrointestinal tract. Vitamin D obtained through the diet must be present for PTH to be effective at these three sites. In the kidneys, PTH acts directly on the renal tubules to increase the reabsorption of calcium and increase the excretion of phosphate in the urine. This maintains a normal serum calcium level. Parathyroid hormone also is necessary for the conversion of vitamin D_3 (cholecalciferol) into its active form in the kidney.

The bones of the skeletal system are the main source of calcium in the body. When serum calcium levels are low, PTH causes the release of calcium from the bone into the circulation. High serum calcium levels reduce PTH secretion, causing either movement of the excess calcium back into the bones or excretion.

In the gastrointestinal tract, PTH directs the absorption of calcium and phosphorus from the duodenum and jejunum through active and passive transport. Vitamin D is essential for this process. Parathyroid hormone also affects the level of phosphorus in the serum. Phosphorus is normally absorbed from the gastrointestinal tract and excreted by the kidneys. Increased levels of circulating PTH stimulate an increase in phosphorus excretion by the kidneys.

Calcitonin counterbalances the effects of PTH by protecting against hypercalcemia through its ability to lower serum calcium levels. This hormone affects the same target tissues as PTH (ie, the bones, kidneys, and gastrointestinal tract) and tends to promote hypocalcemia by the initiation of bone resorption and decreased calcium absorption from the small intestine. Both mechanisms reduce the rate of movement of calcium into the extracellular fluid and thus promote hypocalcemia. In the kidneys, calcitonin initially increases the excretion of calcium and phosphorus.

Gonads

The ovaries produce estrogen and progesterone, which affect reproduction and the development of secondary sex characteristics in the female. The testes produce testosterone, which affects reproduction and the development of secondary sex characteristics in the male. For a discussion of the function and regulation of secretion of the gonadal hormones, refer to Chapter 47.

Pancreas

The pancreas has both endocrine and exocrine functions. For a discussion of the exocrine functions, refer to Chapter 40. The endocrine function of the pancreas involves the secretion of three hormones. The major pancreatic hormones, insulin and glucagon, are secreted by the beta and alpha cells of the islets of the pancreas, respectively. The delta cells of the pancreas secrete a third hormone, somatostatin, also called growth hormone inhibiting factor (GIF).

INSULIN Insulin is a protein secreted by the beta cells of the pancreas that directly affects the metabolism of carbohydrates, proteins, and lipids. This anabolic hormone promotes the synthesis, storage, or both, of carbohydrates, fats, proteins, and nucleic acids. Insulin affects many tissues, but its most important sites of action are fat, muscle, and liver cells. The brain, renal tubule cells, intestinal mucosa, and erythrocytes do not require insulin for the uptake of glucose.

Insulin is thought to act by altering the permeability of the cell membrane, increasing the plasma membrane transport of glucose, other monosaccharides, certain amino acids, certain fatty acids, potassium, and magnesium. Insulin also promotes the movement of potassium and magnesium into the cell. Potassium is an important factor in the regulation of enzymes and affects the membrane potential of the cell. Magnesium is involved in the activation of certain cellular enzymes. Insulin is degraded by the liver, kidney, and pancreas; 80% of this process is accomplished by the liver and kidneys. The major functions of insulin are summarized in Box 30–2.

Many factors inhibit and stimulate the secretion of insulin, including:

- Circulating levels of glucose, amino acids, and fatty acids
- Gastrointestinal hormones
- The sympathetic nervous system
- Other hormones and neurotransmitters
- Drugs

GLUCAGON Glucagon is secreted by the alpha cells of the islets of Langerhans in the pancreas as well as by the cells of the upper intestinal tract. The major site for the action of glucagon is the liver, where it promotes gluconeogenesis (the formation of glucose from noncarbohydrate substances such as fat and proteins), lipolysis, and glycogenolysis. All these actions increase serum glucose levels, which is the major function of glucagon. This hormone also stimulates the release of catecholamines, which increase the serum level of glucose.

Glucagon stimulates the secretion of insulin by a direct effect on the beta cells of the pancreas (Muthe, 1981). This appears to be a contradiction in function but when looked at in its entirety, the process is a mechanism for the control of normal serum glucose levels. For example, in hypoglycemia, the decrease in serum glucose levels caused by insulin stimulates the secretion of glucagon, which then raises glucose levels by stimulating glycogenolysis and gluconeogenesis. Because glucagon has the net effect of raising serum glucose levels, it stimulates the secretion of insulin, which then lowers the level of glucose in the serum. These specific actions of glucagon are under study for the management of insulin dependent diabetes mellitus (see Chapter 32), which is often hard to control. Clients often fluctuate between episodes of hypoglycemia and hyperglycemia, and a glucagon deficiency is thought to play a role.

The secretion of glucagon is stimulated by decreased serum glucose levels, increased levels of amino acids, and decreased serum levels of fatty acids. It is inhibited by increased serum levels of fatty acids. In general, there is an inverse relationship between serum glucose levels and the output of glucagon.

SOMATOSTATIN Somatostatin, or GIF, is secreted by the hypothalamus, the delta cells of the pancreas, and cells in the upper portion of the small intestine and gastric mucosa. Somatostatin's major function is to inhibit the release of GH, and it also inhibits the release of thyrotropin releasing

Box 30–2
Major Functions of Insulin

Carbohydrate metabolism. The major effect of insulin on carbohydrate metabolism is to increase the uptake and utilization of glucose by the muscle and adipose cells. Insulin also regulates the synthesis of glycogen in the liver (glycogenesis) and inhibits the breakdown of glycogen to glucose (glycogenolysis) and of amino acids to glucose (gluconeogenesis). All these actions reduce serum glucose levels.

Fat metabolism. Insulin is required for the transport of glucose across the cell membrane from the circulation into the adipose cell. This hormone enhances the uptake and storage of free fatty acids by the adipose cells and the synthesis of lipids (primarily triglycerides). These actions in turn promote lipogenesis and inhibit lipolysis. Insulin decreases the oxidation of free fatty acids and inhibits ketone formation.

Protein metabolism. Insulin assists the movement of amino acids into the cells and the conversion of amino acids into protein, thereby depositing more protein into muscles. Growth and nitrogen retention are promoted by insulin, whereas proteolysis (the catabolism of protein) is inhibited.

Effect on the liver. The liver plays an important role in the regulation of serum glucose levels. When these levels are elevated, glucose is stored as glycogen in the liver, muscles, or other tissues. When serum glucose levels are low, the liver is able to break down glycogen, lipids, and proteins to glucose and thereby restore the blood glucose levels to normal. It does this through glycogenolysis, lipolysis, and proteolysis.

Effect on fluid and electrolyte balances. Besides decreasing serum glucose levels, insulin decreases the serum levels of potassium by increasing its intracellular transport. Insulin also increases the transport of magnesium and phosphorus into the cell.

Effect of nucleic transformation. Insulin stimulates the formation of DNA, RNA, and adenosine triphosphate (ATP).

factor (TRF). Locally, it appears to inhibit the release of insulin and glucagon by the pancreas and to suppress the secretion of gastrin and other secretions from the gastrointestinal tract, although this role is not clear. Somatostatin is also thought to play a role in body weight, especially in obesity.

Thymus

Although little is known about the thymus, it is thought to produce at least two hormones—thymosin and thymopoietin—which exert their principal effect on the body's immune system. Thymosin stimulates the maturation of T-lymphocytes, which are necessary in the cellular response to infection and influence the production of lymphocytes by peripheral areas of the body. Thymosin also contributes to the development of B-lymphocytes, which are involved in the antigen–antibody response (Muthe, 1981). Thymopoietin is thought to block neuromuscular transmissions and has been implicated as a factor in myasthenia gravis. Decreased or absent circulating levels (specific to age) may be seen in combined immunodeficiency states.

Pineal Gland

The pineal gland secretes melatonin which exerts its effect on the pituitary, hypothalamus, midbrain, and gonads. Other substances associated with the pineal gland are histamine, norepinephrine, dopamine, and serotonin.

Kidneys

The major functions of the kidneys are excretion of urine and the regulation of water, electrolyte, and acid–base balances. The kidneys also perform an endocrine function through production of renin, erythropoietin, and 1,25-dihydroxycholecalciferol. The kidneys control the production of erythropoietin, the hormone that regulates red blood cell production. They also produce renin, an enzyme that functions as an integral part of the renin–angiotensin system. This system is vital to the maintenance of the body's extracellular fluid volume. In the presence of PTH, the kidneys produce 1,25-dihydroxycholecalciferol from 25-hydroxycholecalciferol. The compound 1,25-dihydroxycholecalciferol is the major active form of vitamin D, which is necessary for the maintenance of calcium in the body.

Gastrointestinal Tract

Several hormones work in conjunction with the nervous system to control digestion and the absorption of foodstuffs. These hormones are produced in the walls of the stomach, in the upper intestine, and at various sites throughout the bowel. The hormones that have been isolated and studied are gastrin, secretin, and CCK–PZ. Others currently under study include gut glucagon, somatostatin, and gastric-inhibitory peptide (GIP).

SECTION II

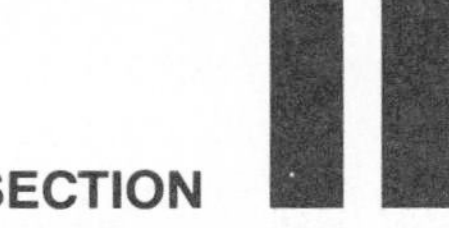

Pathophysiologic Influences and Effects

Pathophysiologic changes commonly seen in endocrine dysfunction are discussed in this section. More specific influences and effects of dysfunction in individual endocrine organs are presented in Chapters 32, 33, and 34.

Anterior Pituitary Gland

Most of the disorders affecting the pituitary gland originate in the anterior lobe. The effects of pathology on the anterior pituitary gland can be broadly summarized as hyperpituitarism and hypopituitarism.

Hyperfunction of the Anterior Pituitary Gland

The most common cause of *hyperfunction* of the anterior pituitary gland is a neoplastic secreting tumor, usually a benign adenoma. Tumors of the pituitary gland exert their effects through two major mechanisms:

- Pressure on structures in the brain (eg, the optic tract), which causes visual symptoms and headaches
- Excessive secretion of one or more of the anterior pituitary hormones, which results in increased stimulation of one or more target glands

One of the pathophysiologic manifestations of these tumors is hypersomatotropism (excess GH), which can result in acromegaly in adults and gigantism in children. Other pathophysiologic effects of excessive GH secretion include **goiter** (from GH stimulation of the thyroid tissues) and diabetes mellitus secondary to the diabetogenic effect of GH. Cardiomegaly and hypertension can also occur. Visual impairment and eventual blindness are possible because of compression of tissue by the expanding tumor. Amenorrhea in women and loss of libido and potency in men may occur because compression from the expanding tumor leads to gonadal deficiencies from loss of healthy gonadotropin-producing cells.

Hypofunction of the Anterior Pituitary Gland

Hypofunction of the anterior pituitary gland can arise from many causes. It can be secondary to pathology of the anterior pituitary gland or to injury to the hypothalamus resulting in a decrease or absence of the hypothalamic releasing factors. Hypopituitarism may be manifested by isolated hormonal deficiencies or by a deficiency of both the anterior and posterior pituitary hormones (panhypopituitarism). The exact hormonal deficit and its etiology are important to an understanding of a client's symptoms and signs. The causes of hypofunction of the anterior pituitary gland are listed in Box 30–3.

The symptoms of hypopituitarism, like those of hyperpituitarism, depend on the number and type of hormones involved. Approximately 70% to 80% of the pituitary gland must be destroyed before symptoms and signs of deficiency are apparent. This loss of function is seen in the gonadal target tissue first; this is followed by signs of thyroid deficiency and, lastly, adrenal cortex insufficiency.

Posterior Pituitary Gland

The two hormones of the posterior pituitary gland are synthesized in the hypothalamus; the posterior pituitary gland simply serves as a site of storage and release. Therefore, damage to the posterior lobe does not affect the synthesis of these hormones. However, if the hypothalamus or hypothalamic–hypophyseal pathways were damaged, changes in the secretions of ADH and oxytocin would result. Only the pathophysiologic influences of ADH will be discussed in this section.

The pathophysiologic effects involving the hypothalamus and posterior pituitary gland can be summarized broadly as a deficiency and inappropriate secretion of ADH hormone. A deficiency of ADH results in diabetes insipidus.

Deficiency of Antidiuretic Hormone

Deficiencies of ADH may be primary or secondary. In primary diabetes insipidus, a defect is thought to be inherent in the posterior pituitary gland itself. The etiology may be congenital or **idiopathic** (accounting for 30% to 40% of cases). In secondary diabetes insipidus, the symptoms are the result of pathology in the hypothalamic–pituitary pathways. Nephrogenic diabetes insipidus arises from an inherited defect in which the kidney tubules are unresponsive to ADH. Its causes include electrolyte disorders, chronic renal disease, and drugs (methoxyflurane, lithium, and demeclocycline). Pathophysiologic changes with diabetes insipidus include copious excretion (5 to 15 L/day) of a dilute urine causing intense thirst and dehydration.

Inappropriate Secretion of Antidiuretic Hormone

Hypothalamic–posterior pituitary pathology also can result in a syndrome of inappropriate ADH (SIADH) secretion. The secretion of ADH normally is controlled by a feedback mechanism that monitors the osmolality of the plasma. For example, as the osmolality of the plasma rises, ADH secretion is stimulated. As it falls (hypo-osmolality), the secretions of ADH is suppressed. In SIADH, a persistent secretion of ADH occurs unrelated to the osmolality of the plasma. Causes of SIADH include tumors, trauma, infections, porphyria, drugs, and stress.

Box 30–3
Causes of Hypopituitarism of the Anterior Pituitary Gland

Nonsecreting primary anterior pituitary tumors (rarely secondary, or metastatic)

Infarctions as seen in sickle-cell disease, temporal arteritis, cavernous sinus thrombosis, atherosclerosis, and Sheehan's syndrome (postpartum pituitary necrosis)

Therapeutic ablation of the pituitary gland by surgery or irradiation

Infiltrative granulomatous disease (eg, hemochromatosis), sarcoidosis, histiocytosis, and idiopathic granulomatous disease

Infection (eg, brucellosis, mycosis, syphilis, or tuberculosis)

Hypothalamic pathophysiology, including congenital malformations (hydrocephalus), trauma, neoplasia, infection, and granulomatous disease

Thyroid Gland

Pathophysiologic influences on the thyroid gland result in hyperfunction, hypofunction, and/or enlargement of the gland. The results are hyperthyroidism, hypothyroidism, or goiter. **Euthyroidism** refers to a normal state of thyroid function.

Hyperfunction of the Thyroid Gland

Hyperfunction of the thyroid gland is characterized by an excessive secretion of thyroid hormone resulting in a condition known as hyperthyroidism. The causes of hyperthyroidism include ingestion of exogenous thyroid hormones; Graves' disease; Hashimoto's thyroiditis; subacute and chronic thyroiditis; nodular hyperthyroidism; ovarian carcinoma; and overproduction of TSH, chorionic gonadotropin, or both. Increased thyroid hormone production affects many body systems as well as the body's basal metabolic rate and energy production. The circulatory, nervous, and endocrine systems are affected, as is the gastrointestinal tract. The pathophysiologic symptoms are generally related to the increase in body metabolism.

Hypofunction of the Thyroid Gland

Hypofunction of the thyroid gland, or hypothyroidism, results in a deficiency of T_3 and T_4 or both. Hypothyroidism can be congenital or acquired. In this condition, the rate of metabolic processes decreases, which affects both mental and physical functions.

Congenital etiologies of hypothyroidism include the absence of the thyroid gland and defects in the enzymes responsible for the synthesis of thyroid hormone. Acquired causes of hypothyroidism include surgical removal of the thyroid gland, chronic thyroiditis, irradiation of the thyroid gland or therapy using radioactive iodine, decreased secretion of TSH from the anterior pituitary gland, and drugs that inhibit the synthesis or release of thyroid hormone. In the adult, a severe deficiency of thyroid hormone results in **myxedema,** which may be primary (from a pathologic condition within the gland itself) or secondary (from a pathologic condition in the anterior pituitary gland).

Enlargement of the Thyroid Gland

An enlarged thyroid gland, or *goiter,* may be fibrous or cystic and may contain nodules or be composed of an increased number of follicular cells. Goiters may be associated with hyperthyroidism, hypothyroidism, or euthyroidism. Goiters associated with normal thyroid function are called *nontoxic goiters.* Goiters are often thought to represent an increase in the size of the thyroid gland to compensate for decreased thyroid hormone synthesis. The stimulus for the enlargement of the gland is the increased secretion of TSH that occurs as a result of the low circulating T_4 levels.

Parathyroid Glands

Pathology of the parathyroid glands results in their hyperfunction and hypofunction. Resulting conditions are *hyperparathyroidism* and *hypoparathyroidism.*

Hyperfunction of the Parathyroid Glands

Hyperfunction of the parathyroid glands leads to an excessive secretion of PTH. This condition, known as hyperparathyroidism, can be classified as primary, secondary, or tertiary. Primary hyperparathyroidism arises from intrinsic pathology in the parathyroid glands. Secondary hyperparathyroidism is the result of a compensatory mechanism to overcome low serum calcium levels (hypocalcemia). Tertiary hyperparathyroidism is caused by an excessive secretion of PTH from an ectopic source.

Hypofunction of the Parathyroid Glands

Hypofunction of the parathyroid, or hypoparathyroidism, results in a deficiency in PTH secretion or a decrease in the peripheral action of PTH. This condition is characterized by low levels of PTH, resulting in low circulating serum levels of calcium (and high serum levels of phosphorus). The elevated serum phosphorus levels maintain the calcium phosphate salts in the bone and bind calcium in the gut. This reduces the absorption of calcium and the effectiveness of vitamin D, which serves to perpetuate the low serum levels of calcium. Causes of hypoparathyroidism include familial or hereditary hypoparathyroidism, autoimmune disorders, and iatrogenic causes.

Adrenal Glands

Pathophysiologic influences on the adrenal glands result in either hyperfunction or hypofunction. The clinical manifestations seen in these clients represent the effects of an excess or deficiency of the adrenal hormones on their target tissues or glands.

Adrenal Cortex

ADRENAL CORTEX HYPERFUNCTION Hyperfunction of the adrenal cortex results in the increased secretion of glucocorticoids, mineralocorticoids, and sex hormones. The overall symptoms and signs are most representative of the excess secretion of cortisol (hypercortisolism). The primary causes of hypercortisolism, originating from within the adrenal cortex itself, include neoplasia and bilateral hyperplasia. In **iatrogenic** hypercortisolism, an exogenous source, such as prolonged use of glucocorticoids or ACTH, is responsible. Increased ACTH production by the pituitary gland due to tumor may cause adrenal hyperfunction. Pituitary tumors or hyperplasia is responsible for approximately 60% to 80% of all cases of adrenal hyperfunction. Ectopic ACTH-producing tumors include carcinomas of the lung or the gastrointestinal tract.

ADRENAL INSUFFICIENCY Hypofunction of the adrenal cortex, or adrenal insufficiency, results in a decreased secretion of glucocorticoids, mineralocorticoids, and sex hormones. The causes of adrenal insufficiency can be grouped into two categories: primary (based on pathology occurring within the gland itself) and secondary (arising from an undersecretion of ACTH from the anterior pituitary gland, which may be due to pathology in the pituitary gland or the hypothalamus). Primary causes may be acute or chronic.

Adrenal Medulla

Pathophysiology of the adrenal medulla is rare and is usually associated with hyperfunction. A pheochromocytoma is the most common cause of adrenal medulla hyperfunction. This tumor secretes excessive amounts of epinephrine and norepinephrine, resulting in increased metabolism, hypertension, and hyperglycemia. Other disorders associated with hyperfunction of the adrenal medualla neurofibromatosis, carcinomas (eg, of the thyroid), and hyperparathyroidism.

Pancreas

In its role as an endocrine gland, the pancreas is responsible for the production of at least three hormones: insulin; glucagon; and somatostatin or growth inhibiting factor (GIF). When there is a deficiency of insulin (diabetes mellitus), the blood glucose level rises. In the diabetic state, the normal insulin mechanism has been disrupted. Factors that may be involved in this include insufficient production of insulin, increased insulin requirements by the body, a decrease in the availability of insulin receptors, a decrease in the effectiveness of the available insulin, and increased destruction of insulin by the liver and other tissues.

Chronic hyperlipidemia often occurs in diabetics because of increased lipolysis. This abnormality, combined with the other derangements of glucose and protein metabolism seen in diabetes mellitus, often results in pathologic changes affecting both large and small blood vessels.

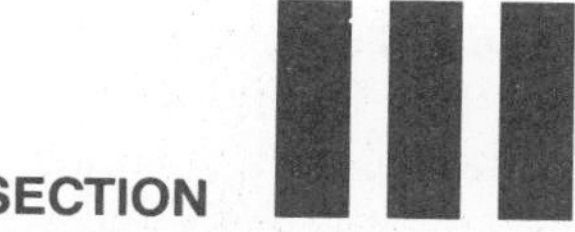

Related System Influences and Effects

The endocrine system affects and is affected by many other organ systems through the action of its hormones. Of special importance is the interrelatedness of the endocrine and central nervous systems mediated through the actions of the hypothalamus and adrenal medulla. The endocrine system also interrelates with the cardiovascular, renal, gastrointestinal, integumentary, musculoskeletal, and reproductive systems. These interactions maintain homeostasis as well as the ability to withstand stress.

The interrelation between the central nervous system and the endocrine system lies between the adrenal medulla and the hypothalamic–pituitary axis. Central nervous system symptoms and signs that may indicate endocrine dysfunction include ataxia, seizures, headache, fatigue, coma, and paresthesia.

Cardiovascular symptoms and signs that may reflect endocrine dysfunction include hypertension, tachycardia or atrial fibrillation, congestive heart failure, deep venous thrombosis, hypotension, bradycardia, and pericardial effusions. Symptoms and signs in the musculoskeletal system possibly related to endocrine problems include fractures, bone pain, arthralgias, and muscle weakness and fatigability. Gastrointestinal symptoms and signs that could be related to endocrine pathology include anorexia, indigestion, weight loss, diarrhea, constipation, peptic ulcer formation, ascites, and abdominal pain.

Renal calculi are sometimes seen in hyperparathyroidism, acromegaly, and Cushing's syndrome. Polyuria and polydipsia can result from pituitary tumors, diabetes mellitus, hypercalcemia, and hyperthyroidism.

Clients with diabetes mellitus, hyperthyroidism, or both often have pruritus. Excessive hair growth may be seen with adrenal hyperplasia or tumor. Clients with acromegaly, hypoglycemia, pheochromocytoma, or hyperthyroidism may exhibit hyperhidrosis. Facial flushing may be seen in clients with pheochromocytoma, and coldness of the skin may be seen with hypothyroidism. Clients with Addison's disease and hyperthyroidism may have hyperpigmentation of the skin, and those with Cushing's syndrome may have ecchymosis and purplish striae on their abdomens.

The endocrine system can cause major changes in an individual's reproductive function. A loss of libido and potency are seen in clients with hypogonadism, diabetes mellitus, acromegaly, and hypothyroidism. Menorrhagia is often associated with hypothyroidism and oligomenorrhea with hyperthyroidism. Amenorrhea can be caused by a pituitary tumor, hyperthyroidism, hypogonadism, acromegaly, or Cushing's syndrome.

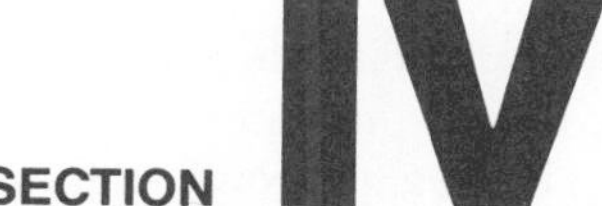

Psychosocial/Lifestyle Influences and Effects

The client with endocrine dysfunction may have to face the reality of coping with chronic illness or an acute life-threatening situation. Anger, fear, guilt, and denial are common initial reactions to a new diagnosis. Individual responses to this challenge vary according to the client's past experiences, attitudes toward health and illness, past coping patterns, and support system strength. It is not unusual to find clients with several years' history of a disease (eg, diabetes mellitus) still working through their anger and denial over the initial diagnosis.

Lifestyle changes may be necessary because of changes in the ability of the client with an endocrine disorder to perform activities of daily living, to tolerate stress, to meet economic obligations, or to continue with usual dietary patterns. The simple fact that these changes are necessary often confirms to the client and significant others that the illness is serious and that all of their lives will be affected.

Self-Concept and Self-Esteem

The client with endocrine dysfunction may have to deal with a change in self-concept and a loss of self-esteem arising from changes in body image, decreased functional abilities, limitations to intimacy, restrictions in autonomy, and limitations in decision-making processes. Changes in self-concept and the loss of self-esteem may interfere with the client's ability to carry through with the treatment plan and accept the diagnosis and its implications. For example, body image significantly affects how people view and feel about themselves. A client who is a pituitary dwarf must adjust to a world structured for taller people. Clients with Cushing's syndrome have to adjust to the cosmetic implications of the moon face, buffalo hump, and truncal obesity seen with that disorder. Those with Addison's disease must protect themselves from stressful situations, and clients with hypothyroidism suffer from easy fatigability and sometimes a slowing in mental functions. These pathophysiologic changes affect the client's ability to function in normal situations, causing further stress and anxiety.

Certain endocrine disorders cause emotional lability and personality change. This presents serious concerns for the client, who often states, "I can't control myself" or "What is the matter with me?" The nurse can help both client and family understand the relation between the physiologic problem and the psychologic changes.

Sexual Expression and Reproduction

Often in thyroid disorders, as well as in disorders affecting the secretion of the adrenocortical sex hormones, clients have concerns about changes in libido and sexual potency. Encourage the client to discuss these concerns with the sexual partner.

Occupational and Economic Factors

Occupational implications of endocrine disorders include the possibility of changing or limiting work because of a physical disability. Clients with visual loss or changes in mentation often must make significant occupational adjustments. The client may have to relocate to be closer to a source of health care, require a special living environment, or need adaptive equipment. Economic factors that might cause a change in lifestyle include the need for lifelong medications and medical supervision along with the burdens of the expense of diagnostic tests and hospitalization.

Dietary Factors

The adjustment to new dietary requirements is a major challenge for clients with endocrine disease. Clients who previously gave little thought to nutrition or balanced meals may now have fluid restrictions, special diets, and dietary supplements. Clients are often asked to weigh and measure each portion of their meals and keep an accurate intake record. These dietary changes not only add extra strain to an already stressful situation but also create an economic burden. In addition, the client who previously gained psychologic satisfaction from eating must now consciously think about not only the content of foods to be ingested but also spacing of meals throughout the day. This is especially true for diabetes, where the variables of nutrition, insulin, and exercise must be balanced carefully.

The nurse must recognize the importance of these psychosocial influences and understand how they affect the client and significant others. Take ample time to explore with clients the effects of these influences on them and their importance for an improved state of health. In planning care for clients with endocrine disorders and for all clients, psychosocial/lifestyle influences of health problems are as important as the pathophysiologic factors.

Chapter Highlights

The major glands of the endocrine system are the anterior and posterior pituitary glands, thyroid gland, parathyroid glands, gonads, adrenal glands, and the pancreas.

The thymus and pineal glands also function as part of the endocrine system, although their exact mechanism of action is still under study. The kidneys and gastrointestinal tract perform an endocrine function, along with other functions.

Hormones are the chemical substances secreted by the endocrine glands directly into the circulation. Their effects may be local or generalized.

Each hormone secreted by an endocrine gland exerts a characteristic effect on its target tissue.

Hormones may be regulated by the hypothalamus, hypothalamic releasing factors, anterior pituitary hormones, the autonomic nervous system, serum nutrient and ion concentrations, feedback mechanisms, autonomous functioning, or diurnal variation.

The effects of pathology on the anterior pituitary gland are hypersecretion or hyposecretion. The symptoms of hyperpituitarism and hypopituitarism depend on the number and type of hormones involved.

Pathologic conditions of the posterior pituitary gland do not affect the synthesis of oxytocin and ADH, because these hormones are produced by the hypothalamus and merely stored and released by the posterior pituitary gland.

The two major endocrine effects related to pathologic conditions of the hypothalamic–posterior pituitary region are deficiency of ADH and inappropriate secretion of ADH.

Pathophysiologic influences on the thyroid gland can produce hyperfunction, hypofunction, or enlargement of the gland.

A goiter is an enlarged thyroid gland and may be associated with hyperthyroidism, hypothyroidism, or euthyroidism. Goiters are thought to represent an increase in the size of the thyroid gland to compensate for decreased thyroid hormone synthesis.

Pathologic conditions of the parathyroid glands

result in hyperfunction or hypofunction of the gland.

The three major disorders resulting from hyperfunction of the adrenal cortex are Cushing's syndrome (adrenal glucocorticoid excess), primary aldosteronism (mineralocorticoid excess), and reproductive disorders related to excessive amounts of adrenal sex hormones.

Hypofunction of the adrenal cortex (adrenal insufficiency) can be primary or secondary. Primary adrenal insufficiency results in Addison's disease.

Pathologic conditions of the adrenal medulla are rare and usually associated with hyperfunction. Pheochromocytoma is the most common cause of adrenal medulla hyperfunction.

The major disorder associated with endocrine dysfunction of the pancreas is diabetes mellitus.

The endocrine system interrelates with many other organ systems of the body to maintain homeostasis and help the organism withstand stress.

Because the endocrine system has far-reaching effects, dysfunction in this system can cause major developmental and sociocultural crises. Lifestyle changes are often necessary because of changes in abilities to perform the activities of daily living; changes in tolerance to stress; economic, environmental, and occupational factors; and special nutritional needs.

Bibliography

Diabetes Mellitus, 8th ed. Indianapolis: Eli Lilly, 1980.

Dimmond M, James SL: *Chronic Illness across the Life-Span.* Norwalk, CT: Appleton–Century–Crofts, 1983.

Hushman JM: *Endocrine Pathophysiology: A Patient-Oriented Approach.* 2nd ed. Philadelphia: Lea & Febriger, 1982.

Kaye D, Rose LF (editors): *Fundamentals of Internal Medicine.* St. Louis: Mosby, 1983.

Miller JF: *Coping With Chronic Illness.* Philadelphia: Davis, 1983.

Muthe NC: *Endocrinology: A Nursing Approach.* Boston: Little, Brown, 1981.

Ryan WG: *Endocrine Disorders: A Pathophysiological Approach.* Chicago: Year Book Medical Publishers, 1980.

Sanford SJ: Dysfunction of the adrenal gland: Physiologic considerations and nursing problems. *Nurs Clin North Am* 1980; 15:481–498.

Solomon BL: The hypothalamus and the pituitary gland: An overview. *Nurs Clin North Am* 1980; 15:435–451.

Taitano–Hoffman JT, Newly–Bond T: Hypercalcemia in primary hyperparathyroidism. *Nurs Clin North Am* 1980; 15:469–480.

Vander AJ, Sherman JH, Luciano DA: *Human Physiology: The Mechanisms of Body Function.* New York: McGraw–Hill, 1980.

Wake–Musante M, Brensinger JF III: The nurse's role in hypothyroidism. *Nurs Clin North Am* 1980; 15:453–467.

Williams RH (editor): *Textbook of Endocrinology,* 6th ed. Philadelphia: Saunders, 1981.

Wilson HS, Kneisl CR: *Psychiatric Nursing,* 2nd ed. Menlo Park, CA: Addison–Wesley, 1983.

CHAPTER **31**

The Nursing Process for Clients With Endocrine Dysfunction

Objectives

When you have finished studying this chapter, you should be able to:

Specify the major components of the health history to be obtained from clients with endocrine dysfunction.

Explain specific assessment approaches in evaluating clients with disease of the endocrine system.

Identify the nursing implications of diagnostic studies commonly used to evaluate clients with endocrine dysfunction.

Determine appropriate nursing diagnoses for clients with disorders of the endocrine system.

Develop, with the client, realistic goals of care.

Anticipate the psychosocial/lifestyle implications of endocrine dysfunction for clients and their significant others.

Develop a nursing care plan for a client with endocrine dysfunction.

Implement nursing interventions specific to clients with endocrine disease.

Evaluate the effectiveness of the nursing care plan and modify it as necessary to meet client needs.

The application of the nursing process to the care of clients with endocrine dysfunction is a challenge because of the complexity of the endocrine system and its interrelation with other body systems. This chapter discusses assessment of the client with suspected endocrine problems, relevant diagnostic studies, and the development of nursing care approaches based on the nursing diagnosis.

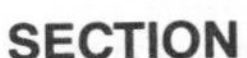

SECTION **I**

Nursing Assessment: Establishing the Data Base

One of the most important nursing responsibilities in working with clients having endocrine dysfunction is the establishment of a comprehensive data base with both subjective and objective information. Because of the widespread effects of endocrine dysfunction, thoroughness and accuracy are essential in the collection of these data.

Subjective Data

Document any history of endocrine disease (eg, thyroid disease or diabetes mellitus). Has the client ever been evaluated for any endocrine disorder? If so, when and where? What was the outcome? Has the client undergone any head trauma, neck surgery, or head and neck radiation? Has the client ever taken any medication for an endocrine disorder? If so, what type, why, and for how long? Obtaining the places and dates of former treatments is invaluable in obtaining medical records later. In addition to specific questions on endocrine dysfunction, ask about related system disorders such as hypertension, seizure disorders, autoimmune dysfunction, reproductive problems, cardiac disease, and central nervous system disorders.

There are specific symptoms and signs in each body system that, when put together with the rest of the history, suggest possible endocrine dysfunction. These include:

- **General symptoms and signs** Sudden or unexplained changes in height or weight; unexplained increase in hand or foot size; change in head size; episodes of weakness or fatigue; fevers or sweats; frequent colds, infections, or illnesses; intolerance to heat or cold
- **Skin and hair** Excessive hair growth or loss, excessive sweating, facial flushing, changes in skin pigmentation and temperature, ecchymoses, pruritus, changes in skin texture, abnormalities in hair distribution, **vitiligo** (skin patches that lack pigment)
- **HEENT** Tinnitus, changes in hearing acuity, visual loss or changes in visual acuity, diplopia, hemianopia, exophthalmos (unilateral or bilateral), changes in size of neck, pressure sensations in throat, difficulty swallowing, goiter
- **Cardiovascular** Hypertension, hypotension, dysrhythmias, tachycardia, atrial fibrillation, bradycardia, congestive heart failure, pericardial effusions, venous thromboses
- **Gastrointestinal** Polyphagia, anorexia, diarrhea, constipation, weight loss or gain, abdominal pain, ascites, indigestion, ulcer
- **Urinary** Polydipsia, polyuria, renal calculi
- **Reproductive** Amenorrhea, oligomenorrhea, dysmenorrhea, menorrhagia, metrorrhagia, changes in sexual function and libido
- **Musculoskeletal** Weakness, fractures, joint and bone pain
- **Neurologic** Headaches, fatigue, changes in cognitive ability, changes in mood or behavior, ataxia, somnolence or coma, seizures, paresthesia

Inherited patterns can occur in some endocrine disorders, so pay careful attention to a family history of pituitary, adrenal, pancreatic, thyroid, parathyroid, or gonadal dysfunction. Question clients about a family history of glucose intolerance. If the family history is positive, determine the nature of the family relationship, as well as the degree of severity of the relative's condition (eg, maternal aunt, age 35, Type I diabetes mellitus, blind × 10 years; paternal grandfather, age 82, Type II diabetes mellitus × 5 years). Knowledge of the family's general state of health gives the nurse an opportunity to identify health problems that may have an immediate or future effect on the client's well-being.

Endocrine dysfunction may produce psychologic as well as physiologic changes. In addition to coping with a possibly life-threatening situation, the client may need to adjust to the probability of living with a chronic disorder that requires major lifestyle changes. A psychosocial history should cover the client's previous responses to ill health, including coping patterns, support system, and cultural and religious influences.

Psychologic problems may arise from the disease process itself and the client's perception of the actual diagnosis and response to it. Although the relation of endocrine dysfunction to psychologic well-being is not well understood, certain psychologic changes have been observed in specific endocrine disorders. For example, clients with hypothyroidism may be lethargic and confused, have slowing of their cognitive processes, and occasionally even experience psychotic episodes. Clients with hyperthyroidism may exhibit increasing irritability, anxiety, and emotional lability. Cognition can be tested formally as part of the mental status examination (see Chapter 5).

Because endocrine disorders can have such widespread effects, the nurse must evaluate clients for the impact of the present problems on their lives. An occupational history should be obtained, including current occupation, type of duties, length of time employed, and ability to perform required tasks. Have any limitations been imposed by the employer because of the client's physical or mental status? How satisfied is the client with his or her present position? Has the client's illness affected the present economic status? Is the client's income adequate to meet current and future needs?

Objective Data

The nurse gathers objective data through a thorough physical assessment of the client and a careful review of all pertinent laboratory data. Assess those systems directly related to the chief concern. The information from the subjective and objective assessments enables the nurse to formulate and rank a list of client problems.

Because the effects of endocrine pathology are so widespread, often several organ systems must be examined. In general, the areas to be assessed in most clients suspected of having endocrine problems include vital signs; general appearance; hair and nails; skin; eyes; neck; heart; lungs; abdomen; genitals; and the musculoskeletal and neurologic systems.

Physical Assessment

VITAL SIGNS Assess the client's height and weight and compare them with growth charts. A careful developmental and familial growth history may help in the interpretation of abnormalities. Assess the blood pressure in both arms initially and in at least two positions (supine and seated). Determine the apical and radial pulse rates, rhythm, and quality along with the client's respiratory rate, rhythm, and depth. Take the client's temperature.

GENERAL APPEARANCE Note whether clients appear to be close to their chronologic age. Are the body parts symmetrical and in proportion? Are any limbs missing or malformed? What is the client's stature and **habitus** (physical appearance)? How is the weight distributed? Are there any abnormal movements of the extremities or face, for example, spasms or twitching of facial muscles (Chvostek's sign)? Does the face appear normal in configuration and color? A **plethoric** (round, erythematous), moon face suggests Cushing's syndrome, whereas puffiness of the face suggests hypothyroidism.

ASSESSMENT OF THE SKIN, HAIR, AND NAILS Endocrine dysfunction often affects the temperature and texture of the skin. Temperature changes are associated with myxedema (cool, dry skin) and pheochromocytoma (increased skin temperature with sweating). It is important to note the presence of any skin lesions. Ecchymoses often accompany Cushing's syndrome, and vitiligo has been seen in clients with adrenal insufficiency, hyperthyroidism, and hypothyroidism. Other skin lesions include skin infections; ulcerations; and, in clients with diabetes, candidiasis, pigmented patches in the pretibial area, and diabetic xanthoma.

What is the texture and distribution of the body hair? Is there **hirsutism** (excessive hair growth) or hair loss? Are the eyebrows present and in a normal distribution? (In hypothyroidism there is often a loss of the lateral third of the eyebrow.) Has the hair prematurely grayed? Are any abnormalities of the nails present (eg, pitting or fungal infections of the nails)?

ASSESSMENT OF THE EYES Pay careful attention to any periorbital swelling, **proptosis, ptosis** of the eyelids, or demonstrable lid lag. Assess the visual acuity and visual fields for any defects.

ASSESSMENT OF THE NECK Inspect the neck for any asymmetry, which can be seen in clients with goiters and other masses. Does the enlargement appear symmetrical or asymmetrical? Carefully palpate the thyroid gland. Note its size, degree of symmetry, and consistency. Assess for the presence of any tenderness or nodules.

CARDIORESPIRATORY ASSESSMENT Evaluate the client's heart rate and rhythm and detect the presence of any murmurs or extra heart sounds. In thyrotoxicosis and pheochromocytoma, elevated blood pressure readings, tachycardia, and atrial fibrillation may be noted. Thyrotoxicosis and Cushing's syndrome often lead to congestive heart failure as manifested by increasing shortness of breath, dyspnea on exertion, paroxysmal nocturnal dyspnea, and cough. Bradycardia and pericardial effusions may result from the insufficient production of T_4 in myxedema. Hypertension can accompany Cushing's syndrome, and hypotension can accompany adrenal insufficiency.

Because of the interrelation between the cardiac and respiratory systems, cardiac pathology often produces changes in the lungs (eg, pleural effusions or congestive heart failure). Therefore, assess the lungs for any abnormal breath sounds, rales, rhonchi, wheezes, or pleural friction rubs.

ASSESSMENT OF THE ABDOMEN AND GENITALS Inspect the abdomen for any asymmetry that might indicate ascites, enlargement of an organ, or a mass. Auscultate the abdomen to detect bruits (especially over the renal arteries).

Assessment of the genitalia is important in the evaluation of clients with endocrine dysfunction, because changes in sexual development and reproductive function often occur. Note the appearance of the client's genitals and any abnormalities. Do the genitals appear appropriate for the client's age and sex? Are there secondary sex characteristics? Does there appear to be agreement between the genital, hormonal, and psychologic sex of the client?

NEUROMUSCULAR ASSESSMENT Examine the musculoskeletal system for bone pain, joint pain, and generalized muscle weakness. The neurologic and endocrine systems work closely together to maintain the homeostasis of the internal environment and to help the person withstand stress. Therefore, pathology in the nervous system often affects endocrine function (eg, a benign tumor of the pituitary gland can cause hypersecretion of anterior pituitary hormones), and pathology in the endocrine system can be reflected in the nervous system (eg, hypothyroidism can dull mentation).

A careful neurologic evaluation should be done including assessment of mental status, cranial nerves, motor and sensory function, cerebellar function, and deep tendon and superficial reflexes. Thoroughness in examination and accuracy in recording findings are essential. Report all abnormal findings to the physician for further evaluation.

Diagnostic Studies

Single measures of endocrine function are rarely sufficient to support a diagnosis but nevertheless should be an integral part of the whole data base. In endocrine testing, be aware of the importance of client preparation and adhere strictly to the testing protocols. Client and environmental influences that might modify the test results are other important nursing considerations. Diagnostic studies common to the endocrine system are summarized in Table 31–1. Specific nursing implications for several of these tests follow Table 31–1.

NURSING IMPLICATIONS FOR SELECTED DIAGNOSTIC STUDIES

THYROID SCANNING Take a thorough history before the administration of ^{131}I. Ask about use of thyroid or antithyroid drugs, estrogen, or barbiturates; the intake of any iodine preparations (eg, saturated solution of potassium

Table 31–1
Diagnostic Studies Common to the Endocrine System

Laboratory Test	Normal Expected Value	Disease State	Expected Abnormal Findings
Anterior pituitary			
Serum growth hormone (GH) RIA	0–8 ng/mL	Increased GH secretion in acromegaly, gigantism, hypoglycemia, exercise, stress	Above 8 ng/mL
		Decreased GH secretion in pituitary dwarfism, hyperglycemia, use of glucocorticoids	Below 8 ng/mL
Insulin tolerance test (ITT or GH stimulation test)	Serum cortisol above 7 μg/dL with peak at 20 μg/dL GH above 20 ng/mL Prolactin above 10 ng/mL (doubling baseline)	Adrenal–hypothalamic–anterior pituitary deficiency	Failure to respond to hypoglycemic challenge indicates a defect in the hypothalamus or anterior pituitary gland
GH suppression test	Basal level 10 ng/mL; suppressed below 5 ng/mL sometime during test	Excess GH (acromegaly, gigantism)	In active acromegaly or gigantism: basal level 5 ng/mL; no suppression below 5 ng/mL during test
		Renal failure, cirrhosis, starvation	Nonsuppression of GH
Radiologic testing			
X-ray and CT scan of skull with attention to sella turcica	Negative	Anterior pituitary dysfunction	Possible widening of sella turcica with anterior pituitary tumor
Posterior pituitary ***Routine screening tests***			
Urine	Specific gravity 1.016–1.022	Diabetes insipidus	Low morning urine specific gravity (below 1.007)
	Urinary sodium (24 h) 100–260 mEq/24 h	SIADH	Increased urinary sodium
		Diabetes insipidus	Increased sodium concentrations in both urine and serum
Serum	Serum sodium 135–148 mEq/L	SIADH	Decreased sodium and chloride concentrations in serum
	BUN 6–20 mg/dL Creatinine 0.6–1.5 mg/dL Potassium 3.6–5.0 mEq/L	Diabetes insipidus	Normal range
	Hematocrit M 40%–54%; F 37%–47% Mean corpuscular volume (MCV) 76–100 fL Mean corpuscular hemoglobin concentration (MCHC) 30%–38%	SIADH	Decreased hematocrit (increased MCV and decreased MCHC) secondary to hemodilution

(continued)

Table 31–1
Diagnostic Studies Common to the Endocrine System (continued)

Laboratory Test	Normal Expected Value	Disease State	Expected Abnormal Findings
Osmolality tests			
Urine	M 390–1090 mOsm/kg or mOsm/L	Diabetes insipidus	Decreased urine osmolality
	F 300–1090 mOsm/kg or mOsm/L	SIADH	Increased urine osmolality
Serum	275–300 mOsm/kg	Diabetes insipidus	Increased serum osmolality
		SIADH	Decreased serum osmolality
Water deprivation test	Urine osmolality over 800 mOsm/kg	Diabetes insipidus (pituitary–hypothalamic etiology)	Serum osmolality greater than 300 mOsm/kg
	Urine osmolality greater than serum osmolality		Urine osmolality less than serum osmolality
	No change in serum osmolality over course of test		**Response to vasopressin**: greater increase in urine osmolality than serum osmolality
	No change in serum sodium levels over course of test	Nephrogenic diabetes insipidus	Serum osmolality greater than 300 mOsm/kg
			Urine osmolality less than serum osmolality
			No response to vasopressin
Water-loading test	Decrease in urinary volume due to stimulation of ADH	Diabetes insipidus (pituitary)	No antidiuresis; no change in urine osmolality (less than 400 mOsm/L)
	Urine osmolality equal or greater than 600 mOsm/L	Nephrogenic diabetes insipidus	No antidiuresis; no change in urine osmolality (less than 400 mOsm/L)
Thyroid gland			
Serum T_4	4–12 μg/dL	Hyperthyroidism	Increase
		Hypothyroidism	Decrease
Serum T_3	80–100 ng/dL	Hyperthyroidism	Increase (greater proportionately than T_4)
		Hypothyroidism	Decrease
Thyroxine-binding globulin (TBG)	10–26 μg/dL	Pregnancy, estrogen administration	Increased TBG and T_4, decreased RT_3U (resin T_3 uptake)
		Hypoproteinemia, androgen therapy, use of salicylates	Decreased TBG and T_4, increased RT_3U
Thyrotropin-stimulating hormone (TSH)	<5 μU/mL	Primary hypothyroidism	Increased TSH and TRF
		Secondary hypothyroidism	Decreased TSH and TRF
Thyroid circulating antibody (thyroid autoantibody, or TAA)	Usually absent	Graves' disease, Hashimoto's thyroiditis	Increased antibody levels
		Most other thyroid disorders; also pernicious ane-	Decreased antibody levels

Laboratory Test	Normal Expected Value	Disease State	Expected Abnormal Findings
		mia, myasthenia gravis, and Type I diabetes mellitus	
Radiologic testing			
Thyroid scanning using radioactive ^{131}I uptake (RAIU) (See nursing implications in the section that follows)	Serum: 2 h, 4%–12% uptake; 6 h, 6%–15% uptake; 24 h, 8%–30% uptake	Hyperthyroidism	Serum: Increased ^{131}I with early high peak
		Hypothyroidism	Decreased ^{131}I with consistent low peak
	Urine: 40%–80% ^{131}I excreted in first 24 h		Urine: Less than 40% excretion (hyperthyroidism)
			More than 80% excretion (hypothyroidism)
Ultrasonography of the thyroid gland	Normal size, shape, and location of thyroid gland	Nonfunctioning thyroid nodules	Can differentiate between cystic and solid nodules; used in following the effect of treatment on thyroid masses
Thyroid stimulation test	Increase in T_4 and RAIU uptake	Primary hypothyroidism	Less than 10% increase in RAIU or less than 1.5 μg/dL increase in T_4
		Secondary hypothyroidism	At least 10% increase in RAIU and 1.5 μg/dL increase in T_4
Thyroid suppression test	25% decrease in second RAIU finding (suppression)	Primary hyperthyroidism (Graves' disease)	No suppression
Serum calcitonin	Undetectable	Medullary carcinoma of thyroid gland	More than 100 pg/mL
Parathyroid glands			
Serum calcium	Adult 8.5–10.5 mg/dL	Primary hyperparathyroidism	Increased serum calcium
		Hypoparathyroidism	Decreased serum calcium
Serum phosphorus	Adult 3.0–4.5 mg/dL	Hyperparathyroidism, rickets, osteomalacia	Decreased serum phosphorus
		Primary and secondary hypoparathyroidism, uremia, alkalosis	Increased serum phosphorus
Serum PTH	Less than 2000 pg/mL	Hyperparathyroidism	Increased PTH
		Hypoparathyroidism	Decreased PTH
Qualitative urinary calcium (Sulkowitch's test)	1+–2+ or negative (scale from negative to positive)	Hyperparathyroidism	Increased urinary calcium
		Hypoparathyroidism	Decreased urinary calcium
Quantitative urinary calcium	50–300 mg/24 h	Hyperparathyroidism	Increased urinary calcium
		Hypoparathyroidism	Decreased urinary calcium
Adrenal cortex			
Serum cortisol	8–10 AM: 5–25 μg/dL 4 PM–midnight: 2–18 μg/dL	Cushing's disease, Cushing's syndrome	Increased serum cortisol
		Addison's disease, hypopituitarism	Decreased serum cortisol

(continued)

Table 31–1
Diagnostic Studies Common to the Endocrine System (continued)

Laboratory Test	Normal Expected Value	Disease State	Expected Abnormal Findings
Serum aldosterone	Normal sodium intake: 8 AM (recumbent) 3–9 ng/dL	Primary aldosteronism (Conn's syndrome), secondary aldosteronism	Increased serum aldosterone
	9 AM (upright) 4–30 ng/dL	Addison's disease, Sheehan's syndrome	Decreased serum aldosterone
Serum ACTH	8 AM (fasting) 20–100 pg/mL 4 PM (nonfasting) 10–50 pg/mL	Primary Addison's disease, ectopic ACTH-producing tumors, stress	Increased serum ACTH
		Cushing's disease secondary to pituitary-dependent adrenal hyperplasia	High-normal to low-normal serum ACTH
		Hypopituitarism, Cushing's syndrome secondary to adrenal adenomas or carcinomas	Decreased serum ACTH
Urinary 17-hydroxycorticosteroids (17-OHCS) (See nursing implications in the section that follows)	M 5–15 mg/24 h F 2–13 mg/24 h	Hyperfunction of the adrenal gland (Cushing's syndrome)	Increased 17-OHCS
		Hypofunction of the adrenal gland (Addison's disease)	Decreased 17-OHCS
Urinary 17-ketosteroids (17-KS) (See nursing implications in the section that follows)	M 8–25 mg/24 h F 5–15 mg/24 h	Hyperfunction of the adrenal gland; testosterone or estrogen-secreting tumors of the adrenal gland, ovaries, or testes; adrenogenital syndromes	Increased 17-KS
		Hypofunction of the adrenal gland	Decreased 17-KS
Urinary free cortisol	0–10 μg/24 h	Cushing's syndrome	Increased urinary free cortisol
Urinary aldosterone	2–26 μg/24 h	Primary and secondary aldosteronism	Increased urinary aldosterone
		Addison's disease, Sheehan's syndrome	Decreased urinary aldosterone
Dexamethasone suppression test (See nursing implications in the section that follows)	Low dose: More than 50% reduction in urinary 17-OHCS levels	Bilateral adrenal hyperplasia (Cushing's syndrome)	Low dose: no change; high dose: more than 50% reduction
	High dose: More than 50% reduction in urinary 17-OHCS levels	Adrenal adenoma or carcinoma	Low dose: no change; high dose: no change
		Ectopic ACTH-producing tumors	Low dose; no change; high dose: no change
ACTH stimulation test (modified Thorn test, ACTH provocative test, ACTH infusion test)	Serum cortisol 40 μg/dL after 24-h infusion	Cushing's syndrome secondary to bilateral adrenal hyperplasia	Increased serum cortisol
		Cushing's syndrome secondary to autonomic	No change in serum cortisol

Laboratory Test	Normal Expected Value	Disease State	Expected Abnormal Findings
		hyperfunctioning adrenal tumors	
		Addison's disease secondary to pituitary hypofunction (secondary adrenal insufficiency)	Serum cortisol 10–40 μg/dL
		Addison's disease secondary to primary adrenal insufficiency	No change in serum cortisol
Metyrapone test	24-h level of 17-OHCS double the baseline	Cushing's syndrome secondary to bilateral adrenal hyperplasia	Double the baseline or higher urinary 17-OHCS
		Cushing's syndrome secondary to autonomous hyperfunctioning adrenal tumors	No change in urinary 17-OHCS
Adrenal medulla			
Serum catecholamines (fractionated) (See nursing implications in the section that follows)	Epinephrine: supine, 0–150 ng/L; standing, 0–150 ng/L Norepinephrine: supine, 103–193 ng/L; standing, 293–489 ng/L	Pheochromocytoma, neuroblastoma, ganglioneuroblastoma, ganglioneuroma	Increased serum catecholamine
Urinary vanillylmandelic acid (VMA)	0.5–8 mg/24 h	Tumors of adrenal medulla (eg, pheochromocytoma)	Increased urinary VMA
Urinary homovanillic acid (HVA)	More than 15 mg/24 h	Neural crest tumor (neuroblastoma or ganglioneuroma)	Increased urinary HVA
		Pheochromocytoma	No increase in urinary HVA
Total urinary catecholamine	Less than 100 μg/24 h (varies with activity)	Tumors of adrenal medulla	Increased total urinary catecholamines
Pancreas (endocrine function)			
Urinary glucose and ketones	Negative	Diabetes mellitus, Cushing's syndrome, acromegaly, stress, HHNK coma	Increased urinary glucose
		Diabetes mellitus, high-fat and low-carbohydrate diet, starvation, febrile and toxic illnesses	Increased urinary acetone
Fasting serum glucose	80–120 mg/dL	Diabetes mellitus, HHNK coma, Cushing's syndrome, acromegaly, stress, acute pancreatitis, and numerous drugs	Increased serum glucose
		Advanced liver disease, Addison's disease, islet cell adenoma, impaired glucose tolerance, spontaneous hypoglycemia	Decreased serum glucose
2-hour postprandial glucose	145 mg/dL; over age 60, less than 160 mg/dL	Diabetes mellitus, HHNK coma, Cushing's syndrome, acromegaly, stress	Increased 2-hour postprandial glucose

(continued)

Table 31–1
Diagnostic Studies Common to the Endocrine System (continued)

Laboratory Test	Normal Expected Value	Disease State	Expected Abnormal Findings
Glycosylated hemoglobin (HbA_{1c})	4.82%–5.09% of total hemoglobin	Hyperglycemia	Increased HbA_{1c}
		Hemolytic states (secondary to loss of hemoglobin)	Decreased HbA_{1c}
24-h urine test for quantitative glucose levels	No glucose in urine in a 24-h period	Diabetes mellitus	Increased urinary glucose
Glucose tolerance test (GTT) (See nursing implications in the section that follows)	Serum glucose levels peak within 30 min to 1 h in a range of 160–180 mg/dL, return to normal range within 2–3 h; urine negative for glucose throughout test	Diabetes mellitus, Cushing's syndrome, pheochromocytoma, CNS lesions, hemochromatosis	Decreased glucose tolerance curve (sharp peak with curve that returns slowly to baseline)
		Insulinoma, Addison's disease, hypothyroidism, hypopituitarism, malabsorption states	Increased glucose tolerance curve (peak at less-than-normal levels)
Serum insulin	4–24 μU/mL	Insulinoma	Increased serum insulin and glucose
		Diabetes mellitus (with insulin resistance), idiopathic functional hypoglycemia, conditions causing reactive hypoglycemia	Increased serum insulin
		Diabetes mellitus (no insulin resistance)	Decreased serum insulin
Tolbutamide tolerance test (TTT, insulin tolerance test, insulin stimulation test) (See nursing implications in the section that follows)	After infusion, serum glucose levels drop to approximately half the fasting level in 30 min and return to pretest levels within 1½ to 3 h	Hyperinsulinism	Results same as in normal individuals
		Insulinoma	Marked drop in glucose with a return to normal in 3 h or more
		Diabetes mellitus	Prolonged time of return to pretest levels; slow initial drop in serum glucose

iodide [SSKI], Lugol's solution, or tolbutamide); a history of any diagnostic studies using an iodine contrast material within the past 5 to 10 years (eg, gallbladder studies or intravenous pyelography); and the intake of any iodine-containing foods (shellfish or fish). The client should not take any iodine or thyroid preparations for 1 week before the test.

URINE TESTS FOR 17-HYDROXYCORTICOSTEROID AND 17-KETOSTEROID Obtain a history to detect consumption of the following products that might influence the test results: aspirin, acetaminophen, paraldehyde, chloral hydrate, nitrofurantoin, coffee, morphine, barbiturates, reserpine, furosemide, thiazides, monoamine oxidase (MAO) inhibitors, colchicine, sulfonamides, quinine, propoxyphene, spironolactone, cloxacillin sodium, and licorice. Because both emotional and physical stress can increase the activity of the adrenal gland, observe the client closely and report any evidence of stress to the physician.

DEXAMETHASONE SUPPRESSION TEST Carefully assess clients for signs of stress, which can affect the test results (stress increases the secretion of ACTH). The administration of dexamethasone with milk or an antacid prevents irritation of the gastric mucosa. Assess the client for factors that might interfere with the normal suppression responses: for example, estrogen therapy, hyperthyroidism, phenytoin therapy, obesity, or mental depression (possibly related to a biochemical phenomenon).

MEASUREMENT OF SERUM CATECHOLAMINE LEVELS (FRACTIONATED) Obtain a careful history of all variables that may affect test results (radioactive scan within 1 week or the ingestion of epinephrine, amphetamines, phenothiazines, levodopa, sympathomimetics, decongestants, tricyclic antidepressants, and reserpine). The client should rest in bed in a quiet environment for at least 30 minutes before the test. Keep the client warm and relaxed. The diet before testing should contain a normal sodium intake.

The client should abstain from amine-rich foods (cheese, coffee, tea, cocoa, beer, bananas, and avocados) for at least 48 hours before testing to avoid distorting the test results. The client should refrain from smoking for at least 15 minutes before the test.

GLUCOSE TOLERANCE TEST Obtain a careful history of all medications that might elevate or depress serum glucose levels (large amounts of salicylates, oral contraceptives, large doses of ascorbic acid, thiazide diuretics, phenytoin, and steroids). A history of other factors that might influence the test results also should be obtained (eg, pregnancy, prolonged inactivity, surgery, trauma, acute illness, and infectious disease). In addition, clients who have been on a low-carbohydrate diet before the test may show an abnormal glucose tolerance curve because of an inability of the pancreas to respond to a high-carbohydrate load.

TOLBUTAMIDE TOLERANCE TEST Obtain a careful history of all substances that might enhance the action of tolbutamide (salicylates, MAO inhibitors, sulfonamides, phenylbutazone, chloramphenicol, and methandrostenolone). False positive test results have occurred in clients with adrenal insufficiency, liver disease, obesity, functional hypoglycemia, alcoholism, and starvation. False negative test results occur in approximately 50% of clients with insulinoma (Treseler, 1982). Use the test with caution in clients in the last trimester of pregnancy; in the elderly; and in clients with a history of heart disease, chronic illness, or severe acute illness.

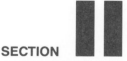

SECTION 

Nursing Diagnosis/Planning and Implementation/Evaluation

Information gathered from the client's health history, physical examination, and diagnostic studies is used to determine nursing diagnoses and the plan of care. Not every client will have the same needs. The Nursing Diagnoses box lists diagnoses **directly related** to endocrine dysfunction along with **potential** nursing diagnoses for clients with endocrine problems. The most common nursing diagnoses for clients with endocrine dysfunction include ineffective individual coping; altered thought processes; altered comfort; disturbance in self-concept: body image; altered nutrition: more than body requirements; altered bowel elimination: diarrhea; and fluid volume deficit. The sample nursing care plan in Table 31–2 focuses on four of these nursing diagnoses: altered nutrition: more than body requirements; fluid volume deficit, actual; knowledge deficit; and activity intolerance. The others are discussed in the narrative.

If the goals of care have not been met, reevaluation is required. The nurse and client should jointly review the nursing care plan. New objectives may need to be formulated; other nursing interventions may be added or modified; or the evaluation may show that more time is required to meet the objectives.

Coping, Ineffective Individual

Because of the profound physiologic and psychosocial stresses on clients with endocrine disorders, it is not unusual for them to be fearful and unable to cope. Their nervousness and anxiety can be directly related to the disorder or exogenous, resulting from vague feelings of unexplained apprehension about the situation.

Endocrine disorders often require the client and significant others to make major changes in lifestyle. Clients with endocrine dysfunction must often depend on medication for life and usually require lifelong medical and nursing supervision. They also may face the possibility of major surgery. The client may have some degree of transitory or permanent sensory loss.

Planning and Implementation

The nurse, although unable to alter the actual disease, can support and reassure clients, as well as educate them about what is occurring. By careful environmental manipulation, the nurse can reduce the internal and external stressors that contribute to a negative outcome. Clients need to be aware that their anxiety is related to what is happening in their bodies and that the treatment is expected to help. Provide opportunities for clients to express what they are feeling and, if appropriate, encourage activities that provide physical release of energy. Organize the environment to provide minimal stimulation and to promote relaxation. Counsel visitors and families to avoid topics that may cause an increase in symptoms. Families or friends need to be reassured that the symptoms and signs they observe in the client reflect the underlying endocrine pathology and are expected to resolve with treatment.

Evaluation

Expected client outcomes following effective nursing interventions for ineffective individual coping include acknowledgment of anxiety, reports of decreased anxiety and fear, and reports by care providers and significant others of the client's improved emotional state.

Thought Processes, Altered

Central nervous system involvement may produce a variety of problems in the endocrine client, ranging from headaches and lethargy (hypoglycemia or pheochromocytoma)

NURSING DIAGNOSES IN
Endocrine Dysfunction

DIRECTLY RELATED DIAGNOSES

- Activity intolerance
- Bowel elimination, altered: diarrhea
- Comfort, altered: pain
- Coping, ineffective individual
- Fluid volume deficit, actual
- Fluid volume deficit, potential
- Knowledge deficit
- Nutrition, altered: more than body requirements
- Self-concept, disturbance in: body image
- Thought processes, altered

OTHER POTENTIAL DIAGNOSES

- Infection, potential for
- Injury, potential for
- Noncompliance
- Nutrition, altered: less than body requirements
- Powerlessness
- Sensory/perceptual alterations: visual, tactile
- Skin integrity, impaired
- Thermoregulation, ineffective
- Tissue perfusion, altered: gastrointestinal, peripheral

to outright psychoses (thyrotoxicosis, Cushing's syndrome, or hyperparathyroidism). Alterations in thought processes and perception pose difficulties not only for clients but for their families and friends as well.

Planning and Implementation

Explain the etiology of the changes in cognitive ability and the mood swings to the client and significant others and provide interventions based on the client's current level of function. For example, for clients with hypothyroidism characterized by mental slowing, interactions should be simple and direct, with explanations geared to the client's present level of understanding. Help clients understand that these changes should be relieved by treatment. Extend teaching and counseling to the client's family or friends, who are often troubled by the dramatic changes they see in their loved one.

The erratic mood swings of cushingoid clients and clients with hyperthyroidism pose another challenge to the nurse. Although the etiology of these fluctuations is pathology in the endocrine system, nursing interventions should be directed toward the symptoms. These clients and their significant others require support and reassurance about the basis of these changes. Clients often respond well to a simple restructuring of their environment to reduce stimulation. For example, turning the lights down, playing soft music on the radio, limiting visitors or avoiding anxiety-producing topics during a visit, and providing soothing baths or back rubs often encourage clients to relax.

Evaluation

Expected client outcomes following effective nursing interventions for alteration in thought processes include orientation to person, place, and time; improved memory; reports of improved cognition and decreased mood swings by care providers and significant others.

Comfort, Altered

Many clients with endocrine dysfunction have problems with thermal regulation. For example, clients with hyperthyroidism often complain of intolerance to heat, and those with hypothyroidism are exquisitely sensitive to cold. Clients with pheochromocytoma, hyperthyroidism, and hypoglycemia often experience excessive sweating. Pruritus is often a problem for clients with diabetes mellitus and hyperthyroidism. Those with hypothyroidism and acromegaly often have joint pain.

Planning and Implementation

The client with hyperthyroidism who is highly sensitive to heat often benefits from a cooler room temperature, fewer blankets with frequent linen changes, and cool back rubs. The client with hypothyroidism generally needs a warmer room temperature, more bed linens, and layers of clothing in cold weather. Clients with excessive perspiration need repeated clothing and bed linen changes, more frequent bathing, and liberal use of deodorants and body powder.

Manage joint pain with rest and heat or cold, depending on which is most effective for the individual client. Aspirin or nonsteroidal anti-inflammatory agents may be ordered if they are compatible with the rest of the client's medical regimen.

Evaluation

Expected client outcomes following effective nursing interventions for alteration in comfort include reports of a decrease in pain, pruritus, heat or cold intolerance; observations by care providers and significant others that the client is more comfortable; and client involvement in relaxation techniques and activities that provide diversion.

Self-Concept, Disturbance in: Body Image

Changes in the skin and hair occur in clients with endocrine dysfunction and frequently contribute to disturbances in body image. Increases in skin pigmentation may occur in clients with Addison's disease. Ecchymoses increase in cushingoid clients because of changes in the fragility of the capillaries. Facial flushing may be seen in clients with pheochromocytoma. Hirsutism is a problem for clients with adrenal tumor or hyperplasia and is an especially troublesome body image problem for women.

Table 31–2
Sample Nursing Care Plan for Clients With Endocrine Dysfunction, by Nursing Diagnosis

Client Care Goals	Plan/Nursing Implementation	Expected Outcomes
Nutrition, altered: more than body requirements related to decreased metabolic requirements secondary to hypothyroidism		
Reduce weight to normal range within 1 yr with consistent initial loss of 1–2 lb/wk; maintain prescribed diet, adequate fluid intake, and exercise regimen	Assess state of control of client's hypothyroidism; weigh and measure client; compare results to actuarial tables to arrive at a proper goal; use skinfold assessment as needed; obtain a 3-day diet diary from client; assess client's food preferences and dislikes; assess client's activity level and general plan of daily activities; assess client's level of understanding regarding hypothyroidism, obesity, and their relation; if client appears to be well controlled on thryoid medication, secure a diet prescription from the physician and nutrition consultant (if available); work with client to plan an appropriate weight-loss regimen based on caloric restriction, adequate fluid intake, and exercise; consider client's food likes and dislikes, as well as any cultural or economic influences; encourage clients to weigh themselves only once weekly at same time of day (usually in morning) while wearing the same amount of clothes; explain that weight may plateau and the reasons for it; encourage client to keep a daily log of what is eaten and any influencing factors (depression, eating out, etc); provide ongoing follow-up (to encourage adherence to diet) via telephone consultation or weigh-ins every 2 wk; refer client to weight-loss or behavior modification groups, if indicated; remember that obesity is often a lifelong disorder and may require considerable lifestyle adjustments; provide support and honestly compliment client for weight loss	Client consistently loses 1 to 2 lb weekly; client within normal range for weight and height within 1 yr; client able to explain the prescribed diet accurately and discuss importance of fluid intake and exercise in successfully meeting the weight goal; client maintains weekly telephone contact with the care provider and weighs in regularly at the prescribed intervals
Fluid volume deficit: actual related to failure of regulatory mechanisms secondary to Addison's disease		
Maintain a normal electrolyte balance; exhibit no signs of dehydration; reduce or eliminate symptoms of weakness; no fluid volume deficit	Monitor vital signs QID or PRN, blood pressure, pulse, respirations, temperature; weigh client daily and report results; measure intake and output and quantify sodium intake; force fluids to 3000 mL/24h; maintain high-sodium, low potassium diet or as ordered (diet may need between-meal supplements). Parenteral therapy may be ordered; provide easy access for frequent urinary elimination; assist with diagnostic tests as ordered, and explain all procedures to client; observe client closely for symptoms and signs of dehydration; administer medications as ordered; teach client to avoid substances that increase diuresis (alcohol, coffee, and tea)	Client maintains a normal electrolyte balance, as shown by laboratory results; no signs of dehydration, as shown by good skin turgor, moist mucus membranes, normal vital signs, normal intake and output, hematocrit, and urine specific gravity within normal limits. Blood pressure and all vital signs in normal range for client's age and body build; serum electrolytes within normal limits; hemoglobin and hematacrit within normal range; client maintains good fluid intake and avoids diuretic substances

(continued)

Table 31–2
Sample Nursing Care Plan for Clients With Endocrine Dysfunction, by Nursing Diagnosis (continued)

Client Care Goals	Plan/Nursing Implementation	Expected Outcomes
Fluid volume deficit: actual related to fluid loss secondary to diabetic ketoacidosis		
Restore normal fluid and electrolyte balance; restore blood glucose to acceptable levels	During acute episode: Obtain electrolyte, serum glucose, carbon dioxide, BUN, hematocrit, and urine specimens stat as ordered; in-dwelling catheter may be inserted; set nasogastric tube to low suction, as ordered; gastric lavage may be done; administer parenteral fluids as ordered (normal saline or sodium lactate solution is usually given initially); replace electrolytes [K] as ordered; administer parenteral sodium bicarbonate as ordered if blood ph 7.0 or below; administer insulin as ordered; monitor client carefully for symptoms and signs of hypoglycemia, especially 12–24 h after treatment has begun; monitor client carefully for hypokalemia, especially if vomiting or diarrhea occurred; obtain ECG as ordered; measure intake and output every hour; test urine hourly for glucose and ketones; check blood pressure, respirations, and apical heart rate every ½–1 h; assess LOC every ½–1 h; observe for symptoms and signs of circulatory collapse (maintain open airway and elevate the lower extremities as needed); be prepared for seizure measures if needed; client is usually more comfortable in Fowler's position; turn and position client every hour; administer skin care as needed	Restoration of normal fluid balance (urine specific gravity 1.016–1.022; urine output 800–2000 mL/24 h; blood pressure, respirations, pulse, and temperature all within normal range; no signs of dehydration); serum electrolytes within normal range; urine negative for glucose and ketones; client alert and oriented; client asymptomatic for symptoms and signs of hyperglycemia, hypoglycemia, hyperkalemia, and hypokalemia
Knowledge deficit related to necessary information regarding diabetic ketoacidosis		
Discuss symptoms and signs of DKA and the factors that produce it	Assess client's understanding of acute episode of DKA; review symptoms and signs of hypoglycemia and DKA; discuss when and how to treat emergency situations and need to call physician immediately; based on client's level of understanding, review diet, medications, exercise, infection management, and self-care skills; involve a member of client's family or a significant other in the client teaching sessions; assess, if possible, the home situation for factors influencing ability to maintain a safe and healthy diabetic regimen. Teach the importance of wearing a Medic-Alert tag	Client able to discuss symptoms and signs of ketoacidosis and the factors that contribute to it; client and significant others seem confident about managing future problems
Activity intolerance related to weakness and fatigue		
Maintain normal activity level; reduce weakness and fatigue; accept limitations in strength and endurance	Provide a quiet, restful, stress-free environment; assess client for generalized weakness and malaise; assess client for ability to tolerate physical activity; counsel client to provide for several rest periods during day to avoid fatigue	Client able to maintain normal activity level

Clients with endocrine disorders are often unable to manage self-care or maintain their home environment. They are at increased risk for injury because of weakness, fatigue, and visual disturbances. Sexual dysfunction may occur as loss of libido or impotence. Menstrual problems such as menorrhagia and amenorrhea are not uncommon.

Planning and Implementation

Many of the body image changes that occur in clients with endocrine dysfunction are amenable to treatment (although the effects often require time to resolve), but some are not. Be sensitive to clients' needs and provide opportunities for them to discuss their feelings and concerns. Although interventions such as makeup or skin creams may have minimal effect, they should not be overlooked, especially if the client and family find them valuable.

Sexual dysfunction and menstrual irregularities often are resolved when the client's specific endocrine problem is brought under control. Remember to ask about changes in these areas, however, because clients are often hesitant to bring them up. If there is no improvement, medications may be contributing to the problem. Bring these concerns to the physician's attention.

Evaluation

Expected client outcomes following effective nursing interventions for a disturbance in self-concept include verbalization of concern about body image and concern about the reaction of loved ones; interest in personal appearance; and requests for specific information about bodily changes and what can realistically be expected in the future.

Chapter Highlights

The carefully collected data base is the foundation for developing nursing diagnoses as well as for the planning, implementation, and evaluation of nursing care for endocrine clients. The data base enables the nurse to use a scientific approach in making judgments about changes in client status.

The areas routinely assessed in a client with endocrine disease are the vital signs; general appearance; skin, hair, and nails; eyes; neck; heart; lungs; abdomen; genitals; and musculoskeletal and neurologic systems.

Studies used to diagnose clients with endocrine dysfunction include screening tests, serum and urine tests, radiologic studies, and special testing procedures.

The nursing diagnoses most relevant to the care of clients with endocrine disease are ineffective individual coping; altered thought processes; altered comfort; self-concept disturbance: body image; altered nutrition: more than body requirements; altered bowel elimination: diarrhea; potential fluid volume deficit; and actual fluid volume deficit.

In planning the nursing care for clients with endocrine dysfunction, consider that clients may have a sensory loss; endocrine disorders often result in significant lifestyle changes for clients and their families; clients often depend on medication and require lifelong medical supervision; and clients may have symptoms that inhibit their coping and adaptation to normal life situations.

The nursing care plan for clients with endocrine problems should be individualized and client centered as well as reflect approaches to meet client care goals arising from nursing diagnoses.

The evaluation of nursing care is an important nursing responsibility keyed to the construction of client-centered goals or objectives. If the objectives have been met, the plan of care is successful. If the objectives have not been met, the nurse and client should review the care plan and make the necessary revisions.

Bibliography

Bates B: *A Guide to the Physical Examination,* 3rd ed. Philadelphia: Lippincott, 1983.

Bolli G et al: Simultaneous central venous and arterial blood sampling for catecholamine assay in pheochromocytoma. *Lancet* 1981; 2(8245):526–527.

Byrne CJ et al: *Laboratory Tests: Implications for Nursing Care,* 2nd ed. Menlo Park, CA: Addison–Wesley, 1986.

Cohen S, Harris E: Programmed instruction: Mental status assessment. *Am J Nurs* 1981; 8:1493–1518.

Diagnostics. Nurse's Reference Library. Springhouse, PA: Intermed, 1983.

Feng CA: Laboratory tests in diabetes mellitus. *New York State J Med* 1981; 81(9): 1328–1331.

Fields WL, McGinn–Campbell KM: *Introduction to Health Assessment.* Reston, VA: Reston, 1983.

Grimes J, Iannopollo E: *Health Assessment in Nursing Practice.* Monterey, CA: Wadsworth, 1982.

Harris E: The dexamethasone suppression test. *Am J Nurs* 1982; 82(5):784–785.

Honigman RE: Deciphering diagnostic studies: Thyroid function tests. *Nurs 82* (April) 1982; 12:68–71.

Kaye D, Rise LF (editors): *Fundamentals of Internal Medicine.* St. Louis: Mosby, 1983.

Malasanos L et al: *Health Assessment.* St. Louis: Mosby, 1981.

Maree SM: The endocrine system. Preoperative evaluation and physical assessment of the patient. *J AANA* 1981; 49:389–404.

Metzger MJ: A new test for blood sugar: Hemoglobin A. *Am J Nurs* 1983; 83(5):763–764.

Most RS et al.: The accuracy of glucose monitoring by diabetic individuals in their home setting. *Diabetes Educator* (Winter) 1986; 12(1):24–27.

Pagana KD, Pagana TJ: *Diagnostic Testing and Nursing Implications: A Case Study Approach.* St. Louis: Mosby, 1982.

Sana JM, Judge RD (editors): *Physical Assessment Skills for Nursing Practice,* 2nd ed. Boston: Little, Brown, 1982.

Saxton DF et al: *The Addison–Wesley Manual of Nursing Practice.* Menlo Park, CA: Addison–Wesley, 1983.

Tamai H et al: Triiodothyronine suppression and TSH-releasing hormone tests before and after ^{131}I therapy for Graves' disease. *J Nuclear Med* 1980; 21:240–245.

Thompson JM, Bowers AC: *Clinical Manual of Health Assessment.* St. Louis: Mosby, 1980.

Treseler KM: *Clinical Laboratory Tests: Significance and Implications for Nursing.* Englewood Cliffs, NJ: Prentice–Hall, 1982.

Watts NB, Keffer JH: *Practical Endocrine Diagnosis,* 3rd ed. Philadelphia: Lea & Febiger, 1982.

Resources

SELF-HELP GROUPS AND OTHER ORGANIZATIONS

American Diabetes Association
National Service Center
1660 Duke Street
PO Box 25757
Alexandria, VA 22313
Phone: (800) 232–3472

A national organization with state and local units that seeks to improve the well-being of persons with diabetes and their families and promotes the search for preventive approaches or a cure for diabetes. Consult the ADA for the address and telephone number of the state affiliates. Consult the state affiliate for addresses and telephone numbers of local chapters.

Division of Diabetes Control
Center for Prevention Services
Centers for Disease Control
Atlanta, GA 30333
Phone: (404) 329–1851

The CDC, a division of the Public Health Service, administers diabetes control programs through the health departments of many states.

International Diabetes Center
5000 W. 39th St.
Minneapolis, MN 55416
Phone: (612) 927–3393

The center conducts educational, clinical care, outreach, and clinical research programs. Its diabetes education programs, print materials, and audiovisual aids are available for health professionals and persons with diabetes.

Juvenile Diabetes Foundation International
432 Park Avenue South
New York, NY 10016
Phone: (800) 223–1138

This international organization focuses on finding a cure for diabetes. The organization actively supports basic medical research.

Michigan Diabetes Research and Training Center
University of Michigan Medical Center
1500 E Medical Center Dr
S2310 Old Main Hospital
Ann Arbor, MI 48109
Phone: (313) 763–5256

The center annually publishes the "Recommended Audiovisual Resources for Diabetes Education" and "Recommended Print Materials for Diabetes Patient Education." These useful catalogs describe diabetes educational materials, including a brief evaluation of current resources and how they can be obtained.

National Diabetes Information Clearinghouse
PO Box NDIC
Bethesda, MD 20892
Phone: (301) 468–2162

The clearinghouse publishes annotated bibliographies on diabetes and the Diabetes Dateline that reports diabetes education and research activities.

Also:

Canadian Diabetes Association
78 Bond St
Toronto, Ontario, Canada M5B 2J8
Phone: (416) 488–8871

Joslin Diabetes Foundation
15 Joslin Rd.
Boston, MA 02215

National Hormone and Pituitary Program
210 W. Fayette St., Suite 510
Balitmore, MD 21201
(301) 837–2552

SPECIALTY ORGANIZATIONS

American Association of Diabetes Educators
500 N. Michigan Ave., Suite 1400
Chicago, IL 60611
Phone: (312) 661–1700

A multidisciplinary organization of health professionals interested in diabetes education. AADE provides educational opportunities for health professionals and promotes quality diabetes education for consumers. Consult AADE for addresses and telephone numbers of local chapters. Many publications available; write for list.

Diabetes Care and Education
American Dietetic Association
208 S LaSalle
Suite 1100
Chicago, IL 60604–1003
Phone: (312) 899–0040

This practice group within the ADA includes registered dietitians involved in diabetes education and management.

HEALTH INFORMATION MATERIAL

Publications of the American Diabetes Association

Diabetes Care. A bimonthly clinical research and care journal for health professionals.

Clinical Diabetes. A bimonthly newsletter for primary care health professionals in clinical practice.

Diabetes Forecast. A bimonthly publication for the person with diabetes that provides up-to-date information on nutrition, clinical advances, and research.

Diabetes. A quarterly newsletter for the person with diabetes that provides basic information.

Goals for Diabetes Education. Outlines the goals and behavioral objectives for education and counseling of persons with IDDM, NIDDM, gestational diabetes, and during pregnancy with prior diagnosis of diabetes. Objectives are given for initial or survival education and continuing education.

Publications of the International Diabetes Center

A complete series of single-concept brochures and booklets is available for use by health professionals for client education. Included in the series are: *What is Diabetes?, Diabetes and Brief Illness, Fast Food Facts, Convenience Food Facts, Diabetes and Exercise, Diabetes and Alcohol, Recognizing and Treating Insulin Reactions, Gestational Diabetes, Meal Planning for Type II Diabetes, Adding Fiber to Your Diet,* and *A Guide to Healthy Eating.*

Publications of the American Association of Diabetes Educators

The Diabetes Educator. A quarterly publication of the association that focuses on educational and clinical issues in diabetes management.

Tupling H et al: *You've Got to Get Through the Outside Layer: A Handbook for Health Educators, Using Diabetes as a Model.* Diabetes Education and Assessment Programme of the Royal North Shore Hospital of Sydney and the Northern Metropolitan Health Region of the Health Commission of New South Wales. Reprinted by the American Association of Diabetes Educators. Available from: Outside Layer, PO Box 802, South Bend, IN 46624. A succinct, well-written, and practical discussion of educational and emotional issues in diabetes and other chronic diseases. Includes examples, case studies, and sample teaching exercises.

Publications of the American Dietetic Association

Wheeler M (editor): *Diabetes Mellitus and Glycemic Responses to Different Foods: A Summary and Annotated Bibliography.* Published by the Diabetes Care and Education Practice Group of the American Dietetic Association, 1983 (and 1985 supplement).

CHAPTER 32

Specific Disorders of Glucose Regulation

Objectives

When you have finished studying this chapter, you should be able to:

Differentiate between Type I and Type II diabetes mellitus, or insulin-dependent diabetes mellitus (IDDM) and noninsulin-dependent diabetes mellitus (NIDDM) on the basis of etiology, clinical manifestations, course, and therapy.

Describe the major goals of diabetes mellitus therapy.

Enumerate the major treatment approaches for IDDM and NIDDM.

Distinguish among the types of insulins by their source, purity, concentration, formulation, and time activity.

Identify the steps in writing a meal plan for clients with diabetes.

Discuss the benefits of exercise in the treatment of IDDM and NIDDM.

Outline the advantages of self blood glucose monitoring.

Specify the goals of client education in diabetes mellitus.

Explain the complications of diabetes mellitus.

Discuss reactive hypoglycemia and its treatment.

The most common disorder of glucose regulation is diabetes mellitus, a chronic disease characterized by abnormal metabolism of carbohydrate, protein, and fat. Reactive hypoglycemia, in which blood glucose concentrations fall to symptomatic levels several hours after a meal, is another glucose regulation disorder. Nursing care is a critical aspect in the control of both conditions.

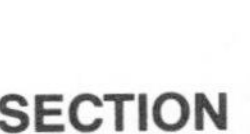

SECTION I

Diabetes Mellitus

Diabetes mellitus results from (1) an absolute lack of insulin, (2) impaired secretion of insulin by the pancreas, or (3) cellular resistance to the action of secreted insulin. Diabetes mellitus is both a metabolic and a vascular disease. Hyperglycemia results from the absolute or relative lack of insulin. Then, as the disease progresses, small blood vessels in the retina and kidney and larger vessels in the heart and peripheral circulatory system deteriorate. Diabetes mellitus is a major health problem, affecting an estimated 66 million people worldwide (Dolan–Heitlinger & Antle, 1983).

Classification of Diabetes Mellitus

For more than a century, two forms of diabetes mellitus have been recognized—one with its onset primarily in childhood and the other beginning primarily in adulthood. In 1979, the National Diabetes Data Group proposed the current classification. The three major categories are diabetes mellitus, impaired glucose tolerance, and gestational diabetes. This revised classification system eliminated such vaguely defined terms as *juvenile-onset, adult-onset,* and *borderline diabetes.*

Diagnostic Criteria

The diagnosis of diabetes mellitus is confirmed by the presence of an elevated serum glucose level. The definition of normalcy for the serum glucose level may depend on factors such as age and pregnancy, however. Therefore, the revised system in Box 32–1 specifies diagnostic criteria for children, pregnant women, and nonpregnant adults. The criteria are stringently defined to prevent overdiagnosis of diabetes mellitus.

This chapter will focus on the two most common clinical types of the disease—Type I, or insulin-dependent diabetes mellitus (IDDM), and Type II, or noninsulin-dependent diabetes mellitus (NIDDM). Although Type I diabetes first appears in childhood, it becomes a disease of adulthood as the person ages. Type II, formerly called *adult-onset diabetes,* is the more prevalent form of the disease and will become even more predominant as the percentage of older adults in the population increases.

Box 32–1
Diagnostic Criteria for Diabetes Mellitus, Impaired Glucose Tolerance, and Gestational Diabetes Mellitus

Nonpregnant Adults

Criteria for diagnosis of diabetes mellitus

Diagnosis of diabetes mellitus in nonpregnant adults should be restricted to those who have *one* of the following:

- A random serum glucose level of 200 mg/dL or greater *plus* classic symptoms and signs of diabetes mellitus including polydipsia, polyuria, polyphagia, and weight loss.
- A fasting serum glucose level of 140 mg/dL or greater on at least two occasions.
- A fasting serum glucose level of less than 140 mg/dL *plus* sustained elevated serum glucose levels during at least two oral glucose tolerance tests. The 2-hour sample and at least one other between 0 and 2 hours after the 75-g glucose dose should be 200 mg/dL or greater. Oral glucose tolerance testing is not necessary if the client has a fasting serum glucose level of 140 mg/dL or greater.

Criteria for diagnosis of impaired glucose tolerance

Diagnosis of impaired glucose tolerance in nonpregnant adults should be restricted to those who have *all* of the following:

- A fasting serum glucose of less than 140 mg/dL
- A 2-hour oral glucose tolerance test serum glucose level between 140 and 200 mg/dL
- An intervening oral glucose tolerance test serum glucose value of 200 mg/dL or greater

Pregnant Women

Screening for gestational diabetes

- By glucose measurement in serum.
- 50-g oral glucose load, administered between the 24th and 28th week and without regard to time of day or time of last meal to all pregnant women who have not been identified as having glucose intolerance before the 24th week.
- Venous serum glucose is measured 1 hour later.
- A value of ≥140 mg/dL (7.8 mmol/L) in venous serum indicates the need for a full diagnostic glucose tolerance test.

Pregnant Women (continued)

Diagnosis of gestational diabetes mellitus

- 100-g oral glucose load, administered in the morning after overnight fast for at least 8 hours but not more than 14 hours, and after at least 3 days of unrestricted diet (≥150 g carbohydrate) and physical activity.
- Venous serum glucose is measured fasting and at 1, 2, and 3 hours. Subject should remain seated and not smoke throughout the test.
- Two or more of the following venous serum concentrations must be met or exceeded for positive diagnosis:
  Fasting, 105 mg/dL (5.8 mmol/L)
  1 h, 190 mg/dL (10.6 mmol/L)
  2 h, 165 mg/dL (9.2 mmol/L)
  3 h, 145 mg/dL (8.1 mmol/L)

Children

Criteria for diagnosis of diabetes mellitus

Diagnosis of diabetes mellitus in children should be restricted to those who have *one* of the following:

- A random serum glucose level of 200 mg/dL or greater *plus* classic symptoms and signs of diabetes mellitus, including polyuria, polydipsia, ketonuria, and rapid weight loss.
- A fasting serum glucose level of 140 mg/dL or greater on at least two occasions *and* sustained elevated serum glucose levels during at least two oral glucose tolerance tests. Both the 2-hour serum glucose and at least one other between 0 and 2 hours after the glucose dose (1.75 g/kg ideal body weight up to 75 g) should be 200 mg/dL or greater.

Criteria for impaired glucose tolerance: The diagnosis of impaired glucose tolerance in children should be restricted to those who have *both* of the following:

- A fasting serum glucose concentration of less than 140 mg/dL.
- A 2-hour oral glucose tolerance test serum glucose level of greater than 140 mg/dL

SOURCE: Reprinted with permission from Rifkin H (editor): *The Physician's Guide to Type II Diabetes (NIDDM): Diagnosis and Treatment.* New York: American Diabetes Association, 1984, p. 10; section on gestational diabetes from the Summary and Recommendations of the Second International Workshop-Conference on Gestational Diabetes Mellitus. *Diabetes* 34, suppl. 2, June 1985, 123–126.

NURSING DIAGNOSES IN
Endocrine Dysfunction

DIRECTLY RELATED DIAGNOSES

- Activity intolerance
- Bowel elimination, altered: diarrhea
- Comfort, altered: pain
- Coping, ineffective individual
- Fluid volume deficit, actual
- Fluid volume deficit, potential
- Knowledge deficit
- Nutrition, altered: more than body requirements
- Self-concept, disturbance in: body image
- Thought processes, altered

OTHER POTENTIAL DIAGNOSES

- Infection, potential for
- Injury, potential for
- Noncompliance
- Nutrition, altered: less than body requirements
- Powerlessness
- Sensory/perceptual alterations: visual, tactile
- Skin integrity, impaired
- Thermoregulation, ineffective
- Tissue perfusion, altered: gastrointestinal, peripheral

General Nursing Implications

The role of the nurse in diabetes mellitus management is to help the client and significant others adapt to the lifelong challenge of living well with diabetes. Few diseases have as many physiologic, emotional, and social implications. Diabetes presents major challenges not only as a multisystem disease but also as a condition that affects issues such as self-image, diet, participation in exercise and sports, sexuality, childbearing, parenting, employment, and insurability.

Diabetes is best approached from a wellness perspective. To best serve diabetic clients, health care providers should help them make decisions that will encourage a full, productive, and healthy life. Client education requires an understanding of the principles of management of the numerous effects of diabetes.

Diabetes education is a lifelong process that can be divided into three phases. Immediate education begins on diagnosis and is designed to provide the basic knowledge necessary for immediate management of diabetes. The second phase, in-depth education, maximizes the client's ability to incorporate diabetes into a healthy lifestyle. The third phase, continuing education, renews previous learning and updates the client's knowledge.

Diabetes Mellitus Type I (IDDM)

Type I diabetes mellitus (IDDM) is distinct from Type II diabetes mellitus (NIDDM) in its etiology, onset, and clinical course. Although IDDM has received more attention from health professionals and the public, it accounts for less than 10% of clients with diabetes. The key difference between IDDM and NIDDM is that in IDDM, the pancreas does not produce enough insulin to sustain life. Therefore, individuals with IDDM depend totally on exogenous insulin. Because of the absence of insulin production, persons with IDDM are prone to **ketosis** secondary to hyperglycemia. In ketosis, the lack of insulin leads to the body's inability to metabolize glucose for energy. As a result, fatty acids are used as a fuel source. Fatty acids are incompletely oxidized, leading to an accumulation of ketones.

The onset of IDDM can occur any time from infancy to middle adulthood as a result of pathogenic causes; it can also occur at any age as a result of traumatic damage to the pancreas. It usually occurs in persons of normal body weight, unlike NIDDM, which is more frequent in the overweight or obese.

The etiology of IDDM is unclear and may be multifactorial. A genetic role is conceivable, because there is an increased frequency of certain antigens of the human leukocyte antigen (HLA) system, part of the body's immune mechanism. There may be an autoimmune mechanism that triggers the production of antibodies to destroy pancreatic islet cells. Such antibodies are found in a large percentage of persons at the time of diagnosis of IDDM. Viral agents, specifically coxsackievirus B, also may damage pancreatic islet cells (Freinkel, 1981).

None of these theories is sufficient to explain the etiology of IDDM. It may be that in the person with a genetic susceptibility, an environmental agent such as a virus may stimulate an autoimmune response, which in turn provokes IDDM.

Clinical Manifestations

The symptoms and signs of IDDM often occur abruptly and include the characteristic three "polys"—polyuria, polydipsia, and polyphagia. The absence of insulin prevents cellular metabolism of glucose. Thus, blood glucose levels rise while fat and protein stores are metabolized for energy, causing weight loss and ketosis. Weight loss continues despite hunger and excessive eating.

Rapid shifts in fluid and acid–base balance also occur. Hyperglycemia produces cellular dehydration and a profound diuresis. Dramatic fluid losses through urination can occur within hours. Hyperglycemia and dehydration accelerate the development of metabolic acidosis. If the disease is untreated, coma and death result.

Medical Measures

Following the diagnosis of IDDM, the immediate and ongoing goal of therapy is the correction of hyperglycemia and the restoration of normal carbohydrate, fat, and protein metabolism to prevent long-term vascular complications. The degree of control over blood glucose levels necessary to prevent the microvascular kidney and retinal complications of IDDM has long been a source of controversy. Proponents of rigorous, or tight, control cite evidence that these complications are directly related to blood glucose levels. Opponents argue that microvascular complications can occur independently of blood glucose control and may be hereditary.

In 1976, after careful review of the evidence, the American Diabetes Association published a position paper that urged optimal control of blood glucose levels, particularly in young and middle-aged persons, who are at greatest risk for developing long-term complications (Cahill, Etzwiler, & Freinkel, 1976). The National Institutes of Health are currently conducting a major 10-year study, the Diabetes Control and Complications Trial, to determine the relation between blood glucose levels and microvascular complications.

INSULIN Insulin is the foremost regulator of energy production, conversion, and storage. It is necessary for the metabolism of carbohydrate, protein, and fat. Metabolism of food carbohydrate begins when it is absorbed across the intestinal mucosa in the form of glucose. Insulin stimulates the entry of glucose into the cells, allowing it to be used for energy. Insulin is also necessary for **glycogenesis**—the synthesis of **glycogen** (stored carbohydrate) from glucose—and for the storage of glycogen in the muscles and liver. When insulin levels are low, *glycogenolysis,* the reconversion of glycogen to glucose, occurs to supply energy.

Food protein is absorbed across the intestinal mucosa as amino acids. Insulin lowers blood amino acid levels along with blood glucose levels. It also facilitates the incorporation of amino acids into tissue protein, allowing for growth and maintenance of body tissues.

Food fat is absorbed across the intestinal mucosa and carried in the lymphatic system in the form of **chylomicrons,** or particles of lipids, which are mostly triglycerides. Excess carbohydrates and amino acids are converted to fat in the liver. Without insulin, the enzyme lipoprotein lipase is not released, and fat cannot be stored. Insulin also inhibits the breakdown of triglyceride from adipose cells.

Hormones that are counter-regulatory to insulin include glucagon, epinephrine, cortisol, and growth hormone (GH). All have the general effect of increasing blood glucose levels. Glucagon stimulates hepatic glucose production through glycogenolysis and gluconeogenesis and inhibits hepatic glucose uptake. It also increases lipolysis, the splitting up of fat.

In the normal state, blood glucose levels are maintained in a limited range by a delicate balance between insulin and the counter-regulatory hormones. In IDDM, this balance is jeopardized. The goal of insulin therapy in IDDM is to replace endogenous insulin so normal blood glucose levels can be maintained.

CLASSIFICATION OF INSULIN Insulin has been greatly improved since it was first administered in 1922. Insulin may be classified by source, purity, concentration, formulation, and time activity:

- *Source and purity.* Bovine and porcine pancreata are the most common sources of insulin. Standard animal insulins have steadily improved in purity. Purified animal insulin contains less than 10 ppm of **proinsulin,** a precursor to insulin that is its chief impurity. Purified animal insulins are indicated for children and adults who are beginning insulin therapy, for short-term insulin therapy, and for situations in which complications arise from the use of standard animal insulin.

  Human insulin, developed in the early 1980s, is produced by recombinant DNA technology or by chemical modification of porcine insulin. It is less antigenic than animal insulin. The DNA generated insulin also provides a continuing supply independent of meat consumption trends. It is indicated for the same reasons as purified animal insulin and may someday replace it.
- *Concentration.* The standard concentration, or number of units per milliliter of fluid, used for insulin therapy in the United States is U100. Several other strengths have been used but discontinued to avoid dosage errors.
- *Formulation and time activity.* Many insulin formulations are available; the common preparations are listed in Table 32–1. Insulin is classified as short, intermediate, or long acting on the basis of onset, peak, and duration of action.

COMPLICATIONS OF INSULIN THERAPY Insulin therapy may involve several complications. Lipoatrophy, the loss of fat at injection sites, occurs more often in women and is thought to be caused by an immune response to insulin impurities. The treatment is injection of purified porcine insulin into affected areas until they fill out, usually in 4 to

Table 32–1
Time Activity of Insulin Formulations

Formulation	Onset	Peak	Duration
Short-acting			
Regular	15–30 min	2–4 h	5–7 h
Semilente	30–60 min	2–8 h	12–16 h
Intermediate-acting			
NPH	1–2 h	6–12 h	24–28 h
Lente	1–2 h	6–12 h	24–28 h
Long-acting			
Ultralente	4–6 h	18–24 h	32–36 h

SOURCE: Adapted from Karam J: Insulins 1983: Overview and outlook. *Clinical Diabetes.* New York: American Diabetes Association, 1983, p. 7.

6 weeks. Lipohypertrophy, the overgrowth of fat at injection sites, occurs more often in men and results from repeated injection into the same site. It can be prevented by rotating injection sites.

Occasionally, local or systemic allergic responses to insulin occur. Local allergies are often transient and may not require treatment. Systemic allergy, ranging from hives to anaphylactic shock (a rare reaction) responds to desensitization. Interrupted therapy with standard animal insulin increases the likelihood of allergy. Therefore, whenever temporary insulin therapy is necessary, as in gestational diabetes mellitus or other stress states, human insulin should be prescribed.

Insulin resistance occurs when blood glucose levels are unaffected by daily doses exceeding 200 units. Obesity is a common cause of insulin resistance, but insulin antibodies may also bind injected insulin and diminish its effect. Treatment in nonobese clients consists of transferring them from standard to human insulin. Hypoglycemia, an acute complication of insulin therapy, is discussed later in this section.

ADMINISTRATION OF INSULIN Insulin regimens meet the body's requirement for insulin at meals and during the remainder of the day. Conventional therapy consists of one daily injection of intermediate-acting insulin alone, or in combination with short-acting insulin, or two daily injections of a combination of short- and intermediate-acting insulin.

When conventional regimens do not result in adequate control, *intensive therapy* is an option. Intensive regimens include multiple daily injections of three or more doses of short-acting insulin in combination with intermediate- or long-acting insulin. Another method of intensive therapy involves continuous subcutaneous insulin infusion (CSII) by a battery-powered external pump (Figure 32–1). The pump delivers a basal level of insulin throughout the day and extra doses, or boluses, before meals. In theory, intensive regimens more nearly mimic insulin secretion of the pancreas.

NUTRITIONAL MANAGEMENT Nutritional management is the foundation of therapy for IDDM (as well as NIDDM). It is essential to convey to the person with diabetes mellitus both the goals and the means of nutritional management through the development of an individualized diet prescription, initial nutrition education, and ongoing nutrition counseling.

The overall goal of nutritional management in both types of diabetes is to normalize blood glucose and blood lipid levels while maintaining good nutrition and health. The nutritional guidelines for achieving this goal are excellent for the whole family, because they are what anyone should eat to remain healthy. With the current focus on control of blood glucose levels, normalization of blood lipid levels must not be forgotten. Approximately 80% of the deaths of diabetic Americans are associated with atherosclerotic lesions.

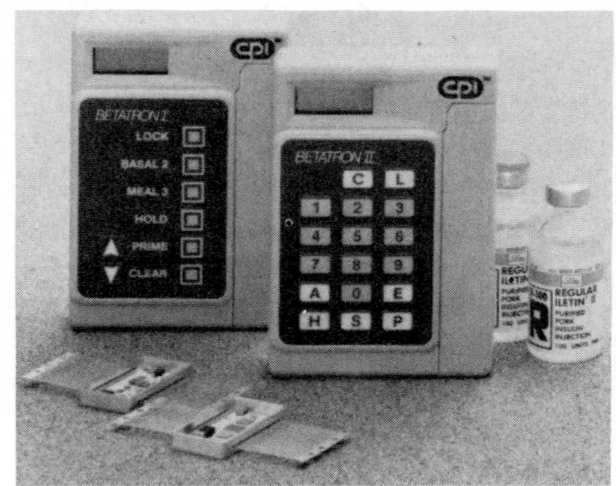

Figure 32–1

Two insulin pumps for continuous subcutaneous insulin infusion (Betatron I, Model 9205; Betatron II, Model 9200). *Courtesy of Cardiac Pacemakers, Inc. St. Paul, MN.*

Specific Nursing Measures

Nursing measures are directed toward client and family education for effective self-management at home.

Home Health Care

NUTRITIONAL APPROACHES The overall nutritional goal is the same for IDDM, and NIDDM, but it is important to understand goals especially important to each type. IDDM, therapy involves three goals:

1. Prevent the acute complications of hypoglycemia and hyperglycemia by balancing food intake with insulin and the client's usual pattern of activity. With conventional insulin therapy of one or two daily injections, the timing of meals and snacks must be consistent from day to day. To prevent hypoglycemia, the client must avoid long periods between meals. Consistency in timing, nutrient content, and caloric level is more important for blood glucose control than the restriction of any specific food item. It is generally more effective to adapt a client's insulin program than to expect major changes in eating habits. Establish a meal plan that is nutritionally adequate and acceptable to the client; then monitor blood glucose levels to integrate insulin therapy.
2. Provide for a normal growth rate in children and the attainment and maintenance of desirable body weight in adults. Any abnormal change in growth rate warrants an assessment of diabetes control and caloric intake. Adults with IDDM also need periodic assessment of weight and, if necessary, help in achieving and maintaining a desirable body weight.

3. Prevent or delay the development of the long-term cardiovascular, renal, retinal, and neurologic complications associated with diabetes mellitus. Epidemiologic evidence suggests that the prevention of hyperglycemia can prevent or mitigate microvascular complications. To attain this goal, clients must be willing and able to monitor their nutrient intake.

DISTRIBUTION OF NUTRIENTS IN THE MEAL PLAN The following percentages of carbohydrate, protein, and fat that make up the meal plan are general recommendations, not rigid requirements. They may be adapted to meet individual eating habits.

Approximately *50%* to *60%* of the total calories in the meal plan should come from *carbohydrates.* There is no need to restrict disproportionately the intake of carbohydrates in the diet as was once common in the management of diabetes. Increased dietary carbohydrate without increased total calories does not increase insulin requirements. Insulin need is more closely related to total caloric intake than to carbohydrate intake, mainly because of the excellent ability of the liver to manufacture glucose from a variety of noncarbohydrate sources.

Research in the mid-1970s demonstrated that increasing the carbohydrate content of the diet actually improved glucose tolerance. In the intestinal wall, in muscle and adipose tissue, and apparently in all tissues involved in glucose utilization and metabolism, a high-carbohydrate diet leads to better metabolism of glucose through enzyme adaptation.

The blood glucose levels produced by various foods are described by the **glycemic index.** This index tells which foods will raise blood glucose levels quickly and which will cause a more moderate rise. Researchers are beginning to learn which foods fall into each category as well as what occurs when foods are eaten separately and when they are eaten as part of a meal.

Many factors affect the glycemic index. The physical form in which food is eaten may affect blood glucose levels. Whole foods, which have a smaller surface area exposed to intestinal enzymes, may be absorbed more slowly than ground foods. Raw foods tend to slow blood glucose response. The meal in which the carbohydrate food is eaten may also be important. Slowly digested carbohydrates eaten in one meal not only cause less blood glucose response after that meal but also lessen the response after the next meal. Finally, carbohydrates taken in small amounts over several hours cause less response than the same amount eaten all at once.

Dietary fiber is another component of food that can affect blood glucose and blood lipid levels. The average daily intake of dietary fiber is 10 to 20 g. A recommended level is between 25 and 40 g, or 20 g per every 1000 calories in the daily meal plan. Table 32–2 lists the fiber content of various foods.

Nursing Research Note

Tallman V: Effect of venipuncture on glucose, insulin, and free fatty acid levels. *West J Nurs* 1982; 4(1):21–29.

The effect of venipuncture on fasting levels of glucose, insulin, and free fatty acids was studied. The author hypothesized that catecholamine release during stress, such as a venipuncture, might alter these levels.

In a sample of 21 inpatients an intracatheter was inserted into an antecubital vein. Blood was drawn immediately after catheter insertion and again 15 minutes after and 30 minutes after insertion.

The glucose levels indicated no significant differences between any test times. Insulin levels dropped significantly after the first drawing and 15 minutes after catheter insertion. At the 30-minute interval, the insulin levels increased somewhat but not significantly. For the free fatty acid levels, there was a significant drop between the first sample and the sample drawn after 30 minutes.

From these results, the author suggested that fasting insulin levels and free fatty acid levels are affected by venipuncture. It was recommended that when accuracy is essential, these blood tests should be drawn 30 minutes after the venipuncture.

The recommended level of *protein* intake is *15%* to *20%* of total daily calories. Protein is usually found in combination with fat in foods. The only foods that contain protein without containing fat are nonfat dairy products such as skim milk and vegetable proteins such as beans, peas, and lentils. Therefore, to keep fat within the recommended limits, protein must be kept at reasonable levels as well.

It is recommended that *fat* intake be reduced from the North American average of 40% to 50% of daily calories to approximately *25%* to *30%*. Dietary fat does not have an immediate effect on blood glucose levels but must be considered for two reasons. First, a gram of fat supplies 9 calories, whereas a gram of carbohydrate or protein supplies only 4 calories. Foods containing large amounts of fat will therefore be high in calories, and counting calories to maintain or attain desirable body weight is a major goal for clients with diabetes. Second, the restriction of foods high in fat, especially saturated fat, reduces blood cholesterol and triglyceride levels and decreases the risk of coronary artery disease (CAD). Because people with diabetes have twice the risk of CAD, such restriction is especially important for them.

Saturated fats are found in animal fats, coconut and palm oils, solid shortenings, and dairy foods that contain fat. As noted, these fats raise blood cholesterol levels. Polyunsaturated fats are liquid vegetable oils such as safflower, sunflower, corn, soybean, and cottonseed oils. They have been shown to lower blood cholesterol levels. Monounsaturated fats are neutral fats that neither raise nor lower blood cholesterol levels. They are found in olives, olive and peanut oil, and most nuts.

Cholesterol is manufactured in the body and is obtained in the diet only from animal foods. Although cholesterol is

Table 32–2
Fiber Content of Various Foods

Food	Portion for Approximately One Exchange of Each Food Grouping	Approximate Dietary Fiber
Vegetables	½ to ¾ cup cooked; 1 to 2 cups raw	2 g
Fruits: fresh or canned	½ cup; 1 small fresh	2 g
Breads: whole wheat breads and crackers	1 slice or 1 oz	2 g
Cereals: dry or cooked bran cereals	Varies Varies	3 g 8 g
Starchy vegetables: potatoes, brown rice, bulgur, green peas	½ cup	3 g
Legumes: peas, beans, lentils	½ cup	8 g
Nuts, seeds, peanut butter	1 oz (¼ cup) or 2 tbsp	3 g

SOURCE: Adapted with permission from Franz MJ: *Exchanges for All Occasions: Meeting the Challenge of Diabetes.* Minneapolis: International Diabetes Center, 1983, pp. 44–48.

usually found in combination with fat, there are a few foods (eg, eggs and liver) that are high in cholesterol without being high in fat.

The following dietary recommendations help reduce fat intake:

- Eat lean meats and pay careful attention to portion size, with a daily limit of 6 oz of meat, fish, poultry, cheese, and eggs. Use poultry and fish whenever possible, avoiding high-fat meats such as cold cuts, bacon, sausage, frankfurters, and prime cuts such as marbled steaks.
- In place of butter, use margarine with a liquid oil listed as the first ingredient on the label.
- Whenever possible, replace hydrogenated or hardened shortenings with liquid vegetable oils. Hydrogenation changes unsaturated liquid fat into a hardened, saturated fat.
- Use nonfat or low-fat dairy products (eg, skim milk and low-fat cheeses) and avoid products that contain dairy fat. Persons with diabetes, starting with children age 2, should use skim milk. Plain yogurt can be substituted for sour cream and mayonnaise.
- Restrict foods containing cholesterol, such as eggs and liver.

Table 32–3
Exchange Lists

Food Groups	Calories	Carbohydrate (grams)	Protein (grams)	Fat (grams)
Starch/bread	80	15	3	trace
Meat and substitutes				
Lean	55	–	7	3
Medium Fat	75	–	7	5
High fat	100	–	7	8
Vegetables	25	5	2	–
Fruit	60	15	–	–
Milk				
Skim	90	12	8	trace
Low fat	120	12	8	5
Whole	150	12	8	8
Fat	45	–	–	5

SOURCE: Summarized from *Exchange Lists for Meal Planning,* Alexandria, VA: American Diabetes Association and Chicago: American Dietetic Association, 1986.

In summary, it appears the ideal diet is high in carbohydrate with an emphasis on fiber; low in total fat, especially saturated fat; and adequate in protein.

EXCHANGE LISTS The most widely used system for translating the previous information into a method for food selection is the Exchange Lists for Meal Planning. These lists were developed by the American Diabetes Association and the American Dietetic Association and revised in 1986. The exchange system divided food into lists (Table 32–3). Each list contains food items similar in calorie, carbohydrate, protein, and fat content. Therefore, any food item on a given list can be exchanged, or substituted, for any other item on the same list.

The 1986 revision includes a symbol for foods that are sources of dietary fiber and a symbol for foods containing 400 mg or more of sodium per serving. The order of the exchange lists was changed to emphasize a higher carbohydrate, higher fiber diet, as well as to better reflect the order of foods in menu planning. Values for the fruit and starch/bread list were changed to reflect more accurately the nutrient composition of these lists.

A meal plan tells how many servings a person may select from each list at each meal and snack. In individualizing such a plan, the best way to start is to take a dietary history to find out what, where, and how much the person would eat if he or she did not have diabetes. Give as much consideration as possible to the person's preferences with respect to types of foods and eating schedules.

Next, the client's caloric needs are determined based on desirable body weight and current activity level. It is not necessary to determine the precise caloric need immediately. An estimate can be used as a starting point, and appropriate adjustments made on the basis of experience. The following generalizations are helpful in determining daily caloric levels:

- Children under 12 require an average of 1000 calories plus 100 calories per year of age. Thus, a 4-year-old would require 1400 calories.
- Boys from ages 12 to 15 usually require all of the above plus 200 calories per year of age after 12. Thus, a 14-year-old needs approximately 2600 calories (1000 + 1200 + 400).
- Girls' caloric requirements begin to drop between the ages of 12 and 15.
- A moderately active young man requires approximately 40 calories per kilogram of body weight daily. Thus, a, 70-kg (154 lb) man requires approximately 2800 calories/day. A relatively inactive young man may require as few as 30 calories/kg (2100 calories), whereas a young man who habitually engages in heavy activity may require as many as 50 calories/kg (3500 calories).
- A typical young woman requires approximately 30 to 35 calories per kilogram of body weight. Thus, a young woman weighing 58 kg (128 lb) who is moderately active needs approximately 1800 to 2000 calories/day.
- Older individuals usually require fewer calories in relation to body size; 30 to 35 calories/kg (or 15 calories/lb) of desirable body weight for the moderately active; 28 calories/kg (13 calories/lb) of desirable body weight after age 55 for the sedentary; and 20 calories/kg (10 calories/lb) of desirable body weight for the very obese or very inactive.

Children and teens with diabetes must have adequate caloric intake to grow normally. Because size and activity levels vary considerably in children of the same age, the formulas given here should be used only as guidelines. Too frequently, inadequate calories are prescribed for children and teens with diabetes.

For lean individuals, an initial diet plan that is generous helps emphasize that the main goal is regulation rather than deprivation. Satiety, appetite, and hunger are usually reliable guides to caloric requirements, but body weight is the definitive long-term guide.

Table 32–4
Sample Breakfast Meal Plan

Exchange	Number of Servings	Carbohydrate (grams)	Protein (grams)	Fat (grams)
Starch/bread	2	30	6	—
Meat	1	—	7	5
Fruit	1	15	—	—
Milk, skim	1	12	8	—
Fat	1	—	—	5
Total		57	21	10

After approximating caloric requirements, design a tentative meal plan based on the diet history and discuss use of the exchange lists with the client. The next step is to total the grams of carbohydrate, protein, and fat in the meal plan. The sample breakfast plan in Table 32–4 contains 57 g of carbohydrate, 21 g of protein, and 10 g of fat. To determine the total calories, multiply the grams of carbohydrate by 4, the grams of protein by 4, and the grams of fat by 9. The total calories for this breakfast plan are approximately 400. After the entire day's totals have been calculated, determine the percentages of calories from carbohydrate, protein, and fat by dividing the calories from each nutrient by the total calories.

After the basic meal plan has been designed, consider the following questions:

- Is it nutritionally adequate?
- Are the total calories appropriate?
- Are the proportions of carbohydrate, protein, and fat appropriate?
- Does the meal plan accommodate activity or exercise patterns?
- Has the client had problems with hypoglycemia at certain times during the day that could be prevented by changes in eating habits?
- Does the client have hypertension, abnormal lipid values, or renal disease necessitating further restriction (eg, sodium)?

The best way to monitor the effectiveness of the meal plan is to have the client try it and report problems to the nutritional counselor.

Children's meal plans should be evaluated at least twice a year, because their schedules and activities change frequently, and caloric needs increase or decrease depending on their growth pattern. Adults' meal plans should be evaluated once or twice a year. If weight gain or loss becomes a problem, changes must be made. Continuing education of all clients is essential for long-term adherence to meal planning.

SPECIAL CIRCUMSTANCES AFFECTING THE MEAL PLAN There is no need to use special or "dietetic" foods. In fact, many so-called dietetic products (ice cream, cookies, cakes, and chocolate candies) are sweetened with sorbitol or fructose and contain as many calories as the products they replace. Clients generally enjoy their food more and spend less when they use regular foods and substitute correctly in their meal plans. Some products with limited calories may be useful, however. Examples are dietetic jams, jellies, soft drinks, and hard candies; fruit canned without sugar; sugarless gums; and artificial sweeteners.

As mentioned, sorbitol and fructose, frequently advertised as being of benefit to people with diabetes, contain the same amount of calories as sucrose (4 calories/g). If used, they must be counted in the meal plan. Saccharin and aspartame (sold as Equal and NutraSweet) are currently available as nonnutritional sweeteners, and when used in moderation they appear safe.

A general rule is: Servings of food that contain 20 calories or less may be considered "free," with a limit of two or three per day. Foods containing more than 20 calories per serving must be included in the meal plan.

Alcohol is a hypoglycemic agent that augments the effects of insulin. The liver is the major organ for alcohol metabolism. Alcohol cannot be converted to glucose or amino acids. However, it can be used as an energy source or converted into fatty acids and triglycerides without requiring insulin.

Clients with diabetes mellitus are more vulnerable to the hypoglycemic effects of alcohol. Two oz of alcohol may produce hypoglycemia in a fasting person with IDDM. Alcohol is high in calories (7 calories/g) and devoid of nutritional value. Many alcoholic drinks (beer and sweet wines) also contain appreciable amounts of carbohydrate. Even so, most clients with diabetes may have an occasional drink. In normal-weight, insulin-dependent individuals whose diabetes is well controlled, moderate use of carbohydrate-free alcohol (2 oz daily) may be regarded as an "extra," best used with or following a meal. If alcohol is used daily, calories from alcohol are added to the total daily caloric intake. No food should be omitted, because of the danger of hypoglycemia.

During pregnancy, the diabetic mother must maintain strict control of her blood glucose level to reduce the likelihood of fetal morbidity and mortality. The diet plan must take into account not only the metabolic requirements of the mother but of the developing fetus as well. A total weight gain of 24 to 30 lb is recommended, with the pattern of weight gain more important than the total amount. Pregnancy is not a time for weight reduction.

Caloric requirements can be met by the addition of 300 calories/day to the prepregnancy meal plan. Additional calories should be supplied by 50 g of carbohydrate and 30 g of protein. The diet should contain approximately 1800 to 2500 calories a day. The importance of regular meals and snacks must be emphasized. In particular, the bedtime snack is essential because of the tendency toward nocturnal hypoglycemia and ketosis.

INSULIN ADMINISTRATION Clients must master several concepts and skills in learning insulin self-administration. To ensure that the same insulin is purchased consistently, the client must know the brand name, formulation, purity, concentration, and species source of insulin. This is difficult because there is a wide array of insulins and because insulin is an over-the-counter item in most states. To avoid confusion, advise clients to show their current insulin vials to the pharmacist at the time of purchase.

Insulin vials in use should be stored at room temperature, away from temperature extremes and direct sunlight. Extra vials should be refrigerated. Insulin should be used before the expiration date printed on the label.

Insulin syringes must match the concentration of insulin, or an incorrect dose will result. If injecting U100 insulin, U100 syringes must be used. Low-dose syringes are available for injections of 50 units or less and usually are more economical.

Consistency in the timing of insulin injections is important in maintaining blood glucose control. In conventional therapy, injections are given approximately 30 minutes before meals. Injection times should not vary more than 1 hour from day to day. Intensive therapy permits more flexibility in the timing of injections.

Insulin dosage changes recommended during a health care visit should be given to the client in writing. Written dosage algorithms that guide the client in making dosage changes based on blood glucose results are also helpful.

Insulin is injected in areas of the body containing sufficient subcutaneous tissue (Figure 32–2). An easy guideline for clients to remember is to inject where they can "pinch an inch" of tissue. Recommended sites are the lateral and dorsal surfaces of the upper arm, abdomen, anterior and lateral thighs, and buttocks. A written plan for rotating sites is helpful in selecting sites and encourages the use of several areas of the body for injection. Site rotation plans should be individualized to account for body size and distribution of subcutaneous tissue, the client's preference for sites, and ease of learning.

A written step-by-step outline of the subcutaneous injection technique for single and mixed formulations of insulin is helpful for the individual who has recently learned the technique as well as for the experienced insulin user. Review of these skills and concepts is an important component of periodic health care visits.

EXERCISE Persons with diabetes experience the same cardiorespiratory, psychologic, and weight control benefits

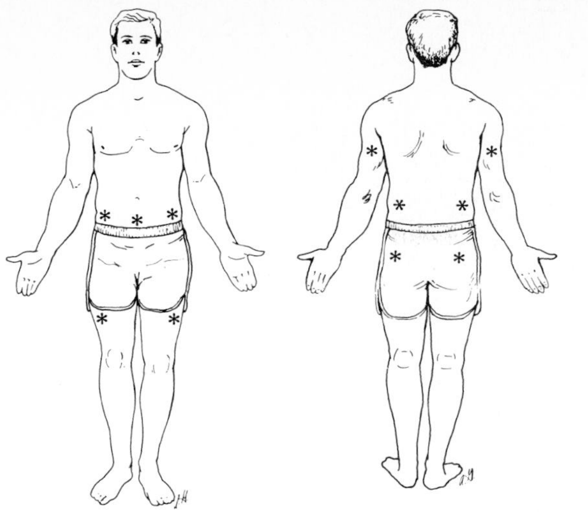

Figure 32–2

Sites for subcutaneous injection of insulin. SOURCE: *Courtesy of Etzwiler DD et al.:* Learning to Live Well With Diabetes. *Minneapolis, MN: International Diabetes Center, 1985.*

that anyone gains from a regular exercise program. In addition, the client with IDDM may benefit from decreased blood glucose levels and improved glucose tolerance. Exercise stimulates glucose uptake in exercising muscles, lowering blood glucose levels and increasing the body's sensitivity to insulin. Thus, regular exercise may decrease the need for injected insulin. Physical training can also help reverse the resistance to insulin that occurs as a result of obesity.

Exercise decreases the levels of very low-density lipoprotein (VLDL) and low-density lipoprotein (LDL). Exercise also is associated with increases in high-density lipoprotein (HDL), which appears to protect against coronary artery disease. Regular exercise also results in lower blood pressure.

To enjoy all the benefits safely, clients with IDDM must take certain precautions before, during, and after exercise. Because exercise adds to the blood glucose-lowering effect of injected insulin, it can increase the likelihood of hypoglycemia. Blood glucose will continue to decrease for up to 24 hours following exercise as muscle and liver glycogen stores are replaced. Food intake may need to be increased before exercising, depending on pre-exercise glucose levels.

Exercise lowers blood glucose levels only when adequate insulin is available. If blood glucose has been chronically higher than approximately 300 mg/dL, especially with mild ketosis, exercise will stress the body and drive blood glucose levels even higher. This occurs because hepatic glucose production increases and peripheral use of glucose decreases. Therefore, when blood glucose levels exceed 300 mg/dL, the client should avoid exercise until better metabolic control is achieved.

Finally, exercise initially may cause unpredictable variations in blood glucose levels. The regular exerciser will have fewer problems with blood glucose instability than the occasional exerciser. The key to safeguarding against instability of blood glucose levels is to test blood glucose levels before, during, and after exercise until a specific level of exercise is well tolerated. It is also wise to avoid injecting insulin into arm and leg sites immediately before exercise. Injecting into the abdomen or buttocks may help avert hypoglycemia.

The most efficient way to improve cardiovascular performance and burn fat with exercise is to (1) exercise at an intensity that results in no shortness of breath, (2) exercise continuously for at least 20 to 30 minutes, and (3) exercise three to five times a week. Aerobic exercise is of low intensity, is of long duration, and uses stored fat as the major energy source. Anaerobic exercise is of short duration (under 2 to 3 minutes), is of high intensity, and uses stored carbohydrate or glycogen as the major energy source. This activity quickly produces exhaustion. Thus, aerobic exercise is best for general fitness and blood glucose control. Aerobic activities require large amounts of oxygen and usually involve movement of the arms and legs, which contain a large part of the body's total muscle mass. Often-recommended aerobic exercises include brisk walking, jogging, swimming, skating, cross-country skiing, bicycling, jumping rope, aerobic dance, and jumping or running in place on a minitrampoline.

Any exercise program should be preceded by a medical evaluation. The program should build gradually in duration and intensity.

FOOT CARE Diabetic foot lesions result from the interplay of peripheral vascular disease and peripheral neuropathy. The primary cause of diabetic foot ulcers is an insensitive foot. Muscle atrophy causes dorsiflexion of toes and creates new pressure points on the plantar surface of the foot. Minor injury often goes undetected until ulceration and infection develop. Treatment is lengthy and includes antibiotics and the elimination or reduction of weight bearing with bed rest or a weight-bearing cast. Amputation is necessary if these treatment measures fail, but long-term survival following amputation is poor.

From 50% to 70% of the nontraumatic amputations in the United States occur in diabetic clients. Most of these amputations are preventable with proper care (Levin & O'Neal, 1983). Therefore, the prevention of foot lesions is a critical aspect of diabetes education and management. Clients should inspect and cleanse their feet daily and use an unmedicated, unscented lubricating cream to prevent the development of skin fissures. Detailed inspection of the feet should be part of the health care visit. Proper footwear stresses comfort over style. As deformities develop, corrective shoes help reduce stress. Corns, calluses, and nails should be trimmed by a health professional skilled in foot care. The client should avoid chemical abrasives. Minor uninfected injuries can be treated with cleansing, daily dressing changes, and rest. Any deviation from normal healing requires prompt medical attention.

SELF MONITORING OF BLOOD AND URINE Clients monitor the effectiveness of nutrition, exercise, and insulin therapy with blood or urine glucose tests. The two types of urine glucose tests are semiquantitative and quantitative. The semiquantitative method tests a small amount of urine with a glucose-sensitive reagent strip or tablet. The result is assumed to reflect the blood glucose level at a specific time. Semiquantitative urine tests correlate poorly with simultaneous blood glucose levels, however. Inaccuracies result from deviations (low and high) from the usual renal threshold for glucose of 160 to 180 mg/dL, the delay between glomerular filtration of urine and collection, and sensitivity and specificity problems with urine test materials.

Despite its disadvantages, however, urine glucose testing is recommended for those who are unable or unwilling to monitor blood glucose levels. Up to four daily preprandial tests are recommended for clients with IDDM. Using fresh second-voided specimens obtained within 30 minutes of emptying the bladder may improve the tests' accuracy.

The success of self blood glucose monitoring (BGM) suggests that it will be the predominant method for self-monitoring of diabetes management in the future. Self BGM is accurate, convenient, and eliminates the disadvantages of urine glucose testing. A drop of capillary blood from a fingertip or earlobe puncture is applied to a glucose-sensitive reagent strip (Figure 32–3). The strip's coloration correlates directly with the blood glucose level and is interpreted visually or by a reflectance meter. Self BGM is recommended for everyone taking insulin. It is mandatory in diabetic pregnancy and intensive therapy, when rigid blood glucose control is necessary.

The frequency of monitoring depends on the type of diabetes, stability of control, degree of control desired, and client preference. Thus, a pregnant diabetic woman may test five to eight times daily, whereas one day of tests a week may be sufficient for the older adult with stable diabetes.

Self BGM does not eliminate the need for urine ketone testing. Ketone testing for the nonpregnant client is suggested whenever preprandial blood glucose levels exceed 240 mg/dL or urine glucose tests exceed 0.5%, especially during illness.

Initial and ongoing client education stressing the importance of blood glucose monitoring is essential. Clients should maintain a written record of test results. Review of the record at each health care visit provides important information on day-to-day control and presents an excellent opportunity for education and support.

Clients should understand whether to test preprandially or postprandially, how frequently to test, what preprandial or postprandial blood or urine glucose targets are, and what action to take if targets are not met. Periodically, the nurse should verify the client's ability to use the testing method. Those using self BGM can compare a capillary blood glucose level with a serum glucose level obtained during the health care visit. The colors of some brands of blood test strips are stable for several days after the reaction if properly stored. Clients can record their visual interpretations on these strips and bring them on their health care visit to verify results.

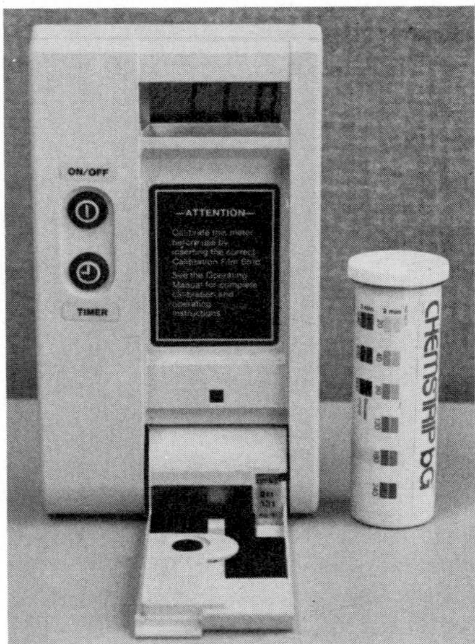

Figure 32–3

One model of a blood glucose monitoring system: The Accu-Chek bG/Chemstrip bG blood glucose monitoring system by Bio-Dynamics.

The random serum glucose level and glycosylated hemoglobin assay are two laboratory determinations commonly used to assess the effect of diabetes therapy. A random serum glucose level rarely reflects overall glycemic status, however, because blood glucose levels can change markedly during the day. In contrast, the glycosylated hemoglobin assay measures long-term blood glucose control over the previous 2 months. It indicates the percentage of hemoglobin attached to glucose (glycosylated). The level of glycosylation depends on the glucose concentration during the 60-day half-life of erythrocytes and hemoglobin. A glycosylated hemoglobin assesses long-term control but cannot be used to make specific changes in day-to-day therapy. Daily blood or urine glucose test results are used for this purpose.

Self BGM enhances the client's role in diabetes self-management. Self-adjustment of conventional insulin therapy is based on the principles of basic pattern control outlined in Box 32–2.

Box 32–2
Principles of Basic Pattern Control in Conventional Insulin Therapy

Blood glucose levels are affected by meal plan, activity, insulin, and emotional or physical stress. Determine whether stressors or inconsistent activity or meal plans exist before adjusting insulin.

Make insulin adjustments on the basis of blood glucose patterns rather than isolated values.

Assess at least 3 days of blood glucose levels to determine a pattern.

Use the time activity of insulin to determine which insulin is responsible for a blood glucose pattern:

- The prebreakfast short-acting insulin affects the prelunch blood glucose level.
- The prebreakfast intermediate-acting insulin affects the predinner blood glucose level.
- The predinner short-acting insulin affects the bedtime blood glucose level.
- The predinner intermediate-acting insulin affects the prebreakfast blood glucose level the following day.

Increase or decrease insulin 1 to 2 units at a time. Monitor the effect for at least 3 days before making another adjustment.

SOURCE: Adapted with permission from Skyler J et al.: Use of insulin in insulin-dependent mellitus. In: Insulin Update: 1982. Princeton, *Excerpta Medica,* pp. 133–139.

Medical and Nursing Approaches to Complications of IDDM

ACUTE COMPLICATIONS Acute complications develop within minutes to days. They include hypoglycemia and diabetic ketoacidosis (DKA).

HYPOGLYCEMIA Hypoglycemia is a serum glucose level below approximately 50 mg/dL accompanied by adrenergic and neurologic symptoms. Normally, catecholamines, glucagon, and GH are released to counteract hypoglycemia. The early symptoms of hypoglycemia, such as palpitations, anxiety, and perspiration, are catecholamine induced. If hypoglycemia persists, cerebral function is impaired, and confusion and irritability result. Severe hypoglycemia produces unconsciousness and seizures.

Because IDDM may impair the usual mechanisms to correct hypoglycemia, this condition should always be treated promptly. Mild symptoms reverse with the ingestion of 10 g of carbohydrate, such as a half cup of fruit juice or nondiet soft drink. If no response occurs within 10 to 15 minutes, treatment is repeated. Overtreatment should be avoided, however, to prevent excessive hyperglycemia. Glucose gel preparations can be administered if the person is uncooperative yet has an intact swallow reflex.

To treat hypoglycemia in an unconscious person in the home setting, administer a glucagon injection. Glucagon produces a transient rise in blood glucose levels, and small, frequent feedings should be started as soon as the person regains consciousness. In the health care setting, severe hypoglycemia is treated with the IV administration of 25 mL of 50% dextrose solution.

Common causes of hypoglycemia include delayed or inadequate food intake, increased activity, and excessive insulin. Snacks and meals scheduled to coincide with the time activity of insulin are important in preventing hypoglycemia. A midmorning snack may be necessary if the client uses prebreakfast short-acting insulin. A midafternoon snack is helpful if the client takes intermediate-acting insulin before breakfast. To prevent nocturnal hypoglycemia, a bedtime snack is essential for everyone taking insulin. Before and during prolonged exercise, extra food is necessary. When hypoglycemia cannot be explained by alterations in food or activity, the client should decrease the insulin taken.

In some individuals, the *Somogyi phenomenon,* or unrecognized hypoglycemia resulting in rebound hyperglycemia, occurs at night. A reduction in insulin or an increase in the bedtime snack is necessary in this case.

Instruct clients with either IDDM or NIDDM to keep a supply of canned fruit juice on hand for hypoglycemic emergencies. One or two cans can be stored in a bedside drawer and in the car glove compartment for ready availability. The calories used to treat the hypoglycemic episode can be subtracted from the day's allowance. Hard candy can be carried in a purse or pocket as a ready source of carbohydrate when traveling.

DIABETIC KETOACIDOSIS DKA is a serious but preventable complication of IDDM that can develop within several hours to days. The mortality rate in severe DKA is 5% to 15% and is usually due to the underlying cause (Barrett & DeFronzo, 1984). Infection is the most common precipitating factor.

DKA results from an insulin deficiency combined with increased secretion of counter-regulatory, or anti-insulin, hormones. Insulin deficiency produces hyperglycemia, because the body's uptake of glucose is reduced and gluconeogenesis is increased. Marked hyperglycemia causes an osmotic diuresis, dehydration, and electrolyte depletion. When insulin is deficient, free fatty acids are mobilized from adipose tissue and converted to ketones in the liver. Serum ketone levels rise, causing metabolic acidosis and compensatory hyperventilation. Ketones are excreted in urine; one form, acetone, is volatile and can be detected on the breath. Acidosis produces peripheral vasodilation and hypotension. Levels of glucagon and other counter-regulatory hormones are elevated and contribute to further gluconeogenesis and conversion of free fatty acids to ketones.

Symptoms and signs that precede DKA are hyperglycemia, ketonuria, polyuria, fatigue, and nausea. When vomiting occurs, dehydration and acidosis can develop rapidly. Listlessness; rapid, deep respirations (Kussmaul's breathing); and severe abdominal pain accompany signs of marked dehydration. A serum pH under 7.2 indicates severe acidosis and results in coma and death if untreated.

DKA can be prevented by having the client take measures such as those listed in Box 32–3 to recognize and treat hyperglycemia and ketonuria. If additional insulin is necessary, usually 20% of the total daily dose is given in the form of short-acting insulin.

The first step in treating moderate or severe DKA is fluid replacement. The rapid IV infusion of 3 to 4 L of isotonic or hypotonic saline within several hours restores tissue perfusion. When serum glucose levels fall below 250 mg/dL, the infusion is changed to 5% dextrose to prevent hypoglycemia.

The second step of therapy is continuous IV infusion or intermittent IM administration of low doses of short-acting insulin. In adults, the dosage generally ranges from 4 to 8 units per hour.

Replacement of potassium may be necessary. Initially, serum potassium may be elevated in DKA, but as ketosis and dehydration are corrected, potassium shifts intracellularly creating hypokalemia. Treatment of the underlying illness that contributed to the development of DKA is also a vital part of therapy.

Box 32–3
Client Guidelines for Brief Illness

Monitor blood glucose and urine ketone levels every 4 hours. Notify your health care provider if blood glucose levels are elevated or if urine ketones develop.

Never omit insulin. The need for insulin continues or increases during illness.

If you are not able to eat regular food, replace carbohydrates with liquids or soft foods. About 50 g of carbohydrate should be taken every 3 to 4 hours. Water, tea, clear broth, or other clear fluids should be taken frequently.

If nausea, vomiting, or diarrhea occur, take small sips of fluids (1 or 2 tbsp every 15 to 30 minutes) and notify your health care provider.

If illness persists beyond 24 hours, notify your health care provider.

SOURCE: Adapted with permission from Franz M, Joynes J: *Diabetes and Brief Illness.* Minneapolis: International Diabetes Center, 1984, pp. 1–7.

INTERMEDIATE COMPLICATIONS The intermediate complications of IDDM develop over several months. Children in whom diabetes is poorly controlled are retarded in growth and delayed in development. In the hyperglycemic state, hundreds of calories may be lost in the urine each day. The lack of insulin decreases protein synthesis and reduces levels of substances that control the effect of GH.

The risks during pregnancy for a diabetic mother and her child have decreased significantly because of the emphasis on control of maternal glycemia and improvements in perinatal and neonatal care. Nevertheless, the incidence of congenital anomalies in diabetic pregnancy is four times the rate in nondiabetic pregnancy. The congenital malformations in children born to diabetic mothers occur in organ systems that develop during the first 8 weeks of life. Thus, optimal diabetes control is ideally established before conception.

LONG-TERM COMPLICATIONS The long-term vascular and neurologic complications of IDDM generally take years to develop and usually become evident in adulthood.

RETINOPATHY Diabetes mellitus affects various ocular structures, but its major impact is on the retina. Approximately 5000 new cases of blindness related to diabetes mellitus are reported annually, and nearly 85% of these are due to retinopathy. More than 80% of diabetic clients have some form of retinopathy 15 years after diagnosis. About 2% of persons with diabetes are legally blind from retinopathy (L'Esperance & James, 1983).

Several factors are associated with the development of retinopathy. Its onset is slower in clients diagnosed as diabetic before age 30. Hypertension and lengthy duration of diabetes are predisposing factors. Finally, some evidence suggests that poor metabolic control, particularly mean blood glucose levels exceeding 200 mg/dL, is associated with retinopathy.

Client education about the detection, prevention, and treatment of visual impairment is a key responsibility of the nurse. Advise clients to have an annual examination by an ophthalmologist beginning 5 years after the diagnosis of IDDM. Eye symptoms warrant prompt medical attention. Encourage and promote the client's efforts to achieve metabolic control and emphasize the importance of early diagnosis and aggressive treatment of hypertension and diabetic renal disease. If visual loss occurs, refer the client to rehabilitation services to support adaptation.

Laser photocoagulation reduces the incidence of severe visual loss by at least 50%. Photocoagulation destroys new blood vessels, leaking blood vessels near the macula, and infarcted areas of the retina. It also produces adhesions that may counterbalance traction from fibrous membranes.

When retinal detachment and massive vitreous hemorrhage develop, vitrectomy restores partial vision in some cases. This procedure removes the blood-filled vitreous and fibrous membranes and replaces them with clear fluid.

NEPHROPATHY Approximately 4000 new cases of diabetic end-stage renal disease occur annually in the United States. Renal failure is the leading cause of death among people with IDDM. Those diagnosed with IDDM before the age of 20 have a 50% chance of developing nephropathy after 20 years. Although the cause of diabetic nephropathy is unclear, the evidence suggests that poor metabolic control is an important factor.

The clinical progression of diabetic nephropathy occurs in three stages, each with specific prevention and treatment objectives. The early or asymptomatic stage may last 10 to 15 years. During this period, prevention and treatment of conditions that might impair renal function are important. For example, hypertension and urinary tract infections should be vigorously managed. Urethral instrumentation and nephrotoxic agents such as certain drugs and radiologic contrast dyes should be avoided. Metabolic control should be encouraged.

Proteinuria is usually the first sign of renal disease. Its presence signals the beginning of the middle stage, which lasts 2 to 10 years. As renal function deteriorates, diuretic therapy and a low-sodium, protein-modified meal plan become necessary. Insulin requirements may decrease up to 50% as nephropathy progresses to end-stage disease. This final stage generally lasts 1 to 2 years and is characterized by chronic renal failure. Dialysis or transplantation is recommended when the creatinine clearance rate is 10 mL/min and serum creatinine exceeds 6 mg/dL.

CARDIOVASCULAR AND PERIPHERAL VASCULAR DISEASE Atherosclerosis occurs earlier and more frequently in clients with diabetes mellitus. Coronary artery disease is the most common complication of the total diabetic population. Longitudinal studies, including the Framingham Study, indicate that diabetes is a significant risk factor in the development of heart disease. Therefore, it is particularly important for diabetic adults to adopt risk reduction strategies recommended for the general population. Meal planning and exercise help the client reduce serum lipid and glucose levels and maintain desirable weight. Hypertension should be treated aggressively to prevent both microvascular and macrovascular disease.

Peripheral vascular disease is the result of both macroangiopathy and microangiopathy. Macroangiopathy, or damage to large and small vessels, is caused by atherosclerotic changes. Microangiopathy involves thickening of the capillary basement membrane. Symptoms and signs of peripheral ischemia include intermittent claudication, cold lower extremities, pain at rest, dependent rubor, diminished or absent pulses, shiny skin with loss of hair, ulcers, infection, and gangrene. Peripheral vascular disease associated with diabetes is often diffuse. Occlusions occur in many segments of vessels, and collateral circulation is involved. The disease usually affects the smaller vessels of both extremities. For these reasons, vascular surgery is difficult.

Glycemic control helps reduce elevated blood lipid levels associated with atherosclerotic changes. Although hyperglycemia alone does not appear to be related to the development of peripheral vascular disease, it should be prevented. Aggressive treatment of hypertension is helpful, and smoking should be discouraged.

NEUROPATHY The effects of diabetic neuropathy have been described for over a century and are among the most common, yet puzzling, complications of diabetes mellitus. The causes are unknown but may include a biochemical imbalance of Schwann's cell metabolism and ischemia. Although the central nervous system is not affected, both the peripheral and autonomic nervous systems may be extensively involved. Peripheral sensory polyneuropathy occurs more often in the lower than in the upper extremities and is usually bilateral and symmetrical. One form is characterized by severe pain that is worse at night. Painful neuropathy often subsides spontaneously after several months.

Treatment is limited and directed at the relief of symptoms. Control of hyperglycemia may reverse symptoms and should be attempted. Analgesic, anticonvulsant, and antidepressant drugs have occasionally proven effective.

The less painful, more insidious form of neuropathy is characterized by proprioceptive disturbances and diminished sensation to touch, pain, and temperature. These sensory deficits increase the possibility that injury will occur and go unnoticed. Peripheral motor involvement results in muscle atrophy and weakness in the upper and lower extremities. The loss of muscle function leads to deformities, particularly in the feet.

Autonomic neuropathies often exist concurrently with peripheral neuropathies. These conditions may include orthostatic hypotension, neurogenic bladder, delayed gastric emptying, and frequent diarrhea. Impotence, one of the most common manifestations of autonomic dysfunction, affects 50% of diabetic men. Diabetic impotence has both neurologic and vascular causes. Treatment consists of the implantation of a penile prosthesis.

Diabetes Mellitus Type II (NIDDM)

Type II diabetes mellitus (NIDDM) is the second major form of the disease. It accounts for approximately 90% of clients and has been diagnosed in more than 5 million adults in the United States.

Type II differs from Type I diabetes mellitus in several ways. It is usually diagnosed after age 40 and is frequently associated with obesity. It results from faulty pancreatic insulin secretion combined with cellular resistance to the insulin produced. Increased hepatic glucose production is also a factor. Because insulin production is sufficient to sustain life, DKA rarely develops.

As with IDDM, the etiology of NIDDM is unknown. Viral and autoimmune causes are unlikely. There is strong evidence that NIDDM is hereditary, but the HLA system is not involved.

Obesity is clearly a risk factor for NIDDM. Insulin resistance is associated with obesity. Many obese persons with NIDDM have abnormally high blood insulin levels. They have a delayed and prolonged release of insulin in response to carbohydrate intake. Insulin secreted in this manner is less efficient in controlling blood glucose levels. The action of insulin depends on the binding of circulating insulin to specific receptors on the cell membrane, followed by intracellular events. Chronically high levels of circulating insulin decrease the number of receptors, resulting in hyperglycemia and, possibly, impairment of intracellular insulin action.

Clinical Manifestations

Unlike the onset of IDDM, the onset of NIDDM is insidious and may go undetected for years. Of the estimated 5 million persons with undiagnosed diabetes in the United States, virtually all have NIDDM. Fatigue, polyuria, polydipsia, delayed healing, chronic infections, and fluctuating vision frequently herald its onset. Occasionally, in long-standing undetected NIDDM, vascular complications are already present at diagnosis.

Medical Measures

The goal of therapy in NIDDM is identical to that in the treatment of IDDM: the restoration of normal blood glucose levels and nutrient metabolism. NIDDM was once regarded as a relatively benign form of the disease. However, as awareness of the morbidity and mortality associated with NIDDM has increased, so have the efforts to improve its detection and management. The three methods of therapy are nutritional management, exercise, and oral hypoglycemic agents or insulin.

NUTRITIONAL MANAGEMENT Sixty to 90% of persons with NIDDM are obese at diagnosis or have a history of obesity. Many produce enough insulin to maintain normal blood glucose levels if they reduce caloric intake, weight, or both. Therefore, the first goal of nutritional management is calorie restriction and increased activity to achieve and maintain a desirable body weight. The calorie-restricted meal plan should be nutritionally adequate.

The second goal is to control hyperglycemia. For some, dietary modification is sufficient to restore normal blood glucose levels. Calorie restriction and weight loss reduce hepatic glucose production, increase the number of insulin receptors, and improve intracellular insulin action.

The third goal of nutritional management is to prevent or treat hypertension, hyperlipidemia, and cardiovascular and renal disease. Often NIDDM coexists with other chronic disease or is diagnosed after the development of a chronic complication. Therefore, nutritional management focuses on treating both diabetes and the related health problem.

ORAL HYPOGLYCEMIC AGENTS AND INSULIN If properly followed nutritional management fails to correct hyperglycemia, oral hypoglycemic agents or insulin are necessary. The oral hypoglycemic agents, or sulfonylureas, have similar mechanisms of action (Table 32–5). They decrease hepatic glucose production, increase insulin secretion, increase the number of insulin receptors, and enhance intracellular insulin activity. In 1970, results of a long-term study, the University Group Diabetes Program, suggested that oral agents increased cardiovascular mortality. Those conclusions were challenged, and in 1979 the American Diabetes Association issued a policy statement indicating that restrictions on the use of oral agents are not valid.

Table 32–5
Sulfonylureas (Oral Hypoglycemic Agents)

Generic Name	Trade Name	Dosage Range (mg/day)	Duration of Action (hour)
Acetohexamide	Dymelor	250–1500	12–18
Chlorpropamide	Diabinese	100–750	60
Glipizide	Glucotrol	5–40	24
Glyburide	DiaBeta, Micronase	2.5–30.0	24
Tolazamide	Tolinase	100–1000	12–24
Tolbutamide	Orinase	500–3000	6–12

SOURCE: Adapted with permission from Rifkin H (editor): *The Physician's Guide to Type II Diabetes (NIDDM): Diagnosis and Treatment.* New York: American Diabetes Association, 1984, p. 41.

Oral agents are appropriate only for those who secrete insulin. Therefore, they should not be used for IDDM. They are most effective in those recently diagnosed as having NIDDM (1) who are at or above desirable body weight and have never received insulin or (2) whose condition has been controlled with fewer than 40 units of insulin daily.

If hyperglycemia persists despite nutritional and oral agent therapy, insulin is used to supplement the body's supply. In contrast to IDDM, control in NIDDM may be achieved with relatively small doses of intermediate-acting insulin given once daily. The lowest dose of insulin necessary to achieve control should be used; overaggressive insulin therapy may increase hunger and promote weight gain, further increasing insulin resistance.

The use of oral agents in combination with insulin has been attempted, but its value is unproven. Therefore, such therapy should be limited to research.

Specific Nursing Measures

Nursing measures are directed toward client and family education for effective self-management at home.

Home Health Care

NUTRITIONAL APPROACHES The steps in creating a meal plan for clients with NIDDM are the same as for those with IDDM. When NIDDM is treated with oral hypoglycemic agents or insulin, the timing of meals is important to prevent hypoglycemia. For those treated with a meal plan alone, the total caloric intake and distribution of nutrients throughout the day are more important than the timing of meals. Snacks are not necessary to prevent hypoglycemia but may help curb the appetite and prevent overeating at meals.

Clients will not follow long meal plans that are unrealistically low in calories. Plans in the range of 1200 to 1500 calories for women and 1500 to 1800 calories for men promote better adherence and allow gradual weight loss. Because 1 lb of body fat contains approximately 3500 calories, weight loss is a slow process. A loss of 1 to 2 lb a week is a reasonable goal.

A major problem for those with NIDDM is maintaining weight loss once it has been achieved. A professionally supervised weight control program that emphasizes individual preferences, long-term behavioral changes, and regular exercise is necessary if clients are to achieve and maintain weight goals.

EXERCISE Exercise is an important aspect of treatment for clients with NIDDM. Physical activity increases energy expenditure and leads to weight reduction. It also can reduce insulin resistance even before weight loss occurs. Exercise promotes cardiovascular health by decreasing serum triglyceride, LDL, and insulin levels. It also results in increased HDL levels, which may prevent cardiovascular disease. These are important benefits, because those with diabetes mellitus are twice as prone to cardiovascular disease as the general population.

SELF BLOOD GLUCOSE MONITORING In assessing the effect of NIDDM therapy, self BGM is especially helpful. The renal threshold for glucose increases with age, so it is not uncommon for older adults with NIDDM to obtain negative urine test results when significant hyperglycemia exists. Semiquantitative urine testing has limited value in NIDDM management.

Testing frequency varies widely. Clients treated with meal plans alone or in combination with oral agents may perform self BGM once a week. Those taking insulin generally test once daily or several times on 1 day each week. Although clients with NIDDM are less likely to develop DKA, urine ketone testing is recommended during illness.

Although blood glucose levels tend to fluctuate less in NIDDM than in IDDM, a random serum glucose level may inaccurately reflect overall control. As in IDDM, the glycosylated hemoglobin assay measures chronic blood glucose status better.

Medical and Nursing Approaches to Complications of NIDDM

ACUTE COMPLICATIONS Acute complications of NIDDM are hypoglycemia and hyperglycemic hyperosmolar nonketotic coma (HHNK). Hypoglycemia is a complication of sulfonylurea therapy. HHNK can be life threatening.

HYPOGLYCEMIA Hypoglycemia is particularly likely with long-acting agents such as chlorpropamide. The symptoms and signs are the same as those in insulin-induced hypoglycemia. Regular meals and snacks protect against hypoglycemia. For clients whose meal patterns are erratic and who have impaired renal or hepatic function, a short-acting agent is preferred. Clients receiving sulfonylureas, especially chlorpropamide, should understand that alcohol consumption may produce a disulfiram (Antabuse)-like reaction. Disulfiram and alcohol in combination cause nausea, copious vomiting, throbbing headache, sweating, dyspnea, weakness, and confusion. This is a side effect rather than a complication of drug therapy.

HYPERGLYCEMIC HYPEROSMOLAR NONKETOTIC COMA HHNK coma is most frequently noted in the elderly. It develops in days to weeks. The pathophysiology of HHNK coma is similar to that of DKA except that ketosis is rarely present. The distinguishing clinical features are severe hyperglycemia in excess of 600 mg/dL; absent or minimal ketosis; profound dehydration with hyperosmolality greater than 340 mOsm/kg; and neurologic abnormalities, including seizures. Confusion and excessive thirst are often present. Precipitating factors may include prolonged therapy with hyperglycemia-inducing drugs, acute infection, and excessive fluid loss. Typically, HHNK coma occurs in the infirm who may not recognize or respond to thirst. Health professionals should observe fluid intake and output patterns in clients with NIDDM.

Treatment of HHNK coma is similar to that for DKA. The rapid IV infusion of hypotonic saline corrects volume depletion. Low-dose insulin, potassium replacement, and correction of the precipitating factor are other facets of therapy.

LONG-TERM COMPLICATIONS Clients with NIDDM are subject to the same long-term vascular and neurologic complications associated with IDDM. The types of diabetes mellitus differ, however, in the likelihood of developing these complications.

Macrovascular complications have a major impact on the health of clients with NIDDM. Coronary artery disease is the major cause of morbidity and mortality in adults, and those over the age of 40 are also at greater risk for diabetic foot problems.

Nephropathy is less likely to develop in NIDDM than in IDDM. Retinopathy, however, may be present at diagnosis. Adults with NIDDM are also more prone to developing cataracts, so annual ophthalmologic examinations for cataracts and retinopathy should begin at diagnosis.

SECTION 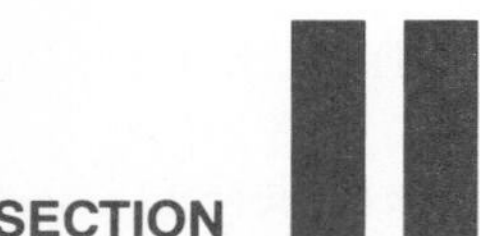

Reactive Hypoglycemia

Reactive hypoglycemia, a fall in blood glucose concentrations to symptomatic levels several hours after a meal, presumably is a response to factors stimulated by food intake. Most clinicians agree that a history of postprandial symptoms that disappear after food intake, reproduction of these symptoms during testing, and a serum glucose level in the hypoglycemic range during the symptoms are necessary to establish diagnosis.

Clinical Manifestations

The etiology of reactive hypoglycemia is unclear, and there is evidence to suggest it is overdiagnosed. The oral glucose tolerance test (GTT) is the most commonly used diagnostic tool, but substantial doubt exists as to its value in detecting reactive hypoglycemia. Hogan et al. (1983) studied 33 persons with a diagnosis of spontaneous reactive hypoglycemia and noted no relation between hypoglycemia during an oral GTT and symptoms. Moreover, many normal individuals experience asymptomatic serum glucose levels in the hypoglycemic range during an oral GTT.

Medical Measures

Nutritional management is the main form of treatment for hypoglycemia, regardless of its cause. The traditional recommendations have included frequent feedings in the form of a low-carbohydrate, high-protein, high-fat diet that avoids simple sugars. Research has demonstrated, however, that a diet high in complex carbohydrates and fiber improves glucose tolerance.

The current nutritional recommendation for clients with reactive hypoglycemia is a diabetic type of diet with 45% to 50% of the calories derived from carbohydrates. Clients should avoid rapidly absorbed sugars such as sucrose. Water-soluble fibers found in fruits and legumes are helpful because they delay gastric emptying by retarding glucose absorption in the gastrointestinal tract. Frequent feedings and moderate alcohol and caffeine consumption also are recommended. Because high-fat diets may interfere with the body's ability to use insulin, reducing dietary fat to improve glucose tolerance and maintain ideal weight is beneficial.

Specific Nursing Measures

Nurses play a significant role in educating the public about reactive hypoglycemia. There is a critical need to disseminate reliable health information substantiated by valid data because there is considerable misinformation about reactive hypoglycemia.

For the client who reports symptoms suggestive of hypoglycemia, recommend a thorough medical evaluation. Whether the diagnosis is confirmed or not, symptoms may persist. The nutritional recommendations outlined earlier are a healthy approach to relieving symptoms.

Chapter Highlights

Diabetes mellitus is characterized by abnormal carbohydrate, fat, and protein metabolism as well as vascular deterioration. It is the most common disorder of glucose regulation.

Approximately 90% of cases of diabetes mellitus in the United States are Type II, or noninsulin-dependent diabetes mellitus (NIDDM), and less than 10% are Type I, or insulin-dependent diabetes mellitus (IDDM).

The key difference between IDDM and NIDDM is that in IDDM the pancreas is unable to produce sufficient insulin to sustain life.

The goals of therapy for both IDDM and NIDDM are the normalization of blood glucose levels and the restoration of normal carbohydrate, fat, and protein metabolism in an effort to prevent long-term vascular complications.

The major approaches to therapy for clients with diabetes mellitus are insulin or oral hypogly-

cemic agents, nutritional management, and exercise. Nutritional management is the foundation of therapy for both IDDM and NIDDM.

Conventional insulin therapy consists of one or two daily insulin injections. Intensive therapy includes three or more daily injections or continuous insulin infusion (CSII) by a pump.

The overall goal of nutritional management in both types of diabetes is to normalize blood glucose and blood lipid levels while maintaining good nutrition and health.

The ideal meal plan is high in carbohydrate, with an emphasis on fiber; is low in total fat, especially saturated fat; and contains adequate amounts of protein.

Regular aerobic exercise reduces insulin resistance, increase HDL, reduces LDL, and lowers blood pressure.

Self blood glucose monitoring (BGM) is preferable to urine glucose testing because it is direct, immediate, and accurate.

The glycosylated hemoglobin assay reflects the preceding 2 months of blood glucose control and is valuable in judging the long-term effectiveness of diabetes therapy.

The acute complications of diabetes mellitus include hypoglycemia, diabetic ketoacidosis, and hyperglycemic hyperosmolar nonketotic coma. Major chronic complications are retinopathy, nephropathy, coronary artery disease, neuropathy, and peripheral vascular disease.

Hypertension accelerates the progression of diabetic retinopathy and nephropathy.

The two primary pathologic conditions leading to diabetic foot problems are peripheral neuropathy and peripheral vascular disease.

Oral hypoglycemic agents increase insulin secretion, reduce hepatic glucose production, increase the number of cellular insulin receptors, and enhance intracellular insulin activity.

Reactive hypoglycemia is a postprandial fall in blood glucose concentrations that results in adrenergic and neurologic symptoms.

Dietary management is the mainstay of therapy for clients with reactive hypoglycemia.

Bibliography

American Diabetes Association policy statement: Glycemic effects of carbohydrate. *Diabetes Care* 1984; 7:607.

Barrett E, DeFronzo R: Diabetic ketoacidosis: Diagnosis and treatment. *Hosp Pract* (April) 1984; 19(4):89–104.

Cahill G, Etzwiler DD, Freinkel N: Blood glucose control in diabetes. *Diabetes* 1976; 25(3):237–239.

Chambers JK: Save your diabetic patient from early kidney damage. *Nurs 83* (May) 1983; 13:58–63.

Dolan–Heitlinger J, Antle M: *Recombinant DNA and Human Insulin: A Source Book*. Indianapolis: Eli Lilly, July 1983.

Etzwiler DD: Education of the diabetic. In: *Clinical Diabetes: Modern Management*. Podolsky S (editor). New York: Appleton–Century–Crofts, 1980.

Etzwiler D et al: *Learning to Live Well With Diabetes*. Minneapolis: International Diabetes Center, 1985.

Forbes K, Stokes SA: Saving the diabetic foot. *Am J Nurs* (July) 1984; 84(7):884–888.

Franz MJ: *Exchanges for All Occasions: Meeting the Challenge of Diabetes*. Minneapolis: International Diabetes Center, 1984.

Franz MJ: Is it safe to consume aspartame during pregnancy? A review. *Diabetes Educator* 1986; 12:145–147.

Fredholm N, Vignati L, Brown S: Insulin pumps: The patients' verdict. *Am J Nurs* (Jan) 1984; 84(1):36–38.

Freinkel N: On the etiology of diabetes mellitus. In: *Diabetes Mellitus*. Rifkin H, Raskin P (editors). Bowie, MD: Robert Brady, 1981.

Funnell MM, McNitt P: Autonomic neuropathy–Diabetics' hidden foe. *Am J Nurs* 1986; 86(3):266–270.

Garcia CA, Ruiz RS: Diabetes and the eye. *Ciba Clin Symp* 1984; 36(4):2–32.

Graham S, Morley M: What "foot care" really means. *Am J Nurs* (July) 1984; 84(7):889–891.

Heins JM, Wylie-Rosett J, Davis SC: The new look in diabetic diets. *Am J Nurs* 1987; 87(2):196–198.

Hogan M et al: Oral glucose tolerance test compared with a mixed meal in the diagnosis of reactive hypoglycemia. *Mayo Clin Proceedings* 1983; 58(8):491–496.

L'Esperance F, James W: The eye and diabetes mellitus. In: *Diabetes Mellitus: Theory and Practice,* 3rd ed. Ellenberg M, Rifkin H (editors). New Hyde Park, NY: Medical Examination Publishing, 1983.

Levin ME, O'Neal LW (editors): *The Diabetic Foot,* 3rd ed. St. Louis: Mosby, 1983.

McCarthy J: The continuum of diabetic coma. *Am J Nurs* 1985; 85(8):878–882.

National Diabetes Advisory Board: National standards for diabetes patient education programs. *Diabetes Care* 1984; 7(1):31–35.

National Diabetes Advisory Board: *Prevention and Treatment of Five Complications of Diabetes: A Guide for Primary Care Practitioners*. US Department of Health and Human Services, 1983.

National Diabetes Data Group, National Institutes of Health: *The Scope and Impact of Diabetes,* Dec 1981.

Rifkin H (editor): *The Physician's Guide to Type II Diabetes (NIDDM): Diagnosis and Treatment*. New York: American Diabetes Association, 1984.

Rizza R, Gerich J: Statement on hypoglycemia. *Diabetes Care* 1982; 5(1):72–73.

Skelly AH, Van Son AR: Insulin allergy in clinical practice. *Nurse Prac* 1987; 12(4):14–23.

Zinman B, Vranic M: Diabetes and exercise. *Med Clin North Am* 1985; 68(1):145–157.

CHAPTER **33**

Specific Disorders of the Thyroid and Parathyroid Glands

Other topics relevant to this content are: Diagnostic studies for clients with disorders of the thyroid and parathyroid glands, **Chapter 31**.

Objectives

When you have finished studying this chapter, you should be able to:

Identify disorders commonly associated with the thyroid gland.

Describe the assessment parameters used to obtain information from clients with possible thyroid dysfunction.

Explain the laboratory studies that might indicate hyperfunction or hypofunction of the thyroid gland.

Discuss the major subjective and objective findings, medical and surgical treatment approaches, and nursing care of clients with hyperthyroidism.

Discuss the major subjective and objective findings, treatment approaches, and nursing care of clients with hypothyroidism.

Compare the common causes of enlargement of the thyroid gland.

Discuss the major subjective and objective findings, medical and surgical treatment approaches, and nursing care of clients with hyperparathyroidism.

Describe causes of hypercalcemia other than hyperparathyroidism.

Discuss the major subjective and objective findings, treatment approaches, and nursing care of clients with hypoparathyroidism.

Anticipate the psychosocial/lifestyle implications of thyroid and parathyroid dysfunction for the client and significant others and outline specific nursing interventions to address their needs.

Disorders of the thyroid gland may be characterized by either an abnormality in the secretion of thyroid hormone or a change in the size or contour of the gland. An excess of thyroid hormone produces hyperthyroidism; a deficiency produces hypothyroidism. *Euthyroidism* refers to normal thyroid function. Disorders associated with changes in size or contour may or may not be accompanied by altered secretion of thyroid hormone; pressure from an enlarged gland may, by itself, produce symptoms.

Similarly, disorders of the parathyroid glands are characterized by abnormalities in the secretion of parathyroid hormone (PTH). Excess PTH produces hyperparathyroidism, whereas a PTH deficiency produces hypoparathyroidism. Changes in the body's PTH levels alter the regulation of calcium and phosphorus.

SECTION 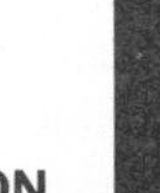

Disorders of Multifactorial Origin

Hyperthyroidism

Hyperthyroidism is characterized by an increase in secretion and plasma levels of the hormones thyroxine (T_4), triiodothyronine (T_3), or both. Symptomatic hyperthyroidism may also be referred to as *thyrotoxicosis.*

Hyperthyroidism associated with diffuse enlargement of the thyroid (goiter) and exophthalmos (protrusion of the eyeballs) is traditionally known as *Graves' disease.* Some clients with exophthalmos may exhibit no clinical or laboratory signs of hyperthyroidism, however. A synonym for Graves' disease is *diffuse toxic goiter.*

Table 33–1
Etiology of Hyperthyroidism

Categories of Hyperthyroidism	Etiology
Graves' disease	Long-acting thyroid stimulator (LATS) in the plasma causing hyperthyroidism, diffuse thyromegaly, exophthalmos
Nodular hyperthyroidism	Increased production of thyroid hormone by an autonomous thyroid nodule
Chronic thyroiditis	Chronic inflammation of the thyroid causing hyperthyroidism
Factitious and iatrogenic hyperthyroidism	Hyperthyroidism induced by the ingestion of exogenous thyroid hormone
Chorionic thyroid-stimulating hormone (TSH)	Hyperthyroidism and thyromegaly seen in women with choriocarcinoma of the placenta and in men with choriocarcinoma of the testes
Struma ovarii	Hyperthyroidism associated with ovarian carcinoma; the tumor is composed of thyroid tissue and secretes thyroid hormone

The etiology of the various categories of hyperthyroidism is shown in Table 33–1. Primary hyperthyroidism (originating within the thyroid itself) and tertiary hyperthyroidism (from exogenous intake) are the most common. Secondary hyperthyroidism, resulting from excessive secretion of thyroid-stimulating hormone (TSH), is rare and usually results from a tumor of the adenohypophysis. Graves' disease, the term often applied to all forms of hyperthyroidism, is classically defined as hyperthyroidism associated with thyromegaly (goiter) and exophthalmos (Figure 33–1).

About 50% of all clients with hyperthyroidism have a positive history of preceding physical or emotional trauma (Kaye & Rose, 1983). The highest incidence of hyperthyroidism is seen in women between the ages of 20 and 40. In Graves' disease, women are affected seven times more frequently than men.

Clinical Manifestations

The clinical manifestations of hyperthyroidism are directly related to the amount of excessive circulating hormone and the length of time it has been circulating, the age of the client, and the client's concomitant disorders. Hyperthyroidism affects almost all the systems of the body. The most common subjective and objective findings are summarized in Table 33–2.

In the elderly, thyroid dysfunction is often called the "great imitator" because it may mimic other disorders. A cardiac dysrhythmia, especially atrial fibrillation, that responds poorly to digitalization may be the first sign of thyroid dysfunction in an older adult. Occasionally, paroxysmal supraventricular tachycardia may be seen. Congestive heart failure that seems not to respond to treatment may also be a presenting sign of hyperthyroidism in the elderly as well as in other clients with a history of cardiac disease.

Hyperthyroidism is diagnosed from the clinical symptoms and signs (Table 33–2), elevated plasma levels of T_4, T_3, or both; and elevated radioactive iodine uptake (RAIU). A thyroid scan may help differentiate diffuse toxic goiter from a toxic multinodular goiter. Plasma levels of T_4 are used as a screening tool. When the diagnosis is uncertain,

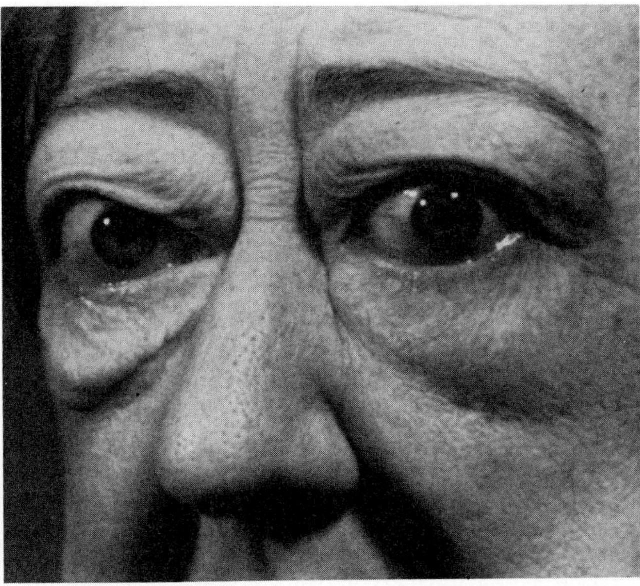

Figure 33–1

Exophthalmos in a client with Graves' disease. *Courtesy of Millard Fillmore Hospital, Buffalo, NY.*

NURSING DIAGNOSES IN Endocrine Dysfunction

DIRECTLY RELATED DIAGNOSES

- Activity intolerance
- Bowel elimination, altered: diarrhea
- Comfort, altered: pain
- Coping, ineffective individual
- Fluid volume deficit, actual
- Fluid volume deficit, potential
- Knowledge deficit
- Nutrition, altered: more than body requirements
- Self-concept, disturbance in: body image
- Thought processes, altered

OTHER POTENTIAL DIAGNOSES

- Infection, potential for
- Injury, potential for
- Noncompliance
- Nutrition, altered: less than body requirements
- Powerlessness
- Sensory/perceptual alterations: visual, tactile
- Skin integrity, impaired
- Thermoregulation, ineffective
- Tissue perfusion, altered: gastrointestinal, peripheral

thyroxine-binding globulin (TBG) may be measured to rule out the possibility of abnormalities in the T_4-binding proteins. These and other tests used in the laboratory evaluation of thyroid disorders are presented in Table 31–1.

THYROID STORM Thyroid storm, or thyrotoxic crisis, is a potentially life-threatening emergency characterized by an increase in all the symptoms and signs of hyperthyroidism. It is a result of a sudden release of thyroid hormone into the bloodstream and may be precipitated by infections, surgery, trauma, radioactive-iodine therapy, aggressive manipulation of the thyroid gland, diabetic ketoacidosis, abrupt withdrawal of antithyroid drugs, or severe stress. With better diagnostic and treatment approaches, thyroid storm now is so rare that it accounts for only 2% of all hospital admissions for hyperthyroidism. Symptoms and signs of thyroid storm include (Kaye & Rose, 1983):

- Marked restlessness and anxiety
- Rise in temperature to 104°F to 106°F (40°C to 41°C)
- Extreme tachycardia (130 to 160 beats per minute)
- Dehydration
- Nausea and vomiting
- Diarrhea
- Delirium and psychosis

Medical Measures

The choice of therapy for the treatment of hyperthyroidism depends on the cause of the disorder. Symptomatic therapy involves the oral administration of an adrenergic blocking agent to treat the increased activity of the sympathetic nervous system that accompanies hyperthyroidism. Propranolol is the agent most commonly used to minimize the sympathetic effects. Others include reserpine, guanethidine, and alpha-methyldopa. Definitive measures for the treatment of hyperthyroidism include antithyroid drugs (eg, propylthiouracil or methimazole [Tapazole]), radioactive iodine, and thyroidectomy.

RADIOACTIVE IODINE (^{131}I) THERAPY Radioactive iodine is an inexpensive and easily administered therapeutic agent used mainly to treat hyperthyroidism in clients ages 40 and above, although the age limit is not an absolute. Pregnant women should not be given ^{131}I.

The thyroid gland cannot distinguish between normal and radioactive iodine and will absorb both isotopes and store them. Concentrated in the thyroid, ^{131}I will destroy cells that store it by localized irradiation, resulting in a decrease in T_4 secretion and a reduction in the size of the gland.

Improvement of symptoms may occur 2 to 4 weeks after treatment, with euthyroidism occurring in about 3 months. Occasionally, if the condition does not resolve, a second dose may be administered.

Radioactive iodine is administered on an outpatient basis in the form of an oral "cocktail." When a large dose of ^{131}I is required, the client may need to be hospitalized and placed on radiation safety precautions.

About 10% of ^{131}I-treated clients may develop hypothyroidism in the first year, and about 3% of them may do so every year thereafter. These clients need hormonal replacement. All clients should have periodic medical follow-up and re-evaluation after attaining a euthyroid state.

CARE OF EXOPHTHALMOS Local care of the eyes includes the use of methylcellulose drops (artificial tears) and steroid ophthalmic drops. For severe inflammation of the eyes, oral prednisone may be necessary. Thiazide diuretics can relieve periorbital and lid edema.

In case of rapid progression of proptosis or development of optic neuritis with changes in visual acuity, irradiation of the retro-orbital tissues or surgical orbital decompression may be instituted. In severe cases of exophthalmos, surgery may correct lid retraction and ophthalmoplegia (eye muscle paralysis).

MANAGEMENT OF THYROID STORM The rare development of thyroid storm poses a serious threat to life. Treatment must be started immediately. The treatment usually includes:

- Propylthiouracil (800 to 1200 mg daily) via a nasogastric tube
- Propranolol (20 to 60 mg q. 4 h PO or 1 to 2 mg IV every 1 to 2 hours)
- Potassium iodide (500 mg q. 6 h or sodium iodide 0.5 g IV q. 8 h)
- Intravenous therapy

Table 33–2
Common Findings in Hyperthyroidism

Subjective Findings	Objective Findings
Clients often note:	*Examiners often observe:*
General: Intolerance to heat, fatigue, insomnia, and hyperactivity; increased anxiety, irritability, restlessness, and nervousness; emotional lability	Hair: Fine, silky Nails: Loosening of the nail from the nail bed (onycholysis)
Skin: Flushing, sweating	Skin: Smooth, soft, thin, moist; excessive sweating (hyperhidrosis); palmar erythema, ankle swelling; a hard, nonpitting swelling over the anterior tibia (pretibial edema)
Eyes: Photosensitivity, diplopia	Eyes: Widened palpebral fissures (stare), exophthalmos, lid lag, lid retraction, diminished convergence, increased lacrimation
Neck: Tightness of collars and necklaces	Neck: Thyromegaly with diffuse or symmetrical enlargement; bruits related to increased vascularity; nodules, thyroid tenderness
Cardiovascular system: Palpitations	Cardiovascular system: Increased systolic blood pressure, tachycardia, wide pulse pressures, systolic flow murmurs, dysrhythmias, peripheral vasodilation with bounding pulses and warm, slightly erythematous extremities
Gastrointestinal system: Weight loss, nausea, diarrhea, abdominal pain	Gastrointestinal system: Weight loss, hyperactive bowel sounds
Neurologic system: Muscle weakness	Neurologic system: Fine tremor of tongue, eyelids, and fingers; hyperactive DTRs with a brisk Achilles reflex; sometimes muscle atrophy
Reproductive system: Impotence, decreased libido, infertility (men); amenorrhea, hypomenorrhea, decreased libido, infertility (women)	Reproductive system: Male: gynecomastia

SOURCE: Adapted with permission from Kaye D, Rose LF (editors): *Fundamentals of Internal Medicine.* St. Louis: Mosby, 1983.

- Measures to reduce hyperthermia (eg, cold packs, hypothermia blanket)
- Oxygen
- Corticosteroids in high doses if the client fails to respond to initial treatment in 12 to 24 hours
- Digoxin with cardiac failure
- Additional measures to lower plasma thyroid levels rapidly (eg, plasmapheresis, exchange transfusions, and peritoneal dialysis)

Hyperthyroidism is often cyclic and may be precipitated by either psychologic or physiologic stress. Recurrence rates are usually in the range of 20% to 30% with any form of therapy except radical thyroidectomy and large doses of ^{131}I. With proper treatment and long-term follow-up, the clinical results are often good, although more as an induced remission than a cure. Hypothyroidism is common in the post-treatment period and may occur several years after a subtotal thyroidectomy or treatment with ^{131}I. Thyroid storm has a poor prognosis and is best prevented by careful preoperative preparation of the client.

Specific Nursing Measures

The nursing care of the client with hyperthyroidism is directed toward ameliorating the symptoms and signs associated with this disorder. Typically, clients with hyperthyroidism are nervous, agitated, slender, often irritable, and subject to emotional lability. They may be hyperactive and restless (because of the increased metabolic rate), have difficulty concentrating for long periods, be intolerant of heat (excessive perspiration), have gastrointestinal problems, and experience sexual dysfunction. In instances of exophthalmos, they may have dryness of the conjunctiva and cornea or visual impairment. These symptoms present a problem not only to the client but also to significant others who are called on to provide support during diagnosis and treatment.

In general, nurses caring for clients with hyperthyroidism should focus on:

- Assessing clients thoroughly
- Maintaining client comfort
- Promoting emotional well-being of client and family

- Monitoring intake and output, diet, and elimination patterns
- Educating clients and their families

Client assessment should include vital signs (temperature, pulse, respirations, and blood pressure) every 4 hours and daily weight. The physician may order a sleeping pulse rate because in hyperthyroidism, the pulse rate often increases during sleep. Especially important is an assessment of the client's mental state, particularly the degree of agitation and restlessness, because increasing restlessness and anxiety may be an early indicator of impending thyroid storm. Also be alert for any symptoms and signs of impending cardiac failure (dyspnea on exertion, shortness of breath, paroxysmal nocturnal dyspnea, dysrhythmias, or rales). Cardiac failure is often a serious complication of hyperthyroidism; it may be seen in the elderly and also in clients with a previous history of cardiac problems.

Clients may require daily baths and frequent linen changes because of profuse perspiration. Give special care to clients who are confined to bed, with attention to bony prominences and other potential areas of skin breakdown. The room temperature should be lowered because of the client's intolerance to heat. Bedding and sleepwear should be lightweight.

In general, clients' activities should be restricted to provide maximum rest and alleviate fatigue. This restriction may further agitate restless, hyperactive clients and provide a challenge for the nurse. To calm such clients, refer them to the occupational therapy department for suitable diversions, alternate the schedule of activity and rest periods, and remove potential sources of stimulation from the environment. Some clients may need to be sedated.

For clients with ocular involvement, elevating the head of the bed may help relieve edema of the periorbital areas. Methylcellulose drops, or artificial tears (0.5% to 1%), alleviate dryness of the eyes and protect against irritation. They should be given as ordered. In clients with severe protrusion of the eyeballs (proptosis), the lids may need to be taped during sleep or a sleeping mask worn to prevent drying of the cornea and conjunctiva. Sunglasses may help minimize the effects of glare. Assess visual acuity and observe for increasing proptosis and ophthalmoplegia.

Clients with hyperthyroidism are often subject to mood swings, which disturb both client and family. In addition, clients are often irritable, restless, easily upset, and distracted. They often benefit from attempts to create a calm, soothing environment in which the routine and primary caretakers change as little as possible. These clients should be assigned to private rooms. Screen visitors and teach them to avoid disturbing or anxiety-producing topics of conversation. Although it is not always possible in practice, attempt to help the client and significant others see the relation between the client's behavior and physiologic state. Because the client may also have some degree of sexual dysfunction, try to provide opportunities to discuss this in a calm, relaxed situation to assure client and family that this, too, is a manifestation of the underlying clinical disorders.

Clients with hyperthyroidism, in spite of an increasing appetite, usually lose some weight because of tissue catabolism resulting from high metabolic rates. They may need 4000 to 5000 calories a day in the form of a high-protein, high-carbohydrate diet. The client should avoid consumption of excessive fiber because of its effect on peristalsis. The amount of caffeine consumed may need regulation to avoid overstimulation. Snacks between meals and at bedtime are beneficial. One of the parameters in assessing the efficacy of a treatment regimen in hyperthyroidism is the maintenance of a stable weight (or weight gain), so weight should be monitored each day or every other day.

Clients with hyperthyroidism often require an increased fluid intake (usually in the range of 4000 mL daily unless there are cardiac or renal contraindications) to overcome excessive fluid loss from increased perspiration due to the high metabolic rate. The increased production of metabolic wastes also requires enough fluid intake to enable their dilution and excretion by the kidneys. This increased fluid intake can be provided in a variety of ways to meet the individual client's needs and tastes. A careful explanation of the purpose of the additional fluid intake may ensure client cooperation.

Clients with hyperthyroidism may also produce stools more often because of the higher rate of peristalsis. This can cause perianal skin breakdown and irritation. Carefully and thoroughly clean the area and apply creams and lubricants as needed.

Client/Family Teaching

Client and family education should focus on the basic self-care essential for the client with hyperthyroidism:

- Symptoms and signs of both hyperthyroidism and hypothyroidism—what to report to the doctor and when and the effect of increased thyroid production on the body
- The client's treatment regimen and its purposes—the name, dosage, action, and side-effects of each medication
- Any dietary prescriptions
- The need for regular medical supervision and its purpose—the data and time of the next medical appointment and a telephone number where client and family can call with questions

In addition, because of the emotional and mental changes, explain to the client and significant others the relation between these behaviors and the overproduction of thyroid hormone as well as to reassure them that medical treatment will ameliorate these changes. Emphasize that the treatment for hyperthyroidism often takes a long time to show an effect. Because subsequent hypothyroidism is also a concern, vigilance is necessary, even after the hyperthyroidism has resolved.

Thyroidectomy

Thyroidectomy, the surgical removal of the thyroid gland, may involve a complete removal of the gland or the removal of a lobe (thyroid lobectomy) or portion (subtotal thyroidectomy). The clinical indications for thyroidectomy are hyperthyroidism (Graves' disease), simple goiter, thyroid nodules, and carcinoma of the thyroid gland. When there is inflammation of the thyroid gland, or thyroiditis, surgery is only indicated to relieve symptoms of obstruction of the trachea or if malignancy is suspected.

In cases of goiter, thyroid nodules, or hyperthyroidism, a subtotal thyroidectomy is performed. This involves resection of about five-sixths of the thyroid gland. The remainder of the gland is usually sufficient to provide the necessary thyroid hormones, so replacement may not be needed. Most cancer of the thyroid, however, is treated with a total thyroidectomy, so the client will require lifelong replacement of thyroid hormone.

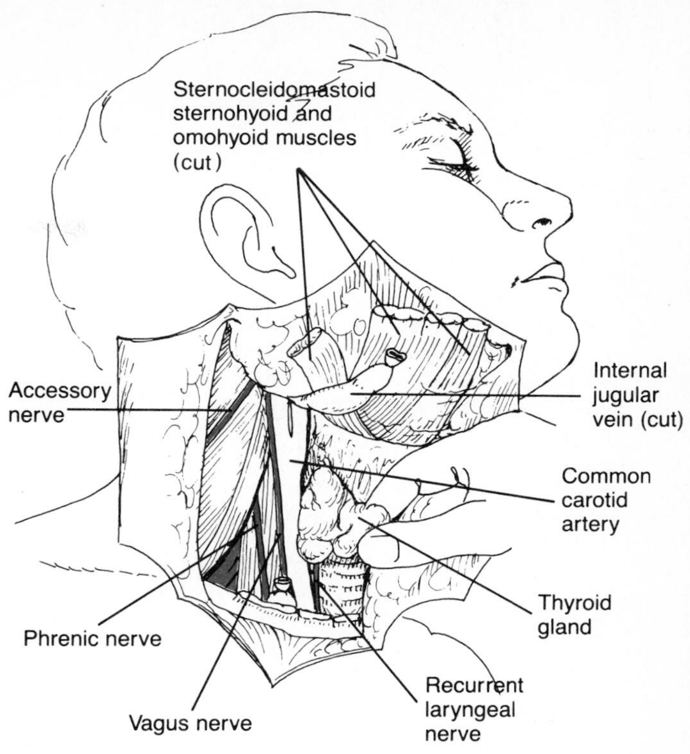

Figure 33–3

Surgical site for removal of the thyroid gland.

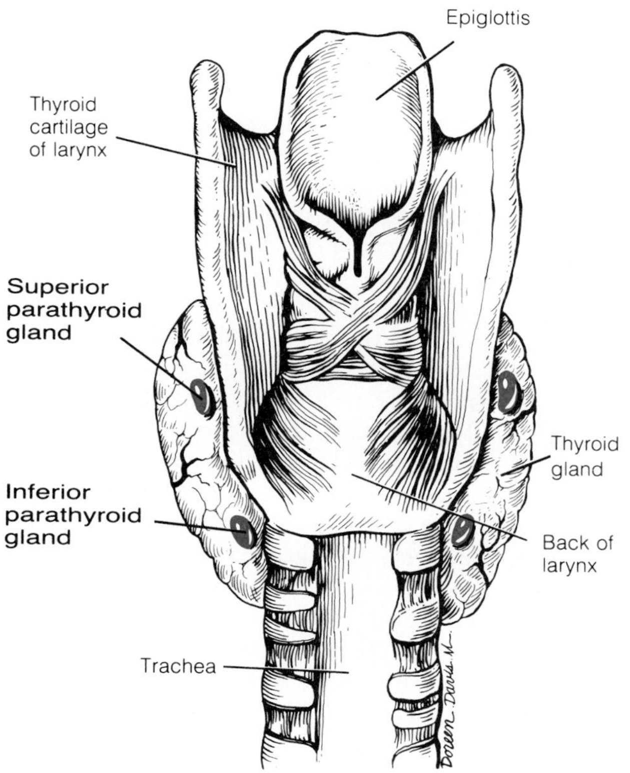

Figure 33–2

Thyroid and parathyroid glands. (Note that this is a posterior view of the thyroid gland.) SOURCE: Spence AP, Mason EB: Human Anatomy and Physiology, *3rd ed. Menlo Park, CA: Benjamin/Cummings, 1987.*

Surgical complications include hemorrhage from the superior thyroid arteries; damage to the parathyroid glands because of their proximity to the thyroid; damage to the trachea during surgery, resulting in the aspiration of blood or the postoperative formation of a tracheocutaneous fistula; perforation of the esophagus; and damage to one or both of the recurrent laryngeal nerves, resulting in hoarseness or total aphonia. Note the relative positions of these structures in Figures 33–2 and 33–3.

The physiologic and psychosocial/lifestyle implications of thyroidectomy are discussed in Table 33–3.

Nursing Implications

PREOPERATIVE CARE Preoperative preparation of the thyroidectomy client depends to a degree on the clinical indications for the surgery. For example, the emotional care for the client who is to undergo thyroidectomy for an undiagnosed mass in the neck must include the possibility of carcinoma. Clients having a thyroidectomy for Graves' disease require a different approach because of their emotional lability secondary to the oversecretion of thyroxine.

The major goal of preoperative care is to help establish as near a euthyroid state as possible. This may require a treatment period lasting between several weeks and 2 to 3 months before surgery. During this time, the client is given antithyroid drugs in an attempt to slow the activity of the thyroid. Ten days before surgery, either in the hos-

Table 33–3
Thyroidectomy: Implications for the Client

Physiologic Implications	Psychosocial/Lifestyle Implications
Immediate postoperative risk for hemorrhage; respiratory complications; tetany from hypocalcemia caused by inadvertent removal of, or injury to, the parathyroid glands; injury to the recurrent laryngeal nerve; and (rarely) thyroid crisis or storm (may develop rapidly in the first 24 hours) Lifelong thyroxine therapy after total thyroidectomy and possibly after subtotal thyroidectomy	Self-management of medication regimen Need to watch for the symptoms and signs of thyroxine overdose (hyperthyroidism), and thyroxine underdose (hypothyroidism), and to seek out health care provider if they occur Visible thyroidectomy scar on the neck for several months until complete healing takes place; in some clients, a disfiguring scar requiring clothing modification and causing alteration in body image

pital or at home, the client is given Lugol's solution to reduce the size and vascularity of the thyroid gland.

Evaluate the client for symptoms and signs of thyroid toxicity and report these immediately to the physician. Assessment parameters include vital signs, body weight, cardiac and respiratory status, bowel elimination pattern, and emotional status.

Specific nursing care during this period is the same as that for the client with hyperthyroidism. Additional preoperative care includes an ECG to establish the client's cardiac status and careful skin preparation before surgery. The client's blood is typed and cross-matched for 2 units of blood before surgery.

Preoperative teaching should include the nature and indication for the procedure and the expected outcome, including the need for lifelong medication and supervision. Tell the client what to expect in the immediate postoperative period (ie, vital signs will be checked frequently, there will be a dressing on the neck, the neck must be kept relaxed and in good alignment avoiding flexion and hyperextension, head movements should be minimized, the throat may be sore for a few days, and medication will be available for discomfort). Give the client an opportunity to express and discuss any fears and anxieties regarding the surgery and its physiologic and cosmetic results.

POSTOPERATIVE CARE Assemble the following equipment at the bedside for use as needed in the postoperative period:

- Emergency tracheotomy tray
- Oxygen equipment
- Suction machine and cannulas

In addition, a humidifier, IV equipment, and ampules of calcium chloride or calcium gluconate should be available. Tubes for the collection of specimens for serum calcium levels should be readily accessible.

Following thyroidectomy, closely observe the client for the first 48 postoperative hours because adverse symptoms may develop quickly and can pose a threat to life. The major complications that may occur in the postoperative period are discussed in the section that follows.

Important observations in the postoperative period include vital signs, which are initially checked every 15 minutes until stabilized. Respiration is carefully monitored with special attention to cyanosis or signs of respiratory distress. Check the client's temperature rectally for the first day or two. Immediately report all fluctuations in vital signs to the physician. In addition, evaluate the client's LOC, including restlessness, apprehension, or anxiety.

Maintain the client in a semi-Fowler's position immediately after surgery to encourage venous drainage from the neck. The head and neck should be in good alignment and may be supported by a small pillow. Flexion and hyperextension of the neck are contraindicated, and the client should keep head movements to a minimum. Place sandbags or small pillows at the sides of the head to aid immobilization. Muscle tension and spasm often develop in the cervical area as a consequence of this immobilization and can be relieved by massage. As clients progress, teach them to assist in the movement of the head and neck by supporting the head at the sides and in the occipital area. After the skin clips or skin sutures have been removed, the surgeon may order gradual active and passive exercises of the neck.

Once the vital signs have stabilized, the client is allowed out of bed, usually on the first postoperative day. During ambulation, remind the client to hold the head in good alignment and to walk erect (the tendency is to flex the neck to minimize tension on the suture line).

Encourage coughing and deep breathing. Coughing may be painful for clients; support and encourage them during this activity. Discourage excessive coughing, however, because it increases throat discomfort and places tension on the suture line. In the early postoperative period, suction may be used to assist the client in clearing the upper airways of excessive mucus secretions. Persistent throat soreness should be reported to the physician, and a room humidifier or medication may be ordered.

Intravenous fluids are usually given until the client can tolerate oral liquids. Liquids are started after nausea subsides and continued until the client can tolerate a soft diet (usually in 2 to 3 days when there is less pain with swallowing). An adequate oral fluid intake will obviate the need for further IV therapy, provide hydration for the client, and maintain renal function.

Usually no medications other than analgesics are ordered in the postoperative period. Meperidine hydrochloride (Demerol) or morphine is given in the first 48 hours to relieve discomfort and apprehension. Postthyroidectomy clients often experience a sense of compression in the neck until the edema subsides. This can be frightening and may make them apprehensive and restless. Careful evaluation of the client before the administration of an analgesic is important to determine the cause of the discomfort.

POSTOPERATIVE COMPLICATIONS

HEMORRHAGE Signs that should alert the nurse to the possibility of hemorrhage include a drop in blood pressure accompanied by a rapid, thready pulse. The nurse may notice either excessive blood on the dressing or behind the neck as well as swelling of the tissues around the dressing. If bleeding is suspected, peel back the outer layers of the dressing carefully and observe the amount of oozing. For clients in the dorsal recumbent position, remember that evidence of bleeding should be assessed laterally and posteriorly to the neck as well as anteriorly. The client may have increased "tightness" of the dressing and difficulty breathing. Wound hemorrhage in a client following thyroidectomy can cause respiratory obstruction by compressing the tissues. Therefore, closely observe the client for cyanosis and asphyxia, which may develop quickly.

If hemorrhage is suspected, the surgeon should be notified immediately and the client placed in the semi-Fowler's position. The dressing may be loosened to promote drainage. An emergency tracheotomy tray, sterile dressings, and oxygen equipment should be brought to the bedside. If the surgeon is not available immediately, the nurse may be instructed to remove the neck skin sutures or clips and separate the skin edges with a Kelly clamp to allow drainage of the accumulated blood. Cover this with a thick sterile dressing until the surgeon arrives.

RESPIRATORY DISTRESS Respiratory distress in the client following thyroidectomy can be caused by hemorrhage, edema of the glottis, or pressure on the trachea from edema. The nurse may note respiratory stridor, "crowing respirations," signs of dyspnea and cyanosis, and the use of the accessory muscles of respiration. The client should be placed in a high Fowler's position and given humidified oxygen by mask. Notify the physician immediately, even for early signs of respiratory distress. Swift nursing interventions are needed to prevent anoxia and cardiac arrest. A tracheotomy tray and endotracheal setup should be at the bedside to use if severe obstruction occurs.

INJURY TO THE RECURRENT LARYNGEAL NERVE Recurrent laryngeal nerve injury and the resultant loss of voice are usually caused by resection of one or both of the nerves, edema, or trauma. Check the client's voice immediately after surgery by asking the client to repeat a few words; excessive talking is not required. Hoarseness or aphonia immediately after surgery is most likely caused by surgical injury to the recurrent laryngeal nerve. If the quality of the client's voice is good in the immediate postoperative period but then becomes hoarse, it is usually a temporary condition caused by edema or pressure from hemorrhage. Hoarseness should not persist more than 3 days. Also be aware of the possibility of paralysis of the vocal cords, which can result in closing of the glottis and respiratory obstruction. Nursing interventions include careful observation and early reporting of symptoms and signs.

HYPOCALCEMIC TETANY Hypocalcemic tetany can be caused by (1) accidental removal of the parathyroid glands during thyroidectomy, (2) injury to the parathyroid glands, or (3) edema of the parathyroid glands. The tetany can occur within the first 24 to 48 hours after surgery as well as up to 6 or 7 days later. The client will have increasing nervousness, tingling in the hands and circumoral areas, painful muscle spasms, and facial spasms and grimaces. Palpitations may also occur.

The nurse may be able to elicit positive Chvostek's and Trousseau's signs. If either of these signs is elicited, the physician should be informed immediately and plasma calcium and phosphorus levels determined. Treatment is often initiated on the basis of these signs even before the laboratory results have been obtained. Keep a tourniquet, a 10-mL syringe, and a 10% solution of calcium gluconate at the bedside.

THYROID STORM OR CRISIS Thyroid storm or crisis is a potentially fatal complication of thyroid surgery rarely seen today because of extensive preoperative preparation of the client and ligation of the blood vessels before the thyroid tissue is handled during surgery. In the surgical client, thyroid storm is caused by a sudden surge of thyroid hormone into the circulation, usually because of excessive manipulation of a toxic gland during the surgical process. The nurse who observes any signs of thyroid storm should contact the physician immediately because this is an emergency requiring prompt medical intervention. Assemble emergency equipment at the bedside while awaiting the physician's arrival.

DISCHARGE PLANNING Because clients are returning home much sooner after surgery than they did in the past, the nurse has a more limited time for client instruction. Some thyroidectomy clients may be discharged on their third or fourth postoperative day. It is helpful if discharge instructions are written as well as verbal so the client and significant others have something to refer to at home.

Discharge instructions for the client include the importance of returning to the physician for further evaluation and follow-up care. This involves evaluation for any recurrent hyperthyroidism or hypothyroidism, as well as for any signs of hypoparathyroidism. Clients should know the symptoms and signs of hyperthyroidism, hypothyroidism, and hypoparathyroidism. They should understand the importance of calling their health care provider if any of these symptoms or signs occurs.

The client should understand the medication regimen, its purposes, and its side effects. Explain any restrictions on activity and diet.

Neck exercises are usually prescribed, and the client should be able to redemonstrate the exercises to the nurse to ensure that they are being performed correctly. Also, the client may be instructed to use a moisturizing cream or emollient on the suture line to prevent contraction of the scar and improve the cosmetic effect.

Hypothyroidism

Hypothyroidism is characterized by a decreased secretion of thyroid hormone. Hypothyroidism may range from a mild state, which is often difficult to diagnose, to myxedema coma. Deficiency of thyroid hormone, which produces the symptoms and signs of hypometabolism, affects almost every system of the body and may be seen in persons of all ages. The major forms of hypothyroidism are cretinism, juvenile hypothyroidism, and myxedema. Cretinism and juvenile hypothyroidism are covered in pediatric texts.

Myxedema, or adult hypothyroidism, is a fairly common disorder that is five times more frequent in women than in men; clients are usually in the 30- to 60-year age range. Symptoms may appear so slowly and insidiously that clients are often unaware of the changes. In severe cases of untreated hypothyroidism, myxedema coma may develop. Myxedema coma is characterized by an intense exaggeration of the symptoms and signs of hypothyroidism, with neurologic impairment leading to loss of consciousness. Myxedema coma occurs in clients of all ages and usually is the result of a precipitating event such as a respiratory tract or other infection; the use of drugs, especially narcotics, tranquilizers, or barbiturates; myocardial infarction or cerebrovascular accident; gastrointestinal bleeding; or exposure to cold. The mortality in myxedema coma has been estimated at 60% to 70%, so prompt recognition of symptoms and early treatment are essential.

Box 33–1
Goitrogens (Foods or Drugs Capable of Causing Goiter)

Dietary goitrogens

- Cabbage
- Rutabaga
- Turnip
- Mustard plant
- Soybeans
- Kale

Drug goitrogens

- Propylthiouracil
- Methimazole
- Perchlorate
- Thiocyanate
- Iodides in pharmacologic doses
- Lithium salts
- Resorcinol ointments
- Aminoglutethimide

The causes of myxedema may be primary (pathology within the thyroid gland itself) or secondary (pituitary insufficiency). Primary thyroid dysfunction is much more common than secondary thyroid dysfunction.

More than 50% of all cases of hypothyroidism are idiopathic. Primary hypothyroidism may also be iatrogenic (ie, may result from thyroidectomy, treatment of the thyroid by ^{131}I or antithyroid drugs such as propylthiouracil or methimazole) or it may be caused by ingestion of goitrogens (Box 33–1) or by chronic thyroiditis. Autoimmunity has been proposed as a cause of primary hypothyroidism, because autoimmune antibodies have been found in the serum of 70% of clients with the disease (Muthe, 1981). Hashimoto's thyroiditis, another cause of hypothyroidism, is also thought to be an autoimmune disorder.

Secondary hypothyroidism usually follows destruction of the pituitary gland by a tumor (chromophobe adenoma) or by postpartum necrosis (Sheehan's syndrome). These conditions cause a decrease in the secretion of TSH by the anterior pituitary gland, resulting in atrophy of thyroid tissue and deficiencies in circulating T_4 and T_3. Because thyroid hormone is necessary for the function of all the endocrine glands, deficiencies in its secretion may result in a secondary hypofunction of the pituitary, adrenal, and other glands.

Clinical Manifestations

The clinical manifestations of hypothyroidism relate directly to the degree of hormonal deficiency and range from mild, often nonspecific symptoms (eg, fatigue, weight gain, or menstrual irregularities) to full-blown myxedema. Symptoms may appear slowly and be characterized by a gradual slowing of both mental and physical processes. Table 33–4 lists the most common subjective and objective findings in hypothyroidism.

In the elderly, symptoms of hypothyroidism are easy to overlook because of the gradual slowing of metabolism that accompanies the aging process. The nurse must be alert for subtle symptoms and signs while assessing older clients.

The onset of myxedema coma, which may be gradual,

Table 33–4
Common Findings in Hypothyroidism

Subjective Findings	Objective Findings
Clients often note:	*Examiners often observe:*
Fatigue, lethargy, generalized weakness	Drooping of the eyelid
Intolerance to cold	Thickened facial tissues
Constipation	Dull facial expression
Anorexia, indigestion, flatulence	Lateral third of the eyebrow thinned or absent
Weight gain (10 to 20 lb)	Enlarged tongue
Deepening or hoarseness of the voice	Slow speech
Dyspnea, chest pain	Decreased hearing
Enlargement of the neck	Abdominal distention
Scalp, axillary, and pubic hair loss	Thyromegaly
Dry, coarse skin; brittle nails	Bradycardia
Numbness and tingling of the hands and feet	Decreased body temperature
Changes in memory and mental ability	Cool, coarse, dry skin
Decreased libido and impotence (men)	Nonpitting edema of the lower extremities
Menorrhagia (women)	Delay in relaxation phase of DTRs (pseudomyotonia)
	On x-ray examination, cardiomegaly, pleural and pericardial effusions

is signaled by a pronounced increase in both the number and magnitude of the findings listed in Table 33–4; there is almost always neurologic involvement as well. Prominent clinical manifestations of myxedema coma include:

- Hypothermia, which can be as severe as 74°F (23.3°C) and is a poor prognostic sign; a normal temperature suggests infection
- Hypotension (50% of clients)
- Intestinal ileus or fecal impaction
- Urinary retention
- Seizures (25% of clients)
- Congestive heart failure or pericardial effusion
- Respiratory failure characterized by hypoxia, retention of carbon dioxide, and respiratory acidosis
- A bilateral positive Babinski's sign

Besides myxedema coma, the major complications of hypothyroidism include cardiac involvement, which is a result of advanced coronary artery disease and congestive heart failure; an increased susceptibility to infection; and organic psychoses with paranoid delusions (the so-called myxedema madness). Infertility is another possible complication of hypothyroidism; it usually responds well to treatment.

The diagnosis of hypothyroidism is made from a careful history including family history of goiter or hypothyroidism, drug use, and previous thyroid surgery or treatment with ^{131}I. Laboratory findings consistent with hypothyroidism include serum T_4 levels under 3.5 μg/dL and low or low-normal T_3 resin uptake.

When the diagnosis of hypothyroidism has been established, radioimmunoassay of TSH levels will help to distinguish between a primary or secondary cause. Plasma TSH levels are elevated in primary hypothyroidism and depressed in secondary hypothyroidism.

Medical Measures

The main approach to the treatment of hypothyroidism is the correction of the underlying cause. Treatment might involve discontinuation of drugs blocking thyroid synthesis, dietary correction, or administration of thyroid hormones to correct the hormonal deficiency. Thyroid hormone replacement drugs are listed in Box 33–2. Clients receive an initial dose of the drug, which is then adjusted to achieve the optimal effect. The client's hormonal levels are then stabilized by a maintenance dose.

Box 33–2
Thyroid Hormone Replacement Drugs

Levothyroxine (Synthroid)
Liothyronine (Cytomel)
Liotrix (Euthroid, Thyrolar)
Thyroglobulin (Proloid)
Thyroid USP (desiccated thyroid)

Myxedema coma is a medical emergency. The immediate steps in treating it are:

- Administration of thyroid hormones
- Administration of glucocorticoids to cover any adrenal insufficiency
- Correction of hypothermia
- Maintenance of ventilation
- Fluid restriction (to less than 1 L/day) if client shows signs of hyponatremia
- Administration of 50% glucose if client shows signs of hypoglycemia
- Treatment of any precipitating causes (eg, infection, myocardial infarction, or gastrointestinal bleeding)

The prognosis for hypothyroidism is good; many clients can be treated easily and effectively with replacement therapy. Restoration of the euthyroid state is possible, but relapse may occur if treatment is stopped. Depending on the type of medication used, the effects of the therapy may not be seen for up to 2 weeks, with complete resolution of symptoms taking several months and more. Share this information with the client and family to avoid discouragement.

Specific Nursing Measures

The nursing care of the client with hypothyroidism can be rewarding because of the satisfaction from seeing successful response to treatment. Remember, however, that the euthyroid state is achieved gradually.

Nursing care includes assessment of the client's response to replacement therapy. Positive results are indicated by a decrease in lethargy and fatigue, decrease in edema, weight loss, improvement in mentation and speech, increased tolerance to cold, improvement in appetite, resolution of constipation, and normalization of the menstrual cycle. Improvements in the hair, skin, and nails are more gradual. Anemia may not be corrected for 2 to 3 months. Monitor elderly clients and those with cardiac problems for increased shortness of breath, dyspnea on exertion (DOE), cough, chest pain, or angina. Cardiac status is monitored by checking vital signs regularly and reporting any symptoms and signs of congestive heart failure, chest pain, increase in angina, or pulse rate over 100. If these occur, discontinue thyroid replacement until the physician is notified.

The client should be kept warm and should be weighed daily to assess fluid loss as an indicator of improvement. Deep breathing and ambulation will improve hypoxia. Lotions and creams will help skin dryness.

Closely monitor the client's drug regimen because the hypometabolic state potentiates many drugs, such as digitalis and insulin, requiring a lower dosage. Dosage requirements will change as the client attains the euthyroid state.

Encourage a diet low in calories and high in protein and fiber. Small, frequent portions may be helpful with the anorexic client. Encourage increased fluids if there is no sign of cardiac involvement. Assess the client for constipation and fecal impaction. Stool softeners may be needed. Clients with hypothyroidism have a decreased response to infection. They must be carefully protected, because infection may precipitate myxedema coma.

Client/Family Teaching

Client and family education should stress not only the favorable prognosis for hypothyroidism with treatment but also the need for clients to remain on medication for the rest of their lives. In teaching clients with hypothyroidism, be aware that their slowed mentation and memory may interfere with their ability to learn and retain new information. Therefore, including a family member or significant other in the teaching sessions is helpful for review of the material with clients after the teaching session. Printed information is useful for this purpose.

Important teaching areas to cover include:

- The symptoms and signs of both hyperthyroidism and hypothyroidism—what to observe and when to call the physician
- The pathophysiology of hypothyroidism, including the role of thyroid hormone in the body
- The need for lifelong medication and medical follow-up
- Any dietary prescriptions
- The drug regimen, including the name and dosage of medications, their expected action and outcomes, and possible side effects

Hypothyroidism can be especially distressing to a family or significant others because of the changes they see in their loved one (weakness, lethargy, and slowing and dulling of mental abilities). An important nursing role is the psychologic support of client and family through the initial diagnosis and treatment period, including reassuring them that most of these observable symptoms and signs will improve and be resolved as treatment progresses.

Another important nursing role in hypothyroidism centers on its prevention, particularly regarding ingestion of goitrogens (see Box 33–1).

Goiter

An enlargement of the thyroid gland is called a *goiter.* A goiter associated with either hypofunction or hyperfunction of the gland is a toxic goiter, whereas nontoxic goiters are associated with euthyroidism. Goiters are classified into three major categories:

- Diffuse goiters (simple goiter)
- Multinodular goiters
- Uninodular goiters

In toxic nodular goiter, the affected thyroid gland usually has one or more nodules that hyperfunction autonomously without the normal feedback control, resulting in clinical symptoms and signs of hyperthyroidism. Hyperfunction of such nodules suppresses TSH levels and consequently suppresses function of the unaffected thyroid tissue. Hyperfunctioning thyroid nodules, also called "hot nodules," concentrate ^{131}I and thus produce a patchy scintiscan.

A nodule must be at least 0.75 to 1 cm to be palpable. Toxic multinodular goiter occurs more frequently in clients between the ages of 50 and 70 , and it is four times more frequent in females than in males.

The causes of nontoxic simple goiter may include iodine deficiency, goitrogens, tissue resistance to thyroid hormone, thyroiditis, or biosynthetic or enzymatic defects. Clients in certain geographic areas, usually away from the seacoast, lack iodine. Insufficiency of iodine in the diet or intrathyroid biosynthetic defects result in a decreased secretion of thyroid hormone. This hypoproduction of hormone results in an increase in TSH secretion by the anterior pituitary gland and a compensatory increase in the size of the thyroid gland. This often returns the thyroid hormone levels to normal but does not resolve the underlying problem. Although iodine deficiency is still common in certain undeveloped areas of the world, it is far less common today in North America because of the prevalence of iodized salt and the use of iodine compounds to preserve foods.

Today, the most common cause of nontoxic goiter is minor intrathyroidal biosynthetic defects (Kaye & Rose, 1983), which appear to occur sporadically and may be acquired or familial. The exact cause of these minor intrathyroidal defects is unknown. Genetic factors are thought to play a role, because 30% to 49% of these clients' relatives show similar goiters or clinical evidence of thyroid disease. Simple goiter may also occur transiently when there is a greater need for thyroid hormone (eg, at the onset of puberty and during pregnancy and lactation). Goitrogens in water, food, and drugs have also contributed to the formation of goiters. Nontoxic diffuse goiters have also been seen in rare cases of tissue resistance to thyroid hormones. Thyroiditis, which is discussed fully in the next section, also causes goiter.

The most common cause of nontoxic multinodular goiter is the long-term changes in the thyroid gland of clients with nontoxic diffuse goiters. These are thought to be degenerative changes that occur in the gland over time. The causes of nontoxic uninodular goiter include thyroiditis, cysts, hemorrhage, and benign or malignant neoplasms.

Clinical Manifestations

The major clinical manifestation of goiter is a visibly enlarged, palpable gland. The enlargement may be diffuse or nodular. The client may be completely asymptomatic or may complain of dysphagia, wheezing, or respiratory distress resulting from compression of structures in the neck or upper chest. A prominent bulge in the neck presents cosmetic problems for many clients.

The diagnosis of simple goiter is made after taking a careful history (investigating place of residence; ingestion of goitrogens; familial history of goiter, thyroid disease, or both; and high-stress states), a physical examination, and laboratory testing. Generally, serum T_4 and T_3 levels and RAIU levels are within normal ranges.

If nodules are present, percutaneous needle or open biopsy may be needed to rule out a malignancy. Ultrasonography can differentiate among solid, cystic, and mixed solid and cystic nodules of the thyroid.

Simple goiters either resolve spontaneously or increase to a point where the client has symptoms of compression. In persons over age 50, long-standing multinodular goiters are likely to become toxic. The incidence of malignancy in these clients has not been established. Simple goiter can be prevented with a dietary intake of 100 to 200 ng of iodine daily. The dosage may be increased to the upper limits during puberty, pregnancy, lactation, or periods of stress. This amount is included in a gram or two of iodized salt. In some geographic areas, iodinated oil has been used as a prophylactic measure for goiter.

Medical Measures

The most common approach to the treatment of goiter is to suppress the further enlargement of the thyroid gland and to reduce it to normal size. Depending on the cause of the goiter, this may be accomplished by nutritional measures; by medical measures; or, in some cases, by surgery.

Levothyroxine (0.2 mg per day) is used to suppress TSH and thyroid hormone production. It should reduce the goiter to normal size in 2 to 6 months. Iodine therapy (Lugol's solution or saturated solution of potassium iodide [SSKI]) is indicated only when iodine deficiency has been established; iodine prophylaxis in other instances may induce hypothyroidism. Medications that promote the formation of goiters (eg, propylthiouracil, methimazole, tolbutamide, and iodine preparations) should be avoided.

Surgery is indicated only to assist in establishing the diagnosis and to rule out potential malignancies. A subtotal thyroidectomy may also be done to reduce the mass of a very large gland in a symptomatic client. Surgery may be followed by medical suppression, because hyperplasia and regrowth of thyroid tissue can occur.

Specific Nursing Measures

Nursing intervention in the care of the client with goiter should focus on client assessment, maintaining client comfort, and client and family education. Client assessment includes reporting and recording symptoms of compression: dysphagia and respiratory distress (increased shortness of breath and wheezing). For clients on thyroid suppression therapy, monitor for symptoms and signs of hyperthyroidism (increased anxiety, tachycardia, palpitations, and diarrhea). These findings should be immediately reported to the physician. Also carefully monitor the client's response to treatment by assessing changes in the size and consistency of the thyroid gland and carefully watching for nodules.

Client/Family Teaching

The client with a large goiter can experience significant alterations in comfort. Assist by positioning the client with the head of the bed elevated; by advising the client to avoid tight, restrictive neckwear; and by making sure the consistency of the client's food facilitates swallowing. For a client with significant **dysphagia,** mealtime should not be rushed. Frequent, small feedings may be helpful. Client and family education should include the nature of the disorder, the relationship of the presenting symptoms and signs to the underlying pathophysiology, the treatment plan, and any specific dietary or lifestyle adjustments necessary. The client and family should be fully familiar not only with the therapeutic regimen but also the overall goals of the treatment plan. Clients should be warned to avoid dietary goitrogens of the sorts listed in Box 33–1.

The nurse's role in the prevention of goiter centers on teaching the necessity of including iodine in the diet. Such teaching is of special importance in geographic areas where goiter is endemic. The early recognition and prompt referral of clients with goiter or thyroid nodules is also an important nursing function. Generally, the smaller a goiter is, the more amenable it is to treatment. Because of the possibility of thyroid carcinoma, the earlier a thyroid nodule is evaluated, the better the prognosis if it is malignant.

Box 33–3
Causes of Hypercalcemia

- Increased gastrointestinal calcium absorption:
  - Vitamin D intoxication
  - Sarcoidosis
  - Tuberculosis
- Increased calcium resorption from bone:
  - Primary hyperparathyroidism
  - Malignancy with bone metastases
  - Malignancy without bone metastases
    - Ectopic parathyroid hormone (PTH) secretion
    - Prostaglandin E production
    - Synthesis of a vitamin D-like substance
  - Multiple myeloma, leukemia, and lymphomas
  - Chronic immobilization
  - Hyperthyroidism
  - Vitamin A intoxication
- Increased renal tubular calcium reabsorption:
  - Therapy with thiazide diuretics
- Unclear mechanism:
  - Milk-alkali syndrome
  - Adrenal insufficiency
  - Renal disease
    - Chronic hemodialysis
    - Renal transplantation
    - Polyuric phase of acute renal failure

SOURCE: Reprinted with permission from Jubiz W: *Endocrinology: A Logical Approach for Clinicians.* New York: McGraw–Hill, 1979, p. 201.

Hyperparathyroidism

Hyperparathyroidism is characterized by a hypersecretion of parathyroid hormone, which brings about an increase in circulating plasma levels of calcium and a decrease in circulating plasma levels of phosphorus. Although one of the major clinical manifestations of hyperparathyroidism is hypercalcemia, it is important to remember that hypercalcemia has several different causes (Box 33–3). Hyperparathyroidism affects women twice as often as men and is more common in persons over age 40. It rarely occurs in childhood.

Hyperparathyroidism can be classified as primary or secondary according to its cause. Primary hyperparathyroidism originates within the gland itself and in about 90% of clients is caused by a single benign adenoma of one gland. Secondary hyperparathyroidism is almost always associated with hyperplasia of all four parathyroid glands and is a compensatory mechanism to combat the hypocalcemia arising from chronic renal disease, rickets, osteomalacia, and acromegaly.

Clinical Manifestations

The clinical symptoms and signs of hyperparathyroidism are related to involvement of the skeletal system, renal system, and hypercalcemia. Certain clients may also have asymptomatic hypercalcemia.

Skeletal symptoms and signs include bone and joint pain; pathologic fractures of the spine, long bones, and ribs, which may lead to progressive kyphosis; bone cysts; giant-cell tumors of the jaw; hypermotility of the joints; and systemic decalcification of the skeletal system. Urinary tract manifestations include polydipsia and polyuria, "sand" or "gravel" in the urine, renal calculi, decreased urine concentration, and secondary renal infection and obstruction that may lead to progressive renal failure and uremia.

Symptoms of hypercalcemia include anorexia, nausea, vomiting, abdominal pain, and polydipsia. In addition, the client may have constipation, anemia, weight loss, and asthenia.

Other clinical manifestations of hyperparathyroidism include hypertension, hypotonia, paresthesia, easy fatigability, and depression of the reflexes. Clients may initially have peptic ulcers and pancreatitis (sometimes recurrent). Changes in the psyche include changes in mentation and personality, depression, apathy, mood swings, and even confusion and coma. Changes in the toenails and fingernails include increased thickening and ridging. Calcium deposits may be observed in the cornea (**band keratopathy**) and, in secondary hyperparathyroidism, in the soft tissues around the joints.

According to Muthe (1981), when renal calculi are the main pathologic condition, bone changes tend not to occur. Conversely, when bone changes are the major symptom, renal calculi tend not to occur. One of the primary concerns in hyperparathyroidism is progressive renal damage from calcium deposits. This may result in hypertension and lead to death from uremia or congestive heart failure. Early detection and intervention are important, because renal lesions tend to progress, whereas bone lesions heal completely.

Hyperparathyroid crisis, although rare, may occur after a parathyroidectomy. The crisis is probably precipitated by the release of excessive amounts of PTH into the circulation during surgery. The symptoms and signs are those of acute hypercalcemia and include anorexia, nausea, vomiting, abdominal pain, weakness, polydipsia, dyspnea, and coma. Hyperparathyroid crisis is potentially life threatening and therefore should be reported immediately to the physician. Prompt intervention and careful observations are needed to restore the balance of calcium and phosphorus in the body.

The most common diagnostic tests used in the evaluation of hyperparathyroidism include measurements of serum and urinary levels of calcium and phosphorus, radioimmunoassays of PTH, assessment of serum alkaline phosphatase, and x-ray examination. In primary hyperparathyroidism, the serum calcium level is usually elevated; serum phosphorus level is low or normal; and urinary levels of calcium and phosphorus are elevated.

Medical Measures

The only treatment indicated for overt primary hyperparathyroidism is parathyroidectomy. Pharmacologic measures may be used to treat hypercalcemia, and medical measures to treat the mild hyperparathyroidism usually found by routine screening procedures. Medical measures in hyperparathyroidism are summarized in Box 33–4.

The surgical treatment of choice is subtotal parathyroidectomy. Sufficient residual tissue is left to preserve function (three glands and a portion of the fourth are resected). The goal of surgery is to remove all affected parathyroid tissue. Surgical intervention is especially indicated in clients with renal and bone involvement, pancreatitis, peptic ulcer, or possible malignancy. Generally, the prognosis for clients with hyperparathyroidism is good if it is identified and treated surgically early in the course of the disease.

Box 33–4
Medical Measures for Treatment of Hyperparathyroidism

For mild hyperparathyroidism (relatively asymptomatic clients):
- Fluids are increased.
- Immobilization is avoided.
- Diuretics are given.
- If renal function is good, phosphorus is prescribed.
- If client is postmenopausal, estrogen is prescribed.

For hypercalcemic crisis (acute):
- IV fluids are increased to facilitate excretion of Ca.
- Phosphorus, calcitonin, mithramycin, sodium chloride, and/or prednisone may be prescribed.

For hypercalcemia (subacute):
- Force fluids—3000 to 4000 mL/day (unless contraindicated by cardiac status)—to combat dehydration arising from severe nausea and vomiting and to prevent renal calculi by diluting calcium concentration.
- Keep accurate I&O record.
- Limit dietary calcium intake, especially of dairy products.
- Maintain an acid urine to prevent renal calculi and incidence of urinary tract infections (alkaline urine enhances precipitation of Ca salts); provide foods high in acid ash (eg, cranberries, prunes, tomatoes, corn, asparagus, grapes, meat, poultry, fish, eggs, and cereals).
- Hypercalcemia may be treated by peritoneal dialysis or hemodialysis, especially in hypercalcemic clients with severe kidney damage.

Specific Nursing Measures

Nursing approaches to the care of the client with hyperparathyroidism should address the potential for renal calculi, ulcers, pancreatitis, constipation, bone fractures, hypertension, depression, confusion, and changes in cognition.

Institute strict and accurate intake and output for all clients with hyperparathyroidism. In the absence of cardiac or renal contraindications, the daily fluid intake should be increased to approximately 3000 to 4000 mL to help prevent the formation of renal calculi. Strain the urine for sediment, and carefully assess the client for symptoms of urinary-tract infections and hematuria, which may occur asymptomatically. The diet should be low in calcium, and dairy products should be limited. A diet high in acid ash is recommended to acidify the urine and prevent the precipitation of calcium salts. Foods high in acid ash include cranberries, prunes, tomatoes, corn, asparagus, grapes, meats, poultry, fish, eggs, and cereal.

Be alert to the symptoms and signs of pancreatitis (epigastric and right-upper-quadrant pain, increased flatulence, nausea, vomiting, prostration) and peptic ulcers (epigastric pain that occurs an hour or two after meals or that awakens the client in the night, hematemesis, and melena). Report and record them immediately. Encourage ambulation unless contraindicated. Fluids should be encouraged and fiber added to the diet. Stool softeners may also be needed.

Assist clients with skeletal involvement with ambulation because of the danger of pathologic fractures. Bear in mind that safety is a prime concern and institute the proper procedures (keep the bed in the low position at all times with siderails up and assist with ambulation).

Confusion, depression, paranoia and other mental problems may be seen in clients with hyperparathyroidism. Report any of these changes and support and reassure both client and significant others. Helpful interventions include organizing the environment to provide rest, a sense of security, and a minimum of disturbances as well as activities to promote interest and involvement.

Because the hypertension in hyperparathyroidism places an additional work load on the heart, carefully assess the client for any signs of cardiac damage or failure. Check vital signs periodically and report any abnormalities. Clients receiving digitalis should be carefully monitored because hypercalcemia has been known to increase the toxicity of digitalis (Muthe, 1981).

Parathyroidectomy

Parathyroidectomy is the surgical removal of all or a portion of the parathyroid glands. The major clinical indications for parathyroidectomy are adenoma of the parathyroid glands and primary hyperplasia of the glands, which produce hyperparathyroidism. About 1% of the adenomas of the parathyroid gland are malignant.

The procedure for parathyroidectomy is similar to that for thyroidectomy except that surgical removal of the parathyroid glands can be more difficult because of their minute size, variability in number, and variability in location (some parathyroid tissue may be found in the mediastinum). The goal of surgery is to remove the required amount of tissue while leaving enough to maintain sufficient PTH levels.

In clients with an adenoma, the gland with the adenoma is removed and sent for a frozen section. The other glands are then inspected and biopsied. Depending on the results of this assessment and the frozen section, the glands may be left in place, or a neck dissection may be performed.

Surgical hazards to these clients are similar to those for clients undergoing thyroidectomy, as discussed in the preceding section. In particular, the client is at risk for either temporary or permanent hypoparathyroidism if the glands have been traumatized or resected.

Physiologic and psychosocial/lifestyle implications of parathyroidectomy are discussed in Table 33–5.

Nursing Implications

PREOPERATIVE CARE The preoperative nursing care of the client with hyperparathyroidism is directed toward the management and stabilization of the symptoms and signs of hypercalcemia. These include weight loss, severe dehydration, nausea and vomiting, bone pain, polydipsia, and polyuria. The nursing care of the client with hyperparathyroidism is discussed above.

Preoperatively, IV phosphate may be ordered to block the absorption of calcium from the gastrointestinal tract. Calcitonin also can be used in some instances to lower the serum calcium levels.

The preoperative preparation of the client is the same as that described for thyroidectomy. Assemble the same equipment as that discussed for the client with thyroidectomy.

POSTOPERATIVE CARE The postoperative care of the client with a parathyroidectomy is essentially the same as the postoperative care of the client with a thyroidectomy. Of primary concern is the observation of the client for any symptoms and signs of tetany. Any of these symptoms and signs should be reported to the physician immediately.

Suction equipment, a tracheotomy set, an endotracheal tube, and oxygen equipment should be available at the bedside.

Be alert for respiratory distress, hemorrhage, and damage to the recurrent laryngeal nerve. Any evidence of these complications also should be reported immediately to the physician.

DISCHARGE PLANNING Discharge planning for the client following a parathyroidectomy is similar to that discussed for clients who have had a thyroidectomy, except the client will be evaluated for any evidence of recurrent hyperparathyroidism or the development of hypoparathy-

Table 33–5
Parathyroidectomy: Implications for the Client 

Physiologic Implications	Psychosocial/Lifestyle Implications
Possible temporary or permanent hypoparathyroidism	Possible need for lifelong medical supervision
Immediate postoperative risk of hypocalcemia and tetany, hemorrhage, respiratory distress, recurrent laryngeal nerve injury, and hyperparathyroid crisis	Possible postoperative medication for months (especially if bone disease is present)
Impeded recovery because of preexisting damage to the central nervous system, heart, skeleton, or kidney from hyperparathyroidism	Self-management of medication regimen
	Dietary restrictions may influence family meal planning

roidism. The client needs to be aware of the symptoms and signs of these two clinical situations.

Hypoparathyroidism

Hypoparathyroidism results from a deficiency in the secretion of PTH hormone or a decrease in the effectiveness of its action. It is characterized by the presence of low serum calcium levels, high serum phosphorus levels, normal levels of alkaline phosphatase, and negative urinary calcium. The most prominent feature of hypoparathyroidism is hypocalcemia. In its most severe form, it is called hypocalcemic tetany. This deficiency of calcium has the potential to affect the function of many bodily systems including the neuromuscular, cardiovascular, integumentary, and gastrointestinal systems. In addition, hypocalcemia may cause changes in the basal ganglia, cerebellum, and eyes (Muthe, 1981).

Remember there are other causes of hypocalcemia that do not involve PTH deficiencies. These include severe renal insufficiency, dietary inadequacies or malabsorption syndromes, insufficiency of vitamin D, and chronic diarrhea. Also remember the relation between vitamin D and calcium; adequate vitamin D is necessary for the proper absorption and utilization of calcium by the body.

Hypoparathyroidism may have iatrogenic or idiopathic causes. The iatrogenic causes of hypoparathyroidism include damage to the parathyroid glands from thyroid surgery; surgery for tumor of the parathyroid, or accidental removal of healthy parathyroid tissue. Idiopathic hypoparathyroidism is thought to arise from either genetic predisposition or an autoimmune failure.

Clinical Manifestations

Symptoms of hypoparathyroidism can appear suddenly or slowly. Hypoparathyroidism can be precipitated by infection, pregnancy, menses, surgery, or other physiologic stresses to the body. Symptoms of acute hypoparathyroidism include muscle cramping, increased irritability, dyspnea, photophobia, diplopia, dysuria, abdominal cramping, nausea, vomiting, and diarrhea or constipation. Symptoms and signs of chronic hypoparathyroidism appear gradually and are often vague. They include increased lethargy, personality changes (depression, agitation, psychosis, delirium), changes in mentation, anxiety, and blurring of vision.

Signs of hypoparathyroidism include convulsions, **carpopedal spasm,** wheezing, respiratory stridor, positive **Chvostek's sign** (twitching of the facial muscles when facial nerve is percussed), positive **Trousseau's sign** (carpopedal spasm with inability to open the hand when a blood pressure cuff is placed on the arm, elevated over the systolic reading, and left in place for 2 to 3 minutes), cataracts, thinness and brittleness of the nails, dryness and scaliness of the skin, increased incidence of candidiasis, loss of eyebrows and patchy alopecia of the scalp, and hyperactivity of the deep-tendon reflexes (secondary to increased neuromuscular excitability).

The major clinical manifestations of acute hypocalcemic tetany include increasing anxiety, tingling in the hands and circumoral area, painful muscle spasms, facial spasms and grimaces, palpitations, and sometimes convulsions. A positive Chvostek's and Trousseau's sign may be present. Acute tetany may be associated with vocal cord paralysis and may lead to respiratory obstruction. In this instance, the presence of stridor should alert the nurse to the need for possible emergency intervention (tracheostomy). Severe hypocalcemia may also precipitate heart failure. A positive Chvostek's sign may be seen in 10% of the normal population. Also, a positive Chvostek's and Trousseau's sign may be elicited in conditions other than hypocalcemia (eg, alkalotic states associated with primary aldosteronism and hyperventilation).

The diagnosis of hypoparathyroidism is based primarily on laboratory tests, supportive x-ray findings (increased density of the long bones), early formation of cataracts, and prolongation of the Q–T interval and a generalized dysrhythmia on the ECG that disappears with treatment if the etiology is hypocalcemia. Specific laboratory findings suggestive of hypoparathyroidism include low serum calcium levels, elevated serum phosphorus levels, normal serum levels of both alkaline phosphatase and magnesium, normal creatinine clearance, low or absent urinary calcium, and low or absent levels of serum PTH (by radioimmunoassay).

Medical Measures

The therapeutic approach to both acute and chronic hypoparathyroidism involves both medical and dietary measures. Although treatment of acute hypoparathyroidism is usually fairly straightforward with good results, long-term treatment is often tedious and expensive for the client and family. Because no effective preparation of PTH is available, periodic assays of serum levels of calcium and phosphorus are required to provide an indicator of possible overtreatment or undertreatment. Medical measures used in the treatment of chronic hypoparathyroidism are listed in Box 33–5.

Specific Nursing Measures

For the client with chronic hypoparathyroidism, important nursing responsibilities include client and family education regarding diet, goals of the medication regimen, and the need for frequent follow-up evaluation. In addition, because clients with chronic hypoparathyroidism often have symptoms involving both the integumentary and gastrointestinal systems, specific nursing measures should be directed toward these problems (eg, using lotions and

Box 33–5
Medical Measures in Chronic Hypoparathyroidism

After the acute phase, the goal of medical treatment is to maintain a normal serum calcium level by means of drugs and diet.

Pharmacologic agents:
- Oral calcium salts
- Dihydrotachysterol
- Calciferol

High-calcium, low-phosphorus diet:
- Increase in milk and milk products (caution: may be restricted because of phosphorus levels)
- Egg yolk (may also be restricted because of high phosphorus levels)
- Green, leafy vegetables (turnip and dandelion greens; spinach avoided because of its oxalate content)

emollients for dryness of the skin, increasing fiber and milk in the diet, and encouraging fluid intake to prevent constipation).

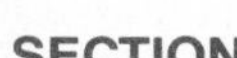
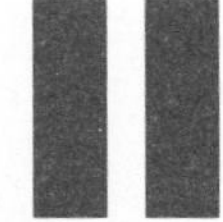

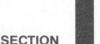

SECTION II

Infectious and Inflammatory Disorders

Thyroiditis

Thyroiditis is an inflammation of the thyroid gland. The three major forms of this disorder are acute suppurative thyroiditis, subacute thyroiditis (also known as de Quervain's thyroiditis), and lymphadenoid goiter (or Hashimoto's thyroiditis). Thyroiditis can be acute, subacute, or chronic. The most common form, Hashimoto's thyroiditis, will be covered here.

Hashimoto's thyroiditis is thought to arise from an autoimmune response of the body. The incidence of this particular form of thyroiditis has been increasing over the past few years. Kaye and Rose (1983) report that it now accounts for 90% of nontoxic diffuse goiters seen in children and 50% of those seen in adults. The incidence is greater in women between the ages of 20 and 50 than in men, and it tends to run in families. Interestingly, the family histories of these clients also show a high incidence of Graves' disease. Hashimoto's thyroiditis can also be seen in clients with other diagnosed autoimmune diseases, such as rheumatoid arthritis, systemic lupus erythematosus, and Sjögren's syndrome.

Clinical Manifestations

In Hashimoto's thyroiditis there is usually a small to medium-sized goiter, especially nontender, with a firm, rubbery consistency on palpation. This goiter enlarges slowly, becoming firmer and more nodular. The enlargement occurs insidiously. Occasionally, a larger goiter compresses the trachea and esophagus, producing localized lymphadenopathy and hoarseness from involvement of the vocal cords.

The diagnosis of Hashimoto's thyroiditis is based on a careful history and physical examination, particularly the finding of a firm, diffusely enlarged goiter. Laboratory studies show:

- Normal T_4 and T_3 levels.
- Increased or normal RAIU levels.
- High titers of thyroid antibodies. In 30% to 50% of clients with Hashimoto's thyroiditis, however, the antibody tests are negative or very low.

A needle biopsy will provide a histologic diagnosis.

Medical Measures

Medical measures for thyroiditis depend on the etiology. Approaches range from the use of antibiotics, to symptomatic support, to the use of thyroid hormone to reduce the size of the gland. Corticosteroids may be used in Hashimoto's thyroiditis to reduce the size of the gland. Permanent destruction of the thyroid cells may result in hypothyroidism in certain clients. Although the prognosis for clients with Hashimoto's thyroiditis is good, this condition has been associated with the later development of carcinoma and lymphoma of the thyroid.

Specific Nursing Measures

For the client with Hashimoto's thyroiditis, the nursing care depends on specific client problems and might include administration of analgesics, thyroid medications to reduce the size of the gland, or corticosteroids. The client may need preparation for surgery.

SECTION

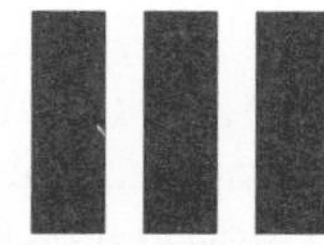

Neoplastic Disorders

Carcinoma of the Thyroid

Carcinoma or malignancy of the thyroid is rare, accounting for fewer than 1% of all malignancies. The incidence is two times greater in women than in men. The average age at diagnosis is 45.

Thyroid cancer can be of four distinct types: papillary, follicular, medullary, and anaplastic carcinoma. These cancer types vary in their degree of malignancy. It is also possible to have metastatic malignancies in the thyroid from other parts of the body. Thyroid carcinoma has been postulated to result from excessive long-standing stimulation by pituitary TSH, seen especially in clients with thyroiditis and certain types of goiter. High levels of TSH have been reported in clients with thyroid cancer (Muthe, 1981). Persons who received x-ray to the head, neck, or upper mediastinum in infancy or childhood are at risk for thyroid carcinoma later in life.

Clinical Manifestations

Thyroid carcinoma occurs as a painless, hard, fixed, irregular nodule on the thyroid. The client is usually euthyroid and asymptomatic at onset. As the tumor progresses, the client may have pressure symptoms such as hoarseness, dyspnea, or vocal cord paralysis. Progression is usually slow, although some types grow rapidly. Metastasis does not often occur; if present, it is usually to the adjacent lymphatic structures, the lungs, or the bones. Certain factors suggest the possibility that a nodule may be a carcinoma:

- Age of client is under 40
- Solitary nodule, rapidly progressive
- History of therapeutic radiation to the head, neck, or upper mediastinum (as seen in childhood treatment of enlarged tonsils, acne vulgaris, or treatment of disorders of the thymus)
- Development of secondary symptoms of hoarseness, paralysis of the vocal cords, or enlargement of the lymph glands
- No change or an increase in the size of the nodule after treatment with a 12-week course of thyroid hormone
- Nonfunctioning or "cold nodule" on thyroid scan

A major diagnostic test in the evaluation of neoplasms of the thyroid is the thyroid scan, which is used to differentiate between "hot" (functioning) and "cold" (nonfunctioning) nodules. Although this test is frequently used, its results are not definitive because the most common cause of cold nodules is not neoplasm but benign thyroid lesions (cysts, goiter, or benign adenomas). In addition, only one out of every five "cold nodules" on scan is malignant.

The use of needle biopsy in diagnosis is controversial. Some consider it valuable in diagnosing thyroiditis and identifying carcinoma. Others cite specific problems with the technique (eg, the needle may miss questionable tissue or may not remove sufficient tissue for a thorough pathologic analysis, and the technique may spread the malignancy to uninvolved tissue). Opponents of needle biopsy recommend surgical excision of the node with pathologic examination. The use of thyroid echograms in the evaluation of cystic thyroid nodules is still under evaluation.

All thyroid function laboratory tests are usually normal unless thyroiditis or a hyperfunctioning nodule is present. Serum thyroglobulin levels may be elevated in clients with thyroid carcinomas and have been found to correlate with the presence of metastases. Return to normal values following thyroidectomy has suggested to researchers that thyroglobulin levels may be of value in the initial evaluation of all clients with thyroid nodules. Elevations of serum thyrocalcitonin are found in medullary thyroid carcinoma, especially in the familial form.

Medical Measures

The approach to treatment of thyroid neoplasms depends on their cause. The main concern is the diagnosis of a client with a single thyroid nodule. For clients with thyroid carcinoma, the approach to treatment must consider the type of tumor, presence of metastases, client's age, and the ability of the tumor to take up radioactive iodine.

For benign nodules in clients at low risk for thyroid carcinoma, thyroid suppression may be started with reevaluations at 3-month intervals. If after 6 months, there is evidence of further growth of the nodule, the client may be referred for surgical excision.

For clients at low risk for thyroid carcinoma who are clinically euthyroid and asymptomatic, close observation for changes in the size or characteristics of the nodule may be all that is indicated. For clients with thyroid cysts, thyroid suppression is started with aspiration of the cysts at 1- to 3-month intervals (Kaye & Rose, 1983). Surgical excision is usually performed if the cyst recurs after the third aspiration.

Surgical approaches in thyroid carcinoma may include total thyroidectomy with or without radical neck dissection or removal of the affected lobe and isthmus. Hypoparathyroidism and vocal cord paralysis can occur following approaches involving radical neck dissection.

Thyroid-suppression therapy may be used in papillary tumors or postoperatively to keep T_4 in a normal range and to suppress TSH. Radioactive iodine has been used with follicular tumors and in treatment of functioning metastases.

Specific Nursing Measures

The nursing care of the client with neoplasms of the thyroid involves the same considerations as care of the client following thyroid surgery (see the section on thyroidectomy in this chapter). If the client has a diagnosis of carcinoma, the nurse should recognize its implications for both the client and family.

Chapter Highlights

The common disorders associated with the thyroid are hyperthyroidism, hypothyroidism, simple goiter, thyroiditis, and neoplasms.

Hyperthyroidism is associated with a hypersecretion of thyroid hormone. Hypothyroidism is

associated with a hyposecretion of thyroid hormone. Simple goiter, thyroiditis, and neoplasms of the thyroid may occur with or without changes in the circulating level of thyroid hormone.

Thyroid storm is a potentially life-threatening emergency characterized by an increase in all the symptoms and signs of hyperthyroidism.

Thyroidectomy, the surgical removal of the thyroid gland, may involve the complete removal of the gland, resection of a lobe, or resection of a portion of the gland because of hyperthyroidism, simple goiter, thyroid nodules, or carcinoma of the thyroid gland.

Closely monitor the thyroidectomy client for symptoms and signs of hemorrhage, respiratory distress, damage to the recurrent laryngeal nerve, hypocalcemia and resultant tetany, and thyroid crisis or storm.

Myxedema coma is a potentially life-threatening emergency characterized by an acute exacerbation of all the symptoms and signs of hypothyroidism.

Thyroid dysfunction in the elderly poses a diagnostic problem and is often called "the great imitator." Congestive heart failure, myocardial infarction, or the worsening of angina may be an initial sign. Early symptoms of hypothyroidism include problems with memory as well as lethargy and fatigue.

Hyperparathyroidism is a clinical state characterized by increases in serum calcium levels and decreased levels of serum phosphorus secondary to increases in the circulating levels of parathyroid hormone (PTH). Its symptoms and signs produce effects primarily in the skeletal, renal, cardiac, and gastrointestinal systems.

Parathyroidectomy, the surgical removal of all or a portion of the parathyroid glands, is performed primarily for a single or multiple adenoma of the parathyroid glands or primary hyperplasia of the glands.

Closely monitor the parathyroidectomy client for symptoms and signs of tetany as well as respiratory distress, hemorrhage, and damage to the recurrent laryngeal nerve.

Hypoparathyroidism is a disorder resulting from a deficiency in the secretion of PTH or a decrease in the effectiveness of its action. It is characterized by low serum calcium levels and high serum phosphorus levels.

Hypoparathyroidism is most often secondary to thyroid disease. Symptoms and signs of acute hypoparathyroidism include muscle cramping, nausea, vomiting, abdominal cramping, increasing lethargy, and personality changes.

The main treatment approaches to hypoparathyroidism are pharmacologic and dietary. The overall goal is to maintain the serum calcium levels and prevent further complications.

Bibliography

Bates B: *A Guide to the Physical Examination,* 3rd ed. Philadelphia: Lippincott, 1983.

Blum M: Thyroid function and disease in the elderly. *Hosp Pract* 1981; 16(10):105.

Entwhistle K: Nursing care study: Thyroidectomy: A strangling feeling. *Nurs Mirror* 1981; 152(16):35–36.

Evangelistic JT, Thorpe CJ: Thyroid storm: A nursing crisis. *Heart Lung* 1983; 12:184–193.

Grimes J, Iannopollo E: *Health Assessment in Nursing Practice.* Monterey, CA: Wadsworth, 1982.

Hahn AB et al: *Pharmacology in Nursing.* 15th ed. St. Louis: Mosby, 1982.

Hoffmann JJ, Newly TB: Hypercalcemia in primary hyperparathyroidism. *Nurs Clin North Am* 1980; 15(3):469–480.

Honigman RE: Deciphering diagnostic studies: Thyroid function tests. *Nurs 82* (April) 1982; 12:68–71.

Jenkins EH: Living with thyrotoxicosis. *Am J Nurs* 1980; 80:956–958.

Kaye D, Rose LF (editors): *Fundamentals of Internal Medicine.* St. Louis: Mosby, 1983.

Kloegman S, Sagor : Nursing care study: A lump in the throat. *Nurs Mirror* 1983; 156(4):54–56.

Klonoff DC, Greenspan FS: The thyroid nodule. *Adv Intern Med* 1982; 27:101.

Levine SN: Current concepts of thyroiditis. *Arch Intern Med* 1983; 143:1952.

Marx IJ: New insights into primary hyperparathyroidism *Hosp Practice* 1984; 19(3):55.

Musante–Wake M, Brensinger JF: The nurse's role in hypothyroidism. *Nurs Clin North Am* 1980; 15(3):453–467.

Muthe NC: *Endocrinology: A Nursing Approach.* Boston: Little, Brown, 1981.

Saxton DF et al: *The Addison–Wesley Manual of Nursing Practice.* Menlo Park, CA: Addison–Wesley, 1983.

Sharkey PL, Myer DA: Hyperthyroidism. *Critical Care Update* 1981; 8(5):12–15, 17–19, 22–24.

Wartofsky L: Guidelines for the treatment of hyperthyroidism. *Am Fam Physician* (July) 1984; 30:199–210.

Williams RH (editor): *Textbook of Endocrinology,* 6th ed. Philadelphia: Saunders, 1981.

CASE STUDY

The Client With Hyperthyroidism

I. Descriptive Data

Mrs Janine Figoerella, age 42, was referred to the endocrine clinic of the university teaching hospital by an occupational health nurse at her place of employment. This is her first visit to the facility, and she is somewhat anxious.

II. Personal Data

Date and Time: March 16, 1988, 11:30 AM
Full Name: Janine A. Figoerella
Address: 14 Deurtt Ave., Detroit, MI
Telephone: Home: 000-0000
Work: 000-0000, ext 714
Sex: Female
Age: 42
Birthdate: 6-8-45
Marital Status: Married
Race: Caucasian
Culture: Italian–American
Religion: Catholic
Occupation: Secretary
Usual Health Care Provider: Leonard Hyzy, MD, who retired from his practice several years ago; she has not found another care provider, nor had need of one until now.

III. Health History

Source of Information: Client
Reliability of Informant: Reliable
Chief Concern: "Nervousness and insomnia for 6 months, increasing in severity."

History of Present Illness: Client states that for the past 6 months she has experienced increasing nervousness and anxiety with frequent verbal outbursts and crying spells. She also has had a difficult time getting to sleep. States family and associates have commented on her irritability and weight loss (17 lb despite an enormous appetite and abundant food intake) as well as her eyes, which she describes as "looking like they're popping out of my head." She first began to notice the changed appearance of her eyes 3 to 4 months ago and feels they are definitely becoming more prominent. She also feels her neck has increased in size. No headache, changes in visual acuity, diplopia, seizures, or blackouts. No sore throat, swollen glands, neck pain. Feels home and work environments are not unusually stressful; family and peer relationships generally good but strained by her outbursts and anxiety. She does not have polyuria, polydipsia, abdominal or epigastric pain, nausea, or change in character of stool.

This is the first occurrence of these symptoms for this client. She has no history of major health problems and takes no medications. She has never been treated for mental health problems.

Past Health History:

Childhood: Rheumatic fever, pertussis
Immunizations: Basic series complete; tetanus booster, 1980
Medical Problems: Pneumonia 1968, not hospitalized; recurrent low back pain since fall on ice in 1977
Surgeries: T&A, 1950; tubal ligation, 1983

(continued)

CASE STUDY (continued)

The Client With Hyperthyroidism

Transfusions: None
Special Diagnostic Procedures: X-ray of the lumbo-sacral spine, 1977; no pathology
Trauma: Fall on ice, winter 1977 c̄ injury to L-S spine
Allergies: None
Medications: Sominex, T to T̈ q. H.S. for sleeplessness; takes no other medications

Family History:
Father, age 73, S/P MI, ASHD
Mother, died age 51, automobile accident
No siblings
Husband, age 48, A&W
Daughters, ages 18 & 20, A&W
MGF, Ca bowel, maternal aunt, thyroid disorder. No known family history of CVA, ↑ BP, TBC, DM

Personal/Social History:
The client resides with her husband of 20 years and two teenage daughters, ages 20 and 18. She has been employed as a secretary in the office of a nearby developmental center for 7 years and expresses enthusiasm for her job and a liking for the developmentally disabled children she comes in contact with. Usual daily schedule: arises at 6:30 AM; works from 8 AM to 4 PM; arrives home around 4:45 PM; fixes dinner and spends evening at home, usually doing household chores. One night a week she bowls with team from developmental center. On weekend, attends church and on Sunday, usually has father and in-laws over to house for dinner and visiting. Occasionally, on weekend will go out with husband for dinner and a movie. Feels she no longer enjoys herself because of her "nerves."

She is a high school graduate and has a 2-year degree from Bryant and Stratton Business Institute. She worked as a secretary for a produce firm for 13 years before taking her current position. She has never traveled outside of North America.

Habits: She eats three to six meals daily to combat weight loss; enjoys bowling and uses her exercise bicycle about three times a week; has never used drugs; has an occasional mixed drink on weekends; smokes one pack of cigarettes per day × 22 years (22 pack years); has no desire to quit, although her husband and children have been urging her to.

Has had difficulty getting to sleep at night for 6 to 7 months; sleeps 3 to 5 hours with much tossing and turning; does not have nightmares or early morning wakening; has "lost interest in sex" since "trouble with nerves"; intercourse one to two times monthly; usually without orgasm.

She and her husband are practicing Roman Catholics and attend mass regularly. They have no major financial concerns. She feels she has good support systems. Her symptoms are worrisome to her; she feels she must be having a nervous breakdown because of her inability to control her emotions. She also verbalizes fear of a brain tumor.

Review of Systems:
General Health: Extremely fatigued; states, "I just know there's something terrible wrong with me."
Skin: Has noted increased perspiration; hair has become finer
Eyes: See HPI

Neck: See HPI
Chest: No DOE, no PND, occasional smoker's cough
Heart: No chest pain; recently has had several episodes of palpitations
Gastrointestinal: Increased frequency of stool (two to three times daily), brown in color, soft
Gynecologic: LMP 3-1-88, 31-day cycle; flow used to be heavy and continue for 3 to 5 days; for past 5 months, has had a very light flow that lasts only 1 to 2 days
Neurologic: Has noted tremors of her fingers, which she never had before

IV. Physical Assessment

Height: 5 ft 7 in
Weight: 108 lb (weight 6 months ago 125 lb)
Vital Signs: BP 160/70 supine rt arm; seated 162/68; apical rate 104 and regular; T, 99.8°F (37.6°C); R, 22

Relevant Organ Systems:

Skin/Hair: Bodily skin very smooth with increased warmth; scalp hair fine and silky; skin feels moist to touch; ō lesions; ō excoriations
Eyes: Eyebrows silky and fine; conjunctivae pink; sclerae white; PERRLA c̄ mild degree of difficulty with convergence; bilateral proptosis; symmetrical; ⊕ lid-lag; fundi: disk margins flat and distinct; A-V ratio 2:3, ō H or E, OU
Neck: Carotids 2 + and equal s̄ bruits; ō lymphadenopathy; thyroid, soft, diffusely enlarged, no bruits, nontender, ō nodules
Heart: Rate 104 and regular with soft grade I–II/VI early systolic murmur heart best at apex to LSB; ō gallops
Lungs: Clear to A & P, ō rales, rhonchi, or wheezes
Extremities: 1 +, nonpitting edema noted bilaterally in pretibial areas, ⊖ Homans' sign; ō erythema; ō warmth; all pulses 2 + and symmetrical
Neurologic:
Mental Status: Demonstrates difficulty concentrating on tasks, decreased attention span
Motor-sensory: Fine tremors of fingers and tongue
Cranial Nerves II–XII: Intact
Cerebellum: Intact
Reflexes:

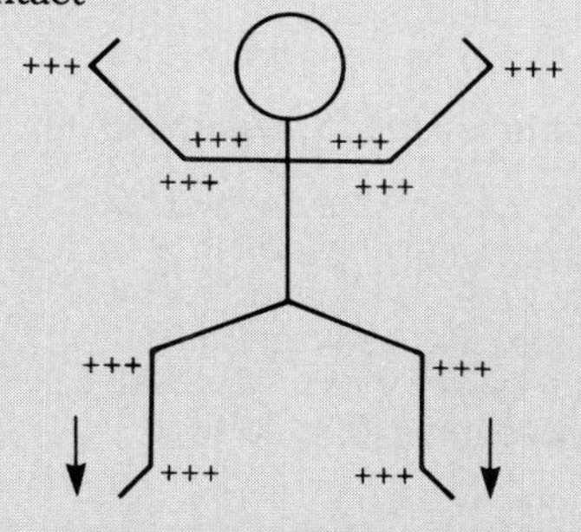

+++ +++
+++ +++
+++ +++
+++ +++
+++ +++

V. Diagnostic Data

Mrs Figoerella was admitted to the hospital and scheduled to have a series of tests. The results are as follows:

ECG: Tachycardia; normal sinus rhythm
Chest X-ray: wnl
T_4: 13 μg/dL (norm: 4 to 12 μg/dL)
T_3 Uptake: Increased, indicating hyperfunction
RAIU Thyroid Scan: Shows increased uptake by gland with an early peak

Mrs Figoerella was diagnosed as having hyperthyroidism (Graves' disease).

(continued)

CASE STUDY (continued)

The Client With Hyperthyroidism

VI. Nursing Care Plan, by Nursing Diagnosis

Client Care Goals	Plan/Nursing Implementation	Expected Outcomes
Comfort, altered related to symptoms of disease		
Maintain client comfort; prevent skin and eye complications	*If diaphoretic:* Change bed linen frequently; provide linen and sleepwear light in weight; frequent sponge baths; attention to bony prominences; observe for signs of skin breakdown and treat immediately; keep room temperature cool *For exophthalmos:* Elevate head of bed to relieve periorbital edema: methylcellulose drops (0.5% to 1%) to alleviate dryness of conjunctiva and cornea as ordered; for severe proptosis, lids may be taped shut during sleep or sleep mask provided; room lighting should be lowered; minimize glare; provide sunglasses if light is bright or client goes outdoors in sunlight	Will experience comfort and relief from diaphoresis and proptotic symptoms; no signs of skin breakdown
Sleep pattern disturbance related to insomnia and hyperactivity		
Obtain sufficient rest to reduce fatigue	Restrict activities to provide for maximum rest and to alleviate fatigue; explain limitations and rationale to client and family; manipulate environment to decrease excessive stimulation (room temperature, lighting, numbers of visitors, radio, television); schedule rest periods between periods of activity; refer to occupational therapy or recreational therapy for diversion; provide sedation as ordered	Client will not be excessively fatigued; will sleep restfully
Nutrition, altered: less than body requirements related to inadequate intake for metabolic needs		
Maintain adequate nutritional status	Weight daily or q. 2 days; diet up to 4000 to 5000 calories per day; diet high in protein and carbohydrate; low in fiber; restrict caffeine; provide snacks between meals and at bedtime; frequently assess visual acuity and measurements of EOMs	Client's weight will remain stable
Anxiety related to unknown outcome of diagnostic work-up		
Maintain minimal exposure to internal and external stressors	Create as calm an environment as possible; decrease external stimuli; provide consistency in caretakers; establish a routine with as little change as possible; provide private room if needed; visitors should be screened and family education provided to avoid topics that will produce anxiety in the client; provide an opportunity for client and family to discuss their concerns and fears; provide client and family education regarding the physiologic and psychologic changes in the client; provide support and reassurance to client and family	Client will experience minimal anxiety

Client Care Goals	Plan/Nursing Implementation	Expected Outcomes
Fluid volume deficit: actual related to fluid loss and increased metabolic rate		
Maintain adequate fluid—electrolyte balance	Increases fluid intake to 4000 mL/day (unless there are cardiac or renal contraindications); monitor intake and output; explain to client and family the need for additional fluids; monitor serum electrolytes and urine values	Client will not experience any deficits in fluid volume: No signs of dehydratrion; specific gravity of urine will remain in normal range; eserum electrolytes will remain in normal range
Injury: potential for related to infection, stress, surgery		
Prevent severe thyroid storm or crisis	Assess client regularly for indications of thyroid storm: marked restlessness and anxiety; fever (104° F to 106°F); extreme tachycardia (30 to 160 beats per minute); dehydration; nausea and vomiting; diarrhea; delirium and psychosis; report these immediately to physician; educate client and family about these symptoms and signs	Symptoms and signs of thyroid crisis will be recognized and treated immediately; severe thyroid storm or crisis will be prevented
Knowledge deficit related to disease process secondary to hyperthyroidism		
Explain the disease and its treatment clearly and accurately	Review hyperthyroidism with client and family or significant others including: symptoms and signs of both hyperthyroidism and hypothyroidism; effects of increased thyroxine production in the body; the treatment regimen and its purposes; name, dosage, action, and side effect of each medication; dietary management; need for regular medical supervision and its purpose; date and time of next medical appointment; what to report to the physician; telephone number where client or family can call with questions	Client and family will understand hyperthyroidism and its management

CHAPTER 34

Specific Disorders of the Pituitary and Adrenal Glands

Other topics relevant to this content are: Diagnostic studies for clients with disorders of the pituitary and adrenal glands, **Chapter 31;** Craniotomy approach for removal of pituitary tumor, **Chapter 29.**

Objectives

When you have finished studying this chapter, you should be able to:

Identify the common disorders of the pituitary and adrenal glands.

Describe the clinical manifestations of disorders of the pituitary and adrenal glands.

Identify medical and surgical measures specific to disorders of the pituitary and adrenal glands.

Specify the common drugs used in treating adrenal and pituitary disorders and discuss their potential side effects.

Explain the specific nursing interventions for clients with problems of the pituitary and adrenal glands.

Anticipate the temporary or permanent lifestyle modifications frequently necessary for clients with problems involving the pituitary and adrenal glands.

Discuss the psychosocial/lifestyle implications of pituitary and adrenal dysfunction for the client and significant others and outline specific nursing interventions to address their needs.

Because of the complex actions of the pituitary and adrenal glands, as well as their interaction with each other and with other bodily systems, their dysfunctions have a variety of causes and clinical manifestations. The nursing process will assist the nurse in understanding and caring for clients with disorders of the pituitary and adrenal glands.

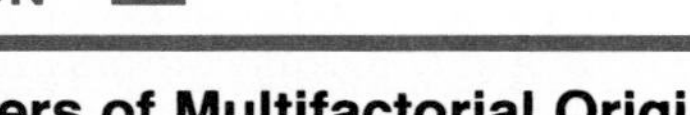

Disorders of Multifactorial Origin

Among the pituitary disorders of multifactorial origin are diabetes insipidus and the syndrome of inappropriate antidiuretic hormone (SIADH) secretion. Adrenal disorders in this category are Cushing's syndrome and Addison's disease.

Pituitary Disorders

Diabetes Insipidus

Diabetes insipidus is a disorder of the posterior pituitary characterized by the excretion of excessively large amounts of hypotonic urine. This leads to increased thirst, the body's compensating mechanism to prevent dehydration.

Diabetes insipidus is idiopathic in about 50% of clients. Secondary diabetes insipidus is pituitary diabetes insipidus arising from a variety of causes: hypophysectomy, tumors (metastatic carcinoma of the breast, craniopharyngioma), trauma (basilar skull fractures), vascular lesions (hemorrhage and aneurysms), infections (syphilis, encephalitis, meningitis), histiocytosis, and granulomatous disease (sarcoidosis, tuberculosis).

If there has been a temporary injury to the hypothalamus, the client may experience a transient episode of polydipsia and polyuria, which can be followed by either complete recovery or permanent diabetes insipidus. The danger in this situation occurs when the client is unable to drink enough fluids to prevent dehydration and/or unable to communicate an increasing sense of thirst. These clients require careful monitoring of their intake and output and blood pressure as indicators of the need for further fluid replacement.

CLINICAL MANIFESTATIONS The two primary clinical manifestations of diabetes insipidus are persistent polyuria and polydipsia. Polyuria may amount to 5 to 20 L/day depending on the degree of pathology; an output of 4 to 5 L is the most common (Muthe, 1981). The urine has an abnormally low specific gravity (1.001 to 1.005) with no other abnormalities. The client may have headache, visual disturbances, muscular weakness, myalgia, anorexia, and weight loss. Symptoms of electrolyte imbalance may be seen. Persistent polydipsia and polyuria can interfere with sleep, causing fatigue, lethargy, and irritability. If the fluid intake is not sufficient to compensate for the amount lost through the urine, profound dehydration and shock may ensue.

Diabetes insipidus is not a life-threatening disorder unless severe electrolyte imbalances occur. These imbalances are not usually seen in individuals who can compensate for the excessive fluid losses by an increased fluid intake.

Diabetes insipidus is diagnosed by routine screening tests such as specific gravity of urine, plasma sodium levels, osmolality tests, and water deprivation and water-loading tests. The diagnosis is confirmed if a deficiency of ADH is demonstrated and the client's kidneys are shown to respond normally to ADH. In response to a water deprivation challenge, clients with diabetes insipidus will demonstrate an inability to increase the specific gravity and osmolality of the urine. These tests are discussed in Chapter 31. The differential diagnosis involves other causes of polyuria. A brain scan, skull x-rays, visual fields testing, and a full neurologic examination may be done to rule out the presence of a tumor.

MEDICAL MEASURES The major therapeutic measure used in diabetes insipidus is replacement therapy. Even though a client may be able to compensate for the excessive loss of fluids by drinking large quantities of liquids, this is often impractical and may involve major adjustments in lifestyle. Administration of exogenous vasopressin (ADH) helps to reestablish a normal fluid balance and relieves the symptoms of polyuria and polydipsia.

SPECIFIC NURSING MEASURES The nursing care of clients with diabetes insipidus involves:

- Measuring intake and output (q. 1 h in certain clients) as a baseline for treatment and as an indicator for fluid replacement.
- Monitoring specific gravity of urine.
- Measuring blood pressure and weight before and after treatment is begun.
- Encouraging increased oral fluid intake:
  Assess client's fluid preference. (Clients with diabetes insipidus often prefer ice water for reasons not well understood.)
  Keep liquids readily accessible to the client.
- Restricting salt and protein to help reduce urinary output.
- Observing the client for symptoms and signs of dehydration and electrolyte imbalance (eg, intense thirst, weight loss, dryness of the oral mucosa, loss of normal skin turgor).
  Look for any signs of skin breakdown due to poor skin turgor.
  Prevent skin breakdown by turning and repositioning q. 2 h, ambulation, skin lotion, and gentle massage.

After replacement treatment has been started, be alert for symptoms and signs of water intoxication secondary to overmedication with vasopressin (change in level of consciousness, confusion, headache, and weight gain). If these symptoms appear, the medication should be stopped, fluids restricted, and the physician notified immediately. Also be alert for diarrhea resulting from increased peristalsis and chest pain, especially in elderly clients with a history of coronary artery disease.

Home Health Care

Before discharge, the client and family should be familiar with the disorder and the need for careful recording of intake, output, and daily weights. Clients should carry an identification card and wear a Medic-Alert bracelet or tag, as should all clients with pituitary dysfunction requiring medication. Clients who are to receive vasopressin parenterally should be skilled in the technique of self-injection; know how to prepare and store the medication, the purpose of the medication, and potential side effects. Clients receiving vasopressin by nasal spray should have practiced the correct administration before discharge from the hospital.

Teach the client and family the symptoms and signs of overdosage and underdosage of medications and when to report these to the physician. Overdosage is indicated by water intoxication; underdosage is indicated by dehydration. The interaction of other medications (epinephrine and heparin) and alcohol and vasopressin should be discussed as well as the importance of regular medical evaluation.

Syndrome of Inappropriate Antidiuretic Hormone Secretion

The syndrome of inappropriate antidiuretic hormone secretion, or SIADH, is a condition characterized by autonomous release of ADH without regard to plasma osmolality. The body is unable to dilute the urine appropriately,

NURSING DIAGNOSES IN

Endocrine Dysfunction

DIRECTLY RELATED DIAGNOSES

- Activity intolerance
- Bowel elimination, altered: diarrhea
- Comfort, altered: pain
- Coping, ineffective individual
- Fluid volume deficit, actual
- Fluid volume deficit, potential
- Knowledge deficit
- Nutrition, altered: more than body requirements
- Self-concept, disturbance in: body image
- Thought processes, altered

OTHER POTENTIAL DIAGNOSES

- Infection, potential for
- Injury, potential for
- Noncompliance
- Nutrition, altered: less than body requirements
- Powerlessness
- Sensory/perceptual alterations: visual, tactile
- Skin integrity, impaired
- Thermoregulation, ineffective
- Tissue perfusion, altered: gastrointestinal, peripheral

so fluid is retained, which expands the extracellular fluid compartment and leads to hyponatremia. SIADH can be caused by release of the hormone from a secreting tumor or from the posterior pituitary from a variety of causes. These etiologic factors are outlined in Box 34–1.

Box 34–1
Etiology of Syndrome of Inappropriate Antidiuretic Hormone (SIADH) Secretion

Central nervous system: Head injury, CVA, brain tumor/abscess, encephalitis, meningitis, Guillain–Barré syndrome, acute intermittent porphyria, seizure disorders, lupus cerebritis, schizophrenia

Intrathoracic causes: Pneumonia, lung abscess, aspergillosis, tuberculosis, cystic fibrosis, positive-pressure respirator (causes sudden release of ADH)

Tumors: Oat cell carcinoma of the lung, adenocarcinoma of duodenum and pancreas, thymoma, Hodgkin's disease, lymphosarcoma, Ewing's tumor, carcinoma of the ureter

Exogenous drugs:
- Drugs that increase release of ADH (nicotine, clofibrate, vincristine)
- Drugs that potentiate ADH (chlorpropramide, thiazide diuretics)
- Drugs that increase renal reabsorption of water (vasopressin, oxytocin)

Other: Surgery, Addison's disease, hypopituitarism, myxedema, emotional stress, idiopathic disorders

SOURCE: Adapted from Kaye D, Rose LF: *Fundamentals of Internal Medicine*. St. Louis: Mosby, 1983, p. 914. Solomon BL: The hypothalamus and pituitary gland: An overview. *Nurs Clin North Am* 1980; 15(3):449.

CLINICAL MANIFESTATIONS Clients with SIADH may gain body weight because of fluid retention. They may also be confused, lethargic, weak, and have convulsions due to their hyponatremia. Clinically, serum sodium levels are below 135 mEq/L, whereas the urinary sodium concentrations are elevated. SIADH is diagnosed by laboratory evaluation of serum and urine sodium and chloride levels and of serum and urine osmolality levels. These tests are discussed further in Chapter 31.

MEDICAL MEASURES Treatment of SIADH is directed toward its underlying cause. The client may be placed on water restriction. The hyponatremia is usually not treated unless the client has severe symptoms.

SPECIFIC NURSING MEASURES Nursing care of the client with SIADH involves:

- Assessing for symptoms and signs related to water intoxication and hyponatremia.
- Measuring and recording intake and output, blood pressure, and weight.
- Assisting clients in managing thirst because clients are often on fluid restrictions:
  Assess fluid preferences.
  Use ice chips rather than water.
  Relieve dryness of mucosa through care of mouth.
  Space fluids over 8-hour time periods.
- Teaching regarding nature of disorder, treatment plan, and procedures.

Adrenal Disorders

Cushing's Syndrome

Cushing's syndrome arises from an excess of cortisol circulating in the plasma. The etiology of Cushing's syndrome may fall into one of three categories, which have in common the oversecretion of cortisol by the adrenal cortex:

- Primary Cushing's syndrome
- Secondary Cushing's syndrome or Cushing's disease
- Tertiary Cushing's syndrome

Primary Cushing's syndrome, also called adrenal Cushing's syndrome, usually results from autonomous secretion of glucocorticoid from a unilateral adrenal neoplasm. About half of these tumors are malignant.

Secondary Cushing's syndrome, also called pituitary-dependent Cushing's syndrome or Cushing's disease, is the most common. It is due to an excess secretion of ACTH that leads to bilateral adrenal hyperplasia.

Tertiary or ectopic Cushing's syndrome arises from the autonomous production of ACTH by at least 25 different extrapituitary malignancies, including carcinoma of the lung and of several organs in the gastrointestinal tract. It is characterized by markedly increased ACTH levels and bilateral hyperplasia of the adrenal glands (Kaye & Rose, 1983).

Cushing's syndrome can also be iatrogenic (ie, occurring in clients who have been given cortisol or ACTH over a period of time). Whatever the etiology, the result of hyperfunction of the adrenal cortex in Cushing's syndrome is an excess of plasma cortisol that produces certain characteristic effects, as described in Table 34–1.

CLINICAL MANIFESTATIONS Hypertension results from the retention of sodium and water. Retained water expands the extracellular fluid volume and increases sensitivity of the vasculature to circulating catecholamines.

Central or truncal obesity, along with a characteristic moon face and buffalo hump, occurs because of deposition of body fat in the abdominal wall, facial, and interscapular areas. The face of the client with Cushing's syndrome is often round and plethoric. Because of a loss of muscle mass resulting from the increased breakdown of protein, the extremities may appear thin, and there may be proximal muscle weakness, especially of the pelvic girdle. Muscle weakness, as well as potential cardiac dysfunction, may be related to hypokalemia resulting from urinary excretion of potassium.

Cutaneous **striae** may be present on the abdomen, breast, perineum, and buttocks. The striae are wide and pinkish purple. The skin becomes thinner and more prone to trauma because of the breakdown of collagen. Clients with Cushing's syndrome are also prone to ecchymosis. If the etiology of Cushing's syndrome is pituitary dysfunction, hyperpigmentation of the skin may be present because of increased plasma levels of ACTH. Hyperpigmentation is not found when Cushing's syndrome is of adrenal origin; therefore, it provides a valuable diagnostic sign to rule out the possibility of an adrenal tumor. Acne, hirsutism, **oligomenorrhea,** and amennorhea may be secondary effects of the overproduction of androgen (Sanford, 1980).

Table 34–1
Common Findings in Cushing's Syndrome

Subjective Findings	Objective Findings
Clients often note:	*Examiners often observe:*
Red, full face	Plethoric moon face
Change in body shape	Truncal obesity with muscle wasting of extremities
Muscle weakness and fatigability	Supraclavicular fat pads
	Pendulous fat pad in chest and abdomen
	Buffalo hump in interscapular area
Skin and hair changes	Loss of skin thickness
Easy bruisability	Skin pigmentation
	Multiple ecchymoses
	Purple abdominal striae
	Acne and hirsutism in women
Susceptibility to infection and bone fractures	Osteoporosis
	Hypertension
Menstrual changes (oligomenorrhea, amenorrhea)	Hypokalemia
Irritability, emotional lability, depression, confusion, sleeplessness	Diabetes mellitus (usually in clients with a family predisposition)
Glucose intolerance	

Oversecretion of cortisol can also increase susceptibility to fractures from osteoporosis (especially of the spine) because of cortisol-stimulated calcium resorption from the bone. Glucose intolerance (hyperglycemia) may develop secondary to the anti-insulin effect of cortisol. Diabetes mellitus may develop in individuals with a predisposition. In addition, there may be emotional symptoms (eg, depression, increased anxiety, euphoria, and frank psychosis). There are increased susceptibility to infection and potential for masking of infection. These symptoms and signs create a typical "cushingoid" presentation (Figure 34–1). The disorder not only causes problems of altered body image and self-esteem but also poses serious potential health concerns.

One of the most important diagnostic findings in the evaluation of Cushing's syndrome is the persistent elevation of serum cortisol levels with loss of the normal diurnal variation. All symptoms and signs are related to this pathophysiologic change. The routine screening tests and other methods used in the evaluation of adrenal dysfunction are discussed in Chapter 31, Table 31–1.

MEDICAL MEASURES The treatment of Cushing's syndrome and disease depends on the etiology. If a tumor is involved, treatment also depends on whether the lesion is benign or malignant. Therapeutic modalities used in the treatment of Cushing's disease are surgical measures, pharmacologic agents, and medical measures such as radiation and diet therapy.

Surgery is the most common modality. Transsphenoidal microsurgery, transfrontal craniotomy, and unilateral or bilateral adrenalectomy are possible approaches to treatment of Cushing's syndrome, depending on the location of the tumor. Surgical procedures used in the care of individuals with endocrine disorders are discussed below.

The use of pharmacologic agents is restricted to situations in which there is an inoperable tumor and radiation has been unsuccessful. Their use generally has been only of short-term value.

When surgery is performed, replacement hormonal therapy is often mandated. It is the responsibility of the nurse to be familiar with the therapeutic use of steroids and their long-term effects and to teach these to the client

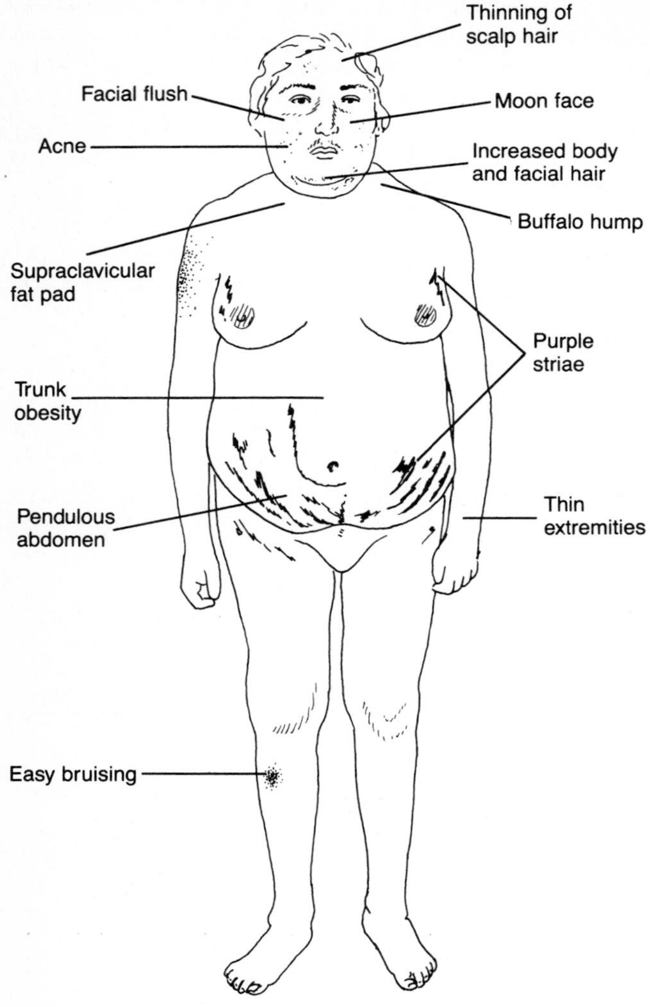

Figure 34–1

A client with typical cushingoid findings.

Table 34–2
Common Side Effects of Long-Term Glucocorticoid Therapy

Side Effects	Physiologic Basis
Retention of sodium; loss of potassium with resulting fluid retention and ↑ BP	Associated mineralocorticoid effect
Increased susceptibility to infection	Suppression of immune system
Muscle weakness, muscle breakdown	↑ Protein catabolism by glucocorticoids
Glucose intolerance, hyperglycemia	↑ Gluconeogenesis by glucocorticoids
Increased deposition of fat in trunk	↑ Lipid synthesis by glucocorticoids
Growth suppression	↓ Of growth hormone action by glucocorticoids
Emotional changes, possible psychosis	Not understood
Osteoporosis, ↑ incidence of fractures	Changes in calcium metabolism leading to ↑ resorption of bone
Gastritis; gastric, peptic ulcers	Direct irritation or protein-wasting effects of protein
Glaucoma	Interference with aqueous outflow in eye; ↑ intraocular pressure
Cataracts	Not understood
Pancreatitis	Possible effect of glucocorticoids on lipid metabolism

SOURCE: Adapted from Clark JB, Queener SF, Karb VB: *Pharmacological Basis of Nursing Practice.* St. Louis: Mosby, 1982, p. 440.

and family. Table 34–2 summarizes the common side effects of long-term glucocorticoid therapy.

SPECIFIC NURSING MEASURES The nursing management of Cushing's syndrome focuses on psychologic support for the client and family or friends, relief of symptoms, protection of the client from possible complications related to the increased production of cortisol, and client and family education. Psychologic support for clients with Cushing's syndrome is especially important because the alterations in body image may affect their self-esteem and their ability to cope with their present life situation. In addition, clients with Cushing's syndrome often have rapid mood changes, which are of concern to both them and their significant others. Provide for a climate of acceptance; create opportunities for both the client and family to express and discuss their questions, feelings, and concerns; and educate the client and family about the nature of the disorder, its clinical course, and the goals of the medical treatment and nursing care plans.

To help relieve the symptoms of Cushing's syndrome:

- Encourage proper diet and fluid intake (eg, low calorie, high protein, high potassium, low sodium) to help correct the metabolic imbalances.
- Monitor vital signs regularly and report any significant elevations in blood pressure immediately.
- Obtain daily weight on the same scale to monitor rate of fluid retention and loss.
- Promote physical and emotional rest; provide emotional support during mood changes, offer explanations as needed, and provide opportunities for verbalization of feelings regarding changes in body appearance and the long-term implications of the disorder.

To help prevent complications related to the increased production of cortisol:

- Check urine periodically for glucose and acetone to screen for the presence of diabetes mellitus.
- Assess the client carefully for infection, remembering that one of the effects of increased cortisol production is the suppression of the immune system and masking of infections.
- Provide protection from injury and trauma because clients' muscle weakness and tendency toward osteoporosis make them susceptible.

Client/Family Teaching

Client teaching should include the nature of the disorder, prognosis, goals of the medical (or surgical) treatment plan, and goals of the nursing care plan. If clients are to receive medications, they and their families should be familiar with their purpose, action, dosage, administration, and side effects. Box 34–2 lists the important nursing implications of long-term glucocorticoid therapy. Actively attempt to create a climate in which both the client and family feel free to discuss the implications of the disorder and its effects on their lives. Consider making a public health nursing referral to evaluate the client's home environment for possible safety factors, assist the family in obtaining adaptive equipment if needed, and monitor the client's progress. Box 34–3 provides a general teaching plan for clients on glucocorticoid therapy.

Adrenalectomy

An adrenalectomy is the surgical removal or resection of one or both of the adrenal glands. A bilateral adrenalectomy involves the removal of both adrenal glands, and a unilateral adrenalectomy is the removal of one adrenal gland. In a subtotal adrenalectomy, a part of an adrenal gland is excised. Bilateral adrenalectomy is more commonly performed for advanced cancer of the breast or prostate. Unilateral or subtotal adrenalectomy is performed for pheochromocytoma.

The major goal of adrenalectomy is to reduce the excessive secretion of the adrenal hormones. The procedure is indicated when there is hyperfunction secondary to a tumor or hyperplasia of the gland, in pheochromocytoma, and in advanced cases of cancer of the breast and prostate. These malignancies are known to be affected by the hormones of the endocrine system; estrogen has an effect on breast carcinomas and testosterone, on carcinomas of the prostate. In certain clients, these hormones are still present after endocrine suppression and have been found to arise from the adrenal cortex. In premenopausal women with cancer of the breast who are to have adrenalectomy, an oophorectomy is performed first. In men with cancer of the prostate who are to undergo adrenalectomy, an orchiectomy is performed first.

The two major surgical approaches to adrenalectomy are the transabdominal and lateral approaches. The transabdominal approach uses a bilateral subcostal or midline incision. The lateral approach involves an incision under

Box 34–2
Nursing Implications of Long-Term Glucocorticoid Therapy

If the course of steroid therapy lasts less than 7 to 10 days, side effects are unlikely.

Monitor the client's weight and blood pressure at frequent intervals.

Check the client's urine regularly for the presence of glucose and acetone.
- For clients who require insulin therapy to treat hyperglycemia, the dosage of insulin varies with the dose of steroids.
- Individuals with diabetes mellitus who require steroid therapy will need adjustment of the insulin dosage.

Assess clients carefully for symptoms and signs of gastric irritation that might indicate an ulcer (dyspepsia, epigastric burning, increased flatulence, hematemesis, coffee-ground emesis, and melena). Ulcers may also develop in clients who receive steroids parenterally.
- Steroids should be taken with meals if possible.
- Physician may prescribe the use of cimetidine (Tagamet) and antacids up to four to six times daily while client is receiving steroids.
- Client may benefit from more frequent, small meals.
- All foods and liquids the client feels contribute to gastric symptoms should be carefully noted and excluded from the diet (eg, coffee, tomato products, alcohol). Aspirin is also contraindicated unless specifically ordered by the physician.

Assess clients, especially postmenopausal females, carefully for symptoms and signs of osteoporosis.
- Client should be taught to report any persistent musculoskeletal pain.
- Client should be advised to avoid strenuous physical activities (eg, contact sports, heavy lifting, and strenuous physical labor).
- Care should be taken in the lifting and transfer of any immobilized client on long-term glucocorticoid therapy to reduce the chance of spontaneous fracture.

Advise clients to consult an ophthalmologist every 3 to 6 months to screen for possible glaucoma and early cataract formation.

Clients with a history of tuberculosis or positive tuberculin reactors who are receiving long-term steroid therapy may also receive antituberculosis medications while they are receiving steroids.

Pregnant women should not take steroids unless they are receiving replacement therapy or are in a potentially life-threatening situation. In this case, close monitoring by the endocrinologist and obstetrician is essential.

The complete return of adrenal function after long-term glucocorticoid therapy may take up to 1 year. The client requires careful assessment during this period and may need corticosteroid treatment if stress or infection occurs or if surgery is to be performed.

SOURCE: Adapted from Clark JB, Queener SF, Karb VB: *Pharmacological Basis of Nursing Practice.* St. Louis: Mosby, 1982, pp. 446–447.

Box 34–3
Teaching Plan for a Client on Glucocorticoid Therapy

A comprehensive teaching plan for any client on glucocorticoids, especially long-term therapy, should cover the following points:

Purpose of therapy (eg, replacement of deficient hormones or treatment of a specific disorder).

Medication: Name, action, dosage, administration, desired effect, side effects.

Importance of taking the medications regularly and of informing the physician immediately when unable to do so. Some clients with adrenal insufficiency may not be able to tolerate taking steroids orally; they must be taught to administer steroids parenterally.

What symptoms and signs to report immediately to the physician:
- Any side effects of the medication (most will resolve when steroid therapy is stopped).
- Any symptoms and signs of infection: Fever, chills, cough, sore throat. (Clients should be encouraged to avoid all other persons who have symptoms and signs of an infection.)
- Any episodes of increased stress (fatigue, infection, emotional upset) that may call for increased dosages of steroids.

Importance of wearing a Medic-Alert tag and carrying a card identifying the client, the diagnosis, and medications. Clients receiving steroid therapy should inform all health care providers.

Rationale for tapering off glucocorticoid therapy and/or rationale for alternative-day treatment. Client should be advised against abruptly stopping the medication.

Importance of diet as a treatment. Diet should include foods high in protein and potassium and low in sodium and carbohydrates. Dietary consultation with nutritionist is often beneficial.

SOURCE: Adapted from Clark JB, Queener SF, Karb VB: *Pharmacological Basis of Nursing Practice.* St. Louis: Mosby, 1982, pp. 446–447.

the twelfth rib in the rear flank area. This incision is similar to that made for a nephrectomy and is used in clients who are obese or at risk for wound dehiscence. Physiologic and psychosocial/lifestyle implications of adrenalectomy are covered in Table 34–3.

Nursing Implications

PREOPERATIVE CARE In addition to general preoperative care, the following points are important in planning preoperative care for clients facing adrenalectomy. The environment should be organized to provide maximum physical and emotional rest for the client. Be aware of the effect of hyperadrenocorticolism on the emotions and provide support and reassurance to the client and family during periods when the client is emotionally labile. Monitor the client for any symptoms and signs of infection, and report these promptly to the physician.

Check the client's blood pressure and vital signs at regular intervals, especially if the client has a pheochromocytoma. Report any marked elevations of the blood pressure to the physician. Check body weight and edema at least daily.

Check serum electrolytes and urinary glucose and acetone levels at regular intervals to screen for hypokalemia and hyperglycemia. All fluid and electrolyte imbalances must be recognized and corrected in the preoperative period because of the profound physiologic changes in the postoperative period. Measure the client's intake and output and weigh the client daily to assess the degree of fluid retention. The potassium-depleted client may receive a solution of potassium chloride. If the client is anemic, transfusion with whole blood or packed cells may be ordered.

Diet in the preoperative period involves a high-protein diet for protein depletion, reduced carbohydrates and calo-

Table 34–3
Adrenalectomy: Implications for the Client 

Physiologic Implications	Psychosocial/Lifestyle Implications
Loss of adrenocortical hormones in pro-proportion to the amount of tissue removed; causes profound physiologic changes Lifelong glucocorticoid and mineralocorticoid replacement after bilateral adrenalectomy In unilateral adrenalectomy, cortisol administration during and after surgery, with gradual adjustment of the dosage until remaining adrenal function is adequate In immediate postoperative period, possible acute adrenal insufficiency or adrenal crisis precipitated by stress	Great effect on psychologic status and lifestyle from the loss of adrenocortical hormones Possible need to arrange life and activities to avoid emotional crises, infections, overfatigue, and extremes of temperature Possible occupational change to avoid stress, because stress may precipitate an adrenal crisis Lifetime medical supervision Dependency on medication and the need to know medication regimen, including the name of the drug, dose, frequency, and side effects Need to watch for the symptoms and signs of medication overdose or hyperadrenocorticolism and underdose, or adrenal insufficiency

ries for hyperglycemia, restrictions of salt intake for hypertension and fluid retention, and increased potassium intake for hypokalemia. An ulcer also requires special dietary planning. In addition, the client with excessive hyperadrenocorticolism may have protein depletion (hypoproteinemia) reflected by a low serum albumin level.

In the immediate preoperative period, an in-dwelling catheter is usually inserted, as well as a nasogastric (NG) tube to reduce vomiting and abdominal distention postoperatively. Corticosteroids are administered preoperatively as well as during surgery to prevent adrenal insufficiency in the postoperative period. Intravenous fluids are usually started and infused slowly to allow prompt administration of corticosteroids and vasopressors if needed.

Because both the transabdominal and lateral approaches involve incisions close to the diaphragm, the client's postoperative respirations tend to be shallow, and coughing is extremely uncomfortable. Therefore, one of the most important preoperative responsibilities of the nurse is to teach clients what to expect and how best to breathe deeply and cough postoperatively (using a pillow to support the incision).

POSTOPERATIVE CARE Postoperative nursing care of the client following adrenalectomy includes frequent monitoring of the vital signs, including LOC and especially blood pressure, for at least the first 48 hours after surgery. Blood pressure is monitored every 15 minutes in the immediate postoperative period until it is stabilized. The client may also have central venous pressure monitoring. Report any unexplained or significant fall in blood pressure to the physician, because it may indicate hypotension caused by the rapid withdrawal of mineralocorticoids and impending adrenal insufficiency. Any complaints of chest pain should also be reported immediately, because they may indicate cardiac involvement or a pulmonary embolus.

Monitor blood chemistry reports and fluid balance regularly until they are stabilized. Serum sodium, potassium, and glucose levels are obtained and possibly, urine sodium levels. Carefully record intake and output, and promptly report any imbalances. In the acute postoperative phase, the client's urinary output is measured hourly. Be alert for symptoms and signs of renal shutdown, such as oliguria, anuria, and increasing BUN and creatinine levels.

Monitor the client for symptoms and signs of adrenal crisis. Adrenal crisis is an emergency and requires prompt intervention with increased corticosteroids, hypertonic saline solutions, or both.

The client may remain on bed rest for 2 to 3 days until the vital signs are stabilized. To prevent complications of immobility, change the client's position and encourage coughing and deep breathing every 2 hours. An NG tube prevents postoperative vomiting and minimizes abdominal distention. After the NG tube is removed, the client progresses to a diet as tolerated.

Administration of corticosteroids is continued by IV infusion until the client is able to tolerate oral doses of cortisol. In some instances, IM injections of desoxycorticosterone may be administered but are usually replaced by oral cortisol when the client can tolerate it. Be alert for symptoms and signs of hyperadrenocorticolism and adrenal insufficiency and report them promptly. When the IV corticosteroids have been discontinued, the IV may be kept open until the client is completely stable. This precaution provides a quick route for the administration of corticosteroids or a vasopressor as needed.

SPECIAL POSTOPERATIVE CONSIDERATIONS WITH PHEOCHROMOCYTOMAS If an adrenalectomy was done because of pheochromocytoma, there are important nursing considerations other than the usual postoperative care. Clients with a pheochromocytoma may require a longer period for their blood pressure to become stabilized than other post-adrenalectomy clients.

Be alert for any sudden elevations of blood pressure in the early postoperative period, which may occur because of the release of epinephrine and norepinephrine from the tumor as it was being excised. Phentolamine or another adrenergic blocking agent may be used intravenously if the blood pressure rises excessively. Severe hypotension may also develop postoperatively in these clients. If untreated, this can lead to shock. Metaraminol bitartrate (Aramine) and norepinephrine bitartrate (Levophed), usually given via IV infusion, may be used to stabilize the blood pressure. The dosage of these vasopressors is titrated to the client's blood pressure. Therefore, accuracy is essential in measuring the blood pressure, as well as in regulating the flow rate of the infusion. The physician prescribes the rate of flow.

Advise all clients with pheochromocytomas to change positions slowly to avoid symptoms of orthostatic hypotension. When the head of the bed is elevated, check the blood pressure to assess the result of position change. Blood pressure is also closely monitored when the client is first allowed out of bed. If a significant drop occurs, the client is placed back on bed rest in a supine position. Elastic stockings may be ordered to prevent pooling of blood in the extremities.

Client/Family Teaching

DISCHARGE PLANNING Clients who have had a bilateral adrenalectomy should understand the significance of the procedure and the fact that hormonal replacement therapy is required for the rest of their lives. They must remain under close medical supervision and should know the indications of adrenal crisis and how it can be precipitated by infection or severe stress. Clients also should be aware of the symptoms and signs of corticosteroid overdose (edema, weakness, hypertension, and hirsutism) and the need to report them to the physician. Those who had hyperadrenocorticolism before surgery should know that these symptoms will slowly subside. Because cortisone tends to mask the symptoms of infection, and adrenalectomy clients are more susceptible to infection, they should be instructed in the subtle signs of illness and encouraged to keep their resistance up and avoid infection whenever possible. They should report early signs of infection immediately to the physician because of the danger of adrenal crisis.

Clients who have a subtotal adrenalectomy should be given the same instructions. They may not need lifelong hormonal replacement but will require careful observation for several months to determine when the remaining adrenal tissue can meet the body's demand. In the meantime, these clients are also at risk for potential adrenal crisis and should be advised to avoid infection, stress, overfatigue, and extremes of temperature. Help clients understand the symptoms and signs of adrenal insufficiency and hyperadrenocorticolism and the importance of reporting them to the physician.

One of the most important nursing responsibilities in discharge planning is to emphasize the need for continued medical care. Emergency medical tags or bracelets will protect clients in emergency situations when they may be unable to communicate. Counsel clients about resuming activities slowly. The proper amount of hormonal replacement may take several months to achieve, and clients should expect frequent dosage readjustments. Many clients who begin corticosteroid therapy will experience a transient insomnia for the first 2 to 3 weeks, but it usually is resolved without treatment. Tell clients who have had an adrenalectomy because of a pheochromocytoma that their blood pressure may not stabilize within an acceptable range for up to 3 months.

Although corticosteroid therapy has been discussed in relation to adrenal and pituitary surgery, it is important to remember that any surgical client could be receiving corticosteroids for a variety of reasons. Box 34–4 reviews the important nursing considerations for any surgical client receiving corticosteroids.

Box 34–4
Influence of Corticosteroids on Any Surgical Client

The nurse caring for any surgical client receiving corticosteroids should be aware of several important facts. Corticosteroids may be given as replacement therapy (in Addison's disease, hypopituitarism, bilateral adrenalectomy), as well as therapeutically for collagen diseases (rheumatoid arthritis, lupus erythematosus, scleroderma, and periarteritis nodosa). They are also used selectively to treat asthma, iritis, and thrombocytopenic purpura. Clients who have received corticosteroid therapy for long periods usually experience a medically induced adrenal insufficiency because of the suppression of pituitary ACTH. The return of normal pituitary and adrenal function following prolonged therapy may take up to 1 year, and during this period the client must be protected by corticosteroids, especially if surgery is necessary.

Surgical candidates receiving corticosteroid therapy should have the dosage of their steroids increased before and during surgery to meet the increased demands of the anesthetic and surgical procedure. If this is not done, acute adrenal insufficiency may result.

Possible complications of corticosteroid therapy for the surgical client are:

- Exacerbation of peptic ulcer (eg, increased bleeding)
- Reactivation of latent tuberculosis
- Cardiac failure
- Increased incidence of fulminating infections

In addition, the client may develop other side effects of corticosteroid therapy such as osteoporosis, hirsutism, psychosis, and acne.

Addison's Disease

Adrenocortical insufficiency may be primary (Addison's disease) or secondary. The primary type arises from pathology occurring within the gland itself; the secondary type arises from pathology of the pituitary or hypothalamus or is iatrogenic. Primary adrenal insufficiency is characterized by insufficient production of all three adrenal hormones. The physiologic manifestations are those of deficiency of the glucocorticoids and mineralocorticoids. (The adrenals are only a secondary source of the sex hormones, so deficiencies of adrenally produced hormones tend to be compensated for by normal ovarian or testicular function.)

It is important to remember that a major difference between primary and secondary causes of adrenal hypofunction is that secondary failure is not usually associated with a marked deficiency of aldosterone. Another differentiating feature is that hyperpigmentation of the skin is only seen in primary adrenal insufficiency. Increased serum levels of ACTH, which is structurally similar to melanocyte-stimulating hormone (MSH), are thought to cause the increased skin tone found in scars, areolae, and skin folds.

CLINICAL MANIFESTATIONS The symptoms and signs of Addison's disease relate directly to the effect of reduced circulating levels of glucocorticoids and mineralocorticoids. Symptoms may appear slowly or as an acute crisis precipitated by stress.

The addisonian client loses sodium in the urine as the distal renal tubules lose the ability to exchange sodium for potassium. This causes hypovolemia and hypotension, which result in decreased renal perfusion and elevated BUN levels as well as hyperkalemia from the retention of potassium. The deficiency of plasma cortisol inhibits the secretion of certain gastrointestinal enzymes; hence, clients with Addison's disease may experience diarrhea, vomiting, anorexia, and abdominal pain, all of which further decrease fluid levels and thus aggravate the hypovolemia and hypotension. Generalized weakness, decreased physical endurance, changes in mental acuity, and weight loss are consistently seen in clients with Addison's disease.

Hypoglycemia occurs in about 50% of the clients diagnosed with adrenal insufficiency. Deficiencies in circulating cortisol cause a decrease in gluconeogenesis by the liver and increased uptake of glucose by the tissues.

ADRENAL CRISIS Some clients with adrenal insufficiency who experience sudden physical or emotional stress or who do not follow their medication regimen may develop an acute and sometimes fatal state of circulatory collapse. Known as adrenal crisis or addisonian crisis, this is characterized by:

- Severe hypotension (the most prominent feature)
- Confusion progressing to coma
- Nausea and vomiting
- Abdominal cramping and diarrhea
- Cyanosis and fever

The symptoms and signs of adrenal crisis are simply the exaggerated symptoms and signs of the disorder. Adrenal crisis is an emergency that requires immediate medical and nursing intervention. Adrenal crisis can also occur following pituitary or adrenal surgery or after trauma to or hemorrhage into the adrenal cortices.

Tests used in establishing the diagnosis of adrenal hypofunction and their implications are discussed in Chapter 31. Briefly, serum cortisol and metyrapone tests are used for screening. For more definitive results, serum ACTH is measured, or the ACTH stimulation test is used.

MEDICAL MEASURES Replacement therapy is the usual treatment for adrenal insufficiency. During periods of physical or emotional stress, shock, or surgery, addisonian clients need careful monitoring of glucocorticoid administration and fluid balance.

SPECIFIC NURSING MEASURES Nurses are actively involved in both the chronic and acute care of clients with adrenal insufficiency. For clients with chronic disease:

- Assess blood pressure, apical–radial pulse, and respirations because addisonian clients are subject to hypotension, especially orthostatic hypotension due to sodium depletion.
- Monitor body weight. Weight loss with adrenal insufficiency is related to gastrointestinal disturbance. Clients should be encouraged to eat a well-balanced, high-protein, high-calorie diet with meals at regular intervals and snacks as required. Advise the client that fasting might precipitate adrenal crisis.
- Assess clients for generalized weakness and malaise. The hyperkalemia, hyponatremia, and loss of the normal diurnal variation in cortisol that accompany Addison's disease may give rise to increased muscular cramping and cardiac dysrhythmias. Clients should be counseled to plan several rest periods during the day to avoid fatigue.
- Avoid clients for possible hypoglycemic symptoms (weakness, diaphoresis, lightheadedness, abdominal cramps). Addisonian clients are highly susceptible to hypoglycemia.
- Assess clients' mental status and ability to tolerate physical activity, because this is affected by depletion of the adrenal hormones.
- Assess clients for symptoms and signs of infection. Counsel clients to call their physician at the first sign of infection. Infection places the body under stress and can precipitate adrenal crisis.
- Screen clients with a tuberculin skin test such as the Mantoux test and/or a chest x-ray before the initiation of steroid therapy. Clients on corticosteroid therapy are considered at high risk for acquiring tuberculosis.
- Teach clients and their significant others the nature of the disorder, its prognosis, and the need for lifelong regular medical treatment and supervision.
- Teach the importance of wearing a Medic-Alert tag and carrying an emergency kit with a syringe filled with 100 mg of hydrocortisone and instructions for use.
- Teach clients and significant others to recognize the symptoms and signs of impending adrenal crisis and of steroid overdosage.
- Teach the importance of maintaining a proper diet to avoid precipitating adrenal crisis.
- Teach the importance of rest periods to avoid fatigue and the need to change position slowly if experiencing vertigo or syncope due to postural hypotension.

The nurse may also be called on to care for clients in adrenal or addisonian crisis. This is an emergency requiring prompt intervention and careful assessment. The immediate goal of medical treatment is to reverse the symptoms of acute deficiency of the adrenal steroids (ie, severe hypotension, vasomotor collapse, and hyperkalemia).

Nurses caring for a client in an adrenal crisis should:

- Monitor blood pressure, apical–radial pulse, respirations, and temperature q. 15 min during the acute phase.
- Administer intravenous fluids and IV and IM medications as ordered.
- Measure fluid intake and output every hour or as ordered.
- Be alert for symptoms and signs of worsening crisis.
- Administer oxygen or plasma as ordered.
- Support the client and family or friends; provide an environment free from additional physical or emotional stressors.
- Attempt to discover what factors (eg, emotional upset, infection, or missed medication dose) might have precipitated the crisis.

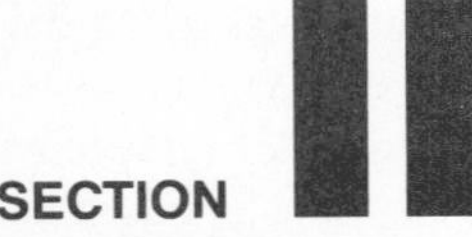

Neoplastic and Obstructive Disorders

Neoplastic and obstructive disorders of the pituitary include gigantism, acromegaly, and Cushing's disease. Adrenal disorders in this category are aldosteronism and pheochromocytoma.

Pituitary Disorders

Gigantism and Acromegaly

Increased secretion of somatotropin by the anterior pituitary results in gigantism (before puberty) or acromegaly (after puberty). The term *acromegaly* refers to enlargement of the acral parts—head, hands, and feet. The crucial factor is the time onset of the disorder. If the hypersecretion of growth hormone occurs during the individual's growth period before the epiphyses of the long bones have closed, gigantism will occur. Acromegaly occurs after epiphyseal closure.

Acromegaly usually starts between the ages of 20 and 50. Physical changes depend on the amount of hormone oversecretion and the age at which the disorder begins. Acromegaly usually develops slowly and insidiously. The disorder is characterized by coarsening of the facial features, enlargement of the extremities, and a high incidence of impaired glucose metabolism. Individuals may also experience impaired vision.

Gigantism starts in infancy or childhood and is characterized by continuous growth of the body until epiphyseal closure occurs. Gigantism in adults is defined as a height over 80 in. Pituitary giants may be as tall as 8 ft (240 cm) and may weigh more than 300 lb (135 kg) (Kaye & Rose, 1983). Individuals with gigantism may develop some associated acromegalic features—very large hands and feet—in adult life (Muthe, 1981).

Both acromegaly and gigantism are traceable to an autonomous hypersecretion of somatotropin caused by an anterior pituitary tumor, usually an eosinophilic adenoma. Eosinophilic adenomas are usually benign; however, they secrete excessive amounts of somatotropin and prolactin, which may create pressure in the brain, causing visual symptoms and headache.

CLINICAL MANIFESTATIONS OF GIGANTISM Clients with gigantism usually live about 20 years. They are subject to a general debilitation, which is progressive, and are likely to die as the result of pituitary failure leading to adrenal cortical insufficiency.

Objective findings include:

- Extremely large size
- Enlargement of the heart, liver, spleen, kidneys, pancreas, thyroid, parathyroids, adrenals, soft tissues, and peripheral nerves
- Increased metabolic rate
- Incomplete or slow development of secondary sex characteristics
- Glucose intolerance with resulting hyperglycemia and diabetes mellitus
- Possible excess secretion of other anterior pituitary hormones (prolactin, MSH, ACTH, TSH)

Advanced signs include extreme muscular weakness and crippling osteoarthritis, which may be associated with a severe kyphosis.

The symptoms of gigantism are usually attributable to the effects of compression of the adjacent tissues by the tumor or by metabolic changes. Symptoms include headache, which may be mild to severe and may be persistent; **bitemporal hemianopia** and other visual field defects (eg, changes in color perception and diplopia) because of pressure in the optic chiasm; and seizures and stroke due to increased intracranial pressure.

CLINICAL MANIFESTATIONS OF ACROMEGALY Clients with acromegaly do not grow especially tall because onset occurs after puberty. However, the hypersecretion of somatotropin stimulates all tissues of the body—including the soft tissues, organs, and bones—to grow wider and thicker. The term *acromegaly* refers to abnormal enlargement of the extremities. The bones formed by intramembranous ossification continue to grow, leading to enlargement of the skull (especially the forehead), jaw, and supraorbital ridges.

The course of the disease varies among individuals: It may be slowly progressive, or it may cause death only a few years after onset. In some instances, progressive increases in the size of the tumor may result in generalized hypopituitarism. Symptoms and signs are due to the pituitary tumor or the excess GH circulating in the plasma.

During the health history, clients may reveal a variety of symptoms. They may report mild to severe persistent headache. Visual changes can include diplopia, changes in visual acuity and color perception, and loss of field of vision. Clients may note an increase in hat, glove, ring, or shoe size over the past year or a change in facial appearance. Clients may complain of paresthesia or arthralgia. Hyperhidrosis (excess sweating) may occur, which can be associated with a disagreeable odor during an active phase of the disorder. Clients may report symptoms related to either hypersecretion or deficiency of the other anterior pituitary hormones (eg, in late stages, clients may have loss of libido or amenorrhea). Because of the diabetogenic effect of GH, symptoms of diabetes mellitus—polydipsia, polyuria, polyphagia, and weight loss—appear. The voice may become deeper as a result of hypertrophy of the larynx.

Objective findings include the characteristic changes in facial appearance: The mandible lengthens, thickens, and protrudes (**prognathism**); spaces between the teeth and overbite may develop; the forehead becomes more prominent; the orbital ridge thickens; the soft tissues of the nose, tongue, ears, and lips become enlarged. The skin appears rough and leathery. The pores become increasingly visible as the amount of connective tissue increases. The amount of body hair and skin pigmentation may increase. The hands and the feet become enlarged; fingers assume a spadelike configuration. Thoracic circumference increases secondary to changes in the costal cartilages. Kyphosis often develops.

In addition to these visible external findings, the disorder produces internal changes such as visceromegaly of the heart, liver, kidneys, spleen, and pancreas; enlargement of the thyroid, parathyroid, and adrenal glands; and joint pathology. Osteoporosis due to loss of calcium may develop in the vertebrae. Hypertension is common, although the exact mechanism is unknown.

The diagnostic measures used to evaluate anterior pituitary dysfunction are discussed in Chapter 31. In general, the history and the physical findings form the basis for the diagnosis of gigantism and/or acromegaly. The laboratory measures simply confirm the diagnosis. Some changes may be noted on x-ray (eg, the sella turcica in 90% of clients with acromegaly will be enlarged).

Clients should be carefully evaluated for any visual field defects. Although the typical presentation is bitemporal hemianopia, other changes in vision may be present as well.

MEDICAL MEASURES Because the usual cause of gigantism or acromegaly is a tumor of the anterior pituitary, the main therapeutic measure is destruction of the tumor by either surgery or radiation. The two major surgical approaches to pituitary tumors are transfrontal craniotomy (transcranial subfrontal hypophysectomy) and transsphenoidal hypophysectomy. These two procedures, their indications, and nursing care are discussed following Cushing's Disease, below. Transsphenoidal hypophysectomy is the treatment of choice for a client with active acromegaly. Somatotropin levels will drop a few minutes after resection of the tumor; over a period of months, soft tissues regress, and the client loses weight and feels less arthritic pain (Muthe, 1981).

Irradiation of the tumor either externally or internally can be used to control the activity of the disease. Conventional high-voltage irradiation has been found to be successful in more than half of the clients treated. High-energy particle radiation, delivered by a cyclotron, requires expert techniques and is applicable only in situations where the tumor is confined to the sella turcica (Kaye & Rose, 1983).

The use of medications in the treatment of gigantism and acromegaly is still being researched. Research centers on agents that will block the release of GH from the tumor. Currently under investigation for clients with acromegaly is a dopaminergic agent, bromocriptine, which has been useful in clients who have received conventional radiotherapy and are waiting for the effects to appear (Kaye & Rose, 1983). A GH release-inhibitor hormone in the hypothalamus has been identified and has been found to act on the anterior pituitary to decrease the output of somatotropin. Its possibilities for therapeutic use are still being evaluated. The use of serotonin receptor antagonists to suppress GH levels in clients with acromegaly is also under investigation.

SPECIFIC NURSING MEASURES Nursing care of the client with acromegaly and gigantism varies with the client's symptoms. Because early recognition and treatment can help reduce the extent of pathologic change, the importance of a thorough history and careful physical assessment cannot be overemphasized. Height, body weight, and length of extremities should be carefully observed and recorded, then compared to growth tables. Any abnormal results in a child or an adult should be reported to the physician for further evaluation. These baseline data also serve as a check on progress after treatment is begun.

Monitor clients for weight loss and for constipation or anorexia, which are common with pituitary dysfunction. Clients may require a high-fiber, high-calorie diet to meet hypermetabolic requirements. Those who are anorexic need smaller, more frequent meals and should be weighed daily. Carefully measure intake and output. Monitor clients for symptoms and signs of diabetes mellitus.

If clients become weaker or increasingly lethargic, help them plan daily activities to alternate periods of rest and activity. Also encourage a slower pace of activities and help with personal care as needed.

Client/Family Teaching

One of the nurse's most important functions is to teach clients about their condition and to allow for client questions. Clients should be made aware of the significance of taking periodic body measurements and accurately recording the results. Because diabetes mellitus can be a complication of both gigantism and acromegaly, instruct clients in its symptoms and signs and teach them to check the urine for glucose. The importance of periodic fasting blood-sugar levels should also be discussed.

Clients should know the symptoms and signs of recurring or expanding tumor. In particular, they should report immediately any changes in vision, any increase in severity or frequency of headaches, or any increasing lethargy or weakness.

Clients receiving medications should be familiar with names, dosages, actions, and side effects. Teach clients the symptoms and signs of overdosage and underdosage and when and what to report to the physician. If there are any special instructions regarding sick days, clients should receive a written copy of these "sick-day rules" and should become thoroughly familiar with them. Sick-day rules are simply instructions for clients to use if they become ill. The instructions are another tool to promote self-care and independence. In addition, clients should be encouraged to wear a Medic-Alert tag or carry a wallet card describing the condition and their medications.

Provide opportunities for clients to discuss and ask questions about the changes in their physical appearance. The child with gigantism or the adult with acromegaly needs to know not only the reason for the changes in physical appearance but what might occur in the future. The physical changes seen in gigantism and acromegaly often cause suffering. Clients must deal with a major change in body image that may threaten their self-esteem.

Provide opportunity for clients to express their feelings about changes in libido, impotence, or the consequences of amenorrhea. Often, nurses, because of their interactions with clients and families over time, are in a position to help clients verbalize and explore their feelings about what is happening to them. Changes in sexual ability and loss of fertility are important concerns to clients and their significant others; these problems should be considered as important as any others in formulating the nursing care plan.

The importance and purpose of ongoing medical supervision and evaluation should be discussed with both client and significant others. They all should be aware of the diagnosis, the symptoms and signs of the condition, and the objectives of the treatment plan.

Cushing's Disease

Hypersecretion of ACTH by the anterior pituitary results in increased stimulation to the adrenal cortex. This causes excessive secretion of glucocorticoids by the adrenal cortex, which in turn produces the characteristic cushingoid features: moon face, truncal obesity, decreased glucose tolerance, supraclavicular fat pads, abdominal striae, abnormal skin pigmentation, and pendulous fat pad in chest and abdomen. This condition is known as Cushing's disease, or pituitary-dependent or secondary Cushing's syndrome, and is characterized by excessive secretion of ACTH, hyperplasia of both adrenal glands, and overproduction of cortisol. If the excessive secretion of glucocorticoids is due to a primary adrenal disorder, as explained earlier in this chapter, the condition is known as Cushing's syndrome.

CLINICAL MANIFESTATIONS The clinical manifestations and diagnostic procedures for all clients with a cushingoid presentation are the same. Refer to the discussion of Cushing's syndrome earlier in this chapter.

MEDICAL AND SPECIFIC NURSING MEASURES The treatment of choice in pituitary-dependent Cushing's disease is destruction of the tumor. The medical measures, surgical measures, and specific nursing measures are the same as those discussed for clients with acromegaly.

Hypophysectomy

Hypophysectomy may involve the resection of a small tumor of the pituitary gland or the complete removal of the gland. The major indications for hypophysectomy are a primary neoplasm of the pituitary gland (adenoma) or the need to retard the growth and spread of such endocrine-dependent malignancies as cancer of the breast, ovary, and prostate. In the last instance, hypophysectomy does not cure the disease but simply removes the source of the gonadotropic hormones that support the neoplasm. This may provide a remission for several months. Hypophysectomy also can be used to relieve pain in these malignancies.

Pituitary ablation has been achieved by external radiation therapy or by using a radioactive implant; by surgical destruction using stereotactic cryosurgery (freezing); or by surgical excision via a transfrontal craniotomy, or a transssphenoidal hypophysectomy. Whether radiation, surgery, or drugs are used depends on the type and amount of hormonal dysfunction, the size of the tumor, and whether it extends outside the sella turcica.

A transfrontal craniotomy is indicated when the tumor extends beyond the pituitary fossa and is impinging on the optic chiasm, because this procedure provides the best view of the operative field. If the tumor does not extend beyond the sella turcica, the surgeon may use a transsphenoidal approach, employing an operating microscope and televised radiofluoroscopy. Because it causes minimal damage to healthy tissue, the transsphenoidal approach has become the procedure of choice.

During a transsphenoidal hypophysectomy, the sella turcica is entered by way of the sphenoidal sinus cavity. The initial incision is a horizontal one made in the gingivae over the maxillary bone, so there is no external incision. Intracranial manipulation is confined to the sella turcica and the area immediately above it. Following surgery, the nasal cavities are usually packed for 48 to 72 hours with petrolatum gauze impregnated with an antibiotic ointment. A gauze sling may be placed under the nasal cavities to absorb secretions. The physiologic and psychosocial/lifestyle implications are discussed in Table 34–4.

Nursing Implications

PREOPERATIVE CARE The preoperative preparation of the client for a transsphenoidal hypophysectomy is similar to that for a transfrontal craniotomy, except the removal of scalp hair is not required. It is important to establish a supportive relationship with the client and significant others, because they may be extremely anxious.

The client and family should understand the need for lifetime hormonal replacement following hypophysectomy. Clients should be informed that in the immediate postoperative period, they will receive IV fluids and nutrients, and the nurse will frequently check their temperature, blood pressure, pulse, and respirations. Clients also should be

Table 34–4
Transsphenoidal Hypophysectomy: Implications for the Client

Physiologic Implications	Psychosocial/Lifestyle Implications
In the client with metastatic disease, relief of bone pain is achieved and further metastases may be arrested or slowed	Following hypophysectomy the lifelong dependency on steroids and hormonal replacement requires lifestyle modification, becomes a financial burden, and may be cause for anxiety
In clients with acromegaly further bony growth will be arrested and a substantial reduction in soft tissue swelling can be expected	For the client with metastatic disease, lifestyle is greatly enhanced by relief of pain and freedom from potent analgesics
Surgical risks are related to the proximity of the optic nerves and chiasm, the carotid arteries, cavernous sinuses, and hypothalamus	For the client with acromegaly, surgery has a positive effect because the gradual but often remarkable improvement in appearance enhances body image; relief of associated symptoms allows for a more normal lifestyle
Visual deterioration or loss can result from direct injury to the optic chiasm, optic nerves, or from compromise to their blood supply	For the client with visual impairment there may be no significant improvement; occasionally vision may be further impaired, requiring significant alterations in lifestyle
Injury to the hypothalamus may occur with radical excision of large suprasella lesions	Sexual dysfunction (infertility, impotence, cessation of menstruation, decreased libido) may cause considerable stress, altered body image, and lowered self-esteem
CSF leaks may be transient after nasal packings are removed	
Diabetes insipidus may occur	

told that their eyes may be ecchymotic and that a nasal drip pad will be used for drainage from the nose.

A corticosteroid preparation is given 1 day before surgery and on the day of surgery to avoid adrenal insufficiency secondary to the removal of the source of ACTH. An in-dwelling catheter may be inserted to enable frequent, accurate determination of postoperative urinary output, which is important in determining the need for ADH replacement. Before surgery, an IV cannula is inserted, and an infusion is started.

Closely monitor clients with diagnosed pituitary tumors for symptoms and signs of *pituitary apoplexy,* which include severe headache, changes in level of consciousness (LOC), diplopia, loss of vision, and shock. Pituitary apoplexy occurs when there is spontaneous hemorrhage into the tumor secondary to rupture of the blood vessels or rapid enlargement of the adenoma with resulting infarction. It is an emergency requiring immediate intervention.

POSTOPERATIVE CARE The postoperative care of a client with a transfrontal craniotomy approach is similar to that for other clients with craniotomies. In addition, observe the client closely for signs of adrenal insufficiency and signs of hypothyroidism (which may develop over several weeks).

Following transsphenoidal hypophysectomy, observe the client closely for leaking of cerebrospinal fluid (CSF) through the nares. This can be differentiated from the normal nasal secretions by special CSF testing materials or a test strip for glucose. Glucose is found only in CSF, not in nasal secretions. Report positive glucose test results to the physician. Place the client on bed rest with the head of the bed elevated to 30° to decrease pressure on the sella turcica.

Most clients recover rapidly from transsphenoidal surgery and are allowed out of bed within 24 hours. Fluids are taken orally the evening of surgery, and the diet is increased as tolerated.

Because of the nasal packs, the client is forced to breathe through the mouth and may report a temporary loss of smell. Oral hygiene—rinsing the mouth with saline or clear water—is important to keep the oral mucosa moist. Brushing the teeth is usually contraindicated because of possible tension on the suture line. The nasal packs are usually removed in 48 to 72 hours. The client may be placed on prophylactic antibiotic therapy in either the preoperative or postoperative period because of the increased danger of infection using the transsphenoidal approach.

Headache may be a problem in the postoperative period and should be reported to the physician immediately because of the danger of meningitis. Headache is usually treated with non-narcotic analgesics or codeine. Because codeine tends to be constipating, carefully monitor the client's bowel status to prevent straining at stool and increased ICP. If analgesics are used, carefully assess the client's LOC and do a neurologic evaluation to monitor the client's progress.

A major complication in the postoperative period is hypopituitarism, which may develop into addisonian crisis and transient or permanent diabetes insipidus. Therefore, observe the client closely for symptoms and signs of addisonian crisis and diabetes insipidus. In the immediate postoperative period, carefully measure the intake and output of all clients as a guide to fluid balance; check the specific gravity of urine after each voiding.

The usual medication regimen is to administer a cortisone preparation preoperatively and continue it intravenously until the client can tolerate an oral dose. This dose is gradually adjusted until a maintenance level is achieved, and a replacement dose of cortisone is continued for the rest of the client's life. In addition, the client may require replacement of thyroid and sex hormones (testosterone and estrogen). A few clients may require ADH to control polyuria. After a total ablation of the pituitary gland, menstruation ceases, and the client becomes infertile.

For men, testosterone may relieve changes in libido and impotence secondary to the surgery. Estrogen may be prescribed for women to relieve atrophy of the vaginal mucosa. Human pituitary gonadotropins have been successful in treating infertility in posthypophysectomy clients, especially women. Be sensitive to the effect of this type of surgery on reproductive capacity and functioning and provide ample opportunity for clients to express their thoughts and feelings. Appropriate referral for counseling has also proven beneficial for both the client and sexual partner.

DISCHARGE PLANNING Two important nursing responsibilities in the discharge of clients following hypophysectomy are instructions regarding (1) medications (cortisone, thyroxine, sex hormones, and ADH), including their purpose and side effects, and (2) the importance of regular follow-up care. The client should also know the proper administration of these hormones, the symptoms and signs of hormonal imbalance, and circumstances under which the physician should be contacted.

Adrenal Disorders

Aldosteronism

Primary aldosteronism, or Conn's syndrome, a condition caused by excessive production of aldosterone by the adrenal cortex, is characterized by hypertension, excessive urinary loss of potassium, and retention of sodium. Primary aldosteronism is thought to be the cause of hypertension in 1% to 2% of all clients with diagnosed hypertension. This is one form of hypertension that is completely curable. Primary aldosteronism originates from one of three sources (Kaye & Rose, 1983): a single adrenocortical tumor (generally a benign adenoma), bilateral hyperplasia of the adrenal cortices, and tumor of the juxtaglomerular (JG) cells of the kidney, which produce renin autonomously. (A secondary form of aldosteronism occurs when increased renal secretion of renin leads to the increased production of aldosterone. The increased renin secretion results from other pathologic processes in the body, such as heart failure, nephrosis, and cirrhosis. The production of aldosterone it triggers in turn initiates a cycle of pathologic changes, resulting in increased fluid retention, further compromising cardiac and hepatic function.)

CLINICAL MANIFESTATIONS The major clinical manifestations of primary aldosteronism are hypertension, excessive urinary loss of potassium resulting in hypokalemia, and retention of sodium (hypernatremia). The hypertension in clients with primary aldosteronism is usually a moderate elevation of the diastolic blood pressure. The client may complain of headaches. On physical examination, early hypertensive retinopathy and cardiomegaly may be noted.

The symptoms attributable to hypokalemia range from mild fatigue to profound weakness. The client may complain of paresthesia, loss of stamina, muscular weakness, and intermittent periods of paralysis. If hypokalemic alkalosis occurs, resulting in tetany, physical examination may elicit positive Trousseau's and Chvostek's signs.

Because of the increased reabsorption of sodium and water, hypernatremia and hypervolemia occur. Generally, edema is not present. The hematocrit may appear abnormally low as a result of the hemodilution. In addition to these major clinical signs, the client with primary aldosteronism may also have severe polydipsia, polyuria, and nocturia resulting from the renal tubules' inability to respond to ADH.

Primary aldosteronism should be suspected in all clients with hypertension, particularly the young. The finding of hypertension, hypokalemia (below 3.5 mEq/L), and excessive mineralocorticoid production (ie, increased serum aldosterone levels) suggest the diagnosis. These findings become more significant if an excessive excretion of urinary potassium is found along with increased serum levels of sodium (hypernatremia) and decreased excretion of urinary sodium.

A spironolactone test may be used in conjunction with determination of serum potassium levels. Other tests to evaluate clients with primary aldosteronism are discussed in Chapter 31.

To localize an aldosterone-producing adenoma before surgery, various techniques may be used. Noninvasive procedures such as nuclear scanning with ^{131}I-19-iodocholesterol, computerized tomography (CT) scanning, and ultrasonography may be employed as well as invasive procedures such as arteriography and retrograde adrenal venography.

MEDICAL MEASURES The two forms of therapy for primary aldosteronism are surgery and drug therapy. Surgery is indicated when there is a unilateral aldosterone-producing tumor. In cases of hyperplasia, a subtotal or total adrenalectomy may be performed. Spironolactone, an aldosterone antagonist, may be given orally over short periods if surgery is contraindicated. Triamterene may also be used.

SPECIFIC NURSING MEASURES The nursing care of clients with primary aldosteronism should include daily weight monitoring and measurement of intake and output to assess degree of fluid retention and loss, as well as frequent assessment of blood pressure, pulse, and respiratory rate. Observe for symptoms and signs of cardiac decompensation and congestive heart failure and irregularities in heart rate and rhythm.

Assess the client for hypokalemia, muscle weakness, cramping, fatigue, and skin breakdown. Also evaluate the client for paresthesia and tetany (related to low serum calcium levels resulting from hypokalemic alkalosis). Provide for adequate rest because the client may have nocturia and may need a daytime nap to make up for lost sleep. The diet should be high in protein, low in sodium, and high in potassium. Calories may be restricted if weight reduction is desired. The preoperative and postoperative nursing care of clients undergoing adrenal surgery are discussed earlier in this chapter.

Client/Family Teaching

Instruct clients with primary aldosteronism on the nature of the disorder; the goals of the medical, surgical, and nursing treatment plan; and how those goals are to be implemented. If they are to be placed on medication, clients should be familiar with its purpose, action, dosage, administration, and side effects. They should know the essentials of their diet and should recognize the need for regular medical evaluation. Postsurgically, clients should be aware that normal endocrine function may take several months to return and that they may need medication during this period. Other clients may not require medications postsurgically or may require lifelong treatment.

Teach clients who are able to take their own blood pressure and pulse regularly, to interpret the findings, and when to report them to the physician. If clients are unable to monitor themselves, family members or friends should be taught to do so.

Pheochromocytoma

Pheochromocytomas are tumors composed of chromaffin cells. The tumors may be found in the adrenal medulla or, less frequently, in the sympathetic ganglia of the abdomen, bladder, or chest. Pheochromocytomas are usually benign and characteristically produce both catecholamines (epinephrine and norepinephrine), although some tumors may release only one of the catecholamines. Hypersecretion of epinephrine elevates the blood pressure by increasing the strength of contraction of the heart, resulting in an increase in cardiac output. Norepinephrine causes arteriolar vasoconstriction, increasing the peripheral vascular resistance to blood flow. Both of these effects result in the marked elevation of both diastolic and systolic blood pressures, which is characteristic of pheochromocytoma. Although clients find its symptoms frightening, pheochromocytoma has a good prognosis.

Pheochromocytomas are thought to occur more often than clinically recognized because they are difficult to diagnose. Pheochromocytomas may be present for varying amounts of time before symptoms occur. Tumors that produce primarily epinephrine are often associated with profuse diaphoresis, palpitations, tremor, anxiety, heat intolerance, and pallor followed by flushing. Tumors that produce primarily norepinephrine are associated with fewer symptoms; the symptoms are similar to those in clients with essential hypertension, hence the difficulty in diagnosis.

Most pheochromocytomas are benign, unilateral adrenal tumors. Men and women are equally affected; the peak incidence is in the fourth and fifth decades of life.

Both epinephrine- and norepinephrine-producing tumors may secrete catecholamines paroxysmally, episodically, or continuously. The most severe symptoms are usually seen in clients with the paroxysmally functioning tumors because of the rapid and marked changes in serum catecholamine levels. About 40% of clients with pheochromocytoma have paroxysmal hypertension, whereas the remainder experience either sustained or labile elevations in the blood pressure (Petersdorf et al., 1983).

The paroxysmal attacks vary in frequency, severity, and duration. Both the onset and resolution tend to be abrupt, with the average attack lasting a few minutes to a few hours. In many clients, these attacks may occur without warning, whereas others may be able to identify a prodrome of dermal paresthesia and increasing anxiety. Paroxysmal attacks are also precipitated by emotional changes, postural changes, and/or physical exertion. Attacks may increase in frequency and duration over time. These attacks may result in pulmonary edema, cerebral hemorrhage, or ventricular fibrillation and hence may be fatal.

CLINICAL MANIFESTATIONS Symptoms of pheochromocytoma include headache, diaphoresis, and intense palpitations. The client may also complain of extreme anxiety, tinnitus, excessive weakness and tremor, blurred vision, vertigo, dyspnea, and anginal chest pain. After the attack, the client may report a feeling of complete prostration.

Signs of pheochromocytoma include marked elevation of the diastolic and systolic blood pressure (which may rise as high as 200 to 300/150 to 175 mm Hg), often with excessive diaphoresis, anxiety, dilation of the pupils, and tachycardia. Orthostatic hypotension due to contraction of the blood volume and hypertensive retinopathy may occur in clients with persistently functioning tumors. Hyperglycemia and glycosuria are also frequently associated with pheochromocytoma because of catecholamine inhibition of insulin and elevation of plasma glucose levels (Blacklow, 1983).

Pheochromocytoma should always be suspected in hypertensive clients who have symptoms and signs of sympathetic hyperactivity, although fewer than 1% of all hypertension is from pheochromocytoma. The diagnosis of pheochromocytoma is based on the demonstration of excessive catecholamine levels in the serum and urine.

After excessive catecholamine secretion has been determined, studies are done to confirm the diagnosis and localize the tumor. Common methods are CT scans of the adrenal glands or radiologic studies such as the intravenous pyelogram with nephrotomograms, abdominal arteriograms, and selective venography.

MEDICAL MEASURES The definitive treatment for pheochromocytoma is surgical excision of the tumor. In the 10% of clients who are not surgical candidates (because of malignant pheochromocytoma with metastases or serious medical problems), control of symptoms is attempted with the use of alpha-adrenergic blocking agents such as phentolamine and phenoxybenzamine hydrochloride. Beta-adrenergic blocking agents may be used in clients with cardiac dysrhythmias or those not responsive to treatment with alpha-adrenergic agents. Clients with pheochromocytoma who are receiving beta-blocking agents should also be receiving alpha blockers to prevent the severe hypertension that can result from unopposed alpha stimulation (Camunas, 1983). Both alpha- and beta-blocking agents should be used with caution because clients can be exquisitely sensitive to them. The surgical approach to pheochromocytoma is discussed in the section on adrenalectomy earlier in this chapter.

SPECIFIC NURSING MEASURES The preoperative and postoperative nursing care for clients with pheochromocytoma is discussed in the section on adrenalectomy. In almost 10% of all clients with this tumor, precise localization of the tumor may not be possible before surgery, creating even more anxiety for the client. Hence, it is important to adopt a confident, supportive approach while ensuring that the client and family have an opportunity to discuss their fears and concerns.

Discharge planning should stress the need for lifelong medical supervision. In pheochromocytoma, there is a 10% to 13% chance of recurrence of the tumor, which may be malignant (Camunas, 1983).

The need for lifelong replacement therapy must be emphasized if a bilateral adrenalectomy has been performed or if the remaining tissue is nonfunctioning. Positive aspects of this disorder that can be stressed in client education are that it is a curable cause of hypertension and has a good prognosis.

Chapter Highlights

Diabetes insipidus is a disorder of water metabolism characterized by the excretion of excessively large amounts of hypotonic urine.

The syndrome of inappropriate antidiuretic hormone (SIADH) is characterized by autonomous release of ADH without regard to plasma osmolality. The body is unable to dilute the urine appropriately. The consequences are fluid retention, expansion of the extracellular fluid compartment, and hyponatremia.

Cushing's syndrome, also known as hypercortisolism, is characterized by an excessive level of cortisol in the plasma.

Adrenalectomy, the surgical removal or resection of one, a portion of one, or both adrenal glands, is performed primarily for hyperfunction secondary to a tumor or hyperplasia of the glands, pheochromocytoma, or advanced cancer of the breast and prostate.

Monitor the adrenalectomy client for symptoms and signs of adrenal insufficiency, hypotension (caused by the rapid withdrawal of mineralocorticoids), electrolyte imbalances, and infection (from suppression of the immune system).

Addison's disease, or primary adrenal insufficiency, is characterized by a deficiency of all three types of adrenal hormones. However, only the effects of deficiencies of the glucocorticoids and mineralocorticoids are usually seen.

Gigantism, defined as a height over 80 inches in an adult, is characterized by an increased secretion of somatotropin before puberty. If the excessive secretion of somatotropin occurs after puberty (ie, epiphyseal closure), the condition is called acromegaly.

Cushing's disease is a disorder characterized by hypersecretion of ACTH, resulting in increased stimulation to the adrenal cortex and excessive secretion of glucocorticoids.

Hypophysectomy, the surgical removal or resection of the pituitary gland, is performed primarily for a neoplasm of the pituitary or when an endocrine-dependent malignancy is present.

Hypophysectomy can be a threatening and anxiety-provoking surgery for clients and their significant others.

Pheochromocytoma is characterized by excessive secretion of the catecholamines (epinephrine and norepinephrine), which produces systolic and diastolic hypertension, profuse diaphoresis, and anxiety.

Pituitary and adrenal disorders, because of their visible physical effects, may cause clients great mental and emotional anguish. Clients often also have a disabling reduction in energy levels and ability to withstand stress. These conditions cause many problems and concerns for clients and their significant others.

Bibliography

Barber LR, Burton JR, Qieve PD (editors): *Principles of Ambulatory Medicine.* Baltimore: Williams & Wilkins, 1982.

Bentley PJ: *Endocrine Pharmacology: Physiologic Basis and Therapeutic Applications.* New York: Cambridge University Press, 1980.

Blacklow D: *MacBryde's Signs and Symptoms,* 6th ed. Philadelphia: Lippincott, 1983.

Bravo EL, Gifford RW Jr: Pheochromocytoma: Diagnosis, localization and management. *New Eng J Med* 1984; 311:1298.

Burch WA: A survey of results with transsphenoidal surgery in Cushing's disease (letter). *N Engl J Med* 1983; 308:103.

Burch WM: Cushing's disease: A review. *Arch Intern Med* 1985; 145:1106.

Burnett J: Congenital adrenocortical hyperplasia: Nursing interactions. *Am J Nurs* 1980; 80:1309–1311.

Camunas C: Pheochromocytoma. *Am J Nurs* 1983; 83(6):887–891.

Clark JB, Queener SF, Karb VB: *Pharmacological Basis of Nursing Practice.* St. Louis: Mosby, 1982.

Fode NC, Laus ER, Northartt RC: Pituitary tumors and hypertension: Implications for neurosurgical nurses. *J Neurosurg Nurs* 1983; 15(1):33–35.

Kaye D, Rose LF (editors): *Fundamentals of Internal Medicine.* St. Louis: Mosby, 1983.

Kruger LB: Complications of transsphenoidal surgery. *J Neurosurg Nurs* (June) 1985; 17:179–183.

Lee KJ, Goodrich I, Pensak M: Pituitary surgery: Current status including transsphenoidal surgery. *Am J Otolaryngol* 1984; 5:138–150.

Malseed RT: *Pharmacology: Drug Therapy and Nursing Considerations.* Philadelphia: Lippincott, 1982.

Mondal BK: Acromegaly: A change in size. *Nurs Mirror* 1981; 153(81):38–39.

Muthe NC: *Endocrinology: A Nursing Approach.* Boston: Little, Brown, 1981.

Paterson AG, Velster DJ: Adrenalectomy for advanced breast cancer: A reappraisal. *Anticancer Res* 1983; 3(2):151–153.

Petersdorf RG et al (editors): *Harrison's Principles of Internal Medicine,* 10th ed. New York: McGraw–Hill, 1983.

Propst CL: Nursing care of a patient undergoing transsphenoidal hypophysectomy. *J Neurosurg Nurs* (Dec) 1983; 15:332–338.

Sanford SJ: Dysfunction of the adrenal gland: Physiologic considerations and nursing problems. *Nurs Clin North Am* 1980; 15(3):481–498.

Saxton DF et al: *The Addison–Wesley Manual of Nursing Practice.* Menlo Park, CA: Addison–Wesley, 1983.

Solomon BL: The hypothalamus and the pituitary gland: An overview. *Nurs Clin North Am* 1980; 15(3):435–451.

Vita JA, Silverberg SJ, Ovlana RS et al. Clinical clues to the cause of Addison's disease. *Am J Med* 1985;78:461.

Volner JS: Endocrine dysfunction associated with pituitary adenomas and pituitary surgery. *J Neurosurg Nurs* (Dec) 1983; 15:325–331.

Williams R (editor): *Textbooks of Endocrinology,* 6th ed. Philadelphia: Saunders, 1981.

UNIT 8

The Client With Gastrointestinal Dysfunction

CHAPTER 35

The Gastrointestinal System in Health and Illness

Other topics relevant to this content are: Care of the client with malnutrition, **Chapter 6**; Endocrine functions of the pancreas, **Chapters 30 and 32**; Diagnostic studies for clients with dysfunction of the gastrointestinal system, **Chapter 36**; Bile secretion, **Chapter 39.**

Objectives

When you have finished studying this chapter, you should be able to:

Identify the major structural and functional components of the gastrointestinal system.

Explain the physiologic mechanisms that regulate the activity of the gastrointestinal system.

Describe some pathologic conditions that lead to gastrointestinal dysfunction.

Discuss alterations in other body systems that result from gastrointestinal dysfunction.

Identify and discuss the psychosocial/lifestyle effects of gastrointestinal dysfunction on the client and significant others.

The gastrointestinal system plays an essential role in maintaining homeostasis by assimilating ingested nutrients and eliminating wastes. Because all bodily functions are ultimately dependent on the nutritional status of the body's individual cells, any dysfunction of the gastrointestinal system necessarily affects all other systems to some degree. No wonder, then, that individuals with disorders of this system make up a large part of the client population in any health care facility and are commonly seen by nurses practicing in outpatient settings and in the community.

SECTION I

Structural and Functional Interrelationships

The gastrointestinal (GI) tract or alimentary canal is essentially a tube through which food is conveyed as it undergoes the process of digestion, that is, conversion into substances the body can use. The canal extends from the mouth through the anorectum (Figure 35–1). The pancreas and the biliary tract, which are considered auxiliary GI structures, are adjacent to the stomach and duodenum, to which they are connected by the pancreatic duct and the common bile duct respectively. These abdominal organs, known collectively as the viscera, are covered by a serous membrane called the peritoneum, which also lines the abdominal cavity.

Swallowing

Before food and fluids can be processed in the alimentary canal, they must be swallowed. The initial phase of the swallowing sequence, which normally occurs after solid materials have been masticated and lubricated by saliva, is voluntary. Once a bolus of food touches the oropharynx, swallowing becomes a reflex controlled by cranial nerves V, IX, X, and XII. As food is forced into the oropharynx, the epiglottis closes over the larynx to prevent aspiration; the soft palate closes off the nasal pharynx; and the tongue rises against the roof of the mouth to prevent food from re-entering and to push it farther along the pharynx. The

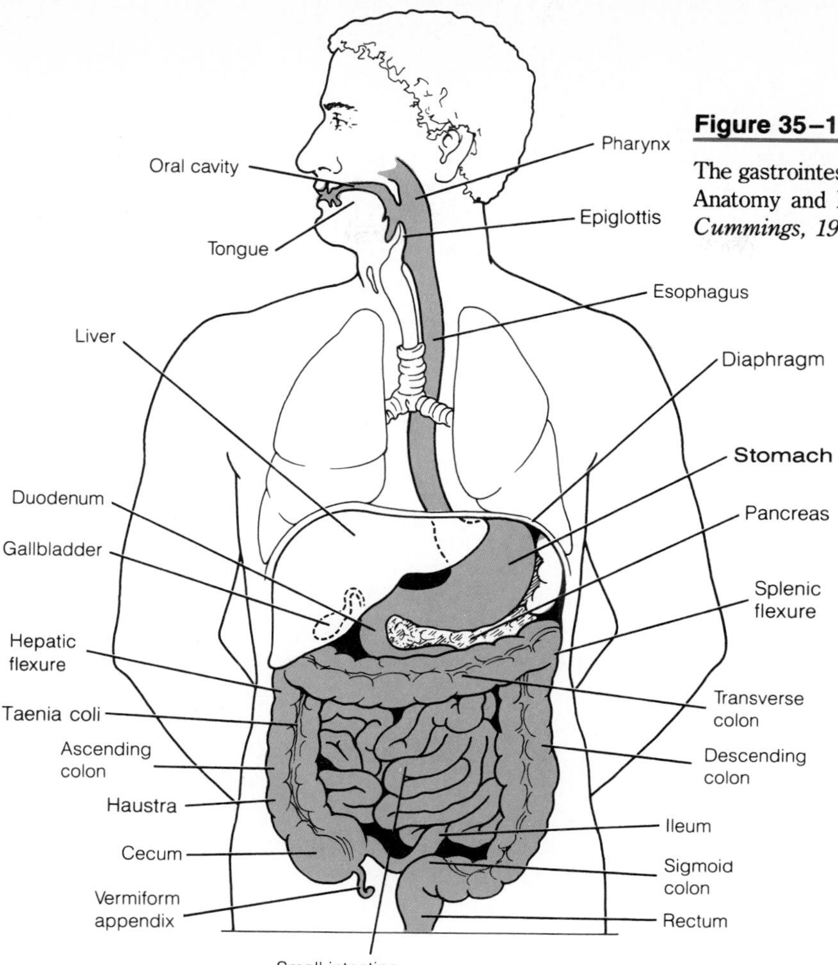

Figure 35–1

The gastrointestinal tract. SOURCE: *Spence AP, Mason EB:* Human Anatomy and Physiology, *3rd ed. Menlo Park, CA: Benjamin/Cummings, 1987.*

upper esophageal sphincter then relaxes, and food moves into the esophagus, where peristalsis and the force of gravity combine to propel the bolus of food toward the stomach.

Secretory Functions

All major structures of the gastrointestinal system produce secretions of some kind—mucoid, digestive, or hormonal. The secretions protect the gastrointestinal mucosa and facilitate digestion and absorption. Secretory activity is initiated in response to neuronal stimulation (primarily from the autonomic nervous system) as well as hormonal and mechanical stimuli.

The Oral Cavity

Most oral secretions are produced by the three pairs of salivary glands. In the normal adult, these glands secrete 1000 to 1500 mL of saliva per day (Spence and Mason, 1987). Saliva is released in response to psychic stimuli (for example, a television commercial featuring a favorite "fast food"), olfactory stimuli (for example, the smell of bread warm from the oven), and/or mechanical stimuli (such as the touch of food on the tongue). Besides acting as a lubricant to facilitate swallowing, saliva helps dissolve dry particles of food. Saliva contains ptyalin, an enzyme that breaks down starches (complex carbohydrates). Clients with conditions that reduce the flow of saliva or dry out the mouth (for example, certain medications or mouth breathing) may have a difficult time chewing and swallowing food.

The Esophagus

Most esophageal secretions are mucoid. They facilitate passage of the food bolus by lubricating it and also protect the esophageal wall by reducing the abrasiveness of swallowed material.

The Stomach

The stomach produces up to 3 L of secretions per day. Some are digestive, some hormonal, and some mucoid. *Pepsinogen*, a proteolytic enzyme, is formed when hydrochloric acid produced by the parietal cells combines with pepsin released by the chief cells. Hydrochloric acid is released in response to a hormone, *gastrin*, which is released into the bloodstream when cells in the lower portion of the stomach are chemically and/or mechanically stimulated by the presence of food. Hydrochloric acid also creates an acidic environment in the stomach. Parasympathetic neuronal pathways—especially the vagus nerve—are also involved in regulating gastric secretions.

Another important gastric secretion is intrinsic factor. This mucoprotein secreted by the parietal cells plays an essential role in the absorption of vitamin B_{12}. Intrinsic factor combines with vitamin B_{12} and is carried through the small intestine. Absorption occurs primarily at the terminal ileum.

Mucoid secretions coat the mucosal wall of the stomach, preventing autodigestion by digestive enzymes and hydrochloric acid. Mucus also coats food particles, facilitating their passage, and is capable of buffering small amounts of acids or alkalis (Guyton, 1981).

The Intestines

The food bolus, now referred to as *chyme,* is gradually released into the small intestine. The wall of the small intestine secretes up to 2 L of fluid per day, including mucus, digestive juices, and hormones in response to mechanical, hormonal, and vagal stimuli. The hormones inhibit gastric secretions and stimulate pancreatic and biliary secretions as the digestive process progresses. As in other portions of the alimentary canal, mucus serves a protective function. Digestive secretions of the small intestine neutralize the pH of the chyme and provide a liquid environment that facilitates absorption of various substances (Guyton, 1981). Many of the digestive enzymes found in the small intestine are intracellular, acting on substances as they are being absorbed.

Secretions of the colon are largely mucoid, which protects the colonic wall and lends cohesiveness to the stool.

The Pancreas and the Duodenum

The pancreas secretes hormones, enzymes, and ions. Its hormonal secretions are discussed in Unit 7. Pancreatic enzymes facilitate digestion of carbohydrates, fats, and proteins. Ionic secretions regulate intestinal pH. Inactive forms of the digestive enzymes are also secreted by the pancreas in response to vagal stimulation.

Bicarbonate ion is necessary to neutralize acidic gastric juices when they enter the intestine, thus providing a pH in which pancreatic enzymes can function. This neutralizing action also prevents damage to the intestinal wall. Release of large quantities of bicarbonate by the pancreas is stimulated by *secretin,* a hormone released by the duodenal mucosa in response to the presence of hydrochloric acid. Secretin is absorbed by the bloodstream and reabsorbed by the pancreas.

Some proteolytic enzymes are released by the pancreas in inactive form and are activated only upon entering the duodenum. Without this mechanism, the pancreas could be consumed by its own enzymes. Release of some of these inactive enzymes occurs in response to stimulation of the pancreas by *cholecystokinin,* a hormone produced and released by the duodenum when products of protein digestion are present. Other inactive pancreatic enzymes are released in response to vagal stimulation.

Motility

The alimentary canal is motile, that is, able to move spontaneously without conscious control. Its motility serves both in mixing and in propulsion of food along the digestive tract.

Once a bolus has been moved into the esophagus by swallowing, it is propelled toward the lower esophageal sphincter by peristalsis, a wave of contraction that passes along the alimentary tract for varying distances and with varying force. In the esophagus, peristalsis is controlled by the vagus nerve. When the bolus reaches the lower esophageal sphincter, which is normally contracted to prevent reflux of gastric contents, the sphincter relaxes in response to the peristaltic wave, allowing passage of the bolus into the stomach.

Gastric motility creates a churning action, moving food that has been longest in the stomach toward the stomach walls, which propel it toward the pylorus. This activity is stimulated by the presence of the hormone gastrin. In response to the pressure exerted by the distended stomach, the pylorus allows small quantities of chyme (about 10 mL/min) to pass into the duodenum. The slow rate of passage permits the duodenum to accommodate to the volume and acidity of the chyme—the inhibitory effect of secretin on gastric motility is in part a means of controlling the rate at which chyme is passed.

The elastic walls of the small intestine distend and contract rhythmically to propel the chyme toward the colon, mixing it to promote contact with the intestinal villi, where digestion and absorption take place. The rate at which chyme passes into the colon is controlled by the ileocecal valve, which also prevents fecal material from flowing back into the ileum.

The mixing contractions of the colon are called *haustrations.* These movements bring the chyme into contact with the intestinal wall to promote absorption. Mass movements (mass peristalsis) are strong periodic contractions that move feces into the rectum several times a day.

Digestion

Digestion is the process by which ingested substances are broken down in the GI tract and converted into absorbable forms. Digestion has both mechanical and chemical aspects. **Mastication** (chewing) and gastric and intestinal mixing of chyme are mechanical activities. The activity of enzymes and other secretions are chemical activities.

Carbohydrates

Digestion of carbohydrates begins in the mouth, where food is chewed and ptyalin begins the breakdown of starches (complex carbohydrates) into simple sugars. As chyme enters the duodenum, pancreatic amylase continues the breakdown of carbohydrates. The wall of the small intestine contains enzymes that further break down carbohydrates into monosaccharides, which are absorbed into the bloodstream.

Fats (Lipids)

Digestion of fats is a complex process that begins in the small intestine, where fats are emulsified by bile salts. Once emulsified, the fat can be broken down by the pancreatic enzyme *lipase*. For example, triglycerides are broken down into monoglycerides, free fatty acids, and glycerol. The monoglycerides and free fatty acids then combine with bile salts, which transport them to the intestinal wall for absorption into the lymphatics. Dietary cholesterol is broken down by pancreatic enzymes; bile salts transport cholesterol to the intestinal wall for absorption into the bloodstream.

Proteins

Digestion of proteins is also a complex process that begins in the stomach, where pepsinogen breaks down the protein into a simpler form. In the small intestine, pancreatic enzymes such as trypsin and chymotrypsin further break down proteins—some of them into amino acids. Intracellular enzymes in the intestinal wall complete the digestion of protein.

Absorption

Absorption occurs in the intestinal tract by means of two mechanisms that are basic to all cellular function: diffusion and active transport. *Diffusion* is movement along an electrochemical gradient from areas of high concentration or charge to areas of lower concentration. *Active transport* is generally *against* a gradient and requires the expenditure of energy as well as the presence of a carrier. Water is absorbed into the bowel by diffusion. Sodium is absorbed by active transport. Sodium absorption is important since the bowel secretes 20 to 30 g/day, reabsorbing all of this plus 4 to 5 g of the dietary intake (Guyton, 1981).

Nutrients and other substances are absorbed at various sites. Concentrated solutions of glucose can be absorbed through the buccal mucosa. The gastric mucosa has minimal absorptive properties—except for absorption of alcohol. The small intestine—the principal site of absorption—absorbs water, nutrients, electrolytes, and vitamins. Major nutrients absorbed by the duodenum include iron, calcium, fat, carbohydrates, and some amino acids. The jejunum absorbs carbohydrates and amino acids. The distal ileum reabsorbs bile salts (see Chapter 39), and the terminal ileum absorbs vitamin B_{12} combined with intrinsic factor.

Both the small and large intestines absorb water and electrolytes; 8.0 to 8.5 L per day are absorbed by the small intestine, and 0.5 to 1.0 L are absorbed by the colon. Under normal circumstances, only 50 to 200 mL of water are lost daily in the feces.

Elimination

Once digestion has taken place and water, nutrients, and electrolytes have been absorbed, solid waste, or feces, is expelled through the anorectum. Fecal matter is first propelled into the rectum by strong contractions of the colon that occur several times a day. A reflex contraction stimulated by these mass movements relaxes the internal sphincter, creating an urge to defecate. Under normal conditions, the external sphincter of the adult is under conscious control, allowing the individual to determine the time and place of defecation. If the urge to defecate is ignored, it subsides until the next mass movement. If sphincter control is lost—for example, due to disease or in cases of sudden, intense fear or stress—stool can ooze involuntarily out of the rectum.

SECTION II

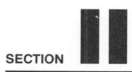

Pathophysiologic Influences and Effects

Pathophysiology of the GI tract can be associated with many conditions, as well as psychosocial factors and disturbances of related organ systems. A general overview of functional alterations is presented here; pathophysiologic and psychosocial factors related to specific disorders are discussed in Chapters 37 and 38.

Alterations in Swallowing

Swallowing is primarily a reflex mechanism. Alterations in swallowing include difficulty in swallowing (**dysphagia**) and backward propulsion of food or gases into the esophagus or through the mouth (reflux, eructation, regurgitation, and vomiting).

Difficulty in swallowing may be related to mechanical, neuromuscular, or psychologic factors. Physical abnormalities, obstruction, or inflammatory responses may cause dysphagia. Interruption of the continuity of the tongue, oropharynx, and esophagus may also be implicated. Difficulty in chewing—because of poor dentition, inadequate dentures, or pain in the temporomandibular joint (TMJ)—may affect the ability to swallow, since food may not be sufficiently mixed with saliva or sufficiently masticated. Injury or paralysis of the cranial nerves and fibrotic disorders may affect the swallowing reflex. In clients under anesthesia or in coma, the gag reflex is suppressed or absent. Various emotional states, such as anxiety, may affect the voluntary phase of the swallowing process.

Dysphagia has several consequences, such as malnutrition and pain. The client may describe the pain as "heartburn," indigestion, or chest pain. Pain can be severe, causing the client to alter eating habits or to seek relief by taking antacids.

Malfunction of the lower esophageal sphincter may cause gastric juices to flow back into the lower esophagus (*gastric reflux*). These highly acid juices may irritate or erode the esophageal mucosa. Belching (**eructation**) is usually associated with swallowing of air—for example, by eating too rapidly or talking while eating. If retained, the swallowed air may cause discomfort associated with distention or may be expelled as "gas" (*flatulence*). *Regurgitation* is reflux of partially digested food into the mouth. It usually causes a sour taste and may occur in association with eructation.

Vomiting is the release of gastric contents through the mouth. It is related to a number of conditions and may be preceded by nausea. The vomiting mechanism is triggered by neurologic stimuli. Vomiting causes a loss of gastrointestinal fluids and electrolytes and can be life threatening if excessive. In clients whose gag reflex has been altered by anesthesia or disease, vomitus may be aspirated into the bronchi, causing *aspiration pneumonia* or even respiratory arrest. Forceful vomiting can tear or rupture the esophagus—a severe complication.

Changes in Secretory Function

The mucoid, digestive, and hormonal secretions of the GI tract protect the integrity of the gastrointestinal wall, promote the passage of food or chyme, and facilitate digestion and absorption. Secretory changes may involve either an increase or a decrease and may be related to many different conditions.

Because secretory activity of the GI system is so complex and so critical to its function, changes in secretory activity may have numerous and far-reaching consequences. A decrease in mucus secretion or alterations in buffering ability (eg, release of bicarbonate ions by the pancreas) can interfere with protective mechanisms, leading to irritation, erosion, and ulceration. Alteration in secretions can also lead to digestion of tissues by their own secretions (**autodigestion**) especially in the stomach and pancreas. Reduced secretion of saliva in the oral cavity can cause dysphagia; elsewhere in the GI tract, a decrease in mucus can interfere with propulsion of chyme through the alimentary canal.

Digestion and absorption may be seriously affected by alterations in secretory activity, leading to serious sequelae. For example, if production of intrinsic factor is impaired or absent, vitamin B_{12} cannot be absorbed. Since vitamin B_{12} is essential to synthesis of erythropoietin, and to the production of red blood cells, malabsorption leads to pernicious anemia.

Absorption of nutrients depends on unimpaired secretion of various hormones and enzymes. For example, pancreatic lipase is necessary for digestion and absorption of both fats and fat-soluble vitamins A, D, E, and K. Conversely, an excess of hydrochloric acid or bile salts may be associated with diarrhea and loss of fluids and electrolytes.

Malnutrition can both cause and result from abnormalities of GI secretions. It causes the intestinal villi to atrophy, diminishing absorption and thus further impairing the client's nutrition. It impairs production of enzymes, which are composed of amino acids. Other sequelae of malabsorption related to malnutrition include loss of muscle mass, changes in skin and hair, impaired wound healing, alterations of immune function, and increase in surgical complications. These and other effects of malnutrition are discussed in Chapter 6.

Changes in Motility

Alterations in motility may be associated with many conditions of mechanical, neurohormonal, or inflammatory origin. Motility may be increased (*hypermotility*) or decreased (*hypomotility*). Mechanical conditions associated with altered motility (usually hypomotility) include ileus (intestinal obstruction) and surgical resection. Neurohormonal conditions include endocrine disorders and reactions to pharmacologic agents. Parasitic infection is one of many inflammatory conditions that alter motility—usually by increasing it.

Gastrointestinal hypermotility has numerous effects. *Dumping syndrome*, rapid emptying of gastric contents accompanied by tachycardia, palpitations, syncope, diaphoresis, cramping, and bloating, is related to changes in the osmolality, acidity, and volume of chyme entering the duodenum. Hypermotility is often associated with pain and discomfort. Moreover, when chyme moves too rapidly through the intestinal tract, digestion and absorption can not be completed. Diarrhea may result, and fluids and electrolytes may be lost, leading to systemic imbalances.

Hypomotility also adversely affects homeostasis. Slowing of peristalsis can cause chyme to reflux. Gastric retention related to hypomotility can cause feelings of fullness, nausea, and emesis. Intestinal hypomotility promotes bacterial overgrowth, leading to flatulence and, eventually, to hypermotility related to inflammation. Hypomotility of the colon may lead to constipation and fecal impaction.

Changes in Digestion

Digestion and absorption are closely linked. Most nutrients cannot be absorbed until digestive enzymes have broken them down to elemental form. Normal digestion depends on availability of food in the GI tract, availability of digestive enzymes, and unimpaired enzymatic function. If no nutrients are available in the GI tract—for example, in a client who is NPO or one whose nutritional intake is from intravenous sources—digestion slows. Enzyme availability may be impaired by disorders affecting the tissues or organs where the enzymes are synthesized—for example, the pancreas or the intestinal mucosa. Alteration in production of bile associated with disorders of the liver and gallbladder may also affect digestion, specifically of lipids.

When enzyme activity is altered, carbohydrates, fats, and/or protein are inadequately digested. If digestion is inadequate, absorption may be impaired or absent. Inadequate absorption may lead to malnutrition which may further impair digestion. Altered digestion and absorption of fat may lead to fatty stools (**steatorrhea**), described as stools that are frequent, frothy, foul, and floating. **Acholic** (clay colored) stools are related to altered secretion of bile.

Changes in Absorption

Most gastrointestinal absorption takes place in the small bowel, where fluids, electrolytes, and elemental nutrients diffuse or are actively transported via the intestinal lumen to the bloodstream and the lymphatic circulation. Malabsorption is frequently related to maldigestion; however, other conditions may be involved, including mechanical insult, neurohormonal disorders, and/or inflammation. Mechanical causes include surgical resection of the intestine, intestinal bypass, proximal ileostomy, and fistula tracts. The consequences of malabsorption include nutrient deficiencies and fluid and electrolyte imbalances. Malabsorption of fats may lead to steatorrhea.

Changes in Elimination

Elimination is the process by which waste products are excreted from the GI tract. Having a bowel movement every day is optimal because the length of time the bowel mucosa is exposed to waste products is reduced and there is less chance for stretching of the bowel mucosa. However, not everyone has this pattern. In assessing "irregularity," the important determination is whether bowel habits of the individual have *changed*, and in what manner. A change in bowel habits is one of the classic "seven warning signals" of cancer. Alteration in elimination may include diarrhea, constipation, and bloody stools. Difficult or painful elimination may also occur.

Diarrhea—loose, watery stools—may be related to many conditions, including hypermotility, inflammation, secretory disturbances, malnutrition, and malabsorption/maldigestion. It may cause loss of fluids and electrolytes and incapacitation of the client due to urgency and frequency. Diarrhea can also be associated with fecal incontinence.

Constipation—passage of hard, dry stools—may be related to hypomotility, dehydration, voluntary postponement of defecation, or immobility. Some drugs (eg, opiates) promote constipation, as do diets low in fiber. Diets high in fiber, or psyllium preparations along with a good water intake, can prevent constipation. Constipation may cause abdominal discomfort, painful defecation, and general irritability. Prolonged constipation may cause hemorrhoids (distended anal veins) to form. Laxatives, enemas, or suppositories may be needed to induce defecation, and impacted stool may have to be removed manually.

Detection of blood in the stool has important implications, and may signal such disorders as ulcers, hemorrhoids, anal fissures, diverticulitis, inflammatory disorders, and malignancy. Stools may appear tarry (**melena**), or frank red blood may be present. Melena is usually associated with bleeding of the upper GI tract; the natural red color is lost during passage through the bowel. Frank red blood is usually seen in disorders involving the distal colon or the anorectum (eg, hemorrhoids).

Anemia is frequently associated with loss of blood in the stools. Severe cases of gastrointestinal hemorrhage may lead to shock or even death. Detection of blood in the stools indicates the need for thorough testing to determine its origin; these tests are discussed in Chapter 36. Hidden blood in the stool (melena or occult blood) or frank blood can each signal cancer and should be investigated without delay, especially in clients over 35 years of age.

Pain or difficulty in defecating is usually related to an abnormality of the anorectum, most commonly anal fissures or hemorrhoids. Both present a potential for blood loss. Hemorrhoids may become strangulated (constricted), although this is uncommon. Fissures may develop into fistulas opening into the skin or, in the female, into the vagina. Rectal fistulas are often associated with Crohn's disease (regional ileitis). Painful defecation may cause the client to try to avoid defecation, worsening any existing constipation.

SECTION III

Related System Influences and Effects

Since body systems are not disparate entities but are part of a functioning organism, disorders affecting any system will affect all to some extent. The GI tract is no exception.

The Nervous System

Because neurologic regulation plays an important part in GI function, any disorder that affects the initiation or transmission of neuronal stimuli, either locally or systemically, affects gastrointestinal homeostasis.

Swallowing, being essentially a reflex, is especially susceptible to conditions affecting the cranial nerves. Among conditions in which dysphagia is a potential complication are Parkinson's disease, cerebrovascular accident, and multiple sclerosis. The client with dysphagia may require alternative sources of nutrients, either intravenous supplementation or total parenteral nutrition.

Alterations in neurologic stimulation may alter motility, secretory activity, or both. Autonomic neuropathy may lead to gastric paresis, correctable by use of gastric stimulants. Intracranial surgery or severe brain injury may be associated with hypersecretion of gastric acids and thus with gastric hemorrhage, perforation, or ulcer formation.

Intestinal motility may be reduced in conditions affecting neurologic stimulation; for example, autonomic neuropathy may lead to hypomotility, proliferation of intestinal bacteria, flatulence, and cramping. Neuropathy may also affect digestion, absorption, and intestinal secretion.

Conditions associated with spinal cord injury, such as paraplegia and quadriplegia, may affect bowel regulation and sphincter control. Incontinence and/or constipation may develop.

The Respiratory System

Alimentary structures lie close to the bronchi, lungs, and diaphragm. Any protrusion from the abdominal cavity (for example, hiatal hernia, gastric distention, ascites, or a neoplasm) can impinge on the movements of the diaphragm or otherwise create pressure on respiratory structures, decreasing vital capacity. Such pressure may create respiratory difficulties ranging from mild dyspnea to severe obstruction. Partially because of proximity, pancreatitis can lead to left pleural effusion and atelectasis because lymph drainage from the pleural space is impaired. Pneumonia and adult respiratory distress syndrome are major complications of pancreatitis.

Several disorders are related to respiratory sequelae. Cystic fibrosis affects the lungs as well as the pancreas since oversecretion of mucus obstructs both organs. Peptic ulcer disease has been associated with chronic obstructive pulmonary disease (COPD), especially when steroids are used to improve ventilatory status. The exact mechanism of the relationship is not clear, although it is thought that increased PCO_2 levels may increase gastric acid secretion. Malignant tumors of the GI tract may raise levels of the neurotransmitter serotonin. Increases in serotonin may be associated with bronchoconstriction and wheezing.

The Cardiovascular System

If arterial circulation is impaired, ischemic damage to GI structures can occur; for example, thrombosis of the mesenteric artery may be associated with intestinal ischemia so extensive that massive resection of the bowel is necessary. Gastrointestinal disorders can affect the oxygenation of tissues to the extent that the client develops shock syndrome—for example, in pancreatitis or massive GI hemorrhage. Impairment of lymphatic drainage may interfere with the body's utilization of absorbed fats, especially if the thoracic duct has been affected.

Gastrointestinal bleeding on any scale can lead to anemia; the volume of blood lost varies with the site of hemorrhage and type of lesion present. Clients receiving anticoagulant therapy or having disorders of coagulation are especially at risk of GI bleeding—as are clients receiving chemotherapy. Anemia also may be related to inadequate nutritional intake, especially of iron, folic acid, or vitamin B_{12}. If the site where these nutrients are absorbed is surgically removed (eg, by resection of the small bowel), deficiencies may occur.

The Hepatic–Biliary System

The hepatic–biliary system is intimately interrelated with the gastrointestinal system and is usually considered an accessory to it. Disorders affecting either system frequently affect both. For example, several GI disorders lead to liver disease; gallstones (**cholelithiasis**) are a potential complication of Crohn's disease. Hepatic lesions can develop in relation to ulcerative colitis or as a complication of jejunoileal bypass surgery.

Any disorder affecting the liver is likely to affect the GI system. Nutrients absorbed by the intestine are transported to the liver for processing; the liver also detoxifies many ingested substances. Normal production and secretion of bile by the liver and gallbladder are necessary to the digestion and absorption of fats and fat-soluble vitamins (A, D, E, and K). Hepatic failure promotes portal hypertension and consequent backup of venous blood into accessory vessels. Eventually, clients develop hemorrhoids and esophageal varices. These clients are prone to gastrointestinal bleeding which is exacerbated by the clotting abnormalities associated with hepatic dysfunction.

Ascites—accumulation of serous fluid in the peritoneal cavity—is related to hepatic disease but affects all abdominal organs. Infectious hepatitis is associated with such gastrointestinal manifestations as anorexia, nausea, vomiting, and diarrhea.

The Urinary System

Since gastrointestinal structures are closely adjacent to structures of the genitourinary tract, a large neoplasm in either system may impinge upon the other. Disorders of the GI system can affect the urinary system, as when large amounts of fluid are lost through diarrhea. If synthesis or absorption of vitamin K by the intestine is impaired, hematuria may occur. Renal calculi (**nephrolithiasis**) are a potential complication of Crohn's disease and ileal bypass surgery.

Conversely, urinary disorders can cause or compound GI disorders. Clients with chronic renal failure may develop pancreatitis, peptic ulcer disease, and other gastrointestinal complications. Renal failure may also be associated with anorexia, nausea, oral ulcerations, and an unpleasant taste in the mouth—major deterrents to optimal nutrition. The dietary restrictions and absorption problems related to renal failure make maintaining adequate nutrition difficult or even impossible.

The Endocrine System

Like the nervous system, the endocrine system is intimately involved with gastrointestinal function and with utilization of absorbed nutrients. Thyroid deficiency may affect GI motility; enlargement of the thyroid gland may feel like a lump in the throat to the client, inducing dysphagia. Hyperparathyroidism is associated with development of peptic ulcer disease and pancreatitis. Tumors of the islets of Langerhans can stimulate increased secretion of gastric acids, leading to ulcer formation and diarrhea.

Pancreatic disorders can have both endocrine and exocrine sequelae. As pancreatitis progresses, disturbances of endocrine function can lead to diabetes mellitus. As diabetes progresses (whether or not related to pancreatitis), autonomic neuropathy can affect GI motility. Impaired motility leads to both gastric and intestinal stasis, which, in turn, leads to proliferation of bacterial flora resulting in diarrhea and flatulence. Many diabetics alternate between constipation and diarrhea because of hypomotility.

SECTION 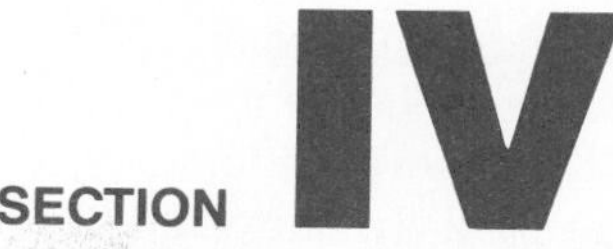

Psychosocial/Lifestyle Influences and Effects

Developmental Influences

Implications for Elderly Clients

Constipation is frequently associated with elderly persons. Although the problem does occur more often among the elderly, it is associated with both degenerative diseases and decreases in some neuronal and hormonal function as people age. Many older people reduce their activity level, whether because of long-term illnesses or, in some cases, because they live in inner cities where they are afraid to leave their homes. Older persons may reduce their consumption of fiber, in some cases because of inadequate dentition or poorly fitting dentures. Mastication may be impaired, leading to digestive difficulties or poor absorption of nutrients. The elderly may also have an inadequate fluid intake. Any of these conditions may lead to constipation and use and eventual overuse of laxatives.

Nurses working with the elderly have many opportunities to help their clients avoid or cope with these problems. Nurses can teach their elderly clients how minor changes in diet, such as eating whole grains, breads and cereals, and fresh fruit, and increasing their fluid intake and activity level can improve overall health as well as alleviate problems of elimination. Encouraging clients to engage in social contact or recreational activities suitable to their physical condition may also direct attention away from concerns about body function.

Psychoemotional Factors

A number of disorders of the GI system—notably peptic ulcer, "irritable bowel syndrome," and ulcerative colitis—have traditionally been considered wholly or partially psychogenic. It is true that mental and emotional states can influence GI function. Fear, anger, anxiety, and other emotional states may increase or decrease intestinal motility. Secretion of hydrochloric acid may increase in states of anger or hostility; secretin production may decrease in clients who are depressed or withdrawn.

The knowledge that some GI disorders are linked to psychosomatic mechanisms, that is, to the physiologic effects of mental states, has sometimes led the general public, and even health professionals, to conclude that such disorders are "all in the client's mind." In recent years, biophysiologic research has unearthed new information that underscores that mind and body are not merely linked: they are essentially one. Unconscious mechanisms such as sphincter control and secretory activity have become better understood, and their link to such previously unknown factors as neurotransmission has been at least partially elucidated.

Accumulating knowledge indicates that GI illnesses thought to be "psychologic" in origin are related less to "neuroses" than to differences in the amount of stress to which individuals are subjected and the vastly different ways in which each individual copes with stress. The nurse who helps clients identify their coping patterns and change maladaptive patterns to health-promoting ones is providing a great service.

Self-Concept and Body Image

Various GI diseases and their treatments have profound psychosocial implications, particularly for body image. Disorders or treatments that alter the route of either ingestion or elimination require tremendous adjustments on the part of clients and significant others.

Although a number of conditions may require temporary alteration in the manner of food intake—for example, intestinal obstruction or major surgery—disorders that require long-term nutritional support present the most problems of coping. For clients who have cancers of the head and neck requiring resections that are often mutilating, ingestion of food and fluids via the oral route may have to be bypassed permanently. Considering how much cultural and social life revolves around food it is not surprising that clients who undergo such profound changes have difficulty in adjusting.

Clients for whom tube feeding and parenteral nutrition require tubes visible to others usually undergo disturbances of body image. Alterations in elimination patterns may be even more distressing. Treatment of some disorders, including cancer of the bowel, inflammatory bowel disease, or trauma to the bowel, require that elimination of waste be diverted to a stoma, a surgically constructed outlet. Having one's feces evacuate through an opening on the abdomen into a collecting bag requires major adjustments in both personal habits and body image. A client may fear rejection by a spouse or interference with sexual relations. A client whose sexual preferences center on the affected structures may experience severe adjustment problems related to sexuality.

Culture and Lifestyle

The cultural beliefs and lifestyles of clients will affect gastrointestinal status and their attitude toward it and will affect whether they consider themselves well or ill when dysfunction occurs. The nurse who fails to take the client's beliefs into account may completely misinterpret the significance of changes in body function to the client.

Eating habits can affect both gastrointestinal function and nutrition. Diets low in fiber have been associated with cancer of the colon; cultures in which many whole grains and fresh fruits and vegetables are consumed have a low incidence of colon cancer. Diets high in fiber promote rapid transit of food and chyme through the alimentary canal. It is thought that intestinal stasis associated with diets low in fiber leads to prolonged contact of carcinogens with the intestinal mucosa.

Cigarette smoking has been linked to development of some gastrointestinal cancers, for example, cancer of the esophagus. Smoking of pipes and cigars and use of chewing tobacco has been correlated with cancers of the oral cavity. Excessive consumption of alcohol affects bowel function and can contribute to the development of gastritis and pancreatitis.

Occupational and Environmental Factors

Occupational and economic effects of gastrointestinal illnesses are similar to those of any illness that may require expensive and prolonged treatment. Occupational stress has been associated with the development of gastrointestinal disorders, especially peptic ulcer.

Environmental sanitation, especially sanitation of food and water supplies, is strongly linked to infectious GI disorders. Water supplies may be contaminated by sewage or by swimmers who defecate or urinate in ponds and lakes. Rural drinking water, which may come from individual wells, is especially vulnerable to contamination by seepage.

Intestinal parasites may be spread by contaminated food. Infectious diseases may be spread by food handlers who are ill or who do not use proper handwashing techniques. Nurses can do much to encourage clients and the public to practice sanitation.

Chapter Highlights

The gastrointestinal system plays an essential role in maintaining homeostasis by assimilating food products and providing for elimination.

Alteration in gastrointestinal function disrupts this homeostatic balance.

Alteration in swallowing may result from mechanical, neuromuscular, or psychologic causes, leading to changes in dietary intake.

Alteration in secretory function can lead to alterations in gastrointestinal wall integrity, digestion, and absorption.

Gastrointestinal motility may be disrupted by mechanical, neurohormonal, and inflammatory causes, interfering with digestion and absorption.

Digestion and absorption may be disrupted by mechanical, inflammatory, or neurohormonal causes, leading to malnutrition.

Alterations in elimination include change in stool character and painful or difficult defecation.

Malnutrition can be caused by alterations of gastrointestinal structure or function and can lead to pathophysiologic changes.

Psychosocial/lifestyle problems can result when the normal route of ingestion and/or elimination is altered.

Normal gastrointestinal function is highly dependent on nervous innervation and vascular supply. Pathophysiology results from alterations.

The physical proximity of the gastrointestinal tract to other body systems makes these systems especially vulnerable when space occupying disorders (eg, tumors, cysts, ascites) occur in the GI tract.

Bibliography

Anderson L et al: *Nutrition in Health and Disease.* Philadelphia: Lippincott, 1982.

Bailey FE, Walker ML: Socioeconomic factors and their effects on the nutrition and dietary habits of the black aged. *Gerontol Nurs* 1982; 8:203–207.

Coleman V: Hidden connections. *Nurs Mirror* 1982; 155:29–30.

Crowley LV: *Introduction to Human Disease.* Monterey, CA: Wadsworth, 1983.

Drossman DA et al: The prevalence of irregular bowel patterns in healthy young adults. *Gastroenterology* 1981; 80:1139.

Drossman DA: The physician and patient. Pages 3–20 in: *Gastrointestinal Disease.* Sleisinger MH, Fordtran JS (editors). Philadelphia: Saunders, 1983.

Edwards GK: Is there a correlation between occupational stress and physical disease and mental symptoms in upper level management? *Occup Health Nurs* 1982; 38:18–28.

Guyton AC: *Textbook of Medical Physiology,* 6th ed. Philadelphia: Saunders, 1981.

Spence AP, Mason EB: *Human Anatomy and Physiology,* 3rd ed. Menlo Park, CA: Benjamin/Cummings, 1987.

Wilson HS, Kneisl CR: *Psychiatric Nursing.* Menlo Park, CA: Addison–Wesley, 1983.

Wolf S: The psyche and the stomach. *Gastroenterology* 1981; 80:605–614.

CHAPTER **36**

The Nursing Process for Clients With Gastrointestinal Dysfunction

Other topics relevant to this content are: The health history and physical assessment, **Chapter 5;** Care of the client receiving TPN, **Chapter 6.**

Objectives

When you have finished studying this chapter you should be able to:

Specify the major components of the health history to be obtained from clients with gastrointestinal dysfunction.

Explain specific assessment approaches in evaluating clients with disease of the gastrointestinal system.

Identify the nursing implications of diagnostic studies commonly used to evaluate clients with gastrointestinal dysfunction.

Determine appropriate nursing diagnoses for clients with disorders of the gastrointestinal system.

Develop, with the client, realistic goals of care.

Anticipate the psychosocial/lifestyle implications of gastrointestinal dysfunction for clients and their significant others.

Develop a nursing care plan for a client with gastrointestinal dysfunction.

Implement nursing interventions specific to clients with gastrointestinal disease.

Evaluate the effectiveness of the nursing care plan and modify it as necessary to meet client needs.

SECTION **I**

Nursing Assessment: Establishing the Data Base

A comprehensive assessment, including a careful health history, is essential regardless of the organ system involved. If the symptoms for which the client sought care suggest a gastrointestinal disorder, or if the existence of a GI disorder has already been established, the assessment should concentrate on data specific to that system. Observations should focus on alterations in swallowing, secretion, motility, digestion, absorption, and elimination, including both subjective symptoms and objective signs reported by the client. Be sure to obtain psychosocial as well as physiologic data. Disorders of the GI system can both affect, and be affected by, psychosocial factors.

Subjective Data

A detailed health history provides a major source of data for the nurse. Remember, though, that limited, spontaneous assessments continually take place in the course of day-to-day nursing care, and much valuable data can be obtained through apparently casual questions.

Nutritional Assessment

Thorough assessment of the client's nutritional state is imperative in evaluating possible origins and potential consequences of gastrointestinal dysfunction. Often, a nutritional problem will precipitate a GI problem, herald its presence, or result from its occurrence. A food intolerance, for example, may be related to malabsorption or may be a cause of diarrhea. Furthermore, malnutrition is associated with many GI disorders. Protein–calorie malnutrition is especially prevalent among clients with gastrointestinal cancer.

DIET HISTORY The diet history includes a thorough assessment of what the client eats, as well as recent changes in intake, food tolerance, energy level, and weight. Are there foods the client cannot tolerate? Have bowel habits changed recently? How? Greater frequency? Less? What about the client's energy level? Diet content can best be assessed by asking the client to describe a typical day's meals and snacks. Nonhospitalized clients may be asked to keep a daily record of food intake on forms the nurse provides. Once client and nurse have determined what is actually eaten, servings per food group can be calculated and problems identified.

Ask the client about indigestion (**dyspepsia**), constipation, and diarrhea, since these conditions may be related to poor nutrition. Be sure that the client describes exactly what he or she means by constipation, since clients may consider any variation from a daily movement as constipation. Note food intolerances and whether they are of recent origin.

Has the client gained or lost weight recently? The thin person being assessed may be a "fat person in disguise" who has recently lost weight with a fad diet; the client who appears fat may be a "yo-yo" dieter who was thin last year. Rapid weight loss or gain may be associated with malnutrition. Does the client seem lethargic or energetic? A low energy level may signal malnutrition.

SOCIOCULTURAL INFLUENCES What is the client's attitude toward food? Everyone has food preferences and prejudices related to psychologic makeup, cultural and family background, and finances. Knowing these is helpful to the nurse, both in assessing the client's condition and in making realistic plans for care. The immediate environment also affects what and how people eat. A client used to eating at home, in the company of friends and family, may find that eating alone from a tray in the tense atmosphere of a hospital promotes anorexia (loss of appetite).

Are there ethnic foods to which the client is especially attached? What about religious restrictions on diet? Ask each individual what his or her preferences are.

DIETARY CONSIDERATIONS WITH THE ELDERLY Older adults should be carefully evaluated for signs of malnutrition. Many psychosocial problems that are especially likely to affect the elderly predispose them to nutritional deficits. In addition to problems such as loneliness or lack of money, older people often become indifferent to food because taste sensation diminishes with age; the number of taste buds declines, and those remaining may atrophy. Deficiencies in protein, calcium, iron, and vitamins A and C are especially prevalent (Kohrs, 1983). Fiber may be missing from the diet. Medications, both prescribed and OTC, may alter intestinal absorption, especially antibiotics and laxatives.

The Mouth and Esophagus

Has the client experienced **aphagia** (inability to swallow) or dysphagia (difficulty in swallowing)? What about difficulty in eating in general? Has the client noticed any oral lesions? Discolorations, vesicles, ulcerations, or growths? Does the client use tobacco or alcohol? Use of these substances often promotes development of leukoplakia—small, elevated, patchy white lesions that may precede oral cancer.

Routine assessment should include noting any reports of bleeding, inflammation, infection, ulceration, or spread of disease already present. Specific therapy may be needed to maintain oral hygiene or to prevent spread of infection. Does the disease process interfere with the client's ability to eat or speak? Alternative methods of eating (ie, tube feeding) or communicating may have to be devised. Box 36–1 gives history-taking suggestions for assessment of the oral cavity.

The Stomach

Has the client experienced nausea or vomiting? Heartburn? Indigestion? Excessive eructation? In older adults, motility of the gut decreases, and fewer digestive enzymes are secreted, often leading to heartburn or indigestion (Tichy & Chong, 1981). If disease is already present, ask the client about any changes in the number, severity, or pattern of symptoms, since this information can be useful in evaluating therapies and nursing care plans.

NAUSEA AND VOMITING If the client reports vomiting, note the odor, color, consistency, and quantity of vomitus. Has the client noticed **hematemesis** (bloody vomitus)? Digested or undigested flood in the vomitus? A fecal odor? A fecal odor may indicate reflux of bowel contents due to intestinal obstruction. A coffee-ground appearance of the vomitus may indicate the presence of partially digested blood. These observations help clarify the course of the client's problem and assist in assessing potential problems related to nutritional and fluid–electrolyte status.

Encourage the client to determine whether symptoms are related to eating any particular food. How long after a meal do symptoms begin? How long do they last? Does

Box 36–1
History-Taking Suggestions: The Oral Cavity

Ask the client about any past or present:

- Severe or persistent pain in mouth or throat
- Recurrent infections, especially streptococcal
- Serious or disabling tooth, gum, or jaw problems
- Chronic hoarseness or laryngitis
- Change in voice
- Pain while chewing
- Difficulty swallowing (dysphagia)
- Impairment of speech (dysphasia)
- Tendency to breathe by mouth
- Sore tongue
- Bloody saliva
- Impaired sense of taste
- Lesions in mouth
- Tonsillectomy or adenoidectomy
- Oral surgery
- Orthodontia work

Also ask about the client's general dental health. Are all the natural teeth present? Any dentures? Partial plates? Any sores or areas of irritation under the dentures? Any problem with toothache or sore, swollen, or bleeding gums? What is the client's daily dental hygiene regimen? How often does the client see a dentist? When was the last appointment?

The following is an example of a write-up *history* for the mouth that could be found under a review of systems:

Mouth—no hx lesions, dysphagia, or hoarseness; frequent sore throats × 2 years; two documented strep throats—6/80, 11/85; has all natural teeth; annual dental exams; brushes and flosses daily; no hx bleeding gums or frequent dental caries; does not smoke a pipe, cigar, or cigarettes; does not chew tobacco

Adapted with permission from: Malkiewitz J: What assessing the mouth can tell you. *RN* (May) 1982; p. 66. Copyright 1982 Medical Economics Company Inc., Oradell, NJ.

eating make symptoms worse or does it alleviate them (as it may, for example, in peptic ulcer)?

Try also to determine whether symptoms are related to emotional states or social situations. Individuals vary in their response to stress and anxiety, but emotional changes can precipitate diarrhea, constipation, nausea, vomiting, indigestion, or other symptoms. In older adults, loneliness, grief, depression, or financial worries can precipitate or worsen gastrointestinal disease.

MEDICATIONS AND VITAMINS Does the client take prescribed or over-the-counter drugs to relieve gastrointestinal symptoms—for example, antacids, antiemetics, or antiflatulents? How often? How well do they work? It is a good idea to use brand names when asking about these products, because clients are often unaware of the generic names of the preparations they are taking. What about vitamins? Vitamin E, for example, may cause nausea if not taken with meals. Fat-soluble vitamins should be ingested with foods to be effectively absorbed; many clients are not aware of this, and asking about vitamins provides opportunity for health teaching. Ask also about aspirin and anti-inflammatory medications, especially in clients of middle age or older, who may be receiving treatment for arthritis. These medications may irritate the gastric mucosa.

The Intestines

Some clients find discussion of bowel function embarrassing and may consider some symptoms undignified or shameful. Asking questions in a matter-of-fact way may help. A surprising number of adults still resort to euphemisms ("number 2") when discussing bowel function. Encourage clients to use any forms of expression that put them more at ease.

Ask the client about anorectal conditions such as hemorrhoids, anal bleeding, or pruritus. Have there been any episodes of fecal incontinence? Although fecal incontinence may have a benign etiology, it may also be a sign of colorectal cancer. Since the association of rectal bleeding with cancer has been so well publicized, the client may need realistic reassurance that other causes are possible or even likely.

Ask the client to describe the odor, color, consistency, and frequency of bowel movements. Have there been any recent changes? Changes in the regularity of bowel movements may be indicative of disease or may be related to therapy. As with nausea or indigestion, try to determine whether dietary or emotional factors are related to any changes. Does the client take laxatives or use enemas to facilitate bowel movements? What kind? How often? Does the client eat fresh fruits and vegetables? Whole grains? Bran? Or "fast foods" and highly refined foods lacking in fiber?

Intestinal obstruction will prevent the passage of stool and flatus, causing the abdomen to become distended. Postoperative clients are especially susceptible to obstruction related to paralytic ileus (intestinal paralysis); therefore, they are checked frequently to determine whether they are passing flatus or stool and whether abdominal distention is present.

COLOR AND CONSISTENCY OF THE STOOL Ask the client about any changes in the color and consistency of the stool. The following findings are especially significant:

- Melena (black, tarry stools), which indicates digested blood from upper GI hemorrhage
- Bloody stools (frank, red blood) which indicate lower GI or anorectal bleeding
- Yellow or green stools, often signifying infectious processes

- Steatorrhea (fatty, foul-smelling, greasy, floating stools), signifying maldigestion or malabsorption
- Loose, frequent stools (diarrhea)
- Hard, infrequent stools (constipation)

Such findings warrant further investigation, in many cases by diagnostic or laboratory tests.

Pain

When asking clients about abdominal pain, remember that visceral pain (pain in specific organs) such as that from the stomach, intestine, or pancreas is poorly localized and may be referred to other parts of the body. The point where the client feels the pain, therefore, may not be the point where the pain originates. Also, because visceral pain is so diffuse, the client may have difficulty describing it. Use open-ended approaches to help clients describe their pain: "Tell me about your pain." If the client finds it hard to describe the quality of the pain, suggest terms such as stabbing, aching, or dull. Remember that in older adults and in persons with some degenerative diseases that affect the nerve endings (for example, diabetes), responsiveness to internal sensations like abdominal distention may have diminished. These clients may not be fully aware of their pain and thus may not report it accurately.

Pain receptors in the visceral organs are most responsive to stretch stimuli. Pain related to distention may thus be more severe than pain associated with other conditions. Pain in the GI tract tends to increase with peristaltic activity and to decrease with elimination. Visceral pain is often intensified with movement that increases pressure. Peritoneal irritation (that is, irritation of the mucous membrane that contains the viscera) is often intensified by movement alone. Pain related to the effect of gastric acid on the gastric mucosa is often associated with a low pH (high acidity) and may therefore be intensified when the stomach is empty.

Objective Data

Objective data are obtained by thorough physical assessment of the oral, abdominal, perianal, and rectal areas. Nutritional status should also be evaluated. Physical assessment is described in detail in Chapter 5. Only those parameters specifically relating to gastrointestinal dysfunction will be mentioned here.

Physical Assessment

ASSESSMENT OF THE ORAL CAVITY The normal mouth is depicted in Figure 36–1. Diseases of the oral cavity include inflammatory and infectious processes, degenerative processes, and abnormal growths. Congenital abnormalities may also be seen in older clients; today these are frequently corrected surgically in childhood. If the presence of disease was established prior to the examination, assess for amelioration or spread of the disease. Note any changes in coloration, odor, or discharge. Also note whether any condition that interferes with eating is present.

Comprehensive assessment includes the teeth, gums, tongue, cheeks, and palate. Note any evidence of neoplasms or lesions, inflammation, discoloration, exudate, swelling, or difficulty in swallowing. Note that sublingual spider nevi are normally present in about 50% of older adults and are not pathologic (Tichy & Chong, 1981).

DENTITION Inspect the teeth (dentition) for caries, which can be painful and may interfere with eating, ultimately affecting nutritional status. Palpate the teeth to determine whether any are painful to touch or loosened from their sockets. Assess for absence or misalignment of teeth. If teeth appear to be missing, ask the client whether they have been extracted. Congenital absence of one or two teeth, often familial, is a fairly common finding (Crowley, 1983).

If the upper (maxillary) and lower (mandibular) dentition do not meet properly—a condition called malocclusion—the client may not be able to chew food properly. Malocclusion may also lead to pain in the temporomandibular joint (TMJ) or in some cases to headaches. Referral to an orthodontist may be indicated. Diseases that affect the jaw such as trauma or arthralgias can impede movement of the mouth or cause anorexia related to fear of pain with eating.

THE GINGIVAE AND THE ORAL MUCOSA The gingivae (gums), tongue, cheek, and palate should be examined for erythema, edema, tenderness, and hemorrhage, which may indicate inflammation or infection. Palpation for neoplasms is essential in assessing for cancerous lesions. Oral inflammation may also indicate nutritional deficiencies. Deficiency of vitamin C may cause edema and hemorrhage of the gums, and folic acid deficiency may cause swelling, redness, and tenderness of the tongue. Deficiency of some B complex vitamins is associated with cracking at the corners of the lips.

In assessing for erythema and pallor, remember that these conditions will be manifested differently in dark-skinned and light-skinned clients. Pallor in a dark-skinned person is usually discernible by absence of the underlying red tones that are normally present. Yellow-brown or ashen coloration of the mucous membranes in dark-skinned persons corresponds to the whitish appearance of pallor in whites. Erythema, which is readily seen in whites, is difficult to detect in dark-skinned clients. Rely on other signs to detect inflammation or infection, such as edema and heat.

THE BREATH When assessing the oral cavity, smell the client's breath. Breath odor is often associated with disease. In diabetic ketoacidosis, for example, the breath

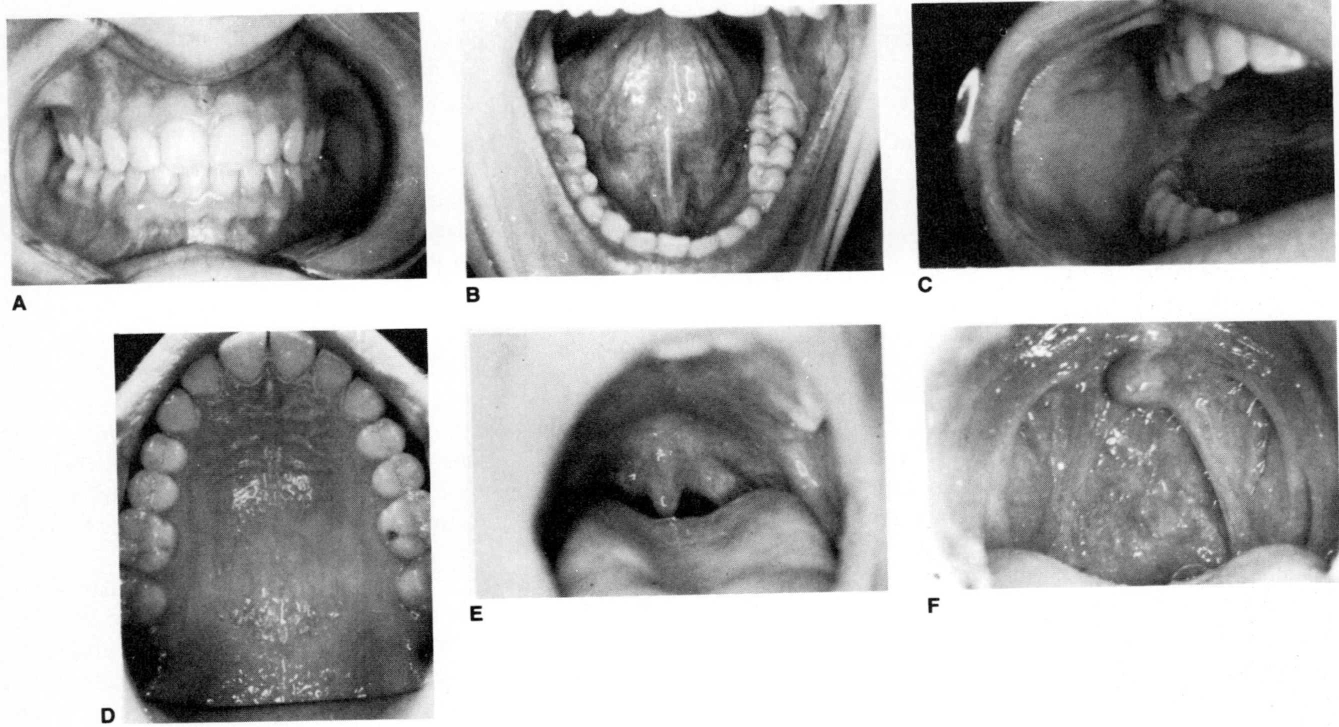

Figure 36–1

The normal mouth. **A.** Healthy gums (gingivae) and teeth. If any teeth are missing, record their location. **B.** The sublingual area, which contains salivary ducts, should always be moist. **C.** Be sure to inspect the buccal mucosa on both sides. **D.** The hard palate is a good place to spot signs of jaundice. Normally, it is pink. **E.** The uvula and soft palate should rise above this position when the client says "A-a-a-h." **F.** The oropharynx should be pink and free of drainage. SOURCE: *Reproduced with permission from Goldman HS, Mardev MZ:* Physicians' Guide to Diseases of the Oral Cavity. *Oradell, NJ: Medical Economics Books, 1982.*

has a fruity or acetone odor. A foul odor may indicate extensive caries, infection, or cancer. Clients with esophageal disorders may also have foul breath; if an esophageal lesion inhibits the passage of ingested food, the action of bacteria on accumulated food creates rancidity. However, a foul odor may simply be related to poor oral hygiene.

ASSESSMENT OF THE ABDOMEN An abdominal assessment, although providing data specific to the gastrointestinal system, is commonly performed in caring for clients with many different disorders. The usual techniques of inspection, palpation, percussion, and auscultation are employed, but in assessing the abdomen, the usual order of examination is changed. Because percussion and palpation may alter the bowel sounds, auscultation is performed first. Inspection always continues throughout the physical assessment.

Inspect the abdomen for contour and symmetry. Masses or enlarged organs will produce bulging and/or asymmetry. Asymmetry of the upper abdomen may be related to disorders of the stomach, pancreas, or transverse colon; asymmetry of the lower abdomen can occur with disorders of the ascending and descending colon.

Distention or asymmetry of the abdomen may be from ascites (fluid in the abdominal cavity), or it may be related to excessive flatus. These conditions must be distinguished from distention related to urinary retention, which is primarily seen in the suprapubic area. In clients with ascites, the abdomen is tense and distended. The skin is tightly stretched, usually shiny, and the flanks bulge. Ascites is commonly associated wih hepatic disorders.

Peristaltic waves, which are not usually visible except in thin people, may be observed in clients with intestinal obstruction. An anteroposterior (AP) aortic pulsation in the midepigastric area is normal in thin clients. When the pulsation is lateral as well as AP, it may be related to aortic aneurysm. Note, however, that the abdominal wall becomes progressively thinner and more flaccid with age, so peristaltic waves and aortic pulsations will be more apparent in older adults, even under normal circumstances (Tichy

& Chong, 1981). Peristalsis can best be visualized by directing a light obliquely over the abdomen while keeping your eyes at abdominal level.

Carefully inspect the abdominal skin, being especially alert for special kinds of changes. Multiple small nodules may herald gastric carcinoma. Localized ecchymoses in the flank may indicate abdominal or periotoneal hemorrhage.

Place the diaphragm of the stethoscope lightly on the abdomen to auscultate for bowel sounds. Bowel motility is likely to be altered in clients with GI disorders, for example, in diarrhea, intestinal obstruction, and paralytic ileus. The high-pitched tinkling sound associated with intestinal obstruction is caused by peristalsis occurring in a bowel that is tensely distended with air. Peristalsis increases above the point of developing obstruction, causing **borborygmi** (hyperactive bowel sounds). Hyperperistalsis, and therefore borborygmi, also occur in gastroenteritis and intestinal hemorrhage. In older adults, louder bowel sounds may occur normally (Tichy & Chong, 1981). Besides auscultating for bowel sounds, assess for arterial bruits with the bell of the stethoscope (see Chapter 5). Aortic bruits may be heard with abdominal aortic aneurysm.

ASSESSMENT OF THE PERIANAL AND RECTAL AREAS This examination may be especially embarrassing for the client. Make sure that privacy and respect for the client are maintained. Observe the perianal area for masses, inflammation, excoriation, ulceration, fissures, and bleeding. If the client has diarrhea, the need for skin care and hygiene may be apparent. Check for the presence of hemorrhoids. Thrombosed external hemorrhoids or prolapsed internal hemorrhoids may appear as painful bluish, shiny, ovoid masses.

Diagnostic Studies

Many alterations in gastrointestinal function can be objectively assessed through analysis of laboratory data and diagnostic studies. Specific findings will usually be associated with particular pathologic conditions. The nurse should understand how various findings relate to the client's gastrointestinal health, and which findings indicate the presence of disease processes. By understanding diagnostic studies, the nurse will be able to prepare clients physically and psychologically for the tests. Understanding how certain diagnostic procedures are done will also help in reinforcing the physician's explanation when legal consent must be obtained.

PANCREATIC ENZYME LEVELS Enzymes produced by the pancreas (amylase, lipase) may escape into tissues and into the bloodstream when acute pancreatic disease is present. With chronic pancreatic disease, amylase levels may be decreased. With these enzymes unavailable to digest fats, steatorrhea occurs.

BILIRUBIN LEVELS Cancer of the head of the pancreas may obstruct the common bile duct, precipitating obstructive jaundice. Serum bilirubin will rise, as will levels of bilirubin in the urine. Levels of bilirubin in the stools will decrease, since flow of bile to the gut has been reduced; stools will be acholic, lacking the bile pigments. These findings may also be associated with a number of hepatic–biliary disorders.

SERUM ELECTROLYTES Serum electrolytes are an important gauge of GI status. Vomiting, diarrhea, malabsorption, and gastric or intestinal suctioning are especially likely to disturb homeostatic balance by depleting the body of electrolytes and fluids. If fluid loss is sufficient to produce dehydration, the hematocrit level will increase. Loss of secretions produced by the pancreas, hepatic–biliary system, or lower bowel may promote metabolic acidosis, since these secretions are alkaline. Diarrhea, mechanical suction, or the presence of a fistula may cause loss of these substances. Conversely, loss of the acidic secretions of the upper GI tract through vomiting or suction may precipitate metabolic alkalosis.

VITAMIN LEVELS Deficiency of vitamin K, which is vital to coagulation of the blood, may be related to malabsorption, diarrhea, ulcerative colitis, intestinal obstruction, or malnutrition. Hepatic–biliary dysfunction may also affect levels of this vitamin. Serum levels of carotene, a precursor of vitamin A, will be depressed in clients with malabsorption syndromes and other GI disorders. Carotene, which is found in green and yellow fruits and vegetables (especially carrots and sweet potatoes), is absorbed from the intestine. If absorption is depressed, serum carotene levels will be low despite ample carotene in the diet.

CARCINOEMBRYONIC ANTIGEN LEVELS Tests for carcinoembryonic antigen (CEA) are performed as an adjunct to other tests in diagnosing GI cancer and monitoring treatment. CEA is a nonspecific test (Kee, 1983).

BLOOD AND URINE STUDIES RELATED TO MALNUTRITION Malnutrition, often associated with GI disorders, depletes protein stores and creates a negative nitrogen balance in the body. Tests that will show evidence of protein depletion include:

- Serum albumin. Albumin, the smallest of the protein molecules, contributes the majority of total protein value.
- Total iron-binding capacity. Measures the amount of iron-transporting protein in the serum.
- Urinary nitrogen and creatinine (a nitrogen-containing compound).
- Serum transferrin. A transporter of protein and a sensitive indicator of visceral protein stores.

Urine ketones will be increased as the body attempts

to provide necessary energy by breaking down lipid tissue. Assessment of urinary ketone levels can be easily performed in the course of daily nursing care.

FECAL ABNORMALITIES Examination of the feces is important in identifying bleeding disorders, malabsorptive and digestive diseases, biliary obstruction, and parasitic and bacterial infections. In infectious processes, the stool must be examined to determine the causative organism. If intestinal infection is suspected, three separate specimens should be collected and tested before the possibility of disease can be ruled out. Sterile containers should be used, and the specimen should be delivered immediately to a laboratory and refrigerated (Byrne et al., 1986).

ROUTINE RADIOGRAPHIC STUDIES Abnormalities of the mouth, such as the presence of a mass, dental caries, or abnormal dentition, can be detected by x-rays. An abdominal x-ray (flat plate) can reveal masses in the stomach, intestine, or pancreas, obstruction of the small bowel, trauma to abdominal tissue, and ascites.

NURSING IMPLICATIONS Testing may be done on an inpatient or outpatient basis. Clients having oral x-rays are usually not restricted in any way. Those having abdominal studies may be asked to fast for 8 hours before the test. Radiographic studies should not be done during the first trimester of pregnancy except in cases of extreme urgency when delay in diagnosis would be dangerous to client and/or fetus. Explain to clients what precautions will be taken to prevent excessive radiation.

FLUOROSCOPIC BARIUM STUDIES Fluoroscopy—visualization with motion—requires use of a contrast agent that can be visualized as it passes through or outlines GI structures. Barium sulfate is the agent used.

UPPER GI SERIES Fluoroscopic examination of the upper GI tract (esophagus, stomach, duodenum, and other portions of the small bowel) is called an upper GI series. The client must swallow barium sulfate (a chalky white substance, sometimes flavored) or another contrast medium. Films are taken sequentially as this material moves through the upper GI tract (Figure 36–2A); the process may also be monitored on a screen similar to a TV screen.

The upper GI series is performed routinely to rule out gastritis; peptic ulcer; neoplasia or strictures of the esophagus, stomach, or duodenum; hiatal hernia; gastric polyps; gastric or duodenal diverticula; or foreign bodies in the tract. A variation of the procedure, known as hypotonic duodenography, involves administration of glucagon, atropine, or propantheline bromide (Pro-Banthine) to slow down small-intestinal peristalsis. It may be used if the client has hyperperistalsis, duodenal spasticity, or a space-occupying lesion such as a tumor of the head of the pancreas (Kee, 1983).

A *long GI series* is used to rule out Crohn's disease, parasitic infection, diverticulitis, or malabsorption. In a long series, the regular test is performed first; the client then swallows additional contrast medium, and more x-rays are taken. A GI series may last from 1 to 6 hours, depending on what part of the alimentary canal is being assessed.

NURSING IMPLICATIONS The client should be NPO for 8 to 12 hours before testing to ensure that the GI tract will be empty. The client should also be advised not to smoke, since smoking stimulates motility. If a long GI series is planned, the client may have to fast for 10 to 12 hours prior to the test. Mouth care is important after upper GI testing to remove the taste of barium.

After the procedure, a laxative should be prescribed and administered. Tell the client to expect light-colored stools for several days. Constipation and fecal impaction may occur, requiring treatment.

LOWER GI SERIES To visualize the lower gastrointestinal tract, barium sulfate is instilled into the colon by means of a rectal tube (barium enema) (Figure 36–2B). Air may be instilled in addition (double-contrast study). The client must retain the enema while x-ray films are taken. Polyps, tumors, lesions, colitis, diverticulitis, and fistulae can be identified in this way.

NURSING IMPLICATIONS Many clients dread this test, often having heard about it from friends or other clients. They expect it to be both painful and embarrassing. Clients may fear that they will be unable to retain the enema during the procedure. The client can be reassured that he or she will most likely be able to retain the contrast material, but that many people are unable to control it entirely and that x-ray personnel are professionals accustomed to this eventuality, should it occur.

The client should be on a clear liquid diet for 18 to 24 hours before testing and NPO from supper the night before. A bowel prep—cleansing of the bowel with laxatives and/or enemas—may be required. As an alternative to laxatives and enemas, GoLYTELY, an oral solution, can be used with minimal fluid and electrolyte loss and greater client convenience. The solution may cause mild cramping and a feeling of fullness. Immediately after the barium enema, the client should attempt to defecate. A laxative and/or enema after the procedure is recommended to facilitate passage of barium from the intestinal tract. Constipation and fecal impaction may occur and require treatment.

ENDOSCOPY Endoscopy involves the visualization of a body cavity or organ by means of an endoscope—an instrument consisting of a combination of lenses and a light source at the end of a long, slender tube. With the development of fiberoptics, a flexible tube can be used since light traveling along these optic fibers can travel around a

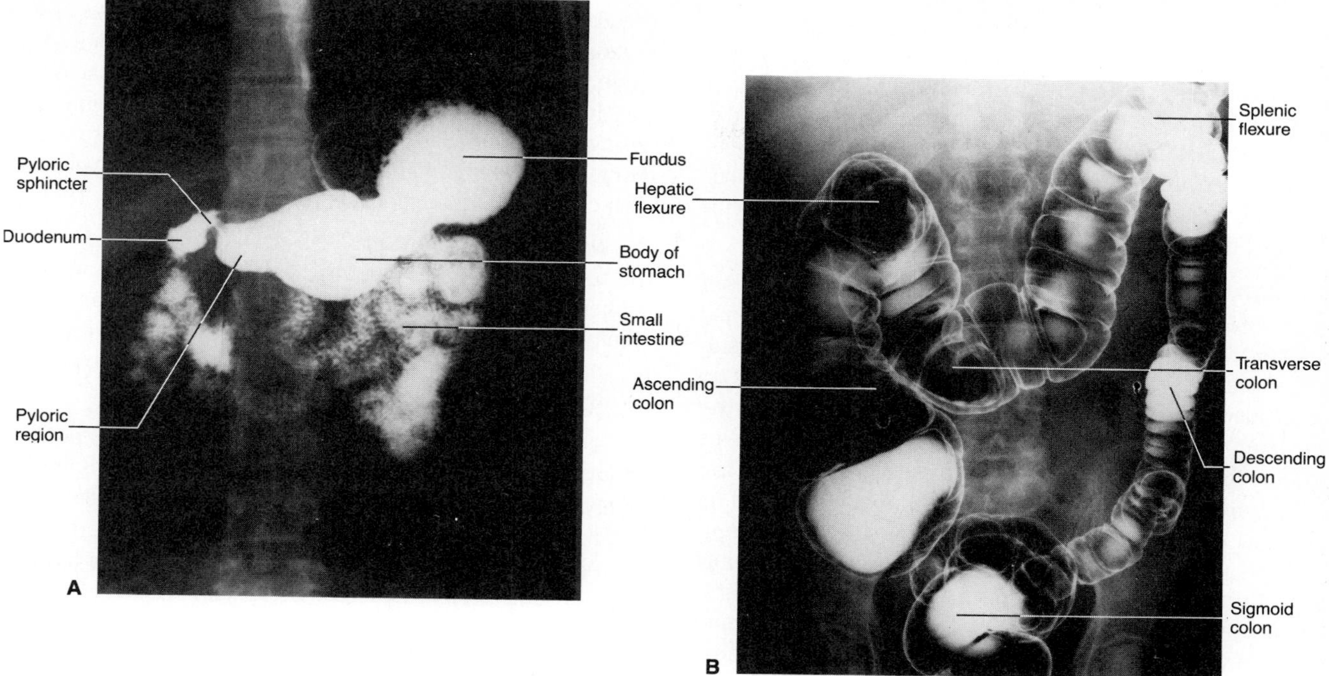

Figure 36–2

A. A normal upper GI series. **B.** A normal barium enema. *Courtesy of Health Care Plan, Buffalo, NY.*

curve. Earlier endoscopes had to employ straight tubes and complex systems of mirrors.

Various forms of endoscopy derive their names from the area viewed. In the case of gastrointestinal endoscopy, these include:

- Esophagoscopy (the esophagus)
- Gastroscopy (the stomach)
- Esophagogastroscopy (the esophagus and stomach)
- Duodenoscopy (the duodenum)
- Esophagogastroduodenoscopy (the esophagus, stomach, and duodenum)
- Proctoscopy (the anus and rectum), from the Greek *proktos,* for anus
- Sigmoidoscopy (the sigmoid colon)
- Proctosigmoidoscopy (the anus, rectum, and sigmoid colon)
- Colonoscopy (the large intestine)

NURSING IMPLICATIONS Endoscopy may be performed in a hospital or clinic. Written consent must be obtained. The procedure is explained to the client, the client's records are consulted to ensure that preparation requirements (NPO status, bowel prep, sedation if any) have been met, baseline vital signs are recorded, and the safety and privacy of the client are ensured.

Draping the client helps alleviate embarrassment. Procedures of the lower tract may produce discomfort and flatus; instruct the client to breathe deeply and slowly to promote relaxation. After endoscopy, whether of the upper or lower GI tract, the client should rest. Vital signs must be taken. Perforation is a rare complication associated with pain, abdominal distention, and hemorrhage (Kee, 1983).

UPPER GI ENDOSCOPY Imflammatory processes, tumors, ulceration, hemorrhage, cancer, and hiatal hernia can be identified by endoscopy of the upper gastrointestinal organs. The client should be NPO for 8 to 12 hours before the procedure. Dentures and jewelry are removed. Sedation may be ordered as premedication, and medication such as atropine prescribed to dry up secretions so that the mucosa may be clearly visualized. A local anesthetic can be applied to the throat before insertion of the endoscope to diminish the gag reflex. The scope is then passed to the desired area. After the procedure, assess the client for return of the gag reflex before giving the client fluids or food.

LOWER GI ENDOSCOPY Polyps, tumors, ulceration, inflammatory and infectious processes, bleeding, hemorrhoids, and fistulas can be detected by visualization of the anus, rectum, sigmoid colon, and large intestine. The lubricated scope is passed to the desired area while the client assumes a knee-chest position (with a rigid scope) or side-lying position (with a flexible scope). The client should have light meals for 1 to 2 days and an 8-hour fast immediately prior to the procedure. A bowel prep involves the use of laxatives the night before the procedure and saline enemas the day of the test. Intravenous meperidine and/or diazepam may be ordered to promote comfort and relaxation. Atropine may be ordered to limit GI tract secretions. After the procedure, the client should be assessed for unusual pain, bleeding, or shock, which could indicate perforation of the bowel.

ULTRASONOGRAPHY Ultrasonography, also called ultrasound, sonography, or echography, involves the use of sound waves to visualize body structures. It is considered a noninvasive technique with no known harmful effects. To produce the image, a transducer is passed over the body area to be assessed; it emits sound waves and receives echoes "bounced" off body structures. These echoes are converted to electrical impulses, which may be viewed on a screen or photographed. In assessing the GI system, ultrasonography can be used to visualize the abdominal aorta to detect aneurysms and to detect tumors, cysts, and inflammation of the pancreas. NPO restrictions should be observed for 8 to 12 hours prior to ultrasonography. Advise the client that the abdomen will be smeared with thick lubricant to facilitate movement of the transducer and that the procedure is painless, although the client will have to remain still for the duration of the examination.

COMPUTERIZED TOMOGRAPHY In computerized tomography scanning (CT or CAT scanning) a narrow x-ray beam is directed at the body from various angles. Esophageal disease, intra-abdominal masses, and organ enlargement can be detected by CT scan, which produces less radiation than standard radiography. Contrast medium is often administered intravenously to enhance visualization.

The client remains alone in a room with his or her body inside a scanner. The test takes about 1½ hours; the client may be asked to take and hold several deep breaths during this time.

NURSING IMPLICATIONS Since contrast medium may be used, question the client about allergy to iodine (including fish and seafood, since the client may not realize that these foods contain iodine). Explain the procedure, and tell the client that a warm, flushed sensation, accompanied by temporary nausea, may occur if contrast medium is injected. Showing the client a picture of the scanner may help, since the size of CT scan equipment is often frightening. Obtain written consent.

ESOPHAGEAL MANOMETRY Esophageal manometry provides an estimate of esophageal motility by measuring pressure under different conditions: the resting esophageal sphincter, the sphincter relaxation response, and esophageal peristalsis. Water-filled catheters, connected to transducers, are passed via the nose or mouth through the esophagus and into the stomach. The catheters are gradually withdrawn, 1 cm at a time, as pressure measurements are taken along the esophagus. Electrodes sensitive to pH can be attached to measure esophageal acidity. This increasingly common test is thought beneficial in diagnosing achalasia (failure of the esophageal sphincter to relax during swallowing) and other esophageal disorders in clients with chest pain and dysphagia (Meshkinpour et al., 1982).

NURSING IMPLICATIONS The client should be NPO from the previous night. Explain that a local anesthetic will be applied topically to the throat to prevent gagging and discomfort. The client should also know that swallowing will be required during the test. Written consent should be obtained.

SCHILLING TEST The Schilling test, which determines the client's ability to absorb vitamin B_{12}, is commonly used to diagnose pernicious anemia. It is also used to diagnose malabsorption syndrome. Adequate uptake of vitamin B_{12} requires the secretion of intrinsic factor by the stomach and normal absorptive capacity of the terminal ileum. For this test, radioactive B_{12} is administered orally, followed by an IM injection of nonradioactive B_{12}. A 24-hour urine sample is collected. A finding of subnormal urinary levels of B_{12} indicates that secretion of intrinsic factor or absorption of vitamin B_{12} is abnormal. The abnormality may be due to malabsorption, renal dysfunction, or lack of intrinsic factor (pernicious anemia). A further test is then done in which intrinsic factor is administered. If excretion remains subnormal, pernicious anemia is ruled out, and malabsorption or renal disease is implicated.

NURSING IMPLICATIONS The client should be NPO for 8 to 12 hours before the test. Written consent should be obtained. Explain that nonradioactive B_{12} is administered parenterally after the radioactive B_{12} is administered orally. The parenteral dose saturates the liver and protein-binding sites so that the oral dose is absorbed and excreted. The urine is collected in a clean container that need not be refrigerated. The client should be cautioned, however, that all urine must be voided or poured into the container, or the test results will not be accurate.

XYLOSE ABSORPTION TEST Xylose is an easily absorbed monosaccharide that requires no digestion. In the xylose absorption test, used to diagnose intestinal malabsorption, the client first fasts for 10 to 12 hours. After voiding, an oral dose of D-xylose is given with water. Urine is collected for 5 hours and tested for the presence of sugar. In malabsorption disorders such as sprue and Crohn's disease, little D-xylose is excreted, since little is absorbed (Given & Simmons, 1984).

LACTOSE TOLERANCE TEST In evaluating a client for lactose deficiency, a lactose tolerance test may be done. This involves drawing a fasting blood sample, after which lactose is given by mouth. Over a period of 2 hours, further blood samples are drawn and tested for blood glucose. Elevated glucose levels in conjunction with the onset of intestinal symptoms signify a positive test. False positive and false negative results can occur, however, because the test is affected by glucose metabolism and gastric emptying time. A breath test for hydrogen before and after the ingestion of lactose is a more sensitive test for lactose deficiency. Unabsorbed lactose is converted to hydrogen by intestinal bacteria, resulting in an elevation of breath hydrogen.

BIOPSY AND CYTOLOGIC EXAMINATION Specimens of tissue for biopsy or cell scrapings for cytologic examination may be obtained during endoscopic examinations, during surgery, or when gastric tubes are inserted. Special instruments (biopsy forceps, cytology brushes) are used by the physician. The specimens obtained are microscopically examined for changes in cellular morphology, as occurs, for example, in malignancy.

NURSING IMPLICATIONS Written consent is necessary. Special postprocedure observation of the client for signs of hemorrhage is indicated. For *biopsy of the small bowel,* a specimen is obtained by passing a tube through the oral cavity. The client should be NPO for 8 hours prior to the procedure, and dentures should be removed. Since hemorrhage is a potential complication of this procedure, vital signs should be taken prior to, during, and afterward. The procedure takes about an hour and may be used in diagnosis of malabsorption disease such as nontropical (celiac) and tropical sprue (Beck, 1981b).

GASTRIC ANALYSIS Gastric analysis (analysis of gastric secretions) is important in the diagnosis of peptic ulcer, pernicious anemia, Zollinger–Ellison syndrome, and achlorhydria (absence of hydrochloric acid in the stomach), which is associated with gastric cancer.

Gastric analysis can be performed in two ways. Nasogastric intubation allows the collection of gastric secretion specimens. The client should be NPO after midnight the evening before and should not smoke the morning of the test until all specimens have been obtained. Gastric secretions are collected every 15 minutes for 1 hour, and labeled consecutively as #1, #2, and so on. These are called basal acid secretion specimens. Once basal acid secretion specimens have been collected, the client is given a gastric acid stimulant, usually histamine, parenterally. Gastric contents are then collected every 15 minutes for 1 hour and labeled appropriately. These specimens are called maximal acid secretion specimens. Monitor the client following histamine administration for adverse side effects such as increased pulse, decreased blood pressure, headache, flushing, dyspnea, vomiting, diarrhea, and shock.

The tubeless method determines the presence or absence of gastric acid without a quantitative measure of acid production. The client must refrain from all foods and medications after the evening meal the night before the test but may have water at any time. The client voids on awakening or immediately before the test is begun, and the specimen is discarded. The client ingests a gastric acid stimulant such as caffeine and is instructed to void again. This specimen is labeled #1. Once the first urine specimen is obtained, the client is given an oral resin–dye complex. This resin–dye complex is excreted in the urine and, in the presence of hydrochloric acid, turns the urine blue. Two hours after ingesting the resin–dye complex, the client voids again; this specimen is labeled #2. Encouraging the client to drink water will facilitate collecting the urine samples. Inform the client that the urine may continue to be blue for several days.

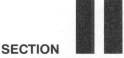

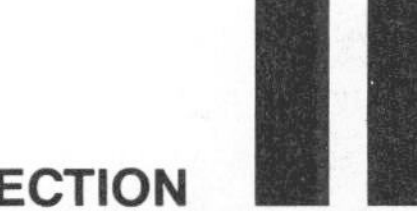

SECTION II

Nursing Diagnosis/Planning and Implementation/Evaluation

Information gathered from the client's health history, physical examination, and diagnostic studies is used to determine nursing diagnoses and the plan of care. Not every client will have the same needs. The Nursing Diagnoses box lists diagnoses **directly related** to gastrointestinal dysfunction along with **potential** nursing diagnoses for clients with gastrointestinal problems. The most common nursing diagnoses for clients with gastrointestinal dysfunction include altered bowel elimination: diarrhea and/or constipation; altered comfort: pain; potential impaired skin integrity; altered nutrition: less than body requirements; potential fluid volume deficit; and self-concept disturbance: body image. The sample nursing care plan in Table 36–1 focuses on five of these nursing diagnoses: altered bowel elimination: diarrhea; altered bowel elimination: constipation; altered comfort: pain; potential impaired skin integrity; and fluid volume deficit. The others are discussed in the narrative.

If the goals of care have not been met, re-evaluation is required. The nurse and client should jointly review the nursing care plan. New objectives may need to be formulated; other nursing interventions may be added or modified; or the evaluation may show that more time is required to meet the objectives.

Nutrition, Altered: Less Than Body Requirements

Disorders affecting the alimentary tract alter swallowing, digestion, and absorption. Singly or in combination, alterations in these functions can leave the client moderately or severely malnourished. Neoplasms or strictures of the

NURSING DIAGNOSES IN
Gastrointestinal Dysfunction

DIRECTLY RELATED DIAGNOSES

- Bowel elimination, altered: constipation
- Bowel elimination, altered: diarrhea
- Comfort, altered: pain
- Fluid volume deficit, potential
- Nutrition, altered: less than body requirements
- Role performance, altered
- Self-concept, disturbance in: body image
- Skin integrity, altered: potential

OTHER POTENTIAL DIAGNOSES

- Adjustment, impaired
- Coping, ineffective individual
- Home maintenance management, impaired
- Infection, potential for
- Knowledge deficit
- Swallowing, impaired
- Tissue integrity, impaired: oral mucous membranes
- Tissue perfusion, altered: gastrointestinal

mouth or esophagus can prevent normal ingestion of foods or fluids. Pancreatic and gastric disorders alter digestive processes; disorders of the bowel alter both digestion and absorption. Moreover, during the course of diagnosis and treatment, the client with GI disease may be subjected to long periods when food and/or fluids are restricted or prohibited. Thus, the client's nutritional state is impaired at a time when the metabolic needs imposed by the body's defense mechanisms, or by the disease itself, actually increase nutritive requirements.

Anorexia, nausea, and/or vomiting are common in GI disease, although these symptoms are also associated with dysfunction of other systems. If ingestion of food is associated with pain or discomfort, the client may be afraid to eat. Secretions and/or odors, such as those from diarrhea or wound drainage, may contribute to a less-than-appetizing atmosphere. Anorexia may also be directly associated with the disease process itself, especially in clients with cancer.

Table 36–1
Sample Nursing Care Plan for Clients With Gastrointestinal Dysfunction, by Nursing Diagnosis

Client Care Goals	Plan/Nursing Implementation	Expected Outcomes
Bowel elimination, altered: constipation related to knowledge deficit regarding nutritional food choices		
Maintain normal bowel elimination; reduce or eliminate constipation	Encourage the client to *"establish a consistent pattern of food intake and elimination; eat breakfast or at least take a hot beverage upon arising; eat foods providing roughage; eat foods such as prunes that contain natural laxatives"; drink more than 1500 mL of fluids each day; establish a pattern of regular exercise; use psyllium instead of laxatives	Client incorporates health teaching into lifestyle that results in daily soft bowel movements that easily pass without straining; should constipation occur, as it often does with traveling and change in usual diet or activity levels, client feels confident to manage problem
Bowel elimination, altered: diarrhea related to increased intestinal motility		
Manage diarrhea effectively	Encourage client to limit intake to liquids initially, gradually adding solids as tolerated; avoid milk and milk products, foods with extremes of temperature, and concentrated sweets, since these may promote diarrhea; eat foods containing pectin, such as bananas and applesauce, since these are naturally acting substances that will limit intestinal activity; eat low-fiber foods initially to avoid stimulating the bowel; clients who tend to have loose stools secondary to life stresses may benefit from regular use of psyllium; relaxation and stress reduction approaches are often helpful	Client incorporates health teaching into lifestyle; bowel elimination is normal: stools are formed, not liquid, and are passed with normal frequency
Comfort, altered: pain related to intestinal inflammation/infection		
Reduce or eliminate pain; explain pain prevention and pain management approaches	Determine the source of pain and eliminate it if possible; provide distraction for the client (ie, reading, television, visitors; encourage relaxation: deep-breathing,	Client understands measures to reduce pain and incorporates them in daily activities; should pain occur, client feels confident to manage pain; knows when to con-

Fatigue is common, especially if vomiting is violent. Large amounts of fluid and electrolytes may be lost in the vomitus and imbalances may occur. Problems associated with deficiencies of particular nutrients may also develop.

Planning and Implementation

If the client has been NPO, make sure an appetizing meal is provided as soon as the client is able to eat. Specific nursing interventions for malnutrition related to anorexia include:

- Determining the client's food preferences and making every effort to provide meals that include them
- Making mealtime a peaceful, appetizing experience
- Keeping the client comfortable and removing unappetizing secretions and odors from the environment
- Providing small, frequent feedings to stimulate appetite

If the client is experiencing nausea and vomiting, determine whether any environmental factors precipitate or worsen the symptoms and try to eliminate them. Oral hygiene may be indicated as well. Antiemetics may also be necessary.

In all clients with altered nutrition, careful intake and output measurements should be kept and used as guidelines in determining nutritional needs. Weigh the client daily. The client may require nutritional support through oral nutritional supplements, gastric or enteral tube feedings, feedings through surgically inserted tubes, or total parenteral nutrition (TPN).

ORAL SUPPLEMENTATION Oral supplements, usually high in protein and carbohydrate, are offered between meals. Standard prepackaged formulas can be used for most clients. Defined or specialty formulas are available for clients with malabsorption or maldigestion syndromes. The supplements should be served cold, in small amounts throughout the day. Flavors can be varied to maintain appetite.

Client Care Goals	Plan/Nursing Implementation	Expected Outcomes
	yoga, etc.); when pain is associated with flatus, encourage the client to avoid: • Foods that produce gas • Carbonated beverages • Air swallowing • High-fat meals • Reclining immediately after meals • Eating rapidly Administer antiflatulents as ordered; when pain is associated with excessive gastric acid secretion, administer prescribed antacids; antacids that contain simethicone help in reducing flatulence; if there are no contraindications, have client assume the knee-chest position, which aids in passing flatus	sult care provider
Skin integrity, impaired: potential related to intestinal drainage		
Remain free from skin breakdown	Keep skin clean and dry; assess skin for signs of breakdown, especially areas most susceptible to breakdown; apply lubricant to areas prone to irritation and skin protectants to areas prone to excoriation; use collection bags around drainage tubes or stomas when excessive drainage is present	Skin integrity is normal: skin shows no signs of breakdown and is smooth, soft, of normal color and moisture, and is not edematous
Fluid volume deficit, potential related to fluid losses		
Remain free from dehydration	Assess the client for symptoms and signs of dehydration; keep accurate weight and intake and output records; encourage oral fluid replacement for lost fluids; careful monitoring of IV infusions and laboratory electrolyte values	Excessive loss of fluid is prevented (eg, diarrhea); fluid and electrolyte balance is within normal limits

*Under Plan/Nursing Implementation column, content on constipation and diarrhea from Suitor & Hunter: *Nutrition: Principles and Application in Health Promotion*. Philadelphia: Lippincott, 1980, p. 267.

Table 36–2
Commercially Available Formulas for Tube Feeding

Classification	Product Names	kcal/mL	mOsm/kg water	Advantages	Disadvantages
Blenderized	Compleat B	1	405	Nutritionally complete*	High viscosity makes
	Compleat Modified	1	300	High residue makes them ideal for elderly or those who have altered bowel function	administration difficult through small-bore tubes
	Vitaneed	1	375		Most contain lactose Not for oral consumption Relatively expensive
Milk-based	Carnation Instant Breakfast	1	615–650	Palatable Good for clients who have increased protein and calorie requirements	High lactose content High osmolality
	Meritene	1	505–690		
	Sustacal Powder	1	644		
	Sustagen	1.7	1110		
Lactose-free	Ensure	1	450	Nutritionally complete*	Protein quality not as high as blenderized or milk-based formulas
	Isocal	1	300	Relatively inexpensive	
	Osmolite HN	1	310	Free-flowing consistency	
	Nutri-Aid	1	300	May be used orally	
	Osmolite	1	300		
	Portagen	1	354		
	Renu	1	300		
	Sustacal Liquid	1	625		
	Travasorb	1	450		
High density lactose-free	Ensure Plus	1.5	600	Nutritionally complete*	Protein quality not as high as blenderized or milk-based formulas
	Isocal HCN	2	740	Relatively inexpensive	
	Magnacal	2	590	Free-flowing consistency	
	Sustacal HC	1.5	650	Ideal for fluid-restricted clients	Must be diluted and advanced slowly
Chemically defined	Citrotein	0.66	500	Require minimal digestion	High osmolality
	Criticare HN	1	650	Lactose-free	Some are relatively unpalatable
	Isotein HN	1.2	300	Low viscosity so easily administered through small bore tubes	Relatively expensive
	Precision Isotonic	1	300		Some contain minimal amounts of long-chain fats
	Precision HN	1	500		
	Precision LR	1	525–545		
	Travasorb HN	1	560		
	Travasorb MCT	1 to 2	300–500		
	Travasorb Std	1	560		
	Vital HN	1	460		
Free amino acid	Vivonex HN	1	810		
	Vivonex Std	1	550		
Specialty formulas	Amin-Aid	1.9	1095	May be given by tube or mouth	High osmolality
	Hepatic-Aid	1.6	1158	Require minimal digestion	High carbohydrate
	Travasorb Hepatic	1.1	690		Some are nutritionally incomplete
	Travasorb Renal	1.35	590		Very expensive
	Trauma-Aid	1	800		Formulas designed for trauma do not meet currently accepted standards for nutritional requirements for increased stress
	Trauma-Cal	1.5	550		
	Vivonex Ten	1	630		
	Stresstein	1.2	910		

Classification	Product Names	kcal/mL	mOsm/kg water	Advantages	Disadvantages
Modules	*Carbohydrate*			Flexible—may be combined to yield specific formula May be added to food	Takes longer to prepare May alter taste and/or texture if added to food
	Moducal	4 kcal/g 2 kcal/mL	(powder) 725		
	Polycose	4 kcal/g 2 kcal/mL	(powder) 850		
	Sumacal	4 kcal/g	(powder)		
	Fat				
	Lipomul	6 kcal/mL	Not applicable for fats		
	MCT (medium chain triglyceride)	7.7 kcal/mL			
	Microlipid	4.5 kcal/mL			
	Protein				
	Casec	4 kcal/g	24 g protein/30 mL		
	Promix	4 kcal/g	24 g protein/30 mL		
	Propac	4 kcal/g	23 g protein/30 mL		
	Nutrisource				

*Nutritionally complete when given in appropriate volumes. SOURCE: Konstantinides NN, Shronts E: Tube feeding: Managing the basics. *Am J Nurs* 1983; 83:1316.

TUBE FEEDINGS Tube feedings may be administered through a gastric tube or through a small-caliber, weighted tube passed to the duodenum or the proximal jejunum (Gramse, 1983). Tubes for feeding may also be surgically inserted into the esophagus (esophagostomy), stomach (gastrostomy), duodenum (duodenostomy), or jejunum (jejunostomy).

Tube feedings into the stomach are usually tolerated well because the stomach has a reservoir capacity, increasing tolerance to volume of feedings. The risk of aspiration is minimized when the esophageal gastric junction is bypassed with a gastrostomy tube. Esophagostomy and nasogastric tubes prevent complete closure of the esophageal–gastric junction, thereby increasing the risk of aspiration.

Many commercial formulas are available for tube feedings. In the past, formulas were compounded by pureeing baby foods or table foods in a blender. This method is impractical, time consuming, vulnerable to contamination, and does not allow for good control of nutritional intake. Table 36–2 outlines many available formulas, most requiring no preparation. The dietitian is important in formula selection for tube feedings and in prescribing the appropriate amount to meet individual needs. Most formulas contain all the necessary nutrients, but some are incomplete and must be supplemented; balanced nutritional intake is essential. Lactose intolerance, a frequent problem, is avoided by using lactose-free formulas for tube feedings.

Feedings may be given intermittently or continuously. The intermittent approach involves administration of formula 5 to 6 times daily given over 30 minutes. This is the most practical and best tolerated method of administering feedings. Giving the formula too rapidly causes cramping, bloating, nausea, vomiting, and diarrhea. Continuous feeding over 24 hours ties the client down, impairing mobility. Feeding pumps are usually used for continuous feeding to control the infusion rate.

When tube feeding is initiated, the client should be allowed 3 to 4 days to acclimate to the feedings, especially if the gastrointestinal tract has been without feedings for 7 days or more. The placement of the tubing should be checked prior to each feeding. Formulas should be started at low concentration and a slow rate, advancing slowly to full strength and full volume. The feeding should be administered with the head of the bed elevated to prevent aspiration. This method will minimize gastrointestinal symptoms and facilitate good nutritional support.

Nursing care with tube feedings entails careful monitoring for complications. Clients who receive tube feedings may experience diarrhea, nausea, abdominal distention, or asphyxia. Increasing the strength and amount of the formula gradually and ensuring that the head of the bed is elevated 30% should prevent these difficulties. Antidiarrheal medications may be necessary. If diarrhea persists, a different formula may be tried.

Natural pectin, such as Certo or Sure-Jel, adminis-

Table 36–3
Common Problems of Tube Feedings

Factors to Assess to Determine How Client Is Tolerating the Feeding	Possible Causes of Problems	Corrective Measures
Gastrointestinal function		
Vomiting	Feeding too soon after intubation	Allow client time to relax and rest after tube is inserted
	Improper location of tip of feeding tube	Repositioning of tube by qualified health professional
	Rapid rate of infusion	Administer slowly
	Excessive volume: (1) Air (2) Formula	Be sure tube feeding container does not run dry before feeding is completed Check with physician regarding number and size of feedings
	Position of client	Position on right side for ½ hr following feeding—reverse Trendelenburg or semi-Fowler's
(Applies to both vomiting and diarrhea)	Food infection or poisoning	Check sanitation of formula and equipment
	Anxiety	Explain procedures; provide reassurance and other needed types of support; provide privacy
Diarrhea	Rapid rate of infusion	Administer slowly—very slowly if formula is cold
	High osmolality of formula or high concentration of formula	Adapt client to formula gradually
	Lactose intolerance	Contact physician regarding change of formula
Constipation	High content of milk in formula Lack of fiber Inadequate fluid intake	Contact physician regarding: (1) Change in formula (2) Laxatives (3) Increasing fluid
Fluid and electrolyte balance		
Dehydration	Rapid infusion of carbohydrate → hyperglycemia → osmotic diuresis → dehydration	Administer slowly; exogeneous insulin sometimes needed
	Excess protein and electrolytes in formula Inadequate fluid intake	Change formula and/or increase fluid according to physician's orders
Edema	Excessive sodium in formula	Check with physician about change in formula
Nutritional adequacy		
Undernutrition (gradual weight loss)	Inadequate number of calories to meet energy requirements	Check to see if client is receiving prescribed amount of formula; estimate client's caloric intake Check with physician regarding increasing the volume, concentration, or number of feedings given
Overnutrition (gradual gain of undesirable weight)	Excessive caloric intake	Check with physician regarding decreasing the volume, concentration, or number of feedings given
Undernutrition (inadequate intake of protein and/or micronutrients leading to biochemical or clinical signs of deficiency)	Amount of standard formula needed to maintain weight is too low to meet requirements for essential nutrients	Check with physician regarding providing appropriate nutrient supplements

SOURCE: Suitor CW, Hunter MF: *Nutrition: Principles and Applications in Health Promotion*. Philadelphia: Lippincott, 1980, p. 371.

tered 2 to 3 times a day helps to prevent diarrhea in clients who are tube fed. When larger bore tubes are used, psyllium is a good source of bulk and can be included in the regimen. Care in administration will prevent clogging of the tube.

To prevent abdominal distention, check the client for residual formula in the stomach before and several hours after a feeding; withhold feeding if more than 150 mL of residual formula is found. A large residual volume implies slow gastric emptying and may require an altered approach to the feeding regimen.

Table 36–3 lists common problems associated with tube feedings as well as measures to correct them. In addition, electrolyte imbalance, alterations in glucose levels, and deficiency of fatty acids may occur; laboratory studies should be monitored for changes in these values.

Specific nursing techniques for insertion, use, and removal of apparatus used for tube feedings may be found in nursing fundamentals texts. Care associated with TPN is described in Chapter 6.

Clients whose nutritional status is compromised are especially prone to infection. Since they are highly susceptible to infectious disease, special precautions should be taken to avoid exposure. Be alert to symptoms of infection.

Evaluation

Expected client outcomes following effective nursing interventions for alteration in nutrition, less than body requirements include acceptance of dietary alteration, freedom from nausea and/or vomiting, absence of aspiration, absence of abdominal distention, maintenance of desired weight, and laboratory values within normal limits.

Self-Concept, Disturbance in: Body Image Role Performance, Altered

Pain, weakness, and poor self-image may interfere with the client's self-care activities. Alterations in body image accompany many treatments, most notably surgical construction of an ostomy. Other disturbances in self-concept may be related to role changes, if, for example, a family breadwinner is immobilized or permanently disabled by disease or treatment, or if the marital partner who has assumed the major responsibility for child care can no longer do so. Sexual dysfunction, while not directly related to gastrointestinal disease, may occur in a client who has a colostomy and avoids sexual contact because of feelings of disgust or shame.

Planning and Implementation

For clients with a disturbance in body image and fears about sexual rejection, nurses should initiate discussion of these fears if the client is unable to do so. Attempt to discover whether the fears are from lack of knowledge about body changes or from concerns about reactions of significant others and/or the sexual partner. Encourage the client to verbalize his/her anger, grief, and/or feelings of despair. Assist the client to become confident in self-management.

Evaluation

Expected client outcomes following effective nursing interventions for disturbance in body image include verbalization of concerns about body image and concerns about reactions of loved ones; interest in personal appearance; interest in maintaining close interpersonal relationships; willingness to adapt lifestyle as necessary; requests for specific information about body changes and what can be realistically expected in the future.

Chapter Highlights

A nutritional assessment is always indicated in caring for clients with gastrointestinal disorders.

Nursing assessments to determine the presence of peristalsis include assessments for abdominal distention, presence of bowel sounds, and the passage of stool or flatus.

Clients with gastrointestinal system disorders often experience symptoms of anorexia, nausea and vomiting, diarrhea, and constipation.

In assessing clients with gastrointestinal disorders, the functions of swallowing, secretion, motility, digestion, absorption, and elimination need to be determined.

Dietary influences include psychologic, social, cultural, and economic factors.

The nurse should ensure the privacy of clients with gastrointestinal disorders, since they may experience embarrassment due to symptoms associated with their disease.

Elderly clients are especially prone to malnutrition and constipation.

Nutritional support is often indicated for clients with gastrointestinal disorders.

Nutritional support includes supplementary oral feedings, gastric and enteral feedings, feedings through surgically inserted tubes, and hyperalimentation.

The client with a gastrointestinal disorder may experience a self-concept disturbance: body image, and altered role performance.

Fatigue is often experienced by clients subjected to the numerous and often lengthy diagnostic procedures associated with gastrointestinal disease.

The client with a gastrointestinal disorder is especially prone to fluid and electrolyte and acid–base imbalances related to the excessive fluid losses that often accompany gastrointestinal disease.

Bibliography

Alterescu KB: What about special procedures? *Am J Nurs* 1985; 85(12):1363–1367.

Anderson BJ: Tube feeding: Is diarrhea inevitable? *Am J Nurs* 1986; 86(6):704–706.

Arnold C: Why that liquid formula diet may not work (and what to do about it). *RN* (Nov) 1981; 35–39.

Baker JP et al: Nutritional assessment: A comparison of clinical judgment and objective measurements. *N Engl J Med* 1982; 306:969–972.

Barisonek K, Newman E, Logio T: My stomach hurts. *Nurs 84* (Nov) 1984; 14:34–41.

Bayer LM, Scholl DE, Ford EG: Tube feeding at home. *Am J Nurs* 1983; 83:1321–1325.

Beck ML: Preparing your patient psychologically for an esophagogastroduodenoscopy. (a). *Nurs 81* (Jan) 1981; 11:28–30.

Beck ML: Two intestinal tests: one oral, one anal. (b). *Nurs 81* (July) 1981; 11:20–22.

Bryne CJ et al: *Laboratory Tests: Implications for Nursing Care,* 2nd ed. Menlo Park, CA: Addison–Wesley, 1986.

Crowley LV: *Introduction to Human Disease.* Monterey, CA: Wadsworth, 1983.

Given BA, Simmons SJ: *Gastroenterology in Clinical Nursing,* 4th ed. St. Louis: Mosby, 1984.

Gramse CA: A review of tube feeding techniques. *Nurs 83* (Feb) 1983; 13:32B–32P.

Grimes J, Iannopollo E: *Health Assessment in Nursing Practice.* Belmont, CA: Wadsworth, 1982.

Hahn AB, Barkin RL, Oestreich SJK: *Pharmacology in Nursing.* St. Louis: Mosby, 1982.

Hui YH: *Human Nutrition and Diet Therapy.* Monterey, CA: Wadsworth, 1983.

Kee JL: *Laboratory and Diagnostic Tests with Nursing Implications.* Norwalk, CT: Appleton–Century–Crofts, 1983.

Kohrs MB: New perspectives on nutritional counseling for the elderly. *Contemporary Nutrition* (March) 1983; 8(3).

Konstantinides NN, Shrouts E: Tube feeding: Managing the basics. *Am J Nurs* 1983; 83:1312–1320.

Meshkinpour H et al: Esophageal manometry: A benefit and cost analysis. *Dig Dis Sci* 1982; 27:772–775.

Metheny NM: 20 ways to prevent tube-feeding complications. *Nurs 85* (Jan) 1985; 15:47–50.

Moghissi K, Boore JRP: *Parenteral and Enteral Nutrition for Nurses.* Rockville, MD: Aspen Systems, 1983.

Moore MC, Guenter PA, Bender JH: Nutrition-related nursing research. *Image* (Spring) 1986; 18:18–21.

Rodman MJ, Smith DW: *Clinical Pharmacology in Nursing,* 2nd ed. Philadelphia: Lippincott, 1984.

Smith CE: Detecting acute abdominal distention. *Nurs 85* (Sept) 1985; 15:34–39.

Stiklorius C: Beginning this month: GI studies. *RN* (March) 1982; 64–65.

Stiklorius C: Preparing for two uncomfortable tests: Gastric analysis and liver biopsy. *RN* (Sept) 1982; 64.

Tichy AM, Chong D: When assessing the aged don't be fooled by these false alarms. *RN* (Sept) 1981; 58–62.

Tuttobene SA: A bowel prep that's easy to follow. *RN* (March) 1984; 52.

Veninga KS: An easy recipe for assessing your patient's nutrition. *Nurs 82* (Nov) 1982; 12:57–59.

Zettel ER: Beaming in on the GI tract. *Am J Nurs* 1986; 86(3):280–282.

Resources

SELF-HELP GROUPS AND OTHER ORGANIZATIONS

American Celiac Society
45 Gifford Ave.
Jersey City, NJ 07304
Phone: (201) 432–1207

The members of this organization are individuals with gluten-sensitive enteropathy and health care professionals (including dieticians and nutritionists) who coordinate and distribute information on celiac sprue, support research into the disorder, and help members locate sources of gluten-free specialty foods. The organization also conducts educational conferences for clients and health care professionals. They publish the American Celiac Society Newsletter.

National Foundation for Ileitis and Colitis, Inc.
444 Park Ave South
New York, NY 10016
Phone: (212) 685–3440

This nonprofit foundation provides information on inflammatory bowel diseases to the public and to professionals and funds related research. Clients and family members can also obtain referrals to government-sponsored services for persons with ileitis and colitis.

United Ostomy Association, Inc.
36 Executive Park
Suite 120
Irvine, CA 92714
Phone: (714) 660–8624

Most members in this organization are ostomates. It provides client mutual-support groups as well as educational programs in ostomy care and management, and assistance in developing and locating ostomy equipment and supplies. It publishes the *Ostomy Quarterly.*

In Canada:
Canadian Foundation for Ileitis and Colitis
21 St. Clair St E
Toronto, Ontario
Canada M5H 1K5
Phone: (416) 920–5038

This foundation for clients with inflammatory bowel disease has 25 chapters in most Canadian provinces and publishes a quarterly, *The Journal.* Specific addresses can be obtained from the headquarters listed here.

HOT LINES

Gutline (American Digestive Disease Society)
Phone: (301) 652–9293, Tues & Thurs, 7:30–9:00 PM, Eastern Time

HEALTH EDUCATION MATERIAL

From:
Patient Information Library
Krames Communications
312 90th St
Daly City, CA 94015–2621
Phone: (415) 994–8800
Pamphlets and booklets related to problems in the GI tract.

From:
National Foundation for Ileitis and Colitis, Inc.
444 Park Ave South
New York, NY 10016
Pamphlets (appropriate for professionals and clients) on Crohn's disease and ulcerative colitis.

From:
American Cancer Society, Inc.
National Headquarters
4 West 35th St
New York, NY 10001
Educational materials, available free, provide information on esophageal, stomach, colorectal, and pancreatic cancer.

From:
US Department of Health and Human Services
Public Health Service
National Institutes of Health
Bethesda, MD 20014

Cancer of the Colon and Rectum. NIH Pub. No. 83–1552, January 1983.

NCI Research Report: Cancer of the Colon and Rectum. NIH Pub. No. 82–95, September 1982.

Cancer of the Pancreas. NIH Pub. No. 82–1560, May 1982.

Cancer of the Stomach. NIH Pub. No. 83–1554, August 1983.

From:
Hoescht–Roussel Pharmaceuticals, Inc.
(Advertising)
Rte. 202–206 North
Somerville, NJ 08876
Phone: (201) 231–2000

What You Should Know About Hemorrhoids and Fissures, 1982.

All the following are available free from:
Blistex, Inc.
1800 Swift Dr.
Oak Brook, IL 60521
Attn: Richard K. Green
Executive Vice-President
Phone: (312) 571–2870

Canker and Mouth Sores, What You Should Know.

Your Lips' Health and Beauty: A Guide From the Lip Care Experts at Blistex.

Mini-Teaching Guide on Lip Care.

From:
General Mills
Attn: Gloria T. Florey
PO Box 1112, Dept 65
Minneapolis, MN 55440
A monthly newsletter, *Contemporary Nutrition,* is available to food and health professionals.

PROFESSIONAL ORGANIZATIONS

International Association for Enterostomal Therapy, Inc.
2081 Business Center Drive
Suite 290
Irvine, CA 92715
Phone: (714) 476–0268
The membership in this organization is limited to enterostomal therapists and other interested individuals who hold licenses in medicine or nursing. Its goal is to provide care and rehabilitation to persons with abdominal stomas, fistulas, draining wounds, pressure sores, and incontinence. Dues: $65.

Society of Gastrointestinal Assistants
1070 Sibley Tower
Rochester, NY 14604
Phone: (716) 546–7241
This association of RNs, LPNs and LVNs develops educational programs in digestive diseases and promotes optimal functioning of clients with digestive diseases.

In Canada:
Canadian Association of Enterostomal Therapy
Catherine Foster
Montreal General Hospital
1650 Cedar Ave.
Montreal, Quebec, H3G 1A4
Phone: (514) 937–6011

CHAPTER 37

Specific Disorders of the Mouth and Esophagus

Other topics relevant to this content are: Assessment and care of the client in pain, **Chapter 3;** Care of the client with cancer, **Chapter 10.**

Objectives

When you have finished studying this chapter, you should be able to:

Identify risk factors associated with disorders of the mouth and esophagus.

Initiate client assessments specific to disorders of the mouth and esophagus.

Discuss the role of the nurse in prevention of disorders of the mouth and esophagus.

Describe medical and surgical approaches to disorders of the mouth and esophagus.

Specify appropriate nursing care for clients with disorders of the mouth and esophagus.

Anticipate psychosocial/lifestyle implications for clients with disorders of the mouth and esophagus.

List oral hygiene measures appropriate for clients with disorders of the mouth.

Plan the dietary modifications most often indicated for clients with disorders of the mouth and esophagus.

The primary significance of disorders of the mouth and esophagus is that they can significantly alter nutritional status by interfering with ingestion, digestion, and/or absorption. Moreover, many of these disorders are associated with considerable discomfort and temporary or permanent alteration in body image.

Clients undergoing surgical treatment of the gastrointestinal system often experience lengthy hospitalizations, altered body image, the need to adjust to a different way of taking in food or eliminating waste products, and embarrassment over the public nature of what are usually, at least in the case of elimination, private functions. The nurse who cares for these clients must be sensitive as well as skilled.

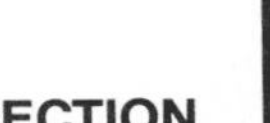

SECTION I

Disorders of Multifactorial Origin

Disorders of multifactorial origin that affect the mouth and esophagus develop during the natural life span of the individual. Some are related to environmental factors, some to lifestyle. Some are preventable, some are not. Teaching preventive measures to clients and the general public is a major nursing responsibility. Once disorders have occurred, dietary instruction and nutritional support may be indicated.

Since these disorders are frequently associated with dysphagia, the client may have to make dietary adjustments to alleviate or compensate for this difficulty. For example, liquid or soft foods may be easier to swallow; small, frequent feedings may be easier to ingest. Oral hygiene measures may prevent the onset or spread of infection and promote the client's personal comfort.

The nurse's support and encouragement will help clients make dietary changes that involve a change from their usual lifestyle, for example, avoiding refined carbohydrates. Referring the client to a dietitian for counseling may be advisable. Some clients with oral and/or esophageal disorders may be undernourished so that providing a well-balanced diet with nutritional supplementation and nutri-

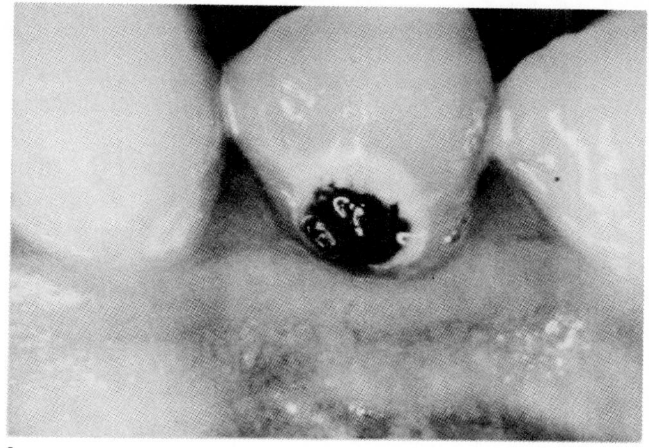

A

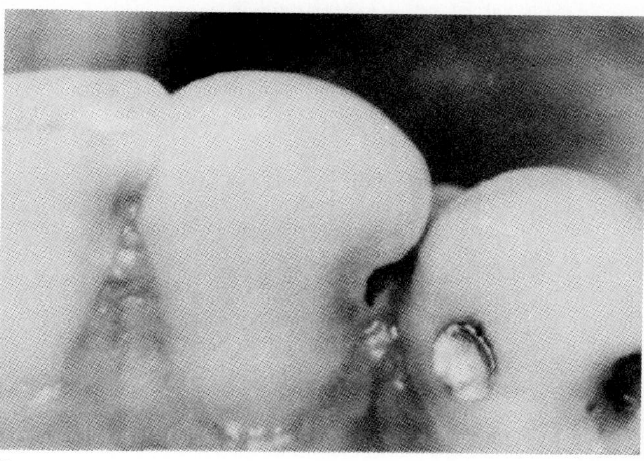

B

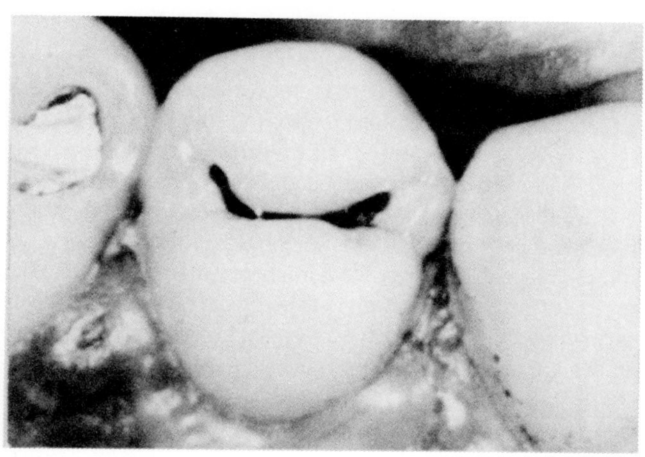

C

Figure 37–1

A. Gumline caries, premolar. **B.** Interproximal caries, lateral incisor and cuspid. **C.** Occlusal caries (chewing surface), premolar. *Courtesy of Gerald Wieczkowski, Jr., DDS, School of Dentistry, State University of New York at Buffalo.*

tional support as needed will be an important nursing responsibility.

Dental Caries

Dental caries, or tooth decay, is the principal cause of tooth loss up to the fourth decade of life (Petersdorf, 1983). Dental caries involves demineralization (decalcification) of tooth enamel and dentin, the main tissue of the tooth (Figure 37–1). Caries can cause pain. The disorder may also interfere with eating, promote halitosis, cause cosmetic changes that embarrass the individual, and lead to loss of teeth. Treatment of dental caries consumes large amounts of money and time.

Caries formation is believed to result from interaction of certain foods (notably refined sugars) and oral bacteria (notably *Streptococcus mutans*) (Schachtele, 1980). Intake of carbohydrates leads to formation of *dental plaque*, a soft, spongy, tenacious material composed of bacteria, protein, and carbohydrate. Bacterial action on ingested carbohydrates produces acids that are destructive to the teeth. Frequent ingestion of carbohydrates, therefore, is of particular significance in the development of dental caries, and numerous studies have linked increased consumption of sugar and sugar-sweetened foods to an increased prevalence of caries.

Clinical Manifestations

The client with caries may not perceive pain until considerable damage has been done to the teeth. Darkening and erosion of the dental surface may be noted on inspection. Accurate assessment of damage to the teeth usually requires x-rays. Once a carious lesion has become extensive, pulpitis (inflammation of the dental pulp) can result. At this point, the client usually notices pain when ingesting cold foods and fluids. Abscesses and more extensive infections may then occur.

Medical Measures

Dental caries is preventable. Meticulous oral hygiene, including brushing and flossing, is recommended. Stannous fluoride, which interferes with bacterial activity on

NURSING DIAGNOSES IN
Gastrointestinal Dysfunction

DIRECTLY RELATED DIAGNOSES

- Bowel elimination, altered: constipation
- Bowel elimination, altered: diarrhea
- Comfort, altered: pain
- Fluid volume deficit, potential
- Nutrition, altered: less than body requirements
- Role performance, altered
- Self-concept, disturbance in: body image
- Skin integrity, altered: potential

OTHER POTENTIAL DIAGNOSES

- Adjustment, impaired
- Coping, ineffective individual
- Home maintenance management, impaired
- Infection, potential for
- Knowledge deficit
- Swallowing, impaired
- Tissue integrity, impaired: oral mucous membranes
- Tissue perfusion, altered: gastrointestinal

teeth, may be used, either by means of fluoridated water supplies or individual application. Since some religious groups and other groups concerned with chemical additives in water have raised questions about the advisability of fluoridating community water supplies, recent emphasis has been on individual application. Fluoride may be applied topically in sprays, gels, and/or toothpaste, or may be taken in capsules or tablets.

Dietary modification has also been recommended. It is generally believed that the incidence of caries may be reduced by:

- Decreasing the frequency of carbohydrate consumption, particularly refined carbohydrates such as those in candy; soft drinks; ice cream; and most cakes, pies, and other baked goods
- Reducing the time sugars remain in contact with the teeth (eg, by prompt brushing or at least rinsing the mouth after eating)

Approaches still being evaluated include combating causative bacteria by topical application of iodine or by introducing nonvirulent bacteria that might inhibit the activity of cariogenic species. Immunization has also been suggested.

Specific Nursing Measures

Prevention is the key factor in management of dental caries. A nurse has many opportunities to teach and encourage preventive measures during interactions with clients, especially during routine physical examinations. Because the etiology of dental caries has been identified rather recently, many adults may not be aware of the role of bacterial action. Has the client been shown how to brush properly? To floss? To use a soft brush? Does the client know what plaque is? A demonstration, using dye, may be revealing, especially to someone whose oral hygiene practices are relatively good.

Changing one's diet is not easy, especially given the American predilection for sugary snacks. Some clients may find it difficult to brush or floss after meals, especially while at work or traveling. Recent studies show that good control can be achieved by thorough brushing and flossing once a day combined with rinsing after meals. Does the client know how to use a Water Pik™ to best advantage? Does the client see a dentist twice a year? All these areas offer opportunities for health teaching.

For clients who are unable to perform their own oral hygiene measures, the nurse will have to do so. It is important to continue brushing and flossing, even if the client is comatose.

Malocclusion

Malocclusion refers to imperfect alignment of teeth that affects how they meet during chewing (the "bite"). Various types have been identified (eg, overbite, underbite, crossbite), and most are discovered and corrected in childhood.

Malocclusion related to abnormal development of the teeth and jaws usually becomes evident in childhood when the permanent teeth erupt. Sometimes malocclusion occurs in adults after oral trauma or with extraction or loss of carious teeth. With improved techniques of correction, more adults are undergoing therapy.

Clinical Manifestations

Malocclusion can cause difficulty in chewing, temporomandibular joint (TMJ) pain, and bone loss. Malocclusion often coexists with TMJ disorders, although the relationship remains unclear. Severe malocclusion may also affect facial appearance as well as the appearance of the teeth.

Medical Measures

Teeth may be brought into alignment by bands and/or wires that exert pressure (braces). The process is long because it relies on changes in the underlying bone that occur over time in response to pressure. Sometimes teeth must be extracted to make room for the remaining teeth. Sometimes oral (maxillofacial) surgery is done; for example, wedges of bone may be removed or inserted to correct the shape of the dental arch. Because correction of malocclusion is a long, usually expensive process, a great deal of commitment is required from the client. Oral hygiene is both crucial and time consuming while the client is wearing braces.

Specific Nursing Measures

Ask the client about pain or difficulty in chewing. Improper chewing can affect digestion; pain may cause the client to avoid eating, promoting malnutrition. Nutritional assessment may be required, and nutritional support may have to be provided.

The client with braces may require instruction regarding their care and reinforcement of the importance of meticulous mouth care. These appliances readily harbor microorganisms. Removable appliances (such as retainers) should be washed daily with soap and water and kept clean. Since braces are so conspicuous and generally associated with adolescence, the adult client may be embarrassed about wearing them and concerned about body image. The late adolescent client may experience intense embarrassment at a time when issues of body image assume great importance.

Hiatal Hernia

A hiatal hernia (sometimes called a diaphragmatic hernia) is the herniation (protrusion) of the stomach through the diaphragm into the thoracic cavity. There are two principal types of hiatal hernia, the sliding or direct hernia and the paraesophageal (rolling or indirect) hernia. In the more common sliding type, the fundus of the stomach and the gastroesophageal junction ride into the thorax. With the rolling type, a part of the stomach separate from the gastroesophageal junction is involved (Figure 37–2A, B).

A hiatal hernia may be related to weakening of gastroesophageal supports, longitudinal contraction of the esophagus, or increased intra-abdominal pressure (Petersdorf, 1983). Intra-abdominal pressure may be increased by pregnancy, obesity, ascites, physical exertion, trauma, coughing, sneezing, or straining at stool.

Hiatal hernia is more common in women, and in both sexes incidence increases with age. Petersdorf (1983) reports that prevalence in persons ages 50 to 59 is approximately 60%.

Clinical Manifestations

Hiatal hernias may be asymptomatic. In cases of sliding hiatal hernia, reflux of gastric contents into the esophagus may be related to incompetence of the lower esophageal sphincter. Reflux produces burning substernal discomfort ("heartburn") and acid regurgitation. Eructation and flatulence may also occur as the client swallows air to reverse the reflux. Reflux and regurgitation may be associated with aspiration, promoting inflammation and/or infection of the respiratory tract.

Continual reflux of gastric contents may cause esophagitis and damage to esophageal tissue. Resulting fibrosis and scarring may cause strictures and decreased esophageal motility, so the client finds it difficult to swallow. Any conditions that increase intra-abdominal pressure may aggravate symptoms, as may the recumbent position. Preventive approaches for gastroesophageal reflux are presented in Box 37–1.

Rolling hernias may incarcerate (become trapped) as the protruding stomach is caught above the diaphragm. Resulting impairment of circulation may cause ulceration of tissue; total ischemia may cause tissue necrosis.

A feeling of fullness after eating is a common symptom of either type of hiatal hernia. Diagnosis is made on the basis of symptoms and diagnostic testing, including radiog-

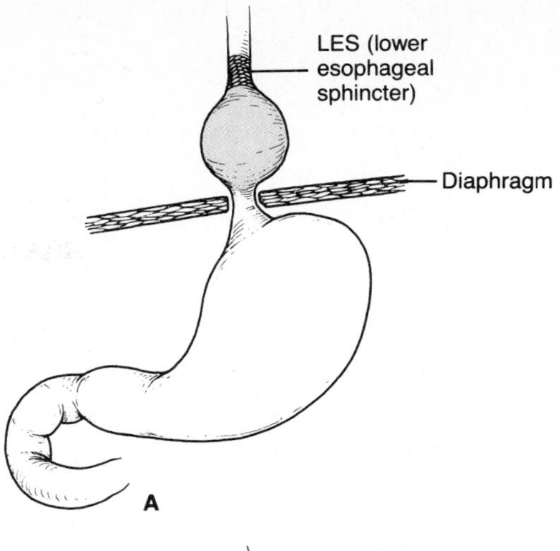

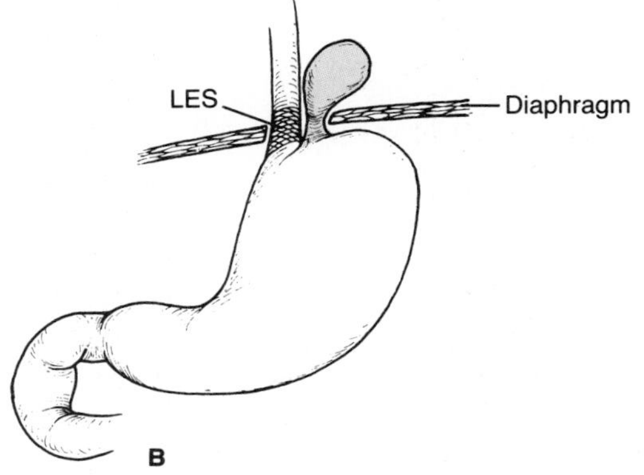

Figure 37–2

Hiatal hernias. **A.** Sliding (direct). **B.** Paraesophageal (indirect or rolling).

Box 37–1
Preventive Approaches for Gastroesophageal Reflux

Avoid bending over or lying down soon after eating.

Elevate the head of the bed on blocks if reflux occurs when lying down.

Eat small, frequent meals to avoid overdistention of the stomach.

Use liquid antacids 1/2 h after meals and at bedtime.

Avoid increased intra-abdominal pressure by:
- Maintaining normal weight
- Wearing nonconstricting clothing
- Stopping smoking to decrease coughing

Avoid alcoholic beverages (alcohol prevents the LES from closing properly).

Avoid foods that may contribute to reflux, including caffeine, spicy or greasy foods, and foods high in acid (eg, tomatoes).

raphy, fluoroscopy, endoscopy, and tests of esophageal motility and pH.

Medical Measures

Antacids are prescribed to reduce acidity and alleviate discomfort. Smoking, which stimulates gastric secretion, should be discouraged. Avoiding the recumbent position for at least 30 minutes after meals may be helpful, and preventive measures for conditions that increase intra-abdominal pressure (eg, straining at stool, obesity) are instituted (eg, increased fiber to prevent constipation, weight loss program). Drinking water after meals may help, as may sleeping on the right side (Given & Simmons, 1984). If these measures fail to control esophagitis and other serious symptoms, surgical repair may be indicated.

Specific Nursing Measures

Relief of symptoms is a high priority. Explain to the client and family the importance of eating slowly and eating small, frequent, nonirritating meals; remaining upright after meals; and avoiding increased intra-abdominal pressure. Try to help the client determine what seems to precipitate symptoms. Heavy meals? Spicy foods such as chili, pizza, ethnic specialties? Acid foods, such as peppers, tomatoes, citrus fruits? Caffeine, which is found in coffee, tea, cola drinks, and chocolate? Are symptoms worse at night when the client is lying down? Is the client swallowing air while eating, while talking or because some life situation is making the client nervous or apprehensive? Once these factors have been identified, nurse and client can work out a plan for avoiding them.

Administer antacids as ordered, and explain how they should be used. Assess for respiratory complications and for esophagitis.

Hiatal Hernia Repair

Hiatal hernia repair is more common than other types of esophageal surgery. When medical treatment is unsuccessful in controlling the symptoms of hiatal hernia, surgical repair may be indicated. Definite indications for surgical repair include obstructive stricture and hemorrhage.

One relatively common surgical approach to the repair of a hiatal hernia is *Nissen fundoplication*. The surgeon wraps the fundus of the stomach around the lower esophagus and sutures the fundus to itself. The fundus prevents the esophageal–gastric junction from slipping into the thoracic cavity so the symptoms of heartburn and pressure will not recur. The physiologic and psychosocial-lifestyle implications for the client are discussed in Table 37–1.

Nursing Implications

Nursing care specific to hiatal hernia repair includes maintaining respiratory status, maintaining gastric suction, and promoting appropriate nutritional intake when the client can begin to eat. Appropriate pain control measures may enhance the ability to aerate the lungs adequately. Clients should not be allowed to smoke for several days and should be encouraged to quit altogether. The nurse should instruct the client in ways of preventing the recurrence of reflux (see Box 37–1).

The client should begin a liquid diet when able to take in fluids. Gas-producing fluids such as carbonated beverages should be avoided because belching may be impaired and gas discomfort may develop. Transient dysphagia may be experienced as a result of edema around the lower esophagus. The client advances to eating solids according to tolerance.

SECTION 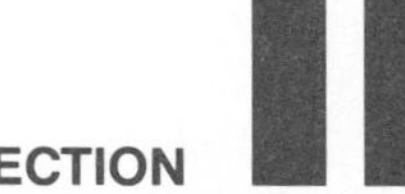

Inflammatory and Infectious Disorders

Inflammation of the mouth and esophagus, whether or not accompanied by infection, may be related to internal or external irritation or to invasion by foreign organisms (bac-

Table 37–1
Hiatal Hernia Repair: Implications for the Client

Physiologic Implications	Psychosocial/Lifestyle Implications
Proximity of incision to diaphragm makes coughing and deep breathing uncomfortable. Eructation may be impaired postoperatively. Postoperative complications include: hemorrhage; infection; pulmonary embolus; dysphagia; esophageal obstruction, perforation, fistula formation.	Abdominal incision may affect body image. To prevent recurrence, tight clothing should be avoided, smoking stopped, normal weight maintained, and emotional stress reduced. Measures to avoid flatulence include eating slowly to avoid excessive air swallowing; avoiding carbonated beverages; and eliminating foods such as beans, broccoli, and cabbage from the diet.

teria, viruses, or fungi). Some of these disorders (eg, periodontitis) are common in the adult population. Others tend to recur in certain individuals (eg, stomatitis). Many may be prevented by oral hygiene.

Periodontal Disease

Periodontal disease, or *periodontitis*, is a chronic inflammatory process that affects the soft tissues and bones that surround and support the teeth. In its advanced stages, periodontal disease promotes degeneration of tissue and separation of teeth from their supports (Figure 37–3A). Gingivitis (inflammation of the gingivae), characterized by red, edematous, bleeding gums, commonly accompanies periodontal disease, which affects over 75% of the US adult population to some extent (DePaola, Alvares, & Etzel, 1982) (Figure 37–3B).

The major etiologic factor in periodontal disease is thought to be plaque. Poor oral hygiene can contribute to excessive plaque formation with subsequent development of periodontitis, and inadequate nutrition may accelerate the process or decrease an individual's resistance to it. Pregnant women, persons with Down's syndrome, and diabetics are especially susceptible to periodontal disease, whereas the use of oral contraceptives and phenytoin (Dilantin) promote development of gingivitis. Increased levels of prostaglandins have been found in inflamed gingival tissue, and it is thought that prostaglandins may be at least partially responsible for the bone resorption that accompanies periodontal disease (Petersdorf, 1983).

Gingival hyperplasia, where the gingiva proliferate and may actually cover the teeth, is an untoward side effect of treatment with phenytoin (Dilantin), nifedipine (Procardia), or cyclosporine. The hyperplasia appears to be plaque related (Figure 37–4).

Clinical Manifestations

The client with periodontal disease will have symptoms of gingivitis: reddened, swollen gums that bleed easily with minimal trauma, such as from brushing the teeth. Pyorrhea (discharge of pus) may occur if the disease is advanced. Gums may recede, and teeth may loosen.

The client with gingival hyperplasia has difficulty chewing. Body image problems often occur because of the unsightly appearance of the gingival overgrowth.

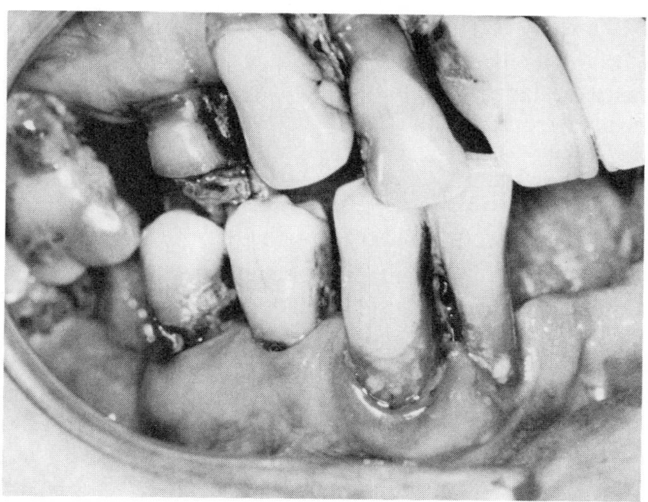

A

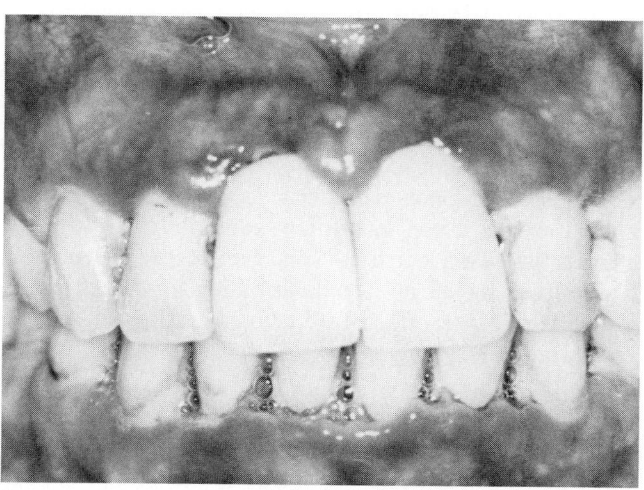

B

Figure 37–3

A. Severe periodontal disease. **B.** Gingivitis related to plaque formation; gums bleed easily. *Courtesy of Sebastian G. Ciancio, DDS, School of Dentistry, State University of New York at Buffalo.*

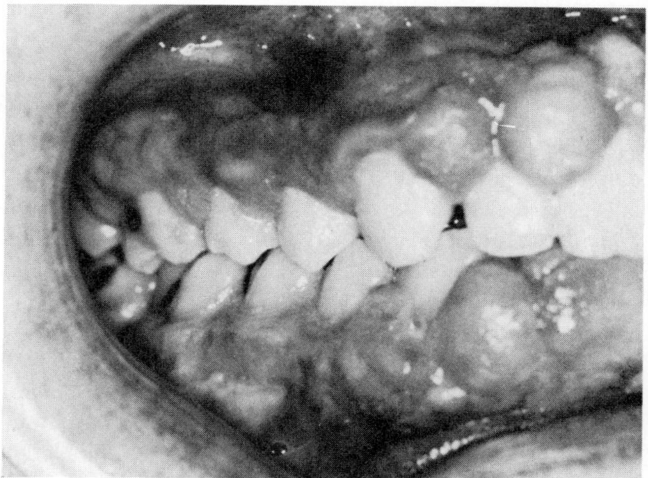

Figure 37–4

Gingival hyperplasia in a client taking phenytoin. *Courtesy of Sebastian G. Ciancio, DDS, School of Dentistry, State University of New York at Buffalo.*

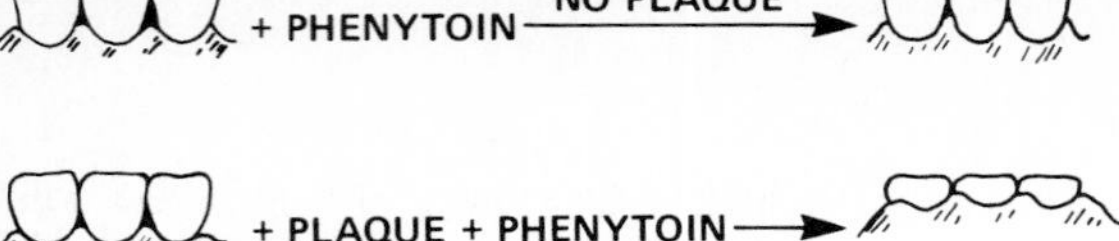

Figure 37–5

Meticulous oral hygiene can reduce dental plaque formation, minimizing gingival hyperplasia in clients taking phenytoin and other drugs. SOURCE: *Reproduced from Ciancio SG, Bourgault PC:* Clinical Pharmacology for Dental Professionals, *2nd ed. Littleton, MA: PSG Publishing, 1984, p. 195.*

Medical Measures

Periodontal disease is more easily prevented than treated. Regular brushing, flossing, and dental examinations are mandatory. Conventional treatment involves control of plaque through rigorous oral hygiene techniques, including scaling and planing the teeth to remove pockets where plaque and bacteria can collect. Dietary counseling may be necessary; the diet should include at least the recommended dietary allowances (RDAs) for basic nutrients, with emphasis on calcium and phosphorus balance. Infection may have to be controlled with antibiotics. If teeth are lost because of periodontal disease, the client may have to wear dentures. In advanced disease, the supporting bone may be so badly affected that denture wear becomes difficult.

Specific Nursing Measures

Since prevention is so important in control of periodontal disease, nurses can help all clients by teaching oral hygiene and dietary measures. If evidence of periodontal disease is seen during a routine examination, refer the client to a dentist or periodontist. Teach clients who are treated with phenytoin, nifedipine, or cyclosporine that regular brushing and flossing can minimize the amount of gingival hyperplasia (Figure 37–5).

Pulpal Infection

Infection of the pulp of a tooth may culminate in formation of an abscess, the most common oral infection (Rose, Hendler, & Amsterdam, 1982). Abscesses that involve the apices of teeth (*periapicular abscess*) or the alveoli—the bony tooth sockets—occur most often. Abscess formation is usually related to death of a tooth's nerve or degeneration of its pulp.

Nerve death or pulpal degeneration is usually due to invasion by caries with resultant pulpitis. Abscesses also occur in relation to physical or chemical trauma. The client with suppression of the bone marrow from chemotherapy or radiotherapy is also susceptible to periodontal infection and abscess formation.

Clinical Manifestations

Sensitivity of the affected teeth is an early sign of abscess formation. Later, moderate to severe pain may predominate. Oral inspection may reveal one or more decayed teeth. Edema and tenderness may be seen in the cheek or at the chin opposite the abscess. Elevated temperature and other signs of systemic infection can occur.

Medical Measures

The infection must first be localized and then removed, usually by a dental specialist at an office or clinic. The diseased pulp may be removed (root canal therapy), or the tooth may be extracted and the abscess drained. Antibiotics are generally given, usually penicillin, since most oral bacteria are sensitive to it (Rose et al., 1982). Prophylactic antibiotic medication is particularly indicated for clients with a history of rheumatic heart disease or valvular disease, since subacute bacterial endocarditis is associated with tooth extraction in these individuals (Petersdorf, 1983).

Preventing spread of bacteria present in the purulent abscess drainage is critical. Drainage secretion precautions must be taken; that is, gowns and gloves must be worn when in contact with infected material. Careful handwashing is important, and affected secretions and materials should be double-bagged.

Specific Nursing Measures

Relief of symptoms is a primary goal for client and nurse. If pain is severe, analgesics should be given as ordered; distraction and promotion of relaxation may be sufficient for less severe pain. Applying hot compresses to the cheek or chin proximal to the abscess relieves pain and speeds removal of toxic products from the infected area by promoting vasodilation. If teeth are painful or sensitive, the client may have difficulty eating; softer foods or a liquid diet may be required. Teach clients to avoid extremely hot or cold fluids, since they may increase discomfort.

Encourage the client undergoing root canal therapy or tooth extraction to take analgesics as prescribed and to apply warm compresses. Rinsing with warm saline solution helps remove debris and can promote comfort.

Any gauze applied to the oral cavity for pressure and/or collection of blood and debris should be sterile. Gauze should remain in the mouth for the period prescribed by the dentist or endodontist. Observe for excessive blood loss. Advise the client to continue taking antibiotics for the entire period prescribed to ensure that all infection has been eradicated.

Parotitis

Inflammation of the parotid glands, or parotitis, is both inflammatory and infectious. Aside from parotitis related to mumps, which occurs most frequently in children, this disorder occurs most often in the elderly and in debilitated clients (Petersdorf, 1983).

Parotitis may be related to poor oral hygiene or may be associated with dryness of the mouth (**xerostomia**) promoted by general anesthesia or medications that dry oral secretions. *Epidemic viral parotitis* (mumps) occasionally occurs in adults; more information about mumps may be found in a pediatric nursing text. Mumps occurring in an adult can cause serious problems, including sterility in men.

Sialolithiasis (formation of salivary calculi) can cause parotitis if a stone lodges in the parotid gland. Pain and edema may be associated with eating if the parotid gland is obstructed by a calculus. This condition is diagnosed by palpation or by x-ray; surgical removal (sialolithotomy) may be required.

Medical Measures

Antibiotic therapy may be combined with hydration, oral hygiene techniques, and massage of the involved gland. Increased hydration facilitates drainage of infected contents. Stimulating salivary secretion, for example, with hard candy, may also promote drainage.

Specific Nursing Measures

The nurse can play an important part in preventing parotitis by maintaining oral hygiene after anesthesia and surgery. Regular brushing and flossing should be carried out, and the lips, tongue, and mucous membranes should be kept moist by rinsing or swabbing. If the client cannot do this, the nurse will have to. A family member can also be taught the importance of maintaining good oral hygiene for the client. If parotitis is present, the client's oral secretions must be aseptically managed. Warm compresses and nursing comfort measures are helpful. Adequate rest and nutrition promote body defenses and healing.

Stomatitis

Stomatitis is a general term referring to inflammation of the mouth. Various oral structures may be involved, including the lips, the tongue (glossitis), the gingivae (gingivitis), the mucous membranes, and/or the palate, depending on the origin of the problem and its extent. Stomatitis may involve ulceration and degeneration of tissue.

Stomatitis can be primary or a symptom of another disease. Chickenpox, melanoma, infectious mononucleosis, syphilis, leukemia, lymphosarcoma, and nutritional deficiency disorders are a few of the disorders with which stomatitis may be associated. Stomatitis is also common with chemotherapy and/or irradiation of the head and neck. Some symptoms of radiologically induced stomatitis may persist for long periods after treatment. For example, taste sensation may be lost for as long as 6 months, and excessive dryness of the mouth (xerostomia) may be permanent (Lane & Forgay, 1981).

Aphthous stomatitis (aphthous ulcers, canker sores) have an undetermined etiology, although a microbial origin has been suggested. Physical and/or emotional stresses are thought to induce changes in body chemistry that promote development of these lesions. Physical stresses include spicy foods, bruising, or poorly fitting oral appliances (for example, orthodontic braces). Emotional stresses can be related to virtually any life change event. Canker sores are more common in women and may appear during menses.

Infection with the herpes simplex (type I) virus may cause *acute herpetic gingivostomatitis*, commonly known as a cold sore or fever blister. This lesion is often seen after stress or at the start of menses.

Bacterial infection of the gingivae, mucous membranes, pharynx, and tonsils may cause *necrotizing ulcerative gingivitis* (trench mouth, Vincent's stomatitis). This form of stomatitis occurs frequently in debilitated clients, especially those with nutritional deficiencies.

The Candida species of fungus can cause *thrush*, also known as oral condidiasis or oral moniliasis. Debilitated clients are especially susceptible, as are those receiving steroids or antibiotics, which may alter the oral pH and the composition of oral flora.

Poor oral hygiene, immunosuppression, and bone marrow suppression can contribute to stomatitis of any etiology. Moreover, oral trauma can provide an easy portal of entry for causative organisms.

Clinical Manifestations

Stomatitis may be characterized by bleeding, painful gums, and ulceration. In *aphthous stomatitis*, clusters of painful ulcers with an inflamed border appear on the mucosa. The lesions heal within 1 to 2 weeks but can cause scarring and may recur.

In *herpes simplex infection*, the lip and oral mucosa are generally affected. Painful vesicles that contain a clear yellow fluid form, rupture, and develop a crust that may ulcerate. Gingivitis and a foul odor may be noted in the oral cavity. A systemic response including elevated temperature and lymphadenopathy can occur. Fever blisters are less common in adults than in children. Uncomplicated lesions heal within 10 to 14 days.

Trench mouth is characterized by gingivitis, foul breath, and a bad taste in the mouth. There may be systemic symptoms such as fever and cervical lymphadenopathy.

Thrush causes white patches in the mouth that reveal a raw, bleeding surface when rubbed. Lesions may occur anywhere in the mouth.

Diagnosis of infectious stomatitis is determined by inspection and smear or culture of lesions.

Medical Measures

Regardless of which type of stomatitis the client has, symptoms must be relieved, infection must be eliminated, and its spread prevented.

In bacterial infections, antibiotic therapy may decrease the severity of ulcerations; antibiotics should be used cautiously, however, since they disrupt normal oral flora and may render the client susceptible to invasion by virulent microbes (Lane & Forgay, 1981). Although topical or systemic steroid therapy can relieve symptoms, it is generally not advisable, since steroids may promote development of candidiasis. Nystatin (Mycostatin) may help control candidiasis. A nystatin suspension may be used as a mouthwash or as flavored ice pops, or vaginal suppositories may be used as lozenges. A new form of treatment for oral candidiasis, clotrimazole (Mycelex) lozenges, has demonstrated a high rate of effectiveness in cancer clients.

Specific Nursing Measures

Local anesthetics, such as lidocaine 2% used as a rinse, may be prescribed prior to meals, since eating can be painful and difficult. A bland liquid or soft diet is indicated and spicy or hot foods should be avoided. The client may be better able to ingest food through straws or syringes.

Local discomfort may be relieved by rinsing with warm saline or bicarbonate of soda solution (1 teaspoon to a glass of warm water). Teach the client that the teeth and oral cavity should be cleansed every 4 hours with a 1:4 solution of hydrogen peroxide and normal saline applied with an Asepto syringe and a soft cloth or toothbrush. Warm saline may be used as a rinse. Normal brushing and flossing and commercial mouthwashes may be too irritating. Water soluble lubricants help alleviate discomfort from dryness and cracking. Ice chips and cool fluids are also helpful. A 1:1 mixture of cough syrup with diphenhydramine hydrochloride, such as Benylin syrup, and Kaotin-pectate used as a mouthwash has also been suggested for pain relief (Nursing Update, 1983).

SECTION 

Neoplastic and Obstructive Disorders

Tumors of the mouth and esophagus may be benign or malignant. Oral and esophageal cancers occur more frequently in men, especially after the fifth decade of life. Smoking and excessive use of alcohol are major etiologic factors.

Cancers of the oral cavity and esophagus and the treatments related to them may cause severe disfigurement and consequent disturbances of body image. Furthermore, these cancers can seriously compromise nutritional status by interfering with ingestion. Malnutrition is a common sequela. Oral and esophageal cancers are associated with significant morbidity and mortality, especially when the diagnosis is made late in the course of the disease.

Cancer of the Oral Cavity

Most cancers of the oral cavity are squamous cell carcinomas. Adenocarcinomas may arise from the mucous and salivary glands, and basal cell carcinoma, malignant melanoma, sarcoma, and lymphoma may also occur. Areas affected, in order of frequency, are the lips, tongue, buccal mucosa, gingivae, floor of the mouth, and the tonsils. Approximately 30,000 new cases of oral cancers and over 9400 deaths related to this disorder in the United States were projected for 1987 (1987 Cancer Facts and Figures). Males, especially those over 40, are more frequently affected.

Heavy use of alcohol and/or tobacco (smoking, chewing tobacco) are identified risk factors; it is thought that irritation by these substances leads to mucosal changes in the mouth. Other factors apparently related to development of oral cancer are chronic irritation from appliances in the mouth (braces, dentures) and poor oral hygiene. Exposure to intense sunlight has been implicated in development of cancer of the lip (Petersdorf, 1983).

Clinical Manifestations

The client may describe sores that do not heal, swelling, difficulty in chewing, dysphagia, difficulty in talking or moving the tongue, and/or drooling. In its late stages, cancer of the salivary gland may be a painful mass associated with neurologic signs such as paresis or paralysis. Pain from cancer anywhere in the mouth may radiate to the face or ear. Lesions may be white, gray, dark brown, or black, and may bleed. An inflammatory response, with erythema and edema, may be seen on inspection.

Early, primary lesions include:

- Leukoplakia (white, nodular patches on the oral mucosa that do not rub off)
- Speckled leukoplakia (white nodular patches interspersed with erythematous areas)
- Erythroplakia (persistent velvety red patches on the oral mucosa)

These early lesions are usually benign but are considered premalignant.

Enlargement of cervical lymph nodes may occur as cancer metastasizes, and underlying bone and muscle may become involved. Prognosis varies, depending on the site of the lesion and its extent.

Medical Measures

Early detection is crucial. Many precancerous lesions are discovered by dentists in routine checkups. Radiation therapy and surgery are the preferred conventional treatments, although chemotherapy is sometimes indicated. Both the primary lesion and any affected lymph nodes are irradiated, and radioactive implants may also be used. Among

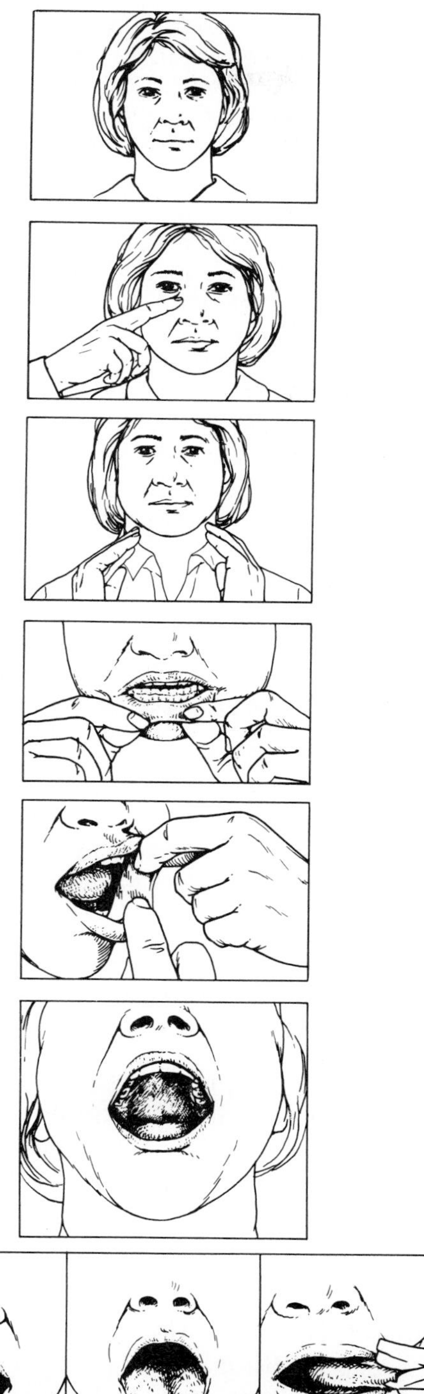

A mirror and adequate lighting are necessary for the self-exam.

Step 1 Symmetry
Look at your face and neck. The right and left sides are normally symmetrical; this means they have the same shape. Any differences in shape, such as a lump or swelling on one side, should be noted.

If similar lumps, bumps or other features are found at the same place on both sides of the face, neck or inside the mouth, they are probably normal.

Step 2 Face
Inspect the skin of the face, neck and lips. Look for changes in skin color, lumps or sores. If glasses are worn, remove them and look closely at the area around the eyes and the bridge of the nose. Replace glasses.

Step 3 Neck
With your fingers press along the sides and front of the neck to detect any lumps or tenderness. (As in Step 1, use symmetry to help identify normal features.)

Any dentures or partial plates should be removed at this point

Step 4 Lips
Pull the lower lip down to view any possible sores or color changes. With your fingers feel for any lump which may not be seen. Repeat procedure for upper lip.

Step 5 Cheek
Use your fingers to expose the left inner cheek surface to observe any white, red or dark patches. Place your thumb on the inside of your cheek and your index finger on the outside. Gently squeeze your cheek between your fingers; check for any lumps or areas of tenderness. Repeat procedure for right cheek.

Step 6 Roof of the Mouth
Tilt the head back and open the mouth wide to observe any color differences or lumps.

Step 7 Floor of Mouth and Tongue
Place the tip of the tongue to the roof of the mouth. Inspect the floor of the mouth and under-surface of the tongue for any color changes or sores. Examine the floor of the mouth by gently pressing with your finger to detect any abnormal lump or swelling.

Extend the tongue and inspect the top surface.

Using a gauze compress or a tissue, gently but firmly grasp the tongue and pull it forward to view the sides. Any swelling or color changes should be noted.

Figure 37–6

Oral self-exam for cancer. *Courtesy of National Cancer Institute.*

the surgical approaches are such radical procedures as glossectomy (removal of the tongue), radical neck dissection, and maxillectomy (removal of all or part of the maxilla).

Nutritional status must be maintained—a formidable problem because of pain, dysphagia, and the effects of radical surgery. Soft or liquid foods of moderate temperature may be given at frequent intervals, or tube feedings or total parenteral nutrition may be required.

Measures to control pain will be necessary, especially in late stages of the disease. Bacterial infection of lesions must be scrupulously avoided.

Specific Nursing Measures

The facial disfigurement and lifestyle changes that can result from oral cancer and its subsequent treatment can be overwhelming to clients and families. Therefore, the importance of early detection cannot be emphasized enough. Advise alcohol and tobacco users of their risk. Teach early warning signs (Box 37–2) and oral self-examination (Figure 37–6).

Clients with oral cancer may have halitosis, a foul taste in the mouth, xerostomia, or drooling. Encourage frequent mouth care and assist as necessary. In addition to brushing and flossing to the extent possible, the client should rinse the mouth with saline solution or dilute hydrogen peroxide. Other antiseptic rinses may be prescribed. A water-soluble lubricant can be applied to dry or cracked lips. if stomatitis occurs, for example, in association with irradiation, it may be treated as described earlier in this chapter.

Excessive dryness of the mouth (xerostomia) may be related to salivary gland dysfunction; fever; administration of atropine, antihistamines, tricyclic antidepressants, or phenothiazines; or surgery or irradiation of the salivary glands. Xerostomia related to radiation may be permanent. Measures to increase moisture in the mouth are indicated. Fluids should be encouraged, irritating foods should be avoided, and lubricants such as mineral oil may alleviate symptoms.

The client may wish to suck on hard candies to stimulate saliva production. Although this may be helpful, sugar-free candies should be used as dental caries can develop. Lemon-flavored candies are especially helpful since their acidity helps stimulate salivation.

Drooling, sometimes related to dysphagia, is embarrassing and uncomfortable to the client. Keep an emesis basin and tissues readily available. Encourage the client to swallow frequently if possible. Suctioning may be necessary. Anticholinergics, belladonna derivatives, or atropine may be prescribed.

Continually assess nutritional status and encourage soft or liquid foods and frequent small feedings. Urge the client to participate actively in meeting nutritional needs; involvement in all activities of daily living is psychologically beneficial. Teach family or significant others how to assist the client with feedings. Both client and family will have problems of adjustment to contend with in addition to the disease itself.

The importance of alleviating pain and discomfort with analgesic therapy and nursing comfort measures cannot be overemphasized. Pain related to cancer is discussed in Chapter 10; a general discussion of pain may be found in Chapter 3.

Box 37–2
Early Signs of Oral Cancer

Oral mucous membranes
- White patches (leukoplakia)
- Red patches (erythroplakia)
- Ulcers
- Masses
- Areas of pigmentation (brownish or black)

Lips
- Fissures
- Ulcers
- Patches of leukoplakia
- Areas of pigmentation

Floor of mouth (under the tongue)
- Leukoplakia
- Masses
- Areas of ulceration

Tongue
- Masses or lesions
- Areas of pigmentation

Asymmetry of the head, face, jaws, or neck

Cancer of the Esophagus

Cancer of the esophagus is relatively uncommon in the United States. Esophageal cancer is common, however, in other parts of the world such as Japan, China, Iran, the Soviet Union, and South Africa. This fact should be considered when examining emigrants from these areas. Males are affected more often than females, and the incidence of esophageal cancer has risen significantly for both male and female American blacks. The disease is most common in individuals ages 50 to 70. Tobacco use and excessive alcohol consumption are major risk factors.

Clinical Manifestations

Symptoms are not usually apparent until esophageal cancer is advanced, accounting for the high mortality rate associated with late-stage detection. The client will experience progressive dysphagia as the tumor obstructs the esophagus. Clients often describe burning or tightness with swallowing, especially with hot liquids. Pain, anorexia, and weight loss may occur, and hoarseness, coughing, regurgitation, and aspiration may be present. By the time esophageal cancer is diagnosed, regional lymph nodes are usually involved, although the involved nodes may not be clinically palpable. Malnutrition, GI hemorrhage, and aspiration pneumonitis are major causes of death in clients with esophageal cancer.

Diagnosis is made by barium swallow, endoscopy, computed tomography (CT) scanning, biopsy, and cytology.

Medical Measures

If tumor growth and/or evidence of metastasis is minimal, an attempt may be made to remove the tumor surgically (*esophagectomy*), although morbidity and mortality are high. If the tumor is inoperable, radiotherapy may be used. Irradiation has been found to relieve symptoms as well as surgery, but it can induce edema that obstructs the esophagus. Chemotherapy has not proved effective (Boyce, 1982).

Esophageal dilation may be performed in combination with radiotherapy to relieve dysphagia and allow more normal eating. Symptomatic relief may indirectly improve compromised nutritional status, but malnutrition may persist despite dilation, and nutritional support may be necessary. Prosthetic devices may be inserted into the esophagus to bypass the tumor, especially in the presence of esophagopulmonary fistulas and associated aspiration of food into the respiratory tract.

Specific Nursing Measures

Emotional support is of high priority. Clients must cope with a grave prognosis or certain expectation of death, as well as many lifestyle changes including alternative methods of feeding. Both client and family will need the nurse's support. Comfort measures and nutritional support as discussed in Chapter 36 will be necessary. Soft or liquid foods must be provided if the client is able to ingest food orally, and foods should be made as appetizing as possible to counteract anorexia. The nurse is in a key position to assess the client's ability to tolerate foods and should continually determine, along with the client, what kinds of food will be best tolerated.

Esophagectomy/Esophagostomy

The entire esophagus or sections of it may be excised because of strictures, esophageal rupture, damage from caustics, or neoplasm. The extent of the resection in an esophagectomy varies, as does the structure to which the remaining esophagus is surgically attached (anastomosed). With a ruptured lower esophagus or other condition that cannot be repaired, the upper esophagus may be diverted to the skin to form an *esophagostomy,* which will drain saliva and any swallowed liquids or foods. When the damage is to the upper esophagus, a feeding esophagostomy (also referred to as a cervical esophagostomy) may be constructed. The esophagostomy tube is inserted in the neck area, threaded through the esophagus, with the end of the tube placed into the stomach. A large bore tube such as the polyvinylchloride nasogastric tube or a rubber tube is usually used. When the lower portion of the esophagus is excised and the remaining portion is sutured to the stomach, the procedure is called an *esophagogastrostomy.* When a significant portion of the esophagus is removed, it may be desirable to construct a conduit for passage of swallowed food and liquid using a portion of the colon or the small bowel. A *colonic interposition* is usually a second-stage procedure performed after a client has sufficiently recovered from an esophagectomy. The physiologic and psychosocial/lifestyle implications are discussed in Table 37–2.

Table 37–2
Esophagectomy/Esophagostomy: Implications for the Client

Physiologic Implications	Psychosocial/Lifestyle Implications
Creation of a stoma changes the physical nature of the feeding; possible skin irritation and breakdown from internal secretions that come in contact with skin	Need for expectoration and an acceptable way to manage accumulated secretions may be embarrassing or result in social isolation
Dryness and cracking of lips from wiping accumulated saliva or frequent licking of lips	Inability to eat normally may interfere with family and social relationships as well as with the client's body image
Drooling from inability to swallow saliva or nasopharyngeal secretions	Possible need to learn to feed self through stoma and to provide skin care
	Client may be facing a terminal diagnosis and all that it involves
	Depression and possible suicidal tendencies may follow the realization of how the client's life has changed if secondary to a suicide attempt

Nursing Implications

PREOPERATIVE CARE Preoperative nursing care for esophageal surgery is the same as for any major surgery, with one exception. If there is a possibility that the esophagus is not to be restored to its normal state, the client may be extremely anxious about the quality of postoperative life.

POSTOPERATIVE CARE Nursing care following an esophagectomy will vary with the approach and with the extent of excision. If the lower esophagus is removed and a stoma created to drain the upper esophagus, a drainage bag will be needed to collect the swallowed material. Skin integrity around the stoma must be maintained. Nursing care for a feeding esophagostomy requires the same care for skin integrity, but in addition requires learning a new method of taking nourishment.

Tell clients that chewing helps maintain oral health and stimulates gastric secretions. Clients who are able may chew food and then expectorate it; this may also have a psychologic benefit. Remind clients to use moisturizing agents to prevent dryness and cracking of lips. Encourage frequent oral care to help maintain integrity of mucous membranes and prevent infection.

Following a partial esophagectomy that includes an anastomosis to the stomach, small intestine, or portion of the colon to make an intact conduit for food, a nasogastric tube is usually used to prevent postoperative gastric retention. It is important to prevent any manipulation of the anastomosis. The nasogastric tube should be taped securely in place and should not be repositioned; a rupture of the esophageal anastomosis can be devastating. Observe the client to make sure the tube is clear of obstructions and draining properly. If the tube is not clear, irrigation may be necessary but should be done very gently to prevent pressure on the suture line. If the esophagectomy is performed through the thorax, the client will require a chest tube to drain the pleural space.

Nursing care following a colonic interposition includes maintaining gastric suction to prevent distention, maintaining chest tube drainage, and maintaining adequate respiration. Tube feedings into the stomach or small bowel may be required temporarily to maintain good nutritional status.

With the excision of the esophagus, either complete or partial, and the formation of an exterior stoma, the client must learn an array of new, often embarrassing, and sometimes frightening procedures. Clients and family members need education and support.

If esophageal damage was secondary to swallowing a caustic substance in a suicide attempt, the life problems that contributed to the self-destructive behavior remain after the surgical intervention. Referral to a mental health professional is essential with these clients as they begin to realize how their lives have been permanently changed by the esophageal damage. Depression and suicidal tendencies may be the aftermath of such knowledge.

SECTION  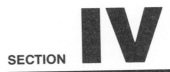

Traumatic Disorders

Trauma to the Oral Cavity and Esophagus

The mouth can be injured in vehicular accidents, falls, fights, or accidents related to employment or recreation. Although esophageal trauma can also have these causes, it is more often caused by ingestion of foreign bodies or burns, especially chemical burns. Suicide attempts may involve ingestion of sharp objects or caustic substances. One source reports that 74% of esophageal perforations are iatrogenic, usually associated with esophagoscopy or dilation (Keszler & Buzna, 1981). Penetrating wounds may be caused by stabbing or gunshot, and crushing injuries may cause stricture or obstruction.

Clinical Manifestations

Oral trauma may consist of puncture wounds, lacerations, or abrasions accompanied by hemorrhage, edema, erythema, and/or pain. With any deep trauma to the cheek, trauma to the parotid gland should be suspected. Injury to the teeth may cause fracture or avulsion; sensitivity to touch and temperature is a sign of dental fracture. Loosened teeth may be painful and movable. An avulsed tooth is completely out of its socket. Edema and debris in the mouth may cause obstruction of the airway.

If the esophagus has been penetrated, the client will experience retrosternal chest pain and fever. Invasion of the respiratory tract by esophageal hemorrhage will result in bloody sputum. Mediastinitis (inflammation of the mediastinum) may occur.

Oral/esophageal trauma with accompanying inflammation can lead to fibrosis of the involved tissue with scarring and loss of function. Difficulty in chewing or swallowing may occur at the time of injury or later.

Any client with trauma to the chest or thoracic cavity should be assessed for possible esophageal injury by x-ray or by cautious passage of an in-dwelling aspirating tube. Additional symptoms of esophageal trauma include dyspnea, cyanosis, upper abdominal pain, hypotension, and subcutaneous emphysema in the cervical or anterior thoracic regions.

Medical Measures

Trauma to the oral cavity requires meticulous cleansing and care of the wound to prevent infection. Suctioning of blood and debris may be necessary. An airway may be inserted. Lacerations may have to be sutured. Injuries to the parotid gland may also be sutured, with insertion of a Penrose drain to drain saliva until healing has occurred. A tetanus booster may be indicated.

Dislodged teeth can be successfully reimplanted if they have been out of their sockets less than 2 hours. The disloged tooth must be held in place in the mouth until dental treatment is begun. Disloged teeth may also be kept alive for up to 12 hours if immersed in cold milk (Johnson, 1983).

Minor esophageal perforations can heal spontaneously. The client is kept NPO and fed by means of a gastrostomy or by total parenteral nutrition, and tubes are inserted in the chest to drain accumulated fluids that may extravasate from the esophagus. The client is usually kept in Fowler's position and placed on antibiotics. Larger perforations should be repaired surgically. If treatment is delayed too long after the injury, surgery may not be possible.

Foreign bodies are removed by fiberoptic endoscopy; a magnet may be attached to the endoscope to remove metallic objects. Perforation is a possible complication of this procedure. Proteolytic enzymes are sometimes used to dissolve dislodged food particles.

Chemical burns of the oral cavity and esophagus should be immediately rinsed with large volumes of water. Steroids may be given to reduce inflammation, and prophylactic antibiotic therapy is generally initiated. Fluids may be given as tolerated, but tube feeding and intravenous fluid replacement are often necessary. Scarring can cause stricture and obstruction.

Specific Nursing Measures

Nursing measures focus on supporting the client and family, preventing infection and complications, promoting comfort, promoting healing, and maintaining nutritional status. Careful assessment of the extent of injury and potential for complication is imperative. Involve the client in care as much as possible.

Chapter Highlights

Clients with disorders of the mouth and esophagus are especially susceptible to malnutrition.

Clients with disorders of the mouth and esophagus often require dietary alterations with soft or liquid foods, given in small amounts frequently.

The nurse can play an important role in prevention of disorders of the mouth and esophagus through teaching clients about associated risk factors.

Cancers of the oral cavity can easily be detected in the early stages during a routine nursing assessment.

With esophageal surgery, manipulation of the nasogastric tube should be avoided to prevent disruption of the surgical site.

In disorders of the mouth, such as stomatitis, nursing comfort measures are of high priority.

Good oral hygiene is imperative in prevention of disorders of the oral cavity.

Bibliography

Bachrach N, Boyce HW, Jackson D: Problems in swallowing and esophageal carcinoma. *Heart Lung* 1981; 10;525–531.

Boyce HW: Approaches to management of cancer of the esophagus. *Hosp Pract* (Nov) 1982; 109–124.

1987 Cancer Facts and Figures. New York: American Cancer Society, 1987.

Ciancio SG, Bourgault PC: *Clinical Pharmacology for Dental Professionals,* 2nd ed. Littleton, MA: PSG Publishing, 1984.

Crowley LV: *Introduction to Human Disease.* Monterey, CA: Wadsworth, 1983.

DePaola DP, Alvares O, Etzel KA: Nutrition and periodontal disease. *Contemporary Nutrition* (Dec) 1982; 7:12.

Given BA, Simmons SJ: *Gastroenterology in Clinical Nursing,* 4th ed. St. Louis: Mosby, 1984.

Johnson R: Milk is a natural. (Letter.) *Nurs 83* (Aug) 1983; 13:66.

Keszler P, Buzna E: Surgical and conservative management of esophageal perforation. *Chest* 1981; 80:158–162.

Lane B, Forgay M: Upgrading your oral hygiene protocol for the patient with cancer. *Canadian Nurs* (Dec) 1981; 27–29.

Larsen G: Rehabilitation of the patient with head and neck cancer. *Am J Nurs* 1982; 82:119–122.

Loustau A, Lee K: Dealing with the dangers of dysphagia. *Nurs 85* (Feb) 1985; 15:47–50.

Nursing update; Nursing implications of cancer chemotherapy. *Nurs 83* (Aug) 1983; 13:64a.

Patient education aid: Help for your dry mouth. *Patient Care* (Feb 29) 1984; 79.

Patient education aid: Relief for gastroesophageal reflux. *Patient Care* (April 15) 1986; 137–138.

Petersdorf RG et al: *Harrison's Principles of Internal Medicine.* New York: McGraw–Hill, 1983.

Rose L, Hendler BH, Amsterdam JT: Temporomandibular disorders and odontic infections. *Consultant* (Dec) 1982; 22(12):110–136.

Sandler RS, Bozymski EM, Orlando RC: Failure of clinical criteria to distinguish between primary achalasia and achalasia secondary to tumor. *Dig Dis Sci* (March) 1982; 27:209–212.

Schachtele CF: Bacteria, diet and the prevention of dental caries. Part I. *Contemporary Nutrition* (July) 1980; 5:7.

CHAPTER 38

Specific Disorders of the Stomach, Intestines, and Pancreas

Other topics relevant to this content are: Infectious gastroenteritis, **Chapter 9;** Care of the client with cancer, **Chapter 10.**

Objectives

When you have finished studying this chapter, you should be able to:

Identify the etiology and risk factors associated with disorders of the stomach, small and large intestines, and pancreas.

Explain the role of the nurse in primary prevention of disorders of the stomach, intestines, and pancreas.

List therapeutic measures, including any medical and surgical treatments, associated with disorders of the stomach, intestines, and pancreas.

Describe specific nursing care for clients with disorders of the stomach, intestines, and pancreas.

Explain the complications of gastrointestinal surgery and the related nursing interventions.

Anticipate the psychosocial/lifestyle impact of disorders of the stomach, intestines, and pancreas on clients and their significant others.

Discuss alterations in body image encountered by clients requiring fecal diversion and their relationship to self-image, sexuality, and role relationships.

Discuss the crucial role of nutritional assessment and support in caring for clients with disorders of the stomach, intestines, and pancreas.

Plan diet regimens appropriate for clients with disorders of the stomach, intestines, and pancreas.

Apply the nursing process in all phases of care for the client with disorders of the stomach, intestines, and pancreas.

Dysfunction of the stomach, small and large intestines, and pancreas can adversely affect an individual's lifestyle and nutritional status. The problem may go almost unnoticed until acute, life-threatening complications—hemorrhage, for example—cause the client to seek professional health care.

Nurses may care for clients with problems of these organs in the home, occupational settings, clinics, or hospitals. Dietary and lifestyle factors are frequently implicated. Nurses are often in a position to identify risk factors as well as counsel the client about preventive approaches. Early detection is another crucial part of the nurse's function, especially when clinical symptoms have not yet become apparent.

SECTION 

Disorders of Multifactorial Origin

Disorders of multifactorial origin primarily affect the stomach and intestines; disorders that affect the pancreas generally have a more specific etiology. Multifactorial disorders develop and manifest themselves during an individual's life span, although some may be familial or hereditary. They often are related to the individual's reaction with the environment, and many are related to dietary intake.

Peptic Ulcer Disease

Peptic ulcer disease has various forms: chronic erosion of the stomach (gastric ulcer), chronic erosion of the duo-

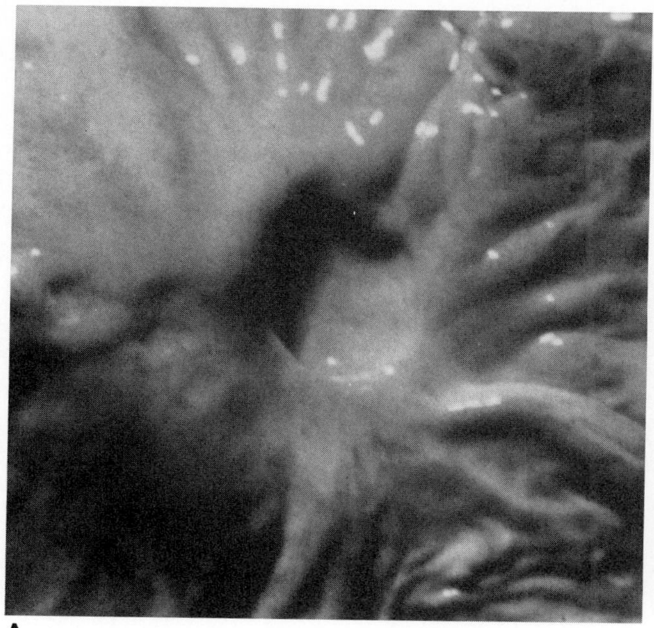
A

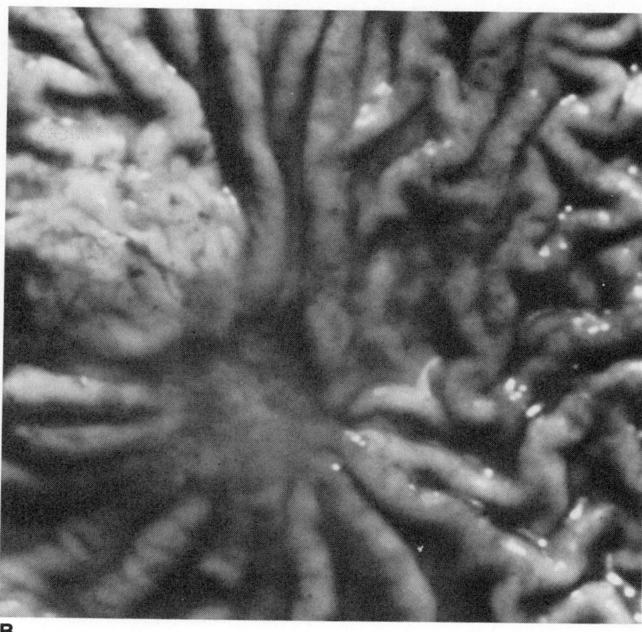
B

Figure 38–1

A. Gastric ulcer. **B.** Healed gastric ulcer. *Courtesy of Millard Fillmore Hospital, Buffalo, NY.*

denum (duodenal ulcer), and acute erosion of the stomach or duodenum (stress ulcer). Duodenal ulceration is most common, affecting up to 10% of the US population, especially men, who are affected 6 to 10 times as frequently as women. Most clients are aged 30 to 50, whereas clients with gastric ulcers tend to be slightly older (40 to 60).

Essentially, peptic ulceration is related to erosion of the gastric or duodenal mucosa by acidic digestive juices (Figure 38–1). In severe and chronic ulcer disease, erosion may penetrate muscle tissue and even the serosa, allowing acidic juices to enter the abdominal cavity.

Although the etiologic pattern of peptic ulcer is not fully understood, it is known to involve intricate interrelationships between (1) secretion of digestive juices and (2) the condition and function of the gastric and/or duodenal mucosa. Individuals who have type O blood and who lack group AB antigens in the saliva are at risk for development of gastric ulcer or duodenal ulcer (Hui, 1983).

With *gastric ulcer,* malfunction of the pyloric valve with subsequent reflux of bile into the stomach, is thought to play a role in ulceration. Chronic inflammation of the stomach (gastritis) is often a causative factor, predisposing the mucosa to breakdown. Smoking has also been implicated in development of gastric ulcer, as have various medications, including steroids, salicylates, indomethacin, phenylbutazone, and reserpine.

Duodenal ulcer disease occurs as a result of excessive gastric acid secretion, as a consequence of an increase in the number of acid-secreting (parietal) cells in the gastric mucosa. In conjunction with more rapid gastric emptying, duodenal contents become more acid, causing ulceration.

Various disorders have been linked with development of duodenal ulcers, including hepatic and pancreatic disorders, endocrine disorders, and Zollinger–Ellison syndrome, which is discussed below. Some studies show an association between duodenal ulcer and ingestion of caffeine, alcohol, and certain medications (salicylates, steroids, indomethacin, phenylbutazone, and reserpine). An increased incidence of duodenal ulcer disease has been noted in cigarette smokers, who respond less well to therapy and have a higher mortality with the disease (Petersdorf, 1983). The role of psychologic factors such as longstanding psychic conflict, anxiety, and stress in ulcer disease remains controversial.

In Zollinger–Ellison syndrome, gastrin-secreting tumors (gastrinomas) are present in the pancreas and other organs. The elevated levels of circulating gastrin lead to excessive secretion of gastric acid and subsequently to ulceration, usually duodenal.

Stress ulcers occur in up to 90% of clients with severe trauma, burns, infection and shock (Petersdorf, 1983). The two basic types of stress ulcers, Cushing's ulcer and ischemic ulcer, may affect either the stomach or the duodenum (Greenberger, 1981). *Cushing's ulcer* is characterized by marked hypersecretion of gastric juices related to profound stimulation of the vagus nerve. It can occur in clients with severe brain injury or those who have undergone neurosurgery. *Ischemic ulcer* is related to ischemia of unknown

NURSING DIAGNOSES IN Gastrointestinal Dysfunction

DIRECTLY RELATED DIAGNOSES

- Bowel elimination, altered: constipation
- Bowel elimination, altered: diarrhea
- Comfort, altered: pain
- Fluid volume deficit, potential
- Nutrition, altered: less than body requirements
- Role performance, altered
- Self-concept, disturbance in: body image
- Skin integrity, altered: potential

OTHER POTENTIAL DIAGNOSES

- Adjustment, impaired
- Coping, ineffective individual
- Home maintenance management, impaired
- Infection, potential for
- Knowledge deficit
- Swallowing, impaired
- Tissue integrity, impaired: oral mucous membranes
- Tissue perfusion, altered: gastrointestinal

cause that renders the gastroduodenal mucosa more susceptible to the action of gastric acids.

Clinical Manifestations

The client with chronic ulcer disease may describe symptoms of "burning" postprandial epigastric pain. The pain of gastric ulcer tends to occur sooner after meals than the pain of duodenal ulcer. Pain may radiate to the back and thorax and may be intensified by stress, tension, fatigue, or exposure to cold (Given & Simmons, 1984). Eating or taking an antacid may relieve symptoms, especially with duodenal ulcer.

Chronic peptic ulcer disease should be suspected whenever a client describes epigastric pain that is relieved by eating or by taking antacids. Diagnosis can be confirmed by an upper GI series, but if a gastric lesion is suspected, endoscopy is usually performed to rule out the possibility of gastric carcinoma. If Zollinger–Ellison syndrome is suspected, serum gastrin levels may be elevated; elevated levels suggest the presence of the disorder.

Complications, which occur in up to 25% of clients with peptic ulcer disease, include hemorrhage, GI obstruction, perforation, or intractable ulcer (an ulcer that responds poorly to treatment and frequently recurs). Elderly clients are at higher risk of complications and mortality (Permutt & Cello, 1982).

Hemorrhage, possibly severe, may occur if the erosion is deep enough to alter the continuity of blood vessels. Hemorrhage may be heralded by hematemesis or melena, depending on its severity.

Gastrointestinal obstruction may be related to fibrotic occlusion secondary to tissue damage and scarring. Abdominal distention, nausea, and vomiting will persist until the obstruction is relieved.

If ulceration is severe enough to penetrate the intestinal lining, gastric or duodenal contents spill into the peritoneum, causing inflammation. Peritonitis (inflammation of the peritoneum) is a serious, life-threatening condition. If the pancreas is affected by spillage, pancreatitis may occur.

Stress ulcers, which develop from 2 to 10 days after the precipitating insult, are not generally associated with any symptoms except bleeding. Bleeding may be scant, or severe hemorrhage may occur. With severe hemorrhage, a mortality rate of over 50% has been reported (Given & Simmons, 1984). Bleeding may be manifested by melena, hematemesis or, if the client has a nasogastric tube, blood may appear in the drainage.

Medical Measures

Therapy in peptic ulcer disease focuses on relieving symptoms, preventing complications, and healing the lesion. Healing may be accomplished in 4 to 6 weeks, but ulcers may recur in a new location.

PHARMACOLOGIC THERAPY The primary drug therapy for peptic ulcer is administration of oral antacid agents, usually taken 1 to 3 hours postprandially and at bedtime. Drugs that inhibit histamine-stimulated gastric acid secretion (H_2 receptor antagonists such as cimetidine) may be prescribed with meals and at bedtime. Sometimes anticholinergic agents are used to decrease gastric acid secretion. Medications are usually given orally, but if the client has severe complications and is NPO, antacids may be given via nasogastric tube, and H_2 receptor antagonists may be given intravenously.

Prophylactic administration of antacids and H_2 receptor antagonists may be successful in clients who are likely to develop stress ulcers (for example, burn clients). Antacids may be given as often as every 30 to 60 minutes through a nasogastric tube, if the client is NPO. If stress ulceration occurs, it is treated similarly to chronic ulceration.

If ulceration is due to Zollinger–Ellison syndrome, surgery must ultimately be performed to remove gastrinomas, although the measures described above may be used temporarily.

DIETARY THERAPY Modification of diet is a cornerstone of peptic ulcer therapy; however, the traditional "ulcer diet" with a high proportion of milk and cream is no longer used. The dietary regimen will depend on the stage of the disease and other factors. Smaller, more frequent meals may be given to prevent exacerbation of symptoms related to an empty stomach. A semibland diet may be prescribed, and the client may be advised to avoid fruits and spicy foods, but this must be decided on an individual basis with the client's condition and preferences in mind. Foods that promote symptoms in that particular client should be eliminated. Frequent offenders include coffee (with or without caffeine), alcohol, and foods containing caffeine, such as chocolate and some soft drinks. Some researchers report that a diet high in fiber appears to prevent recurrence of healed duodenal ulcers (Rydning et al., 1982).

Some clients with peptic ulcer disease will require surgery, especially when persistent hemorrhage, perforation, obstruction, or intractable ulcer are present. Surgical procedures used in gastric ulceration are discussed below.

Specific Nursing Measures

Assessment, especially of food intolerances, is a major nursing responsibility in caring for clients with diagnosed peptic ulcer disease. When caring for surgical clients, burned clients, and those with severe trauma, be alert for signs of bleeding that may signal the development of stress ulcers (eg, black tarry stools). In all clients with peptic ulcer disease, evaluate client comfort and response to therapy on an ongoing basis. Because complications such as hemorrhage or peritonitis can be life threatening, continual assessment of stools, emesis or GI drainage, peristalsis, and pain level are essential.

Home Health Care

Once a plan of care has been developed, help clients integrate it into their particular lifestyle. Explain medication and diet regimens and warn the client about side effects and possible toxicity. Clients should avoid coffee, cola, cigarettes, aspirin, and other irritating drugs. New health care providers should be informed about the client's history of ulcer disease. The client must be instructed about the course of the disease and the nature and signs of possible complications. For example, hematemesis or black tarry stools (melena) should be reported immediately, because they signal the recurrence of bleeding.

Because psychosocial stresses can worsen the disease, the nurse, client, and significant others should work together to reduce stresses in the client's environment. Stress reduction techniques such as relaxation breathing can help the client cope. For hospitalized clients, reduction of stresses associated with the hospital setting is mandatory.

Gastric Resection

A gastric resection may be performed for hemorrhage, perforation, or obstruction resulting from ulcer disease. Gastric tumors are resected for cure or palliation.

The specific surgical procedure performed for ulcer disease or tumor varies with the area and extent of involvement. A *vagotomy,* severing of the vagus nerve, is performed most commonly to decrease gastric acid secretion in duodenal ulcer disease. A *pyloroplasty,* enlarging the pyloric sphincter, is often performed with a vagotomy to control peptic ulcer disease. A pyloroplasty increases the rate of gastric emptying. A *subtotal gastrectomy* is the removal of a portion of the stomach, usually the lower portion. A subtotal gastrectomy may also be performed for gastritis, tumor, or gastric outlet obstruction. A vagotomy is performed along with a subtotal gastrectomy to control peptic ulcer disease.

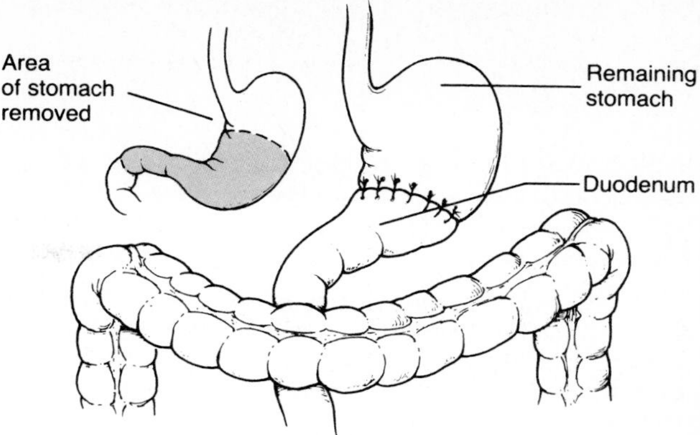

Figure 38–2

Billroth I procedure.

Following the resection of the lower stomach, as with a subtotal gastrectomy, the remaining stomach is sutured end-to-end to the duodenum in a *Billroth I procedure* (Figure 38–2). This is performed primarily for ulcer disease.

Another option for an anastomosis following a subtotal gastrectomy is the *Billroth II procedure,* where the stomach stump is sutured to an opening along the jejunum (Figure 38–3). A blind loop or afferent loop (portion of bowel ending in a dead end) is created that includes the duodenum. This decreases stimulation to the duodenum without interrupting the normal secretion of pancreatic juices into the small bowel.

The entire stomach may be removed as treatment for tumor or Zollinger–Ellison disease, although a subtotal gastrectomy is preferred for localized gastric neoplasms in order to maintain some gastric function. With a *total gastrectomy,* the esophagus is sutured either to the duodenum

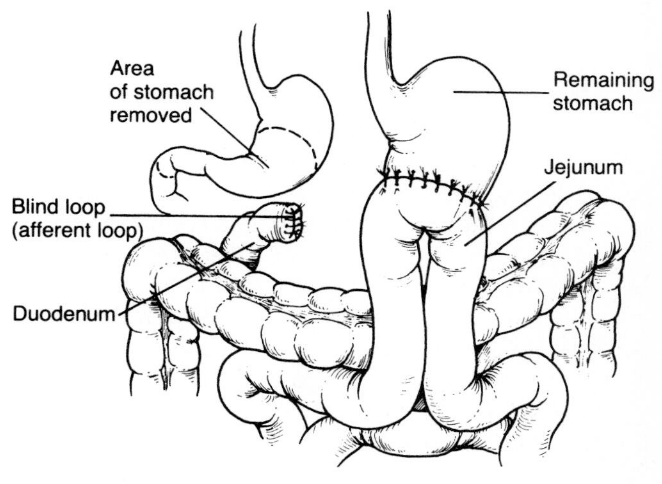

Figure 38–3

Billroth II procedure.

Table 38–1
Gastric Resection: Implications for the Client

Physiologic Implications	Psychosocial/Lifestyle Implications
Vagotomy may decrease gastric motility, causing bloating, pain, and vomiting; may increase gastric emptying, causing diarrhea and symptoms of dumping syndrome; and may be associated with dysphagia, cholelithiasis, and recurrent ulcer.	Partial gastrectomy may lead to early satiety, necessitating a change in eating habits to six small feedings per day.
Achlorhydria following gastric resection and vagotomy may be associated with risk of gastric cancer.	Client should learn to recognize and avoid hypertonic liquids and high carbohydrate foods to decrease dumping syndrome.
Alkaline intestinal secretions may reflux into the stomach, causing gastritis.	If vitamin B_{12} absorption is greatly impaired, the client may need to plan for regular B_{12} injections for life.
Gastric surgery may result in dumping syndrome.	Client may have to learn strategies for coping with dumping syndrome and diarrhea.
Gastrointestinal symptoms of dumping syndrome include bloating, cramping, diarrhea, nausea, and vomiting.	Lifestyle may be altered by the development of osteoporosis.
Vasomotor symptoms of dumping syndrome include flushing, palpitations, lightheadedness, tachycardia, diaphoresis, and postural hypotension.	Chronic anemia may cause fatigue, affecting home life and work.
Long-term complications following gastrectomy may include: 1. Iron and calcium deficiency because these minerals require gastric acid to increase solubility 2. Bone disease—osteoporosis 3. Anemia from maldigestion and malabsorption of iron, vitamin B_{12}, and folic acid 4. Weight loss and malnutrition	

or the jejunum. The physiologic and psychosocial/lifestyle implications are summarized in Table 38–1.

Nursing Implications

Nursing care of the client undergoing a gastric resection will depend partly on the specific procedure. Knowledge of the immediate and long-term complications of gastric surgery is essential for appropriate nursing care.

A nasogastric tube will be in place, connected to suction, for several days postoperatively, to prevent gastric distention (which can produce vomiting and wound separation) and promote drainage of secretions. The secretions will be bloody for the first day and then become brownish to clear. Irrigations may be ordered to keep the tube patent because clots in the bloody secretions may clog the tube. The irrigation should be done gently with normal saline to minimize excess fluid and electrolyte losses. Fluids and electrolytes are given IV to replace the gastric losses.

Inspect the incision line for signs of infection, hemorrhage, and wound separation. Sterile technique should be used when changing the dressing; the first dressing change may be performed by the surgeon. Some remove the original dressing 3 days postoperatively and leave it off. Dressings saturated with fresh blood should be replaced rather than reinforced, since blood can harbor organisms that can infect the site.

The nurse should promote client comfort following gastric surgery. Elevating the head of the bed will facilitate breathing as well as lessen the strain on the suture line. Holding a pillow over the incision may lessen the pain of deep breathing, coughing, and moving. Oral and nasal care can also promote comfort when a nasogastric tube is present. Unless contraindicated, the tape that holds the nasogastric tube in place should be reinforced or replaced when necessary. It is important to avoid changing the tube position when changing the tape to avoid pressure on the internal suture line. The nares should be cleansed if crusted secretions build up around the tube.

The client's nutritional status may be maintained with parenteral nutrition for several days postoperatively (the average is 4 days). Bowel motility will not return until several days after surgery because of the minor degree of postoperative paralytic ileus that normally occurs after abdominal surgery. The nurse should listen for bowel sounds and ask the client if any flatus has been passed. A decrease in nasogastric secretions usually accompanies the return of bowel motility. Oral fluids may be initiated; ice chips are generally well tolerated. The oral intake should be minimal with gastric suction to prevent excess fluid and electrolyte losses. When the nasogastric tube is no longer required, clear liquids can be initiated. The diet is slowly advanced to solid food.

The *dumping syndrome,* caused by rapid flow of chyme into the small intestine, may occur following vagotomy or gastrectomy. Vasomotor symptoms of dumping syndrome include flushing, palpitations, lightheadedness, tachycardia, diaphoresis, and postural hypotension. Gastrointestinal symptoms of dumping syndrome include bloating, cramping, diarrhea, nausea, and vomiting. To avoid the dumping syndrome, high carbohydrate foods and fluids should not be given. With a partial gastrectomy, the client may need six small feedings a day to prevent distention while promoting good nutritional intake. Early satiety with large meals can cause undernutrition. Nutrition is important following a gastrectomy since clients are vulnerable to malnutrition and weight loss.

Surgery for Morbid Obesity

Surgical intervention for obesity is indicated for individuals who weigh 2–3 times their ideal weight for 10–15 years duration with no correctable endocrine causes for the obesity. Such obesity is called *morbid* because it is severe enough to impair activities of daily living as well as to place a tremendous strain on the body. Surgical alternatives are considered when diet, behavior modification, and medications have been unsuccessful in adequately reducing weight. The primary surgical interventions used to control morbid obesity include gastrointestinal bypass and gastroplasty. Jejunoileal bypass is performed less frequently because of its severe metabolic consequences. Most of the desired weight loss occurs within the first year.

In a *gastrointestinal bypass,* the surgeon partitions the stomach to create a pouch with approximately one tenth the capacity of the stomach. The pouch is anastomosed to the jejunum, thus bypassing the lower stomach and the duodenum.

Gastroplasty, also referred to as gastric stapling or gastric partitioning, causes less disruption of the gastrointestinal tract, allowing for normal digestion and absorption. Gastroplasty involves the creation of a small pouch by stapling the stomach together, using the upper portion of the stomach. The capacity of this pouch begins at approximately 50 mL, although stretching eventually increases it. A small channel allows food to pass from the pouch into the remaining stomach, thus maintaining the continuity of the gastrointestinal tract.

The *jejunoileal bypass* is performed to reduce intestinal absorption by bypassing most of the small intestine, thus promoting weight loss by malabsorption of nutrients. The surgical procedure involves the resection of the jejunum 14 inches from its origin and suturing the end nearest to the stomach to the terminal ileum 4 inches from the ileocecal valve. The physiologic and psychosocial implications are discussed in Table 38–2.

Table 38–2
Surgery for Morbid Obesity: Implications for the Client

Physiologic Implications	Psychosocial/Lifestyle Implications
Bowel integrity is disrupted with bypass surgery, causing maldigestion and malabsorption.	Gradual body changes allow for gradual psychologic adaptation.
Gastrointestinal bypass: • Results in malabsorption of iron and vitamin B_{12}, leading to anemia • Results in decreased stimulation of the pancreas since the duodenum is bypassed	Body image will improve with weight loss, improving self-concept. Progress in weight loss may give client hope and a sense of pride, increasing self-esteem.
The pouch created with gastrointestinal bypass and gastroplasty can stretch, rupture, or become obstructed.	Client may experience some frustration in the adjustments because of side effects and limit in ability to splurge because of early satiety from gastrointestinal bypass and gastroplasty (although capacity to eat is altered, desire is not).
The channel created in the gastroplasty tolerates liquids best.	
Jejunoileal bypass: • Results in malnutrition from malabsorption of vitamins, minerals, and amino acids • Results in electrolyte imbalance, worsened with diarrhea, especially loss of potassium, magnesium, and calcium • Can cause bacterial enteritis in the bypassed bowel • Can result in gallstones, renal stones, migratory polyarthritis, liver damage, severe diarrhea	Long-term medical follow-up necessary Reversal or modification of the procedure may be necessary. Necessary to modify dietary intake for life; clients having gastroplasty must drink liquids for 8 to 12 weeks. Clients having gastroplasty and gastrointestinal bypass must eat slowly and chew food well. Need to respond to signs of satiety, to avoid pouch or anastomosis rupture.

Nursing Implications

The nursing care of a client undergoing surgery for morbid obesity is challenging. The nurse needs to know long-term physiologic and psychosocial implications and should be concerned about preventing complications from the surgery and from the obesity. Maintaining pulmonary function is essential since the client has more tissue to oxygenate. The client is vulnerable to hypoventilation in part because fat impairs lung expansion. Facilitate adequate ventilation and lung expansion by frequent position changes, elevating the head of the bed, encouraging early mobility (sitting on the side of the bed, standing, and walking within the first 24 hours following surgery). Assess clients for signs of hypoxia and encourage them to take deep breaths and cough frequently.

The cardiovascular system is already stressed in obesity, causing increased cardiac workload and, in the morbidly obese, hypertension. Often, the usual blood pressure cuff is too small; a thigh cuff used on the arm is a good alternative. Immobility leads to venous stasis and thrombus formation. With prolonged bed rest, these clients often develop thrombophlebitis. Occasionally, clients are given low-dose heparin prophylactically. Assess for thrombophlebitis, which usually occurs in the lower extremities, by checking Homans' sign. Venous stasis can be minimized by encouraging leg exercises in bed, such as pedaling the feet, and performing range-of-motion exercises for the lower extremities. Early ambulation is also beneficial for decreasing venous stasis and improving pulmonary function.

Intestinal bypass, especially the jejunoileal bypass, predisposes the client to fluid and electrolyte losses. Intake and output should be closely monitored. A nasogastric tube will be in place for several days to prevent distention or obstruction, and the resulting fluid loss will cause loss of electrolytes. The gastric secretions should be monitored for color, volume, and pH. Bloody secretions should decrease by the second postoperative day. Check tube patency, irrigating it if ordered. Complaints of abdominal pain and distention may indicate a nasogastric tube obstruction and should be reported promptly.

Diarrhea also promotes fluid and electrolyte losses, particularly of potassium, magnesium, and calcium. Closely monitor for electrolyte losses even after the nasogastric tube has been removed. Clients may require supplementary potassium. Encourage clients to eat foods high in potassium such as oranges, apricots, bananas, baked potatoes, milk and milk products, percolated or instant coffee, tea, or prune juice.

Maintain skin integrity in obese clients. Dampness in skin folds may promote excoriation and fungal infection. Diarrhea may cause anal irritation and skin breakdown. Local application of ointments or sitz baths may be soothing.

Wound management of the obese can be difficult because their wounds heal poorly. Abdominal wounds are particularly vulnerable to separation or dehiscence, and infection may result. The wound site should be handled aseptically and observed for signs of edema, redness, drainage, or separation. A drainage suction device may be used to facilitate removal of secretions from around the wound.

Maintenance of nutrition is essential. Most clients will start sipping liquids within 3 to 4 days of surgery. The diet is slowly advanced to full liquids; however, gastroplasty requires a liquid intake for several months. The transition to food can be frustrating for all clients. Certain foods such as cabbage will worsen bloating, flatulence, and diarrhea; these foods should be discouraged. All clients need to make dietary modifications. Emphasis should be placed on balanced nutritional intake. Working with a dietitian is helpful.

The nurse plays a crucial role in helping clients, their family, and friends adapt to lifestyle changes as well. Help the client identify strategies of dealing with the inability to splurge or binge on food, and with the frustration experienced as a result, by meeting the need for oral gratification in other ways.

Also instruct the client not only to respond to signs of satiety by stopping eating but how to recognize those signs. Remind the client that rupture of the pouch or the anastomosis that spills food into the peritoneal cavity is life threatening, and stretching the pouch excessively not only weakens it but is in opposition to the reason for performing the operation in the first place.

Intestinal Diverticular Disease

Diverticulosis is the asymptomatic presence of herniations or outpouchings of the intestinal mucosa (**diverticuli**). Fecal material may become entrapped within one or more diverticula; the resulting inflammation, which causes symptoms, is called diverticulitis. Diverticulosis may affect either the small or the large intestine. A congenital form (Meckel's diverticulum of the ileum) exists, but most cases of diverticulosis are acquired. Diverticuli of the large intestine are shown in Figure 38–4. The incidence of diverticulosis increases with age; two-thirds of individuals 85 years or older in the United States are believed to have the disorder.

One suggested etiology is increased pressure on the lumen of the intestine that produces herniation at weak areas, for example, where blood vessels penetrate the intestinal wall. Other suggested etiologic factors include atrophy or weakness of the bowel musculature related to aging, obesity, chronic constipation and straining at stool, and abnormalities of intestinal motility.

The role of diet in the formation of diverticuli has received considerable attention. Incidence of the disorder is higher in cultures where highly processed foods low in fiber form a significant part of the diet; it is lower among populations who consume large amounts of fiber. It is known

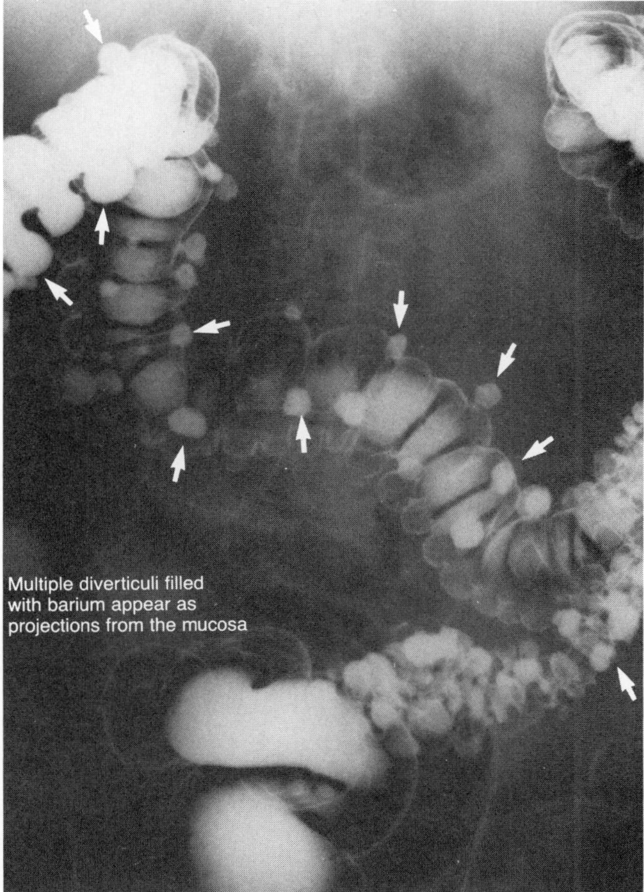

Figure 38–4

Multiple diverticuli of the large intestine as seen on barium enema. The diverticuli filled with barium appear as projections from the mucosa (*arrows*). *Courtesy of Health Care Plan, Buffalo, NY.*

that the presence of fiber (roughage) speeds the transit of the stool; conversely, the stool remains longer in the intestine if fiber is inadequate. More water is reabsorbed from the stool, leaving harder, drier feces and promoting constipation. Accumulation of a hard mass of dry stool (a **fecalith**) in a diverticular sac may cause it to become inflamed.

Clinical Manifestations

Diverticulosis is usually asymptomatic, although constipation, vague abdominal pain and cramping, and abdominal distention may occur. Often the diagnosis is made incidentally during diagnostic evaluation for a different problem.

If diverticulitis occurs, however, the client may report episodic, dull midabdominal or lower-abdominal pain that can radiate to the back. Change in bowel habits, excessive flatulence, bloating, and fever may also occur (Given & Simmons, 1984). Acute symptoms typically follow ingestion of a large meal, alcohol, or a large quantity of roughage. Rectal bleeding may also be noted.

In severe diverticulitis, inflammation may lead to perforation and thus to peritonitis. Edema or fibrosis associated with diverticular inflammation may cause intestinal obstruction. Fistulae may form between the intestine and the urinary bladder, ureter, vagina, abdominal wall, or perineum. These complications increase morbidity and the risk of mortality.

Diagnosis may be confirmed by barium studies, although these are contraindicated in acute diverticulitis, since they may cause further irritation and even perforation. Endoscopy may be used to differentiate diverticular disease from carcinoma, but, like barium studies, this procedure is contraindicated in acute diverticulitis.

Medical Measures

Treatment of diverticular disease depends on whether inflammation (diverticulitis) is present. If it is not, therapy focuses on avoiding increases of intraluminal pressure, which could precipitate diverticulitis. Bulk laxatives such as psyllium and a high-fiber diet are used to prevent constipation and straining at stool.

Diverticulitis can be managed by nonsurgical means in 90% of clients (Given & Simmons, 1984). Treatment is aimed at allowing the colon to rest so the inflamed diverticula can heal. Depending on the severity of symptoms, the client can be treated at home or in the hospital. If hemorrhage, perforation, or obstruction are present, hospitalization is necessary. The client may be NPO, or placed on a low-residue diet. A nasogastric tube may be passed to decompress the intestinal tract. Clients who are NPO may be given intravenous supplementation or, if NPO status is prolonged, total parenteral nutrition (TPN). Antibiotics may be prescribed. Although analgesics are sometimes ordered, caution is indicated since symptoms of complications can be masked. Acute attacks of diverticulitis generally subside within a week.

Specific Nursing Measures

The nursing care plan should focus on promoting comfort, maintaining adequate nutrition, evaluating treatment outcomes, and monitoring for complications. Clients may be apprehensive about the treatment regimen or fear that cancer is present, especially if rectal bleeding has occurred. Once the results of tests and diagnostic studies are known, the nurse can reassure the client and reinforce explanations of the findings. If NPO status and/or intravenous therapy is ordered, the nursing care associated with these therapies is instituted.

Intestinal Hernia

Protrusion of a portion of the intestine through the abdominal walls is called an intestinal (abdominal) hernia. Although the condition may be congenital, it is usually acquired as a result of conditions that increase intra-abdominal pressure and/or cause the abdominal wall to weaken. Increased pressure may be associated with obesity, pregnancy, coughing or sneezing, lifting, constipation, or straining at stool. Weakening of the abdominal wall may be associated with disease or with aging.

Various types of intestinal hernias are given names according to their location: umbilical hernia (at the umbilicus), inguinal hernia (at the inguinal ring), and femoral hernia (at the femoral ring). An intestinal hernia may also occur at the site of an abdominal incision (incisional or ventral hernia). Inguinal hernias are the most common, usually occurring in males.

Clinical Manifestations

An abdominal bulge may be seen on physical examination. Palpation discloses a soft, tender mass. The client may notice that the hernia increases in size during straining or exertion and may feel tenderness at the site.

Major complications of hernia include strangulation and incarceration. In strangulation, the margins of the defect constrict the protruding loop of bowel so severely that blood flow is obstructed, leading to tissue necrosis and/or infection. If a hernia cannot be pushed back into the abdominal cavity (reduced), the condition is called incarceration. Both conditions may be associated with severe pain, nausea, vomiting, and fever. An incarcerated hernia may cause symptoms typical of intestinal obstruction. Figure 38–5 shows the herniation of a loop of intestine through the abdominal wall.

Medical Measures

The client with a hernia is generally advised to avoid any activities that increase abdominal pressure. Stool softeners, psyllium, and a high-residue diet may be prescribed to prevent constipation and straining at stool, which could aggravate the condition. The client is usually told to avoid straining and stretching and to use proper body mechanics. A truss (firm support) may be prescribed; it should be worn as much as possible, especially when the client is ambulating. Temporary reduction of the hernia by pushing it manually back through the abdominal wall may make the client more comfortable and avert strangulation and incarceration. Permanent reduction can be accomplished only by surgery (herniorrhaphy), which is described below. Hernias may recur after surgical repair, so the client will need to learn proper body mechanics and other preventive measures.

Specific Nursing Measures

Observe the client for complications. Instruct the client about the importance of a high-fiber diet with adequate fluids and the avoidance of straining and stretching. Many persons are unaware of proper body mechanics, which the nurse can teach. Clients should also avoid weight gain and should give up smoking to eliminate the problem of smoker's cough.

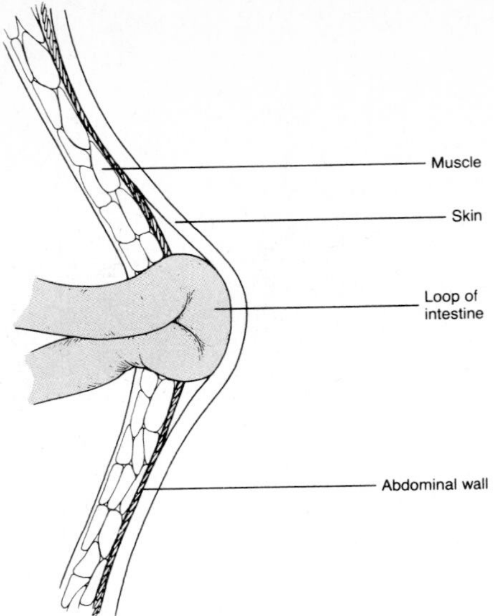

Figure 38–5

Herniation of a loop of intestine through the abdominal wall.

Herniorrhaphy

A herniorrhaphy is the surgical repair of a hernia. Surgery is indicated for repair of an abdominal hernia when medical measures fail to prevent progression or complications. Repair is urgent when a hernia is incarcerated (and thus, irreducible), obstructed, or strangulated. The general principles of repair include surgically replacing the displaced peritoneum, intestines, and omentum through the abnormal opening. The opening is then sutured to prevent further herniation. The physiologic and psychosocial/lifestyle implications are discussed in Table 38–3.

Nursing Implications

Nursing care following a hernia repair depends on the surgical approach and anesthesia. General measures include promoting comfort, preventing straining, assessing urinary status, and observing the incision for signs of infection or hemorrhage and the scrotum for edema. Urination may be somewhat impaired with an inguinal herniorrhaphy because of the pain. Coughing and straining should be avoided to prevent strain on the suture line. The client may ambulate soon after surgery, which will facilitate voiding. There are no special dietary modifications except to avoid constipating foods and to increase bulk and fiber. Explain physical limitations to the client, paying close attention to activities of daily living which need modification to prevent straining. Postoperative discomfort from inguinal hernias may be decreased with the use of a scrotal support with an ice bag. Some hernia repairs are performed on an outpatient basis, limiting the time the nurse has for teaching and postoperative observation.

Table 38–3
Herniorrhaphy: Implications for the Client

Physiologic Implications	Psychosocial/Lifestyle Implications
Hemorrhage, infection, and (for men with inguinal hernia) compromise of the vas deferens or the blood supply to the testes. Scrotal edema and pain possible after inguinal repair.	Physical and sexual activity should be limited for several weeks and heavy lifting avoided for up to 6 weeks. Constipating foods and obesity should be avoided to prevent recurrence. Change in employment or lifestyle that includes heavy lifting may be necessary.

Irritable Bowel Syndrome

Irritable bowel syndrome, the most common functional intestinal disorder, is a disturbance of motility that cannot be attributed to an organic cause. It affects women more often than men and is often first seen when clients are in their twenties or thirties.

Various etiologies have been suggested, including emotional turmoil and food intolerance. Some recent research has suggested that the disorder is related to elevated levels of the hormones gastrin and cholecystokinin, which may excessively stimulate an unusually sensitive GI tract.

Clinical Manifestations

Symptoms of irritable bowel syndrome generally fall into one of three basic patterns (Legerton, 1981):

- Alternating constipation and diarrhea, with or without abdominal pain
- Constipation associated with abdominal pain
- Persistent, usually painless, diarrhea

Symptoms are generally chronic and may be triggered or worsened by stress. Because the intestine is irritated and unusually sensitive, excessive mucus may appear in the stools. Diarrhea, when present, generally occurs in the morning and in clusters. Tests of the stool for signs indicating a known organic cause—blood, pus, excessive fat, parasites, or ova—are usually negative.

Medical Measures

Since no organic cause is known, treatment of irritable bowel syndrome is primarily symptomatic. The client can be helped but probably not cured. Treatment generally occurs outside the hospital.

If constipation is present, a high-fiber diet, adequate fluid intake, and increased activity are indicated. Bulk laxatives may be prescribed. For treatment of diarrhea, antimotility drugs may be indicated, such as anticholinergics or opiates. The client should avoid foods that aggravate symptoms.

The persistent bowel symptoms associated with irritable bowel syndrome can seriously affect the client's lifestyle. Clients frequently suffer from depression (manifested by fatigue, insomnia, and lethargy) and may require psychologic counseling or medication. Because symptoms of irritable bowel syndrome are often stress related, the caregiver should discuss this aspect of the disorder with the client. Stress reduction techniques may be helpful.

Specific Nursing Measures

The client with irritable bowel syndrome needs a great deal of support. Not only are the symptoms unpleasant, inconvenient, and often painful, but the absence of a clear organic etiology for the disorder may lead some caregivers to dismiss the client as "neurotic" and not deserving of serious attention.

The nurse can help the client determine which foods seem to promote or aggravate symptoms. Client, nurse, and dietitian together may plan a dietary regimen appropriate to the client's culture and lifestyle. The relation of stress to the client's symptoms can be explored with a view toward eliminating stressful situations where feasible. The nurse may also teach techniques for stress reduction.

Hemorrhoids and Fissures

Hemorrhoids and fissures are common acquired disorders of the anorectal area. Hemorrhoids are excessively distended veins in the anal area. They may be internal (generally remaining within the anal area and covered with mucous membrane) or external (prolapsing through the anal canal). Fissures are cracks in the skin at the anus. Both conditions are associated with increased pressure in the anal area related, for example, to chronic constipation and straining, obesity, or pregnancy.

Clinical Manifestations

Both hemorrhoids and fissures can be detected on physical examination. External hemorrhoids appear as a cluster of red, blue, or pink tissue at the anal area; internal hemorrhoids may be palpated on digital examination. Fissures are generally apparent on inspection and may be inflamed (Figure 38–6). A fissure causes extreme pain when a digital rectal examination is performed.

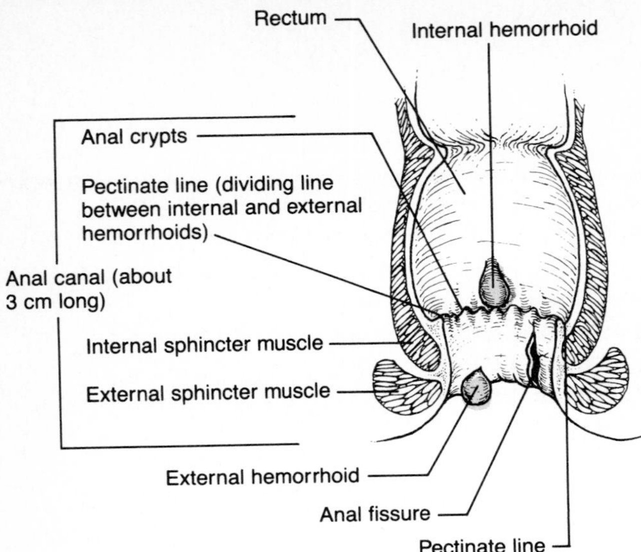

Figure 38–6

Anorectal structures with external and internal hemorrhoids and anal fissure.

The client with hemorrhoids or fissures will generally describe symptoms of pain and bleeding, especially in association with defecation. Pruritus can occur, especially with external hemorrhoids. Hemorrhoids may become thrombosed, and both hemorrhoids and fissures may become infected, with or without abscess formation. Hemorrhoids can also bleed.

Medical Measures

Treatment is generally aimed at decreasing pressure in the perineum and relieving pain and/or itching. If symptoms are acute, a low-residue diet may be prescribed to prevent further irritation and allow the lesion to heal. Generally, however, a high-residue diet, stool softeners, and bulk laxatives are prescribed to prevent constipation and straining.

Symptoms can often be relieved by limiting activity, applying moist heat (sitz baths), and applying local anesthetic agents (usually containing benzocaine), or anti-inflammatory creams (usually containing steroids). Good hygiene is important in preventing infection. Fissures generally heal spontaneously. Hemorrhoids can be alleviated, but acute symptoms may recur.

Specific Nursing Measures

Clients with hemorrhoids and fissures are frequently seen by nurses, often in ambulatory care settings but sometimes in the hospital. In the latter case, the client may have another, more serious disorder that may or may not be related.

Teach measures for preventing constipation and straining at stool. Emphasize the importance of fiber (roughage) in the diet to prevent constipation and consequent straining. Advise the client to keep the legs elevated when sitting to alleviate pressure related to obesity or pregnancy. Teach good hygiene practices: careful cleansing after defecation and use of soft, white, unscented toilet tissue. The client may also need information on preparing and using a sitz bath.

Hemorrhoidectomy

A hemorrhoidectomy is the surgical excision of a hemorrhoid and is frequently performed on an outpatient basis. Several methods are used, including rubber band ligation, sclerotherapy, and excision.

Rubber band ligation, a quick and simple procedure, is performed only on internal hemorrhoids because it is too painful for external hemorrhoids, which have more sensory nerves. Using special equipment, a rubber band is slipped over the base of the hemorrhoid. This will cause the hemorrhoid to shrink from ischemia and slough off or to scar and atrophy. Postprocedural rectal fullness makes it preferable to ligate only one or two hemorrhoids at one time.

Sclerotherapy (injection of a sclerosing agent) is a less common technique used to control internal hemorrhoids. In this procedure, the hemorrhoid is isolated and injected with a sclerosing agent designed to reduce swelling by atrophy of the involved tissue.

Surgical excision, referred to as a closed hemorrhoidectomy, is the preferred procedure for external hemorrhoids where thrombosis has occurred. The physiologic and psychosocial/lifestyle implications are discussed in Table 38–4.

Nursing Implications

Nursing care following hemorrhoidectomy includes promoting comfort, promoting elimination, and observing for complications. Comfort measures include mild oral analgesics and local moist heat. Sitz baths or warm tub baths soothe the inflamed tissue and cleanse the area. Slight bleeding may occur for the first day, but excessive bleeding is of concern. Some clients prefer wearing a protective perineal pad to prevent soiling of clothes and bedding. Instruct the client in dietary modifications to prevent constipation. Increased intake of fluids and high-fiber foods is helpful. Bulk-forming stool softeners such as psyllium mucilloid (Metamucil) can promote normal stooling. Clients should be advised that the first bowel movement may be uncomfortable—some describe the feeling as "passing glass." Clients should be encouraged to avoid straining during a bowel movement.

Upper Gastrointestinal Hemorrhage

Upper GI hemorrhage may occur as a manifestation or complication of a number of disorders of the upper gastrointestinal tract. Hemorrhage can significantly compro-

Table 38–4
Hemorrhoidectomy: Implications for the Client 

Physiologic Implications	Psychosocial/Lifestyle Implications
Complications include infection, hemorrhage, stricture, difficult defecation, and stool incontinence. Hemorrhoids can recur. Client should avoid straining and constipation. If taking anticoagulants or aspirin, the client must be closely observed for bleeding.	Dietary modification is necessary to promote regular bowel movements and avoid constipation. Increased fluid intake and high-fiber foods are helpful. With immediate postoperative fecal or blood oozing, soiling of clothing can be embarrassing. The need to wear protective pads can also be humiliating to some. Weight reduction is advised for the obese client. Regular exercise also helps to maintain normal bowel function.

mise a client's physiologic and psychologic status and can increase the morbidity and mortality associated with the primary disease process.

The most common causes of upper GI bleeding are peptic ulcer disease, erosive gastritis, and esophageal varices (Petersdorf, 1983). Other primary disorders associated with upper GI hemorrhage include esophagitis; esophageal, gastric, and intestinal cancer; and trauma.

Clinical Manifestations

Upper gastrointestinal hemorrhage may be accompanied by hematemesis, melena, hematochezia, and/or occult blood in the stools. Hematemesis (bloody vomitus) may appear red, dark red, brown, or black, depending on how long blood and gastric acids have been in contact. Ordinarily, the longer the contact, the darker the vomited blood. The characteristic "coffee-ground" appearance of the emesis occurs when blood clots have undergone digestion. If blood is not vomited, digestive changes that occur during its passage through the GI tract will promote a characteristic black tarry appearance of the stool (melena).

If the large amount of blood is present in the intestine, however, intestinal motility increases, and blood that originates high in the GI tract will be bright red when it is passed from the rectum (**hematochezia**). Generally, however, hematochezia signifies bleeding from the small or large intestine, or the rectum.

In many instances, bleeding will be less obvious. Hidden (occult) blood in the stool can be identified only by specific testing (eg, Hematest or guaiac testing). Note that stool tests will be positive for up to 3 weeks after a bleeding episode.

Hemorrhage may be acute or long term. Long-term (chronic) blood loss may go undetected until stools are tested for occult blood, often in the course of routine examination, or signs of iron-deficiency anemia appear (weakness, fatigue, lethargy, pallor).

Acute hemorrhage and major blood loss often appear without warning and may be life threatening. It may appear as hematemesis, melena, or hematochezia. If the client has a nasogastric tube to suction, blood will be apparent in the aspirated drainage.

Rapid, acute blood loss of less than 500 mL is rarely associated with systemic signs in adults, except in the elderly and in clients who are anemic. With losses greater than 500 mL, however, the client will experience orthostatic hypotension, syncope, nausea, thirst, and diaphoresis. As blood loss approaches 40% of total blood volume, hypovolemic shock may follow, with pallor; cool, clammy skin; hypotension; and tachycardia (Petersdorf, 1983). A large quantity of blood in the GI tract may cause nausea, abdominal distention, cramping, diarrhea, and borborygmi.

Laboratory studies will reflect hemorrhage and altered hemodynamics. Initially, Hb and Hct readings remain normal. Hemoglobin (Hb) and hematocrit (Hct) readings will eventually reflect a decrease in the number of circulating erythrocytes, although blood loss may not be accurately reflected for up to 36 hours (Greenberger, 1981). An elevated blood urea nitrogen (BUN) level in the presence of a normal serum creatinine level suggests upper GI blood loss in excess of 1000 mL. The BUN level is elevated as a consequence of digestion and absorption of blood protein from the GI tract (Greenberger, 1981).

Medical Measures

Unless anemia is severe, the client with chronic blood loss may be treated as an outpatient. The primary source of the blood loss must be identified and any iron-deficiency anemia corrected. A client with acute, severe hemorrhage is critically ill and must be hospitalized. Treatment priorities include controlling the hemorrhage, preventing shock, and determining the cause of the hemorrhage. A careful history obtained from the client or a reliable significant other helps identify factors that could precipitate hemorrhage (eg, heavy use of alcohol or aspirin, anticoagulant therapy, history of ulcer disease). Endoscopy, angiography, and barium studies may also be used in diagnosing the primary condition.

Immediate intravenous fluid replacement is generally initiated. Normal saline and plasma expanders are infused until the client's blood has been typed and cross-matched and whole blood is available for transfusion.

Strict intake/output measurement is initiated, and an in-dwelling catheter may be inserted to facilitate frequent assessment of blood volume status as reflected in urinary output. A central venous pressure (CVP) line or Swan–Ganz catheter may also be inserted so circulatory volume can be continually assessed. Nasogastric intubation may be necessary so accumulated blood and clots can be aspirated and blood loss measured. Iced saline lavage may also be initiated; the cooled solution promotes vasoconstriction and helps stop hemorrhage.

Pharmacologic therapy is initiated as soon as possible to stop or prevent bleeding. Antacids are generally ordered and instilled via the nasogastric tube. Intravenous cimetidine (Tagamet) is also usually prescribed.

Among the specific procedures that may be implemented to control hemorrhage are selective angiography combined with vasopressin infusion or embolization, or endoscopy with electrocoagulation or laser therapy. Surgery to control hemorrhage may be indicated when hemorrhage requires more than 6 to 8 units of blood, when hemorrhage remains uncontrolled for more than 24 to 48 hours, or when blood transfusion fails to restore circulatory volume.

Specific Nursing Measures

The client with upper GI hemorrhage challenges all the nurse's assessment and intervention skills. Keen observation can be instrumental in detecting signs of anemia in a client with slow, chronic bleeding. Precise assessment is critical in monitoring the client's status during an episode of acute bleeding accompanied by shock and deterioration. Quick thinking and quick action are required.

Intake/output records must be meticulously maintained and transfusions administered safely. If post-transfusion Hct readings are ordered, keep current with the results. Assess hydration and circulatory status frequently; measure output and vital signs every half hour; monitor urine specific gravity and assess skin for pallor and turgor.

If the client has a nasogastric tube to suction, monitor its patency and irrigate the tube (if permitted) as often as necessary to ensure that clots do not obstruct the flow of drainage. Follow antacids or other medications instilled via the nasogastric tube with water, and halt suction temporarily so that the medication can be absorbed and not washed out.

The client's comfort deserves careful attention. If hemorrhage has been severe, the client may be covered with blood and should be washed, provided with a clean gown, and otherwise made comfortable. Losing large amounts of blood is frightening as well as dangerous. Take time to reassure the client and family and to explain briefly what is being done to control the hemorrhage. Family members should be permitted to be at the bedside if at all possible, since the presence of familiar persons may help calm the client.

Positioning is important, especially for clients in shock. The recumbent position with legs elevated is generally recommended. The client may be in pain; prescribed analgesics and nursing comfort measures are indicated.

Lower Gastrointestinal Hemorrhage

Gastrointestinal bleeding distal to the duodenum (ie, from the jejunum, ileum, colon, or rectum) is characterized as lower GI hemorrhage. It may be mild, moderate, or severe. Hemorrhage may be a chronic manifestation of a disease process or may appear spontaneously and be life threatening. Lower GI hemorrhage may be precipitated by a number of disorders discussed in this section. The most common cause is diverticular disease.

Clinical Manifestations

Acute, severe lower GI hemorrhage is usually characterized by hematochezia, but melena may herald the condition if constipation or obstruction is present. The client may have abdominal pain, cramping, distention, and/or diarrhea. *Chronic,* slow blood loss generally presents as iron-deficiency anemia and occult blood in the stool. Like upper GI hemorrhage, bleeding in the lower tract may be accompanied by hypovolemic shock and alteration in laboratory values, depending on the severity of blood loss.

Medical Measures

Treatment is designed to stop bleeding, prevent shock, and determine the underlying cause of the hemorrhage. Sigmoidoscopy and/or colonoscopy is often performed, although the usual bowel preparation is omitted if the client is actively bleeding. Angiography with vasopressin infusion or embolization may be performed to control severe bleeding. Barium studies may be done once active bleeding has ceased, if no diagnosis has been established.

The gastrointestinal tract is generally allowed to rest, and the client is kept NPO and hydrated intravenously. Nasogastric intubation may be used for decompression. Fluid/electrolyte balance must be carefully monitored, and an in-dwelling catheter may be inserted to facilitate input/output measurement and urine studies. Fluid and/or blood replacement is provided as indicated. Prophylactic antacids and cimetidine may be prescribed to prevent stress ulceration.

After an acute episode of upper GI bleeding, or in cases of chronic hemorrhage, a low-residue diet is generally indicated. Iron-deficiency anemia, if present, will require treatment.

Specific Nursing Measures

Supportive therapy will be required, including efficient, accurate, and safe assessment and implementation. Measures used are similar to those discussed under upper GI hemorrhage.

SECTION 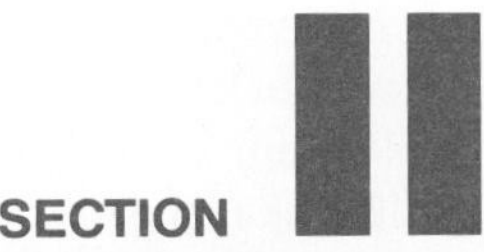

Inflammatory and Infectious Disorders

Inflammatory and/or infectious disorders of the stomach, intestine, and pancreas may be related to internal or external irritation, diet, or proliferation of pathogenic bacteria. These disorders are fairly common in the adult population and therefore pose a significant health problem.

Peritonitis

Peritonitis, an inflammation of the peritoneum, is a potentially life-threatening complication of disorders of the abdominal organs. It is associated with significant morbidity and mortality and is the most common cause of death following abdominal surgery (Given & Simmons, 1984).

Various disorders can lead to peritonitis, including perforated peptic ulcer, ruptured appendix, gangrene of the bowel, perforated diverticulum, trauma, and abdominal surgery (Figure 38–7). Drainage from a perforated or infected area, as well as the introduction of foreign matter (eg, talc in surgical gloves), can chemically or mechanically irritate the peritoneal cavity, stimulating the inflammatory process and fostering the proliferation of pathogenic bacteria.

Clinical Manifestations

The onset of peritonitis is sometimes slow and progressive but more often is acute. The vascular hyperemia

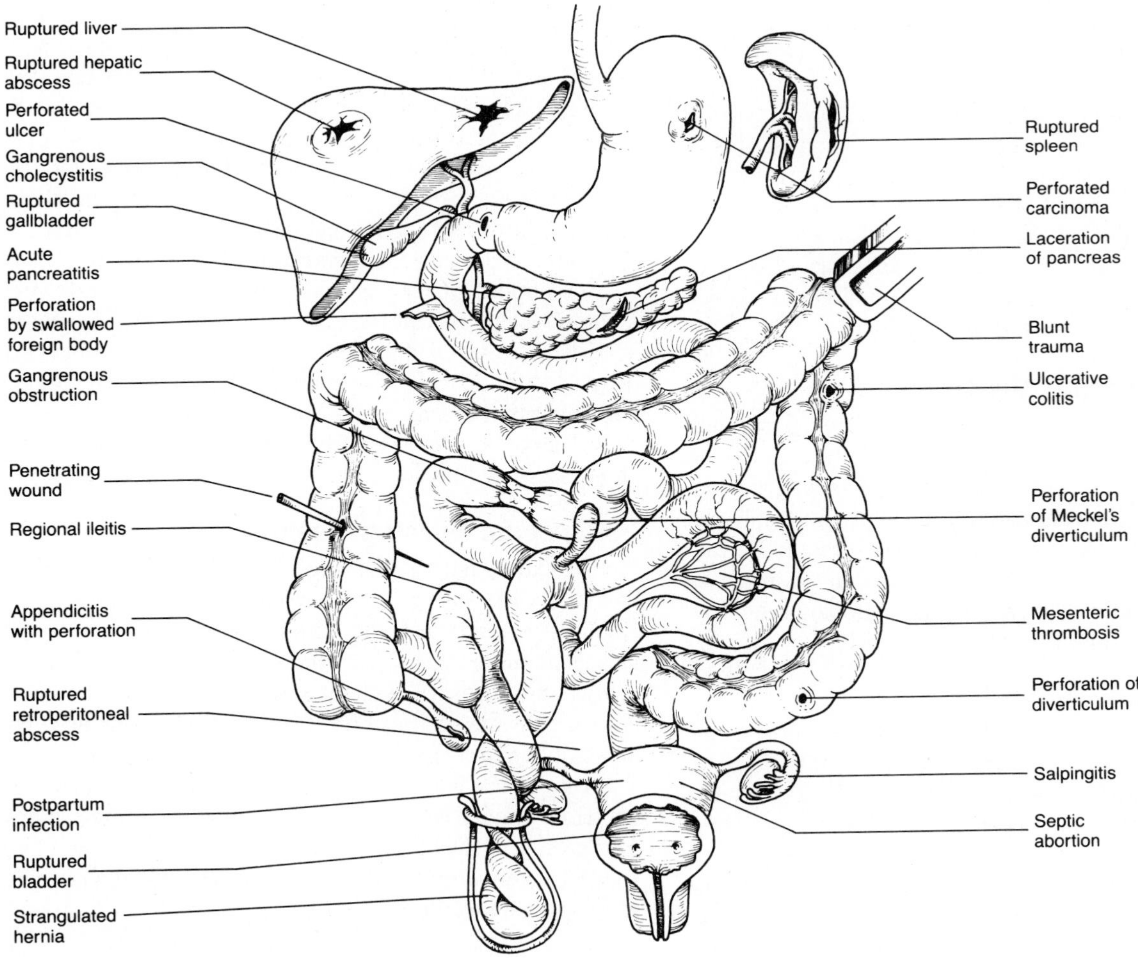

Figure 38–7

Causes of peritonitis.

integral to the inflammatory process causes accumulation of fluid in the abdominal cavity, and thereby abdominal distention and rigidity, pain, anorexia, nausea, and vomiting. The client will often describe pain as severe and report that it intensifies with movement. Muscle guarding is generally noted, and the client may obtain some relief by flexing the knees while recumbent.

Fever and tachycardia will be present, and rebound tenderness will be apparent on palpation. On auscultation, bowel sounds can be diminished or absent, as paralytic ileus may develop. Respiratory function may be seriously compromised, since abdominal distention can inhibit full expansion of the diaphragm. Respirations may become shallow, and hypoxia with signs of tachycardia, restlessness, and cyanosis may occur. Hemodynamics can be seriously affected, leading to shock.

Medical Measures

Septic peritonitis is life threatening and requires prompt and rigorous treatment. The source of irritation must be identified and removed (eg, by appendectomy, gastrectomy, etc.). An exploratory laparotomy will be performed if life-threatening symptoms persist and the source has not been identified. Supportive treatment involves careful monitoring of fluid intake and output; observation for shock; maintenance of circulating fluid volume with intravenous fluids; correction of nutritional, electrolyte, and acid–base imbalances; and administration of antibiotics. Pain relief is also indicated, but analgesics must be used cautiously to prevent masking of diagnostic clues. To alleviate nausea and vomiting, antiemetics are often prescribed.

Specific Nursing Measures

Clients with acute peritonitis are generally frightened and apprehensive. They may have been healthy, only to be suddenly hospitalized with a serious and painful illness. The nurse should be available so the client and family can express fears and ask questions. Therapy should be carried out safely and efficiently, with special attention to nutritional and fluid/electrolyte needs, antiobiotic therapy, and measures to promote comfort and rest.

Gastritis

Gastritis, inflammation of the gastric mucosa, may be acute or chronic (atrophic). The inflammatory changes in the mucosa differ in the two disorders. Self-treatment of this disorder is common, since symptoms may be vague.

Acute gastritis is commonly associated with chemical irritation of the gastric mucosa related to excessive use of alcohol, caffeine, or spices; use of medications such as indomethacin, phenylbutazone, prednisone, or salicylates; food poisoning; systemic infection; or emotional stress. *Chronic gastritis* is often associated with underlying disorders such as gastric ulcer, gastric carcinoma, pernicious anemia, duodenal regurgitation, mucosal injury, or immunologic or endocrine disorders. Incidence of chronic gastritis is high among alcoholics and among clients who have had partial gastrectomies (Given & Simmons, 1984).

Clinical Manifestations

Chronic gastritis is sometimes asymptomatic; acute gastritis is always symptomatic. Symptoms of either disorder include epigastric discomfort, bloating, anorexia, nausea, vomiting, abdominal cramping, diarrhea, and eructation. Hemorrhage may occur and can present as hematemesis, melena, or occult blood in the stool. Iron-deficiency anemia can result from long-term blood loss. Diagnosis is generally based on history, gastroscopy, and biopsy.

Medical Measures

The client with acute gastritis is treated symptomatically. The stomach is permitted to rest and heal while the client is kept NPO and is nourished intravenously until symptoms dissipate. Nasogastric suctioning may be necessary, and, if the client is bleeding, iced saline lavage may be used. Antacids are generally administered, by mouth or by nasogastric tube. Antiemetics may also be prescribed, as may anticholinergics or analgesics. As the inflammation subsides and symptoms diminish, the client gradually returns to a normal diet, although any particularly offensive foods are eliminated.

Treatment of chronic gastritis is aimed at relieving symptoms and preventing acute exacerbations. The client is advised to avoid substances that provoke symptoms (eg, drugs, foods, alcohol). Pharmacologic measures may include administration of antacids, steroids, and/or sedatives. The client must be observed for signs of hemorrhage. Any bleeding should be controlled and anemia corrected.

Specific Nursing Measures

In acute gastritis, nursing therapy should be supportive of the client's needs for fluids, electrolytes, and nutrients. Administer fluids and medications safely as ordered, and closely monitor and report the effectiveness of pharmacologic measures. The client should be made as comfortable as possible and permitted sufficient rest. Observe for signs of hemorrhage, and test stools for occult blood.

Diet counseling is necessary for both acute and chronic gastritis. Advise the client to avoid foods and medications that cause particular difficulties. Encourage the client to read labels on foods and OTC medications. Substances that are especially likely to cause problems include:

- Coffee (regular or decaffeinated)
- Foods containing caffeine (chocolate, soft drinks, tea)
- Spicy foods
- Alcohol

- Salicylates (ie, aspirin and aspirin-containing preparations)
- Ibuprofen (Motrin, Rufen, Advil, Nuprin)
- Indomethacin (Indocin)
- Phenylbutazone (Butazolidin, Azolid)
- Steroids

Pancreatitis

Inflammation of the pancreas, or pancreatitis, may occur in either acute or chronic form. Both forms may be relapsing and, in both cases, inflammation may cause extensive pancreatic tissue changes and/or damage. In some cases tissue regeneration and healing occurs. In others, pancreatic damage may be permanent.

Any disorder that interferes with the flow of biliary or pancreatic secretions or renders secretions more viscous, may precipitate stasis and/or reflux of secretions into the pancreas, leading to inflammation. Autodigestion of pancreatic cells by pancreatic enzymes has also been suggested as a cause of inflammation, degeneration, and, in severe cases, necrosis.

Clinical Manifestations

Both acute and chronic pancreatitis are associated with similar symptoms: anorexia, nausea, vomiting, and upper abdominal pain. The pain is generally steady and may radiate to the upper back. The pain is so severe and intractable, even in chronic pancreatitis, that the client may be unable to eat or to work and may even become addicted to narcotics. Fever is common.

On examination, abdominal rigidity and muscle guarding will be noted, and bowel sounds may be diminished. If the common bile duct is obstructed, jaundice occurs. The client is usually unable to tolerate fatty foods, and diarrhea and steatorrhea commonly occur, because enzymes capable of hydrolyzing lipids are absent or deficient. If symptoms persist, the client may lose weight and develop nutritional deficiencies. Fluid shift related to the inflammatory process may precipitate dehydration, pleural effusion and hypoxia, ascites, peritonitis, and/or shock. Hemorrhage related to tissue damage may also occur.

Blood studies reveal leukocytosis (related to inflammation and/or infection) and elevated glucose levels (related to pancreatic cellular damage or to stress). Hypocalcemia can occur. Chronic pancreatitis can precipitate diabetes. Ultrasound and CT scanning may be useful in diagnosis.

Medical Measures

Therapeutic goals include identifying and, if possible, eliminating the cause, relieving symptoms, and preventing complications. Surgery may be necessary to correct the primary disorder. Symptomatic relief measures include nasogastric intubation to rest and decompress the GI tract, analgesics, antiemetics, and anticholinergics (to reduce pancreatic and ductal spasm). Intravenous fluids and electrolytes and parenteral hyperalimentation are administered as necessary to maintain fluid/electrolyte and nutritional balance.

The client is initially NPO. As symptoms subside and clinical and laboratory data improve, a low-fat diet is prescribed. In chronic disease, degeneration may lead to impaired enzyme production (pancreatic insufficiency). Oral administrations of pancreatic enzymes (eg, pancrelipase, pancreatin) may be necessary.

If glucose metabolism has been seriously altered, insulin may be administered to control hyperglycemia. In severe pancreatitis, the pancreas may be surgically drained or totally or partially resected (pancreatectomy).

Specific Nursing Measures

In acute pancreatitis, the nurse is responsible for assessing the client's symptoms and evaluating the effectiveness of therapy, monitoring for complications, promoting normal fluid/electrolyte and nutritional status, and fostering the client's comfort. Nursing assessments include monitoring the urine for glucose and acetone and observing the client for hypoglycemic or hyperglycemic reactions. Since serum calcium levels may be subnormal, observe for signs of hypocalcemia. Nutritional status warrants special attention; ongoing nutritional assessment and support are essential.

The client recovering from acute pancreatitis or suffering from the chronic form is generally instructed to follow a low-fat diet. Although the diet itself is usually provided by the dietitian, be sure that clients understand the regimen in terms of their own lifestyle and culture. Inform the client about the proper administration of any prescribed medications as well as potential side effects and toxic reactions.

Surgery of the Pancreas

Surgical treatment for disorders of the pancreas is indicated for trauma, neoplasm, inflammation, and obstruction (eg, calculi). A client with pancreatitis may need surgery for such complications as hemorrhage or pseudocyst or when gallstones cause pain or clinical deterioration because of obstruction. The client with pancreatic pseudocyst may need surgery for obstruction, infection, hemorrhage, rupture, or uncontrolled pain. Surgical treatment of pancreatic carcinoma is indicated with localized disease or as a palliative measure. Transplantation of the pancreas is also possible, but not widely performed. The more common surgical procedures are described below.

The pseudocyst can be *drained* internally into adjacent structures such as the stomach, duodenum, or jejunum—the preferred method. However, placing a drainage tube into an external collection device is sometimes necessary. Percutaneous drainage of the pseudocyst can be effective while avoiding risks associated with general surgery. Draining the pseudocyst relieves compression of nearby structures and promotes healing.

The *resection* of the pancreatic tail is indicated to remove disease localized in the distal portion of the organ. With local adenocarcinoma, the tail of the pancreas and the spleen are removed. The spleen is removed because the proximity of this highly vascular organ increases the risk of metastasis. Tail resection is also indicated for chronic calcified pancreatitis.

With chronic recurrent calcific pancreatitis, a *pancreaticojejunostomy* is indicated. This measure is effective when the pancreatic duct is obstructed in the proximal portion of the pancreas. The pancreatic duct and the jejunum are split longitudinally, placed side to side, and sutured together. This drains the pancreatic secretions directly into the jejunum.

When the body and tail of the pancreas are severely diseased with chronic pancreatitis, they can be removed in a *partial pancreatectomy.* This procedure may also be employed when previous surgical procedures have failed to control the pain of chronic pancreatitis.

The *radical distal pancreatectomy* involves the resection of 95% of the pancreas. All but part of the head of the pancreas and the spleen are included in the resection. This procedure is performed when the entire pancreas is involved with chronic pancreatitis.

A *total pancreatectomy* is indicated in some resectable carcinomas, hyperinsulinism, traumatic injury, selected cases of chronic pancreatitis, and in acute fulminant pancreatitis with total pancreatic necrosis.

The *pancreatoduodenectomy,* also referred to as the *Whipple procedure,* is among the most extensive resections for pancreatic disease. The Whipple procedure is indicated for carcinoma of the head of the pancreas, ampulla of Vater, lower common duct, or duodenum. The procedure involves the resection of the right side of the pancreas, distal stomach, duodenum, gallbladder, and (if indicated) the spleen. Reconstruction is necessary, suturing the common duct, pancreas, and stomach to the jejunum. For unresectable carcinomas, palliative measures can be taken to divert biliary and pancreatic secretions.

Physiologic and psychosocial/lifestyle implications of pancreatic surgery are discussed in Table 38–5.

Nursing Implications

Nursing care of the client undergoing pancreatic surgery depends on the procedure performed. The primary nursing responsibilities include preventing complications, promoting comfort, and maintaining fluid/electrolyte and nutritional status.

Following pancreatic surgery, the client should be monitored closely for pulmonary complications. Encourage clients to aerate their lungs fully by deep breathing. Coughing will facilitate removal of secretions. Pulmonary toilet may be indicated. Frequent measures to improve ventilation are essential to prevent pulmonary insufficiency.

Various drainage tubes will be in place to remove secretions and promote healing. A nasogastric tube will be in place for several days to decompress the stomach and prevent distention from putting strain on the suture line. The nurse will also have to care for drainage tubes from

Table 38–5
Pancreatic Surgery: Implications for the Client

Physiologic Implications	Psychosocial/Lifestyle Implications
High level of postoperative pain. Endocrine effects of pancreatic resection include disturbed glucose homeostasis from altered insulin and glucagon production. Exocrine effects of pancreatic resection lead to malabsorption from maldigestion, steatorrhea, diarrhea, and coagulation problems from impaired absorption of vitamin K. Postoperative complications include infection, sepsis, hemorrhage, fistula formation, and necrosis to adjacent structures from leakage of pancreatic enzymes. Resection of the distal stomach as part of the Whipple procedure leads to dumping syndrome. Procedure may fail to control pain of chronic pancreatitis. Proximity to chest increases risk of pulmonary complications postoperatively.	Failure of pain control following surgery can be discouraging and frustrating. Narcotic addiction can result from attempts to control pain of pancreatitis. Dietary modifications may be indicated for extensive excisions and reconstruction (eg, to prevent dumping syndrome following a Whipple procedure). Abdominal incision may affect body image. Clients with pancreatic carcinoma are facing a generally fatal diagnosis. Client and family need time to adjust and assistance with planning approaches to maximize the time the client has left.

the incision. These may be attached to suction devices, to facilitate removal of secretions. A T-shaped tube may be in place to drain bile from the common duct. Skin care is crucial with external pancreatic drainage, because pancreatic secretions are highly irritating to the skin. Observe the wound for signs of infection or hemorrhage and ensure aseptic handling of dressings to prevent infection. Assess the client's temperature frequently for elevations due to infection and check vital signs for any indication of hemorrhage. Blood transfusions are frequently required because of operative blood loss.

The client will require frequent doses of narcotics to control pain following pancreatic surgery. Adequate pain control facilitates cooperation with efforts to cough and deep breathe and to change position. However, doses large enough to cause sedation may result in respiratory depression, further increasing the chance of pulmonary complications.

Following pancreatic surgery, fluid and electrolyte balance must be restored. The specific requirements will vary from individual to individual.

Maintenance of nutritional status is essential in pancreatic surgery. Often, these clients show poor nutritional status, either because of chronic disease or alcohol abuse. Preoperative parenteral nutrition, continued postoperatively, will reduce morbidity and mortality. The parenteral nutrition should be tailored to individual needs and is generally administered with a central venous catheter. Monitor blood sugar levels closely. Exogenous insulin may be required to promote cellular uptake of glucose for metabolism and to prevent hyperglycemia. Parenteral nutrition should be continued until oral intake can safely be started. When oral intake is initiated, the nurse should make sure that the client tolerates clear liquids well before introducing solid food. Clients may require supplementation of oral pancreatic enzymes and subcutaneous insulin to promote absorption and utilization of nutrients.

Clients undergoing pancreatic surgery often have numerous psychologic needs requiring great understanding from the nurse. The client may be physically and psychologically worn down from chronic disease and unrelenting pain. The client may be facing a terminal diagnosis. There may be a long history of drug or alcohol abuse with all the accompanying personal and family difficulties. These problems, compounded by the discomfort of surgery, require a consistent and caring approach that can pose a challenge for the nurse.

Appendicitis

Appendicitis is acute inflammation of the vermiform appendix, thought to be related to ulceration at the area. It may occur as a single attack or as repeated episodes. Appendicitis occurs most often in the second and third decades of life (Petersdorf, 1983).

Several etiologic factors have been suggested for appendicitis, including viral infection and obstruction of the lumen of the appendix. Obstruction may be related to a primary inflammatory process associated with edema, development of fecaliths, the presence of foreign bodies or worms, or an infectious process with enlargement of lymphatic tissue.

Clinical Manifestations

Ulceration and inflammation at the appendix commonly cause anorexia, nausea, vomiting, bowel changes, and pain that begins as diffuse midabdominal pain and eventually localizes in the right lower quadrant of the abdomen. An elevated temperature and leukocytosis are generally noted. Physical examination will reveal rebound tenderness, shallow respirations, and guarding. Pain will also be noted on rectal or vaginal examination.

Infection, with or without abscess formation, may occur, as may necrosis and gangrene. Rupture of the inflamed appendix with perforation of the intestinal wall and consequent peritonitis is a serious potential complication.

Early diagnosis of appendicitis is important to limit possibly life-threatening complications such as perforation and peritonitis. Diagnosis may be delayed in the elderly, since older persons are less likely to develop a temperature, or in the pregnant client, in whom symptoms may be mistaken for a side effect of pregnancy. Hospitalization and observation are generally indicated when any suspicion of appendicitis exists.

Medical Measures

The client with acute appendicitis requires prompt, effective treatment to eliminate inflammation and infection and to prevent complications. To rest the bowel, NPO status is instituted and the client is given fluids intravenously. A nasogastric tube is passed to decompress the GI tract. Enemas and cathartics must be avoided, since they may irritate an already inflamed area and promote perforation. Antibiotics, an important component of treatment, are generally administered intravenously. Analgesics may be given, but caution is indicated, since they may mask symptoms. Surgery (appendectomy) is generally performed as soon as possible.

Specific Nursing Measures

Accurate nursing assessments are crucial to the client's well-being. Any increase in abdominal pain and rigidity may herald life-threatening perforation and/or peritonitis and must be reported promptly. The nurse is responsible for the timely and accurate administration of antibiotics, for monitoring fluid/electrolyte balance, and for administering intravenous solutions. Nursing comfort measures are especially important if analgesics are withheld or kept to a minimum. Explaining that pain medication may mask crucial symptoms may help the client in coping with pain. Keep the client and family informed about tests and treatments. The client will probably require surgery, so preoperative preparation should begin promptly.

Appendectomy

An appendectomy is the surgical removal of the appendix. An appendectomy may be performed in the presence of infection (appendicitis), to allay symptoms and prevent perforation (ruptured appendix), or as a prophylactic measure in clients having other abdominal surgery.

The appendix is not known to have an important physiologic role, and its removal produces no known physiologic consequences, aside from the possible complications of the surgery itself. Abdominal adhesions in later years may be secondary to a ruptured appendix or to the appendectomy.

An appendectomy has few psychosocial implications; the scar is small and inconspicuous, except for those with major wound infections. It may be hard for some young adults to accept that activities must be limited for several weeks until the wound has healed completely. Older clients may find that it takes longer for them to resume their normal lifestyle.

Nursing Implications

The postoperative course of an uncomplicated appendectomy includes a hospital stay of 3 to 4 days. Incisional care is similar to that for other postoperative wounds. If there was excessive preoperative vomiting, fluids and electrolytes are monitored and replaced parenterally if needed.

Inflammatory Bowel Disease

Although the term "inflammatory bowel disease" could be applied to any inflammatory disorder of the small intestine or colon, it is generally used to designate two conditions: ulcerative colitis and Crohn's disease (regional enteritis, regional ileitis, granulomatous colitis). Both are chronic, recurrent diseases that pose significant health problems.

Ulcerative colitis, the more common, primarily affects the superficial mucosal layers of large areas of the colon. Crohn's disease affects all layers of the ileum and/or the colon and frequently causes patchy lesions interspersed with normal tissue. Both disorders occur equally in both sexes and occur more commonly in Caucasians, especially those of Jewish origin (Petersdorf, 1983).

Various factors have been implicated in the etiology of inflammatory bowel disease. Its familial tendency suggests a hereditary component. Infection, immune factors, and psychosocial factors have been proposed.

Clinical Manifestations

ULCERATIVE COLITIS The inflammation associated with ulcerative colitis destroys tissue, causing ulceration and necrosis that, in turn, precipitate abdominal pain and diarrhea. The stool may contain blood and/or mucus, or may be watery. Symptoms can occur as an isolated attack, may be intermittent or recurrent, or may be continuous. In severe or prolonged episodes, fever, leukocytosis, infection, fluid/electrolyte imbalance, and malnutrition can occur. Fissures, hemorrhage, and formation of abscesses or fistulas are possible complications. Scarring associated with healing of tissue may obstruct the bowel at a later time. Toxic megacolon (severe dilatation of the colon) is a serious complication that can predispose the client to perforation and peritonitis.

CROHN'S DISEASE (REGIONAL ENTERITIS) The client with Crohn's disease will experience symptoms similar to those of ulcerative colitis, but the course of the disease is generally more slowly progressive. Fever, abdominal pain, and diarrhea frequently occur, as well as anorexia, nausea, and vomiting. Malabsorption and steatorrhea as well as fluid/electrolyte and nutritional disturbances may also be encountered. Potential complications include intestinal perforation, obstruction, infection, fistula formation (Figure 38–8), fissures, and hemorrhage, although bleeding is generally less severe than with ulcerative colitis.

Chronic, frequent, and/or prolonged episodes of inflammatory bowel disease subject the client to serious, long-standing nutritional imbalances and to weight loss. These clients often appear thin, even emaciated. The chronic aspect of the disease, and the symptoms associated with it, may make the client anxious and/or depressed. The client's lifestyle is greatly altered, especially if bowel resection becomes necessary. Diagnosis is confirmed through the use of barium studies, endoscopy, biopsy, and stool analysis.

Medical Measures

Treatment for ulcerative colitis and Crohn's disease is essentially the same. If symptoms are severe, if complications occur, or if nutritional status is greatly impaired, the client is often hospitalized. In acute episodes, the intestinal tract is allowed to rest. The client is kept NPO and nourished intravenously until symptoms subside. If the client's intake is restricted for a long period, TPN may be indicated to replace nutritional losses. Gradually, a low-residue diet is introduced, as tolerated. Any anemia precipitated by blood loss is corrected.

Pharmacologic measures may include use of anti-inflammatory agents, steroids, anticholinergics, and antispasmodics to control diarrhea, and antibiotics (especially sulfasalazine) to prevent or control infection. Counseling may assist the client in coping with stresses associated with chronic illness. Although ulcerative colitis often subsides (at least temporarily) with treatment, Crohn's disease may persist and progressively worsen.

In severe, intractable inflammatory bowel disease,

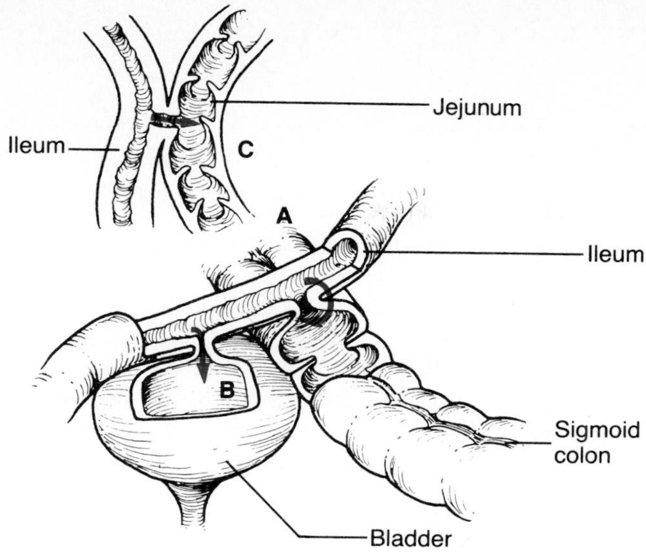

Figure 38–8

Fistula formation in Crohn's disease. **A.** Ileosigmoid fistula. **B.** Internal fistula between ileum and bladder. **C.** Ileojejunal fistula.

surgical intervention may be necessary. Surgery involves resection of the diseased portion of the bowel with a temporary or permanent ileostomy. Surgery is curative in ulcerative colitis.

Specific Nursing Measures

The client with inflammatory bowel disease requires a great deal of physiologic and psychosocial support. Ongoing nutritional assessment is imperative, and long-term diet counseling may be necessary. The client may find that certain foods are especially likely to provoke acute episodes and should eliminate them from the diet. The health history can pinpoint offensive dietary items. Supplementary feedings are often indicated. Encourage the client to take them as ordered and suggest ways to make these feedings more palatable. Consultation with the nutritionist can be helpful.

Assessments should also focus on fluid/electrolyte needs. Observe stools for blood and mucus and report observations accurately. Due to diarrhea, the skin in the anal area may become excoriated and susceptible to infection. Use aseptic technique in performing perineal hygiene and demonstrate the technique to the client. Clients are often severely stressed. Consulting a mental health nurse clinician can assist the nursing staff in working with the client and significant others.

Infectious Gastroenteritis

Inflammation and infection of the GI tract, causing diarrhea among other symptoms, is usually related to invasion or overgrowth of microbes. Serious morbidity can be associated with these infections (especially among the elderly or malnourished), but most clients can be treated on an outpatient basis. Viral gastroenteritis (also known as infectious diarrhea) is the second leading cause of illness in the United States (Petersdorf, 1983).

Infections are commonly associated with situations in which bacteria, viruses, or parasites gain entry into the GI tract and then proliferate. Infectious gastroenteritis may follow ingestion of contaminated food or water, an upper respiratory infection, or oral/anal or anal/genital contact. Factors that decrease the acidity of gastrointestinal fluids (eg, gastric ulcer, gastric surgery), depress motility, or diminish or destroy normal flora (eg, antibiotic therapy) increase the client's risk of GI infection. Infectious gastroenteritis caused by food poisoning is discussed in Chapter 9.

Clinical Manifestations

The client with gastroenteritis may experience vomiting, diarrhea, abdominal cramping, respiratory symptoms, otitis media, and pharyngitis. Malabsorption often characterizes the infection, and steatorrhea may appear. These symptoms combine to make the client fatigued and susceptible to fluid/electrolyte imbalance, nutritional deficiencies, and weight loss. Symptoms generally persist for a week or more. Diagnosis is based on symptoms and stool culture.

Medical Measures

Treatment is supportive. The client is rehydrated as necessary; oral electrolyte–glucose mixtures are available for this purpose. A low-residue diet is prescribed until symptoms dissipate. Pharmacologic therapy commonly includes bismuth subsalicylate (Pepto-Bismol) administered at half-hour intervals for 4 hours. Sometimes antibiotics are necessary.

Specific Nursing Measures

Nursing care is also supportive. Encourage the client to comply with the low-residue diet, emphasizing the need for fluids. Advise the client to rest and to resume activities as symptoms permit. Assess for dehydration and explain to the client how to do so. Explain the medication regimen. Since many of these disorders can be spread through the fecal–oral route, advise the client to follow enteric precautions and explain how to do so.

Pilonidal Cyst

A pilonidal cyst is a foreign body reaction to ingrown hair that develops in the upper end of the cleft between the buttocks in the sacrococcygeal region. Affected clients usually have a deep intergluteal cleft and heavy hair growth in the area. Obesity and jobs that require considerable sitting contribute to the friction, warmth, and moisture that exacerbate the problem.

There are often several openings (sinus tracts) to the skin. The client may only become aware of the cyst when purulent drainage occurs through the sinus tracts from secondary infection in the area. Pain, localized erythema, and swelling may accompany the drainage.

In the past, pilonidal cysts were believed to be of embryologic origin. Currently, foreign body reaction with secondary infection is thought to be the predominant etiology.

Medical Measures

Initial treatment involves probing the sinus tracts under local anesthesia with removal of all hair and debris. The wound is packed open and is kept packed until healing takes place. If the cyst recurs, surgical excision of the sinus tract is required. Primary closure is attempted. If the excision is too wide, the wound is packed and allowed to heal by granulation.

Specific Nursing Measures

Since most clients are discharged early, nursing care mainly involves teaching client and family about protection of the surgical site from trauma and from contamination by urine and feces. For promoting comfort and relieving strain on the surgical area, the side-lying position with the upper leg supported by pillows is often the most comfortable.

Rectal Abscess

A localized infection of the perirectal area (rectal abscess) may be caused by chronic inflammation and eventual infection of hair follicles, contamination of rectal fissures, or thrombosed hemorrhoids.

Clinical Manifestations

The primary manifestation of rectal abscess is pain, especially with defecation. The abscess may be apparent with inspection and can generally be felt with palpation. An abscess high in the rectum generally produces additional symptoms of pain and malaise. Pelvic discomfort may be present. Fistulas can form between the abscess and other body areas, especially the bladder and vagina.

Medical Measures

Analgesics and sitz baths often relieve symptoms. Antibiotics may be prescribed. Incision and drainage are usually necessary and are discussed below.

Specific Nursing Measures

Nursing care is supportive and is aimed at relieving symptoms. Assist the client with the use of the sitz bath, and stress aseptic hygienic practices.

Surgery for Anorectal Infection

Surgery may be indicated for infectious disorders of the anorectum. Infections can result from traumatic fissures (cracks or ulcers) or infected anal glands. An infected anal gland can progress to form an acute abscess, which can progress further to form a fistula (sinus tract). Disorders that predispose to the development of anorectal infection include Crohn's disease, trauma, radiation therapy, and cancer.

A wide variety of surgical procedures may be used. Selection of a procedure depends upon the extent of the anorectal infection. *Incision and drainage* involves a surgically created opening that allows for passage of secretions. Removing purulent secretions promotes internal healing and decreases discomfort from pressure. This procedure is often preferred for fistulas and abscesses. *Fistulotomy* is the incision and drainage of a fistula. This may be preferred to an excision, which may leave a gaping wound. *Fistulectomy* is the surgical excision of the involved tissues around a fistula. This creates a wound that requires meticulous care to prevent reinfection. *Fissurectomy* is the surgical excision of a fissure. Since a fissure can be more superficial than a fistula, the area of excision is not as large. If the excised area becomes reinfected, a fistula or abscess

Table 38–6
Surgery for Anorectal Infections: Implications for the Client

Physiologic Implications	Psychosocial/Lifestyle Implications
Complications include wound infection, hemorrhage, stricture, difficult defecation, fecal impaction, fecal incontinence, and urinary retention.	Dietary modifications are necessary to promote passage of soft stool. Increased fluid intake, increased high-fiber food intake, and bulk-forming stool softeners are indicated.
Anorectal infections have a high rate of recurrence.	Fecal or pus incontinence can be embarrassing and demoralizing. Perineal pads may be necessary.
Crohn's disease, trauma, radiation therapy, and cancer can predispose to recurrence.	The potential of recurrence can be frustrating and discouraging.
Lesions can extend into the vagina, causing drainage and dyspareunia.	Anorectal sexual activities may need to be modified to control recurrence or complications.
With prior radiation therapy, healing will be impaired, possibly necessitating a diverting colostomy to prevent fecal contamination.	Dyspareunia may persist.

can result. *Sphincterotomy* is an opening or excision to enlarge the sphincter to prevent further tearing and promote healing of an anal fissure. See Table 38–6 for physiologic and psychosocial/lifestyle implications of surgery for anorectal infections.

Nursing Implications

The nursing care following surgery for anorectal infections includes promoting comfort, promoting wound healing, promoting elimination, and preventing complications. Anorectal procedures may be performed in outpatient or inpatient settings, modifying the general nursing approach. Local anesthetic ointments or oral analgesics are used for pain control. Comfort measures include providing cushion pads to sit on to minimize the direct pressure on the affected area. Warm baths or sitz baths are soothing and promote cleansing of the incision; the warm water may also promote the drainage of purulent secretions.

Wound management varies. Open wounds may be packed with sterile gauze. Gauze soaked in solutions designed to draw out purulent secretions or with bacteriostatic action may be packed or applied to the lesion. Close attention to wound management is essential, since anorectal infections tend to recur.

Proper elimination is promoted by ingestion of high-fiber foods, increasing fluid intake, and administering bulk-forming stool softeners. Defecation should be encouraged to prevent fecal impaction.

SECTION 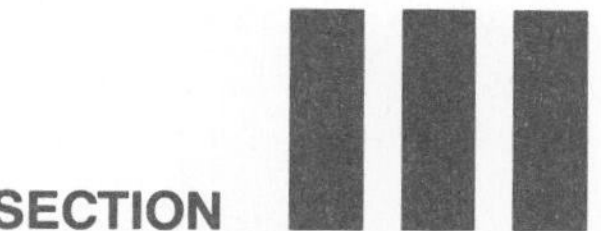

Neoplastic and Obstructive Disorders

Neoplasia of the stomach, intestine, and pancreas may be benign or malignant; in either instance, the client may experience significant morbidity with altered digestion, absorption, and elimination. Nutritional deficiencies and weight loss are common. The nurse is often in a position to detect early symptoms or signs of neoplastic and obstructive disorders of the stomach, intestine, and pancreas. Whether taking a history, performing a physical assessment, or providing routine care, the nurse should be alert for:

- Any history of continuing anorexia, nausea, and/or vomiting
- Weight loss without dieting
- Epigastric or abdominal pain that persists
- Changes in bowel habits
- Blood in the stool or black tarry stools in a client who does not take iron or Pepto-Bismol

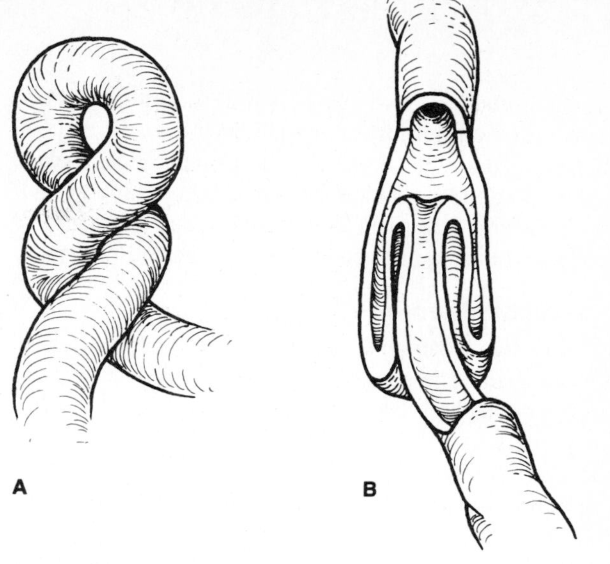

Figure 38–9

A. Volvulus, twisting of the bowel. **B.** Intussusception, small bowel telescopes into itself.

Intestinal Obstruction

Obstruction of the small or large intestine, with inhibition of the passage of intestinal contents, may occur as an acute or chronic problem. Adhesions or hernias cause a majority of small bowel obstructions. These may be a consequence of previous trauma, intestinal or pelvic surgery, or appendectomy.

Obstruction of the large intestine is commonly related to cancer, diverticulitis, volvulus (twisting of the bowel), or intussusception (invagination of the bowel) (Figure 38–9). Paralytic (adynamic) ileus may also be considered a form of intestinal obstruction. Paralytic ileus occurs to some degree after any peritoneal insult (for example, abdominal surgery). Usually, it persists for 2 or 3 days and gradually subsides without treatment.

Clinical Manifestations

Symptoms are precipitated when fluid (gastric, pancreatic, or biliary secretions), gas, and ingested substances accumulate proximal to the site of obstruction. The client generally has abdominal pain and distention and may vomit. If the obstruction is near the lower end of the intestinal tract, vomiting can occur late and may have a foul, fecal odor caused by bacterial overgrowth in the intestinal tract. The client will probably report being unable to pass stools or flatus. In partial obstruction, diarrhea may be noted. **Singultus** (hiccups) is common.

Borborygmi may be noted on physical examination, except in cases of ileus or peritoneal irritation, in which bowel sounds are diminished or absent. Peristaltic rushes (periodic loud bursts of sounds) are common. Low-grade fever may also be present.

Fluid/electrolyte and acid/base imbalances are common, since fluid shift and absorption in the intestines are abnormal, and output losses may be extreme. Nutritional deficiencies and weight loss also occur. Complications include peritonitis and strangulation (impaired blood supply) and/or incarceration (impaired blood supply and necrosis) of the bowel, which may also promote infection and/or sepsis.

Medical Measures

Supportive treatment is given while the primary cause of the obstruction is sought. The client is kept NPO, and fluid/electrolyte and nutritional needs are met with intravenous fluids and TPN as necessary. A nasogastric or intestinal (Cantor, Miller–Abbot) tube to suction decompresses the intestinal tract and alleviates nausea and vomiting.

Intake and output are carefully measured, and an indwelling catheter may be inserted to facilitate this process. Replacement of fluid losses is imperative. Antibiotics may be prescribed to prevent infection. Analgesics are ordered for pain relief but must be used with caution, since they can mask diagnostic symptoms. Surgery (exploratory laparotomy) is performed as soon as possible to identify and/or treat the primary disorder.

Specific Nursing Measures

The client with intestinal obstruction requires efficient, accurate measurement and recording of intake and output. Carefully describe intestinal-tract drainage. Assess skin turgor, urine specific gravity, and the client's thirst frequently to determine hydration status. Measure abdominal girth to monitor distention.

Explain why NPO status is necessary and provide mouth care frequently to make the client more comfortable. If analgesics are being withheld for diagnostic reasons, explain why this is being done. Ensure the patency of the nasogastric or intestinal tube and irrigate it as necessary (unless this is contraindicated).

If the client has an intestinal tube, understand that it is intended to advance along the intestinal tract to provide for distal decompression. Often the physician will order that the tube be advanced a few inches at a time by the nurse. Passage of the tube through the pylorus into the duodenum is facilitated by having the client lean forward with arms extended. When advancing the tube a prescribed distance, have the client change position, alternating the supine and side-lying positions (Swearingen, 1984).

Throughout the course of care, be available to provide psychologic support when needed and encourage the client and family to express any fears about the diagnosis, which may be uncertain.

Polyps

A **polyp** is a projection of the mucosal surface of the lumen of an organ. Polyps may occur in the stomach or intestine and may be single or multiple, benign or malignant. The most common form is the adenomatous polyp (adenoma), which may originate in the benign form and then undergo malignant changes (Petersdorf, 1983).

Familial colonic polyposis, which generally appears in childhood or adolescence, is a hereditary disorder characterized by numerous polyps. It has a 100% association with cancer of the colon by age 40 (Petersdorf, 1983). Polyps are generally diagnosed by digital examination, endoscopy, and biopsy.

Clinical Manifestations

Polyps may produce hemorrhage, diarrhea, and, if large, symptoms and signs of intestinal obstruction. Polyps can also be asymptomatic.

Medical Measures

Once identified, polyps are generally removed by colonoscopy, sigmoidoscopy, or gastroscopy as an outpatient procedure or during hospitalization. A low-fiber diet is generally prescribed prior to polypectomy to inhibit inflammation and bleeding. In familial colonic polyposis, prophylactic colectomy, with or without formation of a colostomy, is generally indicated.

Specific Nursing Measures

Nursing care of the client with a GI polyp is primarily supportive. Explain any treatment such as polypectomy and support the client throughout the experience. Counsel the client about the relationship of polyps to the incidence of cancer, stressing the importance of routine checkups and prompt reporting of symptoms.

Polypectomy

A polypectomy is the surgical removal of a polyp. The safest and therefore the most common method for removing colon and rectal polyps is to snare them through an endoscope, either a flexible colonscope or a rigid sigmoidoscope. Laser surgery may also be used. This may be an outpatient procedure. The surgeon can also approach the lesion through an abdominal incision when the polyp cannot be reached or appears to be malignant.

Nursing Implications

PREOPERATIVE CARE The bowel is prepared for a polypectomy by restricting oral intake and using cathartics, enemas, and possibly antibiotics to clear normal colon flora. Prepare the client for the fact that the procedure may be somewhat painful and embarrassing. With the rigid sigmoidoscope, the endoscopy procedure is done in the knee–chest position on a sigmoidoscopy table. Many clients find the position (and the procedure) uncomfortable and may become dizzy, nauseated, or feel faint during endoscopy. Provide the client with the opportunity to discuss any fear of malignancy.

POSTOPERATIVE CARE Preprocedure sedation wears off in several hours. Postprocedure care involves evaluating vital signs and checking for rectal bleeding. The client should be observed for a day or two for signs of hemorrhage. Slight bleeding from the rectum is not uncommon. The client who is returning home shortly after the procedure should be prepared for the possibility of some mild bleeding and assessed to be sure the client is not dizzy or faint, and can ambulate safely. Regular follow-up is important, including colonoscopy or sigmoidoscopy every 2 to 3 years to detect recurrence.

Cancer of the Stomach

Malignant tumors of the stomach affect males more often than females and usually appear after the fourth decade of life. The incidence of gastric cancer has steadily declined in the United States in recent years although it is still a major potentially lethal health problem, especially if detected late in its course.

Dietary factors have been implicated in the etiology of gastric cancer, notably a diet high in starches, smoked foods, and preservatives. Cancer of the stomach has also been associated with achlorhydria, group A blood type, chronic (atrophic) gastritis, adenomatous polyps, and pernicious anemia (Petersdorf, 1983).

Clinical Manifestations

Unfortunately, symptoms are generally slowly progressive and appear late in the course of the disease. The client may report anorexia, nausea, vomiting, weight loss, bloating, and epigastric discomfort. An abdominal mass may be palpated and occult blood may be present in the stool. Anemia can occur as a late manifestation. Diagnosis is made on the basis of barium studies, gastroscopy, biopsy, and gastric analysis.

Medical Measures

Gastric cancer is treated by surgery (gastrectomy), chemotherapy, and sometimes radiation. Nutritional support and fluid/electrolyte maintenance are generally indicated. The client with severe symptoms may have to be NPO, and nasogastric intubation may be used to decompress the digestive tract.

If the client is permitted to eat, small, frequent feedings are helpful. Antiemetics may be ordered for nausea, and analgesics for pain. Any anemia is treated as well. Metastasis, if it occurs, usually involves the liver, bones, or lungs.

Specific Nursing Measures

The client with cancer of the stomach requires consistent nutritional assessment and support. Nursing measures to promote the client's nutritional status are indicated. Often, the client will require TPN to maintain nutritional and fluid/electrolyte needs.

Pain control requires the nurse to use comfort measures and to administer analgesics as necessary. Careful assessment of pain is indicated, and any signs or suspicions of metastasis should be brought to the physician's attention.

Cancer of the Pancreas

Cancer of the pancreas is the fourth most common cause of cancer-related death in the United States, occurring more commonly in men (Petersdorf, 1983). It generally appears in the sixth or seventh decade of life. The head of the pancreas is most often affected.

The etiology of pancreatic cancer remains unclear. Increased incidence, however, has been associated with diabetes, smoking, and pancreatitis.

Clinical Manifestations

Cancer of the pancreas is associated with significant morbidity and mortality. Its course is painful and progressive. Abdominal pain, anorexia, nausea, vomiting, and weight loss frequently occur, although symptoms may be vague until the disease is well advanced.

Malabsorption related to pancreatic enzyme insufficiency may occur, accompanied by steatorrhea. If symptoms interfere significantly with ingestion and absorption, the client may be severely malnourished and emaciated. Fluid/electrolyte disturbances are often seen, and the client may become hyperglycemic as insulin production is impaired. Laboratory findings can include elevated serum lipase and amylase levels as well as hyperglycemia.

Diagnosis is determined by sonography, endoscopy, CT scan, angiography, and/or percutaneous aspiration, which may be performed with ultrasound guidance.

Medical Measures

The client with cancer of the pancreas requires supportive treatment to help alleviate symptoms. The client may be more comfortable if kept NPO with nasogastric intubation to decompress the bowel. Nutritional support, often with hyperalimentation, is imperative. Antiemetics and analgesics are indicated.

Most pancreatic tumors are inoperable, but sometimes the pancreas and duodenum are surgically resected. A *Whipple procedure,* involving removal of the head of the pancreas, a portion of the stomach, the duodenum, and the common bile duct, is an alternative. After pancreatic surgery, replacement of insulin and pancreatic enzymes is necessary.

Radiation and chemotherapy may also be used. In general, survival rates are poor, and the disease is often fatal within a year of onset of symptoms.

Specific Nursing Measures

The client with cancer of the pancreas requires tremendous physiologic and psychologic support from the nurse. Monitor nutritional and fluid/electrolyte status continuously. Check fractional urines q.i.d. to detect glucose abnormalities. Nursing measures to promote nutrition and comfort are of high priority. Monitor all symptoms and evaluate the effectiveness of any measures to control them. The client receiving radiation treatment or chemotherapy requires specialized care as discussed in Chapter 10.

Throughout the course of the client's illness, be available to answer questions from the client and significant others. Both client and family need opportunities to express their feelings about the symptoms of the disease and its grave prognosis.

Cancer of the Colon and Rectum

Primary neoplasms of the intestinal tract usually affect the large intestine or rectum. Excluding skin cancer, the incidence of colorectal cancer is second only to cancer of the lung. Male and female incidence is equal. Colorectal cancer most often appears in the fifth to seventh decades of life.

Low-fiber diets, which promote slow stool transit time and stasis of bowel contents, are thought to be related to possible carcinogenic changes in the GI tract. A high intake of fats and meats may also be related. Colorectal cancer is also associated with familial colonic polyposis and inflammatory bowel diseases. Recent research indicates that some colon cancers arise from genetic defects, traced to a specific chromosome.

Clinical Manifestations

Clients frequently describe changes in bowel habits, black tarry stools, or bleeding from the rectum. Pain may also be present. Unfortunately, the client may not report these symptoms as soon as they are detected.

As the disease progresses, bleeding may increase, and symptoms of obstruction may occur as the neoplasm grows. Anemia can develop as a consequence of bleeding. Location and occurrence of major symptoms associated with colorectal cancer are summarized in Table 38–7.

Early detection is possible. The American Cancer Society recommends that digital examination, stool guaiac testing, and proctosigmoidoscopy be performed as noted in Box 38–1. Barium studies and biopsy are also useful in diagnosis.

Medical Measures

A combination of surgery, chemotherapy, and radiation therapy may be used for treatment. Surgery generally involves resection of the malignant area, and a temporary or permanent colostomy.

Prior to surgery, the bowel is thoroughly cleansed with enemas, laxatives, and/or irrigations to prevent operative contamination. Antibiotics are usually prescribed preoperatively to decrease bacterial flora in the GI tract. Symptoms are relieved with analgesics, and nutritional and fluid/electrolyte imbalances and anemia are corrected as necessary. A low-residue diet is indicated prior to surgery. The prognosis for survival is good with early detection and treatment, but the outlook is more grave if metastasis has occurred.

Table 38–7
Location and Occurrence of Major Symptoms of Cancer of Large Intestine

Symptom	Right Colon	Left Colon	Rectum
Abdominal mass	Right lower quadrant: 69%	Left lower quadrant: 29%	
Pain	Vague, dull, uncharacteristic (aggravated by walking): 89%	Gas pain, cramps: 82%	Late feature: 65%
Blood in stool	Dark or mahogany red mixed in stool: 30%	Bright red, coating surface of stool: 49%	Bright red, coating surface of stool: 80%
Flow of stool	No alteration	Decrease in caliber of stools, tendency toward constipation	Sense of incomplete evacuation; tenesmus
Weight loss (>5 kg)	50%	35%	7%
Obstruction	Acute: 7%	Causes progressive abdominal distention, pain, vomiting, and constipation: 16%	7%
Changes in bowel habits	54%	69%	71%

SOURCE: Given BA, Simmons SJ: *Gastroenterology in Clinical Nursing*. St. Louis: Mosby, 1984, p. 366.

Specific Nursing Measures

Since early diagnosis is so crucial to the outcome of colorectal cancer, the nurse alert to early symptoms and signs may literally save a client's life. Encourage clients to have periodic examinations as recommended by the American Cancer Society.

Once a diagnosis has been established, physiologic and psychologic support and nutritional assessment and support are ongoing nursing responsibilities. Monitor the client's weight and observe stools for signs of bleeding. Nursing comfort measures and analgesics promote comfort and relief from pain.

If the client is to receive chemotherapy or radiation therapy, be prepared to support the client throughout the experience and to provide symptomatic relief as necessary. If a colostomy is performed, the client will need teaching about colostomy care and assistance in adjusting to a new body image. Since a diagnosis of cancer is so frightening to many clients, encourage verbalization of feelings by client and family. If the client is expected to die, the nurse can work with the client and family as they go through the grieving process.

Bowel Resection

A bowel resection is the surgical excision of any portion of the small or large intestine or rectum. There are numerous indications for a bowel resection, including trauma, ischemic injury, obstruction, fistula, neoplasm, inflammation, and conditions that benefit from temporary or permanent fecal diversion (eg, rectovaginal fistula). The most common indications are obstruction, carcinoma, and inflammatory bowel disease.

Preservation of the continuity of the intestinal tract is desirable but not always possible with bowel resection. The construction of a stoma for fecal elimination through the abdominal wall may be necessary for cancer of the rectum or sigmoid colon, or for inflammatory bowel disease. With diverticulitis, a temporary diverting colostomy may be necessary to allow time for healing of excised areas.

The *small bowel resection* is indicated primarily for Crohn's disease, ischemic damage, and obstruction. The area and extent of resection are variable. The small bowel can be anastomosed to another portion of the small bowel, to the colon, or to the anorectum. The small bowel may be used to form an ileostomy.

A *colectomy* is the surgical excision of all or part of the colon with or without removal of the rectum. An external ostomy stoma may be constructed as a result of partial or total colectomy, or the colon may be anastomosed to another portion of the colon or to the rectum.

A *proctectomy* is the surgical excision of the rectum. The surgical excision of the entire colon and rectum, *total proctocolectomy,* is indicated for ulcerative colitis and multiple polyposis. The total removal of the colon and rectum makes an ileostomy necessary.

Box 38–1
Recommended Protocol for Early Detection of Colorectal Cancer

The American Cancer Society (1987) recommends the following tests:

Digital rectal examination: once every year for a client over 40 years of age

Stool guaiac test: once each year for the client over 50 years of age; can be done by the client at home

Proctosigmoidoscopy: following two negative annual examinations, once every 3 to 5 years for the client over age 50

Clients who are at higher risk (eg, personal history of polyps or family history of cancer of the colon or rectum) should receive more frequent, thorough examinations beginning at an earlier age

Several surgical procedures require the construction of a stoma. These procedures are compared in Table 38–8 and discussed below. An *ileostomy* involves bringing the ileum (usually the terminal ileum) onto the abdominal surface to form a stoma. An ileostomy can be either temporary or permanent. The *conventional ileostomy* is constructed by pulling the proximal end of the ileum through the abdominal wall and turning it over itself to form a cuffed stoma. Fecal contents drain from the stoma into a collection pouch, which is worn continuously. The *loop ileostomy* involves pulling the intact ileum through the abdominal wall, placing a rod underneath the resulting loop to support it above the abdominal cavity, and making an opening on the top of the loop to permit fecal passage into a collection pouch. This procedure is used when a temporary ileostomy is necessary to promote healing of an anastomosis of the ileum to the anus. A *continent ileostomy* involves the construction of an internal reservoir pouch for stool to control stool output. With the continent ileostomy, wearing an external collection device is unnecessary. *Cecostomy,* a rarely performed procedure, is an opening into the cecum, usually placed temporarily for decompression prior to a colectomy or an ileal–rectal anastomosis. The cecostomy usually has a tube in place for drainage.

A *colostomy* is a surgical opening of some portion of the colon onto the abdominal surface. The colostomy is constructed with either the proximal end of the remaining bowel or with a loop of colon. The loop colostomy is generally a temporary measure performed on the transverse colon. The loop may be kept intact with both proximal and distal openings together, or the loop may be severed to form two stomas (a double-barrel colostomy). The double-barrel colostomy prevents fecal passage into the distal bowel. Consistency of stool changes in the colon; therefore, the

Table 38–8
Types of Ostomies

Type	Indication	Usual Location of Stoma	Consistency of Stool
Conventional ileostomy (Brooke ileostomy)	Ulcerative colitis; fecal diversion; temporary bowel rest; Crohn's disease; familial polyposis	Right lower quadrant	Liquid to pastelike
Continent ileostomy	Ulcerative colitis; familial polyposis	Right lower quadrant	Liquid to pastelike
Ascending colostomy	Fecal diversion	Right upper or lower quadrant	Liquid to semiformed
Transverse colostomy, single barrel	Fecal diversion; trauma; unresectable obstructing carcinoma	Right lower quadrant	Liquid to semiformed
Transverse colostomy: • Double barrel • Loop	Fecal diversion; trauma; unresectable obstructing carcinoma	Proximal in right lower quadrant Distal on left side	Liquid to semiformed
Descending colostomy	Colorectal cancer; diverticulitis	Left lower quadrant	Semiformed to solid
Sigmoid colostomy	Colorectal cancer; fecal diversion	Left lower quadrant	Semiformed to solid

more distal the colostomy, the more formed the stool (Figure 38–10).

A *mucous fistula* is a stoma constructed from a dormant portion of bowel following a bowel resection. In this procedure, a colostomy or ileostomy is constructed leaving the rectum intact; the proximal end of the rectum is brought up to the abdominal wall for drainage, thus forming the mucous fistula. This procedure prevents intraperitoneal leakage from the rectal suture line where healing may be impaired (eg, after radiation therapy).

Construction of an ileal–anal reservoir is optimal for multiple polyposis and ulcerative colitis because it preserves the rectal sphincter and no permanent stoma is needed. The ileal–anal reservoir requires an intact anus and functional rectum. The entire colon is resected and a reservoir is constructed with two or three loops of the terminal ileum and is stapled to the anus. The reservoir acts to slow the passage of stool, although the client will experience diarrhea three to eight times per day. To promote healing of the reservoir and suture line, a temporary loop ileostomy is usually constructed for fecal drainage for about 3 months to allow time for healing the anal anastomosis.

The surgical procedure most widely used for rectal cancer is the *abdominal-perineal resection.* Through abdominal and perineal incisions, the rectum and local tissue likely to be tumor bearing are removed, including skin, muscle, fat, and lymphoid tissue. A descending or sigmoid colostomy is constructed.

An alternative to the abdominal–perineal resection is the low *anterior resection* for proximal rectal carcinomas. The involved rectum is resected, leaving the lower rectum intact. A colostomy is avoided by constructing a colorectal anastomosis using a stapling device.

Table 38–9 discusses physiologic and psychosocial/lifestyle implications of ostomies, abdominal–perineal resection, and ileal–anal reservoir for the client.

Nursing Implications

Appropriate and adequate nursing care for a client undergoing bowel resection depends on the specific surgical procedure, extent of reconstruction, and the likely pathophysiologic and psychosocial/lifestyle consequences.

PREOPERATIVE CARE Preoperative management includes both physical and psychologic preparation. The client will be restricted to oral fluids only for 2 to 3 days to control fecal accumulation. Cathartics, enemas, and/or suppositories are given to empty the intestines of feces to minimize fecal contamination of the operative site. Systemic broad-spectrum antibiotics may be used immediately preoperatively to reduce bacterial flora, especially in the colon, and continued postoperatively to control infection.

Clients may enter the hospital with fluid and electrolyte imbalances that need to be corrected before surgery. Anemia may also need correction (by iron or blood administration) to improve oxygen transport. Debilitated clients may need several weeks of parenteral nutrition to improve nutritional status.

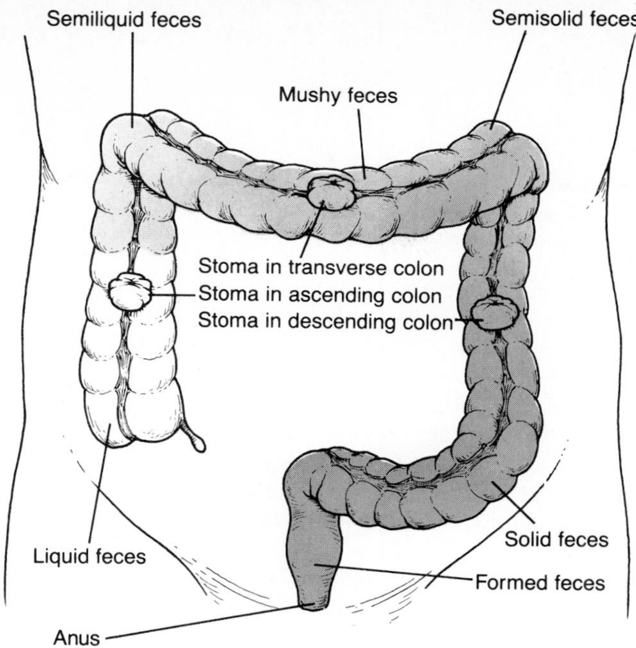

Figure 38–10

Colostomy stoma site and fecal consistency.

For clients who will have an ostomy performed, the enterostomal therapy (ET) nurse plays a crucial role in the client's physical and psychologic care both preoperatively and postoperatively. The client's nurse should work with the ET nurse in the preoperative psychologic preparation. The client's knowledge and perception of life with an ostomy should be assessed and any misconceptions corrected. The client should be taught the basics of gastrointestinal physiology, how the ostomy will alter the normal physiology, and what strategies are available to compensate for the changes. The client's anxieties should be addressed and support system and coping mechanisms evaluated. This knowledge will help in understanding and planning for postoperative reactions. Clients and their families must be encouraged to share their feelings and concerns. Good preoperative rapport with client and family will facilitate postoperative adjustment.

The ET nurse can also arrange for the client to meet someone who already has had an ostomy—an ostomate. Discussion with a well-adjusted ostomate can relieve anxiety and helps both client and family to feel they are not alone. The ostomate often continues the relationship with client and family and may play an important role in facilitating postoperative adjustment and return to home and society.

POSTOPERATIVE CARE Postoperative nursing goals include preventing complications, promoting wound healing, monitoring bowel function, promoting comfort, and maintaining adequate nutritional status. Specific care needs for the client with a conventional ileostomy, continent ileostomy, or colostomy are discussed later in this section.

PREVENTING COMPLICATIONS Decompression of the bowel will help to prevent complications. The bowel may be decompressed with a nasogastric tube, an intestinal tube, a cecostomy tube, a rectal tube, or a tube placed into the continent ileostomy reservoir. A long intestinal tube, similar to a nasogastric tube, can be advanced into the small bowel (usually by a mercury bolus attached to the tube), where it decompresses the small bowel generally by attachment to low suction.

The cecostomy tube, rectal tubes, and continent ileostomy tubes are relatively short tubes with wide lumens. Stool can plug these tubes, which may require periodic gentle irrigation to maintain patency. The continent ileostomy drainage tube is left in place for 2 weeks to promote healing.

Monitor drainage from all tubes carefully for amount, consistency, and characteristics. This information should be recorded every 2 hours.

PROMOTING WOUND HEALING The nurse's role in wound management following bowel resection begins with observing the incision line for infection, hemorrhage, or separation. Sterile technique must be observed in changing dressings. Drainage tubes may be placed into the wound or along the incision to promote drainage of fluids, which may otherwise impair healing. Drainage tubes may drain by internal pressure or by externally applied suction. Portable vacuum collection devices are frequently used when drainage is expected. These collection devices should be emptied regularly and the drainage characteristics and amount recorded.

The stoma should be observed for warmth, moisture, and normal pink or red color, indicating adequate blood supply. The skin around the stoma (peristomal skin) should be protected by a skin barrier such as karaya gum (a protective resin) or a pectin wafer product (eg, stomadhesive, Hollihesive) soon after surgery before stool output begins. The stoma should be covered with a transparent collection pouch to protect the skin, to protect the incision from contamination by drainage from the stoma, to allow observation of the stoma and assessment of bowel function, and to decrease odor and increase client acceptance.

Perineal wound management presents a challenge to the nurse. When the entire rectum is removed, an empty space remains, which will eventually fill with granulation tissue. To promote drainage and healing, the perineal wound may be left open with gauze dressings packed inside, may be partially closed with a drainage tube in place, or may be completely closed. The perineal wound is also uncomfortable for clients, making positioning and sitting difficult. Pain management is essential.

MONITORING BOWEL FUNCTION Continually monitor the client's bowel function following bowel resection. For several days, bowel motility will be minimal. Observe for return of bowel activity by auscultating for bowel sounds,

Table 38–9
Bowel Resection: Implications for the Client 

Physiologic Implications	Psychosocial/Lifestyle Implications
Colostomy and ileostomy	
Inappropriate stoma placement can lead to difficult appliance management; too wide a stoma opening can lead to hernia or prolapse; stoma too small can lead to stenosis or obstruction; stoma that does not protrude enough makes successful pouching difficult. Obesity may interfere with constructing the stoma and may contribute to decreased blood supply to the stoma or to a flush or retracted stoma. Pregnancy may lead to obstruction or prolapse, although this is uncommon. Complications of an ileostomy include fluid loss (usual output 500 to 1500 mL/day); electrolyte, vitamin, and mineral loss (especially sodium, magnesium, zinc, and vitamin B_{12}); obstructions from food blockage or adhesions. Complications of an ileostomy and of a colostomy include skin irritation, stomal edema, stomal necrosis, and stomal recession or prolapse. Continent ileostomy advantages include no appliance necessary, little potential for skin excoriation. Complications of continent ileostomy include incontinence, difficult intubation, fistula, abscess, obstruction, perforation by catheter; may have malabsorption of fat, iron, folate, and vitamin B_{12}; fluid and electrolyte imbalance; pouchitis—inflammation due to bacterial overgrowth.	Adjustment is difficult when the client has unrealistic expectations (eg, ostomy will solve all problems) or perceives it as only temporary if it is permanent. Client should be able to resume previous activities including recreation, social life, and work. Procedure involves a complex psychosocial adjustment. May initially feel frustrated, discouraged, isolated, or depressed. May feel they have lost control and become dependent. Client may have many fears, including rejection by significant others; loss of job; loss of role and status; interference with sexual relations; fear others will notice appliance under clothes, hear gas passing, and smell foul odors. Continent ileostomy requires intubation for drainage two to four times daily. A public restroom may be necessary for drainage. Fewer problems with gas and noise. Body image and self-esteem alterations occur because of body changes and loss of sphincter control. Client may be concerned about ability to bear children. When learning physical skills, client may initially feel a lack of confidence and frustration. Clothing preferences do not have to change. Dietary changes may be necessary, including need to increase fluid intake to prevent dehydration and avoiding foods that increase gas and odor of feces (eg, baked beans, onions, eggs, fish).
Abdominal–perineal resection	
Perineal wound healing may be prolonged with complications such as infection, wound separation, and hemorrhage. This wound may require drains. Denervation in the perineal resection may lead to bladder and sexual dysfunction. The abdominal wound has the potential complications of infection, hemorrhage, and wound separation.	Psychologic reactions are related to having cancer, fear of recurrence, and adjustment to mutilating nature of surgery. Body image and sexual expression are affected by having an ostomy and having had perineal resection with closure of anus.
Ileal–anal reservoir	
A sphincter-preserving surgery with no ostomy required and no appliance. May require a two- or three-stage procedure with a temporary ileostomy. Diarrhea will persist and can be excessive. May take 6 to 12 months until adequate bowel function is established. May need to use drugs or bulk agents for adequate control. Complications include excessive diarrhea, anastomotic leak, incontinence, urgency, pouchitis, perineal skin irritation.	Procedure may fail if disease recurs in rectal stump, necessitating an ileostomy. Need to learn self-intubation of anus with S pouch. May have to deal with incontinence or soiling, especially at night. May need to irrigate reservoir to promote stool evacuation and prevent reservoir inflammation. Regular follow-up with sigmoidoscopy and biopsies to detect recurrence or malignant changes associated with ulcerative colitis necessary.

asking clients if they have passed flatus, and monitoring any ostomy output. With an ostomy, stool output is expected within 4 to 7 days after surgery, but can occur as soon as 1 to 2 days.

MAINTAINING ADEQUATE NUTRITIONAL STATUS When oral intake is delayed for up to a week or longer, parenteral nutrition is indicated. Parenteral nutrition is best administered through a central venous catheter. The client should be maintained on parenteral nutrition until oral intake reaches more than half of the required intake for 3 consecutive days. Specific nutritional considerations with ostomies are discussed in the following section.

OSTOMY CARE The principal goals of ostomy care include facilitating self-care and psychosocial adaptation, maintaining peristomal skin integrity, and promoting appropriate bowel elimination.

Ostomy clients can live a completely normal life. They need to be helped to manage their ostomy in a caring, supportive, and practical manner. Because each client is unique and each lifestyle different, the nurse should understand as much as possible about the client's lifestyle—diet, exercise, bathroom facilities, travel, sexual preferences, work situation, and support systems. Instruction can be individualized to meet the client's unique needs.

CARE OF THE CONVENTIONAL ILEOSTOMY The conventional ileostomy will drain serosanguineous fluid within 24 hours of surgery. Stool output begins with the return of bowel function in 3 to 5 days. The drainage is involuntary and frequent, especially at first. The stool is liquid, and may approach 1500 mL per day, but as the body adapts to the ileostomy, the drainage becomes pasty and about 500 mL per day. Because feces contain enzymes that are irritating to the skin, skin protection is critical.

The ileostomy appliance (drainage device) used postoperatively should be disposable, drainable, adhesive backed, and odorproof. A skin barrier must be used as well. When the postoperative stomal swelling subsides, the client and ET nurse can discuss appliance alternatives. There are two basic types, disposable and reusable. The many criteria to be considered in appropriate appliance selection include stoma construction, character of the peristomal skin, cost, client preference, and the client's manual dexterity.

Appliances without a skin barrier will require the addition of a skin protector prior to application. The peristomal skin should be cleansed with mild soap and water when the appliance is changed. The frequency of change depends on the type of appliance and the construction of the stoma. The appliance is easiest to change when the output is minimal, generally early in the morning. All equipment necessary for change should be organized and ready. The new appliance should be prepared before the old one is removed. The collection pouch should be drained as soon as it is one third full of gas and/or stool. The nurse should measure the output. Care should be taken when handling the pouch so client acceptance is enhanced. For example, a facial expression while changing the pouch may say more to the client than words ever could.

Nursing Research Note

Gloeckner MR: Perceptions of sexual attractiveness following ostomy surgery. *Res Nurs Health* 1984; 7:87–92.

This research evaluated feelings of sexual attractiveness in four groups of ostomy clients: those with colostomies, ileal conduits, ileostomies, and the Kock pouch.

The results suggest that in the first postoperative year, feelings of sexual attractiveness are lower than feelings preoperatively. After the first year, feelings of sexual attractiveness increased. Clients with Crohn's disease and ulcerative colitis had increased feelings of sexual attractiveness in subsequent postoperative years, surpassing preoperative feelings.

These findings may assist nurses in educating clients undergoing ostomy surgery regarding changes in body function and body image. Nurses should openly discuss issues of sexuality with the client and sexual partner, encouraging verbalization of feelings and sharing of perceptions, concerns, and fears between partners.

With a new ileostomy, introduction of food into the diet should be gradual. Clients will slowly learn which foods cause increased drainage, odor, or gas. Cabbage and onions are common odor offenders. Yogurt may be eaten to control odor. When there is considerable air in the pouch, it should be emptied to prevent leakage. There are a number of deodorizers on the market, which can be swallowed or put into the bag. Blockage of the ileostomy should be avoided as far as possible by diet manipulation. Chewing food well, avoiding high-fiber foods, and adequate hydration will help to keep the ileostomy patent.

Clients and a family member, if possible, need to learn ileostomy care prior to discharge. Teaching must include emotional support and discussion of client concerns; skin care; equipment care; emptying, preparing, and applying the appliance; where to obtain supplies; odor management; and dietary modifications. The client should be encouraged to resume all previous activities.

CARE OF THE CONTINENT ILEOSTOMY For several weeks postoperatively, the ostomy is intubated continuously with a catheter set at low suction. This prevents distention of the new pouch and therefore promotes healing. After 2 to 3 weeks, the ostomy is periodically and gently intubated, two to four times daily, with a soft catheter to drain the contents of the pouch. The frequency of intubation can be decreased as the pouch capacity increases. Fibrous food is avoided to prevent blockage. The client can drink grape juice as a mild laxative to keep stool liquid. Skin integrity is maintained with daily cleansing, and the stoma, which produces mucus, is kept covered with an absorbent dressing between emptying. The nurse teaches the client proper intubation and how to detect signs of obstruction. Irrigations may be necessary to remove stool and decrease pouchitis.

CARE OF THE COLOSTOMY The most common colostomy is the sigmoid or descending colostomy. Transverse loop colostomy is less common and presents more difficulties in maintaining skin integrity and proper appliance fit. The sigmoid colostomy will usually drain formed stool on a relatively regular schedule, making care easier than ostomies with frequent, liquid drainage. Many clients prefer a closed and odorproof pouch and are willing to use irrigations to maintain regularity. If irrigations are not desired or are inappropriate, a drainable pouch is indicated. Skin barriers are optional, but a correctly fitting appliance is essential to prevent breakdown of peristomal skin.

Colostomy irrigations may give the client with a low descending or sigmoid colostomy some control over elimination. The procedure takes approximately 1 hour, and it is usually performed in the bathroom. The client fills a container with 500 to 1000 mL of warm, not hot, tap water; hangs the container at shoulder level; and flushes water through the tubing to remove the air. A cone tip is attached to the irrigating tubing and lubricated. The colostomy appliance is removed, and the belted irrigating sleeve is applied. The cone tip is inserted gently into the stoma. This device fits snugly into the stoma and prevents backflow. The water is infused slowly over 3 to 5 minutes to prevent cramping and distention. The client then removes the cone, and fecal material drains directly through the irrigating sleeve into the toilet. When drainage is complete, the client cleans and dries the peristomal skin. The appropriate appliance is applied with or without skin barrier.

The client should be adequately prepared for discharge. Time is needed to recover from surgery and develop confidence in colostomy management. Teach the client site care; emptying, preparing, and applying the pouch; equipment care; proper irrigations; and dietary modifications. Provide emotional support. Discharge planning should include what supplies are necessary, where to obtain them, and where to obtain home help. Referral to a home health agency may be needed.

PSYCHOSOCIAL SUPPORT WITH AN OSTOMY The psychologic reaction to having an ostomy varies. An effect on body image and self-esteem is expected. Clients experience many fears—realistic and unrealistic. The nurse can support clients by helping them to express their feelings and anxieties. Many clients worry about the impact of an ostomy in social interactions. Some fear that the stoma will be obvious to others, and many fear it will interfere with sexual relations. If appropriate to the client's situation, the significant other should be included in discussions regarding resumption of normal activities, including sexual relations. There are times when ostomy surgery, or any surgery, may cause a person to feel less desirable sexually or may cause the partner to view the loved one in that way. Helping clients accept the alteration as a minor change in bodily appearance or function that has not decreased their worth as a person, and helping them feel good about themselves, will assist them most when working out their own relationships with loved ones.

Gastrostomy

A gastrostomy is an opening into the stomach. Generally, a tube is inserted into the opening, externalizing the gastrostomy for drainage or feedings. A gastrostomy for drainage is used with longstanding or progressive obstruction of the gastric outlet or intestine. This method is used, for example, as palliation when metastatic carcinoma causes bowel obstruction.

A gastrostomy can also be used for feeding in conditions where oral feeding is contraindicated for relatively long periods of time but the gastrointestinal tract is functioning. Examples are some head and neck carcinomas, esophageal rupture or massive resection, conditions with impaired swallowing such as advanced multiple sclerosis, or amyotrophic lateral sclerosis (ALS). Physiologic and psychosocial/lifestyle implications of gastrostomy on client and family are discussed in Table 38–10.

Nursing Implications

Nursing care includes site care to maintain skin integrity, prevent infection, and maintain tube patency. The

Table 38–10
Gastrostomy: Implications for the Client

Physiologic Implications	Psychosocial/Lifestyle Implications
See also Table 37–2.	External feeding tubes may affect the client's body image.
Skin irritation and breakdown possible around the gastrostomy tube from gastric secretions.	Inability to taste and chew food may be upsetting to the client.
Cramping, bloating, nausea, vomiting, and diarrhea are possible complications of tube feeding.	Situations where food and drink are served may be uncomfortable for the client as well as for others.

gastrostomy site should be observed daily for drainage and the area cleansed with the appropriate solution, usually hydrogen peroxide, povidone–iodine, or alcohol. A dressing should be placed over the site to prevent contamination. The tube should be securely taped to the skin to prevent stress on sutures or accidental tube dislodgement.

A surgically inserted gastrostomy tube has a psychosocial impact on the client. The presence of a tube, especially when exposed to others, affects the client's body image. The inability to eat in the normal oral way will greatly affect a client who places much value on oral consumption—tasting the food, chewing, swallowing. Altered eating methods may affect the social practices of mealtime, leaving the client feeling isolated. If long-term feedings are required, the client will have to learn how to administer them at home and how to obtain the necessary supplies. The client and family members will require time to adjust to the altered eating style. The nurse can help by suggesting strategies to keep the client integrated into the family group. When insurance does not cover these expenses, the client may feel guilt about the financial burden to the family.

Feeding Jejunostomy

A feeding jejunostomy is an adjunct to major abdominal surgical procedures of the esophagus, stomach, duodenum, pancreas, or biliary tract, or is used in the presence of an enterocutaneous fistula when feeding into the esophagus, stomach, or duodenum is undesirable. A feeding jejunostomy is established by inserting a feeding tube or catheter through an abdominal incision into the jejunum. The physiologic and psychosocial/lifestyle implications are similar to those for gastrostomy discussed in Table 38–10.

Nursing Implications

Nursing care includes flushing the catheter to keep it open; small-caliber catheters are especially vulnerable to clogging. The catheter should be well anchored to the abdominal wall to prevent its being dislodged; feeding into a dislodged catheter could deliver formula into the peritoneal cavity.

Site care is similar to that of any postoperative drainage tube. Cleanse the area daily (usually with hydrogen peroxide, povidone–iodine, or alcohol), inspect the tube site for infection, and cover it with a sterile dressing. An antimicrobial ointment may be applied to the site.

Feedings should be initiated at dilute strengths and low volumes to avoid problems such as discomfort or diarrhea, and should be administered with an enteral infusion pump to control the rate. Feedings administered continuously are best tolerated. The best formula for a feeding jejunostomy is partially predigested, low in viscosity (to avoid clogging the catheter), and isotonic.

Home jejunostomy feedings require education of both client and family, including a method for obtaining supplies. Because this may initially be disruptive to a client and family, the nurse has an important role in helping them to adapt.

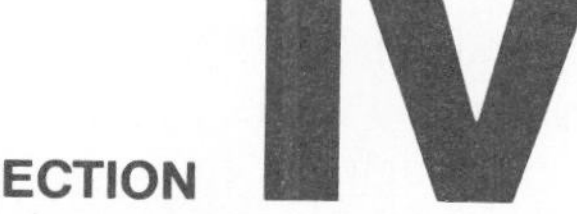

SECTION IV

Traumatic Disorders

Trauma to the Stomach, Intestines, and Pancreas

The stomach, intestines, and pancreas are often traumatized when abdominal injuries are sustained. Major or minor contusions, lacerations, and perforations are frequently encountered. Often, internal injury may be present without overt signs of trauma. These injuries may be fatal if left undiagnosed and untreated.

Trauma to these organs may be blunt or penetrating. Blunt trauma is frequently related to motor vehicle accidents, falls, and fights. Vehicular seatbelts may cause blunt abdominal trauma if worn incorrectly or if an accident is severe. Penetrating wounds are frequently caused by bullets, knives, or stones. Trauma from gunshot wounds is usually more extensive than wounds caused by other penetrating objects, because of the high velocity of the bullet.

Clinical Manifestations

Blunt abdominal trauma may or may not be associated with external injury. When external bruises, lacerations, and contusions are present, however, they frequently correlate with the site of internal involvement. Although external trauma is apparent with penetrating wounds, it may not accurately reflect the extent of internal injury. The angle of entry of a penetrating object may be helpful in localizing internal damage.

Abdominal distention, inhibition of respirations, and guarding may occur. Crepitation (subcutaneous emphysema) may be noted as crackling sounds as the fingertips palpate an area where extravasation of air has occurred (eg, from an injured colon or diaphragm). Bowel sounds may be diminished or absent if intestinal trauma or irritation has occurred. If an organ has ruptured, causing fluids to leak into the abdominal cavity, peritonitis will result.

Hemorrhage may accompany trauma. Injury to the stomach or intestine may cause bleeding into the GI tract, evidenced by hematemesis or, in severe bleeding, hematochezia. If a nasogastric tube is in place, drainage will contain blood. Frequently, blood from damaged organs seeps into the peritoneal cavity. Cullen's sign (ecchymosis at the umbilicus) and Turner's sign (ecchymosis at the flank) indicate retroperitoneal bleeding and internal injury.

To check for intra-abdominal injury, paracentesis or abdominal lavage may be performed. In lavage, the preferred procedure, a catheter is inserted into the peritoneal cavity through a short umbilical incision, and a small sample of fluid is aspirated and inspected for blood. The presence of blood confirms internal injury and indicates the need for surgery. If the sample of fluid shows no gross evidence of blood, irrigation fluid is instilled through the catheter and allowed to drain. Drainage is inspected for gross signs of blood and is also sent to the laboratory for analysis.

Perforation, peritonitis, and sepsis may follow intestinal trauma. Trauma to the rectum may also have occurred and should be evaluated. Complications of pancreatic trauma may include formation of abscesses or fistulae, enzyme insufficiency and malabsorption (with steatorrhea), and hyperglycemia related to abnormal insulin production or secretion.

Medical Measures

The client with suspected or apparent internal injury is immobilized and made comfortable. Any open wounds should be protected and cleansed. Protruding objects should be left in place. An IV is generally started immediately to provide a route of administration for fluids, blood, and medications. When internal injury is apparent, an exploratory laparotomy is performed to determine the extent of injury and to repair damaged organs.

Supportive care includes analgesics, fluid/electrolyte and/or blood replacement, and treatment for shock. Antibiotics are given to prevent or control infection, and tetanus prophylaxis is also administered. The client gradually resumes normal activity as tolerated.

Specific Nursing Measures

The client with trauma to the stomach, intestine, or pancreas may be cared for in the community, the hospital, or an emergency facility. In an emergency situation, the nurse may give care at the scene of the accident as a bystander. Wherever the trauma occurs, the nurse must be knowledgeable about care and possible consequences.

In caring for the client with abdominal trauma, the nurse must be alert to:

- Symptoms and signs that will localize the injury
- The extent and seriousness of the injury
- Early signs of complications

Obtain a history to determine the exact cause of the injury and the presence of any pre-existing disease. It is especially important to determine whether the wound is dirty (contaminated), since aggressive therapy is needed to prevent infection of a contaminated wound. A medication and immunization history should also be obtained. If the client is unable to provide the necessary information, another reliable source should be sought. An accurate description of the location and nature of pain is especially important.

Since abdominal trauma may be associated with trauma to other body areas, evaluate and monitor the function of all body systems. Once therapy is instituted, the nurse is responsible for ongoing assessment of the client's symptoms and the effects of therapy. Assess the client's psychologic status, since injured clients are often anxious and fearful.

Use sterile technique in caring for any open wounds. Blood and debris should be removed, but any protruding objects (eg, a knife) should be left in place initially, since removal could cause hemorrhage. During the process of wound healing, carefully evaluate the area for any signs of infection, with each dressing change. These should be reported promptly to the physician.

Pay particular attention to maintaining fluid/electrolyte balance and measuring intake and output frequently and precisely. If the client is permitted to eat, observe how food is tolerated. With intestinal trauma, bowel status must be monitored. Administer medications as ordered and explain the rationale for their use to the client.

In the course of nursing care, involve the client and family to the greatest extent possible. Trauma to the body, mild or severe, is accompanied by trauma to the spirit. Answer questions and provide information as necessary, encouraging expression of feelings.

Chapter Highlights

Disorders of the stomach, small and large intestines, and pancreas can significantly alter the nutritional status of a client through interference with the digestion and absorption of nutrients.

Clients with disorders of the stomach, intestines, and pancreas frequently have symptoms and signs of bleeding and/or obstruction, each requiring prompt and efficient medical and nursing care.

Complications of surgery on the gastrointestinal system include infection, sepsis, hemorrhage, wound separation, and paralytic ileus.

Respiratory effort may be impaired when gastrointestinal surgery close to the thoracic cavity affects abdominal muscles used in breathing and coughing or produces incisional pain on breathing or coughing.

Drainage via a nasogastric tube is frequently used with gastrointestinal surgery to decompress the stomach, intestine, or both.

Parenteral nutrition is often provided before and after gastrointestinal surgery to maintain nutritional status through the period of intestinal paralysis that follows gastrointestinal surgery.

When surgery results in drainage of gastrointestinal fluids, careful replacement of fluids and electrolytes is essential.

The change in elimination status and bowel regimen that may accompany intestinal disorders can have significant impact on the self-esteem, body image, and lifestyle of an affected client.

Preoperative evaluation for stoma placement is essential to assure a proper fit of a drainage appliance.

Psychosocial adjustment to an ostomy includes knowledge of the altered physiology, psychologic comfort in managing the ostomy, and a realistic understanding of the impact on lifestyle.

Some disorders of the stomach, intestines, and pancreas may be prevented through dietary discretion.

The nurse can play an important role in the prevention and early detection of disorders of the stomach, intestines, and pancreas through teaching about associated risk factors and symptoms to report such as bleeding, stool changes, and epigastric discomfort.

Pancreatic surgery can affect both exocrine and endocrine functions of the pancreas.

Early detection of cancers of the stomach, intestines, and pancreas is imperative, since survival rates increase with early treatment.

Bibliography

Alterescu V: The ostomy: What do you teach the patient? *AJN* 1985; 85:1250–1253.

Boehmer VW, Turk MF: Caring for the gastroplasty patient. *AORN J* 1981; 34:1036–1042.

Bordley DR et al: Early clinical signs identify low-risk patients with upper-GI hemorrhage. *JAMA* (June 14) 1985; 253(22):3282–3285.

Broadwell DC, Jackson BS: *Principles of Ostomy Care.* St. Louis: Mosby, 1982.

Deters GE: Managing complications after abdominal surgery. *RN* (March) 1987; 27–32.

Dusek JL: Nursing rules—fact or myth? Iced gastric lavage slows bleeding in gastric hemorrhage. *Crit Care Nurse* (July/Aug) 1984; 8.

Everett WG: Hemorrhoidectomy without tears—or not too many. *Nurs Times* 1982; 78:526.

Fazio VW: Regional enteritis (Crohn's disease): Indications for surgery and operative strategy. *Surg Clin North Am* 1983; 63:27–48.

Gilman CJ: Improving survival in patients with rectal cancer. *Am Fam Physician* (Jan) 1984; 29:165–169.

Given BA, Simmons SJ: *Gastroenterology in Clinical Nursing.* St. Louis: Mosby, 1984.

Gloeckner MR: Perceptions of sexual attractiveness following ostomy surgery. *Res Nurs Health* 1984; 7:87–92.

Goldberg SM, Gordon PH, Nivatvongs S: *Essentials of Anorectal Surgery.* Philadelphia: Lippincott, 1980.

Goligher JC: Alternatives to conventional ileostomy in the surgical treatment of ulcerative colitis. *J Enterostom Ther* 1983; 10:79–83.

Greenberger NJ: *Gastrointestinal Disorders.* Chicago: Yearbook Medical Publishers, 1981.

Greifzu S: Colorectal cancer: When a polyp is more than a polyp. *RN* (Sept) 1986; 23–30.

Groszek DM: Promoting wound healing in the obese patient. *AORN J* 1982; 35:1132–

Hui YH: *Human Nutrition and Diet Therapy.* Monterey, CA: Wadsworth, 1983.

Infectious diarrhea? What's the cause? *Patient Care* (May 15) 1983; 79–115.

Johnson S: A safer gastrostomy for the high risk patient. *RN* (March) 1986; 49:29–33.

Jones VA et al: Food intolerance: A major factor in the pathogenesis of irritable bowel syndrome. *Lancet* (Nov 20) 1982; 1115–1117.

Kobza L: Impact of ostomy upon the spouse. *J Enterostom Ther* 1983; 10:54–57.

Kodner IJ, Fry RD: Inflammatory bowel disease. *Clin Symp* 1982; 34(1):3–32.

Kosel K et al: Total pancreatectomy and islet cell autotransplantation. *Am J Nurs* 1982; 82:568–571.

Lamphier TA: Small-bowel obstruction: Think of it early. *Consultant* (Jan) 1981; 165–172.

Lamphier TA, Lamphier RA: Upper GI hemorrhage: Emergency evaluation and management. *Am J Nurs* 1981; 81:1814–1816.

Legerton CW: Current thinking on irritable bowel syndrome. *Consultant* (June) 1981; 25–29.

Lewicki LJ, Lesson MJ: The multisystem impact on physiologic processes of inflammatory bowel disease. *Nurs Clin North Am* 1984; 19(1):71–80.

Maingot R: *Abdominal Operations.* Vols 1 and 2. New York: Appleton–Century–Crofts, 1980.

Miller BK: Jejunoileal bypass: A drastic weight control measure. *Am J Nurs* 1981; 81:564–568.

Mojzisik CM, Martin EW: Gastric partitioning: The latest surgical means to control morbid obesity. *Am J Nurs* 1981; 81:569–572.

Myer SA: Overview of inflammatory bowel disease. *Nurs Clin North Am* 1984; 19(1):3–9.

Nostrant TT, Wilson JAP: How good is screening for colorectal cancer? *Postgrad Med* (June) 1983; 73:131–139.

Parks AG, Nicholls RJ, Belliveau P: Proctocolectomy with ileal reservoir and anal anastomosis. *Br J Surg* 1980; 67:533–538.

Patient education aid: Care of the perianal area. *Patient Care* (March 15) 1986; 178.

Patient education aid: Caring for your ulcer. *Patient Care* (April 30) 1986; 125.

Patras AZ: The operation's over, but the danger's not. *Nurs 82* 1982; 12:50–56.

Patras AZ, Paice JA, Lanigan K: Managing GI bleeding: It takes a two-track mind. *Nurs 84* (July) 1984; 14:26–33.

Patterson RS, Andrassy RJ: Needle-catheter jejunostomy. *Am J Nurs* 1983; 83:1325–1326.

Permutt RP, Cello JP: Duodenal ulcer disease in the hospitalized elderly patient. *Dig Dis Sci* (Jan) 1982; 27:1–6.

Penninger JI, Moore SB, Frager SR: After the ostomy: Helping the patient reclaim his sexuality. *RN* (April) 1985; 48:46–50.

Petersdorf RG et al: *Harrison's Principles of Internal Medicine.* New York: McGraw-Hill, 1983.

Petlin AM, Carolan JM: Getting your patient through a lower GI bleed. *RN* (Feb) 1982; 42–45.

Rucker RD Jr et al: Searching for the best weight reduction operation. *Surgery* 1984; 96:624–631.

Rydning A et al: Prophylactic effect of dietary fiber in duodenal ulcer disease. *Lancet* (Oct 2) 1982; 736–738.

Schaefer KM: Easing the torment of an irritable bowel. *RN* (April) 1986; 34–38.

Schumann D: Wound healing in your abdominal surgery patient. *Nurs 80* 1980; 10:34–40.

Scott HW: Metabolic consequences of jejunoileal bypass for morbid obesity. In: *Advances in Gastrointestinal Surgery.* Najarian JS, Delaney JP (editors). Chicago: Year Book Medical Publishers, 1984.

Segal HL: Clues to cancer of the digestive system. *Consultant* (Dec) 1981; 101–103.

Simmons MA: Using the nursing process in treating inflammatory bowel disease. *Nurs Clin North Am* 1984; 19(1):11–25.

Simplifying diagnosis of malabsorption. *Patient Care* (Oct 15) 1981; 128–178.

Sleisinger MH, Fordtran JS: *Gastrointestinal Disease.* Philadelphia: Saunders, 1983.

Smith CW Jr: The irritable bowel syndrome. *Female Patient* 1985; 10:81–90.

Smith DB: The ostomy: How is it managed? *AJN* 1985; 85:1246–1249.

Soballe PW: Peritoneal lavage in blunt abdominal trauma. *Am Fam Physician* (March) 1984; 29:193–198.

Stotts NA, Fitzgerald KA, Williams KR: Care of the patient critically ill with inflammatory bowel disease. *Nurs Clin North Am* 1984; 19(1):61–70.

Stout K: The surgical treatment of morbid obesity. *Nurs Clin North Am* 1982; 17:245–250.

Suitor CW, Hunter MF: *Nutrition: Principles and Application in Health Promotion.* Philadelphia: Lippincott, 1980.

Supporting the patient with Crohn's disease: Nursing grand rounds. *Nurs 83* (Nov) 1983; 13:46–51.

Swearingen PA: *Addison–Wesley Photo Atlas of Nursing Procedures.* Menlo Park, CA: Addison–Wesley, 1984.

Thomson NA: Convert your assessment into a lifesaving care plan for the patient with abdominal trauma. *Nurs 83* (July) 1983; 13:26–33.

Utsunomiya J et al: Total colectomy, mucosal proctectomy and ileal anal anastomosis. *Am Society of Colon and Rectal Surg* 1980; 23:459–466.

Watt R: The ostomy: Why it is created. *AJN* 1985; 85:1242–1245.

Weakley FL: Cancers of the rectum. *Surg Clin North Am* 1983; 63:129–135.

Zettel ER: Beaming in on the GI tract. *AJN* 1986; 86:280–282.

1987 Cancer Facts and Figures. New York: American Cancer Society, 1987.

CASE STUDY

The Client With Bowel Obstruction and Possible Malignancy

I. Brief Description Data

Mr John Jones, a 50-year-old engineer, has been admitted to the surgical unit from the emergency room. He has had persistent symptoms of anorexia, nausea, vomiting, and tenderness in the abdomen for the last 24 hours. His wife accompanies him.

II. Personal Data

Data and Time: Jan 26, 1988
Full Name: John Henry Jones
Social Security Number: 000-00-0000
Address: 42 Scott St, Martysville, Maine
Telephone: Home: 000-0000
Business: 000-0000
Sex: Male
Age: 50
Birthdate: 8-18-37
Marital Status: Married
Race: Black
Religion: Catholic
Occupation: Electrical engineer
Usual Health Care Provider: Katharine Keith, MD

III. Health History

Source of Information: Client and wife
Reliability of Informant: Reliable
Chief Concern: "I started to vomit yesterday, and my stomach feels full and sore."

History of Present Illness:

Twenty-four hours prior to admission, Mr Jones noted the onset of anorexia and nausea. Soon after, he began vomiting dark green liquid and undigested food. He limited his intake to toast and tea but continued to vomit. He has been unable to sleep, although he feels exhausted from all the discomfort and vomiting. At the urging of his wife, he came to the emergency room for examination.

In January 1983, he had a colon resection for a small benign tumor of the descending colon. He has experienced no problems with his bowels since the surgery until now. He has not had a BM or passed gas in 3 days. Prior to this, stools have been well formed, brown, and were passed easily without straining. He has noted no black tarry stools nor blood in the stool. Annual checkups since the surgery have all been normal.

He eats a well-balanced diet, including fruits, vegetables, and bran cereal. Since his surgery, he has avoided fatty foods, quit smoking, and maintained a regular exercise program. He takes no medications. Family history is positive for malignancy of breast, prostate, colon. Brother with benign colon polyp.

Past Health History:

Childhood: Usual childhood diseases
Immunizations: Last Td 1978
Medical Problems: None
Surgeries: Colon resection 1/83, benign tumor descending colon

CASE STUDY (continued)

The Client With Bowel Obstruction and Possible Malignancy

Transfusions: None
Special Diagnostic Procedures: Sigmoidoscopy, Ba enema 12/82
Trauma: None
Allergies: Sulfa (rash)
Medications: None

Family History:

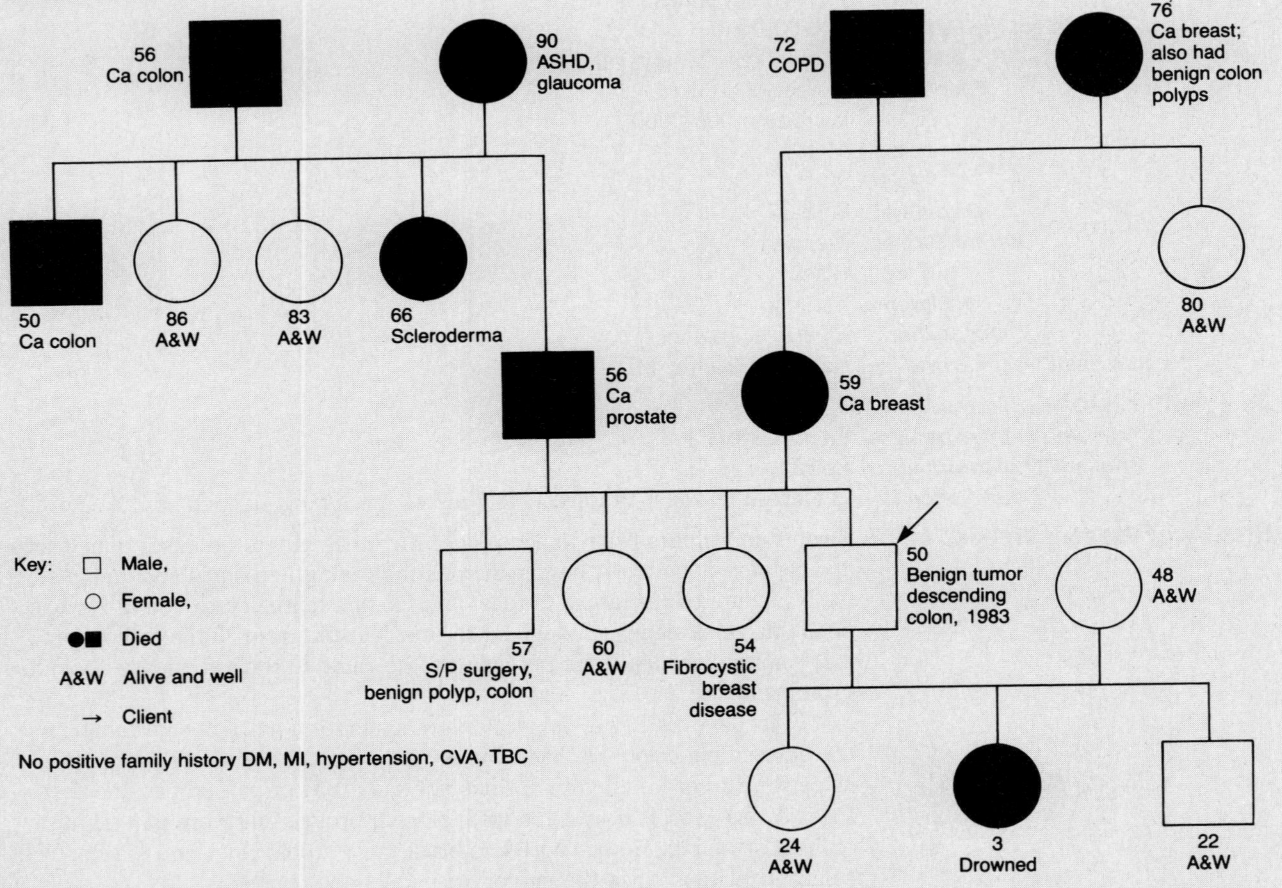

56
Ca colon

90
ASHD,
glaucoma

72
COPD

76
Ca breast;
also had
benign colon
polyps

50
Ca colon

86
A&W

83
A&W

66
Scleroderma

80
A&W

56
Ca
prostate

59
Ca breast

57
S/P surgery,
benign polyp, colon

60
A&W

54
Fibrocystic
breast
disease

50
Benign tumor
descending
colon, 1983

48
A&W

24
A&W

3
Drowned

22
A&W

Key: □ Male,
○ Female,
●■ Died
A&W Alive and well
→ Client

No positive family history DM, MI, hypertension, CVA, TBC

Personal/Social History: Has worked as electrical engineer for past 25 years. Lives with wife in home they own. Daughter and son both in graduate school out of town, return home for holidays. He maintains a good relationship with them. Leaves for work at 7:45 AM and returns home at 5:30 PM. Recreation includes health club activities 2 evenings per week and playing cards 1 evening per week. Eats three meals per day (states they are well balanced with fresh fruit and vegetables). Sleeps well (7 to 8 hours per night), except for recent problem. Financially stable with adequate medical coverage. States he is generally relaxed and not a highly anxious person, although now he is worried about the possiblity that cancer is causing his problem.

Review of Systems: States overall health is excellent, energy level good, weight stable.

Chest: No cough; no SOB; no history of pneumonia, TBC, or chest trauma

Heart: No chest pain, no palpitations, no DOE, no PND; ECGs always wnl; no history of murmur, dysrhythmia

Gastrointestinal: See HPI.

Genitourinary: No nocturia, dysuria, hematuria, polyuria, hesitancy, urgency, frequency, or problems with urinary stream; no history of UTI, renal calculi; able to maintain erection; no pain with intercourse or problem with ejaculation

IV. Physical Assessment

Height: 5 ft 9 in

Weight: 180 lb

Vital Signs: BP 120/80; apical P 86; R 20; rectal temperature, 100°F (38°C)

Relevant Organ Systems:

Skin: Brown; poor skin turgor

Eyes: Sclerae without jaundice

Mouth: Dry, cracked lips; oral mucous membranes and tongue dry

Neck: Without nodes

Chest: Expansion = bilaterally; resonant to percussion, clear to auscultation

Heart: Apical rate, 86, regular; S_1, S_2 nl; ō Ⓜ

Abdomen: Distended; midline vertical scar extends from 2 in below xyphoid to suprapubic region; ō bruits; bowel sounds hyperactive with peristaltic rushes; slightly tender all quadrants; no masses palpable; ↑ tympany all quadrants

Rectal: No external lesions or masses; sphincter tone good; prostate nl; no masses or areas of tenderness; small amount hard dark brown stool in rectum; stool heme ⊖

Urine: Dark amber, concentrated; SG 1.033.

V. Medical Regimen

An N/G tube was passed and 300 mL of dark green gastric contents were drained immediately; IV fluids were started. A preliminary diagnosis of intestinal obstruction was made, and Mr Jones is tentatively scheduled for an exploratory laparotomy tomorrow. The following orders were written:

- NPO
- Bed rest
- IV 5% dextrose in 0.45 normal saline at 150 mL/hr
- NG to low Gomco suction, irrigate p.r.n.
- Intake and output
- Monitor specific gravity of urine q.8h.
- Prochlorperazine (Compazine), 10 mg q.6h. p.r.n. for nausea
- Ampicillin, 500 mg q.6h. IV
- Morphine sulphate 2–4 mg IV q.10 min. Not to exceed 10 mg in 2 hr.

VI. Nursing Care Plan, by Nursing Diagnosis

Client Care Goals	Plan/Nursing Implementation	Expected Outcomes
Fluid volume deficit: actual related to excessive losses		
Maintain normal fluid balance	Administer IVs as ordered; monitor for symptoms and signs of normal hydration and dehydration (thirst, check skin turgor, check mouth and lips for dryness); monitor urine SG; strict intake and output; determine if balanced and report inconsistencies	Client's hydration status should show improvement as therapy is instituted; skin turgor should be normal; mouth should be moist; urine SG should be normal; and I&O should be balanced

CASE STUDY (continued)

The Client With Bowel Obstruction and Possible Malignancy

VI. Nursing Care Plan, by Nursing Diagnosis (continued)

Client Care Goals	Plan/Nursing Implementation	Expected Outcomes
Maintain electrolyte balance	Alleviate nausea and vomiting through use of nasogastric tube; maintain patency with irrigation p.r.n.; give prochlorperazine as needed; provide fluid and electrolyte replacement as ordered; observe for symptoms and signs of electrolyte imbalance; monitor laboratory values; report problems to MD promptly; monitor client's weight daily	Electrolyte status remains normal; no further weight loss
Tissue integrity, impaired: oral mucous membranes related to dehydration		
Reduce or eliminate dryness of mouth and lips	Allow client to suck on gauze pad moistened with water or use ice chips, as permitted; provide materials for frequent mouth rinse; lubricate lips with sterile jelly or use Chapstick; continue mouth care with attention to flossing and brushing of teeth; instruct client and wife in mouth care	Condition of client's mouth will improve; lips and mouth will be moist and not cracked and dry; wife will demonstrate involvement in husband's care
Self-care deficit: toileting related to weakness and bed rest		
Promote hygiene	Assist client p.r.n. with use of bedpan, urinal; keep within easy reach; provide materials and water for hygiene; assist p.r.n.; should client and wife desire, teach wife management of urinal and bedpan and where to save urine for I&O	Client with be clean, with all needs for hygiene and elimination met; urine will be measured and discarded promptly
Bowel elimination, altered: constipation related to probable obstruction		
Maintain bowel elimination status	Monitor bowel elimination status frequently; check frequently for bowel sounds, change in abdominal distention, passage of stool or flatus; report any improvement or deterioration of bowel status promptly	Client's elimination status improves (passes stool or flatus, bowel sounds normal) or remains status quo
Fear; related to uncertainty of diagnosis		
Express fears of malignancy, colostomy because of strong positive family history of cancer	Encourage client to verbalize fears and feelings; keep client and wife informed about his status; encourage family to ask questions and verbalize their feelings as well; encourage family to visit and participate in care; if any possibility of colostomy exists, urge the surgeon to discuss this fully with client and spouse; remain with client after this discussion to clarify any questions	Client appears calmer; expresses his fears more readily; does not manifest signs of severe anxiety
Comfort, altered: pain related to mechanical obstruction		
Reduce or eliminate discomfort	Assess pain level; administer pain medication as ordered; provide comfort measures	Client reports decrease in or elimination of discomfort

UNIT 9

The Client With Hepatic–Biliary Dysfunction

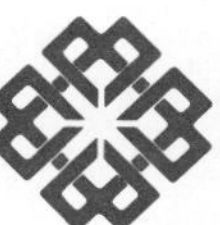

CHAPTER 39

The Hepatic–Biliary System in Health and Illness

Other topics relevant to this content are: Care of clients who abuse alcohol, **Chapter 8;** Hepatotoxic substances, **Chapter 40;** Care of the client with cholelithiasis, **Chapter 41.**

Objectives

When you have finished studying this chapter, you should be able to:

Identify the major structural and functional components of the hepatic–biliary system.

Explain the physiologic mechanisms that regulate the activity of the hepatic–biliary system.

Describe some pathologic conditions that lead to hepatic–biliary dysfunction.

Discuss alterations in other body systems that result from hepatic–biliary dysfunction.

Identify and discuss the psychosocial/lifestyle effects of hepatic–biliary dysfunction on the client and significant others.

The liver and gallbladder perform several regulatory functions essential to maintenance of homeostasis. The liver synthesizes substances, including coagulation factors, that are vital to life. The gallbladder plays an important role in the digestive process, in particular, the digestion of fats. Although the human body can survive loss of the gallbladder—for example, by surgical removal—survival without a liver is not possible.

SECTION I

Structural and Functional Interrelationships

The hepatic and biliary systems are both structurally and functionally interrelated. The liver, the largest of the internal organs, performs the following functions:

- Storage and filtration of the blood—a vascular function
- Production of bile—a regulatory function
- Removal of bilirubin from the body—an excretory function
- Metabolism of carbohydrates, fats, and proteins—a metabolic function
- Storage of vitamins A, D, B_{12}, and iron
- Synthesis of coagulation factors
- Detoxification of chemicals

The Liver and Gallbladder

The normal liver of an adult weighs about 1500 g. The wedge-shaped organ lies in the right upper quadrant of the abdominal cavity, where it is protected by the rib cage. The superior surface underlies the diaphragm. The posterior and inferior surfaces together are generally referred to as the *visceral surface.* The right visceral surface is in contact with portions of the colon, the kidneys, the adrenal glands, and the duodenum; the left visceral surface is bordered by the stomach and spleen.

The liver is divided into 50,000 to 100,000 liver lobules. These tiny structures, a few millimeters in length and 1 to 2 mm in diameter, are the functional units of the liver. Each liver lobule is composed of platelike "spokes" of hepatic cells that radiate from a "hub" or central vein that passes through the connective tissue between lobules. The central veins are branches of the portal vein that, together with the portal artery, furnish the blood supply of the liver. Bile is manufactured in the hepatic plates. Tiny bile canaliculi, or bile channels, lying between the hepatic plates carry the bile to bile ducts. Like tributaries forming ever larger streams, the bile ducts merge to form larger ducts. Eventually, they form two hepatic ducts, one from the right lobe and one from the left. These in turn join to form a single hepatic duct that merges with the cystic duct to form the common bile duct. Bile manufactured by the liver, together with bile stored and later secreted by the gallbladder, leaves the hepatic–biliary system via the common bile duct.

The septa between lobules contain venules and arterioles, both of which drain into the hepatic sinusoids, where venous and arterial blood mingle. This mingling is related to the detoxifying and metabolic functions of the hepatic system. Plasma, including proteins, can diffuse out of the blood. For example, nutritive or toxic substances carried from the intestine in the blood diffuse through the epithelial lining of the sinusoids into the hepatic cells, where they are metabolized, stored, or altered. The sinusoids are also lined by Kupffer cells, phagocytic cells that remove bacteria and other foreign substances from blood that passes through the liver (Spence & Mason, 1987).

The liver is richly supplied with both arterial and venous blood. Each minute approximately 1100 mL arrives from the hepatic portal vein and 400 mL from the hepatic artery to mix in the sinusoids before returning to the heart via the inferior vena cava. Portal venous blood coming from the intestines has a low concentration of oxygen but a high concentration of substances absorbed by the intestine during digestion. Blood coming from the hepatic artery is high in oxygen but low in nutrients. The pressure of blood in the portal and hepatic veins is low, allowing easy diffusion of nutrients and other substances along the concentration gradient. Oxygen-rich blood from the hepatic artery maintains the integrity of the liver; if perfusion is absent or diminished, necrosis of hepatic cells will occur (Spence & Mason, 1987).

The gallbladder is a pear-shaped, hollow, saclike organ about 7 to 10 cm long that lies in a fossa on the inferior surface of the liver. The *cystic duct,* which drains the gallbladder, joins with the hepatic duct of the liver to form the *common bile duct* (Figure 39–1). Pancreatic secretions also enter this duct via the pancreatic duct. Bile in the common bile duct enters the duodenum through the sphincter of Oddi. When this sphincter is relaxed, bile can enter the duodenum; when the sphincter is contracted, bile manufactured by the liver is stored in the gallbladder. The function of bile is discussed in the following section.

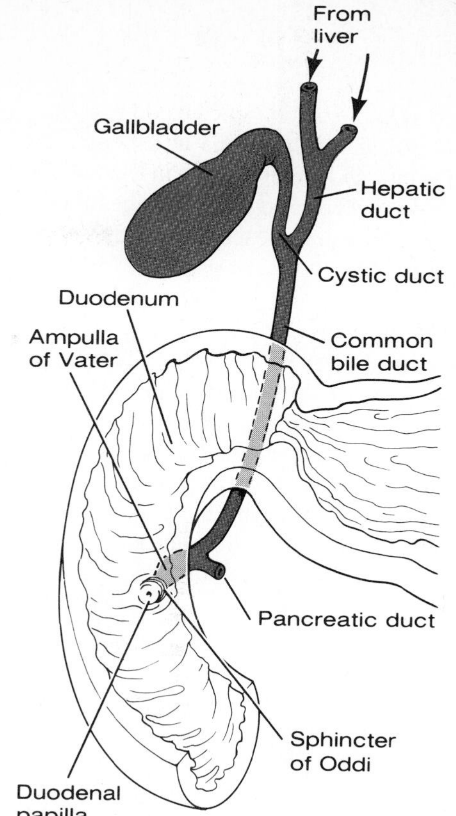

Figure 39–1

The gallbladder and bile ducts. SOURCE: *Spence AP, Mason EB:* Human Anatomy and Physiology, *3rd ed. Menlo Park, CA: Benjamin/Cummings, 1987.*

Regulatory Functions of the Hepatic–Biliary System

Vascular Functions

The liver is capable of storing a considerable quantity of blood, the amount depending on the pressure relationships in the arteries and veins. If pressure in the hepatic veins increases by a few millimeters of mercury, for example in the presence of congestive heart failure, cirrhosis, or hepatic congestion, as much as 300 to 400 mL may be stored. If hemorrhage occurs anywhere in the body, the liver releases this stored blood into the circulatory system to maintain circulatory volume (Guyton, 1986).

The phagocytic Kupffer cells lining the sinusoids normally remove 99%–100% of bacteria from blood entering the liver. Kupffer cells multiplv in response to increased levels of foreign particles in the blood. Since blood entering the liver through the portal vein contains intestinal bacteria, the Kupffer cells play an important role in the body's defense against infection. Any condition that damages these cells or inhibits their replication increases the body's susceptibility to infection.

Secretory Functions

The hepatic cells of each liver lobule continually secrete small amounts of bile, a thick, greenish yellow, slightly alkaline fluid. When first secreted from the liver through the canaliculi, bile is composed of water, bile salts, bilirubin, cholesterol, fatty acids, and lecithin as well as sodium, potassium, calcium, chloride, and bicarbonate ions.

Bile is concentrated in the gallbladder, which contracts during digestion to squirt it into the duodenum, where it functions as a kind of "biologic detergent" to emulsify fat particles (Crowley, 1983). The bile salts decrease the surface tension of fat particles so the agitation of the intestinal tract can break them into small globules easily acted on by digestive enzymes. Lecithin acts similarly. Fat is digested much more slowly if bile is not present.

Bile salts also improve absorption of lipids. The salts combine with fatty acids and monoglycerides to form small complexes called micelles. The ion charges provided by the bile salts enhance diffusion of the micelles across the intestinal mucosa into the bloodstream.

If absorption of fats is diminished because of absence of bile, vitamins A, D, E, and K, which are fat-soluble, cannot be absorbed.

Bile salts are "recycled" from 15 to 20 times in a process known as enterohepatic circulation (Guyton, 1986). From 90%–95% of bile salts secreted are reabsorbed in the distal ileum and carried in the portal vein back to the hepatic cells, which reabsorb and then resecrete them.

Excretory Functions

Bilirubin (bile pigment), a major waste product of hemoglobin metabolism, is excreted by the liver. Normally, erythrocytes have a life span of about 120 days. They are then broken down by the reticuloendothelial cells, and the iron (heme) from the worn-out red cells is conserved for reuse in the synthesis of fresh hemoglobin. The remaining iron-free pigment is free (unconjugated) bilirubin, which is continually present in the bloodstream in small quantities. As blood passes through the liver, unconjugated bilirubin is removed. It is then combined (conjugated) with other substances and excreted via the bile ducts. (A small amount of conjugated bilirubin returns to the blood.)

Conjugated bilirubin is more soluble and less toxic than unconjugated bilirubin. In the intestines, conjugated bilirubin is converted into a highly soluble substance called *urobilinogen,* which is excreted primarily in the feces in an oxidized form known an *stercobilin.* Some 5% of urobilinogen is absorbed into the bloodstream and excreted via the kidneys in an oxidized form called *urobilin.* Since stercobilin gives feces their brownish color, acholic (clay-colored) stools are a classic sign of biliary tract abnormalities.

Metabolic Functions

CARBOHYDRATE METABOLISM The liver plays a major role in carbohydrate metabolism. One aspect of this role is a glucose buffer function that contributes to maintenance of normal blood sugar levels. The liver can remove excess glucose from the blood, store it as glycogen, and reconvert and release it as glucose in response to hypoglycemia. If blood glucose concentrations fall and glycogen is not available, the liver can convert proteins or amino acids to glucose—a process known as glyconeogenesis. The liver is also capable of converting galactose to glucose.

FAT (LIPID) METABOLISM Synthesis of fat from carbohydrates and proteins occurs primarily in the liver. The lipoprotein produced in this process is transported in the bloodstream to the body's adipose tissue for storage. The liver is also capable of rapid metabolism of ingested fat in response to energy requirements. The liver can also synthesize lipoproteins, cholesterol, and other phospholipids.

PROTEIN METABOLISM Before amino acids can be converted into carbohydrates or fat or used to supply caloric needs, a process known as *deamination* (liberation of ammonia) must occur. The liver is the principal site of deamination and the only site where ammonia is detoxified by conversion into urea. In addition, nearly all the plasma proteins are synthesized in the liver, as are several nonessential amino acids.

Storage Functions

VITAMIN STORAGE The liver is capable of storing up to a four-months' supply of vitamins B_{12} and D and up to a ten-year supply of vitamin A for release as needed. Because of this storage capacity, excessive ingestion of vitamins A or D can have toxic effects on liver function.

IRON STORAGE Except for the iron stored in hemoglobin, most of the body's iron is stored in the liver as *ferritin.* Stored iron is released when blood levels of iron fall, a process known as *iron buffering.*

Synthesis of Coagulation Factors

Prothrombin and factors VII, IX, and X, necessary for effective blood coagulation, are synthesized in the liver. Vitamin K is necessary to promote synthesis of these clotting factors, but if bile secretion is inadequate, absorption of this fat-soluble vitamin cannot occur. The liver also synthesizes fibrinogen, another clotting factor.

Detoxification

Many chemicals are detoxified in the liver, including such medications as barbiturates, antidiuretic hormone (ADH), amphetamines, aldosterone, and estrogen. If these substances were not detoxified, they could be fatally toxic to body tissues or organs or could have other adverse effects such as, for example, feminization of males or masculinization of females.

Concentration and Storage of Bile

The hepatic cells can produce from 600 mL to 1000 mL of bile in 24 hours—over ten times the 50 mL to 75 mL storage capacity of the gallbladder. The mucosa of the gallbladder concentrates bile by absorbing water and electrolytes. This leaves a solution of bile salts, cholesterol, lecithin, and bilirubin that is five to ten times as concentrated as bile secreted by the liver.

Bile Secretion

When ingested fat enters the small intestine, a hormone called cholecystokinin is released from the intestinal mucosa. The cholecystokinin travels to the gallbladder via the bloodstream, initiating contraction of the smooth muscle in the wall of the gallbladder and relaxation of the sphincter of Oddi. Vagal stimulation also contributes to contraction of the gallbladder. While the hormone secretin, produced by the jejunal and duodenal mucosa, weakly stimulates bile secretion by the liver, peristalsis stimulated by food further relaxes the sphincter of Oddi. These factors combine to produce squirting of bile into the duodenum with each gallbladder contraction and peristaltic wave. The gallbladder empties poorly in the absence of ingested fat but empties completely within an hour if fat is present. Approximately 94% of the bile salts released into the duodenum are reabsorbed and returned to the liver via the bloodstream.

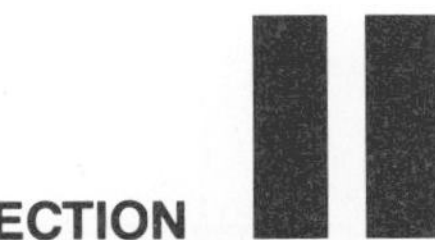

SECTION II

Pathophysiologic Influences and Effects

Liver Enlargement

Under normal circumstances, the liver is capable of regeneration once an acute condition (eg, drug toxicity, abscess, or inflammation) has been alleviated. If the pathogenic influence persists, however, regeneration will be of fibrotic origin.

When dead or diseased cells are replaced by fibrous tissue, the liver becomes enlarged **(hepatomegaly).** Fibrotic scar tissue may impede emptying of blood from the hepatic veins, causing the liver lobules to become engorged. This engorgement leads to further enlargement. Pressure exerted on abdominal nerves by the enlarged liver or displacement of other abdominal organs may cause discomfort or pain. Hepatomegaly may also be related to invasion and multiplication of neoplastic cells.

Liver Atrophy

Although the liver may be enlarged during the early stages of hepatic pathology, it eventually atrophies if the pathogenic influence is not removed. In the alcoholic client, for example, continued ingestion of alcohol combined with malnutrition cause scar tissue to replace the dead cells. In time, the scar tissue shrinks, and the liver becomes smaller than normal. Adjacent organs tend to encroach on the space formerly occupied by the liver. (For this reason, a liver from a donor smaller than the recipient is best for transplant purposes.)

Portal Hypertension

As hepatic tissue becomes increasingly fibrotic, the portal venules become compressed. This compression increases back-pressure as portal venous blood volume rises. Portal hypertension results, with pressures in the portal vein as high as 20 mm Hg. This contributes to the development of **ascites,** the accumulation of protein-rich serum in the peritoneal cavity.

Collateral pathways develop between the portal and systemic circulation in areas where tributaries of portal and systemic veins are in close approximation. The most common collateral pathways are shown in Figure 39–2. As portal pressure increases, all collateral pathways between the portal and systemic circulation enlarge.

Collateral vessels in the lower esophagus dilate because they are not anatomically structured to carry the extra blood shunted via the azygos system. These dilated veins, called esophageal varices, may rupture causing massive hemorrhage. Hemorrhoids (rectal varices) can result from the increased pressure in hemorrhoidal veins. Splenomegaly can develop secondary to engorgement of the splenic veins.

When esophageal varices hemorrhage, treatment is complicated by abnormalities in blood coagulation related to impaired hepatic function. As bile production becomes impaired, absorption of vitamin K is also impaired. Insufficiency or lack of vitamin K leads to decreased production of prothrombin and coagulation factors VII, IX, and X. Insufficiency of clotting factors, in turn, is related to increased clotting times. This pathogenic sequence may be signaled by ecchymoses all over the body, bleeding of the gums, or blood in the stool.

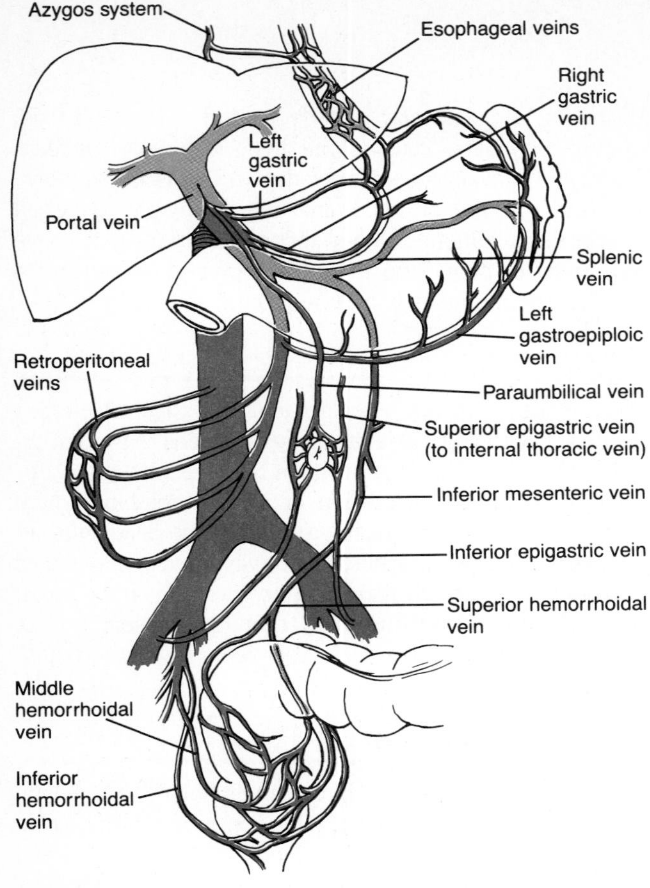

Figure 39–2

Common collateral pathways in portal hypertension.

Impaired Gas Exchange

Although the vascular dehydration seen in hepatic failure may mask erythrocytopenia, red blood cell deficiency does occur in relation to several factors. For instance, the impaired liver cannot store sufficient vitamin B_{12} and iron for erythrocyte synthesis. In alcohol-related pathologic states, ingestion of large quantities of alcohol inhibits renal synthesis of erythropoietin; the blood contains a higher proportion of immature erythrocytes and fewer mature red cells. This deficit may be manifested as dyspnea, increased cardiac output, cardiomegaly, and clubbing of the fingers (Schearman and Finlayson, 1982).

Box 39–1
Principal Causes of Jaundice

- Impaired bilirubin conjugation
- Obstruction of the common bile duct (choledocolithiasis, neoplasia)
- Cholecystitis
- Spasms of the sphincter of Oddi
- Overproduction of bilirubin related to hemolysis
- In newborns, deficiency of glucuronyl transferase
- Inherited disorders

Increased Susceptibility to Infection

Injury to the liver is accompanied by damage to or destruction of the Kupffer cells. Phagocytosis is impaired. Microorganisms enter the general circulation and may form abscesses in the liver tissue itself. Whereas the normal liver accounts for 25% of the body's production of lymphocytes, the diseased liver is incapable of lymphocyte production. Lymphocytopenia increases the body's susceptibility to infection.

Impaired Bilirubin Excretion

In a compromised liver, absorption and conjugation of bilirubin are impaired. Increased levels of unconjugated bilirubin in the blood and body fluids lead to jaundice, or icterus. The skin becomes yellowish and pruritic, renal excretion of unconjugated bilirubin causes the urine to become mahogany colored, and the stools are clay colored (acholic) due to the absence of stercobilin.

Jaundice is not always related to impairment of bilirubin conjugation. If the common bile duct is obstructed by gallstones **(choledocolithiasis)** or a neoplasm, bilirubin that has been conjugated by the liver cannot be excreted into the duodenum. Levels of bilirubin rise, and the symptoms of jaundice occur. Icterus may also be related to **cholecystitis** (inflammation of the gallbladder) or to spasms of the sphincter of Oddi, often associated with cholelithiasis. These conditions are discussed in Chapter 41.

Overproduction of bilirubin related to hemolytic states is another cause of jaundice. Reaction to a blood transfusion can induce a hemolytic state. Some hereditary disorders are also associated with jaundice. Principal causes of jaundice are summarized in Box 39–1.

Ammonia Toxicity

As the functional capacity of the liver diminishes, the ability to convert ammonia to urea for excretion by the kidney is impaired. Moreover, the collateral circulation caused by portal hypertension allows ammonia formed in the intestines to bypass the liver and enter the general circulation. The combined effect of these phenomena is ammonia toxicity. This toxicity manifests itself in hepatic encephalopathy, an altered mental state that begins with confusion and progresses to combative states and ultimately to hepatic coma. Another characteristic symptom of ammonia toxicity is **asterixis** ("liver flap"), a flapping tremor of the hand.

Altered Nutrition

Injury to hepatic cells compromises bile production and interferes with other hepatic functions such as synthesis of glycogen. The decrease in appetite that often occurs in liver disease is followed by weight loss, subnormal body temperature, fatigue, and the metabolism of body fat and muscle to meet caloric requirements. Impairment of bile secretion leads to fat intolerance and decreased fat absorption. The use of muscle mass as an energy source combined with decreased capacity for urea formation lead to a negative nitrogen balance. The limbs become emaciated while the abdomen swells with ascites. Skin breakdown is common. Inability to metabolize the amino acid methionine adequately produces **fetor hepaticus,** a sweet breath odor resembling acetone or old wine.

Deficiencies of folic acid and the B complex vitamins often occur in clients with alcoholic liver disease. Alcohol increases the demand for B vitamins, impairs absorption of folate and the B vitamins, and generally contributes to an inadequate consumption of all nutrients. Folic acid deficiency is manifested by a macrocytic anemia, glossitis, and diarrhea. Lesions of the oral mucosa and tongue, fissures at the corners of the mouth (**cheilosis**), and peripheral neuropathies result from lack of B complex vitamins.

Diminished fat absorption leads to deficiencies of the fat-soluble vitamins A, D, E, and K. Night blindness is associated with deficiency of vitamin A. Osteoporosis may occur in relation to vitamin D deficiency, putting the client at risk for fractures. Vitamin E deficiency can cause impaired red blood cell survival in adults. Coagulation disorders associated with vitamin K deficiency have already been discussed.

Altered Fluid Volume

Among the substances synthesized by the normal liver is the plasma protein albumin, which is necessary for maintaining the colloidal osmotic pressure of the plasma. If plasma albumin is insufficient or absent the normal colloidal osmotic pressure of the blood is not maintained. Plasma seeps into the interstitial spaces, causing peripheral and dependent edema. Pulmonary edema may lead to right-sided congestive heart failure. Ascites may be related to hypoalbuminemia and failure of the liver to detoxify aldosterone, as well as to portal hypertension. Accumulations exceeding 2 L can lead to difficulty breathing from pressure on the diaphragm, decreased appetite, feeling of fullness, constipation, flatulence, and umbilical hernia. The weight and bulk of the fluid may also restrict activity.

Impaired Detoxification

The diminished detoxification capacity of the compromised liver may compound the problems related to hypoalbuminemia. Increased levels of circulating aldosterone and ADH increase retention of sodium and water, respectively, further complicating the client's edema. Intravascular dehydration—lack of plasma in the blood vessels—related to the hypoalbuminuria may mask erythrocytopenia, because the dilution state of the blood has been altered.

Alteration in detoxification may also induce other problems related to excessive levels of hormones, chemicals, or drugs. Changes associated with an excess of estrogen may occur: loss of axillary, pubic, and body hair; soft skin; and gynecomastia and testicular atrophy in males. Decreased libido, impotence, spider angiomas, and palmar erythema are also associated with increased estrogen levels. Alcohol, antibiotics, psychotropic drugs, and some antihypertensive medications can also accumulate in toxic levels when liver function is impaired.

SECTION 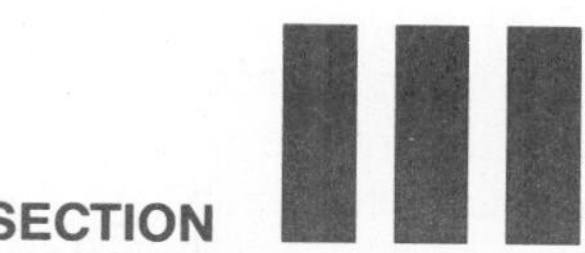

Related System Influences and Effects

Integumentary System

Yellowing of the skin is characteristic of jaundice. **Pruritus** (itching) associated with jaundice can become so severe that clients scratch until they bleed. The break in skin integrity increases the client's susceptibility to infection.

Xanthomas and **xanthelasmas** can occur in clients with biliary problems in whom serum cholesterol levels are high. These foamy cholesterol-filled cells may appear anywhere on the body but are commonly seen on the hands and around the eyes.

Edema and poor nutritional status also may make the skin highly susceptible to breakdown. Decubitus ulcers may form within hours in clients who are not frequently repositioned. White nails, where 80% of the proximal nail bed is white leaving a distal band of normal pink, are often associated with cirrhosis.

Cardiovascular System

Fluid overload or congestive heart failure may occur in response to excessive levels of aldosterone and ADH. Reduced oxygen-carrying capacity from erythrocytopenia may lead to increased cardiac output as the heart labors to deliver oxygen to starved tissues. Increased portal vein pressure related to hepatic fibrosis increases pressures within adjacent vessels and thereby leads to esophageal varices, splenomegaly, and periumbilical dilation. Hemorrhage of esophageal varices may further reduce the erythrocyte count. Increased clotting time because of deficiency in coagulation factors can produce hemorrhage and hypovolemic shock.

Neurologic System

Ammonia toxicity is related to alteration in mental states ranging from confusion to hepatic coma. The client who is confused or combative has a high potential for injury.

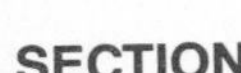

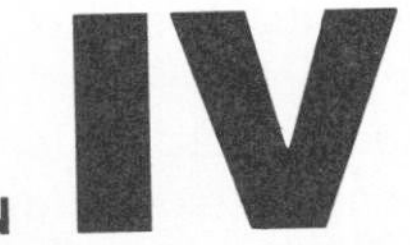

SECTION IV

Psychosocial/Lifestyle Influences and Effects

Developmental Influences

Cholelithiasis (gallstones) occurs in women four to five times as often as it does in men. This increased incidence is thought to be related to the action of the female hormones estrogen and progesterone, which increase the cholesterol saturation of bile. The higher the cholesterol saturation, the greater the risk that gallstones will form. Pregnant women and those taking contraceptive pills are at even higher risk of developing cholelithiasis, especially those who have had several pregnancies or who have been on oral contraceptives for several years.

Cholelithiasis is more common in persons over 40 years of age. It can occur at any age, however, especially in association with risk factors such as high fat intake, obesity or diabetes, multiple pregnancies, or an oral contraceptive regimen.

Young adults and elderly individuals are at greater risk of contracting viral hepatitis. This increased risk may be associated with poor nutrition or with crowded or unsanitary living conditions.

Implications for Elderly Clients

Elderly persons are susceptible to problems of drug toxicity, in part because renal and heptic function declines with age. At age 70, renal and hepatic efficiency may be half what it was at age 20, yet prescription of medications for elderly clients often do not reflect this fact. A drug may be prescribed at twice the dosage actually needed. The elderly often have multiple health problems. Several different health care providers may inadvertently prescribe medications that interact unfavorably. Self-medication with over-the-counter remedies may compound the overdosage.

Substance Abuse

Abuse of alcohol is a factor in many, though by no means all, conditions that damage the liver. Drug abuse, especially of injected substances, is associated with a high risk of contracting hepatitis. Cultural and psychologic aspects of alcohol and drug abuse are discussed in Chapter 8.

Lack of Sanitation

Drinking water or water used in preparation of foods such as fresh fruit or salad greens may become contaminated by secretions or fecal material from persons with viral (type A or type B) hepatitis. Shellfish caught in waters contaminated by untreated or inadequately treated sewage may also transmit the virus of hepatitis A. Sanitation is an important factor in control of hepatitis. Nurses, especially those working in community settings, can help inform their clients of the importance of washing hands before handling food and after using toilet facilities.

Dietary Factors

High-fat diets can contribute to the development of cirrhosis of the liver as well as to gallbladder disease. Biliary diseases are more common in cultures where food is prepared mostly by frying or where large amounts of fat are used in cooking. Conversely, the incidence of gallbladder disease is low in African and South American countries where fat consumption is low. Due in part to the popularity of fast food chains and fried snack products, the American diet is currently high in fat. A high intake of alcohol and associated malnutrition also contribute to the development of hepatic and biliary disease.

Economic Factors

Although malnutrition is usually associated with poverty, a high income does not ensure a balanced diet. Reliance on fast foods and snack foods and consumption of a fat-laden diet occur in all socioeconomic classes. Poor sanitation and high alcohol consumption may also occur at any income level.

Occupation and Avocation

Exposure to all types of hepatitis is a special risk of health care professionals, who may be exposed to virus-contaminated blood or secretions. Laboratory and operating room personnel and those who work in hemodialysis units risk contamination through exposure to body fluids. Nurses administering intravenous therapy or disposing of secretions may be exposed to hepatitis if strict asepsis and isolation principles are not followed. Dentists may be exposed to the hepatitis virus in the saliva of a hepatitis carrier or a person with active disease.

Exposure to toxic chemicals may be related to occupation, leisure-time hobbies, or a pharmaceutical regimen. Halothane and chloroform, to which operating room personnel are exposed, are hepatotoxic. Carbon tetrachloride, used in dry cleaning and in various industrial processes, is hepatotoxic, as are toluene and other chemicals used in paint thinners and other compounds used by both professionals and hobbyists. Gold, used in the jewelry trade and in fabrication of some electronic components, is also hepatotoxic. Among the medications that may have a toxic effect on the liver are a number of antibiotics (including erythromycin, oxacillin, and clindamycin), some psychotropic medications, and oral contraceptives. (A more extensive list of hepatotoxic substances appears in Chapter 40.) Highly stressful occupations or those that require a great deal of socialization may contribute to alcohol abuse.

Chapter Highlights

The liver is essential to life and functions as a regulator for many homeostatic systems.

Principal functions of the liver include (1) storage and filtration of blood, (2) secretion of bile, (3) conjugation and excretion of bilirubin, (4) metabolism of carbohydrates, fats, and proteins, (5) storage of vitamins and iron, (6) synthesis of coagulation factors and lymph, and (7) detoxification of ingested substances.

The basic functional unit of the liver is the liver lobule, of which there are 50,000 to 100,000 in the adult liver.

The principal function of the gallbladder is concentration and storage of bile.

Fibrotic enlargement of the liver is characteristic of most liver disorders; eventually, scarring may result in atrophy in late stages of liver disease.

Increased back-pressure in the portal venous system related to hypertrophy and fibrosis of the liver is the principal cause of periumbilical dilation, esophageal varices, and ascites, and may be related to splenomegaly and hemorrhoids.

Erythrocyte production decreases when the liver is compromised, owing to inadequate storage of vitamin B_{12} and iron (heme).

The client with impaired hepatic function is at risk for hemorrhage related to diminished production of clotting factors due in part to deficient absorption of vitamin K.

Destruction of phagocytic Kupffer cells and impairment of lymph production in a diseased liver increases the client's susceptibility to infection.

Jaundice associated with liver disease is related to impairment of bilirubin conjugation and excretion.

Inability of the compromised liver to convert ammonia to urea for excretion leads to ammonia toxicity, a condition that causes impairment of mentation sometimes leading to coma, as well as asterixis.

Hypoalbuminemia and impaired detoxification of ADH and aldosterone can lead to development of ascites and peripheral edema as well as vascular dehydration, which may mask erythrocytopenia by altering blood viscosity.

Lifestyle factors contributing to hepatic disease include alcohol abuse and work-related exposure to hepatotoxic substances.

Women are more susceptible to cholelithiasis than men, especially those who have had multiple pregnancies and those taking oral contraceptives; obesity, diabetes, high fat intake, and age over 40 are additional risk factors.

Bibliography

Briem F: Review of the anatomy and physiology of the gallbladder. *Society of GI Assistants* 1986; 8(3):40–41.

Crowley LV: *Introduction to Human Disease.* Monterey, CA: Wadsworth, 1983.

Fredette SL: When the liver fails. *Am J Nurs* 1984; 1:64–67.

Groer ME, Shekleton ME: *Basic Pathology: A Conceptual Approach,* 2nd ed. St. Louis, MO: Mosby, 1983.

Guyton, AC: *Textbook of Medical Physiology,* 7th ed. Philadelphia: Saunders, 1986.

Newton MP et al: The anatomy and physiology of the liver. *Society of GI Assistants* 1986; 8(3):42–43.

Petersdorf RG et al (editors): *Harrison's Principles of Internal Medicine,* 10th ed. New York: McGraw–Hill, 1983.

Ramsey JM: *Basic Pathophysiology: Modern Stress and the Disease Process.* Menlo Park, CA: Addison–Wesley, 1982.

Schearman DJC, Finlayson, ADC: *Diseases of the Gastrointestinal Tract and Liver.* London: Churchill Livingstone, 1982.

Sherlock S: *Diseases of the Liver and Biliary System,* 7th ed. Oxford: Blackwell, 1985.

Spence AP, Mason EB: *Human Anatomy and Physiology,* 3rd ed. Menlo Park, CA: Benjamin/Cummings, 1987.

Taylor DL: Gallstones: Physiology, signs, and symptoms. *Nurs 83* 1983; 13(6):44.

Taylor DL: Jaundice: Physiology, signs and symptoms. *Nurs 83* 1983; 13(8):52–54.

Vick RL: *Contemporary Medical Physiology.* Menlo Park, CA: Addison–Wesley, 1984.

Wimpsett J: Trace your patient's liver dysfunction. *Nurs 84* 1984; 14(8):56–57.

CHAPTER 40

The Nursing Process for Clients With Hepatic–Biliary Dysfunction

Other topics relevant to this content are: Care of clients who abuse alcohol, **Chapter 8;** Care of the client undergoing hepatic-biliary surgery, **Chapter 41.**

Objectives

When you have finished studying this chapter you should be able to:

Specify the major components of the health history to be obtained from clients with hepatic–biliary dysfunction.

Explain specific assessment approaches in evaluating clients with disease of the hepatic–biliary system.

Identify the nursing implications of diagnostic studies commonly used to evaluate clients with hepatic–biliary dysfunction.

Determine appropriate nursing diagnoses for clients with disorders of the hepatic–biliary system.

Develop, with the client, realistic goals of care.

Anticipate the psychosocial/lifestyle implications of hepatic–biliary dysfunction for clients and their significant others.

Develop a nursing care plan for a client with hepatic–biliary dysfunction.

Implement nursing interventions specific to clients with hepatic–biliary disease.

Evaluate the effectiveness of the nursing care plan and modify it as necessary to meet client needs.

The nursing process for clients with hepatic and biliary dysfunction encompasses a wide range of assessments and interventions. Nursing responsibilities generally applicable to hepatic and biliary disorders are discussed in this chapter.

SECTION I

Nursing Assessment: Establishing the Data Base

Subjective Data

This chapter discusses assessment data related specifically to the hepatic and biliary system. The client should be questioned about any recent loss of weight, change in appetite, or changes in bowel patterns. What color are the client's stools? What color is the urine? Clay-colored stools or mahogany-colored urine suggest obstruction of the common, hepatic, or cystic duct or an abnormality of bilirubin excretion. Was a change in color of stool or urine accompanied by yellowing of the sclera or the skin? Did pruritus occur when these changes were noticed? Associating these symptoms may help the client remember when they began.

Has the client lost weight or lost interest in food? A positive reply might suggest development of hepatitis or hepatic cancer, depending on other symptoms and signs elicited during the assessment.

What does the client usually eat? High fat intake might suggest cholelithiasis. Does the client bruise easily or bleed for a long time after a minor cut? Decreased absorption of vitamin K—possibly associated with hyperbilirubinemia—can affect blood coagulation.

Edema of the ankles, difficulty breathing, and collection of fluid in the abdomen could indicate right-side heart failure, hypoalbuminemia, portal hypertension, or inadequate detoxification of antidiuretic hormone (ADH) and aldosterone. The client may not remember when such changes began, but asking when clothing became tight around the waist or shoes no longer fit might jog the memory.

Has the client had frequent infections? Increased incidence of infection may be related to destruction of Kupffer cells. Has the client been exposed to hepatitis or mononucleosis? Has the client had any recent blood transfusions? A positive answer may be correlated with other evidence suggesting hepatitis. Impotence or loss of libido may related to impaired estrogen detoxification. Questioning about this sensitive subject might best be postponed until rapport has been established with the client. Tactful questioning of the client's sexual partner may elicit data suggesting sexual dysfunction.

Determining whether alcohol abuse might be related to liver dysfunction also requires discretion and tact. One should not presuppose that the client is an alcohol abuser, even if the suspected disorder is commonly associated with consumption of alcohol. The client who does have an alcohol problem may be reluctant to answer, may evade questions, or may deny any drinking problems. Sometimes significant others will verify unexplained changes in behavior that may suggest alcohol abuse. Psychosocial changes related to alcohol abuse are discussed at length in Chapter 8.

Specific, nonjudgmental questions are most likely to yield useful data about drinking habits:

- What do you like to drink?
- How often do you drink? Every day? Several times a day? A week? A month? Such specifics are more useful than generalities such as "rarely" or "often."
- How much do you drink? One drink? Three or four?
- How many shots do you put in a highball? Do you order drinks "up" or with ice? Does wine with dinner mean a glass or a carafe? By "a few beers" do you mean a couple of cans? A six-pack?

Remember that alcohol in any form (wine, beer, or hard liquor) has the same effect. A 12 oz bottle of beer, a 4 oz glass of wine, and a 1 oz shot of Scotch contain the same amount of alcohol. Other questions related to drinking habits might be:

- When you drink, how much do you consume in 24 hours?
- What is the most you've drunk in 24 hours?
- Do you drink in the morning? At or after work? With friends? Alone?
- Have you ever blacked out?
- Does drinking make you sick or does it make you feel better? Gastritis related to alcoholism will be alleviated by a drink (Hawks, 1983).

Remember not to concentrate on alcohol while ignoring other clues. What is the client's occupation? Does it involve exposure to solvents, dry-cleaning solutions, anesthetic agents, or other hepatotoxic substances? Does the client have hobbies such as furniture refinishing that might have hepatotoxic side effects? A list of common substances causing hepatic damage is presented in Box 40–1.

Box 40–1
Drugs and Chemicals Capable of Causing Hepatic-Biliary Dysfunction

Drugs

- *Acetaminophen (Tylenol, Datril)
- Acetohexamide (Dymelor)
- Allopurinol (Zyloprim)
- Aminosalicylic acid (PAS)
- Androgens and anabolic steroids
- *Azathioprine (Imuran)
- Chlorpromazine (Thorazine)
- Chlorpropamide (Diabinese)
- Clindamycin (Cleocin)
- Erythromycin estolate (Ilosone)
- Ethionamide (Trecator SC)
- Gold salts
- Imipramine (Tofranil)
- *Isoniazid (INH)
- Methimazole (Tapazole)
- Methotrexate
- Methyldopa (Aldomet, Aldoril)
- Monoamine oxidase inhibitors
- Nitrofurantoin (Furadantin, Macrodantin)
- Oral contraceptives
- Oxacillin (Prostaphilin)
- *Phenacetin
- Phenazopyridine (Pyridium)
- Phenylbutazone (Butazolidin)
- Phenytoin (Dilantin)
- Propoxyphene (Darvon)
- *Rifampin
- Sulfonamides
- Tetracyclines

Inhalation Anesthetics

- Halothane (Fluothane)
- Methoxyflurane (Penthrane)

Industrial Inhalants

- *Arsenic
- *Carbon tetrachloride
- *Yellow phosphorus

*Hepatotoxins (dose related)

Objective Data

Physical Assessment

Physical assessment of the client with hepatic–biliary dysfunction involves careful inspection of the skin, nails, and hair. Physical findings that suggest cirrhosis include:

- Ascites
- Ankle edema

- Muscle wasting
- Dilated periumbilical veins (caput medusae)
- Ecchymoses
- Spider angiomas
- Loss of body hair
- **Gynecomastia** (breast enlargement in men)
- **Jaundice** (yellow coloration to skin and sclerae)
- Clubbing of the fingers

If the client is in a late stage of liver dysfunction, asterixis related to ammonia toxicity will be observed—the hands rapidly clench and unclench. Inflating a blood pressure cuff on the arm will worsen the tremor. Asterixis may also be seen in clients with cancer of the liver. In clients with hepatitis, however, only ecchymoses and jaundice will be apparent unless the condition is long standing. Bruising and jaundice may sometimes accompany hepatic abscess; however, diminished appetite may be the only sign of this disorder. As mentioned previously, jaundice may also be secondary to an obstructive condition or an abnormality affecting bilirubin conjugation.

Diminished bowel sounds are common in clients with ascites. Listen for hepatic bruits, which may be heard with hepatic carcinoma.

Hepatomegaly and splenomegaly can be present in clients with hepatitis, cholecystitis, hepatic abscess, mononucleosis, cirrhosis, or cancer of the liver. *Because of the danger of damaging or rupturing these organs, the inexperienced nurse should not palpate the liver or spleen.* Swollen lymph nodes may be palpable in the neck or in the groin with an infectious disorder such as mononucleosis.

Three assessment techniques can be used to determine whether fluid is present in the abdomen.

1. With the client supine, both flanks may be percussed for dullness, which indicates the presence of fluid.
2. When the client assumes a side-lying position, fluid will fall toward the side on which the client is lying, where it may be percussed for dullness.
3. The presence of a fluid wave may be determined as follows: Have the client lie flat and place his or her hand, ulnar side down, along the abdominal midline and apply pressure to anchor the fat in the mesentery. (If the client is too ill to participate, an assistant can do this.) Place one hand on one flank to detect signs of a fluid wave while tapping the opposite flank with the other hand (Figure 40–1). There will be a short time lag between the tap and receipt of the impulse.

Abdominal girth should be measured daily with a tape measure. Measurements taken at the same location (eg, at the level of the umbilicus) assist in evaluating progression and/or treatment of ascites.

Diagnostic Studies

HEMATOLOGIC STUDIES Blood samples for determination of white blood cell count (WBC), prothrombin time (PT), hemoglobin level (Hb), and hematocrit (Hct) may be drawn at any time. Hemoglobin and hematocrit values are unaffected by early stages of hepatic disease but may drop if there is hemorrhage from esophageal varices and in response to malnourishment. Prothrombin time will increase with vitamin K deficiency, for example, in cirrhosis, hepatitis, cholecystitis, cholelithiasis, mononucleosis, or cancer of the liver. Leukocyte levels increase in clients with mononucleosis, hepatitis, and abscesses.

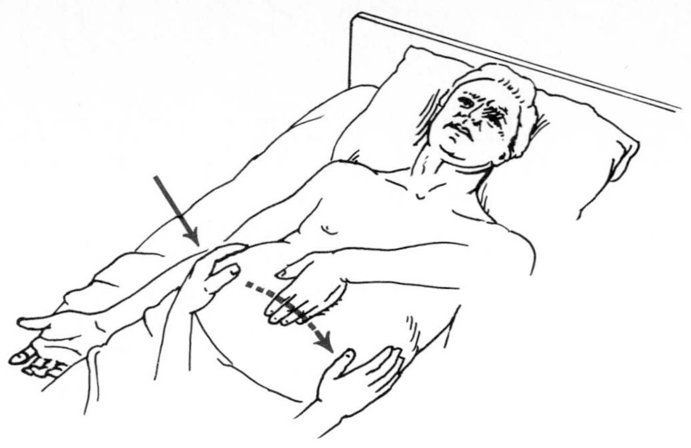

Figure 40–1

Assessing for ascites by checking for a fluid wave.

SERUM ENZYME STUDIES Elevated serum enzyme levels occur when hepatic cells are damaged and enzymes are released into the blood. Values that are likely to be elevated with liver or gallbladder disease include:

- Lactic dehydrogenase (LDH)
- Serum glutamic oxaloacetic transaminase (SGOT); also called aspartate aminotransferase (AST)
- Serum glutamic pyruvic transaminase (SGPT); also called alanine aminotransferase (ALT)
- Alkaline phosphatase
- Gamma-glutamyl transpeptidase (GGT)

LDH, SGOT, and SGPT values are significantly increased in obstructive jaundice and mononucleosis; they are also markedly elevated in acute and toxic hepatitis, cirrhosis, and hepatic neoplasia. Alkaline phosphatase levels, important in measuring biliary obstruction, are extremely elevated in obstructive jaundice, significantly elevated in cancer of the liver and mononucleosis, and slightly elevated in hepatitis (viral or toxic) and cirrhosis. Elevation of gamma-glutamyl transpeptidase is the most accurate enzymatic indicator of hepatic disease. Enzyme levels will rise as the disease progresses, peaking at the time of maximum cell death, and then begin to fall.

BILIRUBIN VALUES Studies of bilirubin values are important in determining the cause of jaundice and hyperbilirubinemia. Direct or conjugated bilirubin levels will be elevated if biliary ducts are obstructed and conjugated bilirubin cannot be excreted. Indirect or unconjugated bilirubin levels will be high if parenchymal (liver lobule) cells have been damaged.

Elevated levels of urobilinogen in the urine indicate parenchymal liver disease such as cirrhosis, toxic or infectious hepatitis, or infectious mononucleosis—or they may indicate cholelithiasis. By impairing excretion of bilirubin in the stool, these conditions lead to increased excretion by the kidneys. Urine that contains bilirubin develops a yellow foam when shaken. Fecal levels of urobilinogen are decreased if the bile ducts are obstructed, but this test is rarely performed because of the difficulty in obtaining accurate values.

BLOOD AMMONIA VALUES Blood ammonia levels rise when cirrhosis is present because the disease impairs conversion of ammonia to urea for renal excretion. Bleeding esophageal varices exacerbate ammonia toxicity, since the ammonia produced by the action of intestinal bacteria on the protein in blood adds rapidly to already elevated serum ammonia levels. Hepatic coma can result.

OTHER LABORATORY TEST VALUES Changes in serum protein levels are common in hepatic and biliary disorders. Serum albumin levels drop (hypoalbuminemia) and gamma globulin levels rise when parenchymal cell damage occurs. Serum antigen–antibody levels are helpful in evaluating hepatitis (Table 40–1). For example, hepatitis B surface antigen (HBsAg) is present in the blood of persons who have hepatitis B and also in those who are carriers of the disease. Clients with hepatitis B surface antibody (anti-HBs) in their blood have immunity to hepatitis B.

ULTRASOUND Ultrasound is used for diagnosis of gallbladder disease before more invasive techniques such as oral cholecystogram or intravenous cholangiogram are used (Fishbein, 1985). Ultrasound is cheaper than an oral cholecystogram and has a diagnostic accuracy of 96% (Sherlock, 1985). Ultrasound can show gallstones of 3 mm in size and larger (Figure 40–2), as well as increasing thickness of the gallbladder wall. It is useful in differentiating benign cysts and tumors from malignancies. Liver abscesses, dilation of intrahepatic ducts, and biliary tumors can also be identified.

NURSING IMPLICATIONS To ensure that the gallbladder is at maximum size for the test, the client must be kept NPO after midnight on the day of testing. Were the client to eat, contraction and emptying of the gallbladder would reduce its size, making it more difficult to visualize. NPO orders are not necessary for visualization of the liver. If barium contrast studies have been performed prior to the ultrasonography, a laxative will be ordered to cleanse the bowel of residual contrast medium.

In explaining the procedure to the client, the nurse can offer reassurance that the study is not painful. The client should be prepared for the copious amount of lubricant that will be applied to the skin to enhance transmission of the sound waves. The rationale for any NPO order should be explained. The procedure will take from 20 minutes to 2 hours if more than the liver and gallbladder are being evaluated.

Table 40–1
Immunologic Antigen–Antibody Tests for Viral Hepatitis A and B

Antigen/Antibody Tests	Comments
anti-HAV (antibody to hepatitis A virus)	Early antibody is of IgM class; convalescent antibody of IgG class; clients with anti-HAV in serum are immune to reinfection.
HBsAg (hepatitis B surface antigen)	Specific for hepatitis B infection; appears about 4 weeks after exposure to hepatitis B; originally called Australian antigen.
anti-HB_s (antibody to hepatitis B surface antigen)	Its presence in the blood indicates immunity to hepatitis B.
HB_cAg (hepatitis B core antigen)	The core of the Dane particle; core antigen is difficult to identify.
anti-HB_c (antibody to hepatitis B core antigen)	In the absence of Hb_sAg and anti-Hb_s, a high titer of anti-HB_c reflects ongoing viral replication.
HB_eAg (hepatitis B "e" antigen)	Found in HB_sAg positive serum only; an indicator of relative infectivity of the client with hepatitis B; persistent positives may be associated with chronic hepatitis.
anti-HB_e (antibody to hepatitis B "e" antigen)	Its presence is associated with a lower degree of infectivity.

HAV (hepatitis A virus): RNA virus, present in serum and stool.
HBV (hepatitis B virus—Dane particle): DNA virus, present in serum, saliva, semen, breast milk.

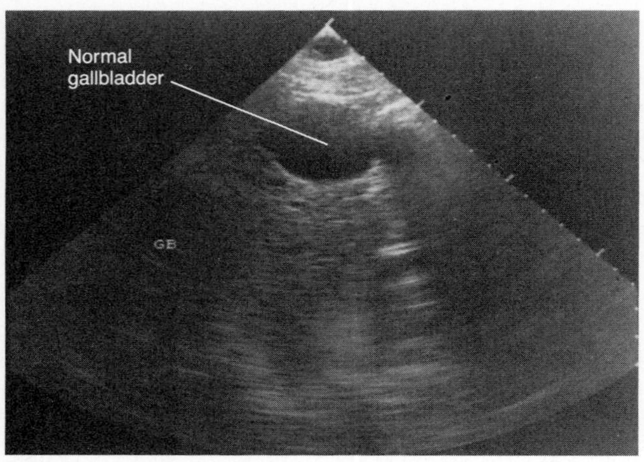

A

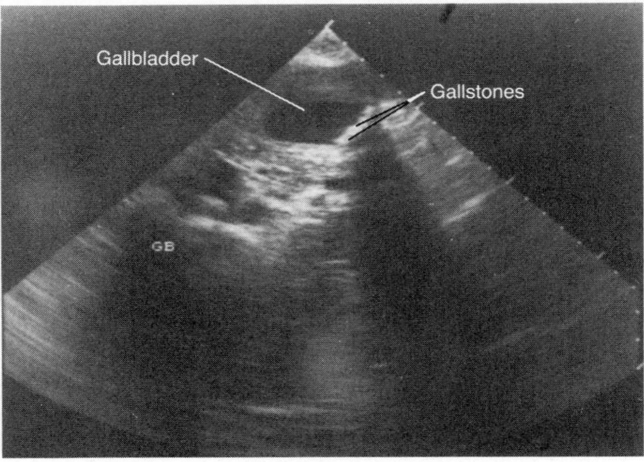

B

Figure 40–2

A. Ultrasound of a normal gallbladder. **B.** Ultrasound of a gallbladder containing gallstones. *Courtesy of Health Care Plan, Buffalo, NY.*

LIVER SCAN A radionuclide is administered intravenously. Thirty minutes later a detecting device is passed over the client's abdomen to record the distribution of radioactive particles in the liver. Although this technique exposes the client to far less radiation than x-rays, it can only demonstrate filling defects greater than 2 cm in diameter. It is contraindicated for pregnant clients and those who might have difficulty lying still during the scan, which takes about one hour.

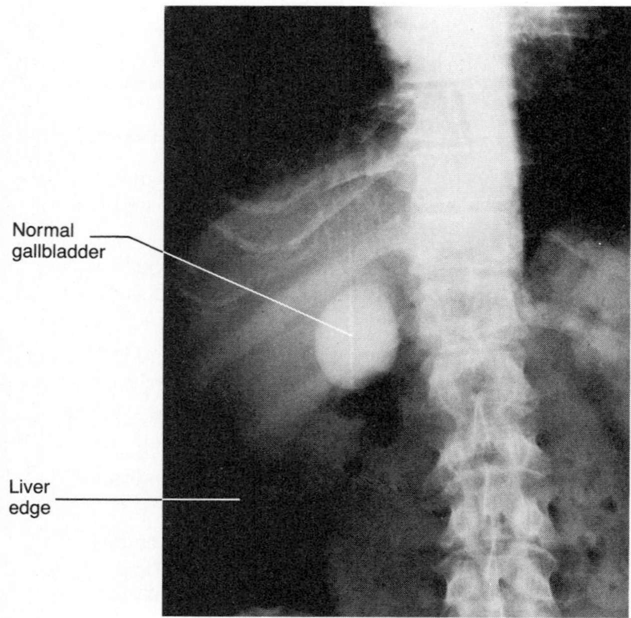

Figure 40–3

A normal oral cholecystogram. The gallbladder is filled with contrast dye. *Courtesy of Health Care Plan, Buffalo, NY.*

NURSING IMPLICATIONS No special preparation is required for this study. The nurse should explain the procedure and explain that small amounts of radioactive substances are used. Some clients are apprehensive about the amount of time required for the scan, and it is helpful to explain that the scanning device does not emit radiation but rather records radiation emanating from the injected radioisotope. Pregnant health care providers should not be assigned to the client for at least 24 hours after the radionuclide injection.

DYE CLEARANCE STUDIES For this procedure, the client fasts for 12 hours prior to the test. Dye is injected intravenously (about 5 mg/kg of body weight). Blood is drawn 45 minutes after the injection and inspected for the presence of dye. Normally, less than 5% of the dye will be found in the serum; the presence of a greater proportion of the dye indicates liver cell damage—the impaired cells cannot absorb the dye from the blood. If hepatic damage is known to exist, lower dosages of dye are administered. Either indocyanine green (ICG) or Bromsulphalein (BSP) is used for this study.

ORAL CHOLECYSTOGRAPHY An oral cholecystogram, or "gallbladder series," provides visualization of the gallbladder following oral ingestion of a radiopaque iodinated dye. Figure 40–3 shows a normal cholecystogram. In the first test of the series, gallstones when present may be visualized as dark shadows in a dye-filled gallbladder. Satisfactory visualization of the gallbladder can be obtained only if the gallbladder has concentrated the dye. Adequate concentration depends on correct dosage of the dye, adequate absorption of the dye from the gastrointestinal tract (ie, no nausea or vomiting), and absence of food in the digestive tract (ie, NPO after midnight). If nonvisualization occurs, the test is repeated the next day with a doubled dosage of dye. Hepatocellular dysfunction, cystic duct obstruction, or inflammation of the biliary mucosa will prevent visualization.

In the second phase of the series, the client is given a fatty meal immediately following the first phase, and x-rays are taken to determine how well the gallbladder empties. The x-rays are repeated every 30 minutes until the dye is gone and the gallbladder can no longer be visualized. This may take one to five hours but usually takes no more than three.

Oral cholecystography is contraindicated for pregnant women, clients too ill to swallow the dye tablets or to eat a meal, and persons allergic to iodine. Ultrasonography may soon replace oral cholecystography because it is less invasive, more accurate in diagnosing cholelithiasis, and can be used with pregnant clients and those who cannot take the oral contrast agent.

NURSING IMPLICATIONS The client will have to swallow seven or eight tablets of absorbable iodine dye (Telepaque, for example) the evening prior to the test. Once the tablets are swallowed, only water may be given until midnight; after midnight the client is kept NPO. Nursing implications include:

- Verifying that no iodine allergy exists. The client should be questioned about seafood allergies, since not all clients are aware of what foods contain iodine.
- Ascertaining that the client is given a low-fat meal on the evening before the test.
- Verifying that serum bilirubin is less than 1.8 mg/dL (so that visualization will be possible).
- Explaining the procedure to the client.
- Administering the tablets at five-minute intervals.
- Observing for adverse effects of the dye. (Anaphylactic reactions have occurred.)
- Maintaining NPO status.

INTRAVENOUS CHOLANGIOGRAPHY Intravenous cholangiography allows visualization of the hepatic and common bile ducts in addition to the gallbladder and cystic duct. It is used for clients with acute inflammatory disorders, those with proven gallstones, and those who are NPO or unable to tolerate the orally ingested dye used in cholecystography. It is contraindicated for clients with serum bilirubin levels higher than 3.5 mg/dL, for those allergic to iodine, and for pregnant clients. While supine, the client is given an intravenous infusion of iodinated contrast medium. X-rays are then taken at intervals for up to eight hours.

NURSING IMPLICATIONS No special diet is required for this procedure. Usually, bisacodyl (Dulcolax) is ordered to be given on the morning of the examination. In explaining the procedure to the client, mention that it is normal to feel heat with the administration of the contrast medium. Verifying that the client is not allergic to iodine is an important precaution. The nurse is also responsible for administering the cathartic, verifying bilirubin level, and maintaining NPO status. The client should be kept as comfortable as possible; for example, oral hygiene may be administered during the intervals between films.

INTRAOPERATIVE CHOLANGIOGRAPHY Cholangiography may be performed during a surgical procedure to ascertain that all calculi have been removed from the common bile duct, reducing the probability of complications or follow-up surgery. Dye is injected to enhance visualization.

T-TUBE CHOLANGIOGRAPHY A T-tube cholangiogram may be taken seven to ten days following a cholecystectomy. The T-tube is placed during surgery. Later, dye is injected via the T-tube so the common bile duct may be visualized and its patency ascertained.

ENDOSCOPIC RETROGRADE CHOLANGIOPANCREATOGRAPHY The icteric client with bilirubin levels above 3.5 mg/dL cannot be evaluated by oral cholecystography or intravenous cholangiography. Endoscopic retrograde cholangiopancreatography (ERCP) and percutaneous hepatic cholangiography (PTHC—see following section) are alternative techniques for these clients. ERCP studies allow visualization of the bile ducts as well as benign masses, cysts, and malignant neoplasms.

A type of fiberoptic endoscope (a duodenoscope) is inserted into the duodenum via the esophagus. Intravenously administered secretin immobilizes the duodenum, facilitating visualization of the ampulla of Vater. Contrast material combined with a broad-spectrum antibiotic are administered through a small cannula inserted into the ampulla, and films are taken periodically for approximately an hour. The antibiotic is given to prevent gram-negative sepsis that may occur if bacteria are forced into the bloodstream by the pressure of the dye injection. Perforation of the esophagus, stomach, or duodenum is another possible complication of ERCP (Pagana and Pagana, 1982).

NURSING IMPLICATIONS A consent form is necessary for this procedure. In teaching the client about the procedure, explain that an impulse to gag will be felt when the tube is passed. The client is kept NPO after midnight. Meperidine and atropine are administered intramuscularly before the client is taken to the radiology department. Emotional support should be given as needed. After the procedure, the client's pulse, temperature, and blood pressure are monitored for signs of shock that may arise from perforation or hemorrhage and for signs of septicemia. Pancreatitis may occur in response to the pressure exerted on the pancreatic duct during the procedure; therefore, a serum amylase test should be performed on the day following an ERCP.

PERCUTANEOUS TRANSHEPATIC CHOLANGIOGRAPHY Like ERCP, percutaneous (through the skin) transhepatic cholangiography (PTHC) is used for icteric clients with serum bilirubin levels above 3.5 mg/dL. During this procedure, a combination of contrast medium and antibiotic is injected into the intrahepatic bile duct to visualize the biliary system. The area below the right costal margin is locally anesthetized, and a spinal needle is inserted directly into the liver guided by fluoroscopy. When bile appears through the needle, it is withdrawn by syringe. Radiopaque dye is then injected directly into the biliary tree. Fluoroscopy is used to determine filling of the biliary tract.

The client is intravenously sedated during the procedure, which takes about one hour. If obstruction is found, a catheter may be left in place for drainage of bile. A PTHC is contraindicated for clients who have prolonged clotting times or iodine allergy, for clients who have had recent gastrointestinal contrast studies or are unlikely to tolerate surgery, and for combative clients. Bile peritonitis, hemorrhage, and septicemia are possible complications.

NURSING IMPLICATIONS A consent form is necessary for this procedure, and coagulation studies as well as information regarding possible iodine allergy must be verified. The client is kept NPO after midnight. A laxative may be prescribed if gastrointestinal studies using barium have been recently administered. An intravenous infusion is started for venous access, and the client is premedicated with meperidine and atropine before leaving the unit. After the procedure, the client is kept NPO and in bed for 12 to 24 hours or, if very ill, until the condition improves. Vital signs must be monitored as for a postsurgical client. A sterile closed system must be maintained if a catheter has been left in place.

LIVER BIOPSY The purpose of a liver biopsy is to obtain a sample of tissue for histologic examination. Prior to the procedure, a liver scan may be done to determine the precise location of the liver, and a coagulation profile must be obtained so the risk of hemorrhage can be calculated. The client's blood is typed and cross-matched in case a transfusion is needed.

For the study, the client is assisted into a supine or left lateral position. The skin is aseptically cleansed and anesthetized, and a small incision is made to allow insertion of a specialized needle into the liver. A small core of hepatic tissue is then withdrawn and sent for microscopic evaluation (Figure 40–4).

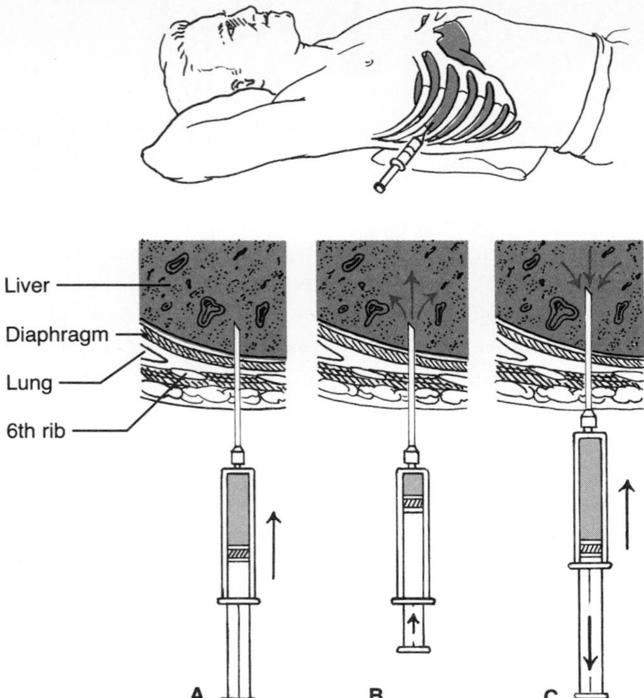

Figure 40–4

Liver biopsy procedure. **A.** Have the client hold his or her breath at the end of expiration to bring the liver and diaphragm to the highest position; the physician then inserts the biopsy needle into the liver. **B.** Approximately 1 mL of saline is injected to clear the needle of blood and tissue. **C.** The needle is pushed farther into the liver. Liver tissue is aspirated, the needle withdrawn, and pressure applied to the injection site. The liver specimen is expelled into formalin to preserve it for analysis.

NURSING IMPLICATIONS This procedure requires a consent form. The client is kept NPO after midnight. Nursing responsibilities include:

- Checking coagulation studies and consent form.
- Maintaining NPO status.
- Recording preprocedure vital signs.
- Providing emotional support for the client; this procedure can be frightening and uncomfortable.
- Explaining the procedure to the client, emphasizing the importance of lying still.
- Immediately prior to needle insertion asking the client to inhale deeply, exhale completely, and hold the breath at the end of expiration. This immobilizes the chest wall and keeps the diaphragm at its upper level during the procedure (which takes 5 to 10 seconds).
- Applying pressure to the biopsy site after needle removal.
- Turning client onto right side with a pillow under the costal margin to maintain pressure to the site.
- Assisting the physician as indicated.
- Monitoring postprocedure vital signs (q. 15 min $\times 4$, q. 30 min $\times 4$, then q. 4h), and administering comfort measures after the procedure.

The client should remain immobile on the right side for several hours and be closely observed for signs of hemorrhage, extravasation of fluid from the biopsy site, peritonitis, and pain. Pain in the right upper quadrant and right shoulder area is common. The client should be reassured about this while being encouraged to report any change in pain level. Analgesics, if given, must be nonhepatotoxic and must not affect clotting.

SECTION 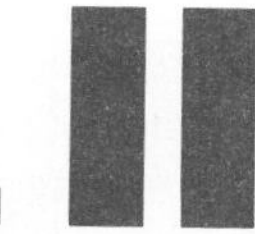

Nursing Diagnosis/Planning and Implementation/Evaluation

Information gathered from the client's health history, physical examination, and diagnostic studies is used to determine nursing diagnoses and the plan of care. Not every client will have the same needs.

The Nursing Diagnoses box lists diagnoses **directly related** to hepatic-biliary dysfunction along with **potential** diagnoses for clients with hepatic-biliary problems. The most common nursing diagnoses for clients with hepatic-biliary dysfunction include altererd comfort; impaired skin integrity; self-concept disturbance: body image; self-concept disturbance: self-esteem; altered thought processes; altered nutrition; impaired gas exchange; fluid volume deficit; fluid volume excess; and altered tissue perfusion. The sample nursing care plan in Table 40–2 focuses on altered comfort, potential impaired skin integrity, and self-concept disturbance: body image. Altered thought processes, altered nutrition, impaired gas exchange, fluid volume deficit, and altered tissue perfusion are discussed in the narrative.

If the goals of care have not been met, re-evaluation is required. The nurse and client should jointly review the nursing care plan. New objectives may need to be formulated; other nursing interventions may be added or modified; or the evaluation may show that more time is required to meet the objectives.

Thought Processes, Altered

Ammonia toxicity is related to the inability of the compromised hepatic cells to convert ammonia to urea for excretion in the urine. The ammonia interferes with brain

Table 40–2
Sample Nursing Care Plan for Clients With Hepatic–Biliary Dysfunction

Client Care Goals	Plan/Nursing Implementation	Expected Outcome
Comfort, altered related to pruritus		
Maintain comfort. Reduce or eliminate jaundice and pruritus. State cause of pruritus.	Be sure itching is not related to allergy. Ensure rest, good diet, ventilation, cotton clothing, distraction, no alkaline soaps, infrequent baths, whirlpools, emollients. Keep nails short, have client wear gloves to decrease breaking skin integrity from scratching, provide distraction, change wet sheets, diphenhydramine as ordered. Teach about pruritus.	Performs ADL without scratching; rests comfortably without scratching; relief from itching; describes cause of pruritus.
Comfort, altered related to pain		
Ambulate without undue discomfort; rest comfortably.	Avoid hepatotoxic drugs; use drugs broken down and excreted by kidney; Brompton's cocktail or morphine infusion drip for intractable cancer pain; meperidine, nitroglycerin, or phenobarbital for cholelithiasis pain; nursing comfort measures.	Performs ADL without undue pain; rests comfortably without severe pain; relief from pain.
Skin integrity, impaired: potential related to pruritus		
Maintain skin integrity. Understand need for eating diet high in protein.	Teach about and provide high protein diet; relieve itching; turn every one to two hours; relieve pressure on edematous areas with positioning; prevent infection with good skin care.	Normal skin integrity; evidence client is eating high protein diet.
Self-concept, disturbance in: body image related to disease		
Accept body image changes.	Instruct about causes of body changes; allow client to ventilate feelings; encourage family support.	Describes causes of body changes; discusses feelings openly.

NURSING DIAGNOSES IN
Hepatic-Biliary Dysfunction

DIRECTLY RELATED DIAGNOSES

- Comfort, altered: pain, pruritus
- Fluid volume deficit
- Fluid volume excess
- Gas exchange, impaired
- Nutrition, altered: less than body requirements
- Self-concept, disturbance in: body image
- Skin integrity, impaired: potential
- Thought process, altered
- Tissue perfusion, altered: cardiopulmonary

OTHER POTENTIAL DIAGNOSES

- Breathing pattern, ineffective
- Coping, ineffective family disabled
- Coping, ineffective individual
- Knowledge deficit
- Self-concept, disturbance in: self-esteem
- Sleep pattern disturbance
- Sexuality, altered patterns

metabolism, leading to alterations of mentation ranging from slight confusion to coma. Initially, clients may be somewhat confused or disoriented—unable, for example, to remember their names or where they are. Asterixis may also be apparent. Clients may then progress through lethargy to combativeness and abusiveness before lapsing into coma. Gastrointestinal hemorrhage further increases serum ammonia levels due to bacterial action on blood in the gut. Wernicke–Korsakoff syndrome, characterized by confusion, disorientation, and amnesia with confabulation, is sometimes seen in alcoholics. The syndrome is thought to be related to thiamine deficiency.

Planning and Implementation

Evaluate the client's mental status, promote safety, and monitor for decreasing ammonia toxicity. Mentation can be monitored by assessing the client's orientation to person, place, and time. One convenient technique for detecting changes in ammonia toxicity levels is having the client write his or her name daily and comparing the signatures. Severity of asterixis can be evaluated by pumping up a blood pressure cuff on the client's arm; the more rapidly the hand clenches and unclenches, the higher the serum level of ammonia. The client's breath should be assessed for fetor hepaticus, which is similar to the odor of acetone or old wine.

As the person who administers most medications, the nurse must be alert to the possibility that a hepatotoxic drug or dosage has been inadvertently prescribed. (See Box 40–1.) Detoxification capacity declines in older individuals, even under normal conditions; this impairment will be worsened in hepatic disease.

Safety measures such as padded siderails or restraints may be necessary to protect clients who are confused or combative as a result of hepatic encephalopathy. The client must be reminded not to get out of bed unassisted. Activities of daily living should be supervised, as should smoking.

Various therapeutic measures may be prescribed to decrease serum ammonia levels. Intravenous administration of glucose may provide protein-conserving carbohydrates. Rest can decrease release of ammonia associated with muscle contraction.

Pharmacologic measures may also be used. Potassium is sometimes given to improve cerebral metabolism of ammonia. Antibiotics such as neomycin may be administered orally or by enema to reduce the number of ammonia-synthesizing bacteria in the gut. Since neomycin is poorly absorbed from the intestine, its bactericidal action in the intestine is prolonged; however, this antibiotic may cause ototoxicity or nephrotoxicity if administered for more than six days (Malseed, 1982).

Lactulose (Cephulac, Duphalac) may be given orally or by nasogastric tube. This drug acts by acidifying the colon so ammonia couples with hydrogen ions and is excreted in the feces. Improvement may be seen within 24 hours, with serum ammonia levels being reduced by 25%–50% in most clients. Diarrhea is common with lactulose therapy, so electrolyte levels must be monitored. Sometimes hemodialysis may be necessary to reduce serum ammonia levels.

Check stools for occult blood and monitor vital signs for changes that might indicate gastrointestinal hemorrhage. Bacterial action on blood in the gut may cause ammonia levels to rise. If esophageal varices are bleeding, tap water enemas may be ordered to cleanse the intestines of all contents, including protein-rich blood.

Evaluation

Orientation to person, place, and time, absence of asterixis, and the ability to write one's name the same way on sequential days are evidence that support maintenance of thought processes. If asterixis develops or changes in handwriting are noted, the nurse may need to modify plans and interventions.

Nutrition, Altered: Less Than Body Requirements

Hepatic dysfunction is associated with impaired metabolism of proteins, fats, carbohydrates, and vitamins. Weight loss, fatigue, negative nitrogen balance, vitamin B deficiency, and deficiencies of fat-soluble vitamins A, D, E, and K are common. Abdominal pressure from ascites can cause a constant feeling of fullness as well as flatulence or constipation. These conditions may also diminish appetite, further depleting nutritional status.

In cholelithiasis or cholestasis, a low-fat diet should be consumed because fat metabolsim is reduced by disturbances in biliary function. Deficiency of vitamin K may also accompany these disorders.

Planning and Implementation

Unless ammonia toxicity is present, the client with hepatic dysfunction should receive a diet high in protein to promote hepatic healing and prevent loss of muscle mass. The diet should be low in salt and high in vitamins, carbohydrates, and calories. If ammonia toxicity is present, low-protein, potassium-rich foods should be provided. The client with biliary dysfunction should reduce the quantity of fats consumed.

Promoting a well-balanced diet with a client who often has no appetite is a challenge. Appetite may be improved by providing oral hygiene and fresh air, minimizing movement, and administering prescribed antiemetics. The nurse can work with the dietitian in providing appetizing meals, perhaps in small frequent feedings supplemented by nourishing snacks. Protein supplements may be used if not contraindicated by ammonia toxicity. It is helpful if the mealtime environment is pleasant and free of unpleasant odors. Food preferences elicited in the nursing history should be considered. Explaining the rationale for the diet may encourage the client to eat more.

If the client is unable to eat enough to meet caloric needs, feeding via nasogastric tube or total parenteral nutrition may be prescribed.

Evaluation

Expected outcomes for improving nutritional status and knowledge of nutrition include the ability to list foods high in protein and potassium and low in salt and fats, evidence of increasing intake of well-balanced foods, and signs that nutritional deficiencies are being corrected. This will be a slow process, but if a client is eating half the food on the tray instead of nothing, improvement has been shown. Consulting with the client to make a list of favorite foods and seeing that those foods are served may improve consumption. Cultural and ethnic preferences should be considered in planning the diet.

Gas Exchange, Impaired

Several conditions related to hepatic and biliary disease impair exchange of oxygen and carbon dioxide. Retention of sodium and water is associated with pleural effusion and ascites. Ascites exerts pressure on the diaphragm, interfering with inspiration. Inadequate oxygenation of body tissue related to erythrocytopenia also impairs gas exchange.

Planning and Implementation

Several measures may be prescribed to improve oxygenation. If dyspnea occurs at rest or on exertion, oxygen therapy may be initiated. Oral iron supplements or a transfusion of packed red cells may be given to improve hemoglobin and hematocrit levels. Intramuscular injections of vitamin K_1 (AquaMEPHYTON) improve clotting. Diuretic therapy or administration of albumin may be prescribed to reduce pleural effusion, which hinders gas exchange, or to decrease ascites, which exerts pressure on the diaphragm.

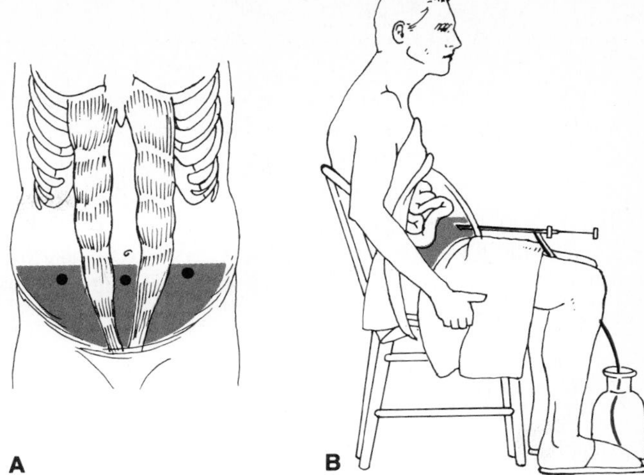

Figure 40–5

Paracentesis in a client with ascites. **A.** The preferred sites for trocar insertion are indicated to avoid injury to the deep inferior epigastric vessels. **B.** Assist the client to a comfortable seated position with the chest and abdomen draped. In this position the intestines will float away from the paracentesis site.

The nurse may be called upon to assist with paracentesis (Figure 40–5) to remove ascitic fluid from the abdomen. The client is assisted to a sitting position. The abdomen is cleansed with an antiseptic solution and draped. Local anesthesia is administered, and a trocar is inserted and tubing attached. Fluid drains via gravity into a sterile container. Up to 2 L of fluid may be removed; removal of a larger quantity may lead to shock. The nurse documents the amount and color of ascitic fluid removed before sending a sample of the fluid for laboratory evaluation. Paracentesis may be repeated periodically as fluid reaccumulates.

Ascites may also be controlled by a LeVeen or Denver shunt procedure; these are discussed in Chapter 41.

Evaluation

One expected outcome might be the client's ability to ambulate without oxygen supplementation. Another is return of the hemoglobin level to normal. Others might be absence of dyspnea on exertion; absence of cyanosis; or increased energy shown by knitting, working a crossword puzzle, or writing a letter. If these data can be observed, the nursing plan may be considered successful.

Fluid Volume Deficit
Fluid Volume Excess

Alterations in fluid volume may be either deficits or overloads. For example, when the compromised liver can no longer detoxify ADH and aldosterone, retention of sodium and water contributes to circulatory congestion and hypertension. Conversely, fluid volume deficit can be related to hemorrhage of esophageal varices (leading to shock) or to overuse of diuretics. If plasma colloidal osmotic pressure is reduced because of hypoalbuminemia, fluid extravasation into the interstitial space will cause edema despite intravascular dehydration.

Planning and Implementation

Edema related to hepatic dysfunction is misleading because vascular dehydration frequently accompanies it. Diuretic therapy alone can worsen dehydration. Diuretics should not be overused and should be given in conjunction with albumin. Aldosterone antagonists are the diuretics of choice since edema is related to inadequate detoxification of aldosterone. Intake–output records should be maintained and electrolyte values and skin turgor assessed. The client should be weighed and girth measured daily to assess fluid volume status; weight loss should not exceed half a pound (0.23 kg) a day. Greater losses may result in a shift of fluids into the abdominal cavity, may promote electrolyte imbalance, and may precipitate hepatic encephalopathy.

In the client with ascites, accumulated fluid may stretch the skin so tightly that it tears. The client should be urged to avoid restrictive clothing, take good care of the skin, and change positions frequently. Place a pillow under the costal margin for support if the client is lying on his or her side.

Support hose should be worn and the limbs elevated frequently to minimize peripheral edema. When seated, clients should be warned to support their legs, not to cross them or let them dangle.

A fluid deficit may occur, for example, during episodes of variceal hemorrhage. Lost blood must be replaced and vital signs closely monitored.

Evaluation

Expected outcomes related to fluid volume include good skin turgor, decreased circumference of edematous extremities or abdominal girth, and intake and output measurements indicative of correction of a fluid volume alteration. Correction of fluid volume alterations may take a long time, and several plans and revisions may be required.

Tissue Perfusion, Altered: Cardiopulmonary

Increased cardiac output associated with hypertension is related to fluid volume alterations. Erythrocytopenia can lead to increased cardiac output as the heart attempts to compensate for tissue oxygen needs.

Planning and Implementation

Tissue perfusion may be improved by correcting anemia; iron supplements, vitamins B_{12} and K, and blood transfusions can be administered. When hemoglobin and hematocrit values are restored to normal levels, the heart pumps blood throughout the body more efficiently. Ecchymoses and gingival hemorrhage may indicate vitamin K deficiency. If the client has coagulation disorders, injections—especially intramuscular injections—should be avoided whenever possible, and pressure should be applied after any injection is given. Decreasing fluid overload, if present, will improve cardiac output.

Evaluation

A blood pressure no greater than 140/80 mm Hg and normal hemoglobin and prothrombin time are indications of adequate tissue perfusion. Hemoglobin and hematocrit values and blood pressure readings can be deceiving if vascular dehydration is present.

Chapter Highlights

When interviewing the client to assess for hepatic or biliary dysfunction, ask about bowel habits, yellowing or itching of the skin, swelling of the ankles, diet patterns, drinking habits, and exposure to hepatitis or toxic chemicals.

Diagnostic studies used for clients with known or suspected hepatic or biliary dysfunction include ultrasound, radionuclide scanning, dye clearance studies, oral cholecystography, intravenous cholangiography, endoscopic retrograde cholangiopancreatography (ERCP), percutaneous transhepatic cholangiography (PTHC), and T-tube and operative cholangiography.

For the client with alteration in comfort related to pruritus, promoting comfort includes ruling out allergy, encouraging rest and a well-balanced diet, providing ventilation and dry clothing and linen, avoiding frequent baths and alkaline soaps, applying emollients, and keeping fingernails short.

Nursing measures related to relief of pain for the client with hepatic–biliary dysfunction include administering analgesics appropriate to the source and severity of pain, avoiding hepatotoxic analgesics, and providing nursing comfort measures.

Nursing measures related to maintenance of skin integrity include providing a high-protein diet

(unless ammonia toxicity is present), relieving pruritus, repositioning and turning the client with edema every one to two hours, and providing good skin care.

Helping the client with hepatic or biliary disease maintain satisfactory mentation involves assessing for changes in mental status; instituting safety measures; providing a low-protein diet; preventing aspiration of blood from variceal hemorrhage; giving tap water or neomycin enemas; and administering potassium, neomycin, or lactulose as prescribed.

Nursing measures to overcome nutritional deficiencies include encouraging intake of a well-balanced diet high in potassium, vitamins, carbohydrates, and protein (if appropriate), and low in sodium.

Promoting adequate O_2/CO_2 exchange in the client with hepatic or biliary dysfunction involves proper positioning for adequate expansion of the diaphragm; administering diuretics and albumin to correct edema; assisting with paracentesis; and administering iron, vitamin K, and blood transfusions as ordered.

Nursing measures to promote normalizing of fluid volume include administering albumin and diuretics, weighing the client and measuring abdominal girth daily, recording intake and output, and monitoring skin turgor and possible hemorrhage of esophageal varices.

Nursing measures to promote adequate tissue perfusion in clients with hepatic and biliary disorders include correction of fluid overload by administering diuretics as ordered and correcting low hemoglobin and hematocrit values by administering iron, vitamins K and B_{12}, and transfusions of packed red cells as prescribed.

Bibliography

Byrne CJ et al: *Laboratory Tests: Implications for Nursing Care.* 2nd ed. Menlo Park, CA: Addison–Wesley, 1986.

Fishbein RH: What the nonsurgeon should know about cholecystectomy. *Hosp Medicine* 1985; 21(1):197–201.

Gannon RB, Pickett K: Jaundice. *Am J Nurs* 1983; 83(3):404–407.

Gever LN: Lactulose: A crucial element in treating hepatic encephalopathy. *Nurs 82* 1982; 12(8):76–78.

Hawks JEH: Alcoholism: An overview. *Plast Surg Nurs* 1983; 3:49–52.

King DE: How to give your portal hypertension patients a fighting chance. *RN,* July 1983: 31–37.

Laing F: Diagnostic evaluation of patients with suspected cholecystitis. *Surg Clin NA* 1984; 64(7):3–22.

Malseed RT: *Pharmacology: Drug Therapy and Nursing Considerations.* Philadelphia: Lippincott, 1982.

Pagana KD, Pagana TJ: *Diagnostic Testing and Nursing Implications.* St. Louis, MO: Mosby, 1982.

Quinless F: Portal hypertension: Physiology, signs and symptoms. *Nurs 84* 1984; 14(1):52–53.

Sherlock S: *Diseases of the Liver and Biliary System,* 7th ed. Oxford: Blackwell, 1985.

Smith CE: Assessing the liver. *Nurs 85* 1985; 15(7):36–37.

Resources

ORGANIZATIONS AND SELF-HELP GROUPS

American Digestive Disease Society
(Includes gallbladder disease; see Resources in Chapter 41.)

American Liver Foundation
998 Pompton Ave
Cedar Grove, NJ 07009
Phone: (201) 857–2626

This volunteer-run agency funds research, education, and training programs for the public and professionals and programs for detecting and treating liver disease.

For clients with cancer refer to the resources list at the end of Chapter 10.

For alcoholic clients refer to the resources list at the end of Chapter 8.

HEALTH EDUCATION MATERIALS

Krames Communications
312 90th St.
Daly City, CA 94015–1898
Phone: (415) 994–8800

This organization provides the following client education materials:

The Gallbladder Book, in English or Spanish

Abdominal Sonogram, in English or Spanish

Oral Cholecystogram, in English or Spanish

CHAPTER 41

Specific Disorders of the Hepatic–Biliary System

Other topics relevant to this content are: Care of the client undergoing paracentesis, **Chapter 40.**

Objectives

When you have finished studying this chapter, you should be able to:

Identify nursing, medical, surgical, and pharmacologic measures for clients with cirrhosis.

Compare and contrast type A; type B; type non-A, non-B; toxic; drug-induced; and chronic active forms of hepatitis.

Discuss risk factors, symptoms and signs, and pharmacologic, surgical, and nursing management of cholecystitis and cholelithiasis.

Explain the complications of hepatic–biliary system surgery and the related nursing interventions.

Explain the circumstances associated with carcinoma of the hepatic–biliary system and interventions for these clients.

Specific disorders of the hepatic–biliary system include some life-threatening illnesses with long-term implications, for example, cirrhosis. Viral hepatitis is a disease with increasing incidence, and one for which health care providers are at risk. Disorders of the hepatic–biliary system can be generally classified as multifactorial in origin, infectious, neoplastic and obstructive.

Surgical procedures involving the hepatic–biliary system have serious implications related to the compromised status of the client. Impaired synthesis of coagulation factors, often associated with poor absorption of vitamin K in the absence of bile, renders the client susceptible to hemorrhage. Moreover, impaired hepatic function is generally associated with metabolic imbalances. For these reasons, the client undergoing any surgical treatment for hepatic or biliary disease must be closely observed to avert and treat complications.

SECTION 

Disorders of Multifactorial Origin

Disorders of multifactorial origin are those for which no single, specific etiologic agent has been identified. For the hepatic–biliary system, cirrhosis is the major disease process of multifactorial origin.

Cirrhosis

Cirrhosis is a chronic process in which the normal configuration of liver lobules is disrupted. Cell death occurs, and regeneration is associated with scarring. Nodular cells formed during regeneration distort the morphology of the liver and obstruct hepatic flow of blood and lymph. Eventually, cirrhosis leads to hepatic failure and portal hypertension.

Cirrhosis may be classified as (1) Laennec's cirrhosis, (2) biliary cirrhosis, or (3) postnecrotic cirrhosis. Laennec's cirrhosis is usually caused by chronic alcohol abuse. Biliary cirrhosis is related to prolonged obstructive jaundice or to an infection that ascends from the gallbladder to the small bile ducts by way of the hepatic duct. Postnecrotic cirrhosis is related to formation of scar tissue following hepatitis or hepatic abscess.

Clinical Manifestations

With histologic examination of the cirrhotic liver, fatty infiltration, cellular necrosis, and disruption of the lobes are seen. Gross inspection reveals a "hobnail" appearance; the hepatic surface is often stippled and nodular, somewhat like a football.

Portal hypertension results in compensatory development of collateral blood vessels in the esophagus. These vessels, called esophageal varices, dilate as portal hypertension increases. Because such vessels are inadequate to accommodate the increased blood flow, hemorrhage may occur. The client with cirrhosis has a characteristic appearance: The skin is orange-yellow, the eyes are sunken, and the facial bones are prominent. The limbs are emaciated, whereas the abdomen is enlarged due to ascites.

Medical Measures

Therapeutic measures in treatment of cirrhosis include those discussed in Chapter 40: analgesic, antiemetic, and diuretic therapies; nutritional interventions; and treatments directed at controlling variceal hemorrhage and ascites. Pharmacologic therapies commonly used in cirrhosis are listed in Box 41–1.

Esophageal variceal hemorrhage may be controlled temporarily by administering infusions of vasopressin (Pitressin) to promote diffuse arterial vasoconstriction and to lower portal pressure by constricting the splanchnic arterial bed. The infusion may be given systemically or via the superior mesenteric artery. Either method provides only temporary control and is associated with complications, including systemic arterial hypertension and coronary vasoconstriction possibly leading to myocardial infarction.

Box 41–1
Pharmacologic Agents Commonly Used in Treatment of Cirrhosis

Albumin	Lactulose
Aldosterone antagonist diuretics	Neomycin
Anticholinergics	Potassium
Antiemetics	Propranolol (Inderal)
Diphenhydramine (Benadryl)	Vitamin K
Emollients	

If vasopressin administration is unsuccessful, gastric lavage with ice-cold saline, use of the Minnesota tube or Sengstaken–Blakemore tube, or portal-systemic shunting may be implemented to control bleeding temporarily. A Sengstaken–Blakemore tube has three lumens: one suctions gastric contents, one inflates a gastric balloon, and one inflates an esophageal balloon (Figure 41–1). The Min-

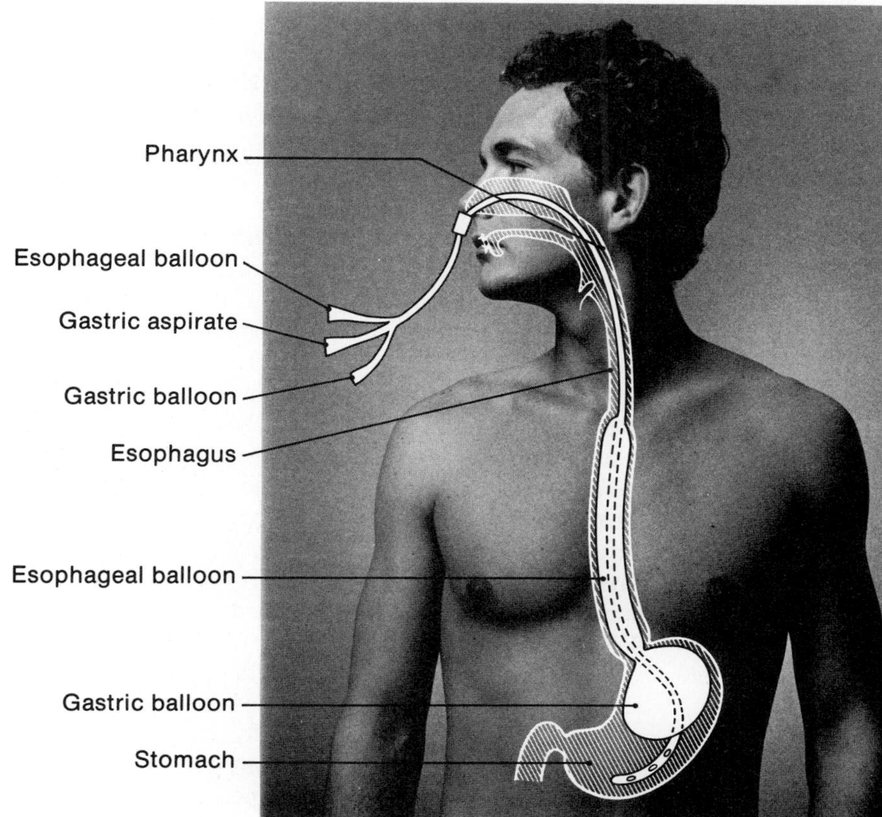

Figure 41–1

Triple-lumen esophageal–nasogastric (Sengstaken–Blakemore) tube. SOURCE: *Swearingen PL:* The Addison–Wesley Photo-Atlas of Nursing Procedures. *Menlo Park, CA: Addison–Wesley, 1984, p. 228.*

NURSING DIAGNOSES IN
Hepatic–Biliary Dysfunction

DIRECTLY RELATED DIAGNOSES

- Comfort, altered: pain, pruritus
- Fluid volume deficit
- Fluid volume excess
- Gas exchange, impaired
- Nutrition, altered: less than body requirements
- Self-concept, disturbance in: body image
- Skin integrity, impaired: potential
- Thought processes, altered
- Tissue perfusion, altered: cardiopulmonary

OTHER POTENTIAL DIAGNOSES

- Breathing pattern, ineffective
- Coping, ineffective family disabled
- Coping, ineffective individual
- Knowledge deficit
- Self-concept, disturbance in: self-esteem
- Sleep pattern disturbance
- Sexuality, altered patterns

nesota tube has a fourth lumen used to aspirate esophageal contents. Shunts are discussed later in this chapter.

Injection sclerotherapy, an alternative long-term control measure, may be performed as a bedside procedure with the client sedated with diazepam (Valium) or meperidine hydrochloride (Demerol). Sclerosing solutions are injected directly into the bleeding varices by means of fiberoptic endoscopy. Various solutions are used; an example is 5% sodium morrhuate, alone or with bovine thrombin. Complications include chest pain, transient fever, ulceration of the injection sites, and formation of strictures. Most are self-resolving; strictures may be treated by dilatation. Perforation, a major complication, is rare, since the instruments used are flexible. If perforation does occur, it is treated by keeping the client NPO, suctioning gastric contents, and administering antibiotic therapy; surgery is seldom required.

Specific Nursing Measures

Nursing care for the client with cirrhosis generally requires interventions for all the nursing diagnoses identified in Chapter 40. It is important to emphasize that clients with cirrhosis must abstain from alcohol. They are plagued with jaundice and associated pruritus, ammonia toxicity, ascites, edema, and hemorrhagic tendencies, especially in the gastointestinal tract. Because cirrhosis is a chronic condition, most nursing interventions will be related to the client's comfort. Teaching clients and the public about the effects of alcohol may have preventive benefits. A case study of a client with cirrhosis is presented at the end of this chapter.

Nursing measures for clients with esophageal hemorrhage include explaining treatments to the client and assessing frequently to determine whether hemorrhage has ceased. As with any hemorrhage, the nurse is responsible for monitoring blood replacement therapy. Bleeding esophageal varices create a crisis for client and family. Timely explanations of ongoing interventions and anticipated results will help the client cope with panic and fear of death. Providing nursing care in a decisive, supportive manner helps the client regain control and participate in the therapy. To provide optimum crisis care, assess the family support structure and provide information and support to significant others as well as to the client.

Portacaval and Portal–Systemic Shunts

The purpose of these shunt procedures is to decompress esophageal varices and maintain optimal portal perfusion. Clients with portal hypertension are poor surgical risks; however, continued episodes of variceal hemorrhage are associated with an equal or higher mortality rate than the surgery.

A *portacaval shunt* permits blood to flow directly into the inferior vena cava so it no longer needs to circumvent the scarred hepatic cells by way of the collateral circulation. A *portal–systemic shunt* (such as splenorenal shunt) connects the splenic vein to the renal vein also bypassing the scarred hepatic cells. Since pressure in the portal system is reduced, dilation of the esophageal varices is also reduced, decreasing the risk of hemorrhage. Various types of shunting procedures may be performed, depending on the pathologic condition.

Schematic illustrations of some shunt procedures are presented in Figure 41–2. Indications for various shunt procedures and their advantages and limitations are compared in Table 41–1. Implications for the client are summarized in Table 41–2.

Nursing Implications

PREOPERATIVE CARE Nutritional, fluid, and coagulation abnormalities should be corrected before surgery. Laboratory studies include serum albumin, serum bilirubin, electrolyte values, and prothrombin time. Diagnostic studies such as endoscopy, arteriography, upper gastrointestinal series, and esophagography may be ordered to locate esophageal varices. Prepare the client for these procedures physically and psychologically and explain how they are done. Also prepare the client and family for temporary memory loss, confusion, and lethargy from decrease in hepatic function. Assessment of the course of the client's illness, possible substance abuse, behavioral patterns, nutritional status, and sexual function will aid the nurse in determining the client's needs.

Immediately prior to surgery, effective plasma volume should be established, a nasogastric tube inserted, a central venous line started, and prophylactic antibiotics and steroids administered. Transfusions are almost always required, so the client should be typed and cross-matched for several units of whole blood and packed cells.

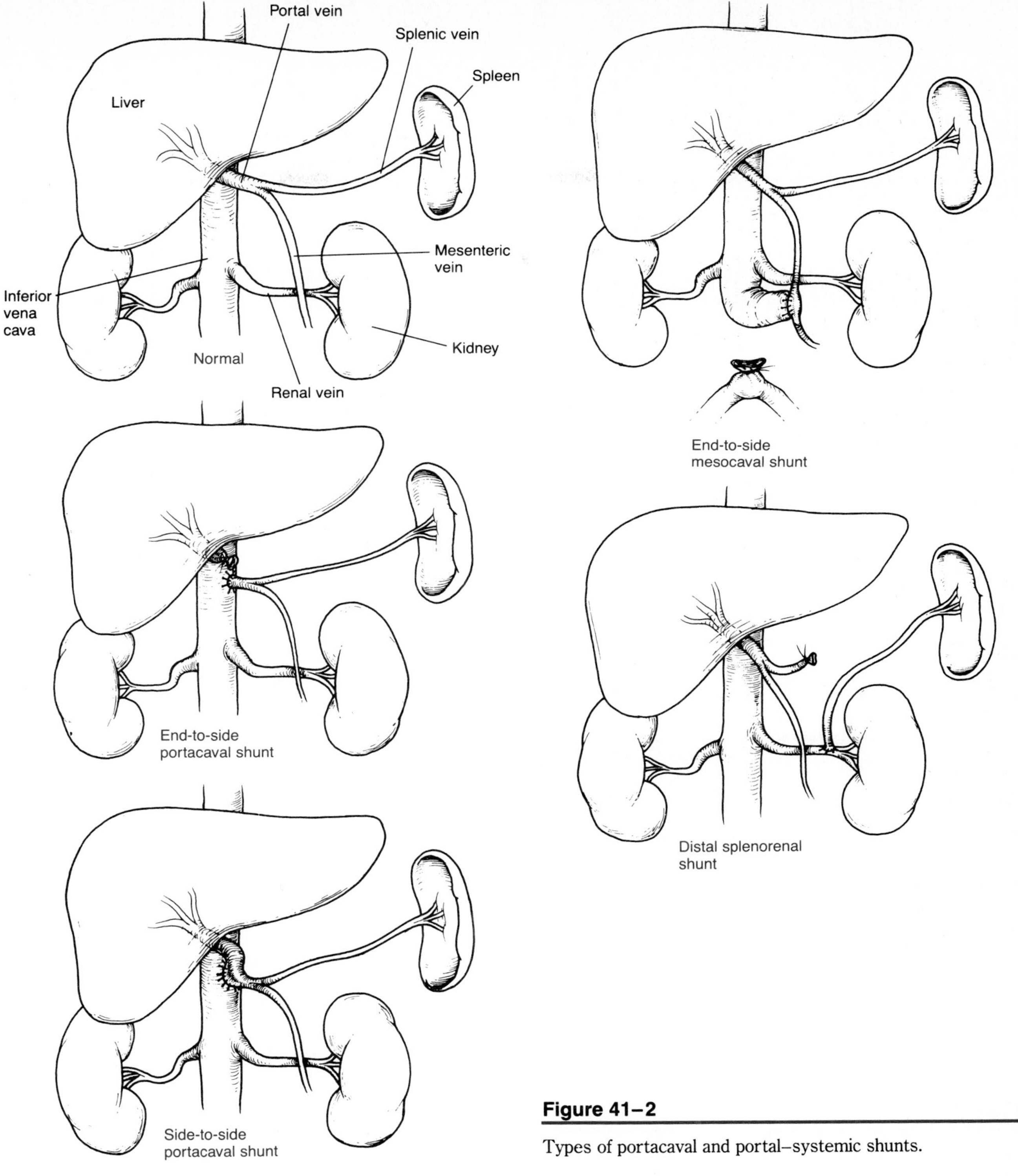

Figure 41–2

Types of portacaval and portal–systemic shunts.

POSTOPERATIVE CARE The client will be kept in an intensive care unit for several days for observation and management of complications. For the confused, restless client with encephalopathy, assess neurologic status every 4 hours, provide a safe environment, reorient often to reality, see that protein intake has been restricted, and administer neomycin and lactulose as prescribed.

If injections cannot be avoided, small-gauge needles should be used. Vitamin K administration may be ordered to decrease the risk of hemorrhage. Both stools and secretions from the nasogastic tube should be regularly tested for indications of internal hemorrhage; platelets may have to be administered. Blood glucose levels should be monitored since it may be necessary to administer glucose if hypoglycemia occurs. Total parenteral nutrition with amino acid solution (Travasol) and 25% dextrose with added vitamins, minerals, and trace elements may be used to maintain blood glucose levels and to correct nutritional defi-

Table 41–1
Comparison of Portacaval and Portal–Systemic Shunt Procedures

Procedure	Purpose	Indications	Advantages	Limitations
End-to-side portacaval shunt	Joins inferior vena cava with portal vein	Emergency Little ascites Portal vein patent	Decreases portal pressure and probability of variceal rebleeding	Interrupted portal perfusion Encephalopathy Toxins not detoxified
Side-to-side portacaval shunt	Joins inferior vena cava with portal vein	Problem ascites Hepatic vein thrombosis	Decreases portal pressure and probability of variceal rebleeding	Interrupted portal perfusion More difficult to construct
End-to-side mesocaval shunt	Joins inferior vena cava and mesenteric veins	Problem ascites Portal vein obstruction	Useful when portal vein not available	Reversal of hepatic artery flow Decreased venous drainage of lower limbs
Distal splenorenal shunt	Joins splenic vein and left renal vein	No ascites Normal hepatic function Idiopathic portal hypertension	Shunt usually stays patent	Difficult to construct Diminished portal flow

Table 41–2
Portacaval and Portal–Systemic Shunt Procedures: Implications for the Client

Physiologic Implications	Psychosocial/Lifestyle Implications
Nutritional imbalances Decreased oxygenation Peripheral edema after mesocaval shunt Decreased fluid volume Increased clotting time Hepatic encephalopathy is a possible complication	Nutritious diet required Abstention from alcohol Encephalopathy and temporary decrease in hepatic function may cause memory loss, confusion, and lethargy in early postoperative period Altered sexual function Limitation of activity as for any abdominal surgery

ciencies. A low-sodium diet or intravenous infusions may be prescribed to minimize peripheral edema and ascites formation.

LeVeen Shunt

The *LeVeen shunt* provides a route for reinfusion of ascitic fluid into the venous system. It operates according to a simple principle of physics: *Matter flows along a pressure gradient from areas of high pressure to low.* When properly positioned, the shunt runs from the abdominal cavity through the peritoneum and under the subcutaneous tissue into the superior vena cava. Figure 41–3 illustrates a shunt in place, showing its main components—a perforated peritoneal tube, a valve consisting of a one-way diaphragm supported by rubber struts, and a venous catheter.

The valve remains open only so long as pressure in the peritoneal cavity is at least 3 cm H_2O higher than pressure in the superior vena cava. (Thus, if the client's vascular system is overloaded, the valve remains closed, avoiding further overload.) At this pressure, the valve struts flex, moving the diaphragm away from the tube to allow ascitic fluid to pass into the venous catheter.

During inspiration, pressure in the intraperitoneal cavity usually rises to about 5 cm H_2O higher than pressure in the vena cava, and ascitic fluid moves along the pressure gradient from the abdomen into the venous circulation. On expiration, the pressure drops, and the valve closes.

A modified version of the LeVeen shunt is the *Denver shunt.* With the Denver shunt, an internal bulb is positioned so it can be felt externally and pumped to increase intraperitoneal pressure and force fluid into the vena cava.

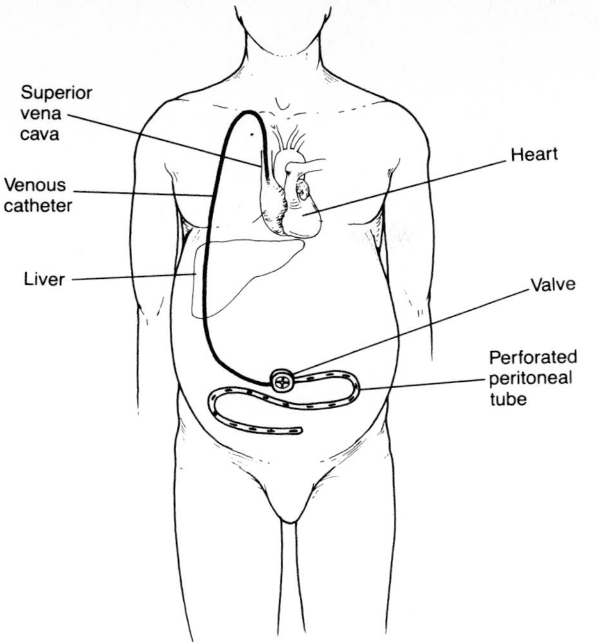

Figure 41–3

Anterior view of client with LeVeen shunt in place.

The Denver shunt may be used for clients who are unable to practive breathing exercises to enhance fluid movement. It is the preferred shunt for treatment of ascites related to a malignancy. The physiologic and psychosocial/lifestyle implications of the LeVeen shunt for the client are discussed in Table 41–3.

Nursing Implications

PREOPERATIVE CARE The client's weight must be checked and recorded daily before breakfast. Comparison of daily weight will identify any fluid gain and will provide a baseline for measuring fluid loss after the procedure. Measure abdominal girth at the umbilical level daily for the same reasons. Accurate intake–output records are also necessary to establish a baseline for determining fluid loss after surgery. Prophylactic antibiotic therapy is started 24 hours before surgery.

Several laboratory tests are done before surgery: 24-hour urine collections to test for electrolyte imbalances; ascitic fluid is chemically analyzed; and liver function tests, bilirubin, BUN, creatinine, serum protein and electrolyte studies, a complete blood count (CBC), and prothrombin time. If CBC values show anemia, the client should receive a transfusion of packed red cells to bring hematocrit levels up to normal before surgery. Vitamin K is indicated if prothrombin times are too long.

POSTOPERATIVE CARE Several preoperative measures are continued postoperatively. Weigh the client immediately after the operation and then daily. Measure and record abdominal girth daily. Urine output is recorded hourly.

Furosemide may be administered immediately after surgery and again if urine output falls or peripheral edema is evident. Hematocrit values are monitored every 4 hours during the first postoperative day so the extent of hemodilution can be evaluated. A transfusion of packed red cells may be ordered. A vein is kept open for quick access if complications arise. To prevent fluid overload, a minidrip tubing setup is preferred, although infusion pumps may also be used. The amount infused should not exceed 125 mL per 8 hours.

After the first 24 hours, tightly apply an abdominal binder to promote removal of fluid. Intake–output records, prophylactic antibiotic therapy, and 24-hour urine collections are also continued. Ascitic fluid for analysis is drawn once daily for 2 days and then weekly.

Teach the client how to inhale against resistance to facilitate the flow of ascitic fluid through the shunt. Having the client use a blow bottle will make instruction easier. The client begins eating a regular low-salt diet. If signs of ammonia toxicity are present, the diet may also be low in protein. Potassium supplementation may be ordered

Table 41–3
LeVeen Shunt: Implications for the Client 

Physiologic Implications	Psychosocial/Lifestyle Implications
Hemodilution during the first postoperative week results in decreased hematocrit	Abstention from alcohol
Cardiac overload, congestive heart failure, and renal overload are possible complications	Low-salt diet
Septicemia, wound infection can occur	Breathing exercises to facilitate flow of ascitic fluid through shunt
Hemorrhage, occlusion of the shunt, disseminated intravascular coagulation (DIC), and extravasation of ascitic fluid from incision sites are other possible complications	Resumption of ADL and self-care as ascites is gradually reduced
Relief of dyspnea	Improved appearance

if hypokalemia develops. Monitoring for complications such as those listed in Table 41–3 is a continuing responsibility.

Discharge planning includes dietary instuction, which may reinforce the dietitian's teaching or may originate with the nurse. Clients should demonstrate ability to do the breathing exercises and must be shown how to maintain records of daily weights and temperatures. Reassure clients that daily living activities, including sexual relations, can be resumed as tolerated.

SECTION II

Infectious and Inflammatory Disorders

Viral Hepatitis

Hepatitis is an inflammation of the liver. The viral forms of hepatitis may be classified as type A, type B, or non-A, non-B. The viruses responsible for hepatitis A and B have been identified; the virus or viruses responsible for non-A, non-B hepatitis are not yet known (Table 41–4). Hepatitis A and B are characterized by three stages: prodromal, icteric, and recovery. (Non-A, non-B hepatitis is often not associated with icterus.) The prodromal (preicteric) stage lasts 1 to 3 weeks; the icteric or jaundiced stage lasts 6 to 8 weeks, and the recovery stage may last from 3 to 4 months. The three types of viral hepatitis are discussed separately.

Hepatitis A (Infectious Hepatitis)

Hepatitis A, an infectious hepatitis associated with brief incubation (3 to 5 weeks) and low mortality (1% or less), is known to be caused by an RNA virus. Outbreaks of hepatitis A have occurred in institutional settings in association with poor sanitation and a large population. The virus is found in blood, feces, saliva, and urine of infected individuals, and transmission is usually by the fecal–oral route. Raw shellfish from polluted waters may also carry the virus. The type A virus may be transmitted from person to person or by way of contaminated water or food. Young adults (15 to 29 years), middle-aged adults, and persons living in crowded conditions appear more susceptible to the type A virus. Washing hands after bowel movements and before eating, and environmental sanitation are the most effective means of preventing the spread of hepatitis A.

CLINICAL MANIFESTATIONS Flulike symptoms may occur in the preicteric stage, including headache, fatigue, malaise, anorexia, pruritus, weakness, fever, and aversion to cigarettes. Sometimes, however, the client is asymptomatic. At the end of the preicteric stage, the urine appears mahogany colored and the stools are acholic. During the second (icteric) stage, the urine remains dark, the stools light. The skin usually appears jaundiced, and the liver and spleen are swollen and tender. Laboratory studies will show elevated white blood count (WBC), SGOT, SGPT, alkaline

Table 41–4
Comparison of Types of Viral Hepatitis

	Hepatitis A	Hepatitis B	Non-A, Non-B Hepatitis
Cause	Type A virus	Type B virus	Unidentified virus
Incubation period	3–5 weeks	5–25 weeks	2–23 weeks
Carrier	No	Yes	Yes
Chronicity	No	Yes	Yes
Type of virus	RNA	DNA	Unknown
Transmission	Feces, blood	Blood and body fluids (semen; vaginal, oral, and nasal secretions; breast milk, CSF)	Blood
Symptoms	May have none. Flulike, headache, fatigue, anorexia, fever, dark urine, jaundice, hepatomegaly, aversion to cigarettes	More severe than hepatitis A. Fever, rash, arthralgia, headache, aversion to cigarettes, hepatomegaly, dark urine, jaundice, fatigue, anorexia	Similar to hepatitis B. Often no jaundice
Prevention	Immune serum globulin after exposure	Hepatitis B immune globulin after exposure; hepatitis B vaccine before exposure	None

phosphatase, and indirect bilirubin levels. Serum protein and lipid values will be slightly below normal.

MEDICAL MEASURES Medical measures are directed at relieving symptoms. Vitamin K may be prescribed if coagulation abnormalities are found. Frequent high-calorie meals, intravenous fluids, and restricted physical activity are common treatment approaches.

Anyone who comes in contact with hepatitis A should receive intramuscular administrations of immune serum globulin (ISG) or gamma globulin within 1 week. Gamma globulin or ISG provides immunity for 6 to 8 weeks. The usual dosage is 0.02 mL/kg of body weight. Smaller dosages are sometimes administered prophylactically every 2 to 3 months to persons at high risk—for example, health care personnel who work with many clients with hepatitis.

Home Health Care

SPECIFIC NURSING MEASURES Persons with hepatitis A may often be cared for at home. Hospitalized clients will require interventions for alterations in comfort (pruritus and pain), nutritional intake, and fluid volume; impairment of skin integrity and O_2/CO_2 exchange; and disturbances in self-concept. (See Chapter 46.) In addition to these measures, the client with hepatitis A is placed in enteric isolation. The nurse must wear gloves when in contact with fecal matter, bedpan, or linens soiled with stool. Persons giving care in the home should also wear gloves if contact with feces is possible. Gloves should be worn in any situation where gross soiling occurs. Careful attention to handwashing is essential for clients and for those giving care.

Discharge planning for hospitalized clients includes encouraging the client to get ample rest, ingest a well-balanced diet, drink at least 3000 mL of fluid per day, and avoid alcohol and OTC medications for at least 6 months. These clients should be told they will have a lifetime immunity to hepatitis A virus. There is no chronic carrier state with hepatitis A. The client will not progress to chronic hepatitis or cirrhosis.

Hepatitis B (Serum Hepatitis)

The hepatitis B virus, a DNA virus, usually causes a more serious form of the disease. The incubation period for hepatitis B (also called serum hepatitis or long-incubation hepatitis) is long—5 to 25 weeks, and the mortality rate is 1% to 10% (Gurevich, 1983). Incidence of hepatitis B is higher in populations of individuals who have received blood transfusions, in recreational drug users who may share infected needles or syringes, and in homosexuals. All ages are affected, but young adults appear most susceptible.

The virus may be found in blood, saliva, tears, nasal secretions, breast milk, semen, and vaginal secretions of infected individuals and in blood-sucking insects that have ingested the virus from infected persons. The disease may be contracted via the parenteral route (eg, during blood transfusion, by injection, or during hemodialysis), by intimate contact with carriers or persons acutely ill with the disease, from contaminated instruments, or by transmission from mother to infant. Hepatitis B carriers may be asymptomatic.

Less than 1 mL of blood is required to transmit infection. Health care personnel who have any break in skin integrity can readily contract the disease from contaminated secretions. Tattooing and ear piercing have been associated with hepatitis B.

CLINICAL MANIFESTATIONS Hepatitis B is characterized by many of the same symptoms as hepatitis A, but in more virulent form. Clients who recover sometimes develop chronic hepatitis. Development of a subclinical carrier state is also possible with hepatitis B. General malaise, arthralgia, rash, pruritus, gastrointestinal symptoms, and hepatomegaly are common in the prodromal stage. Severe nausea and vomiting accompany jaundice in the icteric stage. Common laboratory findings include elevated WBC, SGOT, andf SGPT levels as well as elevated alkaline phosphatase and indirect serum bilirubin. The presence of hepatitis B surface antigen (HBsAg) is diagnostic of the disease.

MEDICAL MEASURES Medical measures for treatment of hepatitis B may include intravenous fluids and electrolytes, since the anorexia associated with the disease can cause dehydration and electrolyte imbalance. Vitamin K is given to most clients, and various measures for relief of symptoms may be prescribed such as antihistamines for pruritus and antiemetics for nausea and vomiting.

PREVENTIVE MEASURES Persons at high risk for exposure to hepatitis B include health care professionals working in dialysis units, emergency rooms, and operating rooms. Also at increased risk are intravenous therapy nurses, oral surgeons, dental hygienists, and medical technolo-

Nursing Research Note

James AM et al: A survey of hepatitis B vaccination programs for hospital employees. *Am J Infect Control* 1985; 13(1):32–34.

A survey of county hospitals in Los Angeles determined community practice regarding hepatitis B virus screening and immunization of employees. Only 33% of the hospitals had an immunization policy, and 73% of these planned to screen their employees. The hepatitis B virus vaccine became available in June 1982, and policies were left to the discretion of the individual hospitals because risks varied among hospitals.

The vaccine continues to be controversial because of the cost of the screening and the vaccination serum itself. Nurses who work in high-risk areas where exposure to hepatitis B virus is prevalent should read the literature about its efficacy. Nurses should also inquire about their hospital's policies regarding hepatitis immunization.

gists. All nurses are at some risk by being in health care environments.

Passive immunoprophylaxis is available against hepatitis B via hyperimmune globulin or hepatitis B immune globulin (HBIG). For example, with a needle-stick injury, passive immunoprophylaxis may be given with HBIG. HBIG must be given as soon as possible after exposure, preferably within seven days. The recommended prophylactic dose of HBIG is two IM injections—0.06 mL/kg of body weight, given 30 days apart.

Until recently, no safe active vaccine was available against hepatitis B. Now there is a live vaccine, which enables recipients to develop antibodies against the disease. It is given in 3 IM dosages (initial dose, second dose one month later, third dose 6 months after initial dose) in the deltoid muscle. Gluteal IM administration should not be used because of erratic absorption of vaccine. It is known to be effective for up to 5 years and perhaps much longer. There seem to be no major risks from hepatitis B vaccine. The question has been raised whether AIDS can be contracted from the vaccine because the vaccine is made from the plasma of human hepatitis B carriers, who may be gay men. To date there are no known cases of AIDS resulting from hepatitis B vaccine.

Home Health Care

SPECIFIC NURSING MEASURES Rest, frequent high-calorie meals, and at least 3000 mL of fluid per day are important to recovery. Hepatotoxic medications must be avoided. Whether the client is hospitalized or at home, caregivers should avoid direct contact with any of the client's bodily fluids. Gloves should be worn when handling the client's eating utensils, soiled tissues, linens, wash cloths, bath towels, and underwear. The nurse should be particularly careful when giving injections, drawing blood, or removing intravenous tubing to avoid needle-stick injuries or direct contact with the client's serum. For protection of other health care workers and housekeeping personnel, extreme care must be observed in disposal of needles and IV equipment.

Discharge teaching includes cautioning clients not to donate blood, informing them that they will have lifetime immunity to hepatitis B following recovery, and encouraging them to get adequate rest. Clients must be cautioned not to engage in sexual relations until serum liver function tests return to normal (which could be as long as 3 to 4 months) because semen and vaginal secretions will infect others. If sexual contact does occur, clients should use protective barrier measures such as condoms, although there is no guarantee that these are totally protective. The client should abstain from hepatotoxins such as alcohol and avoid OTC medications such as acetaminophen.

Non-A, Non-B Hepatitis

Non-A, non-B hepatitis affects all ages. It has been seen most often in persons who have had fifteen or more blood transfusions and in drug abusers who use injected substances. The incubation period is 14 to 160 days, with the mean being about 50 days. Non-A, non-B hepatitis is more lethal than hepatitis A and B and may progress to chronic hepatitis.

CLINICAL MANIFESTATIONS As with other types of hepatitis, there are inflammation of hepatic cells, hypertrophy of Kupffer cells, and bile stasis. During the prodromal phase, the client experiences malaise, anorexia, headache, and lassitude and is febrile. Later, hepatomegaly, liver tenderness, and arthralgia occur. The client is often without icterus.

MEDICAL AND SPECIFIC NURSING MEASURES Adequate hydration, nutrition, and rest are essential for recovery. The client with non-A, non-B hepatitis is usually hospitalized because of the need for intravenous fluid replacement, tube feedings or total parenteral nutrition, relief from pruritus, and rest. Vitamin K is prescribed to correct coagulation abnormalities.

Extreme care must be taken with needle punctures to avoid hemorrhage or spread of the disease. Blood isolation precautions are observed, but enteric isolation is not necessary, since the disease is blood borne. Other nursing activities are similar to those already described.

Since blood transfusions are associated with risk of contracting non-A, non-B hepatitis, nurses may wish to suggest to clients planning to have elective surgery that they donate their own blood for use if transfusions are necessary.

Toxic and Drug-Induced Hepatitis

Certain agents, including carbon tetrachloride, yellow phosphorus, and acetaminophen (in large doses) are hepatotoxins. When ingested or inhaled they cause necrosis of hepatic cells. Hepatitis related to these substances is called toxic hepatitis.

Varying patterns of hepatic dysfunction are seen in response to use of other drugs and anesthetic agents. For example, halothane, methyldopa, and isoniazid can produce a reaction indistinguishable from viral hepatitis. Chlorpromazine, erythromycin estolate, and methimazole can cause intrahepatic cholestasis with jaundice. Phenylbutazone and the sulfonamides can produce granulomas within the liver. (A list of drugs and other agents associated with hepatic damage is found in Box 40–1.)

Clinical Manifestations

Both drug-induced and toxic hepatitis are manifested by inflammation of hepatic cells, hyperplasia of Kupffer cells, and bile stasis; however, toxic hepatitis is associated with acute cellular necrosis. The onset of both forms is similar to that of viral hepatitis, from which they must be quickly distinguished if detoxification is to be initiated to save the client's life. Anorexia, jaundice, and hepatomegaly are common. In *toxic hepatitis,* the illness may progress rapidly, with rising fever, subdermal hemorrhage, and severe vomiting. Delirium, coma, and convulsions develop, and the client dies within a few days. If the toxin is promptly identified and exposure is discontinued, however, the client may recover quite rapidly. Cirrhosis sometimes develops after recovery.

Drug-induced hepatitis may develop after repeated exposures have sensitized the client to a drug. For this reason, any medication that causes pruritus or other symptoms of sensitivity should be immediately withdrawn and the sensitivity noted on the client's record. Chills, fever, rash, pruritus, arthralgia, and nausea are early signs of drug-induced hepatitis. Icterus, hepatomegaly, and hepatic tenderness follow. The urine is dark. Symptoms may subside once the drug is withdrawn, but drug-induced hepatitis may be fatal, and postnecrotic cirrhosis also may develop. The anesthetic agent halothane has been linked to episodes of drug-induced hepatitis; therefore, anesthetics should be rotated for clients undergoing repeated surgical procedures.

Medical and Specific Nursing Measures

Treatment is directed at removal of the toxin or sensitizing agent, if known. There are no antidotes.

Early diagnosis is important. The health history taken by the nurse yields data indicative of toxic or drug-induced hepatitis. Attention should focus on occupational history, possible exposure to hepatotoxins during hobby activities (for example, furniture refinishing), and medication history, including OTC medications and self-prescribed vitamin therapy. (Large doses of vitamins A and D may be hepatotoxic.) Once the disease has been diagnosed, nursing care focuses on comfort measures and the replacement of blood, fluids, and electrolytes.

Chronic Active Hepatitis

Chronic active hepatitis, or chronic active liver disease (CALD), is related to active inflammation with associated hepatic necrosis. Usually the person has had hepatitis B or non-A, non-B hepatitis before development of the chronic condition. CALD is usually fatal within a few years. Remissions may occur, but the client usually develops cirrhosis.

Clinical Manifestations

The client is fatigued, icteric, anorexic, anemic, and has a low-grade fever. Arthralgia and abdominal pain are common, and women may be amenorrheal. There is speculation that CALD may be related to interaction with the immune system because IgG, IgM, and IgA values are elevated. Antinuclear antibodies are also found in the serum of persons with CALD.

Medical and Specific Nursing Measures

Rest and adequate nutrition are required, and steroids may be prescribed to lessen the intensity of the immune reaction.

Cholecystitis

Cholecystitis is an inflammation of the gallbladder. It may be either acute or chronic. An acute inflammation may begin in the mucosal layer as a primary infection. More often it is superimposed on a chronic infection initially related to cholelithiasis. The gallbladder becomes dilated and filled with bile, pus, and blood. Common infective organisms include staphylococci, streptococci, and enteric organisms.

Clinical Manifestations

Major symptoms of cholecystitis are intense pain, tenderness, and rigidity in the right upper quadrant of the abdomen associated with nausea, vomiting, and the usual signs of inflammation. Jaundice may be present if there is an obstruction. If the gallbladder is filled with frankly purulent matter, the condition is called empyema of the gallbladder. Although chronic cholecystitis may be related to an acute attack, it is almost always associated with cholelithiasis.

Medical and Specific Nursing Measures

The gallbladder is usually resected after acute inflammation has been relieved by medical intervention. Surgical removal of the gallbladder (cholecystectomy) is discussed below. Because cholecystitis and cholelithiasis are closely associated, medical and nursing measures are discussed in the section on obstructive disorders.

SECTION 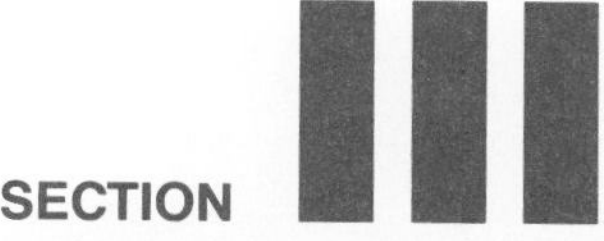

Neoplastic and Obstructive Disorders

Although hepatic and biliary neoplasia and cholelithiasis may both be classified as obstructive, the two types of obstruction have little in common. Nursing measures will therefore be discussed for each disease process.

Cancer of the Gallbladder

Cancer of the gallbladder is rare. Malignant tumors are usually columnar cell carcinomas that cause symptoms of inflammation and obstruction (Groer and Shekleton, 1983). In part because of its rarity, biliary carcinoma may be overlooked or confused with cholelithiasis.

Cancer of the Liver

Most hepatic cancer in the United States is metastatic in origin. Primary carcinoma of the liver is rare in the United States and Canada but common in Asia and Africa. The frequency of primary hepatic cancer in parts of the Third World is thought to be related to the large number of hepatitis B virus carriers in these populations. Chronic carriers are at increased risk of developing liver cancer.

Primary malignant neoplasia of the liver generally is an adenocarcinoma arising from hepatic cells or bile ducts. The larger right lobe is more often involved than the left. The lesion develops most frequently in persons aged 60 to 79, with males having 6 to 10 times the incidence of females. In addition to hepatitis B, factors associated with primary hepatic carcinoma are cirrhosis, intestinal parasites, hemochromatosis, and schistosomiasis (liver flukes).

Metastatic carcinomas are seen in over 50% of end-stage cancers. Often the tumors will enlarge the liver to seven times its normal size.

Clinical Manifestations

Symptoms and signs are not pathognomonic of cancer; instead, symptoms are related to the extent of hepatocellular damage and functional failure of the liver. Initially, the client may lose weight; later, increase in weight may be associated with ascites and fluid retention. Other manifestations are cachexia, anemia, abdominal fullness and pain, fever, hemorrhage, obstructive icterus, splenomegaly, and hepatomegaly. Liver function test results will show abnormalities.

Box 41–2
Pharmacologic Agents Commonly Used in Treatment of Hepatic Carcinoma

Chemotherapeutic agents:
- Doxorubicin HCL (Adriamycin)
- Methotrexate
- 5-fluorouracil

Aldosterone antagonist diuretics

Antiemetics

Diphenhydramine (Benadryl)

Emollients

Potassium

Brompton's cocktail

Morphine drip

Medical Measures

Severe, intractable pain frequently is associated with hepatic carcinoma; morphine drip or Brompton's cocktail may be prescribed. A low-sodium diet, tube feedings, or total parenteral nutrition may be necessary, as well as measures to alleviate other manifestations of hepatic dysfunction (for example, paracentesis; see Chapter 46). Pharmacologic agents commonly used in treating hepatic carcinoma are listed in Box 41–2.

Nonmetastatic solitary localized tumors are surgically resected. Because of the liver's capacity for regeneration, as much as 90% of liver tissue has been successfully removed. Chemotherapy is usually instituted to promote regression of the tumor and prolong client survival. Methotrexate, 5-fluorouracil, or other agents may be administered systemically or by *intrahepatic arterial line*. Arterial lines are used with increasing frequency because the drug reaches the tumor at full strength, yet partial detoxification within the hepatic cells minimizes systemic side effects. The client is kept NPO and sedated prior to intrahepatic arterial line insertion, which is done under fluoroscopic guidance. Once the catheter is inserted, it is sutured in place. X-rays are used to verify proper placement of the catheter and may be taken daily for the duration of treatment.

Insertion of the line through the abdomen into the hepatic artery or through the antecubital fossa into the brachial artery allows the client more freedom of movement. Insertion of the line via the groin into the femoral artery requires that the client be on bed rest. Chemotherapeutic agents are administered through the line for a period of about 5 days, and the catheter is removed when the chemotherapy is completed. Hemorrhage and arterial occlusion are possible complications.

Specific Nursing Measures

Preoperative care for the client having intrahepatic arterial line insertion includes instructing the client and significant others about the procedure and reviewing the results of coagulation studies. If bleeding times are prolonged, vitamin K therapy may be ordered for several days prior to the procedure.

Postoperative care includes maintaining the patency of the arterial line and monitoring for complications. A pressurized infusion containing heparin, usually in 5% dextrose and water, is continued while the line is in place. Pressure is necessary to keep the solution running and to prevent thrombosis. Check pedal or radial pulses, depending on the catheter site, every 1 to 2 hours to determine that circulation is adequate in the immobilized limb. Take vital signs every 2 to 4 hours to monitor for hemorrhage or infection. Secure all tubing connections and be sure there is no tension on the tubing. If continuity of the tubing is interrupted, hemorrhage, air embolism, or infection can occur. If the catheter is displaced, chemotherapeutic agents, most of which are toxic or caustic, might be misdirected. As a precaution, a hemostat should be kept near the client, and the client and significant others should be taught how to clamp the tubing.

Cholelithiasis

Cholelithiasis, the formation of gallstones, can lead to obstruction of the bile ducts associated with obstructive icterus and severe colicky pain. An estimated 20 million Americans have cholelithiasis, and almost 1 million new cases are diagnosed each year.

Several predisposing factors are related to development of cholelithiasis:

- Women are affected four times as frequently as men.
- Persons over 40 are affected more often than younger persons.
- Women taking oral contraceptives are twice as likely as other women to develop gallstones.
- Cholelithiasis occurs more often in multigravidas than in childless women.
- High fat intake and cholesterol saturation of bile predispose a person to cholelithiasis.
- Obesity and diabetes are associated with increased risk of gallstone formation.

Gallstones are classified as either cholesterol or pigment stones. Cholesterol stones are usually of mixed composition and contain more than 70% cholesterol plus calcium salts, bile pigments, fatty acids, and proteins. There is a high incidence of cholesterol stones in North America. Pigment stones are primarily calcium and bilirubin and contain less than 10% cholesterol. Pigment stones are less common in North America but have a high prevalence in Japan.

Clinical Manifestations

Calculi formed in the gallbladder may move into the cystic duct, the common bile duct, or even into the liver via the hepatic ducts. Calculus obstruction of the pancreatic duct can cause pancreatitis.

The most common symptom of cholelithiasis is colicky pain believed to be related to spasms of the sphincter of Oddi. Pain may also be related to obstruction and distention of a bile duct. Usually, the pain is felt in the epigastrium or the right upper quadrant of the abdomen, but it may radiate up the back between the scapulae to the right shoulder or around the abdomen to the back, making it difficult for the client to assume a comfortable position. Biliary colic may occur at varying intervals following meals or may awaken the client from sleep. Usually, symptoms occur at progressively shorter intervals after ingestion of almost any food. Occasionally, however, a single pain episode will never be repeated.

In addition to the characteristic pain, nausea and vomiting are common, as is elevated temperature. Distention of the bile ducts stimulates the vomiting center. If the common bile duct is obstructed by a calculus, greenish-yellow jaundice develops. Pruritus often develops before the jaundice is visible in the sclerae. Icterus is accompanied by acholic stools and dark, frothy urine. Ecchymoses may be evident.

Laboratory and diagnostic studies assist in confirming the diagnosis. WBC levels, direct bilirubin levels, prothrombin time, and alkaline phosphatase and serum lipid levels will be elevated. Urine urobilinogen levels will decrease, but bilirubin will be found in the urine. Cholecystography, cholangiography, or endoscopic retrograde cholangiopancreatography (ERCP) may be ordered.

Medical Measures

If symptoms are mild, a low-fat diet may be sufficient to control them. The diet should be high in proteins and carbohydrates. Depending on the client's nutritional status, intravenous glucose and protein supplementation may be indicated. A nutritious diet promotes healing and helps prevent hepatic damage. Vitamin K may be required if coagulation abnormalities are demonstrated.

If the client's serum cholesterol and triglyceride levels are markedly elevated, antilipemic agents may be prescribed. One such agent, cholestyramine (Questran), combines with bile so it is excreted and lipids are not absorbed; this drug can cause constipation. Because cholestyramine may impair absorption of other medications, they should be given 1 hour before cholestyramine. Clofibrate (Atromid-S) and niacin have also been used to reduce serum lipid levels but are associated with severe side effects.

Medications that dissolve gallstones have been used experimentally. One such agent, chenodeoxycholic acid or chenodiol has been in clinical use in many countries for some time. It is effective only for calculi formed of cholesterol; gallstones containing large amounts of calcium do not respond. The treatment is currently expensive, involving a 2-year regimen for dissolution of the calculi and maintenance therapy thereafter. Chenodiol has recently been approved for use in the United States for clients who have radiolucent pure-cholesterol stones.

Side effects may include diarrhea, hepatotoxicity, and an elevation in serum cholesterol levels. Because chenodiol may affect fetal growth and development, it should not be given to women capable of conception unless they have adequate contraceptive protection. Persons with chronic liver disorders or biliary obstruction should not receive chenodiol because of possible hepatotoxity.

If gallbladder function is impaired or if the bile ducts

Box 41–3
High-Fat Foods to Be Avoided by Clients With Cholelithiasis

- Cream and artificial creamers
- Whole milk
- Rich rolls, doughnuts, pancakes, and waffles (especially with added butter)
- Pastries
- Ice cream
- Cookies, cakes, and pies
- Fried foods
- Mayonnaise
- Avocados
- Cheese (except low-fat cottage cheese or ricotta)
- Cream soups and sauces
- Peanut butter
- Nuts
- Chocolate
- High-fat snack foods such as potato chips
- Butter, margarine, and cooking oils
- Bacon, sausage, and other fatty meats

are obstructed, surgical intervention is required. Surgical approaches to biliary obstruction are discussed below.

Specific Nursing Measures

In addition to comfort measures and administering analgesics and other prescribed medications, the nurse can consult with the dietitian and the client to work out a palatable low-fat diet. The client may find a list of foods useful (Box 41–3).

Cholecystostomy

A *cholecystostomy* is the surgical formation of an opening in the gallbladder. Calculi, bile, and purulent matter are removed and a drainage tube is sutured into place. A cholecystostomy is performed to relieve acute or chronic cholecystitis in clients who would be at great risk if cholecystectomy were performed. Implications related to cholecystostomy are summarized in Table 41–5.

Nursing Implications

PREOPERATIVE CARE Preoperative care is similar to that for any surgical procedure, including instructing the client in coughing and deep breathing.

POSTOPERATIVE CARE A major nursing responsibility in the postoperative period is connecting the drainage apparatus and ensuring its patency, sterility, and preventing dislodgment. The client will require intravenous therapy, and vitamin K may be prescribed if clotting abnormalities occur. Administration of medications and nursing measures for relief of pain, nausea, and vomiting will be required.

Pneumonia is a common complication. Assist the client with turning, coughing, and deep breathing by helping the client splint the incision and administering analgesics. Discharge instructions should include information about required medications (vitamins, anticholinergics, antispasmodics), low-fat diet, skin care, and aseptic technique for dressing changes around the drainage tube. The client should also know symptoms and signs of potential complications such as infection or dislodgement of the drainage tube, which generally remains in place until the client is well enough to tolerate a cholecystectomy.

Cholecystectomy and Choledochostomy

A *cholecystectomy* is a resection of the gallbladder. A *choledochostomy* involves incision of the common bile duct for removal of biliary calculi and the insertion of a T-tube (Figure 41–4) to allow drainage of bile and to maintain the patency of the common duct during the postsurgical period, when edema develops at the operative site. These operations are performed on some clients who have acute or chronic cholelithiasis and cholecystitis. Implications of these procedures are summarized in Table 41–6.

Nursing Implications

PREOPERATIVE CARE In addition to the usual preoperative concerns, the nurse has several further responsibilities for the client undergoing cholecystectomy and cho-

Table 41–5
Cholecystostomy: Implications for the Client 

Physiologic Implications	Psychosocial/Lifestyle Implications
Relieves pain and infection	Fat in diet restricted
Client may have problems related to deficiency of bile: coagulation problems, inadequate absorption and digestion of fats and fat-soluble vitamins	Client usually too ill to work or perform all ADL
Pneumonia and hemorrhage are possible complications	Drainage tube in place until client is well enough to tolerate surgical removal of gallbladder

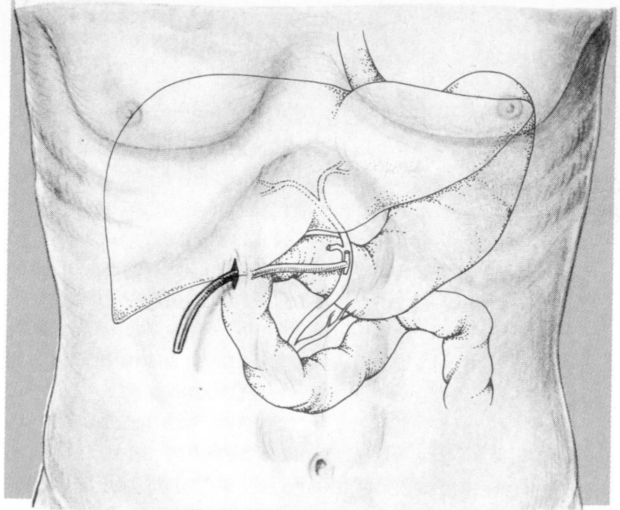

Figure 41–4

T-tube placement. The arms of the T are inserted into the hepatic duct (leading from the liver) and the common bile duct (leading into the duodenum). The tail of the T exits from a stab wound in the abdomen.

ledochostomy. Vitamin K will be prescribed if clotting abnormalities are found. A prolonged prothrombin time or positive results of reagent strip tests (Hemastix) performed on emesis should alert the nurse to coagulation problems. Intravenous infusions are started 24 to 48 hours before surgery to hydrate the client, correct electrolyte imbalances, and increase hepatic glycogen stores.

Relieving the client's pain is another nursing goal. Meperidine (Demerol) may be used, although some physicians prefer to prescribe nitroglycerin or phenobarbital to relieve pain by relaxing smooth muscle. Morphine is not used because it is believed to increase spasms at the sphincter of Oddi. Nursing comfort measures such as repositioning, providing distraction, and removing noxious stimuli from the environment to reduce nausea may also be employed.

A nasogastric tube and suction are often prescribed to relieve abdominal distention and remove gastric juices that stimulate the secretion of cholecystokinin. Antiemetics are also prescribed.

In addition to the teaching accompanying any major surgical procedure, preoperative teaching includes explanation of the nature and function of the T-tube. The client should expect to be given intravenous infusions for several days following the operation, until oral ingestion of food and fluid can be tolerated. Because of the location of the incision, teaching the client how to splint the incision during coughing and deep breathing is especially important.

POSTOPERATIVE CARE As with any abdominal surgery, the goal is to prevent complications. Taking vital signs and assessing for hemorrhage are important responsibilities. Pneumonia is a common complication of gallbladder surgery; because of the subcostal location of the incision, coughing and deep breathing are painful. Encourage the client to take ten deep breaths per hour and to cough. Assist the client in splinting the incision to reduce pain when coughing.

CARE OF THE T-TUBE Care of the T-tube is primarily the responsibility of the nurse. The tube must remain attached to the drainage collection bag, it must not be kinked, and the contents of the bag should be measured at least once during each shift. During the initial 24-hour postsurgical period, drainage of 200 to 500 mL is normal; the amount of drainage then diminishes. When a few days have elapsed, such amounts may indicate obstruction of the common bile duct.

Placement of the T-tube is important. Its purpose is to form a passage so bile can drain out under pressure. Make sure the tube is not kinked. It should be taped on the abdomen slightly below the T-tube wound site. Taping it too low creates too much drainage. Taping it too high prevents free drainage and allows fluid to flow back into the common bile duct.

Once the client resumes eating, the T-tube may be clamped to aid digestion. It is usually removed 7 to 10 days following surgery if the findings of a T-tube cholangiogram are normal. Some clients are discharged with a T-tube in place to drain excess bile or to remove small stones that could lodge in the common bile duct.

ASSESSING FOR COMPLICATIONS The appearance of icterus may indicate injury to the ducts or obstruction of a duct by a calculus. Acholic stools may also be related to duct injury or obstruction. Excessive T-tube drainage several days after surgery might suggest obstruction of the common bile duct. Excessive loss of bile may necessitate

Table 41–6
Cholecystectomy and Choledochostomy: Implications for the Client

Physiologic Implications	Psychosocial/Lifestyle Implications
Relieves pain and inflammation	Low-fat diet for 4–6 weeks
Fat absorption impaired; flatulence common	Heavy lifting, some ADL restricted for about 8 weeks
Complications may include pneumonia, hemorrhage, or thrombosis	May have T-tube in place when discharged

recycling the client's bile by straining it and adding it to juice for oral ingestion. Fever and abdominal pain may be symptoms of infection, whether wound infection or bile peritonitis. These symptoms may also be related to pancreatitis from trauma to the pancreas during surgery. Hemorrhage is a possible complication related to decreased absorption of vitamin K and decreased synthesis of prothrombin.

DISCHARGE PLANNING General discharge teaching is similar to that for any abdominal surgery. Special points to emphasize include avoiding fatigue, lifting, and excessive exercise during the first 8 weeks. Fat intake should be limited.

Home Health Care

Clients who are to be sent home with a T-tube in place should be instructed in its care. Remind the client to be sure the tube is not kinked or obstructed, to tape it securely, and to place it correctly. Although a daily shower provides adequate cleansing of the T-tube site, additional cleansing with an antiseptic solution helps prevent infection. A dry, sterile dressing is placed over the wound and tube and then taped into place. It should be changed daily and more often if it becomes soiled or wet. Povidone–iodine ointment may be applied to the wound site. Zinc oxide may be applied where the tube exits and on nearby skin to prevent skin irritation from bile.

Being discharged with a T-tube may cause considerable anxiety. Drawing a picture of the biliary system with the T-tube in place, explaining the function of the tube, and teaching the client how to unclamp the tube and measure drainage may alleviate fears. Sometimes the tube is kept clamped at all times. Clients should also be prepared for the possibility of a repeat cholangiogram after discharge.

Tell the client to consult a health care provider regarding signs of possible complications, such as infection, obstruction, or dislodgement of the tube. A list of signs is provided in Box 41–4. Before the client is discharged, measure the length of the T-tube from the wound site to the connecting tube. The client who uses this measurement as a baseline will be able to tell whether the tube has moved or been dislodged.

Box 41–4
Signs of Possible Complications of Cholecystectomy and Choledochostomy

Signs of Infection

Redness, Warmth, Swelling — at incisional area, site of drainage tube, or site of previous intravenous infusions

Temperature higher than 100°F (37.7°C)

Purulent drainage at T-tube site

Signs of Obstruction

Tenderness or pain in right upper quadrant of abdomen

Bile drainage around T-tube if clamped

Nausea and vomiting

Acholic (clay-colored) stools

Jaundice

Mahogany-colored urine

Signs of Tube Dislodgement

Decreased drainage

Evidence that tube has shifted position

Liver Resection

A liver resection, or lobectomy, is a serious operation performed only when a lesion—usually a neoplasm—can be totally excised. Resection is not indicated for metastasized malignancies. Occasionally, a large hepatic abscess may be resected if antimicrobial therapy and percutaneous drainage have been unsuccessful in eradicating an infection.

A client can survive with only 10% of the liver functioning; complete destruction or removal of the liver is not compatible with life. The liver has unique regenerative capacities. Some sources have reported regeneration within 6 months of a successful resection of 90% of liver tissue. Resection is most successful, however, when less tissue is removed.

Liver resections involve considerable risk of massive hemorrhage followed, within minutes, by death. To reduce this risk, hypothermia is commonly employed to slow down metabolism and restrict circulation.

For a right lobectomy, a large thoracoabdominal incision is required to expose the right lobe. Hemorrhage and pulmonary complications commonly accompany this type of incision. A large abdominal incision is made for a left lobectomy; evisceration is a possible additional complication of this approach. Client implications of liver resection are summarized in Table 41–7.

Nursing Implications

PREOPERATIVE CARE The nurse is the key person in helping the client meet physical and emotional needs. Abnormalities related to nutrition, fluid and electrolyte levels, and coagulation must be corrected before surgery. Several laboratory and diagnostic studies will need to be done. Prepare the client for these procedures and explain why and how they are done. Also prepare the client for the monitoring and supportive instrumentation that will be in place following the surgery and for the possibly frightening and disorienting atmosphere of the intensive care unit. Usually, a bowel preparation procedure of cathartics,

Table 41–7
Liver Resection: Implications for the Client

Physiologic Implications	Psychosocial/Lifestyle Implications
Risk of hemorrhage leading to shock	Emotional support needed
Pneumonia; other pulmonary complications	Good nutrition required
Cardiac complications	Must avoid alcohol and hepatotoxins
Hypoglycemia common	Activities limited postsurgically as for any abdominal operation
Susceptibility to hepatotoxins	With diagnosis of malignancy, client and family require guidance, explanation, and support; coping strategies should be planned
Pain for first 3–7 days	
Rapid regeneration of hepatic tissue	

enemas, and intestinal antibiotics is begun 2 days before surgery.

POSTOPERATIVE CARE Clients are often assigned to the intensive care unit during the immediated postoperative period. Constant attention is needed to correct metabolic abnormalities and prevent complications, especially during the first 72 postoperative hours. Hypoglycemia is common, requiring close monitoring of blood glucose levels and administration of intravenous glucose. Drugs that are toxic to the liver must be avoided. Postoperative care also includes measures appropriate for any abdominal or thoracic procedure.

Pain is a major problem for the client for the first 3 to 7 postoperative days. Its control is more challenging because of medication restrictions related to hepatotoxicity. Coughing and deep breathing may be so painful that pneumonia develops or other pulmonary problems, such as pneumothorax or collapse of a lung, occur because of accumulated secretions. A chest tube may have to be inserted to re-expand the lung.

The family and significant others may require the support of the nurse as they cope with the critical diagnosis and serious surgery. Discharge planning is consistent with that for any abdominal or thoracic procedure. Emphasize the importance of -2voiding alcohol and hepatotoxins.

Liver Transplantation

Liver transplantation is a relatively new technique that may be considered for persons with irreversible liver dysfunction who are free of infection, malignancy, severe atherosclerosis, or cardiopulmonary disease. Although infants with potentially fatal hepatic and biliary disorders are prime candidates, adult clients with biliary sclerosis or sclerosing cholangitis are also potential candidates. It is less commonly used for alcoholic cirrhosis and primary liver malignancy (Gordon et al, 1986).

Two transplantation techniques are possible: (1) The diseased liver can be removed and a donor liver placed in the same area of the right upper quadrant of the abdomen. (2) The diseased liver is left in place and the donor liver placed in the groin or pelvis. Both techniques require reconstruction of the biliary drainage system. Immunosuppressive therapy is usually instituted prior to surgery and continued after revascularization and total hemostasis have been achieved. Client implications related to liver transplantation are summarized in Table 41–8.

Nursing Implications

PREOPERATIVE CARE Transplant candidates must undergo rigorous physiologic tests, including liver function studies, coagulation studies, and hemoglobin and electrolyte profiles. They are also given psychologic tests and interviewed to determine if they are capable of coping with the stress of the surgery, possible rejection, and the concept of having a part of someone else's body. Offer support during this testing phase and explain the need for the tests to the client and significant others.

The nurse is also the key person in providing information about the surgical procedure, the mechanisms of rejection, and postoperative monitoring and medications. The nurse also helps prepare the client and significant others for the lifestyle changes that will occur once the surgery is successfully completed.

POSTOPERATIVE CARE Intensive postoperative nursing care is required for the transplant recipient. This is best provided in a transplant unit, where nurses are accustomed to caring for transplant clients and have specialized knowledge of the unique problems associated with transplantation. Mechanical ventilation and constant ECG, hemodynamic, and arterial pressure monitoring will be required for the first 48 to 72 hours. Signs of rejection are monitored through liver function tests such as the SGOT, bilirubin studies, liver scans, and cholangiography. Coagulation studies, electrolyte levels, and hemoglobin profiles are also watched closely.

Table 41–8
Liver Transplantation: Implications for the Client

Physiologic Implications	Psychosocial/Lifestyle Implications
Improved condition (ascites diminishes and liver function returns to normal)	Experience is emotionally draining for client and significant others
Rejection of transplant, infection, and occlusion of vessels are possible complications	Average hospital stay is about 2 months
Cushing's syndrome and other side effects associated with steroid therapy	Immunosuppressive drug regimen must be meticulously followed without interruption
Renal failure from nephrotoxic drugs (gentamycin, cyclosporine) possible	Alterations in body image
	Fear of organ rejection and death
	Exposure to crowds must be limited, particularly at the height of the cold and flu season

Bed rest for 24 to 48 hours is important. Intravenous fluids, antibiotics, and immunosuppressive drugs are administered by the nurse. The nurse must also be alert for signs of rejection such as an elevated temperature, enlarged and tender liver, hypertension, tachycardia, and abnormalities of coagulation or liver function (icterus, mahogany-colored urine, acholic stools). If signs of rejection occur, dosages of immunosuppressants are increased.

Considering the many responsibilities of physical care, the nurse must be creative in finding time to attend to the client's need for human interaction, especially in the early postsurgical hours when the client is alone and separated from family and familiar stimuli.

Family members must be kept informed of the client's condition. Their need for encouragement and support often can best be met by nurses who are caring for their loved one. As the client's condition improves, visiting time can be extended. Client and significant others will need to know what medications will be prescribed, what their purpose is, and how important it is to follow instructions conscientiously. In most units, clients take their medications and keep logs of important information, such as temperature, before they are discharged. These practices assist the nurse in evaluating the client's comprehension and enhance the client's chances for success as an outpatient.

The importance of never missing a single dose of immunosuppressive agents must be stressed repeatedly. Discharge teaching should include instructions for obtaining an intravenous or intramuscular administration of the immunosuppressant if nausea or vomiting prevent taking of oral medication. Since a health care provider may not be immediately available, teach the client and a family member how to give an intramuscular injection. The technique of giving an injection can be practiced with sterile saline prior to discharge.

Discharge planning should also include the importance of avoiding crowds and fatigue and information about a special diet, if one has been prescribed.

Chapter Highlights

Care for the client with cirrhosis includes promoting comfort; maintaining skin integrity, tissue perfusion, and thought processes; improving nutritional intake; and correcting fluid volume alterations.

Hemorrhage of esophageal varices may be controlled with vasopressin therapy, gastric lavage with iced saline, placement of a Sengstaken–Blakemore or Minnesota tube for temporary control, and injection sclerotherapy or portal–systemic shunting for long-term control.

Hepatitis A, also known as short-incubation or infectious hepatitis, is associated with a lower mortality rate than other forms, is transmitted via the fecal–oral route, and provides lifetime immunity for persons who have had the disease.

Hepatitis B, also known as long-incubation or serum hepatitis, is transmitted via all bodily fluids with the possible exception of feces; it can progress to chronic hepatitis or to a subclinical carrier state.

Immune serum globulin (ISG) for hepatitis A and hepatitis B immune globulin (HBIG) for hepatitis B are given prophylactically within one week of exposure. Hepatitis B vaccine is available for persons continually exposed to this disease and to high-risk individuals such as dialysis clients.

Non-A, non-B hepatitis, seen in persons with multiple transfusions and in abusers of parenterally administered drugs, is more lethal than hepatitis A and B.

Toxic hepatitis, caused by drugs or chemicals that induce cell necrosis, and drug-induced hepatitis, caused by drugs that sensitize the liver, can be completely reversed if the sensitizing or toxic agent is removed.

Chronic active hepatitis, seen in persons who have previously had hepatitis B or non-A, non-B hepatitis, is believed to involve an immune interaction because IgG, IgM, and IgA values are elevated.

Metastatic cancer of the liver is 25 times as common as primary liver cancer. Hepatic carcinoma is associated with weight loss, ascites, cachexia, anemia, abdominal fullness and pain, fever, hemorrhage, obstructive icterus, splenomegaly and hepatomegaly.

A liver resection, or lobectomy, is done only if the lesion, an abscess or tumor, can be totally excised.

The client who receives a liver transplant will require lifelong immunosuppression. The nurse will teach client and family about medications, daily records, and signs of transplant rejection and verify their comprehension before the client with a liver transplant is discharged.

Cholecystitis is inflammation of the gallbladder frequently associated with cholelithiasis and characterized by intense pain, tenderness, and rigidity in the right upper quadrant of the abdomen.

During a cholecystostomy, the gallbladder is opened, and calculi, bile, and purulent matter are removed. A bile drainage tube is usually inserted.

During a cholecystectomy, the gallbladder is excised. This procedure is often done in conjunction with a choledochostomy, in which the common and hepatic bile ducts are explored and obstructions are removed.

Postoperative care for the client with gallbladder surgery includes (1) preventing complications including hemorrhage, thrombus formation, abdominal distention, and especially pneumonia; (2) promoting relief from pain and nausea; (3) caring for the T-tube apparatus; and (4) providing discharge teaching.

Bibliography

Anderson FD: Portal-systemic encephalopathy in the chronic alcoholic. *Crit Care Q* 1986: 8(4): 40–52.

Cooperman AM (editor): Liver, spleen, and pancreas. *Surg Clin North Am* (Feb) 1981; 61:1.

Decker SI: The life-threatening consequences of a GI bleed. *RN* (Oct) 1985; 18–27.

Dodd RP: Ascites: When the liver can't cope. *RN* (Oct) 1984; 26–33.

Dong B et al: Viral hepatitis. *Nurse Pract* (March) 1984; 9:27–32.

Epstein M: Renal complications of liver disease. *Clin Symp* 1985; 37(5):3–32.

Fishbein RH: What the nonsurgeon should know about cholecystectomy. *Hosp Med* 1985; 21(1): 197–201.

Garvey EC, Manganaro M: Nursing implications of hepatic artery infusion. *Cancer Nurs* 1982; 5:51–55.

Gillham MB, Southworth K, Dollahite J: Nutritional treatment for the alcoholic patient. *Crit Care Q* 1986; 8(4): 20–28.

Goldenberg DA: Management of bleeding esophageal varices. *Crit Care Q* 1982; 5(2): 33–46.

Gordon RD et al: Indications for liver transplantation in the cyclosporine era. *Surg Clin North Am* 1986; 66(3): 541–556.

Groer ME, Shekleton ME: *Basic Pathophysiology: A Conceptual Approach,* 2nd ed. St. Louis, MO: Mosby, 1983.

Gullatte MM, Foltz AT: Hepatic chemotherapy via implantable pump. *Am J Nurs* 1983; 83(12):1674–1676.

Gurevich I: Viral hepatitis. *Am J Nurs* 1983; 83:571–586.

Jackson BS, Carlisle PM: How post-op complications can burgeon into crisis. *RN* (Jan) 1981; 44:26–32.

Jermier BJ, Treolar DM: Bringing your patient through gallbladder surgery. *RN* (Nov) 1986; 18–25.

Keith JS: Hepatic failure: Etiologies, manifestations, and management. *Crit Care Nurs* 1985; 5(1):60–86.

Kirkman–Liff B, Dandoy S: Hepatitis B: What price exposure? *Am J Nurs* (August) 1984; 84:988–990.

Klopfenstein ML: Hepatic artery cannulation. *AORN J* 1981; 34:956–964.

Klopp A: Shunting malignant ascites. *Am J Nurs* 1984; 84:212–213.

LaSala C: Caring for the patient with a transhepatic biliary decompression catheter. *Nurs 85;* 15(2): 52–55.

Malony JP: Surgical intervention in the alcoholic patient with portal hypertension. *Crit Care Q* 1986; 8(4):63–73.

Miller B, Gavant ML: Biliary catheter care. *Am J Nurs* 1985; 85:1115–1117.

Munoz E et al: Surgonomics: The cost of cholecystectomy. *Surgery* 1984; 96:642–647.

Newell J: Portal systemic encephalopathy. *Nurse Pract* (July) 1984; 9:26–37.

Petersdorf RG et al: *Harrison's Principles of Internal Medicine,* 10th ed. New York: McGraw–Hill, 1983.

Pimstone NR, French SW: Alcoholic liver disease. *Med Clin North Am* 1984; 68(1): 39–56.

Quinless F: Portal hypertension: Physiology, signs and symptoms. *Nurs 84* 1984; 14(1): 52–53.

Quinless F: Teaching tips for T-tube care at home. *Nurs 84* 1984; 14(5):63–64.

Sanowski RA: Nondrug treatment of bleeding esophageal varices. *Geriatric Consultant* (July/Aug) 1986; 24–25.

Sherlock S: *Diseases of the Liver and Biliary System,* 7th ed. Oxford, Blackwell, 1985.

Smith SL: Liver transplantation: Implications for critical care. *Heart Lung* 1985; 14:617–627.

Solomon J, Harrington D, Gogel HK: When the patient suffers from esophageal bleeding. *RN* (Feb) 1987;24–27.

Tarter RE et al: Neuropsychiatric status after liver transplantation. *J Lab Clin Med* 1984; 103:776–782.

Taylor PD: Liver transplantation. *Am J Nurs* 1981; 81:1672–1673.

Vargo J: Viral hepatitis: How to protect patients and yourself. *RN* (July) 1984; 22–29.

Wimpsett J: Trace your patient's liver dysfunction. *Nurs 84* 1984; 14(8):56–57.

CASE STUDY

The Client With Cirrhosis

I. Brief Descriptive Data

Mr Morton Smith, age 55, has been admitted to the hospital with a diagnosis of prehepatic coma secondary to Laennec's cirrhosis. His skin and sclerae are slightly jaundiced, and he has itching skin. Ascites, peripheral edema, multiple bruises, confusion, and drowsiness are apparent.

II. Personal Data

Date and Time: Sept. 25, 1987: 7:00 PM
Full Name: Morton Smith
Social Security Number: 000-00-0000
Address: Box 28956, Branston, Colo
Telephone: Work: 000-0000
Home: 000-0000
Sex: Male
Marital Status: Married
Age: 55
Birthdate: 5-1-32
Religion: Protestant
Race: Caucasian
Occupation: Carpenter
Usual Health Care Provider: Earl Taylor, MD

III. Health History

Source of Information: Client and wife
Reliability of Informant: Client confused at times; wife is reliable but apathetic
Chief Concern: Itching, confusion, and drowsiness off and on

History of Present Illness:

Has been admitted several times during the past ten years for problems associated with cirrhosis—ascites and peripheral and pulmonary edema. Bleeding esophageal varices, 1981. LeVeen shunt placed, 1982. Was also hospitalized in 1960, 1966, for alcohol-related automobile accidents. Sustained fx rt femur, 1960; mild concussion, 1966.

Current main concern of client is itching skin and being "tired" much of the time, no fatigue pattern identified. Wife identifies recent confusion and forgetfulness as most significant concern. Ten days ago wife noted husband's increased episodes of confusion and decreased appetite. No vomiting, but has been nauseated on occasion late in afternoon; bowel movements twice a day—some stools are tarry, black, while others are lighter in color, flatulence has increased and caused some cramping discomfort, epigastric discomfort accompanies nausea at times. Still ingests alcohol—one to two beers per evening prior to dinner; continues to drink 5–6 cups caffeinated coffee per day; stays on low roughage diet. Concerned about loss of job because of worsening condition and financial difficulties.

Past Health History:

Childhood: Childhood diseases—measles, mumps, chickenpox
Immunizations: Polio, 1961; Td, 1982; influenza and pneumonia, 1982
Medical Problems: Hepatitis B, 1948; cirrhosis, 1978; congestive heart failure, 1980; esophageal variceal hemorrhage, 1981
Surgeries: Appendectomy, 1961; paracentesis, 1980, 1981; LeVeen shunt, 1982
Blood Transfusions: 1974, 1976, 1978, 1981, 1982
Trauma: Auto accidents, 1960 (fx femur); 1966 (mild concussion); minor auto accidents, 1971, 1974, 1977

Past Health History:

Allergies: None

Medications: Furosemide, 40 mg PO b.i.d.
Propranolol, 20 mg PO t.i.d.
Spironolactone, 25 mg PO t.i.d.

Family History:

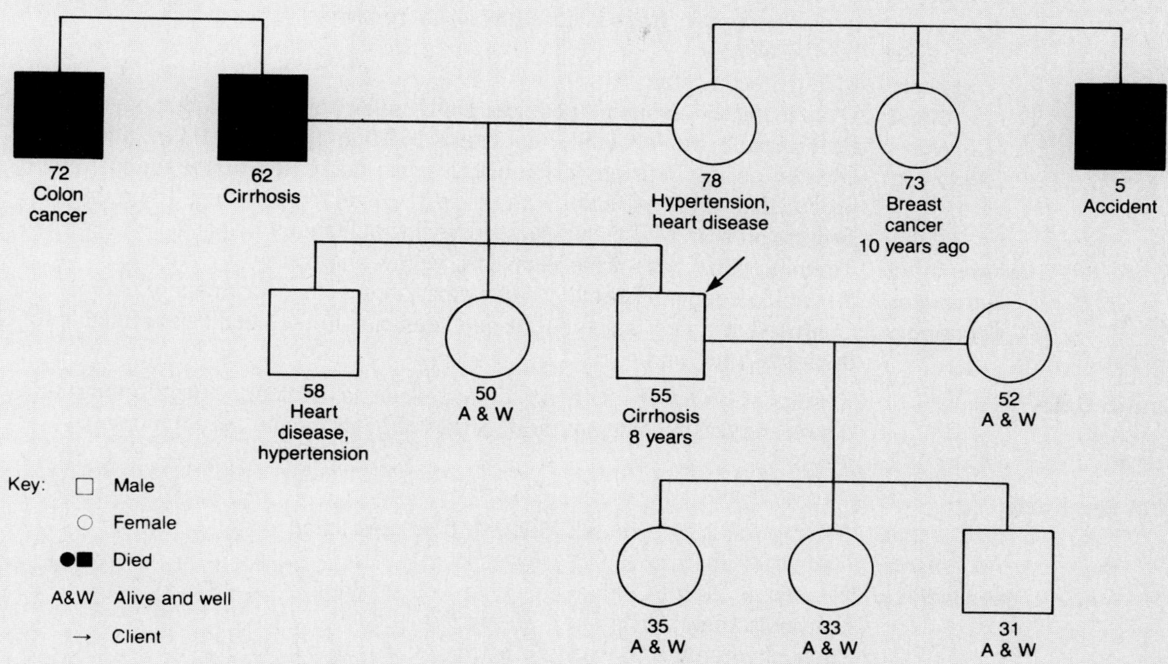

Personal and Social History: Currently works about 20 hours per week as a carpenter; condition has prohibited more than that for last 5 years; children are all away from home and doing well; wife works full time as secretary for local attorney; very little exercise as tolerates it poorly; likes to build wagon wheel lamps and tables in spare time; 3-pack-a-day smoker × 30 years, quit 3 years ago; wife is supportive; children call often.

Review of Systems: General health has deteriorated over past 2 years.

Skin: Frequent itching

Mouth: States, "Gums bleed when brushing"

Respiratory: Has shortness of breath on exertion

Gastrointestinal: See HPI

Urinary: Voids approximately 10 times per day, nocturia × 2 at night; denies dysuria, urgency, hesitancy

Genital: Unable to achieve erection for two years; both client and wife find this upsetting

Endocrine: Denies polydipsia, polyphagia

Psychologic: Believes he will get well; becomes frustrated when unable to remember things

IV: Physical Assessment

Height: 6 ft, 0 in

Weight: 200 lb

Vital Signs: BP 160/96; pulse 105; respirations 28; temperature 98.2°F (36.8°C). Tall, ill-appearing, obviously jaundiced, somewhat confused 55-yr-old w/m

(continued)

CASE STUDY (continued)

The Client With Cirrhosis

Relevant Organ Systems:

Skin: Orange–yellow discoloration, spider angiomas on anterior chest; no breaks in skin integrity; bruises noted on all extremities

Eyes: Sclerae yellow

Breasts: Mild gynecomastia

Chest: Dyspnea noted in supine position; DOE; rales both lower lobes posteriorly

Heart: PMI palpable 5th left ICS, 2 cm lateral to MCI; apical rate 98, regular

Abdomen: Obvious ascites, dilated periumbilical veins; decreased bowel sounds, no bruits; liver edge palpable 5 cm below rt costal margin; liver 15 cm by percussion at rt MCL; fluid wave present; spleen not palpable

Genitourinary: Thinning pubic hair; urine very dark yellow and frothy

Extremities: 3+ ankle edema bilaterally; limbs emaciated except for areas of edema

Neurologic: Confused at times; some decreased sensation in toes and hands (unable to distinguish hot and cold)

V. Diagnostic Data

Results of laboratory data include hypokalemia, prolonged prothrombin time, decreased plasma albumin, and increased bilirubin and serum ammonia levels.

VI. Medical Regimen

Diet: 500 mg Na, 15 g protein, 1500 mL fluid restriction

Treatments: Tap water enema

Medications: Neomycin, 20 g PO q.i.d.
Spironolactone (Aldactone), 25 mg PO t.i.d.
Diphenhydramine (Benadryl), 50 mg PO h.s. p.r.n. for itching
Vitamin K (AquaMEPHYTON), 2 mg IM, MWF
Furosemide (Lasix), 40 mg PO b.i.d.
Propranolol HCL (Inderal), 20 mg PO t.i.d.
Potassium, 20 mEq PO t.i.d.

VII. Nursing Care Plan, by Nursing Diagnosis

Client Care Goals	Plan/Nursing Implementation	Expected Outcome
Comfort, altered: related to pruritus		
Reduce or eliminate pruritus; increase comfort; sleep throughout the night	Rest, good diet, ventilation, cotton clothing, change wet sheets, distraction, no alkaline soaps, infrequent baths, whirlpool, emollients, keep nails short, diphenhydramine 50 mg p.r.n., have client wear gloves	Performs ADL without scratching; rests comfortably; relief of itching
Skin integrity, impaired: potential		
Change position frequently; take in well-balanced diet; understand efffects of prolonged pressure on skin integrity	Well-balanced diet (low protein, low Na because of diagnosis); relieve itching; frequent turning, use of air or water mattresses, and position change to relieve pressure on edematous areas; keep skin clean, dry; keep sheets wrinkle-free; teach about effect of pressure on skin	Normal skin integrity; avoids staying in same position more than 1 hour; client and family understand mechanism of skin breakdown

Client Care Goals	Plan/Nursing Implementation	Expected Outcome
Thought processes, altered: related to substance abuse		
Regain satisfactory thought processes	Have him write name daily, check extent of asterixis by pumping BP cuff, assess for orientation: date, time, place, and person. Do not reinforce disorientation. Provide safety measures.	Writes name daily without changes; oriented to date, time, place.
Fluid volume, excess: related to ascites and portal hypertension		
Improve fluid volume balance	Potassium 20 mEq t.i.d., furosemide 40 mg b.i.d., 500 mg Na diet, spironolactone 25 mg t.i.d.; intake and output; monitor esophageal varices, daily weight, abdominal girths; assess patency of LeVeen shunt; measure circumference of extremities; 1500 mL of fluid restriction	Good skin turgor, decreased abdominal girth and circumference of extremities, increased output in comparison to intake
Fluid volume, deficit: related to potential for hemorrhage		
Decrease bruising, possibility of other bleeding problems	Vitamin K 2 mg IM, MWF; monitor prothrombin time and observe for bleeding; check stool hemoccults; explain that caffeine, alcohol are irritants to the GI tract and can cause gastritis and ulcer disease Sengstaken–Blakemore or Minnesota tube if esophageal varices bleed; may assist with ice lavage; neomycin sulfate 1 g o.i.d., potassium 20 mEq t.i.d.; tap water enema, assess for fetor hepaticus, rest	Prothrombin time within normal limits; absence of bleeding or further bruising; avoids GI irritants such as caffeine, alcohol
Health maintenance, altered: related to lack of ability to make deliberate and thoughtful judgments		
Understand effects of alcohol use on body; describe other common substances that can cause hepatic damage	Explain that cirrhosis and portal hypertension are related to history of alcohol use; also explain need to avoid substances that may further damage the liver (drugs, chemicals)	Abstinence from alcohol and other hepatotoxins; does not use over-the-counter drugs without checking with care provider
Understand need to maintain low sodium diet and fluid restriction	Instruct in 15 g protein, 500 mg sodium, 1500 mL fluid restricted diet	Client and family aware of diet and fluid restrictions and adhere to them
Sexual dysfunction: related to disease process		
Understand how cirrhosis leads to hormonal imbalances, causing impotence	Explain hormonal imbalances that accompany cirrhosis to client and wife; discuss alternative approaches to meeting sexual needs if couple is interested	Both partners understand effects of cirrhosis on sexual function and can talk about the situation with each other

UNIT 10

The Client With Musculoskeletal Dysfunction

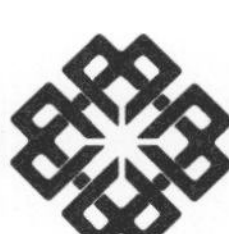

CHAPTER 42

The Musculoskeletal System in Health and Illness

Objectives

When you have finished studying this chapter, you should be able to:

Identify the major structural and functional components of the musculoskeletal system.

Explain the physiologic mechanisms that regulate the activity of the musculoskeletal system.

Describe some pathologic conditions that lead to musculoskeletal dysfunction.

Discuss alterations in other body systems that result from musculoskeletal dysfunction.

Identify and discuss the psychosocial/lifestyle effects of musculoskeletal dysfunction on the client and significant others.

The musculoskeletal system is composed of many anatomical structures that work together to move, support, and protect the body and its parts. These structures include the bones and joints of the skeletal system; the skeletal muscles; and the tendons, ligaments, and other elements that connect muscle to bone or bone to bone.

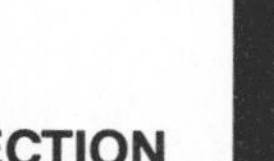

SECTION I

Structural and Functional Interrelationship

Bone Tissue

The human skeletal system has several functions that are reflected in the structure of the bones. The skeleton as a whole provides a framework for supporting the other body tissues. Individual bones may protect vital organs and soft tissues or serve as levers that are moved by attached muscles. Bones are also responsible for hematopoiesis, or production of blood cells, and serve as storage sites for minerals such as calcium and phosphorus. Bones differ from one another in form and in tissue type.

Bones are classified into four major groups according to shape:

- Long bones, consisting of two knobs connected by a shaft, are the major bones of the limbs.
- Short bones make up the wrist and ankles.
- Flat bones form the ribs and sternum, as well as much of the braincase.
- Irregular bones include the vertebrae and some of the bones of the face and pelvic girdle.

A less common type, called a sesamoid bone, develops within a tendon; the most prominent example of a sesamoid bone is the patella.

The parts of a long bone, such as the femur, are shown in Figure 42–1. The knobby ends of the bone are called epiphyses or heads. The proximal epiphysis is the end closer to the trunk; the distal epiphysis is farther from the trunk. The epiphyses are covered with articular or hyaline cartilage, which is resilient and provides padding for the opposing joint surfaces. The shaft of the bone is known as the diaphysis. Periosteum, a dense white fibrous membrane, covers the diaphysis, providing a surface for the attachment of tendons and ligaments. The inner layer of the periosteum, richly supplied with blood vessels and nerves, contains bone-forming cells called osteoblasts, necessary for repair and for increase in growing bone diameter. Between the epiphysis and diaphysis of growing bones is the epiphyseal plate, responsible for growth in length. When growth stops, the epiphyseal plate is replaced

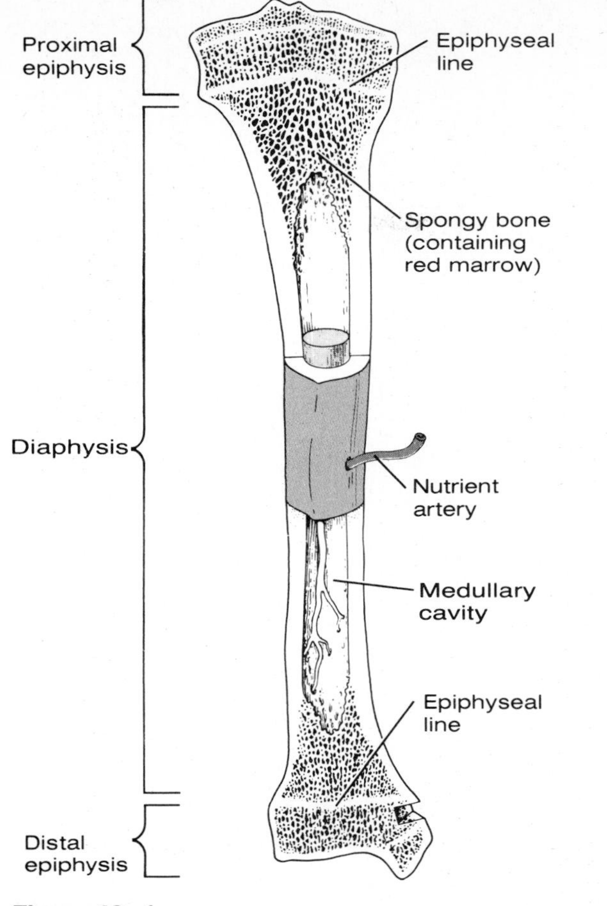

Figure 42–1

Structure of a long bone. SOURCE: *Spence AP, Mason EB:* Human Anatomy and Physiology, *3rd ed. Menlo Park, CA: Benjamin/ Cummings, 1987.*

by bone. Inside the shaft of a long bone is the medullary canal or cavity, which is filled with yellow bone marrow. The canal is lined with a layer of osteoblasts.

Bone Growth and Turnover

Bones grow in length at the epiphyseal plates. In a growing long bone cartilage, cells proliferate rapidly in the epiphyseal plates and are gradually replaced by bone cells through a process called **ossification.** In this manner, the shafts of the long bones continue to increase in length until a person is about 20 to 25 years old, when the epiphyses close and ossification is complete. A process called *remodeling*—selective bone resorption and formation that maintains the epiphyses at a relatively constant size—occurs as the bone increases in length.

Bones grow in circumference as bone-forming *osteoblasts* deposit new layers of bone tissue around the outside. At the same time, bone-destroying cells called *osteoclasts* dissolve away bone cells on the inner aspect of the bone, increasing the size of the medullary cavity.

Bone is a dynamic structure that is continuously remodeled by bone cell activity. Old bone is removed and new bone is formed through the processes of *resorption* (eating away) and *deposition,* performed by osteoclasts and osteoblasts respectively. The replacement of bone tissue through resorption and deposition is called *turnover.* The process of resorption may be more active in the elderly, the inactive, and in some disease states. In the normally active adult, the two processes are generally balanced.

Bone formation and remodeling occur in response to the stresses exerted on the bone. During prolonged periods of bed rest, the forces applied to bones are changed, and the bones may become fragile and lose structural mass.

Healing of Disrupted Bone Tissue

A break in the continuity of bone tissue is called a **fracture.** Fracture healing occurs by formation of new bone tissue and can be described in four stages, as diagrammed in Figure 42–2.

1. *Procallus (hematoma) formation.* Bleeding occurs at the broken ends of the bone just as it does in other injured tissues. The bleeding, which is from damaged vessels in the bone, the bone marrow, the periosteum, and surrounding soft tissues, forms a hematoma at the fracture site. Initial healing actually begins with the formation of a hematoma called a procallus. The hematoma becomes a fibrin network. New capillaries form, fibroblasts invade the clot, and granulation tissue is formed. Dead cells and tissue debris are moved by phagocytosis.
2. *Callus formation.* The fibroblasts differentiate into cells, which lay down a new matrix for bone formation. A collar of soft fibrocartilaginous tissue known as callus surrounds the fracture site, bridging the gap. The callus is much wider than the bone's diameter and extends above and below the fracture line.
3. *Ossification.* Mineral salts are deposited in the new matrix, and the callus eventually becomes bone. The fracture ends are firmly bound together but are not yet strong enough for weight bearing.
4. *Consolidation and remodeling.* The callus is remodeled by osteoclastic and osteoblastic activity according to the stresses placed on the bone by muscles and weight bearing. The excess callus is eventually absorbed and the bone assumes a more normal shape.

The rate of healing depends on several factors, such as the person's age and the type and location of the fracture. A child's bone heals much faster than an adult's bone. Favorable conditions for healing include good circulation, adequate nutrition, absence of infection, and proximity and immobility of the fracture ends. In some cases fracture healing can take a year or longer.

Joints

Bones are bound together at joints, which allow the bones varying degrees of mobility. Together with the muscles,

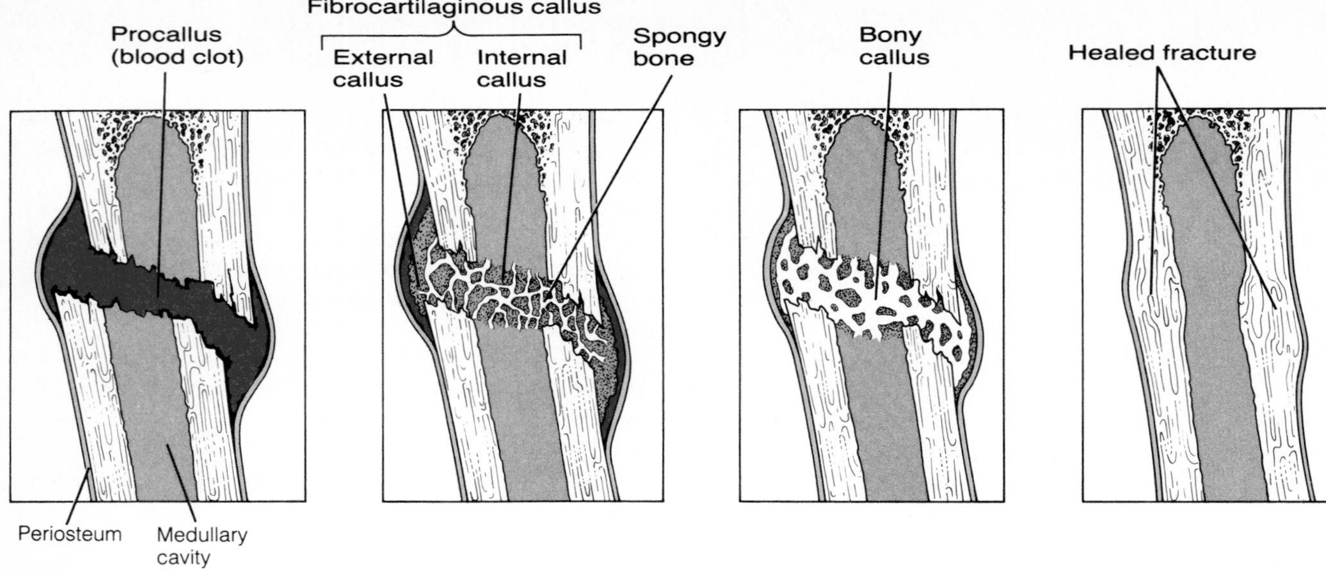

Figure 42–2

Healing of a fracture. **A.** Initial repair begins with formation of a blood clot called a procallus. **B.** Connective tissue invades the procallus, replacing it with a fibrocartilaginous callus. **C.** The fibrous callus is eventually replaced by bone that develops from cells of the periosteum. **D.** Healed fracture. SOURCE: *Spence AP, Mason EB:* Human Anatomy and Physiology, *3rd ed. Menlo Park, CA: Benjamin/Cummings, 1987.*

ligaments and tendons, the movable joints provide stabilization and permit motion of the body parts. The many joints of the body allow for a variety of movements that can be coordinated into agile or skilled activities.

The joints of the body are classified into three types:

- *Synarthroses,* or immovable joints, such as those in the sutures of the skull
- *Amphiarthroses,* slightly movable joints, such as the symphysis pubis
- *Diarthroses,* or freely movable joints, such as those in the knee and hip

The structure of the diarthroses will be discussed because changes in this type of joint most often affect health. A diarthrotic joint (Figure 42–3) has a *synovial cavity* and is, therefore, also known as a synovial joint. The cavity is surrounded by a *joint capsule* of strong fibroelastic tissue, which is attached to the periosteum of the articulating bones. The capsule allows movement while resisting dislocation. The inner surface of the joint cavity is lined with *synovial membrane,* which secretes *synovial fluid.* The cartilage-covered bone ends and the synovial fluid reduce friction as joint surfaces rub against each other. The amount of synovial fluid is small but is enough to lubricate the joint and provide nourishment for the articular cartilage. The synovial membrane can also secrete antibodies to protect the joint from disease.

Some diarthrotic joints have *articular discs (menisci)*

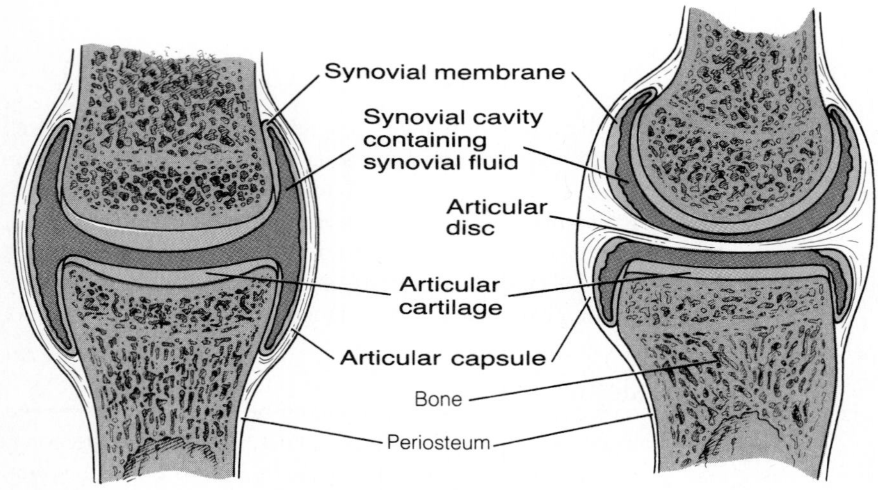

Figure 42–3

Structure of diarthrotic (synovial) joints. **A.** Synovial joint without articular disc. **B.** Synovial joint with articular disc. SOURCE: *Spence AP, Mason EB:* Human Anatomy and Physiology, *3rd ed. Menlo Park, CA: Benjamin/Cummings, 1987.*

made of fibrocartilage (Figure 42–3B), which lie between the articulating bone surfaces and act as shock absorbers. In the knee, these are known as *semilunar* cartilages. Many diarthrotic joints have ligaments inside and outside the joint capsules to bind the bones together and give additional stability.

Skeletal Muscles

Contraction of skeletal muscle is responsible for moving the bones of the skeleton. The bone serves as a lever, the joint serves as a fulcrum upon which the bone pivots, and the muscle provides the force that moves the lever. A second function of skeletal muscles is maintenance of body posture. There is a residual amount of contraction in the muscles, known as *muscle tone,* which serves to keep the body erect and ready for action. A third function is heat production. When a person is cold, small rapid contractions of skeletal muscle, called shivering, produce body heat.

A typical skeletal muscle is anchored at each end to bone by a fibrous connection called a tendon. The muscle often stretches across a joint. The muscle's attachment to the less movable bone is called its *origin,* and its attachment to the more movable bone is called its *insertion.* When the muscle contracts, one bone remains more or less stationary, forcing the other bone to move.

Most skeletal muscles work in groups. The *prime mover* is the muscle that contracts to produce the movement. *Synergists* are muscles that work together with prime movers to assit in performing the movement. *Antagonists* are muscles that work opposite prime movers by relaxing during their contraction or by acting to produce an opposite effect. An **isotonic contraction** occurs when a muscle shortens during contraction. An **isometric contraction** occurs when a muscle becomes tense while remaining the same length.

Other Structures Related to Movement

Tendons are cords of connective tissue that attach muscles to the periosteum of the bones. During muscle contraction, the muscle pulls the tendon, which pulls the bone to which it is attached, producing movement. *Ligaments,* made of fibrous connective tissue, connect bones to one another. They have the ability to stretch while providing stability.

A *bursa* is a fluid-filled sac that facilitates motion of structures that move against each other. It can be found between skin and bone, muscle and bone, tendons and bone, ligaments and bone, and between muscles. The bursae function as padding between structures to reduce the friction caused by moving parts.

Connective tissue, in the broad sense of the term, includes all tissues made up of cells in a matrix: bone, cartilage, blood, and lymph, for example. The term is used in a more limited sense, however, when discussing diseases of the connective tissues. In this sense, connective tissue means the binding and covering tissues of the body, including tendons, ligaments, muscle fascia, and the deep layers of the skin. This kind of connective tissue (sometimes called "connective tissue proper") is essential in holding together all the components of the musculoskeletal system.

Regulatory Functions of the Musculoskeletal System

Skeletal muscle contraction begins with the stimulus of a muscle fiber by a motor neuron. Every motor neuron ends in many fine branches, each branch connecting with an individual muscle fiber.

When a nerve impulse reaches the end of a motor neuron, small vesicles in the ends of the nerve branches release acetylcholine, which increases the permeability of the muscle cell and causes an influx of calcium ions into the cell. The calcium ions cause structural changes in the myofilaments that allow them to slide past each other, causing contraction. The structural changes also allow breakdown of ATP (adenosine triphosphate) to ADP (adenosine diphosphate) to provide energy for the contraction. The muscle relaxes as a result of the action of the enzyme cholinesterase, which breaks down acetylcholine, allowing the muscle to return to its resting state.

At the beginning of muscle contraction, ATP is formed from creatine phosphate stored in the muscle. The supply of creatine phosphate is limited, however, and even with mild muscle activity, additional ATP must be formed from ADP. The energy for forming this additional ATP is supplied by respiration—the breakdown of fats and carbohydrates by the cell. The first step in respiration is glycolysis, or anaerobic respiration, which produces lactic acid and small amounts of ATP. Under normal conditions, the lactic acid is broken down further by aerobic respiration, which requires an oxygen supply; the final products of aerobic respiration are carbon dioxide, water, and large amounts of ATP.

During sustained strenuous exercise, however, the blood cannot supply enough oxygen to keep pace with glycolysis, and lactic acid accumulates in the muscle, causing an oxygen debt. Muscle contractions continue for a short time using the small amount of ATP produced by glycolysis, but soon the demand exceeds the supply and the muscle is fatigued. The contractions decrease in strength and then stop. The pain of muscle fatigue is associated with the presence of accumulated lactic acid. The oxidation of the excess lactic acid occurs after the exercise, when the person breathes deeply to pay off the oxygen debt (Silverstein, 1980). Exercise involving bursts of strenuous activity, which require the muscles to operate anaerobically (ie, on glycolysis alone), is called *anaerobic exercise.* Gentler, sustained exercise that stimulates rapid aerobic respiration without outstripping the oxygen supply is called *aerobic exercise.*

SECTION 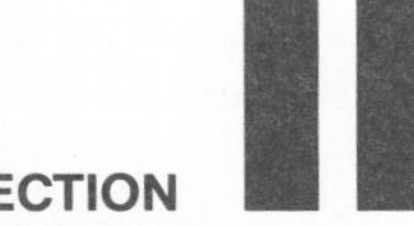

Pathophysiologic Influences and Effects

Metabolic Alterations

The structure of bone may be disrupted by inadequate calcium content. Since calcium gives bone its hardness, a deficiency causes bone to be soft and deformed. Pain is caused by stresses on the bone from weight bearing or when a considerable pull is exerted by muscles. The structure of bone is also altered when bone resorption exceeds bone formation. The bone is decreased in mass and becomes porous, causing it to be weak and susceptible to fractures. Pain also occurs as a result of fractures. Vertebrae that are affected become deformed, altering the spinal curvature.

Joints can be damaged by deposits of urate crystals resulting from abnormal uric acid metabolism, or gout. An inflammatory reaction occurs, causing pain that restricts motion. If the inflammation is severe and untreated, crippling deformities may occur.

Inflammation

The diarthrotic (synovial or movable) joints of the body are affected by the inflammatory disease rheumatoid arthritis, which causes changes in the synovial membrane. As the disease progresses, there is erosion of the articular cartilage, the joint capsule, and ligaments. The destruction of articular cartilage exposes the bone so that fibrous adhesions and bony fusion can occur. The effects of the disease include pain, limited joint mobility, and joint deformity. Inflammation may occur in other musculoskeletal structures from excessive or repeated strain as well as bacterial invasion. Restricted motion and pain usually result.

Degenerative Changes

The joint is the musculoskeletal structure most frequently influenced by degenerative disease. Changes are most often associated with aging, obesity, trauma, and inflammatory conditions. The degenerative process is a wearing out of the joint surfaces. The articular cartilage softens, thins, and ulcerates, and the joint surface becomes rough. There may be a narrowing of the joint space, swelling of adjacent soft tissue, and formation of bone cysts (Koerner & Dickinson, 1983). The normal smooth-gliding joint action is diminished. The periosteum becomes irritated by friction, stimulating the growth of bone spurs at the joint margins (Silverstein, 1980). The effects of this destruction include joint pain, stiffness, and joint deformity, which result in slight to moderate limitation of movement.

The intervertebral disks are also affected by degeneration. The water content of the disks decreases with age, causing them to become thinner. The surrounding fibers (ligaments) also change with age, so the disk becomes unstable. These changes cause decreased height and painless restriction of spinal movement. Sometimes the condition becomes more severe, with pressure on nerves causing pain and neurologic deficits.

Somewhat akin to degeneration is the process of **atrophy,** or wasting away. Muscle and bone can atrophy as a result of disuse. The normal strain on muscles and bones contributes to their development and to the maintenance of their size, shape, strength, and composition. Through disuse, muscle cells become reduced in size and weakened, the muscle mass becomes more fibrous, and bone cells become demineralized. Inactivity can also lead to joint **contracture.** The muscle fibers are shortened and fixed, and the joint's range of motion is limited. These conditions are reversible if the person resumes normal activity. Contractures can progress to an irreversible state without treatment, however. Ligaments can also lose their ability to maintain joint stability.

Nursing Research Note

Lambert VA: Study of factors associated with psychological well-being in rheumatoid arthritic women. *Image* (Spring) 1985; 17:50–53.

This research identified and described factors associated with well-being in women afflicted with rheumatoid arthritis. Social support, severity of the illness, and demographic characteristics were examined in relation to each other and to the level of psychologic well-being. The study sample consisted of 92 women ranging in age from 21 to 80 years with a mean age of 55 years. Data were collected by a structured interview.

Under the category of severity of the illness, pain was the single significant predictor of psychologic well-being (ie, psychologic well-being decreases as joint pain and difficulty in carrying out tasks increase). Dependence on others was significantly correlated with difficulty in performing tasks.

Clients with rheumatoid arthritis need to understand pain prevention and joint preservation approaches to optimize their quality of life. Nurses have a responsibility to provide this kind of information to clients. Because many older women with rheumatoid arthritis have limited support systems, nurses can assist clients in locating support services.

Infection

Bone can become infected by pathogens entering the bone by way of the circulation or through open wounds, including surgical incisions. The proliferation of bacteria causes pressure, bone destruction, and eventual bone necrosis. The resulting pain usually limits mobility. Some infections become chronic, with perpetual draining abscesses.

Other musculoskeletal structures, such as joints and bursae, can be infected by pathogens entering from penetrating wounds or via the circulation. Pain and restricted motion are common.

Neoplasia

Neoplastic growths in the musculoskeletal system can be benign or malignant. Benign tumors grow slowly or not at all and usually are encapsulated. They may cause mild pain, tenderness, and sometimes an abnormal prominence on the bone. Malignant tumors grow rapidly, causing intermittent to persistent pain (especially at night), tiredness, limited movement, swelling, and spontaneous fractures. Other effects may occur as a result of a tumor pressing on other structures (eg, nerves, blood vessels, or organs).

Malignant lesions may be from growths originating in musculoskeletal tissue (primary) or to metastatic lesions (secondary). The most common are bone lesions due to metastasis, from the lung, breast, intestine, thyroid, kidney, and prostate. Since the malignant cells can spread via the circulation, and the bones have a rich blood supply, the cells easily migrate to the bone. This is especially true for bones with large amounts of red marrow such as the spine, pelvis, and ribs. Cellular activity in the tumor may be osteolytic (bone destroying) or osteoblastic, forming abnormal new cells.

The effects of neoplastic growths can range from treatable conditions with no residual problems to death from tumor growth or resulting complications. Depending on the specific neoplasm, the client may experience a temporary limitation in mobility (due, for example, to surgery for tumor removal) or permanent limitation due to mutilating surgical excision, such as amputation of a limb.

Trauma

Trauma to a bone can cause a fracture. A person with a fracture has limited mobility, if not from instability or deformity then from the pain movement would cause. Soft tissue adjacent to a fracture, such as blood vessels, nerves, muscles, and adjacent organs may be damaged from the actual traumatic event or from the sharp edges of the broken bone. If the skin has been broken because of the fracture, the opening becomes a potential site for infection. The wound and the generous blood supply of the bone provide an excellent medium for bacterial growth. Muscle spasm at the fracture site can pull on the segments of the bone, holding the bone in an angulated position or causing side-by-side displacement of the bone fragments. A displaced segment of bone must be repositioned so the bone can heal in proper alignment.

Skeletal muscle can be injured by trauma. Fortunately, skeletal muscle fibers can regenerate, but when the damage is extensive, the fibers are replaced by scar tissue. Trauma to the musculoskeletal structures supporting the joints is common. Muscle fibers may be injured due to overuse, overstretching, forcible twisting, and other abnormal movements. The fibers may be torn, or stretched too far, and joint surfaces may dislocate, that is, separate partially or completely. Associated blood vessels and nerves may be damaged in the process. Pain and limited motion are the result.

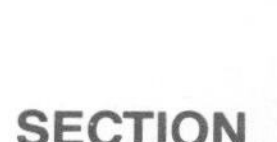

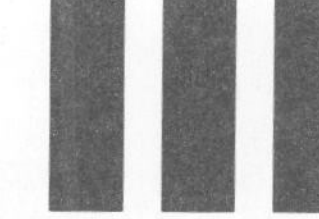

SECTION III

Related System Influences and Effects

Systemic Effects of Immobilization

Musculoskeletal disease can lead to immobilization; immobilization is also a method of treatment for many musculoskeletal conditions. Immobilization affects every system in the body to some extent, including the musculoskeletal system itself. Although immobility may help some musculoskeletal conditions heal, it may give rise to others. The effects of immobility on the body systems are summarized in Table 42–1.

Neurologic and Vascular Systems

Neurologic and vascular problems can cause or contribute to musculoskeletal disorders. Since muscle function is the result of the combined effect of muscle fibers and motor nerves, damage to or interference with the nerves can impair muscle function. Decreased function can cause muscles to atrophy, and paralysis can occur. Likewise, disruption of the vascular supply to bones or muscles can limit the nutrients and oxygen supplied to the cells and interfere with removal of cellular waste products. Prolonged interruption of circulation leads to necrosis of the tissues ordinarily supplied by the vessels.

Musculoskeletal disorders can also give rise to neurologic or vascular problems, which may in turn cause further musculoskeletal damage. Pressure from bandages, traction equipment, casts, tumor growth, and poor positioning are a few problems that can hinder nerve and blood vessel function. Trauma to muscles causes edema and hemorrhage in soft tissues, increasing the pressure within a confined space. Pressure on nerves and blood vessels in the area can become so great as to produce irreversible necrosis of the muscle tissue. An ugly, crippling, permanent contracture of the limb may occur, as well as loss of motor and sensory function.

Table 42–1
Summary of Effects of Immobility on the Body System

System	Results
Musculoskeletal	Demineralization of bone; decreased muscle mass and strength; joint stiffness; contractures; instability
Cardiovascular	Orthostatic hypotension; increased thrombus formation; increased workload on the heart
Respiratory	Decreased respiratory efficiency due to: decreased respiratory muscle movement, decreased movement of respiratory secretions, change in CO_2 and O_2 exchange; hypostatic pneumonia
Gastrointestinal	Anorexia; change in bowel habits (eg, constipation)
Urinary (especially from prolonged supine position)	Stasis of urine in kidney pelvis; formation of renal calculi; urinary retention; urinary tract infection
Integumentary	Abrasions; decubitus ulcer formation
Psychologic	Loneliness; boredom; depression; sensory deprivation

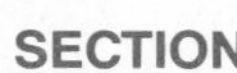
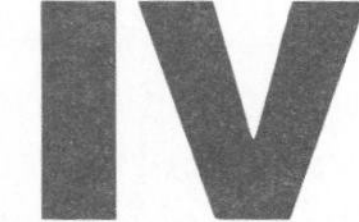

SECTION IV

Psychosocial/Lifestyle Influences and Effects

Developmental Influences

The aged person is more prone to injuries because of vision problems, loss of balance, and falls. With osteoporosis, which is common in postmenopausal women, fractures are more likely. Men also have a moderate decrease in bone density and muscle mass as they age because of a reduction in testosterone secretion.

Dietary Factors

Nutritional intake can affect the function of the musculoskeletal system in several ways. Nutritional excesses leading to obesity can cause stress fractures and excessive wear on joints. Vitamin deficiencies can cause bones to be deformed during growth, affect the turnover of bone in adulthood, and cause bones to be thin and porous. Vitamin D is especially important because it enhances the absorption of calcium and phosphorus from the intestinal tract. Musculoskeletal effects of vitamin deficiency diseases are uncommon in developed countries because an ordinary diet is usually adequate to prevent these symptoms. However, people with poor eating habits, such as alcoholics, occasionally develop vitamin deficiency diseases. Vegetarian diets that exclude all animal foods including dairy products and eggs require careful planning to ensure there are enough nutrients to prevent deficiency states.

Mineral deficiencies can also cause problems. Calcium imbalances affect the musculoskeletal system because calcium is essential for bone growth and turnover and for muscle contraction. A calcium deficit can result in increased neuromuscular excitability and bone demineralization, whereas calcium excess can cause muscle weakness. Low-calcium intake is often a contributing cause of osteoporosis, a disease involving bone demineralization that is common in the elderly. Bone demineralization can also occur from a deficiency of phosphorus.

Occupation and Recreation

A person's occupation can contribute to alterations in the musculoskeletal system, especially alterations resulting from trauma. Constant stress on joints, as from the use of a jackhammer, for example, can cause arthritic changes. Jobs involving heavy lifting and working with machinery have a high risk of traumatic injuries, including injuries to bones, joints, and muscles. People who work on assembly lines with dangerous machinery are susceptible to hand injuries. Today employee health and safety measures are reducing the incidence of such accidents in many countries.

Some musculoskeletal conditions require long-term or permanent changes in a client's way of life. Clients with an amputation, for example, may need to change their occupations. Various musculoskeletal disorders can reduce the number of hours clients can stay on their feet on the job.

The current interest in physical fitness has prompted many people to become active in athletic endeavors. While more and more people are becoming aware of the conditioning and training necessary to participate in physical activities, numerous injuries still occur.

Sports injuries are of two kinds, those that are acute and those that result from overuse. Acute injuries occur most often in contact sports and include breaks, strains, sprains, and dislocations. Overuse injuries are usually a result of repetitive motions common to a particular sport or of a sudden change in the sport, such as increasing the distance run, using different equipment, or playing on a different surface. The most common overuse injuries are inflammation of tendons and stress fractures. Ankle and foot injuries, dislocated hips, strains, and sprains of the back and neck have been seen in breakdancers. Engaging in high-risk sports such as race car driving increases the potential for personal injury.

With musculoskeletal disorders, clients may have to abandon recreational activities because they can no longer perform them or because the activities will cause further damage. Roles within the family may change; for example, a housewife may go out to work while her husband assumes the child-rearing responsibilities. Occasionally, it is necessary to modify a client's home, such as lowering the kitchen cupboards and work spaces. These changes require a period of adjustment for the entire family.

Economic Factors

Lengthy hospitalization, numerous surgical procedures, and the need for appliances and adaptive devices may be an enormous expense for the client and family. Those injured on the job frequently receive worker's compensation, but many injuries are not job related. Persons with health insurance coverage may have all or most of their medical expenses covered, but they usually are not compensated for income lost from not working.

Roles and Relationships

Conditions of the musculoskeletal system particularly affect a person's emotions because these conditions usually affect independence and mobility. A person who is temporarily or permanently dependent on others for assistance with activities of daily living may have feelings of powerlessness, loss of security, and a decrease in self-esteem. Being placed in a cast or in traction increases feelings of powerlessness. The chronic nature of many musculoskeletal problems may make clients wonder if they are becoming a burden on their families. They may no longer feel needed or useful to others because of their limitations. Some elderly people fear that they will be judged incapable of caring for themselves and be sent to a nursing home.

The nurse will see orthopedic clients in various phases of the grieving process. The grief may be for a lost body part or lost function, or even for lost loved ones who were killed in the same accident in which the client was injured. Other clients are uncertain about the outcome of their conditions and may have fears of deformity, disfigurement, or paralysis.

Body image may be altered as a result of a deformity or from devices used in treating the condition. Client self-perception will include anything connected to the body, such as a traction apparatus, cast, crutches, or even the bed. Confinement to a bed or room for an extended period of time may cause sensory deprivation, resulting in such manifestations as boredom, anxiety, and confusion.

With all this change, grief, fear, and doubt, changes in behavior are not surprising. Clients may seem unreasonable, demanding, frustrated, or depressed. They may realize a new source of power in voicing their anger. Musculoskeletal pain exacerbates clients' emotional reactions, making them feel even worse.

Sexual Expression

Some treatments for musculoskeletal conditions may provide obstacles to sexual activity. Examples are casts, traction, and long confinement in the hospital. The client's feeling of freedom to engage in sexual activity may be affected by fear of causing pain or of disrupting a healing injury or surgical repair.

The individual's sexual self-concept may be altered by changes in role or body image or by feelings of dependence and inadequacy. Sexual dysfunction may be related to feelings of depression and anxiety. The partner's perception of the client as a sexual being may be altered, affecting their sexual relationship. The couple may need to find new approaches for intercourse or other methods of sexual satisfaction.

Chapter Highlights

Normal development and function of muscles and bones requires the usual physical stresses and strains of daily activities.

Alterations in anatomy and physiology of the musculoskeletal system can result in limited motion, pain, and deformity.

Bone structure can be disrupted by vitamin and mineral deficiencies, altered bone metabolism, infection, tumors, and trauma.

Muscular structure and function can be altered by degenerative changes, inactivity, trauma, and abnormal calcium levels.

Joints can be damaged by degenerative changes, inactivity, infection, inflammation, and trauma.

Musculoskeletal conditions can result in long-term problems requiring lengthy medical treatment and adaptation to changes.

The emotional status of a client with limited mobility may be affected because of loss of independence and self-esteem, changes in body image, and alterations in sexual function.

Irreparable damage can occur to muscle and

bone tissues when there is interference with their nerve or blood supply.

Immobilization for treatment of musculoskeletal conditions can have adverse effects on all body systems.

Bibliography

Crelin ES: Development of the musculoskeletal system. *Clin Symp* 1981; 33(1):2–36.

Garrick JG: The sports medicine patient. *Nurs Clin North Am* 1981; 16:759–766.

Koerner ME, Dickinson GR: Adult arthritis: A look at some of its forms. *Am J Nurs* 1983; 83:254–262.

Lentz M: Selected aspects of deconditioning secondary to immobilization. *Nurs Clin North Am* 1981; 16:729–737.

Porth C: *Pathophysiology: Concepts of Altered Health States.* Philadelphia: Lippincott, 1983.

Price SA, Wilson LM: *Pathophysiology: Clinical Concepts of Disease Processes,* 2nd ed. New York: McGraw-Hill, 1982.

Rosse C, Clawson DK: *The Musculoskeletal System in Health and Disease.* New York: Harper & Row, 1980.

Silverstein A: *Human Anatomy and Physiology.* New York: Wiley, 1980.

Spence AP, Mason EB: *Human Anatomy and Physiology,* 3rd ed. Menlo Park, CA: Benjamin/Cummings, 1987.

Turner P: Caring for emotional needs of orthopedic trauma patients. *AORN J* 1982; 36:566–570.

CHAPTER 43

The Nursing Process for Clients With Musculoskeletal Dysfunction

Other topics relevant to this content are: Care of the client having a lumbar puncture, **Chapter 28;** Care of the client having a myelogram, **Chapter 28.**

Objectives

When you have finished studying this chapter, you should be able to:

Specify the major components of the health history to be obtained from clients with musculoskeletal dysfunction.

Explain specific assessment approaches in evaluating clients with disease of the musculoskeletal system.

Identify the nursing implications of diagnostic studies commonly used to evaluate clients with musculoskeletal dysfunction.

Determine appropriate nursing diagnoses for clients with disorders of the musculoskeletal system.

Develop, with the client, realistic goals of care.

Anticipate the psychosocial/lifestyle implications of musculoskeletal dysfunction for clients and their significant others.

Develop a nursing care plan for a client with musculoskeletal dysfunction.

Implement nursing interventions specific to clients with musculoskeletal disease.

Evaluate the effectiveness of the nursing care plan and modify it as necessary to meet client needs.

Orthopedics is the branch of medicine that studies and treats conditions of the bones, muscles, joints, and associated structures. An orthopedic nurse is one whose practice is primarily concerned with orthopedic clients. Almost all nurses, however, deal with at least some clients who have orthopedic problems, whether in the emergency department, surgical suite, intensive care units, ambulatory care settings, nursing homes, or medical and surgical units. This chapter discusses application of the nursing process to clients with musculoskeletal disorders in general.

SECTION I

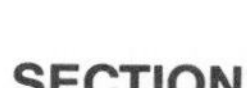

Nursing Assessment: Establishing the Data Base

The nursing assessment of the orthopedic client requires special emphasis on the musculoskeletal, neurologic, and vascular systems. In emergencies, nurses must deal first with life-threatening conditions such as hemorrhage and breathing difficulties; broken bones can usually wait until more urgent problems are treated. Assessing the emergency client for spinal injury is also important before attempting assessment of range of joint motion.

Subjective Data

Pain

Pain, sometimes severe, is a common manifestation of musculoskeletal problems. Ask clients to describe their pain thoroughly, including location, intensity, quality, duration, radiation, precipitating factors, and successful relief measures. Ask the client to point to the location where it hurts most; point tenderness (a highly localized sensitivity to touch) may be the site of a fracture. Some clients ache all over and need to indicate each of the areas involved.

Knowing the quality of pain may help pinpoint a specific problem, but the client may need help in describing the pain. A burning pain under a cast may indicate pressure sore formation or skin irritation, whereas pain radiating down a leg may indicate pressure on spinal nerves. All these data are helpful in making a nursing diagnosis and may also aid the physician with the medical diagnosis.

Some orthopedic clients experience pain so severe they cannot tolerate moving or being touched. Others have learned to live with chronic pain for so long that they may require less postoperative analgesia than usual. Pay attention to descriptions of pain that seem unusual or excessive for the client's condition. The pain may indicate a new or undiagnosed condition (eg, pain in the calf several days postoperatively may be the result of a complication such as thrombophlebitis).

Paresthesia

The client may describe abnormal sensations, or paresthesia, such as tingling, numbness, and diminished or absent sensation. The affected area should be defined as precisely as possible. Paresthesia is an indication of a neurologic problem and requires an in-depth assessment by the nurse.

Changes in Activities of Daily Living and Mobility

The nurse can obtain additional subjective data by asking the client how the problem affects activities of daily living (ADL) and mobility. Changes in normal activities may be from pain alone or from additional causes such as fatigue, weakness, stiffness, or decreased mobility of a particular body part. One client may report an inability to sleep at night because of leg pain, whereas another may say pain begins after walking as far as the bus stop. A client may have made adjustments to maintain independence ("I have to ride the elevator for just one floor now") or abandoned certain activities ("I can't serve a tennis ball any more because my shoulder hurts so much"). Encouraging clients to discuss their view of the situation helps to bring insights and misconceptions to the surface. Clients might also reveal feelings such as fear of dependence or of being a burden, or worries about being unable to support or care for a family.

Assistive Devices

The nurse should ask the client about any assistive devices used to help maintain independence. The client may use aids for walking, eating, dressing, bathing, toileting, or all of these. Some people are creative and adaptive in finding new ways to meet their daily needs.

Trauma History

Subjective data are particularly helpful when an injury is caused by trauma. The health care team will want to know:

- What was the client doing when the injury occurred?
- How long ago did the injury happen?
- What caused the injury?
- What position was the limb in at the time of injury?
- Did the client hear a crack or pop when the injury occurred?
- What initial symptoms (bleeding, deformity, bone protrusion, change in sensation, bruises, swelling, pain) did the client notice?
- What action (elevating the limb, applying ice, applying heat, continuing to use the limb, immobilizing the limb) did the client or someone else take in response to the injury?
- Was alcohol or drugs involved in the accident?
- Was any medication given?

This information can help the health care team determine what tissues and structures were injured as well as anticipate potential problems. If the client is unconscious or unable to supply the information because of shock, pain, or emotional distress, the health team needs to obtain a description of the accident from someone who accompanied the client to the hospital. It is important to ask people who bring in trauma clients to stay until someone can question them.

Objective Data

Physical Assessment

Objective data include the results of physical assessment and of laboratory and other diagnostic tests. In assessing clients with musculoskeletal disorders, the nurse considers vital signs, posture, muscle strength and tone, ability to ambulate, and neurologic status.

VITAL SIGNS An assessment of the vital signs is of particular importance in musculoskeletal trauma. Be alert to signs of shock. A temperature elevation may accompany inflammation and is common with an infection such as osteomyelitis (infection of the bone). Observing respiration is essential when injury occurs to the face, neck, or chest. Clients with spinal or chest deformities may also have abnormal respirations.

INFLAMMATION AND SWELLING Inflammation results from injury to tissues caused by physical trauma or by chemicals, bacteria, or foreign substances. Swelling occurs as inflammatory exudate forms to defend the tissues from the injury. Edema (usually resulting from circulatory problems) may also be present. Inspection and palpation are used when assessing clients for swelling and inflammation and comparing one extremity to the other for size, warmth, and erythema (redness). A joint will appear swollen when there is an increase in synovial fluid or when blood or purulent material is present in the joint capsule. This swelling is known as **effusion.** Effusion in the knee is detected by displacing the fluid with an upward stroke along the medial side of the knee and then pressing on the lateral side. The fluid will return and form a bulge (the bulge sign). Be gentle when assessing inflamed areas because they are usually tender. It is best to start palpating at a distance from the obvious tender area and work toward it, letting clients know when and where they will be touched and reassuring them that the touch will be gentle. Describe the amount of any swelling, and take note of how the injury was first treated. The latter is important for determining the significance of the amount of swelling. For example, after the same initial damage, an extremity that was iced and elevated after injury will have less swelling than one that was held in a dependent position while being soaked in warm water.

SKIN INTEGRITY Injury or disease processes may cause changes in the skin. Discoloration results when trauma to soft tissues causes **ecchymosis** (bruising). The skin may be broken or torn as a result of injury. Describe any lesions completely; include the location, length, depth, and appearance of the involved tissue. If there is any drainage, describe the amount, color, type, and odor.

Rashes are common in connective tissue disorders. Look for changes in the skin such as discoloration, dryness, scaliness, and lesions. Areas to observe are the face (including the eyes and mucous membranes), trunk, and extremities. Also assess the hair and nails because alopecia (hair loss) and nail changes can accompany some types of arthritis. Discoloration, usually redness, may occur in the palms, over joints, and at the distal ends of toes and fingers. Normal pigmentation may also be altered. Observe for thickening or thinning of the skin. Thin skin is especially susceptible to skin tears. Nodules characteristic of some arthritic conditions may be noted when palpating and observing the skin.

Other skin changes may be the result of treatment such as immobilization, casts, and traction. The nurse must therefore assess the skin condition of clients receiving such treatment. Pressure sores can occur readily at any point of pressure. Assess the skin around cast edges frequently and any areas touched by the traction apparatus. If the client cannot be turned, take advantage of any opportunity to view normally hidden areas. For example, check the skin of the heels and sacrum when the client is raised for back care.

DEFORMITIES Assess joints for deformities by observation and palpation. Compare joints in one extremity with those in the corresponding extremity, checking for symmetry, position, and changes in alignment. See Box 43–1 for the major points in general joint assessment.

When there is a joint dislocation, the normal shape of the joint is lost. There may be an abnormal bulge or mass in the joint area (as when the patella is displaced to the side, for example), or the two extremities may differ in length. Leg length discrepancy can be determined by measuring from the anterosuperior iliac spine to the medial malleolus when the client is lying down, as shown in Figure 43–1.

Assess the spine for abnormal curvature. A lateral

Nursing Research Note

Southwick JR, Callahan DJ: A study of blood-drainage patterns on synthetic cast materials. *Orthop Nurs* (March-April) 1985; 4:72–75.

This study investigated blood drainage in five types of fiberglass casting materials and one type of plaster of Paris. The fiberglass cast material did not absorb blood. The blood was drained to the outside of the cast or was absorbed into the casting pad. With plaster of Paris, however, blood was absorbed into the plaster material.

The authors stated that, with fiberglass casts, wound drainage will be found on bed linen or on the cast pad. Clients must be alerted to the possibility of bleeding and what to expect. This visible drainage is a method for assessing client status and wound status postoperatively.

Box 43–1
General Joint Assessment

Examine all joints in sequence from head to toe.

Examine painful joint last so less pain and fewer muscle spasms are induced.

Compare joints from one side to the other for symmetry.

Note size and contour of joints.

Observe for joint deformity, swelling, contractures, subluxation (partial dislocation), ankylosis (fixation).

Inspect color of overlying skin.

Palpate for temperature.

Touch gently to locate areas of tenderness in surrounding skin, muscles, bursae, and ligaments.

Palpate synovial membrane. Normally, the membrane is about the thickness of paper; the abnormal membrane feels boggy or doughy. Test for bulge sign.

Evaluate range of motion (ROM), active and passive.

Palpate for crepitation (a grating sound) on motion.

Assess muscle strength.

Observe for muscle atrophy.

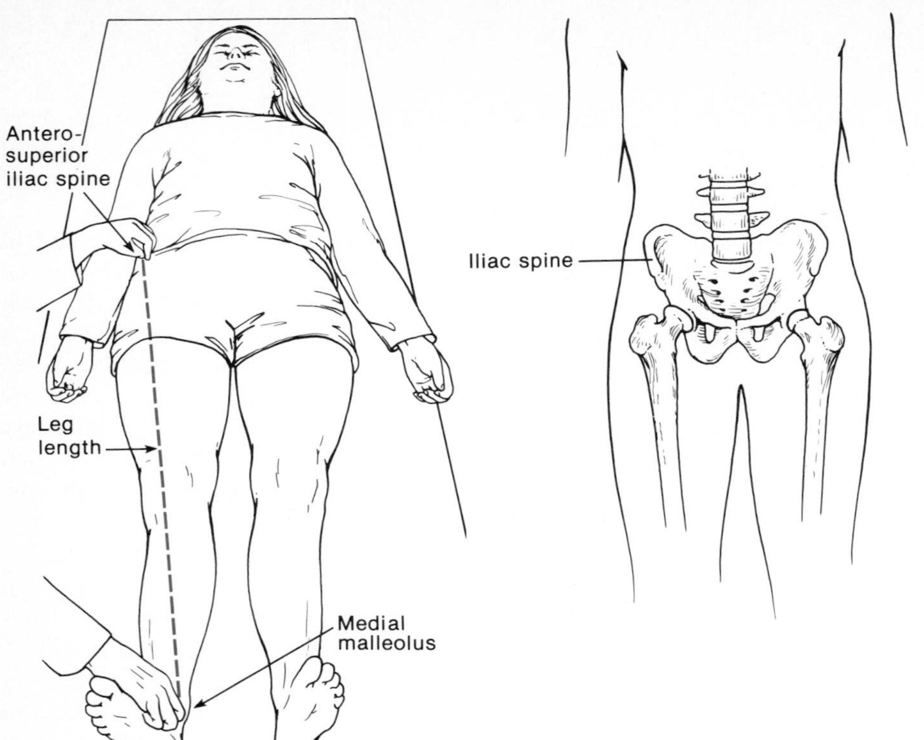

Figure 43–1

Measurement of leg length with client supine.

curve is known as **scoliosis.** An increased convex curve of the thoracic spine (hunchback) is called **kyphosis,** whereas an increased concave curve of the lumbar spine (swayback) is known as **lordosis.** With a deformity, the client may shift another body part in the opposite direction to compensate for the imbalance (eg, the pelvis may tilt to compensate when one leg is shorter than the other). Look for these compensatory changes.

RANGE OF MOTION Range of motion (ROM) is measured with an instrument called a goniometer (Figure 43–2). Placing the arms of the goniometer parallel to the axis of the bones that form the joint, the examiner measures the angle for the typical positions of the joint. The elbow's normal flexion, for example, is 160°, whereas its normal extension is 0° (Rodts, 1983). To determine what is normal for a client, compare a joint with an apparently abnormal ROM to the corresponding joint in the other extremity. Elderly people are likely to have some normal decrease in ROM, so it would be incorrect to use the average range as the standard for them.

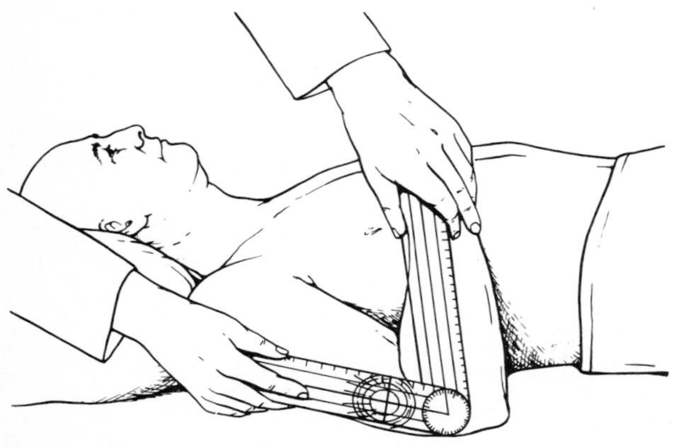

Figure 43–2

Use of a goniometer to measure the range of motion of a joint.

Ask the client to do ROM actively during evaluation. If the client is unable to move the extremity because of paralysis, determine ROM through passive movement. Do not move a joint beyond the point of comfort, and do not assess ROM in an acutely inflamed joint because it will be tender.

During the assessment of ROM, note joint stiffness, instability, and deformity. A grating sensation may be heard or felt during movement when there is a rough surface on the articular cartilage or when broken bone ends rub together. This grating is known as bony **crepitation.** A limitation of motion may be due to a *contracture* (permanent muscle shortening). The nurse who detects early signs of limitation of movement can implement measures to improve the ROM and prevent further limitations.

POSTURE Observe the client's standing posture for abnormalities. Posture can be affected by deformities, anomalies, muscle weakness, trauma, and pain. Clients may hold themselves in positions that relieve or decrease pain. Observe the symmetry of the body parts. Deformities of the spinal column may affect posture, causing exaggeration of any of the normal spinal curves. Posture is also an indication of energy and muscle tone. Normally posture is erect but not as rigid as a soldier standing at attention.

Box 43–2
Grading Muscle Strength

Grade 0: no evidence of contractility

Grade 1: trace of contractility

Grade 2: active movement with gravity eliminated

Grade 3: active movement against gravity

Grade 4: complete motion against gravity and some resistance

Grade 5: normal, complete motion against gravity and full resistance

MUSCLE STRENGTH, SIZE, AND TONE Muscle strength, size, and tone help diagnose disease conditions and also give the nurse information about the amount of assistance a client may need when ambulating and participating in activities. The examiner tests muscle strength by asking the client to resist movements or to move against resistance applied by the examiner. Strength is graded on a scale of 0 to 5 (see Box 43–2).

Observe and palpate muscles bilaterally to check their size and any asymmetry. If there seems to be a discrepancy in size, measure the limb circumferences with a tape measure to see if there are significant differences.

Muscle tone is assessed by moving the extremities passively. While the client is relaxed, the examiner moves the extremity through the range of motion, noting resistance to movement. A muscle with diminished tone is described as *flaccid.* When the muscle is tight and tense from involuntary contraction, it is said to be *spastic.*

ABILITY TO AMBULATE To assess ability to ambulate, ask the client to get up to walk across the room, turn around, and come back. Note whether the client has any difficulty getting up from the chair or bed. Normally when a person walks, the feet are about 2 to 4 in. apart, and the body shifts from side to side about 1 in. Posture is erect, with toes pointed straight ahead and shoulders in a straight line; the arms swing back and forth at the person's side, and movement is smooth with good balance.

There can be a variety of irregularities in walking. A limp can occur from abnormalities of leg length, joint motion, muscle strength, or other causes. The gait may appear stiff, unsteady, or wide-based; the feet may drag, or the steps may be very short. The body may lurch to the side as the individual shifts weight from one leg to the other. An irregular gait may cause fatigue because of the extra energy needed for walking. Ambulation may also be affected by discomfort, fear of falling, and loss of balance and coordination. As adults age, walking speed and balance may decrease. Steps may be short and shuffling, without the confidence and poise of youth.

The nurse should also evaluate the client's use of ambulatory aids such as crutches and canes. It is important to be aware of any difficulties the client is having and of potential safety hazards. Assistive devices must be in good repair.

NEUROVASCULAR STATUS Assessment of neurovascular status in the extremities is important for clients with traumatic injuries, surgery, casts, and traction. Perform the assessment regularly (more frequently initially), comparing the involved extremity to the other one to detect changes. The acronym CMTS is a reminder to check color, motion, temperature, and sensation in the limb. A variation of this is CMS, which stands for circulation, movement, and sensation. *Abnormalities in neurovascular status should receive immediate attention to prevent complications and irreversible damage to the limb.*

The color of the extremity or of the toes or fingers extending from the cast is an indication of the adequacy of circulation. If the color is white, there may be inadequate arterial blood flow; if it is blue, there may be venous stasis. Perform the *test for blanching* (or capillary refill) to check circulation to the toes or fingers. Press the nail firmly until it turns white, then release the pressure quickly; the normal pink coloring should return in 3 to 5 seconds. If the color is slow to return, there may be reduced arterial blood flow to the extremity.

Interference with the nerves supplying the extremity can cause a decrease in motion and change in sensation. To check motion, ask the client to move (flex, extend, abduct, and adduct) all the toes or fingers of the involved extremity within the limitation imposed by pain (or cast). Observe for diminished or absent motion. Assess all toes or fingers of the extremity for changes in sensation because some digits are innervated by one nerve and some by another. Test sensation by pricking the toe or finger with an object such as the end of a straightened paper clip. The client should describe the sensation, such as numbness, tingling, burning, dull pain, or no sensation.

Temperature is assessed by feeling the extremity and comparing to the other one. Take into consideration that a wet cast or ice bag application can make the extremity cold.

Peripheral pulses should be assessed, especially those distal to an injury, an operative area, or a cast or traction apparatus. When a pulse is difficult to locate, it is helpful to mark the spot with ink. Also observe for edema of the extremity, which is a sign of poor venous return.

Diagnostic Studies

SERUM ENZYME TESTS Alkaline phosphatase is an enzyme that can give an indication of new or active bone formation, because osteoblasts secrete large quantities of this enzyme when they are actively depositing bony matrix. Extreme elevations are common with Paget's disease of the bone, metastatic tumors to bone, and osteogenic sarcoma. (This enzyme is also elevated in liver disease.)

SERUM TESTS FOR ANTIBODIES AND ANTIGENS Antinuclear antibodies (ANA) are autoantibodies, produced against components of one's own cell nuclei. They are often present in clients with inflammatory connective tissue diseases, such as systemic lupus erythematosus or rheumatoid arthritis. The antibodies are detected by immunofluorescence, which is used as a screening test for clients with symptoms of such conditions. When ANA is present, the fluorescent dye used as a stain reacts within the antibodies and shows up under ultraviolet light (a positive result). The dye forms certain patterns that have been associated with disease. ANA results may also be positive with advancing age, but otherwise the test should be negative in the absence of connective tissue disease. After the presence of ANA is established, specific tests are done to identify particular antibodies such as anti-DNA (specific for systemic lupus erythematosus) and anti-RNA (specific in mixed connective tissue disease and systemic lupus erythematosus).

The test for the rheumatoid factor (RF) is specific for rheumatoid arthritis. The test, also called latex fixation, is frequently negative in the early stages of the disease but is usually positive in advanced rheumatoid arthritis. RF is also present in some chronic inflammatory diseases, including connective tissue disorders, but the titers are lower.

The test for the presence of human lymphocyte antigen B27 (HLA-B27) is used to help diagnose or rule out ankylosing spondylitis and Reiter's syndrome. This antigen is present in 90% of those with these diseases (Tilkian, Conover, & Tilkian, 1983). The antigen can also be found on tissue cells of those without these diseases, however, so its presence is not sufficient for a diagnosis.

SERUM CALCIUM AND PHOSPHORUS The level of calcium in the blood is used to detect bone disease and parathyroid gland disorder. A test for calcium is usually ordered along with serum phosphorus level because their concentrations are interrelated. Generally, when one level is elevated, the other is lowered. Conditions that increase bone resorption (osteoclastic activity) such as hyperparathyroidism, invasive bone disease, bone atrophy, osteoporosis, and osteomalacia cause an increase in the level of serum calcium.

SERUM URIC ACID Serum uric acid is elevated during an acute episode of gout but may be normal during remission. The serum uric acid level is also used as an indication of kidney function.

LE CELL PREPARATION The LE prep (lupus erythematosus cell preparation) is useful in diagnosing systemic lupus erythematosus (SLE). It is positive in 90% of untreated SLE; however, false positive and false negative results do occur. Since negative results do not eliminate the diagnosis of SLE, and since results may be positive in other diseases, this test is not used as much today as it has been in the past. The anti-DNA test is more specific for diagnosing SLE.

ERYTHROCYTE SEDIMENTATION RATE The erythrocyte sedimentation rate (ESR or sed. rate) is a test in which the settling of red blood cells in uncoagulated blood is timed. It is not a specific test for any particular disease, but elevations occur during inflammatory conditions and tissue necrosis. Changes in the ESR give an indication of improvement or worsening of the condition.

SYNOVIAL FLUID ANALYSIS Synovial fluid may be analyzed to detect inflammatory joint conditions, arthritis, and joint infection. The fluid is removed from an involved joint by aspiration (arthrocentesis). The procedure is done with aseptic technique, including skin preparation, local anesthetic, and use of a sterile needle and syringe. Normal joint fluid is clear and straw colored, with high viscosity and a white blood cell count (WBC) of less than 200/μL. In disease conditions, the fluid may appear cloudy, turbid, green, gray, or red, with decreased viscosity and an elevated WBC. The fluid may be used for a mucin clot test: A drop of synovial fluid normally forms a firm clot when added to an acetic acid solution, but in some inflammatory conditions, the clot will be soft and friable. When joint infection is suspected, Gram's stain and culture of the fluid are done to detect the causative organism.

X-RAYS Examination by x-ray helps diagnose bone and joint problems; it also allows following of the progress of a condition and its response to treatment. Abnormalities of bones that can be detected by x-ray include fractures, changes in density, and changes of position. X-rays also show joint changes such as erosion of joint margins, joint space narrowing, bone spurs, loose bodies, and dislocation. Specific injuries to soft tissues such as tendons and ligaments do not show on x-rays, but soft tissue swelling may be obvious. There is no special preparation for x-rays, but the client should be instructed to remain still when asked. When a fracture is suspected, clients should be moved cautiously to and from the x-ray department as well as on and off the cart and x-ray table to prevent further injury. It is essential to splint an extremity before the client is moved.

Special x-rays requiring injection of radiopaque substances are sometimes used for further study. Question the client before the procedure to determine any allergy to radiopaque dyes or iodine (because many dyes contain iodine). An *arthrogram* is an x-ray of a joint following the injection of radiopaque dye; the injection requires sterile technique. The internal structure of the injected joint can be visualized on the x-ray because the dye outlines the intracapsular joint space. Changes in the joint structure, such as injury to the ligaments and meniscal tears, show on the x-ray as patterns taken by the dye.

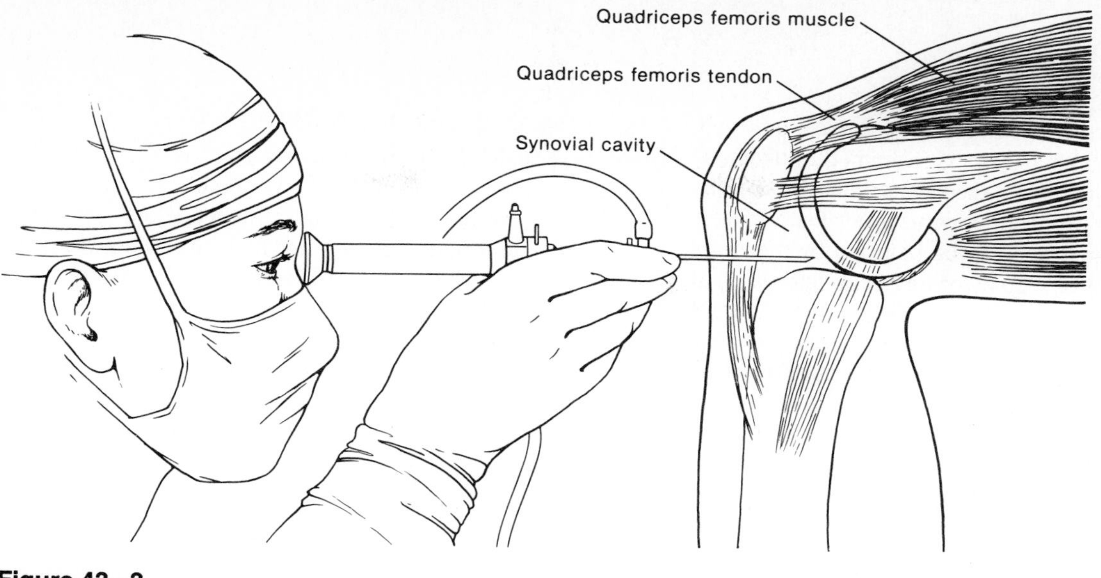

Figure 43–3

Use of an arthroscope to view interior of the knee.

A *myelogram* is an x-ray and fluoroscopic exam of the spinal cord and subarachnoid space following the injection of a contrast medium, which is introduced by way of a lumbar puncture (see Chapter 28). Abnormalities such as a herniated disk can be localized when filling defects are seen on the x-ray. When Pantopaque medium is used, the postprocedural care is like that following a lumbar puncture. A newer medium, metrizamide (Amipaque), is being used for lumbar myelography. It provides the advantages of better visualization and use of a smaller needle. The medium does not need to be withdrawn. When Amipaque is used, the postprocedural care includes prevention of nausea, vomiting, headache, and seizures. The head of the bed must be elevated 30–40° for 8 hours, followed by flat bed rest with bathroom privileges for the next 16 hours. Oral fluids are encouraged. Phenothiazines, MAO inhibitors, and tricyclic antidepressants should be withheld 48 hours prior to the myelogram to decrease the possibility of seizure activity. Phenothiazines must also be avoided for 24 hours after the procedure (Branson, 1982).

BONE SCAN A bone scan provides a picture of radioactivity in bones after intravenous injection of a radioactive isotope, usually technetium 99. The radioactive substance accumulates in areas of increased osteoblastic activity, which then show up as dark spots on the screen. Since some malignant bone tumors have accelerated osteoblastic activity, the bone scan is useful in diagnosing these tumors. A bone scan may be done when bone metastasis from other tumor sites is suspected. A bone scan can detect lesions at an earlier stage of disease than a routine x-ray. Tell clients that the injection may be a little uncomfortable and that they must remain still during the scan itself.

ARTHROSCOPY **Arthroscopy** is the examination of a joint through a special fiberoptic endoscope called an arthroscope (Figure 43–3). The knee is the joint most commonly examined by this means. The instrument has lenses and a light source permitting photography and surgical procedures through it. The procedure is done in the operating room using aseptic technique, usually with the use of a local anesthetic, although a general anesthetic may be given. A tourniquet helps to reduce blood flow to the area. A cannula is inserted into the joint, through which the scope is introduced, and normal saline is instilled to provide a viewing medium. The technique can be used for biopsy of the synovium or cartilage, as well as removal of loose bodies from the joint. After the procedure, a compression dressing, such as an Ace bandage, is applied. The client may be allowed to bear weight, avoiding excessive use for a few days, or may be directed to avoid use for 24 hours, depending on the surgeon's preference and the nature of the procedure. Teach the client to observe for signs of infection. The procedure is frequently done on an outpatient basis (Farrell, 1982).

ELECTROMYOGRAM The **electromyogram** (EMG) is a test to measure the electric currents produced by muscles, at rest and during contraction. Small needle electrodes are inserted into the muscles being tested and then connected by wires to an electromyograph machine. The results are recorded, displayed on a screen, and heard on a speaker. Changes in muscle electrical activity may be helpful in diagnosing neuromuscular disease. The test is particularly useful in differentiating muscular disease from neurologic disease. There is no special preparation before the test. Inform the client that small needles will be inserted into skin and muscle, causing some discomfort but that there is no danger of electrical shock.

BIOPSY Various biopsies may be performed on the musculoskeletal system. Bone may be obtained by open or needle biopsy to diagnose or follow a bone disease or lesion. Skin, obtained by a punch biopsy, is examined to diagnose some of the connective tissue disorders. Muscle biopsies are usually operative procedures done to evaluate muscle disease. Synovial membrane can be biopsied by means of an arthroscopy, a needle biopsy, or an open incision. Synovial membrane analysis is useful in diagnosing different types of arthritis. Buccal mucosa may be biopsied to help diagnose Sjögren's syndrome, and the temporal artery may be biopsied to diagnose temporal arteritis.

SECTION 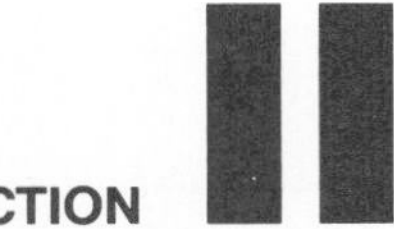

Nursing Diagnosis/Planning and Implementation/Evaluation

Information gathered from the client's health history, physical examination, and diagnostic studies is used to determine nursing diagnoses and the plan of care. Not every client will have the same needs. The Nursing Diagnoses box lists diagnoses **directly related** to musculoskeletal dysfunction along with **potential** nursing diagnoses for clients with musculoskeletal problems. The most common nursing diagnoses for clients with musculoskeletal dysfunction include impaired physical mobility, impaired skin integrity, altered bowel elimination: constipation, ineffective breathing pattern, altered tissue perfusion, altered comfort: pain, potential for injury, self-care deficit, and altered sexuality patterns. The sample nursing care plan in Table 43–1 focuses on the immobilized client and includes discussions of impaired skin integrity, altered comfort, urinary retention, altered bowel elimination: constipation, altered breathing pattern, potential for injury, altered tissue perfusion: peripheral, impaired social interaction, activity intolerance, and self-care deficit. The narrative content discusses altered comfort, potential for injury, self-care deficit, and altered sexuality patterns.

If the goals of care have not been met, re-evaluation is required. The nurse and client should jointly review the nursing care plan. New objectives may need to be formulated; other nursing interventions may be added or modified; or the evaluation may show that more time is required to meet the objectives.

Comfort, Altered: Pain

Clients with musculoskeletal dysfunction often have pain, swelling, and inflammation. Whether the client's discomfort is related to trauma, arthritis, low back pain, or degeneration, the plan of care may share common features.

Planning and Implementation

Pain and discomfort should be assessed thoroughly before attempting nursing interventions. Because some orthopedic problems are chronic, dependence can occur with prolonged drug use. Comfort measures and relaxation approaches should be attempted and not abandoned because they were not effective initially.

Rest is particularly useful in treating inflammatory conditions of the joints, especially during the acute phase, because it helps relieve pain and prevent further destruction of joint tissues. Rest is also helpful after musculoskeletal trauma because it helps minimize pain and swelling and promotes healing of injured tissues. A fractured bone is rested by use of a splint, cast, or traction after the bone is placed in good alignment. Rest is also used to relieve muscle spasms.

When the weight of covers causes discomfort, a foot cradle or footboard may be helpful. Check for dressings that might be too tight, causing pain. Crumbs in a cast can be removed by a portable vacuum.

Bed rest may be helpful during joint inflammation and is necessary with traction. Because prolonged bed rest can result in many complications, specific nursing measures are necessary to prevent their occurrence (see Table 50–1). Splinting joints provides stability, relieves pain caused by movement, and maintains the joint in a functional position. Rest may also be achieved by restricting weight bearing on an injured extremity, thus resting it.

A balance between rest and activity is desired so that function can be maintained while additional disability is prevented. Clients with arthritis need extra rest periods and extra hours of sleep at night. Teach the importance of planning for this additional rest to control fatigue and restore energy.

APPLYING HEAT OR COLD The use of either hot or cold applications provides temporary relief of pain and increased range of joint motion. It used to be common to apply heat only to arthritic joints, but cold has also been found to be helpful for many people. Alternating application of heat and cold can be effective in some. Physicians suggest using whatever works for the arthritic client. Contraindications for heat or cold include poor circulation, decreased temperature sensation, and hypersensitivity to heat or cold. Use is limited in those who are not alert enough to note abnormal sensations from the heat or cold, including those who are sedated.

Heat specifically causes vasodilation, thereby increasing blood flow. It relaxes muscles, relieves morning stiffness, and provides analgesia. Heat is not used on acutely inflamed joints but is useful in subacute or chronic joint problems (Simpson, 1983). Many forms of heat, including dry and moist heat, are used for arthritic conditions. *Moist heat* is more penetrating and can be applied by a shower; by foot, hand, or tub baths; and by hot packs or compresses. *Dry heat* can be administered at higher temperatures than moist heat. Methods of dry heat include diathermy (electromagnetic waves) and ultrasound (high frequency sound waves), usually administered by a physical therapist. Heating pads, lamps, and hot water bottles also provide dry heat.

Heat is often applied before exercise and massage. The exposure should last about 15 to 30 minutes, depending on the method used. Prolonged use of heat causes vasoconstriction. The need for safety measures in applying heat cannot be overemphasized. The area should be checked frequently (every 5 minutes, at least) for redness and discomfort. Clients should be instructed to get attention immediately if the application feels too hot. Clients should be taught not to adjust the heat source themselves.

Cold applications cause vasoconstriction, decreasing blood flow and helping to decrease or prevent swelling after injury. Pain may be relieved because cold raises the pain threshold. In some people, stiffness is relieved by cold. Cold is more useful in those with acute pain or acutely inflamed joints. It can be applied by cold compresses, ice bags, or a cold bath. Ice is applied to traumatic injuries for the first 24 hours after the accident to decrease fluid accumulation, control bleeding by vasoconstriction, and decrease pain. Prolonged use of cold, however, causes vasodilation. Therefore, cold is applied for 15 to 30 minutes, removed for 10 to 15 minutes, and then reapplied in a cyclical pattern. In between, dry the skin and check for untoward signs such as paleness, cyanosis, mottling, and secondary vasodilation. At times, ice is applied continuously to reduce swelling. If continuous cold is ordered, check the client frequently (every 5 minutes, at least) for undesired effects.

Evaluation

Expected client outcomes following effective nursing interventions for alteration in comfort include statements by the client and significant others of a decrease or absence of pain, an increase in comfort, and adequate rest and sleep. Care provider observations confirm the reports of client and family.

Injury, Potential For

Clients with musculoskeletal dysfunction are at risk for serious complications. The plan of care must include careful attention to preventive measures. Loss of muscle strength and joint mobility, contractures, and falls are some potential complications.

Planning and Implementation

Proper positioning and body alignment, exercise, and ambulation are the major considerations in restoring full mobility. Teach the client and significant others the underlying rationale and involve them in the plan of care.

POSITION AND BODY ALIGNMENT The client with an injured extremity or who has had surgery on an extremity will usually have the extremity elevated on pillows; the foot of the bed may also be elevated. When elevated, the entire length of a cast or splint should be supported to avoid strain on the unsupported area. When the client is lying on one side, the uppermost limb should be supported with pillows along its entire length to avoid adduction. Particular attention should be given to avoid pressure over nerves and bony prominences.

The normal curves of the back should be supported with small pads when the client is supine. Use of only a small pillow under the neck helps prevent neck flexion contracture. Trochanter rolls are used to prevent external hip rotation when supine. The prone position should be included in the positioning schedule when the client's condition allows.

A client with an inflamed or painful extremity will hold it in the most comfortable position. Often that position involves flexion of a joint. Without exercise and changes in position, a contracture will develop. When joints are acutely inflamed or painful, a splint may be applied to rest the joint in a *functional position* (one that would be most useful if the joint became frozen in that position). Make sure splints fit properly, are removed periodically for skin care, and are reapplied. When handling painful extremities, the least distressing method is to support the limb above and below the affected area, handling it gently.

A firm mattress is especially important for the client confined to bed for an extended period of time, for those having back problems, and for those with heavy casts requiring support. A trapeze on the bed is useful to allow clients to shift their body weight periodically.

EXERCISE AND AMBULATION The benefits of exercise include increased circulation, maintenance of joint mobility, improvement in joint mobility, preservation of muscle strength, and improved muscle strength. ROM exercises, whether active or passive, help prevent contractures.

Isometric or muscle-setting exercises are done when a muscle contracts without movement, thereby maintaining strength, increasing tone, and aiding circulation. The client should be taught to contract or tighten the muscle, holding it until the count of 10, then relax. This should be done 10 to 15 times every 3 to 4 hours when awake. To instruct clients in isometric quadriceps exercises, tell them to try pushing the back of the knee against the mattress while sitting in bed. If this is done properly, the thigh muscle tightens and the heel raises off the mattress. Encourage clients to try it on the unaffected leg first to demonstrate the method. Quadriceps atrophy begins in 1 week if the muscle is not exercised (Farrell, 1982). Isometrics should be done on quadriceps, gluteal, and abdominal muscles to prepare the client for ambulation.

Isotonic exercises are done with uninvolved extremi-

NURSING DIAGNOSES IN Musculoskeletal Dysfunction

DIRECTLY RELATED DIAGNOSES

- Activity intolerance
- Bowel elimination, altered: constipation
- Breathing pattern, ineffective
- Comfort, altered: pain
- Health maintenance, impaired
- Injury, potential for
- Mobility, physical impaired
- Self-care deficit
- Sexuality, altered patterns
- Skin integrity, impaired
- Social interaction, impaired
- Tissue perfusion, altered: peripheral
- Urinary retention

OTHER POTENTIAL DIAGNOSES

- Bowel elimination, altered: incontinence
- Comfort, altered: chronic pain
- Diversional activity deficit
- Home maintenance management, impaired
- Incontinence, functional
- Post-trauma response
- Role performance, altered
- Self-concept altered: body image
- Sensory/perceptual alterations: tactile

ties. When the client will be using crutches, the arms can be strengthened by push-ups when prone, lifting the buttocks off the bed by pushing the palms against the mattress while sitting, weight lifting, and use of the trapeze. Commercial weights may be used, but objects such as sandbags or books can also serve as weights for lifting.

Exercises beneficial to arthritics include ROM and isometrics. Acutely inflamed joints are not exercised. Studies have shown that rest and splinting of inflamed joints cause minimal or no permanent joint mobility loss. Arthritic clients should not use isotonic or weight-lifting exercises that stress affected joints. They should also limit the number of repetitions of each movement (Simpson & Dickinson, 1983).

All clients should be encouraged to move all unrestricted body parts. Participation in ADL provides some exercise and should be encouraged. Those with a cast or splint should exercise the joints above and below the appliance, unless contraindicated. Clients with an arm cast tend to hold their shoulder in one position. For them, the sling should be removed and ROM exercises performed to keep the shoulder free.

Physical therapists usually are consulted to help the client with ambulation. They also measure and fit the client for ambulatory aids such as crutches, canes, walkers, and wheelchairs. However, physical therapists are not readily available in most ambulatory care settings or emergency departments, where a majority of musculoskeletal injuries are treated. Therefore nurses should familiarize themselves with this information, in case they are called upon to measure crutches and teach crutch-walking. In most inpatient settings, an appropriate gait is taught and practiced in physical therapy. Nurses are responsible for assisting the client on the unit during ambulation, so they must be familiar with proper crutch posture and crutch-walking gaits. Proper posture includes: head held high, feet under the pelvis, crutches about 10 inches in front and slightly to the sides of the feet, and weight carried on the wrists and palms, not the axilla. If the weight rests on the axilla, the radial nerve may be injured, causing paralysis of the elbow and wrist extensor muscles. When the client is standing upright with shoulders relaxed, the axillary bar should be one to two fingers below the axilla. Both client and nurse should be aware of the amount of weight bearing allowed on the affected leg or legs: full, partial, or none.

Measuring a client for crutches can be done in bed or standing, with the shoes on. Measure from the axillary fold to a point 6 to 8 in. lateral to the heel. Another method is to subtract 16 in. from the height. The hand bar should be placed so that the elbow has 30° flexion (see Figure 43–4) when resting. The elbow extends when a step is taken. The crutches should be assessed for safety. Bolts should be tightened; rubber tips should not be worn down.

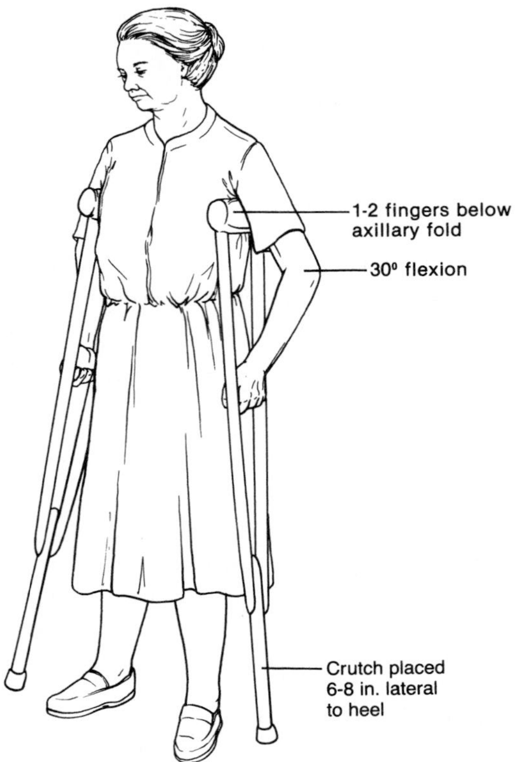

Figure 43–4

Correctly fitted crutches.

Table 43–1
Sample Nursing Care Plan for Clients Who Are Immobilized, by Nursing Diagnosis

Client Care Goals	Plan/Nursing Implementation	Expected Outcome
Mobility, impaired physical related to muscle atrophy		
Actively exercise the involved mucles within the limits of prescribed therapy; understand the causes of muscle wasting and the benefits of active exercise	Assess muscle size, strength, symmetry; ambulate as much as possible; encourage participation in ADL; teach isometric exercises when isotonics are not possible; active ROM, at least b.i.d.; teach how active exercise prevents muscle wasting	Muscle symmetry, size, strength will be equal to those of uninvolved extremity; will ambulate and participate in ADL with minimal assistance; will describe reason for active exercise
Mobility, impaired physical related to joint contracture		
Perform ROM exercises of the involved joints within the limits of prescribed therapy; understand the causes of joint contracture and the benefits of exercises and correct alignment; maintain proper body alignment when sitting or lying	Assess the client's ROM; ROM at least b.i.d.; position in correct body alignment; change position frequently; use assistive devices that maintain position, such as hand cones, footboard; encourage participation in ADL; teach ROM exercises, correct positioning; teach how mobility prevents contractures; rest in a functional position (ie, avoid hip rotation, wrist drop, footdrop)	Will retain normal range of joint motion; will describe reasons for exercises and correct alignment
Health maintenance, altered related to potential for bone demineralization (osteoporosis)		
Change position frequently; carry out daily weight-bearing exercises and activities; understand the effects of immobility on the bone; eat a well-balanced diet	Encourage weight bearing as much as possible including standing, sitting, ambulation; encourage resistive exercises; encourage participation in ADL; teach how mobility helps prevent bone demineralization; implement frequent position changes; encourage eating a well-balanced diet with adequate intake of calcium, vitamin D, and protein	Will perform weight-bearing exercises regularly; will describe reasons for activity, weight bearing, and balanced diet; will show no evidence of bone pain or porous bones (on x-ray)
Skin integrity, impaired: potential related to immobility		
Change position frequently; take in a well-balanced diet and 3000 mL of fluids per day; understand the effects of prolonged pressure on skin integrity; observe own skin for pressure sores where possible	Encourage position changes q. 1 h; assess and teach client to assess skin for signs of potential skin breakdown; redness, edema, pain; keep skin clean, dry, and lubricated; check every 4–8 h; keep sheets wrinkle free; use special devices to decrease pressure such as air or water mattresses; teach client to shift weight periodically; encourage a well-balanced diet with 3000 mL of fluids per day; teach how prolonged pressure causes decubitus ulcer formation	Will avoid staying in the same position for more than 1 h; skin will show no signs of breakdown; will describe how skin breaks down from prolonged pressure
Comfort, altered: pain related to calculi formation		
Take in 3000 mL of fluids per 24 h; understand relationship between immobility and stone formation; change position frequently and ambulate when able	Encourage fluid intake of 3000 mL per 24 h; I & O; ambulate as much as possible; change position frequently; especially use an upright position periodically; teach that mobility helps decrease stone formation; observe for signs of stone formation such as hematuria, flank pain, dysuria; check urine pH daily; check serum Ca^{++} values	Will show no signs of urinary calculi formation; will ambulate and change position regularly; will describe reason for activity and increased fluid intake; fluid intake is 3000 mL per 24 h; urine pH will remain slightly acidic

(continued)

Table 43–1
Sample Nursing Care Plan for Clients Who Are Immobilized, by Nursing Diagnosis (continued)

Client Care Goals	Plan/Nursing Implementation	Expected Outcome
Urinary retention related to potential for calculi formation		
Empty bladder adequately, voluntarily; understand the relationship between decreased activity, decreased muscle tone, and difficulty voiding; change position frequently	Note voiding pattern (frequency, amount); assess for signs of urinary retention, such as inability to void, abdominal distention; I & O; use a sitting (or standing) position to void; provide privacy; encourage activity and ambulation as much as possible; teach that mobility aids the ability to void normally; use methods to facilitate voiding, such as running water within hearing distance	No signs of bladder distention or incontinence; will describe how activity aids voiding
Bowel elimination, altered: constipation related to decreased activity		
Ambulate and exercise regularly; understand the causes of constipation; take in 3000 mL of fluids per 24 h; include roughage in diet	Question client regarding a BM daily; I & O; ambulate as much as possible; encourage fluids, at least 3000 mL per 24 h; encourage foods containing fiber; use a sitting position for BM; provide privacy; consult with physician as needed for orders for laxatives, stool softeners; teach relationship between mobility, fluids, fiber, and constipation	Will maintain usual bowel pattern; will describe how constipation is related to immobility
Breathing pattern, ineffective related to decreased expiratory effort		
Practice coughing and deep-breathing exercises (C & DB); ambulate and change position frequently; understand the effects of immobility on respiratory system	Assess rate, depth, rhythm of respirations q. 4 h; assess the chest for abnormal breath sounds; assess skin color for hypoxia; teach and encourage C & DB excercises q. 2 h; encourage ambulation as much as possible; encourage frequent position changes, especially upright; observe for obstructions to respirations, such as a tight cast or bandage; teach about the relationship between immobility and respiratory problems	Will show no signs of respiratory problems; will explain how inactivity affects the respiratory system; will perform C & DB exercises q. 2 h
Injury, potential for related to unsafe ambulation		
Safely ambulate or assume upright position regularly; understand the relationship between immobility and postural hypotension	Encourage regular exercise and ambulation; encourage the upright position; have client wear elastic stockings; teach and encourage client to get up slowly; check BP while dangling, before standing, and q. 4 h; observe for light-headedness when upright; teach the relationship between hypotension and immobility	Blood pressure will remain stable when upright; will explain the cause of postural hypotension and the reason for rising slowly; will engage in regular activity including ambulation
Tissue perfusion, altered: peripheral related to impaired venous circulation to lower extremities		
Exercise the extremities actively; understand the tendency for clot formation during inactivity; increase fluid intake to at least 3000 mL per 24 h	Observe for signs of thrombus formation, such as tenderness, edema; check Homans' sign; have client wear elastic stockings; encourage active leg exercises regularly, such as pedaling the feet, drawing imaginary circles with the toes; avoid positioning with acute angle flexion of the knees, such as using the knee gatch on the bed or pillows under the knees; change position q. 2 h; encourage fluid	No signs of thrombus formation; will explain relationship between thrombus formation and immobility; will carry out active leg exercises at least q. 2 h

Table 43–1
Sample Nursing Care Plan for Clients Who Are Immobilized, by Nursing Diagnosis (continued)

Client Care Goals	Plan/Nursing Implementation	Expected Outcome
	intake of at least 3000 mL per 24 h; avoid trauma to the limb; avoid positioning with one limb leaning on the other, causing pressure; teach about the relationship between immobility and blood clot formation	
Social interaction, impaired related to prolonged bedrest		
Express feelings about condition and situation; use all senses; remain oriented; maintain independence as much as possible; interact with others regularly; participate in activities as able	Encourage participation in ADL; encourage independence; exercise and ambulate frequently; change position frequently; encourage client to be out of room, socializing with others; encourage visitors and phone calls; orient or reorient as necessary (calendar, clock, familiar objects); encourage participation in usual hobbies and activities, when possible; provide opportunities for decision making; encourage expression of feelings; allow client to vent feelings about immobility, role change, restrictions; assess for changes in emotional reactions, orientation, motivation, body image, and self-concept; provide a change of scenery or encourage family to do so; use sensory stimuli such as touch, radio, TV	Will show proper orientation to person, place and time; will demonstrate normal psychosocial status, as indicated by family; will display emotional reactions that are appropriate to the circumstances; will maintain maximum independence; will actively participate in interactions and activities; will share feelings and frustrations
Activity in tolerance related to medically imposed restrictions		
Exercise the muscles to be used in ambulation; use any ambulatory aids correctly; understand safety measures for ambulation; adjust home environment to facilitate ambulation, as needed	Teach exercises appropriate for ambulation: (1) isometrics of the quadriceps, abdominal, and gluteal muscles (2) doing pushups when prone (3) lifting buttocks off bed while sitting by pushing down on bed with hands Teach use of trapeze appropriate for client (ie, bending knees and raising back and buttocks off the bed; shifting weight periodically, without holding breath when lifting); try the upright position a few times before ambulation for those who have been flat; use sturdy shoes when ambulating; get help when ambulating the first time and as needed; dangle feet first; teach transfer acitivites (eg, lock wheelchair wheels, elevate head of bed); teach correct use of ambulatory aids (physical therapist may do this but nurse should be familiar with methods to aid ambulation on the unit); make sure ambulatory aids are correct height, size; teach client to keep head up, looking forward (not down) when walking; assess balance; provide a safety belt for client's waist, for nurse to hold when walking; remove clutter, loose rugs, wet spots on floor, other items that may cause falls; also teach client and family; observe that client is using proper gait for	Will ambulate with minimal assistance; will describe safety measures necessary for ambulation; will use ambulatory aids correctly; will participate in appropriate exercises; will use trapeze as taught; there will be no accidents or injuries in either hospital or home environment

(continued)

Table 43–1
Sample Nursing Care Plan for Clients Who Are Immobilized, by Nursing Diagnosis (continued)

Client Care Goals	Plan/Nursing Implementation	Expected Outcome
	aids used; make sure client can ambulate well enough to maneuver up and down stairs and in and out of bed before discharge; have someone assess client's home environment for safety and possible necessary alterations to assist ambulation; have family member make necessary adjustments before discharge	
Self-care deficit: bathing/hygiene, dressing/grooming, toileting, feeding related to intolerance to activity		
Participate in ADL, as able; learn new ways to perform ADL when necessary and able; adjust to changes in ADL abilities	Assess ability to perform ADL; assess need for assistive devices; encourage participation in ADL; give reinforcement (acknowledgment, reward) for good performance and effort; place objects client will use nearby to facilitate self-help; teach alternative methods for achieving ADL; consult with physician, OT, PT for additional intervention as needed; consult for financial aid through social services, when needed for assistive devices, etc.; encourage family involvement when client will need assistance at home; encourage resourcefulness and creativity when trying adaptive techniques (buying a tool for every activity is not necessary); allow expression of feelings, (eg, of discouragement or anger); give encouragement as needed and encourage family to do so	Will function with as much independence as possible; will cope with necessary adjustments in performing ADL; client and family will creatively adapt usual life activities to client's impairment in mobility

A pad may or may not be used on the axillary bar. The client should wear low-heeled shoes with nonskid bottoms.

The most common crutch-walking gait is the three-point gait. The crutches are moved forward first, then the involved leg, and then the uninvolved leg. This gait is used when partial or no weight bearing is allowed on the involved leg. The two-point gait is used when some weight bearing is allowed on both feet. The client advances one crutch and the opposite leg simultaneously, then the other crutch and remaining leg together. The four-point gait is also used when some weight bearing is allowed on both feet. One crutch is advanced, then the opposite leg, then the remaining crutch, and finally, the other leg. This gait is harder to learn but provides more stability because three "points" are always on the floor.

The nurse can assist the client to gain confidence in walking on crutches by having the client wear a belt that the nurse can grasp as needed to keep the client from falling. The nurse should walk slightly behind and to the affected side. For crutch-walking on stairs, the affected leg should move together with the crutches. When the stairs have a railing, the client can put both crutches under the arm opposite the railing while the near hand holds the rail. When climbing, the client advances the unaffected leg first, then the crutches (while standing on the unaffected leg, as the affected leg dangles). When descending, the client moves the crutches first, and the unaffected leg last. Going down the stairs with crutches is particularly frightening; clients should practice with supervision until they gain skill in this maneuver.

A cane is used to lessen weight bearing on a hip or knee. It provides a wider than normal base of support and aids balance. The client should hold the cane on the side opposite the involved leg, taking part of the weight off the sore leg. Canes with three (tripod) or four (quad) legs are also available and provide added stability. A properly fitted cane allows slight (15° to 30°) flexion of the elbow when it is being held and extension of the elbow during weight bearing.

A walker is often used by elderly people because it provides greater support and a feeling of security. It is useful for clients with an unsteady gait and when partial weight bearing is necessary. The client can pick up and move the walker or push it forward. Walkers come in different sizes or can be adjusted. They are the correct height when the client's elbows are flexed 15° to 30° while holding the handles. Walkers are not very useful on stairs unless the tread is very deep, so the client may require assistance when navigating stairs.

Safety precautions are necessary with all types of aids

to ambulation. At home, the family should remove clutter and loose rugs. Clients should wear sturdy shoes. A three-in-one over the toilet/bedside commode provides the support of sidearms for transfers as well as the elevation some clients need when using the toilet. Clients should be assisted until they are ambulating well without help. It is important to plan ahead by instituting an exercise program to prepare the client for ambulation. Ambulation should begin with plenty of time available for practice before the client is discharged.

Evaluation

Expected client outcomes following effective nursing interventions for potential for injury include optimal client mobility without complications. The client demonstrates an understanding of limitations on activity as well as the need for continued efforts at prescribed exercise and ambulatory activities. Significant others report that safety precautions have been taken in the home (eg, throw rugs removed, cords relocated to avoid tripping).

Self-Care Deficit

Some clients with musculoskeletal dysfunction will have difficulty with eating, dressing, toileting, and/or bathing. The nursing care plan should address the problem and develop approaches for maximizing client independence.

Planning and Implementation

Many self-help devices are available to assist the disabled client in maintaining independence. It is not always necessary to purchase these items; suitable devices can be made at home. Clients and their significant others can often improvise to meet their needs.

Home Health Care

Various modified eating utensils are available, some with built-up handles, others with long handles, and some with handles at a different angle than is usual.

Clients who cannot reach their feet adequately can use elastic shoelaces and various long-handled appliances such as shoehorns and stocking holders. Those who cannot raise their arms can use reachers and long-handled combs. The use of Velcro fasteners, rather than buttons, aids those with difficulty in fine motor skills. In the bathroom, an elevated toilet seat, handrails, a shower chair, nonskid mats, and a long-handled bath sponge can be helpful.

The occupational therapy (OT) department can assist the client in developing self-care abilities and make recommendations for easier, safer methods to do many tasks. In some facilities, the nurse can make referrals to OT; in others, the nurse must consult with the physician.

When a client normally uses special devices for self-care at home, encourage continued use when hospitalized. Any methods that keep clients independent should be encouraged, even if doing a task themselves takes longer or creates a mess. A nursing care plan for encouraging self-care is provided in Table 43–1 under "change in ability to perform ADL."

Evaluation

Expected client outcomes following effective nursing interventions for self-care deficit include observations by client, care providers, and significant others that the client is able to perform self-care activities to an optimal level. The client initiates self-care activities, asks for assistance as appropriate, and takes pride in resuming independence.

Sexual Dysfunction

Sexual dysfunction can result from obstacles created by casts, traction, or prolonged hospitalization or immobility. Pain, deformity, altered body image, or role change can also lead to sexual dysfunction.

Planning and Implementation

Discuss with the client the possible effects of pain, immobility, and change in role on sexuality. Consider the effects on the sexual partner also. Encourage communication about sexual needs between the client and sexual partner. If the client is hospitalized, allow time alone and privacy for the couple. Encourage verbalization of sexual concerns by both client and partner. Teach the client which positions are prohibited (eg, acute hip flexion after total hip replacement). Support any sexual activity that is gratifying to the client without causing discomfort or disrupting treatment.

Evaluation

Expected client outcomes following effective nursing interventions for sexual dysfunction include client verbalizations of concern about sexual function, willingness to discuss sexual issues with sexual partner, and requests for information from care providers as necessary.

Chapter Highlights

Subjective data on the client with musculoskeletal dysfunction can be gathered by inquiring about pain, paresthesia, changes in ADL and mobility, use of assistive devices, and any trauma.

Essential objective data to be gathered on clients with musculoskeletal problems include vital signs; skin integrity; range of motion; posture; strength, size, and tone of muscles; ability to ambulate; neurovascular status; and abnormalities such as swelling, inflammation, and deformity.

In addition to other routine diagnostic tests, the musculoskeletal system can be assessed by specific x-rays; by blood tests for muscle and bone enzymes, bone components, and autoantibodies; analysis of synovial fluid, and tissue biopsies; arthroscopy and electromyography.

The most important nursing diagnosis for clients with musculoskeletal problems is impaired physical mobility.

Other nursing diagnoses common to clients with musculoskeletal dysfunction include impaired skin integrity, altered bowel elimination, ineffective breathing pattern, altered tissue perfusion, altered comfort: pain, potential for injury, self-care deficit, and altered sexuality patterns.

Nursing measures common to musculoskeletal problems include rest, positioning in correct alignment, comfort measures, hot or cold applications, good skin care, exercise, ambulation, introducing assistive devices, diversional activity, and nutritional support. The effectiveness of nursing interventions is evaluated by determining if musculoskeletal function and ADL are maintained and if pain, deformity, and complications of immobility are absent. Clients should understand their condition and be able to give or obtain necessary care and cope with any limitations.

Bibliography

Baird SE: Development of a nursing assessment tool to diagnose altered body image in immobilized patients. *Ortho Nurs* 1985; 4(1):47–54.

Bates B: *A Guide to Physical Examination,* 3rd ed. Philadelphia: Lippincott, 1983.

Branson KA: Patient management following Amipaque myelography. *Ortho Nurs* 1982; 1(6):38–40.

Campbell EB, Williams MA, Mlynarczyk SM: After the fall—Confusion. *Am J Nurs* 1986; 86(2):151–154.

Cohen S, Viellion B: Patient assessment: Examining joints of the upper and lower extremities. *Am J Nurs* 1981; 81:763–786.

Dickinson GR, Gorman TK: Adult arthritis: The assessment. *Am J Nurs* 1983; 83:262–265.

Drinker PA, Phipps MA, Gannon JJ: Air bags: An uplifting idea. *Am J Nurs* 1985; 85(2):150–151.

Dunn BH: Components of musculoskeletal examination. *Ortho Nurs* 1982; 1(6):33–36.

Farrell J: Arthroscopy. *Nurs 82* (May) 1982; 12:73–75.

Farrell J: *Illustrated Guide to Orthopedic Nursing,* 2nd ed. Philadelphia: Lippincott, 1982.

Farrell J: Orthopedic pain: What does it mean? *Am J Nurs* 1984; 84:466–469.

Fischbach F: *A Manual of Laboratory Diagnostic Tests,* 2nd ed. Philadelphia: Lippincott, 1984.

Johnson LL: Diagnostic and surgical arthroscopy. *Clin Symp* 1982; 34(3):2–32.

King PA: Foot problems and assessment. *Geriatr Nurs* (Sept/Oct) 1980; 182–186.

Maher AB: Early assessment and management of musculoskeletal injuries. *Nurs Clin North Am* 1986; 21(4):717–724.

Patterson DC: Musculoskeletal examination. *Occup Health Nurs* (July) 1984; 356–367.

Rodts MF: An orthopedic assessment you can do in fifteen minutes. *Nurs 83* (May) 1983; 13:65–73.

Self-help devices: When hand function is compromised. *Patient Care* (April 30) 1984: 48–99.

Shannon ML: Five fallacies of pressure sores. *Nurs 84* (Oct) 1984; 14:34–41.

Simpson CF: Heat, cold, or both? *Am J Nurs* 1983; 83:270–273.

Simpson CF, Dickinson GR: Exercise. *Am J Nurs* 1983; 83:273–274.

Taylor SL: Lower back pain assessment: Part I—History-taking. *Ortho Nurs* 1983; 2:4, 11–16. Part II—Defining range of motion. 2:5, 39–44. Part III—The physical examination. 2:6, 21–27.

Tilkian SM, Conover MB, Tilkian AG: *Clinical Implications of Laboratory Tests,* 3rd ed. St. Louis: Mosby, 1983.

Treseler KM: *Clinical Laboratory Tests: Significance and Implications for Nursing.* Englewood Cliffs, NJ: Prentice–Hall, 1982.

Tucker JB, Marron JT: The qualification/disqualification process in athletics. *Am Fam Physician* (Feb) 1984; 29:149–154.

Vanderbeck KA: Getting the facts: a guide to orthopaedic assessment. *Ortho Nurs* 1984; 3(5):31–34.

Wassel A: Nursing assessment of injuries to the lower extremity. *Nurs Clin North Am* 1981; 16:739–748.

Wells R, Trostle K: Creative hairwashing techniques for immobilized patients. *Nurs 84* (Jan) 1984; 14:47–51.

Resources

SELF-HELP GROUPS AND OTHER ORGANIZATIONS

American Alliance for Health, Physical
Education, Recreation, and Dance
Promotions Unit
1900 Association Drive
Reston, VA 22091
Phone: (707) 476–3400

This voluntary educational organization answers questions about recreation and fitness opportunities for the handicapped.

American Lupus Society
23751 Madison St.
Torrance, CA 90505
Phone: (213) 373–1335

Volunteer workers promote public awareness of lupus, obtain funds for lupus research, and sponsor programs where clients and their families can meet to exchange information and offer mutual support.

Arthritis Foundation (National Headquarters)
1314 Spring St. NW
Atlanta, GA 30309
Phone: (404) 872–7100

This foundation funds research and provides information to the public and professionals for education and training. Local chapters throughout the United States support clinics, home care programs, rehabilitation services, and mobile consultation units for clients with arthritis.

Muscular Dystrophy Association
810 Seventh Ave.
New York, NY 10019
Phone: (212) 586–0808

This voluntary health agency provides comprehensive client care programs in local chapters throughout the country to persons with muscular dystrophy and related disorders, group recreation programs, and personal counseling by trained volunteers.

National Amputation Foundation
12-45 150th St.
Whitestone, NY 11357
Phone: (718) 767–8400

This membership organization of both civilian and veteran amputees offers information and support, a program of social rehabilitation, and referrals to centers throughout the country for the manufacture of prosthetic devices and training in their use (they maintain a prosthetic device center in New York City). Their "Amp-to-Amp" program offers person-to-person counseling.

National Lupus Foundation
5430 Van Nuys Blvd., Suite 206
Van Nuys, CA 91401
Phone: (818) 885–8787

This nonprofit organization run by volunteers raises funds to support research and distribute literature to the public and professionals.

United Scleroderma Foundation, Inc.
PO Box 350
Watsonville, CA 95077-0350
Phone: (408) 728–2202

HOT LINES

Athritis Medical Center
Phone: (800) 327–3027

Sponsored by Arthritis Medical Center. A physician will answer telephone questions; printed literature is also available.

Medical Advice for Jogging Related Problems
Phone: (202) 667–4150

Sponsored by the American Running and Fitness Association. Advice is given to members for problems related to jogging.

HEALTH EDUCATION MATERIAL

Patient Information Library
Krames Communications
312 90th St.
Daly City, CA 94015-2621

Provides health and safety booklets related to numerous musculoskeletal problems at low cost.

NURSING ORGANIZATIONS

National Association of Orthopedic Nurses
Box 56
Pitman, NJ 08071
Phone: (609) 582–0111

Members of this organization are nurses involved in the care of orthopedic clients. The association's goals are to enhance personal and professional growth through continuing education and the promotion of research.

CHAPTER **44**

Specific Disorders of Connective Tissue and Muscles

Objectives

When you have finished studying this chapter, you should be able to:

Describe the clinical manifestations and significance of disorders of connective tissue and muscle.

Identify therapeutic measures specific to disorders of connective tissue and muscles.

Specify the common drugs used in muscle and connective tissue disorders and discuss their potential side effects.

Formulate specific nursing interventions for clients with disorders of connective tissue and muscles.

Anticipate the temporary or permanent lifestyle modifications frequently necessary for clients with problems involving muscles and connective tissue.

Explain necessary health teaching for clients with specific disorders of connective tissue and muscles.

Injury to connective tissue and muscle may arise from acquired disease or from trauma. Diseases and traumatic injuries that primarily affect the joints are discussed in Chapter 46; this chapter deals with injury to muscles and connective tissues surrounding the joints or in other parts of the body.

SECTION I

Inflammatory Disorders

Bursitis and Tendinitis

Many pathologic conditions involve inflammation of connective tissue. Most inflammatory conditions covered in this chapter are related to alterations in the immune system and are discussed in the next section. This section deals only with bursitis and tendinitis, inflammatory conditions not usually associated with immunologic disorders.

Bursitis is an inflammation of the synovial membrane lining a bursa; *tendinitis* is an inflammation of a tendon. These inflammations may result from trauma, or they may be secondary to disease. Although both conditions are usually acute, they can become chronic and quite disabling with repeated injury or inadequate care.

Bursitis and tendinitis develop from prolonged overuse of a particular muscle group that can eventually damage a bursa or tendon. Overuse may be due to repetitive work movements or to a sports activity. Since the vascular supply of tendons is poor, their healing is limited, and inflammation can become chronic, resulting in tissue damage and persistent pain. Often a person with a chronic condition is unable to continue performing the movements that led to the problem and must seek other employment. Calcium deposits in tendons or bursae may also be the cause of inflammation. Tendon sheaths may become inflamed secondarily to systemic diseases such as gout, rheumatoid arthritis, or scleroderma. Since bursitis and tendinitis have similar causes, symptoms, and treatments, they will be discussed together.

Clinical Manifestations

The major symptom of bursitis/tendinitis is pain, often so severe that the client is unwilling to move the affected part. Swelling may be present, and this alone may keep the client from moving the joint. The pain may awaken the client at night, especially when turning onto the affected area during sleep. Any of the body's many bursae and tendons can become inflamed, but some joint areas are more commonly affected than others and will be discussed here.

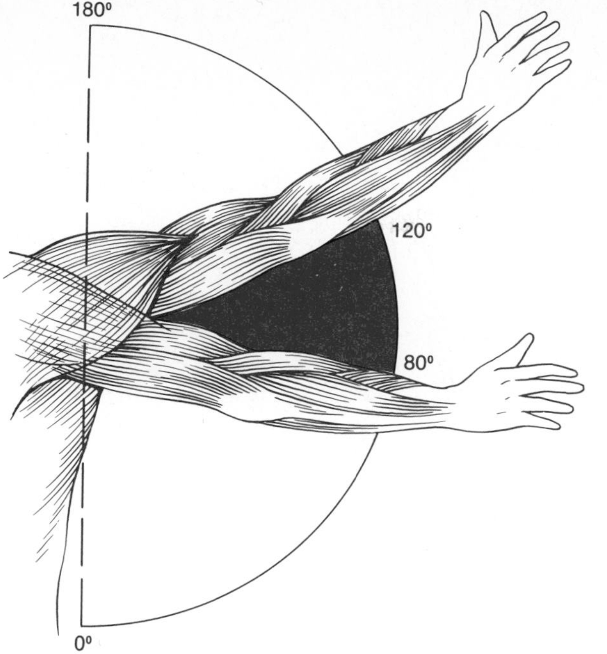

Figure 44–1

The painful arc in tendinitis and bursitis of the shoulder.

Note, however, that acute pain and erythema in joint areas may also be due to infection, gout, or rheumatoid arthritis.

Bursitis and tendinitis of the *shoulder* involve the subacromial and subdeltoid bursa (which are different sections of the same large bursa) and the tendon of the supraspinatus muscle. The onset of bursitis or tendinitis in the shoulder usually follows activities involving repetitive movements of the whole arm, such as sanding, painting, sawing, or repeated lifting. Pain in the deltoid area increases when the client lies on the shoulder or actively abducts the arm. A classic sign of bursitis or tendinitis of the shoulder is the "painful arc" between 80° and 120° of active arm abduction as shown in Figure 44–1; the client is unable to support the weight of the arm at these angles. Further abduction causes no pain, and the examiner can perform passive range of motion (ROM). If passive ROM causes pain, suspect capsulitis, or inflammation of the joint capsule, rather than a periarticular disorder.

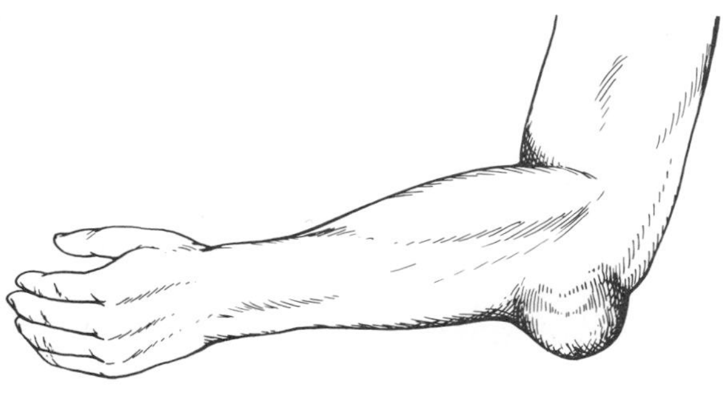

Figure 44–2

Localized swelling of the olecranon bursa.

Inflammations of the *elbow* region most often involve the olecranon bursa and the medial and lateral epicondyles. Tennis elbow is generally lateral epicondylitis, and pitcher's elbow is medial epicondylitis. These inflammations cause pain that radiates from the elbow down to the forearm. The client may drop heavy objects because of a feeling of decreased strength, although no real loss of strength actually occurs. Palpation of the involved epicondyle causes pain. There is no loss of motion of the joint. Activities involving lower arm movement, such as tennis or hammering, may precipitate an attack. Olecranon bursitis usually is caused by leaning or falling on the elbow. There may not be severe pain, but swelling is often extensive and alarming to the client (Figure 44–2).

Inflammation of the tendon sheath (tenosynovitis) is common in some of the tendons of the *hand*. "Trigger finger," an inflammation of the sheath of the flexor tendon of the finger, can occur from either excessive use of the finger involved or from diffuse connective tissue disease. The examiner can feel a "click" when the joint is moved actively or passively.

Tenosynovitis stenosans (de Quervain's disease) is an inflammation of tendon sheaths of the wrists common in women. The client usually has pain with the use of the thumb or wrist. The pain will radiate along the radial aspect of the forearm and thumb; adduction of the thumb across the palm also causes pain.

The most common inflammatory problem of the *hip* is trochanteric bursitis. Pain, which is distributed over the lateral aspect of the hip and thigh, may inhibit ambulation. An increase in pain is seen with abduction and internal rotation against resistance. The client feels tenderness with palpation over the greater trochanter. Clients who have leg length discrepancy may develop this inflammation in the hip of the longer leg.

Four bursa in the *knee* (Figure 44–3) can cause significant discomfort for the client when inflamed:

- Prepatellar bursa
- Superficial infrapatellar bursa
- Deep infrapatellar bursa
- Pes anserine bursa

Prepatellar bursitis (housemaid's knee) results from the combined action of excessive kneeling and leaning forward as in washing floors or gardening. Superficial infrapatellar bursitis (clergyman's knee) can result from excessive kneeling in a prayerful position. Deep infrapatellar bursitis and pes anserine bursitis are secondary to excessive weight bearing or unusual heavy exercise.

Achilles tendinitis is a painful inflammation of the tendon of the *ankle* with or without swelling. This painful injury often results from a single episode of overuse such as a weekend bicycle ride. It can also occur in runners who wear shoes with rigid soles. Recurrent episodes of Achilles tendinitis, when a client resumes activity before complete

NURSING DIAGNOSES IN Musculoskeletal Dysfunction

DIRECTLY RELATED DIAGNOSES

- Activity intolerance
- Bowel elimination, altered: constipation
- Breathing pattern, ineffective
- Comfort, altered: pain
- Health maintenance, impaired
- Injury, potential for
- Mobility, physical impaired
- Self-care deficit
- Sexuality, altered patterns
- Skin integrity, impaired
- Social interaction, impaired
- Tissue perfusion, altered: peripheral
- Urinary retention

OTHER POTENTIAL DIAGNOSES

- Bowel elimination, altered: incontinence
- Comfort, altered: chronic pain
- Diversional activity deficit
- Home maintenance management, impaired
- Incontinence, functional
- Post-trauma response
- Role performance, altered
- Self-concept altered: body image
- Sensory/perceptual alterations: tactile

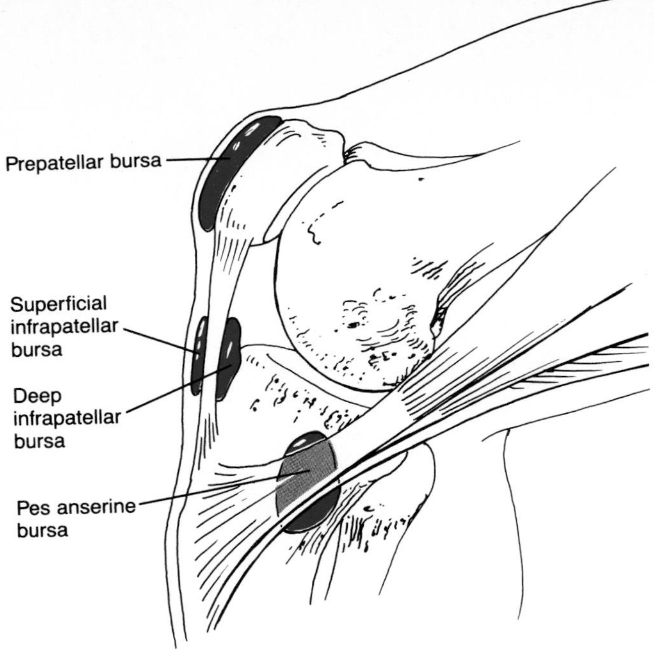

Figure 44–3

Clinically significant bursae of the knee.

healing has occurred, can result in progressive scar formation, which may require surgical repair.

Medical Measures

The measures employed for relief of bursitis and tendinitis vary according to the client's age and the location, cause, and severity of the injury. Recommendations usually include:

- Immobilization for 48 hours, with use of a splint or sling
- Ice packs applied to the affected area as often as possible for 15 to 30 minutes at a time (ice should not be applied directly to the skin)
- Exercise after the initial period of rest
- Anti-inflammatory medication (salicylates, nonsteroidal anti-inflammatory drugs)
- Occasionally, local corticosteroid injections into the inflamed bursa or tendon area

Exercise is crucial in the rehabilitation process, and active movement is started early. For example, in bursitis of any bursa of the knee, quadriceps-setting exercise is begun as soon as pain allows (Figure 44–4). When pain and tenderness have completely subsided, range of motion and full quadriceps activity are initiated. Physical therapists are often involved in designing exercises for clients, according to their individual needs. Occupational therapists may also participate if the nature of the problem involves a modification or change in job.

Fluid may be aspirated from the bursal space to relieve the symptoms. Fluid obtained should be cultured and inspected microscopically. Heat therapy by means of hot packs, ultrasound, or diathermy is used following cold therapy with some clients. *X-rays* of joints are usually normal, but in some instances calcium deposits can be identified as the precipitating factor. *Arthrography* is indicated in specific types of shoulder trauma to rule out any disruption of the joint capsule. *Surgery* is rarely used for bursitis or tendinitis unless rupture of the tendon occurs.

Specific Nursing Measures

Nurses are most likely to encounter clients with bursitis or tendinitis in ambulatory care or in emergency rooms. Goals of nursing care are to relieve the client's pain, maintain maximum mobility, and prevent joint contracture. Assessment of pain and range of motion is important both initially and after treatment to measure the effectiveness of the treatment. Reassurance and support can contribute to the relief of pain, so assure the client that the pain of bursitis or tendinitis is usually of short duration. Muscles tend to go into spasm under stress and aggravate the underlying condition, so it is important to take measures to relieve the client's stress.

Instruct the client in the use of ice therapy as well as heat therapy, if appropriate. The client should understand the reasons for using a splint or sling as directed; explain the importance of resting the joint while movement is painful. The client may be in considerable pain and therefore

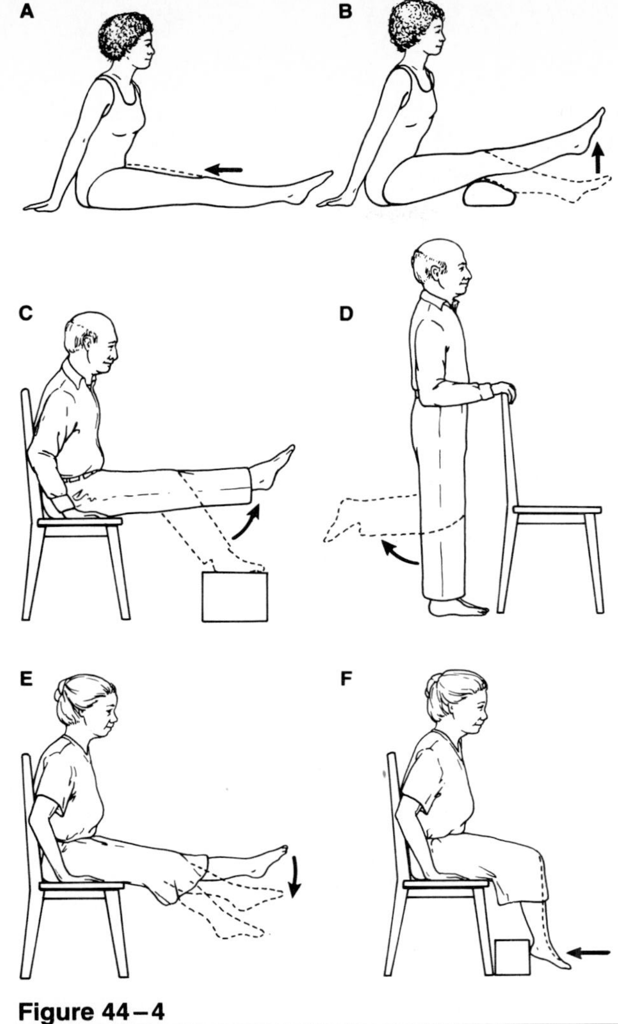

Figure 44–4

Exercises for rehabilitation of the knee. **A.** Isometric quadriceps exercise. **B, C.** Isotonic quadriceps exercises. **D.** Gravity-resisted isotonic flexion exercise. **F.** Isometric flexion exercise.

not concentrating when the treatment is explained, so written instruction should also be provided. Include information about medications: dosage, frequency, route, and major side effects. Clients may get prompt pain relief from medications and be tempted to use the affected area too soon. Caution them to refrain from early resumption of activity to avoid reinjury.

Exercises for rehabilitation of the affected area are initiated as ordered by the physician. Some simple shoulder exercises are illustrated in Figure 44–5. The first, the gravity-assisted pendulum exercise, can usually be initiated very early. As pain allows, the arc of the pendulum swing should increase. Figures 44–5B and C illustrate walking the fingers up the wall in two positions. Figure 44–5D demonstrates the use of a pulley to raise the affected arm as high as possible, and Figure 44–5E shows the client using a towel to simulate the motion of drying the back with alternating arm movements. Provide a good deal of encouragement because exercises will be uncomfortable at first. If physical therapy is needed, be sure the client has an appointment with the therapist and understands the importance of keeping it.

SECTION 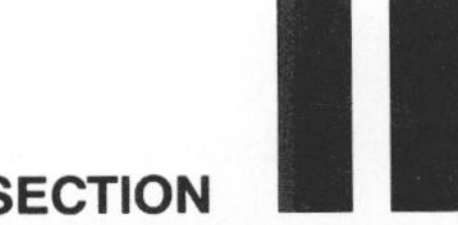

Immunologic Disorders

Systemic Lupus Erythematosus

Systemic lupus erythematosus (SLE), is a chronic systemic inflammatory disease that may affect the connective tissue of one or more organ systems at any given time.

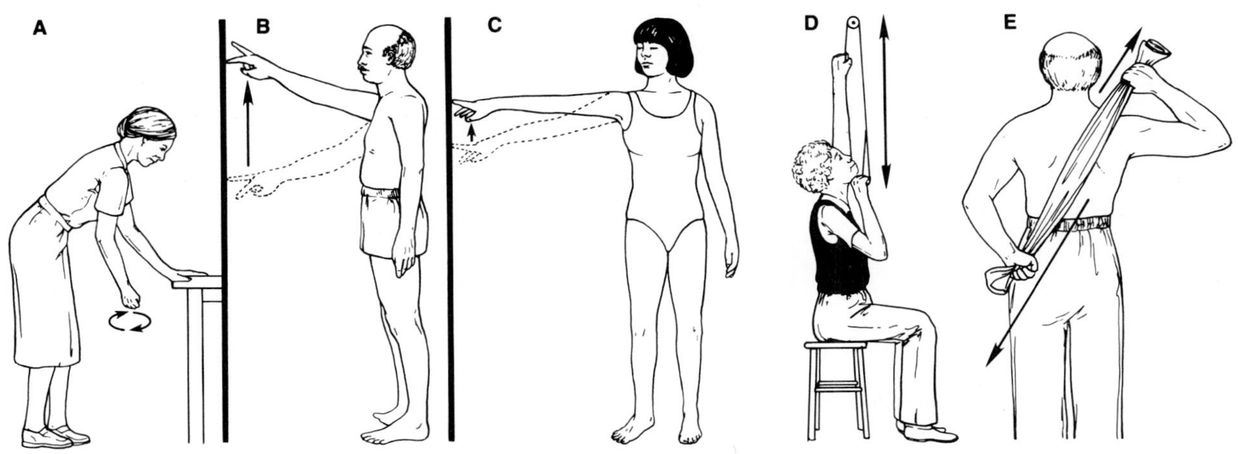

Figure 44–5

Exercises for rehabilitation of the shoulder. **A.** Gravity-assisted pendulum swing. **B, C.** Wall-walking exercises in two positions. **D.** Use of pulley to raise arm. **E.** Drying-of-back motion to exercise shoulder.

Joints, skin, blood, heart, lungs, and glomeruli can be involved, although usually not all are involved in the same individual. Occasionally, the disease is fulminating and rapidly fatal. For the most part, however, SLE follows an irregular course with exacerbations and remissions. Women of childbearing age are most often affected.

Of the many theories regarding the etiology of SLE, none is proved. All researchers are confident that the immune system is somehow involved. The role of slow or latent viruses, genetic factors, hormones, and drugs are all being investigated. It is postulated that SLE may not be a single disease entity but several closely related disorders with different genetic, immunologic, and pathogenic causes. The hallmark of SLE is the presence of antinuclear antibodies (ANA) in the serum. ANA forms immune complexes with specific antigens, and these complexes penetrate the cell membrane, causing diffuse damage in various organ systems. The complement system is also implicated in the tissue damage.

The diagnosis of SLE is established by the presence of at least four of the clinical criteria listed in Box 44–1. The presence of ANA or other abnormal laboratory results is not diagnostic unless accompanied by clinical symptoms. (This is true of all immunologic disorders of the muscle-connective tissue system.) Absence of ANA does not rule out a diagnosis of SLE. A negative ANA decreases the likelihood of this diagnosis, however.

Clinical Manifestations

The *joints* are the most common areas of involvement in SLE, and many clients are misdiagnosed as having rheumatoid arthritis. In the arthritis of lupus, the affected joints often appear normal, although they can be hot, swollen, and tender as in typical rheumatoid arthritis. The most commonly affected joints are the proximal interphalangeal (PIP) joints, knees, wrists, and metacarpophalangeal (MCP) joints. Most people also have morning stiffness. Deformities and bone erosions are rare, but aseptic necrosis of the hip sometimes occurs because of high steroid dosage. Infectious arthritis of one or more joints may appear because of the client's decreased resistance to infection.

The *skin* is the second most common area of involvement. Malar (cheekbone area) rash in butterfly distribution is a classic sign of SLE although not frequently seen. In clients with skin involvement, exposure to sunlight often brings on the skin eruptions. Patchy alopecia, oral or nasal ulcers, and Raynaud's phenomenon may also be present.

The pleura and pericardium may be involved. Clients may experience pleuritic-type chest pain, and a pleural friction rub may be heard on auscultation, with pleural effusion visible on x-ray. Pericarditis may be present, as evidenced by a pericardial friction rub on auscultation, pericardial effusion on x-ray, and ECG changes.

Kidney involvement occurs in approximately 50% of clients and is one of the most serious manifestations of SLE, since it can lead to renal failure and death. The first signs of renal damage are proteinuria, hematuria, and cellular casts. Monitor the client's blood pressure closely because an increase in blood pressure may herald renal involvement.

Central nervous system manifestations sometimes occur and are varied. Seizures, psychosis, emotional lability, cranial nerve abnormalities, migraine headaches, and major motor weakness may occur. Psychologic changes must be evaluated carefully however, because they may be from high-dose steroid therapy rather than SLE. The highest SLE mortality rates are in clients with central nervous system and/or renal involvement.

SLE can affect *blood elements*. Possible hematologic problems include hemolytic anemia, leukopenia, lymphopenia, and thrombocytopenia; these can occur even in the absence of drug therapy.

Other common clinical manifestations are fever, malaise, arthralgia, myalgia, lymphadenopathy, anorexia, weight loss, nausea and vomiting, and abdominal pain. Extreme fatigue may be an early symptom of SLE.

Menstrual abnormalities are not uncommon in the early stages of SLE. Pregnant clients usually do well with careful management if they have no active renal disease. An exacerbation of the disease may occur in the last trimester or in the postpartum period. It is best for a client to become pregnant while in remission and taking no medications. Miscarriages, premature births, and stillbirths do occur.

Box 44–1
Criteria Indicative of Systemic Lupus Erythematosus

- Facial erythema (butterfly malar rash)
- Hemolytic anemia, leukopenia, or thrombocytopenia
- Photosensitivity
- Oral or nasopharyngeal ulceration
- Arthritis without deformity
- LE cells or anti-DNA
- ANA
- Profuse proteinuria (>3.5 g/day) or urinary cellular casts
- Discoid rash
- Pleuritis or pericarditis
- Psychosis, convulsions, or neurologic deficits

SOURCE: Rodnan GP, Schumacher HR (editors): *Primer on the Rheumatic Diseases*, 8th ed. Atlanta: Arthritis Foundation, 1983.

Medical Measures

The goal of treatment is to control symptoms and suppress the disease activity as much as possible. Specific measures vary depending on the clinical manifestations in each client. Although there is no known cure for SLE, proper treatment may decrease the number of exacerbations and prolong life. Much of the treatment is supportive and educational and is described under Specific Nursing Measures.

Various drugs are used, separately or in combination, to treat the symptoms of SLE. *Salicylates* are used for arthralgia, arthritis, myalgia, and fever. If skin problems are also present, *antimalarials* may be used. These are administered in low doses because of the chance of causing retinopathy. Clients taking antimalarial drugs should have ophthalmologic exams every 6 months. Clients with skin manifestations are advised to avoid the sun and to use sunscreens when exposure is unavoidable.

Corticosteroids, when indicated, usually have a dramatic effect. They are never used prophylactically, however, because they do not prevent serious manifestations. Indications for corticosteroid therapy are CNS or renal involvement, pericarditis, pleurisy, severe myositis, hemolytic anemia, clotting problems, leukopenia, and thrombocytopenia. Corticosteroids are often given every other day so symptoms of persistent SLE activity can be detected on the off day. Alternate-day therapy can also preserve or restore the hypothalamic–pituitary–adrenal axis and causes fewer side effects than daily doses.

With severe nephritis, cytotoxic agents are sometimes used in addition to corticosteroids. These drugs are used with extreme caution because of their serious side effects of marrow toxicity, hemorrhage, alopecia, and sterility. The full effects of long-term use of these drugs are still unknown.

Although plasmapheresis has been used in some clients, it has no proven effect on the symptoms of SLE. Dialysis and renal transplantation have been used in renal failure with some success (Decker, 1982). A low-sodium, low-protein diet is prescribed for renal failure.

Table 44–1
Assessment for Complications of Systemic Lupus Erythematosus

System Involved	Subjective and Objective Findings
Cardiopulmonary	Chest pains, tachypnea, dyspnea, orthopnea, tachycardia
Renal	Increased weight, decreased urinary output, edema, hematuria, proteinuria, cellular casts, elevated BP
Gastrointestinal	Nausea and vomiting, diarrhea, pain, distention, decreased or absent bowel sounds
Neurologic	Diplopia, ptosis, nystagmus, ataxia, seizures, personality change, paranoid or psychotic behavior
Hematopoietic	Malaise, weakness, fever, chills, petechiae, epistaxis, hematemesis, positive stool for occult blood

Specific Nursing Measures

Nurses may see clients with SLE in both inpatient and ambulatory care settings. Discovering early symptoms and signs of exacerbations and complications is important in prolonging the life of clients with SLE. Table 44–1 lists assessment priorities in identifying complications. Carefully monitor all diagnostic study reports to remain well informed about the client's progress.

Client/Family Teaching

The nurse can instruct clients and their families about preventing exacerbations. Discuss medications with them: dosage, actions, side effects, and scheduling. Clients can buy their medications in bulk to save money, and they may want to shop around for the best buy. Clients should not change the dosage of the drugs they are taking without consulting the physician and should continue to take their medications even when they are feeling well. Clients taking steroids should wear a medical alert bracelet because they may need an increased dosage in case of a major accident or surgery. Clients should know that drugs such as birth control pills, antibiotics, hydralazine, procainamide, and tetanus toxoid may trigger or exacerbate symptoms. Advise clients to avoid over-the-counter drugs and hair dyes or cosmetics, except those approved by their physician.

Suggest that clients try to avoid stress-producing people and situations. Clients and their families may undertake a stress management program of their own. Stress management groups may also be beneficial. Clients should rest periodically throughout the day; midmorning and midafternoon naps are advisable in addition to a full 8 hours of sleep at night. Clients should try to adjust their activities so a low level of activity follows a high level and should discontinue any activity before becoming tired. Because clients with SLE are susceptible to viral and bacterial infections, they should avoid crowds and people with infections and colds during seasons when upper respiratory infections are common. Clients who develop an infection should be evaluated by their health care provider.

Clients with skin manifestations should apply skin cream as directed. If exposure to the sun causes exacerbations, clients should wear protective clothing and broad-brimmed hats or use sunscreens. If oral ulcers are present, clients should eat soft foods and take meticulous care of their mouths. Clients with Raynaud's phenomenon should keep their hands warm; they should wear gloves in cold weather and when putting their hands into a freezer. They should also try to avoid air-conditioned rooms because in some cases this can precipitate a Raynaud's attack.

Teach clients with troublesome arthritis ROM exercises and methods for applying ice and heat. Also demonstrate proper body alignment and postural techniques to preserve function and decrease deformities. Stress the importance of regular health care even when feeling well for early detection of exacerbations or complications.

Encourage clients to maintain a positive self-image through careful attention to dressing and grooming. If makeup is used, it should be hypoallergenic. Maintaining independence and usual role routines is usually possible except during acute exacerbations.

The Arthritis Foundation publishes helpful literature on SLE. Discussion groups of people with SLE have been helpful for both clients and families. Nurses should be familiar with resources in their own local areas for client referral.

Progressive Systemic Sclerosis

Progressive systemic sclerosis, also called PSS or *scleroderma,* is a connective tissue disorder. It causes fibrous changes in the skin, synovium, and small arteries of the digits, as well as in various internal organs, most notably the esophagus, intestines, heart, lungs, kidney, and thyroid. The disease occurs in various forms, ranging from a skin condition (localized scleroderma) to the CREST variant of PSS (Box 44–2), which is thought to be a more benign type, to involvement of visceral organs (systemic scleroderma). Some clients with the CREST syndrome have subsequently developed visceral and more extensive cutaneous lesions of PSS.

In all forms of the disease, there is vascular injury at the level of small arteries and capillaries, and the resulting decrease in circulation is the cause of the tissue changes. What precipitates the vascular damage is unknown, although investigations show that immunologic mechanisms may be involved. Collagen also increases, which causes fibrosis of the affected organ. There is no laboratory test to diagnose PSS. Autoantibodies occur in this disorder, and the ESR may be elevated.

Clinical Manifestations

The most frequent presentation in PSS is the clinical triad of *skin changes, Raynaud's phenomenon,* and *esophageal hypomotility.* However, other organs must be continually monitored for involvement.

The most typical changes in PSS occur in the skin. (Scleroderma means "hard skin.") Typically, skin changes begin with swelling of the hands and gradual thickening, tightening, and hardening of the skin of the fingers (sclerodactyly). The fingers become tapered and eventually even clawlike. Ulcers may develop on fingertips and over knuckles as the skin becomes taut. Sometimes the skin changes progress proximally at a slow rate, eventually affecting the face. The skin of the face becomes tight and shiny with a loss of normal wrinkles and skin folds. The nose may become beaked, and sometimes radial furrowing is seen around the mouth. The person cannot open the mouth completely. Sometimes the face becomes expressionless.

Box 44–2
The CREST Syndrome of Scleroderma

C • Calcinosis (subcutaneous calcifications)
R • Raynaud's phenomenon
E • Esophageal hypomotility
S • Sclerodactyly
T • Telangiectasia

SOURCE: Rodnan GP, Schumacher HR (editors): *Primer on the Rheumatic Diseases,* 8th ed. Atlanta: Arthritis Foundation, 1983.

Most clients with PSS have *Raynaud's phenomenon,* and this is often the first symptom to appear. With Raynaud's there is diminished blood flow to the digits secondary to vasoconstriction of the digital arteries, triggered by cold, vasoconstricting drugs, or emotional states. The initial sign is digital pallor. The digits then become blue as a result of cyanosis and later become red secondary to erythema on rewarming.

The client may have pain and stiffness in both small and large peripheral joints. Occasionally, a client develops arthritis and synovial effusion. Contractures and atrophy of the fingers may eventually occur.

Hypomotility of the *esophagus* occurs in a majority of clients with PSS. There is gastroesophageal reflux, with resulting heartburn and stricture. The client may have difficulty swallowing. Esophageal dilation is sometimes needed, and the client's nutrition may be impaired. Gastrointestinal involvement can progress to the intestine and colon, with development of hypomotility of the small intestine and wide-mouth diverticuli.

The systemic disease can also cause cardiopulmonary problems. Dyspnea may develop because of pulmonary hypertension and interstitial fibrosis. The examiner may hear fine dry rales or crackles at the bases of the lungs, and spirometry is often abnormal. Manifestations involving the heart are primarily the result of lung complications. Dysrhythmias, conduction disturbances, pericarditis, and pericardial effusions sometimes occur.

The *kidneys* are sometimes seriously affected, with malignant hypertension rapidly producing renal failure. Renal failure is the leading cause of death in PSS. Clients with affected kidneys have high renin levels and proteinuria.

Hematologic problems, in addition to a mild normochromic, normocytic anemia, include vitamin B_{12}/folic acid deficiency anemia, which may occur secondarily to bacterial overgrowth because of atony of the small intestine. There also may be some GI bleeding and resultant iron deficiency.

Medical Measures

Treatment of PSS is symptomatic, and much of it will be described under nursing measures. Drugs such as corticosteroids are used if there is accompanying disabling myositis or severe mixed connective tissue disease.

If skin ulcers develop, soaks and debridement along with topical antibiotics may be necessary. Physical therapy for the hands is important to prevent contractures. For clients with Raynaud's phenomenon, biofeedback is sometimes useful for controlling temperature in the hands and feet.

Some clients with esophageal dysmotility require intermittent esophageal dilation. When malabsorption occurs in the small intestine, absorption often improves with the use of tetracycline, which destroys the bacterial overgrowth that occurs with hypomotility.

Hypertension is treated aggressively with drugs to prevent irreversible renal damage. Propranolol, clonidine, and minoxidil, drugs that block the renin–angiotensin pathway, are most often used. Dialysis may be necessary with progressive renal failure.

Arthritis responds to NSAIDS, and the dry eyes (sicca syndrome) of Sjögren's syndrome are helped by artificial tears. A client with dry mouth (xerostomia) should have frequent dental exams because this condition predisposes people to severe dental caries.

Specific Nursing Measures

Assess the client's skin and joints and cardiovascular, pulmonary, and gastrointestinal status. Evaluate the eyes and mouth for adequate lacrimal and salivary gland secretion. Monitor blood pressure closely and review laboratory results. Venipuncture in the antecubital area may be difficult because of skin changes. Avoid finger sticks because of the client's compromised circulation; the earlobe may afford the best site if only a capillary tube of blood is needed.

Client/Family Teaching

Explain the nature and course of PSS to client and family and help them become knowledgeable about signs of more serious involvement. Teach them about prescribed medications and demonstrate ROM exercises to prevent joint contracture. Encourage the liberal use of skin lotions to decrease dryness.

Advise clients with Raynaud's phenomenon to avoid cold, ergotamine, and amphetamines. They should wear gloves and socks in winter and whenever their hands and feet are exposed to cold. Smoking should be avoided since nicotine causes pronounced peripheral vasoconstriction, which markedly aggravates Raynaud's.

Clients with esophageal dysmotility should eat small, frequent meals; chew their food thoroughly; and follow meals with water. They should avoid any foods that cause them particular problems. Antacids after meals and at bedtime help to relieve gastric irritation. Raising the head of the bed on blocks will decrease nocturnal esophageal reflux.

The nurse who has established a relationship of trust with clients may be able to help them express their thoughts and fears. These clients are dealing with a diagnosis with a varied prognosis that causes significant body image changes. The possible loss of hand function may be more stressful than the facial changes to many clients because of potential loss of independence. The mental health clinical nurse specialist can be of considerable assistance to these clients and also to the nursing staff caring for them.

Dermatomyositis and Polymyositis

Dermatomyositis and polymyositis are closely related disorders involving degenerative and inflammatory changes in connective tissues. Dermatomyositis involves skeletal muscle and skin; polymyositis, skeletal muscle alone. The rate of onset and progression of symptoms are varied. There is evidence that these disorders may be caused by a viral infection or by an autoimmune response.

Clinical Manifestations

The most outstanding symptom of dermatomyositis and polymyositis is extreme muscle weakness. Clients experience weakness in the proximal limb muscles making it difficult for them to raise their arms, go up and down stairs, or get out of a bathtub or a chair. They may be unable to raise their heads from the pillow or to squat. Often the client feels no pain, but the muscles may be tender to palpation. Occasionally, there is aching pain in the buttocks, thighs, and calves. The pharyngeal and laryngeal muscles may be affected, resulting in dysphagia and dysphonia (difficulty in speaking or hoarseness). Raynaud's phenomenon and arthritis may also be present.

Occasionally, cardiac abnormalities such as dysrythmias occur. With severe cardiac involvement, there may be necrosis of the myocardial fibers resulting in death. Cough and dyspnea may be an indication of interstitial pneumonitis and fibrosis.

The skin lesions in dermatomyositis consist of diffuse erythema of the face, neck, and anterior chest and a purple-hued maculopapular rash that occurs periorbitally and on the nose, cheeks, forehead, and fingernails. Pruritus and periorbital and perioral edema may also be present.

Laboratory findings include elevated muscle enzymes including SGOT, SGPT, CK, and aldolase. Positive ANA, rheumatoid factor, and elevated ESR are common. The EMG reveals inflammation, and muscle biopsy findings show tissue changes such as muscle necrosis and regeneration. The muscle biopsy should be taken from muscle that is involved but not atrophied. The diagnosis is based on the clinical picture, along with an abnormal EMG, elevated muscle enzymes, and a positive muscle biopsy. Evaluation of muscle enzymes is helpful in monitoring the client's response to treatment.

Medical Measures

Corticosteroids are the cornerstone of therapy, and their effects can be determined by monitoring the muscle enzyme levels. Decreasing or discontinuing the steroid too soon may cause an exacerbation that may be difficult to control. If clients respond poorly to steroids, immunosuppressive drugs such as azathioprine may be added to the regimen.

Clients who do not respond to corticosteroids should have a workup for a malignancy. If a malignancy is found and treated, the muscle weakness should resolve.

Specific Nursing Measures

Clients with dermatomyositis or polymyositis present a challenge for the nurse because their severe muscle weakness and inability to move against gravity make them almost immobile. If the initial phase, clients will need complete care and meticulous attention to prevention of the complications of immobility.

The dysphagia resulting from pharyngeal weakness can cause numerous problems such as choking and aspiration pneumonia. Anyone offering food or fluids to the client should be fully aware of the client's difficulty in swallowing and offer oral medications, fluids, and food slowly with the client in a comfortable upright position. A gastrostomy tube or hyperalimentation is sometimes necessary.

Continuous assessment of the client is important to monitor response to corticosteroids. Muscle weakness can be evaluated by the client's ability to move the limbs against resistance. Assessment of the skin, lungs, and cardiovascular system are important nursing responsibilities.

In helping clients and families with the psychosocial problems that inevitably arise from such a disabling condition, reinforce the fact that most clients make a full recovery. Clients with skin manifestations may find it hard to accept their altered appearance; the nurse should encourage them to express their feelings and assist them to look as good as possible. Gently encourage independence even if it is in the smallest task. Praise for small accomplishments is essential.

Teaching the family gentle massage and ROM activities is beneficial to the client, not only to prevent complications of immobility but also for the touching involved. Resistive exercises can be added as enzyme levels drop. Both client and family should understand the medication regimen prior to discharge. Community health nursing visits to the home may be helpful as well as referral to relevant community agencies.

SECTION III

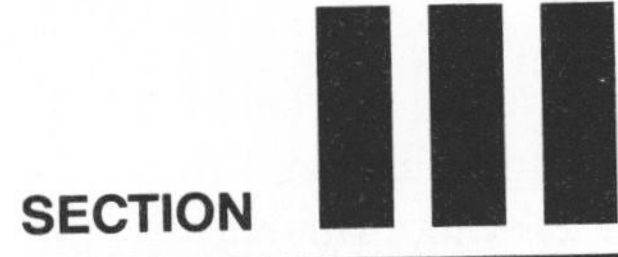

Traumatic Disorders

Sprains and Strains

Traumatic injuries to the soft tissues surrounding joints—muscle, ligaments, and tendons—are called sprains and strains. The injury may arise from blunt trauma to the muscle or joint; excessive exercise; or twisting, stretching, or forcible extension of a joint. Surgery is seldom needed unless complete rupture occurs, but the pain of such an injury can be severely limiting. Serious sprains or strains can be more debilitating than fractures or internal knee derangement

A *sprain,* an injury to a ligament, is the result of forcing a joint beyond its normal ROM. The ligament may be stretched or actually torn. Often a blunt blow to the joint can sprain it. Sprains usually occur during sports activities or falls. A *strain* is an injury to a muscle and/or tendon at any location from origin to insertion. Strains are associated with excessive stretching of a muscle or muscle unit; they usually do not occur because of a blow or direct trauma. Poor conditioning, improper warm-up before activity, muscle fatigue or weakness, and strength imbalance can all contribute to muscle strain. Precipitating events include lifting improperly, sudden straining motions, and falls. Intermittent joggers and weekend sports buffs often have strains; well-conditioned athletes are usually spared. Strains have a high incidence of recurrence.

Table 44–2
Grading and Treatment of Sprains

Degree of Injury	Treatment
First degree: tenderness and swelling over the ligament; the joint is stable	P • Protection R • Rest I • Ice C • Compression E • Elevation and NSAIDs
Second degree: partial ligament disruption with some joint instability in addition to tenderness and swelling *Third degree:* complete tearing of the ligament with loss of joint stability on the side of the ligament rupture	PRICE, immobilization, NSAIDS, x-rays to determine need for further treatment

Clinical Manifestations

A *sprain* causes pain, swelling, local hemorrhage, spasm of the muscle that moves the joint, and disability (Table 44–2). The pain occurs with passive movement of the joint, and there is intense pain over the involved ligament itself. Sprains are graded according to damage to the ligaments and the resultant joint instability.

Ankle sprains, the most common, occur when inversion of the foot tears a ligament, usually the anterior talofibular ligament. *Knee sprains* cause swelling, hemarthrosis, significant decrease in the range of motion, and joint laxity. The injured person is usually unable to bear weight. Often the person hears a "pop" when the injury occurs and later describes the knee as feeling as if it is going to "give way." The medical collateral ligament is most commonly involved.

Strains cause pain, swelling, muscle spasm, and hemorrhage into the muscle (Table 44–3). Discoloration and weakness may also be present. Pain increases with active flexion or passive stretching, which helps in differentiating strains from sprains. Strains are graded according to loss of muscle strength.

Medical and Specific Nursing Measures

Treatment is basically the same for strains and sprains. The nurse should take a thorough history to determine the nature and cause of the injury as well as any significant health problems that may influence the treatment. When a suspected strain or sprain occurs, the PRICE treatment is initiated. Cold compresses should immediately be applied to minimize swelling and to decrease spasm and pain. The extremity is then wrapped with an elastic bandage, which is soaked first in cold water to aid the cooling process, and elevated above heart level to limit the amount of dependent edema and swelling. The PRICE regimen is usually continued for the first week after injury, although there is some controversy about whether cold or heat is used after the first 24 hours. Cold is usually recommended for 5 to 7 days because of its anti-inflammatory and analgesic effect. Then wet heat is encouraged to aid in relaxation of muscles and to promote blood flow to the area. Sometimes heat is used immediately after the first 24 hours of injury.

With a second or third degree sprain, an x-ray is always taken to rule out a fracture (Table 44–2). Clients with sprains are usually immobilized for 1 week. When all pain on motion has ceased, clients can begin active ROM and muscle-strengthening exercises. Nonsteroidal anti-inflammatory drugs are the treatment of choice (Box 44–3).

The PRICE regimen and NSAIDs are also appropriate for management of a strain (Table 44–3). Emphasis is placed on prevention of recurrence through the use of muscle-strengthening and stretching exercises. The importance of doing warm-up exercises before engaging in strenuous activity is stressed. For example, recurrent ankle sprains are often associated with tight Achilles tendons. Daily slow stretching of the Achilles tendon can effectively reduce the incidence of ankle sprain (Figure 44–6). Should complete muscle rupture occur, surgical intervention is needed. Many professional athletes elect to have surgery even for partial rupture because this promotes faster healing.

Table 44–3
Grading and Treatment of Strains

Degree of Injury	Treatment
First degree: local pain, tenderness, swelling with pain on active flexion or passive stretching; no loss of strength or motion	PRICE, NSAIDs
Second degree: partial disruption resulting in some loss of strength	PRICE, NSAIDs, splinting
Third degree: complete disruption with a functionless muscle-tendon unit	Surgical repair

Box 44–3
Nonsteroidal Anti-Inflammatory Drugs (NSAIDS) for the Treatment of Sprains and Strains

Indomethacin (Indocin)
Ibuprofen (Motrin)
Tolmetin sodium (Tolectin)
Sulindac (Clinoril)

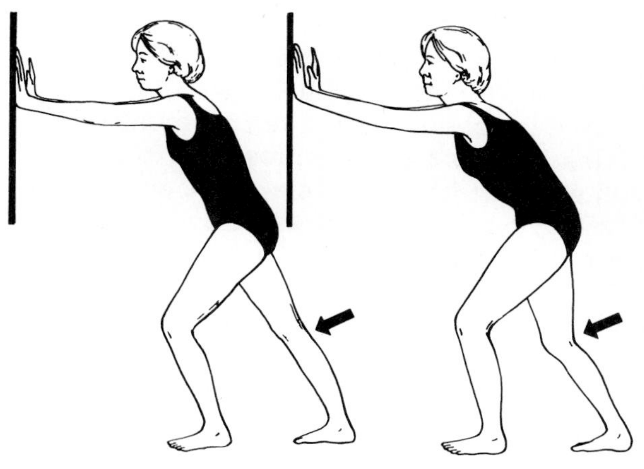

Figure 44–6

Achilles tendon stretch.

Chapter Highlights

Pain is the most important symptom in evaluating bursitis and tendinitis. Therefore, a careful pain assessment is an important part of the data base.

The most common sites for bursitis and tendinitis are the shoulders, elbows, hands, hips, knees, and ankles.

Therapeutic measures for bursitis and/or tendinitis consist of rest, ice, exercises, analgesics, and anti-inflammatory drugs, and local injections of corticosteroids.

Medications used in immunologic disorders are toxic. Therefore, the nurse, client, and family should be familiar with symptoms and signs of toxicity.

Systemic lupus erythematosus is now thought to be a number of closely related, but separate illnesses that have different immunologic, genetic, and pathogenic causes.

Clinical manifestations of immunologic disorders of muscles and connective tissue may include arthritis, myositis, integumentary changes, gastrointestinal changes, nephritis, CNS disturbances, and cardiopulmonary abnormalities. Fever, malaise, anorexia, and weight loss may also be among the primary symptoms.

Therapeutic goals for clients with immunologic disorders are to control symptoms and suppress the disease activity. Various medications such as salicylates, NSAIDS, antimalarials, corticosteroids, and immunosuppressives are used.

Serious sprains and strains can be more debilitating than fractures and have a high incidence of recurrence. Therefore, education for prevention is the primary nursing concern.

General therapeutic measures for sprains and strains include protection, rest, ice, compression with Ace bandages, elevation, and immobilization to minimize pain, decrease edema, and prevent further injury.

Bibliography

Birrer RB: *Sports Medicine for the Primary Care Physician.* New York: Appleton–Century–Crofts, 1984.

Brody DM: Running injuries. *Clin Symp* 1980; 32(4):2–36.

Decker JL: The management of systemic lupus erythmatosus. *Arthritis Rheum* 1982; 7:891–894.

Garrett WE: Sprains and strains in athletes. *Postgrad Med* 1983; 73(3):200–209.

Hoffman GS: Tendinitis and bursitis. *Am Fam Physician* 1981; 23(6):103–110.

Krupp MA, Chatton MJ: *Current Medical Diagnosis and Treatment,* Los Altos, CA: Lange, 1981.

Lewis KS: Systemic lupus erythematosus: The great masquerader. *Nurs Prac* 1981; 9:13–22.

Petersdorf RG et al: *Harrison's Principles of Internal Medicine,* 10th ed. New York: McGraw–Hill, 1983.

Phillips RM, Wasner CK: Scleroderma: Current understanding of pathogenesis and management. *Postgrad Med* (Sept) 1981; 70:153–168.

Rodnan GP, Schumacher HR (editors): *Primer on the Rheumatic Diseases,* 8th ed. Atlanta: Arthritis Foundation, 1983.

Roy S, Irvin R: *Sports Medicine.* Englewood Cliffs, NJ: Prentice–Hall, 1983.

Sheon RP et al: The hypermobility syndrome. *Postgrad Med* 1982; 71(6):199–209.

Simkin PA: Tendinitis and bursitis of the shoulder. *Postgrad Med* 1983; 73(5):177–190.

CHAPTER **45**

Specific Disorders of the Bones

Other topics relevant to this content are: Care of the client with cancer, **Chapter 10;** Preoperative and postoperative care, **Chapter 11;** Care of the client with a fracture of the nose or jaw, **Chapter 15;** Care of the client with rib fracture, **Chapter 16;** Care of the client with vertebral fracture, **Chapter 29;** Care of the client with hyperparathyroidism, **Chapter 33;** A sample nursing care plan to prevent disuse osteoporosis, **Chapter 43.**

Objectives

When you have finished studying this chapter, you should be able to:

Describe the clinical manifestations and significance of disorders of the bones.

Identify therapeutic measures specific to skeletal disorders.

Explain the use of casts, traction, and internal and external fixation in fracture management.

Define the surgical procedures presented involving the musculoskeletal system.

Discuss the nursing implications of caring for these clients in the preoperative and postoperative periods.

Explain the complications of orthopedic surgery and the related nursing interventions.

Discuss appropriate nutritional management for conditions of the skeletal system.

Specify nursing interventions appropriate for clients with disorders of the bones.

Identify evaluation criteria for determining effectiveness of nursing care given to clients with specific bone disorders.

Conditions affecting the bones usually interfere with a person's mobility, comfort, and independence and sometimes require prolonged treatment and rehabilitation. The disorder may leave the client with a deformity, which may cause numerous physiologic and psychosocial consequences. Some conditions affecting bone can be life threatening, particularly those caused by malignancy. This chapter will cover the specific disorders that affect bones in adults; these can be classified as disorders from metabolic alteration, infection, neoplasm, or trauma.

The care of clients undergoing orthopedic surgery is similar in many respects to that of other surgical clients with a few special considerations. Additional preoperative laboratory tests may be done including erythrocyte sedimentation rate, serum calcium, phosphorus, and alkaline phosphatase. Coagulation studies and typing and cross-matching of blood are usually done because bones are highly vascular, and hemorrhage is possible.

Orthopedic clients may go to surgery in their beds so traction can be maintained or so they can be placed in the bed right from the OR table, eliminating possible complications from additional moves. Elastic stockings may be applied preoperatively to prevent thrombus formation.

Infection can occur more readily in bone than in soft tissue. A bone infection will interfere with healing or bone union and can become chronic. Therefore, special skin preparation may be done, such as sterile prep and wrapping with sterile bandages or drapes. Antibiotics may be started preoperatively and continued postoperatively as a prophylactic measure. The prevention or early detection of postoperative infection is an important nursing function.

Many orthopedic clients have been immobilized by their condition before surgery. Assessing for, and preventing complications of, immobility are other very important nursing functions.

For those who face orthopedic surgery, common fears are of pain, loss of body parts, and in some cases the possibility of paralysis. In addition to psychologic prepa-

NURSING DIAGNOSES IN
Musculoskeletal Dysfunction

DIRECTLY RELATED DIAGNOSES

- Activity intolerance
- Bowel elimination, altered: constipation
- Breathing pattern, ineffective
- Comfort, altered: pain
- Health maintenance, impaired
- Injury, potential for
- Mobility, physical impaired
- Self-care deficit
- Sexuality, altered patterns
- Skin integrity, impaired
- Social interaction, impaired
- Tissue perfusion, altered: peripheral
- Urinary retention

OTHER POTENTIAL DIAGNOSES

- Bowel elimination, altered: incontinence
- Comfort, altered: chronic pain
- Diversional activity deficit
- Home maintenance management, impaired
- Incontinence, functional
- Post-trauma response
- Role performance, altered
- Self-concept altered: body image
- Sensory/perceptual alterations: tactile

ration for surgery, the nurse must plan for postoperative psychologic support. Many orthopedic clients undergo body image alteration along with a lengthy recovery period that may require extensive rehabilitation. For clients who go into surgery directly after trauma, the nurse may have to plan for postoperative psychologic assistance in facing a sudden and permanent change in lifestyle or a long and unexpected confinement.

SECTION 

Metabolic Disorders

Metabolic disorders affecting bone interfere with bone formation, weakening the bone. The metabolic disorders *osteoporosis, osteomalacia,* and hyperparathyroidism all cause demineralization and loss of bone mass. The first two disorders are discussed in this section; hyperparathyroidism, an endocrine disorder, is covered in Chapter 33. *Paget's disease of the bone,* also discussed in this section, involves deposition of weak bone and has symptoms similar to those caused by bone loss.

Because the onset of metabolic disorders is insidious, clients with metabolic bone disorders may not be hospitalized until their condition is severe or a fracture occurs. If ambulatory care nurses and community health nurses are aware of the conditions contributing to these diseases, they may be able to detect them in their early stages and encourage clients to seek medical intervention. They can also intervene for those at risk by teaching about the benefits of a nutritionally balanced diet, regular exercise, and good body mechanics.

Osteoporosis

Osteoporosis is a condition in which the rate of bone resorption exceeds the rate of bone formation, reducing bone mass. An osteoporotic hand and wrist is compared to a normal one in Figures 45–1A and B. Osteoporotic bones become porous, brittle, and subject to fracture from minimal trauma or normal stress. Bones most often affected are the vertebrae, ribs, and wrist and hip bones.

All people lose some bone as they grow older, beginning at about age 30, but when bone mass is less than normal for someone's age, the person is considered to have osteoporosis. Several factors contribute to excessive bone loss. Osteoporosis is much more common in postmenopausal women than in men and appears to be related to the *diminished levels of estrogen* occurring after menopause, whether natural or surgically induced. *Immobility* or lack of exercise is also associated with increased bone resorption. The bones need the usual stress of weight bearing and activity to continue normal bone turnover; otherwise, demineralization occurs. Elderly people who become less active with age are subject to *disuse osteoporosis.* Astronauts in space experience osteoporosis related to *lack of gravity,* despite the exercises they perform.

Osteoporosis is sometimes associated with *inadequate nutrition,* such as deficiencies in calcium and vitamin D, and excess phosphorus. High-protein diets for weight reduction may increase bone resorption because the increased acid resulting from increased nitrogen is buffered by calcium taken from the bones. Osteoporotic changes occur secondarily to several endocrine problems such as Cushing's disease, hyperthyroidism, hyperparathyroidism, diabetes mellitus, and acromegaly. Medications associated with osteoporotic changes are corticosteroids, when used for long periods, and heparin.

Clinical Manifestations

Osteoporotic changes may go on a long time before they are noticed; Lukert (1982) states that 50% of women past 65 years of age have asymptomatic osteoporosis. Initial symptoms include weakness, unsteady gait, stiffness, and poor appetite. The symptom that brings the client to the physician is commonly back pain, usually in the lower thoracic or lumbar region. The onset of the pain may be sudden or insidious. Changes in the spine cause loss of height, rounded back (kyphosis), and pressure on nerves.

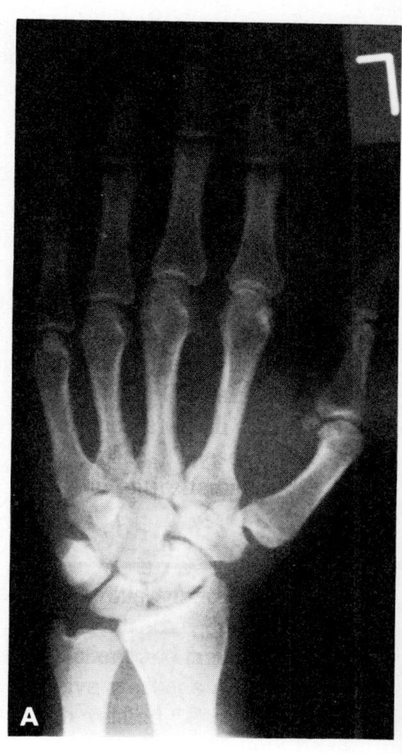

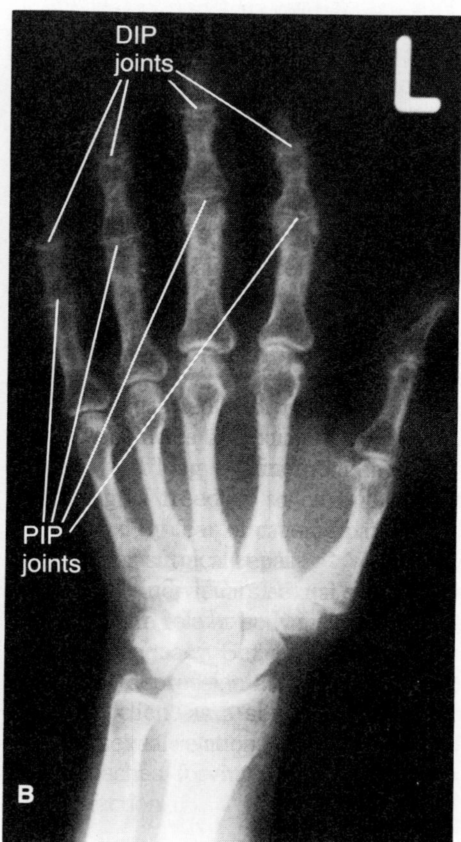

Figure 45–1

A. X-ray of a normal hand. **B.** X-ray of a hand with osteoporotic changes and degenerative joint disease. Note the loss of bone matrix in the phalanges and the joint space narrowing, especially the DIP joints. *Courtesy of Health Care Plan, Buffalo, NY.*

Spinal deformity may also decrease the size of the thorax, causing changes in respiratory function. Other areas that are often painful are the hips, pelvis, and legs. Elderly people often experience pathologic fractures in weight-bearing or other stress-bearing areas such as the hips, wrists, and vertebrae due to osteoporosis; in fact, over two-thirds of clients with hip fractures are found to have osteoporosis.

The serum calcium, phosphorus, and alkaline phosphatase levels of osteoporotic clients are usually normal. On x-ray, the affected bones appear thin, porous, and radiolucent; fractures may also be obvious.

Medical Measures

The best strategy for osteoporosis is prevention through regular activity, exercise, and an adequate calcium intake throughout life. Women over 35, who do not have sufficient calcium in their diets, should probably begin oral calcium supplements. Exercise reduces the rate of normal bone loss. If osteoporosis does develop, treatment is prescribed according to the contributing factors. Exercise and a well-balanced diet with foods from the four food groups are recommended for anyone with osteoporosis; calcium and vitamin D supplements are prescribed for clients with dietary deficiencies.

The use of estrogen is controversial. Studies have shown that estrogens retard the rate of bone loss, but the long-term benefits have been questioned. There is also an increased risk of endometrial carcinoma when estrogens are used to treat a postmenopausal woman with an intact uterus. Lindsay (1982) suggests giving progestogen (synthetic progesterone) once a month or every 3 months to a woman with a uterus who is taking estrogen to help decrease the incidence of endometrial shedding. The combined estrogen–progesterone regimen can cause the woman to have cyclical uterine bleeding. The side effects of this hormone combination are the same as those for birth control pills, including phlebitis and emboli. A woman taking these hormones needs an annual gynecologic examination. The question of whether there is greater risk from endometrial cancer or from the significant morbidity and disability that may accompany osteoporosis remains unanswered. Women may have to answer that question for themselves in terms of their own quality of life.

Specific Nursing Measures

Osteoporosis is one of the hazards of immobility, so a nurse caring for any client requiring prolonged immobilization or bed rest must be concerned with its prevention. A sample nursing care plan for preventing disuse osteoporosis is given in Chapter 43. Since the nursing measures for prevention of osteoporosis are similar to those for its treatment, this section will discuss them together.

NUTRITION Proper nutrition is essential for both prevention and treatment of osteoporosis. The recommended dietary ratio of calcium to phosphorus is 1:1. The American diet, however, has much larger percentages of phosphorus than calcium. Those over 45 years of age consume about half the recommended dietary allowance (RDA) of calcium (Gorrie, 1982). High phosphate intake stimulates parathyroid activity and thus increases bone resorption. A dietary history is helpful in assessing deficient intake; the client may need dietary changes or supplements to meet recommended allowances. In general, a diet adequate in vitamin D, calcium, and protein, will provide the nutrients necessary for bone formation. The nutritional management for osteoporosis is summarized in Table 45–1.

Client/Family Teaching

Milk products usually are recommended for increasing calcium intake, but some elderly clients do not tolerate milk because of discomfort from intestinal lactase deficiency. For these people, the nurse should recommend cottage cheese, aged or extra sharp cheddar cheese, and green leafy vegetables. Also make suggestions for preparing vegetables such as collards, kale, and turnip greens because some people may have never tried them. Clients can take preparations of lactase with milk products to prevent the cramping and diarrhea of lactase deficiency (Wolanin & Phillips, 1981).

People with osteoporosis should not consume high-protein diets because a diet excessively high in protein (more than 100 g/day) may increase urinary excretion of calcium. Since many high-protein foods are also high in phosphorus, decreasing protein intake also aids in maintaining a lower phosphorus intake.

EXERCISE The nurse and client should plan a program of exercises in which movement and weight bearing are emphasized. All clients who are able should engage in regular exercise, such as walking 30 to 60 minutes at least 3 times a week. Other beneficial exercises are bicycling, stationary cycling, and aerobic dancing. The client should avoid activities that would add pressure to or jar weight-bearing joints and vertebrae, such as jogging.

Other measures the nurse can discuss with the client include safety precautions; good posture and body mechanics; a firm mattress (or a bedboard under a sagging mattress) to provide adequate support to the spine; and corsets for back support. A client with acute back pain should have a few days of bed rest on a supportive mattress, with ice applied intermittently to reduce muscle spasm.

Osteomalacia

Osteomalacia is an adult form of *rickets*, a disease in which bone tissue fails to calcify and becomes soft and flexible. Instead of affecting bone growth, as rickets does in a child, osteomalacia affects the turnover of bone because bone growth is completed in the adult.

Osteomalacia results from vitamin D deficiency, which depresses calcium absorption, causing bone demineralization. Vitamin D deficiency occurs with:

- Inadequate dietary intake of vitamin D
- Deficient vitamin D synthesis in the skin because of lack of exposure to sunlight
- Malabsorption of vitamin D or calcium from the intestine (as occurs in any intestinal disorder associated with steatorrhea)
- Chronic renal failure interfering with metabolism of vitamin D
- Hepatic disorders or anticonvulsant therapy that impairs absorption and conversion of vitamin D
- Gastrectomy, which contributes to diminished intake or defective absorption of vitamin D secondary to the rapid passage of stomach contents past the duodenum

In osteomalacia, normal bone is replaced with osteoid tissue, which is structurally weak and subject to deformity and fracture with stress. Osteomalacia, although not common in North America, does occur in the household elderly, in women who have little sun exposure and who undergo repeated pregnancies and prolonged lactation, and in over 50% of clients with chronic renal failure.

Clinical Manifestations

In addition to the changes mentioned earlier, clients with osteomalacia have severe muscle weakness, nagging pain resulting from strain on the soft bone, and decreased height because of kyphosis. Softening of bone also leads to angulation of the sternum and deformities of the pelvis and femoral necks. On x-ray, diminished bone density and bone deformities are seen. Laboratory findings include decreased serum calcium and phosphorus levels and elevated alkaline phosphatase levels. The diagnosis of osteomalacia can be confirmed by bone biopsy.

Medical and Specific Nursing Measures

Osteomalacia caused by dietary deficiency can be prevented by supplying the adult with adequate vitamin D, calcium, and phosphorus. See Table 45–1 for nutritional management in osteomalacia. The nurse should determine

Table 45–1
Nutritional Management in Osteoporosis and Osteomalacia

Nutrient	Recommendation in Osteoporosis	Recommendation in Osteomalacia	Sources
Calcium	↑ to 1500 mg q.d.	At least 800 mg q.d.; add 400 mg more in pregnancy and lactation	Dairy products; collards; kale; turnip, dandelion, and mustard greens; canned sardines and salmon eaten with bones; oysters
Vitamin D	Maintain usual level if frequent sun exposure; if house-bound, increase intake	↑ intake	Exposure to sunlight, fortified milk and cereals, eggs, butter, fish liver oils
Phosphorus	↓ intake	800 mg q.d.; add 400 mg more in pregnancy and lactation; ↓ use of antacids containing aluminum hydroxide, which interfere with phosphorus absorption	Beef, poultry, fish, soft drinks
Protein	Avoid excessive intake	Avoid excessive intake	Meat, poultry, fish, dairy products, eggs, cheese, grains, beans, peas, nuts

the reason for dietary deficiency so that the cause can be treated: Is it due to poor eating habits, lack of knowledge of a balanced diet, or lack of available foods? Does the client use antacids? Many clients ingest large amounts of antacids containing aluminum hydroxide, which interfere with phosphorus absorption. Explain that antacid use can lead to phosphorus deficiency. The client may need help in planning and selecting a balanced diet based on financial resources, food preferences, and the availability of foods.

If osteomalacia develops, it is treated with high doses of vitamin D: 25 to 125 μg daily, increasing to 1250 μg daily if malabsorption is evident. Calcium and phosphorus supplements may also be given. When a client is taking such large doses of vitamin D for an extended time, serum and urine calcium levels should be monitored for hypercalcemia and hypercalciuria. Signs of vitamin D toxicity are excessive calcification of bones and soft tissues and symptoms of hypercalcemia such as malaise, headache, anorexia, nausea, vomiting, weakness, constipation, polyuria, and polydipsia (Krause & Mahan, 1984).

Encourage clients to expose their skin to sunlight so they can synthesize their own vitamin D. A client with osteomalacia will also benefit from a firm mattress and a brace or corset for support.

Paget's Disease of the Bone

Paget's disease (osteitis deformans) of the bone is mentioned here because it has some similarities to metabolic bone diseases, although it does not cause a decrease in bone mass or demineralization of bone. In the early stages of Paget's disease, increased osteoclastic resorption of bone occurs. As the disease progresses, normal bone is replaced by immature woven bone, the haversian system disappears, and bone architecture becomes highly disorganized. These changes lead to a mosaic structure that is weak and fractures easily. The bone remodeling leads to swelling and deformity of bones; for example, the long bones become thicker and bow. The number of affected bones ranges from one to many; commonly involved are the vertebrae, pelvis, long bones, and skull.

The cause of Paget's disease is unknown, although a viral etiology is suspected. The disease is uncommon before the age of 40 but incidence increases steadily with each subsequent decade. Often there is a positive family history. Osteogenic sarcoma is a rare but usually fatal complication of Paget's disease.

Clinical Manifestations

Some clients are asymptomatic; others have pain and aching. Manifestations vary with the location of the lesion and the extent of the condition. Enlargement of the skull may cause facial pain, headaches, and need for a larger hat size. Hearing loss may occur secondary to direct involvement of the ossicles of the inner ear or to compression of cranial nerve VIII, the vestibulocochlear nerve. Long bones such as the femur or tibia may appear swollen, deformed, or bent, and the skin over the affected bone will be warm due to increased vascularity. There may be changes in gait. The serum alkaline phosphatase level is extremely elevated, an indication of the increased bone activity. X-rays show opaque and radiolucent areas.

Medical and Specific Nursing Measures

Most clients require no treatment because the disease is localized and causes no symptoms. Otherwise, treatment is supportive and symptomatic, with emphasis on good body mechanics. Ambulatory aids may be necessary for a client with an altered gait. Analgesics or nonsteroidal anti-inflammatory agents are given for pain. A person with an extremely high rate of bone turnover may be given drugs to suppress bone activity—for example, calcitonin, mithramycin, or etidronate disodium (see Table 45–2).

The nurse must explain the importance of good body mechanics. Emotional support is essential, because this is a chronic condition with no definitive treatment, and the client may become discouraged and frustrated. If the client is inactive, hypercalcemia may occur. A hypercalcemic client needs a low calcium diet and high fluid intake to help prevent urinary calculi. The client should drink about 3 to 4 L/day, unless this high intake is contraindicated for other reasons. Fluids to offer, in keeping with the low calcium requirement, are water, tea, coffee, and cranberry or prune juice.

Table 45–2
Pharmacologic Approaches to Paget's Disease

Drug	Action
Aspirin and nonsteroidal anti-inflammatory agents	Analgesia
Steroids	Suppress the disease, but only in large doses, so are not recommended
Sodium fluoride	Decreases symptoms, but may lead to poorly mineralized bone
Salmon, porcine and human calcitonin	Inhibits bone resorption, decreases serum alkaline phosphatase levels; given subcutaneously
Cytotoxic drugs, (eg, mithramycin)	Inhibits bone resorption, decreases serum alkaline phosphatase levels; given intravenously
Etidronate disodium (EHDP)	Inhibits bone resorption, decreases serum alkaline phosphatase levels; can be taken orally

SECTION 

Infectious Disorders

Osteomyelitis

Infections of the bone, bone marrow, and surrounding soft tissues by *pyogenic* (pus-forming) bacteria are called *osteomyelitis*. Such infections, which usually involve the long bones, can be acute or can progress to a chronic state; in either case, they cause bone destruction, limited mobility, and severe pain.

The organism most often responsible for osteomyelitis is *Staphylococcus aureus*; hemolytic *Streptococcus* is the second most common; *Neisseria gonorrhoeae, Hemophilus influenzae,* and *Salmonella* may also infect bones. The bacteria enter the bone by way of the bloodstream (bacteremia), by extension of a local soft tissue infection, or from open wounds.

Osteomyelitis can be divided into three types: acute infectious, acute localized, and chronic. In *acute infectious* osteomyelitis, also known as *hematogenous*, the infection enters the bone from another site in the body. This type of bone infection is most common in children, usually affecting the metaphysis (the area in the shaft next to the epiphyseal plate) of long bones. However, it can occur in adults as a more localized infection, especially of the vertebrae. There is often a history of mild, local trauma, which causes decreased resistance in the bone. A systemic infection already present in the body may then move via the bloodstream into the area of decreased resistance. The ends of long bones are usually affected because they are highly vascularized, with sluggish circulation. *Acute localized* osteomyelitis, also known as *exogenous*, occurs when there is direct invasion of bacteria from open fractures, septic surgery, or penetrating wounds. The infection usually remains localized. *Chronic* osteomyelitis is a dreaded condition that can follow the other types because of inadequate or ineffective treatment during the acute phase. It is characterized by remissions and exacerbations; the client may be asymptomatic during the remission phase, but pain and inflammation occur during exacerbation as the body tries to rid itself of necrosed bone fragments, called *sequestra*. Sinuses form, drain purulent material, heal over, and form again.

After bacteria enter the bone, they multiply and destroy cells, and macrophages enter to kill the bacteria. The collection of debris and resulting edema cause a rise in pressure in the rigid bone structure. When the pressure reaches arteriolar pressure, blood (and the antibiotics it carries) cannot enter the area. Eventually, the pus leaks out of the bone and the pressure elevates the periosteum, stripping the bone of its surrounding blood vessels and causing necrosis. The pocket between the periosteum and the bone surface is called a subperiosteal abscess; sequestra are found beneath such abscesses. The bone lays down new bone cells over the sequestrum in an attempt to heal itself, forming a new bone covering called an *involucrum.* The involucrum encloses the bacteria in the bone, interferes with normal phagocytosis, and acts as a barrier to antibiotics, thus causing a chronic condition. Sinus tracts may form between the sequestra and the skin or into an adjacent joint, draining the purulent material contained in the abscess.

Infections of the bone are extremely difficult to eradicate. An acute infection can progress into a chronic one involving many hospitalizations and prolonged disability. An infection that is present when a fracture is trying to heal will result in poor healing, nonunion, or malunion. If an infection occurs involving a prosthesis used for joint replacement, the prosthesis frequently must be removed, leaving the client with a significant disability.

Clinical Manifestations

Acute osteomyelitis is characterized by an abrupt onset of severe pain in the involved extremity. Edema, redness, and heat occur locally, Clients may have muscle spasms and hold the extremity in flexion, resisting any attempts to touch it. Other manifestations include fever, chills, diaphoresis, malaise, headache, and nausea. The white blood cell (WBC) count is very high, and the erythrocyte sedimentation rate (ESR) is elevated. X-rays are negative until about 2 weeks after the onset, when the bone will have areas of density and radiolucency.

In the chronic phase, an exacerbation may be characterized by low grade fever, pain, and persistent drainage from a sinus tract. A *sinogram,* an x-ray in which dye is injected into the open sinus, reveals the course of the sinus tract.

Medical Measures

Since it is essential to begin antibiotic therapy before the infection becomes isolated, multiple antibiotics are given as soon as blood or wound culture specimens are obtained. When the culture results are available, inappropriate antibiotics are discontinued, and others, specific to the causative organism, are begun. Antibiotics are continued for several weeks. In acute infectious osteomyelitis, abscesses are incised and drained if the response to the antibiotics is slow. In acute localized osteomyelitis, I&D (incision and drainage) allows removal of any hardware (metal used for bone repair) as well as drainage of the wound. Chronic conditions may require surgical removal of the sequestra followed by continuous wound irrigation with antibiotic solutions, in addition to prolonged systemic treatment with antibiotics. Bone grafting may be done to provide stability after repeated infections.

Specific Nursing Measures

Prevention of bone infection is of utmost importance when caring for orthopedic clients. Strict aseptic technique and meticulous hygiene measures are essential. The nurse who is aware of the symptoms and signs of osteomyelitis can aid in early diagnosis and treatment, to prevent an acute infection from becoming chronic. The nurse should appreciate the extraordinary pain caused by acute disease and the ordeal caused by the chronic condition in planning appropriate nursing measures. The client with osteomyelitis requires good body alignment, regular position changes, prevention of the complications of immobility, assistance with ambulation, sedentary diversional activities, comfort measures, and application of heat if ordered. A high-calorie, high-vitamin C diet is recommended for both acute and chronic osteomyelitis, and a vitamin C supplement may be helpful in promoting healing, Encourage generous intake of fluids, particularly when fever is present. Vital signs should be taken every 4 hours when the client's temperature is elevated; antipyretics may be needed.

PAIN RELIEF AND IMMOBILIZATION Dealing with the client's pain may be a challenge. When moving the client, give analgesics first, get help, and support the limb well so that the joints above and below the painful area are stabilized. All movements should be gentle and smooth, to prevent pathologic fractures as well as pain. Sometimes, just touching the bed causes the client pain, so it is a good idea to post signs warning others to avoid bumping or touching the bed. Treatment will involve some method of immobilizing the limb, such as a splint, cast, or traction. The extremity should be maintained in a functional anatomic position. The extremity is often elevated. Do not allow continued flexion of the limb; prevent footdrop by means of a splint. A bed cradle may be useful for keeping sheets off the painful limb.

ANTIBIOTICS AND HYDRATION The client will be receiving antibiotics intravenously, and the nurse must see that these are given on time to assure sustained blood levels. It is essential that the client receive proper hydration if IVs are interrupted to give antibiotics; intake and output should be measured. Since antibiotics are given in high dosages and for prolonged periods, the nurse must watch for side effects of the medications.

WOUND CARE When the client has an open wound, the nurse must use strict sterile technique for dressing changes. The infection will also require wound and skin precautions. Sometimes isolation technique is indicated. Observe and chart the wound drainage. A continuous wound irrigation apparatus may be used. Usually, an IV-type setup drips antibiotic or detergent solution into the wound while tubing connected to a Hemovac or low-suction machine collects the wound drainage; the wound is covered with a dressing. At times the dressing gets soaked and drips onto bed clothes, or the solution runs along the client's leg; provide waterproof absorbent pads and skin care to keep the client dry. The irrigation must be maintained—the physician should be called when it is not working properly. Handle the apparatus and dressings using aseptic technique. It is a good idea to have change-of-shifts review of the apparatus to maintain continuity.

Client/Family Teaching

Health teaching includes methods for preventing the spread of infection by clients, visitors, and staff. Clients with chronic conditions may need to learn dressing care before discharge. Caution them to avoid weight bearing until instructed, to prevent fracture. Clients should also know about the drugs they will be taking at home: their action, correct dosage, and possible side effects.

Clients with chronic disease require emotional support. They may be faced with intermittent pain, an unsightly limb because of scars from draining wounds, and foul-smelling drainage. They may fear loss of the limb. Allow clients to verbalize their feelings and help correct any misconceptions. Encourage continuing medical supervision. The nurse may want to make a referral to a community health nurse to be certain that the client is managing wound care properly at home. In addition, the nurse can assess the client's mental status and overall adjustment to the disease.

SECTION 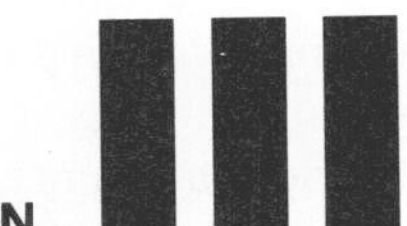

Neoplastic Disorders

Tumors of the bone can be of three types: benign, primary malignant, and secondary malignant (metastatic). A benign bone tumor originates in bone tissue, as does a primary malignant tumor. A secondary malignant bone tumor occurs as a result of metastasis from primary lesions elsewhere in the body.

Bone tumors cause pain, sometimes severe, and interfere with mobility. They may cause permanent limitation and disfigurement if amputation of a limb is necessary. These tumors frequently occur in young people and pose a threat to body image and self-concept, which are extremely important in the adolescent and young adult years.

Clients with malignant bone tumors have a poor prognosis, but early detection of such a tumor may promote early treatment and prevent metastasis. The nurse should be aware of the symptoms and signs of bone cancer and encourage the client to seek medical attention without delay.

Osteogenic Sarcoma

Osteogenic sarcoma, also known as osteosarcoma, is the most common malignant primary neoplasm of bone, occurring primarily in young people 10 to 25 years old. It also can occur later in life secondarily to Paget's disease of the bone, chronic osteomyelitis, or previous bone irradiation. The areas affected most often are the ends of long bones (especially around the knee) including the distal femur, proximal tibia, and proximal humerus. The etiology of this disease is unknown, and the prognosis is generally poor.

The lesions of osteogenic sarcoma may vary in appearance. Osteolytic osteogenic sarcomas dissolve the bone and invade adjacent soft tissues. Osteoblastic osteogenic sarcomas form new bone. The bone may become weak and fracture, particularly when the tumor grows slowly. The tumor may metastasize, most often to the lung, resulting in a poorer prognosis.

Clinical Manifestations

Clients usually have pain at night, sometimes intermittently. They may experience sudden onset of pain, perhaps after minor trauma. As with other bone tumors, clients are likely to have a local swelling or mass and may walk with a limp. In addition, the client with osteogenic sarcoma may complain of fatigue.

The lesion is visible on x-ray; a bone scan shows increased activity at the tumor site. Serum alkaline phosphatase is elevated in 50% of clients. When initial alkaline phosphatase levels are very high, the course is often rapidly fatal. Analysis of a biopsy of the lesion will confirm the diagnosis. Candidates for limb salvaging procedures should have needle biopsy under fluoroscopy. An open bone biopsy may disrupt the tumor, making limb salvage difficult.

Medical Measures

The tumor must be removed or destroyed. The location of the tumor dictates the extent of the surgery. The most satisfactory surgical procedure is amputation, but sometimes the tumor and the area around it can be removed without amputation. Limb salvaging procedures have been made possible by advances in chemotherapy and endoprosthetics. Clients must have achieved most of their bone growth to be candidates for these procedures. Therefore amputation remains the procedure of choice in younger children. The client may be given chemotherapy preoperatively and postoperatively.

Specific Nursing Measures

Most of the nursing interventions appropriate for bone tumor clients are discussed elsewhere in this text. Measures for preventing deformity, assisting with ambulation, providing comfort, and changing position are included in Chapter 43. Routine preoperative and postoperative care are covered in Chapter 11. Nursing care related to surgical procedures such as amputation and internal fixation will be covered later in this chapter. Measures to deal with the specific problems of cancer, radiation therapy, chemotherapy, and surgery for cancer clients are covered in Chapter 10, as are measures used to encourage nutrition for those receiving radiation therapy and chemotherapy.

Help with emotional problems is likely to be as important as any other nursing intervention. The client, who may be young, may be grieving over loss of a limb or impending death. Encourage expression of feelings, and accept expressions of anger and frustration. The entire family will need emotional support. A referral to a mental health or religious counselor may be helpful.

Amputation

An amputation is the removal of all or part of a limb because of disease or injury. An amputation can also occur traumatically as the result of an accident, requiring surgery to care for the resulting wound.

Most lower extremity amputations are necessary due to peripheral vascular diseases (PVD), such as diabetes mellitus and arteriosclerosis. Upper extremity amputations are rarely done for PVD, but they may be necessary as a result of trauma, such as that occurring in explosions or crushing injuries. Other indications include: infection, such as osteomyelitis or gas gangrene; tumor, such as osteosarcoma; thermal injury, such as frostbite or burns; and congenital deformity. Limbs that seriously interfere with function or are extremely painful and have not responded to other treatment may require amputation also.

The surgeon tries to save as much of the limb as possible, while providing for the best fit and function of a prosthesis. The higher the level of the amputation, the greater the energy expenditure for ambulation with a prosthesis. Some common amputation sites are:

- Transmetatarsal: part of the foot is removed; does not usually require a prosthesis
- Ankle: foot is removed at the ankle
- Below the knee (BK): 10 to 14 cm of the tibia should be preserved; allows for a more natural gait than at or above the knee, because the knee is preserved
- At the knee (knee disarticulation): lower leg is removed at the knee joint
- Above the knee (AK): leg is removed about 6 cm above the knee joint
- Below the elbow: lower arm is removed to about 14 cm below the elbow
- Above the elbow: lower arm is removed; all possible length is preserved down to 5 cm above the distal end of the humerus

There are two types of amputation—open (guillotine) and closed (flap). The open technique leaves the wound edges open; the skin, muscle, and bone are all cut at the same level (similar to the way a guillotine would cut). The open wound is necessary when infection is present so purulent material can drain. A bulky soft compression dressing is applied. Skin traction may be utilized to prevent skin and muscle retraction, which would interfere with fitting a prosthesis. Four traction strips of adhesive or rubber are applied above the dressing and attached to 5 lb of traction weight. When the infection has cleared, the wound may be surgically closed or allowed to heal by granulation.

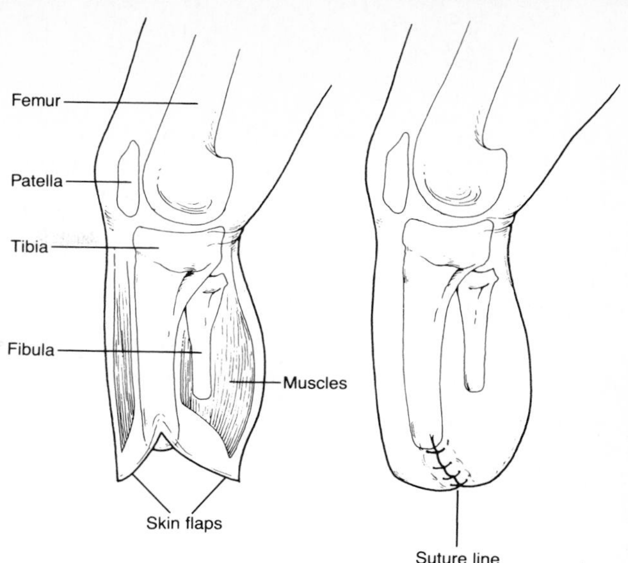

Figure 45–2

Amputation using closed technique.

In the closed technique, the bone is cut 2 in. shorter than the skin and muscles so the tissues can cover the end of the bone (Figure 45–2). The muscles may be sutured to the bone or to their antagonistic muscle group. Penrose drains are inserted and brought out through the incision, and a Hemovac may be inserted to prevent accumulation of fluid and blood under the tissues. The skin is sutured so the suture line is placed in a nonweight-bearing area.

The surgeon decides whether to use an early or a delayed prosthesis fitting. If a delayed prosthesis fitting is used (the conventional method), the stump is covered with fluffy absorbent dressing followed by a compression bandage. Elastic bandage is used to decrease swelling and to begin shaping the stump for the future prosthesis.

If the surgeon chooses the early fitting (also called immediate postoperative fitting or rigid dressing), the stump is covered with an absorbent dressing and padding followed by a plaster cast. For a lower extremity amputation, a suspension strap is attached to the cast so it can be connected to a waist belt. A temporary prosthesis, made of a pylon tube and prosthetic foot, is attached to the cast either immediately or a few weeks after surgery (Figure 45–3). Another method employs an air splint over the dressing to provide compression for controlling edema. The client can ambulate while wearing the splint, which is covered with a metal cylinder.

After the amputation, it may seem to the client as if the missing limb is still there. This feeling, known as *phan-*

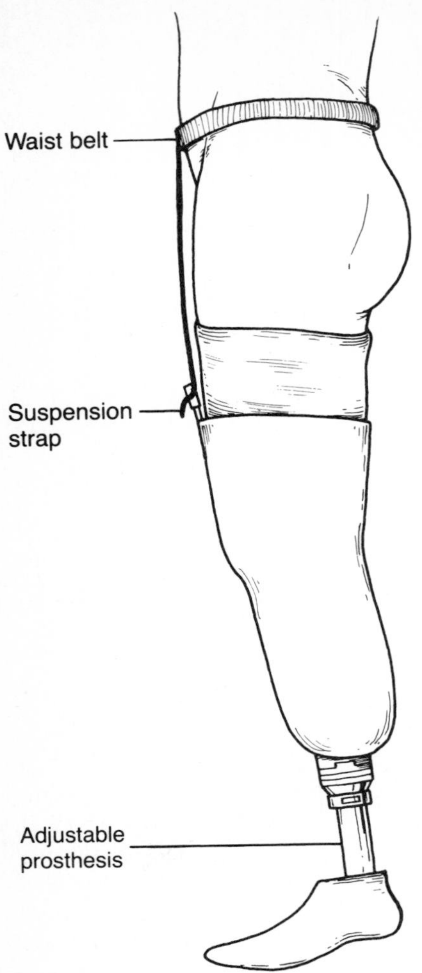

Figure 45–3

Immediate postoperative prosthetic fitting (rigid dressing).

tom limb sensation, may occur briefly or may continue for years; there are instances of reported phantom limb sensation for as long as 20 years after amputation. Exactly why this experience happens is not completely known. It may happen because cut nerve endings that formerly innervated the limb have been stimulated or because the remaining neurons in the stump continue to send impulses to the same area of the brain as before.

Phantom limb sensation eventually disappears. It may diminish by a process known as telescoping, in which the limb actually seems to be receding or shrinking toward the stump. The thumb, index finger, and great toe are usually the final parts to "disappear." Phantoms of the upper extremity seem to last longer than phantoms of the lower extremity.

Not to be confused with phantom limb sensation is another event called *phantom limb pain.* Clients have described this pain by using words such as *acute, crushing, grinding,* and *burning.* Fortunately, painful phantoms are relatively rare and occur in only 1% to 2% of all amputations. Why painful phantoms occur is also not clear. Phantom limb pain may result from inflammation or regrowth (neuroma formation) of the cut nerve endings and may occur soon after the amputation or not until many years later. Persistent pain has been treated by nerve block, anti-inflammatory drugs, neuroma excision, electrical nerve stimulation, and psychotherapy. Carpamezapine (Tegretol), an anticonvulsant and analgesic drug, and amitriptyline (Elavil), an antidepressant drug, have also been used. All approaches to treatment of persistent phantom limb pain have met with limited success. The implications of amputation for the client are summarized in Table 45–3.

Nursing Implications

PREOPERATIVE CARE In addition to the usual preoperative orthopedic preparation, the client may be taught specific muscle strengthening exercises to prepare for rehabilitation.

A type and cross-match of blood is necessary so blood is available for surgery. Any chronic diseases, such as diabetes mellitus must be under control. Encourage the client to express fears and anxieties, and explain the possibility of phantom limb sensation. When the amputation is necessary because of an accident, the client may be taken directly to surgery from the emergency department. There is no time to prepare such a client psychologically, to bring a chronic disease under control, or to teach exercises before surgery, so it is necessary to perform these activities postoperatively.

Some religions require burial of the amputated part. Try to find out whether the client wants the limb to be buried and help to make the necessary arrangements with the family.

POSTOPERATIVE CARE Postoperatively, routine nursing care is necessary, particularly comfort measures, positioning, body alignment, skin care, exercise, and ambulation. The dressing is checked frequently along with the vital signs, to detect any sign of hemorrhage. A large tourniquet is kept at the bedside; if hemorrhage occurs, apply the tourniquet and notify the physician immediately. Drainage from the dressing is to be expected because Penrose drains are used; however, bright red drainage is a sign of fresh bleeding. The client should do coughing, deep breathing, and incentive spirometry every 1 to 2 hours. Antibiotics are given to prevent infection. Nursing measures to prevent urinary retention, constipation, and skin problems are described in Chapter 43. The diet is advanced as tolerated. Range of motion exercises are necessary for all joints. Do not underestimate the client's pain or discomfort; provide adequate pain relief and comfort measures.

POSITIONING Assist the client to change position every 2 hours, avoiding positions that would encourage contracture formation. For the client with a lower extremity amputation, the foot of the bed may be elevated for 24 to 48 hours to decrease stump edema. Thereafter, continuous elevation of the legs is avoided to prevent hip flexion con-

Table 45–3
Amputation: Implications for the Client 

Physiologic Implications	Psychosocial/Lifestyle Implications
May provide relief of pain, prevent metastasis of a tumor, arrest a life-threatening infection, eliminate persistent ulceration of extremity, or remove a useless or bothersome limb.	May provide relief of chronic pain, or freedom from a useless limb, improving quality of life.
Temporary local pain and edema occur in the stump; may have severe pain in stump with upper extremity amputation.	A permanent handicap occurs that requires changes in many areas of the client's life.
A compression dressing is necessary to shape the stump for delayed prosthesis fitting.	The grieving process may occur over loss of a limb.
The advantages of early over delayed prosthetic fitting are that the early fitting controls edema, shapes the stump, allows earlier ambulation and permanent prosthesis fitting, and decreases phantom limb pain.	Body image is altered.
An extensive physical therapy program is necessary to build strength and learn prosthesis use.	May require abandoning previous activities and learning new ways of doing things.
Upper extremity prostheses cannot reproduce fine motor movements of the hand.	Change in occupation may be necessary.
Ambulatory aids may be necessary for lower extremity amputee.	May become dependent on others.
Potential complications: hemorrhage and shock, phantom limb pain, joint contracture, wound infection, and skin breakdown on stump.	Lengthy hospitalization and rehabilitation may cause financial problems.
	Fear and anxiety about self-worth and being a burden may occur.
	Adjustment after traumatic amputation may be more difficult than after a planned amputation.
	Persistent phantom limb pain may be discouraging.
	Motivation and hard work are necessary for rehabilitation.

tracture. No pillow is allowed under the operative leg or between the legs; a flexion or abduction contracture would interfere with use of a prosthesis. A firm mattress is necessary to prevent hip flexion. The client should assume the prone position for 30 minutes 3 to 4 times a day. For part of the time the client is supine, the bed should be completely flat. Trochanter rolls can be used to prevent rotation of the leg. Discourage continuous knee flexion when the client is in bed or sitting in a chair. The client should begin isometric exercises of the quadriceps, gluteal, and abdominal muscles on the first or second postoperative day and perform them 4 to 5 times a day to maintain strength.

STUMP CONDITIONING AND BANDAGING With the delayed fitting amputation, the client carries out stump conditioning exercises by pushing the stump against an object, beginning with a towel or soft pillow and progressing to harder surfaces. The amputation stump is further prepared for the prosthesis by molding it into a conical shape with elastic bandaging. The nurse begins doing this the first or second postoperative week and should eventually teach the client how to do it. The elastic bandage is wrapped so the greatest compression is at the distal end of the stump, with decreasing compression as the bandage ascends the limb. The bandaging should be rewrapped about five times a day to maintain the compression and checked frequently to note slipping or tightening of the bandages. Check also for complications of skin healing on the end of the stump from pressure, poor circulation, or infection.

The AK amputation stump is wrapped so the bandage is anchored around the hips in figure-eight turns. Oblique turns are used on the limb rather than circular turns, which could be constricting. The bandaging should be smooth, so no skin is exposed and the edges of the bandage do not flap. It should not be so tight as to cause pain or discomfort or interfere with circulation. The BK amputation stump is wrapped using the same principles, with figure-eight turns about the knee.

An elastic stump shrinker may be used instead of the bandage. Two sets of bandages should be available, so one can be washed and dried daily as the other is worn. The bandage should be laid flat to dry, to prevent stretching.

The rigid dressing must remain in place on an amputation stump using immediate postoperative fitting. If it falls off, wrap the stump with elastic bandages immediately and call the physician to replace the dressing; otherwise, the stump will swell and lose its desired shape.

REHABILITATION AFTER LEG AMPUTATION The client with a leg amputation will be out of bed in 1 or 2 days postoperatively. The client can stand on the unaffected leg to transfer to a chair. The physical therapist will teach exercises and ambulation technique, which the nurse can reinforce when the client is back on the unit. When a temporary prosthesis is first used for ambulation, only limited weight bearing is allowed. The client progresses from parallel bars to crutches or a walker, then to a cane, and finally to no aids. The rate of progress varies with the individual. An AK amputee eventually uses a prosthesis with a knee joint that locks when weight is applied. The physical therapist is responsible for gait training and teaching the client how to maneuver on stairs.

REHABILITATION AFTER ARM AMPUTATION People usually experience more pain with arm amputation than with leg amputation, so comfort measures are especially important for a client who has lost an arm. The client wears a sling when out of bed. Range of motion exercises are necessary to prevent contracture; physical therapists teach arm exercises. The client will need to have someone wrap the arm because it is impossible to wrap with one hand.

Use of the arm prosthesis is difficult. Skilled use requires long training with the physical therapist and a great deal of practice; the fine movements of the hand are never replaced. One type of prosthesis for the arm is made with a split hook, which opens voluntarily by means of control cables activated by arm or shoulder movement. Other devices work by electrical power. A cosmetic prosthesis provides less function but is more pleasing to the eye. There have been many improvements in prostheses in recent years, and improvements should continue. Research is currently focused on developing methods of computer-assisted mobility.

FITTING AND CARE OF THE PROSTHESIS A prosthetist measures and fits the client for the prosthesis. Prostheses are made of wood, metal, and plastic. Some prostheses are held on by a belt around the waist; some stay in place by suction (air is forced out as the stump is placed in the socket).

The prosthetist teaches the client how to care for the appliance. A prosthesis is an expensive item and requires conscientious care. The socket should be cleaned daily with mild soap and water and dried thoroughly; the hinges should be lubricated; mechanical parts should not get wet. The client should not alter the prosthesis in any way. The prosthetist should be seen immediately when problems occur with the prosthesis, and a yearly checkup may be recommended.

STUMP CARE WITH A PROSTHESIS The nurse teaches the client stump care so the limb can be maintained in optimal condition. Clients should inspect the stump thoroughly before and after using the prosthesis. They may need a mirror to see all areas of the stump. If there are irritated or sore areas, the prosthesis should not be worn, and the physician should check the stump to avoid development of a more serious problem. The client should wash the skin with mild soap and water, rinse it thoroughly, and dry it well. If a stump sock is worn, it should be washed daily. The client should have enough stump socks to wear a clean, dry sock every day. Stump socks should be discarded if they develop rough spots or holes; they should not be mended because mending causes rough areas. Tell the client that the stump may shrink and require refitting.

BODY IMAGE AND SEXUAL FUNCTION A visit from an amputee who has adjusted well to a similar amputation and prosthesis may help the client. Clients may find it hard to use the word "stump" at first, so the nurse can encourage discussion about their "limb" or "leg." A client may become discouraged with the amount of work necessary to learn new skills, especially a client with an arm amputation. Help clients to set realistic goals and to progress steadily toward self-care. Accomplishments should be praised by the health team. Encourage the family to do the same.

Although an amputation should not seriously affect a person's ability to engage in sexual activity, clients may perceive themselves as less attractive or may worry about what their partner thinks or feels. Some changes may be necessary because of the presence of the prosthesis, or because the person no longer has a limb that was once used for sexual activity. A client who has lost a hand will need to use the other one for touching. Assess for potential difficulties and encourage the client and sexual partner to discuss their feelings.

PREPARATION FOR DISCHARGE Clients may be discharged from the hospital as soon as the wound heals and they can do the prescribed exercises, wrap the stump correctly, and ambulate as directed. Training with the prosthesis is not usually done on an inpatient basis. Urge the client to continue follow-up visits to the physician, prosthetist, and physical therapist and teach care specific to the underlying condition, such as PVD or diabetes mellitus, before client discharge. A referral to a community health nurse may be helpful, to reinforce teaching and assess progress. The client may also be referred to a social worker, to help with financial problems, and to the local Office of Vocational Rehabilitation, which can provide occupational assistance.

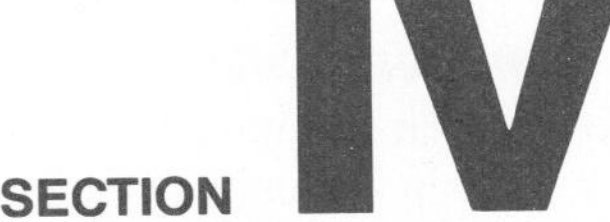

SECTION IV

Traumatic Disorders

Traumatic conditions affecting the bones include fractures and amputations. Amputations are treated surgically and are covered earlier in this chapter.

Fractures

A **fracture** is a break in the continuity of a bone. Many terms are used to describe types of fractures. A fracture in which the skin over the injury remains intact, so there is no connection between the bone and the skin surface, is known as a *closed* fracture (formerly called a simple fracture). An *open* fracture (formerly known as compound) is one in which the skin surface over the injury is broken and the surface wound connects with the fracture. The open wound may have been caused by the fracture fragments piercing the skin or by a force from outside the body, such as a bullet which pierced the skin, hit the bone, and caused the fracture. Fracture fragments that break through the skin may protrude from the wound or they may move back inside; in the latter case, the examiner does not know whether the wound communicates with the fracture. A person who administers first aid should note whether the bone protruded. An open fracture is more complicated than a closed one because of the potential for infection. The fracture can be described further by indicating the area of bone involved. Long bones are divided into thirds: proximal, middle, and distal. Various kinds of fractures are diagrammed and described in Table 45–4.

Fractures occur when a bone is unable to absorb or transmit a stress placed upon it. The stress can occur from a direct force such as a blow, falling, or crushing, or from an indirect force like twisting or extreme muscle contraction. Minimal stress can break a weakened bone (pathologic fracture). A *stress fracture* can occur in normal bone that is subjected to repeated stresses, such as strenuous activity. Jogging can cause stress fractures, for example, in experienced as well as inexperienced joggers.

Fractures can cause disruption of more than the bone. Surrounding soft tissues and adjacent organs can be damaged either from the injury itself or from sharp bone fragments. For example, fractured ribs may puncture the lung, or a fractured pelvis may injure the bladder. Nerves or blood vessels may be damaged or severed. Therefore, management of fractures includes thorough assessment for related problems. Fractures interfere with bodily movements such as ambulation and ADL and may also be painful. If untreated, fractures may heal in deformed positions, affecting the future use of the part, or they may not heal at all. Many complications can occur as a result of fractures, including complications resulting from treatments such as casts, traction, and immobilization.

Clinical Manifestations

The manifestations of a fracture depend upon its type and location and on the other tissues involved. A history of the traumatic event may suggest the possibility of a fracture. Severe pain usually occurs immediately, and there may be *point tenderness* at the fracture site. There may be obvious *deformity:* The limb may be bent, shortened, or twisted, or the contour of bones in the skull may be changed. Protrusion of bone fragments through an open wound is an obvious sign of fracture.

Swelling may be caused by bleeding into the tissues and accumulated serous fluid at the site of injury. *Ecchymosis* may also occur due to bleeding, but this usually takes a few days to be apparent. Involuntary and painful *muscle spasm* may occur around the site of injury; spasm is sometimes caused by attempts to move the limb. Spasm also occurs with the loss of normal tension on the muscle from the fracture. The examiner may hear or feel *crepitation*, a grating caused by bone fragments rubbing together; do *not* try to elicit this sign, however, because movement of sharp bone fragments may cause further damage to surrounding tissues. The limb may display abnormal motion; for example, a long bone fractured along the shaft may bend at the point of fracture, where it would normally be rigid. There may be loss of function due to displacement of bone fragments, muscle spasms, instability, or pain; injury to a nerve may cause *paralysis*. A final manifestation of fracture is *shock*, which may occur as a result of hemorrhage or extensive traumatic damage. X-rays confirm the diagnosis and provide the physician with information about the type of fracture and the displacement of fragments.

Occasionally, a client may have an impacted fracture or one without displacement of fragments and will be able to use the limb. The only symptoms may be pain with direct pressure and some swelling. When medical care is finally obtained, an x-ray will reveal the fracture line.

Medical Measures

Some specific types of fractures and their treatment are covered in other units in this textbook. Fractures of the jaw, nose, and ribs are covered in Chapters 15 and 16. Fractures of the vertebrae are covered in Chapter 24. The general objectives of fracture management are:

- Realigning the bone fragments, a process called *reduction*
- Maintaining the alignment by *immobilization*
- *Restoring function* to the part

Reduction of a fracture can be accomplished in three ways. *Closed reduction* is the manipulation of the bone fragments until the bone is realigned. Some manual traction and rotation of the limb may be necessary. This type of reduction is done on closed fractures with or without a local or general anesthetic. Sedation may also be used. The realigned bone is then immobilized by application of a cast or splint. *Open reduction* is a surgical procedure in which the fracture fragments can be directly visualized to place them back into alignment. The bone is immobilized by use of nails, rods, plates, screws, or pins, which hold the bone fragments together, a procedure known as *open reduction internal fixation* (ORIF). These surgical approaches will be covered later in this chapter.

The third type of reduction is *traction*. **Traction** is pulling force applied to the limb to overcome muscle spasm and realign the fracture. The traction pull maintains the bone in alignment, so traction is also a means of immobilization. X-rays are taken after application of traction to

Table 45–4
Types of Fractures

Type	Description	Illustration
Closed (simple)	The skin over the fracture remains intact.	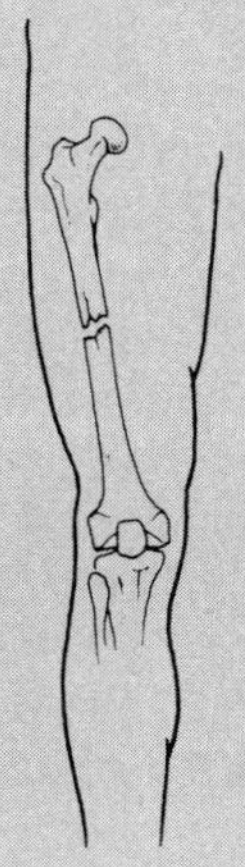
Open (compound)	The skin surface over the fracture is broken, and the surface wound connects with the fracture.	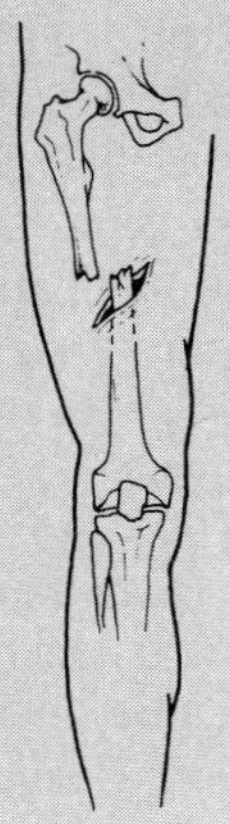
Comminuted	The bone is broken into three or more fragments.	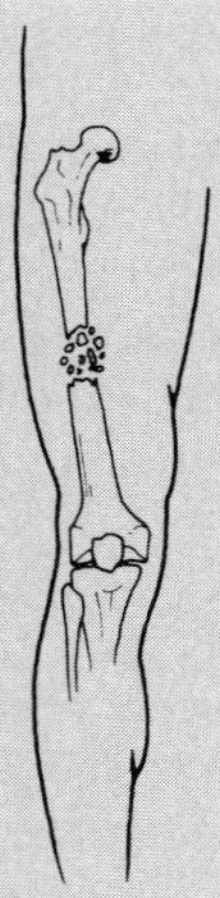
Transverse	The break runs straight across the bone (ie, perpendicular to the bone's long axis).	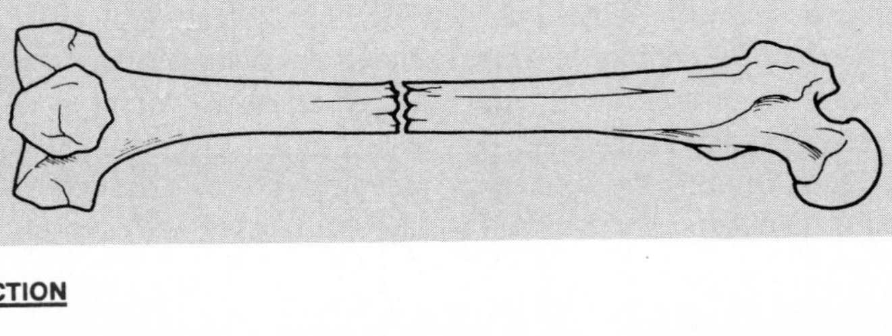

Type	Description	Illustration
Oblique	The break runs at an angle, or slanted, across the bone.	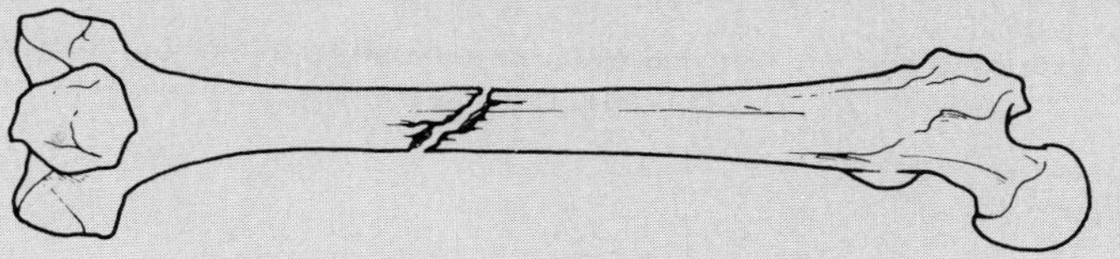
Spiral	The break coils around the bone. This usually occurs from torsion (twisting) of the limb such as occurs in a skiing accident when the foot is stuck in one position while the leg continues to turn.	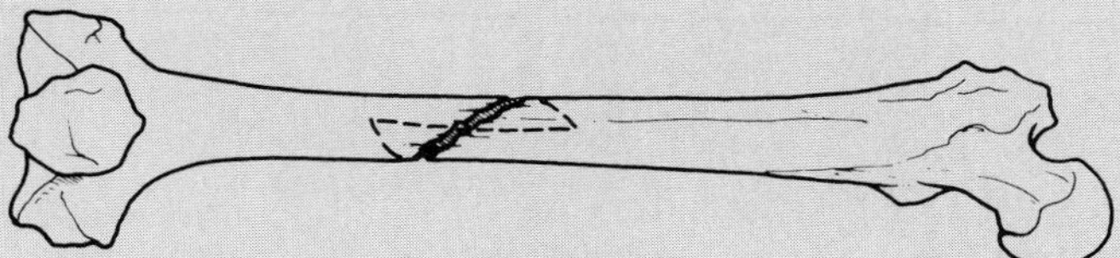
Impacted	The fracture fragments are pushed into each other (telescoped). This can occur when a person falls straight down, landing on the feet.	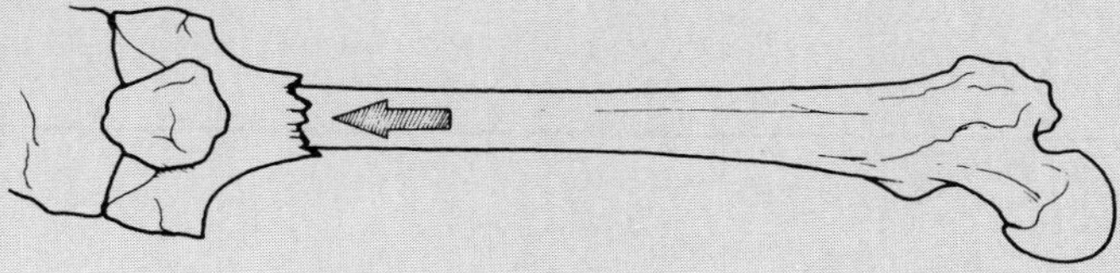
Greenstick	The fracture does not go all the way through the bone; rather it splinters on one side. This occurs in children because their bones are soft, much like the flexible green limb of a tree, which does not break through completely when one tries to snap it in two. These fractures heal rapidly.	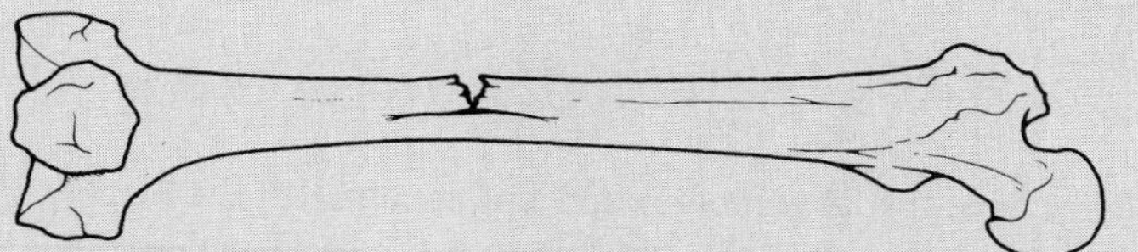
Pathologic	The fracture occurs at a point in the bone weakened by disease, such as with tumors or osteoporosis. The break may occur from only a small force or normal activity such as sneezing or twisting.	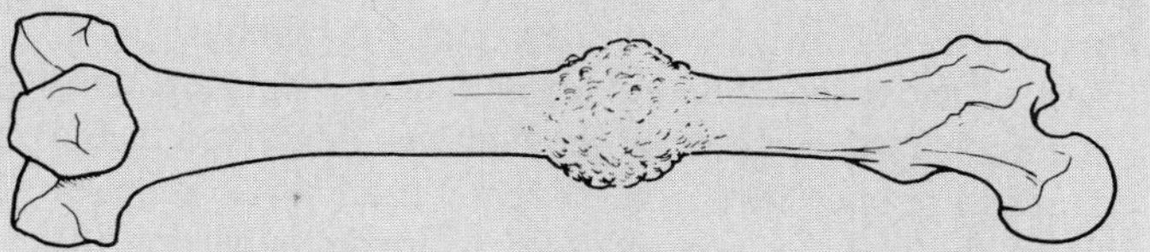
Avulsion	A fragment of bone connected to a ligament breaks off from the rest of the bone.	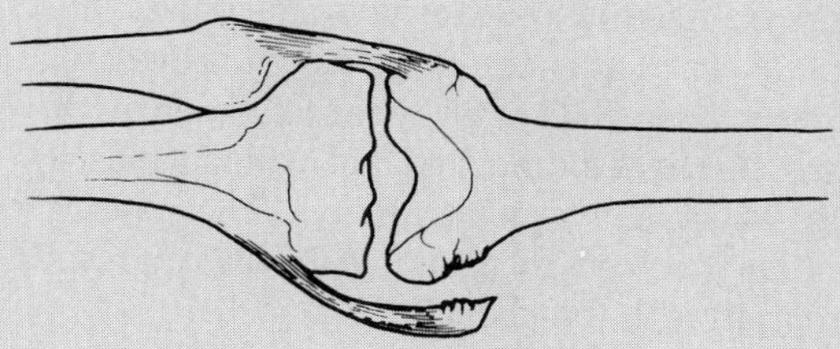

(continued)

Table 45–4
Types of Fractures (continued)

Type	Description	Illustration
Extracapsular	The fracture is close to a joint but remains outside the joint capsule.	
Intracapsular	The fracture is within the joint capsule.	

determine that alignment is appropriate and that the pieces are not too far apart. In addition to fracture management, traction may be used to correct deformities, to reduce muscle spasms, and to rest injured or diseased joints.

Immobilization is essential after the fracture fragments are realigned. If the fragments are not immobilized, hematoma and callus formation will be disrupted and the bone will heal slowly or in poor alignment. Splints, casts, traction, and internal and external fixation tools are used for immobilization. Internal fixation was described in the discussion of open reduction. External fixation also requires surgery but uses an external device for immobilizing the fracture fragments. During surgery, pins are inserted into the bone above and below the fracture; these extend through the skin and are clamped to an external framework.

Restoration of function is accomplished by preventing complications during immobility and by rehabilitation methods that prepare the client for mobility and maintain muscle strength, tone, and range of joint motion. The physical therapist is often involved in planning an exercise and ambulation program with the client.

THE USE OF CASTS IN FRACTURE MANAGEMENT Casts are used to immobilize fracture fragments after they have been reduced. Casts can also be used to correct deformity; to rest weak, injured, or diseased parts; and to immobilize parts after such surgeries as joint fusion or reconstruction. Some common types of casts are described and illustrated in Table 45–5. The pressure points are also shown.

APPLYING THE CAST The most common casting material is mesh bandage impregnated with *plaster of paris*, a powder made from gypsum. The bandage is supplied in various-sized rolls or strips (splints). When the rolls or splints are immersed in water, a chemical reaction takes place between the water and the powder, giving off heat and forming crystals. The crystals interlock and produce a strong, firm cast as the material dries. When wet, the bandage can be molded to fit the contour of the body part. The strength of the cast depends on the number of layers of plaster bandage applied.

Casts can be applied in the physician's office, the emergency room, a special cast room, or the operating room. The plaster is messy, so the person applying the cast wears an apron and rubber gloves and covers the client's clothing. The client may need analgesics before the cast is applied, and the client should be helped to relax. Clients should be told that the cast will be heavy and will

Table 45–5
Types of Casts

Type	Description	Illustration and Pressure Points
Short arm cast	Extends from below the elbow to the palm or fingers. The thumb may or may not be included in the cast, depending on the location and type of fracture. Used for fractures of the distal forearm, wrist, carpals, or metacarpals.	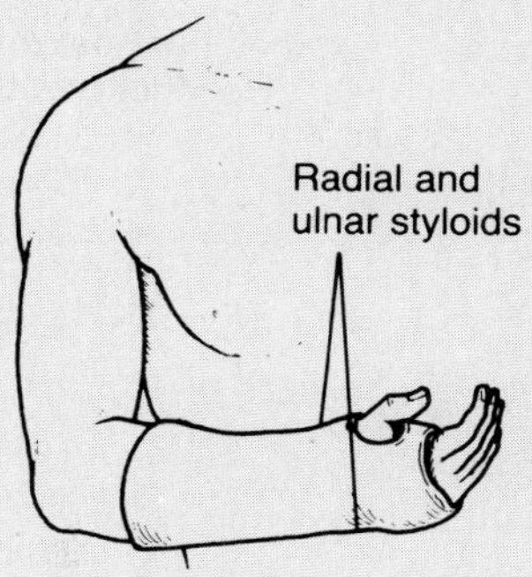 Radial and ulnar styloids
Long arm cast	Extends from above the elbow to the palm or wrist. Used for fracture of the distal humerus, forearm, or carpals.	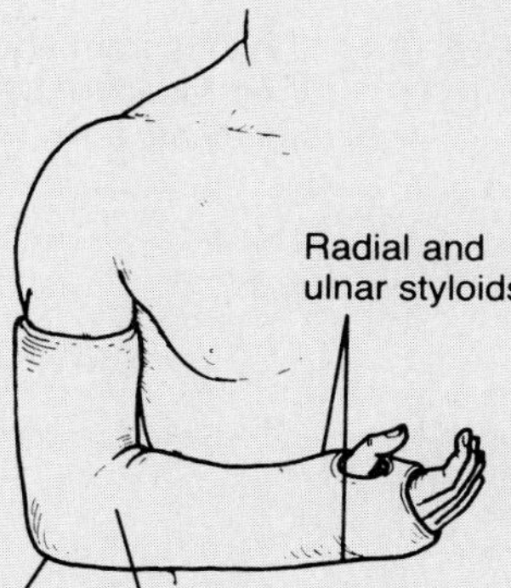 Radial and ulnar styloids; Olecranon; Epicondyles
Hanging long arm cast	Cast hangs from a special sling attached to the cast and looped around the client's neck. As it hangs, the weight of the cast provides traction to realign a fracture of the humerus. This combines the principles of casting and traction. The cast must remain hanging, unencumbered to maintain the traction force (ie, the cast should not be supported or rested on anything).	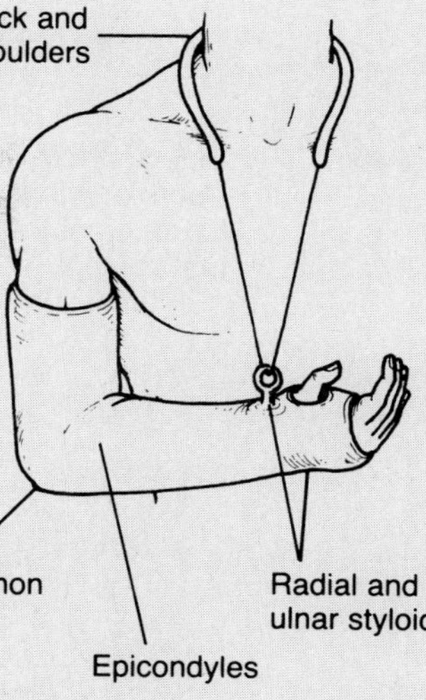 Neck and shoulders; Olecranon; Radial and ulnar styloids; Epicondyles

(continued)

Table 45–5
Types of Casts (continued)

Type	Description	Illustration and Pressure Points
Short leg cast	Extends from below the knee to the toes. Used for fractures of the ankle or foot.	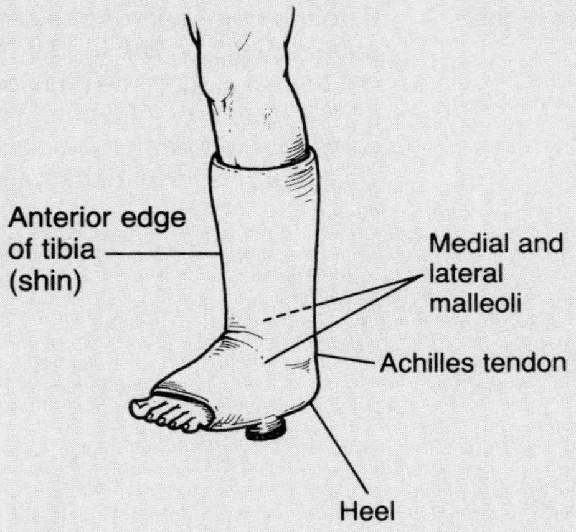 Anterior edge of tibia (shin); Medial and lateral malleoli; Achilles tendon; Heel
Long leg cast	Extends from above the knee to the toes. Used for fractures of the femoral condyles, tibia, fibula, or ankle.	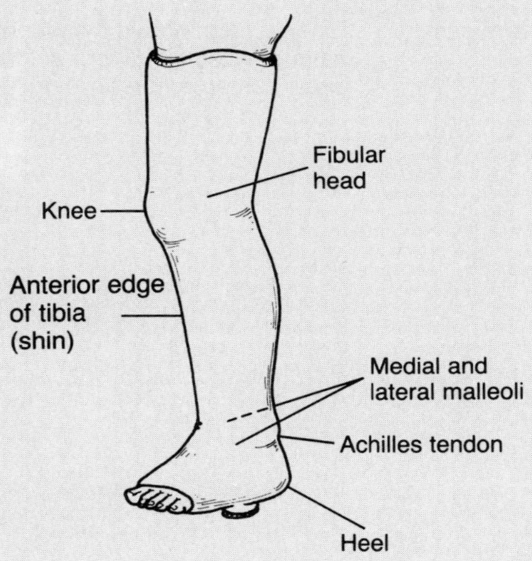 Fibular head; Knee; Anterior edge of tibia (shin); Medial and lateral malleoli; Achilles tendon; Heel
Cylinder cast	Extends from the ankle to the thigh. Used for injuries to the knee and stable fractures of the distal femur and proximal tibia.	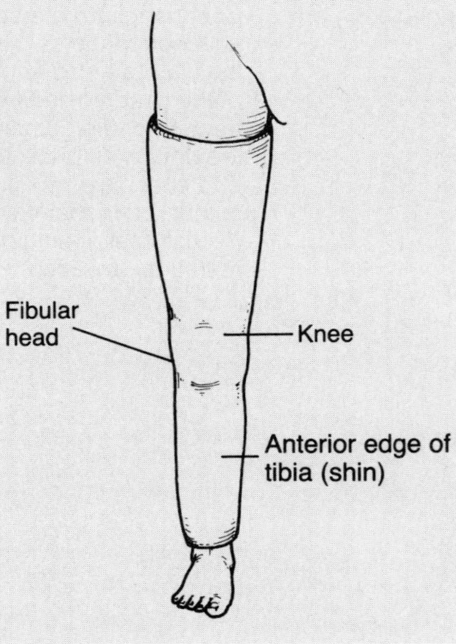 Fibular head; Knee; Anterior edge of tibia (shin)

Type	Description	Illustration and Pressure Points
Body cast	Covers the trunk; it may include the upper chest or start below the axillae. A window is cut over the abdomen to prevent pressure on the internal organs. Used for fractures or dislocation of the spine, for scoliosis, or after spinal surgery.	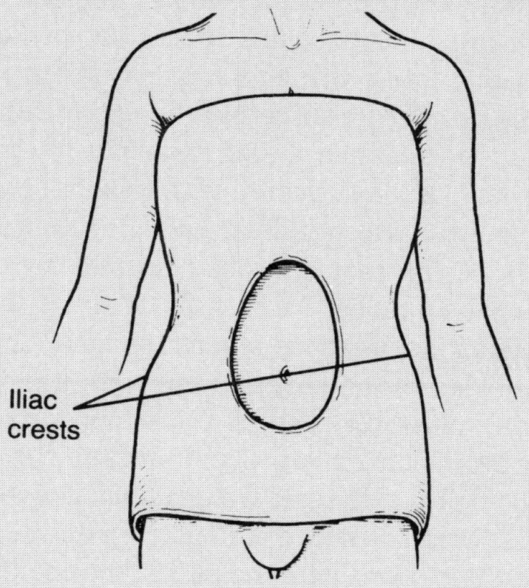 Iliac crests
Hip spica cast	A *spica cast* is applied with a figure-eight turn of the plaster rolls between the body and an appendage. There are shoulder spica and thumb spica casts, but the hip spica cast is the one most often referred to as a spica cast. The hip spica may include the trunk and both legs (double spica), one leg (single spica), or a one-and-a-half spica, which extends to the toes of one leg and the knee of the other. A window is cut over the abdomen, and an opening is left in the groin area. Used for fractures of the femoral shaft, the upper femur, or the hip and for hip dislocations. It is also used for immobilization of the hip after special reconstructive surgery or joint fusion.	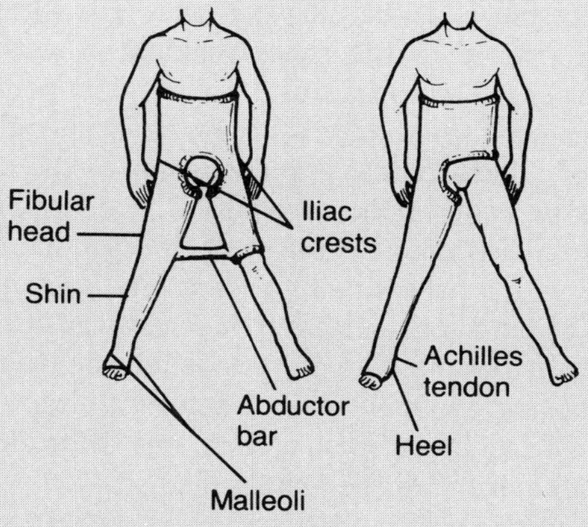 Fibular head Shin Iliac crests Abductor bar Malleoli Achilles tendon Heel
Cast brace	A device used to immobilize a fracture while permitting joint mobility. It is most frequently used to treat fractures of the femoral shaft after a few weeks of skeletal traction. A snug thigh cast of plaster is applied from the high upper thigh to above the knee joint. Another cast is applied to the lower leg; it may be a walking cast or a cylinder cast. The two casts are connected by two hinges at the knee joint. Sometimes the thigh area includes a minispica cast around the pelvis. Allows early ambulation and weight bearing, which facilitate healing and shorten the rehabilitation period. (Recall that the stresses placed on a bone stimulate bone formation.) The hinges can be locked for walking and unlocked for exercising the knee. Problems with this type of appliance include pressure sores at the edges of the thigh cast, swelling of the knee, and difficulty sitting on the bedpan or commode. The extremity should be elevated when the client is not walking.	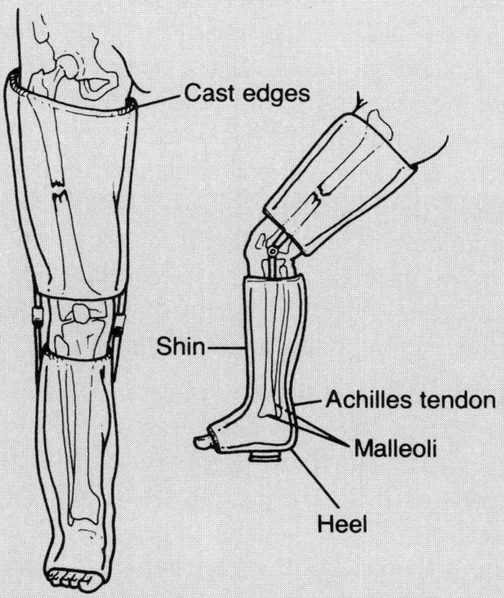 Cast edges Shin Achilles tendon Malleoli Heel

give off heat for 10 to 30 minutes while drying because of the chemical reaction. Frequently, the nurse holds the limb in position as the cast is applied.

First, the skin over which the cast will be placed is inspected well to note any redness, abrasions, open areas, or bruises. These areas may require special care before casting and evaluation after, through a cast window and during cast change, to see that the skin is not breaking down. The skin is cleansed and dried. After the fracture is reduced, the limb is usually covered with tubular stockinette. The stockinette, which is long enough to extend beyond both ends of the cast, is rolled up and applied smoothly, to prevent wrinkles. Next, rolls of sheet wadding, a feltlike material, are wrapped around the limb. Sheet wadding can be molded to the shape of the limb; it is layered to provide a comfortable padding and wrapped sufficiently over bony prominences to prevent pressure. A roll of plaster bandage is placed in tepid water until it is evenly soaked, and excess water is squeezed out. Tepid water is used because hot water (along with the heat of the chemical reaction) may cause burns on the client's skin, whereas cold water may cause delayed drying time. The plaster bandage is wrapped over the sheet wadding in smooth layers and molded to the shape of the limb. The person holding the limb must use the flat palms of the hands rather than fingertips, which can cause indentations in the cast and thus pressure areas on the extremity. The ends of the stockinette are folded over the edges of the cast and fastened in place with a final wrap of plaster. The cast is *set* in a few minutes but is still subject to indentations. It may take 24 to 48 hours or longer to dry completely, depending on its thickness and the humidity and temperature of the air. The finished cast is placed on pillows, and the extremity is x-rayed to make sure the bone is aligned.

Pressure points must be avoided in the application of any immobilizing device. With cast application, bony prominences such as the head of the fibula, the malleoli of the ankle, or the epicondyle of the distal humerus are protected by padding. However, the proper molding of the cast around bony prominences following the normal contour of the extremity is more important in preventing pressure areas than is the application of excessive padding.

Pressure areas can form under the cast at any time because of muscle spasms causing continued friction over joints, toys or other objects dropped down the cast, or rolling up of the padding material under the cast.

ALTERNATIVE CAST MATERIALS Materials other than plaster of paris have been used for casts recently (eg, fiberglass and plastic). Casts made of these materials are lighter and more porous than plaster casts, yet they are strong. They are also easier to clean and do not deteriorate when wet, as a plaster cast does. The client may be allowed to immerse a cast made from such materials in water, as long as the cast and skin are thoroughly dried afterward to prevent skin maceration. A blow dryer set on medium is used for drying after immersion, which may take up to a few hours. The material used for padding under the cast is made of a synthetic that dries quickly.

Fiberglass and plastic casts become hard and strong in about 15 minutes or less. One type, called a light-cured fiberglass cast, is applied from a roll and then exposed to ultraviolet light for a few minutes until it hardens. Other lightweight materials are softened in hot water or immersed in cool water before application and then are molded to the extremity. These newer casting materials are more expensive than plaster, so they are not used on clients who require frequent cast changes. They also are inappropriate for an injury where bleeding may occur because the drainage will not be absorbed as it would be with plaster.

CAST ALTERATIONS Occasionally, alterations are made in casts. A cast *window* may be formed by cutting out a small section of the cast. A cast cutter is used to cut a rectangular area in the cast, the plaster is removed, and the sheet wadding is cut to expose an area of skin that requires observation or care. There may be a wound requiring dressings, a pressure area causing discomfort, or stitches needing removal. The plaster square that is cut out should be saved because it is frequently put back to prevent the limb from swelling into the opening. The window plug may be taped in place with adhesive or wrapped with an elastic bandage. When wound care is given through the window, it is important to avoid getting the cast wet.

In another cast alteration, known as *bivalving*, the cast is split by the cast cutter along both the entire lateral and medial cast surfaces. This may be done to relieve edema or to change the cast into a half-shell splint. The splint is formed by removing the upper (or lower) half, allowing the limb to rest in the other half. A half-shell splint allows access to the joints and limb, but still provides support. The removed half of the cast is saved, and it is put back in place when the client is turned. The two shells are fastened together with straps, adhesive, or elastic bandaging (Figure 45–4).

A *walking heel* may be applied to a leg cast to allow weight bearing. If a client wonders why he or she does not have a walking cast, explain that this is only used when the type of fracture and position of the limb allows walking before healing is complete. Sometimes a walking heel is added later, when sufficient callus formation occurs, to allow weight bearing. The client must wait until the plaster dries before trying to walk on it. An alternative to the heel is a cast shoe worn over the cast (Figure 45–5).

REMOVING THE CAST When the fracture is healed, the cast is split with an electric cast cutter, which has a blade that oscillates rather than cuts. The vibrating blade is raised quickly as it breaks through the plaster (or synthetic cast) so it does not cut through the padding underneath. The

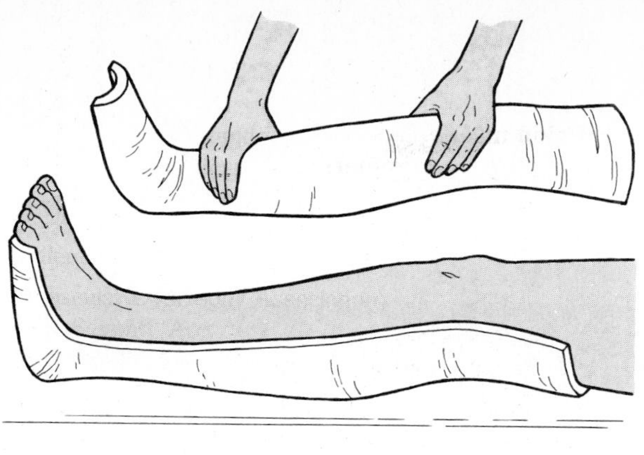

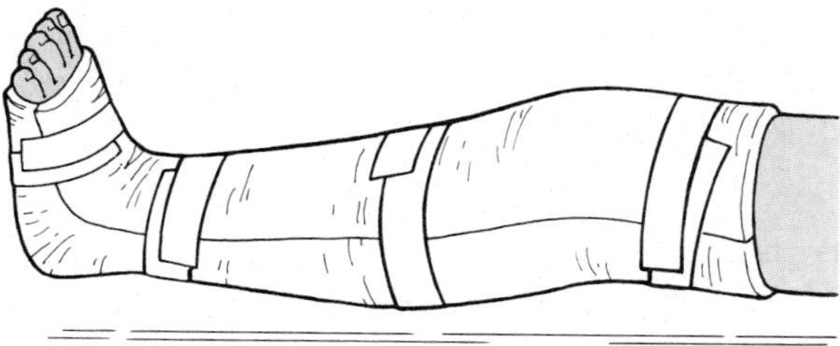

Figure 45–4

A bivalved cast. *SOURCE: Kozier B, Erb G:* Techniques in Clinical Nursing: A Nursing Process Approach, *2nd ed. Menlo Park, CA: Addison–Wesley, 1986.*

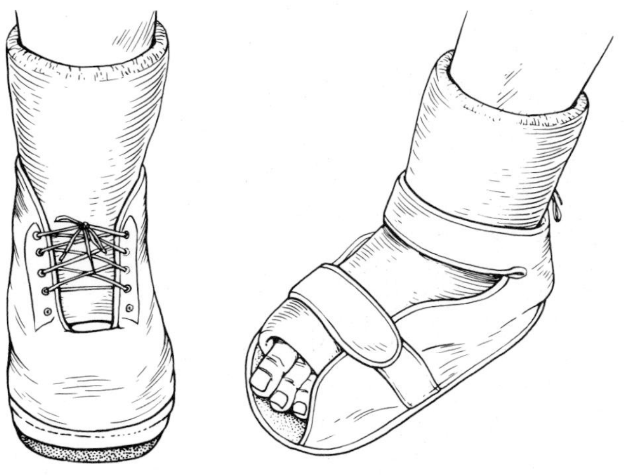

Figure 45–5

Cast shoe.

cutter is noisy, and the client may feel some pressure and heat. All this can be frightening; the client will need reassurance that the cutter will not go through to the skin. After the cast is split, the cut edges are spread apart with tools, and the sheet wadding is cut with bandage scissors.

THE USE OF TRACTION IN FRACTURE MANAGEMENT Traction is applied by ropes, pulleys, weights, and an apparatus that connects them to the body part. The traction is adjusted to hold the fracture fragments in the proper alignment while healing takes place. When a force pulls in one direction, it is necessary to have a counterforce pulling in the opposite direction to keep the client from being pulled off the bed. Usually the countertraction is the client's body weight and the position of the bed (eg, the foot of the bed may be elevated). It is important to note the position of the client and the bed when traction is set up and to maintain these: otherwise the traction pull may be changed, altering the bone alignment.

Placing a person in traction means confinement to bed and usually a lengthy hospitalization (unless this is a temporary measure, for example, until a cast is applied). The bed should have a firm mattress, bedboard (if there are springs on the bed), and an overhead trapeze. An overbed frame is frequently necessary to connect traction equipment. An alternating air mattress or egg-crate-type foam rubber on the mattress is helpful in preventing pressure sores. A water mattress may be used as long as the limb remains in alignment on it. The physician, or someone trained in traction application, sets up the apparatus. X-rays are taken to see that the fracture fragments are in alignment. The client's condition should be assessed well before traction application, including neurovascular status and skin condition. Then it can be determined if changes are from the injury or the traction. The apparatus should not be applied over open wounds, if possible.

GENERAL TYPES OF TRACTION Traction can be either skin or skeletal traction. *Skin traction* is usually used for comfort and to decrease muscle spasm. It may be used intermittently, allowing access to the skin for good skin care. In skin traction, a material such as strips of foam rubber, moleskin, or tape adheres to the skin of the body part, applying a pull indirectly to the bone and muscle. The material is held in place by wrapping the limb with elastic bandaging. Skin traction can also be applied by use of a halter around the head for cervical traction or a pelvic belt for traction of the lower vertebrae. In Buck's extension (described later), a foam boot is used and fastened with Velcro straps. Skin traction is used for a shorter length of time than skeletal traction (up to 4 weeks) and uses small weights. The skeleton is capable of tolerating more weight than the skin.

Skeletal traction is applied directly to the bone. It is used for long-term alignment of fracture fragments. Under local or general anesthesia, a pin or wire is inserted aseptically through the skin and bone so traction weights can be applied to it. The pin extends through both sides of the limb and is attached to a U-shaped metal spreader, or bow, to which the traction ropes are tied. When skeletal traction is applied to the cervical vertebrae, the pull is applied by means of tongs inserted into the skull. The pin or wire is inserted distal to the fracture, not through the fracture area itself. For example, when the femur is fractured, the pin may be inserted through the proximal tibia. Skeletal traction is applied usually for a prolonged period of time

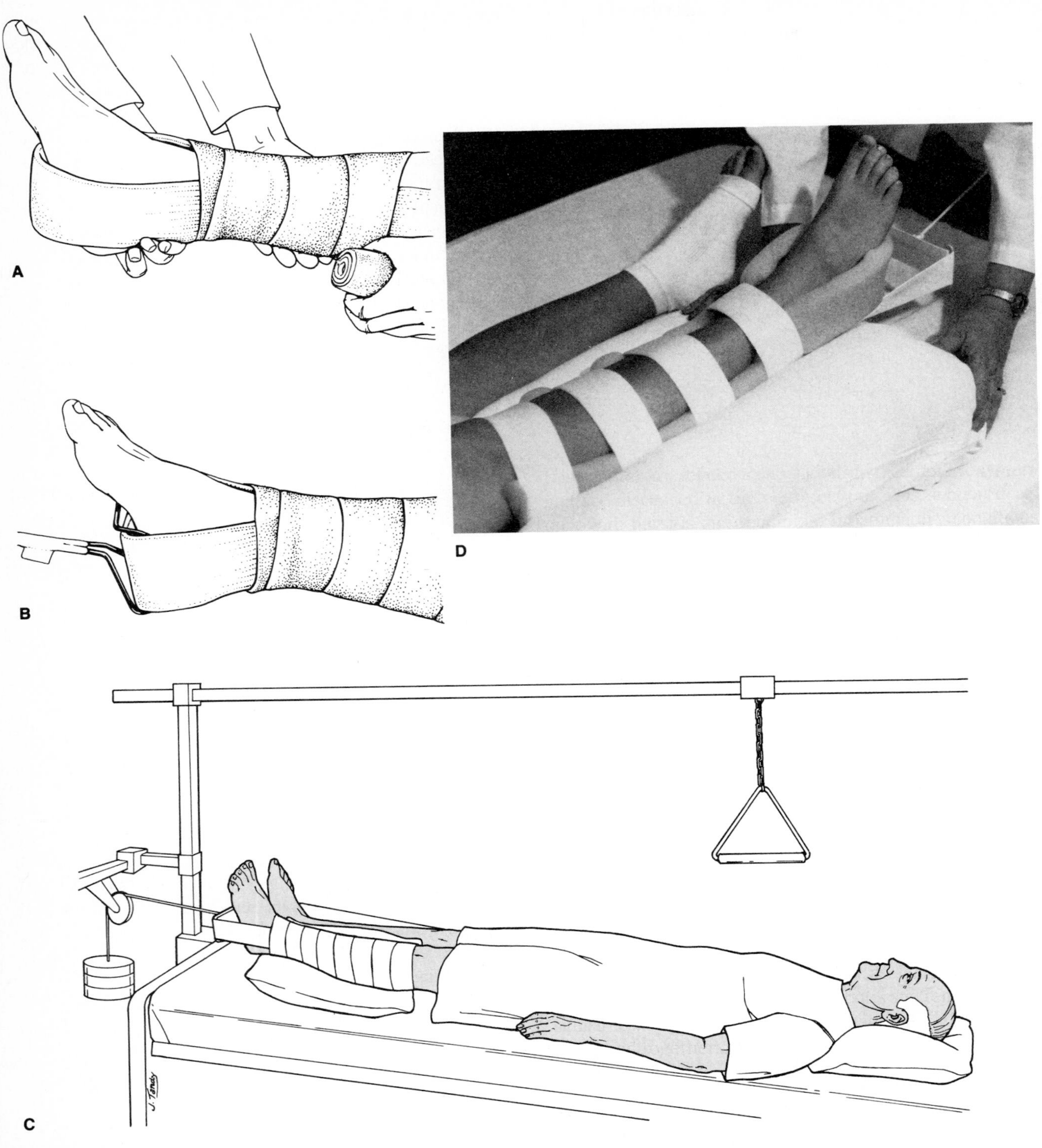

Figure 45–6

Applying Buck's extension. **A.** The leg is supported while being wrapped. The strips are placed along the medial and lateral aspects of the calf. Elastic bandage is applied smoothly and evenly from above the ankle to the knee. **B.** The spreader keeps the strips away from the malleoli. **C.** Buck's extension traction in place. **D.** A Buck's boot for extension traction. SOURCE: *C, Kozier B, Erb G:* Techniques in Clinical Nursing: A Nursing Process Approach, *2nd ed. and* ***D****, Swearingen PL:* Addison–Wesley Photo Atlas of Nursing Procedures. *Menlo Park, CA: Addison–Wesley, 1984.*

and uses weights of up to 40 lb. The insertion of pins into the skeleton may be a sourse of infection, which could develop into osteomyelitis.

Both skin and skeletal traction can be applied as *straight (running)* or *balanced (suspension)* traction. In straight traction, the body weight and bed position are used as countertraction. In balanced traction, the pull is exerted while the limb is supported by use of a sling, splint, or hammock, and weights provide the countertraction. The limb is suspended rather than lying on the bed, and movement is permitted because the weights move when the client moves, maintaining constant traction. Any slack that would otherwise occur in the ropes during movement is taken up by the suspension apparatus. This type of traction permits greater activity for clients and aids the nurse in giving care because clients can be moved slightly to relieve pressure on the back. They can raise to use the bedpan and receive back care without changing the pull of the traction.

SPECIFIC TRACTION DEVICES Some specific types of traction are described below. Readers wanting more information should consult orthopedic nursing textbooks.

Buck's extension is an example of straight skin traction (Figure 45–6 A-C). It is applied to the lower leg:

- To relieve muscle spasm
- For preoperative immobilization of a fractured hip or femur
- For maintaining alignment after hip surgery
- To reduce hip or knee contractures
- To rest a diseased hip or knee

It can be used on one or both legs. Frequently, the nurse applies Buck's extension. Various types of apparatus are used to apply this type of traction. When adhesive tapes are used, the nurse may shave and cleanse the leg and coat it with protective skin spray such as tincture of benzoin. Opinions differ about the advisability of shaving and use of tincture of benzoin because shaving may cause skin abrasion, and benzoin is not as useful for protecting against infection or adhering the tape as was once believed (Farrell, 1982). Nonadhesive strips require skin care and assessment but not shaving. The nurse places the tape or strip along the medial and lateral aspects of the calf (and sometimes the thigh also), leaving space at the bottom for inserting the spreader or footplate used for attaching the traction rope. Folded or rolled stockinette can be placed just above the malleoli to keep the tapes off the ankles. Elastic bandaging is wrapped *smoothly* over the tapes, from above the ankle to the knee, to secure them. Particular care is taken to avoid pressure over the fibular head (the lateral side of the calf below the knees), to prevent pressure on the peroneal nerve. The traction rope and weight are applied to the spreader or footplate; the spreader should be wide enough to keep the tapes off the malleoli. A boot-type of apparatus with Velcro straps may be used instead of tapes and bandages (Figure 45–6D). The weights for this type of traction should not exceed 8 to 10 lb; otherwise, the skin will break down. A pillow may be placed under the lower leg with the heel extending over the end of it. The foot of the bed may be elevated to provide countertraction. The physician should let the nurse know if the traction can be removed for skin care; however, the adhesive-tape type is not removed. Problems that can occur from this type of traction are skin breakdown or neurovascular damage from constriction (eg, peroneal nerve palsy), allergy to the materials, pressure sores on the heels, or slipping of the traction apparatus so traction is not maintained.

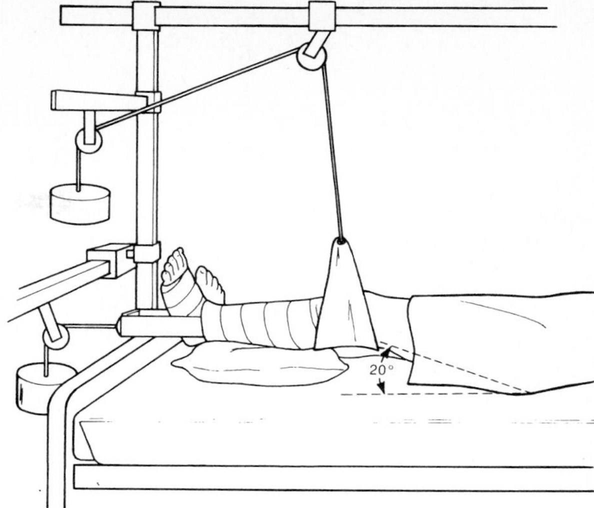

Figure 45–7

Russell's traction. SOURCE: *Kozier B, Erb G:* Techniques in Clinical Nursing: A Nursing Process Approach, *2nd ed. Menlo Park, CA: Addison–Wesley, 1986.*

Russell's traction is a type of skin traction (Figure 45–7) applied to treat fractures of the shaft of the femur and to correct knee and hip deformities. It can also be used bilaterally to treat back pain. The lower leg is wrapped as in Buck's extension to provide horizontal pull. In addition, a sling is placed under the knee to provide vertical lift. The back of the knee is padded with thick felt or foam rubber to prevent pressure. A pillow may be placed under the knee and lower leg, depending on the physician's preference. This helps keep the heel off the bed. The angle of the knee bend is determined by the desired alignment. The foot of the bed is elevated by gatching the knee or using "shock" blocks. This type of traction allows the client more freedom of movement because the limb is suspended. The same type of setup can be used with skeletal traction when heavier traction weights are required. The pins may be placed through the distal fibula and tibia or the calcaneus. Skin traction is used mostly in children; adults usually require heavier weight, and therefore skeletal traction, to treat fractures of the femur. In addition to the problem areas mentioned above for Buck's extension, Russell's traction can cause pressure sores in the popliteal area.

Pelvic traction is a type of running skin traction used to treat pelvic fractures and low back pain. A pelvic belt is applied around the body over the iliac crests (Figure 45–8). The belt has straps that connect to a spreader bar, ropes, and weights. The weights may be up to about 20 lb. The foot of the bed is elevated or knees gatched. Problems occurring from this type of traction include pressure sores on the iliac crests, sore elbows from shifting in bed, and slipping of the pelvic belt due to improper fit or application. If the head of the bed is elevated too high, the client may slip down in bed, negating the traction.

The *Thomas* or *Harris splint* and *Pearson attachment* are used when balanced skeletal traction is applied to treat fractures of the shaft of the femur. The splint is placed along the thigh, and slings are attached to the rods to support the thigh from underneath. The slings may be made of cloth or sheepskin or padded with foam rubber. The Pearson attachment supports the knee in a flexed position and has slings on which the lower leg rests. This attachment allows the knee to be moved actively and passively. A foot support is used to prevent footdrop. The skeletal pin is inserted into the distal femur or the proximal tibia and connected to a U-shaped bow, ropes, and a weight. The foot of the bed may be elevated. Changing the height of the head of the bed should not be done because it alters the traction. A similar form of suspension can be used with skin traction.

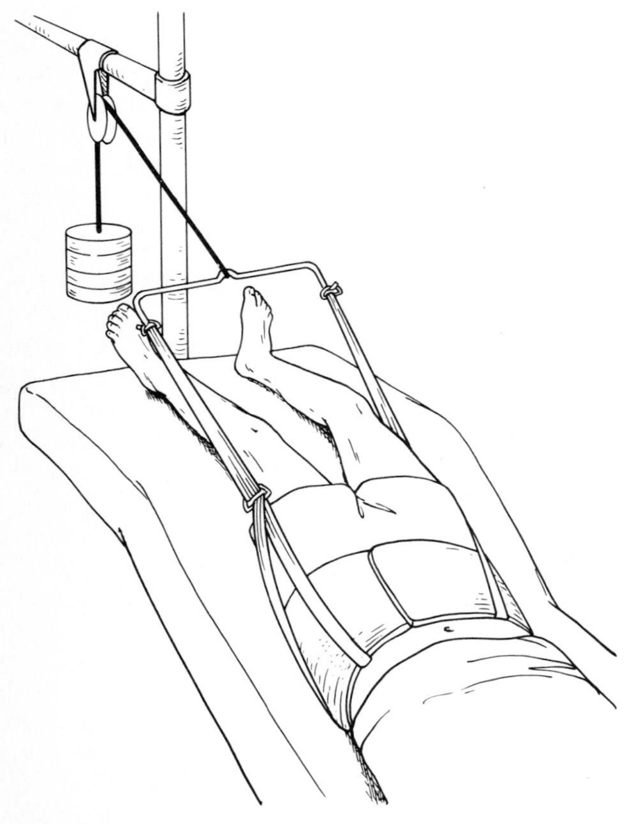

Figure 45–8

Pelvic girdle traction.

There are other types of splints for traction known by various trade names. The upper-thigh end of the splint may have a full ring or half ring that fits around the thigh. Some physicians apply the half ring so it is across the anterior thigh, and some place it under the posterior side. The ring is made of metal covered with padding and moisture-proof material or leather. It can cause pressure in the groin and skin irritation, and is difficult to keep clean and dry with use of the bedpan and bathing. Other problems with this type of skeletal traction include infection from insertion of skeletal pins and pressure sores in the ischial area and the areas of skin that touch edges of the slings.

Crutchfield tongs are used for skeletal traction to treat fractures and dislocations of the cervical vertebrae (Figure 45–9). The pins are inserted about a half inch into the skull after the area is shaved, scrubbed, and anesthetized, and tongs are attached to ropes and weights. The weight may be as much as 35 lb. The head of the bed may be kept elevated slightly by physician's order. Frequently, a special turning bed such as the Roto Rest kinetic treatment table, Circo-electric bed, or Stryker frame is used. This type of apparatus and treatment are used for clients with neurologic problems.

Halo traction may be used for cervical fractures. The traction headpiece is attached to a vest, maintaining head and neck immobilization. This allows early ambulation of the client.

REMOVING THE CLIENT FROM TRACTION When the client is removed from traction, a cast or surgical fixation device may be needed. Skeletal wires are removed after the surrounding skin and exposed wires have been scrubbed with antiseptic solution. The physician depresses the skin around the wire, cuts the wire beneath the skin surface, then pulls it out the opposite side. Small sterile dressings are applied to the skin.

After all immobilizing devices have been removed, the involved part will be weak and its muscles atrophied. The client will need physical therapy to help regain strength and balance and to learn to walk again.

Specific Nursing Measures

A nurse, paramedic, or other trained person should apply first aid as soon after the injury as possible to prevent further injury and to help prevent complications from fractures. First aid measures include splinting, elevation, ice application, and rest. The client should be assessed for the 5 Ps—pain, paresthesia, paralysis, pallor, and pulses. With an open fracture or dirty wound area accompanying the

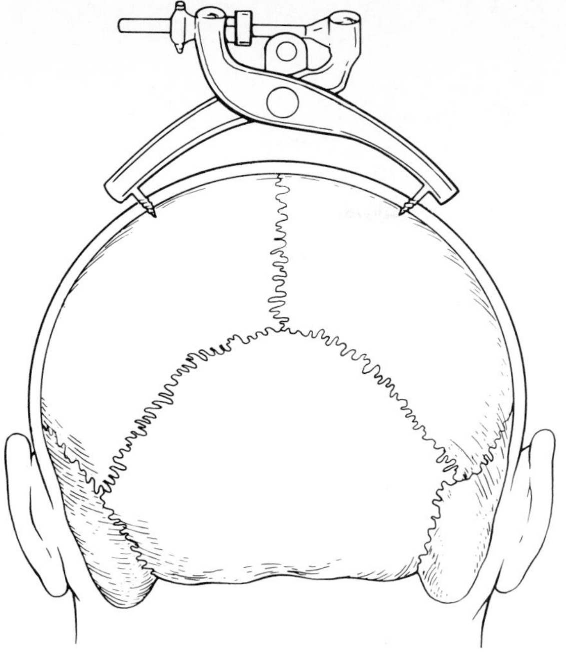

Figure 45–9

Crutchfield tongs.

fracture, the client requires administration of tetanus toxoid if immunization has not been done within the past 5 years.

The general nursing care for musculoskeletal disorders covered in Chapter 43 applies to fractures, especially measures related to rest, positioning and body alignment, comfort, skin care, exercise, ambulation, and diversional activity. Some forms of fracture treatment involve lengthy hospitalization and/or limited mobility after the client is discharged. Clients undergoing such treatment need considerable emotional support and encouragement to participate in the activities necessary for rehabilitation. A nurse who feels sorry for clients and does not encourage the exercises necessary to maintain strength may delay return of mobility. Clients must be partners in their own care; the nurse can elicit cooperation by teaching clients what to do and the reasons for doing it.

NEUROVASCULAR ASSESSMENT Frequent neurovascular assessment of the client with a fracture is ongoing from the onset through surgical intervention or immobilization with a cast or traction, to rehabilitation. If neurovascular impairment is not recognized early, irreversible damage can result with loss of function or even loss of the extremity.

Precast or pretraction neurovascular assessment provides a basis for comparison following immobilization. Following application of the cast or traction, assessments should be made on all clients every hour for the first 24 hours. If normal, assessments may be done every 4 hours for the duration of the immobilization.

Neurovascular assessment includes evaluating the following aspects of the extremity:

- Circulatory status—color, temperature, capillary refill, edema, and pulse(s)
- Neurologic status—sensation, mobility, presence of numbness and tingling

When evaluating sensation on the hands or feet, check all five digits on both medial and lateral aspects because of nerve distribution. For example, in the hand, the median nerve innervates the thumb, index, third, and medial half of the fourth fingers. The ulnar nerve innervates the fifth finger and the lateral half of the fourth finger.

The physician should be notified immediately if signs of neurovascular impairment are present. Clients should be taught to monitor their own neurovascular status so they can alert health care providers and family to the need for prompt intervention.

PAIN MANAGEMENT Fractures can be extremely painful, and narcotics should be given as soon as the possibility of a concomitant head injury has been ruled out. Throughout the client's hospitalization, alterations in the intensity of pain are carefully evaluated and the appropriate actions taken. For example, pain from muscle spasms can be treated with frequent change of position and muscle relaxants.

In some instances, the underlying cause of the pain should be aggressively investigated and analgesics should be withheld until the source of the pain is known. For example, pressure areas under the cast cause a burning pain. Cutting a window over the affected area is the treatment of choice. Ischemic pain, such as occurs with impaired neurovascular status or compartment syndrome, is managed by bivalving the cast to relieve pressure.

AVOIDING HAZARDS OF IMMOBILITY All measures to prevent the hazards of immobility are essential. Encourage the client to exercise all uninvolved extremities every 4 hours while awake. Joints not confined by a cast or traction need ROM, and the client should do isometric exercises to maintain muscle strength in unaffected extremities. The physician should prescribe specific exercises for the affected limb. Encourage self-care, and place articles and the call bell where they can be reached. The client will need help with ADL, especially when the hand or arm is confined in a cast or traction. Diversional activities are necessary. Remember that casts and traction also affect the client's body image and sexual needs.

The client with a leg cast or with traction will be able to maneuver in bed better with use of an overhead *trapeze.* Clients will need instructions on how to use the trapeze (eg, bend the good leg to help lift, pull the body upward, and avoid breath-holding while lifting). When holding the breath to lift, a person performs the Valsalva maneuver, which increases the intrathoracic pressure, decreasing blood flow to the heart. When the person exhales, the intrathoracic pressure decreases, causing a sudden surge of blood to the heart. A client with heart problems may not be able to compensate for the sudden increase of blood flow.

Skin areas susceptible to pressure should be assessed hourly for 48 to 72 hours after a cast or traction is first applied. Care to obvious pressure areas should begin before any problems are noted. Elbow and heel protectors are useful in preventing soreness to these areas, which are easily irritated from shifting the body weight around in bed.

NUTRITION Metabolic needs are greatly increased following trauma. Extensive fracture healing may require an intake of 3000 to 4000 calories per day. Additional fiber and fluids help prevent constipation caused by immobility. The client whose intake is inadequate may receive vitamin and protein supplements. Increased calcium is usually discouraged because calcium is mobilized from the bones during immobility (disuse osteoporosis), and excesses can cause urinary calculi. Therefore, the client's fluid intake should be at least 3000 mL per day, if not contraindicated.

CARING FOR A CLIENT WITH A CAST

DRYING THE CAST A finished cast is placed on pillows, both to elevate the extremity and to avoid placing the cast on a hard surface, which could flatten it as it dries. Pillows should provide support along the entire length of the cast, except a leg cast should be positioned so the heel hangs over the edge to prevent pressure on the heel. It is best to use pillows *without* plastic or rubber covering because airtight pillows trap the heat and may cause burns to the skin (Farrell, 1982). If plastic-covered pillows must be used, place several layers of toweling or a bath blanket between the cast and pillow to allow the heat to dissipate.

The nurse may need extra help to move a client with a fresh cast into a bed while supporting the cast. Be sure to handle the wet cast with the palms, not the fingertips. Plaster that got on the surrounding skin during cast application should be removed with plain water. Turn the client to expose all surfaces of the cast while it is drying. If the client feels cool or chilled during the drying, cover uncasted areas of the body for warmth. Occasionally, lights or cast dryers are used to help dry the cast. Take care to place the lamp far enough away from the cast (15 in.) and to prevent intense heating. Cast dryers can cause uneven drying with a dry outside and an unstable interior. When the cast is completely dry, it is hard and odorless. Weight bearing is not allowed until then (if it is a weight-bearing cast). When the cast is dry, the client may be turned to any comfortable position because the fracture fragments are immobilized by the cast.

EDEMA Ice bags may be applied to the fracture site intermittently (on for 20 to 30 minutes, off 10 to 15 minutes, as described in Chapter 43) for the first 24 to 48 hours. Place the ice bags along the sides of the cast rather than on top. The ice bags should be only about half full so they are not heavy enough to cause indentation. Swelling under the cast may impair circulation. Therefore, it is important to elevate the cast higher than the heart, if possible, unless compartment syndrome exists. Occasionally, a change in position will relieve pressure from the cast.

SKIN CARE Skin care along the cast edges includes washing and drying every day, being careful not to get the cast wet. The skin can be massaged with alcohol but not with lotion, which tends to soften the skin and may cause maceration. Run the fingers under the cast edge to remove plaster crumbs, which may irritate the client's skin. A portable vacuum cleaner may also be helpful. Also inspect the skin for signs of breakdown. Care of the skin should be taught to both client and family.

Clients in a cast or traction should use a fracture bedpan. Sometimes people are afraid to use such a small bedpan, thinking they will overfill it, as indeed they do occasionally if the foot of the bed is elevated. Disposable underpads and good skin care after bedpan use are important. Those unfamiliar with the fracture bedpan tend to insert it backwards so the client is sitting in the deepest part. The shallow, flat end of the pan should be pointed toward the head of the bed.

CAST CARE The nurse should inspect the cast for fit and for softened areas, which would tend to cause changes in alignment of the fracture fragments. Initial swelling that has subsided may cause the cast to be too loose. If the cast does not have a stockinette finished edge, the edges can be finished by placing "petals" along them after the swelling and pain subside. This is done by cutting strips of adhesive tape, rounding one end, and tucking the other end under the cast smoothly so it adheres to the sheet wadding inside the cast, being careful not to roll the tape edges. The free end of the tape is brought over the cast edge and secured to the outside cast surface. The petals should overlap to cover the entire cast edge; they help keep it from breaking down and prevent skin irritation from rough edges. Casts can be protected from soiling in the perineal region by tucking waterproof material under the cast and fastening it to the outside with adhesive. A dirty cast can be cleaned a little with scouring cleanser and a slightly moistened cloth. A cast should not be painted or varnished, because it must remain porous so evaporation can take place.

INFECTION AND DRAINAGE The nurse should assess the cast for unusual odors, which can be an indication of infection under the cast. This means sniffing right next to the cast. Hot spots along the cast may also be an indication of infection. Drainage coming through the cast is a sign of infection or bleeding underneath. Expect bleeding to occur through the cast for the first few days after surgery. Most nurses circle the drainage area with ink and label the date and time on the cast; later checks will show if the area extends. However, some think visible drainage is a poor indication of amount of drainage, and some physicians do not want anything drawn on a client's cast. Excessive drainage should be reported. Remember to check the undersurface of the cast, as drainage will flow downward.

SPECIFIC TYPES OF CASTS The client with an *arm cast* usually wears a sling to support the arm when not lying down. The hand should not hang off the end of the sling, and it should be higher than the elbow. If the physician permits, the client should remove the sling at least four times a day and put the arm, and especially the shoulder, through ROM exercises. If the client does not use a sling, the arm should be kept elevated unless the cast is specifically meant to hang (eg, to provide traction for a fractured humerus). A hanging arm cast should not rest on pillows, and the client must sit upright to provide proper alignment of fracture fragments. Areas to assess for pressure with arm casts include bones of the wrist and elbow.

The client with a *leg cast* will need to learn to use some type of ambulatory aid to get around. Warn clients that their toes may swell when the cast is lowered, and encourage them to elevate the extremity when sitting or lying back supine. The cast may be heavy, and extra help may be needed to move the leg when getting in and out of bed. When up in a wheelchair, the client's leg should be elevated and tied to the footrest along with a supporting pillow so it does not fall. Areas to assess for pressure with a leg cast include the head of the fibula on the lateral surface of the leg, which is near the peroneal nerve; the anterior tibia; the kneecap; the heel; and both sides of the ankle.

The client in a *hip spica cast* is usually confined in the cast for several months. Clients need to be turned regularly and require assistance for this in addition to helping themselves with the overhead trapeze. Clients usually turn onto the unaffected side while the nurse supports the cast. When on their sides, position clients with pillows between the legs and against the back. While the cast is still wet, the client must be turned frequently from supine to prone because this cast takes a few days to dry. It is important to support the wet cast as the client rolls and to place pillows for supporting the cast. If the cast has an abductor bar between the legs, the bar should not be grasped to move the client. If the client begins to ambulate with the cast, it is done gradually, first trying the upright position by use of a tilt table (Figure 45–10). The cast requires sitting in a reclining-type position, which hinders client participation in personal care.

HEALTH EDUCATION AND SUPPORT A list of points to cover when teaching the client about cast care is provided in Table 45–6. The client should be taught not to tamper with or alter the cast and not to scratch under it with any object. The client will experience frequent itiching under the cast, and the temptation to poke something under the cast for scratching will be great. If scratching occurs, the skin underneath can become injured or irritated, causing sores under the cast. Forcing air under the cast with a bulb syringe or a hair dryer on cool setting may be helpful for soothing an itch.

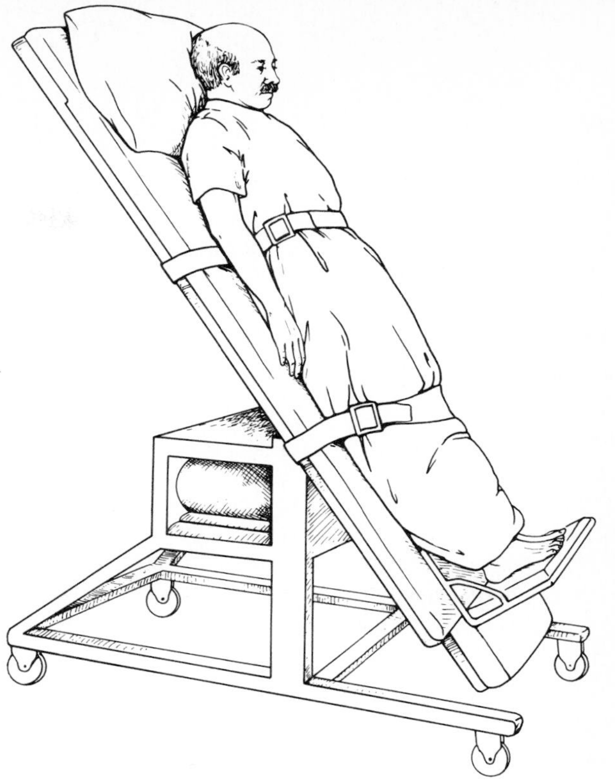

Figure 45–10

A tilt table is used to aid the client in gradually adjusting to the upright position.

Wearing a cast can be frustrating because it is heavy and clumsy and restricts independence. The client needs encouragement to try new methods of performing tasks to remain independent or to accept temporary dependence on others.

CARE AFTER CAST REMOVAL When the cast is removed, the casted extremity will appear thin and flabby, and the skin will be scaly and may be foul smelling. The nurse should prepare the client for this ahead of time. The limb will also be weak and may be painful to use; balance may be unstable. The scaly skin requires gentle cleansing followed by application of oil or lanolin; the skin is tender and should not be scrubbed. Some physicians recommend soaking the limb to remove the scales. The weak limb should be supported when moved. The limb will swell when held in a dependent position; instruct clients to continue to elevate the extremity and reassure them that with activity and exercise, the tendency for swelling will subside. The physician will prescribe exercises and instruct the client in the amount of activity or weight bearing allowed. A physical therapist may assist in the rehabilitation program.

Table 45–6
Instructions for Clients Going Home in a Cast

1. Check the color, temperature, movement, and sensation of all toes or fingers exposed from the cast at least twice a day (more often for a new cast).
2. Elevate the limb (toes higher than the knee; hand higher than the elbow). For an arm cast, wear a sling when not lying down.
3. Do not alter the cast in any way (except adhesive tape petals can be applied over sharp edges).
4. Keep the cast clean and dry. Plastic over the cast will help when going out in bad weather. The cast can be cleaned a little by using a slightly damp cloth and scouring cleanser. Avoid soaking.
5. Wash the skin along the cast edges and dry well every day. Skin can be massaged with alcohol, but do not use lotion at cast edges.
6. Inspect the skin along cast edges every day; run fingers under the edges to remove cast crumbs.
7. Inspect the cast for drainage, odors, cracked or softened areas, and hot spots.
8. Do not scratch under the cast or poke any objects under the cast.
9. Exercise the joints above and below the cast at least four times a day, if permitted by your physician.
10. Notify your physician if:
    - You have a fever.
    - The cast is loose, cracked, or softened.
    - There is a foul odor from the cast.
    - There is drainage coming through the cast.
    - Swelling does not go down when the cast is elevated.
    - Fingers or toes are changed compared to those on the other limb (for example, cold, numb, no feeling, pale, or unable to move).
    - There is pain or burning under the cast.
    - The skin around the cast edges becomes broken and sore.
11. Continue to see your physician for scheduled appointments.

CARING FOR THE CLIENT IN TRACTION

MAINTAINING THE TRACTION The traction pull should be in alignment with the axis of the long bones. During the first week of traction, the physician may make traction adjustments as the muscle spasms decrease and the bone position changes. After the traction apparatus is set up, the nurse should study it, know what it is supposed to look like, and keep everything the same, even the placement of pillows. It may be a good idea to take a picture of the bed and hang it at the bedside for reference. The traction should never be altered without the physician's order. Instructions from the physician should be clear about how much movement is allowed, for example, in raising and lowering the head of the bed, or in turning, and to which side. If the traction can be removed temporarily, as is sometimes done, that should be made clear in the physician's orders. The nurse should instruct the client about the positions allowed, especially if there are electric controls on the bed.

Assess the traction apparatus at least once every shift. Weights should hang freely without touching or resting on anything. The traction would not be maintained if, for example, the client slid toward the foot of the bed so the weight sat on the floor. The footplate or spreader should not touch the foot of the bed or frame. The rope should be examined to see that it is not frayed, that the knots are secure, that it is not rubbing against the overbed frame, and that it is resting in the groove of the pulley. Sometimes the rope gets caught at the edge of the wheel in the pulley, changing the traction pull. The ends of the rope can be taped to the rope to prevent knots from slipping. The weights should be fastened securely and hung so they are not jarred or hit by traffic going by.

MAKING A TRACTION BED It is usually easier to make the bed from top to bottom when the client is in traction and cannot be turned. The nurse must get sufficient help. The client assists by lifting with the trapeze; an assistant can help lift the client as allowed. The dirty linens are removed as the clean ones are pulled into place; top linens are not tucked under the mattress. While the helper is available, give back care. Observe the back and sacral area for pressure sores. If the client cannot be lifted enough for good skin observation and care, depress the mattress with a hand to make more room. Back care may be necessary every few hours. Use the same method to administer the bedpan. It is important to get extra help when lifting the client and giving care so as not to cause the client needless pain and to keep the pull of the traction constant.

EXERCISE Isometric exercises can be done to the involved extremity in many kinds of traction but it is best to check with the physician to see if exercises are permitted because they are contraindicated for some people.

PIN CARE The care of skin around skeletal pins (Figure 45–11), known as *pin care,* varies according to physician preference. Frequently, the physician places a sterile gauze pad around the pin, with an iodine or antibiotic ointment applied to the site. Some physicians do not apply any dressing. Some want the skin cleansed around the pin to remove the drainage that accumulates; others do not. Therefore, the physician must order pin care, and it should not be done otherwise. One method is to clean around the pin with half-strength hydrogen peroxide solution on a cotton swab, then apply a gauze pad with povidone–iodine (Betadine) ointment, using aseptic technique. Cut a slit in the pad with sterile scissors so the pad can be placed around

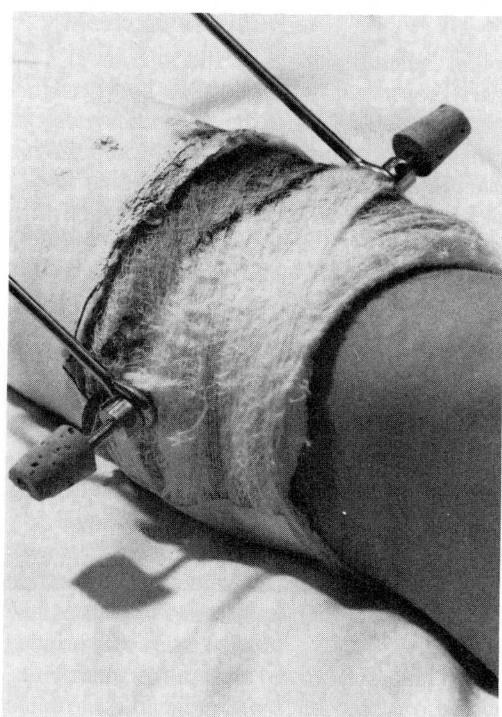

Figure 45–11

Skeletal traction: a pin through the bone with corks covering the ends. *SOURCE: Swearingen PL:* Addison–Wesley Photo-Atlas of Nursing Procedures. *Menlo Park, CA: Addison-Wesley, 1984.*

the pin, or use drain sponges with a slit already made in them. Inspect the skin around the pin at least once a day, and check the pin to see that it is not loose or slipping to one side. Bring any changes to the physician's attention. Indications of infection include redness, tenderness, and purulent drainage. Cover the pin ends with cork (the rubber stoppers from venipuncture tubes also work well) to keep from getting scratched or catching the linens.

CARE AFTER TRACTION REMOVAL Confinement in traction can be a source of emotional stress. The client may be afraid to move, so the nurse should provide clear explanations of the amount of movement and activity allowed, with assurance that the traction apparatus will maintain the bone in alignment.

When clients are removed from traction and begin ambulation, they must slowly acclimate to the upright position. This can be done with a few sessions on a tilt table or by slow elevation to a seated position and eventually to the upright position, with each attempt progressing as far as tolerated. Observe the client for signs of orthostatic hypotension such as pallor, a lowering of blood pressure, faintness, or dizziness with position change. Explain to clients that the limb will be weak and unsteady at first, and encourage them to follow the physician's instructions concerning the amount of weight bearing and activities permitted. The criteria to evaluate the effectiveness of nursing interventions in fracture care are listed in Box 45–1.

Complications of Fractures

Infection as a complication of fracture healing was described earlier in this chapter under osteomyelitis. The *complications resulting from immobility* are also possible with fracture treatment. Prevention and treatment of these complications are covered in Chapter 43. This section discusses other complications that can arise during healing of fractures.

PROBLEMS OF BONE UNION *Delayed union* of the fracture occurs when the bone does not unite in the usual amount of time. This delay can have various causes, including infection, inadequate reduction or immobilization, poor circulation to the bone, and metabolic disturbances that affect the protein and vitamins available for healing. *Nonunion* is the failure of healing so firm union does not take place. The causes of nonunion include those listed for delayed union, as well as separation of the bone fragments so that callus cannot span the gap, massive loss of bone from the injury, or soft tissue between the fracture fragments. Delayed union and nonunion are treated by discovering and correcting the underlying problems.

For nonunion, surgical revision of the fracture ends or bone grafting may be helpful. A new method of treatment that is proving effective is electrical stimulation to promote bone formation (Bassett, Mitchell, & Gaston, 1981). One method uses noninvasive equipment that can be placed

Box 45–1
Criteria to Evaluate the Effectiveness of Nursing Interventions in Fracture Care

The client with a fracture will:

Demonstrate good body alignment and good posture

State that pain is relieved

Describe and comply with the prescribed restrictions in activity

Demonstrate recommended exercises and ambulation techniques correctly

Adjust to the temporary body image changes

Cope with the limitations imposed by the injury and treatment

Describe symptoms and signs of complications that can occur from fractures and their treatment

Display no signs of infection, deformity, skin breakdown or other hazards of immobility

Display no signs of complications such as those from neurovascular impairment or fat embolism

Use ambulatory aids effectively and safely

Describe and correctly demonstrate care required after discharge over the skin or cast surface. The client takes the equipment home and uses it about 10 to 12 hours a day, usually during sleep. The treatment may be continued about 3 to 8 months. Another method uses a semi-invasive technique in which insulated electrodes are inserted percutaneously into the medullary canal of the fracture, using image-intensified fluoroscopy to determine placement. The electrodes are connected to a battery pack outside the cast. The client must avoid weight bearing to prevent pulling out the electrodes and should be seen by the physician once a month. The electrodes are removed after 12 weeks of treatment (Connolly, 1981).

Malunion is a complication in which union occurs in a deformed or angulated position. This can occur from inadequate reduction and immobilization. If the condition is severe, it may be treated by remanipulating the bone or by surgical intervention.

COMPARTMENT SYNDROME *Compartment syndrome* occurs when swelling or pressure develops within a confined space, or compartment, in an extremity. A compartment is a normally occurring area in which a muscle group is enclosed in tough fascial tissue. Small openings allow blood vessels and nerves to enter and exit the compartment. Little room remains for swelling. Tight bandages and casts may cause pressure from outside the compartment, or inflammation and resulting edema or hemorrhage may cause pressure from within, compromising circulation in the extremity. *Ischemia* (lack of blood supply) of the muscle occurs if enough pressure builds up, and ischemia leads quickly to nerve damage. The first symptom of compartment syndrome is pain that increases in severity, especially with passive stretching, and is unrelieved by narcotics. Other symptoms and signs include paralysis, paresthesias, decreased or absent pulses, and tense skin over the limb. Farrell (1982) states that irreversible damage begins in muscles and nerves after 6 hours of ischemia, and the extremity becomes useless in 24 to 48 hours. Ischemic muscle tissues are replaced by fibrotic tissue, forming contractures. For example, Volkmann's contracture can occur with injuries in the elbow region. The hand and forearm become permanently disabled, and motor and sensory function are lost.

Preventive measures for compartment syndrome include elevation of an injured extremity and intermittent ice application; frequent, regular neurovascular assessment for early detection; avoiding tight dressings, splints, or casts and IV infiltration; and listening to the client's concerns and seeking prompt medical attention when complications are suspected. The importance of frequent, regular assessment of neurovascular status after injury cannot be stressed enough. Immediate treatment is necessary when compartment syndrome is suspected. The heart may attempt to increase blood flow to the extremity in response to ischemia. This will exacerbate swelling. Keeping the extremity at heart level, rather than elevated, may circumvent this compensatory increase in blood flow. The front half of the cast or any occlusive bandages are removed. If there is no improvement in 1 hour, the physician performs a *fasciotomy,* in which the skin and fascia over the muscle group are incised to allow release of the tight compartment. A damaged or bleeding vessel can also be repaired. Sterile dressings are applied without encircling the extremity to minimize the pressure. Eventually, the incisions may be closed or skin grafts performed.

NERVE DAMAGE *Nerve damage* can result from the injury itself (eg, from sharp bone fragments) or from the treatment. The peroneal nerve runs along the lateral side of the lower leg below the head of the fibula where it is superficial and can easily be affected by pressure from a cast or traction apparatus. Damage to this nerve can result in footdrop. Peroneal nerve function can be checked by asking the client to dorsiflex the ankle and to extend the toes. Sensory function is checked by pricking the lateral side of the great toe and the medial side of the second toe. The damage may be permanent but is sometimes temporary. Wristdrop can occur from injury to the radial nerve. To test for motor function, the client is asked to hyperextend the wrist or thumb. To test the sensory status, prick the skin in the web between the thumb and index finger. When nerve damage is impending or suspected, treatment includes splitting the cast or adjusting the traction apparatus.

FAT EMBOLISM *Fat embolism* can occur as a complication of fractures or surgery of the long bones, from multiple trauma, or from other conditions unrelated to trauma. The cause of fat embolism is not completely understood but is probably at least partly related to a release of bone marrow fat into the circulation, a change in the fat composition in the circulation after trauma, or both. Apley and Solomon (1982) state that circulating fat globules occur in most adults with closed fractures of long bones, but only a small portion of these people develop problems.

Measures to prevent fat embolism are prompt immobilization of fractures and avoidance of manipulation of the fracture fragments. Symptoms and signs usually occur 12 to 72 hours after surgery or injury and include steadily rising pulse, respiratory rate, and temperature; cyanosis and respiratory distress; petechiae on the upper anterior chest, axillae, and conjunctiva; and mental confusion, agitation, and apprehension. Frequently, a change in sensorium is the first sign. It may be a subtle change such as a feeling that something is wrong. The condition is a serious one that can progress to convulsions, coma, and death; it requires prompt diagnosis and management. Treatment is supportive and includes managing the particular symptoms, such as treating shock, raising the head of the bed to aid breathing, or administering oxygen. Bed rest helps prevent release of more fat into the circulation. Clients may be instructed to cough and deep breath to improve oxygenation and may even require intubation and use of a respirator. The client may receive corticosteroids to decrease inflammation and edema or heparin to decrease the clotting of serum lipids and platelets. Sometimes a blood transfusion is necessary to maintain blood volume and oxygen-carrying capacity. Encourage the client to rest and remain calm, and provide both client and family with emotional support during this crisis.

AVASCULAR NECROSIS *Avascular necrosis,* also known as *aseptic necrosis,* occurs when a bone is deprived of its blood supply, causing bone death. This is a common complication of fractures, especially fractures of the femoral neck. Vessels within the joint capsule that supply the head of the femur may be damaged from the trauma; without the normal blood supply, the bone becomes osteoporotic and necrotic. Avascular necrosis can also occur with joint dislocation; high-dosage, long-term steroid therapy; and other conditions. The client experiences pain and limited movement. Treatment is usually surgical removal of the femoral head and replacement with a hip prosthesis.

CAST SYNDROME *Cast syndrome,* a complication of body casts, is caused by compression of part of the duodenum by the superior mesenteric artery, resulting in obstruction. The symptoms and signs of cast syndrome include prolonged nausea and vomiting, abdominal distention (seen through a cast window cut over the abdomen), and vague abdominal pain. The condition can be fatal if allowed to progress. Treatment includes gastrointestinal decompression, NPO, fluid and electrolyte replacement, and removal of the cast (Farrell, 1982).

Internal Fixation of Fractures

Internal fixation immobilizes reduced fractures by means of nails, rods, plates, screws, pins, or even unabsorbable sutures. The metals being used today, such as Vitallium and stainless steel, are less likely to cause a foreign body reaction than those used in the past. Occasionally an individual does develop a tissue reaction, however, due to sensitivity to metals in the alloys.

Internal fixation is used to maintain reduction when closed treatment is unsuccessful, impossible, or contraindicated. For example, it is useful for fractures that are prone to nonunion, such as fractures of the femoral neck, and for those that will be pulled apart by the action of muscles, such as transverse fractures of the patella. Surgical fixation of fractures is a good treatment method for elderly clients, because it preserves the range of joint motion and often permits earlier mobility than treatment by traction alone, thus avoiding the hazards of immobility. Open fractures should not be treated with internal fixation devices because incidence of complications such as wound or bone infection is higher for open fractures than closed ones.

An intramedullary (IM) rod, nail, or pin is used to treat a fracture of the shaft of a long bone, such as that shown in Figure 45–12. A similar procedure known as closed nailing uses image-intensified fluoroscopy. An incision over the fracture site is not required, because fluoroscopy replaces direct viewing.

Some other fixation devices are shown in Figure 45–12. Combinations of devices are also used. The hardware may be removed after complete healing, according to the physician's preference and the client's response to it; if it is not causing a problem, it may be retained. The implications of internal fixation procedures for the client are summarized in Table 45–7.

Nursing Implications

PREOPERATIVE CARE The preoperative preparation for internal fixation is the same as for other orthopedic surgical clients. Sometimes clients are taken directly from the emergency room to the operating room with little time to prepare them for what to expect. Such a client may need postoperative instructions on topics that normally would be taught preoperatively, such as exercises, coughing, and deep breathing.

POSTOPERATIVE CARE Postoperative positioning in correct body alignment is important for maintaining the integrity of the fixation device. After an intramedullary rod is inserted, traction may be used to keep the limb from rotating until the client regains muscle control. Otherwise, sandbags may be placed along the sides of the limb to prevent external rotation.

The affected limb is elevated postoperatively. Check the dressing or cast for bleeding and assess the client's neurovascular status regularly to detect signs of complications. Dressing changes require sterile technique. Care will be needed to prevent the hazards of immobility. Provide analgesics and comfort measures to relieve pain. Isometric exercises help maintain muscle strength and stimulate callus formation. For an intramedullary rod, the isometrics press the bone fragments together and help prevent them from pulling apart.

After surgical fixation of a lower extremity, clients must stay in bed until they can move the limb well. When they are allowed out of bed, the physician specifies how much, if any, weight bearing is allowed. The client must use crutches until bony union is evident on x-ray.

Before discharge, teach the client the symptoms and signs of infection, how much weight bearing is allowed, wound care, and cast care and ambulation techniques when these are appropriate. Encourage follow-up visits with the physician. A sample home care handout is shown in Box 45–2. It is general enough to be used for postoperative clients after other surgical orthopedic procedures. Also,

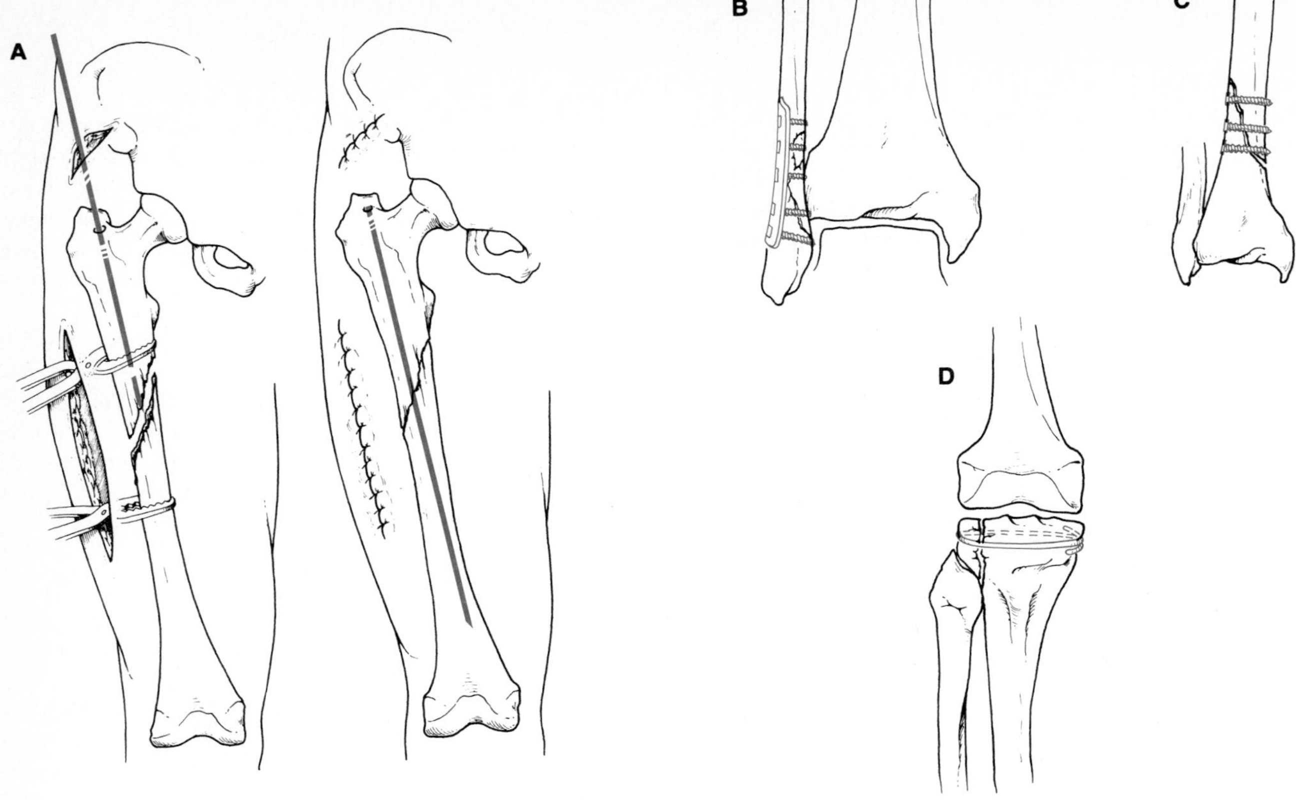

Figure 45–12

Internal fixation devices. **A.** Intramedullary rod insertion. An incision is made at the top of the trochanter to insert the rod. Another incision is made over the fracture so the rod can be manipulated across the fracture line. **B.** Plate and screws holding together a comminuted fracture of the distal fibula. **C.** Screws used to hold an oblique fracture of the tibia. **D.** Wire used to secure a fragment of the tibial plateau.

Table 45–7
Internal Fixation: Implications for the Client

Physiologic Implications	Psychosocial/Lifestyle Implications
Alignment maintained so bone healing can occur. Earlier mobility than with traction alone may decrease the chances of immobility hazards. Temporary pain and local swelling occurs. Potential complications: wound infection, bone infection, vascular or nerve injury, metal plate may break, device may loosen or migrate.	Earlier mobility provides greater independence; client may be discharged sooner. Casts, splints, or traction may be used after internal fixation, causing alterations in independence. May require the use of an ambulatory aid.

for a client in a cast, refer to the teaching described in Table 45–6.

External Fixation of Fractures

External fixation is a method of holding fracture fragments in alignment so healing can take place. Pins inserted into the bone above and below the fracture are attached to an external metal framework, which exerts pressure on the pins to stabilize the fragments in the proper position (Figure 45–13).

External fixation is used for complicated fractures that are difficult to repair by the usual methods of casts, traction, or internal fixation. Such fractures include open fracture with extensive soft tissue damage; comminuted fractures; fractures in which part of the bone is lost (eg, from a bullet wound); infected fractures; fractures complicated with burns; and severe open fractures, possibly with neu-

Box 45–2
General Home Health Care Handout for Postoperative Orthopedic Clients

1. Elevate the limb (toes higher than the knee; hand higher than the elbow). For arm surgery, wear a sling when not lying down.
2. Your surgical wound should be cared for as follows: ______
3. Exercise your arms and legs as instructed: ______
4. The amount of activity you are allowed with your involved limb is ______
5. Activities not allowed (check those appropriate):
   ______ Tub bath
   ______ Shower
   ______ Driving
   ______ Sexual intercourse
   ______ ______
6. Continue to use (walker, crutches, cane) as taught until instructed otherwise by your physician.
7. Notify the physician if:
   - You have a fever
   - The area of your incision appears reddened, swollen, hot, or has a foul odor
   - You have any drainage from the incision
   - You have numbness or loss of feeling in your leg or arm
   - You are unable to move your fingers or toes
   - You have severe pain at the incisional area
8. Continue to see the physician for scheduled appointments.

rovascular damage, which might otherwise result in amputation of the limb. External fixators are most commonly applied to fractures of the leg but are also used on fractures of the forearm and pelvis. The implications of an external fixation device are summaried in Table 45–8.

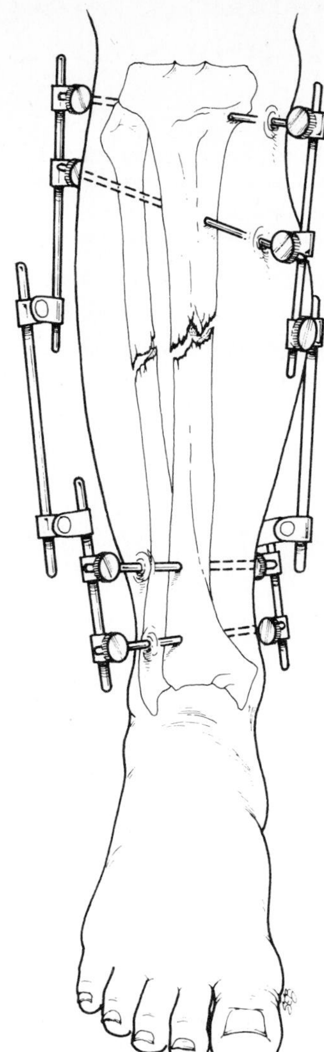

Figure 45–13

External fixation devices.

Nursing Implications

PREOPERATIVE CARE Preoperatively, the nurse should describe the appearance and function of the external fixation device to the client and family. A picture of such a device or seeing another client with one is more helpful than a verbal description. Since this type of treatment has been uncommon in the past, most people have never seen the apparatus. Explain to the client that the device holds the bone together to permit healing while allowing care of the open wound. Clients should understand that they must not adjust the apparatus in any way, since that would alter the bone alignment.

POSTOPERATIVE CARE Postoperatively, the limb is elevated to reduce swelling. This is frequently done by means of balanced suspension traction, applied by tying traction ropes directly to the fixator. If traction is not used, elevate the limb on pillows or by raising the foot of the bed. Move the limb by grasping the frame rather than the limb itself. The sharp pin ends can be covered with cork, Vacutainer plugs, or the plastic ends that come with some pins. Assess the client's neurovascular status regularly, and provide comfort measures as necessary to relieve pain. Antibiotics are given to prevent infection.

EXERCISE AND AMBULATION Help the client maintain joint mobility by doing range of motion (ROM) exercises at least twice a day and maintain strength by doing frequent isometric exercises, as allowed. When clients are ambulating, the physician should specify whether they can bear weight on the affected leg. The physical therapist can prepare clients for ambulation and teach them the use of ambulatory aids, usually crutches. Encourage clients to move slowly and smoothly because the heavy, awkward fixator may affect balance and coordination. It is important for someone to help clients get in and out of bed and move around until they can manage safely on their own.

Table 45–8
External Fixation: Implications for the Client 

Physiologic Implications	Psychosocial/Lifestyle Implications
Provides stability of fracture fragments.	Alters body image.
Allows visualization and care of open wound.	Device is heavy and awkward.
Allows movement of unaffected joints and muscles and permits earlier ambulation in many cases.	Hospitalization and/or recuperation may be lengthy.
Decreases risk of fat embolism.	Client must learn use of ambulatory aid.
Prevents bone shortening by maintaining gaps between bone fragments so that bone healing occurs between them.	Client or family member needs to learn to give wound and pin care for home care.
Local swelling and pain for a few days postoperatively.	The type of clothing that can be worn with the device may require adjustment after discharge.
Potential complications: wound infection, bone infection, nerve or vascular damage.	The device may interfere with return to work.

WOUND AND PIN CARE Wound care is a challenge with the external framework in the way. The fixator is not sterile, but wound care requires *strict* aseptic technique. Sterile gloves and/or sterile forceps are necessary, and the nurse must avoid touching them on the framework. The dressings may be maneuvered into place by use of sterile instruments or sterile tongue blades. These dressing changes take longer than others.

Daily pin site care is necessary to prevent infection. The type of pin care should be specified by the physician. Serous fluid will normally drain around the pin sites and form crusts. The fluid forms as a result of the soft tissues sliding over the pins. Pin site care requires cleansing of each site with a separate sterile cotton-tipped applicator to remove the crusts. Crust removal is important because crusts can harbor bacteria when left in place. Usually, hydrogen peroxide is used for cleansing, followed by normal saline. Observe the skin for redness, pain, tenderness, odor, or skin tension. An antibacterial agent such as iodophor ointment or foam may be applied, or antibiotic ointments are sometimes used. Sterile technique requires the use of many sterile cotton-tipped applicators, one per site. Sterile dressings are sometimes applied.

As soon as clients are able, they should be involved in pin site and wound care. Involvement in care helps prepare clients for discharge. Teach sterile technique and observe until clients perform satisfactorily. Instruct clients to notify the physician of any abnormal symptoms or signs, or if a pin becomes loose. Loose pins contribute to destabilization of the fracture, and may enhance development of infection by irritation of soft tissue. Clients can keep the fixator clean by wiping it with a clean damp cloth.

Sometimes the external rods are removed and a cast is applied over the pins, incorporating them into the cast. Then the nurse needs to teach the client cast care before discharge. Wearing clothing over the device may take simple tailoring so that sleeves or pantlegs can be snapped over the fixator. Velcro fasteners are helpful.

To help clients adjust to changes in body image, encourage expression of feelings about the wound and external fixator, and involve them in their own care. Encourage them to discuss their situation and their feelings about it. The fixator may interfere with the client's return to work. A referral to a social worker may be necessary if prolonged hospitalization or recuperation causes worries about financial matters.

Hip Pinning

Hip pinning (or nailing) is a type of internal fixation procedure used for repair of fractures of the proximal femur that cannot be treated by rest alone.

Hip fractures are most common in the elderly; the average age of occurrence is 73. Seventy percent of hip fractures occur in women (Connolly, 1981). Hip fractures may occur from falls, a twisting motion, direct trauma, or stress on diseased bone. Characteristics of the elderly that probably contribute to falls and hip fracture include poor vision; slowed reflexes; problems with balance; weak muscles; postural hypotension; and weak, fragile bones from osteoporosis.

Since hip pinning is a type of internal fixation, the implications summarized in Table 45–7 apply here. In addition, the specific implications of a fractured hip and surgical hip repair are summarized in Table 45–9.

Nursing Implications

Implications for Elderly Clients

PREOPERATIVE CARE Since hip fracture clients are usually elderly, their condition may be complicated by the chronic diseases that accompany old age. The client's condition must be stabilized before surgery is attempted; as

Table 45–9
Hip Pinning: Implications for the Client*

Physiologic Implications	Psychosocial/Lifestyle Implications
Aseptic necrosis may occur if the blood supply to the femoral head is damaged; may require hip prosthesis	Former level of independence may be decreased temporarily or permanently.
Procedure usually causes pain, local swelling, ecchymosis.	Client may require a change in living accommodations.
Hemorrhage and shock may occur.	Client may be depressed.
Full weight bearing is not permitted until healing occurs (possibly as long as 5 months).	Early mobility may have a positive effect on the client.

*See Table 54–1 for implications of internal fixation.

with any preoperative client, fluid and electrolyte balance and nutritional status should be optimal. An elderly client is particularly susceptible to the hazards of immobility, and the longer stabilization is delayed, the longer the client is immobile. Surgery should be done within 48 hours of injury if the client is medically stable.

On admission, the nurse and several assistants transfer the client gently to the bed. An egg crate or air mattress should be applied to the bed first. A thorough preoperative assessment is necessary to plan care that will help get the client in optimal condition for surgery. Include assessment for other injuries. Buck's extension or Russell's traction may be applied to reduce pain and muscle spasm, or the client may be allowed to assume a position of comfort without traction. Do not attempt to align the leg as long as the neurovascular status is satisfactory (Farrell, 1982). Turning the client should be done with pillows between the legs.

In addition to the usual preoperative preparation a type and cross-match is done to have blood available for surgery. The nurse may start an intravenous (IV) infusion to give preoperative antibiotics. Prepare the client to expect the following postoperatively: an IV, Hemovac, antibiotics, a dressing in the trochanteric region, and analgesics for pain. Explain the positions that will be allowed, exercises that will need to be done, and use of the trapeze.

POSTOPERATIVE CARE In general, assess the client's neurovascular status and the condition of the dressing each time vital signs are taken. Observe the part of the dressing under the client carefully, since drainage will flow downward and may be missed from a side view. A Hemovac is usually used for a few days postoperatively and should be kept collapsed. Measure the drainage each shift; the amount should decrease with time. An IV is usually used to give intravenous antibiotics. Provide comfort measures and analgesics after a thorough assessment of the client's pain. Good skin care and observation of common pressure areas are important.

Coughing, deep breathing, and incentive spirometry are necessary to prevent respiratory problems. The client wears elastic stockings; remove these at least twice a day to give skin care and to observe the heels for signs of breakdown. Range of motion exercises are necessary for all uninvolved joints, and the client should do isometric exercises to maintain strength in the quadriceps, abdominal, and gluteal muscles.

A fracture bedpan prevents unnecessary flexion of the operative hip and pain. Incontinence of urine or stool may soil the nearby dressing, requiring prompt dressing change to prevent wound contamination. To prevent constipation, encourage adequate intake of fluids and roughage; exercise, stool softeners, and laxatives may also be helpful. The client is often able to tolerate regular foods the day after surgery. Nutritional management for those with fractures is covered earlier in this chapter.

POSITIONING AND TURNING Physicians' postoperative orders vary mostly in regard to positioning the client. Some physicians use traction (Buck's or Russell's) or a cast to reduce muscle spasm and maintain alignment. Turn the

Nursing Research Note

Williams M et al.: Predictors of acute confusional states in hospitalized elderly patients. *Res Nurs Health* 1985; 8(1):31–40.

Acute confusion is often a problem for elderly individuals admitted to the hospital following a sudden event such as a fall. This study examined the factors that put elderly clients with hip fractures at risk for development of confusion. These clients were mentally alert, physically well, and independent before the traumatic fall. It was found that increased age, a lower level of preinjury physical activity, and increased errors on an admission mental status test were valid predictors of confusion.

Nurses can assess for these predictive factors when admitting elderly clients for hip repair. Nursing care can enhance orientation and provide a supportive environment. This study also suggested that certain hospital events and treatments may be related to confusion. These include urinary elimination problems, slow mobilization, pain, and pain relief. These treatments and events must be closely monitored by the nurse and assessments of their effects documented.

client only as ordered. In general, the client can and should be turned very 2 hours. The doctor may have a preference for which direction the client may be turned (toward the operative or unoperative side). Whenever the client is moved, avoid extreme positions and movements such as acute angle flexion of the operative hip. Adduction and external rotation should also be avoided. Tell the client to keep toes pointing toward the ceiling while resting in bed. Trochanter rolls or covered sandbags placed beside the leg are helpful in preventing rotation, but avoid pressure on the upper lateral calf to prevent peroneal nerve injury. Place pillows between the client's legs to maintain abduction. Whenever the client is turned, assistance will be needed to support the uppermost leg in abduction. Be sure pillows have been placed between the client's legs to prevent a strain on the operative area.

With pinning, the risk of displacement of the surgical device is less than with a hip prosthesis (see next section), but gentle handling and proper positioning are still necessary. Assess frequently for maintenance of good body alignment. Do back care and skin observation when the client is in the side-lying position.

AMBULATION When clients are allowed out of bed, the nurse should know specifically how to get them up and what positions are allowed. Most clients are allowed out of bed the first or second day after surgery, with no weight bearing on the operative leg. Assess how well the client will follow directions. If the ability to follow directions is questionable, it is better to lift the client int the chair. The chair should be firm, not low, and should have armrests. It should be placed parallel to and touching the bed, positioned so the client can move toward the strong (unoperative) side. The client should wear firm, nonskid shoes, and the chair and bed wheels should be locked. Give clear instructions, with the assurance that the staff will be there to assist at all times.

To get up, the client turns to the side, swivels into a sitting position, dangles until stable, stands with weight on the unoperative leg only, pivots, and eases into the chair by grasping the armrests. All this is done with the assistance of the nurse, using good body mechanics. The physician should specify if the leg should remain elevated when the client is in the chair. The first time out of bed should be only about 15 to 20 minutes, unless the client wants to be up longer. While up, personal hygiene, hair care, and oral care can be done, or the client can eat a meal, as long as there is no discomfort. Prolonged sitting in a chair should be avoided to prevent pelvic vein thrombosis. The client returns to bed by reversing the order of the actions used to get up.

Walking begins according to the client's readiness and the physician's preference. A physical therapist instructs the client in the use of a walker, usually without weight bearing on the operative leg. The walker and no weight bearing are necessary until the fracture is healed—about 4 months.

SAFETY MEASURES Evaluate the client's mental status for planning interventions according to the level of orientation. Elderly clients may become confused, jeopardizing safety and surgical repair. When the client is confused, interventions to maintain safety are necessary. Siderails should be up, and a small light may be left on in the room at night. A confused client may try to get out of bed, especially at night. Use restraints only as a last resort. Interventions to control pain and maintain hydration may help combat some of the causes of confusion. It will be necessary to repeat instructions and supervise the elderly or forgetful client's activities at times. Providing orientation and encouraging family visits may help the client's mental status. Encouraging independence and participation in self-care is helpful for the client who is depressed because of feelings of helplessness.

Home Health Care

Consult the family when preparing the client for discharge. The home should be made safe for use of a walker (eg, by removing throw rugs, clutter, and electric cords from traffic areas). Families will need to obtain a walker and perhaps an elevated toilet seat. The client should use a firm chair with armrests. The client and family may be referred to social services to plan for help in the home or to plan discharge to a specialized facility when necessary. Encourage follow-up visits to the physician, who will use x-rays to evaluate healing and to detect signs of complications, such as avascular necrosis.

Hip Prosthesis

Insertion of a hip prosthesis is a surgical procedure used to treat certain hip fractures. A metal device consisting of a ball-shaped head attached to an intramedullary rod is used to replace the head and neck of the femur (Figure 45–14). Use of a hip prosthesis is indicated for hip fractures that are prone to development of avascular necrosis. A hip prosthesis may also be used for comminuted femoral neck fractures and other fractures that are difficult to reduce.

The implications of hip pinning summarized in Table 45–9 apply here as well. Table 45–10 lists those implications that are different for hip prosthesis clients.

Nursing Implications

The nursing care for clients with hip pinning, described in the previous section, is pertinent here also. The positioning of the client is important to prevent hip dislocation and strain on the incisional area. Postoperative positioning is specified by the surgeon. As with hip pinning, avoid acute flexion and adduction of the hip. To maintain the operative leg in an abducted position, use a wedge-shaped

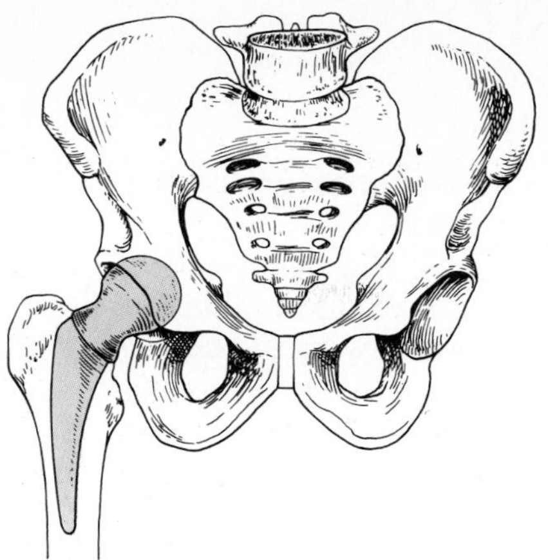

Figure 45–14

A hip prosthesis in place. The ball fits into the acetabulum; the stem is inserted into the femoral medullary canal.

abductor pillow or a splint (Figure 45–15). The pillow fastens with Velcro straps. It is important to prevent circulatory problems from tight straps and to prevent pressure ulcers from pressure of the appliance. The straps should not be placed over the upper fibula where the peroneal nerve lies. Remove the appliance to provide skin care and to observe the skin condition while the client keeps the leg in the required alignment. The length of time the abduction device is used depends upon the physician's preference and the client's progress. Some physicians use ordinary pillows or sandbags to position the leg in abduction instead of the abduction devices.

The client is allowed to turn only with physician's orders because some physicians prefer the supine position only. When clients are not allowed to turn, teach them to use the trapeze to help lift themselves for linen changes and frequent back care. Lifting the client in this way is much easier and safer with extra assistance. The operative leg must be kept in the desired alignment while lifting.

If the client is allowed to turn to a side-lying position, the specific side is ordered by the surgeon. Generally, the client turns onto the operative hip, since the bed can splint the limb and maintain alignment. Pillows (or the abductor

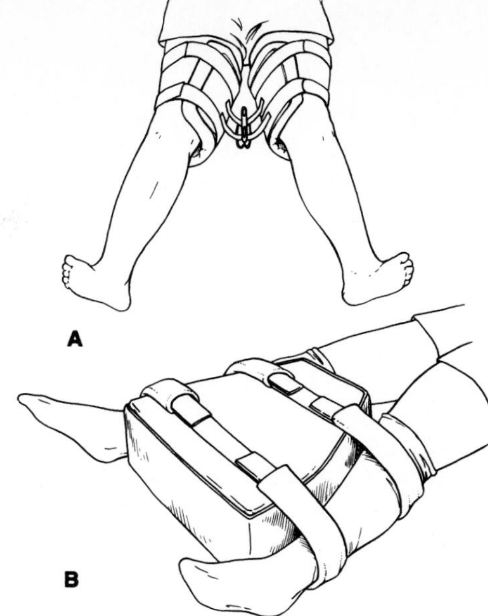

Figure 45–15

Abductor splint (**A**) and pillow (**B**).

device) must be kept between the legs. No matter how the client is turned, the desired position of abduction must be maintained, and the hip should not be acutely flexed. Elevation of the operative limb on one or two pillows may be ordered; otherwise it should be kept flat. The surgeon may also specify how high the head may be elevated.

The client may be allowed out of bed 1 to 3 days after surgery to sit in a chair; no weight bearing is allowed on the operative leg. Physical therapy helps the client progress to ambulation; weight bearing with the use of a walker may begin about 3 days postoperatively. The client may find the walker helpful for 6 to 8 weeks and then begins to use a cane. Using an elevated toilet seat postoperatively prevents strain on the hip. Explain to clients that legs must not be crossed because it causes adduction. The reason for all these positioning specifications is to prevent the prosthetic head from dislocating out of the acetabulum. Symptoms and signs of hip dislocation include sharp pain and

Table 45–10
Hip Prosthesis: Implications for the Client* 

Physiologic Implications	Psychosocial/Lifestyle Implications
Provides a functioning hip joint without the chance of avascular necrosis. Earlier weight bearing is allowed than with hip pinning. Chances of hip dislocation related to adherence to specific preventive positioning orders. Complications are loosening of the prosthesis and erosion of the prosthetic head through the acetabular cartilage.	Postoperative positioning may be restrictive and interfere with comfort. Use of walker may be easier than with hip pinning because weight bearing is allowed earlier.

*See Table 45–9 for implications of hip pinning.

abnormal limb position, such as shortening and external rotation. The client should notify the physician immediately if these things happen and may have to return to surgery for treatment.

Chapter Highlights

Metabolic disorders of the bone include hyperparathyroidism, osteoporosis, and osteomalacia. These conditions may result in bone pain, weakness, deformities, and pathologic fractures.

Paget's disease of the bone leads to swelling and deformity of bone with weakness and potential for fracture.

Osteomyelitis is an acute or chronic infection of the bone and surrounding tissues, causing pain, bone destruction, and limited mobility.

Prevention of bone infection is of utmost importance because an acute infection may progress into a chronic one.

Symptoms and signs of bone cancer include pain, tenderness, local swelling, a mass, and walking with a limp. Medical attention should be sought without delay upon detection.

Bone tumors must be surgically removed or destroyed by chemotherapy or radiotherapy.

A fracture is a break in the continuity of a bone. It causes pain, swelling, limited movement, and possibly damage to surrounding tissues and organs.

A fracture heals best when the bone fragments are realigned in close proximity, immobilized to maintain alignment and when circulation is good, infection is absent, and nutrition is adequate.

Methods used to immobilize a realigned fracture include casts, splints, internal fixation, external fixation, and traction.

Potential complications of musculoskeletal surgery include nerve or blood vessel disruption, wound infection, bone or joint infection, hemorrhage, shock, phlebitis, pulmonary or fat embolism, and loosening or breaking of hardware.

Abnormalities noted upon neurovascular assessment must be brought to the attention of the surgeon immediately.

The client will need some assistance with ADL postoperatively especially when mobility is limited.

To prevent changing the contour of a wet cast, it must be handled with flat palms and placed on pillows to support its entire length. Casted extremities should be elevated above heart level when possible.

Traction equipment must remain in the position set by the physician to maintain the alignment and immobilization of the bone fragments.

Traction should be assessed at least every shift to evaluate alignment and maintain the intended pull. The ropes should be in the pulley grooves, and weights should be hanging freely.

General nursing interventions for clients with bone disorders include measures to prevent the hazards of immobility; comfort measures such as analgesics and position changes; exercising unaffected extremities; encouraging self-care; providing diversional activities; giving emotional support; encouraging a nutritionally balanced diet; and assisting with the use of ambulatory aids and ADL.

Any concerns of a client treated with a cast or traction should be investigated fully and promptly to avoid complications.

Nerves and skin can deteriorate from pressure of casts, splints, and traction apparatus. Areas to assess for pressure include: area over the fibular heads; both malleoli; anterior tibia; heels; knees; radial and ulnar styloids; elbows; epicondyles of the elbow; iliac crests; and skin touching the edges of casts and traction equipment.

Complications of fractures include delayed union, nonunion, malunion, infection, the hazards of immobility, compartment syndrome, nerve damage, fat embolism, avascular necrosis, and cast syndrome.

The surgical treatment may alter the body image because of disfigurement, impaired musculoskeletal function, and the use of orthopedic appliances or ambulatory aids.

Lengthy hospitalization and recovery period may be an emotional and financial burden for clients with fractures and for their families.

Before discharge, the nurse teaches the client about cast care; wound care; symptoms and signs of complications; ambulation restrictions; good body mechanics; and necessary rest, exercise, nutrition, and follow-up care.

Bibliography

Apley AG, Solomon L: *Apley's System of Orthopaedics and Fractures,* 6th ed. London: Butterworth, 1982.

Bassett CAL, Mitchell SN, Gaston SR: Treatment of ununited

tibial diaphyseal fractures with pulsing electromagnetic fields. *J Bone Joint Surg* 1981; 63:511–523.

Blake SA: Noncemented femoral prosthesis: Intraoperative focus. *Ortho Nurs* 1985; 4(1):40–42.

Brown SL: Avoiding postoperative pitfalls with hip fracture patients. *RN* 1982; 45(5)48–54.

Brunner NA: *Orthopedic Nursing,* 4th ed. St. Louis: Mosby, 1983.

Burg ME: Compartment syndrome. *CCQ* 1983; 6(1):27–32.

Connolly JF (ed): *DePalma's the Management of Fractures and Dislocations: An Atlas,* 3rd ed. Philadelphia: Saunders, 1981.

Crowther HT: New perspectives on nursing lower limb amputees. *J Adv Nurs* 1982; 7:453–460.

Doheny MO: Porous coated femoral prosthesis: Concepts and care considerations. *Ortho Nurs* 1985; 4(1):43–45.

Farrell J: *Illustrated Guide to Orthopedic Nursing,* 2nd ed. Philadelphia: Lippincott, 1982.

Geier KA, Hesser K: Electrical bone stimulation for treatment of nonunion. *Ortho Nurs* 1985; 4(2): 41–49.

Gorrie TM: Postmenopausal osteoporosis. *JOGN Nurs* 1982; 11:214–219.

Hay BK, Karas CB: External fixation: Option for fractures. *AORN J* 1981; 34:417–426.

Kaplan FS: Osteoporosis. *Clin Symp* 1983; 35(5):2–32.

King JP: Bones: How to grow new ones. *AORN J* 1982; 35:968–975.

Kostuik JP: *Amputation Surgery and Rehabilitation.* New York: Churchill Livingstone, 1981.

Krause MB, Mahan LK: *Food, Nutrition, and Diet Therapy,* 7th ed. Philadelphia: Saunders, 1984.

Kryschyshen PL, Fisher DA: External fixation for complicated fractures. *Am J Nurs* 1980; 80:256–259.

Kuska BM: Acute onset of compartment syndrome. *JEN* 1982; 8(2):75–79.

Lane JM, Vigorita VJ: Osteoporosis. *Ortho Clin North Am* 1984; 15(4):711–728.

Lane PL, Lee MM: New synthetic casts: What nurses need to know. *Ortho Nurs* 1982; 1(6):13–20.

Lindsay R: The role of sex hormones and synthetic steroids in prevention of post-menopausal osteoporosis. *Clin Invest Med* 1982; 5(2/3):189–194.

Lukert BP: Osteoporosis: A review and update. *Arch Phys Med Rehabil* 1982; 63:480–487.

Mather MLS: The secret to life in a spica. *Am J Nurs* 1987; 87(1):56–58.

McWilliams N: *Manual of Orthopedic Surgery for Nurses.* Bowie, MD: Brady, 1982.

Merkow RL, Lane JM: Current concepts of Paget's disease of bone. *Ortho Clin North Am* 1984; 15(4):747–763.

Milazzo V: An exercise class for patients in traction. *Am J Nurs* 1981; 81:1842–1844.

Mourad L: *Nursing Care of Adults With Orthopedic Conditions.* New York: Wiley, 1980.

Notelovitz M, Ware M: *Stand Tall: The Informed Women's Guide to Preventing Osteoporosis.* Gainesville, FL: Triad Publishing, 1982.

Powell M: *Orthopaedic Nursing and Rehabilitation,* 8th ed. London: Churchill Livingstone, 1982.

Richards M: Osteoporosis. *Geriatr Nurs* 1982; 3(2):98–102.

Robinson JE, Mar LO: A nail-safe method. *Am J Nurs* 1985; 85(2):158–161.

Searls K et al: External fixation: General principles of patient management. *CCQ* 1983; 6(1):45–54.

Southwick JR, Callahan DJ: A study of blood drainage patterns on synthetic cast materials. *Ortho Nurs* 1985; 4(2):72–75.

Sproles KJ: Nursing care of skeletal pins: A closer look. *Ortho Nurs* 1985; 4(1):11–19.

Trigueiro M: Pin site care protocol. *Can Nurse* 1983; 79(8):24–26.

Voluz JM: Surgical implants. *AORN J* 1983; 37:1341–1352.

Walters J: Coping with a leg amputation. *Am J Nurs* 1981; 81:1349–1352.

Wolanin MO, Phillips LRF: *Confusion: Prevention and Care.* St. Louis: Mosby, 1981.

CHAPTER 46

Specific Disorders of the Joints

Other topics relevant to this content are: Laminectomy/disk-ectomy to treat disease or injury of the spinal cord or the spinal nerves, **Chapter 29.**

Objectives

When you have finished studying this chapter, you should be able to:

Discuss joint problems of multifactorial origin, including gout, low back pain, scoliosis, and carpal tunnel syndrome.

Identify the clinical manifestations and medical and surgical treatments for degenerative joint disease.

Describe the articular and extra-articular manifestations of rheumatoid arthritis (RA) and the various approaches to treatment of this disease.

Explain the nursing interventions for Sjögren's syndrome.

Recognize the circumstances leading to infectious disorders of the joints, describing the kinds of pathogens involved, their differential diagnosis, and treatment measures.

Specify the nurse's role in the therapeutic and preventive care of traumatic disorders of the joints.

Discuss alterations in body image encountered by clients undergoing orthopedic surgery and their potential impact on self-image, sexuality, and role relationships.

A joint is the point of articulation between two bones. Because of their location and constant use, joints are susceptible to stress, injury, and inflammation. This chapter discusses the major disorders affecting the joints.

SECTION I

Disorders of Multifactorial Origin

Joint problems of multifactorial origin include a wide variety of conditions, including gout, low back pain (low back strain and intervertebral disk disease), scoliosis, and carpal tunnel syndrome.

Gout

Gout is a disease that produces joint inflammation because of the deposition of uric acid crystals (monosodium urate crystals) in the articular tissue. Deposition occurs either because of an increased production of uric acid or a decrease in uric acid excretion. Gout can be classified as either primary or secondary. In primary gout, an unknown metabolic defect is responsible for increased serum uric acid. Men are most often affected, and the disease seems to run in families.

The reason for the increase in serum uric acid in secondary gout is either an excessive turnover of cells, as in leukemia, Hodgkin's disease, or myeloma, to name a few, or impaired excretion of uric acid by the kidney because of chronic kidney failure or the effects of drugs on the kidney, especially diuretics. Some other problems that may precipitate attacks of secondary gout are alcohol, starvation, psoriasis, and sarcoidosis.

Clinical Manifestations

There are four stages of gout (Kelley, 1981):

- Stage 1—asymptomatic hyperuricemia
- Stage 2—acute gouty arthritis
- Stage 3—intercritical gout
- Stage 4—chronic tophaceous gout

In stage 1, the uric acid level is elevated, but there are no arthritis symptoms, tophi (nodules that contain monosodium urate crystals), or calculi. About 5% of these clients will develop gouty arthritis. In men, hyperuricemia is defined as a uric acid level of 7.0 mg/100 mL or greater, and in women as 6.0 mg/100 mL or greater. A value greater than 7.0 mg/100 mL increases the risk of renal calculi or gout attacks. Gout usually occurs after 20 to 30 years of sustained hyperuricemia. However, some people will have renal colic before their first episode of arthritis.

The primary manifestation of the acute gouty arthritis stage (stage 2) is an extremely painful arthritis, usually monoarticular, beginning at night. Later the joint is so swollen, red, and tender that the client cannot even tolerate the pressure of bedclothes. There can be polyarthritis and fever. The attacks are of short duration, and intervals are completely free from pain. Ninety percent of individuals experience their acute attack in the great toe (podagra—involvement of the first metatarsophalangeal joint). The acute attack can be caused by minor trauma, surgery, or excessive alcohol consumption.

Stage 3, intercritical gout, refers to the intervals between attacks. After an acute attack of gout, 7% of clients will never have a second episode. Most, however, will have another attack within 1 year, although the interval may be as long as 10 years. The second attack is polyarticular and more severe, lasts longer, and may occur with fever.

If untreated, individuals progress to stage 4, chronic polyarticular disease, and develop tophi. These are difficult to differentiate from rheumatoid nodules on physical examination. Tophi occur in cartilage, synovial membrane, and soft tissue. If they ulcerate, a white, chalky, pasty material containing uric acid crystals is found.

Other manifestations of gout include renal dysfunction (which occurs in 90% of clients with a history of gouty arthritis) and albuminuria (a possible initial manifestation). Renal calculi occur in 10% to 25% of clients with gout, sometimes before joint symptoms appear. Obesity, elevated triglyceride levels, and hypertension may also accompany gout.

Initially, there are no x-ray abnormalities, but later bone erosions with an overhanging margin may be seen. This helps differentiate gout from rheumatoid arthritis (RA).

Diagnosis is made by using a polarized light microscope to visualize uric acid crystals within the white blood cells found in synovial fluid from the inflamed joints. It is important to culture synovial fluid to rule out infection.

Medical Measures

Acute attacks of gout respond to rest and NSAIDs such as naproxen (Naprosyn) and indomethacin (Indocin). Colchicine can also be given orally; however, since the higher doses needed cause abdominal cramps and diarrhea, it is not usually used. Colchicine is also available for IV use but is used rarely because it is an irritant and causes severe pain and necrosis if it infiltrates. The drug should be diluted in normal saline and infused in no less than 5 minutes. Other side effects are bone marrow depression, seizures, alopecia, hepatocellular failure, mental depression, ascending paralysis, respiratory depression, and death. Toxic effects are greater in those clients with hepatic, bone marrow, and renal disease.

According to Kelley (1981), indomethacin is the treatment of choice in clients with an established diagnosis of gouty arthritis. If a single joint is involved, aspiration and intra-articular injection of steroids are beneficial. The acute symptoms usually resolve in a few days.

The long-term management of gout includes measures to lower serum uric acid levels; these should be initiated after the acute attack subsides for clients who continue to be hyperuricemic. Small doses of colchicine (1 to 2 mg q.d.) may be used prophylactically. In addition, antihyperuricemic agents are often used to lower serum uric acid levels to less than 7.0 mg/100 mL. These either increase the renal excretion of uric acid or decrease uric acid production.

Drugs that increase the renal excretion of uric acid include sulfinpyrazone (Anturane) and probenecid (Benemid). Their long-term use promotes resorption of tissue deposits and tophi. Aspirin should not be given with these drugs since it blocks the uricosuric effect.

Allopurinol (Zyloprim) decreases uric acid production. The usual dose is 300 mg q.d., although it is used in a lower dose if there is renal dysfunction. Significant side effects include gastrointestinal distress, skin rashes, fever, alopecia, bone marrow suppression, hepatitis, jaundice, and vasculitis.

Other measures that may improve the client's symptoms are weight reduction, joint rest, joint protection, heat or cold therapy, and a decreased purine diet. Diet restriction is usually limited to alcohol and glandular meats. Strict purine restriction is unrealistic since most foods contain purines.

Specific Nursing Measures

Assess joints frequently for erythema, tenderness, tophi, and swelling. Bed cradles are used in the hospital so bedclothes will not press on painful joints, and clients at home can improvise similar protective devices. Resting the affected joint is important, and nonpainful joints should be put through frequent ROM exercises. As the acute

NURSING DIAGNOSES IN
Musculoskeletal Dysfunction

DIRECTLY RELATED DIAGNOSES

- Activity intolerance
- Bowel elimination, altered: constipation
- Breathing pattern, ineffective
- Comfort, altered: pain
- Health maintenance, impaired
- Injury, potential for
- Mobility, physical impaired
- Self-care deficit
- Sexuality, altered patterns
- Skin integrity, impaired
- Social interaction, impaired
- Tissue perfusion, altered: peripheral
- Urinary retention

OTHER POTENTIAL DIAGNOSES

- Bowel elimination, altered: incontinence
- Comfort, altered: chronic pain
- Diversional activity deficit
- Home maintenance management, impaired
- Incontinence, functional
- Post-trauma response
- Role performance, altered
- Self-concept altered: body image
- Sensory/perceptual alterations: tactile

symptoms subside, the affected joint should also be exercised. Apply heat or ice as ordered.

Maintain fluid intake at 2 to 3 L per day to decrease the chance of renal calculi. Clients should understand the rationale for increased fluids, which is even more important for those taking uricosuric medications. Monitor intake and output carefully. If a renal calculus is suspected, urine must be strained in an attempt to trap the calculus for laboratory evaluation. For the hospitalized client, the nurse should monitor all laboratory reports for uric acid and albuminuria. Also, be alert for gout attacks 24 to 96 hours after any surgical procedure on a client with gout.

Client/Family Teaching

Client education includes instructing the client and significant others in the use of heat and cold for joint symptoms and the importance of increased oral fluids. Because many clients with gout are overweight, a condition that stresses the joints, weight reduction is important. Teach clients with gout to avoid rich foods, which are high in purines and contribute to elevated triglyceride levels and obesity. Other purine-rich foods are organ meats (eg, liver and sweetbreads), alcohol, and fried foods. Base-forming foods, such as milk, cream, vegetables (except corn and lentils), fruits (except cranberries, plums, and prunes), molasses, carbonated beverages, and baking soda and baking powder, may be helpful. They will alkalinize the pH of urine.

The client should understand the action of all medications taken. Provide written instructions that include the amount, dose, frequency, route of administration, and potential side effects. Tell the client taking probenecid or sulfinpyrazone to avoid aspirin.

Low Back Pain

Low back pain is one of the major causes of disability in North America and is, therefore, of extreme importance. Two common disorders causing low back pain will be discussed in this section: low back strain and intervertebral disk disease.

Erect posture and a sedentary lifestyle predispose people to low back pain. Certain stressors that put unequal pressure on the spine also contribute (eg, congenital anomalies, leg length discrepancy, asymmetrical development of the spine, weak abdominal muscles, obesity, and trauma).

There is some evidence that cigarette smoking increases the incidence of low back pain, possibly by interfering with oxygen delivery to the disk (Kelsey, 1984). In addition, gradual degeneration of the intervertebral disks does occur with the normal process of aging.

Clinical Manifestations

Low back strain is the most common cause of low back pain. There is usually a history of injury, most often a minor injury followed by an immediate or delayed pain in the lower back. Pain can radiate into the buttocks and posterior thigh. Any motion of the spine causes pain. Clients often assume distorted positions to be comfortable. Lack of exercise, weak abdominal muscles, and obesity all contribute to the problem. Additional influencing factors include improper reaching, lifting, or bending; sitting too long in overstuffed, nonsupportive chairs; lying on soft, lumpy mattresses; or riding in a car for long periods in low bucket seats. History taking should include information about these aspects of the client's life. Carrying a large wallet or credit card case in a rear pants pocket, causing asymmetrical pressure on the lower back when sitting, also contributes to low back pain.

Physical examination of a client with low back strain reveals tenderness and spasm of the paravertebral muscles. The ROM of the lower lumbar spine decreases, and tender areas may be palpated at the posterosuperior iliac spines. There may be a discrepancy in leg length.

The straight leg raising test to differentiate low back strain from herniated intervertebral disk is done with the client supine. Raise the leg on the affected side straight up until pain is experienced, then lower the leg slightly and dorsiflex the foot, which stretches the sciatic nerve (Figure 46–1). If pain occurs in the back or along the sciatic

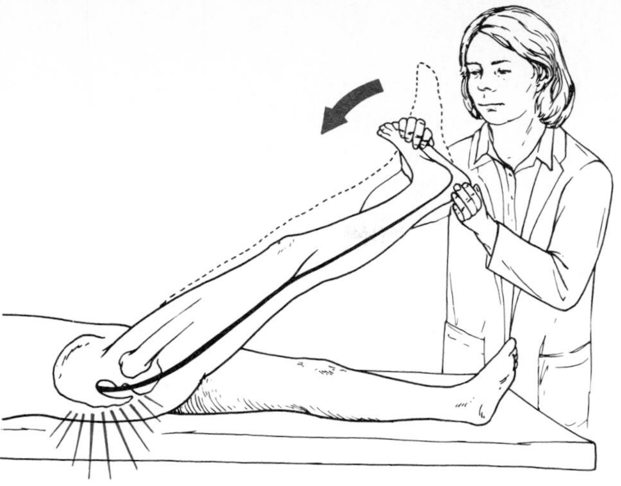

Figure 46–1

Straight leg raising exam in which dorsiflexion of the foot produces sciatic pain.

nerve distribution with dorsiflexion of the foot, herniated disk is suspected. In low back strain, there is no pain on dorsiflexion of the foot and no sensory, motor, or reflex changes noted in the legs.

With intervertebral disk disease, there is severe low back pain with radiation into the buttocks, legs, and feet, usually on one side. *Sciatica* is the term used to describe the pain in the posterior thigh and lateral calf, occasionally extending to the foot, that occurs with herniated lumbar intervertebral disk disease. Coughing, sneezing, bending, and riding in a car will increase the pain. Disk disease is common in elderly people, because compression fractures of the vertebrae increase from osteoporosis. Steroid therapy compounds the problem.

Physical examination of a client with lumbar intervertebral disk disease usually reveals sensorimotor loss and, later, weakness and muscle atrophy. The straight leg raising test induces sciatic pain rather than low back pain. The most common location is the disk between L4-L5 or L5-S1. Pain is relieved with rest and increased with motion. Disk disease can also affect the cervical area, C5-C6 or C6-C7. Usually, a chronic aching pain radiates to the shoulders and into the neck or goes down to the arm and into the hand. The hands and fingers may be numb.

Diagnosis of a herniated disk can be determined by history and physical examination. A computerized tomography (CT) scan confirms the diagnosis and can be used to monitor treatment.

Diagnosis of low back pain should include a full blood count; ESR; a biochemical profile including serum calcium, phosphate, alkaline phosphatase, and serum protein levels; and electrophoresis. Men should have a serum acid phosphatase drawn and a thorough rectal examination to rule out cancer of the prostate. Spine x-rays are not taken routinely but should be ordered if physical examination suggests even a remote possibility of ruptured disk.

Myelograms are only necessary if surgery is being considered. A CT scan is ordered if spine x-ray results are within normal limits but the client's condition does not improve with treatment.

Medical Measures

Low back strain is usually self-limiting. Bed rest, analgesics, muscle relaxants, heat or ice therapy, and flexion exercises can relieve the initial spasm. After severe pain subsides, abdominal muscle-strengthening exercises and back exercises can prevent recurrences. Lumbar girdle support also can be helpful to younger clients.

The conservative treatment of intervertebral disk disease involves bed rest, sometimes for as long as 1 to 3 months. Traction, lumbar corset support, analgesics, physical therapy, and exercises are all potentially helpful approaches to treatment. Epidural injections with steroids can sometimes help clients who are not responsive to other measures. Transcutaneous electrical nerve stimulation (TENS) also helps relieve pain in some clients. Because not everyone responds, clients are advised to rent the unit for 2 weeks and use it at home before purchasing it.

Chemonucleolysis, a procedure with some risk, may be considered for clients who do not do well with other treatment. The enzyme chymopapain is injected into the disk to shrink it, thereby relieving pressure. Serious neurologic problems have been reported following chemonucleolysis with chymopapain, including paraplegia, cerebral hemorrhage, and transverse myelitis. It is currently recommended that chemonucleolysis be limited to the one disk producing the client's symptoms (Smith, 1984). The other option is surgical intervention; laminectomy is the most common procedure. Laminectomy is discussed in Chapter 45.

Specific Nursing Measures

The primary function of the nurse in the management of low back disorders is prevention. Therefore, the main thrust is toward client education. Tell clients that active people have less back pain and fewer injuries. Swimming, aerobics, and physical fitness approaches of almost any kind are good. Being out of shape contributes to the incidence of back problems. Include instruction about proper lifting technique, muscle-strengthening exercises, and posture (Box 46–1).

Client/Family Teaching

Most people lift incorrectly, using a straight back and flexed knees. This technique throws people off balance, and they either fall or incorrectly straighten their legs and flex their back to avoid falling, straining the lumbar area (Owen, 1980).

In addition to poor lifting techniques, weak lumbar muscles, weak abdominal muscles, prolonged sitting, poor

Box 46–1
Approaches to the Prevention of Low Back Pain

Proper Lifting Technique

The best height for lifting a load is when it is already placed 2 feet off the floor. Therefore, having loads consistently placed at this level in the workplace aids in proper lifting.

Always position the load close to the body.

Position the body so that muscle groups can work together.

The weight to be lifted is excessive if it is 35% or more of the lifter's body weight.

If the object is bulky (30 in or more to a side) do not attempt to lift it if it is more than 20 lb.

Always avoid twisting; try to pivot with the entire body.

Make several trips; use a mechanical apparatus when possible; and do not hesitate to ask for help if needed.

Do not bend over at right angles.

Make sure no obstacles are in the way and that the feet are secure.

Exercise

Flexed-knee sit-ups to strengthen the abdomen

Bent-knee leg lifts to strengthen the abdomen

Knee–chest leg lifts to stretch the lower back and tighten the abdomen

Back flattening to stretch the lower back and tighten the abdomen

Posture

Sleep on the back or side with a small pillow. Keep the knees flexed while in bed. A small pillow under the knees may help, but a pillow should be used cautiously if there are joint problems with the knees, since flexion contracture of the knees can occur quickly.

Sleep on a supportive mattress.

Use a straight-back chair when sitting.

Do not cross the legs or sit with the legs straight out on a footstool.

Wear flat-heeled shoes.

When standing, use a small stool to rest one leg at a time; shift the weight from one leg to the other when standing for long periods.

posture, and obesity all contribute to back insults. Therefore, the strengthening of abdominal and lumbar muscle groups, along with proper lifting techniques, proper posture, and weight reduction, reduces the risks of back injuries. All exercises should be done gently and slowly to build up endurance. In addition, exercises should always be done with the knees flexed.

Teach clients about the side effects of medication; for example, muscle relaxants may cause some drowsiness, and NSAIDs may exacerbate ulcer problems. Explain the proper and discriminate use of analgesics, because back pain can be a long-term problem. If the client is hospitalized, explain procedures and therapies before they are encountered to allay anxiety. Before myelography, ask the client about allergies; the radiopaque dye contains iodine, and people who are allergic to seafood are usually allergic to the dye. Explain that myelography is an uncomfortable procedure and that sedation will be given beforehand. Following myelography, the client must remain supine for 6 to 9 hours to prevent headache and must drink adequate fluid. Postprocedure care includes monitoring vital signs and assessing neurologic function.

Help the obese client formulate a nutritional and realistic diet. Refer the client to an accessible weight reduction program or begin one.

Urge smokers to stop smoking. Have material available on support groups and quit-smoking commercial programs in the area. Tell smokers about nicotine gum that is available by prescription.

Offer supportive care for emotional ramifications of back injuries. In addition to the costs from lost wages, medical expenses, and insurance premiums, the costs to the client and family or significant others can be great in psychologic trauma.

Explain to the client with a back injury that complete bed rest is essential initially, and that the more activity, the longer it will take to improve. Apply heat and cold therapy safely and instruct the client in home use. Take advantage of massage and other comfort measures to help relieve pain.

Laminectomy

Laminectomy, the removal of one or more vertebral bony arches (laminae), may be done when the severe back and leg pain of a herniated intervertebral disk has not responded to conservative treatment. The portion of the protruding disk (nucleus pulposus) that is pressing on the nerve root is removed through the opening provided by the laminectomy. This procedure is called a *diskectomy* (also discectomy). When the surgery is done as part of a procedure to treat disease or injury of the spinal cord, it is usually performed by a neurosurgeon, rather than an orthopedic surgeon (see Chapter 29).

The procedure is most common in the lumbar region but may also be necessary in the cervical or thoracic spine. Spinal fusion may be done at the same time if the spine is unstable as a result of either the laminectomy or the under-

Table 46–1
Laminectomy: Implications for the Client 

Physiologic Implications	Psychosocial/Lifestyle Implications
Successful surgery provides relief of pain and improves ambulation.	Chronic pain and disability may be relieved, improving the quality of life.
Local pain and edema occur as a result of surgical manipulation.	Temporary limitation in activity and positioning is necessary; spinal fusion may require wearing a back brace for a few months.
Neurologic manifestations may occur immediately postoperatively due to operative area edema.	Good body mechanics and posture are a lifelong necessity.
Nerve damage can occur, causing permanent neurologic deficits.	Recurrence of symptoms is discouraging.
Diskectomy is not always successful in relieving the symptoms; symptoms may recur.	Failed surgery may result in disability or a change in occupation.
A complication of cervical spine surgery is respiratory distress.	Recurrence of condition may cause others to think client is malingering.
Spinal fusion eliminates movement in the involved vertebrae; the recuperation period is lengthy.	A lengthy disability period may cause discouragement and financial problems.

lying condition. The implications of laminectomy are summarized in Table 46–1.

Nursing Implications

PREOPERATIVE CARE Routine preoperative orthopedic care is necessary. In addition, teach the client how to logroll (described under "Positioning and Turning") and how to get out of bed postoperatively (described under "Ambulation"). Assess the client's neurovascular and comfort status for comparisons to postoperative condition. Many clients fear that paralysis could occur as a complication of back surgery. Encourage clients to verbalize their apprehension and correct any misconceptions. Explain that swelling from surgery may cause the pain and numbness experienced before surgery to remain for some time afterward. Collect several pillows before surgery for positioning the client afterward.

POSTOPERATIVE CARE Routine postoperative care includes comfort measures, neurovascular assessment, and prevention of the hazards of immobility. When moving the client back into bed from the recovery room cart, at least four people should lift the client gently, keeping the spine in good alignment. The bed should have a firm mattress.

The client's neurovascular status must be assessed with vital signs and any loss of sensation or deterioration in ability to move reported promptly to the physician. Stress respiratory status assessment in the client with cervical spine surgery. Observe the dressing for signs of hemorrhage or leaking cerebrospinal fluid, either of which should be reported to the physician.

The physician may order elastic stockings. Clients should move their arms, dorsiflex and plantarflex their feet, and cough and deep breathe every 2 hours. Use comfort measures and analgesics to relieve pain. If the client is discouraged because the preoperative symptoms are still present, explain that edema may be responsible.

Observe for difficulty with voiding because position limitations may be a hindrance. Use a fracture bedpan, and roll, rather than lift, the client onto it.

The diet is advanced as tolerated; foods to prevent constipation are encouraged. Initially, the client will have to eat in the side-lying position. Clients should be positioned on the side that allows them to use the dominant hand to feed themselves.

POSITIONING AND TURNING Positioning varies with the physician's preference and the surgical procedure done. When the spinal fusion client is supine, the bed is completely flat. For diskectomy, the physician may prefer to have the client's legs elevated on pillows along their entire length or in a position with knees and hips flexed. Either of these positions relaxes the back muscles and provides comfort. The head of the bed may be elevated with physician's order only; it is usually elevated after cervical vertebrae surgery. When elevated, the client should be positioned in the bed so bending occurs at the hips, not somewhere along the back; it is important not to slouch. A sign above the client's bed indicating which positions are allowed or forbidden is helpful.

Turn the client every 2 to 3 hours. At first, two nurses are needed for turning to maintain perfect body alignment. The method for turning, known as *logrolling,* involves turning the client all at one time, without twisting the spine. The client will eventually be able to turn unassisted by logrolling, after healing has begun and instruction has been given. The client is moved to one side of the bed, a pillow is placed between the legs, and the arms are crossed over the chest. The nurse places one hand on the client's far shoulder and one on the hip and rolls the client toward her/him while another nurse supports the back in alignment. Place pillows at the client's back for support, a pillow under the head, another between the knees, and one in front of the chest to support the arm. The uppermost knee should be flexed for balance.

A doubled-thickness drawsheet can also be used as a turning sheet for logrolling. Back rubs should be given and the skin inspected with each position change. Avoid rubbing the operative area. Place the call light and other needed objects near the bed so the client can avoid excessive reaching, which may strain the back.

AMBULATION Progressive ambulation usually begins with dangling, possibly the evening of surgery. Some surgeons prefer to be present when the client dangles for the first time. Two methods are used. In the first, the head of the bed is elevated, and the nurse brings the client's legs over the edge of the bed, swiveling the client's body at the same time without twisting the spine. In the second method, the client begins in the side-lying position, then pushes the upper body into the upright position using one or two hands as nurses move the legs over the edge of the bed and support the back. Observe for postural hypotension, especially if the client has been supine for several days. Begin teaching the client how to ambulate early in the postoperative period.

Getting out of bed is done in the same manner and may begin from 1 to 5 days postoperatively, or in the case of spinal fusion, perhaps 2 weeks postoperatively. Some clients are allowed only to walk, not stand in one spot. The nurse should encourage good posture when walking. If the client is allowed to sit in a chair, the chair should be firm, with a straight back. Encourage good sitting posture, with the feet flat on the floor. In some cases, sitting is not allowed for several weeks.

Home Health Care

The length of hospitalization varies, but is typically about 1 to 2 weeks. Before discharge, the physician informs the client about restricted activities, such as driving and sexual activity. The restrictions usually apply for about 4 to 6 weeks postoperatively. The nurse should teach the client good posture and principles of body mechanics. The client's return to work depends on the type of activity the job requires. The prolonged absence from work (which often begins before surgery, when the client is undergoing conservative treatment) may create financial problems. A social worker may help find financial assistance.

Scoliosis

Scoliosis is a lateral curvature of the spine, most commonly in the thoracic area with convexity to the right and compensatory convex curves to the left in the cervical and lumbar areas. Scoliosis can be functional (a result of poor posture or leg length discrepancy) or structural (a result of deformity of the vertebral bodies, paralysis, congenital malformations, or idiopathic causes). Idiopathic causes are the most common and appear when the growth spurt begins in adolescence.

Clinical Manifestations

Symptoms of backache, fatigue, and dyspnea occur only after scoliosis is well established. Screening and early referral of children during their elementary school years are essential to prevent long-term problems. Untreated scoliosis can result in pulmonary insufficiency from decreased lung capacity, back pain, degenerative arthritis of the spine, intervertebral disk disease, and sciatica.

The older adult client, most often female, may exhibit kyphosis, a postural curvature of the spine that is due to aging, disk degeneration, atrophy of spinal muscles, osteoporosis, or vertebral collapse. Adults with kyphosis have a rounded back and possibly weakness and generalized fatigue. Kyphosis rarely produces local tenderness except in severe osteoporosis with compression fractures.

Medical Measures

Early treatment of scoliosis consists of exercises, bracing, surgery, or a combination of these. If the client is untreated in adolescence, problems that develop in adulthood can only be treated symptomatically. These clients have severely compromised lung capacity, and any upper respiratory tract infection must be treated aggressively to prevent pooling of secretions, pneumonia, and atelectasis.

Specific Nursing Measures

Clients with scoliosis often have body image problems related to the deformity. They have trouble finding clothes that fit properly and difficulty finding comfortable positions in which to sit or lie. When the older adult with severe kyphosis or scoliosis is hospitalized for any problem, careful attention to positioning is essential (eg, on x-ray tables, operating room tables, and carts, as well as for gynecologic examinations); improper positioning is not only extremely uncomfortable for the client, but it can precipitate a vertebral fracture, especially in a client with osteoporosis.

School nurses are in an ideal position to monitor adolescents for scoliosis with yearly screening. If scoliosis is detected early, exercises and bracing usually can correct the problem. Some adolescents will require surgical intervention, however. With vigilance on the part of school nurses and active programs to instruct parents about signs of scoliosis, adults with scoliosis will be a problem of the past.

To prevent abnormal spinal curvature in older women, usually resulting from osteoporosis, regular exercise and calcium supplements are important. Some sources suggest that women begin calcium supplementation as early as age 35 to prevent the numerous complications of osteoporosis, one of which is vertebral collapse.

Carpal Tunnel Syndrome

Carpal tunnel syndrome is an entrapment neuropathy resulting from pressure on the median nerve as it passes through the space formed by the bones of the wrist and the transverse carpal ligament (Figure 46–2). A variety of problems can cause entrapment of the median nerve, including tenosynovitis, trauma, rheumatoid arthritis, gout, edema of pregnancy, and premenstrual edema. Carpal tunnel syndrome, which is much more common in women than men because women's carpal tunnels are smaller, occurs most often in the age range of 40 to 50 years. The dominant hand is affected most often, but the condition can be bilateral. Median nerve paralysis can occur if the nerve entrapment is not treated.

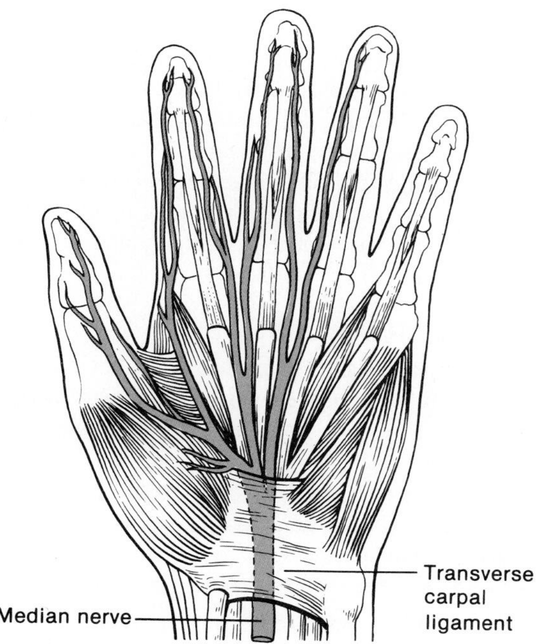

Figure 46–2

Carpal tunnel: anatomic relation of median nerve.

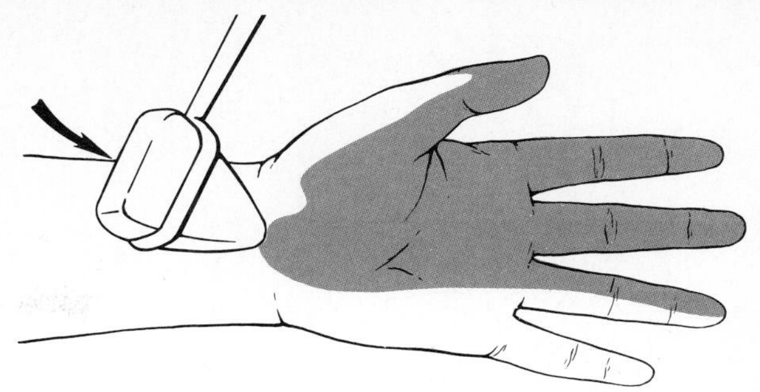

Figure 46–3

Tinel's sign.

Clinical Manifestations

Paresthesia occurs in the areas supplied by the median nerve: the thumb, the index and middle fingers, and the adjacent side of the ring finger. Pain may radiate up the arm and is worse at night. Some fine motor movements may be difficult. There may be atrophy of the thenar eminence (fleshy eminence at the base of the thumb) as time progresses, and abduction of the thumb weakens. A positive Tinel's sign is elicited by light percussion over the median nerve on the flexor surface of the wrist. Normally, there is no response, but in carpal tunnel syndrome the percussion elicits a tingling sensation in the 3½ digits innervated by the median nerve (Figure 46–3). Electromyography can confirm the diagnosis.

Medical Measures

Diuretics and a low-salt diet may be helpful if edema is a factor in carpal tunnel syndrome. Splinting of the wrist at night as well as during the day helps avoid flexion. Local injections of steroids may provide relief for some clients. Surgical release of the transverse carpal ligament may be necessary.

Specific Nursing Measures

Explain the nature of carpal tunnel syndrome to the client, and encourage the use of a low-salt diet. Discuss the rationale for diuretic therapy and frequent follow-up with the care provider when diuretics are given on a long-term basis. The potassium levels of clients on diuretic therapy should be checked every 3 months.

Instruct the client to inspect the skin of the wrist frequently when using the splint. The hands should not be overused, and rest is essential when symptoms are present. The client can remove the splint several times a day to expose the skin and do gentle ROM exercises.

Bunionectomy

Bunionectomy is a surgical procedure done to remove a *bunion,* a bony prominence and bursa on the medial side of the first metatarsal head of the great toe. A bunion is

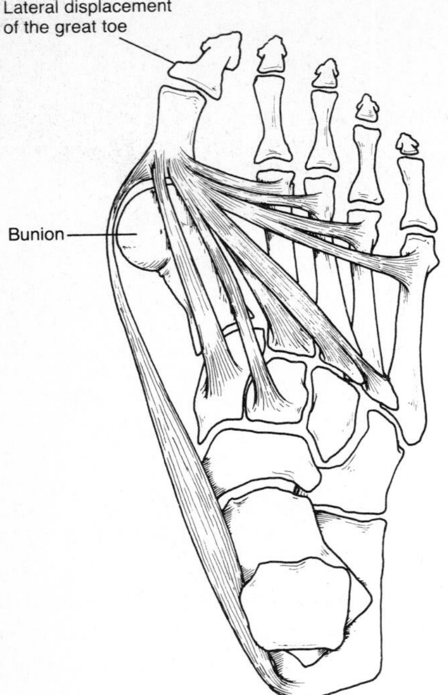

Figure 46–4

Bunion and hallux valgus.

commonly associated with an abnormal position of the great toe known as hallux valgus, in which there is lateral displacement of the great toe at the metatarsophalangeal joint (Figure 46–4). Various procedures are done to remove the bunion, the bony overgrowth, and to realign the great toe if necessary.

The indication for bunionectomy is pain unrelieved by conservative measures, which may become severely disabling. Bunions are more common in women than men; they are usually bilateral; and they may be caused by congenital deformity. The influence of footwear as a cause of bunions is disputed; however, improperly fitted shoes do contribute to the worsening of hallux valgus when the deformity exists (Apley & Solomon, 1982). The client implications of bunionectomy are summarized in Table 46–2.

Nursing Implications

Routine preoperative and postoperative orthopedic care are necessary. Check neurovascular status, vital signs, and cast or dressing frequently. The operative foot is elevated. Comfort measures and analgesics are given to relieve pain. The amount of weight bearing allowed depends upon the procedure done, so the postoperative orders should be specific. Some clients are allowed to walk on their heel at first and progress to weight bearing as tolerated. If realignment of the great toe is required, the client may not bear weight for 3 to 6 weeks. Physical therapy teaches clients the use of ambulatory aids.

SECTION II

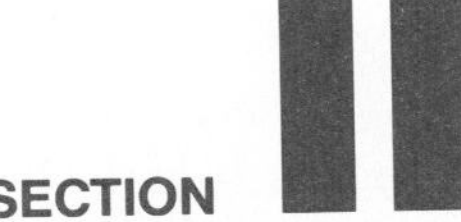

Degenerative Disorders

Degenerative Joint Disease

Degenerative joint disease (DJD), also known as *osteoarthritis*, is the only disease to be discussed in this section. One of the most common joint problems seen in clinical practice, it is primarily a disorder of the articular cartilage. Aging seems to be the most important factor in the development of DJD.

In DJD, the bony tissue near the cartilage becomes more dense, and overgrowth (osteophytes or spurs) occurs near the joint edges. The joint space eventually becomes severely narrowed, and ultimately bone rests on bone, resulting in a deformed joint (Figure 46–5).

Degenerative joint disease may be classified as primary or secondary. Primary DJD occurs in the older age group without evidence of predisposing abnormality. It is essentially a wear-and-tear phenomenon. Secondary DJD results from previous joint damage and may begin at any age. Clinical findings are similar in primary and secondary DJD.

Clinical Manifestations

The onset of pain in DJD is gradual. Local pain in the affected joint or joints is usually worse after activity and

Table 46–2
Bunionectomy: Implications for the Client 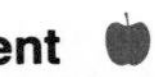

Physiologic Implications	Psychosocial/Lifestyle Implications
Provides relief of pain; alleviates disability.	Relief of chronic pain should improve quality of client's life.
Temporary local swelling and pain occur from the procedure.	Appearance of the foot is improved.
Potential complications: nerve or blood vessel damage, wound infection.	Ambulatory aids will be necessary temporarily.

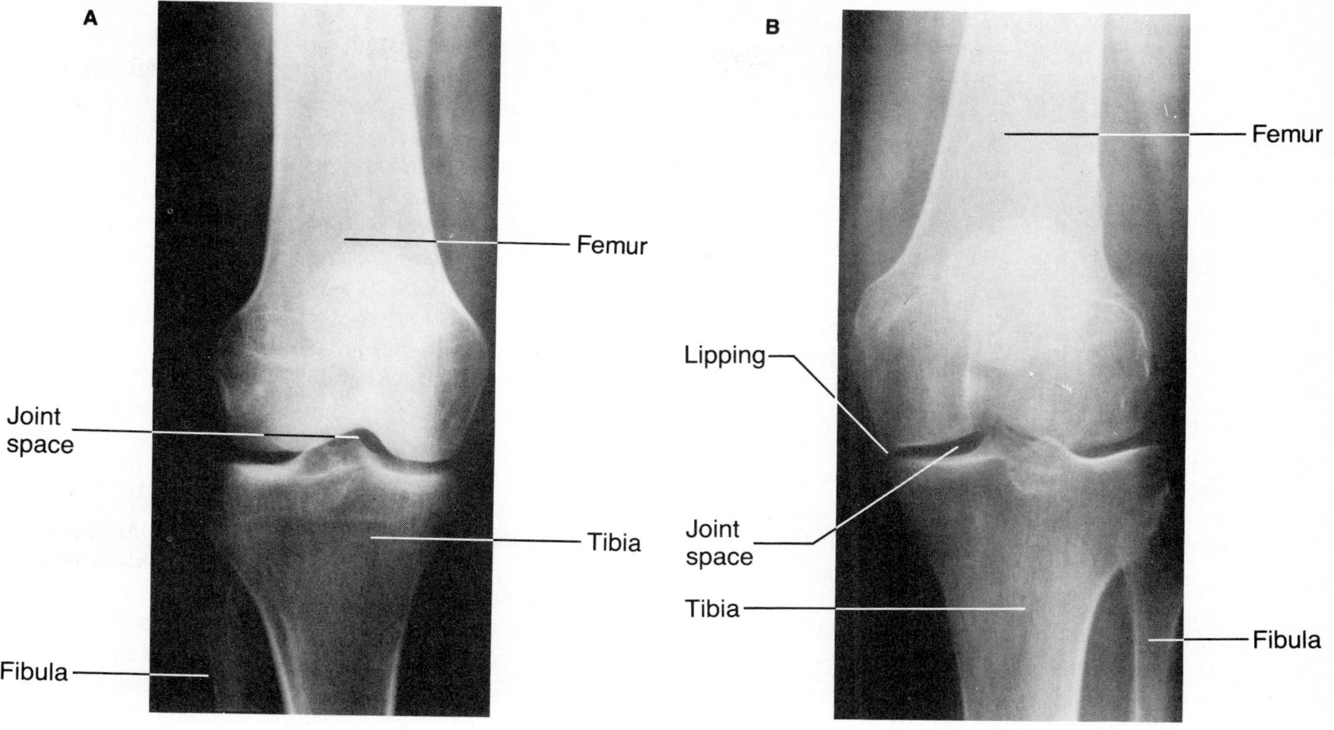

Figure 46–5

A. X-ray of a normal right knee. Note the joint space. **B.** X-ray of the left knee in a client with DJD. Note the joint space narrowing, sharpened articular margins, and the marginal osteophyte formation (lipping). *Courtesy of Health Care Plan, Buffalo, NY.*

relieved with rest. There may be a history of some morning stiffness, but this usually lasts for only a brief period. Because DJD is not a systemic disorder, fatigue is mild and not incapacitating. As time goes by, the joint becomes restricted in motion, and surrounding muscles may atrophy. Pieces of cartilage that break off can irritate the synovial lining, and inflammation and swelling may occur.

Joints most affected by DJD are distal interphalangeal (DIP) joints, proximal interphalangeal (PIP) joints, carpometacarpal joint of the thumb, cervical and lumbar spines, metatarsophalangeal (MPT) joint of the big toe, acromioclavicular joints, knees, hips, and temporomandibular joints. Although DJD is usually asymmetrical, generalized DJD may occur; it mimics a more systemic arthritis when numerous joints are affected at once.

Physical assessment may reveal crepitation on movement of the joint, limited range of motion, and atrophy of surrounding muscles. Bony overgrowths may be seen on the DIP joints of the fingers (Heberden's nodes) (Figure 46–6) and the PIP joints of the fingers (Bouchard's nodes).

X-rays of various joints involved confirm the diagnosis of DJD. Although cartilage itself cannot be seen on x-ray film, DJD involves a narrowing of joint space. There may also be osteophytes and bone cysts as the disease progresses, along with joint deformity. If erosive, inflamma-

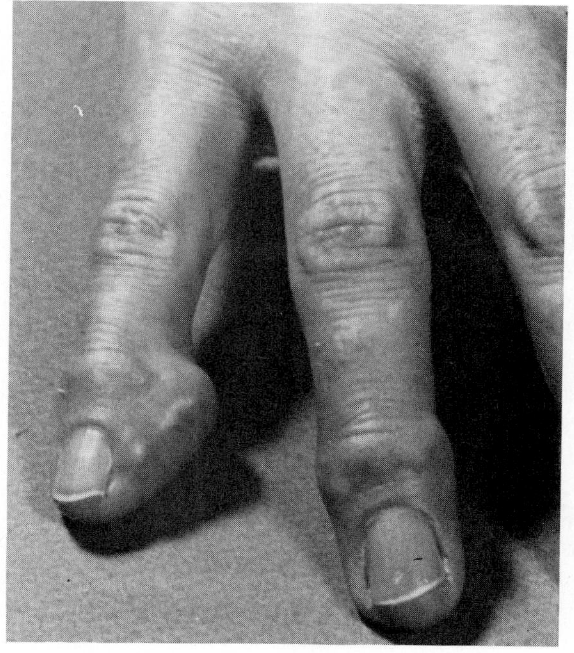

Figure 46–6

Heberden's nodes as seen in DJD. *Courtesy of Millard Fillmore Hospital, Buffalo, NY.*

tory arthritis is present, the x-ray film may show erosions of the bones that may be difficult to distinguish from RA.

Laboratory analysis of the blood is not diagnostic in DJD, but various tests can rule out the other types of arthritis, which may occur simultaneously. If a joint is aspirated, culture and analysis of the fluid are mandatory to rule out infection. Joint fluid in DJD usually appears normal.

Medical Measures

The goal of treatment in clients with DJD is to relieve pain, decrease swelling, increase joint function, improve muscle strength, and allow the client to pursue a more active lifestyle. Aspirin, usually enteric coated, relieves pain and, in higher doses, decreases inflammation. Because aspirin can irritate the stomach, it is usually given with food. If aspirin is not acceptable, many NSAIDs can be used to treat DJD. Sometimes trials with different medications are necessary to find one acceptable for the individual client. The addition of analgesics can help control pain.

Oral corticosteroids are not helpful in DJD. However, aspiration of joint fluid and intra-articular injections of corticosteroids do effectively relieve pain and increase function. These injections must be infrequent because increased cartilage degeneration can occur if corticosteriods are used too often.

Ice can be applied to relieve swelling for 10 minutes 2 to 4 times a day. If the client prefers heat, it can be applied to reduce muscle spasm but always with the heat source on a medium setting for a maximum of 20 minutes at a time. Ultrasound therapy also has brought relief to some clients.

Various isometric exercises improve muscle strength. The quadriceps exercise improves knee function. Have the sitting client extend the leg and hold for 6 seconds; repeat 5 times. While watching television, the client can do this each time a commercial comes on—a handy way to remember to do the exercise. Elastic bandages, canes, and walkers also can protect the joint from stress.

When clients do not respond to conservative treatment, surgery and possibly total joint replacement can be an option. Joint replacement of a hip or knee is most common, but prosthetic implants are possible for other joints as well.

Specific Nursing Measures

Instruction about pain relief is an important nursing responsibility. Explain the need for rest and paced activities. The client should understand that activity causing pain that lasts for hours is too strenuous. Instruct the client to begin slowly and add activities gradually.

Administer ice or heat therapy—whichever is most effective—and instruct the client in its use. Place a towel between the skin and the therapeutic agent (eg, heating pad, ice bag). Pillows should not be placed under the knees. Although they are comfortable, they can cause contractures. Provide other comfort measures, such as massage and topical analgesic creams, to help relieve pain. Although topically applied analgesic creams may not relieve pain entirely, they are soothing and comfort some clients.

Administer medications as prescribed, and explain their dosage, route, and side effects to the client. Instruct clients to write down the pertinent information about each medication and carry it in their wallets. This step will help clients remember, as well as make the information accessible to other health professionals, if necessary.

Perform passive ROM exercises on the joint, and demonstrate the types of isometric exercises to strengthen muscles. Also provide instruction regarding the proper use of canes, crutches, and walkers, if applicable. Have the client redemonstrate their use. Tell the client using elastic bandages to wrap toward the heart. The bandages should not be too tight or too loose and generally should not be worn during sleep.

The joints of the hips, knees, and back can benefit from weight reduction, because stress from added weight can cause more rapid cartilage breakdown. If the client is overweight, help plan a realistic weight loss program. Urge clients of normal weight to be conscientious about maintaining that weight level. Instruct the client about safety measures to be taken at home to prevent injury, especially from falls.

Implications for Elderly Clients

Elderly clients with DJD face additional problems. Some have other disease processes with which to cope. Also, their support groups may be more limited, because spouses and friends may be deceased, and children may live far away or be involved in their own lives. Older persons may also be at a disadvantage financially, because their incomes may be fixed and they cannot afford needed medications. These clients need a great deal of emotional support to relieve anxiety and decrease muscle tension, which may contribute to their pain. Suggestions of support groups, referral to specific agencies, or arranging for community health nursing visits are possible approaches nurses should pursue.

SECTION 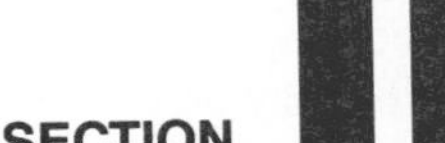

Immunologic Disorders

Rheumatoid Arthritis

Rheumatoid arthritis (RA) is a systemic disease characterized primarily by chronic inflammation of the synovial lining of the joints. Joints are usually symmetrically affected.

The most commonly involved joints are the wrists, PIP joints, metacarpophalangeal (MCP) joints of the hands, and MTP joints of the feet. Extra-articular involvement of RA includes muscle atrophy; anemia; osteoporosis; and skin, ocular, vascular, pulmonary, and cardiac symptoms. The course of the illness is variable, with a few or every joint in the body invaded. The long-term results are also unpredictable in regard to remission and exacerbation. Although classified in the 1983 *Primer on the Rheumatic Diseases* as a diffuse connective tissue disorder, RA is discussed in the chapter on joints because its major manifestation is joint inflammation. Women develop RA three times more often than men.

The etiology of RA is unknown. Whatever the cause, it releases various chemical mediators of inflammation (antigen–antibody complexes) into the joint. These chemicals cause synovial lining proliferation and cell lysis, a destructive process that eventually heals in a way that leaves a particular kind of scar tissue called *pannus*. Pannus generally tightens as other scar tissue does and pulls on structures already weakened by the destructive process. This results in flexion contractures and fibrosis, with possible calcifications.

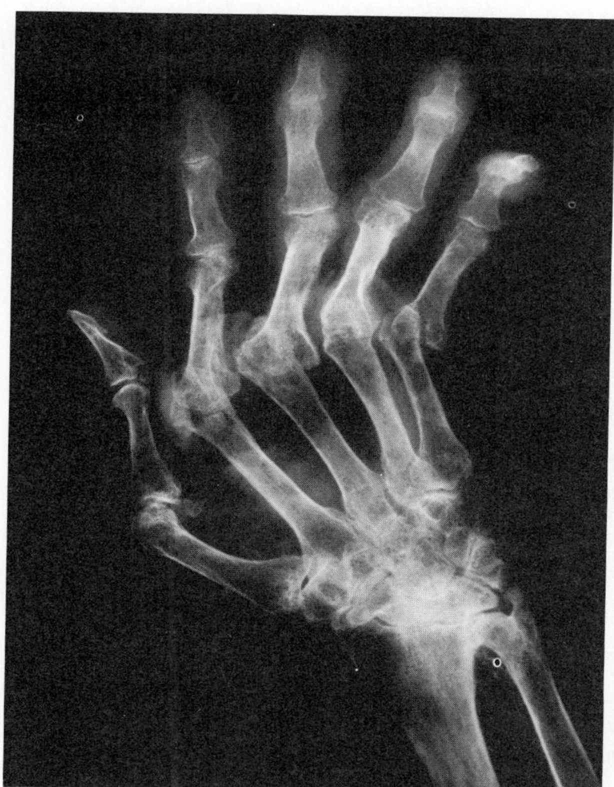

Figure 46–7

X-ray of the hand of a client with rheumatoid arthritis. Note the ulnar deviation of the fingers and the enlarged DIP joint in the ring finger. SOURCE: *Spence AP, Mason EB:* Human Anatomy and Physiology, *3rd ed. Menlo Park, CA: Benjamin/Cummings, 1987.*

Clinical Manifestations

ARTICULAR MANIFESTATIONS Swollen joints develop, especially the PIPs, MCPs, MTPs, and wrists, in bilateral symmetrical distribution; monoarticular involvement is also possible. The swelling is caused by proliferation of the synovial membrane that produces increased synovial fluid. Joint symptoms usually are insidious over weeks to months. Morning stiffness lasting from 30 minutes to several hours is characteristic of RA because of the synovial congestion, increased synovial fluid, and capsule thickening.

Deformities may occur later in the course of the disease because of soft tissue weakness and joint destruction. Ulnar deviation of the fingers is most common in RA (Figure 46–7). Swan-neck deformity of the fingers occurs when there is hyperextension of the PIP joints in conjunction with flexion of the DIP joints. Similarly, a boutonnière deformity of the fingers results from a flexion deformity of the PIP joints and extension of the DIP joints. Carpal tunnel syndrome with paresthesia of the thumb and the second, third, and radial aspects of the fourth digit may occur secondary to synovitis of the wrist, which compresses the median nerve beneath the transverse carpal ligament.

EXTRA-ARTICULAR MANIFESTATIONS Fatigue, weakness, anorexia, and weight loss may be present because of the systemic effect of the inflammatory process. Anemia, which is associated with a chronic arthritis, also may develop.

Rheumatoid nodules—firm rounded or oval nodules that occur in subcutaneous or deeper connective tissue—may be present over the extensor surface of the elbows or Achilles tendons. These benign lesions are uncomfortable, mainly because they have been produced by friction and pressure.

Vasculitis of the coronary, cranial, and mesenteric vessels has been reported, as well as vasculitis of small peripheral vessels. Myocardial infarction, neuropathy, skin necrosis, and leg ulcers may also result. Pericarditis appears more often in males and is unrelated to the duration of the disease. The course of the pericarditis varies from mild and self-limiting to cardiac tamponade and death. Lung involvement includes pleurisy with or without effusion, pulmonary fibrosis, and rheumatoid nodules of the lung.

DIAGNOSIS Diagnostic study data to be gathered include blood work, synovial fluid analysis, and x-rays. The ESR is elevated, parallel to the disease activity. There may be a normocytic, monochromic, or hypochromic anemia. The rheumatoid factor is present in 70% of adults with RA but is not specific for the disease. Complement levels are depressed. Five to ten percent of clients with RA have false positive tests for syphilis. Antinuclear antibody (ANA) test results are positive in 25% of cases, with a diffuse pattern.

Synovial fluid analysis can help establish the diagnosis when polymorphonuclear leukocytosis is present. X-rays early in RA show soft tissue swelling and periarticular osteoporosis. As the disease progresses, joint space narrowing and bony erosions are seen. In late RA, malalignment and ankylosis can be visualized.

Diagnosis of RA is made over time, as the disease settles into a bilateral, symmetrical, polyarticular arthritis usually by the end of 1 to 2 years. At that point, laboratory tests help confirm the diagnosis, and x-ray changes are usually present.

Medical Measures

In spite of the variable course of RA, client care plans should include the following goals:

- Involve the client and family in all aspects of therapy planning and decision making to preserve a sense of personal value and control.
- Decrease pain and joint inflammation, and suppress the systemic disease process.

PHARMACOLOGIC APPROACHES Aspirin, which is inexpensive and well tolerated, is used as an anti-inflammatory agent in doses of 2.4 to 4.0 g/day. Failure of aspirin therapy is often the result of noncompliance, gastric intolerance, or tinnitus.

For clients who are unable to tolerate aspirin or who require more potent anti-inflammatory medication, NSAIDs are indicated. These work by blocking the production of local inflammatory mediators such as prostaglandins and kinins, thereby reducing pain and inflammation and promoting joint mobility. Ibuprofen (Motrin), indomethacin (Indocin), naproxen (Naprosyn), and tolmetin (Tolectin) are but a few of the NSAIDs available today. Each has a similar action, but clients are unique in their response to them. At least a 2-week trial of each drug is recommended before discontinuation because clients may initially do well on a drug, and then the effect may dissipate. When this occurs, another NSAID should be tried. Because the main side effect of all NSAIDs is gastrointestinal distress, all clients should take them with food or milk, and they should be given cautiously to people with ulcers. Analgesics can be used in conjunction with anti-inflammatory agents when necessary. These include acetaminophen (Tylenol), propoxyphene hydrochloride (Darvon), and codeine.

Gold is used as a suppressive agent in RA to potentiate remission. Gold therapy is presently available in either injectable or oral forms. Both are equally effective. Toxic effects of injectable gold include mild skin rash, proteinuria, exfoliative dermatitis (a rare complication), mouth ulcers, and aplastic anemia. Oral gold, auranofin (Ridaura), is similar in action to injectable gold, but smaller doses are effective. Diarrhea is the most common side effect, but this may be controlled by decreasing the dosage. Both oral and injectable gold must be monitored closely with blood and urine samples. Prescriptions for auranofin should be written for one month at a time to maintain client–physician contact for adequate monitoring.

Penicillamine (Depen, Cuprimine) is similar to gold in its action and percentage of remission produced, but it has the benefit of being an oral agent. The medication is given in increasing increments monthly. Toxicity to penicillamine may be as high as 50%, and clients should be monitored for proteinuria or bone marrow depression. A common benign side effect of the drug is a blunting of taste sensation, which usually disappears as the client continues taking the medication. Chemically related to penicillin, this drug usually should not be administered to individuals with a known penicillin allergy.

Steroids are seldom used to treat RA except in a severe exacerbation or for intra-articular injections. Cytotoxic agents are used in rare cases for immunosuppression. They are effective but dangerous because of their toxicity.

Methotrexate, however, is one immunosuppressive that has been effective in the treatment of RA. Studies have shown that 70% of clients tested improve significantly in a short period of time on both oral and injectable forms. Methotrexate should only be used for clients who have been refractory to conventional therapy.

ACTIVITY, REST, AND EXERCISE Exercise is always indicated for clients with RA to strengthen and preserve muscle groups affecting the involved joints. The client should never approach exercise too aggressively, however. If pain is present for longer than 2 hours after exercise, the client has done too much and should decrease the amount of activity at the next session. During acute exacerbations, performing passive ROM exercises twice a day is optimal therapy. When the disease course is stable, exercise is best done in divided doses three to four times per day. Water exercises are excellent for arthritics, because the buoyancy allows easier joint movement.

Heat and cold therapy raise the client's pain threshold and help decrease muscle spasms. It is useful to use heat or cold in conjunction with exercise to increase joint range of motion and decrease stiffness. Contraindications to heat include poor circulation, decreased sensation, skin infection, heat hypersensitivity, and decreased alertness. Contraindications to cold include vasculitis and Raynaud's phenomenon.

Cold is often more effective for acute pain, whereas heat works better for subacute chronic pain. An easy method of applying cold therapy to a joint is to use a bag of frozen peas. The bag retains its temperature while molding to the involved joint. Methods of heat application include paraffin baths, diathermy, ultrasonography, hydrotherapy, saunas, or showers. Determining factors for this treatment include client preference, ease of use, and cost.

Rest is a necessary therapy for clients with both acute and chronic RA. In acute stages of the illness, the client may have to maintain bed rest for 1 to 2 weeks to allow joint rest and muscle relaxation. Too much rest can result in contracture and permanent damage to the joint, however. Encourage clients with chronic stable RA to alternate activity with rest, allowing 1 to 2 hours of rest during the day and 10 to 12 hours of sleep each night.

SURGICAL APPROACHES Fusions performed in wrists or ankles may increase stability and decrease pain, although joint function is lost. Surgical implants or repair work can increase joint function. Implant procedures generally give good results. Total joint replacements are most effective in the hip, although finger, shoulder, and knee replacements also can be done. Early synovectomy is not beneficial in RA; long-term results show no lasting positive outcome. Arthrodesis and arthroplasty are covered later in this chapter.

Nursing Research Note

Burckhardt C: The impact of arthritis on quality of life. *Nurs Res* 1985; 34(1):11–16.

The quality of life experienced by individuals with arthritis was investigated. The results suggest that positive self-esteem, belief in internal control over health, positive perceptions regarding support, and low negative attitudes toward the illness contributed to a higher quality of life. The severity of the arthritis and subsequent impairment indirectly affected the quality of life through the mediator variables of self-esteem and internal control over health.

Because self-esteem, a sense of personal control over health, supportive relationships, and a low negative attitude toward the illness result in higher levels of perceived quality of life, nursing care should be aimed toward enhancing these variables. Education, and client and family involvement in decision-making and care requirements are possible approaches.

Specific Nursing Measures

Monitor the client's vital signs, level of pain, and other joint symptoms and signs. Continuously evaluate the client for new joint involvement and extra-articular manifestations of RA by assessing all joints, the chest and heart, the eyes, and skin. Follow laboratory results, especially ESR, rheumatoid factor, and x-rays. Monitor the client's weight, and encourage a balanced diet. There is no diet therapy in the treatment of RA except for ensuring good nutrition and ideal weight to decrease stress on joints.

Prepare the client thoroughly for all procedures. Administer medications as ordered, explain their side effects, and evaluate the client's response to the drugs. Watch for gastrointestinal distress when aspirin or NSAIDs are used. Observe for proteinuria, skin rash, and bone marrow depression with gold or penicillamine therapy.

Medicate the client for pain before each exercise session when necessary, and evaluate results. Apply heat or cold therapy, especially after exercise sessions. Encourage the client to manage activities of daily living, and provide enough time to accomplish tasks. Schedule periods of activity alternating with periods of rest. Apply splints as indicated.

Evaluate the client for problems with self-esteem, body image, and depression. Referral to mental health professionals can help clients who are having problems coping with a disease that will markedly alter their lives. Social workers can help clients who face a change in occupation. Inform the client and family about the Arthritis Foundation and its activities, particularly the client support groups and education classes.

Discharge planning involves careful instruction regarding all therapeutic measures to be used at home (eg, exercises and heat or cold treatments). Both client and family or significant others should know all medications to be used and their potential side effects. Emphasize the importance of frequent follow-up visits with the health care provider. There is a case study of a client with RA at the end of this chapter.

Arthrodesis

Arthrodesis is the surgical fusion of a joint to provide stability or relief of pain. Bone grafts and internal fixation devices are used to fuse the joints together. Joint movement is no longer possible after bony union takes place. Arthrodesis is indicated when joint movement causes severe pain or instability, and other measures have failed to relieve it. Such a condition may result from joint disease, such as tuberculosis or arthritis; fractures with nonunion; congenital defects; muscle imbalance from neuromuscular disease; or may follow failure of total joint replacements.

If the joint can be fused in a functional position, it may be more useful to the person than before. That is, a fixed position may allow use of an extremity that otherwise would be impossible because movement is so painful or the joint is unstable. Joints on which arthrodesis is performed include the hip, wrist, spine, ankle, knee, interphalangeal joints, and shoulder. The implications of arthrodesis are summarized in Table 46–3. The implications of internal fixation (see Table 45–7) are pertinent here also.

Nursing Implications

PREOPERATIVE CARE Preoperatively, the nurse should assess the client's understanding of the procedure. Since the intended result is an immobile joint, it is particularly important that the client be aware of the outcome and that any misconceptions be clarified before surgery.

POSTOPERATIVE CARE Postoperatively, check the client's vital signs frequently along with neurovascular status. Any problems with circulation should be reported immediately so the cast can be cut and spread. The extremity

Table 46–3
Arthrodesis: Implications for the Client*

Physiologic Implications	Psychosocial/Lifestyle Implications
Provides relief of pain. Joint is fused into one position, providing joint stability. Weight bearing is not allowed until bony union occurs. Nonunion at the site of attempted fusion is a possible complication.	A pain-free, stable joint should improve the quality of life. The postoperative cast and restricted weight bearing may limit general mobility. A stiff joint may cause a limp or alter the client's ability to move or sit. Body image may be altered because of limited movement; however, the stability may improve body image.

*See Table 45–7 for implications of internal fixation.

should be elevated and ice bags applied intermittently for 24 to 48 hours. There may be a moderate to large amount of bloody drainage on the cast the first few days postoperatively. No weight bearing is allowed until union occurs. Exercises and ambulation are ordered according to the client's progress and the procedure done.

Arthroplasty

Arthroplasty is a type of joint repair in which the diseased articulating surfaces of a joint are replaced by artificial components. In general, the indication for an arthroplasty is a painful, poorly functioning joint. The condition may be the result of rheumatoid, traumatic, or osteoarthritis. In addition, instability, tumors, and pathologic fractures in the joint area may be treated by joint replacement. Hip and knee arthroplasties are the most common. Other joints for which replacement surgery is done include the shoulder, elbow, wrist, fingers, ankle, and toes. The procedures are not as common or as advanced as the hip and knee arthroplasties.

In a total hip replacement, the head and neck of the femur are replaced with a metal femoral component, usually made from stainless steel or Vitallium. The acetabular surface is replaced with a cup-shaped component usually made from high density polyethylene, although sometimes made of metal (Figure 46–8). Both pieces are secured by a bone cement, methyl methacrylate.

There are two general types of knee prostheses, condylar and hinged (Figure 46–9). The condylar type consists of a metal femoral component and a high density polyethylene tibial component. They are concave and convex to fit together. The hinged type is a metal prosthesis with components that fit into the distal femoral shaft and proximal tibial shaft; the two components are connected by a hinge. The hinged type is used mostly for unstable knees with faulty supporting ligaments. Both types are usually cemented into place with methyl methacrylate.

To decrease the chance of wound infection during hip replacement surgery, special precautions are used in the operating room. The number of personnel in the room or moving in and out is limited. A clean air or laminar air flow room may be used to reduce the amount of particles and contaminants in the air. Gowns and drapes made of impervious materials may be used; surgeons may double glove. Antibiotic solutions are used to irrigate the wound. These precautions are taken because the foreign material placed in the body may restrict the body's defense mechanisms, increasing the chances for infection.

Large amounts of IV fluids (typically 2000 to 3000 mL) may be given during surgery to increase the blood volume. This is done so that the blood pressure is maintained when the methyl methacrylate is inserted because the substance causes hypotension (Farrell, 1982). Clients may be placed directly into their bed from the OR table so they will be in the desired postoperative position and not require further transfer. The implications of hip and knee replacement are summarized in Table 46–4.

Nursing Implications

PREOPERATIVE CARE In addition to providing the usual preoperative care for orthopedic surgery, teach the client about the specific restrictions and exercises to be followed postoperatively. In some hospitals, the physical therapist assesses the client preoperatively and teaches some exercises needed for recuperation. An overhead frame and trapeze are placed on the client's bed to teach how to lift.

The client's blood is cross-matched. The nurse may scrub the operative area twice a day with antibacterial soap, and antibiotics may be started prophylactically before surgery, either orally or IV. Clients may start wearing elastic stockings before going to surgery and may go to the operating room in their bed.

POSTOPERATIVE CARE AFTER HIP REPLACEMENT Postoperatively, nursing interventions such as neurovascular assessment, good body alignment, comfort measures, exercises, ambulation, skin care, and preventing the hazards of immobility will be necessary. Complications to watch for and try to prevent are shock, wound infection, thrombophlebitis, pulmonary emboli, and fat emboli.

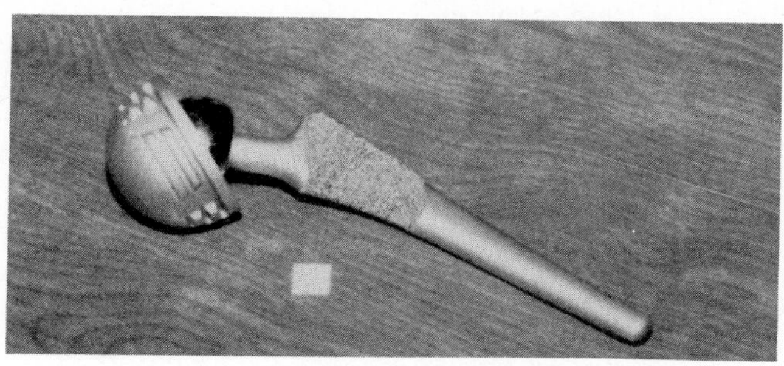

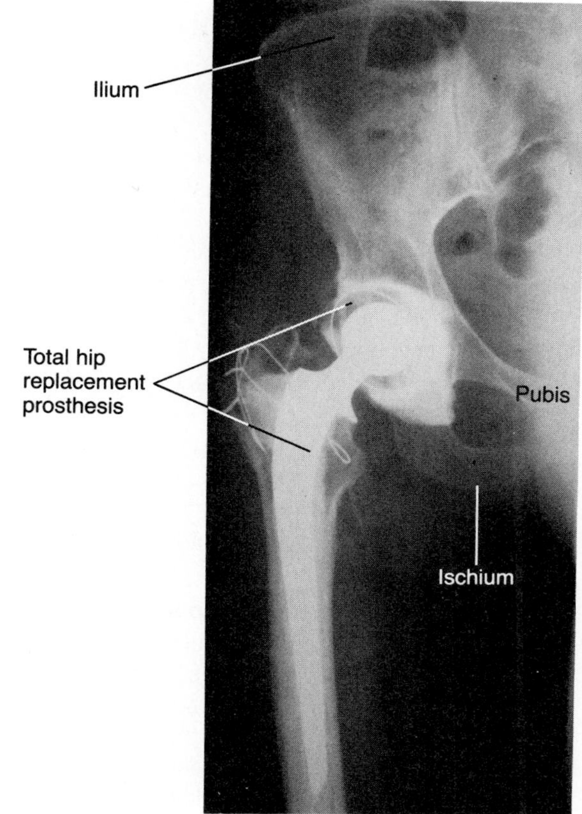

Figure 46–8

Total hip replacement prosthesis. **A.** A standard total hip prosthesis with plastic acetabular component and metal femoral head and neck component. **B.** X-ray of a client with a total hip replacement. *Courtesy Health Care Plan, Buffalo. NY.*

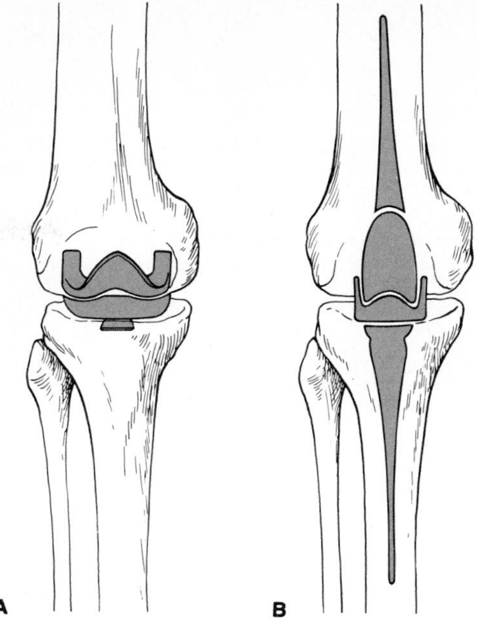

Figure 46–9

Total knee replacement prosthesis. **A.** Condylar type with metal femoral component and plastic tibial component. **B.** Hinged type with hinge connecting femoral and tibial components.

POSITIONING, LIFTING, AND TURNING The position of the client postoperatively is important to prevent hip dislocation. Clients may be placed directly into their beds from the OR table so that they will be in the desired postoperative position and not require further transfer. Required positions vary, depending on the surgical approach as well as the surgeon's preference. The postoperative orders should be clear, and the nurse and client should follow them exactly. The operative hip must be kept in abduction. An abductor pillow or splint may be used, or traction may be applied. Buck's traction, or sometimes Russell's traction may be used to reduce muscle spasm and maintain abduction. The traction may be used continuously for a few days and then applied only at bedtime or discontinued. Rotation of the hip is not generally allowed; the hip should remain in neutral alignment unless specified (some surgeons order slight external rotation). The hip should not be flexed to less than a 90° angle. If elevation of the head of the bed is allowed, it should be only 30° to 45°. Some surgeons allow head elevation only for short periods; the client should be flat some of the time to prevent hip flexion contracture.

The client maintains bed rest for about 2 to 5 days. If turning is not permitted, the staff performs back care and top-to-bottom linen changes by lifting the client straight up in bed. The client lifts with the trapeze and at least three staff members should assist with lifting, one doing the back care. If turning is allowed, orders should specify to which side, because some surgeons prefer turning onto the operative side only. Never turn the client without placing pillows or an abductor splint between the legs. Check a confused client frequently to see that the desired position is maintained.

MONITORING VITAL SIGNS AND DRAINAGE Check the vital signs, the neurovascular status, and the dressing routinely, being careful to observe the part of the dressing under the client. A Hemovac will be in place for about 2 days; keep it deflated and empty it every shift, using aseptic technique to prevent wound infection. Measure and record the nature of the drainage accurately.

MEDICATIONS The client is on IV broad-spectrum antibiotics for about 2 days postoperatively and then receives

Table 46–4
Arthroplasty: Implications for the Client 

Physiologic Implications	Psychosocial/Lifestyle Implications
Provides relief of pain and a functioning, stable joint. Nerves and blood vessels may be damaged during surgical manipulation or by cast or immobilizer. Blood loss may be extensive and require replacement. Specific exercises are necessary to regain strength and function. Temporary local swelling and pain occur from the surgical procedure. Early ambulation is allowed. Complications in the hip itself: wound infection, hip dislocation, loosening of the cement or breaking of the prosthesis. Complications in the knee itself are possible, such as: wound infection, loosening or breaking of the prosthesis, ligament instability, damage to the surrounding bone. Prophylactic antibiotics are necessary when undergoing invasive procedures or dental surgery.	A pain-free, functioning joint should improve quality of life. May be able to resume activities previously impossible due to pain and instability. Positioning restrictions after hip replacement may be an inconvenience. Wearing a cast or immobilizer may be a temporary inconvenience. The recovery period may be lengthy. Use of ambulatory aids is necessary for an extended period of time. Having someone to assist at home is necessary after hip replacement. Caution is required to prevent falls. May return to work in 4–6 months, depending on occupation and progress. Should not become overweight. Habits need to be adapted to prevent hip dislocation (eg, use caution when sitting and standing; avoid soft, low chairs; avoid leg crossing).

oral forms. Prophylactic anticoagulants are sometimes ordered to prevent formation of emboli, and the client may wear elastic stockings on one or both legs. Clients on steroids will need to have increased doses during surgery and for a few days afterward.

COMFORT MEASURES Analgesics and comfort measures are necessary to relieve pain for the first few days. Pain is mostly from muscle spasms and decreases daily. The client returns to a normal diet according to tolerance and should take plenty of fluids. A Foley catheter may be in place; the client uses a fracture bedpan. It may be difficult for clients to void in the restricted position, so the nurse should watch for urinary retention and bladder distention.

SKIN CARE AND EXERCISE Heel protectors and possibly an air mattress are used to protect the skin. The operative thigh is often edematous and tends to develop blisters under the tape; be very careful when changing the dressing. The client's heels, elbows, and sacral region should be observed frequently for signs of breakdown. Heels can be elevated off the bed by means of padding under the calf or with leg troughs.

The client should exercise all unaffected extremities routinely. Isometric exercises and plantar flexion and dorsiflexion on both legs can be done. Incentive spirometry with coughing and deep breathing exercises are also important.

AMBULATION, DISCHARGE, AND HOME CARE. Ambulation begins according to the surgeon's preference and the client's progress. Various routines are used; for example, the physical therapist or the nurse may assist the client out of bed for the first time or a tilt table may be used to help the client into the upright position at first. However it is done, hip flexion should be kept to a minimum. The chair used for sitting should be firm and not low, and it should have arms. Physical therapy may begin anywhere from the second to the sixth day postoperatively. The client progresses from parallel bars to crutches or a walker, then to a cane. The amount of weight bearing allowed varies. The physical therapist teaches exercises used for strengthening muscles and gives the client a regimen to follow. The client learns to go up and down stairs and how to put shoes and socks on without acutely flexing the hip. An elevated toilet seat is used for the same reason.

When preparing clients for discharge, instruct them about all restricted activities, such as those listed in Box 46–2. A printed sheet with prescribed exercises for reference is given to the client. Explain the importance of wearing the elastic stockings for another 6 weeks. The occupational therapist may teach clients how to dress without flexing the hip more than 90°. Explain the need for

Box 46–2
General Home Health Care Guidelines for the Total Hip Replacement Client

Bend the hip only to a 90° angle (right angle), *not less!*

Use a firm chair with arms; seat should be high enough so your hips are not lower than your knees.

*Keep your knees about 12–18 in apart when sitting.

*Do not use a rocking chair; soft, low seats; anything that creates a hammocklike effect.

*Use an elevated toilet seat.

Do not sit for more than 30 minutes at a time. Get up and take a few steps at least every half hour when sitting.

*Do not cross your legs when sitting, standing, or lying.

If allowed to lie on your side, keep a pillow between your legs.

Have someone help with bathing and dressing (eg, putting on your socks) or use special devices.

*Women should avoid high heels.

Use a reacher to pick up objects from the floor or get someone to do it for you. Do not squat or bend way over.

Continue to exercise as instructed by the physical therapist.

Sexual activity may be resumed as long as restricted positions are avoided, such as bending your hip less than a 90° angle and crossing your operative leg beyond your body's midline.

Do not drive a car until your physician permits.

Continue to use whatever aids (walker, crutches, cane) you have learned until instructed otherwise.

Inform your physician if you have a fever; severe pain; redness, swelling, or drainage from your incision; or inability to use your leg.

Keep appointments with your physician for follow-up.

Your physician will instruct you if and when changes in these activities can be made.

*Recommended as lifetime habits.

prophylactic antibiotics during future surgical procedures. Clients should have someone at home to assist them after discharge. The length of hospitalization is about 2 to 3 weeks.

POSTOPERATIVE CARE AFTER KNEE REPLACEMENT With knee replacement surgery there are different restrictions on positioning; traction is not used; and ambulation follows a different course.

The client remains on bed rest for about 1 to 2 days postoperatively, with the operative leg in extension by use of a plaster cast, splint, or knee immobilizer, and elevated on pillows. The head of the bed may be elevated to the level of comfort. If the client is wearing a knee immobilizer, check to see that it is neither too tight nor so loose that it slips downward when the client is ambulating. Depending on the procedure done and the surgeon's preference, the immobilizer may be removed from the second to the tenth day postoperatively, may be replaced at bedtime, and/or used for ambulation only. The client may get out of bed to a chair on the first to second postoperative day. The client stands on the unoperative leg, placing limited weight or no weight (as specified by the surgeon) on the operative leg. When the client is in the chair, the leg must be elevated on pillows at first; eventually, clients will be able to bend their knees and lower their legs.

Exercises may begin 1 to 2 days postoperatively to increase strength and function. Straight leg raising and quadriceps setting exercises are important so the client can begin ambulating when the muscles are strong enough to control leg movement. Passive knee flexion and extension exercises progress to active. Clients need encouragement and reinforcement when exercising because it is difficult and may be exhausting. In physical therapy, they progress from standing between parallel bars to walking with a walker or crutches and learning to climb and descend stairs. Discharge from the hospital occurs about 2 weeks after surgery. Clients will walk with crutches or a walker for about 2 more months. They may progress to a cane and eventually walk unassisted. After discharge, clients must follow a prescribed exercise regimen and may increase their activity as tolerated; progress varies from one client to another.

More recently, continuous passive motion (CPM) has been used postoperatively on clients with total knee replacement. Knee movement is provided by a stationary, electrically powered machine or by a dynamic apparatus of suspended ropes and pulleys. The advantages of this treatment include: greater range of motion, faster relief of postoperative pain, earlier discharge, greater muscle strength maintenance, reduced incidence of adhesions, and stronger fixation of the prosthesis due to stimulation of healing. Mobility is restricted since the client must remain supine the greater portion of the day; therefore, the complications of immobility must be prevented (Strang & Johns, 1984).

Sjögren's Syndrome

Sjögren's syndrome (SS) is a chronic inflammatory disorder characterized by a sicca syndrome—decreased lacrimal gland secretions, which causes dry eyes (keratoconjunctivitis), and decreased salivary gland secretions, which causes a dry mouth (xerostomia)—that occurs along with a connective tissue disease. Originally, SS was most commonly associated with RA, but now it is also linked to systemic lupus erythematosus, progressive systemic sclerosis, polyarteritis nodosa, and polymyositis. There is even a form of SS that is a distinct process in itself with no associated disorder. Sjögren's syndrome is more prevalent in women, with an average age of onset of 50 years.

The etiology of SS is unknown. As with other immune

disorders, 50% of SS clients appear to have an autoimmune response of the body—on the exocrine organs in this instance.

Clinical Manifestations

A slowly developing dryness of the eye occurs that clients often describe as a sensation of a foreign body in the eye or as a sandy or gritty feeling. The client may experience a burning sensation, decreased tearing, and redness of the eye. Thick, ropy strands of discharge may be present at the inner canthus, especially in the morning. Little or no saliva present in the mouth leads to lip cracking; dental caries, and ulcerations of the mouth, tongue, and lips. The client may also have difficulty in chewing, swallowing, and phonation. Nasal dryness results in epistaxis or abnormalities of taste and smell. Lower respiratory tract involvement can cause chronic bronchitis, tenacious sputum, and a dry mouth.

Dyspareunia or a burning sensation in the perineal region may occur because of vaginal dryness. Generalized skin dryness is common. One half of SS clients may develop parotid or submandibular salivary gland enlargement. This is symmetrical and may occur with fever, tenderness, and erythema.

Diagnosis of SS is made when keratoconjunctivitis, xerostomia, and a connective tissue disease are present. When xerostomia and keratoconjunctivitis alone occur, sicca syndrome is the diagnosis.

Medical Measures

Therapeutic measures for SS largely treat its symptoms. Artificial tears (0.5% methylcellulose) help decrease ocular symptoms and prevent local complications. Increasing fluid intake is the primary treatment for xerostomia, although artificial lubricants and sugar-free lozenges may also relieve symptoms. Careful brushing and dental flossing of the teeth are mandatory to maintain oral health. Saline soaks can relieve nasal dryness, and water-soluble lubricants applied at the introitus and into the vagina help prevent dyspareunia. Eucerin cream or any other nonalcohol-based moisturizer is recommended for dry skin therapy.

Specific Nursing Measures

Explain the nature and management of the illness to the client and significant others. Maintain a fresh container of water and other fluids within reach for the hospitalized client to drink. Teach proper oral care. Monitor the client's eyes frequently for infection and other eye symptoms. Explain the importance of avoiding oil-based lubricants for the nose or vagina to avoid lipid pneumonia or vaginitis. Teach the client proper skin care: Little or no soap should be used, and the skin should be lubricated frequently.

SECTION IV

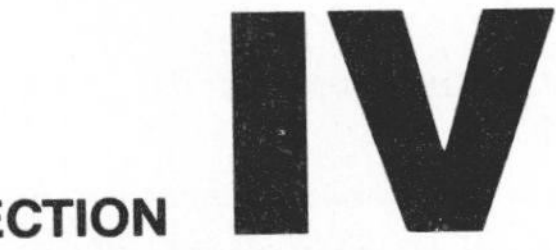

Infectious Disorder

Infectious Arthritis

Infectious arthritis is the inflammation of a joint resulting from an invading organism that attacks the synovium and synovial fluid. Viral, bacterial, and fungal infections all predispose susceptible people to arthritic involvement. Pathogens present in the host circulate freely in the bloodstream and become trapped in the richly perfused synovial membrane, leading to the inflammatory and subsequent degenerative changes. Infectious arthritis is an opportunistic disease that takes advantage of people who are immunocompromised by chronic illness or medication, or who already have joint destruction from an immune disorder such as RA. Diabetics, clients receiving steroids, and the elderly are prime candidates for such joint involvement. Swift diagnosis and treatment can prevent serious degenerative changes.

Clients with infectious arthritis undergo repeated arthrocentesis, which is stressful for people afraid of needles and medical procedures. Clients may require hospitalization for the duration of therapy, which ranges from 2 to 4 weeks in acute disease to as long as 1 year in subacute or chronic infections. Financial difficulties may result for clients and their families through the loss of wage earner's salary and added hospitalization expenses.

The nurse should be available to both the client and significant others for psychologic support, physical care, health education, and monitoring of the client's response to therapy. The control of pain and protection of the involved joint or joints are priorities of nursing care. The nurse who is familiar with the pathophysiology of the infections and the differences between the various invading organisms will know when aggressive therapy is needed to prevent destruction versus when the disease is self-limiting and will lead to little or no residual damage.

Bacterial Arthritis

Bacterial infections most commonly affect clients who are unable to resist invading organisms. The old, young, and those who have compromised defense mechanisms because of chronic illness or immunosuppressive drugs are especially susceptible. A primary bacterial source of infection, such as pneumonia, endocarditis, or a simple urinary tract infection, is prerequisite for the arthritis.

Gram-positive cocci such as staphylococci, gram-positive rods, mycobacteria, and *Treponema* present a clinical picture of similar arthritic and systemic components. Onset of the arthritis is usually abrupt, and the client has a single hot, erythematous, swollen joint, usually the knee. X-rays demonstrate soft tissue swelling soon after onset. After several weeks of disease activity, osteomyelitis may be visualized. In general, the client feels ill and is febrile with shaking chills. Leukocytosis is present in 50% of clients.

Gonococcal infections, the most common cause of bacterial arthritis, are the exceptions to the rule. This gram-negative coccus usually affects young, healthy, sexually active adults (women more often than men). People who develop gonococcal arthritis usually experience fever at its onset, with migratory polyarthralgias and polyarthritis. Tenosynovitis is common in the upper extremities, expecially in the wrists and small joints of the fingers. A generalized rash occurs two-thirds of the time and may involve maculopapular, pustular, vesicular, or bullous lesions. Of clients with gonococcal arthritis, 30% to 50% have a purulent joint effusion; the rest have a sterile effusion.

Tuberculosis (TBC) arthritis, caused by the bacillus *Mycobacterium tuberculosis,* was common in the past and still must be considered in a differential diagnosis for infectious arthritis. Its onset is insidious, usually monoarticular, and primarily affecting the hips or knees. The client may not have concurrent active TBC but has a positive tuberculin skin test and usually shows evidence of previous TBC on chest x-ray. Tubercle bacilli will be present in the synovial fluid.

Viral Arthritis

Arthritis of viral origin is an interesting subunit of infectious arthritis. Its transmission, like that of any other infectious agent, is through the bloodstream. The viral arthritic process may have all the signs of a much more harmful process, such as RA, but will resolve of its own accord. Viral arthritis is a self-limiting infection in which the potential for joint damage is minimal. The viral illnesses most commonly responsible for secondary arthralgias include rubella, mumps, herpes, mononucleosis, and hepatitis A or B. Viral arthritis also can be acquired after immunization with live rubella virus.

Fungal Arthritis

Four fungal diseases are most commonly associated with the development of fungal arthritis: coccidioidomycosis, sporotrichosis, blastomycosis, and candidiasis. In general, arthralgias occur with the primary infection from the fungi without residual joint damage. However, joint destruction is possible when the organism disseminates into a secondary arthritis. Treatment of fungal arthritis is the same for all fungal organisms.

Medical Measures

The invading organism in infectious arthritis should be identified as quickly as possible to prevent joint destruction. Isolating the organism will guide in the selection of antibiotics and the level of aggressiveness needed to control the infection. Pathogens are identified through the aspiration of synovial fluid, synovial fluid cultures, and synovial biopsy. Appropriate antimicrobial medications are then instituted. For example, isoniazid or rifampin may be given for TBC arthritis, and amphotericin B may be used to treat fungal arthritis.

Depending on the severity of the arthritis, the client may be kept in bed and given aspirin or an NSAID in addition to the antimicrobial agent. The client with a viral arthritis will be on aspirin or NSAIDs alone, because there are currently no effective antiviral agents.

A key diagnostic and therapeutic point with gonococcal arthritis compared with other kinds of bacterial arthritis is the rapid resolution of symptoms upon the administration of penicillin or other appropriate antibiotic therapy. Within 24 to 48 hours, the joint effusion begins resolving, making routine aspirations unnecessary. This rapid recovery after drug therapy initiation helps provide a diagnosis in cases where the bacterium *Neisseria gonorrhoeae* has not been isolated from either the involved joint or the genitourinary tract.

Other therapeutic measures for infectious arthritis include surgical excision of the affected synovium in instances where destruction of the joint cartilage, tendons, or both appears imminent.

Specific Nursing Measures

In taking the client's history, the nurse should realize that it is a key to diagnosis. Has the client recently had a viral illness (eg, rubella, mumps, or hepatitis)? Has the client had a urinary tract infection, pneumonia, or other bacterial infection? Has the client received any recent immunizations? Question the client about sexual activity and whether the partner has any known infection. Ask about dysuria and urgency or frequency related to urination because gonorrhea may cause urinary symptoms. Since fungal infections are often endemic to certain areas of the country, ask about recent travel. Is the client taking immunosuppressants? Does the client have a history of TBC or positive tuberculin test? Has the client had any recent invasive diagnostic studies or treatments (eg, hyperalimentation, venipuncture, or cystoscopy)? Also investigate thoroughly the onset of the arthritis using the seven dimensions discussed in Chapter 5.

To protect the intra- and extra-articular structure from future damage and reduce the client's discomfort, immobilize the involved joint during the acute arthritic stage. Because the client is usually on complete bed rest, active and passive ROM exercises for uninvolved joints are essential. Apply warm compresses to the involved joint.

Assess the involved joint frequently for drainage and any change in condition. Use sterile technique with any dressing changes. Administer antimicrobials, anti-inflammatory agents, and analgesics as ordered, and observe the client carefully for side effects.

For the client receiving parenteral fluids, measure intake and output accurately. Promote cooling for the client with fever by frequent sponging, encouraging fluids, and using a hypothermia blanket, if necessary. Monitor laboratory test results daily, especially the results of culture and sensitivity tests. Assist with joint aspirations or synovial biopsy using proper aseptic technique.

Home Health Care

The education of the client and significant others for home care should include instruction about ROM exercises to maintain joint mobility; dressing change techniques and wound care, if appropriate; and the names, dosages, actions, and potential side effects of all medications to be taken at home. The client and others involved should be aware of symptoms and signs of repeated infection (eg, increased pain, fever, swelling, redness, and drainage). They must take care to avoid any trauma to the joint.

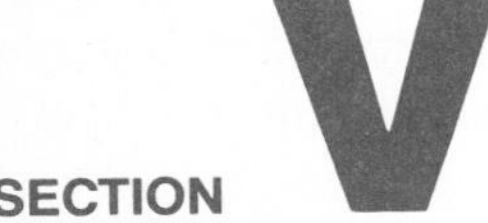

SECTION V

Traumatic Disorders

Permanent structural changes may occur in a joint as a result of cartilage and capsular tears, detachment of menisci, hemorrhagic effusions, articular fractures, or repetitive trauma. Because of the realignment of involved bone, bursa, and tendons, a mechanical deterioration of articular cartilage results in DJD.

Acute traumatic arthritis may result from unexpected force, such as sports or automobile accidents. Repetitive trauma is an internal occurrence—a chronic injury resulting from repeated smaller stresses to a joint through vibrations, blows, abnormal strain, or position. This type of injury is related to occupation and lifestyle (eg, the stress placed on the MTP joints of a ballerina or the knees of a jogger). Over time, repetitive trauma may realign the joint and lead to the same result as an acute injury.

The client with traumatic arthritis must make lifestyle changes. The football player who has developed DJD of the knees as a result of multiple tackles may need to wear special equipment or stop playing. The factory worker exposed to repeated vibratory trauma may need a different job assignment. As obvious as these solutions are, they may not be popular with the client, and the decision to make a lifestyle change must come from the client. The responsibility of the care provider is to give the client accurate information about the alternatives available.

The nurse plays an important role in the therapeutic and preventive care of traumatic disorders. As the first person on the scene of an accident, the nurse may be able to prevent any residual damage by protecting the limb by splinting, elevating the area, applying ice, and not allowing weight on the area. At the workplace, the nurse can evaluate jobs for injury and health risks. It may be possible to identify tasks that expose employees to repetitive trauma; employees then can rotate through these jobs rather than be assigned permanently to potentially harmful tasks.

Joint Effusions

Joint effusions can occur as a result of simple trauma or secondary fractures, internal derangements, or severe sprains. Within 24 hours after a blow to the joint, synovial fluid accumulates. If blood vessels in the synovium are broken, a hemarthrosis also occurs. The knee is most commonly affected by this injury.

Clinical Manifestations

In simple traumatic synovitis, joint swelling with mild pain occurs. Aspiration of the joint produces clear fluid with elevated protein content and decreased viscosity. Hemarthrosis, which usually develops from 15 minutes to 2 hours after the trauma, is usually more painful than a clear effusion and is accompanied by low-grade fever. Aspiration of the joint produces bloody fluid. Diagnosis of traumatic synovitis is primarily by physical examination, but x-ray examination is done to rule out fracture.

Medical and Specific Nursing Measures

Apply ice initially for 30 minutes q.i.d. to reduce swelling and relieve pain. After the first 24 hours, apply moist heat to the area for 30 minutes q.i.d. Repeated joint aspirations are necessary if fluid reaccumulates. Assist the physician with joint aspirations. Compression dressings applied to the joint, along with bed rest or limited weight bearing, may be necessary, depending on the severity of the injury.

Instruct the client in the application of cold and heat. Emphasize the need to protect the joint while pain is present to prevent reinjury. Teach the use of crutches, if necessary.

Dislocation and Subluxation

When a joint's articulating surfaces are completely displaced because of trauma, it is termed a dislocation. Partial displacement of the articulating surfaces results in a subluxation. Both subluxations and dislocations can damage soft tissues, nerves, or blood vessels if not attended to promptly. The joints most often affected are shoulders, wrists, elbows, fingers, hips, knees, and ankles.

Clinical Manifestations

After injury, the joint appears deformed; it is tender, and motion is limited. The involved extremity is shortened. Joint pain may be intense, especially if articular surface fractures are present. With immediate treatment, there is good prognosis. However, bone necrosis can result if reduction of the subluxation or dislocation is delayed.

The diagnosis is made through physical examination and client history. X-rays are taken to evaluate joint displacement and to determine whether fractures are present.

Medical Measures

The longer the delay in correcting a joint displacement, the more difficult the procedure becomes because of edema and muscle spasms. Two types of procedures can correct this injury. Closed reduction is manual traction done under local or general anesthesia. Narcotics may be given for analgesia, and tranquilizers are administered for their antispasmodic effect. Open reduction is done where wire fixation of the joint or repair of torn ligaments is necessary. A splint, cast, or traction is used for 3 to 6 weeks after reduction.

Specific Nursing Measures

At the accident site, the nurse should splint the joint as is—even if crooked—to prevent further damage. Apply ice to decrease pain and swelling.

The hospitalized client requires immediate orthopedic examination. Observe the area distal to the injury for evidence of vascular damage (pallor, absent pulse, or abnormal coolness) and nerve damage (paresthesia or paralysis).

After reduction, monitor respirations and keep a ventilating bag and airway at the bedside, since the narcotics and tranquilizers administered can depress respirations. Check the dressing or cast for pressure that may impair blood flow. Instruct the client regarding gradual mobilization of the joint when the dressing or cast is removed.

Tendon Surgery

Tendon surgery is indicated for laceration or rupture of a tendon and for an avulsion fracture, in which a tendon tears away still attached to a fragment of the bone. Traumatic damage to a tendon causes loss of function and pain. Other indications for tendon surgery are recurrent dislocation and deformity from congenital or neuromuscular conditions.

Various methods of surgical restoration are used. A tendon may be transplanted, (ie, repositioned to alter motion); or it may be lenghtened or divided to achieve the desired result. A tendon that is torn or ruptured may be sutured back together or reinserted into the bone. Tendons can also be transferred from elsewhere in the body, possibly to restore movement to a paralytic limb. An avulsion fracture may need open reduction and internal fixation. The implications of tendon surgery are summarized in Table 46–5.

Nursing Implications

PREOPERATIVE CARE The preoperative care is like that for other orthopedic clients. The client should be taught the exercises necessary for recovery, such as straight leg raising and quadriceps setting exercises for patellar tendon surgery.

POSTOPERATIVE CARE Routine postoperative care is necessary, as well as checking neurovascular status frequently, elevating the extremity, and applying ice intermittently for 24 to 48 hours. Observe the dressing or cast when checking vital signs. Postoperative pain may be severe and require analgesics and comfort measures. The client with upper extremity surgery will need assistance with ADL and should have the bedside stand placed within reach of the unaffected arm.

The surgeon should specify limitations in weight bearing and use of the limb. A physical therapy program will help restore functioning and teach the use of ambulatory

Table 46–5
Tendon Surgery: Implications for the Client 

Physiologic Implications	Psychosocial/Lifestyle Implications
May provide normal function and stability.	Return to previous activity level.
Temporary local swelling and pain occur from the procedure.	For a congenital condition, new movement may be possible allowing greater independence.
An extensive exercise program may be necessary to regain strength and function.	Assistance with ADL is necessary for those with upper extremity surgery.
Ambulatory aids will be necessary for lower extremity surgery.	Exercise program may require a great deal of work.
Potential complications: joint instability, recurrent weakness, movement difficulty, failure of the surgery, nerve or blood vessel damage, and wound infection.	Wearing a cast or immobilizer may be necessary for 3 to 8 weeks, depending on the tendon involved.
	Learning the use of ambulatory aids is necessary for lower extremity surgery.

Table 46–6
Meniscectomy: Implications for the Client 

Physiologic Implications	Psychosocial/Lifestyle Implications
Provides relief of pain, eliminates locking.	Diminishes the fear of the knee locking.
Produces mild rotary instability of the knee.	The closed procedure (arthroscopy) allows faster recovery than the open procedure.
Exercises strengthen the muscles to overcome this.	Crutches required for about 10 days after arthroscopic surgery, and 6 weeks after open meniscectomy.
Partial regeneration of the meniscus may occur.	

aids. The allowed movement, required exercises, and ambulatory aids will be determined by the specific procedure. The client should have a good understanding of all these when discharged from the hospital.

Meniscectomy

A meniscectomy is a surgical procedure in which a torn or damaged meniscus (semilunar cartilage) is removed from the knee joint. The torn part alone or the entire meniscus may be removed. Meniscectomy is performed through an arthroscope (described in Chapter 43) whenever possible because it is less traumatic than open surgery.

When a meniscus is torn, it causes symptoms such as pain, tenderness, limited motion, mild effusion, and possibly locking. The knee locks when the torn cartilage locates between the femur and tibia and interferes with motion. When locked, it can be flexed but not extended. A torn meniscus commonly occurs from a twisting motion of the knee as in athletic injuries. Ligaments of the knee are often injured at the same time.

The medial meniscus is torn most often. A torn meniscus will not heal and must be removed if it is causing difficulty. Surgery is not always necessary, but it is performed if conservative treatment is not successful. The general implications of meniscectomy for the client are summarized in Table 46–6.

Nursing Implications

PREOPERATIVE CARE Preoperatively, the care is like that for other orthopedic surgery clients. Teach quadriceps setting and straight leg raising exercises preoperatively.

POSTOPERATIVE CARE Postoperatively, the nurse assesses vital signs, neurovascular status, and the dressing frequently. The leg is elevated, and ice may be applied intermittently for about 24 hours. All other joints should be exercised. A physical therapy program is necessary to help the client strengthen the muscles. Exercise begins with quadriceps setting and straight leg raising, progressing to crutch walking. The progress depends on how well muscle strength is regained.

Chapter Highlights

Gout is a disease that produces joint inflammation as a result of deposition of uric acid crystals in the articular cartilage.

Low back pain can have a multiplicity of causes including congenital anomalies, leg length discrepancies, asymmetrical development of the spine, weak abdominal muscles, acquired injuries, sedentary lifestyle, and/or obesity.

Low back strain is the most common cause of low back pain. It is a self-limiting condition treated with bed rest, analgesia, muscle relaxants, heat or ice, and flexion exercises.

The nurse's main role in back disorders is prevention. Clients should be taught proper lifting techniques, muscle strengthening exercises, and the importance of proper posture.

Screening for and treatment of scoliosis is important in early adolescence, because untreated, it can lead to decreased lung capacity, back pain, degenerative arthritis of the spine, intervertebral disk disease, and sciatica.

Carpal tunnel syndrome is an entrapment of the median nerve due to tenosynovitis, trauma, rheumatoid arthritis, gout, edema of pregnancy, or premenstrual edema. Paresthesia of the thumb, index, middle, and medial side of the ring finger occur.

Degenerative joint disease (DJD), also called osteoarthritis, is primarily a disorder of articular cartilage resulting from "wear and tear" (primary) or traumatic causes (secondary). The pain of DJD is gradual in onset, most severe after activity, and relieved with rest.

The treatment goals of DJD are to relieve pain, decrease swelling, increase joint function, and allow the client to lead a more active lifestyle. Aspirin or NSAIDs, heat or ice, exercise, and possibly surgery can help to relieve the discomfort and achieve treatment goals.

Rheumatoid arthritis (RA) is a systemic disease characterized primarily by chronic inflammation of the synovial lining of joints. Symmetrical swelling of joints occurs most commonly in the MCPs, PIPs, MTPs, and wrists.

Because of the systemic nature of RA, clients should temper activity with periods of rest to avoid fatigue.

Exercise is indicated for clients with RA to strengthen and preserve muscle groups around involved joints.

Sjögren's syndrome is a chronic inflammatory disorder characterized by decreased lacrimal gland and salivary gland secretions. Treatment for Sjögren's syndrome is mainly symptomatic.

Infectious arthritis can occur due to bacterial, viral, or fungal invasion of the richly perfused joint synovium and synovial fluid. The invading organism must be identified early in the course of the arthritis so that appropriate therapy can be initiated. Joint destruction occurs swiftly with fungal and certain bacterial infections, whereas viral arthritis is a self-limiting illness.

Traumatic arthritis may occur from a sudden, unexpected force, or from repeated trauma. Joint effusions, dislocations, and subluxations occur as a result of acute trauma. If not attended to promptly, long-term damage occurs to the joint and its surrounding soft tissue.

Bibliography

Agee BL, Herman C: Cervical logrolling on a standard hospital bed. *Am J Nurs* 1984; 84(3):315–318.

Bartell L: Bunionectomies. *Ortho Nurs* 1985; 4(1):21–28.

Burckhardt CS: The impact of arthritis on quality of life. *Nurs Res* 1985; 34(1):11–16.

Chaffman M, Brogden RN, Heel RC: Auranofin—A preliminary review of its pharmacological properties and therapeutic use in rheumatoid arthritis. *Drugs* 1984; 27:378–424.

Clegg DO, Ward JR: Slow-acting anti-rheumatic drug therapy for rheumatoid arthritis. *Nurse Prac* 1987; 12(3):44–52.

Cohen LM, Killian PJ: The spondyloarthropathies: The spondylitis associated disorders. *Postgrad Med* 1982; 72(5):127–136.

Delany P: Neurologic complications of systemic lupus erythematosus. *Am Fam Physician* (July)1983; 28(1):191–193.

Dickinson GR: A home care program for patients with rheumatoid arthritis. *Nurs Clin North Am* 1982; 25(9):1048–1053.

Dickinson GR, Gorman TK: Adult arthritis: The assessment. *Am J Nurs* 1983; 83(2):262–265.

Gallagher LL: Shoulder arthroplasty. *Nurs 80* 1980; 10(7):46–49.

Harris CJ: Rheumatoid arthritis and the pregnant woman. *Am J Nurs* 1985; 85(4):414–417.

Hawley DH (editor): Symposium on arthritis and related rheumatic diseases. *Nurs Clin North Am* (Dec) 1984; 19(4):565–725.

Kelley WN et al: *Textbook of Rheumatology.* Philadelphia: Saunders, 1981.

Kelsey J et al: Acute prolapsed lumbar disc: An epidemiologic study with special reference to driving automobiles and cigarette smoking. *Spine* 1984; 9:608.

Koerner ME, Dickerson GR: Adult arthritis. *Am J Nurs* 1983; 83(2):255–262.

Laborde JM, Powers MJ: Life satisfaction, health control orientation, and illness related factors in persons with osteoarthritis. *Res Nurs Health* 1985; 8(2):183–190.

Lambert VA: Study of factors associated with psychological well-being in rheumatoid arthritic women. *Image* (Spring) 1985; 17(2):50–53.

Lorig KR: Arthritis self-management: A patient education program. *Rehabil Nurs* 1982; 7(4):16–19.

Meenan RF et al: The arthritis impact measurement scales: Further investigation of a health status measure. *Arthritis Rheum* 1982; 25(9):1048–1053.

Miller BK, Gregory M: Carpal tunnel syndrome. *AORN J* 1983; 38:525–532.

Owen BD: How to avoid that aching back. *Am J Nurs* 1980; 80(5):894–897.

Owen BD, Damron CF: Personal characteristics and back injury among hospital nursing personnel. *Res Nurs Health* 1984; 7:305–313.

Petersdorf RG et al: *Harrison's Principles of Internal Medicine,* 10th ed. New York: McGraw–Hill, 1983.

Phillips KF: The use of gold therapy with rheumatoid arthritis. *Ortho Nurs* (July/Aug) 1983; 2(4):31–34.

Rodman GO, Schumacher HR, Zvaifler NJ: *Primer on the Rheumatic Diseases.* Atlanta: Arthritis Foundation, 1983.

Simpson CF: Heat, cold or both. *Am J Nurs* 1983, pp 270–273.

Smith WS: Letter to doctors and pharmacists dated July 19, 1984, regarding the neurologic complications following use of chymopapain. Smith Laboratories, Inc. 1984.

Steinberg FU: *Care of the Geriatric Patient.* St. Louis: Mosby, 1983.

Strang EL, Johns JL: Nursing care of the patient treated with continuous passive motion following total knee arthroplasty. *Ortho Nurs* 1984; 3(6):27–32.

Strodthoff C: Pathophysiology of rheumatoid arthritis. *Nurse Pract* (June) 1982; 7:34–35.

Walsh CR, Wirth CR: Total knee arthroplasty: Biomechanical and nursing considerations. *Ortho Nurs* 1985; 4(1):29–34, 70.

Waxman J: Localized rheumatologic diseases. *Postgrad Med* 1983; 75(2):189–196.

Weinblatt ME et al: Efficacy of low dose methotrexate in rheumatoid arthritis. *N Engl J Med* 1985; 312:818–822.

CASE STUDY

The Client With Rheumatoid Arthritis

I. Descriptive Data

Mr David Watts, a 45-year-old black male who has had rheumatoid arthritis (RA) for 5 years, was seen by his primary physician at the HMO 1 month ago for a pruritic, generalized skin rash and given a tentative diagnosis of "gold reaction." He comes to the HMO's Rheumatology Department today for further evaluation and recommendations.

II. Personal Data

Date: Oct 2, 1987
ID Number: 00000-00-0
Full Name: David Ernest Watts
Address: 35 Beach St., Hanover, NY 14002
Telephone: Home: 000-0000
Work: None
Sex: Male
Marital Status: Married
Age: 45
Birthdate: 12-12-41
Religion: Baha'i
Race/Culture: Black
Occupation: Presently on disability. Formerly employed as a millwright.
Primary Health Care Provider: Paul Marine, MD

III. Health History

Source of Information: Client and medical records
Reliability of Informant: Client is reliable but reticent to reveal information unless specifically questioned
Chief Concern: "My wrists, hands, knees, and feet are swollen and hurt all the time. The pain even wakes me up when I try to roll over at night."

History of Present Illness:

Mr Watts joined the HMO in 1979. Shortly thereafter, he developed migratory joint pains, which involved his hands, his wrists, shoulders, knees, and metatarsals of his feet. These acute problems were unifocal and resolved following application of moist heat, rest, and nonsteroidal anti-inflammatory (NSAID) therapy. Laboratory studies were within normal limits. X-rays of the hands showed soft-tissue swelling.

In March 1980, Mr Watts developed a symmetrical painful swelling of his MCPs, PIPs, wrists, knees, and metatarsals. He experienced morning stiffness, which would gradually lessen by afternoon and lost 20 lb in 6 weeks. He also developed anorexia and chronic fatigue. A rheumatoid factor was positive with a titer of 1:1640. An ANA was positive with a diffuse pattern and a titer of 1:20. ESR was 60 mm/h. At this point, he was diagnosed as having RA.

His symptoms became progressively worse as he continued to work. Finally, he took a disability leave from his job with a local car manufacturer, per his physician's advice. ASA and NSAIDs were not sufficient to control Mr. Watts's inflammation and arthralgias, and he was given intermittent oral steroids to control symptoms. Since this therapy is not recommended long-term, gold therapy was initiated 12/83. A considerable improvement in his condition was noted by the spring of 1984, and he was maintained on gold salts (Myochrysine) 50 mg IM q.4 weeks, sulindac 200 mg b.i.d., and acetaminophen p.r.n.

Five weeks ago, a maculopapular, pruritic rash started on the client's anterior and posterior thorax, arms, and legs. It was determined that the gold injections were the probable cause, and the drug was discontinued. With questioning, Mr Watts admits to morning stiffness lasting approximately 3 hours. He has increased pain and swelling of his MCPs, PIPs, wrists, and knees. He is currently taking sulindac 200 mg b.i.d., ASA gr X q.4 h, and diphenhydramine 25 mg t.i.d. p.r.n. for pruritus (has not needed any for past 1 week). He appears discouraged with this present setback and voices fear that he will never be as well again as he was with the gold injections.

Past Health History:

Childhood: Mumps, measles, chickenpox

Immunizations: Tetanus toxoid, 1979; unsure of other immunizations

Medical Problems: No other problems but RA

Surgeries: Tonsillectomy, 1946; appendectomy, 1958

Transfusions: None

Special Diagnostic Procedures: None

Trauma: Fracture right radius age 10 with no sequelae

Medications: Diphenhydramine (Benadryl), 25 mg PO t.i.d. p.r.n.
Sulindac (Clinoril), 200 mg b.i.d.
ASA gr X q.4 h p.r.n.

Family History:

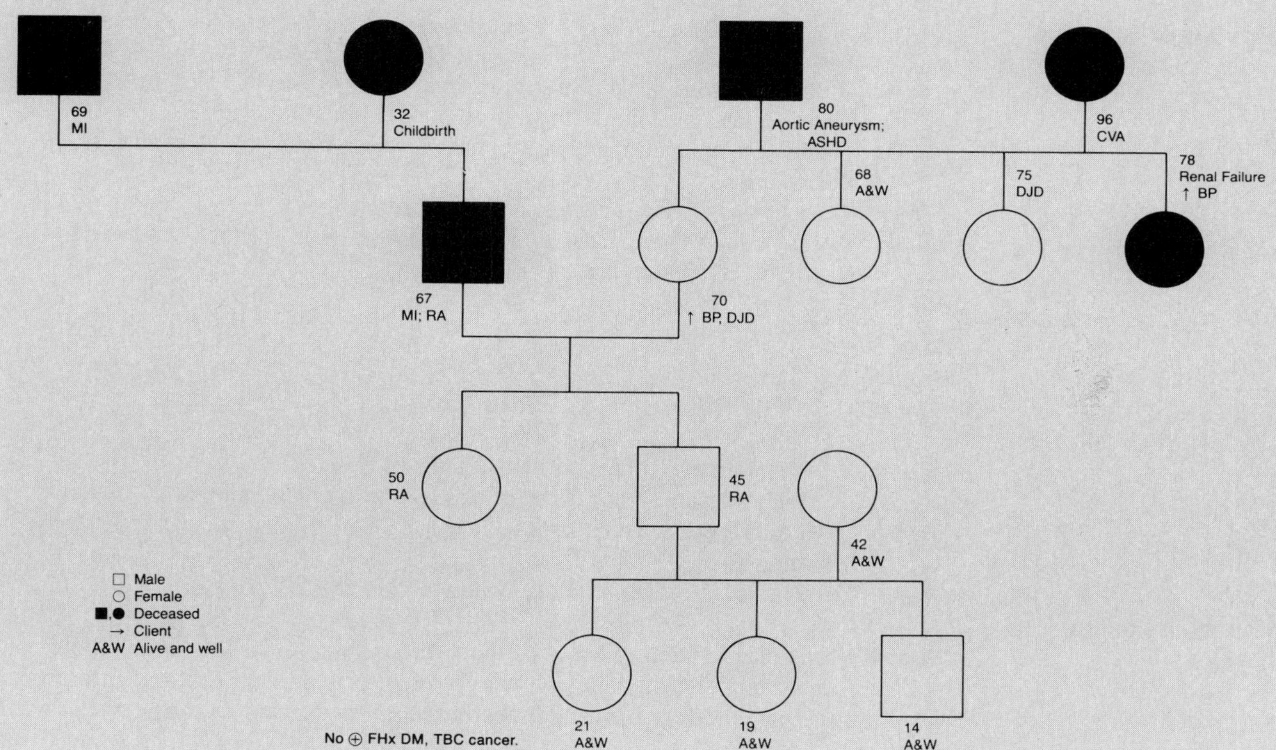

Personal/Social History: Lives with spouse and children in a modest split-level home, which they own. Mr Watts spends his time on a woodworking hobby that he hopes to turn into a full-time business. At present, he sells his wood name plates,

(continued)

The Client With Rheumatoid Arthritis

sconces, and wall hangings at craft shows and fairs to supplement his family's income. Drives his own car. Son and Mr Watts care for outside home maintenance.

High school graduate. Worked as a millwright for 22 years before taking disability leave. There are no current financial problems because he had good personal disability coverage.

Habits: Eats three balanced meals a day. Loses weight whenever RA is in severe exacerbation. Has not felt capable of exercising regularly. Most of exercise comes from walking when RA is in remission. Smokes 1½ packs of cigarettes a day for 28 years. Has rare ETOH intake. Attempts to sleep 7 hours a night, but pain has been waking him; he then watches late night television for distraction. He will rest for 1 to 2 hours in the afternoon if arthritis is in exacerbation.

Sexual Functioning: Sexually active with wife without difficulties.

Coping Pattern: Tends to ignore or deny the chronicity of RA; alters medications on his own and misses appointments with the physician when he feels well. Wife and children are supportive to client; family is close-knit; outside support systems limited.

Review of Systems: States overall health is good, but fatigue is a chronic problem that interferes with activities.

Skin: Rash has resolved; no current pruritus.

Eyes: Requires glasses for reading but otherwise has good vision.

Mouth: Has noted dry mouth and lack of saliva, which makes swallowing difficult periodically.

Lungs: No cough, dyspnea, or pain with deep breath.

Vascular: Notes numbness and blanching of fingers with cold weather, followed by erythema of involved areas with warming.

IV. Physical Assessment

Weight: 148 lb

Height: 6 ft 2 in.

Vital Signs: T.98°F(36.7°C); P. 88; R. 20; BP 120/76

Relevant Organ Systems:

Skin: Brown, warm to touch, without lesions or nodules

Lungs: Normal resonance with percussion; clear to auscultation A & P

Heart: PMI at 5th LICS, medial to MCL; apical pulse 88/min, regular; no rub, ⓜ, or gallop

Vascular: 2 + brachial, radial, femoral, popliteal, DP, and PT pulses

Musculoskeletal:

Hands: Bony enlargement of MCPs, PIPs with swelling, erythema; areas warm to touch, tender, with "boggy" texture on palpation; ulnar drift and interthenar wasting noted; grip strength decreased; 2 cm ganglion cyst on dorsum of left hand

Wrists: 1 + effusion of right wrist; bilaterally tender radial styloids; limitation of motion noted bilaterally

Shoulders: 45° lateral abduction of right arm with tenderness

Knees: 3 + effusion of right knee; 1 + effusion of left; crepitation palpable with ROM; "doughy" texture to joints on palpation

Posture and balance are within normal limits. Client limps, favoring right leg.

V. Diagnostic Data

- Bilateral x-ray of hands and knees show joint space narrowing and bony erosions.
- CBC: WBC 5.9, RBC 4.8, Hgb 13.4, Hct 39.8%, MCV 84, MCHC 33.8
- Urinalysis: Color: yellow; clarity: clear; specific gravity: 1.013; protein, glucose, ketones, blood: negative; 0–2 WBCs, O–1 epithelial cells
- Erythrocyte sedimentation rate (ESR): 68 mm/h
- ANA positive—1:40 titer with diffuse pattern
- Rheumatoid factor—1:640
- Serum complement—within normal limits

VI. Summary

After evaluating Mr Watts, his rheumatologist concurred with the diagnosis of gold toxicity rash and decided to change to penicillamine. Penicillamine 250 mg $\bar{\dot{\text{i}}}$ q.d. for 2 weeks and then b.i.d. after that time was prescribed. Mr Watts was advised of the toxic effects of the medication and told to return for a follow-up appointment in 1 month.

VII. Nursing Care Plan, by Nursing Diagnosis

Client Care Goals	Plan/Nursing Implementation	Expected Outcomes
Mobility, impaired physical related to chronic pain and stiffness		
Reduce or eliminate pain and diminish joint stiffness and swelling	Suggest keeping a time chart for medications; stress importance of maintaining a blood level for medications; encourage to alternate rest with periods of light activity	Will take NSAIDs and acetaminophen on a regular schedule; will begin penicillamine as directed; will avoid activities that cause further joint pain/stiffness or swelling
Activity intolerance related to weakness and fatigue secondary to exacerbation of disease		
Decrease fatigue	Plan with client a realistic rest schedule (eg, 2 hours midmorning and midafternoon) until acute flare-up resolves	Client will moderate activities and maintain a specific rest schedule to decrease fatigue
Role performance, altered related to chronic illness		
Share feelings and frustrations	Allow time at appointment sessions for client to discuss feelings, share frustrations; organize a group session of clients who have RA to allow mutual support	Acceptance of present physical situation; improved coping ability
Health maintenance, altered related to necessity for major lifestyle change		
Understand importance of following medication regimen and activity modifications	Instruct in pathophysiology of RA and in the importance of long-term management, including compliance with medication regimen, proper joint rest, and follow-up care	Client will continue medication as instructed; client will plan rest and activity periods carefully; client will keep follow-up appointments
Knowledge deficit related to current drug therapy		
Recognize signs of adverse drug reactions	Instruct in benign and serious side effects of penicillamine (pruritic rash, abnormal taste sensation, renal damage)	Will competently manage penicillamine therapy and will contact physician if a problem occurs

(continued)

CASE STUDY (continued)

The Client With Rheumatoid Arthritis

Knowledge deficit related to complications of RA		
Explain need for joint exercise to prevent contracture	Instruct client in ROM exercises to be done when joint is not acutely inflamed; explain contracture formation; refer to physical therapy if available	Client will demonstrate more joint ROM and express confidence in managing his condition
Nutrition, altered related to inadequate intake during exacerbations of disease		
Discuss proper nutrition and importance of keeping up nutritional status when exacerbations of RA occur	Discuss food likes and dislikes with client and offer suggestions for adding more calories to diet	Maintains present weight during acute flare-ups; gains 5 to 10 lb when feeling good

UNIT 11

The Client With Reproductive System Dysfunction

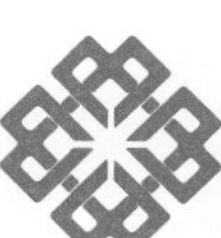

CHAPTER **47**

The Reproductive System in Health and Illness

Objectives

When you have finished reading this chapter, you should be able to:

Describe the structures of the external and internal genitalia and discuss their function.

Trace changes in hormone secretion and their effects in women and men from puberty to mature adulthood.

Describe the four phases of sexual response.

Compare the parallels between the female and male reproductive systems.

Identify the variations in bleeding in women and the major causes and characteristics of pelvic pain and the gonadal endocrine disturbances of men.

Discuss the interrelatedness of the reproductive system with the other body systems.

Explain the psychosocial influences on the well-being and dysfunction of the reproductive system in adolescence, young and middle adulthood, and menopause.

The purpose of any reproductive system is propagation of the species. In human beings, the reproductive organs are also a means for obtaining sexual satisfaction and pleasure. In accomplishing these primary tasks, the reproductive system has significant effects on growth, cellular metabolism, general well-being, and other body systems.

Although the structures of the reproductive system are localized, the system's functions depend on and affect many other structures and systems. The reproductive system operates in a feedback relation to the neurologic and endocrine systems, and the hormones involved affect many other parts of the body.

Both the normal variations and the dysfunctions of the reproductive system may produce great anxiety because of the relation of the system to women's and men's sexual identity, social roles, and body image. Although failure within the system usually does not have life-threatening effects on the individual, it can result in serious physical and emotional alterations in well-being.

The nurse who can integrate a knowledge of anatomy and physiology with an understanding of the emotional and social experiences and needs of clients with reproductive system dysfunction can offer competent, caring, and comprehensive health services.

SECTION 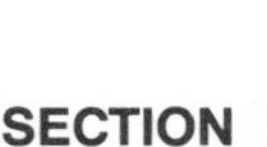

Structural and Functional Interrelationships

Structure and Function of the Female Reproductive System

The female external genitalia provide protection, enhance sexual arousal and pleasure, and are the site of urination. The internal genitalia are the sites of major biologic events in a woman's life, including **menarche** (the onset of menstruation), premenstrual changes, pregnancy, and **menopause** (the cessation of the menstrual cycle).

External Genitalia

The term *vulva* refers to the female external genitalia. Refer to Figure 47–1 in the following discussion of the vulva's specific structures.

MONS PUBIS At the top of the external genitalia is the mons pubis, or mons veneris. This rounded pad of fatty

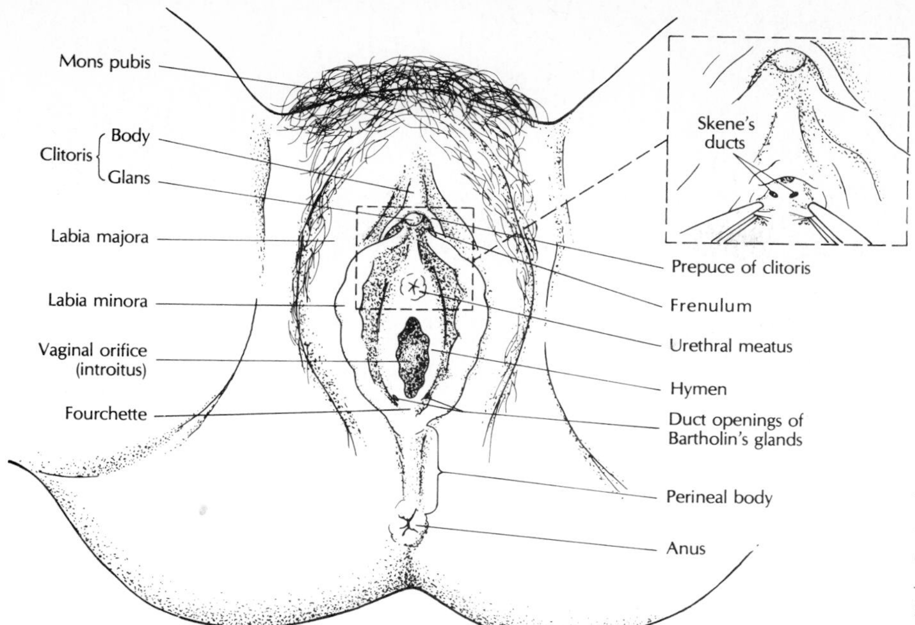

Figure 47–1

Female external genitals, longitudinal view. SOURCE: *Olds SB, London ML, Ladewig PA:* Maternal–Newborn Nursing: A Family-Centered Approach, *2nd ed. Menlo Park, CA: Addison–Wesley, 1984, p. 71.*

tissue becomes fuller in adolescence, and pubic hair appears in the area around 11 or 12 years of age. In menopause, there is a loss of fatty deposits, so the mons pubis becomes less prominent, and the pubic hair thins and decreases. The mons pubis has three functions: protecting the pelvic bones, making coitus more comfortable; distinguishing the female by its rounded contour; and enhancing arousal. Stimulation of the mons pubis causes orgasm for some.

CLITORIS The clitoris, from the Greek word for key, is considered the most erotically sensitive part of the female genital tract. The clitoris is visible between the folds of the labia minora at the anterior juncture. The external portions are the body and the glans. The glans consists of a mucous membrane with an enormous number of free nerve endings; this makes the clitoris a sensitive area of the body requiring, in some women, only light stimulation to bring an orgasm.

LABIA MAJORA The labia majora, or "lips," originate in the mons pubis and end in the perineum, forming the lateral boundaries of the vulva. The labia majora contain fatty tissue, sweat glands, hair, blood vessels, lymphatic vessels, and nerves. The labia majora function mainly as a protective covering for the genitals, but they also serve as a source of erotic pleasure. The area is extremely sensitive to touch, pressure, pain, and temperature.

Pregnancy causes the labia to lose tone, producing a loose appearance. At menopause, the labia atrophy and appear less prominent. There are many normal variations in the appearance of the labia from woman to woman, throughout life.

Because the labia majora have much loose connective tissue, the structure is especially susceptible to edema. The lymphatic drainage of the labia majora is shared with other structures of the vulva. Therefore, labial congestion or swelling can be a clue to malignancies in a number of other areas.

LABIA MINORA The labia minora are two thin longitudinal folds of tissue lying inside the labia majora. Their surface is shiny and has no hair follicles. Posteriorly, the labia merge to form the fourchette, the fold of skin immediately posterior to the vaginal orifice that is often traumatized during childbirth.

The tissue of the labia minora is erectile. Because of many tactile nerve endings, a vaginal discharge is potentially irritating. By a rich supply of sebaceous glands, the labia minora lubricate the vulvar skin. The labia minora also provide bactericidal secretions and heighten sexual arousal and pleasure. After menopause, the labia minora atrophy, losing fat tissue and becoming flatter as the labia majora do, although to a lesser degree.

URETHRAL MEATUS The urethral meatus, or external urethral opening through which urine flows, usually is about 2 to 3 cm inferior to the clitoris but may be located at other nearby points where it is more difficult to see. The meatus is slightly elevated and has depressed areas on each side. The opening may be stellate or crescent shaped.

PARAURETHRAL GLANDS The paraurethral glands (Skene's ducts) are located bilaterally and open into the posterior wall of the urethra. Skene's ducts do not appear to have a specific function in the female. They are susceptible to gonococcal infection, however.

VESTIBULE, INTROITUS, AND HYMEN The vestibule, visible upon separation of the labia majora, is the elliptical space bordered by the labia minora laterally, the urethra and clitoris superiorly, and the fourchette inferiorly. The vaginal introitus (the opening into the vagina) sits within the vestibule. The hymen (also called the hymenal ring) is

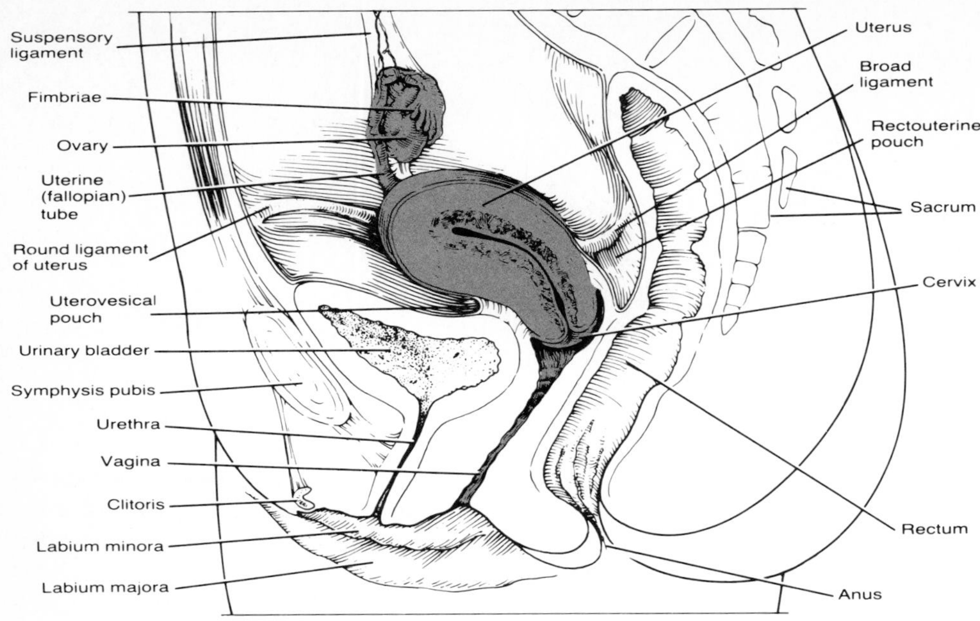

Figure 47–2

Median view of the female pelvis. SOURCE: *Spence AP, Mason EB:* Human Anatomy and Physiology, *3rd ed. Menlo Park, CA: Benjamin/Cummings, 1987, p. 825.*

an irregular membranous fold of epithelium and fibrous tissue that surrounds and covers the vaginal introitus to varying degrees. The strength and size of the hymen vary among individuals and in the individual at different times. If the hymen is thick, surgery may be necessary to perforate it to allow intercourse, pelvic examination, and menstrual flow. The hymen can be broken through strenuous physical activity, masturbation, or the use of tampons. It may remain intact, however, even in parous women.

BARTHOLIN'S GLANDS Just inside the middle to lower vaginal introitus are Bartholin's glands, whose ducts appear as two small papular elevations just at the base of the vestibule and external to the hymenal ring. These glands are thought to secrete mucus that keeps the vaginal mucosa moist.

PERINEUM The term *perineum* is often misused to refer to the vulva or external genitalia. The perineum actually includes the skin and tissues between the vaginal introitus and the anal orifice.

The muscles of the perineum collectively anchor and protect the pelvic viscera and external genitalia and provide the sphincter activity of the urethra, vagina, and rectum. The contractions of these muscles serve as a major stimulus of orgasm.

Internal Genitalia

The internal organs both respond to hormonal stimulation and secrete hormones, profoundly affecting biopsychosocial responses such as premenstrual stress reactions and postnatal feelings of well-being. The structures of the internal genitalia are the sites of the most common health problems related to the female reproductive system, such as dysmenorrhea and vaginitis. Refer to Figures 47–2 and 47–3 in the following discussion.

VAGINA The vagina is like a tunnel, tube, or passageway open at its anterior end and extending inward to the center of the pelvis. This musculomembranous structure accommodates menstrual discharge, the penis in coitus, and the fetal head during delivery.

The cervix of the uterus projects into the upper part of the anterior wall of the vagina, making the anterior wall shorter than the posterior wall by 2.5 cm.

The lining of the vagina is noncornified stratified squamous epithelium that proliferates under estrogenic stimulation. The rugae vaginales are transverse ridges of mucous membrane in the posterior and anterior vaginal walls. The lateral walls are smoother. The surface appears this way from menarche to menopause. After stretching from pregnancies and decreased estrogenic stimulation with menopause, the rugae vaginales smooth out and the lining becomes thinner and drier, or atrophic.

The pudendal nerve innervates the lower third of the vagina, and there are no special nerve endings. This explains why vaginal sensations during coitus and sexual excitement are minimal, as well as why pain during the second stage of labor is manageable. Recent research has revealed a dime-sized area just above the anterior surface of the vaginal wall about one-third to one-half the way into the vagina—the Gräfenberg spot, or G-spot. Women and their partners report that continued stimulation of the G-spot may result in an intense orgasm and the expulsion of a fluid (Bullough et al., 1984). Because of methodologic problems, no definitive study has yet proven that the ejaculate is different from urine or vaginal secretions (Heath, 1984).

The vagina is acidic from menarche to menopause, and its surface is moist from fluid secreted by the vaginal epithelium. Döderlein's bacilli, which produce lactic acid, and the vaginal contents exist symbiotically. Ovarian hormones regulate the glycogen content and the sloughing and renewal

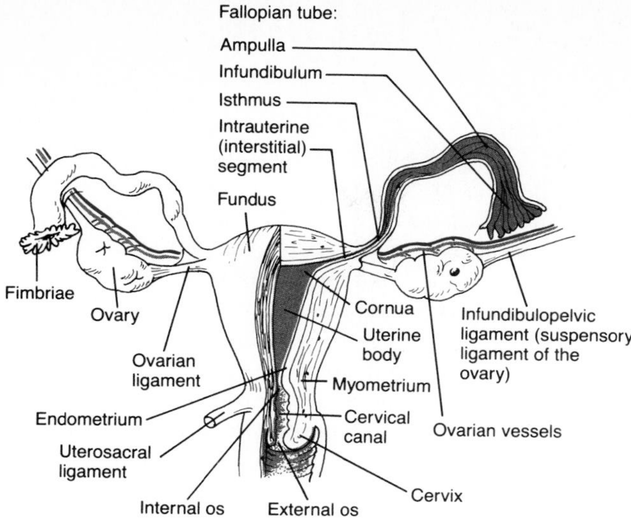

Figure 47–3

The fallopian tubes (oviducts or uterine tubes) and ovaries. *SOURCE: Adapted from Olds SB, London ML, Ladewig PA:* Maternal–Newborn Nursing: A Family-Centered Approach, *2nd ed. Menlo Park, CA: Addison–Wesley, 1984, p. 82.*

of vaginal epithelial cells. The interaction of the bacilli with this process by enzymatic breakdown of glycogen to lactic acid maintains the acidity of the vagina. Douching interrupts this natural protective process and can make the vagina more susceptible to infection.

Muscular and ligamentous support of the vagina is provided by the levator ani muscle and the transverse cervical, pubocervical, and sacrocervical ligaments at the level of the upper vagina. The urogenital diaphragm supports the middle vaginal portion and the perineal body, the lower segment. The levator ani is the principal muscle that closes the vagina.

CERVIX The cervix of the uterus provides much information about menstruation, the presence of infection, pregnancy, and the stages of labor. The cervix is highly elastic. The many folds in its surface increase its potential surface area, as does its 10% muscle composition.

The openings of the cervix are the external os at the vaginal end and the internal os at the uterine end; the area between the two is the cervical canal. The cervix is partly vaginal and partly supravaginal. The vaginal cervix appears pink, whereas the supravaginal cervix is redder. Squamous stratified epithelium covers the vaginal cervix, and tall columnar ciliated cells with mucus-secreting glands line the supravaginal cervix. These two linings meet at the squamocolumnar junction, the area from which cells are taken in a Papanicolaou (Pap) test to screen for cervical cancer.

Mucus-secreting cells in the cervical canal produce mucus, which provides lubrication and acts as a bacteriostatic agent. The character of cervical mucus is affected by the level of estrogen.

UTERUS The uterus, or womb, is an organ with great significance in health and culture. As a symbol of reproductive ability, it is described in myths and endowed with symbolic meanings. Uterine changes occur at each developmental stage of a woman's life. The shedding of the lining signifies menarche and the possibility of reproductive capability, and the cessation of the shedding signifies menopause. The uterus endows a woman with the capacity to reproduce and sometimes it is the source of discomfort or disease as well.

The uterus is located at the center of the pelvic cavity between the base of the bladder and the rectum and above the vagina. The uterus is held in position by the broad and round ligaments in the upper area; the cardinal, pubocervical, and uterosacral ligaments hold it in place in the middle area and at the pelvic floor inferiorly.

The uterus actually consists of two unequal parts. The corpus, or body, forms the upper two-thirds and consists mainly of myometrium. This pear-shaped portion is larger during the reproductive years. The portion of the corpus above where the fallopian tubes attach is the fundus. The neck or cervix (discussed previously) forms the lower part. The isthmus, the slight constriction or narrow part, constitutes the division of the cervix and the corpus.

The corpus of the uterus has three layers: the perimetrium, myometrium, and endometrium. The perimetrium, the serous membrane covering the uterus, is composed of the peritoneum that runs continuously over the anterior abdominal wall, the bladder surface, the fundus, and the posterior part of the corpus. The myometrium, which lies beneath the perimetrium, is continuous with the fallopian tubes, the vagina, and some ovarian ligaments and is composed of three layers of involuntary muscle. The endometrium, the innermost layer of the corpus, is a single layer of columnar epithelium, glands, and stroma. This is the layer that is shed and then rebuilt from menarche to menopause in the absence of pregnancy. Hormonal effects, which are discussed later, stimulate the shedding and rebuilding.

FALLOPIAN TUBES From the sides of the uterus arise the fallopian, or uterine, tubes, which extend almost to the side walls of the pelvis. The tubes are 8 to 13.5 cm long and are moveable, not rigid. The fallopian tubes form a passageway that connects the peritoneal cavity with the external environment via the uterus and vagina, creating the potential for the spread of infection between these areas. The tubes enable transport of the ovum from the ovary to the uterus and provide a favorable, nourishing environment for fertilization.

Depending on the section of the tube, its size or diameter varies from 1 to 4 mm. The uterine opening into the tube is about the size of a hairbrush bristle; the rest of the tube size varies but is approximately the size of a strand of spaghetti. At its funnel-shaped distal end, the infundibulum, the tube fans out to a trumpetlike shape. Around the small orifice of the infundibulum are fimbriae (folds of tissue).

More proximal to the uterus is the ampulla, which has a wide lumen and distensible wall. The isthmus of the tube is closer to the uterus. This portion is straight and narrow and has a muscular wall. This is the point where tubal ligation is done.

The fallopian tubes are rich in blood supply and innervated by sympathetic and parasympathetic motor and sensory nerves. Women experience pain from the tubes in the area of the iliac fossa.

OVARIES The ovaries, almond-shaped organs positioned on each side of the uterus, are approximately 1.5 to 3.0 cm wide, 2 to 5 cm long, and 1 to 1.5 cm thick. The ovaries' size increases at adolescence and decreases during menopause.

Each ovary is supported by the mesovarium, which attaches it to the broad ligaments; the ovarian ligament, which connects it to the uterus; and the suspensory ligament, which attaches it to the lateral pelvic wall. An ovary is composed of the medulla (the inner portion, which contains nerves and lymph vessels) and the cortex (the functional outer portion, which contains follicles and ova). Germinal epithelium covers each ovary. The peritoneum does not cover the ovary; this allows the release of ova but also permits the spread of neoplastic cells.

The ovary usually releases one ovum each month (ovulation). The functional unit of the ovary is the follicle, which changes as it matures and again with ovulation. This process is described more fully in the later discussion of the menstrual cycle.

The surface of the ovary, once tense, shiny, and elastic, becomes scarred and pitted by the development of fibrous tissue that forms at the site of the follicle rupture in the absence of pregnancy. This process, repeated with each menstrual cycle, results in an ovary progressively more scarred and pitted with age.

Pelvis

The female bony pelvis has many functions. It supports the upper torso, protects the organs of the lower pelvis, and forms an axis through which the fetus passes at delivery. Viewed from the top, the pelvis is like a basin open at its base. It is formed by the ischial, iliac, and pubic bones on the sides, with connection in the front by a cartilage "joint," the symphysis pubis. The two iliac bones are joined by a cartilage "joint" with the sacrum and coccyx. The spines of the ilium are what people sit on. The pelvic outlet is formed by the ischial spines and the tip of the coccyx.

Breasts

The female breast is a cutaneous gland that is an accessory of the reproductive system. It is cone shaped and has a "tail" of breast tissue extending into the axilla.

The breast is a tightly woven, complex structure composed of a glandular and ductal network, fat, connective tissue, fasciae, blood vessels, nerves, and lymph (Figure 47–4). In the center of the breast are the nipple and the areola, which are pigmented more darkly with puberty, pregnancy, and exogenous estrogen use. The nipple varies from 0.5 to 1.3 cm in diameter. Its erectile tissue responds to sexual excitement, cold, friction, pregnancy, and menses by becoming more rigid and prominent. The surface of the areola is irregular and papillary because of the presence of Montgomery's tubercles, which secrete a liquid that protects the breasts during infant sucking.

The glandular portion of the breast can be visualized as a series of lobes radiating from the nipple, extending anteriorly to posteriorly, separated by adipose tissue. The lobes consist of lobules formed by alveoli, clusters of saclike structures that are the termination of collecting ducts whose anterior ends store milk during lactation. Progesterone, along with estrogen, is responsible for alveolar and lobular development. The growth of the ductal epithelium is regulated by estrogenic hormones (Tyler & Woodall, 1982).

The veins of the breast connect with the superior vena cava and are part of a low-pressure system susceptible to change in intra-abdominal pressure. These veins form a pathway for metastasis of neoplastic cells from the breast to the lungs, pelvis, vertebrae, or skull. Lymph flows mainly toward the axilla, then travels medially, and finally empties into the jugular and subclavian veins—a short route that makes it easy for cancer cells to metastasize into the general circulation.

Breast development occurs in stages beginning in the neonatal period. About the time of menarche, the breasts develop a cone shape and increase in size. Changes in breast size and structure also occur during pregnancy. In early menopause, women often experience uncomfortable breast sensations such as fullness and tenderness because of fluctuations in estrogen levels. Later in menopause, hormone levels stabilize. Overall estrogen levels decrease during menopause, resulting in a decrease of fat tissue in the breast and the replacement of fat tissue by fibrous cords.

Female Sexual Response

Female sexual responses, like those of the male, are determined by both psychologic and tactile stimuli of either the genital organs or other areas of the body. Both sympathetic and parasympathetic autonomic nerves carry the

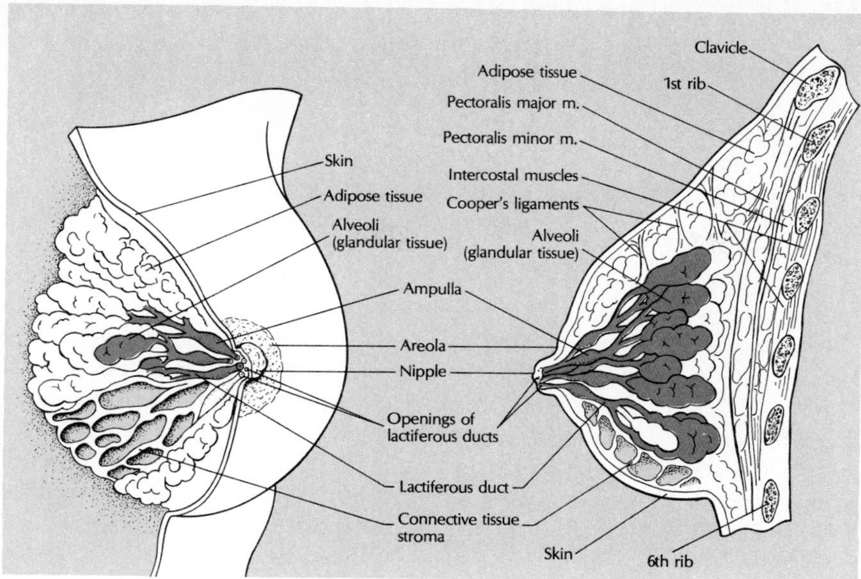

Figure 47–4

Anatomy of the breast. **Left.** Anterior view of partially dissected left breast. **Right.** Sagittal view. *SOURCE: Olds SB, London ML, Ladewig PA:* Maternal–Newborn Nursing: A Family Centered Approach, *2nd ed. Menlo Park, CA: Addison–Wesley, 1984, p. 84.*

motor impulses that result in the responses to stimulation. The phases of sexual response are excitement, plateau, orgasm, and resolution. Although the phases of sexual response are named the same for both men and women, the durations vary. Male sexual response is discussed later in this chapter.

EXCITEMENT PHASE The excitement phase can be initiated by many different types of stimuli, including sight, sound, touch, or smell, and its intensity may increase rapidly. The first physical sign of response in women is vaginal lubrication, equivalent to a sweating reaction, which may occur in 10 to 30 seconds. Vasocongestion around and in the vagina causes a transudate to pass through the tissue of the vaginal walls. Other reactions during the excitement phase are: vasocongestion of the labia minora and majora, increase in size of the glans of the clitoris and elongation of the shaft, upward and backward movement of the cervix and uterus, erection of the breast nipples, and increase in alveolar size. The breasts and the labia minora may also become flushed.

PLATEAU PHASE If adequate stimulation continues and distraction does not interfere, the plateau phase follows the excitement phase. In this intensification of the excitement phase, the outer third of the vagina becomes engorged, decreasing the opening and forming the orgasmic platform; the labia minora's color deepens to a bright red; the clitoris retracts; and heart rate and blood pressure increase.

ORGASM PHASE The orgasm phase is characterized by rhythmic contractions of muscles, including those of the clitoris, vagina, and uterus. Muscle tension is released, and blood vessels become engorged. Vaginal contractions occur at 0.8-second intervals and vary from 3 to 15 contractions per orgasm (Hogan, 1984). Stimulation of the clitoris results in the same orgasmic changes as those caused by stimulation of the vagina. Women's descriptions of orgasm vary from a slight pleasurable movement sensation to intense throbbing. During orgasm, the respiratory rate increases to as high as 40 respirations per minute and the heart rate to 180 beats per minute. Blood pressure becomes elevated as well.

RESOLUTION PHASE The resolution phase is characterized by a return to the pre-excitement phase. The clitoris returns to normal as swelling disappears. The labia also return to normal size, and in 3 to 4 minutes the vagina loses its distention.

Regulatory Functions of the Female Reproductive System

Regulation of the phases of female development is an interactional process occurring along the hypothalamic–pituitary–gonadal axis. The anterior pituitary gland is controlled by secretions from the anterior hypothalamus, which is under the feedback control of hormones secreted by the ovaries. Gonadotropins are substances produced by the anterior pituitary gland and placenta that have an affinity for acting on the ovaries and control their function. Three hierarchies of hormones in the female endocrine system are part of the axis described: (1) luteinizing hormone releasing factor (LRF), secreted by the hypothalamus; (2) follicle stimulating hormone (FSH) and luteinizing hormone (LH), secreted by the anterior pituitary gland in response to stimulation by LRF; and (3) estrogen and progesterone, secreted by the ovaries in response to FSH and LH.

Puberty and Menarche

The regulatory mechanisms in the timing of the onset of puberty are not yet fully understood. Research has shown that the onset of puberty is related not only to maturity of the hypothalamic–pituitary–gonadal axis but also to genetics, the environment, body fat, and other endocrine phenomena.

The hypothalamus seems to be become less sensitive to estrogen as it matures. The immature hypothalamus inhibits the secretion of LRF and, in turn, the secretion of FSH and LH, which are necessary for the development and release of an ovum. As the hypothalamus matures, the low levels of circulating estrogen no longer inhibit the secretion of LRF, so LRF is secreted and stimulates the pituitary gland to produce FSH and LH.

Menarche occurs in response to these higher levels of FSH and LH that ultimately cause follicular growth and development in the ovary. Levels of estrogen also increase, which causes the endometrium of the uterus to proliferate. A cyclic pattern emerges, with feedback to LRF in the hypothalamus resulting in cyclic menstrual bleeding that is caused by sloughing of the endometrium.

At first uterine bleeding may occur without ovulation, called an anovulatory cycle. These anovulatory cycles are common in the first 2 years of menstruation as well as later. As the system matures, a two-phase positive feedback system develops within the hypothalamus; a rise in estrogen levels late in the follicular phase of the menstrual cycle triggers an FSH-LH surge, resulting in the development and release of an ovum.

The effects of increased estrogen levels during puberty include the development of the ductal part of the breasts; the growth of the external genitalia; and the development of a female body configuration, including fat definition at the hips and thighs. The increased estrogen levels also stimulate sebaceous gland secretions that may result in acne. Testosterone, which is present in small amounts in women, is produced by the interstitial cells and stroma in the ovary. Testosterone is thought to be responsible for an increase in sex drive, hair growth in a masculine pattern, and the development of acne resulting from an increase in the production of sebum by the sebaceous glands.

Menstrual Cycle

OVARIAN CYCLE The ovarian cycle has three phases: the follicular, ovulatory, and luteal phases. Day 1, the first day of bleeding, marks the beginning of the *follicular phase.* During this phase, FSH and the LH levels increase. The FSH acts on the primary follicle, increasing the number of granulosa cells and the production of estradiol, the most potent estrogen. As the estradiol level increases, FSH levels begin to fall, and LH levels begin to rise. The LH present promotes the production of more estradiol. By Days 5 to 7, a dominant follicle develops, and estradiol has increased the number of cells and stroma in the uterine endometrium (Emans & Goldstein, 1982). The organs are preparing for pregnancy or menstruation. As the estradiol level increases, so does the LH level. Follicles other than the dominant follicle undergo atresia, and less FSH is needed. As the LH level rises, progesterone production increases, and the granulosa cells are luteinized.

The *ovulatory phase* is much briefer. Approximately 1 day before ovulation, estradiol secretion decreases as progesterone secretion begins to rise. As a result of the rise in LH and progesterone levels, the theca interna forms enzymes that cause it to dissolve, which is followed by more swelling of the wall. As the theca and granulosa cells are luteinized, new blood vessels grow into the follicle wall, prostaglandins are secreted into the follicular tissues, and more plasma seeps into the follicle. This results in more swelling, as well as rupture and release of the ovum. This is what is referred to as **ovulation.**

The *luteal phase* of the cycle involves an increase in the size of the granulosa cells and an accumulation of lutein to form the corpus luteum. The corpus luteum is highly vascular and secretes progesterone and estrogen. About 8 days after ovulation, it is functionally at its peak. Unless pregnancy occurs, at 10 to 12 days after ovulation, the corpus luteum begins to regress and the secretion of estrogen and progesterone decreases. The decreased levels of estrogen and progesterone cause the pituitary gland to again produce LRF and then FSH and LH.

UTERINE CYCLE The uterine cycle has two phases: the proliferative and secretory phases. The *proliferative phase* coincides with the follicular phase of the ovarian cycle just described. Under the influence of estrogen, the endometrium proliferates and increases in thickness. During this phase, there is tortuosity of the endometrial glands, lengthening of the endometrium itself, and mitotic activity in the epithelial cell lining of the endometrial glands. The length of this phase is variable.

The *secretory phase* coincides with the luteal phase of the ovarian cycle and occurs in response to increasing levels of progesterone, which cause swelling and secretory development of the endometrium. In the stromal cells, cytoplasm, liquid, and glycogen increase greatly. The blood supply increases as well, and the endometrium doubles in thickness. Should an ovum implant in the endometrium, it is now adequately prepared to nourish the development into an embryo.

Menopause

The depletion of follicles caused by their monthly release from the ovaries over the years results in low levels of estrogen and progesterone. Without estrogen and progesterone feedback to the hypothalamus, releasing factors continue to stimulate pituitary gland secretion of FSH and LH (Olds et al., 1984; Tyler & Woodall, 1982). When the ovaries become unable to respond to the FSH and LH, ovarian activity diminishes.

Menopause generally occurs at about age 50. The

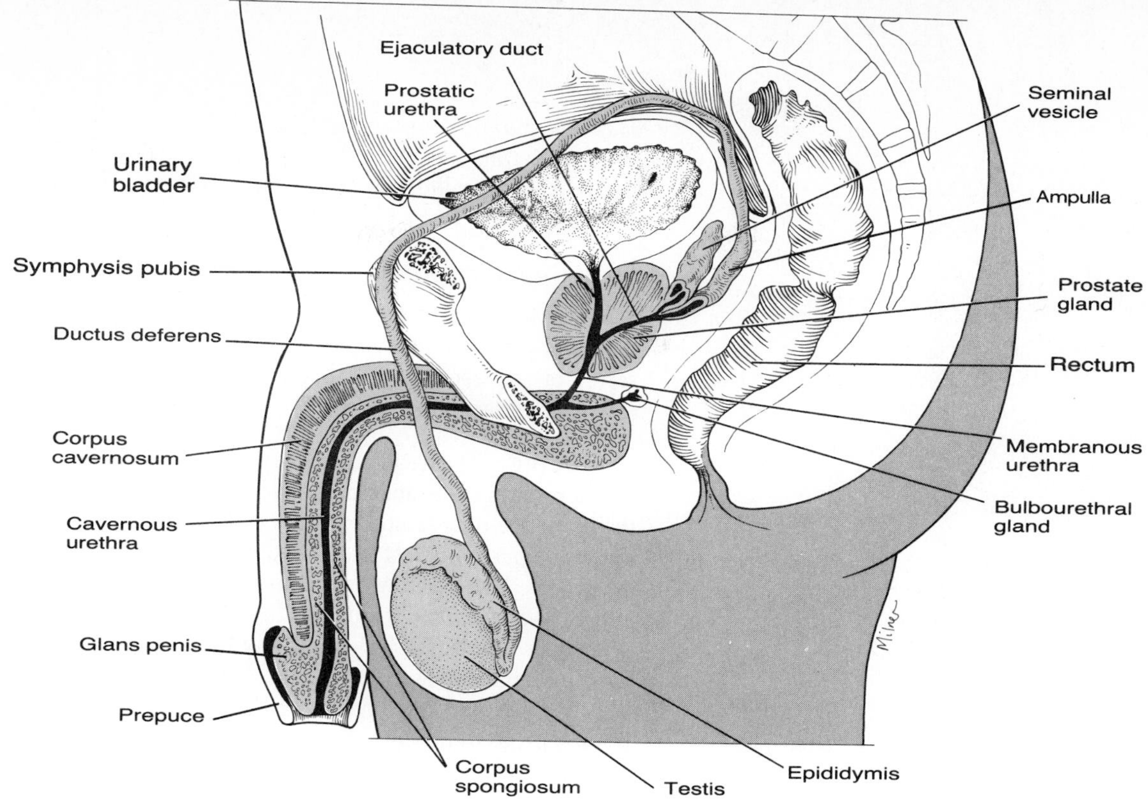

Figure 47–5

Sagittal section of the male pelvis with a portion of the left pubic bone attached to illustrate the path of the left ductus deferens. SOURCE: *Spence AP, Mason EB:* Human Anatomy and Physiology, *3rd ed. Menlo Park, CA: Benjamin/Cummings, 1987, p. 817.*

ovarian and menstrual cycles gradually become irregular, and many menstrual cycles are anovulatory. The period of premenopausal changes is called the **climacteric.**

Vasomotor instability in the form of hot flashes is a common premenopausal symptom. Although estrogen replacement therapy seems to alleviate vasomotor instability, it is not clear whether decreased estrogen levels are the etiologic basis for the instability. Many other physical changes that occur during menopause, however, are the result of decreased estrogen. Among these are atrophy of skin, subcutaneous tissue, and mucous membranes, along with osteoporosis or excessive calcium loss. Menopause is discussed more fully in Chapter 49.

Structure and Function of the Male Reproductive System

Organs of the male reproductive system play complementary roles in the system's functions. The external organs serve primarily to protect the testes and to propel sperm and urine from the body. For the internal structures, the principal functions are spermatogenesis and testosterone production. Refer to Figures 47–5 and 47–6 in the following discussion of the male reproductive system.

External Genitalia

The penis and scrotum are designed to deposit sperm in the vagina, accomplish urination, contain and protect the testes, and function in sexual activities.

PENIS The penis is a pendulous soft-tissue structure attached to the anterior and lateral walls of the pubic arch by muscle and suspensory ligaments. It is composed of three longitudinal columns of erectile tissue: a central column containing the urethra and two encompassing columns that provide the organ's main structural support. The lateral columns, the corpora cavernosa penis, are divided into cavernous spaces that become blood-filled sinuses during erection. The central column, the corpus spongiosum urethra, is also divided, but the spaces are smaller and the walls thinner owing to its support of the penile urethra. At the distal end, the corpus spongiosum urethra expands and becomes the glans penis, which surrounds the urethral meatus. The skin covering the penis is continuous from the base of the penis at the pubic arch to the glans penis, where it folds inward and backward upon itself and is called the prepuce, or foreskin. Usually, only the base of the penis is covered with hair.

Blood supply to the penis is via pudendal arteries that

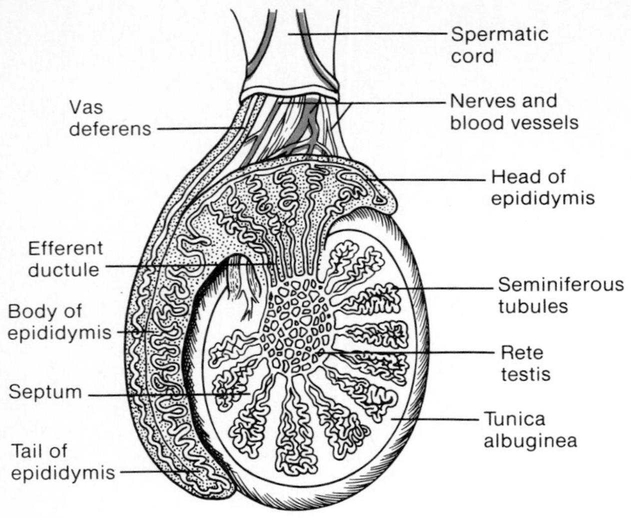

Figure 47–6

Sagittal section of the ductus deferens, the epididymis, and the testis. SOURCE: *Adapted from Spence AP, Mason EB:* Human Anatomy and Physiology, *3rd ed. Menlo Park, CA: Benjamin/ Cummings, 1987.*

form a complex network terminating in the cavernous spaces. The connection between blood supply, innervation, and psychic stimulation in the sexual response is discussed later.

The penis is a functional part of the urinary system that transports the urethra to its external oriface, the meatus. It is also a crucial part of the reproductive system, serving to deposit sperm in the female vagina, as well as an organ of considerable psychic importance in conveying sensations of sexual pleasure and well-being.

SCROTUM The scrotum, a thin-walled sac continuous with the abdominal wall, hangs suspended from the perineal region posterior to the penis. The scrotal wall is composed of deeply pigmented skin and a complex of fascial connective tissue and smooth muscle fibers called the tunica dartos.

The scrotum keeps the testes at a lower temperature than the abdominal cavity would, which is more conducive to sperm viability. The fibers of the tunica dartos layer contract readily with temperature or tactile stimulation. This action draws the scrotum and its contents protectively up toward the body and gives the structure a wrinkled appearance. These soft linear folds are called rugae. At warm temperatures, the scrotum is smooth and pendulous. The surface of the scrotum is supplied with sebaceous glands and is sparsely covered with hair.

The interior of the scrotum is divided by tunica dartos fibers into two compartments, each of which contains a testis, an epididymis, and a ductule system that passes through the inguinal canal. The scrotum is innervated by sacral (S-3) and lumbar fibers and is sensitive to pressure, pain, and temperature. Consequently, it can perform its protective function while serving as an organ of sexual pleasure. In later life, the scrotum stays more relaxed and pendulous.

Internal Genitalia

The function of the testes is to produce sperm and testosterone. The ductal system conveys sperm, and the series of accessory glands secretes a medium for sperm nourishment and transport.

TESTES The testes are two small, oval organs that develop within the abdominal cavity of the fetus. Under the influence of testosterone, the testes descend into separate compartments of the scrotum at 24 to 35 weeks of gestation. The peritoneum actually precedes the testes into the scrotum and forms the tunica vaginalis, the outer covering of the testes. Beneath the tunica vaginalis is the tunica albuginea, and fibroelastic connective tissue containing some smooth muscle cells. The tunica albuginea sends fibrous septa into the body of the testis, dividing it into many wedge-shaped lobes.

Within each of the 200 to 300 lobes of the testis are seminiferous tubules tightly coiled into position. Here the male gamete (the sperm) is formed and undergoes a portion of its maturation process. Also within the lobes and dispersed around the seminiferous tubules are supportive nutritive cells called Sertoli's cells and the interstitial Leydig's cells, which produce testosterone.

The seminiferous tubules unite within each lobe and generally within each testis to form a duct system that in turn forms the rete testis. This network throughout the testis ultimately forms several common ducts that leave the internal testis, penetrate the tunica albuginea, and empty into the epididymis.

The testes are well supplied with blood and lymphatic vessels. They are innervated by parasympathetic fibers from the vagus nerve (cranial nerve X) and by sympathetic fibers from the thoracic cord. Visceral fibers transmit afferent impulses.

DUCTAL SYSTEM The epididymis is the first part of an efferent ductal system leading from each testis through the inguinal canal and finally opening into the prostatic portion of the urethra. The epididymis consists of a continuous tube that is coiled and forms a head (attached to the top of the testis), a body (which descends along the posterior aspect of the testis), and a tail (which straightens and turns away from the testis and begins the ascent to the vas deferens). The tail of the epididymis provides a reservoir where spermatozoa mature over several days.

The vas deferens, or ductus deferens, is a long simple tube capable of peristaltic motion that propels sperm through the system. The duct travels from the epididymis through the scrotum (where it is innervated with sensory receptors), through the inguinal canal, and over the bladder. It then joints a duct that dilates at its terminal to an ampulla just before it opens into the prostatic portion of the urethra. The ampulla serves as the main reservoir for sperm and tubular secretions.

The vas deferens is suspended and contained within the spermatic cord through most of its length. This connective tissue structure suspends the testis, epididymis, and vas deferens as well as the complex of blood vessels, lymphatics, and nerves that supplies these structures. It extends from the tail of the epididymis to the abdominal inguinal ring and is enclosed by the cremaster muscle and layers of fascia coming from the abdominal wall.

ACCESSORY GLANDS AND URETHRA Seminal vesicles, the urethral and bulbourethral glands, and the prostate gland make up the male accessory glands. Two seminal vesicles—lobulated glands lined with secretory epithelium—lie posterior to the bladder at the base of the prostate. They secrete a thick, nutritive, alkaline fluid that mixes with sperm on ejaculation. The fluid contains fructose and proteins, which are essential to sperm mobility and metabolism. The seminal vesicles each have a duct that joins the vas deferens to form an ejaculatory duct about 1 in. long, where sperm from the vas deferens and nutritive fluid from the seminal vesicles mix and are discharged into the prostatic portion of the urethra.

The urethra is a shared pathway for urine and semen and the final link from the testes to the exterior. This tubelike organ extends from the internal urethral orifice at the bladder to the tip of the glans penis, where it emerges, forming an external meatus. The urethra is lined with a large number of small glands (Littre's glands) along its surface, which produce and contribute mucus. The urethra has an internal sphincter that forms a smooth muscle valve at the outlet of the bladder and responds to parasympathetic and sympathetic stimulation. The external urethral sphincter lies at the point where the urethra penetrates the urogenital diaphragm and is composed of skeletal muscle; hence, it is under voluntary control. Each portion of the urethra is named for the structures it passes through. Thus, there is the prostatic urethra, the membranous urethra (which passes through the urogenital diaphragm), and the penile urethra (or cavernous urethra).

The bulbourethral glands are two pea-sized glands located on either side of the urethra and opening into it. They produce a lubricating alkaline mucus that is expressed into the urethra during ejaculation, reducing its usually acidic state and creating a more hospitable environment for sperm.

The *prostate gland* is a spherical body that surrounds a portion of the urethra and lies adjacent and inferior to the neck of the urinary bladder. A capsule of muscle fibers encases this lobulated gland, which contains 30 to 60 branched, ducted segments opening ultimately into the ejaculatory ducts, which in turn open into the prostatic urethra. The gland secretes a thin, milky, slightly acidic fluid containing few nutrients, some minerals, and fibrinolysin. Under both endocrine and neural control, the prostate gland is subject to hyperplasia, which is most common in older men but occurs in men of all ages.

Male Gamete

The male gamete is the sperm, which is produced under the influence of gonadotropic hormones in all the seminiferous tubules of the testis beginning at sexual maturation and continuing throughout life. The gamete's function is to contribute one-half of the genetic material to a new life.

Each spermatozoon has a head, neck, body, and tail, each with a highly specialized function. The oval head contains the nucleus and, thus, the genetic message. A structure called the acrosome sits like a helmet on the head of the sperm and contains digestive enzymes used to penetrate the surrounding investment of the ovum. The neck is the site of the centrioles, and mitochondria are arranged in the body. Extending out from the body is a long tail containing large quantities of adenosine triphosphate (ATP) necessary to sustain the continued movement of the tail as it propels the sperm through the female reproductive tract once it is deposited at the mouth of the cervix.

During a 2-week passage from the testes to the vas deferens sperm undergo maturation and capacitation; that is, they become capable of penetrating the investment of the ovum and fusing with its yolk.

Newly formed sperm are transported through the system in a seminal plasma, or **semen,** which is the collective product of the male accessory sex glands. Each accessory gland contributes an exocrine secretion to the seminal plasma, which provides the correct environment for sperm at each portion of passage: Seminal vesicles, bulbourethral glands, and urethral glands secrete a mucoid, alkaline fluid, whereas the prostate gland secretes a slightly acidic, milky fluid. The combined products result in a hospitable seminal plasma pH. Although exquisitely sensitive to elevated temperatures, sperm can survive freezing indefinitely and be viable upon their return to normal temperatures.

Male Sexual Response

As a physiologic event, the male sexual response consists of two distinct components: a genital vasocongestive reaction (which produces penile erection) and reflex clonic muscular contractions (which result in orgasm). The two components involve different anatomic structures and are innervated by different parts of the nervous system. This distinction becomes important in recognizing and treating sexual dysfunctions.

The male sexual response cycle parallels the female's in its four phases: excitement, plateau, orgasm, and resolution.

EXCITEMENT PHASE The erectile component of the sexual response transforms the flaccid penis into a firm phallus that makes insertion into the vagina possible. The response is initiated in the excitement phase with local stimulation of the genitals, psychic stimulation such as erotic thoughts or viewing a desirable partner, or a combination of these experiences. Parasympathetic fibers from sacral cord segments S-2, S-3, and S-4 control the diameter and valves of penile blood vessels; these fibers permit the engorgement of sinuses to produce erection and then the emptying of these vessels and loss of erection. These parasympathetic fibers are the same sacral fibers that innervate the rectum and the detrusor muscle of the bladder. Consequently, diseases, injuries, and surgeries that affect these fibers also affect bowel and bladder function and possibly erectile function.

PLATEAU PHASE Once attained, erection can be maintained for long periods in the plateau phase. This permits the man to engage in seduction activities with the female partner, who is usually more slowly aroused. Erection may be achieved and lost several times during lovemaking as a normal pattern. Men over 50, however, frequently find they are less likely to regain an erection for several hours once the penis is flaccid.

ORGASM PHASE The male orgasm has two phases, emission and expulsion or ejaculation. Emission, the first orgasmic response, entails contraction of the internal reproductive organs (vas deferens, prostate, seminal vesicles, and urethra) and discharge of their secretions into the reproductive tract. Ejaculation, the second phase of orgasm, is the convulsive contraction of the bulbocavernous muscles that results in spurts of semen being forced outward from the penis. Although this is an involuntary reflex, it is mediated by voluntary fibers, so a certain amount of voluntary control is possible. Once emission has occurred, ejaculation is essentially inevitable and difficult for the male to postpone for even a few moments. In this phase, the man experiences the intense pleasures of orgasm.

RESOLUTION PHASE Following ejaculation is a refractory period during which the man cannot respond physiologically to further sexual stimulation. Younger men have shorter refractory periods and a greater frequency of ejaculation, whereas older men experience longer refractory periods and decreased frequency of ejaculation. There is no such alteration in the capacity for erection, however, and older men can continue to enjoy sexual play with simply a decrease in the frequency of ejaculation.

Regulatory Functions of the Male Reproductive System

Both the male and female reproductive systems are controlled by the hypothalamic–pituitary–gonadal axis. In the male, LH stimulates the interstitial Leydig's cells to secrete testosterone, and FSH stimulates the seminiferous tubules to spermatogenesis. When there is a high level of testosterone to stimulate hypothalamic receptors, the body responds by slowing or ceasing its production of the hormone. When there is a low level of the hormone present, the body responds by increasing its production of testosterone.

A small amount of testosterone is also secreted by the male and female adrenal cortex. Under normal conditions, this testosterone is insufficient to stimulate masculinization.

Reproductive Effects of Testosterone

In males usually between the ages of 11 and 13, the level of testosterone begins to rise in response to LH and FSH. The exact cause for this change in previous levels of hormones is not yet known. As gonadotropin levels rise, the testosterone secretion increases many times, and the ducts and accessory glands of the reproductive tract enlarge and become active. Testosterone is also necessary for the secretion of fructose by the seminal vesicles for the nourishment of sperm. Spermatogenesis initiation and maturation depend on adequate levels of testosterone, along with FSH. After puberty, testosterone influences the length and width of the penis, scrotal rugae, and genital pigmentation.

Testosterone also directly mediates secondary sex characteristics in the male during and after puberty. Many of these effects are logical consequences of testosterone's metabolic effects and incude the appearance and distribution of pubic and auxillary hair, lengthening and thickening of the vocal cords, increased activity of sebaceous glands, broadening of the shoulders, and general increase in muscle mass. The maintenance of all these effects requires continued adequate levels of testosterone.

General Effects of Testosterone

Testosterone is an anabolic hormone capable of placing the body into positive nitrogen balance (a state in which less nitrogen leaves the body than was consumed in the form of protein and so can be retained for tissue building). This action of testosterone is responsible for the more heavily muscled body and thicker skin of the postpubertal male.

Testosterone has profound metabolic effects, many of which are easily observable at puberty. It can increase the metabolic rate up to 15%. It improves calcium absorption and retention, as well as increases the deposition of calcium salts in bones. Bones grow in thickness, and their matrix density increases. This results in an initial spurt of height, but testosterone also ultimately causes the epiphyses to unite, limiting longitudinal growth. Skeletal muscle increases in quantity and density, and the vocal cords thicken and lengthen. Epithelial cells respond with proliferation, thickening, and coarsening; body hair increases, especially in pubic and axillary areas. All these effects result in the heavier, more densely muscled, deeper voiced, and hairier male of the species.

Puberty, when testosterone effects are at peak level, creates the familiar pattern of the adolescent male with a voracious appetite, burgeoning height, and alto-to-soprano voice who is trying to get accustomed to his rapidly changing body and new psychic drives. Male adulthood is physiologically calmer.

Effects of Diminishing Testosterone

Maintenance levels of testosterone gradually decrease with time but never cease abruptly as ovarian secretions in the female do. Indeed, spermatogenesis and testosterone secretion continue with aging and decline only slightly. Even this slight reduction in testosterone secretion, however, results in a moderate decrease in muscle mass, bone density, and skin thickness, as well as a change in vocal timbre. Although every man's general appearance changes with age, the extent of the change varies with the individual. A decrease in muscle mass is evident in large muscles responsible for postural changes as well as in small muscles, such as those that contribute to facial contours. The skin loses its elasticity, hair growth slows, subcutaneous fat deposits regress, and the characteristic appearance of the older man becomes established. Calcium is lost from bone and not redeposited at the former rate, resulting in a more brittle skeleton.

Diminishing testosterone levels are directly related to all these changes, but they are probably not the only responsible factor. For example, testosterone increases the deposition of calcium in bones but so does weight-bearing stress. The older man has traditionally engaged in less physical activity, such as running and lifting; therefore, the weight-bearing stress on the skeleton is lessened. This fact, along with the diminished testosterone levels, is probably a more complete explanation of skeletal fragility.

The reduction of testosterone production—whether from age or disease state—also affects sexual responses and performance. Adequate testosterone levels are considered crucial to libido and orgasm. Although the older man may remain sexually active, orgasms are usually less frequent than in the younger years.

Although testosterone clearly has a significant influence on behavior, in humans it is probably not possible to separate psychosocial factors from biologic factors in sexual behavior. Although testosterone can affect the sexual drive and its intensity, it can be assumed that testosterone does not affect how sexual desire is expressed through behavior toward the self and others (Vick, 1984). Behavior is influenced by individuals' psychosocial experiences and choices as they interact with others throughout life.

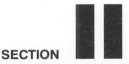

SECTION 

Pathophysiologic Influences and Effects

The reproductive system, like all the body's systems, is vulnerable to deterioration, infection, and neoplasia. Immune responses and chemical exposures can cause a variety of problems. Congenital defects, although not life threatening, can greatly restrict adequate function. Although influences on the system are many and varied, the most common pathophysiologic changes are discussed below.

In Women

Variation in bleeding and pelvic pain are the two most common pathophysiologic changes related to the female reproductive system. Women's visits to health care providers are often the result of problems with menstrual cycles. Clients may notice either that they do not bleed, bleed irregularly, bleed too little, bleed too much, or experience painful menstruation.

Amenorrhea

Amenorrhea, the absence of menses, can be primary or secondary. The less common primary amenorrhea is a condition in which the woman has never menstruated. Causes include congenital obstruction, testicular feminization, and adrenal or ovarian tumors. Secondary amenorrhea is the cessation of menses for over 6 months after menarche. In most women, this is caused by the lack of the LH surge at midcycle (Ellis & Beckmann, 1983). Common causes include severe illness, major life changes or high anxiety, and changes in exercise and dietary habits. The use of phenothiazines, reserpine, or oral contraceptives also may induce secondary amenorrhea (Fogel & Woods, 1981). Amenorrhea after discontinuing oral contraceptive use usually does not last more than 6 months. Other less common causes of secondary amenorrhea include pituitary tumors, ovarian cysts, uncontrolled diabetes, hyperthyroidism and hypothyroidism, and Cushing's syndrome. Secondary amenorrhea also occurs in pregnancy and menopause.

Variations in Cycle Length

Variations in cycle length include bleeding at intervals of 18 to 21 days or less, uterine bleeding at times other than the normal menstrual flow, or bleeding at intervals greater than 35 days. Increased frequency of menstrual periods is caused by a shortening of either the follicular or luteal phases of the menstrual cycle. Increased frequency is more common during premenopause and just after menarche. Intermenstrual bleeding may occur with cervicitis, malignancy, or at the time of ovulation. Bleeding at intervals greater than 35 days occurs because there is a prolonged proliferative phase of the menstrual cycle, the cause of which is often unclear. Possible causes include obesity, malnutrition, emotional factors, ovarian disease, and systemic disease (Ellis & Beckmann, 1983). In addition to causing anxiety about possible pregnancy or pathologies, bleeding at longer intervals decreases fertility and increases the risk of endometrial cancer.

Variations in Amount or Duration of Bleeding

Variations in the amount or duration of bleeding include excessive or prolonged menstrual flow and bleeding at times other than the usual menstrual period and at irregular intervals. Excessive menstrual flow may occur because of ectopic pregnancy or spontaneous abortion. In cycles in which ovulation occurs, other causes of a heavy flow include fibroids, adenomyosis, and erosion into an endometrial vessel by an intrauterine device (IUD) (Fogel & Woods, 1981). Hypothyroidism and blood dyscrasias are possible systemic causes. Medications that can be responsible are anticoagulants, diuretics, anticholinergics, and phenothiazines.

Anovulation (absence of ovulation) leads to excessive endometrial buildup followed by heavy bleeding and, usually, prolonged menses. Progesterone deficiency is the basis for the process. A dysfunction of the hypothalamic–pituitary–ovarian axis is often associated with anovulatory cycles.

In ovarian failure in the perimenopausal years, either little progesterone is secreted or the endometrium becomes so proliferated that sloughing occurs. If progesterone production returns or the endometrium "reaches its limit," bleeding is outside the usual pattern, prolonged, and heavy. In the postmenopausal woman, any bleeding must be considered serious until proven otherwise. The incidence of malignancy in women with postmenopausal bleeding is high.

Pelvic Pain

Although a common problem of women, pain in the pelvic area is often hard to diagnose. At times, the pain's origin is never found even though the pain is definitely present. It is particularly difficult for women to localize pelvic pain. Pain can originate from cutaneous and muscle fibers or from visceral innervations. The former is experienced as acute pain; is more easily localized; and is more likely to arise from the labia, vagina, and abdominal wall. Visceral pain is more likely to be burning, aching, or chronic; is often referred pain; and is likely to originate in the uterus, tubes, ovaries, or bladder (Fogel & Woods, 1981).

In Men

Men's visits to health care providers are often the result of gonadal endocrine disturbances. The adrenal gland and peripheral tissues produce some testosterone, but the amount is insufficient to affect any of the reproductive functions. The testes are the main source of testosterone; consequently, any disease process affecting the testes profoundly affects the reproductive endocrine status. Problems occur with either overproduction or underproduction of the hormone.

Hypogonadal Endocrine Responses

Hypogonadal endocrine responses occur primarily because of a developmental or destructive lesion of the testes. They occur secondarily by failure in the production of the gonadotropins or their releasing factors.

In primary hypogonadal response, an injury may be present at birth; in this case, puberty will not occur. Primary hypogonadism can also be acquired at any time later in life. Acquired conditions resulting in testicular tissue damage can cause either complete or partial failure of function. For example, the testes are especially sensitive to high temperatures, and exposure to high environmental temperatures or fevers secondary to any illness may compromise testosterone production and spermatogenesis. Failure of the testes to descend from the abdomen (cryptorchidism) where the temperature is higher results in testicular atrophy that is usually irreversible beyond puberty. Many infectious diseases, especially viral diseases, also can cause testicular failure. Examples include mumps, tuberculosis, leprosy, gonorrhea, brucellosis, and syphilis.

Neoplastic diseases of the testes may result in either underproduction or overproduction of hormone, usually the latter. This can affect both sperm and testosterone production. Radiation and chemotherapy for testicular neoplasms can result in diminished androgen levels and *oligospermia* (diminished number of sperm in the semen) or *azoospermia* (absence or failure of formation of sperm in the semen). Many therapeutic or recreational drugs affect plasma levels of testosterone. Antiandrogens (eg, cyproterone acetate) oppose the action of testosterone, and other drugs suppress its production. Chronic marijuana use, for example, has been correlated with decreased plasma testosterone levels, oligospermia, and impotence. Secondary hypogonadism, the result of insufficient gonadotropins, can result from pathologic conditions of the pituitary gland or lack of releasing hormones from the hypothalamus.

When testicular failure occurs congenitally or any time before the normal onset of puberty, puberty does not occur. In this case, the adolescent growth spurt does not take place; the infant genital morphology persists; body hair remains fine and does not increase on the face, axilla, and pubic areas; and the voice does not deepen. Although the growth spurt does not occur, total height may increase because the epiphyses do not unite. A lack of the signs of puberty past ages 15 to 17 should alert the clinician to a possible pathologic condition.

In younger adults, testicular failure or removal results in some regression of the secondary sex characteristics, such as beard growth, skin texture, voice timbre, and genital pigmentation. The accessory glands often get smaller, especially the prostate gland. Sperm count and motility decrease, and fertility is compromised. Libido will most likely diminish, and **gynecomastia** (enlarged feminine-appearing breasts) may appear. In the older male, some of these regressive changes may not be noticeable because of expected developmental changes.

Hypergonadal Endocrine Responses

Primary hypergonadism is caused by an androgen-producing testicular tumor, usually a trophoblastic tumor or tumors of Leydig's or Sertoli's cells. These pathologic changes usually result in palpable testicular masses and are most common in an undescended testis. Lymphoma, leukemia, and carcinomas of other tissues sometimes produce secondary tumors in the testis (Griffin & Wilson, 1983).

Secondary hypergonadism, the result of increased levels of gonadotropins, may be familial, pituitary, or hypothalamic in origin. Tumors in the region of the third ventricle are commonly the cause. Results of the hypersecretion are the same as for hypersecretion of primary origin, but the treatment differs.

Regardless of its cause, the overproduction of testosterone has various consequences depending on the client's age. In the adult male, few somatic changes are observable with testosterone excess. Some clinicians believe that high levels are associated with behavioral changes, including increased libido and aggression. Often, however, the only demonstrable sign is the palpable testicular mass in the case of testicular disease.

The prostate gland is especially sensitive to androgen stimulation. In cases of androgen excess, the gland can become greatly enlarged, even to pathologic proportions. The gland is also sensitive to estrogen stimulation and responds with similar enlargement. This hypertrophic response can have severe consequences for the urinary tract because of the prostate's anatomic position. The hypertrophy of prostatic tissue can actually obstruct the urethra, leading to the inability to void and the eventual destruction of kidney tissue. It also can signal a premalignant state.

In Both Women and Men

Infertility

Infertility is a diagnosis that can be applied to an individual but is most appropriately applied to a couple attempting conception. In primary infertility, there is failure to achieve pregnancy after 1 year of unprotected intercourse. Review of data by Lipshultz and Howards (1983) found that of couples attempting a first pregnancy, 15% fail to conceive within a year. In 30% of all cases significant male pathology exists, and in 20% of cases both male and female pathology exists. Thus, in 50% of infertile couples, the male is at least in part the cause of the failure to conceive.

Sperm can meet ovum for conception only if viable, mature, and motile sperm with an unimpeded route from the testes to the fallopian tubes meet a viable ovum. Many factors can compromise this process. Any infectious, endocrine, congenital, neoplastic, or immunologic disease that affects the reproductive organs can cause infertility. Many chemicals and drugs may also cause or contribute to infertility.

Infertility is often situational to the couple. The woman's reproductive tract and the man's sperm may or may not be compatible. For example, the contour of a particular female's reproductive tract may slightly prolong the time required for the ascent of sperm. If her partner also has a borderline low sperm count, their pairing may result in infertility. Quite possibly, either partner paired with another person might conceive without difficulty. Some women have an immune response to certain sperm and actually form antibodies that destroy them.

The frequency of ejaculation is another situational factor that affects sperm quality. Sperm lose motility and viability with prolonged storage, whereas frequent ejaculation can force sperm through the duct system with inadequate time for maturation. The most effective frequency of intercourse for adequate sperm is every 48 hours.

The timing of intercourse is the simplest situational cause of infertility but also the most frequent. Many couples do not understand the significance of the menstrual cycle nor the life expectancy of sperm, which is approximately 2 days in cervical mucus and only hours in the vagina. They also may not understand the importance of position during intercourse. Depositing of sperm deep in the female reproductive tract at the cervical os can compensate for low sperm counts by improving sperm survival. In some positions, sperm are not as likely to be placed at the cervical os. The female superior position, for example, permits gravity to work against the deposition of sperm at the cervical os; for some couples, this simple fact can affect fertility.

Sexual Dysfunctions

A sexual dysfunction is a physical impairment of the sexual response. In the male, this includes problems with erection, emission, ejaculation, sexual desire, genital muscle spasm, and dyspareunia (painful sexual intercourse). Among women, problems with sexual desire and dyspareunia are among the most common sexual dysfunctions. The cause of these dysfunctions may be physical or psychosocial, but the altered response is a physical impairment.

SECTION III

Related System Influences and Effects

Endocrine system infuences and effects have been discussed earlier in this chapter. Because the reproductive and endocrine systems relate so closely, it is impossible to discuss the structure and function of the female reproductive system without discussing hormonal function as well.

Neurologic damage from disease (multiple sclerosis, myasthenia gravis, or Parkinson's disease) or trauma (such as spinal cord injuries) interrupts the autonomic control of the sexual response. Dysfunction in the central nervous system, such as endogenous depression, tumors, and epilepsy, can cause sexual dysfunction from these higher centers.

Respiratory and cardiovascular problems affect the reproductive system through diminished ability to respond to stimuli and compromised tissue integrity. Dysfunction may cause specific reproductive system difficulties. For example, arteriosclerosis in penile arteries impairs the vascular mechanism leading to erection.

Trauma and diseases of the musculoskeletal system can pose a special problem to the reproductive system. Pain, immobility, or disfigurement may make it difficult to find a comfortable position for sexual response. Postmenopausal women are at risk of osteoporosis (a decrease in bone density), which is thought to be caused by an increased rate of bone resorption as estrogen levels decline. The rate of decline in skeletal mass is much more rapid in women than in men. In men, the decline in testosterone is more gradual and less overall.

Older women may develop a rectocele—a prolapse of the posterior vaginal wall and rectum into the vaginal canal—from past obstetric trauma resulting in muscle weakness. Constipation may be a side effect of this weakness. Constipation and even bowel obstruction also may occur as uterine fibroids exert pressure on the intestines.

Estrogen decline in menopause may result in urethral atrophy, leading to a distal urethritis and stricture formation. This may result in some bladder obstruction and symptoms of urinary frequency and dysuria.

In men, prostatic neoplasms cause urinary tract obstructions. Renal dialysis clients and those with severe liver disease are commonly impotent and are frequently infertile. Fixed incontinence may be caused by neurologic damage, pelvic relaxation secondary to obstetric trauma, and urethral narrowing.

The turgor, elasticity, and color of skin are all affected by ovarian function. Decrease in estrogen causes skin to dry and lose its elasticity. Hormonally induced pigmentary changes occur in pregnancy, oral contraceptive adminstration, menopause, and in the presence of ovarian or testicular tumors.

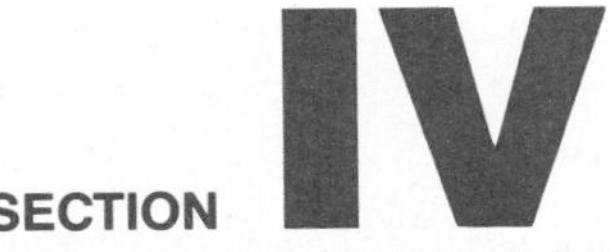

SECTION IV

Psychosocial/Lifestyle Influences and Effects

The well-being and dysfunction of the reproductive system are determined by both biologic and psychologic factors. Thus, not only anatomic and physiologic details but also the psychosocial/lifestyle factors affecting women and men should be an important part of the data used to plan for and give nursing care.

Developmental and Cultural Influences

Females mature from 2 to 2½ years faster than males. They become taller than males at age 7, but by adulthood males are 6% taller and 20% heavier. In general, though, females grow up faster, enter puberty sooner, and then cease to grow earlier than males. The onset of adolescence, or puberty, marks a major change in the life cycle of children. Puberty is more easily identified in girls than in boys because of menarche. The sequence of physical changes in adolescence is much the same for all persons, although the age of onset varies among individuals and cultures.

Learning and behavior theorists recognize the significance of learning in the early years. For this reason, experiences of reproductive or urogenital dysfunction and painful or privacy-violating experiences can affect an individual throughout life. Associations can form between the fear-ridden, painful episode and the individual's own use of the reproductive system. Physiologic risks to the system in the early years are primarily those of genetic and congenital anomalies. Except for these occurrences, trauma (to the system or the child in general) poses the biggest problem.

Cultural impact on the reproductive system includes the interpretations that adults make to the child concerning the use and meaning of the genitals in that culture. The child also observes the adults' behavior in regard to privacy, respect, and the use of genitals and forms personal attitudes and behaviors from these experiences. The 2-year-old who is told that the genitalia are "dirty" may have difficulty later in learning to handle or let sexual partners handle the genitals for pleasurable purposes. After biologic maturity, changes in reproductive status are minor. Throughout adult life, however, psychosocial influences may provoke a wide range of sexual behaviors and habits.

Pressures and stresses felt in adult life directly influence reproductive functioning as well as the sexual response and the energy available for sexual activity. Simple fatigue, such as that experienced by a man or woman working two jobs or engaged in highly competitive and demanding employment, may be sufficient to impair sexual response. Life crises such as job change, death in the family, marriage, separation, and divorce are stressful experiences.

During early and middle adulthood, many persons make major life transitions by making choices regarding work, social supports, marriage, and children. To many women and men, sexual and reproductive concerns are paramount in the 20s and 30s.

Biologic events associated with aging—for example, loss of reproductive function in women—make biologic reproductive boundaries obvious. In later years, subtle changes in sexual performance may cause the man to believe he is too old for sexual activity. Although this is not physiologically true, cultural expectations may strongly prejudice his attitudes. The most common disease conditions in older males include hydrocele and prostate problems, which do affect both reproductive status and sexual response.

Religious and cultural factors also strongly affect reproductive status and the frequency of sexual activity and the number and variety of partners. Religious and cultural convictions that limit the number and choices of partners can have a protective effect; research has shown an increased incidence of reproductive system diseases among people with a number of partners (Nass, Libby, & Fisher, 1984).

Dietary Habits and Medication Regimen

Good nutrition is particularly important for females during adolescence, pregnancy and lactation, middle age, contraceptive use, and menopause. The effect of nutrition on the male reproductive system is primarily on general well-being and tissue integrity.

Oral contraceptives seem to affect nutritional status by altering the metabolic need for several nutrients. Carbohydrate metabolism is altered because estrogen causes increased insulin secretion, increased secretion of growth hormone (GH), and elevated serum glucose levels. Serum levels of cholesterol, triglycerides, phospholipids, and lecithin are also elevated. The nutrients thought to be needed in increased amounts by women taking oral contraceptives include vitamins B_6, B_{12}, and C and folic acid. Heavy blood loss during a menstrual period can cause anemia. This is particularly true for women with IUDs.

In middle age, the main nutritional problem is a decreasing need for calories; if not respected, this leads to obesity. Women are more prone to obesity than men. Obesity increases a woman's vulnerability to cancers of the breast and endometrium, degenerative joint disease, and cardiovascular disorders.

Throughout history, various foods and drinks have been believed to be aphrodisiacs. There is no evidence that any nutritional preparation has a major effect on the reproductive system. Nevertheless, good nutrition is essential for sexual energy and tissue health, just as it is essential to the well-being of other body systems.

Drug-induced sexual dysfunction is irreversible while the use of the drug continues. When the drug is being used to treat a disease condition, an alternative drug might treat the disease satisfactorily but have fewer effects on the reproductive system. Some drugs that adversely affect male sexuality are drugs to treat hypertension, drugs that affect mental and emotional function, and the cholinergic-blocking drugs that are used in the treatment of Parkinson's disease and peptic ulcer.

Sexual Expression

Sexuality is the psychosocial expression of the reproductive system. The biologic developmental changes covered in the previous discussion have a powerful effect on sexuality. In addition, however, each developing person has certain sexual experiences that profoundly affect orientation to sexuality and pleasure. Cultural interpretations can enhance or diminish the sexual experience and lead to patterns of seeking or avoiding certain sexual activities thoughout life. Even chance experiences, such as a perfect first experience, rape, or incest, can radically change an individual's appreciation of sexual activities. Psychic phenomena are powerful facilitators and inhibitors of sexual response and greatly affect the development of sexual preferences.

Sexual dysfunction can be caused or exacerbated by many interpersonal variables. Libido, or sexual drive, can be altered by psychosocial factors such as rejection or acceptance by peers, as well as by general wellness and energy levels. Anxiety about performance, difficulty with self-esteem and trust, and feelings about the sexual partner strongly influence sexual function. Poor communication as a result of negative self-perception, attitudes, or both is a frequent source of unsatisfactory sexual experiences. People are more likely to be stimulated pleasurably if they let partners know what works for them. Unfortunately, many people are not skilled at asking directly for what they want. Compounding the problem is the fact that although societal attitudes and public education are changing, it is not uncommon for adults to know little about their anatomy and how it relates to the sexual response cycle.

The contraction of a sexually transmitted disease is a major risk of coitus, and the risk increases for the person who has multiple sex partners, engages in intercourse impulsively, or who is uncomfortable discussing the risk or possibility of venereal disease with a partner. Also, the use of oral contraceptives instead of condoms increases the risk of STD contraction for two possible reasons: Oral contraceptives provide no physical barrier and result in extrusion of the squamocolumnar junction of the cervix, making it more susceptible to invasion by foreign organisms that cause STDs. Lack of knowledge, which results in an unknowing transmission of infections, is another contributing factor.

When a pathologic condition has severe and irreversible effects on sexual expression, some further options remain. Reconstructive plastic surgery of the genitals is achieving acceptable results. Penile implants to achieve erection are available and, for many men, provide satisfying and acceptable results.

Body Image and Self-Concept

The resolution of body image problems in adolescence is important if a person is to develop into an adult who accepts the body and its natural processes. Developing other abilities while valuing unique physical attributes contributes to the adolescent's successful movement from issues of identity to issues of intimacy.

Later, during young and middle adulthood, physical characteristics remain essentially stable. Major body image changes are likely to occur in women during pregnancy when the effects of reproductive system alterations are experienced in all body systems.

How people encounter aging varies. Attitudes toward aging and involvement in adult roles strongly determine adjustment in older age. The importance one places on changes in body image and cessation of reproductive capacity or alterations in sexual response is influenced by previous experiences and cultural attitudes. For the individual whose self-esteem is broader than physical beauty alone or who does not believe that youth equals physical beauty, the effects of body changes may be slight.

Gender identity and sexual identity are important components of the self-concept. Gender identity is that part of the self-concept that recognizes maleness and femaleness and composes an acceptable profile of a male or a female for the self. Although this identity includes sexuality, it also encompasses all the learned cultural expressions of what males and females do. In North American society, these definitions are changing. Fifty years ago, few people would have disagreed with the idea that adult males work to support families and adult females care for those families in the home. Today such a statement would not necessarily be accurate. There is no confusion about biologic gender, but the role identify of the genders is taking on new definitions. Sexual identity is that part of the self-concept that defines the expression of reproductive drives unique to the individual. This aspect of self-concept is also totally affected by cultural and life experiences.

Occupation and Avocation

Increasing numbers of women over age 16 are joining the labor force in North America. The ability to delay childbearing has contributed to this trend. The effect of working on women's health is under study, but not many conclusions have been drawn. In general, women employed outside the home have neither more nor fewer physical complaints than those who work at home; this could be because sick women do not seek employment, or if they do look for jobs, they are not hired.

Some employers believe that, because of hormonal variations in menstruation and menopause, women's emotions are too labile for them to be reliable and to perform consistently. This attitude places women under more stress than men in similar jobs and hampers women's efforts to achieve their full potential. Recent publicity about premenstrual syndrome (PMS) has drawn added attention to the impact of hormonal variations on women. It is important that studies be done on the impact of the information about PMS on employers' hiring, firing, and promotional practices. Studies also are needed on the actual impact of variations in estrogen and progesterone levels on behavior and performance.

Some occupations can pose a hazard to the male reproductive system. Jobs that require prolonged sitting or standing are associated with an increased incidence of prostate problems. Jobs that require heavy lifting increase the risk of hernia, hydrocele, and varicocele. Many farm accidents, especially with bailers and mechanized pickers, involve trauma to the external organs of reproduction. Truck drivers who sit over motors may experience heat injuries to the testes or infertility problems because of the heat. Men who manufacture or use hazardous substances are also at risk.

Even recreational activities can pose hazards. Hot tubs

and spas have been implicated in heat-induced infertility problems that are usually temporary. Tight-fitting clothing holds the scrotum close to the body, creating temperatures that may be too high for adequate testicular function.

Environmental hazards may exist on the job or elsewhere. Society is only beginning to learn of the risks of disease from exposure to toxic chemicals and waste from a variety of agents. Such exposure may have adverse effects on fertility or even cause chromosomal or fetal damage. A few of these substances are (Mann & Lutewak–Mann, 1981):

- Organochlorine compounds (dichlorodiphenyltrichloroethane or DDT, some defoliants, and components of plastic) are easily absorbed through the skin and can damage DNA in the germ cell.
- Dibromochloropropane, a soil fumigant, has antispermatogenic properties. Its inhalation or oral administration causes severe degenerative changes in the testes.
- Organophosphorus (including many insecticides) inhibits cholinesterase, transiently affecting autonomic response but possibly also affecting spermatogenesis.
- Paraquat (a herbicide used extensively on marijuana) has mutagenic and antifertility properties.

Infertility and fetal damage have been associated with exposure to halogenated hydrocarbons, carbon monoxide, benzene, and radiation. Health workers such as nurses are also exposed to hazardous substances such as anesthetic gases and chemotherapeutic agents in health care environments. The list of hazardous substances continues to grow as dysfunctions are identified and epidemiologically associated with environmental exposure.

Chapter Highlights

The purpose of any reproductive system is continuing the species and providing a means of sexual pleasure and satisfaction.

The external organs of the female reproductive system include the mons pubis, clitoris, labia majora and minora, and several accessory structures; the internal organs are the vagina, uterus, fallopian tubes, and ovaries.

The external organs of the male reproductive system are the penis and scrotum; the internal organs are the testes, epididymis, vas deferens, and several accessory glands.

Both female and male sexual response involves four phases: excitement, plateau, orgasm, and resolution. Causes of sexual dysfunction can be biologic or, more commonly, psychosocial.

The reproductive system is structurally and functionally responsive to the hormonal variations controlled by the hypothalamic–pituitary–ovarian axis.

Three major developmental points for women are puberty and menarche, pregnancy, and menopause. There is a definite biologic change in the male at puberty, but only a moderate and gradual biologic change with aging following middle age.

Each major biologic alteration in the reproductive system affects social roles, interpersonal relationships, and body image.

Sexual dysfunctions are impairments of the sexual response.

Any disease or drug that affects the autonomic nervous system, respiratory system, or cardiovascular system can impair the sexual response. General well-being compromised by disease in any system is also likely to affect the sexual response. Some drugs and toxic chemicals also can impair fertility and sexual response.

Gender identity is the self-image of maleness or femaleness constructed by the individual, whereas sexual identity is that part of the self-concept that defines the unique expression of reproductive drives.

Bibliography

Bullough B et al: Subjective reports of female orgasmic expulsion of fluid. *Nurse Pract* 1984; 8:55–58.

Crooks R, Baur K: *Our Sexuality.* Menlo Park, CA: Benjamin/Cummings, 1983.

Ellis JW, Beckmann CRB: *A Clinical Manual of Gynecology.* Norwalk, CT: Appleton–Century–Crofts, 1983.

Emans SJH, Goldstein DP: *Pediatric and Adolescent Gynecology.* Boston: Little, Brown, 1982.

Fogel CI, Woods NF: *Health Care of Women: A Nursing Perspective.* St. Louis: Mosby, 1981.

Fromer MJ: *Ethical Issues in Sexuality and Reproduction.* St. Louis: Mosby, 1983.

Griffin E, Wilson J: Disorders of the testes. In: *Harrison's Principles of Internal Medicine,* 10th ed. Petersdorf RG et al (editors). New York: McGraw–Hill, 1983.

Griffith–Kenney J: *Contemporary Women's Health: A Nursing Advocacy Approach.* Menlo Park, CA: Addison–Wesley, 1986.

Guyton AC: *Textbook of Medical Physiology.* Philadelphia: Saunders, 1981.

Heath D: An investigation into the origins of a copious vaginal discharge during intercourse. *J Sex Res* 1984; 20:194–209.

Hogan RM: *Human Sexuality: A Nursing Perspective,* 2nd ed. Norwalk, CT: Appleton–Century–Crofts, 1984.

Horwith M, Imperato–McGinley J: The medical evaluation of disorders of sexual desire in males and females. In: *The Evaluation of Sexual Disorders.* Kaplan HS (editor). New York: Brunner/Mazel, 1983.

Kolodny RC et al: *Textbook of Human Sexuality for Nurses.* St. Louis: Little, Brown, 1979.

Lipshultz L, Howards S (editors): *Infertility in the Male.* New York: Churchill Livingstone, 1983.

Mann T, Lutewak–Mann C: *Male Reproductive Function and Semen.* New York: Springer–Verlag, 1981.

Masters WH, Johnson VE: *Human Sexual Response.* Boston: Little, Brown, 1966.

Moses AE, Hawkins RO: *Counseling Lesbian Women and Gay Men: A Life-Issues Approach.* St. Louis: Mosby, 1982.

Nadelson C, Marcotte D (editors): *Treatment Intervention in Human Sexuality.* New York: Plenum, 1983.

Nass GD, Libby L, Fisher M: *Sexual Choices: An Introduction to Human Sexuality,* 2nd ed. Monterey, CA: Wadsworth, 1984.

Olds SB, London ML, Ladewig PA: *Maternal Newborn Nursing: A Family Centered Approch,* 2nd ed. Menlo Park, CA: Addison–Wesley, 1984.

Porcino J: *Growing Older, Getting Better: A Handbook for Women in the Second Half of Life.* Reading, MA: Addison–Wesley, 1983.

Shephard DL: Sex differentiation and the development of sex roles. In: *Handbook of Developmental Psychology.* Wolman BB et al (editors). Englewood Cliffs, NJ: Prentice–Hall, 1982.

Spence AP, Mason EB: *Human Anatomy and Physiology,* 3rd ed. Menlo Park, CA: Benjamin/Cummings, 1987.

Turner BF: Sex-related differences in aging. In: *Handbook of Developmental Psychology.* Wolman BB et al (editors). Englewood Cliffs, NJ: Prentice–Hall, 1982.

Tyler SL, Woodall GM: *Female Health and Gynecology Across the Life Span.* Bowie, MD: Brady, 1982.

Vick RL: *Contemporary Medical Physiology.* Menlo Park, CA: Addison–Wesley, 1984.

Woods NF (editor): *Human Sexuality in Health and Illness,* 3rd ed. St. Louis: Mosby, 1984.

CHAPTER **48**

The Nursing Process for Clients With Reproductive Dysfunction

Other topics relevant to this content are: Technique of testicular self-examination, Figure 5–18 in **Chapter 5;** Resources available on AIDS, Resource list in **Chapter 22;** Care of the client undergoing breast aspiration, breast biopsy, or laparoscopy, **Chapter 49.**

Objectives

When you have finished studying this chapter, you should be able to:

Specify the major components of the health history to be obtained from clients with dysfunction of the reproductive system.

Explain specific assessment approaches in evaluating clients with disease of the reproductive system.

Identify the nursing implications of diagnostic studies commonly used to evaluate clients with dysfunction of the reproductive system.

Determine appropriate nursing diagnoses for clients with disorders of the reproductive system.

Develop, with the client, realistic goals of care.

Anticipate the psychosocial/lifestyle implications of reproductive dysfunction for clients and their significant others.

Develop a nursing care plan for a client with reproductive dysfunction.

Implement nursing interventions specific to clients with reproductive system disease.

Evaluate the effectiveness of the nursing care plan and modify it as necessary to meet client needs.

The nursing process for clients with reproductive system dysfunction includes both general and specialized assessment skills and interventions. This chapter discusses the planning of individualized client care related to disorders of the female and male reproductive systems.

SECTION 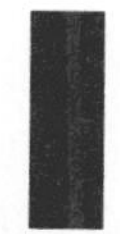

Nursing Assessment: Establishing the Data Base

Assessment of the female and male reproductive systems can be the most difficult part of a history and physical examination. The examiner, the client, or both may experience anxiety or embarrassment when discussing sexuality and sexual function. Clients are often reluctant to seek medical attention until the symptoms are advanced. This may be because of difficulty in acknowledging the existence of the problem, anxiety, embarrassment, or false hope that the symptoms will disappear.

Subjective Data

The nurse is often the health team member who must elicit primary assessment data and review previous nursing and medical treatment records. Variations in lifestyles and the definitions of acceptable behavior necessitate that the interviewer be nonjudgmental. Phrase questions about social or sexual habits so the client will not feel threatened or defensive.

When collecting data about the client's chief concern, recognize that many reproductive system problems are multifaceted. Disorders of other body systems, such as the urinary and gastrointestinal systems, may produce concerns similar to those caused by reproductive problems. Furthermore, clients' own interpretations of the meaning of pain influence their ability to describe it. For example, pelvic pain—one of the most common female problems—is often difficult to describe. The pain site the client identifies may be a referred site instead of its source. Thus, the examiner must gather information about all body systems suggested by the symptoms.

A detailed health history is essential in assessing reproductive health. Examine current lifestyle, recent significant changes, and stress level. Explore the client's medical and surgical history to determine whether previous illnesses or treatments and current problems are related.

Asking specific questions helps determine the usual characteristics of the presenting symptoms. Information on the onset and frequency of the symptoms is important, because the timing of the symptoms often suggests their cause. If a symptom is not continuous, question what seems to make it worse or better. Associated symptoms or signs, such as pruritus or discharge should be investigated. The effect the problem has on activities of daily living and self-prescribed treatments needs to be determined.

The Female Health History

PAIN Pain may be associated with genital lesions or discharge, inflammatory disease, congestion, muscle spasm, obstruction, and irritation. The timing of the pain's onset in relation to previous normal function is important. For example, spasmodic primary dysmenorrhea in women begins with cramping on the first day of flow and is rarely associated with physical abnormalities or pathologic conditions. Secondary dysmenorrhea, in contrast, is the onset of painful menses after a previously established pattern of relatively comfortable periods. The cause of secondary dysmenorrhea often is traced to organic problems, frequently endometriosis. Unilateral lower quadrant pain may suggest an ectopic pregnancy, **mittelschmerz** (ovulatory pain), or an ovarian cyst. Breast pain may indicate premenstrual fluid retention, neoplasms, cysts, or inflammation.

Dyspareunia (pain associated with intercourse) may have a physiologic or psychogenic cause. Vulvar or vaginal infections or a rigid hymen can cause pain on immediate penetration, whereas pain associated with deep penile penetration can be caused by endometriosis, tumors, or pelvic inflammatory disease (PID). A client may experience dyspareunia from decreased vaginal lubrication because of normal low estrogen levels, such as during postpartum, lactation, or menopause.

VAGINAL DISCHARGE A troublesome vaginal discharge is often caused by infection or irritation. Occasionally a contraceptive agent or disease process is the underlying cause. Consider the possibility of a sexually transmitted disease (STD) in all clients. Clues to this possibility are often found in the client's reasons for seeking care. Gonorrhea may be characterized by a yellow purulent discharge, dysuria, and lower abdominal pain. Herpes simplex infections can cause exquisitely painful genital lesions.

A detailed history assists in the determination of the cause, which may be multifactorial and influenced by stress, hygiene, and lifestyle. Ask the client when the symptoms began and the character and color of the discharge. Copious, frothy discharge is characteristic of *Trichomonas vaginalis*. *T. Vaginalis* and *Hemophilus vaginalis (Gardnerella)* are also associated with a foul-smelling discharge. Collect data concerning associated symptoms such as pruritus, burning, or tingling. Pruritus of the vulva with a discharge resembling cottage cheese indicates *Candida albicans* infection.

Look beyond the initial cause of vaginal discharge to rule out other contributors such as systemic disease, frequent douching, or the concurrent use of medications. Unless these are addressed, the treatment is not likely to be effective, and the problem will recur.

BLEEDING Unusual bleeding or lack of normal menstrual bleeding is not an uncommon problem. The client's menstrual history is essential in assessing her chief concern. Elicit information about the age of menarche and the frequency and duration of the menses. A description of the amount of flow is highly subjective among women. Try to obtain an accurate picture of how much blood is lost and the character of the bleeding. Ask the client how many pads or tampons she uses during her menstrual period as a whole, as well as on specific days. For example, are panty liners sufficient, or must she use maxipads or superabsorbent tampons? Also determine whether there have been any changes from the client's usual pattern and character of menstruation, including pain.

The Male Health History

General questions when evaluating male reproductive system problems should elicit information about prostatic problems, sexually transmitted diseases, benign or malignant lesions, and overall sexual function.

Enlargement of the prostate is common in males over age 50 and usually causes no problems. If the prostate is markedly enlarged it can interfere with urinary function. Ask the client if he has any difficulty starting or stopping his urinary stream. Has there been a change in the force of the stream? Does he feel he does not empty his bladder completely? Is there any urinary dribbling? These symptoms can indicate prostatic problems.

Does the client have any penile discharge? If he does, ask about the color, odor, and amount. Does he have any sores, ulcers, blisters, rashes, or lesions on the penis or scrotum? Has he had any known contact with an STD? Does his partner have any discharge or lesions?

Does the client practice testicular self-exam? Has he

noted any swelling or lumps in his testicles? Is there any pain in the testicles?

Does the client have a satisfactory sexual relationship? Does he have any problem achieving and maintaining an erection? Is he able to ejaculate? Does he have pain with intercourse? Has there been any change in his libido? Is he willing to use condoms to protect a partner from pregnancy or a partner or himself from disease?

Objective Data

Physical Assessment of the Female

After the history has been completed, the client is prepared for a physical examination. It is recommended that women over 20, as well as younger sexually active clients, have an annual pelvic examination. Ask the client to empty her bladder and undress before the examination. Drape her adequately to protect her modesty, but to still allow for eye contact with the examiner. Placing a mirror so that the client is able to observe her own cervix facilitates teaching. Explain in advance each step of the physical examination.

The examination begins with a general assessment to determine the development of secondary sex characteristics and overall client health. Examination of the breasts usually follows the examination of the heart and lungs. The breasts are inspected for size, shape and symmetry, the appearance of the skin, and the presence of any masses or dimpling. The nipples are inspected for size and shape, as well as for redness, ulceration, and discharge. A uniform palpation pattern of the breast is necessary to note tenderness or nodules. The examiner should describe any nodules palpated by their location, size, shape, consistency, mobility, and tenderness. This is a good time to teach the client how to perform breast self-examination (BSE) or, if she already does BSE, to review the proper procedure.

After the breast examination, the examiner generally inspects, auscultates, and palpates the abdomen. In the gynecologic examination, the health care provider is alert for abdominopelvic masses. A mass associated with severe pain, fever, or hemorrhage demands immediate action. A careful history and physical examination can usually determine whether the mass originates in the reproductive organs, bowels, or urinary tract.

As the examination progresses, the client assumes the lithotomy position. The examiner inspects the external genitalia for normal development and signs of inflammation, swelling, ulceration, discharge, or nodules. In older women or those who have had vaginal deliveries, it is important to assess perineal support. The examiner will ask these women to strain downward, and will note any bulging of the vaginal walls, which indicates weakening.

Internal examination of the vagina and cervix is next. Examination is accomplished by the use of a speculum of the appropriate size and shape, which should be warmed and lubricated with warm water. Other lubricants should be avoided if cytologic studies are planned. The cervix and its os are inspected for color, position, ulcerations, nodules, masses, discharge, and bleeding. Slowly withdrawing the speculum allows inspection of the vaginal tissues for lesions or inflammation.

After withdrawing the speculum, the examiner proceeds with a bimanual examination. Two gloved lubricated fingers of one hand are inserted into the client's vagina while the other hand simultaneously palpates the abdomen. This allows examination of the uterus and the adnexa (adjacent structures, including ovaries, fallopian tubes, and uterine ligaments). The size, shape, consistency, and mobility of the uterus are noted, as well as any tenderness or masses. To palpate each ovary, the abdominal hand applies pressure in the right or left lower quadrant, pushing the ovary toward the palmar surface of the intravaginal fingers (Figure 48–1). The ovaries are examined for size, shape, consistency, and degree of tenderness (the normal ovary is somewhat tender). Ovaries of women 3 to 5 years past menopause have usually atrophied and should not be palpable.

Ovarian and other adnexal masses generally can be differentiated from lesions on the body of the uterus during palpation and bimanual examination. The examiner carefully palpates any mass for size, position, configuration, and mobility. In the premenopausal woman, any ovarian cyst less than 5 cm in diameter is usually functional, whereas cysts larger than 6 cm in diameter are suggestive of neo-

Nursing Research Note

Ewald BM, Roberts CG: Contraceptive behavior in college-age males related to Fishbein model. *ANS* 1985; 7(3):63–69.

Beliefs, attitudes, and intention to use condoms as a contraceptive method were studied in male college students aged 18 to 20. Fishbein's Belief-Attitude-Intention Behavior (BAIB) model was used as a theoretical framework. The BAIB model shows specific behavior is a function of intention to perform that behavior. The intention to perform is seen as a function of an attitude toward a behavior and the person's perception of what significant others think about a behavior. The attitude is a function of belief about the consequences of a behavior and personal evaluation of these consequences. The model attempts to predict and understand particular behaviors.

Positive beliefs about condom use were significantly correlated with positive attitudes about condom use. Attitudes about condom use were also related to intention to use condoms. The result indicated that intention to use condoms was positively associated with use in the past month during the study. Therefore, this study supports the Fishbein model in that positive beliefs and attitudes combined with intention to use were positively associated with utilization of this birth control method.

The Fishbein model indicates that beliefs result in particular behaviors. Altering beliefs may alter behaviors. Therefore, teaching birth control use may be more effective if it is aimed at altering beliefs rather than behaviors.

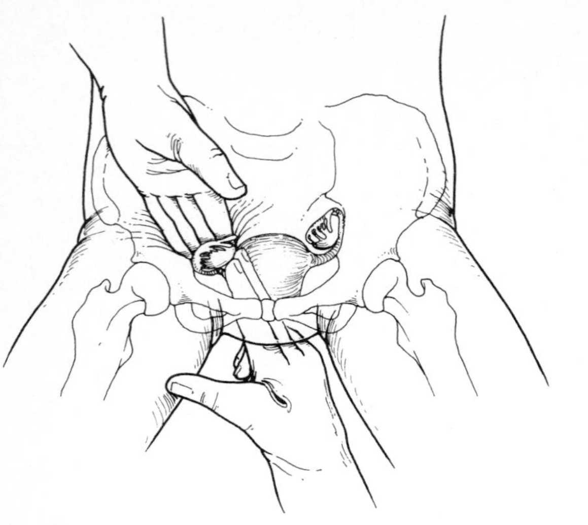

Figure 48–1

Bimanual abdominovaginal palpation of the adnexa.

plasms. Any palpable structure in the adnexa of postmenopausal women is suggestive of cancer because the ovaries normally are atrophied and nonpalpable.

A rectal and rectovaginal examination is the last phase of the pelvic examination. The examiner places one finger in the rectum and one finger in the vagina. The procedure for the bimanual examination is repeated. The examiner palpates the posterior vaginal wall, giving special attention to the region behind the cervix (where a bowel mass can be more readily felt) and the posterior uterine surface, because this is the only time it is available for examination. The rectal examination makes it easier to detect abnormalities of the deeper structures and the posterior surfaces of the reproductive organs.

Following the pelvic examination, a gentle wiping of the perineal area removes secretions and lubricant. The client may need some assistance in removing both feet from the stirrups at the same time to reduce strain on the perineal muscles. Some clients experience orthostatic hypotension if they sit up too quickly, so the examiner should evaluate the client for symptoms and signs of dizziness before letting her get off the examining table using a stool. Allow adequate time for dressing, and be available to answer questions or interpret collected data.

Physical Assessment of the Male

For inspection of the male genitalia, the client should stand facing the examiner. General observation includes assessment for the presence of secondary sex characteristics (pubic hair and appropriate testicular and penile development), which should be present in the normally developed adult man. The testes are generally symmetrical, although the left testis is slightly lower than the right.

Further inspection includes observing the condition of the integument, noting whether the skin is intact and whether there are any lesions or ulcers. Common lesions on the penis include the chancre and condylomata acuminata, or venereal warts. Chancres, usually caused by syphilis, are painless, reddened, rounded, eroded ulcers with induration at their bases. Venereal warts have a cauliflower, wartlike, pedunculated, reddened, moist appearance. Carcinoma of the penis is rare in North America but is a significant worldwide health problem. It most often occurs in uncircumcised men as a nodule or ulcer on the glans penis or the inner aspect of the prepuce. Because the prepuce may cover this type of lesion, the client should retract the prepuce, if possible, for inspection. These lesions are usually painless. As with any other potential cancer, any sore that does not heal must be investigated further.

When the prepuce is retracted, the glans is inspected for leukoplakia (white patches that could be precancerous) and smegma (a cheeselike secretion of sebaceous glands that builds up if hygiene is poor). In phimosis the prepuce cannot be retracted; in paraphimosis, the retracted prepuce cannot be returned.

To inspect the distal end of the urethra, the client is asked to squeeze the penis between his fingers near the head. If discharge is present, a smear and gonococcal culture are obtained. The location of the urethral opening should be central. An opening on the inferior surface is known as hypospadias. Some degree of hypospadias is common, but more pronounced conditions are usually corrected in childhood. Epispadias, a urethral opening on the anterior part of the penis, is less common.

Next, the scrotum is inspected. For good visualization, the client is asked to hold the penis up and to the side so it is out of the way. Both the anterior and posterior surfaces of the scrotum are inspected. The groin is observed for swellings or bulges that could indicate an inguinal hernia. This observation is made with the client at rest and as he bears down.

Gloves are worn during palpation if lesions or an infection is present. The penis is palpated for any signs of inflammation, tenderness, and changes in size and contour. The testes are most easily palpated if the skin is warm and relaxed. The testes are gently rolled between the thumb and fingers. Normally, they are smooth, mobile, bilaterally consistent in size, and somewhat sensitive to pressure.

If any swelling or irregularities are noted in the scrotum, the scrotum is transilluminated. The room is darkened and a flashlight placed behind the scrotum. Normally, a red glow is present as the light shines through serous fluid (tissues and blood will not transilluminate). Any hard, irregular masses that do not transilluminate should be reported.

Early detection and treatment are critical for the client with testicular cancer. All adolescent males should be taught TSE and should perform it monthly. (TSE is described and illustrated in Chapter 5.) Tell clients to examine themselves after a warm shower, when scrotal muscles are relaxed. They should hold their scrotums in their hands and palpate for hardenings or lumps by gently rolling the testes between the thumb and forefingers. Any lumps, hardenings, or lack of symmetry should be promptly reported.

Thorough assessment of the male reproductive system also includes palpation of the prostate. Techniques for this examination vary according to the client's health status. The ambulatory client is best examined while standing. He should bend at the waist, turn his toes in, and rest his upper body across an examining table. In this way, the gluteal muscles relax, the buttocks flatten, and the rectum and anus become more accessible. A client unable to tolerate this position is placed on his left side, his right knee flexed and his buttocks close to the edge of the table.

The examiner uses a gloved lubricated index finger to palpate the posterior prostate, which protrudes about 1 cm into the anterior rectal wall. The lateral lobes and median sulcus can be identified. The size, shape, consistency, and symmetry should be noted. In a client with benign prostatic hyperplasia, the prostate may be soft, smooth, and symmetrically enlarged, protruding more than 1 cm into the rectal wall. The enlargement may obliterate the median **sulcus** (a midline groove that separates the two lobes). Tenderness, edema, and bogginess may indicate prostatitis. If this condition is suspected, the prostate can be massaged to force discharge into the urethra for culture. Any irregular, hard, fixed nodules might indicate cancer of the prostate. Because cancer of the prostate frequently begins in the posterior lobe and is easily palpable on rectal examinations, this procedure is recommended annually for all males over age 40.

During palpation, the examiner also should feel for the presence of an inguinal hernia. To palpate for an indirect hernia, have the client slightly bend his knee on the same side. The examiner's little or index finger then follows the inguinal canal inward as far as it goes. At that point, the client is asked to bear down. A bulging mass indicates a hernia. This same examination is then done on the opposite side. The examiner should use the left hand on the left side and the right hand on the right side. A direct hernia is palpated by asking the client to bear down while two fingers are placed bilaterally over the inguinal rings. A bulge indicates a direct inguinal hernia.

Diagnostic Studies—Female

PAPANICOLAOU AND OTHER CYTOLOGIC TESTS The *Papanicolaou* (Pap) *test* has been used since the 1950s to screen for cervical cancer. Most gynecologists recommend that women receive the test annually, and women over 40 and those at high risk may be advised to have semiannual exams. This relatively painless cytologic test can detect precancerous and cancerous cells among the cells shed from the cervix. Occasionally, adenocarcinoma cells of the endocervix or the endometrial lining of the uretus also will be discovered. Atypical cells discovered in the cytologic screening may be from cervicitis.

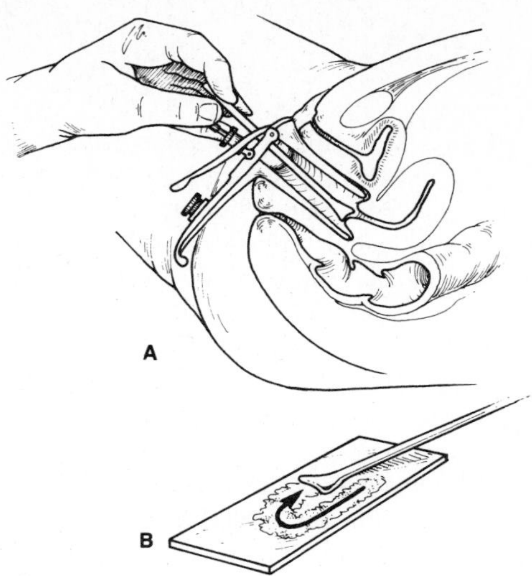

Figure 48–2

The Papanicolaou (Pap) test. **A.** The curve of the wooden spatula allows it to scrape the cervix and the endocervix simultaneously. **B.** Transferring the specimen to a glass slide.

The Pap test should be scheduled between the client's menstrual periods. Advise the client to avoid douching, vaginal medications or deodorants, and sexual intercourse for at least 24 hours before the test. Douching will wash away cellular deposits, and vaginal medications or deodorants may confound the cytology. Semen also can confound the cytology.

At the time of the examination, give the client assistance and support as needed. Relaxation techniques, including deep breathing and concentrating on a visual focus point, may be valuable to the apprehensive client. Explain all procedures to the client prior to their performance.

The Pap test takes just a few minutes after the woman is in the lithotomy position. After the cervix is visualized through the speculum, a wooden spatula is used to scrape the cervix and endocervix (Figure 48–2A). The specimens are immediately transferred to glass slides and either sprayed or immersed in a fixative solution (Figure 48–2B). If the smear is allowed to dry on the slide before the fixative has been applied, accurate diagnosis will be impossible. A pathologist examines and interprets the smears, and the test results are usually received in 2 to 3 days.

The accepted (Papanicolaou's) classification of the cytologic findings is:

- Class 1: Absence of atypical or abnormal cells
- Class 2: Atypical cytology but no evidence of malignancy
- Class 3: Cytology suggestive of, but not conclusive for, malignancy
- Class 4: Cytology strongly suggestive of malignancy
- Class 5: Cytology conclusive for malignancy

A finding of abnormal cytology, with the exception of Class 5, does not necessarily mean a diagnosis of cancer. Additional studies should be ordered to confirm the test results. These commonly include colposcopy, biopsy and conization, and dilatation and curettage (D and C).

When informing a client that her specimen showed atypical cells, emphasize that only Class 5 is conclusive for malignancy. Provide support and honest answers to the client's questions, and encourage her to return to the clinic for follow-up testing to validate the test results.

Cytologic examinations can also detect viral, fungal, and parasitic disorders and evaluate the client's endocrine status. The vaginal mucosa cells respond cyclically to the monthly fluctuation of steroid hormones, and cell scrapings of the lateral vaginal walls permit easy study of these fluctuations.

SCHILLER'S IODINE TEST Schiller's iodine test is an outpatient procedure to identify unhealthy cervical epithelium. A positive test is only suggestive of neoplasms. To perform the test, the client is placed in a lithotomy position, and the cervix is visualized through a speculum. The entire surface of the cervix is painted with Schiller's iodine solution (1 part aqueous iodine, 2 parts potassium iodide, and 300 parts water).

Normal cervical cells contain glycogen, which reacts with the iodine solution to stain the cells a mahogany brown. Thus, brown staining over the entire squamous epithelial surface of the cervix is interpreted as a negative test result. A positive test, the absence of staining in some sites, indicates that immature cells are present; this is suggestive of neoplasms. Because cancer depletes the epithelial cells' store of glycogen, they cannot react to the stain. Any sites that appear pale in comparison to the surrounding cervical tissue should be biopsied, even though the majority of these sites will be noncancerous.

VULVAR STAINING (COLLINS' TEST) Skin changes of the vulva can be stained and identified for biopsy by a procedure similar to Schiller's test. In Collins' test, a 1% solution of toluidine blue O is painted over the entire vulva. After the skin has dried briefly, it is washed with 1% acetic acid, which removes the blue stain from normal cells. Any areas that retain the dark blue stain are considered positive and should be biopsied.

COLPOSCOPY AND COLPOMICROSCOPY The colposcope and colpomicroscope provide three-dimensional magnification (from 10 to 20 times and up to 400 times, respectively) of the cervical epithelium. Colposcopy is also suited for inspection of the vagina and vulvar epithelium. Either stained or unstained cells may be visualized.

The examiner visualizes the cervix with a speculum and cleans secretions from it. A cotton swab moistens the cervix with saline to allow better visualization of vascular patterns and the squamocolumnar junction. The cervix may be painted with 3% acetic acid, which acts as a mucolytic agent to draw moisture from the tissue and accentuate important morphologic features. The colposcope provides intense illumination and magnification to visualize tissue areas under question. A biopsy is still required, however, for accurate diagnosis of questionable sites.

Colposcopy is recommended for any women suspected of having diethylstilbestrol (DES) changes (such as daughters of women who took DES) and for clients with precancerous and malignant lesions to localize the exact site for biopsy. A combination of cytology and colposcopy is recommended.

CERVICAL BIOPSY A biopsy is the examination of choice to remove cervical tissue for cytologic study. The type and extent of the biopsy vary. If a lesion is clearly visible with a colposcope, a punch biopsy may be used to extract a small column of tissue. Cervical specimens preferably include a portion of the squamocolumnar junction (the area of most cervical malignancies). Cervical punch biopsy can be done as an office procedure without anesthesia, because the cervix has few pain receptors. The biopsy specimen need not cause excessive bleeding; light cauterization with a silver nitrate stick usually is sufficient to control light bleeding. All biopsy specimens are immediately placed in a formalin solution for transport to the cytology laboratory.

The client should be scheduled for the biopsy during the middle of the menstrual cycle, when the cervix is the least vascular. Explain the procedure to the client, paying attention to the physical sensations she might expect. Because cervical biopsy is performed to evaluate areas that could be cancerous, most women are anxious and need time to explore feelings and fears. The use of relaxation techniques often facilitates comfort and expedites the procedure.

Advise the client to rest for 24 hours after the procedure and to avoid heavy lifting. Although some oozing is considered normal, the client should report any excessive bleeding (more than a regular menstrual period flow). The client should avoid douching and sexual intercourse until the biopsy site has healed completely.

ENDOMETRIAL BIOPSY AND ASPIRATION Both endometrial biopsy and aspiration are techniques to obtain cells directly from the uterine lining of women at risk for cancer of the endometrium. Endometrial biopsy is also of significant value in assessing functional menstrual disturbances (especially anovulatory bleeding) and infertility. The biopsy should be performed during the immediate premenstrual period to serve as an index of progesterone influence and ovulation. Biopsies done in the last half of the menstrual cycle (approximately Days 21 and 22) can evaluate corpus luteum function and the presence or absence of a secretory endometrium.

An endometrial biopsy is often performed as an office

procedure using a small amount of intrauterine anesthesia. After the cervix has been dilated, a curet is passed through the cervix and pressed firmly against the uterine wall, and a portion of the endometrium is withdrawn by either the cuplike end of the curet or by suction. A specimen that contains malignant cells confirms the diagnosis of endometrial cancer. A negative test result does not rule out the diagnosis, however; it only provides evidence that there are no malignant cells in the limited site of the biopsy, and carcinoma may be present in other areas of the endometrium. Women with symptoms suggestive of endometrial cancer need a diagnostic curettage for accurate diagnosis.

A disposable unit is often used to obtain cytologic specimens by irrigating the entire uterine cavity with saline solution. Negative pressure systems, such as the Gravlee Jet Washer, prevent potentially malignant cells, forced from their implantation site in the uterus, from being pushed into the fallopian tubes.

CULDOSCOPY AND LAPAROSCOPY Culdoscopy, a method of pelvic endoscopy, is the simplest procedure for direct visualization of the pelvic cavity, organs, and ligaments in women who may not require surgical intervention. Culdoscopy is highly accurate and useful in women with suspected ectopic pregnancy, primary ovarian disorders and infertility, unexplained pelvic pain, and pelvic masses of undetermined nature.

The knee-chest position is essential to provide the best view of the pelvis during the procedure. The majority of culdoscopies are done with only local anesthesia in the vaginal cul-de-sac. The culdoscope, a tubular instrument with a lamp and lens near its tip, is inserted through the cul-de-sac into the pelvic cavity (Figure 48–3). Inspection combined with abdominal palpation provides a detailed view of the pelvic contents. The examination site heals easily without sutures, but the client is advised not to douche or have intercourse for approximately 2 weeks after the procedure.

A second method of pelvic endoscopy is laparoscopy (pelvic peritoneoscopy). It is frequently used as a diagnostic procedure when minor surgery is anticipated. In addition to the indications previously listed for culdoscopy, laparoscopy provides a route for procedures such as tubal sterilization, ovarian biopsy, cyst or graafian follicle aspiration (to retrieve ova for in vitro fertilization), and lysis of adhesions around the fallopian tubes. Laparoscopy is discussed in Chapter 49.

METHYLENE BLUE TEST The location of a vesicovaginal fistula is facilitated by the instillation of methylene blue into the client's bladder. Dye will not appear in the vagina if the woman has a ureterovaginal fistula or a rectovaginal fistula. A test with negative results is followed by the IV injection of indigo carmine. This dye appears in the vagina of clients with a ureterovaginal fistula. An intravenous pyelogram (IVP) and cystoscopy may also be performed to determine the location and number of fistulas.

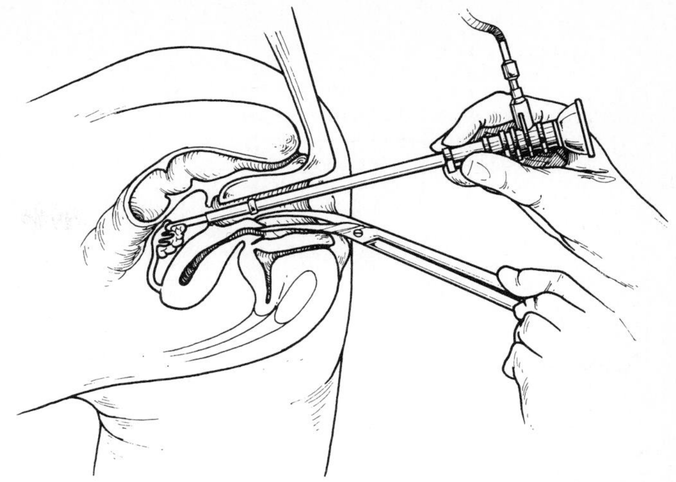

Figure 48–3

Culdoscopy. The culdoscope is inserted through the cul-de-sac. Note that the client is in the knee-chest position for this procedure.

INFERTILITY STUDIES The woman typically seeks treatment for infertility. Because the problem is complex and multifactorial, however, the health care provider should see both partners to obtain a more complete history. It is important to listen to the couple's separate and joint concerns. The period when the couple admits their infertility to themselves and outsiders is particularly stressful. The initial work-up and probing of the couple's intimate life threatens their maleness and femaleness and can affect their personal relationship. Having both partners available facilitates their ability to process information given to them and makes the treatment a joint concern.

Unless the couple has extenuating circumstances such as advanced maternal age, the infertility work-up is generally not begun until 1 year without conception. The initial investigation consists of a thorough medical, sexual, and social history of each partner. A physical examination and routine laboratory tests are performed for both man and woman to determine their general state of health.

The women's infertility work-up includes a detailed history of menstruation, previous pregnancies, use of birth control techniques, and any STDs. The man's history includes questions about any previous impregnations, history of STDs, and his ability to achieve and maintain an erection and produce an ejaculation. Because infertility can be multifactorial, finding one cause in one partner does not exclude the possibility of other causes in the same partner or other partner.

BASAL BODY TEMPERATURE CHARTING A basal body temperature chart is a simple graph used as a part of infertility studies to indicate ovulatory function. Immediately on awakening each morning, the woman takes her temperature with a basal body thermometer. This thermom-

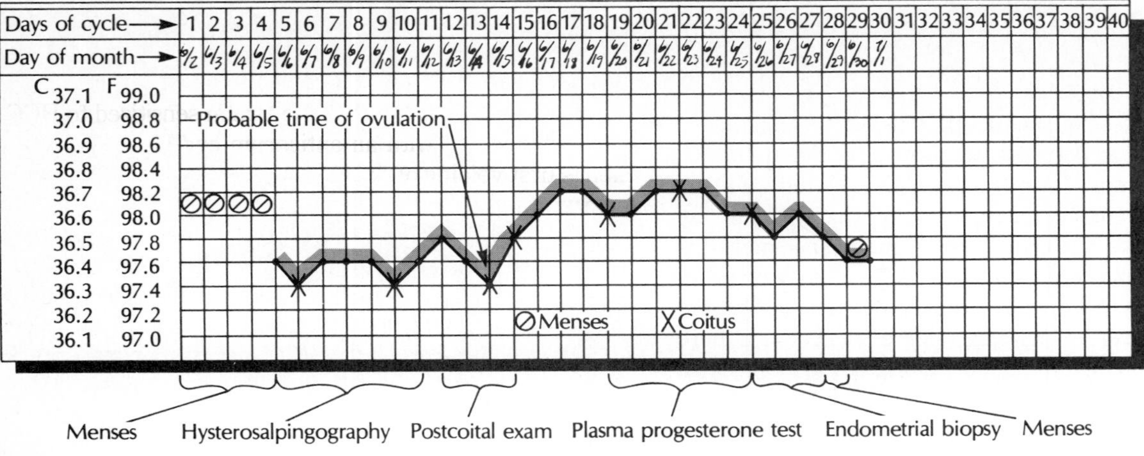

Figure 48–4

Basal body temperature chart with different types of testing and the time in the cycle that each would be performed. *SOURCE: Olds SB, London ML, Ladewig PA:* Maternal Newborn Nursing: A Family-Centered Approach. *Menlo Park, CA: Addison–Wesley, 1984, p. 115.*

eter is similar to a standard oral thermometer, except the markings between degrees are easier to read. The client must take her temperature before getting out of bed to determine the body temperature at total rest. The client records the temperature on a graph that plots the degrees Farenheit for each day of the menstrual cycle. The client should keep the chart for four or more menstrual cycles to be able to identify recurring patterns. She should indicate on the chart the days when intercourse occurred and any reasons for an elevated temperature, such as illness. The charts are useful in planning optimal times for intercourse and future infertility testing (Figure 48–4).

The normal temperature chart shows a biphasic curve for each menstrual cycle. Normally, the basal body temperature is lower in the preovulatory phase. In the second phase, progesterone affects the temperature curve by causing a sustained increase of 0.4°F or more from the point of ovulation until menses begins. An irregular, low, monophasic pattern indicates anovulation with absent or inadequate progesterone production. A graph that shows a biphasic pattern with a sustained temperature elevation through the first missed period suggests pregnancy.

Keeping the basal body temperature chart can be stressful to the couple, because it calls specific attention to their infertility every day and removes spontaneity from intercourse. The couple may feel as though the chart dictates when they may express desire for each other and when they should have coitus.

FERN TEST (CERVICAL MUCOUS ARBORIZATION TEST) The fern test is a second simple way to assess whether a woman ovulates. Cervical mucus under the influence of increasing estrogen production has a high concentration of sodium chloride shortly before ovulation, so it forms crystal patterns when drying. The characteristic fern pattern is seen in dried cervical mucus only when there is adequate estrogen. Ovulation and the secretion of progesterone inhibits or completely abolishes this pattern even though estrogen is still being produced. During pregnancy, when there is continuous progesterone influence, this pattern also does not occur. The cervical mucus of a menopausal woman will not show ferning because of the absence of sufficient estrogen.

The fern test is easily performed by the health care provider. The client is prepared for a pelvic examination, and her cervix is exposed with a speculum and gently swabbed clean. A sample of endocervical mucus is obtained and smeared on a glass slide. If the sample is spread too thinly or blood is present in the specimen, ferning will not occur. The slide is allowed to air-dry completely for at least 10 minutes before it is read under a microscope.

A positive fern test indicates a predominant estrogen state. The fern test also can help determine ovulation if the cervical mucous smear is inspected twice during the menstrual cycle, once during the preovulatory stage and later after the last date on which ovulation could have occurred in a menstrual cycle.

SPINNBARKEIT TEST The quantity and quality of the cervical mucus respond to the effects of estrogen and progesterone in other ways as well. At the beginning of the menstrual cycle, the mucus is scant and viscid. By midcycle, the mucus is copious, clear, slippery, and stretchy. The watery midcycle mucus has been compared to raw egg white and exhibits the characteristic spinnbarkeit.

The spinnbarkeit test evaluates the stretchability of endocervical mucus. The mucus is stretched between two glass slides or by placing the mucus on the end of a sponge forceps and gently opening it (Figure 48–5). At midcycle, the mucus will stretch for at least 5 cm (about 2 in.) into a string or thread without breaking. After midcycle, when progesterone is dominant, the mucus tends to become thick and cloudy. Therefore, the absence of strings is a good indication that ovulation has occurred.

POSTCOITAL CERVICAL MUCOUS TEST The postcoital cervical mucous test (Sims' test or P–K test) provides both

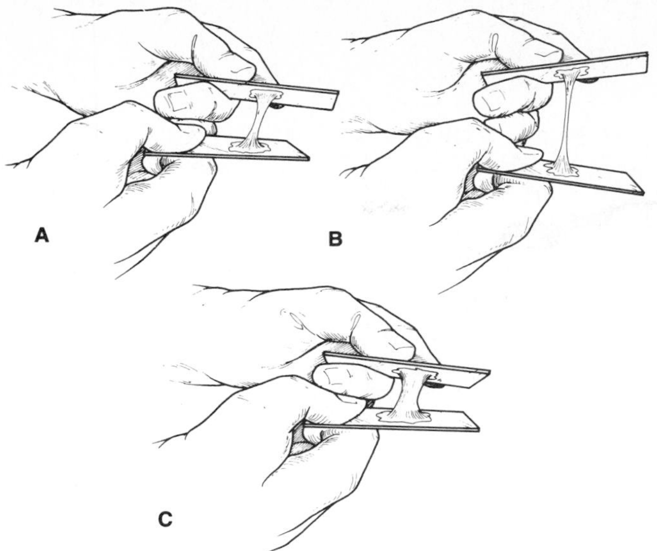

Figure 48–5

Spinnbarkeit test. **A.** Beginning of cycle. Mucus is sparse and viscid. **B.** Midcycle. Mucus is copious, resembles raw egg-white, clear, stretchy, slippery; spinnbarkeit is present. **C.** End of cycle. Mucus becomes thick and cloudy white or yellow with no spinnbarkeit.

male and female reproductive system assessment data. The couple is advised to abstain from intercourse for 48 hours before the test. The test usually is scheduled on or within 24 hours of the day on which other tests (such as the basal body temperature test) predict that ovulation should occur. The couple ideally has intercourse 4 to 8 hours (some authorities recommend as few as 2 hours or as many as 8 hours) before the woman is to be examined, and she must not tub bathe or douche after intercourse.

The woman is prepared for a pelvic examination, with the cervix exposed using a nonlubricated speculum. Samples of the endocervical mucus and secretions from the vaginal pool are examined separately under a microscope. Sperm in the cervical mucus indicates that the coital technique is adequate. If the mucus shows midcycle changes, the pH and quality of the mucus will facilitate sperm transport. A cervical mucus sperm count should show 5 to 20 sperm per high-powered field. Normally, 4 hours after intercourse 50% of the sperm will still be active. At 12 hours after intercourse, the number of active sperm normally drops to 25%.

PREGNANCY TESTS Pregnancy tests are all based on the detection of human chorionic gonadotropin (HCG) in blood or urine. They rule out or confirm pregnancy, and also aid in the diagnosis of retained placental tissue, hydatidiform mole, and choriocarcinoma. Furthermore, because many drugs and interventions for preventive or tertiary treatment are teratogenic (causing birth defects in the fetus), it is essential to determine that the client is not pregnant.

Biologic tests that employ laboratory animals for pregnancy testing have been abandoned in favor of immunologic tests that use a latex particle preparation sensitized to HCG. This is combined with an antiserum and a sample of the client's first voiding of the day, and the mixture is observed for clumping of the latex particles (positive result). Other pregnancy tests produce color changes if results are positive. The most accurate immunologic test results are usually available in 2 to 3 hours, but commercially available tests can provide fairly accurate results in 2 minutes. These tests can detect or rule out HCG reliably in urine specimens of women 10 to 14 days after their first missed period. Some can even detect positive samples 4 to 5 days after a missed period.

The most accurate tests for the presence of HCG in serum are radioimmunoassay and radioreceptorassay. Both use radioactive iodine and are capable of detecting small amounts of HCG in the blood. These tests approach 100% accuracy within the first days after a missed period.

PITUITARY GONADOTROPIN DETERMINATION Determination of the quantitative levels of follicle-stimulating hormone (FSH) and prolactin help in the differential diagnosis of reproductive tract disorders. Most of these tests are now done by radioimmunoassay. The FSH and LH (luteinizing hormone) levels are important in the evaluation of subfertile women. Determination of the level of prolactin helps in the investigation of women with galactorrhea (breast discharge) with or without amenorrhea.

STEROID HORMONE DETERMINATION In the diagnosis of female reproductive system disorders, the ability to determine the levels of the steroid hormones estrogen and progesterone is extremely important. The client's 24-hour urine sample can be screened for estradiol and pregnanendiol (urinary by-products of estrogen and progesterone). The radioimmunoassay technique can detect both plasma estrogen and progesterone at any given time in the menstrual cycle. Progesterone levels can be indicative of ovulation and pregnancy, whereas falling serial levels of progesterone in pregnancy may indicate impending abortion.

HYSTEROSALPINGOGRAPHY Hysterosalpingography is an x-ray examination following the injection of a constant substance to highlight the interior of the cervix, uterus, and fallopian tubes. The test is useful in the evaluation of tubal anatomy and patency and the detection of uterine abnormalities (fibroids, tumors, or fistulas).

This examination should be scheduled for the second to fourth day after the end of the client's normal menstrual flow. Scheduling is important to prevent the accidental flushing of a fertilized ovum from the fallopian tube or the exposure of a fetus to radiation. The client is usually prepared with a cathartic the evening before the test followed by an enema the morning of the examination to reduce distortion of the x-rays by gas shadows.

The client signs a consent form before the procedure. The nurse confirms the date of the client's last menstrual period and records it in the progress notes. The woman may be premedicated to promote comfort and decrease apprehension. The nurse should inform her that she may experience some nausea and vomiting, abdominal cramping, or faintness. Explain that although these are all normal, the client should inform the examiner of any severe, continuous cramping. Listen attentively to the client's concerns, and encourage her to ask questions before and after the procedure.

The client assumes the lithotomy position, and her cervix is exposed by a speculum. A few milliliters of radiopaque dye or an oil-based medium is injected through a cannula into the uterine cavity by the radiologist. Usually, only two to three x-rays are taken to show the path and distribution of the contrast medium. If the fallopian tubes are patent, the dye enters the peritoneal cavity within 10 to 15 minutes.

The phrenic nerve may be irritated by the dye and cause shoulder pain following the procedure. The dye also may drain from the cervix, so the woman should be given a perineal pad to wear for several hours following the test to prevent soiling her clothes. Inform her that she may have some bloody discharge, but if it continues for 4 days or more, she should contact her physician. The client also should contact her physician to report any signs of infection, such as lower quadrant pain, fever, malodorous discharge, and tachycardia.

ULTRASONOGRAPHY The use of ultrasonography as a diagnostic technique is becoming routine in most obstetrics and gynecology clinics. It involves no exposure to ionizing radiation and is considererd safe for use during pregnancy.

In gynecologic practice, the pelvis and abdomen are scanned in a linear fashion to outline and define soft tissue masses and differentiate tumor types, ascites, and encapsulated fluid. Ultrasonography also can locate escaped intrauterine devices (IUDs) and monitor progress or tumor regression following medical treatment. The technique is especially useful in obese clients when bimanual examinations are not satisfactory to make differential diagnosis.

TESTS TO IDENTIFY PATHOGENS

WET PREP A sample of the secretions in the vaginal pool (those that collect in the vagina when the client is on her back) can be obtained at the beginning of an examination that uses a nonlubricated speculum. The wet prep (simple fresh or wet smear), a standard vaginal test, is useful in the diagnosis of Gardnerella, trichomonal or candidal vaginitis, as well as nonspecific vaginitis or cervicitis. The test also can evaluate atrophic vaginitis. Curdy white plaques seen on the vaginal wall should be scraped and examined to rule out candidal vaginitis.

To perform this test, the specimen is placed on a glass slide, and a drop of saline and a coverglass are applied. The slide is examined under the microscope using both low and high power to confirm or rule out the presence of pathogens.

POTASSIUM HYDROXIDE PREPARATION Preparation of a vaginal smear with potassium hydroxide (KOH) greatly facilitates the diagnosis of candidal vaginitis. If possible, the specimen is obtained from the white patchy areas on the vaginal walls. If the vaginal patches are unavailable, the specimen is obtained from the erythematous area on the labia or vulva. The specimen is placed on a glass slide and combined with one drop of 10% to 20% KOH solution; this dissolves cellular debris, leaving the stained hyphae (threads or filaments) and yeast forms visible. Because it is often difficult to get a good specimen, even a single spore confirms the diagnosis.

TZANCK TEST The Tzanck test is used to detect genital herpesvirus Type II. Scrapings from the base of a lesion are placed on a slide, fixed, stained, and examined under a microscope. Findings typical of *herpesvirus* are giant multinucleated cells or acidophilic intranuclear inclusion bodies.

VAGINAL AND CERVICAL CULTURES Vaginal cultures are indicated to identify the pathogenic organism and determine the appropriate antibiotic therapy. Culture media are available for growing *Trichomonas,* but a culture is rarely necessary, because the differential diagnosis is readily made by examination of a wet prep. An inexpensive, accurate culture method uses Nickerson's medium to grow *Candida* in 1 to 5 days in slated tubes. This method is especially helpful, because the identification of candidal vaginitis by wet prep alone is often difficult. When a nonspecific bacterial vaginitis is suspected, routine bacteriologic cultures and antibiotic-sensitivity studies are ordered. Viral culture mediums are available for suspected herpetic infections of the vagina, vulva, or cervix.

One of the most important cultures in gynecologic practice is the culture to detect *Neisseria gonorrhoeae.* A culture is essential for confirming the diagnosis of gonococcal infection in women, because a large number of clients that harbor the organism are asymptomatic. Specimens also can be obtained from the urethra, rectum, and oropharynx.

DARK-FIELD EXAMINATION FOR SYPHILIS A dark-field examination of the clear serum from the surface of the ulcerated lesions aids in the identification of *Treponema pallidum* in primary or secondary syphilis. The spirochete cannot be seen under direct light because it is translucent, and it cannot be stained with the usual dyes. The dark-field method of microscopic examination reflects light through the organism instead of directly onto it. A positive test identifies the spirochetes moving back and forth. If the client has applied alcohol to the lesion or used systemic or local antibiotics, the surface spirochetes will be killed, and the test will yield a false-negative result. If this is suspected, the dark-field examination should be repeated later.

VENEREAL DISEASE RESEARCH LABORATORY TEST The Venereal Disease Research Laboratory (VDRL) test is a nontreponemal antigen test used to detect, confirm, and follow cases of syphilis. This test is not absolutely specific or sensitive for syphilis, because both false-positive and false-negative results are possible, but it is economical and highly indicative. Some acute and chronic conditions that cause false-positive results are tuberculosis, infectious mononucleosis, recent smallpox vaccination, rheumatoid arthritis, subacute bacterial endocarditis, and hepatitis.

The normal range is nonreactive, and other results may be weakly reactive or reactive. A titer of 1:8 or greater indicates syphilis. A titer above 1:32 can indicate the secondary stage of syphilis.

BREAST SCREENING

MAMMOGRAPHY Mammography is a soft tissue x-ray study of the breast that is helpful as a screening tool for women at higher-than-normal risk of developing breast cancer. Mammograms are used to detect differences in the density of the breast tissue and are especially helpful in the evaluation of breasts with poorly defined masses, multiple masses or nodules, nipple changes or discharge, skin changes, and pain. Mammography can detect many cancers that are not palpable by physical examination, but some cancers appear benign on mammography. Thus, mammography should not take the place of biopsy when there is a single, dominant lump in the breast.

The National Cancer Institute recommends that mammograms not be used in the routine screening of women younger than 35 years but should be provided for any woman with a suspected neoplasm or at high risk for breast cancer. The American Cancer Society suggests that women between the ages of 35 and 39 have a baseline mammogram, those between 40 and 49 should have a mammogram every 1–2 years, and all women should have annual mammograms after age 50, although many physicians and nurse practitioners believe this is too frequent. Mammograms are rarely done on pregnant women because, although shielding of the abdomen is possible, it is impossible to stop the radiation from internal scattering. Biopsy of a suspicious lump is preferred.

As with other nursing interventions, explain or reinforce the purpose and procedure to the client. Mammography can be painful when the breast is compressed during the x-ray. The actual test takes approximately 15 minutes; ask the client to wait until the x-rays have been developed in case a view needs to be repeated. Caffeine restriction prior to the mammogram may make the breast compression more comfortable. Ask the woman not to use creams, powders, or deodorant on the breasts or underarm areas before the x-rays; these products contain aluminum chlorhydrate and may show up as white on x-rays, mimicking calcium clusters.

XEROMAMMOGRAPHY The xeromammogram uses a much lower dose of radiation than the low-dose mammogram to provide a xerogram of the soft breast tissue. A special selenium-coated plate is placed under the breast exposed to the x-rays, and the xerogram is photoelectrically recorded on paper without the use of film.

THERMOGRAPHY Once thought to be a boon for the routine screening of clients for breast disease, thermography has dropped from favor because it requires expensive equipment and is difficult to interpret accurately. A thermogram is a picture of the surface temperature of the skin that does not use ionizing radiation. Infrared photography detects the circulation pattern of different areas of the breasts. Areas of increased blood supply (eg, around tumors) produce more heat than normal breast tissue. Thermography can accurately detect large cancers but often fails to detect small or deep neoplasms.

BREAST ASPIRATION AND BIOPSY Aspiration and biopsy of suspicious breast nodules are integral parts of the diagnosis of breast masses. These procedures are discussed in Chapter 49.

Diagnostic Studies—Male

The Tzanck test for genital herpes, the dark-field examination for syphilis, and the VDRL discussed in the previous section are also applicable to men. The following tests are specific to male reproductive problems.

SERUM ACID PHOSPHATASE TEST Serum acid phosphatase levels are studied to detect prostatic cancer. Acid phosphatase is an enzyme found in many body tissues, including the kidney, red blood cells, platelets, liver, spleen, and bone. The major concentration is in the prostate, where it is 100 times more concentrated than in other tissues.

The normal values for serum acid phosphatase are 0 to 1.1 Bodansky units/mL, 1 to 4 King–Armstrong units/mL, and 0.13 to 0.63 Bessey–Lowry units/mL, depending on the method of measurement. An increase in acid phosphatase levels indicates the metastasis or extension of a tumor, and a decrease indicates a response to treatment. Prostatic massage will cause a false elevation of acid phosphatase levels; to avoid this, the test should be performed before a rectal examination or at least 24 hours afterward. A false increase also can occur if the client has received clofibrate (Atromid-S), or ingested fluorides, oxalates, or phosphates. After the specimen is drawn, it must be sent to the laboratory immediately.

SERUM HUMAN CHORIONIC GONADOTROPIN TEST The presence of human chorionic gonadotropin (HCG) in the serum may indicate testicular choriocarcinomas or other testicular tumors. Radioimmunoassay to measure HCG levels is invaluable for the early detection of testicular tumors. With effective treatment, the HCG levels decrease to normal.

ALPHA-FETOPROTEIN TEST Another testicular tumor marker is alpha-fetoprotein (AFP), which is also measured by radioimmunoassay. AFP is produced in the liver, yolk sac, and gastrointestinal tract of the fetus and is the major circulating protein. The normal level for males and non-pregnant females, less than 25 ng/mL, increases in 70% of clients with embryonal testicular cancer. AFP levels should decrease with effective treatment. AFP is measured before and after orchiectomy (removal of the testis). Elevated AFP levels after orchiectomy suggest metastasis.

TESTOSTERONE ANALYSIS In a client with fertility problems, serum or plasma testosterone levels are determined. Abnormally low levels may be found in infertility. In males, the normal level is 406 to 954 ng/dL.

SEMEN ANALYSIS Semen analysis, a part of fertility testing, identifies abnormalities in one of the following areas:

- *Sperm motility.* Normally, at least 60% to 70% of sperm are moving forward.
- *Morphology and quality of sperm.* More than 70% should be motile and normal in appearance.
- *Volume/density.* There should be at least 20 million sperm per mL of ejaculate. Ejaculatory volume should be between 2 and 6 mL.

Before the semen analysis, the client should be sexually abstinent for at least 48 hours. Abstinence should not be longer than 5 days, however, because the quality and motility of the sperm will decrease. Heat and cold will destroy the sperm, and the specimen must be delivered to the laboratory within 2 hours; thus, the client should masturbate in the physician's office while wearing a condom to collect the specimen. Some male clients are uncomfortable with the request to masturbate to obtain semen because of religious beliefs or personal reasons (Orthodox Judaism and Roman Catholicism have sanctions against masturbation). These clients can be instructed to collect semen in a condom during sexual intercourse and to take the specimen to the laboratory immediately. The semen analysis is performed at least twice. If the sperm count is less than 20 million/mL, endocrine testing and testicular biopsy are indicated (Pagana & Pagana, 1982).

GONOCOCCAL CULTURE If gonorrhea is suspected, a urethral gonococcal culture is usually obtained. Both a culture and Gram's stain can be performed, but a culture is particularly important because of gonococcal resistance to antibiotics.

BIOPSY OF THE PROSTATE OR TESTIS To detect cancer, a prostatic biopsy may be performed. First, a cystoscopy is performed, and the area of the biopsy is identified by rectal examination. A needle is then inserted into the perineal skin, and prostatic tissue is aspirated. Usually, a biopsy is performed on more than one area. A small dressing is placed on the site of needle insertion using aseptic technique (Lerner & Khan, 1982).

A testicular biopsy can be performed to check for a testicular abnormality if no sperm are obtained on semen analysis. The biopsy is done bilaterally; an incision is first made into the scrotal skin, and separate incisions are then made into each testis. Testicular biopsy specimens should not be placed in a preservative because it will alter cellular structure and kill live sperm, making the results inaccurate. Afterward a dressing is applied, and a scrotal support is used to prevent scrotal edema. The client may feel mild pain (Lerner & Khan, 1982).

SECTION 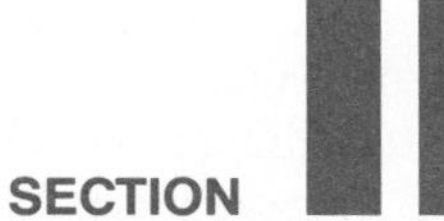

Nursing Diagnosis /Planning and Implementation/Evaluation

Information gathered from the client's health history, physical examination, and diagnostic studies is used to determine nursing diagnoses and the plan of care. Not every client will have the same needs. The Nursing Diagnoses box lists diagnoses **directly related** to reproductive dysfunction along with **potential** nursing diagnoses for clients with reproductive problems. The most common nursing diagnoses for clients with reproductive dysfunction include self-care deficit, impaired skin integrity, altered nutrition: less than body requirements, knowledge deficit, sexual dysfunction, and altered sexuality patterns. The sample nursing care plan in Table 48–1 focuses on knowledge deficit in the following areas: early cancer warning symptoms and signs, conception and sexual function, and STDs. Altered sexuality patterns related to loss of a body part or a body function are also discussed. Knowledge deficit related to female perineal hygeine, impaired skin integrity related to vaginal discharge, altered nutrition: less than female body requirements, and other aspects of sexual dysfunction, including infertility, are discussed in the narrative.

If the goals of care have not been met, re-evaluation is required. The nurse and client should jointly review the nursing care plan. New objectives may need to be formulated; other nursing interventions may be added or modified; or the evaluation may show that more time is required to meet the objectives.

Table 48–1
Sample Nursing Care Plan for a Client With Reproductive Dysfunction, by Nursing Diagnosis

Client Care Goals	Plan/Nursing Implementation	Expected Outcome
Knowledge deficit related to early cancer warning symptoms and signs		
State warning symptoms of gynecologic or testicular cancer and accurately perform monthly BSE or TSE; annual Pap test	Teach cancer warning symptoms and BSE or TSE; use return demonstration; encourage client to return for periodic examination	Client states cancer warning symptoms; demonstrates correct technique for breast or testicular self-examination; performs examinations at regular monthly intervals; returns annually for Pap test
Knowledge deficit related to conception and sexual function		
Understand normal menstrual cycle physiology, determine approximate time of ovulation, conceive only when desired, have no pain during intercourse, follow medical orders about sexual relations, experience satisfaction with sexual function	Establish nonjudgmental, supportive relationship; explain normal menstrual cycle physiology; teach techniques for approximating time of ovulation; teach contraceptive methods and help with decision making; provide information on coital techniques to decrease discomfort; provide information on nongenital methods of mutual satisfaction; administer prescribed medications; encourage discussion of feelings with partner	Client states menstrual physiology; indicates approximate time of ovulation; has no unplanned pregnancies or pain with intercourse; states satisfaction with sexual function
Knowledge deficit related to STDs		
Understand symptoms of, mode of transmission of, and means of protection from STDs; no recurrence of STD after teaching; accept and comply with complete course of STD treatment if appropriate	Establish nonjudgmental, supportive relationship; teach symptoms and transmission of STDs; teach means of protection from STDs; encourage compliance with complete treatment	Client states symptoms of major STDs, mode of transmission, and means of protection; completes total treatment; has no recurrence of STD after treatment
Sexuality, altered pattern related to loss of body part or body function (eg, mastectomy, orchiectomy)		
Demonstration of movement toward acceptance of loss; ability to discuss meaning of loss; resumption of sexual relations	Establish trusting relationship; encourage discussion of meaning of loss; encourage sharing of concerns with partner; role play through fear of rejection; encourage discussion of strengths of relationship; give permission for resumption of sexual relations	Client views and discusses loss with less discomfort; discusses meaning of loss to self and relationship; states sexual relations have resumed

Knowledge Deficit Related to Female Perineal Hygiene

Because of the proximity of the female urethral, vaginal, and rectal openings, the gynecologic client may be seen for vaginal infections precipitated by incorrect perineal wiping techniques. Infections from *Escherichia coli* from the colon attributed to posteroanterior perineal wiping usually are labeled nonspecific vaginitis.

Planning and Implementation

The nurse should advise clients on the correct technique to wipe the perineum: from front to back, disposing of the tissue after a single wipe. This technique prevents inadvertent contamination of the urethra and vagina by rectal flora. During foreplay and intercourse, the client should take care to avoid cross-contamination from the rectal area to the vagina. Intercourse can encourage the development of cystitis by friction and the spread of vaginal bacteria to the urethra. Voiding immediately after intercourse can prevent bacteria from ascending into the urethra.

Evaluation

Following effective teaching, the client should be able to state the correct method of wiping the perineum and its importance. Her perineum will remain clean, and there will be no occurrence of urinary or vaginal infection secondary to fecal contamination.

NURSING DIAGNOSES IN
Reproductive Dysfunction

DIRECTLY RELATED DIAGNOSES

- Knowledge deficit
- Nutrition, altered: less than body requirements
- Sexuality, altered patterns
- Sexual dysfunction
- Skin integrity, impaired: actual

OTHER POTENTIAL DIAGNOSES

- Anxiety
- Comfort, altered: pain
- Coping, ineffective individual
- Fear
- Health maintenance management, impaired
- Hopelessness
- Knowledge deficit
- Infection, potential for
- Self-concept, disturbance in: self-esteem, body image, personal identity

Skin Integrity, Impaired

Excessive vaginal discharge facilitates the growth of organisms that thrive in a warm, moist environment. Irritation of the vulva with redness, edema, and general malaise often follows. Lesions of the vulva from *Candida albicans* or herpes simplex virus may be associated with intense itching and lead to further skin breakdown attributed to scratching and secondary infections. Mechanical irritation from tight or nonabsorbent clothing and chemical irritants such as deodorants and douches also can cause skin alterations.

Planning and Implementation

The improvement of skin integrity depends on the prevention of further skin breakdown. In female reproductive disorders, the genital skin is often compromised because of the continually warm, moist environment. Normal skin integrity requires cleanliness of the perineum, but some vaginal discharge is normal and nonoffensive. Some women have difficulty accepting this physiologic phenomenon, however, and routinely use strong alkaline soaps, douches, and deodorants to keep themselves "clean." This assists in the destruction of normal flora, predisposing the client to further skin breakdown.

Client/Family Teaching

The client with pruritus should be informed about its causes. Since moist clothing may aggravate pruritus, the client should attempt to stay as clean and dry as possible by frequently changing perineal pads. Distraction can prevent itching, and fingernails should be kept short if the client is inclined to scratch the area. Control of the offending organism by appropriate medication resolves the itching.

In health teaching, recommend undergarments that provide ventilation through natural fibers. Nonrestrictive clothing prevents chafing. Women with heavy vaginal discharge should use and frequently change pads or tampons.

Women being treated for a vaginal infection should complete the total treatment even after the initial symptoms subside. If vaginal tablets or suppositories are prescribed, the woman should remain recumbent for approximately 30 minutes after application to allow for some absorption and dispersal of medication in the upper vaginal area. She should expect some drainage of the medication, which is best coped with by wearing a perineal pad. (Tampons should be avoided because they absorb too much of the medication.) The client should continue treatment even if she begins to menstruate, and she should avoid intercourse until treatment has been completed. If the vaginal irritation is an allergic response, the offending substance must be removed. If the external genitalia are swollen and uncomfortable, sitz baths with warm water can promote comfort and speed healing by increasing circulation to the area. Air drying and exposing the area to a heat lamp also can provide relief.

Evaluation

Absence of lesions and discomfort result from a successful plan of care. The woman is able to state the correct method of perineal hygiene and refrains from irritants that may alter normal vaginal pH. She also completes the total medically prescribed treatment and is able to rest and sleep without disturbance from perineal discomfort.

Nutrition, Altered: Less Than Female Body Requirements

Health care providers are seeing an increasing number of young women with menstrual irregularities. A low percentage of body fat has been associated with amenorrhea and anovulation. With the social emphasis on physical fitness, many young women are participating in prolonged, strenuous exercise such as long-distance running. Studies have documented the return of normal ovulation in long-distance runners when they decreased their amount of running time and increased their percentage of body fat. Additionally, some women with anorexia nervosa or bulimia experience amenorrhea.

Planning and Implementation

Health care providers must have insight into why a client consumes amounts inadequate to meet nutritional requirements. The possibility of pathologic conditions should be eliminated through medical screening. If no such condition exists and adequate food is available, the client may need to seek psychologic counseling. Women with inadequate body fat levels to support normal menstrual function should be counseled about a balanced daily diet and appropriate caloric requirements. The nurse may suggest alternative meal plans that might work better in the client's lifestyle. Support and encouragement need to be given through follow-up counseling. Social programs should be explored to assist women who do not have the means to purchase adequate foods. These can provide low-cost foods and preparation guides to maximize the client's food-value intake. Teach women who have been trying unsuccessfully to become pregnant that their inability to conceive can be caused by anovulation secondary to low body fat content.

Evaluation

Expected outcomes for a female client whose reproductive function is inhibited due to failure to meet minimum nutritional requirements include the ability to state the recommended daily amounts of each of the basic food groups, to choose appropriate foods, and to show an increase in body weight and fat. The resumption of normal menstrual function is not expected immediately. The client should understand that the initiation of menstruation may be delayed for some time.

Sexual Dysfunction

There are many possible causes of sexual dysfunction including infertility, STDs, knowledge deficit, fear, anxiety, grief, altered body image, altered self-concept, role change, or altered physiologic states. To determine when a diagnosis of sexual dysfunction is appropriate, look for some of the following characteristics:

- Expression of sexual problems or lack of sexual satisfaction
- Physical alterations that indicate a potential or actual dysfunction
- Significant role changes
- Feelings of shame or guilt
- A violation of cultural or religious sexual taboos
- A loss of privacy
- A loss of power or control
- Ingestion of recreational or therapeutic drugs that affect sexual function

Planning and Implementation

Infection can cause sexual dysfunction. The overall goal of nursing care is to relieve symptoms of the infection and prevent its spread to others. To prevent the infection's spread, clients must understand its cause and mode of transmission. They must understand the need for appropriate antibiotic treatment and for identifying and treating sexual contacts if the infection is an STD. Clients should understand that they must take the full course of antibiotic therapy and not resume sexual activity without protection until both they and any partners have been treated. Wearing a condom will provide a barrier to the spread of infection for those who resume sexual activity before treatment is completed. Infection control by the nurse includes proper hand-washing techniques, the use of sterile technique with dressing changes, and the timely administration of antibiotics.

Clients often perceive infertility as a blow to their self-esteem and sense of identity. The overall nursing goals are to assist the client in identifying possible correctable contributing factors by encouraging evaluation by a physician expert in infertility, if that has not already been done, and in coping more effectively with the problem. Encourage open communication between partners. The infertile couple may choose to accept being childess or may choose such alternatives as adoption, artificial insemination, in vitro fertilization, or surrogate parenting.

Clients with altered cardiovascular function often need to reduce the work load of the heart and the chance of pain during sexual activity. They can achieve this goal through position changes; both the female-superior and side-lying positions are less exerting for the male. The appropriate use of medications is also important. For example, taking a nitroglycerin tablet before intercourse can relieve anginal pain. If needed or desired, the client can use alternative means of sexual satisfaction.

Evaluation

Successful outcomes for clients with sexual dysfunction include increased sexual satisfaction, relief from infection, the resolution of or acceptance of infertility, and a decrease in fatigue or pain during intercourse.

Chapter Highlights

When interviewing clients with reproductive system dysfunction, it is important to assume a supportive and nonjudgmental attitude.

Reproductive system disorders can be multifaceted and produce symptoms similar to disorders of other body systems.

Female reproductive disorders often cause pain, vaginal discharge, or bleeding. Diagnosis may be possible from a complete history of the timing, character, and location of the symptoms. The physical examination is used to confirm the diagnosis.

Sensitive support from the nurse will help clients cope with the wide variety of invasive and noninvasive laboratory and diagnostic studies used.

The nurse should instruct clients about the early warning symptoms of reproductive system cancer and self-examination procedures to promote early detection.

The client's knowledge deficit related to ovulation, sexual function, or STDs can be overcome

by supportive, nonjudgmental, and informative nursing consultation and advice.

Proper female perineal hygiene is necessary to prevent urinary and vaginal contamination from fecal material.

The improvement of skin integrity depends on the prevention of further skin breakdown. Health teaching is important to promote normal vaginal flora, control pruritus, and help clients understand and follow treatment regimens for vaginal infections.

Teaching the female client with an inadequate percentage of body fat about good nutrition, and providing her with support and proper food choices, will help promote the return of her menstrual function.

For the client with sexual dysfunction, nursing interventions to promote satisfactory sexual function begin with establishing effective communication between nurse and client and between the client and sexual partner.

Bibliography

Beal MW: Understanding cervical cytology. *Nurse Pract* 1987; 12(3):8–22.

Bell R (editor): *Changing Bodies, Changing Lives: A Book for Teens on Sex and Relationships.* New York: Random House, 1980.

Boston Women's Health Book Collective: *The New Our Bodies, Ourselves: A Book by and for Women.* New York: Simon & Schuster, 1985.

Byrne JC et al: *Laboratory Tests: Implications for Nursing Care,* 2nd ed. Menlo Park, CA: Addison–Wesley, 1986.

Cancer Facts and Figures: 1987: New York: American Cancer Society, 1987.

Carpenito LJ: *Nursing Diagnosis: Application to Clinical Practice.* Philadelphia: Lippincott, 1983.

Casey MP: Testicular cancer: The worst disease at the worst time. *RN* 1987; 50(2):36–40.

Crooks R, Baur K: *Our Sexuality,* 2nd ed. Menlo Park, CA: Benjamin/Cummings, 1983.

Fischbach F: *A Manual of Laboratory Diagnostic Tests,* 2nd ed. Philadelphia: Lippincott, 1984.

Fogel CI, Woods NF: *Health Care of Women: A Nursing Perspective.* St. Louis: Mosby, 1981.

Frank DI: Counseling the infertile couple. *J Psychosoc Nurs* 1984; 22(5):17–23.

Griffith–Kenney J: *Contemporary Women's Health.* Menlo Park, CA: Addison–Wesley, 1986.

Haggerty BJ: Prevention and differential of scrotal cancer. *Nurse Pract* 1984; 8(10):45–52.

Jensen MD, Bobak IM: *Maternity and Gynecologic Care: The Nurse and the Family.* St. Louis: Mosby, 1985.

Lerner J, Khan Z: *Mosby's Manual of Urologic Nursing.* St. Louis: Mosby, 1982.

McConnell EA, Zimmerman MF: *Care of Patients With Urologic Problems.* Philadelphia: Lippincott, 1983.

Malasanos L et al: *Health Assessment,* 3rd ed. St. Louis: Mosby, 1985.

Muhlenkamp A, Waller M, Bourne A: Attitudes towards women in menopause: A vignette approach. *Nurs Res* 1983; 32(1):20–23.

Olds SB, London ML, Ladewig PA: *Maternal–Newborn Nursing,* 2nd ed. Menlo Park, CA: Addison–Wesley, 1984.

Pagana KD, Pagana TJ: *Diagnostic Testing and Nursing Implications.* St. Louis: Mosby, 1982.

Pearson JC et al: Radioimmunoassay of serum acid phosphatase after prostatic massage. *Urology* 1983; 21:37–41.

Peckman BM, Shapiro SS: *Signs and Symptoms in Gynecology.* Philadelphia: Lippincott, 1983.

Roseman D, Ansell JS, Chapman WH: Sexually transmitted diseases and carcinogenesis. *Urol Clin North Am* 1984; 11(1):27–44.

Ruby EB, Estok P: Intensity of jogging: Its relationship to selected physical and psychosocial variables in women. *West Nurs Res* 1983; 5(4):325–335.

Siemens S, Brandzel RC: *Sexuality: Nursing Assessment and Intervention.* Philadelphia: Lippincott, 1982.

Resources

SELF-HELP GROUPS AND OTHER ORGANIZATIONS

For resources on acquired immune deficiency syndrome (AIDS), see the resources list in Chapter 23.

American Fertility Society
2131 Magnolia Avenue
Birmingham, AL 35256
Phone: (205) 251–9764

Responds to written requests for referral to infertility specialists in local communities.

Association for Voluntary Surgical Contraception
122 E. 42nd St.
New York, NY 10168
Phone: (212) 351–2500; for information only, call (213) 351–2555

This association can refer clients considering tubal ligation or vasectomy to specialists and treatment centers for consultation. It also offers information and sponsors educational programs.

DES–Action
PO Box 1977
Plainview, NY 11803
Phone: (516) 433–7070

This organization is for women who took the hormone DES during pregnancy and for their offspring. It conducts workshops, training courses, and seminars and publishes a newsletter. Also provides referrals to physicians who are specialists in DES exposure and to "rap" groups.

ENCORE (Contact a local YWCA)

This is a national YWCA program for postoperative breast cancer clients. It includes floor and pool exercises and group discussions.

HELP
PO Box 13827
Research Triangle Park, NC 27709
Phone: (919) 361–2742

This organization provides information about herpes genitalis and advice on coping with it.

Impotents Anonymous
119 S. Ruth St.
Maryville, TN 37801
Phone: (615) 983–6064

This organization, founded in 1981, offers information about the causes of impotence, treatments available, and emotional support. Meetings are held once or twice a month, and no dues or fees are collected. An associated organization, I-Anon (modeled after Al-Anon) gives impotent men's partners the chance to share their concerns and to benefit from the experience of others. Both organizations guarantee anonymity.

J2CP Information Service
PO Box 184
San Juan Capistrano, CA 92693
Phone: (714) 496–J2CP [recording only]

Clients who are considering a sex change operation or who have questions about transsexualism can obtain information from this facility. Requests for information must be accompanied by a contribution of at least $25.00 to cover costs of materials, handling, and postage.

Fund for Human Dignity
80 Fifth Ave., Suite 1601
New York, NY 10011
Phone: (212) 529–1604 (5-10 PM)

Offers information and support to gay persons or to those interested in personal and social issues affecting same-sex intimate relationships

National Woman's Health Network
224 Seventh St., SE
Washington, DC 20003
Phone: (202) 347–1140

This feminist health advocacy and resource group offers addresses of local women's health services and is concerned with women's health issues such as maternal and child health during pregnancy and birth, conception control, abortion, breast cancer, and toxic shock syndrome.

Reach to Recovery
American Cancer Society, Inc.
19 W. 56th St.
New York, NY 10019
Phone: (212) 586–8700

An American Cancer Society visitor program that offers support for women who have breast cancer. Volunteers who have breast cancer demonstrate exercises and provide information and a temporary breast form.

Resolve, Inc.
5 Water St.
Arlington, MA 02174
Phone: (617) 643–2424

This national organization provides support, counseling, and referral services for infertile couples through trained telephone counselors. Referrals to artificial insemination and adoption facilities are also offered.

Sex Information and Education Council of the United States (SIECUS)
New York University
32 Washington Place, Room 52
New York, NY 10003
Phone: (212) 673–3850

This organization maintains an information clearinghouse on all aspects of human sexuality and will help clients locate information.

HOT LINES

Genetic and Teratogen Hot Line
Phone: (212) 270–2072 from 10 AM to 4 PM weekdays

Genetics counselors from the State University of New York Downstate Medical Center respond to calls about infectious, environmental, and genetic hazards. This hot line also provides information to expectant parents who may want to know the effects of a specific drug on the unborn fetus.

VD National Hot Line
Phone: (800) 227–8922 (nationwide, except CA) from 8 AM to 8 PM weekdays and from 10 AM to 6 PM weekends.

This toll-free number offered by the American Social Health Organization provides confidential answers about sexually transmitted disease and the locations of over 5000 free or low-cost treatment services in the continental United States.

HEALTH INFORMATION MATERIAL

From: American Institute of Cancer Research
Washington, DC 20069

"Questions and Answers About Breast Lumps and Breast Cancer" and "BSE Exam" are two free brochures written for women clients. The first includes treatment options and a list of US cancer centers, and the second explains how and when to do breast self-exam. Instruct clients to send a stamped, self-addressed business envelope with their request.

From: National Cancer Institute
Bethesda, MD 20205

The Breast Cancer Digest is an excellent 212-page book for professionals. It covers the psychosocial as well as the physiologic aspects of breast cancer with a comprehensive guide to audiovisual materials and professional and client educational materials.

Teaching Breast Self-Examination: A Guide for Nurses is a brochure and a pocket-sized card of the basic points to be covered in BSE instruction.

SPECIALTY ORGANIZATIONS

American Association of Sex Educators, Counselors and Therapists
11 Dupont Circle, NW, Suite 220
Washington, DC 20036
Phone: (202) 462–1171

This organization is involved in sex education, research, and therapy and certifies qualified sex educators and counselors. Provides client referrals.

Nurses Association of the American College
of Obstetricians and Gynecologists (NAACOG)
600 Maryland Ave., SW, Suite 22 East
Washington, DC 20024
Phone: (202) 638–0026

The goals of this organization are to stimulate interest in and promote high standards in gynecologic, obstetric, and neonatal nursing. Membership comprises RNs and allied health workers with primary job responsibilities in these specialty areas. Dues, $60.

CHAPTER **49**

Specific Disorders of the Reproductive System

Other topics relevant to this content are: AIDS, **Chapter 25**; Sexually transmitted parasitic infestations, **Chapter 55**; Urinary system dysfunction, **Unit 5**.

Objectives

When you have finished studying this chapter, you should be able to:

Identify common disorders affecting the female and male reproductive systems.

Discuss medical and surgical measures for common reproductive system disorders.

Explain the complications of reproductive surgery and the related nursing interventions.

Help the client explore changing sexual and reproductive roles in the presence of reproductive system disorders.

Instruct clients in measures to prevent or reduce the risk of infectious vaginitis or sexually transmitted disease (STD).

List risk factors in the development of reproductive system neoplasms

Discuss alterations in body image encountered by clients having surgery of the external or internal genitalia or the breasts.

Develop general nursing interventions for clients with disorders of the reproductive system.

Anticipate the psychosocial/lifestyle implications of reproductive system disorders for clients and their significant others.

Conditions that affect the reproductive system include congenital, multifactorial, degenerative, infectious and inflammatory, and neoplastic disorders as well as traumatic disorders from surgery, irradiation, and injury. This chapter discusses the etiology, significance, clinical manifestations, therapeutic measures, and specific nursing measures for these disorders. Clients with reproductive system disorders often undergo changes in body image and sexual dysfunction. Therefore, emotional support is among the most important nursing interventions.

Some clients have advanced reproductive system disease because they failed to seek early medical care. Often these delays are caused by inability to recognize the symptoms as pathologic or by embarrassment. Furthermore, most people fear sexual disfigurement and may fail to have early symptoms evaluated to avoid confronting the possibility of surgery. Clients can be informed about new surgical technologies that result in less tissue destruction and disfigurement. It is hoped that these delays can be reduced by sensitive health care personnel and accurate health education.

The nurse who cares for a person undergoing reproductive surgery must be sensitive to both the physiologic and the psychosocial/lifestyle impact the procedure may have. Thus, nursing clients with reproductive disorders requires a broad knowledge base. The ability to give postoperative care is not enough. Sensitivity to the psychologic issues associated with reproductive surgery, an understanding of the medical conditions that can be unique to these clients, and an assessment of the client's knowledge of reproductive and sexual function are also essential.

SECTION **I**

Congenital Disorders

Congenital disorders affecting the female reproductive system involve some abnormal process in the embryonic development of the fetus at the time of sexual differentia-

NURSING DIAGNOSES IN
Reproductive Dysfunction

DIRECTLY RELATED DIAGNOSES

- Knowledge deficit
- Nutrition, altered: less than body requirements
- Sexuality, altered patterns
- Sexual dysfunction
- Skin integrity, impaired: actual

OTHER POTENTIAL DIAGNOSES

- Anxiety
- Comfort, altered: pain
- Coping, ineffective individual
- Fear
- Health maintenance management, impaired
- Hopelessness
- Knowledge deficit
- Infection, potential for
- Self-concept, disturbance in: self-esteem, body image, personal identity

tion. Because they affect internal structures, some congenital disorders may not manifest themselves until menarche or when they delay or prohibit menarche. Problems manifested at birth are treated in childhood.

A congenital disorder usually is identified when the client has difficulty with menstruation or fertility. The disorder alters the client's body image because of a conflict between reality and what she anticipates as normal in the reproductive system. The more severe the disorder, the greater its potential to alter body image.

Most significant congenital disorders of the male reproductive system are corrected during childhood. Failure to treat them early can seriously affect a person's psychosocial development, contributing not only to possible physiologic dysfunction but also to severe body image problems. Three examples are hypospadias (the condition in which the urethra opens on the underside of the penis or the perineum), epispadias (the absence of the upper wall of the urethra, and cryptorchidism (undescended testes) which contributes to infertility and greatly increases the risk of testicular cancer in the adult male. Complete information on these problems can be found in maternal health, women's health, and pediatric nursing textbooks.

SECTION 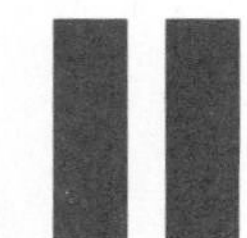

Disorders of Multifactorial Origin

Primary Dysmenorrhea

Dysmenorrhea is painful menses. Primary dysmenorrhea occurs when there is painful menses in the absence of a pelvic pathologic condition. In secondary dysmenorrhea, the pain's cause is some pathologic condition such as endometriosis, pelvic inflammatory disease (PID), or congenital abnormalities of the reproductive tract. The causes of secondary dysmenorrhea are discussed elsewhere in this chapter, so this section will cover only primary dysmenorrhea.

Primary dysmenorrhea is caused by an excess of prostaglandin, which is formed in the endometrium following ovulation and reaches a peak at menstruation. The increased prostaglandins are thought to result in three conditions: (1) an increase in uterine contractions, (2) ischemia from the decrease of uterine blood flow, and (3) a lowering of the pain threshold of the nerves in the uterus.

Clinical Manifestations

The onset of symptoms in primary dysmenorrhea is usually within 12 months of menarche. Lower abdominal cramps in waves radiate to the lower back, upper thighs, or both. The pain is most intense during the first 3 days of the menstrual cycle and usually subsides within the first 24 to 48 hours. The accompanying symptoms may include headache, nausea and vomiting, and diarrhea. It is most common in women up to 25 years of age.

Medical Measures

The most frequent treatment for primary dysmenorrhea is the use of nonsteroidal anti-inflammatory drugs (NSAIDs). Aspirin, although an NSAID, has little effect on painful menstruation, and not all NSAIDs are recommended for dysmenorrhea. Some specific NSAIDs that help reduce dysmenorrhea are ibuprofen (Motrin, Advil, and Nuprin), mefenamic acid (Ponstel), and naproxen sodium (Anaprox). These medications are given when the dysmenorrhea occurs and do not need to be given before the onset of menstruation.

Another treatment is the use of oral contraceptives if the client desires birth control. Oral contraceptives decrease the amount of prostaglandins in the menstrual flow. Because of the side effects associated with their use, oral contraceptives should be given only when the client desires birth control. Primary dysmenorrhea often markedly decreases after pregnancy.

Specific Nursing Measures

When primary dysmenorrhea is treated with NSAIDs, the nurse should discuss the possibility of gastrointestinal upset and headache. Less common side effects include peripheral edema, reversible alteration of liver enzymes, urticaria, angioneurotic edema, and bronchospasms in clients with asthma. The side effects of oral contraceptives vary, depending on the type of agent used. The more serious side effects include gallbladder disease, hepatic adenoma, thrombophlebitis, myocardial infarction, stroke or hypertension, and migraine headaches. Caution the client to contact her health care provider if these side effects occur.

Instruct the client that the medication may not relieve the discomfort for several months. Physical exercise, including swimming and the pelvic rock exercise (see Box 49–2) may help decrease the pain. Other measures for relieving discomfort include the use of heat in the form of tub baths, showers, or heating pads as well as increased sleep during menstruation. Instructions in personal hygiene may help alleviate some misconceptions about how the body functions during the menstrual cycle. Finally, good nutrition can impart a sense of well-being.

Dysfunctional Uterine Bleeding

Dysfunctional uterine bleeding (DUB) is caused by a hormonal imbalance in the hypothalamic–pituitary–ovarian axis, without an organic pathologic condition of the organs of reproduction themselves. The menstrual cycles are usually anovulatory, which interferes with the usual menstrual pattern. The bleeding may be caused by excessive growth of the vascular tissue of the endometrium; this tissue breaks down sporadically, leaving the vascular channels exposed. The diagnosis of DUB is made after the following conditions are found not to be the cause: pregnancy, malignancy, myomas, cervical erosion, polyps, vaginal infection or trauma, ovarian dysfunction, systemic disease, and medication.

Clinical Manifestations

Characteristic abnormal patterns of bleeding are **menorrhagia** (excessive profuse menstrual flow), **metrorrhagia** (bleeding between menstrual periods), prolonged menstrual flow, and **oligomenorrhea** (markedly diminished menstrual flow. The interval between menstrual periods and the length of the menstrual period may also be shortened or increased. The client with anovulatory DUB is usually an adolescent or a woman in her 50s.

Medical Measures

There is no single method for treating DUB. Pharmacologic measures include the administration of estrogens, progesterones, androgens, and ergot derivatives; ovulation induction; and antiprostaglandin therapy.

Specific Nursing Measures

Any bleeding can concern the client. Because multiple treatments are used for DUB, the client may become concerned about the number of procedures being used. Provide support and instruct the client to keep a record of her bleeding to determine the effectiveness of each treatment.

Cervical Dilatation and Uterine Curettage

Cervical dilatation and uterine curettage (D and C), the most frequent gynecologic surgery, can be done for diagnostic or therapeutic purposes. The indications for the procedure include dysfunctional uterine bleeding (DUB) (to determine the histologic composition of the endometrium); infertility (to determine the presence of ovulation); and the need to diagnose endometrial cancer or tuberculosis, remove uterine polyps, and remove early products of conception (to eliminate hemorrhage or other complications when a spontaneous incomplete abortion has occurred or when an elective abortion is desired). A D and C is also performed prior to other gynecologic surgeries to ensure that intrauterine pathology does not exist.

The physician uses a uterine probe to determine the length and direction of the uterine cavity. Next, dilators that gently stretch the muscles and fibers of the cervix gradually enlarge the cervical canal and internal os. After this dilatation has been completed, the uterine cavity undergoes systematic curettage (scraping). Table 49–1 summarizes the client implications of a D and C.

Nursing Implications

PREOPERATIVE CARE The D and C often is conducted in an outpatient setting, so the nurse should provide the client with clear instructions for preliminary preparation. Specific information regarding dietary restrictions, arrival time, and arrangements for postoperative transportation will facilitate a successful outcome.

When the client arrives for surgery, ascertain that she has complied with the preoperative instructions, obtain vital signs, explain the procedure, orient the client to the surgical surroundings, and instruct the client to empty her bladder. When the D and C is performed as an inpatient procedure, the preoperative preparation is similar. A mild sedative may be given prior to the procedure.

POSTOPERATIVE CARE The client will remain in a recovery area until fully reacted (approximately 1 hour). Monitor the vital signs every 15 minutes until stable. A falling blood pressure with a rapid pulse should alert the nurse to the possibility of hemorrhage from a cervical laceration or uterine perforation.

Table 49–1
Cervical Dilatation and Uterine Curettage: Implications for the Client

Physiologic Implications	Psychosocial/ Lifestyle Implications
Possible complications are perforation of the uterus or cervical laceration, leading to hemorrhage Occasional vasovagal effects at the time of cervical dilatation Uterine cramping Bleeding for 5–7 days	Normal activities, including intercourse, may be resumed in 2–3 weeks

Assess the client's perineal pad frequently. Vaginal bleeding should not be heavier than that of a normal menstrual period. A woman in a dorsal recumbent position can have significant undetected bleeding, because gravity allows the blood to flow in the direction of her buttocks and sacrum. Therefore, check not only the perineal pad but also the area under the buttocks.

Discomfort is generally mild. The client may experience uterine cramping, which is readily alleviated with mild analgesics and rest. Pain not relieved by these measures must be brought to the physician's attention.

Discharge instructions should include information on when the pathology report will be available, the recommended method of contraception, when the client may resume normal activities, and the time of her next appointment. Remind the client that symptoms or signs such as fever, heavy bleeding, or severe uterine cramping require emergency care.

Endometriosis

Endometriosis is the presence of functioning endometrial tissue outside the uterus. The common sites of endometriosis are shown in Figure 49–1. The cause of the disease is not known. It is speculated that endometrial tissue refluxes from the uterus into the pelvic cavity at menstruation or that the condition is congenital. The incidence of the disease is not known because it can be present without any symptoms. Some research studies have identified endometriosis in 5% to 50% of gynecologic surgery clients (Duenhoelter, 1983). Endometriosis is most often found in women who have delayed childbearing.

Clinical Manifestations

The symptoms are based on the location of the lesions. The most common symptoms are dysmenorrhea, deep dyspareunia, and sacral backache. The client may also have infertility and menstrual abnormalities. Pain develops gradually and increases in intensity over time. The location of the pain depends on where the lesions are located. The extent of the endometriosis and the severity of the pain and symptomatology are not necessarily related.

Medical Measures

Treatment is highly individualized and depends on the symptoms and the client's desire for childbearing. The medical management of choice includes the use of the antigonadotropin, danazol (Danocrine), a synthetic androgen, which is prescribed for a 6- to 9-month period. High-dose birth control pills may also be used to shrink endometrial tissue. High-dose progesterones are no longer recommended by the Food and Drug Administration (FDA). Pregnancy is encouraged because it may cause the disease process to regress and because of the increased risk of infertility as the disease progresses.

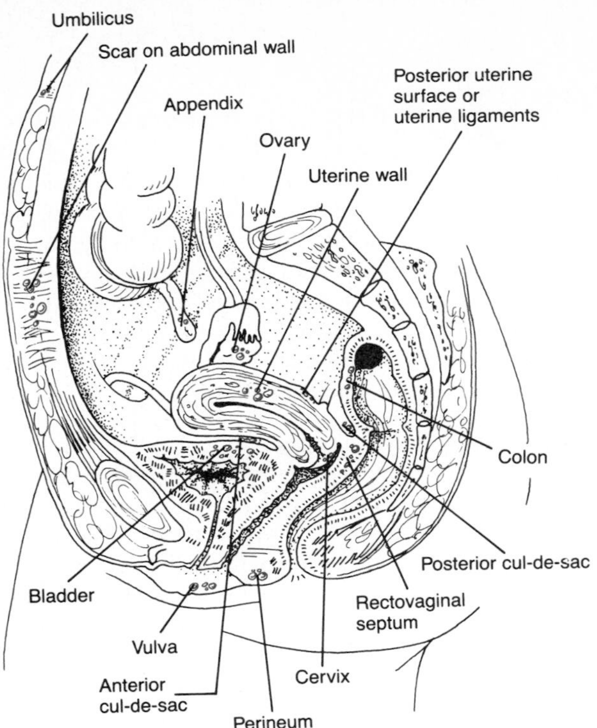

Figure 49–1

Possible sites of endometriosis.

Surgical treatment includes total hysterectomy and bilateral salpingo-oophorectomy (TAH-BSO) if no further childbearing is desired. An option is to leave part of an ovary intact for hormonal production if there are no apparent lesions on it. If childbearing is desired, conservative surgery that involves the removal of active implants by excision, as well as lysis of adhesions, is carried out.

Specific Nursing Measures

Because endometriosis often results in infertility, the client will need the nurse's emotional support. If pain has been a major factor, the client may be relieved to find its cause. The encouragement not to delay childbearing may necessitate a different family-planning schedule for the client and her partner. Provide support and be an effective listener as the client discusses these concerns and possible changes in plans.

Premenstrual Syndrome

Premenstrual syndrome (PMS) is a collection of symptoms that occur in the luteal phase of the menstrual cycle and alter the client's normal physiologic and emotional states. They are not present once the menstrual period is over. According to different studies, the incidence of the syndrome varies from 5% to 95%. The onset of PMS is from 2 weeks to a few days before menses.

No specific cause is known. The peak time for the occurrence of PMS is ages 30 to 40. Environmental stress may play a role in the development of PMS, as may expectations about the menstrual cycle's being a time of distress.

Clinical Manifestations

The symptoms must recur for at least 3 cycles before a diagnosis of PMS is made. The list of PMS symptoms can be divided into physical and psychologic. The physical symptoms include edema of the legs and fingers, a bloated feeling in the abdomen, weight gain, breast tenderness, headaches and dizziness, heart palpitations, excessive thirst and appetite, excessive sleeping, constipation, back pain, craving for sweets, and acne. The psychologic symptoms include sadness, depression, crying easily, tenseness, anxiety, irritability, restlessness, mood swings, increased or decreased sexual desire, and feelings of irrationality. The symptoms vary with individuals; however, they increase in severity just prior to the onset of menstruation and subside as the menstrual flow starts.

Medical Measures

There is no standardized treatment for PMS. Diuretics can relieve edema, and anxiolytic agents (or minor tranquilizers) can treat symptoms on a short-term basis. Vitamin B_6 also may bring some relief. Bromocriptine mesylate (Parlodel), a prolactin-suppressing drug, may help in the management of breast tenderness, edema, and weight gain. Progesterone may be used to counter estrogen's sodium-sparing actions and may provide a calming effect; however, progesterone works sporadically and can actually worsen symptoms. Some experts think that psychologic counseling may be helpful in returning the feeling of bodily control to the client.

Specific Nursing Measures

Nursing measures depend on PMS symptoms and the treatment the physician prescribes. The nurse can direct the client to keep a diary of her symptoms to help better understand them and thus increase her feeling of control over herself. Help the client realize that PMS is a disorder and that individualized treatment is necessary. It is also helpful to include the client's family or significant other in the management of PMS.

Proper nutrition is important in relieving some of the symptoms, so nutritional counseling should include instructions to consume food high in vitamin B_6 and magnesium, and to avoid refined sugars, caffeine, or red meat. Smoking is also discouraged. Exercise should be encouraged. A health teaching guide for women with PMS is in Box 49–1.

Diethylstilbestrol-Exposed Clients

The in-utero exposure of offspring to diethylstilbestrol (DES) may cause various reproductive tract abnormalities. In the 1950s and 1960s, DES was used to prevent abortion and was given to pregnant women with diabetes, toxemia, premature labor, and other conditions. In 1971, a link between reproductive system abnormalities and DES exposure in utero was found.

Clinical Manifestations

The clinical manifestations of in-utero DES exposure depend on when the exposure occurred. In females, it may include epithelial changes, a cock's comb–appearing cervix or a cervix with clefts or pseudopolyps, and inelastic fornices. There may be changes in the uterus. The typical T-shaped uterus found in DES-exposed clients may predispose them to infertility and spontaneous abortion.

In males, abnormalities may include epididymal cysts, hypospadias, an abnormally small penis, testicular varicoceles, testicular calcifications, sperm and semen abnor-

Box 49–1
A Self Checklist for Women With Symptoms and Signs of PMS

1. Lessening frequency of headaches, cravings and/or fatigue by keeping the blood sugar level up:
   a. Eating at least 45 grams of protein daily
   b. Eating six meals daily, not more calories but more frequent meals
   c. Eating fruits for snacks, not sweets
   d. Decreasing fluid retention
2. Lessening or controlling depression/irritability by:
   a. Getting 7–8 hours of sleep nightly
   b. Exercising the equivalent of 2 miles of walking daily
   c. Getting with a support group/person to express your feelings
   d. Increasing Vitamin B_6 foods in diet (corn, liver, wheat, yeast, tomatoes, unsalted sunflower seeds, peanuts) or 200 milligrams of Vitamin B_6 daily prior to menses
   e. Increasing foods high in magnesium in diet (whole grain, dried beans, seafood)
   f. Decreasing stress (exercise, meditation, yoga, relaxation, stop talk—keep mind from unnecessary worries—assertiveness training)
   g. Decreasing fluid retention (no salt at table, 1 lemon in water daily, no more than 1 carbonated beverage a day, Rule of S's—avoid salt, soup, sauces, etc)
3. Decreasing swelling/bloating, breast tenderness by decreasing fluid retention through:
   a. Using no salt at the table
   b. Eating frozen, not canned foods
   c. Avoiding salty foods (pickles, potato chips, pork, Rule of S's)
   d. Using natural diuretics (1 lemon or tbsp 100% lemon juice in 8 oz water daily, caffeine, if acceptable
4. Other measures commonly recommended follow:
   a. Avoiding nutritional irritants by:
      1. Avoiding coffee, chocolate (if one finds these to worsen the symptoms)
      2. Decreasing use of refined sugar by using sweeteners, honey, fruits instead of sweets for snacks
   b. Attaining or maintaining recommended body weight
   c. Using primrose oil capsule for breast tenderness

SOURCE: Kirkpatrick MK, Grady TR: PMS: A self-help checklist. *Occup Health Nurs* (Feb) 1985; 33:92.

malities, and undescended or hypoplastic (unusually small) testicles. Urethral strictures and other urinary tract abnormalities may also occur. There is an increased risk of developing cancer for both males and females.

Medical Measures

In past years, female clients exposed to DES in utero underwent the administration of progesterone, skinning of the cervix, or other aggressive procedures such as surgical excision, cauterization, cryotherapy, or laser evaporation of abnormal tissue. Currently, the plan of care includes routine Papanicolau (Pap) tests and careful pelvic examinations yearly. If there is a change in the Pap test or the appearance of the vaginal mucosa, the client is followed more closely.

Male clients exposed to DES in utero should undergo periodic physical examination and perform testicular self-examination (TSE) regularly.

Specific Nursing Measures

Nursing care involves screening for clients who have been exposed to DES. The nurse is also responsible for informing the client about the necessity of routine follow-up examinations. The nurse provides emotional support through therapeutic communication skills. Nursing care for the client who develops cancer is described in the later section on neoplastic disorders.

Phimosis and Paraphimosis

Phimosis, which is seen in the uncircumcised male, is the inability to retract the prepuce over the glans penis (Figure 49–2A). Phimosis most often is secondary to infection that has resulted from poor hygiene. The infection leads to scarring and fibrosis, which in turn lead to more infection and further scarring. *Paraphimosis* is the inability of the uncircumcised retracted prepuce to be returned easily (Figure 49–2B). Like phimosis, it is usually the result of recurrent chronic infections.

Clinical Manifestations

The clinical manifestations of phimosis include scarring; the inability to retract the prepuce; and signs of infection such as swelling, warmth, and exudate under the prepuce. Penile constriction and urethral obstruction are possible complications.

In paraphimosis, the retracted prepuce forms a constrictive ring around the penis, the penis becomes edematous and the foreskin becomes even more difficult, if not impossible, to return. Bluish discoloration of the penis results from obstruction of the blood supply; gangrene is possible.

Medical Measures

The administration of antibiotics and warm soaks to the penis relieves the infection. Creating a dorsal slit in

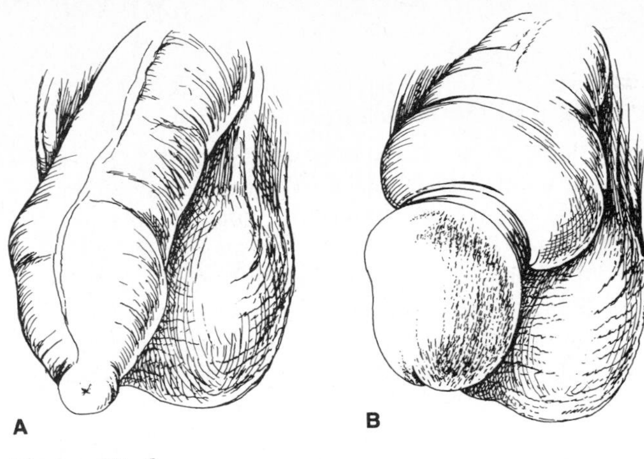

Figure 49–2

A. Phimosis. Note pinpoint opening of prepuce. **B.** Paraphimosis. Retracted prepuce has become a constricting band around the penis.

the prepuce relieves any constriction or urethral obstruction the phimosis is causing. After the infection is resolved, a circumcision is performed.

Manual reduction is the initial treatment measure for paraphimosis. The glans penis is squeezed for 5 minutes in an attempt to decrease penile size. The penis is then pushed back while the prepuce is pulled forward. If this is unsuccessful, a surgical dorsal slit into the constricting ring relieves the pressure. Any infection is treated prior to a circumcision, which prevents the recurrence of paraphimosis.

Specific Nursing Measures

Preventive health teaching about basic hygiene is particularly important to prevent infection and resultant phimosis. The uncircumcised client should retract the prepuce daily and wash the penile shaft with soap and water to remove smegma from the penis and prevent infection. Instruct the client with phimosis to administer warm soaks and give him information on the proper administration of antibiotics.

The most important nursing intervention for the client with paraphimosis is providing information and emotional support because the constriction of circulation to the penis causes severe anxiety. As in the case of the client with phimosis, it is important to prevent infection with basic hygiene. The client facing circumcision needs information about the procedure as well as emotional support.

Circumcision

A circumcision, the removal of the prepuce, is often performed in infancy because of religious or cultural reasons. In the adult, a circumcision is usually performed for a problem such as phimosis, paraphimosis, or carcinoma in situ on the prepuce. Adult clients may delay seeking treatment because they fear penile damage or sexual dysfunction as a result of surgery. The implications for the adult client undergoing circumcision are summarized in Table 49–2.

Table 49–2
Circumcision: Implications for the Client

Physiologic Implications	Psychosocial/Lifestyle Implications
Hemorrhage and edema are possible complications	No sexual intercourse until healing complete
Pain, usually minimal	Fear of damage to penis or impaired sexual function
Potential skin grafting if large area of prepuce removed	Altered body image and changes in sensation depending on extent of surgery
Increased comfort	Fear of cancer progression or extension
Enhanced ability to maintain hygiene	

Nursing Implications

PREOPERATIVE CARE Circumcision is not minor surgery to the client facing it. The client needs complete information about the circumcision procedure, and the nurse should allow him to verbalize his fears.

POSTOPERATIVE CARE The client will return from surgery with a pressure dressing of petroleum jelly gauze and a dry sterile dressing on top. Carefully assess for bleeding, a potential postoperative problem. The dressing and wound site must remain clean and dry, so the dressing should be changed after voiding. Carefully observe for and document the first voiding to ensure that the urethra is patent. If the client is discharged with a dressing in place, he should be taught to care for the operative area until it heals.

Hydrocele, Spermatocele, and Varicocele

A *hydrocele* is accumulation of fluid in the tunica vaginalis testis (Figure 49–3A). Hydrocele is frequently a congenital anomaly associated with an inguinal hernia. It can also occur after injury or irradiation to the scrotum. A *spermatocele* is a cyst of the epididymis or rete testis that contains dead sperm (Figure 49–3B). Spermatoceles occur at the upper pole of the testis adjacent to the epididymis. A *varicocele* is a varicosity in the pampiniform plexus (a complex of veins from the testis and the epididymis that constitutes part of the spermatic cord). A varicocele usually results from incompetent vein valves (Figure 49–3C). It is far more common on the left side, where the veins drain at a right angle.

Clinical Manifestations

A hydrocele usually appears as a transilluminating, painless, oblong, soft mass in the scrotum. A spermatocele is usually small, asymptomatic, and painless. If the mass becomes large, it may be mistaken for a hydrocele. If a spermatocele is firm, it should be distinguished from a tumor; unlike a tumor, a spermatocele is freely moving

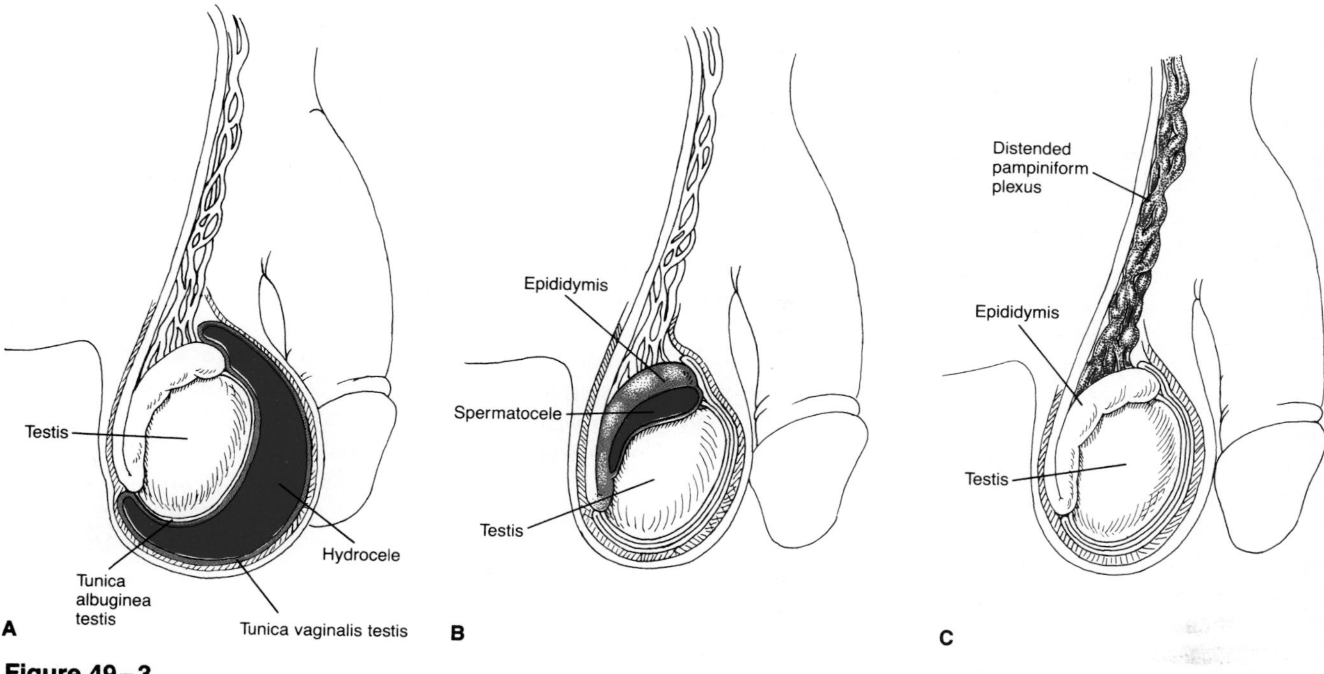

Figure 49–3

A. Hydrocele. **B.** Spermatocele of the epididymis. **C.** Varicocele.

and will transilluminate. On aspiration, a white opaque liquid with dead sperm cells is observed.

The client with a varicocele may complain of an aching, pulling feeling in the scrotum. Semen analysis may show decreased sperm production, more immature sperm, and decreased sperm motility. The swelling formed by the varicocele feels like a "bag of worms" and appears bluish through the skin of the scrotum. To detect a varicocele, the client stands and performs Valsalva's maneuver. If there is a varicocele, the examiner will feel a rush of blood in the scrotum and will hear it with the Doppler stethoscope.

Medical Measures

If the hydrocele is neither large nor causing discomfort, treatment is not required. Treatment is indicated, however, if physical or emotional discomfort occur because of the hydrocele's appearance or if circulation to the testis is impaired by pressure from the hydrocele. At times, it is important to reduce the size of the hydrocele so the testes can be examined carefully because a hydrocele can occur as a complication of testicular cancer.

Conservative treatment involves aspiration of the fluid. Hydroceles tend to recur, and the fluid may need to be reaspirated every 6 to 20 weeks. Surgical excision (hydrocelectomy) may be necessary.

Usually no treament is needed for a spermatocele. A large spermatocele requires spermatocelectomy, however. Varicoceles usually are not treated unless the client has a problem with infertility or discomfort. The semen quality improves in most clients after variococelectomy.

Specific Nursing Measures

Be sure the client understands the reason for aspirating the hydrocele, and explain that reaspiration may be necessary. A scrotal support may decrease discomfort caused by the weight of the hydrocele. Provide emotional support as needed for the client's altered body image or concern over the cause or effect of the hydrocele or spermatocele.

Inform the client with a varicocele about the relationship between varicoceles and infertility. Make the client comfortable so he can ventilate feelings and anxiety. Give information and support the client so that he can make an informed decision about surgery. Be sure he is not inadvertently raising his intrascrotal temperature by wearing tight pants or underwear. A scrotal support may help the client bothered by a heavy, pulling feeling.

Varicocelectomy, Spermatocelectomy, and Hydrocelectomy

A *varicocelectomy* is the removal of a varicocele in the channels of the spermatic cord. The major indications for the procedure are client discomfort and infertility. A *spermatocelectomy* is the removal of a sperm-filled sack in the scrotum (spermatocele). Because spermatoceles are usually small, they usually do not require surgery unless the client experiences pain or is embarrassed by the scrotum's appearance. A *hydrocelectomy* is the removal of a fluid-filled sac in the scrotum (hydrocele). If no underlying pathology is present, hydroceles are usually removed only if they are large enough to be uncomfortable and embarrassing. Client implications for these three procedures are given in Table 49–3.

Table 49–3
Varicocelectomy, Spermatocelectomy, and Hydrocelectomy: Implications for the Client

Physiologic Implications	Psychosocial/Lifestyle Implications
Possible increased fertility	Possible increased fertility
Relief from pain, discomfort, or feeling of heaviness	Need to wear scrotal support and use ice pack until edema subsides
Scrotal edema	Improved appearance
Scrotal drain likely with hydrocelectomy	Self-care of incision site and dressing

Nursing Implications

The nurse should provide preoperative emotional support to the client, as well as information on the procedure and postoperative implications. Postoperatively, the client having a varicocelectomy or a spermatocelectomy will have an ice pack on the scrotum for the first 24 hours. He should wear a scrotal support after surgery until edema subsides. A scrotal drain will be in place for 24 to 48 hours after a hydrocelectomy, and an absorbent dressing and scrotal support will be necessary for several days. Usually, the client will receive an oral anti-inflammatory drug for 1 week postoperatively to prevent edema.

Vasectomy

A vasectomy is the removal of all or part of the vasa deferentia. Approximately 500,000 elective vasectomies are performed each year in the United States (Kessler, 1982). The wish to be sterile is the major reason clients have vasectomies. The other reason is to prevent epididymitis after a prostatectomy. Anyone about to undergo a vasectomy should fully realize that the procedure may be permanent. The client should not expect that this procedure can be reversed at a later date.

A vasectomy usually can be performed in an outpatient setting using local anesthesia and a scrotal incision. A variety of surgical procedures is used. The success rate is generally high, but each technique has some failures. Some techniques combine both excision and fulguration with

Table 49–4
Vasectomy: Implications for the Client

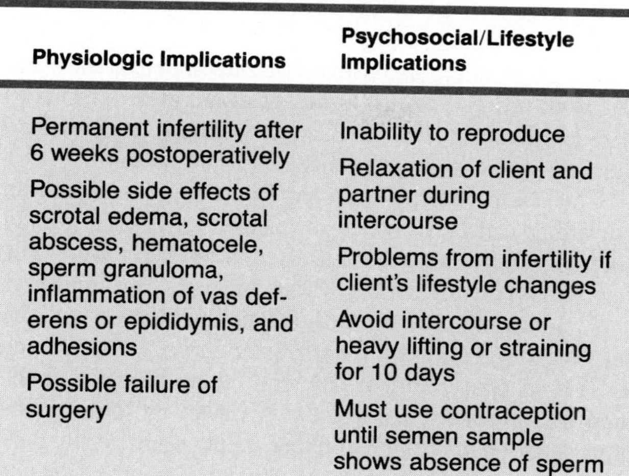

Physiologic Implications	Psychosocial/Lifestyle Implications
Permanent infertility after 6 weeks postoperatively	Inability to reproduce
Possible side effects of scrotal edema, scrotal abscess, hematocele, sperm granuloma, inflammation of vas deferens or epididymis, and adhesions	Relaxation of client and partner during intercourse
Possible failure of surgery	Problems from infertility if client's lifestyle changes
	Avoid intercourse or heavy lifting or straining for 10 days
	Must use contraception until semen sample shows absence of sperm

electrocautery. The physiologic and psychosocial/lifestyle implications for the vasectomy client are summarized in Table 49–4.

Nursing Implications

PREOPERATIVE CARE The major preoperative nursing role is to ensure that the client fully understands the implications of the vasectomy procedure. He must understand that he will be rendered permanently sterile (unless reversal is possible) and that his wish not to have children must be firm. The client may feel anxious about the surgery and will require appropriate emotional support.

POSTOPERATIVE CARE This surgery is usually performed in an outpatient clinic, so the client must clearly understand postoperative instructions. He should remain on bed rest for 24 hours with ice applied to the incision site. Once ambulatory, he should wear a scrotal support and refrain from intercourse or heavy lifting and straining for 7 days.

The client must understand that he is still fertile and must continue to use contraception until a semen sample (which is first taken 6 weeks postoperatively after 20 ejaculations) shows no sperm in 20 × magnification under high power. If any sperm—even immotile ones—are in the ejaculate, the client is still not sterile (Kessler, 1982).

Vasovasostomy

A vasovasostomy is surgery on the vasa deferentia to reverse the effects of a vasectomy. A scrotal incision is used, scar tissue is excised, and one of several methods of reanastomosis is performed. The high rate of divorce and remarriage in the United States has resulted in an increase in requests for reversal of vasectomy (approximately 2 requests in 1000 vasectomies). Client implications for a vasovasostomy are listed in Table 49–5.

Table 49–5
Vasovasostomy: Implications for the Client

Physiologic Implications	Psychosocial/Lifestyle Implications
Semen again present in ejaculate	Ability to reproduce after successful surgery
Ability to impregnate if surgery successful	Grieving and regret if ability to impregnate not reestablished
Possible failure of surgery	No heavy lifting, straining, or intercourse for 3 weeks
Possible side effects of scrotal edema, scrotal abscess, hematocele, sperm granuloma, inflammation of vas deferens or epididymis, and adhesions	

Nursing Implications

PREOPERATIVE CARE Support the client preoperatively as he verbalizes his concern about the outcome of the surgery. Regret over ever having chosen to have a vasectomy is common.

POSTOPERATIVE CARE The client should wear a scrotal support for 10 days after surgery. Ice packs will be used for the first 24 hours to decrease edema. Discharge instructions include no heavy lifting, straining, or intercourse for 3 weeks. A semen analysis is performed 1 month postoperatively. Sperm may be present but are commonly abnormal in appearance and motility. Motility usually peaks at 6 months. Clients and their partners will need a great deal of emotional support as they wait and hope for a successful outcome, as will those whose surgery is unsuccessful.

Penile Implant

A penile implant is the insertion of a prosthesis into the corpora cavernosa so the client can achieve an erection and thus improve his sexual performance and satisfaction. An implant is one means of treating impotence. Clients with organic impotence not amenable to endocrine therapy are candidates for this surgery. This group can include diabetics, clients with spinal cord injuries, and those on antihypertensive medications. Some clients with psychogenic impotence who have not been responsive to psychologic counseling also can benefit from penile implants.

Two basic types of implantable penile prostheses are the solid-rod (noninflatable) and inflatable types. The solid-rod prosthesis consists of paired semirigid rods inserted into the corpora cavernosa through a small incision in the suprapubic, scrotal, or perineal area in a 30-minute procedure.

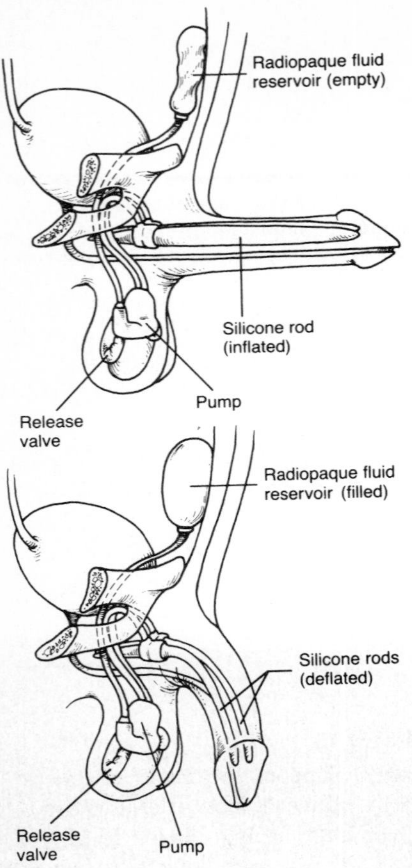

Figure 49–4

Inflatable penile prosthesis.

The inflatable prosthesis is usually inserted via an upper scrotal approach, which allows direct access for both cylinder and pump placement. Tunnels are created in the corpora cavernosa on both sides of the penis, and an appropriate-sized cylinder is inserted into each tunnel. The pump used to inflate and deflate the cylinders is implanted in the most dependent portion of the scrotum. The fluid-containing reservoir is placed beneath the rectus muscle in front of the bladder (Figure 49–4). Table 49–6 summarizes the implications for the penile implant client.

Nursing Implications

PREOPERATIVE CARE The nurse's first priority in preoperative care is to be sure the client is well informed about the types of procedures available and that he is given sufficient time to think through his options before making a decision about this elective procedure. When possible, the client's sexual partner should participate in the decision making. The nurse may also administer preoperative prophylactic antibiotic therapy (usually an aminoglycoside or cephalosporin).

POSTOPERATIVE CARE The antibiotics administered preoperatively are continued during the postoperative period. In addition, postoperative pain is first relieved by a parenteral narcotic, and then an oral agent. The need for analgesics usually decreases about 48 hours after surgery.

Blood loss is generally minimal, but for the first 24 hours, check the dressing every 2 hours and change it as needed. Some surgeons insert a wound drain into the scrotum. With a drain, up to 30 mL of drainage a day is considered within normal limits (Googe & Mook, 1983). Wound drains are usually removed after 24 to 48 hours.

The client returns from the operating room with an in-dwelling catheter, which is usually removed after 24 hours. Carefully check voiding after catheter removal. The client should be ambulating within 24 hours after surgery.

An inflatable prosthesis should not be inflated until the first visit to the surgeon 1 week after surgery. Starting on the second postoperative day, the client should pull the pump to the lowest part of the scrotum by locating the pump between his thumb and index finger and gently pulling it downward. The client is usually discharged on the third postoperative day. He has no dressing and can shower or bathe. Because some manual skill is involved, it is important for the client to practice using the prosthesis to avoid embarrassment when first attempting intercourse.

SECTION III

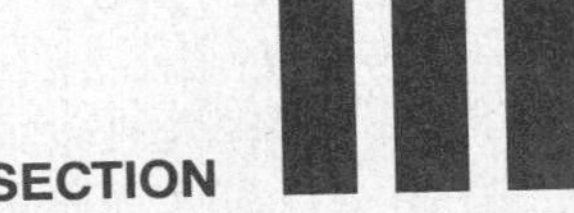

Degenerative Disorders

Uterine Prolapse

Prolapse of the uterus may result in the descent of the cervix to the vaginal introitus (first-degree prolapse), protrusion of the cervix through the introitus (second-degree prolapse), or prolapse of the entire uterus through the introitus (third-degree prolapse or procidentia).

Clinical Manifestations

The general symptoms of uterine prolapse may include sacral backache, a feeling of the "insides falling out," a feeling of "sitting on a ball," and a bearing-down sensation. There may be bleeding if the cervix is exposed, as well as cervical erosion caused by congestion and trauma.

Medical Measures

Preventive measures include performing Kegel exercises in the postpartum period. Lacerations of the perineum and episiotomies should be sutured carefully with good approximation of the structures. Unnecessary traction should not be applied to the cervix and uterus during obstetrical or surgical procedures.

Treatment involves the use of exercises to help strengthen the muscle floor. Surgery, usually hysterec-

Table 49–6
Penile Implant: Implications for the Client 

Physiologic Implications	Psychosocial/Lifestyle Implications
Solid-rod prosthesis	
Small–Carrion prosthesis: penis always semirigid	Embarrassment from continual erection for some; improved cosmetic appearance for others
Jonas prosthesis: positional shaping of penis possible because of malleable core	Possible need to manipulate penis manually during intercourse
Flexi-rod: perineal hinge allowing for folding into perineum	General satisfaction with sexual function
Penis neither as large nor as rigid as with a physiologic erection	No strenuous activity for 3 weeks
Less penile rigidity and decreased girth on erection	No intercourse for 6 weeks
Possible interference by cylinders in voiding, cystoscopy, or TUR	
Temporary scrotal edema (7–10 days) and discoloration (2 weeks)	
Inflatable prosthesis	
Simulation of normal physiologic erection	General satisfaction with improved potency
No change in external appearance	Possible reproduction ability
No interference in cystoscopy or TUR	Embarrassment if mechanical failure occurs
Maintenance of intercourse, orgasm, and ejaculation	No strenuous activity for 3 weeks
Decrease in client's own partial erection	No intercourse for 6 weeks
Possible allergic reaction to fluid	
Need to be able to activate pump	
Temporary scrotal edema (7–10 days) and discoloration (2 weeks)	

tomy, is performed when there are significant symptoms such as pain and bleeding and when a second-degree or third-degree prolapse is present. Pessaries, hard rubber or plastic devices placed in the vagina to support the uterus, may be used by clients who refuse surgery or are not suitable candidates for surgery.

Specific Nursing Measures

If surgery is not indicated, instruct the client in how to perform pelvic tilt and Kegel exercises to tighten the pubococcygeal muscle, improving support to the pelvic organs. Nurses caring for female clients should teach them to perform Kegel exercises to avoid or decrease the severity of uterine prolapse. The exercise can be taught to all women of childbearing age before pregnancy. Instructions for Kegel and other related exercises are given in Box 49–2.

Explain the care of the pessary if one has been inserted. The device must be removed and cleaned with mild soap and water about every 6 weeks, and regular douching may be necessary. Discuss hygiene measures that help decrease the risk of infection. Clients with pessaries are at increased risk for infection due to trauma from the pessary itself and the long-term presence of material foreign to the body. Instruct the client to notify her health care provider if she experiences pain, changes in the urinary pattern, unusual vaginal discharge or if the pessary is expelled.

Cystocele and Rectocele

A *cystocele* is the herniation of the posterior aspects of the bladder into the vagina through the cervicopubic fascia of the anterior vagina. A *urethrocele* is a herniation of the urethra into the vagina. *Rectocele* results when the rectovaginal fascia weakens and the rectum herniates into the posterior vaginal wall. An *enterocele* is the herniation of the intestine into the vagina. All of these conditions are caused by the same conditions as uterine prolapse, usually childbearing, obesity, or chronic lung conditions.

Clinical Manifestations

The most common manifestation of cystocele is urinary stress incontinence. A cystocele may cause an increased incidence of bladder infections because of congestion in

Box 49–2
Exercises for Pelvic Relaxation and Stress Incontinence

Do all exercises slowly on a firm surface several times daily.

1. *Kegel exercise*
   a. When lying on your back, tighten the pelvic floor muscles as hard as you can, holding for the count of 5 seconds, squeeze tighter, then release. As you learn to do this, it can be done many times daily, while sitting or standing. Repeat at least 10 times in a row.
   b. When you are urinating, do exercise 1a, using the muscles to stop the flow of urine. Hold for 5 seconds, then relax. Do this each time you use the toilet to check to see if you are doing the procedure correctly.
   c. Lie on your back with a pillow under your knees. Cross your ankles. Squeeze your buttocks together drawing in the anus, as if to prevent a bowel movement. Grip your knees together. Hold for 5 seconds, squeeze tighter, then relax. Remember to breathe normally. Repeat at least 10 times.
2. *Pelvic tilt*
   a. Lie on your back with your knees partly bent and feet flat on the floor. Pull in your abdomen and tighten your buttocks, so the small of your back presses against the floor. Remember to breathe normally. Hold for 5 seconds and relax. Repeat 10 times.
   b. Repeat exercise 2a while on your hands and knees, using the abdomen and buttock muscles to make your lower back flatten out. Hold 5 seconds and relax. Repeat 10 times.
   c. Practice pelvic tilts standing with your back against a wall. Pelvic tilts strengthen the abdomen and are the basis for many postural exercises.
3. *Partial curl-up*. Lie on your back with your knees bent and feet on the floor. Have your arms at your sides, just off the floor. Do a pelvic tilt (exercise 2) and then lift your head and shoulders off the floor. Slowly lie back down. You do not have to do a full sit-up to get the benefits of this exercise. Full sit-ups are not recommended for people who may have back problems. Repeat 5 to 20 times.
4. Tighten your stomach muscles while sitting and standing. Hold for count of 10, breathing normally. Repeat 5 times.

the base of the bladder as well as a herniation in the anterior wall of the vagina from the weakened supports. Specific manifestations of rectocele include rectal fullness and incomplete evacuation of stool. At times, the client may need to reduce the posterior wall of the vagina manually to evacuate her stool.

Medical Measures

Conservative management for stress incontinence includes the Kegel exercises. Alpha-adrenergic receptor stimulants may increase the tone of the bladder and the urethral smooth muscle. Estrogens in small doses may be prescribed for postmenopausal clients. Urinary tract infections should be treated promptly. Surgical management for cystocele includes anterior colporrhaphy and various uterine and bladder suspension procedures.

Because rectoceles are present in all parous women to some extent, it is necessary to treat only those with symptoms. Perineal exercises such as Kegel exercises can help premenopausal clients and those without major symptoms. Stool softeners will help prevent constipation and reduce the instances of incomplete evacuation of stool. Surgical management for rectocele includes posterior colporrhaphy.

Specific Nursing Measures

Explain the Kegel exercises and review the importance of taking prescribed medications. Be aware of the embarrassment the client may feel if she has stress incontinence or if she must wear pads or plastic protective underpants. Garments that fit well will prevent leaking. Encourage the client to void frequently. The nursing measures for clients with rectoceles are the same as those for clients with cystoceles, except rectocele clients are not prone to bladder infections.

Anterior Colporrhaphy

Cystocele and urethrocele are the indications for anterior colporrhaphy. Anterior colporrhaphy repairs the weakness of the anterior vaginal wall. When a cystocele occurs without stress incontinence, a simple anterior colporrhaphy corrects the vaginal weakness and returns the bladder to its anatomic position. If stress incontinence was a problem, the surgeon can modify this procedure with added sutures to draw the suburethral ligaments under the urethra and restore the vesicourethral angle. Anterior colporrhaphy is often performed in conjunction with posterior colporrhaphy, vaginal hysterectomy, or both. See Table 49–7 for a summary of implications for the client of anterior colporrhaphy.

Nursing Implications

Preoperative care is similar to care for clients undergoing vaginal hysterectomy. After surgery, the client returns to the unit with vaginal packing, which is removed in 24 to 48 hours. Because packing can mask overt signs of bleeding, monitor vital signs frequently. Instruct the client to report dizziness or light-headedness, symptoms indicating acute blood loss.

Voiding is difficult because of urethral narrowing, edema, and postoperative discomfort. Urinary drainage is accomplished by a Foley catheter or suprapubic cystostomy tube. Foley catheters are removed in 2 to 4 days. If the client has small frequent voidings, suspect urinary retention. Residual urine volumes greater than 100 mL usually neces-

Table 49–7
Anterior Colporrhaphy: Implications for the Client

Physiologic Implications	Psychosocial/Lifestyle Implications
Relief of stress incontinence Reduction in number of bladder infections Possible complications of urinary tract infection, voiding difficulties, dyspareunia, hemorrhage Recurrence of cystocele in 10% of clients	Reduction in embarrassment from incontinence Decreased sexual pleasure from dyspareunia in some instances

sitate the reinsertion of the Foley catheter. When the suprapubic drainage system is used, the tube is clamped for voiding. Residual urine can be directly measured after each voiding by unclamping the cystostomy tube.

Posterior Colporrhaphy

Rectocele or enterocele are the indications for posterior colporrhaphy. Posterior colporrhaphy repairs the posterior vaginal wall. This procedure is often performed along with an anterior colporrhaphy, vaginal hysterectomy, or both. The client implications of posterior colporrhaphy are summarized in Table 49–8.

Nursing Implications

Preoperative nursing care of posterior colporrhaphy clients is similar to that of clients undergoing other vaginal surgeries. Assess postoperative clients for bleeding and infection. If operative oozing was excessive, it may be necessary to place a drain in the incision; this reduces the possibility of infection by lessening the risk of hematoma formation. An in-dwelling Foley catheter will initially resolve the problem of urinary retention. Sitz baths are helpful in promoting healing and relieving discomfort. Stool softeners are used to prevent straining.

Assess the client's dietary habits and instruct her to include foods that contain bulk and fiber. A high-residue diet is thought to facilitate defecation, preventing recurrence of the rectocele.

Table 49–8
Posterior Colporrhaphy: Implications for the Client

Physiologic Implications	Psychosocial/Lifestyle Implications
Resolution of symptoms of rectocele Delay in return of complete rectal strength for at least 6 weeks Possible bleeding, infection, dyspareunia, urinary retention	High-fiber diet to prevent constipation and musculature weakening Possible need for stool softeners and laxatives Decreased sexual pleasure from dyspareunia possible in some instances

Menopause

Menopause is the cessation of ovarian activity with a concurrent cessation of the menses and a decrease in the ovarian hormones estrogen and progesterone. In the premenopausal state, the menses become irregular, and the flow may decrease. This occurs at different ages between 35 and 60 years; the average age in North America is 51. Although menopause is a natural state, not a disorder, it is included here because it may require treatment for uncomfortable symptoms.

Clinical Manifestations

The clinical manifestations of menopause result in part from the loss of estrogen and in part from aging. The transitional period, the climacteric, occurs over a period of time as the ovaries gradually decrease in size and function, the menstrual cycles become further apart, and the blood flow decreases in amount. This period of time is referred to as the *premenopause* and usually lasts for a few months, or sometimes for a few years. Most women experience these as mild changes and adapt with minimal disruption to their usual lifestyle during this premenopausal period.

The symptoms and physical signs involve many areas of the body. In the genital area, the vulval tissue thins. The vagina becomes shorter and narrower; the tissue thins, leading to atrophic vaginitis and perhaps an increase in irritation and infection. In the urinary tract, atrophic distal urethritis and stricture formation may occur. The ovaries and uterus markedly decrease in size.

The skin loses its elasticity. There may be muscle loss with fibrotic tissue formation. Bone mass peaks at age 35, after which it is either maintained or lost. This depends, in part, on the ratio of calcium to phosphorus. Osteoporosis, found mainly in small boned, thin, fair women, may result from the loss of estrogen. Family history of osteoporosis also increases the risk.

Vasomotor instability results in hot flashes, the sensation of overwhelming warmth that starts in the chest and rises upward. The skin becomes flushed, and the client may perspire profusely. Night sweats may interfere with sleep. Hot flashes stop when the body becomes adjusted to the new estrogen levels. Vasomotor symptoms may also include dizziness and numbness and tingling in the fingers and toes.

Psychologic symptoms may include irritability and depression. The cause of depression has not been pinpointed, but if it occurs, it is probably due to a combination of factors. Some of the physiologic factors are biochemical and are related to aging and changes in hormone production. Others may be related to psychosocial factors such as the loss of youth and childbearing potential, children having grown up and left home, and anxiety about job security and life accomplishments.

Medical Measures

Conservative treatments of menopausal symptoms include vitamins and herbs. Vitamin therapy includes the use of calcium supplements and a decrease in the consumption of phosphorus found in foods such as breads, cereal, and soft drinks. Because older persons have a decreased ability to absorb calcium from the intestine in the presence of a high phosphorus level, the maintenance of the calcium–phosphorus ratio will help prevent bone loss.

Herbs and vitamins may alleviate vasomotor instability. Ginseng is thought to normalize the metabolic rate. Vitamin E may promote energy and a feeling of well-being; it also may alleviate leg cramps and relieve hot flashes by decreasing FSH. The vitamin B complex also may aid in the control of hot flashes (Fogel & Woods, 1981; Jensen & Bobak, 1985).

Estrogen replacement therapy (ERT) is indicated for osteoporosis; severe vasomotor instability; and, in local application, for atrophic vaginitis. The major risk of prolonged ERT is an increased risk of endometrial cancer (American Cancer Society, 1987). The lowest effective dose of estrogen should be used for only short periods—a few months or, at most, only a year—when the physical discomforts associated with menopause are at their peak. The estrogens used for ERT are ethinyl estradiol, estradiol (Estrace), or conjugated estrogens (eg, Premarin). It is recommended that ERT be given on a cyclic schedule of 3 weeks on and 1 week off (Rodman & Smith, 1984). An increased incidence of blood clotting episodes has been seen in women who are on ERT for longer periods or who take larger doses. Vitamins B and C may be depleted in clients on ERT.

Bellargal tablets (a combination of phenobarbital, ergotamine tartrate, and belladonna) have also been used for hot flashes. Because the drug contains a barbiturate, it produces a sedative effect and may be addictive.

Specific Nursing Measures

It is important to stress the normalcy of menopause. Most women do not have difficulty with the climacteric. If serious effects are present, however, either vitamin therapy or ERT may be considered. The nurse can instruct the client in keeping a diary of her menstrual pattern.

● Educate the client on the types of food to avoid, such as those high in phosphorus (see Box 19–1 in Chapter 19). Encourage a diet rich in calcium and vitamins E and B. Calcium can be found in cheese, milk, sesame seeds, and seaweed. Vitamin E is found in vegetable oils, wheat germ, soybeans, peanuts, and spinach; this vitamin takes from 2 to 4 weeks to begin decreasing FSH and effectively preventing hot flashes. Vitamin B is found in wheat germ, yogurt, whole grains, brewer's yeast, liver, and milk. The client should avoid a high-protein diet.

Discuss the risks of ERT with the client. Prepare the client for the possibility of side effects with low-dose ERT such as breast tenderness, occasional gastrointestinal upset, and spotting. Inform the client that bleeding is normal when estrogens are withdrawn. Reassure the client that bleeding does not indicate a renewal of menstruation nor the possibility of becoming pregnant in postmenopausal women.

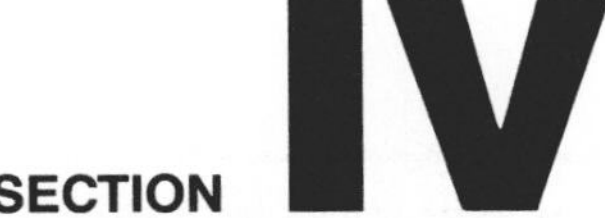

Infectious and Inflammatory Disorders

Infectious Vaginitis

Infectious vaginitis is one of the most frequent reasons female clients seek medical attention. A number of different agents such as yeasts, bacteria, and protozoa can produce symptoms and signs of infectious vaginitis.

The most common type of yeast infection is that from the overgrowth of *Candida albicans*. Yeast infections are most common in diabetic and pregnant women because of their high blood glucose level. The overgrowth of *Candida albicans* also can occur with the use of broad-spectrum antibiotics, which decrease the normal vaginal flora.

The hemophilus bacterium *Gardnerella vaginalis* can cause vaginal infection. The bacteria can be transmitted sexually but can also exist normally in the vagina in small amounts without causing symptoms. When vaginal acidity is decreased, the bacteria will overgrow.

Trichomonas vaginalis infections are caused by the protozoan of that name. This one-celled parasite is transmitted sexually and possibly by contact with objects contaminated by vaginal or urethral discharge from an infected person.

Chlamydial vaginitis is caused by some of the organisms in the genus *Chlamydia*. Chlamydia are also a major cause of nongonococcal urethritis (NGU). It is the most prevalent STD in the United States.

Clinical Manifestations

The vaginal discharge in yeast infections is thick, white, and cheesy. There is also perineal pruritus, and severe infections may cause dysuria from vulval, perineal, and periurethral excoriation. Diagnosis is made by microscopic evaluation of the discharge using saline or potassium hydroxide for slide preparation or by culture of the discharge.

The vaginal discharge in *Gardnerella vaginitis* is profuse and has a pronounced fishy odor. Microscopic examination shows characteristic epithelial cells covered with bacteria, referred to as *clue cells,* as well as a large number of leukocytes. A general bacterial culture can also confirm the presence of *Gardnerella vaginalis.*

A *Trichomonas vaginalis* infection has symptoms that include a profuse thin, foamy, yellow-green discharge with an unpleasant odor. The vagina or cervix may have a strawberry color from small petechiae. The protozoan can be easily identified by microscopic examination using a saline preparation.

The vaginal discharge in chlamydial vaginitis is thin, white, and bubbly, with little odor. The diagnosis is made by culture using a special medium or by excluding other possible causes.

Medical Measures

Therapeutic measures for yeast infections include the insertion of miconazole nitrate (Monistat) or clotrimazole (Lotrimin) suppositories or cream into the vagina nightly for 5 to 7 days. These pharmacologic agents treat the infection effectively. The partner should also be treated because the yeast may be present on the prepuce, the folds of skin on the penis, and the scrotum.

Therapeutic measures in gardnerella vaginitis include tetracycline or metronidazole (Flagyl). If the client is allergic to these pharmacologic agents, erythromycin or ampicillin may be used. Treatment of the client's sexual partner will prevent reinfection. Ampicillin should be used to treat pregnant women.

Treatment by metronidazole effectively eradicates the *Trichomonas vaginalis* infection if the sexual partner is also treated. If not, the client will become reinfected. Pregnant clients should not take metronidazole. A povidone–iodine gel can help to decrease the discharge; however, it does not eradicate the infection.

Treatment for chlamydial vaginitis involves either tetracycline or doxycycline. For those clients in whom tetracycline is contraindicated or not tolerated, erythromycin is recommended. Sexual partners should also be treated.

Specific Nursing Measures

Instruct the client with a yeast infection to avoid a high-carbohydrate diet. Test the client for possible diabetes because the organism thrives in a high-carbohydrate environment. It also grows in warm, moist environments. Advise the client to take off her bathing suit after it becomes wet and to avoid tight jeans and nylon underwear.

Tell the client with gardnerella vaginitis or chlamydia to avoid intercourse or use condoms until the treatment has been completed.

Specific nursing measures for the client with *Trichomonas vaginalis* vaginitis should include the identification of pregnancy because pregnant women should not be treated with metronidazole. Because the organism can live in moist environments outside the body for up to 6 hours, clients should be cautioned against sharing towels or other personal items with others.

Gonorrhea

One of the most common STDs is caused by *Neisseria gonorrhoeae,* a gram-negative diplococcus. Of the approximately 1 million cases of gonorrhea reported annually, the large majority are in men, with a peak incidence in young adults (20 to 24 years old) and the next highest incidence in teenagers between the ages of 15 and 19.

The organism survives poorly outside its host and is destroyed by both heat and drying. *N. gonorrhoeae* is transmitted via sexual contact, although Harrison (1984) notes rare reports of viable organisms being recovered from toilet seats after 18 hours and from wet towels between 10 and 24 hours after contact. The organism has become increasingly resistant to penicillin since the 1950s. A strain referred to as PPNG (penicillinase-producing *Neisseria gonorrhoeae*; resistant to all forms of penicillin) was first identified in 1976 on US military bases and cities in the Philippines. Since then, this strain has been identified in approximately 30 countries in North America, Europe, Asia, Africa, and the Pacific islands (Krieger, 1984).

Clinical Manifestations

The reproductive organs are most commonly affected in gonorrhea. If anal or oral sex has occurred, rectal inflammation and pharyngitis can be present.

It is estimated that between 50% and 75% of women with gonorrhea are asymptomatic or have mild symptoms, including transient vaginal discharge, dysuria, low abdominal discomfort, or a change in menstrual patterns (Miles, 1984). The endocervix is the primary site of infection in women. The infection can spread up the reproductive system and cause pelvic inflammatory disease (PID) as it spreads into the fallopian tubes, possibly during menstruation. It also can spread downward, leading to a urethral infection that causes dysuria, discharge, and urinary frequency. Gonorrhea can also be present in Bartholin's glands, causing infection with signs of labial pain and edema. A disseminated gonococcal infection causes symptoms of fever;

skin lesions that begin as maculae and progress to vesicles and hemorrhagic pustules; and joint pain with or without swelling, erythema, and heat.

In men, the gonococcus usually causes gonococcal urethritis. Manifestations of gonorrhea in men include dysuria and a white or yellowish green cloudy urethral or rectal discharge. These symptoms range from severe to minimal. A client can also be asymptomatic and spread the organism without knowing it. Without treatment, the inflammation subsides within 2 to 4 weeks, and the individual may become a carrier.

Medical Measures

Diagnosis is made by culturing the urethra, endocervix, rectum, and pharynx, depending on the type of sexual involvement. It is essential to identify penicillin-resistant gonococci. The PPNG strain is often also resistant to other antibiotics, such as tetracycline. The key to the treatment of gonorrhea is effective antibiotic administration. Treatment is usually based on the recommendations of the Centers for Disease Control (CDC) (1985).

All clients treated for gonorrhea should have follow-up cultures performed 4 to 7 days after treatment is completed. All sexual partners must be identified, examined, cultured, and treated. Ineffective treatment can result in epididymitis, genital abscesses, proctitis, pharyngitis, and infertility or pelvic inflammatory disease in women.

Specific Nursing Measures

Prevention is the key in the nursing management of the client at risk of developing gonorrhea. Education about the risk of developing gonorrhea as well as other STDs must be emphasized and imparted in a straightforward, matter-of-fact, nonjudgmental way. Give the facts, and allow clients to form their own value judgments based on these facts.

Information given to clients should include facts about the incidence, risk, and transmission modes of gonorrhea. Clients should understand that all contacts must be identified and treated. Using a condom during intercourse and limiting sexual contacts to one of a few known sexual partners can help prevent the transmission of the disease. Teach good hand-washing techniques to prevent the infection's spread to the conjunctiva. Other important information includes making sure clients realize that they can become reinfected by having contact with an untreated partner. Clients being treated for gonorrhea should refrain from intercourse until the follow-up cultures are negative. A client who has had intercourse with a high-risk individual should begin an antibiotic regimen.

Before administering antibiotics, check for any drug allergies. Give instructions for taking oral medication if necessary, and warn the client not to share medication with partners. Explain the importance of returning for a follow-up culture, and make an appointment for the client.

Finally, the client should be allowed to express any feelings of anxiety, shame, or guilt. If telling a partner presents particular difficulty, the nurse may help by being a supportive listener as the client works through this problem.

Syphilis

Syphilis is caused by the spirochete *Treponema pallidum.* The incidence of syphilis has dropped sharply recently. The CDC attributes the declining syphilis rate to a major change in sexual behavior in homosexual men because of fear of AIDS. In past years, gay men have accounted for more than half of the syphilis cases in the United States.

Clinical Manifestations

The incubation period of primary syphilis is 10 to 90 days, with an average of 21 days. *Treponema pallidum* thrives in a warm, moist environment. As the organism incubates, there are no symptoms. The primary stage involves the formation of a lesion. The chancre (the painless lesion of syphilis) is a papule that progresses to a reddened, indurated, painless ulcer (Figure 49–5).

Diagnosis is hindered by the fact that the chancre may appear on the rectum, lips, tongue, or pharynx rather than on the more typical place, the genitalia. If treatment is not begun, the ulcer will heal in about 3 to 9 weeks. The regional lymph nodes also may be enlarged at this time.

The causative agent, the *Treponema pallidum,* is detected by dark-field examination of the chancre during the first stage of the disease after the incubation period of 10 to 90 days. The routine serologic test for syphilis is the VDRL test, which is positive after about 3 months of exposure.

Secondary syphilis occurs when the organism enters the bloodstream. On the average, this occurs about 6 to 8 weeks after the infection begins. The client has a generalized maculopapular rash, fever, aches, sore throat, hair loss, and lymphadenopathy. In blacks, the rash appears annular with a clear center (Drusin, 1984).

Between 4 and 12 weeks after the initial infection, syphilis becomes latent. If untreated, it manifests itself as tertiary syphilis about 18 to 20 years after the initial infection. Tertiary syphilis often involves the neurologic and cardiovascular systems.

Medical Measures

The treatment for syphilis in the primary and secondary stages is the administration of penicillin G benzathine IM in a single dose. Probenecid is given 30 minutes before the injection. Aqueous penicillin G procaine also may be administered. Clients allergic to penicillin may be given tetracycline hydrochloride. If a pregnant client has a penicillin allergy, erythromycin should be given instead of

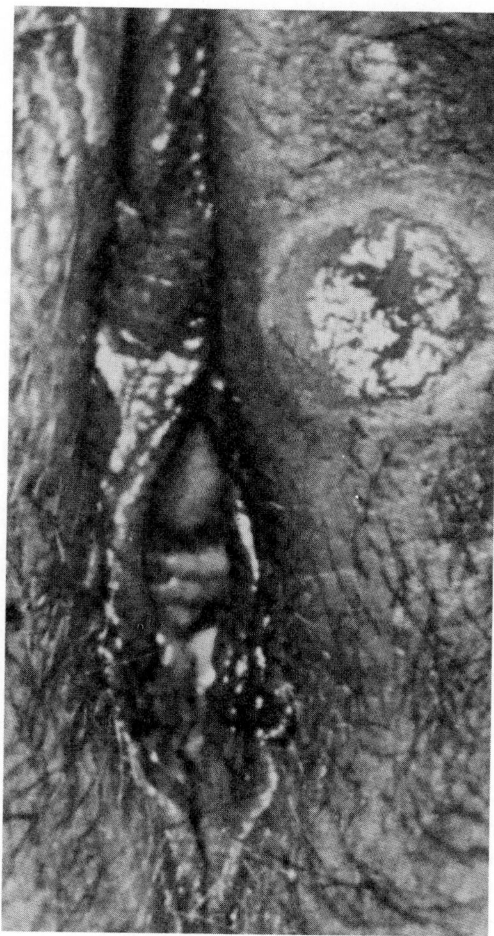

Figure 49–5

Syphilitic chancre on the labia. *SOURCE: Crooks R, Bauer K:* Our Sexuality, *2nd ed. Menlo Park, CA: Benjamin/Cummings, 1983.*

tetracycline. Erythromycin is also given to those allergic to both penicillin and tetracycline.

Specific Nursing Measures

The basic preventive measures that apply for other types of STDs also apply to syphilis. These include limiting intercourse to one or a limited number of known partners and using a condom to help prevent the disease's spread. The nurse should assist the client in identifying all contacts of the last 3 months, who will require treatment.

Warn the client that the administration of high doses of penicillin can create soreness at the injection site.

Tell the client who is being treated during the secondary stage that a post-treatment reaction may occur approximately 4 hours after treatment. This reaction, the *Jarisch–Herxheimer reaction,* results from the sudden massive destruction of spirochetes by antibiotics. It is characterized by chills, elevated temperature, general body aches, headache, malaise, and increased skin lesions. The reaction usually peaks in about 8 hours and lasts for about 16 hours. If this reaction occurs, clients are less likely to be made anxious by it if it is explained to them and they anticipate its possibility. Offer the client symptomatic relief and reassurance during this uncomfortable period. Treatment should not be discontinued unless the symptoms are severe or threaten to be fatal, or if laryngitis, auditory neuritis, or labyrinthitis is present since these may signify the possibility of irreversible damage.

Encourage the client to contact the sexual partner or partners so that they can receive effective therapy. The client should return for repeat serologic tests 3, 6, and 12 months after treatment. Finally, clients with syphilis should understand that they are at risk of developing the disease any time they are exposed to the organism; there is no immunity to syphilis.

Herpes Genitalis

Infections with herpes simplex viruses (HSVs, or *Herpesvirus hominis*) are common STDs. The majority of genital infections are caused by *Herpesvirus hominis* Type II, although at least 15% are caused by *Herpesvirus hominis* Type I, the virus that causes cold sores (a reflection of the increase in oral–genital sex). Herpes genitalis can be transmitted via a genital or oral–genital route. The incubation period is 2 to 10 days.

The exact incidence and prevalence are not known because herpes genitalis is a nonreportable disease, and some individuals are asymptomatic. Herpes genitalis seems to rank after gonorrhea and chlamydia infections as a leading STD.

The infection is found most often in the age group of 15 to 30 years. The virus causes serious complications to the newborn who contracts it during delivery or after the membranes rupture. HSV has been linked to cancer of the cervix and vulva.

Clinical Manifestations

Generally, herpes genitalis is less severe in men than women. The first episode is the worst and may last about 3 weeks. The client usually has multiple bilateral painful pustules or yellowish-gray ulcerative lesions on the penis (Figure 49–6), genital area, groin, or rectum in men, and on the medial aspects of the labia minora and the clitoris, vagina, urethra, and cervix in women. The lymph nodes are tender, and generalized symptoms of malaise and fever may appear. As some vesicles form pustules, ulcerate, crust, and heal, new vesicles appear. During the period of open lesions, the virus sheds from the lesions, and the infection can be spread to sexual contacts. Half the males infected with *Herpesvirus hominis* complain of dysuria, and the virus can be isolated from the urethra. In fact, herpes simplex without external lesions can cause NGU. The herpesvirus may be simultaneously present in other areas of

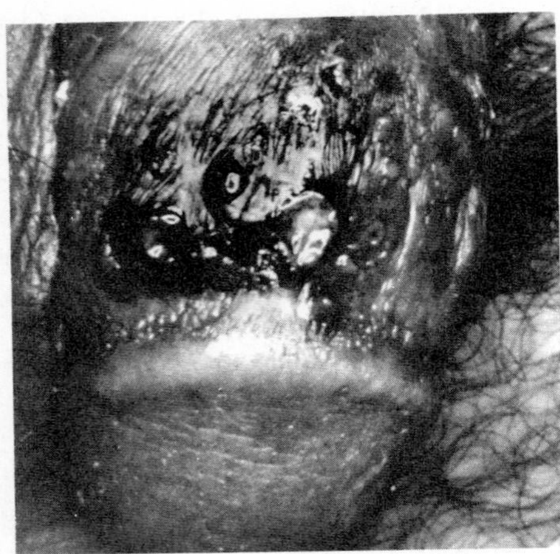

Figure 49–6

Genital herpes blisters on the penis. *Courtesy of Centers for Disease Control, Public Health Service, US Department of Health and Human Services, Atlanta, GA.*

the body. Mertz and Corey (1984) report that 10% of clients with primary herpes genitalis have pharyngitis and lesions on their buttocks and fingers.

The herpesvirus lies dormant in the spinal root ganglia and can reactivate at any time. The exact cause of recurrence is not known, but it is believed that emotional stress or tight clothing that increases warmth in the genital area may be factors. Recurrent infections are usually not as severe as the first infection, but they occur more often in men than women. There are fewer systemic manifestations, the lesions cover a smaller area, and usually they heal more quickly. Urethritis does not usually recur. Fifty percent of clients have a prodromal period with an itching, tingling sensation before the lesions break out (Mertz & Corey, 1984).

The disease can cause neurologic complications such as aseptic meningitis and sacral radiculopathy, an inflammation of the roots of the sacral nerves. It also can cause proctitis and prostatitis.

Diagnosis of herpes genitalis is made by microbiologic smear by touch preparation on a slide; multinucleated giant cells are usually found. The Pap test also may be used.

Medical Measures

There is no cure for herpes genitalis, and researchers are seeking a cure or a vaccine. The major breakthrough so far has been the drug acyclovir, a nucleoside analogue. Treatment during the initial episode includes acyclovir for 7–10 days, begun within 6 days of the onset of lesions. Acyclovir can be given IV to clients with severe symptoms. Treatment in severe recurrent infections will shorten the mean clinical course of the disease by about one day. Continuous treatment will reduce the frequency of the disease. The long-term effects of the drug are not known. It is not recommended during pregnancy.

Alcohol and other drying agents can be used to dry lesions. The client may need sedation during the first week of the disease when the lesions are the most painful. Hospitalization may be necessary if extensive lesions prevent normal voiding.

Specific Nursing Measures

During the painful primary stage, evaluate the client's need for pain medication and inform the client that recurrences of the disease will not be as incapacitating. Instruct clients to refrain from intercourse when lesions are present. Close follow-up during pregnancy is necessary because of the risk of the unborn child's contracting a highly fatal neonatal infection or congenital deformities.

Herpes genitalis causes psychologic pain and suffering in addition to physical discomfort. The client may feel stigmatized and ashamed. A client with herpes genitalis should tell future sexual partners about the condition. These clients need complete information and emotional support as they work through the changed self-concept the diagnosis generates.

Herpes genitalis is prevented by avoiding intimate contact with an individual with active lesions. Condoms do not necessarily provide protection. Teach the client to avoid touching other parts of the body because autoinoculation is possible and to keep the blisters clean and dry. The client needs to know that acyclovir treatment must be started early in the outbreak. All lesions should be covered with the ointment every 3 hours six times a day for 7 days (Centers for Disease Control, 1985).

Condylomata Acuminata

Condylomata acuminata (veneral warts) are considered a "minor" STD. According to Margolis (1984), however, they account for 1 million office visits per year and can undergo carcinogenic changes.

Clinical Manifestations

Clients may have cauliflowerlike warts that appear in masses or clusters on the shaft of the penis, on the scrotum, in the anorectal area, on the labia, in or near the urethral meatus, and on the vaginal or cervical mucosa. The incubation period is 1 to 2 months.

Medical Measures

The area where the warts occur must be kept dry to prevent their spread. One common treatment is the topical application of 10% to 25% podophyllin solution in tincture of benzoin (four weekly applications). It is important to avoid normal tissue to prevent irritation and scarring. Normal tissue should be protected with petrolatum jelly or other protective covering and the solution removed in 1 to 4 hours. Other treatments include cryotherapy, electrosurgery, and surgical excision. The warts should be biopsied to check for cancer. The removal of warts in the urethral meatus may cause stricture formation.

Specific Nursing Measures

The nurse must support the client as he or she undergoes the treatment regimen. Be sure the client is fully informed about the possible treatment options.

Nongonococcal Urethritis

The client with nongonococcal urethritis (NGU) has symptoms of urethral inflammation, but the gonococcus is not present on culture. There are many causes, but the most common are *Chlamydia trachomatis* and *Ureaplasma urealyticum.* This disease can occur at any age, and its incidence is increasing. Clinics treating STDs report that over half of the urethritis seen is NGU (Bowie, 1984). The greatest incidence is in the young adult age group (20 to 24 years). The incubation period varies between 1 and 5 weeks.

Clinical Manifestations

The manifestations of NGU are similar to those of gonococcal urethritis but often less acute. Dysuria and a thin, watery discharge are early symptoms. Later, the discharge may be thick, white, and creamy. For definitive diagnosis, the urethra should be milked and a Gram's stain and culture performed. Nongonococcal urethritis is more difficult to treat than gonococcal urethritis; penicillin is not effective, and the discharge is slow to clear. Between 30% and 40% of cases recur within 6 weeks (Bowie, 1984). The diagnosis and treatment may be further confounded because a client can have NGU and gonorrhea at the same time.

Inflammation of the epididymis, or ***epididymitis,*** is the major complication of NGU. One-sided scrotal pain, redness, and swelling are typical of epididymitis. When it occurs in a man under 35 years of age, epididymitis is usually caused by the gonococcus or *Chlamydia trachomatis.* In clients who practice anal intercourse, it may be caused by the *Escherichia coli.* The likely cause in those over age 35 and in preadolescent males is either a coliform or pseudomonas bacteria; rather than being sexually transmitted, the infection is usually caused by urinary tract disease.

Medical Measures

Tetracycline hydrochloride effectively eradicates *Chlamydia trachomatis.* Doxycycline is more effective against *Ureaplasma urealyticum* and will also treat gonorrhea. For the client unable to take tetracycline hydrochloride, treatment with erythromycin is recommended.

Antibiotic treatment for epididymitis is similar. An anti-inflammatory agent such as indomethacin (Indocin) may be given, and analgesia is necessary.

Specific Nursing Measures

Prevention of NGU is difficult, because the causative organisms are prevalent, the affected individuals are frequently asymptomatic, and the organisms commonly are resistant to the prescribed drugs. As with other STDs, the nurse can teach the client that having one or a limited number of known partners will help control the disease's spread. The use of condoms or spermicides also may be helpful.

The client should be taught to avoid alcohol during the treatment phase. He should not resume intercourse for 4 weeks after treatment because recurrence is common; if he does resume intercourse during this time, the client should be sure to use a condom. It is important that the client comply with the treatment regimen because untreated cases usually have complications, the major one being epididymitis. Partners need to be identified and treated.

The exquisite pain caused by epididymitis makes pain relief a priority in the early period. Assess the client frequently for pain and the effectiveness of the analgesic. The client probably will take an oral analgesic such as oxycodone with acetaminophen (Percocet) every 4 hours; be sure the medication is administered on time and is given before the pain cycle begins so the client is spared intermittent painful episodes.

The client's activity is limited to either bed rest or bed rest with bathroom privileges. Ice applied to the scrotum for the first 24 hours and scrotal elevation may reduce inflammation. When the client is out of bed, he should wear an athletic supporter. Further nursing interventions include monitoring the client's temperature every 4 hours and forcing fluids to maintain hydration and keep the temperature down.

Prostatitis

Prostatitis, inflammation of the prostate gland, is the most common complication of STDs in men. Acute bacterial prostatitis is usually not sexually transmitted. It is caused by *Escherichia coli, Klebsiella pneumoniae, Proteus mirabilis,* or *Pseudomonas aeruginosa.* Chronic nonbacterial prostatitis is more common in 30- to 45-year-olds and is thought to be caused by the sexually transmitted organisms *Chlamydia trachomatis, Ureaplasma urealyticum,* and *Trichomonas vaginalis.*

Clinical Manifestations

The symptoms of prostatitis include dysuria, suprapubic and perineal pain, urethral discomfort, rectal fullness, nocturia, urgency and frequency of urination, and blood in the ejaculate. With acute bacterial prostatitis, the client has severe symptoms of a systemic and prostatic infection. On rectal examination, the prostate feels enlarged, tender, and boggy. Massage should not be attempted because it can cause septicemia. The symptoms of chronic nonbacterial prostatitis are generally similar but subacute.

Medical Measures

Acute prostatitis is usually treated with tobramycin given intramuscularly until the client is afebrile. Afebrile clients usually receive a drug such as trimethoprim or sulfamethoxazole orally for 30 days. If the infection becomes chronic, treatment is more difficult.

Specific Nursing Measures

If the cause of the prostatitis is sexual transmission, the client should be urged to identify contacts so they can be treated. Explain to the client the mode of transmission and possible preventive measures. Be sure the antibiotics are administered in a timely manner, and closely monitor the renal function of clients taking tobramycin. Alcohol, caffeine, and spicy foods aggravate prostatitis, so instruct the client to avoid them.

Toxic Shock Syndrome

Most cases (97%) of toxic shock syndrome (TSS) coincide with tampon use during the menstrual cycle (Cibulka, 1984). It can occur without tampon use in association with infected wounds, deep abscesses, lacerations, and insect bites. The causative agent is usually toxin secreted by strains of *Staphylococcus aureus,* but the mechanisms are not clearly understood. In cases involving tampon use, there seems to be a correlation between the chemical fibers used in superabsorbent tampons and the incidence of TSS. Fibers that bind the magnesium in the vagina were demonstrated to increase strikingly the amount of toxin produced (Mills et al., 1985). The incidence of TSS in the United States is 6.2 cases per 100,000 menstruating women per year.

Clinical Manifestations

The toxin can affect almost any body system. The symptoms include a rapid onset of fever of 102°F (38.9°C) or higher, nausea and vomiting, and a diffuse rash followed by desquamation of the skin of the palms and soles about 1 to 2 weeks after the disease's onset. Hypotension with a systolic blood pressure less than 90 mm Hg is also a symptom. Clients may also have severe myalgia, hyperemic mucous membranes, impaired renal function, and central nervous system symptoms of confusion, alterations in consciousness, and possible combative behavior.

Medical Measures

The tampon should be removed and the client placed in isolation. Treatment for TSS includes bed rest and antibiotic therapy with beta-lactamase–resistant antibiotics such as nafcillin and gentamicin. Cultures from the nasopharynx, blood, urine, stool, and open sores should be obtained. Intravenous infusion can prevent shock from hypotension and electrolyte loss. If the infusion does not prevent hypotension, a vasopressor drug may be used. Oxygen may be needed if the client shows signs of respiratory distress.

Specific Nursing Measures

Administer antibiotics and assess the client's temperature frequently; a hypothermia blanket may be needed. Nausea and vomiting may necessitate a nasogastric tube. Administer medication for nausea and vomiting as ordered. Because of prolonged bed rest, assess the client's skin frequently and help eliminate areas of pressure. Provide passive ROM and turn the client frequently. Encourage coughing and deep breathing.

Monitor fluid intake and output for signs of circulatory overload (headache, flushed skin, a rapid pulse, venous distention, coughing, and shortness of breath). Also monitor arterial blood gases for signs of adult respiratory distress syndrome.

If necessary, protect confused and combative clients with soft restraints, and frequently orient them to time, person, place, and events. Prevent sensory overload by ensuring a quiet environment.

Support the client's family or significant others by explaining procedures and answering questions. Clients who have had TSS should know that they are at risk for TSS in the future and should probably avoid tampon use.

SECTION V

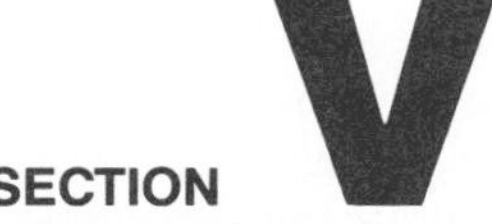

Neoplastic Disorders

Uterine Leiomyomas

A uterine leiomyoma is a benign tumor, known to many clients as a fibroid, that is composed of smooth muscle cells and some connective tissue. It compresses the normal uterine muscular tissue as it grows and may involve the submucosa layer or be intramural in origin (Figure 49–7).

Clinical Manifestations

The clinical manifestations of uterine leiomyomas include an enlarged, irregular uterus. The client may experience prolonged and heavy or painful menstruation. Depending on the location or size of the tumor or on the number of tumors, the client may also experience other symptoms such as a feeling of heaviness in the lower abdomen or pelvic region, constipation, frequency of urination, or var-

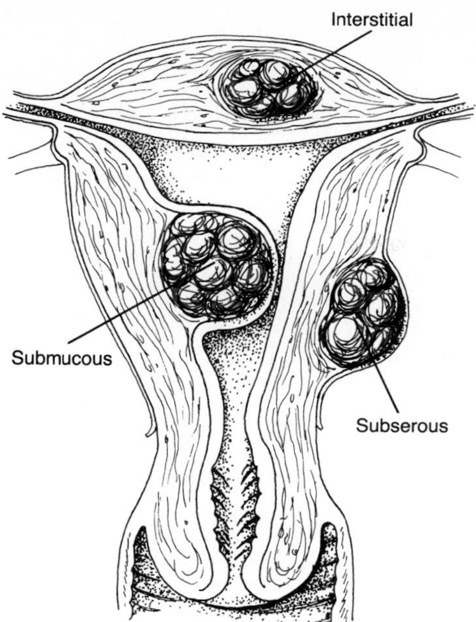

Figure 49–7

Uterine leiomyomas.

icosities of the lower extremities or vulva. There may be no symptoms, however, and the tumor may be found on pelvic examination.

Medical Measures

Treatment depends on the client's symptoms and desire for future childbearing. The client with no symptoms does not require treatment. She is instructed to report any changes in her bleeding pattern, such as prolonged or heavy menses.

Myomectomy (removal of the tumor) is performed if the leiomyoma interferes with maintaining a pregnancy. A total hysterectomy is performed when heavy and prolonged menstruation results in anemia. A hysterectomy is also performed if the tumor results in a uterus larger than one of a 12-week gestation or when the woman cannot carry out activities of daily living because of excess bleeding. After menopause, the tumor will decrease in size; however, if the uterus continues to enlarge, a TAH–BSO is performed.

Specific Nursing Measures

Before the pelvic examination, have the client void so the bladder is not confused with a tumor. Pregnancy testing also should be performed if there is a possibility of conception. The preoperative and postoperative nursing care for the hysterectomy client is reviewed later in this chapter.

Benign Ovarian Neoplasms

More neoplasms arise from the ovary than from any other reproductive organ, and the ovary is the most frequent site of a pelvic mass in the female reproductive tract. Most of the benign neoplasms manifest themselves during the reproductive years. They include functional cysts such as follicle cysts, corpus luteum cysts, and theca lutein cysts. Benign neoplasms of the ovaries also include tumors derived from the germinal epithelium such as the benign cystic teratoma (dermoid cyst) and ovarian fibroma.

Clinical Manifestations

Follicle cysts are usually small and may rupture upon pelvic examination. They usually disappear spontaneously during the menstrual cycle either by absorption or rupture.

Corpus luteum cysts are less common. The client has delayed menstruation with an irregular and prolonged onset of menses. Pain is usually associated with the cyst because of intraluminal bleeding. The cyst may rupture on its own or regress slowly.

Theca lutein cysts, the least common of the ovarian cysts, are usually associated with trophoblastic disease of pregnancy. They are bilateral and may reach 20 to 25 cm in diameter.

Benign cystic teratoma occurs in clients from 20 to 30 years old; they may be either cystic or solid in structure. Unilateral involvement is more common. The cysts contain fatty, viscoid sebaceous material, matted hair, and teeth. The cystic tumors are pedunculated and may twist and cause lower abdominal pain. If the cysts rupture, the material inside them can cause chemical peritonitis. A tumor of the solid type can grow larger than the cystic type and may adhere to surrounding structures.

Ovarian fibromas have no unique symptomatology. They may produce estrogen and are usually unilateral and pedunculated (thus, they may undergo torsion). Ascites usually accompanies the larger lesions.

Medical Measures

Follicle cysts are managed conservatively and observed over a number of menstrual cycles. Gonadotrophic suppression may cause regression of the cyst. If it enlarges beyond 6 cm in diameter, laparoscopy is performed, at which time the cyst may be aspirated.

Corpus luteum cysts must be differentiated from ectopic pregnancy by ultrasonography or laparoscopy. They may regress slowly, or rupture and cause intraperitoneal bleeding and require surgical intervention. The preservation of ovarian tissue is the goal of treatment.

Theca lutein cysts usually completely regress after evacuation of the trophoblastic tissue. They should not be removed or drained.

If clients with a benign cystic teratoma or ovarian fibroma desire preservation of fertility, management involves preserving as much of the ovary as possible. Hemorrhage, torsion, rupture, or infection may necessitate removal of the ovary and fallopian tube, however.

Specific Nursing Measures

If the client has a cyst that will be observed over the menstrual cycle, instruct the client to note any symptoms and to return for follow-up care. If the client will undergo surgery, she and her family or significant other may find the potential diagnosis of cancer traumatizing. Nursing care of the client undergoing ovarian surgery is discussed later in this chapter.

Laparoscopy

Within the last decade, laparoscopy (pelvic peritoneoscopy) has become widely used to visualize the pelvic cavity (Figure 49–8). Laparoscopy enables the surgeon to perform many diagnostic and therapeutic procedures that otherwise would require major abdominal surgery. The technique is often preferable to traditional laparotomy, which requires an abdominal incision, because laparoscopy requires less operative time, less hospital confinement, less discomfort, less cost, and less time lost from normal activities.

The diagnostic uses include exploration of the pelvic cavity and reproductive organs, tissue biopsy, aspiration of pelvic cysts, and the evaluation of infertility. It is usually combined with a diagnostic D and C. The therapeutic uses are for surgery on pelvic adhesions, tubal sterilization, removal of an intrauterine device (IUD), aspiration of pelvic cysts, aspiration of ova (for in vitro fertilization), and the removal of an early ectopic pregnancy. Physiologic and psychosocial/lifestyle implications for the client undergoing laparoscopy are listed in Table 49–9.

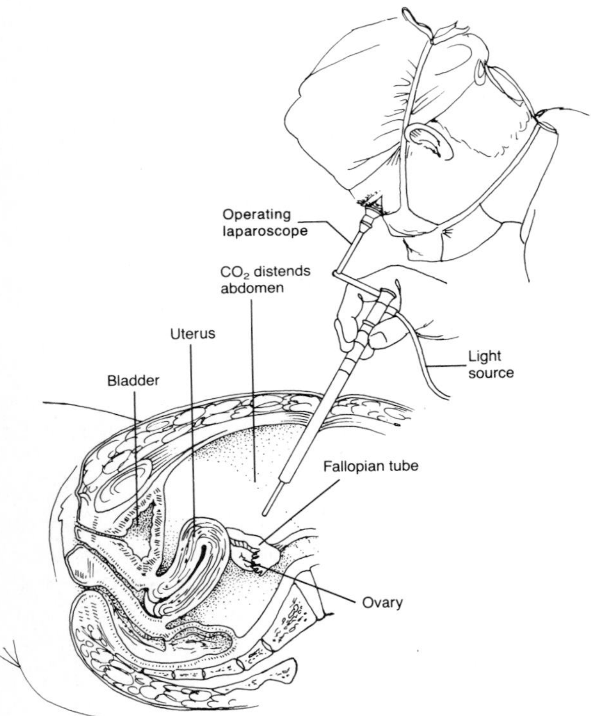

Figure 49–8

Laparoscopy. The laparoscope is inserted through a small (3–4 cm) infraumbilical incision. Gas distends the abdominal wall lifting it away from the pelvic organs (pneumoperitoneum).

Table 49–9
Laparoscopy: Implications for the Client

Physiologic Implications	Psychosocial/Lifestyle Implications
Rare complications of peritonitis, necrosis of the bowel, catastrophic hemorrhage, cardiopulmonary impairment	Same-day surgery reduces lifestyle limitations
Mild abdominal discomfort	Minimal restrictions on activity for 5–7 days
Referred sudden intermittent sharp shoulder pain from pneumoperitoneum for a few days	Avoid tub bathing until incision heals
	Change own dressing (plastic bandage)

Nursing Implications

PREOPERATIVE CARE Preoperative nursing care is similar to that for a D and C. Discussing postoperative discomforts at this time might help to minimize the client's anxiety.

POSTOPERATIVE CARE Postoperative nursing care is similar to that for a D and C but also includes assessment of the infraumbilical incision for drainage or hematoma formation. Mild analgesics may be helpful in the first few postoperative days to alleviate the shoulder pain caused by irritation of the phrenic nerve by residual gas from the pneumoperitoneum. Only oral analgesics are necessary if the client's anxiety has been reduced by preoperative preparation. Discharge instructions in addition to these are similar to those given for a D and C. Because clients are often discharged the same day of the surgery, provide instructions on wound care and dressing changes.

Oophorectomy

Oophorectomy is the surgical removal of one or both ovaries. The indications include ovarian malignancy, unresolved benign ovarian neoplasm, tubo-ovarian abscess, and the need for prophylaxis in perimenopausal and menopausal clients having hysterectomies. Client implications for oophorectomy are listed in Table 49–10.

Nursing Implications

Preoperative and postoperative nursing care are similar to that for abdominal hysterectomy clients. Complica-

Table 49–10
Oophorectomy: Implications for the Client 

Physiologic Implications	Psychosocial/Lifestyle Implications
If malignancy is found, possible removal of fallopian tubes and uterus In bilateral procedure, sudden climacteric and sterility In unilateral procedure, ability of remaining ovary to meet physiologic needs Complications similar to abdominal hysterectomy (see Table 58–5)	In bilateral procedure, sterility and possible need for hormonal replacement in premenopausal women Possible body image change Fears associated with malignancy See also Table 58–5

tions are also similar to those that may be expected with abdominal hysterectomy.

Endometrial Cancer

Endometrial cancer effects mostly mature women between the ages of 55 and 69. The conditions that put women at risk for the development of endometrial cancer are history of infertility, failure of ovulation, prolonged use of ERT, and obesity (American Cancer Society, 1987).

Clinical Manifestations

The major symptom of endometrial cancer is some form of abnormal bleeding. Any vaginal bleeding in a postmenopausal client should be evaluated. A D and C is performed to assess the uterine lining for signs of endometrial hyperplasia or carcinoma. The Pap test, although highly effective in detecting early cervical cancer, is only 50% effective in detecting endometrial cancer. An endometrial biopsy at menopause is a more accurate method of detection.

Medical Measures

Surgery combined with radiation therapy is usually the treatment of choice for endometrial cancer depending on the stage of the disease and the individual health characteristics of the client. Small tumors may be treated surgically without irradiation. Preoperative radiation therapy either by radium implants or external irradiation may also be used. In more extensive carcinomas, the TAH–BSO is performed along with lymph node dissection. In those clients with inoperable tumors and those with postoperative recurrences, treatment includes external and/or intracavitary irradiation.

Clients with tumors that are positive estrogen and progesterone receptors usually respond to hormonal therapy. Progestins or megestrol acetate may be used in premenopausal clients who do not choose to have a TAH–BSO because they wish to preserve childbearing potential. For clients with advanced disease (extended outside the uterus) or recurrent disease, hydroxyprogesterone caproate (Delalutin) may be effective. Tamoxifen citrate (Nolvadex) may be effective in clients whose disease has progressed after therapy with progestins.

There is no specific combination of chemotherapy agents used in advanced disease. Combinations of vincristine, dactinomycin and cyclophosphamide, or dacarbazine and doxorubicin, have been shown to be somewhat effective.

Specific Nursing Measures

Nursing measures for endometrial cancer clients is also discussed in Chapter 10.

Hysterectomy

A hysterectomy is the surgical removal of the uterus. The various types of hysterectomy procedures and the organs involved are listed in Table 49–11. The indications for this operation include large leiomyomas, adenomyosis, malignancy, uterine prolapse, severe pelvic infection, endometriosis, and DUB that is unresponsive to conservative measures.

The surgical approach can be through the abdomen or vagina. The abdominal route is indicated when the pelvis must be explored for pelvic malignancy or severe infection and when the uterus is too large to remove vaginally. The vaginal approach is indicated for prolapse of the uterus and cancer in situ of the cervix. This route allows more rapid recovery because there is less restriction of mobility, less postoperative discomfort, and no abdominal incision. Implications for the hysterectomy client are summarized in Table 49–11.

Nursing Implications

PREOPERATIVE CARE The routine preoperative preparation common to other abdominal surgery is also indicated for a hysterectomy. In addition, the physician may order an antiseptic vaginal douche the evening before surgery. A Foley catheter may be inserted prior to the client's going to the operating room. If the hysterectomy is performed through the vagina, the client will be given prophylactic antibiotics before the operation.

Although the client should have been informed by the physician of the exact nature of the hysterectomy procedure and its implications, it is a nursing responsibility to make sure the client understands the procedure and the implications.

POSTOPERATIVE CARE The postoperative nursing care for the hysterectomy client is determined by her previous

Table 49–11
Hysterectomy: Implications for the Client

Type of Surgery	Organs Removed	Physiological Implications	Psychosocial/Lifestyle Implications
Subtotal hysterectomy	Uterine body	Possible hemorrhage, infection, thromboembolic disease; cessation of menses in premenopausal women (except in rare instances when sufficient endometrial tissue remains); sterility; possible continuation of cyclic premenstrual symptoms; continued cervical cancer screening	Sterility; possible body image problems
Total hysterectomy	Uterine body; uterine cervix	More postoperative pain with abdominal approach than vaginal approach; possible hemorrhage, infection, thromboembolic disease; cessation of menses in premenopausal women; sterility; possible continuation of cyclic premenstrual symptoms	Sterility; possible dyspareunia if vaginal shortening was part of the procedure; possible body image problems
Total abdominal hysterectomy with bilateral salpingo-oophorectomy (TAH–BSO)	Uterine body; uterine cervix; fallopian tubes; ovaries	More postoperative pain because of abdominal approach; possible hemorrhage, infection, thromboembolic disease; sudden climacteric in premenopausal clients; sterility	Sterility; possible dyspareunia if vaginal shortening was part of the procedure; possible body image problems; possible need for hormonal replacement
Radical hysterectomy	Uterine body; uterine cervix; upper third of vagina; supportive structures; pelvic lymph nodes; may also include ovaries and fallopian tubes	More postoperative pain because of abdominal approach; possible hemorrhage, infection, thromboembolic disease; risk of hypokalemia and hypoalbuminemia; wound drains inserted at time of surgery and remaining for 4 to 5 days; cessation of menses in premenopausal women; sterility; possible continuation of cyclic premenstrual symptoms; sudden climacteric if ovaries removed in premenopausal women; possible disrupted innervation to bladder and rectum	Sterility; possible dyspareunia if vaginal shortening was part of the procedure; possible body image problems; possible nerve damage to bladder requiring that client be discharged with Foley catheter or cystostomy tube; need to use Credé's maneuver every 2–3 hours to empty the bladder completely when urinary drainage apparatus is removed (see Chapter 25); need for laxatives for adequate bowel function

health status, the indications for surgery, and the surgical approach. In general, nursing interventions involve the promotion of healing through adequate nutrition, the alleviation of discomfort, the prevention of complications, and the promotion of a positive self-concept.

Initially, hydration is maintained and electrolytes are replaced by supplements and IV fluid therapy. Clients with abdominal hysterectomies are NPO for 24 hours or until nausea subsides and bowel sounds return. They are then placed on a diet that progresses from clear liquids to solid food. Vaginal hysterectomy clients can consume food earlier, because there has been less bowel manipulation. Flatulence, a common problem in gynecologic surgery, can be relieved by simethicone (Gas-X, Mylicon), a rectal tube, the left lateral Sims' position, and increased physical activity.

The amount of postoperative discomfort varies

according to the placement of the surgical incision, the surgical approach, the amount of tissue manipulation, and the client's level of anxiety. As a rule, clients with vaginal hysterectomies experience less discomfort and are mobile sooner than those who have had abdominal procedures. Clients with transverse abdominal incisions may have more discomfort than those with midline incisions. For pain control, narcotics are ordered every 4 to 6 hours if appropriate during the first 48 hours. Nursing comfort measures include proper positioning and splinting of the incisional area with movement.

Hemorrhage can occur with any type of hysterectomy but is more frequent with the vaginal approach. Monitor vital signs every 15 minutes until stable. Any fall in blood pressure associated with unusual postoperative pain should alert the nurse to the possibility of occult hemorrhage. Observe perineal pads for bright red blood; a small amount of serosanguineous discharge is expected. Clients with vaginal procedures may have vaginal packings for the first 24 hours to put mild pressure on the suture line and control postoperative oozing. The abdominal dressing should remain dry, and the nurse should report significant discharge or bleeding.

Pulmonary atelectasis, bronchitis, and pneumonia are complications that can be minimized by nursing intervention. Encourage mobility and pulmonary exercises. Incentive spirometry should be used for clients at increased risk for pulmonary infection because of obesity, smoking, or chronic lung disorders.

Wound infections, abscesses, or cellulitis can occur at both abdominal and vaginal incision sites. Infections of the vaginal cuff (the closed-off portion of the upper vagina after removal of the cervix) are more common, because the nonsterile environment encourages growth of pathogens. Be alert for foul-smelling discharge on the client's dressing or perineal pad. Again, a small amount of serosanguineous drainage is expected. Report temperature elevations to the surgeon. Therapy consists of systemic antibiotics.

Because of its proximity to the reproductive organs, the urinary system is susceptible to trauma and infection. Clients return to the unit with in-dwelling urethral catheters, which the nurse must evaluate for patency. Urinary drainage should be assessed for hematuria. In the absence of complications, the catheter is removed in 12 to 24 hours. Some clients have difficulty voiding after catheter removal because of the edema and discomfort from surgery. Check for frequent small voiding as a clue to residual urine. Distention of the bladder requires repeat catheterization. Once adequate voiding has been established, remind clients to wipe from front to back to prevent fecal contamination of the urethra and vagina. Avoid bacterial concentration in the bladder by encouraging fluids that flush the urinary tract.

Manipulation and trauma of the pelvic vessels predispose the gynecologic client to thromboembolic disease, and a prior history of thromboembolic disease, pelvic malignancy, and obesity accentuates the risk. Exercises while in bed, early postoperative ambulation, and the use of antiembolic stockings are thought to minimize these complications. Encourage women to avoid positions that obstruct venous return from the lower extremities.

Pelvic Exenteration

Total pelvic exenteration is the removal of the entire female reproductive tract, along with both urinary and fecal diversion. Modifications of this procedure involve removal of the reproductive organs with only urinary diversion or removal of the reproductive organs with only fecal diversion. This surgery is performed on clients with invasive cancer of the uterine cervix.

Deep pelvic node and groin node excision are likely to be part of the surgical procedure. It may not be possible to approximate the wound edges, and some of the area may be left to heal by secondary intention. Drains attached to suction are often inserted at the inguinal areas. Some of the operative area may be covered with either light dressings or pressure dressings, whereas other parts may be left exposed to the air. Client implications of pelvic exenteration are summarized in Table 49–12.

Nursing Implications

PREOPERATIVE CARE Preoperative nursing for pelvic exenteration is similar to the care of clients undergoing vulvectomy and those having urinary and fecal diversion. The nurse must devote considerable time toward allowing these clients to verbalize their anger and fears.

POSTOPERATIVE CARE The long surgical procedure and a fluctuating blood volume predispose pelvic exenteration clients to hemorrhage and shock. Clients need to be monitored carefully so corrective measures can be taken

Table 49–12
Pelvic Exenteration: Implications for the Client

Physiologic Implications	Psychosocial/Lifestyle Implications
Prolonged healing	Severe disruption of body image
Possible fecal and urinary diversion	Sexual intercourse no longer possible unless vagina is reconstructed
Complications of hemorrhage, shock, fluid and electrolyte imbalances, infection, thromboembolic disease	Need to adapt to both urinary and fecal diversion
Stay in intensive care unit	
High mortality rate (15%)	

immediately. Fluid maintenance and electrolyte balance are major concerns. Because of the radical surgery, infection is a major cause of death. The postoperative care for bladder and fecal diversion are discussed in Chapters 26 and 38. These clients may also be receiving chemotherapy or radiation.

Cervical Cancer

There are two types of cervical cancer. The most common type, squamous cell carcinoma, is believed to be viral in origin and almost never occurs in virgins. The other type, adenocarcinoma, may be present in virgins as well as nonvirgins.

Cervical cancer begins as a change in the epithelial covering of the cervix and eventually involves the epithelial layer. This change can be considered premalignant and is called cervical intraepithelial neoplasia (CIN); at this stage, there is no metastasis of the cells. The Pap test is highly effective in detecting these early changes. Invasive carcinoma extends beyond the surface, involves the body of the cervix, and from there can spread to the lymphatic system and extend to surrounding structures such as the vagina, bladder, and rectum. The 5-year survival rate is 66%. For clients diagnosed early the rate is 80–90% (American Cancer Society, 1987).

Early age at first intercourse and multiple sex partners are factors associated with increased risk.

Clinical Manifestations

The client is symptom-free in the early stages, although early changes in cellular structure can be diagnosed by the Pap test. Therefore, regular examination of the cervix, vagina, and vulva are necessary along with a complete pelvic examination.

Medical Measures

Treatment depends on the extent of the disease, the state of the client's general health, her age, and whether or not she wishes to have her reproductive potential preserved. The treatment of premalignant lesions can consist of cryotherapy, electrocautery, laser therapy, or conization. Hysterectomy is performed for carcinoma in situ. Early carcinoma can also be conservatively managed by cervical conization, transvaginal roentgentherapy, and laser treatment. Clients who are conservatively managed should be closely evaluated at least yearly for further appearances of cancer.

The surgery for more advanced cancer may involve a TAH, or a TAH with removal of the upper vagina, depending on the tumor depth. Radical abdominal hysterectomy and bilateral pelvic lymphadenectomy are also performed. Irradiation alone or pelvic exenteration, although rarely used, may be performed in advanced disease.

Radiotherapy is effective in the treatment of cervical cancer and is often used in combination with surgery. In early stages, intracavitary applications of radium are used. In the operating room, vaginal cylinders are placed in the lateral vaginal fonices. Once the client returns to her room, the applicators are loaded with the radioactive material. The dose and time are calculated by a computer; the usual insertion length is 48 to 72 hours. During this period of time, the client remains on bed rest with a catheter and a low residue diet.

In advanced tumors, external radiation is beneficial in reducing the symptoms. External and internal radiation may be used together. Interstitial radiation, the direct insertion of radioactive needles into the tumor, is another treatment modality.

Chemotherapeutic agents that have been used with some success include methotrexate, cyclophosphamide, and combinations of hydroxyurea or doxorubicin and radiotherapy. Combination chemotherapy is used for late and recurring carcinomas and includes such drugs as bleomycin, mitomycin C, and cisplatin.

Specific Nursing Measures

A discussion of preoperative and postoperative nursing care for the various procedures follows below. Chapter 10 discusses chemotherapy, radiation therapy, and general nursing care of the cancer client.

Cervical Cryosurgery

In gynecology, cryosurgery frequently is used to destroy areas of cervical dysplasia or chronic cervicitis. It is also used to remove small vulval lesions. Cervical cryosurgery has basically replaced cervical cauterization as a surgical treatment.

Cryosurgery is an ambulatory procedure often performed in the physician's office. It requires no anesthesia and is almost painless. The freezing agent is applied with a cryoprobe applied directly to the involved tissue. Total treatment time is about 2 minutes.

Laser treatment for treating cervical dysplasia or chronic cervicitis is also available. Because it requires special equipment and skills, it is not as readily available as cryosurgery. The discussion in this section can also be applied to cervical laser surgery. The client implications for cryosurgery are found in Table 49–13.

Nursing Implications

PREOPERATIVE CARE Preoperative nursing care is similar to that for other outpatient gynecologic procedures. Nursing care has been described under D and C.

POSTOPERATIVE CARE After cryosurgery is completed, instruct the client regarding the implications in Table 49–13. Stress the importance of returning to the health

Table 49–13
Cervical Cryosurgery: Implications for the Client

Physiologic Implications	Psychosocial/Lifestyle Implications
Profuse watery discharge Possible spotting Necrotic tissue sloughs in about 10 days Complete healing may take 2 to 3 months Possible complication of cervical stenosis requiring dilation	No intercourse for 2 weeks Return visit to health care provider in 2 weeks Regular cytologic exams (Pap smear)

care provider regularly for cytologic follow-up examinations, because dysplasia can recur in other areas of the cervix.

Cervical Conization

Conization is the surgical removal of a cone-shaped piece of tissue from the uterine cervix for diagnostic or therapeutic purposes. In past years, many women who were found to have abnormal cervical cytology underwent this procedure. Conization now has been replaced by the less traumatic cryosurgery and laser techniques. Surgical conization is still indicated, however, when the pathologic lesion cannot be visualized via the colposcope or when cervical dysplasia persists despite repeated conservative therapies. Table 49–14 summarizes the client implications of conization.

Nursing Implications

PREOPERATIVE CARE Explain the conization procedure to the client, including physical sensations. Fear of cancer also should be discussed.

Table 49–14
Cervical Conization: Implications for the Client

Physiologic Implications	Psychosocial/Lifestyle Implications
Possible hemorrhage Possible infertility Some discharge Cervical packing possible	No intercourse, douching, or tampon use for at least 3 weeks Rest for 24 hours No heavy lifting for 2–3 weeks Need for regular cytologic examinations

POSTOPERATIVE CARE Postoperative nursing care is similar to that for a D and C. Later hemorrhage can be a significant complication, so discharge instructions must be directed toward preventing this problem. The client should report immediately to the physician any bleeding heavier than a normal menstrual period or associated with the passage of clots. Remind the client of the implications in Table 49–14.

Ovarian Cancer

Ovarian cancer is more difficult than endometrial cancer to detect in its early stages, and therefore the disease has often spread by the time it is detected. The overall survival rate is only about 38% (American Cancer Society, 1987). Ovarian cancer occurs in all age groups but is more common in women 40 to 65 years old. By 55 years, it is the fourth most common cause of cancer deaths in women.

Clients at high risk are those who have never had children, and those with ovarian imbalance as demonstrated by infertility, nulliparity, and early menopause. There is also a correlation between a diet high in animal fat and an increased incidence of ovarian cancer. Clients with breast or endometrial cancer, and clients with colorectal cancer are also at increased risk. Incidence rates are higher in North America and Northern Europe, and in nuns, Jewish women, and women who have never married.

Clinical Manifestations

Most ovarian cancers are not diagnosed until the lesion has metastasized outside the pelvis. The client may have an increase in abdominal girth from the growth of the tumor, ascites, or both. Any adnexal mass after menopause should be evaluated by laparoscopy or laparotomy. Other symptoms that should be evaluated are an adnexal mass 6 cm in diameter or greater in a woman of any age, a mass less than 6 cm in diameter that persists through one menstrual cycle, and any solid mass that cannot be diagnosed as a uterine leiomyoma.

Medical Measures

Evaluation of the tumor determines what type of surgery is indicated in premenopausal clients. If the cancer is a dysgerminoma (derived from the germ cells of the embryonic gonad), only the affected ovary need be removed. In postmenopausal clients, a TAH–BSO is performed. The omentum and lymph nodes may also be removed if there is evidence of metastasis.

Radioactive phosphorus (P^{32}) may also be installed at the time of surgery. Chemotherapeutic agents are thought to be responsible for remissions in some instances. The chemotherapeutic agents used include alkylating agents, cisplatin, doxorubicin, and various combinations of these agents.

Specific Nursing Measures

Nursing measures for surgical care of the client are discussed under the various procedures in this chapter. Care of the client with cancer is discussed in Chapter 10.

Vulval Cancer

Cancer of the vulva is usually found in elderly women, with the highest incidence between ages 70 and 80. Those most at risk have had chronic vulvitis treated by various methods without biopsy. The disease progresses from a dysplasia through intraepithelial neoplasia to invasive cancer. The premalignant dysplasia and epithelial involvement may be present for 10 years or longer, and the invasive lesion may extend locally for a time before it metastasizes.

Clinical Manifestations

The most common symptom of vulval cancer is vulval pruritus. There may also be a history of chronic vulvitis (chronic inflammation of the vulva). A neoplasm should be suspected in any woman with a chronic irritation that fails to heal with treatment, or when an ulceration develops. A raised, grayish white hypertrophic patch on the vulva, referred to as **leukoplakia,** may precede invasive cancer in up to 50% of cases (Kase & Weingold, 1983). Fewer than 10%, however, become malignant.

Medical Measures

The treatment for vulval cancer is surgical removal of the vulva (vulvectomy) and the superficial inguinal lymph nodes. Radiation therapy is not performed because of the high probability that it will cause extensive tissue necrosis.

Specific Nursing Measures

The elderly woman may hesitate to have a vulvectomy because of embarrassment. She will need the nurse's support during both diagnosis and treatment.

Vulvectomy

Vulvectomy involves excision of the external female genitalia. The indications for this surgery include premalignant vulvar lesions, cancer in situ, or invasive carcinoma. *Simple vulvectomy* usually involves the clitoris, labia majora, labia minora, and tissues between them. With invasive carcinoma, a *radical vulvectomy* may be performed to remove the entire vulva, lymphatics, subcutaneous fat, and skin portions from the abdomen and groin. Table 49–15 summarizes the physiologic and psychosocial/lifestyle implications for the client.

Table 49–15
Vulvectomy: Implications for the Client

Physiologic Implications	Psychosocial/Lifestyle Implications
Complications of infection, hemorrhage, edema, thromboembolic disease, hypokalemia, hypoalbuminemia	Alteration in body image because of genital mutilation
Healing is prolonged with radical procedure	Decreased sexual pleasure in intercourse after removal of clitoris
Possible need for skin grafting after radical procedure	Fear related to diagnosis of malignancy
Vaginal stenosis requiring surgical intervention	

Nursing Implications

PREOPERATIVE CARE Preoperative preparation of the vulvectomy client is similar to that for a vaginal hysterectomy client. The nursing care also should be directed toward helping the client adjust to changes in body image and sexual function.

POSTOPERATIVE CARE Prevention of infection, hemorrhage, and edema are primary postoperative nursing concerns with the simple vulvectomy. These complications can be prevented by pressure bandages, the use of sterile technique in dressing changes, and the use of wound drains. Prophylactic antibiotics initiated prior to the surgery are continued for 48 hours postoperatively to prevent infection. Poor healing with wound dehiscence can result from poor circulation and infection. Sitz baths are controversial; although they provide generalized heat, they also may contribute to infection. Heat lamps promote circulation and thus the supply of oxygen at the wound site. In many instances, healing occurs by secondary intention—a long and uncomfortable process that requires meticulous attention to preventing infection. The nursing care for clients with skin grafts is described in Chapter 55.

Fluid and electrolyte management is essential in these clients to prevent hypokalemia and hypoalbuminemia. Older clients may require wedge pressure monitoring by a Swan–Ganz catheter to regulate fluid replacement.

Benign Breast Disease

Benign breast disease includes the majority of breast masses that develop in women. These include fibrocystic disease, also referred to as *cystic hyperplasia* and *chronic mastitis;* fibroadenomas; and intraductal papillomas. The reactions of a woman who palpates a breast lump may be fear of cancer, denial of the possible significance of the lump, and anxiety. The diagnosis of benign breast disease involves evaluation to rule out cancer.

Clinical Manifestations

Fibrocystic disease usually first occurs at the median age of 30. A painful and tender mass decreases and increases in size in relation to the menstrual cycle, becoming larger and more painful as menses approaches. The mass is characteristically firm, mobile, and regular in shape and is usually found in the upper outer quadrant of the breast. Aspiration of the mass usually produces a gray-green fluid. The disease usually regresses after menopause as the ovarian hormones decrease.

Fibroadenomas are usually found in the younger client but may occur between the ages of 15 and 60. Fibroadenomas are usually painless and do not change in size in relation to the menstrual cycle. They are mobile, spherical, firm, and usually 2.0 to 2.5 cm in diameter when discovered.

Intraductal papilloma occurs most often in women between the ages of 35 and 45 years. The primary symptom is a serous or serosanguineous nipple discharge. There is usually no palpable mass.

Medical Measures

A mass reported to have cyclic changes is first followed over a menstrual cycle to verify those changes. The primary surgical measure used in fibrocystic disease is aspiration biopsy for diagnosis. The medical treatment of fibrocystic disease includes the promotion of a diet low in fat and substances with methylxanthine such as chocolate, coffee, tea, and cola products. The daily use of vitamin E (600 units) also may help decrease the symptoms.

Fibroadenomas are treated by surgical excision. Intraductal papillomas are surgically treated by excision of the involved duct by wedge resection.

Specific Nursing Measures

The nurse has an important role in providing the client with necessary support during the diagnostic procedures by explaining the procedures and their implications. The client diagnosed as having benign breast disease may still feel apprehensive about changes in her body image caused by scarring from the surgical procedure. She may worry about the effects of radiation exposure to her breasts in mammography. Provide the opportunity for the client to discuss her fears and concerns to aid adjustment.

Breast Cancer

About one out of every 10 women in the United States will develop breast cancer (American Cancer Society, 1987). As a woman ages, her risk of developing breast cancer increases. Breast cancer is most often found in women over the age of 50, but the incidence has increased in women aged 20 to 30. A personal history of breast cancer and a family history of the disease—especially if it occurs before menopause and is bilateral—increase the risk. Women who have never had children or delayed pregnancy until after the age of 30 are also at an increased risk. The onset of menses and menopause influence the risk of developing breast cancer: If menses occurs before the age of 14 and menopause occurs later than age 55, the risk of breast cancer development is higher. Some nutritional factors also have been linked to the development of breast cancer, including being overweight by more than 40% and consuming a diet high in fat.

Breast cancer usually develops in the epithelial breast tissue. The most common sites are the ducts (90%) and the lobules (5%), with the remaining 5% being other types, including Paget's disease of the nipple and inflammatory carcinoma (USDHHS, 1984). The epithelial cells undergo hyperplasia, which may or may not gradually progress to carcinoma in situ and then to invasive carcinoma. The most common type is invasive ductal carcinoma, which often spreads to the axillary nodes. About half the tumors develop in the upper outer quadrant of the breast.

Breast cancer can be detected by breast self-examination (BSE), mammography, thermography, ultrasonography, computerized tomography (CT), and magnetic resonance imaging (MRI). At this time, mammography is the most widely used method for detecting small tumors and distinguishing between benign and cancerous conditions. The most definitive method of diagnosis of cancer is biopsy of the tumor. The best hope for recovery from breast cancer lies in early treatment. The 5-year survival rate has risen to 90% (American Cancer Society, 1987).

Clinical Manifestations

The early clinical manifestations of breast cancer may be the appearance of a lump upon palpation, routine mammography screening, or other technique. Most excised breast lumps (70%) are benign (Sheehan, 1984).

A unilateral increase in breast size may signify a breast tumor. A change in the shape of the breast also can be a warning sign. The most important change in shape is dimpling of the skin, which can be from the retraction of a fibrous strand from an underlying tumor.

Nipple changes include retraction, ulceration, scaliness, or discharge. Any pain or tenderness of the nipple may also be a sign of breast disease. Blood-stained discharge from the nipple may be a sign of a duct papilloma.

Edema of the skin, which may be caused by lymphatic drainage failure, gives the breast a *peau d'orange* ("orange peel") appearance. Lesser degrees of edema may be palpable as an increase in the thickness of the skin. Other skin changes may include the appearance of prominent subcutaneous veins and, with advanced tumors, infiltration by direct extension of the tumor.

Pain is not a frequent symptom in cancer of the breast,

and severe pain is usually a symptom of inflammation. When cancer is present, the client usually perceives the pain as a pricking sensation. Clinical manifestations of the metastasis of breast cancer most often occur in the chest wall and lymph nodes. Advanced disease involves metastasis to the bone, lung, liver, and brain.

Medical Measures

The treatment of breast cancer is based on the recognition that breast cancer is not strictly a localized disease, but is instead a systemic one. Both localized and systemic treatments are used. The treatment for breast cancer depends on the stage of the disease among other factors. Today the decision about the type of treatment considers the woman's desire for preservation of the breast. Even when surgery is required to remove the breast, later reconstruction can provide a breast mound that enables the client to look normal in clothes and eliminates the need for a breast prosthesis.

Several radiotherapeutic techniques are used to treat breast disease. In the early stage of the disease, simple excision of the tumor and sampling of the axillary nodes are followed by a course of radiation therapy, the dose and length of treatment depending on the axillary node involvement. A "booster" dose of radiation may supplement the external radiation; this is accomplished by an implant of radioactive material or by an electron beam from a linear accelerator. Iridium is typically implanted in breast tissue. Small tubes are threaded through the breast tissue, usually under local anesthesia, and then filled with seeds of the radioactive material. The tubes are left in place for approximately 50 to 60 hours and deliver approximately 2000 rads to the surrounding tissue. Radiation therapy also can be used in the advanced stage of breast cancer, when metastasis has occurred. It then is often used with other methods of treatment, which are combined to decrease symptoms and provide remission of the disease.

The medical management of breast cancer also includes the use of hormonal therapy, chemotherapy, and immune system stimulants such as bacillus Calmette–Guerin (BCG) or Levamisole, used in combination. These methods are most often used in advanced breast disease, when surgery and radiation have been unable to destroy the cancer growths, but they also can be used to prevent metastasis, which may occur from a few months to 30 years later. The mean interval for recurrence is 3 years.

The goal of the various methods of hormonal therapy is to reduce the amount of estrogen produced in the body. This can also be accomplished surgically by oophorectomy or adrenalectomy. Adrenalectomy can be replaced by hypophysectomy or the use of aminoglutethimide to inhibit adrenal steroid synthesis (these procedures are discussed in Unit 7). The antiestrogen used is tamoxifen citrate to assess the level of effectiveness. Diethylstilbestrol is given to women with metastatic disease, who are postmenopausal for at least 5 years, to assess the level of effectiveness and then is continued until relapse occurs.

A universally effective chemotherapeutic regimen has not been demonstrated, so various drug combinations are used, depending on such factors as the stage of the disease, the client's age, and the type of tumor. The most common chemotherapeutic agents include cyclophosphamide, methotrexate, fluorouracil, and doxorubicin.

Specific Nursing Measures

Specific nursing measures are reviewed below for the various surgical diagnostic and therapeutic procedures for breast cancer, as well as for reconstructive surgery. Specific nursing measures related to chemotherapy and radiation therapy are reviewed in Chapter 10.

It is important to remember that the client may have many decisions to make after the diagnosis of breast cancer. Her coping mechanisms may be overwhelmed at this time, so she will need the nurse to provide support in the decision-making process and to explain alternative types of treatment. The nurse can anticipate questions clients have regarding the treatment process and provide information. It is also important to assess the support systems available to the client. The family or significant others will also need the support of the nurse during this critical time.

Breast Biopsy

The breast biopsy is performed by aspiration of the fluid or tissue from the tumor, incisional removal of a portion of the tumor, or excision of the whole tumor. Any breast mass should be evaluated for the possible diagnosis of cancer. Biopsy can differentiate whether a fibrocystic lesion is (1) a simple cyst or cysts caused by a change in the cells lining the ducts and the secretion of fluid or (2) a premalignant condition that is caused by hyperplasia of the cells. Biopsy also can identify fibroadenomas and intraductal papillomas. A histologic examination is performed on the discharge or fluid, and a biopsy is performed on the duct involved. If no mass is present with nipple discharge, as in mammary duct ectasia, diagnosis is made by histologic examination of the discharge. Client implications of breast biopsy are summarized in Table 49–16.

Nursing Implications

PREOPERATIVE CARE Preoperative instructions to the breast biopsy client vary according to the type of anesthesia used and the type of biopsy performed. Needle aspiration of a potential cyst is usually performed in a primary care setting, whereas excisional and incisional biopsy procedures may be performed in the hospital. Give instructions on dietary restrictions to the client undergoing general anesthesia. Tell all clients about arrival time,

Table 49–16
Breast Biopsy: Implications for the Client

Physiologic Implications	Psychosocial/Lifestyle Implications
Sensations of pulling or probing during the procedure	Anxiety and fear of cancer
Mild postoperative discomfort	Alterations in body image because of scar and absence of breast tissue
Breast usually continues to function if client is in her reproductive years	Need for emotional support
	Decisions about type of treatment if cancer is diagnosed
	Dietary changes: elimination of methylxanthine substances, increase in fiber, decrease in fats
	Monthly BSE

preoperative laboratory work, and the need for transportation postoperatively. Information about the sensations to expect during the biopsy is also important. Provide emotional support by listening to the client's fears and providing information on the procedure. Tell the client when the results of the histologic test will be available.

POSTOPERATIVE CARE Immediate postoperative nursing care includes assessment of the site for bleeding and monitoring of vital signs. Ice applied to the incisional area may decrease swelling. A supportive bra may provide comfort and should be worn at night. Mild analgesics may relieve incisional pain.

Provide emotional support for the client and significant others. Discharge teaching will include information on nutrition, incisional care, and scheduling of a return visit to the health care provider for removal of sutures if appropriate. Teach or review monthly BSE procedures.

Nursing Research Note

Scott D: Anxiety, critical thinking, and information processing during and after breast biopsy. *Nurs Res* 1983; 32(1):24–28.

Critical thinking ability, anxiety, and information processing were examined in a group of women 18 through 60 years of age undergoing breast biopsy for the purpose of diagnosing a carcinoma. The sample was tested during hospitalization and retested again 6 to 8 weeks after biopsy when results were known.

The findings suggest that critical thinking abilities are reduced during hospitalization compared with 6 to 8 weeks postbiopsy. Anxiety levels during hospitalization before a benign test result were extremely high. The anxiety was reduced 6 to 8 weeks after hospitalization. The anxiety level was correlated with difficulty in the reasoning process and decision-making abilities. Information processing was not significantly reduced in the hospitalized group, but information processing declined somewhat with high anxiety levels.

Because anxiety diminishes critical thinking abilities and impairs information processing, nurses must pay special attention to clients and monitor health teaching. These clients also need intense nursing support to cope with immediate stressors.

Mastectomy

A mastectomy, or removal of the breast, is the most common surgical procedure performed when a malignant tumor is found. The mastectomy procedure is controversial; many women are demanding more conservative and less destructive surgery for breast cancer, a move supported by many cancer authorities. The smaller the tumor in the absence of metastasis, the greater the survival rate and the number of alternatives for treatment. When the cancer involves the muscle or interpectoral node, more muscle and tissue must be removed.

In the United States, the standard surgical procedure for treatment of breast cancer has been the *modified radical mastectomy.* This aggressive procedure removes the involved breast tissue as well as the nipple and areola, surrounding skin, lymph nodes of the axillary region, and possibly the smaller pectoral muscle. The greater pectoral muscle is left intact. A *simple mastectomy,* or *total mastectomy,* involves removal of the breast only and is indicated for Paget's disease of the nipple and other localized cancers. Lymph nodes and the pectoral muscles are left intact. It is also used as a palliative measure when a large tumor has metastasized and may cause ulceration and draining.

In the *quadrantectomy,* the excision includes the entire quadrant of the breast containing the tumor, the fascia covering the greater pectoral muscle, and the entire smaller pectoral muscle. *Partial mastectomy* (also called segmental resection) involves an excision of the tumor and a 2- to 3-cm wedge of tissue surrounding it. A portion of the overlying skin and the underlying fascia are also excised. Both procedures usually include nodal dissection to determine the need for chemotherapy. *Lumpectomy* or tylectomy is similar to excisional biopsy, discussed earlier; it removes the tumor and the near surrounding tissue but leaves the skin and fascia intact. Axillary lymph nodes may or may not be removed through a separate incision. These procedures are illustrated in Figure 49–9.

The *Halsted radical mastectomy,* a more extensive and destructive surgical dissection, removes the breast, nipple and areola, axillary nodes, and both pectoral muscles. Variations of this procedure have also included removal of part of the rib cage to excise the internal mammary lymph nodes as well as removal of the supraclavicular lymph nodes. The

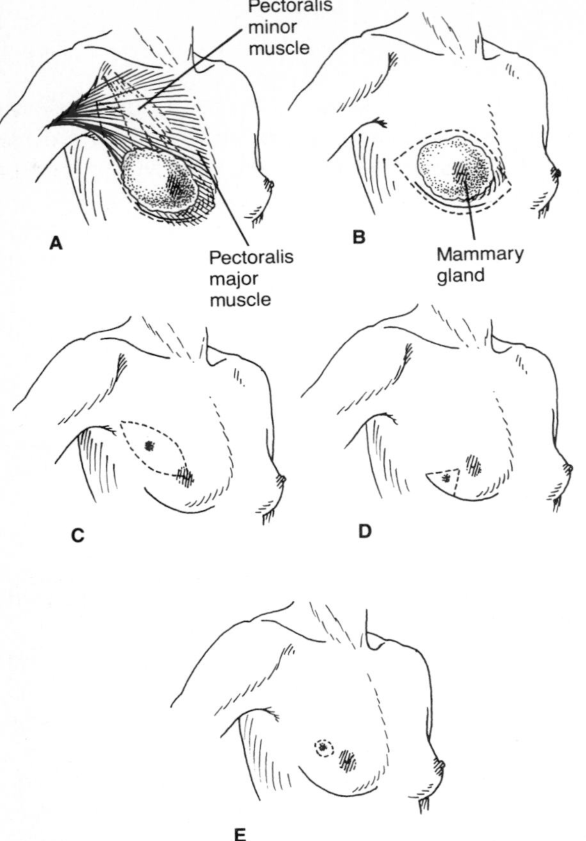

Figure 49–9

Mastectomy procedures. **A.** Modified radical mastectomy. **B.** Simple or total mastectomy. **C.** quadrantectomy. **D.** Partial mastectomy (segmental resection). **E.** Lumpectomy (tylectomy).

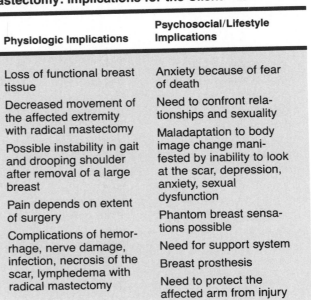

Table 49–17
Mastectomy: Implications for the Client

Physiologic Implications	Psychosocial/Lifestyle Implications
Loss of functional breast tissue	Anxiety because of fear of death
Decreased movement of the affected extremity with radical mastectomy	Need to confront relationships and sexuality
Possible instability in gait and drooping shoulder after removal of a large breast	Maladaptation to body image change manifested by inability to look at the scar, depression, anxiety, sexual dysfunction
Pain depends on extent of surgery	Phantom breast sensations possible
Complications of hemorrhage, nerve damage, infection, necrosis of the scar, lymphedema with radical mastectomy	Need for support system
	Breast prosthesis
	Need to protect the affected arm from injury

Halsted procedure is rarely used today. Client implications of mastectomy are summarized in Table 49–17.

Nursing Implications

PREOPERATIVE CARE The nurse is in a position to offer both instruction and emotional support before the mastectomy. Preoperative teaching includes the need for deep-breathing exercises because of a restrictive dressing that may decrease chest expansion. Emphasize the need to move the affected extremity after surgery to increase circulation, decrease edema, and reduce arm and shoulder stiffness and numbness. Explain that a suction apparatus will be placed in the wound, discuss its purpose, and inform the client that removal can be anticipated about 3 days after a modified radical mastectomy.

POSTOPERATIVE CARE

EMOTIONAL SUPPORT Emotional support by the nurse and other members of the health care team is of paramount importance in the postoperative period. The nurse can describe the incision to the client who cannot initially look at it, share the experience of looking at the incision with her, and let her express her fears concerning her body image changes. The services of an American Cancer Society Reach to Recovery volunteer, a woman who has had a mastectomy, also can assist the client in adjusting to her surgery and her new body image. In this program, knowledgeable and well-adjusted breast cancer clients visit new clients to demonstrate how they are coping with their illness and the effects of their surgery. Emotional support and an exercise program are offered by the ENCORE program of the YWCA. Clients participate in floor and swimming pool exercise sessions and group discussions. Both programs are in the resources list in Chapter 48.

The client should be consulted about her involvement in physical care and treatment to reduce her feelings of vulnerability. Help the client identify support systems and discuss her usual coping mechanisms.

Both the client and her partner can view the wound postoperatively if they wish. Affection can be encouraged by hand-holding and touch. Concerns about returning to sexual relations should be discussed before the client is discharged. Discussing potential sexual problems or the partner's response to the woman's loss of her breast may be difficult for the client. During hospitalization, she may be more concerned initially about physical care. Clients' feelings about their disease and its treatment are not easily resolved, and it may take months to years for them to work out their feelings. During this period, the woman may avoid sexual intimacy because she fears her partner's reaction to her changed body.

The partner may also experience a wide range of emotions, such as fear that sexual overtures will be rebuffed or that lovemaking that included the breast may have somehow caused the cancer. The partner may fear that facial expressions may betray his or her difficulty in coping with the client's changed appearance. Although some partners may be physically repelled by a missing or disfigured breast, most adjust quickly. A partner's facial expression of concern, sadness, or anxiety may stem from distress about what the surgical procedure represents—a threat to life. When the client interprets such facial expressions as rejection, her worst fears may be validated. Box 49–3 has guidelines for initiating a discussion on sexuality with a client and her partner.

PHYSICAL CARE Pain is controlled by analgesics, depending on the severity of the surgical procedure and the client's pain tolerance. The client can also be made more comfortable with proper positioning. Check the dressing and the bedclothes beneath the client for bleeding. Also check the affected arm for warmth, color, edema, and feeling. Care of the suction catheter includes accurate measurement of output, the possible application of povidone–iodine (Betadine) ointment around the site, and daily sterile dressing changes. Assist the client out of bed on the day following surgery if not before. Diet can be as tolerated.

EXERCISE INSTRUCTION The client should begin exercising the extremity immediately after surgery with encouragement to move the fingers. Range-of-motion (ROM) exercises are crucial to maintain joint mobility, maintain circulation, and reduce edema. Mobility is essential in resuming everyday activities, such as fastening a bra, pulling up a zipper, grooming, cooking, and engaging in sports. Assisted ROM exercises for the involved shoulder may be started as soon as the client returns to her room. Exercise is progressive and follows a routine format: sets of ten performed three times daily. Clients who have had a modified radical mastectomy should be encouraged to undertake self-care activities by the next day; these include washing the face and upper body, applying cosmetics, and combing or brushing their hair using the involved arm.

Some clients, especially those who have had a Halsted radical mastectomy, may be unable to lift the involved arm without assistance. Help the client lift her arm rather than taking over self-care activities for her. When the client is able to lift the involved arm without help, she is ready for a more complex exercise such as that illustrated in Figure 49–10.

Assistive devices will also help maintain joint flexibility and can be adapted for home use during the later recovery period. They include using a rope end pulley, "climbing a wall," and pulling down on a rope held behind the back (Figure 49–11).

The client should perform more exercises as she can tolerate them. In planning exercises, consider the amount of discomfort the client experiences. Usually, the more muscles that are cut and the more tissue removed, the greater the discomfort. Clients are often apprehensive and worry that exercises may delay healing or disrupt the sutures. Explaining the purposes of the exercises, the resilience of the body, and the strength of the sutures, as well as assuring the client that she will not be required to perform exercises beyond her level of tolerance, will all help reduce the client's apprehension.

PREVENTION OF INFECTION AND LYMPHEDEMA Removal of the axillary nodes and lymphatic channels predisposes the client to infection and lymphatic obstruction. To prevent these complications, it is important not to take the blood pressure and blood samples on the involved side.

Box 49–3
Guidelines for Initiating a Discussion on Sexuality

Be comfortable with the topic of sexuality. The client and her partner should not be embarrassed or slighted because their needs surpass the nurse's limits. A nurse who feels uncomfortable in helping a couple with sexual concerns is responsible for consulting another health care professional who feels comfortable in this area.

Designate one nurse on a unit to discuss the feelings, beliefs, and attitudes pertaining to breast cancer, the surgery, and sexuality with a given client and her partner. In this way, the psychosexual aspects of the woman's care are included in the care plan, but the client and her partner will not be bombarded with a host of well-intentioned nurses.

Arrange for the discussion to take place in a relaxed and quiet area.

Include the client's partner in the discussion. Other family members may be included if the client desires or it is seen by the nurse to be of therapeutic value.

Initiate the discussion by starting with less threatening items, such as instructions on breast forms or range-of-motion exercises. Essentially, the more physical or external topics provide a basis for delving into the emotional aspects of the surgery.

Exhibit a caring, supportive, nonjudgmental attitude throughout the discussion. Any signs of disgust or horror will only lower the client's opinion of herself.

Be certain that the words used in discussion are not only familiar but also are interpreted similarly by all involved.

Keep in mind the client's cultural and religious beliefs as well as the effects of other medicines and/or illnesses upon her level of sexual functioning.

Do not force the client and her partner to divulge their concerns about sexuality. However, they need to know that a concerned individual is there to listen and guide them when they are ready.

Do not overwhelm or rush the couple during the discussion period. Instead, it is important that the nurse keep pace with the needs and interests of the couple.

Do not assume that all breast cancer clients have or want a sexual partner or that the sexual partner is male.

SOURCE: Adapted from *The Breast Cancer Digest.* US Department of Health and Human Services, NIH Publication No. 84–1691. Bethesda, MD: National Cancer Institute, 1984, p. 149.

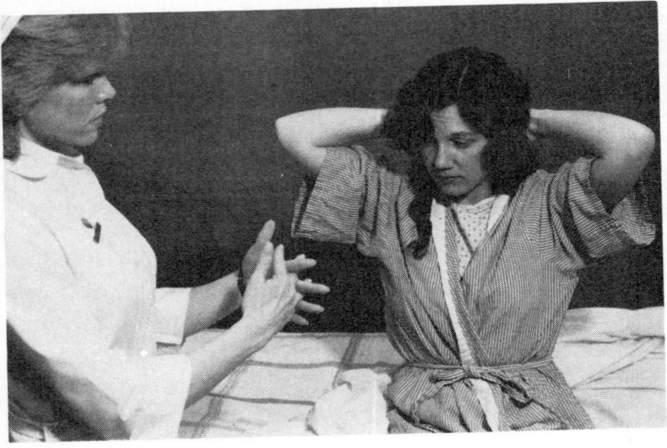

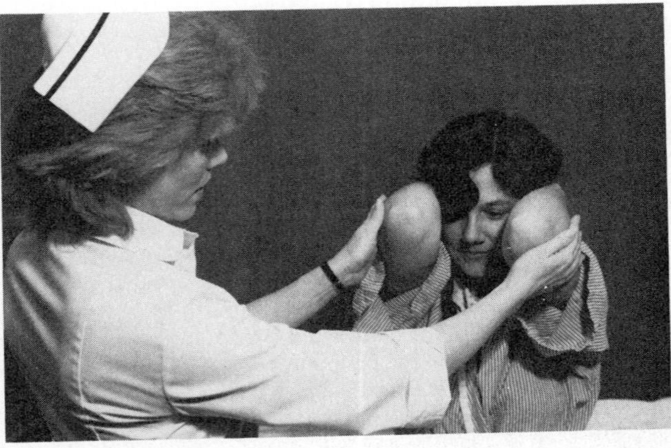

Figure 49–10

Exercise after mastectomy. **Top.** When the client is able to lift her involved arm actively without assistance, instruct her to clasp her hands behind her head (as shown). **Bottom.** She should then attempt to touch her elbows together, or to bring them as close together as possible. This movement will flex, externally rotate, and adduct the involved shoulder. SOURCE: *Swearingen PL:* Photo-Atlas of Nursing Procedures. *Menlo Park, CA: Addison–Wesley, 1984.*

Medications should not be injected into the affected arm. Heavy objects, including purses, should not be carried on the affected side. Instruct the client to use a protective glove when doing chores, avoiding injuries and exposure to strong detergents and chemicals. Any breaks in the skin should be promptly treated. The client should apply lanolin-based hand cream daily or more often if necessary. Instruct the client to report pain, redness, increased swelling, or hardness to her health care provider.

A collateral lymphatic drainage system usually develops within 3 or 4 weeks postoperatively. In the interim, elevating the involved arm so the elbow is higher than the shoulder and the hand is higher than the elbow helps prevent or reduce edema. Massaging the arm from the hand toward the shoulder is another useful technique. Women who exercise, elevate, and massage the involved arm for at least 3 months after surgery are less likely to have severe lymphedema. Severe lymphedema that occurs many months, or sometimes even years, after surgery should always be promptly assessed for infection and related treatment if appropriate. The client may wear a supportive elastic sleeve similar to an antiembolic stocking to reduce lymphedema. This should be applied in the morning before the client sits or stands. Lymphedema is much less frequent after modified radical mastectomies than after Halsted radical mastectomies.

BREAST PROSTHESES Most women who have had a mastectomy are concerned about restoring their normal appearance as soon as possible. A temporary breast prosthesis is usually provided by a Reach to Recovery volunteer before the client is discharged from the hospital. This lightweight, soft prosthesis is used while the incisional area is healing and until tenderness and edema dissipate in about 6 weeks. By that time, most clients are ready to be fitted for a more natural-looking prosthesis.

Commercial breast forms are available in a wide variety of sizes and shapes and are sold in most large department stores (where specially trained fitters help the client select an appropriate prosthesis), surgical supply stores, and some pharmacies, or by mail order. Like natural breasts, the weight and consistency of prostheses vary; they may be filled with foam rubber, chemical gel, water, ceramic particles, or silicone gel. Silicone prostheses are the heaviest and most expensive (from $100 to $200). Their advantage is that their weight provides better balance and reduces problems such as muscle strain caused by asymmetry. Some forms are available with a modified nipple; nipple prostheses can be purchased to augment prostheses without nipples or can be used by women who have had reconstructive surgery that did not replace the nipple. In some locations, it is possible to purchase a custom-designed prosthesis made from a mold of the breast before surgery; these cost about $400.

Reach to Recovery volunteers and fitters in department stores can often recommend bras that fit comfortably and can be adapted to suit each woman's individual needs. Specially designed clothing is also available in department stores and by mail order.

Insurance companies may fully or partially reimburse clients for prostheses and specially designed or altered bras. This information is usually supplied by Reach to Recovery volunteers or is available through the American Cancer Society. In many instances, clients will need a physician's prescription and receipts to take the medical deduction from federal income tax.

BREAST RECONSTRUCTION Breast reconstruction does not fully restore the normal appearance of the breast but creates a breast mound, which helps the woman look normal in clothes and eliminates dependence on a prosthesis.

Figure 49–11

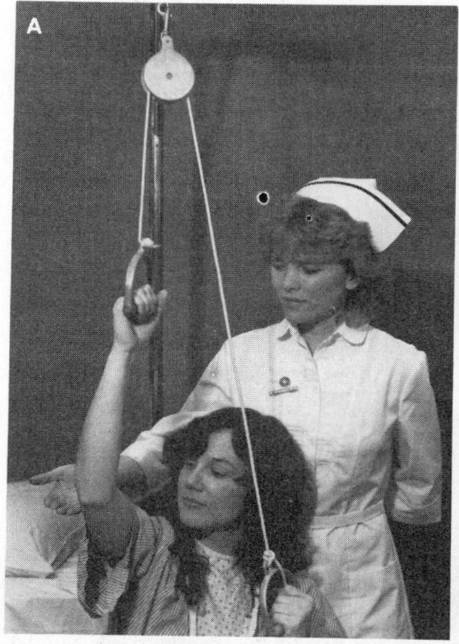

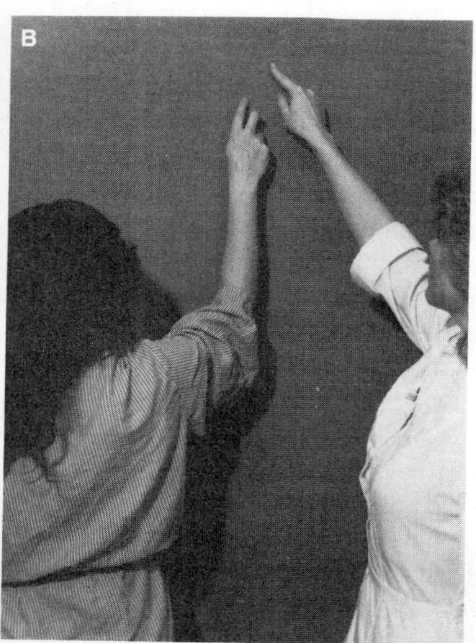

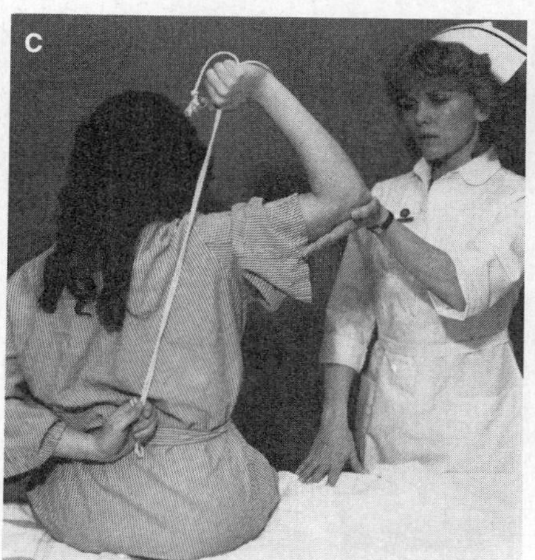

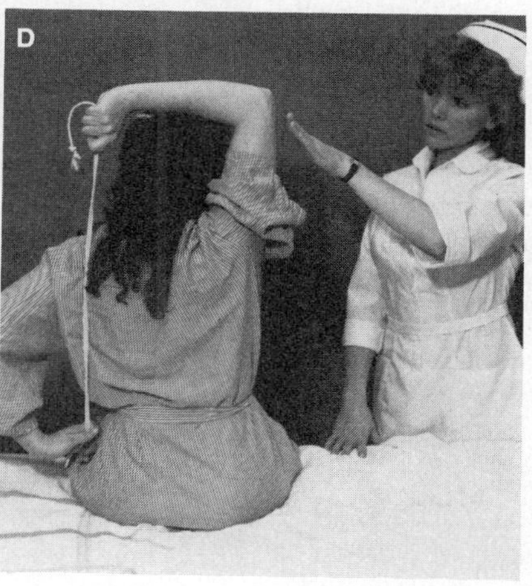

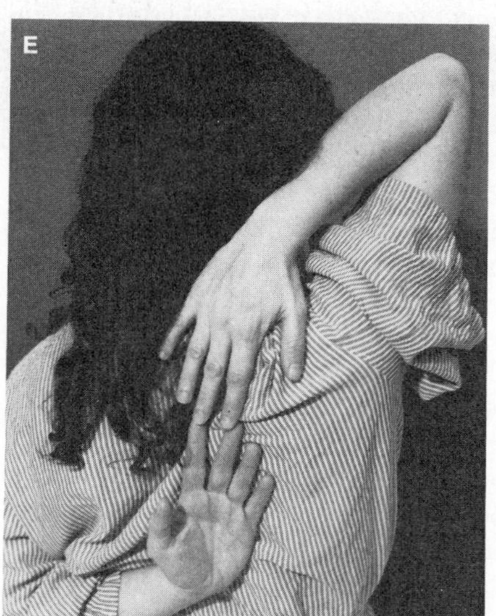

A. The client can also use assistive devices to achieve shoulder flexion. With physician approval, assemble a rope and pulley system onto an overhead trapeze bar. The client should grasp the hand grips and begin the exercise with the involved arm in the lower position. Instruct her to pull down gently with the hand of the uninvolved arm, allowing the involved arm to be raised gradually (as shown). Explain to the client that some discomfort and a sensation of stretching the incision is normal, but that to achieve maximum shoulder range, she should flex the shoulder as much as possible. *Note: The client may adapt this exercise at home by placing a rope over a stable shower curtain rod or over a wall hook.* **B.** Teach the client how to "climb a wall," which will promote shoulder flexion without the use of an assistive device. The client should face the wall and position her involved arm at shoulder level. Gradually, she will scale the wall by "walking" her fingertips upward (as shown). Encourage her to achieve maximum shoulder ROM. *Note: Place a tape marker on the wall to indicate her progress after each exercise. This will give her a goal to strive for with each new attempt.* **C.** Around the second postoperative week, usually after the sutures have been removed, the client can begin exercises that will maximize external rotation and abduction of the shoulder. A 75-cm (30-in.) rope can be used to assist the client in achieving maximum range. Instruct her to grasp the rope, holding the lower end in her uninvolved hand in the back at the level of her waistline. The top of the rope should be held in the hand of her involved arm at about the level of her head. **D.** She should very gently pull down on the rope with the hand of her uninvolved arm, guiding the involved arm through abduction and external rotation. This exercise should be performed at least three times daily in sets of ten each. **E.** Just prior to discharge, show the client how to achieve maximum shoulder flexion by touching her fingertips behind her back with the involved arm uppermost. This exercise simulates the range required for zipping back zippers and fastening brassieres. *SOURCE: Swearingen PL:* Photo-Atlas of Nursing Procedures. *Menlo Park, CA: Addison–Wesley, 1984.*

There is no medical need to replace the lost breast; however, for many women, the psychologic benefit of a restored self-image is sufficient justification for undergoing the procedure. Reconstruction requires further consideration or might be contraindicated where the client needs extensive skin grafting or extensive irradiation or when the client has unrealistic expectations for the reconstructed breast.

Breast reconstruction surgery is performed either after the mastectomy has healed, which takes a minimum of 3 months, or at the same time as the mastectomy. Immediate reconstruction may have poorer cosmetic results because of the effects of radiation therapy or chemotherapy, and it increases the risk of complications such as fibrous capsular contracture.

The breast reconstruction procedure depends on the type of mastectomy and the type of deformity. When the muscle is not damaged, the reconstruction can be accomplished by the placement of a silicone gel implant beneath the pectoral and serratus muscles. Another type of simple breast reconstruction is accomplished by using an expander implant with a built-in filler port that allows it to be injected with sterile normal saline. The injections are repeated several days to a week apart until the implant has expanded beyond the desired size. Overstretching the skin and muscle by overfilling the expander implant creates a more normal drape, with a more natural appearance, over the smaller implant. After the implant has been in place for several weeks or months, it is replaced with a permanent silicone gel implant of appropriate size. Figure 49–12 shows the good results that are possible with this procedure.

When soft tissue, muscle, and skin are inadequate for placement of an implant alone, reconstruction using grafts from the rectus abdominis muscle, or the latissimus dorsi muscle, abdominal tissue, and skin is possible. (Skin grafting and tissue transfer are discussed in Chapter 55.)

If the client wants a nipple on the reconstructed breast, it can be created, once the desired contour has been attained, from the opposite nipple, inner thigh, buttock, or labia majora or minora.

The most common postoperative problem is fibrous capsular contracture, the formation of a fibrous capsule around the implant; this contracts, makes the breast round and hard, and may displace it upward. To decrease the risk of fibrous capsular contraction, the client should perform breast massage as illustrated and described in Figure 49–13. This also keeps the implant mobile and stretches the surrounding tissue to help achieve a more natural appearance; this, in turn, positively affects the client's self-image.

Breast Augmentation and Reduction Mammoplasty

Breast augmentation mammoplasty is the surgical method of increasing the breast size. The client requests the surgery to improve her body image. Breast augmentation also may be used as a reconstructive procedure after mastectomy.

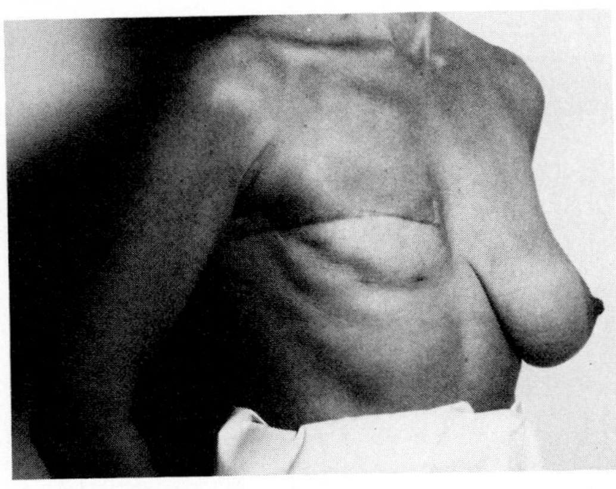

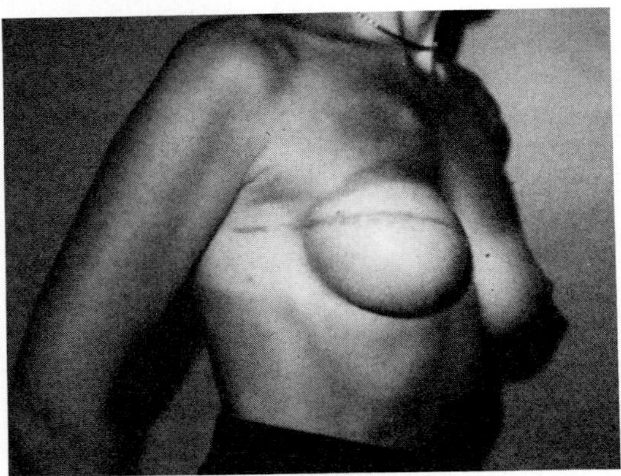

Figure 49–12

Pre- and postoperative views of a client who underwent breast reconstruction with an expander implant on the right. A later breast reduction on the left brought the breasts into better symmetry. SOURCE: Woods JE: *Current state of the art in breast reconstruction.* Plast Surg Nurs *1984; 4:86.*

Breast reduction mammoplasty is performed when the breasts have hypertrophied, are very large, or are asymmetrical. Large breasts may cause back pain and shoulder discomfort from bra straps. Both breast augmentation and reduction give women important opportunities to make choices about their bodies.

In the breast augmentation procedure, the surgeon makes an inframammary or periareolar incision, and places a silicone sac (usually filled with either silicone gel or saline solution) in a subpectoral or subcutaneous submuscular pocket.

The reduction procedure is more involved. Excess tissue and skin are removed, and the nipple is transplanted to its proper position on the reconstructed breast. Physiologic and psychosocial/lifestyle implications for the client after breast reduction and augmentation are summarized in Table 49–18.

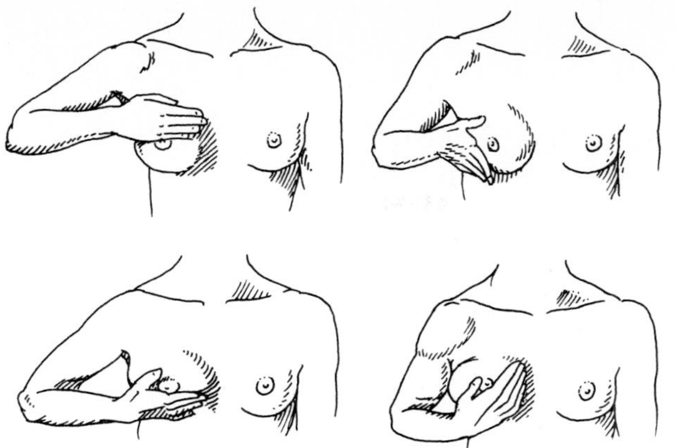

Figure 49–13

Postoperative breast massage technique to help the breast soften and become more natural in contour. Gently press the breast with the palm of the hand on each side for a count of five. Move from superior to lateral, to inferior, and to medial aspects, and repeat the sequence five times. Perform the exercise at least three times daily or more often as directed for 3 to 6 months postoperatively.

Nursing Implications

PREOPERATIVE CARE The nurse should support the client's decision for breast size change and be available to discuss possible guilt and anxiety over the procedure. Preoperative teaching should include techniques of manual breast massage.

POSTOPERATIVE CARE Manual massage should be performed to prevent fibrous capsular contracture. If fibrous capsular contracture occurs, it is treated by the plastic surgeon with manual rupture or surgery to release the fibrotic tissue. Discharge teaching involves wound care, signs of infection, and the techniques and importance of monthly BSE.

Table 49–18
Breast Augmentation and Reduction Mammoplasty: Implications for the Client

Physiologic Implications	Psychosocial/Lifestyle Implications
Possible fibrous capsular contracture after breast augmentation	Positive body image change
Complications of hematoma, infection, hypertrophy of the scar	Satisfaction with procedure influenced by expectations
Possibility of silicone seepage into the body with breast augmentation	Improved social interaction
Relief of backache and shoulder discomfort after breast reduction (no excess weight of large breasts)	Monthly BSE
Loss of breast function after breast reduction	Need to wear a support bra by day and an Ace bandage at night for about the first 2 weeks after breast augmentation
Pain for 7–10 days	

Benign Prostatic Hyperplasia

Benign prostatic hyperplasia (BPH) is caused by an increased production of prostatic cells (Figure 49–14). The term *hypertrophy*—an increase in the size of the cells—is commonly misapplied to BPH. The prostate gland increases in size because the number of prostatic cells (not their size) increases. BPH is the most common neoplastic growth in men; at least 50% of men over age 50 have some degree of hyperplasia. The progressive increase in size of the prostate gland can obstruct urine flow and lead to urinary tract infections, hydronephrosis, and the eventual destruction of renal parenchyma. Exactly why prostatic hyperplasia occurs is not known. It may be related to aging or an unexplained hormonal mechanism.

Clinical Manifestations

Early in BPH, the increasing obstruction causes compensatory hypertrophy of the detrusor muscle of the bladder wall (see Figure 49–14) to overcome urethral resistance. The symptoms at this point may depend on the compensatory ability of the bladder, but ultimately diver-

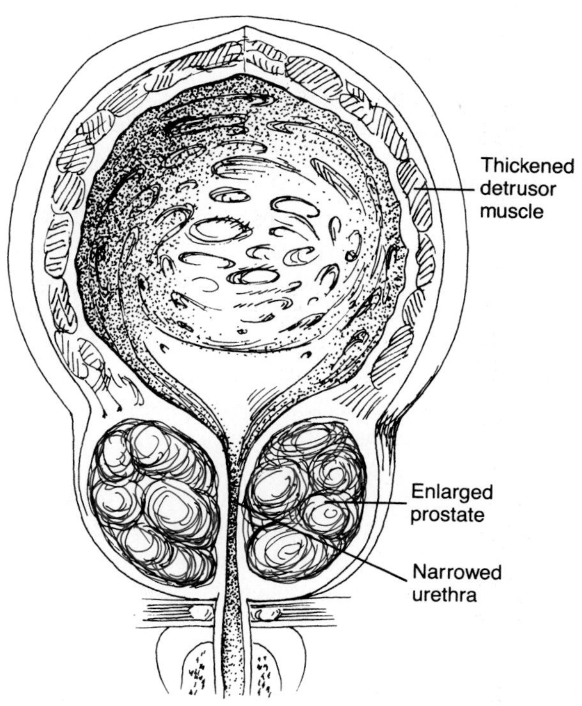

Figure 49–14

Benign prostatic hyperplasia.

Nursing Research Note

Scott DW, Oberst MT, Bookbinder MI: Stress-coping response to genitourinary carcinoma in men. *Nurs Res* 1984; 33(6):325–329.

Stress responses were studied in males undergoing periodic evaluation of genitourinary carcinoma. All subjects had previously been diagnosed as having a noninvasive chronic bladder cancer.

The results demonstrated that anxiety levels of the subjects were within normal range for a general outpatient population and lower than in most medical–surgical clients. It was also determined that as anxiety levels increased, critical thinking abilities declined. Additional stressors and other unresolved problems were found to increase anxiety levels in this sample. Subjects exhibiting higher anxiety levels had lower educational levels, lower critical thinking skills, and were unable to resolve major problems. This group with higher anxiety levels exhibited greater behavioral responses, such as depression and helplessness.

This research suggests that assisting clients to cope effectively with life stressors is an important nursing responsibility. Coping skills can be enhanced through client education, active involvement of both family and client, adequate preparation for discharge, and follow-up.

ticula may form in the bladder wall and lead to residual urinary stasis and urinary tract infection. Later, when the bladder can no longer undergo hypertrophy, signs of decompensation include acute urinary retention, bilateral hydroureter and hydronephrosis, and infection because of urinary stasis. Typical symptoms of BPH include hesitancy, frequency, nocturia, urgency, decreased urinary stream, and difficulty starting the stream. Sexual function, sexual frequency, and quality of erection may decline.

Medical Measures

A drug history is first obtained. Any of the following drugs can cause urinary symptoms: parasympatholytics, bronchodilators, antispasmodics, antihistamines, muscle relaxants, tranquilizers, and ganglionic blocking agents. Discontinuing the drug may correct the problem. An infection must be treated before any manipulative procedure such as cystoscopy is performed because these procedures carry a high risk of sepsis.

The client with acute urinary retention has a small Foley catheter inserted to relieve pain, prevent the loss of bladder tone from distention, and prevent further hydronephrosis. Usually, once careful, controlled decompression has been performed, the client is treated surgically by prostatectomy. The client who is not a good surgical candidate will have a small in-dwelling catheter that remains in place. The urine is usually kept acidic to decrease the chance of infection by giving methenamine mandelate (Mandelamine) or vitamin C. Antibiotics are administered only if the client develops epdidymitis. Complications of long-term catheterization include stricture, recurring epididymitis, and periurethral abscess. If these occur, a suprapubic catheter is indicated.

Specific Nursing Measures

Nursing interventions for BPH clients include keeping the client well informed and preparing him for catheterization and surgery. Maintain continuous catheter drainage and perform catheter care every shift using aseptic technique. For further interventions, see Chapter 25 for catheter care and below for care after prostatectomy.

Cancer of the Prostate

Cancer of the prostate ties with lung cancer as the most common cancer in the US male population and the third leading cause of cancer deaths in men (American Cancer Society, 1987). It represents a significant health problem for men over 50, and its incidence peaks at age 70. Although its cause is not known, a familial tendency suggests the possibility of a genetic basis. The incidence is higher in blacks than whites and in clients who have received androgenic hormones. It is hypothesized that prostatic cancer is caused by hormonal changes, but neither the exact cause nor the relationship between host and tumor factors is clear. Dietary fat may be a factor.

Clinical Manifestations

The early clinical manifestations of prostatic cancer are similar to those of BPH, including obstructive urinary symptoms and blood in the ejaculate. The obstruction may progress more rapidly than with BPH.

Metastasis is common in prostatic cancer, and the diagnosis is often not made until this stage. Metastatic symptoms include bone pain, low back pain radiating down the legs, weight loss, and anemia. The major site of metastasis is the bone, and other common sites include the lung, liver, and lymph nodes. With metastasis, serum acid phosphatase levels are elevated. Hematuria is a late symptom.

Rectal palpation of the prostate is recommended yearly for all men over 40 years old because this screening examination may detect the tumor in its early stages. A hard, fixed nodule may be palpated in later stages. Cystoscopy, intravenous pyelography, ultrasonography, and computerized tomography (CT) scans also may be performed as part of the diagnostic work-up. Regional lymph nodes are not usually symptomatic. Peripheral edema may occur with massive pelvic lymph node involvement.

Medical Measures

Early prostatic cancer may be treated either by surgery or radiation therapy. Advanced disease is usually treated with a radical prostatectomy, possible lymph node dissection, and supplemental external beam radiation. Some physicians treat more advanced stages with interstitial radiation therapy using implants of radioactive iodine (^{125}I), radioactive gold (^{198}Au), and radioactive iridium (^{192}Ir). These implants are usually performed in conjunction with pelvic lymphadenectomy.

A palliative approach is taken with metastatic disease. Treatment usually includes estrogen therapy, bilateral orchiectomy, or both. In most clients, the initial response to estrogen therapy is dramatic, with a disappearance of bony metastasis and bone pain as well as a shrinkage of the prostate. Hormonal failures are usually treated with chemotherapeutic agents. Fluorouracil, cyclophosphamide, cisplatin, doxorubicin, and mitomycin-C alone or in combination are administered to clients with metastatic prostatic cancer.

Specific Nursing Measures

Early detection of prostatic cancer improves the prognosis, so the nurse should teach men over age 40 to have yearly checkups that include rectal examination. Furthermore, because there is a significant correlation between gonococcal infection and later prostatic cancer, the prevention and prompt treatment of gonorrhea may help decrease the incidence of prostatic cancer.

The client with prostatic cancer feels anxious and fearful, and his body image is threatened. Not only does the client view the diagnosis of cancer as life threatening, the location in this case includes a threat to his sexual potency and overall masculinity. All nursing interactions stem from the client's need for clear, accurate information about his condition and for emotional support as he works through this massive disruption in his life.

External radiation therapy usually decreases the obstructive symptoms and increases client comfort. Proctitis, diarrhea, and urinary frequency can result, however. The client who undergoes radiation therapy in the genital area faces possible temporary or permanent sterility or impotence. Approximatley 30% of these clients have problems with impotence, so for most it is realistic to believe that potency can be maintained. Chromosomal damage is also a risk. The client needs clear information about these risks as well as a good deal of emotional support as he faces these significant life changes. If the client is concerned about fertility, his sperm may be placed in a sperm bank before radiation therapy is begun.

The client receiving antiandrogen therapy (estrogen or orchiectomy) should be informed about the side effects of this therapy, including a decreased libido and impotence; feminization, including tender gynecomastia; and edema of the ankles. Teach the client to reduce his salt intake to help control the edema. Furosemide (Lasix) also may be prescribed.

These clients have an increased incidence of thromboembolism and of death from this complication. Attempt to prevent this through the use of antiembolic stockings, ambulation, and ankle pushes when in bed. Because the client may be debilitated and in great pain, mobility may be difficult to maintain.

Transurethral Resection

The transurethral resection (TUR) of the prostate, or transurethral prostatectomy (TURP), is by far the most common type of prostatic surgery. Between 85% and 95% of clients needing prostatectomies are treated with TUR, which involves removal of the prostate gland via the urethra (Figure 49–15). The major indication for performing a TUR is obstructive benign prostatic hyperplasia that no longer can be managed medically. This approach requires no surgical incision, which makes it particularly useful for the elderly client needing relief of obstructive symptoms, such as from malignant prostatic nodules. Very small cancerous lesions also can be removed transurethrally. The procedure is contraindicated for clients with hip joint problems because it requires a lithotomy position. One major disadvantage of the TUR is that prostatic tissue remains, so hyperplasia can occur again.

The physiologic and psychosocial/lifestyle implications of clients undergoing TUR are similar to those for clients undergoing other prostatectomy approaches. An overview of all client implications, with an emphasis on TUR, is in Table 49–19.

Nursing Implications

PREOPERATIVE CARE Clients facing any type of prostatectomy have many concerns that the nurse should

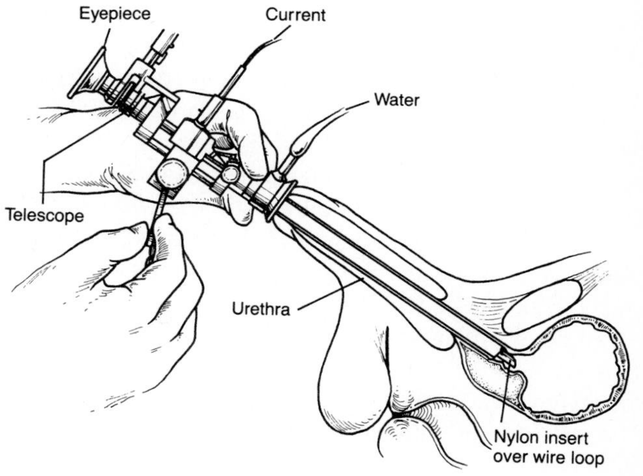

Figure 49–15

Transurethral prostatectomy. The telescope and lamp assist the surgeon in locating and resecting the prostatic tissue. A rotating wire loop at the end of the resectoscope connected to a cutting current shaves off the enlarged prostatic tissue, which is then flushed away.

Table 49–19
Prostatectomy: Implications for the Client 

Physiologic Implications	Psychosocial/Lifestyle Implications
Retrograde ejaculation (backflow of ejaculate into the bladder)	Impaired relationship as a result of impotence
Urinary incontinence (usually temporary)	Social isolation as a result of incontinence
Postoperative hemorrhage and clot formation	Infertility secondary to retrograde ejaculation
Atelectasis, pulmonary embolism, and other respiratory complications	No strenuous activity or heavy lifting for 6 weeks; avoid all driving and riding on bumpy roads
Postoperative deep vein thrombosis, especially if exaggerated lithotomy position required	No intercourse for 4 to 6 weeks
Urinary tract infection	Body image and self-esteem changes with altered sexual functioning
Bladder spasms	Maintain daily fluid intake of 2–3 L
Urethral stricture	Take stool softeners if necessary to avoid straining that occurs with constipation
Electrolyte system imbalances (especially hyponatremia)	
Risk of impotence, especially with perineal prostatectomy	
Scrotal and leg lymphedema after radical prostatectomy	
Urinary and fecal incontinence from sphincter damage during perineal prostatectomy	

address. Clark and O'Connell (1984) list clients' major concerns as: Will I be impotent? Will I be less masculine? Will I be sterile? Will I be able to go back to work? Will I lose control of urination?

Providing full information to the preoperative client facing a prostatectomy is a critically important nursing function, not only because the client needs accurate information to help allay his fears but also because the client has a right to this information. Explain, for example, any activity limitations the client will face postoperatively. Besides giving information, provide the opportunity for the client to verbalize his concerns so his preoperative anxiety can be kept at a manageable level. For example, fears of cancer are common and not unrealistic.

Standard preoperative preparation includes a general preoperative work-up, blood typing and cross-matching, renal function tests (BUN and serum creatinine tests), an intravenous pyelogram, voiding cystograms, and cystometric evaluation. The client with a urinary tract infection should have a culture and sensitivity study done, and specific antibiotic therapy should be started before surgery. Surgery is delayed until the urinary tract infection is under control. Some surgeons administer antibiotics prophylactically, although this use of broad-spectrum antibiotics is controversial. If the client has a urinary catheter in place preoperatively, strict aseptic technique is essential. The maintenance of catheter drainage is an important aspect of nursing care.

A client facing a prostatectomy should come to surgery well hydrated, so encourage drinking of fluids and monitor the client being hydrated with preoperative IV fluids. Because prostatic surgery is usually performed on elderly clients, overhydration must be avoided.

Preoperative preparation also should include a careful history to check for any prior respiratory or vascular problems that may contribute to postoperative complications. Clients should be informed about what tubes and drains to expect postoperatively. After a TUR, a client will have a two- or three-way Foley catheter with a 30 mL balloon in place. He also may have continuous bladder irrigation. Tell the client that this may cause him to feel the urge to void, but caution him that bearing down as if to void will contribute to bladder spasms. Bladder spasms will be relieved with antispasmodics.

Elastic bandages are usually placed on the legs preoperatively and are also used intraoperatively and postoperatively. Anticipate the need for antiembolic stockings and take calf measurements preoperatively so stockings will be available as soon as possible postoperatively.

POSTOPERATIVE CARE The usual nursing care given any client after surgery also applies to the postprostatectomy client. Take vital signs every 15 minutes until they are stable, then progress to every hour and then every 4 hours. Intake and output, level of mobility, and consciousness also should be assessed. Monitor electrolyte, BUN, and creatinine levels.

Generally, ambulation and hourly deep breathing and

coughing are performed on the first postoperative day. Frequent turning, toe wiggling, and gentle leg exercises should be done with assistance the night after surgery. Fluids are administered intravenously until the first postoperative day, and the client may take fluids orally the night of surgery. Thereafter, the client may take a diet as tolerated.

Fluid intake of 2 to 3 L/day should be encouraged while the urinary catheter is in place, usually 2 to 5 days after a TUR. If the client has continuous bladder irrigation, carefully record intake and output, making sure to account for the irrigating fluid. If the urine is bloody, the catheter stays in longer, and the rate of irrigating fluid should be increased. Restraints may be required because clients confused after surgery may try to get out of bed and pull out their catheters. If clots form in the single-lumen catheter, manual irrigation may be required to remove them.

Venous bleeding is common in the initial postoperative period. The surgeon usually applies traction by pulling the retention catheter so that the 30 mL balloon lodges against the bladder neck, applying pressure on the bleeding prostatic fossa.

The 30 mL balloon and traction used after a prostatectomy contribute to the postoperative problem of painful bladder spasms. These spasms are made worse if clotting obstructs the catheter or the client attempts to void around the catheter. The spasms can be recognized by the client's subjective sensation of pain, by palpation of the contracted bladder, and leakage of urine around the catheter. Instruct the client not to attempt to void around the catheter even though he may feel an intense urge to do so. Explain that this urge is caused by the feeling of fullness created by the large balloon and the traction. Maintaining catheter patency will reduce the frequency of spasms. Belladonna and opium (B and O) suppositories or other antispasmodics are used to relieve spasms.

The risk of infection increases when an in-dwelling catheter is present. Forcing fluids to prevent stasis of urine is one means to help prevent infection. Strict asepsis and maintaining a closed drainage system are also important. Report any signs of urinary tract infection, such as fever; cloudy, foul-smelling urine; or mucous shreds in the urine. The high risk of infection after prostatectomy usually necessitates the administration of prophylactic antibiotics.

If delayed bleeding occurs after the catheter has been removed, the catheter is reinserted, the clots are flushed out, traction is reinstituted, and diuresis is instituted. The clues that indicate that clots are forming are an urgent feeling of the need to void and leakage of urine around the catheter. Clients are usually given stool softeners to prevent straining at stool, which may cause bleeding.

The client may experience urinary incontinence for a few days after catheter removal. Teach the client to do exercises designed to increase sphincter tone, such as Kegel exercises. Starting and then stopping the urinary stream also helps strengthen the sphincter. Medications such as propantheline bromide (Pro-Banthine) or ephedrine may be used. Propantheline bromide relaxes the bladder, thus decreasing the voiding reflex. Ephedrine increases sphincter tone. The client with incontinence that continues for 6 months after surgery may require external drainage or the insertion of an artificial sphincter. Straining to void and a decrease in the urinary stream could indicate the development of urethral stricture. Observe for these signs and report them to the physician.

Assess the client for signs of hypervolemia and hyponatremia by watching for signs of cerebral edema (changes in level of consciousness, notable confusion, twitching, irritability, convulsions, and coma) within the first 24 hours. The irrigating fluid used for continuous bladder irrigation should be isotonic. A client with water intoxication may be placed on restricted fluids and given sodium.

Positioning during surgery may affect postoperative recovery. Because clients who have had a TUR will have been in the lithotomy position, which predisposes them to deep vein thrombosis and subsequent pulmonary embolism, they may be treated with prophylactic heparin.

If elastic bandages or antiembolic stockings have been used, they should be removed each shift and the condition of the underlying skin checked. Early ambulation, hourly coughing and deep breathing, and ankle exercises while in bed also can be helpful preventive measures. Avoid applying pressure on the popliteal and calf areas. The client should not cross his legs, and the bed should not be gatched. Because of the risk of pulmonary embolus, calf massage should be avoided.

Most persons over age 60 still have active sex lives, so postoperative impotence is a serious concern. Impotence is more likely to occur after perineal prostatectomy. The impotent client needs time to grieve and verbalize his feelings postoperatively because the impotence will threaten his masculine identity and body image. The client may be a candidate for a penile implant, or alternatives to genital sex can be explored. If impotence presents a problem for the client after a simple prostatectomy, the possible psychosocial sources of this problem should be explored.

A case study of a client undergoing TUR is at the end of this chapter.

Suprapubic Prostatectomy

In the suprapubic approach, the prostate gland is removed through an incision in the bladder via the lower abdomen. The details of this procedure are illustrated in Figure 49–16. This procedure can relieve the symptoms of obstructive prostatic hypertrophy and is often used when surgical removal of bladder calculi or diverticula is also needed. It also may be used when the prostatic enlargement is too

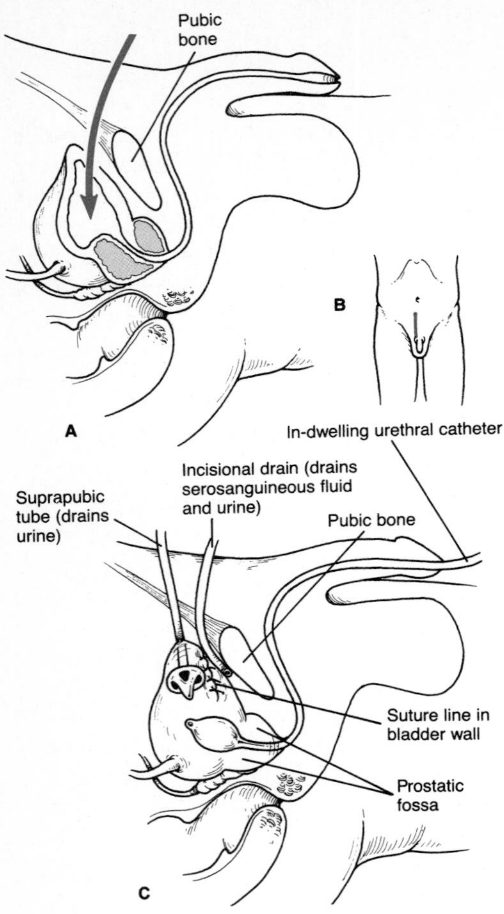

Figure 49–16

Suprapubic prostatectomy. **A.** Side view. **B.** Incision line. **C.** Suture lines and drainage tubes.

great for TUR. A summary of the client implications for suprapubic prostatectomy are in Table 49–19.

Nursing Implications

PREOPERATIVE CARE Preoperative care for the client having a suprapubic prostatectomy is similar to that for a client having a TUR. Major nursing activities include providing information about implications of the procedure, maintaining catheter care, monitoring hydration, and taking a history to assess the risk of postoperative complications.

POSTOPERATIVE CARE The recovery period after a suprapubic prostatectomy is generally longer than after a TUR. The nurse should perform routine daily catheter care and maintain accurate intake and output measurements. Assess vital signs every 4 hours. A sudden temperature elevation may indicate infection. Urine may leak around the suprapubic tube, so frequent dressing changes using aseptic technique are important. B and O suppositories may be ordered for bladder spasms.

After the first or second postoperative day, the surgeon usually removes one of the catheters (usually the Foley catheter) to reduce the possibility of urethral stricture from inflammation and subsequent scarring. The suprapubic catheter is usually clamped for 24 hours before removal to be sure the client can void. Residual urine volume not greater than 50 to 75 mL should be achieved before suprapubic catheter removal, which usually occurs between the seventh and tenth postoperative day.

Usually, the abdominal drain is advanced by the surgeon and removed between the fourth and sixth days. The drainage may contain urine and serosanguineous material, and frequent dressing changes are needed to prevent skin irritation and infection.

After a suprapubic prostatectomy, the client may have a nasogastric tube in place until peristalsis returns. Keep the tube on low suction and maintain its patency, irrigating with normal saline as needed. To assess for the return of peristalsis, check for the presence of bowel sounds and the passage of flatus.

Discomfort from the abdominal incision is another postoperative condition requiring nursing intervention. Narcotic analgesics can relieve incisional pain. Other applicable postoperative nursing interventions are discussed in the section on TUR.

Retropubic Prostatectomy

In the retropubic approach (also called a retrovesical prostatectomy), a low abdominal incision is made, and the prostate gland is entered directly. The retropubic approach, which totally removes all prostatic tissue, is used when the prostate is larger than 100 g (too large for TUR) or when malignant tissue needs to be surgically excised.

A radical retropubic prostatectomy involves the total removal of the prostate, ejaculatory ducts, seminal vesicles, and fascia. Frequently, a radical lymphadenectomy is performed prior to the removal of the prostate.

Nursing Implications

PREOPERATIVE CARE Clients undergoing radical prostatectomy often have a bowel preparation preoperatively to be sure the bowel is cleared in case of bowel injury. This consists of enemas, the administration of an antibiotic such as neomycin, and a low-residue diet. For other nursing implications of retropubic prostatectomy, refer to the discussion of TUR.

POSTOPERATIVE CARE After a retropubic prostatectomy, the client has an in-dwelling catheter in place. Assess its patency and measure intake and output. A major postoperative nursing goal is the prevention of urinary tract infection; thus, the nurse should maintain the integrity and sterility of the drainage system. After a simple prostatectomy, the catheter is usually removed on the sixth postoperative day. After a radical retropubic prostatectomy, the catheter may have traction applied for 1 week, and the catheter may remain in place for as long as 3 weeks.

The drain inserted around the incision site is usually advanced by the surgeon on Day 6 and removed on Day 7. After a radical retropubic prostatectomy, however, the drains are advanced after 1 week and removed in 10 days if no urine leakage is present.

Like the suprapubic prostatectomy client, the retropubic prostatectomy client may have a nasogastric tube in place until peristalsis returns. Keep the tube on low suction, and maintain its patency by irrigation with normal saline as necessary. IV fluids are required at this time.

Incisional pain can be controlled by narcotic analgesics. The skin is kept dry by a change of abdominal dressing at least twice daily. If scrotal and leg edema occur, the legs and scrotum should be elevated, and the nurse should carefully observe the client for increasing edema. Chronic edema may become a problem after lymphadenectomy, especially if the client has had postoperative pelvic irradiation. Another common serious problem after lymphadenectomy is thromboembolism. Elastic bandages or antiembolic stockings help prevent venous stasis as well as edema. Other postoperative procedures are described in the discussion of TUR.

Perineal Prostatectomy

The perineal approach is useful when the prostate is enlarged beyond 40 to 60 g and when the abdominal approach is contraindicated, as it may be in a severely obese client or a client at risk of suffering postoperative respiratory complications. The surgical time is short, so fewer cardiopulmonary complications are associated with perineal prostatectomy. This approach also is used for removal of a prostate with calculi. The perineal approach carries the risk of rectal injury and urinary fistula to the perineum or rectum. This approach also necessitates placing the client in the lithotomy position, which is a contraindication for some clients. A summary of client implications appears in Table 49–19.

Nursing Implications

PREOPERATIVE CARE A bowel preparation before perineal prostatectomy minimizes the chance of postoperative wound infection. The nurse should give the client opportunities to express feelings related to threatened loss of normal sexual function, loss of masculinity, and changes in self-esteem and self-worth. See the discussion of TUR for other aspects of preoperative nursing care.

POSTOPERATIVE CARE After a perineal prostatectomy, the client usually has a Foley catheter in place for 2 weeks, and a closed drainage system is essential to prevent infection. A drain also will be present in the perineal area. This drain is usually removed on the seventh postoperative day.

Pay strict attention to keeping the incision clean and dry to promote healing and prevent infection, change the dressing at least twice daily, and cleanse the incision with soap and water after each bowel movement. Incisional pain, although mild, may require analgesics. To prevent rectal perforation or fistula development, the client should receive nothing by rectum. This includes no rectal thermometers, enemas, suppositories, rectal tubes, or any other rectal procedure during the postoperative recovery period.

Encourage the client to communicate with his spouse or sexual partner feelings of loss of masculinity and self-esteem. Alternate methods of sexual expression or penile implants may also be discussed.

Urinary incontinence may take longer to resolve than with other prostatic surgeries. Dribbling can be corrected by Kegel exercises and gluteal exercises performed five to ten times per hour. See the section on TUR for additional postoperative nursing measures.

Testicular Cancer

Testicular cancer affects otherwise healthy young men between the ages of 15 and 40, and it is one of the leading causes of cancer death in that age group. Marked advances in diagnosis and treatment have increased the potential for cure, even when metastasis is present. Risk factors associated with testicular cancer include a history of cryptorchidism, a possible genetic predisposition (incidence is much higher in whites than blacks), and carcinoma in situ (malignant changes in the epithelial tissue).

More than 90% of testicular cancer arises from the germ cell epithelium of the testis. There are two main classifications of these tumors—seminomas and nonseminomas—depending on the tissue type. Nonseminomas are further subdivided into teratomas, embryonic carcinoma, and choriocarcinoma. The type of tumor affects both treatment and prognosis.

Clinical Manifestations

The earliest manifestation of testicular cancer is a smooth, painless lump. It usually does not adhere to the scrotal wall, so scrotal shape is maintained. If the tumor is large, the scrotum is taut and glistening. Often, the client discovers the tumor as a lump or hardening in the testes. The tumor will not transilluminate. More advanced signs include general abdominal and inguinal aching and heaviness. Pain is a late sign. When first seen by the physician, 35% of clients have either lymph node or distant metastasis.

The client with metastasis may have symptoms and signs of a supraclavicular or abdominal mass from lymphatic spread—abdominal pain, bowel or urinary obstruction, a cough from lung metastasis, and general weight loss and anorexia. Any testicular tumor may cause gynecomastia, especially if the tumor is from choriocarcinoma.

The HCG level is often elevated in clients with

embryonal cancer and is always elevated in clients with choriocarcinoma (Javadpour, 1980). Alphafetoprotein levels are often elevated in clients with teratoma and embryonal cancer.

Medical Measures

Therapy for testicular cancer is based on the stage of the disease. Staging classifications vary, but there is general agreement on progression (Javadpour, 1980): in stage I or A, the tumor is limited to the testis; in stage II or B, there is metastasis to regional lymph nodes; and in stage III or C, there is metastasis to distant organs.

An orchiectomy with high ligation of the spermatic cord is performed upon the initial discovery of the tumor. Seminomas, the most common type of testicular tumors, are radiosensitive; postoperative radiation therapy to the lymph drainage areas of the testes is employed to treat this type of tumor. Javadpour (1980) reports that radiation therapy results in a 5-year survival rate of more than 90%. In stage I, supervoltage radiation is given to the inguinal, aortic, and caval lymph areas. In stage II, the medastinal and supraclavicular lymph nodes are also included. Stage III disease is treated with chemotherapy (usually cyclophosphamide and cisplatin).

Nonseminomatous tumors with negative tumor markers (HCG and AFP are not elevated) and nodes are treated postoperatively with x-rays and followed with tumor markers for 2 years. Clients who have stage II disease showing either positive nodes or markers are treated with chemotherapy. Those with stage III disease are treated with node dissection and chemotherapy (usually vinblastine sulfate, cisplatin, and bleomycin).

Specific Nursing Measures

Early detection and treatment are critical for the client with testicular cancer. Therefore, all adolescent males should be taught TSE and should perform it monthly.

The client with testicular cancer should be informed that prompt treatment holds the promise of cure. He requires a great deal of emotional support as he faces surgery, radiation, or chemotherapy. Most men maintain sexual function after surgery, although retrograde ejaculation may cause infertility problems. Artificial insemination using the client's sperm is possible if sperm is obtained, frozen, and banked before treatment. For further nursing care related to the client receiving radiation therapy or chemotherapy, see Chapter 10.

Orchiectomy

An orchiectomy is the removal of the testis. Simple orchiectomy involves removal of the testis alone, whereas radical orchiectomy involves high ligation of the spermatic cord and may include retroperitoneal lymphadenectomy. A simple orchiectomy is performed for recurrent epididymo-orchitis when more traditional medical treatment has failed. It also is used as palliative treatment for cancer of the prostate. A radical orchiectomy is performed whenever there is cancer of the testis, epididymis, or spermatic cord. Bilateral orchiectomy may be performed for metastatic cancer of the prostate. Implications for the orchiectomy client are summarized in Table 49–20.

Table 49–20
Orchiectomy: Implications for the Client

Physiologic Implications	Psychosocial/Lifestyle Implications
Potency and fertility maintained after unilateral orchiectomy	Fear of cancer
Potential for postoperative phlebitis	Fear of emasculation from surgery
After lymphadenectomy, possible respiratory, vascular, and abdominal complications	Possible improvement in appearance with a prosthesis

Nursing Implications

PREOPERATIVE CARE The major preoperative preparation of the client is psychologic preparation. The nurse needs to provide emotional support to the client as he verbalizes his concerns about cancer, emasculation, and lifestyle changes.

POSTOPERATIVE CARE Recovery is rapid for the client who has had an orchiectomy without retroperitoneal lymphadenectomy. A general diet and ambulation are usually started the day of surgery; as with other types of genitourinary surgery, early ambulation usually can avert phlebitis. An ice pack applied to the scrotum for 24 hours after surgery reduces edema and bleeding. Analgesia may at first be accomplished by parenteral narcotics, but usually after the first 24 hours oral analgesics are sufficient.

The extent of the surgery and incision necessitate bed rest for the first 24 to 48 hours after an orchiectomy with retroperitoneal lymphadenectomy. Respiratory and vascular complications are likely to follow, so the nurse should help the client with ankle pushes, turning, deep breathing, and coughing every 2 hours. The extensive abdominal manipulation in this surgery leads to paralytic ileus, and the client will have a nasogastric tube set to suction until bowel sounds return and flatus is passed.

Cancer of the Penis

Although rare in Northern America, cancer of the penis is a significant worldwide health problem. Its highest incidence is in men in their 60s and 70s. A contributing causative factor is poor hygiene.

Clinical Manifestations

Lesions considered to be precancerous are leukoplakia and painful velvety red plaques (erythroplasia of Queyrat) on the dorsal aspect of the uncircumcised penis. The most common cancerous lesion is squamous cell carcinoma, which usually is seen as a visible lesion on the glans or prepuce. Penile discharge also may be present.

Medical Measures

If the disease is on the prepuce, a circumcision is performed. If the lesion is on the distal shaft, a partial penectomy is performed. A total penectomy is done for more advanced disease. Lymphadenectomy is indicated if the nodes are diseased. In a young client with a small lesion, external radiation may be used instead of surgery. A client with inoperable nodes or metastatic disease is treated with systemic chemotherapy (usually bleomycin or methotrexate).

Specific Nursing Measures

Teaching clients the importance of basic hygiene is important in the prevention of penile cancer. The uncircumcised client must understand that daily retraction of the prepuce and washing the penis are essential. The client and his partner require a great deal of emotional support as they face disfiguring surgery that directly threatens male identity, sexual performance, and fertility.

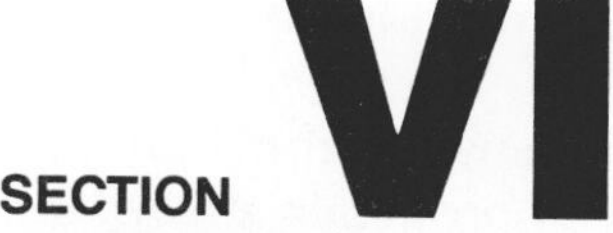

Traumatic Disorders

Lacerations, Hematomas, and Fistulas in the Female

Traumatic disorders of the female reproductive tract occur either by direct injury to the vulva, vagina, or breasts, or as the result of surgery or irradiation. Trauma to the vulva, although rare, may result in a laceration or in hematoma formation. Trauma to the vagina usually results from an intercourse injury or the insertion of foreign bodies into the vagina. Trauma from surgery or irradiation can result in fistula formation.

The majority of fistulas are the result of surgery to the bladder or the reproductive tract. Fistulas between the bladder and vagina are known as vesicovaginal fistulas. There are also ureterovaginal, urethrovaginal, rectovaginal, perineal–vaginal, vesicouterine, and vesicocervical fistulas (Figure 49–17).

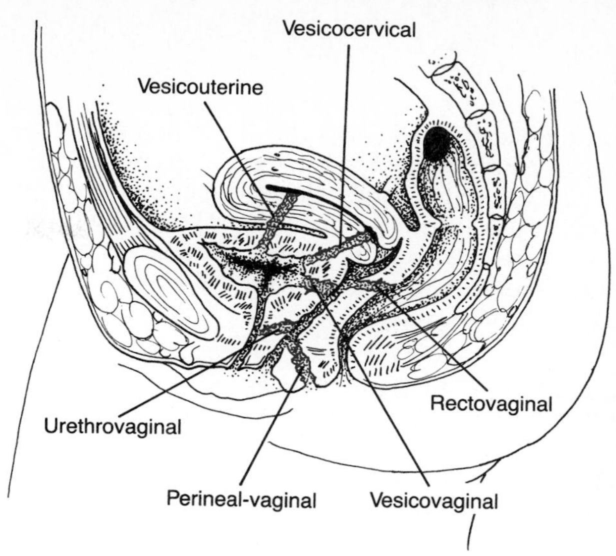

Figure 49–17

Fistulas that may develop in the female reproductive system.

Clinical Manifestations

Symptoms of vulval or vaginal trauma include pain, possible bleeding, and the presence of lacerations or hematomas. The client with a fistula has involuntary leakage of urine or involuntary leakage of stool from the vagina. When the fistula is located between the bladder or ureter and the vagina, there is involuntary leakage of urine from the vagina. Urine may leak intermittently if the urethra is involved. When the fistula is between the rectum and vagina, there is leakage of stool from the vagina.

Medical Measures

To repair minor lacerations of the vulva or vagina, a local anesthetic can be used before suturing; this is usually an outpatient procedure. Extensive lacerations should be repaired in the operating room with adequate anesthesia.

Hematomas of the vulva may need to be drained, depending on the size, type, and location of the vessel involved. If the hematoma is small or of moderate size and is not expanding, close observation is all that is necessary.

Fistulas are surgically managed; techniques depend on their extent and site. A vaginal approach is often used to repair postoperative vesicovaginal fistulas. Surgeons may use the abdominal approach if tumors and radiation therapy caused the fistulas. With very large fistulas, urinary or fecal diversion may be necessary.

Specific Nursing Measures

If direct injury caused the trauma, nursing care involves observation of the laceration and hematoma. Ice can reduce pain and edema with a hematoma. The client will need emotional support during the emergency situation. This can be accomplished by staying with the client, answering her questions, and reassuring her. If surgery is needed for repair, the client should receive preoperative and postoperative care individualized to her specific needs.

The client with a fistula will need long-term physical care and help in adjusting to her changed body image. The lack of control over body functions can cause her to feel helpless. Therefore, the nurse is a needed source for venting feelings and frustrations.

Trauma to the Penis or Scrotum

Trauma to the penis can result from a bullet or stab wound or can be caused by catching the clothing in a power tool. Circulation to the penis can be impaired as a result of strangulation from a twisted condom catheter, a string wrapped around the penis, a tight ring, or a worker's tool. A blunt injury to an erect penis can lead to corporeal or urethral rupture. Scrotal injuries are not common, because the scrotum is mobile and the scrotal muscles retract reflexively. Blunt or penetrating objects can injure the scrotum, however.

Clinical Manifestations

Discoloration of the penis or scrotum may indicate trauma, impaired circulation, or both. If major blood vessels have been damaged, life-threatening hemorrhage can occur; the client may be in shock.

Medical Measures

Treatment depends on the cause of the trauma. Damage from a penetrating missile must be surgically repaired as soon as possible. The management of a strangulation injury includes removal of the object.

Trauma to the scrotum usually requires surgical exploration and treatment for the particular problem. Prompt surgical intervention minimizes damage to the testes. Nonsurgical intervention includes elevating the scrotum and applying ice. Neither measure preserves the testes, however.

Specific Nursing Measures

Provide the client with specific information about the extent of injury and treatment. Most clients will need substantial emotional support in dealing with disfigurement and surgery.

Bed rest and scrotal elevation are quite important after a scrotal injury. Whenever the client is ambulatory, the client should wear a scrotal support and should avoid strenuous activity, lifting heavy objects, or climbing stairs for several days after the injury.

Chapter Highlights

The client with a reproductive system disorder may undergo an altered body image and altered sexuality patterns. Thus, emotional support is a key nursing intervention.

The in-utero exposure of offspring to DES may cause various reproductive tract abnormalities.

Any disturbance in reproductive bleeding may produce fear and anxiety.

Major gynecologic surgeries are often preceded by laparoscopy, D and C, or both.

Although clients are sterile after all forms of hysterectomy, some procedures cause a sudden climacteric and others do not. An important nursing responsibility is to be sure the client understands the implications.

Penile implants can be used to correct organic impotence as well as some forms of psychogenic impotence. Clients are usually satisfied with solid-rod and inflatable prostheses.

Perineal exercises, such as Kegel exercises, can help prevent or reduce the severity of pelvic relaxation problems.

Anterior and posterior colporrhaphy correct problems that result from relaxation or weakness of the pelvic musculature.

Infectious vaginitis is one of the most frequent reasons women seek medical attention.

An important nursing role in caring for STD clients is teaching them about the disease's incidence, mode of transmission, preventive measures, and treatments.

The best hope for recovery from breast cancer lies in early treatment.

Most breast masses in women are from benign breast disease, including fibrocystic disease, fibroadenomas, and intraductal papillomas.

Breast biopsy, mastectomy, and breast reconstruction often involve the diagnosis of cancer, which necessitates additional nursing support and information. Monthly BSE becomes especially important for these clients.

Breast reconstruction, augmentation mammoplasty, and reduction mammoplasty are performed at the client's request to improve her body image. The procedures usually have positive effects.

Benign prostatic hyperplasia is the most common neoplasm in men. Transurethral resection (TUR) is the most common therapeutic measure.

Early detection of prostatic cancer improves the client's prognosis, so the nurse should encourage yearly rectal examinations for men over age 40.

Testicular self-examination is a simple means of early detection of testicular cancer. This should be taught to all adolescent males and practiced throughout adulthood.

Vasectomy is a safe and effective means of birth control. It should be performed only if the client is sure he does not want more children, however. Vasovasostomy can reverse vasectomy, but does not guarantee the ability to impregnate.

Trauma to the penis or scrotum can constitute an emergency and can result in serious damage to urinary and sexual function.

Bibliography

Aitken DR, Minton JP: Complications associated with mastectomy. *Surg Clin North Am* 1983; 63(6):1331–1349.

American Cancer Society: *1987 Cancer Facts and Figures.* New York: American Cancer Society, 1987.

Babian R: Malignant tumors of the urogenital tract. In: *Conn's Current Therapy.* Pakel RE (editor). Philadelphia: Saunders, 1984.

Barber H: Ovarian cancer. *CA-A Cancer J Clin* (May/June) 1986; 36(3):149–183.

Benson R: *Current Obstetric and Gynecologic Diagnosis and Treatment,* 5th ed. Los Altos, CA: Lange, 1984.

Bernhard LA: Endometriosis. *JOGN Nurs* 1982; 11(5):300–304.

Bowie WR: Nongonococcal urethritis in sexually transmitted disease. *Urol Clin North Am* 1984; 11(1).

Brown M, Zimmer P: Personal and family impact of premenstrual symptoms. *JOGN Nurs* 1986; 15(1): 31–37.

Busch D, McBride A, Benaventura S: Chemical dependency in women: the link to OB/GYN problems. *J Psychosoc Nurs* 1986; 24(4): 26–30.

Caffee H. The effects of hematoma on implant capsules. *Ann Plast Surg* (Feb) 1986; 16(2):102–105.

Centers for Disease Control: Sexually transmitted disease treatment guidelines. *MMWR [Suppl]* (Oct 18) 1985; 34:778–948.

Cibulka NJ: Toxic shock syndrome and other tampon related risks. *JOGN Nurs* 1984; 12(2):94–99.

Clark N, O'Connell P: Prostatectomy: Answering your patients' unspoken questions. *Nurs 84* (April) 1984; 14:48–51.

Couch RB et al: Genital herpes: An epidemic disease. *Heart Lung* 1983; 12:320–324.

Cramer D et al: Dietary animal fat in relation to ovarian cancer risk. *Obstet Gynecol* 1984; 63:833–838.

Crawford ED, Borden TA: *Genitourinary Cancer Surgery.* Philadelphia: Lea & Febiger, 1982.

Danforth D, Scott J (editors): *Obstetrics and Gynecology,* 5th ed. Philadelphia: Lippincott, 1986.

Datta PK: The post-prostatectomy patient. *Nurs Times* 1981; 77:1759–1761.

Del Regato J, Spjut H, Cox JD: *Ackerman and Del Regato's Cancer Diagnosis, Treatment, and Prognosis,* 6th ed. St. Louis: Mosby, 1985.

De Vita VT, Hellman S, Rosenberg S: *Cancer Principles and Practice of Oncology,* Vol I, 2nd ed. Philadelphia: Lippincott, 1985.

Dinner MI, Dowden RV: Breast reconstruction: State of the art. *Cancer* 1984; 53:809–814.

Drusin LM: Syphilis: Clinical manifestations, diagnosis and treatment. *Urol Clin North Am* 1984; 11(1):121–130.

Duenhoelter JH: *Greenhill's Office Gynecology,* 10th ed. Chicago: Year Book Medical Publishers, 1983.

Dugan KK: The bleak outlook on ovarian cancer. *Am J Nurs* 1985; 85(2):144–147.

Fogel CI, Woods NF: *Health Care of Women: A Nursing Perspective.* St. Louis: Mosby, 1981.

Glenn JF: *Urologic Surgery.* Philadelphia: Lippincott, 1983.

Glenn JF, Werneth JL: The male genital system. In: *Textbook of Surgery,* 12th ed. Sabiston D (editor). Philadelphia: Saunders, 1981.

Goldberg P, Stolzman M, Goldberg H: Psychological considerations in breast reconstruction. *Ann Plast Surg* 1984; 13:39–42.

Googe MC, Mook TM: The inflatable penile prosthesis: New developments. *Am J Nurs* 1983; 83:1044–1047.

Gregory JG: Impotence: The surgical approach. *Surg Clin North Am* 1982; 62(6):981–998.

Griffith–Kenney J: *Contemporary Women's Health: A Nursing Advocacy Approach.* Menlo Park, CA: Addison–Wesley, 1986.

Haggerty BJ: Prevention and differential of scrotal cancer. *Nurse Pract* 1983; 8(10):45–52.

Harris J, Hellman S, Silen W: *Conservative Management of Breast Cancer: New Surgical and Radiotherapeutic Techniques.* Philadelphia: Lippincott, 1983.

Harrison WO: Gonococcal urethritis. *Urol Clin North Am* 1984; 11(1):45–54.

Hassey M, Bloom LS, Burgess SL: Radiation alternative to mastectomy. *Am J Nurs* 1983; 83:1567–1569.

Hogan R: *Human Sexuality: A Nursing Perspective.* New York: Appleton–Century–Crofts, 1980.

Holmes KK, Bell TA, Berger RE: Epidemiology of sexually transmitted disease. *Urol Clin North Am* 1984; 11(1):3–12.

Ireton RC, Berger RE: Prostatitis and epididymitis. *Urol Clin North Am* 1984; 11(1):83–93.

Javadpour N: Germ cell tumor of the testes. *CA* 1980; 30:242–255.

Jensen MD, Bobak IM: *Maternity and Gynecologic Care: The Nurse and the Family,* 3rd ed. St. Louis: Mosby, 1985.

Jones H, Rock J: *Reparative and Constructive Surgery of the Female Generative Tract.* Baltimore: Williams & Wilkins, 1983.

Kase N, Weingold A (editors): *Principles and Practice of Clinical Gynecology.* New York: Wiley, 1983.

Kessler R: Vasectomy and vasovasostomy. *Surg Clin North Am* 1982; 62(6):971–980.

Kirkpatrick MK, Grady TR: PMS: A self-help checklist. *Occup Health Nurs* (Feb) 1985; 33:90–92.

Knobf MK: Breast cancer: The treatment revolution. *Am J Nurs* 1984; 84:1110–1117.

Kramer SA: Circumcision. In: *Urologic Surgery.* Glenn JF (editor). Philadelphia: Lippincott, 1983.

Krieger JN: Biology of sexually transmitted disease. *Urol Clin North Am* 1984; 11(1):15–25.

Lauerson NH: Recognition and treatment of PMS. *Nurs Pract* 1985; 10:11–12.

Lauver D: Irregular bleeding in women: Causes and nursing interventions. *Am J Nurs* 1983; 83:396–401.

Lerner J, Kahn Z: *Mosby's Manual of Urologic Nursing.* St. Louis: Mosby, 1982.

Levitt D et al.: Group support in the treatment of PMS. *J Psychosoc Nurs* 1986; 26(1):23–28.

Lierman LM: Support for mastectomy. *AORN J* 1984; 39:1150–1157.

Margolis S: Genital warts and molluscum contagiosum. *Urol Clin North Am* 1984; 11(1):163–170.

McConnell EA, Zimmerman MF: *Care of Patients With Urologic Problems.* Philadelphia: Lippincott, 1983.

McDougal WS, Persky L: *Traumatic Injuries to the Genitourinary System.* Baltimore: Williams & Wilkins, 1981.

Mertz G, Corey L: Genital herpes simplex virus infections in adults. *Urol Clin North Am* 1984; 11(1):103–117.

Miles PA: Sexually transmitted diseases. *JOGN Nurs* 1984; 13 (Suppl):102s–124s.

Mills JT et al: Control of toxic-shock-syndrome toxin-1 (TSST-1) by magnesium ion. *J Inf Dis* 1985; 151:1158–1161.

Molitar P: Transurethral resection. *Nurs Mirror* (Oct 5) 1983; 153:22–27.

Northouse LL: Coping with the mastectomy crisis. *Top Clin Nurs* 1982; 4(2):57–65.

Olds SB, London ML, Ladewig PA: *Maternal–Newborn Nursing: A Family Centered Approach,* 2nd ed. Menlo Park, CA: Addison–Wesley, 1984.

Paritzky JF, Overby BA: Preoperative teaching on a gynecologic unit. *JOGN Nurs* 1982; 11(6):384–386.

Parker M: Psychological problems in the treatment of gynecological malignancy. *Nurs Times* 1983; 79(10):56–57.

Pitkin R, Zlatnik F (editors): *The Yearbook of Obstetrics and Gynecology.* Chicago: Year Book Medical Publishers, 1984.

Pfeiffer CH, Mulliken JB: *Caring for the Patient With Breast Cancer: An Interdisciplinary/Multidisciplinary Approach.* Reston, VA: Reston, 1984.

Reichman RC et al: Treatment of recurrent genital herpes simplex infections with oral acyclovir: A controlled trial. *JAMA* 1984; 251:2103–2107.

Reynolds M: *Gynaecological Nursing.* Boston: Blackwell, 1984.

Riddle L: Augmentation mammoplasty. *Nurs Pract* 1986; 11(3):30–40.

Ridley JH: *Gynecologic Surgery. Errors, Safeguard, Salvage,* 2nd ed. Baltimore: Williams & Wilkins, 1981.

Ritchie JP, Garnick MB: Changing concepts in the treatment of non-seminatous germ cell tumors of the testes. *J Urol* 1984; 131:1089–1092.

Rodman MJ, Smith DW: *Clinical Pharmacology in Nursing.* Philadelphia: Lippincott, 1984.

Roseman D et al: Sexually transmitted disease and carcinogenesis. *Urol Clin North Am* 1984; 11(1):27–44.

Rutledge DN: Nurses' knowledge of breast reconstruction: A catalyst for earlier treatment of breast cancer? *Cancer Nurs* 1982; 5:469–473.

Schmidt JD: Treatment of localized prostatic carcinoma. *Urol Clin North Am* 1984; 11(2):305–309.

Schwartz GF: Benign neoplasms and "inflammations" of the breast. *Clin Obstet Gynecol* 1982; 25:373–385.

Senie RT, Rosen PP, Kinne DW: Epidemiologic factors associated with breast cancer. *Cancer Nurs* 1983; 5:367–371.

Shafer M et al: Self-concept in the diethylstilbestrol daughter. *Obstet Gynecol* 1984; 63:815–819.

Sheahan SL: Management of breast lumps. *Nurse Pract* 1984; 2(2):19–22.

Spirnack PJ, Resnick ML: Disturbed sexual function due to spermatocele. *Med Aspects Hum Sexuality* 1984; 18(1):221–236.

Stanfill PH: The psychosocial implications of hysterectomy. *JOGN Nurs* 1982; 11(5):318–322.

Stewart BH: *Operative Urology.* Baltimore: Williams & Wilkins, 1982.

Sullivan LD: Benign prostatic hyperplasia. Pages 534–538 in: *Conn's Current Treatment.* Pakel RE (editor). Philadelphia: Saunders, 1984.

US Department of Health and Human Services: *The Breast Cancer Digest.* NIH Publication No. 84-1691. Bethesda, MD: National Cancer Institute, 1984.

Veenema RJ, Wechsler M: Commentary: Radical retropubic prostatectomy. In: *Current Operative Urology,* 2nd ed. Whitehead ED, Leiter E (editors). New York: Harper & Row, 1984.

Vogel CH: Sex after radical prostatectomy. *Nurs 80* (June) 1980; 10:90–91.

Weatherley–White RC: *Plastic Surgery of the Breast.* New York: Harper & Row, 1980.

Weisenthal M: Reach-to-Recovery Program of the American Cancer Society. *Cancer* 1984; 53:825–827.

Whettam J: Update on toxic shock: How to spot it and treat it. *RN* 1984; 47(2):55–56, 58, 60.

Whitehead ED, Leiter E: *Current Operative Urology,* 2nd ed. New York: Harper & Row, 1984.

Wilhelm–Hass E: Premenstrual syndrome: Its nature, evaluation, and management. *JOGN Nurs* 1984; 13(4):223–229.

Woods JE: Current state of the art in breast reconstruction. *Plast Surg Nurs* 1984; 4:85–88.

Zinike H, Utz DC: Surgical management of prostatic cancer. In: *Principles and Management of Urologic Cancer,* 2nd ed. Javadpour N (editor). Baltimore: Williams & Wilkins, 1983.

CASE STUDY

The Client With Benign Prostatic Hyperplasia

I. Descriptive Data

Mr Charles Egan, age 68, arrives at the emergency department of the local hospital because he has been unable to void for 24 hours and is quite uncomfortable. He is accompanied by his wife. This is the first time Mr Egan has been hospitalized.

II. Personal Data

Date and Time: Nov 19, 1987, 6 AM
Name: Charles Egan
Social Security Number: 000-00-0000
Medicare Number: 000000000
Supplemental BC/BS Number: 0000000000
Address: 1816 Fulton St, Melton, NH 00040
Telephone: 000-0000
Sex: Male
Age: 68
Birthdate: 10-15-19
Marital Status: Married
Race: Caucasian
Religion: Catholic
Occupation: Retired railroad worker
Usual Health Care Provider: Stephen Riley, MD

III. Health History

Source of Information: Client
Reliability of Informant: Alert, oriented, and reliable
Chief Concern: "I haven't been able to pass water since yesterday and it sure does hurt."

History of Present Illness:

Mr Egan has noticed that over the past 10 years he has had increasing difficulty starting his urinary stream and in stopping it once it starts. His urinary stream has decreased in force, and he usually wakes up twice a night to void. During the past week, he has noticed increased frequency, burning on urination, and nocturia up to five times a night. It has been increasingly difficult for him to start the stream. Yesterday he was totally unable to void; he has not voided since.

He has no history of UTIs, STDs, or any abdominal surgery. He has not noted any lumps, lesions, or bulging in the genital area. He has had no trauma to the perineal area. He has a soft, brown, formed stool every morning without difficulty, His stools have never been black. He takes no medication.

Client is married; his wife of 40 years has been his only sexual partner; sexually active but reports frequency has decreased from weekly to once or twice a month. Last had intercourse 2 weeks ago without difficulty.

Past Health History:

Childhood: No major health problems
Immunizations: Has not had a shot in 30 years
Medical Problems: None
Surgeries: None
Trauma: None

(continued)

CASE STUDY (continued)

The Client With Benign Prostatic Hyperplasia

Past Health History, (continued):

Allergies: None

Medications: None

Family History:

Father, died age 70 from pancreatic carcinoma
Mother, age 90, A&W; has cataracts
Sisters × 2, ages 64 and 62, A&W
Wife, age 65, A&W
Sons × 3, ages 39, 37, and 34, all A&W

No ⊕ FHx DM, MI, CVA, hypertension, or malignancy except for his father; states that he comes from a family of "long livers," and that his father was the first and only one to have cancer.

Personal/Social History:

Lives with wife on a small farm in New Hampshire. They enjoy a good relationship and are active in the Catholic church and local Grange. In summer, client spends his time caring for a productive vegetable garden and taking care of his two cows, three goats, and ten chickens. At harvest time, he sells his produce at the farmer's market and participates in the county fair. During the winter, he cares for his animals and otherwise busies himself inside or with church activities.

Completed eighth grade. He reads a lot and is well informed on current events. Retired 4 years ago as a railroad conductor on a commuter train between Boston and New Hampshire. He has not traveled outside New England except for serving with the Marines in the Pacific during World War II.

He feels the family is financially stable. They own their own farm. He makes extra income on vegetables and eggs, receives a railroad pension, and has $20,000 in savings.

Habits: States he is a meat-and-potatoes man; eats eggs and bacon every morning for breakfast. Walks at least 2 miles every day. Cares for garden and animals. Has never smoked. Drinks one shot of whiskey every night. States, "It warms me up and keeps my motor going."

Review of Systems:

General: Weight stable; no symptoms of fatigue, anorexia, or difficulty sleeping

Eyes: Wears glasses for reading; no eye pain or decreased vision

Ears: States he "doesn't hear the wife as well as he used to"; also has difficulty hearing in a crowded room with many voices in the background

Cardiopulmonary: No chest pain, no cough, no DOE; last chest x-ray 20 or 30 years ago; no TBC exposure; never had a TBC skin test; no PND, no ankle edema; never had an ECG

GI: No food intolerance, no dysphagia, no hx of ulcer disease, no reflux, no abdominal pain

M-S: Occasional low back pain with excessive bending and lifting; relieved by rest and ASA

Psychologic: No major worries except about current symptoms; usual coping pattern is to walk or tend the garden if upset

IV. Physical Assessment

Client is tanned with well-developed shoulder, abdominal, and leg muscles. Appears younger than stated age and overall health seems to be good.

Height: 5 ft 11 in.

Weight: 185 lb

Vital Signs: T: 99°F (32.2°C), P: 84, R: 20

BP: 130/80 (L) arm, sitting

Relevant Organ Systems:

Cardiovascular:	Apical rate 84, regular; no murmurs or gallops; pedal pulses 3 + and equal bilaterally
Abdomen:	No scars or bruits, muscular, nontender; no CVA tenderness; L-S-K not palpable; bladder dull to percussion and palpated to 4 cm below the umbilicus
Genitals:	Penis circumcised; no lesions, masses, or discharge; scrotum without masses or lesions; no inguinal or femoral hernias
Rectum:	No perianal lesions, no ext hemorrhoids; sphincter tone good; rectal walls without lesions; prostate, enlarged symmetrically, soft, smooth, slightly tender to palpation

V. Summary

Mr Egan was admitted to the hospital as an emergency. An 18 F Foley catheter was inserted, 1000 mL of urine was drained, and the catheter was clamped. One hour later, the catheter was unclamped, and another 800 mL of urine was drained; the catheter was left open to straight drainage.

Urine was sent to the laboratory for urinalysis and urine culture and sensitivity. Mr Egan was scheduled for an IVP, a voiding cystogram, and cystometric evaluation. Routine blood work, an ECG, and a chest x-ray were done in anticipation of surgery.

Mr Egan was placed on ampicillin to treat a urinary tract infection. Five days after admission, with the UTI under control, Mr Egan was taken to the operating room for a transurethral resection of the prostate gland.

VI. Nursing Care Plan, by Nursing Diagnosis

Client Care Goals	Plan/Nursing Implementation	Expected Outcome
Fluid volume deficit: potential related to possible postoperative hemorrhage		
Remain free of hemorrhage and hypovolemic shock	Assess skin temperature, skin color; check vital signs q. 15 min; progress to q. 30 min and to q. 1h as they become stable; assess for large amounts of bright red bleeding through and around the catheter; maintain catheter traction; administer stool softeners to prevent straining	Client's vital signs will remain stable; any untoward bleeding will be discovered early so hypovolemic shock is prevented; client will have a postoperative course free of active hemorrhage and clots
Urinary retention related to urethral obstruction secondary to formation of blood clots		
Remain free of urinary retention and obstruction	Maintain catheter patency by gravity drainage; no dependent loops; maintain continuous bladder irrigation as ordered; teach perineal exercises to decrease dribbling after catheter is removed; force fluids to 3000 mL/day	Catheter will remain patent and free of obstruction
Infection, potential for related to urinary tract infection		
Remain free of urinary tract infection	Administer antibiotics as ordered; maintain sterile closed system; practice strict asepsis; give catheter care q. 12h	Urine will remain clear and free of infection
Comfort, altered: pain related to bladder spasms		
Remain relatively pain-free	Maintain continuous bladder irrigation to prevent formation of clots; teach client not to try and void around catheter even though he may have that sensation; administer B and O suppositories for relief of bladder spasms	Client will remain free of bladder spasms and comfortable

(continued)

CASE STUDY (continued)

The Client With Benign Prostatic Hyperplasia

VI. Nursing Care Plan, by Nursing Diagnosis

Client Care Goals	Plan/Nursing Implementation	Expected Outcome
Sexuality, altered patterns related to medically imposed restriction		
Verbalize an understanding of temporary sexual dysfunction	Tell client that usual intercourse may be resumed 6 weeks after surgery but that he should check with his doctor before resuming; explain that impotence is not expected after TUR; encourage nongenital touching to express caring until intercourse can be resumed	Client expresses understanding of need for a temporary restriction on sexual intercourse; client and partner are able to express caring to each other; satisfactory sexual relations will be reestablished
Knowledge deficit related to home care post-discharge regimen		
Verbalize an understanding of post-discharge instructions	Instruct client in activity limitations, including avoiding heavy lifting and riding on bumpy roads; taking medications as prescribed by his physician; to expect blood-tinged urine; maintain fluid intake of at least 2000 mL/day	Client expresses understanding of post-discharge instructions

UNIT

12

The Client With Visual or Auditory Dysfunction

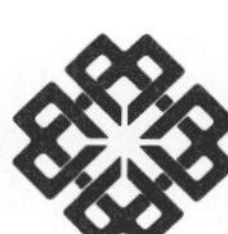

CHAPTER **50**

The Visual and Auditory Systems in Health and Illness

Other topics relevant to this content are: Close-up view of anterior chamber angle in normal eye and in glaucoma, Figure 52–4 in **Chapter 52;** Decibel levels of common noises and effects on hearing, **Chapter 52** and Table 52–12; Visual field defects, **Chapter 29** and Figure 29–1

Objectives

When you have finished studying this chapter, you should be able to:

Identify the anatomic structures of the eye and ear.

Describe the functions of the visual and auditory systems.

List pathophysiologic influences that can adversely affect the function of the eye or ear.

Describe alterations in other body systems that can affect vision and hearing.

Discuss psychosocial influences that have some relationship to vision, hearing, and balance.

The eyes and ears, sole sensory organs for gathering visual and auditory data, are complex anatomic and physiologic structures. The data they gather allow a person to detect changes in the environment and to direct a variety of activities. In addition, vision and hearing contribute to feelings of self-worth and self-concept. They provide pleasure and the ability to share human experiences. Mobility, communication, financial security, independence, career, and self-image—in other words, all of life—frequently depend on the normal structure and function of the eyes and ears.

Although sensory organs, the eyes and ears are also part of the central nervous system (CNS). Their major functions, vision and hearing and the maintenance of equilibrium, interface closely with the CNS. The eyes and ears are the most important sources of information that we have about the world we live in and the space we occupy.

SECTION 

Structural and Functional Interrelationships

Structure and Function of the Eye

The eye is approximately 1 inch in diameter and nearly spherical with the anterior portion slightly more convex.

The eye can be divided anatomically into the protective structures; the external, middle, and inner layers; and the refracting media. The muscles, nerves, and blood supply of the eye interrelate to the main structures.

Protective Structures

Only one-sixth of the eye is exposed; the rest is recessed and protected by the *orbits* (bony sockets) formed by the cranial bones. Posteriorly, the eye is cushioned by fat pads and connective tissues. In addition to protecting the eye, the orbit provides a pathway for the nerves and blood vessels that supply the eye.

The *eyelids* protect the eye from external irritation and can prevent about 99% of light from entering. (Note, however, that the eyelids will *not* prevent retinal damage from ultraviolet rays, as when a person lays face up in the sun.) The eyelids' protective function is mediated by three mechanisms: movement of the eyelids (blinking), the screening and sensing action of the cilia (eyelashes), and lubrication of the cornea and the conjunctiva by the secretions of the meibomian glands (sebaceous glands). The skin of the eyelids, the thinnest in the body, is loose and elastic. This gives the eyelids a great potential for swelling.

Tears, secreted by the lacrimal glands, bathe the anterior surface of the eye, cornea, and conjunctival epithelium. The tears drain into the lacrimal sac through the *puncta* (small openings located on the medial aspect of the eyelid), and from there to the nasal cavity. Blinking spreads tears over the surface of the eye. Tears prevent friction between the eyelids and conjunctiva, inhibit the growth of microorganisms, rid the eye of cellular debris and foreign bodies, and provide oxygen and small amounts of glucose necessary for corneal metabolism and for the maintenance of corneal transparency.

The *conjunctiva* provides a protective lubricating environment between the eyelid and eyeball when the eye blinks or moves. The conjunctiva is composed of a thin, transparent, avascular mucous membrane that covers the inside surfaces of the eyelids and the anterior surface of the sclera.

External Layer

The outermost layer of the eye is composed of two structures: the sclera and the cornea.

SCLERA The *sclera* is the white, opaque, and fibrous outer protective coat of the eye (Figure 50–1). It is continuous with the cornea anteriorly and with the dural sheath of the optic nerve posteriorly. Because the sclera is composed of dense connective tissue and many collagen fibers, it helps preserve the shape of the eye and protect the more delicate internal structures. The sclera forms five-sixths of the external layer of the eye.

CORNEA The *cornea,* a transparent avascular tissue, makes up one-sixth of the external layer of the eye and is situated in front of the iris. It functions as a refracting and protective window through which light rays pass en route to the retina. The cornea's greater curvature causes it to protrude from the sclera (see Figure 50–1).

The cornea has five distinct layers. The outer layer or epithelium, which is continuous with the conjunctiva, serves as a barrier to microorganisms and has an abundance of nerve fibers. Thus, abrasions to the corneal epithelium are very painful and may lead to infection of the deeper layers. The curve of the cornea bends light rays, producing approximately 50% of the focusing power of the eye.

Middle Layer

The middle layer of the eye, the *uveal tract,* is a vascular layer composed of three structures: the choroid, the iris, and the ciliary body and ciliary muscles.

CHOROID The *choroid,* a layer of tissue that lies between the retina and the sclera, extends from the edge of the optic nerve posteriorly to the ciliary body anteriorly (see Figure 50–1). It is composed largely of blood vessels that supply oxygen and nutrients to the outer portion of the underlying retina.

IRIS The *iris* is the pigmented circular membrane behind the cornea and in front of the lens that gives the eye its color (see Figure 50–1). It contains a central aperture or hole, the *pupil,* which regulates the amount of light entering the eye and increases the eye's depth of focus. Sphincter and dilator muscles within the iris regulate these processes by either dilating or constricting the pupil. Although changes in the size of the pupil are most often related to how much light enters the eye, drugs and changes in emotional states or attitudes also can affect pupil size.

CILIARY BODY AND CILIARY MUSCLES The *ciliary body* is anterior to the choroid and extends to the root of the iris (see Figure 50–1). A circular array of tiny spiderweb-like fibers, the *zonules,* stretches from the ciliary body to the lens to hold it in place. The *ciliary muscles* contract and relax the zonular fibers to the lens to put images upon the retina, adjusting focus between far and near objects (**accommodation**). The ciliary body also manufactures a steady flow of aqueous humor (discussed later in this chapter).

Inner Layer: The Retina

The *retina* is a thin structure with a neural tissue layer and a pigmented layer covering the inside of the back of the eye (see Figure 50–1). The pigmented layer stores vitamin A, an important precursor to the photosensitive pigment, *rhodopsin.* The neural layer contains more than 125 million photoreceptor cells, called *rods* and *cones* because of their respective shapes.

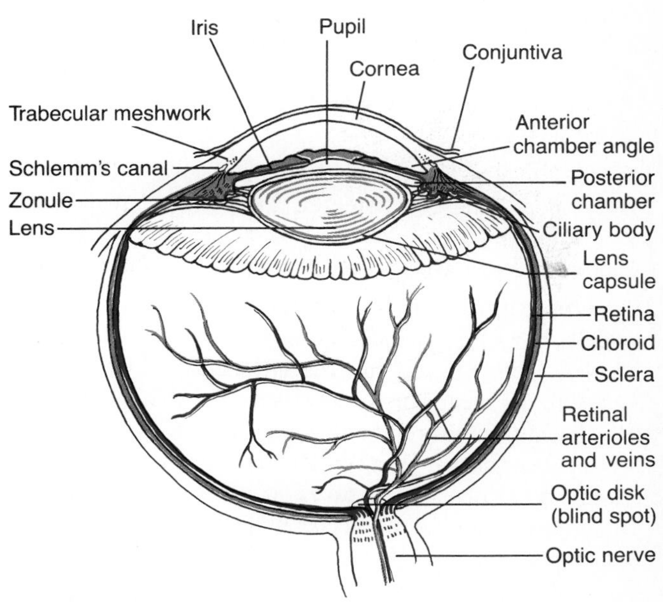

Figure 50–1

Internal structures of the eye.

Cones are specialized for fine visual discrimination and color perception. They are stimulated by medium and high levels of illumination. (That is why color cannot be detected by moonlight.) Cones are most densely concentrated in the yellow central portion of the retina, or *macula*. The center of the macula is the *fovea centralis*. Visual acuity is the greatest in this portion of the retina. Because of the high concentration of cones in the center of the retina, central vision has far better acuity than peripheral vision.

Rods, in contrast, are located peripherally to the fovea centralis. More sensitive to light than cones, rods can be stimulated by dim light. Rods also allow perception of shapes and movement in dim light and aid in peripheral vision.

The prime function of rods and cones is to absorb light. The energy from this absorbed light initiates a chemical reaction within the rhodopsin stored in the rods, causing electrical impulses to flow from the rods and cones into the neural layer of the retina. Axons from the neural layer converge at the back of the eyeball to form the optic nerve (Figure 50–1). The point at which the nerve fibers leave the eye to form the optic nerve is called the *optic disk*. Because it is free of photoreceptors and is light insensitive, the optic disk is called the *blind spot*. The optic nerve dispatches electrical impulses initiated in the retina to the brain for interpretation.

Diverging blood vessels emerge from the optic disk—usually in pairs of an artery and vein—and spread over the retinal surface.

Refractive Media

The *refractive media* are the transparent parts of the eye having refractive power, the ability to bend light rays at the surfaces of two transparent media. The eye has four refractive media: the cornea (already discussed), the lens, the aqueous humor, and the vitreous humor. Refraction is discussed in detail in the section, "Regulatory Functions of the Eye."

LENS The *lens*, a biconvex, avascular, transparent body about 8 mm in diameter, focuses light rays on the retina (see Figure 50–1). It is composed of a *cortex* and a central *nucleus* and is encased in a supportive elastic *capsule*.

VITREOUS HUMOR The *vitreous humor* is a clear, jellylike fluid that maintains the transparency and form of the eye. The vitreous fills the intraocular space from the retina to the posterior lens. Because the vitreous does not regenerate, its loss in any significant quantity as a result of trauma or surgery may create tension within the eye and distort other ocular structures. The vitreous may also disintegrate with age, allowing pigment or blood cells to become suspended in it and cast shadows (**floaters**) on the retina.

AQUEOUS HUMOR The *aqueous humor* is a clear watery fluid that provides nutrients to the lens and cornea, and contributes to the maintenance of intraocular pressure. It is secreted by the ciliary body into the *posterior chamber* of the eye (the area behind the iris and in front of the lens). Aqueous humor flows through the pupil into the *anterior chamber* of the eye, a narrow space between the cornea and iris, toward the trabecular meshwork and Schlemm's canal. The *trabecular meshwork* is a series of small openings or perforations in the connective tissue. Aqueous humor flows through and is filtered by the trabecular meshwork on its way to Schlemm's canal. *Schlemm's canal* is a large outflow channel that leads into the venous circulation.

Extrinsic Muscles of the Eye

Extrinsic muscles originate in the orbit and insert on the outside surface of the eyeball. These extrinsic muscles move the eyeball in various directions; so sensitively is their action adjusted that each fovea centralis normally is directed at the same object. There are six **cardinal directions of gaze**—directions in which the globe can move depending on which muscle is acting predominantly. These are illustrated in Figure 50–2.

Innervation of the Eye

The eye is supplied with motor and sensory nerves. The abducens (cranial nerve VI), trochlear (cranial nerve IV), and oculomotor (cranial nerve III) nerves are the three main motor nerves that innervate the extrinsic muscles of the eye.

The optic nerve (cranial nerve II), a "trunk" consisting of approximately 1 million axons arising from the retina, is the chief sensory nerve of the eye. It serves as a pathway for vision. The optic nerve emerges from the back of the globe and passes through a circular opening in the sclera to the optic chiasm, the area at the base of the brain just anterior to the pituitary gland where the left and the right optic nerves come together, and where one half of the fibers then cross to the opposite sides of the brain. The fibers then form the left and right optic tracts, which continue to the primary visual cortex, or visual area of the brain, in the occipital lobes. Each optic tract contains fibers from both retinas—the lateral retina of the same side and the medial retina of the opposite side (Figure 50–3). This anatomic structure has diagnostic significance because specific defects in the visual fields help to pinpoint the location of tumors or damage to the retina, optic nerve, or optic pathway. This is further discussed and illustrated in Chapter 29.

Another sensory nerve of the eye is the ophthalmic nerve, a branch of the trigeminal nerve (cranial nerve V). It carries sensations of pain, touch, and temperature to the eye. The facial nerve (cranial nerve VII) innervates the orbicularis muscle, which closes the eyelid.

Blood Supply to the Eye

The eye receives its main blood supply from the ophthalmic artery, a branch of the internal carotid artery. The ophthalmic artery in turn branches into several smaller

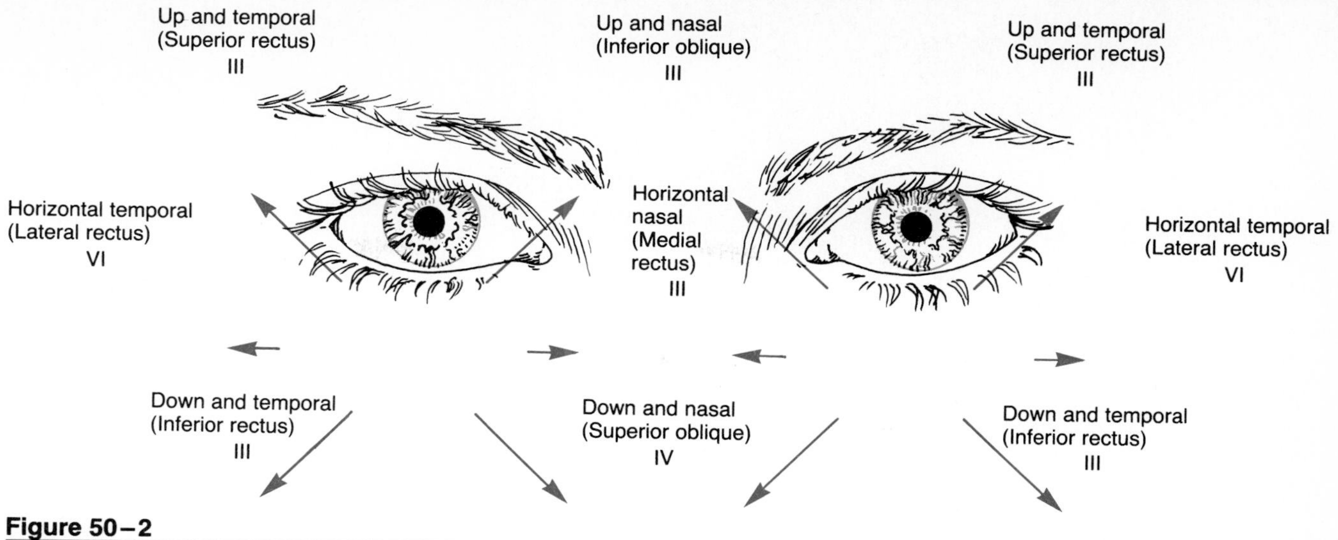

Figure 50–2

The six cardinal directions of gaze. The muscles that act predominantly are given in parentheses. The cranial nerves responsible for innervation are also listed.

arteries that supply blood to specific portions of the eye. The external carotid artery, in addition to the internal carotid artery, contributes to the blood supply of the eye and eyelids.

Regulatory Functions of the Eye

For normal binocular vision to occur (see Figure 50–3), the two eyes must simultaneously focus images on the same points of the two retinas. This provides a larger visual field and the ability to perceive depth. A coordinated process of refraction, accommodation, regulation of pupil size, and the meeting of visual lines (convergence) makes normal binocular vision possible.

Refraction

Refraction involves the passage of light rays from a transparent medium (such as air) into a second transparent medium with a different density (such as water). Refraction bends light rays at the surface of the two media. The light rays entering the eye are bent as they pass through the cornea and the lens on their way to the retina. If an object is 20 ft or more from the viewer, the reflected light rays are nearly parallel to one another and are sufficiently bent to fall on the fovea centralis, where sharpest vision takes place. However, objects closer to the viewer have reflected light rays that are divergent rather than parallel to each other. These divergent light rays must be refracted (bent) more toward each other for them to fall on the fovea centralis. This change in refraction ability is the responsibility of the lens.

Accommodation

The lens, through accommodation, can change shape; it becomes more convex or concave, thereby changing its focusing power. The more a lens curves outward, the more acutely it bends the light rays toward each other. When the eye is focusing on a close object, the reflected light rays are more divergent; thus, the lens curves greatly to bend the rays toward the fovea centralis. During accommodation, the ciliary muscle contracts and releases the tension on the lens, allowing it (because of its elasticity) to shorten, thicken, and bulge outward. In near vision, the ciliary muscle is contracted, and the lens is bulging. In far vision, the ciliary muscle is relaxed, and the lens is flatter. With aging, the lens loses elasticity and thereby loses some of its ability to accommodate; this condition is known as **presbyopia.** Any abnormalities related to improper refraction, such as **myopia** (nearsightedness), **hyperopia** (farsightedness), **astigmatism** (irregularities in the surface of the lens or cornea), or a lens opacity (cataract) may produce blurred or distorted visual images.

Regulation of Pupil Size

The regulation of pupil size is another crucial process in the formation of clear retinal images. The contraction of the circular muscle fibers of the iris causes pupil constriction, which narrows the diameter of the hole through which light rays enter the eye. This prevents light rays from entering the eye through the periphery of the lens. (These rays would not be focused on the retina and would result in blurred vision.)

Convergence

Convergence of the eyes—the medial movement of the two eyeballs so they are both directed toward the object being viewed—also is associated with focusing images on the retina. Convergence allows light rays to fall on and stimulate identical spots on the two retinas, resulting in the perception of a single image. If the extrinsic eye muscles are weak, damaged, or uncoordinated, light rays from an object fall on different points of the two retinas, and two objects are perceived (**diplopia**).

After an image has been formed on the retina by refraction, accommodation, constriction of the pupil, and

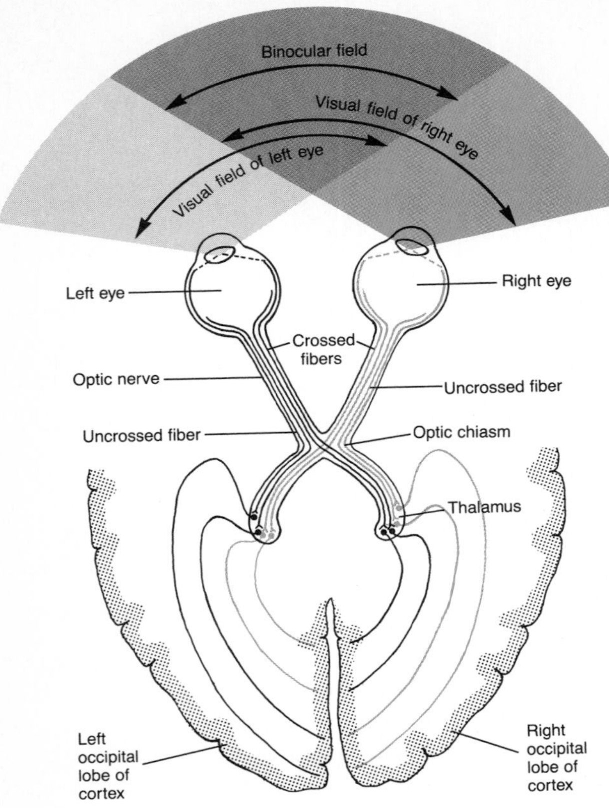

Figure 50–3

The pathway for visual impulses showing the visual fields. The colored arrows indicate the left portions of the visual field of each eye. The black arrows indicate the right portions. Binocular vision occurs when these visual fields overlap.

convergence, light impulses must be converted into nerve impulses by rods and cones. The light breaks down the photosensitive chemicals in either rods and cones (depending on the degree of illumination), which stimulates electrical impulses to be conducted to the brain for interpretation. The exact mechanism by which this occurs is not clear.

Regulation of Intraocular Pressure

Pressure in the eye is controlled by minute structures in the anterior chamber of the eye (the trabecular meshwork and Schlemm's canal) located at the *anterior chamber angle* between the cornea and the iris. Normally, this is where aqueous humor leaves the eyeball and enters the venous circulation. Essentially, the trabecular meshwork functions as release valves. If the intraocular pressure (IOP) is too low, outflow decreases; if the pressure is too high, outflow increases. In glaucoma, the fluid fails to flow normally into Schlemm's canal, and the accumulation of fluid causes IOP to rise. Increased IOP may cause atrophy of the optic nerve and result in loss of vision.

Structure and Function of the Ear

The ear can be divided anatomically according to external, middle, and inner structures.

External Ear

The external ear consists of two structures: the auricle, or pinna, and the external auditory canal, sometimes called the external acoustic meatus or external auditory meatus.

AURICLE The *auricle* (Figure 50–4) is the visible funnel-shaped part of the ear that is attached to the skull by muscles and ligaments. The auricle, with the exception of the lobule, consists of a thin layer of elastic fibrocartilage (more pliable in children than in adults) covered with closely adherent skin. The lobule consists of fatty tissue, which facilitates ear piercing. The auricle is the receptor for the mechanical vibrations of sounds—it catches sound waves and helps direct the sound waves through the concha to the external auditory canal.

EXTERNAL AUDITORY CANAL The *external auditory canal* (see Figure 50–4), which is only about 2.5 cm (1 in.) in length, bends downward and forward from the concha to the tympanic membrane (eardrum). The outer third of the canal consists of elastic cartilage, whereas the inner two thirds is bone. Skin lining the canal is continuous with the auricle and tympanic membrane. The thick skin lining the cartilaginous area contains numerous hair follicles, as well as sebaceous and apocrine glands. The hairs help prevent dirt, dust, and foreign bodies from entering the canal. Secretions from the sebaceous and apocrine glands form a yellowish-brown wax, **cerumen,** which serves a number of useful functions. First, it provides a self-cleaning system for the ear; second, it is bacteriostatic because of its acid pH; and third, its enzyme activity prevents drying of the epithelium in the canal (Marshall & Attia, 1983). The bony portion of the canal is lined with thin skin that is extremely sensitive to touch.

At the inner end of the external auditory canal is the *tympanic membrane,* a concave, shiny, pearly gray, translucent membrane that separates the external ear from the middle ear. When sound waves funnel through the canal and reverberate off the sides, they cause the tympanic membrane to vibrate.

Middle Ear

The middle ear, or *tympanic cavity,* is situated within an air-filled cavity of the temporal bone (see Figure 50–4). An opening in the posterior wall, the *tympanic antrum,* connects the middle ear with the mucous-membrane–lined mastoid sinuses of the mastoid portion of the temporal bone. The mastoid portion is located just posterior to the external auditory canal. The middle ear also connects with the nasopharynx through the eustachian tube, which enters

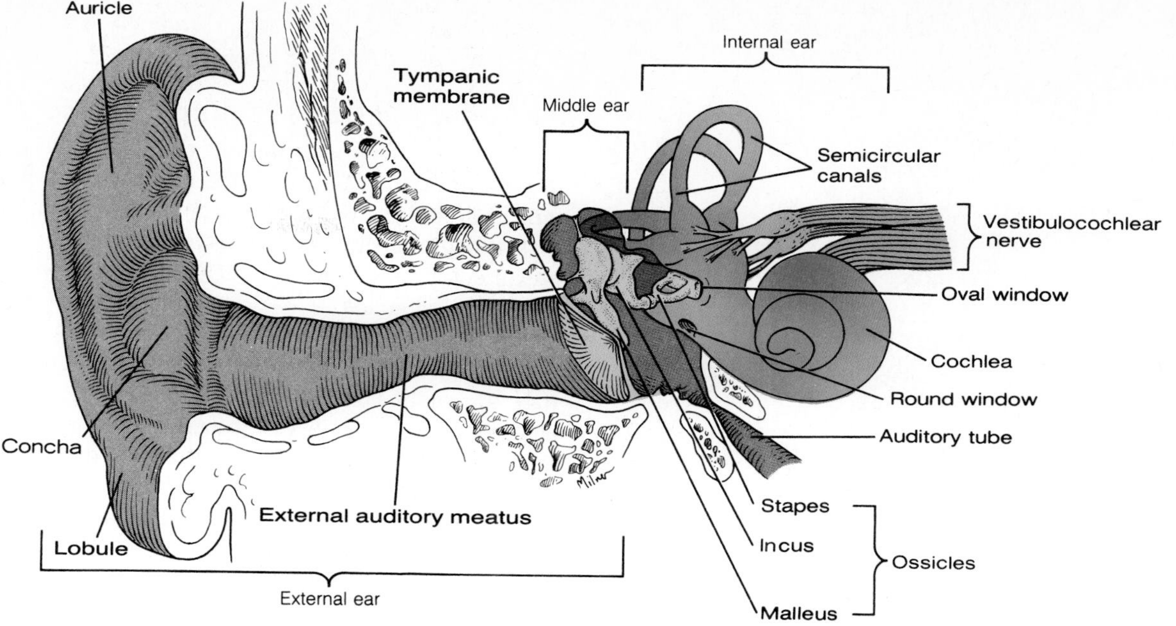

Figure 50–4

The ear. SOURCE: *Spence AP, Mason EB:* Human Anatomy and Physiology, *3rd ed. Menlo Park, CA: Benjamin/Cummings, 1987.*

the middle ear through an opening in the floor of the temporal bone. This anatomic feature makes it possible for microorganisms to enter the middle ear through the eustachian tube and even to move into the mastoid sinuses through the tympanic antrum, causing infections in either location. Because of the close proximity of the mastoid sinuses to the brain, infections there can spread to the meninges of the brain.

Because it connects the middle ear with the nasopharynx, the eustachian tube equalizes the pressure in the middle ear with atmospheric pressure. Swallowing and yawning open the eustachian tube, and high atmospheric pressure closes it.

Attached to the tympanic membrane is the ossicular chain, or ossicles, a set of three bones—the *malleus* (hammer), *incus* (anvil), and *stapes* (stirrup)—with freely movable synovial joints. The ossicles are the smallest bones in the human body. Figure 50–5 is a close-up view of the ossicles and their relationship to one another. The handle of the malleus is attached to the tympanic membrane. The incus is attached by ligaments to both the malleus and the stapes. The footplate of the stapes fits against the *oval window,* a membrane-covered opening of the temporal bone into the inner ear. These bones act as a chain of levers across the middle ear, transmitting and amplifying vibrations received at the tympanic membrane to the oval window and from there into the inner ear. The middle ear has a second membrane-covered opening into the inner ear called the *round window.*

Inner Ear

In the base of the skull between the sphenoid and occipital bones lies the petrous portion of the temporal bone, the most compact bone in the body. Within this petrous bone lie the inner ear and the internal auditory meatus, an opening through which the facial nerve (CN VII) and vestibulocochlear nerve (CN VIII) transmit their impulses to the brain.

The inner ear consists of two parts: the bony labyrinth and the membranous labyrinth. The bony labyrinth is a series of interconnecting passageways within the petrous portion of the temporal bone. The membranous labyrinth is similar in shape but smaller than the bony labyrinth and lies within it, much like the inner tube of a tire. The space between the bony labyrinth and the membranous labyrinth is filled with a watery fluid called *perilymph,* which separates them. The membranous labyrinth is filled with a similar fluid called *endolymph.*

The bony labyrinth consists of the cochlea (the anterior part); the vestibule (the central part); and the superior, posterior, and lateral semicircular canals (the posterior part). Correspondingly, the membranous labyrinth consists of the cochlear duct within the cochlea, the utricle and the saccule within the vestibule, and the semicircular ducts within the semicircular canals (Figure 50–6).

The organ of hearing, the *cochlea,* is a spiral, snail-shaped structure. On the basilar membrane of the cochlear duct is the spiral *organ of Corti,* which is responsible for converting mechanical energy (sound) into a form that stimulates the auditory nerve endings. The organ of Corti contains *hair cells* (the receptor cells of the nerve fibers of the auditory nerve) that rest on the basilar membrane. Hairlike projections from the hair cells are in contact with an overhanging gelatinous membrane called the tectorial membrane. These sensory hair cells are innervated by sensory fibers from the cochlear division of CN VIII.

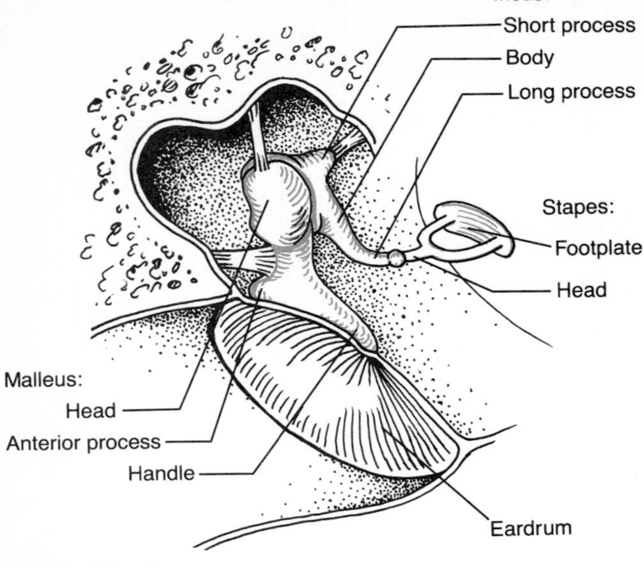

Figure 50–5

The ossicles. The handle of the malleus attaches to the tympanic membrane, through which it receives sound wave vibrations. The vibrations travel through the incus to the stapes and through its footplate to the membrane covering the oval window.

When the ossicles vibrate, causing the oval window to move inward, a fluid wave is created in the perilymph. This fluid wave causes the round window to bulge outward into the middle ear and moves the basilar membrane of the cochlear duct, causing the hairlike projections of the hair cells to move against the tectorial membrane and release chemical transmitter substances onto the afferent endings of the cochlear division of CN VIII. The result is a discharge of electrochemical impulses to the auditory fibers of the cochlear division of CN VIII, which transmits the electrical impulses to the brain.

The vestibule and three bony semicircular canals make up the vestibular system within the ear (refer to Figure 50–6). The *semicircular canals* are arranged at right angles to one another—much like the floor and two adjacent side walls in the corner of a room. Floating within the semicircular canals are three semicircular ducts. On the end of each duct is an enlargement called an ampulla, which contains a group of receptor hair cells, called cristae, embedded in a gelatinous mass. In response to turning the head, movement of the endolymph bends the hair cells. Consequently, these hair cells fire impulses to the nerve fibers of the vestibular portion of CN VIII.

The saccule and utricle, two enlargements of the membranous labyrinth within the vestibule, contain maculae (similar to cristae) covered with particles of calcium carbonate; these are known as *otoliths*. The otoliths press on the hair cells in response to different positions of the head, sending impulses to the vestibular branch of CN VIII. How equilibrium is maintained is discussed later in this chapter.

Blood and Nerve Supply to the Ear

Blood is supplied to the ear through branches of the internal and external carotid, the maxillary, the superficial temporal, and the occipital arteries. Veins drain into corresponding branches. Lymph from the ear drains into the preauricular, postauricular, occipital, and superficial and deep cervical nodes.

Nerve supply to the ear includes branches of the facial nerve (CN VII), vagus nerve (CN X), trigeminal nerve (CN V), vestibulocochlear nerve (CN VIII), and glossopharyngeal (CN IX) nerve. Stimulation of the vagus nerve accounts for reflex coughing or sneezing during examination of the ears, and stimulation of the trigeminal, facial, and glossopharyngeal nerves accounts for earaches with referred pain from the teeth, tongue, or pharynx. The auditory nerve is the vestibulocochlear nerve (CN VIII), which has two separate divisions—the cochlear and vestibular nerves. The two divisions join to form a common trunk, termed the vestibulocochlear nerve. The *cochlear division* innervates the hair cells of the organ of Corti and transmits impulses related to hearing to the cortex of the temporal lobe of the brain. The *vestibular division,* which supplies the vestibules and ampullae of the semicircular canals, maintains equilibrium. It transmits impulses to motor areas of the medulla and cerebellum.

Regulatory Functions of the Ear

The two primary regulatory functions of the ear are hearing and maintenance of equilibrium. Each of these functions is described here.

Hearing

To hear a sound, the ear must perceive sound waves that travel through the air, pass through the external auditory canal, are transferred to the inner ear, and are transmitted to the brain via the cochlear branch of CN VIII. Thus, hearing is a complex process involving the structures and fluids described earlier.

Two qualities of sound—pitch and intensity—are important in understanding hearing. *Pitch* is related to the frequency of the sound wave (the number of cycles per second, called hertz, or Hz). Sounds can be high pitched (a soprano voice) or of lower pitch (alto or bass). High-pitched sounds stimulate different portions of the basilar membrane than low-pitched sounds. High-pitched sounds stimulate the basilar membrane near the base of the cochlea; low-pitched sounds stimulate the basilar membrane near the apex of the cochlea.

Intensity is related to the loudness of the sound and is measured in decibels (dB). Each 10-decibel increase in the intensity of sound is actually a tenfold increase in loudness. A ticking watch makes a sound of about 20 dB. A noisy restaurant usually registers at a sound level of about 70 dB. This means that the noisy restaurant is 100,000 times

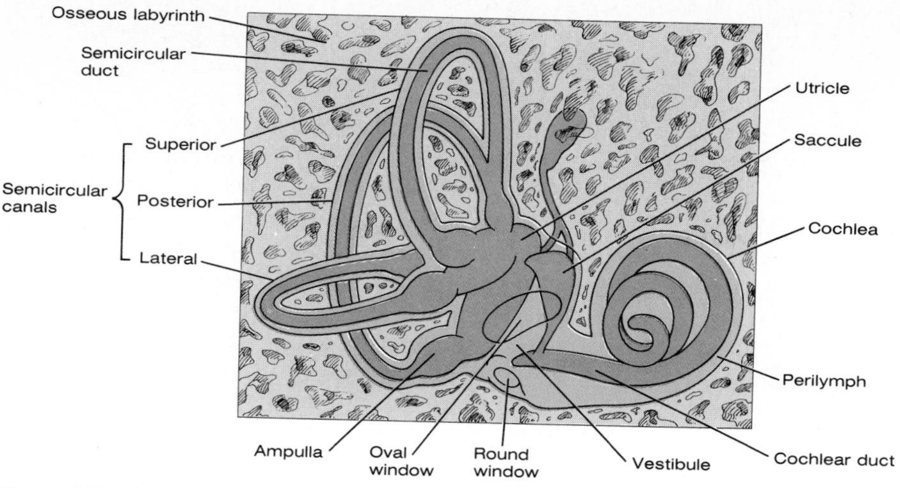

Figure 50–6

Structures of the inner ear. SOURCE: *Spence AP, Mason EB:* Human Anatomy and Physiology, *3rd ed. Menlo Park, CA: Benjamin/Cummings, 1987.*

as loud as a ticking watch. Both pitch and intensity are important in interpreting sound.

Equilibrium

The inner ear provides information about the movement and position of the head. The saccule and utricle inform us about position when the head is still, whereas the semicircular canals provide information about changes in position. We use this information to coordinate movements and to maintain balance. In these three organs of balance, receptor structures composed of hair cells with hairlike projections in contact with a gelatinous substance are sensitive to stimulation and movement of endolymph caused by changes in position. Displacement of the hairs alters the pattern of nerve impulses transmitted to the medulla and the cerebellum by the vesicular branch of CN VIII. The receptors in the ampulla, the *cristae,* help maintain balance during starting, stopping, or turning movements.

SECTION 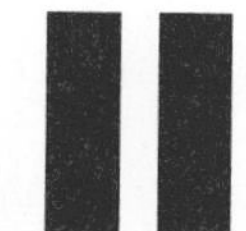

Pathophysiologic Influences and Effects

The Eye

Many pathophysiologic influences can alter the normal function of the eye. They may cause mild, temporary effects such as blurred vision and itchy eyes, or more severe and permanent afflictions such as blindness.

Congenital Alterations

Congenital alterations are genetically determined and are present at or before birth. They tend to occur in families and are usually bilateral. **Abiotrophic diseases,** which also are genetically determined, are not present at birth. Retinitis pigmentosa is an example of an abiotrophic disease that can lead to progressive visual impairment.

Refractive errors, motor anomalies (eg, ptosis and nystagmus), and congenital cataracts interfere with the normal development of sight unless corrected. Congenital metabolic disorders frequently associated with other anomalies also may contribute to a variety of alterations to the eye. The lens, the cornea, or both may be clouded; the nervous system may be affected; **photophobia** (ocular discomfort induced by bright light) may occur; and a number of other alterations may be present. In short, they all impair vision, and they may all be associated with pain, psychologic adjustments, and even blindness.

Multifactorial Alterations

Syphilis or rubella of the mother, premature birth, infant oxygen intoxication, trauma, and drugs ingested by the mother during pregnancy all have been associated with dysfunctions of the eye and reduced vision. Retinal detachment, refractive errors, and glaucoma are other conditions that have a range of possible etiologies during adulthood.

Degenerative Alterations

The aging eye undergoes many normal degenerative processes. The eyelids may wrinkle or droop because of decreased skin elasticity. Senile plaques and infiltrates are occasionally found on the conjunctiva or cornea and produce distorted vision. The lens may lose its transparency and its ability to change shape with ciliary muscle constriction, thereby producing blurred vision and decreased accommodation. Arteriosclerosis of vessels supplying the choroid and retina may result in decreased central vision, night blindness, or complete blindness.

Degenerative alterations also may occur as a secondary phenomenon resulting from other diseases. These may be either monocular or binocular. Inflammations of the cornea, conjunctival disease, and chronic glaucoma may lead to degeneration of the cornea, epithelial tissue, and lens, respectively. These, along with many other degenerative alterations, can affect the eyes with varying degrees of severity.

Immunologic Alterations

Allergens such as pollen, dust, hay, and cats may cause rapid vascular congestion (edema), itching, tearing, and burning of the eyes. These symptoms are usually temporary and have no residual effects. Inherited allergenic diseases are termed atopic diseases and are antibody mediated.

Nonatopic immunologic (cell-mediated) diseases of the eye include corneal allograft reactions and corneal ulcers formed in response to bacteria. Systemic immunologic diseases such as multiple sclerosis, rheumatoid arthritis, and systemic lupus erythematosus can also adversely affect the eye, causing disorders such as optic neuritis, glaucoma, cataracts, or corneal lesions that in turn cause pain, mental anguish, and loss of vision.

Infectious Alterations

Bacterial, viral, or fungal microorganisms can infect the external eye structures (eyelids, lacrimal glands, and conjunctiva) relatively easily and cause swelling, redness, pain, tearing, discharge, and blurred vision. Hordeola (styes) and cysts are common problems associated with infection of the cilia or meibomian glands. The loss of the corneal epithelium, which acts as a barrier to most infections, may result in corneal ulcers that cause pain and impaired vision. Infectious involvement of the central nervous system may give rise to muscle palsies and optic neuritis.

Neoplastic Alterations

A wide variety of both benign and malignant tumors occurs in the eye, eyelid, and orbit. These tumors may destroy important structures, interfere with their function and cause mild to severe effects, or both. Intraocular lesions may obstruct vision, interfere with aqueous humor drainage, displace the lens, or cause retinal detachments. Corneal lesions produce decreased vision. Retrobulbar and orbital tumors may displace the eye forward and cause diplopia and exophthalmos. Like any neoplasm, a neoplasm in the eye may invade blood vessels, become dispersed in surrounding tissues, and eventually lead to death.

Traumatic Alterations

Despite the many protective mechanisms of the eye, the incidence of eye injuries is high. Whether the effects of trauma are long- or short-term depends on the extent and type of injury incurred and which tissues are damaged. Corneal abrasions, burns, and perforations cause pain, scarring, photophobia, and possible infections. Contusions can affect all eye structures and elicit edema, vitreous hemorrhages, retinal detachments, hyphema (blood in the anterior chamber of the eye), lens dislocation, glaucoma, and optic nerve damage. The effects of these conditions include pain, photophobia, decreased acuity and vision, blindness, ecchymoses (a "black eye"), and body image changes. Penetrating injuries frequently cause ocular infections and may lead to blindness. All eye injuries carry the potential for further injury and increased chances of permanently impaired vision.

The Ear

A person with a hearing loss, or **hypoacusia,** has a functioning, though defective, auditory system and can respond to amplified sounds. Hearing loss can be classified as *conductive* (or peripheral), *sensorineural* (or perceptive), or *mixed* (or combined). Conductive hearing loss results from defective transmission of acoustic energy (sound) from the auricle to the hair cells of the organ of Corti. Conductive hearing loss generally occurs in the external ear, the middle ear, or both. Modern microsurgical observations have broadened the concept to include the cochlear fluid system in the inner ear (eg, a loss of perilymph fluid would also affect the transmission of energy). Sensorineural hearing loss results from dysfunction occurring anywhere in the neural pathway from the organ of Corti to the auditory cortex of the brain. Sensorineural hearing loss is sometimes referred to as central hearing loss. A combination of conductive and sensorineural hearing loss is called mixed, or combined, hearing loss.

Congenital Alterations

Congenital hereditary disorders can cause structural malformations or missing parts of the ear, which can lead to deafness or conductive, sensorineural, or mixed hearing loss. Congenital acquired disorders, in contrast, result from the following:

- Trauma incurred during pregnancy or during delivery
- Syphilis and bacterial or viral infections of the mother during pregnancy
- Certain drugs taken by the mother during pregnancy
- Rh incompatibility
- Prematurity or prolonged anoxia of the infant

Degenerative Alterations

Degenerative changes in the ear from aging are similar to those seen in other parts of the body. Loss of elasticity, thinning of the epidermis, and a decrease in secretions from the sebaceous glands result in dryness and pruritus of the external ear and narrowing of the auditory canal. Degenerative changes in the bones and joints of the ossicles can result in conductive hearing loss. Narrowing of blood vessels and the resulting decreased circulation to the inner ear can cause **tinnitus** (ringing, buzzing, or hissing in the ear or head), **vertigo** (sensations of disturbed motion), or hearing loss. A decrease in the number of hair cells and nerve fibers with aging results in presbycusis, a gradual sensorineural hearing loss.

Immunologic Alterations

Contact dermatitis evidenced by pruritus and pain in the external ear is caused by an allergic reaction to earrings, hair dyes, cosmetics, or shampoos. Pollens, dusts, and other allergens can increase mucous secretions in the eustachian tube and the middle ear. These sticky secretions cause malfunctions of the eustachian tube and decreased mobility of the tympanic membrane and ossicles, resulting in conductive hearing loss.

Infectious Alterations

Bacteria, yeasts, and fungi are the usual causes of infections of the external ear. These can result in excruciating pain or obstruction of the external auditory canal that leads to mild conductive hearing loss. Upper respiratory tract infections transmitted through the eustachian tube are usually responsible for middle and inner ear infections. These can cause fever, pain, and mild conductive hearing loss.

Neoplastic Alterations

Basal and squamous cell carcinomas as well as melanomas can affect the skin of the external ear. Benign or malignant tumors can affect the middle ear, inner ear, or auditory and facial nerves as they pass through the internal auditory canal. Middle ear tumors may be accompanied by extreme pain associated with otorrhea (discharge) and conductive hearing loss. Inner ear and nerve involvement can lead to vertigo, tinnitus, sensorineural hearing loss, and facial paralysis.

Obstructive Alterations

The amount of cerumen within the ear canal varies from individual to individual; some tend to produce large amounts, which often obstruct the external canal. Foreign bodies include vegetable objects, such as peas or beans; beads; flying insects; or cotton. Attempts to remove such objects often result in trauma and infection, which lead to edema, pain, and temporary conductive hearing loss. Polyps in the external auditory canal may also obstruct the passage of sound waves.

Edema from an upper respiratory tract infection also occurs in the eustachian tube. Obstructions in the eustachian tube prevent air from entering the middle ear, causing an imbalance of pressure on either side of the tympanic membrane. Decreased pressure in the middle ear can disrupt the transmission of sound to the inner ear. Other obstructions resulting from trauma or neoplastic disorders cause pain as well as hearing loss.

Traumatic Alterations

Frostbite, lacerations, and bruises to the external ear, although painful, usually do not result in hearing loss. Direct blows to the head, however, can result in fractures of the temporal bone, dislocation of ossicles, lacerations in the mucous lining of the middle ear, rupture of the oval window and tympanic membrane, and damage to the auditory nerve. Trauma can lead to vertigo, pain, bleeding from the ear, nausea, vomiting, nystagmus, tinnitus, and conductive and sensorineural hearing losses. Hearing loss also can result from continued exposure to loud noise or sudden but limited exposure to a loud explosive sound.

SECTION 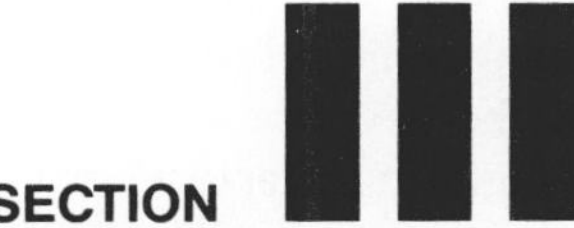

Related System Influences and Effects

Function of the eyes and ears, like that of many structures of the body, is related to the normal function and processes of other body systems.

Nervous System

CNS disorders such as meningitis and encephalitis may alter the function of the optic nerve or motor nerves or interfere with the visual pathways. Guillain–Barré syndrome may lead to corneal ulceration if facial paralysis results in the inability to close the eyelids. Clients with multiple sclerosis may have blurred vision when paralysis of the extrinsic muscles occurs. The auditory pathways may also be affected by multiple sclerosis, resulting in hearing loss. Ocular symptoms also occur with cerebral palsy, head trauma, and brain abscess. These alterations may result in a variety of symptoms (eg, the loss of peripheral or central vision or vision loss in one eye) and can affect vision permanently or temporarily.

Cardiovascular and Respiratory Systems

Blood vessels of the eye are subject to the same changes from diseases such as arteriosclerosis, atherosclerosis, and hypertension as vessels of the same size elsewhere in the body. A decrease in cardiac output, vascular occlusions, and thrombi all may impair blood supply to the eye. Increased intraocular pressure may result from an obstruction to the superior vena cava. Hypertension may potentiate *retinopathy* (noninflammatory degeneration of the retina) or intraocular hemorrhages. It is also possible that hypertension results in increased production of aqueous humor, thus contributing to glaucoma. Again, the conditions may temporarily or permanently impair vision, and a variety of symptoms may occur. Ischemia of the internal carotid artery frequently causes **amaurosis fugax** (a transient loss of vision in one eye). Aneurysms within the blood vessels of the brain or within the circle of Willis may cause pain above the eye, diplopia, and ptosis.

Bacterial and viral infections of the upper respiratory system affect the middle ear through the eustachian tube. Decreased circulation or vascular occlusion can result in vertigo; however, more research is needed to show the relationship with hearing losses.

Endocrine System

Diabetes mellitus is the most common cause of blindness in young people and in older people who have had diabetes for more than 10 years. Diabetes mellitus often causes retinopathy and, less frequently, the development of cataracts, optic neuropathy, and changes in refractive error.

Hyperthyroidism is frequently accompanied by prominent ocular changes such as exophthalmos because of an increase in the volume of orbital contents and eyelid retraction. Although no definite proof can be found, there appears to be a relationship between hearing loss and hypothyroidism (Goodhill, 1979).

Musculoskeletal System

Most autoimmune diseases, such as systemic lupus erythematosus and rheumatoid arthritis, influence ocular functions. The predominant effects of systemic lupus erythematosus are inflammation of the sclera (scleritis) or conjunctiva, the simultaneous inflammation of the cornea and conjunctiva, and retinal hemorrhage. The eyelids may sometimes be involved in facial lesions. Rheumatoid arthritis may herald scleritis and episcleritis (superficial scleritis) from circulating antigen–antibody complexes. These antigen–antibody complexes cause systemic inflammation and nodule formation in various body structures, including the sclera of the eye. Drugs used to treat diseases such as arthritis are toxic to the ear and may cause hearing loss (see Renal System below).

Just as many systemic diseases affect the function of the eye, so can alterations of the eye affect other body systems. For example, holding the head in a certain position to see, as is sometimes necessary with extraocular muscle dysfunctions, can lead to musculoskeletal problems such as stiffness of the neck or contractures.

Renal System

With impairment of the renal system, drugs such as acetylsalicylic acid (aspirin) that are mainly or entirely excreted by the kidneys can accumulate within the bloodstream. Ototoxic drugs (drugs with a noxious effect on CN VIII) may accumulate in the inner ear and cause tinnitus and a gradual sensorineural hearing loss. The exact cause of ototoxicity of acetylsalicylic acid is unknown. The hearing loss is usually bilateral but is reversible 7 to 10 days after acetylsalicylic acid use is discontinued. Hemodialysis and renal transplantation are frequently accompanied by sensorineural hearing loss and vestibular lesions. The administration of high doses of drugs may be a factor in this relationship.

Hepatic–Biliary System

Many other systemic diseases will not affect vision but may alter the eye's appearance. For example, liver diseases such as hepatitis cause icteric (jaundiced) sclera from the excess bilirubin in the blood. Such nonfunctional alterations are important clues in the diagnosis of other disease processes in the body. In this way, the eye serves as a window to the rest of the body.

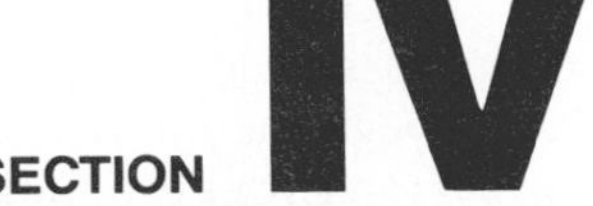

SECTION IV

Psychosocial/Lifestyle Influences and Effects

Impaired vision or hearing has both psychosocial and lifestyle influences and effects. Because vision and hearing are such an integral part of life, anything that affects them will affect the person's human relationships, self-concept, self-confidence, physical integrity and activity, communication, and career and financial security.

The way in which a person reacts to the loss of vision or hearing varies with the severity of impairment, the age at which the handicap occurred, the available support systems, and the way in which the person has dealt with other stressors in life. A loss of sight or hearing mandates many changes in learned behavior and in activities of daily living, presenting difficulties in meeting basic needs, including security, safety, nutrition, activity, and self-esteem.

Developmental Influences

People blind from birth seem to experience increased learning difficulties throughout life, because they have no memory of objects, color, or the environment. In addition, they suffer disturbances in proprioception and in achieving various social and developmental milestones. People who become blind later in life may have difficulty with developmental milestones that occur after sight has been lost.

Problems of hearing also affect psychosocial development. Those who do not hear well often find that their ability to communicate verbally is impaired, making it more difficult to resolve the psychosocial tasks successfully at various developmental stages and to meet the challenges of education and job preparation.

Sex and Age

With normal aging comes degenerative changes in the eyes' structures and, commonly, a gradual decrease in vision. These degenerative changes that accompany aging and result in impaired vision include presbyopia, dry eyes, glaucoma, macular degeneration, and cataract formation. Reduced vision leads to many psychosocial and behavioral changes in older people. For example, increased anxiety is prevalent among the elderly with impaired vision as their world becomes a confusing place. Visual loss, especially in the elderly, increases susceptibility to illusions, withdrawal, disorientation, and interpersonal isolation. People first experiencing presbyopia sometimes deny it and refuse to get glasses. Feelings of insecurity and isolation intensify for the aged driver with night blindness.

Other emotions experienced by the elderly with visual impairments include boredom, fear, depression, resentment, grief, anger, and lability of affect. Dry eyes (lack of tear secretions) are not only annoying; they also may evoke fear of further damage to the eye, such as ulceration. Artificial tears help this problem, but the frequent instillation required is often difficult for older people.

Other ocular changes occur well before old age. Adolescents generally experience mild hyperopia, because accommodative power can no longer counteract the hyperopic error. At about age 50, a further hyperopia tends to develop that is caused by lens changes. Myopia can be manifested early in life, occasionally at birth. It also can occur during periods of rapid growth and may continue to advance through adult life when degenerative changes occur. Thus, age plays a role in progression, and treatment varies accordingly.

More men than women have hearing impairment. This may be due largely to the fact that men are more likely to have been exposed to harmful levels of noise in the workplace than have women. Now that more women work outside the house, however, there is an increase in their reported instances of hearing problems that can be traced to the work environment. One genetic disorder, otosclerosis, is more common among women.

The instances of hearing loss increase with age (US Public Health Service, 1982); some degree of hearing loss is first noticed around age 50. It is one of the top three chronic conditions among the aging population, occurring in 25% over age 65, in 50% over age 75, and in 90% of the residents in nursing homes (Porcino, 1983).

Dietary Habits

Poor nutrition adversely affects all body systems. Vitamin A deficiency is most commonly associated with night blindness. Vitamin A is required for the regeneration of rhodopsin. Thus, a deficiency in vitamin A leads to a delay in darkness adaptation. Vitamin A deficiency also may contribute to a loss of integrity of the epithelial structures. The conjunctiva and cornea may become dry, keratoconjunctivitis (simultaneous inflammation of the cornea and conjunctiva) may occur, and corneal ulcers may develop.

Although no other specific vitamin deficiencies have been conclusively identified as a cause of specific eye conditions, many associations are being researched. Disorders of galactose metabolism are thought to contribute to the development of cataracts. Other associations are vitamin B deficiency with retrobulbar neuropathy and intraocular hemorrhage with clinical scurvy (vitamin C deficiency) (McLaren, 1980). These associations are most common in less developed rice-dependent countries.

Osteomalacia and sensorineural deafness are thought to be associated (Brookes & Morrison, 1981). Deficiencies of vitamin D and ionized calcium are thought to affect the transmission of action potentials generated by the cochlea. Lohle (1982) found a correlation between vitamin A deficiency and auditory thresholds in both animal and human experiments. More research on the role of nutrition in hearing impairment is needed.

Culture and Lifestyle

The eyes and ears and things associated with them, such as makeup, glasses, earrings, and hearing aids, have different significance and implications to various cultures and individuals. Some people think eye makeup brings attention and adds beauty to the eyes, whereas others feel it is unnatural and hides true beauty. Many in this culture equate the use of eye makeup with maturity and sophistication, because it is used mostly by adults. However, eye makeup is a common source of eye infections and allergies, so it should be used with care.

People also vary in their perception of correctional lenses (glasses or contacts) and hearing aids. Many stereotypes are associated with glasses or types of glasses. For example, thick, horn-rimmed glasses are frequently associated with studious people. Some people see the need for glasses or a hearing aid as an imperfection or a signal that they are getting older. To people of economically deprived countries, glasses and hearing aids may express a form of affluence; many individuals cannot afford them, let alone vision and hearing examinations.

Economic Factors

Economic situations may also indirectly affect the function of the eye and ear. Insufficient financial resources of families or societies often contribute to nutritional deficiencies of individuals. In addition, the lack of education and poor sanitation and housing conditions associated with the financially deprived may lead to increased eye and ear infections and a decreased resistance to other diseases. People often avoid health care (eg, routine eye and ear examinations and corrections) because they lack money to pay for the care received, there is a lack of health care facilities, or they are unable to pay for transportation to health care facilities. Some may not know of special provisions in income tax laws or insurance reimbursement for the vision- and hearing-impaired.

Vision- and hearing-impaired people may be forced into early retirement, reducing their income. In addition to its effects on individuals, early retirement under these circumstances also hurts society as a whole because it cannot benefit from the contributions of this segment of the population.

Occupation and Avocation

Various occupations increase the risk of ocular trauma and irritation, and occupational causes account for approximately 80% of all eye injuries (Voke, 1982). Chemical burns can damage the cornea and conjunctiva, causing pain, ulcers, and possible blindness or permanent visual loss. Chemical or thermal burns also can cause external scars to form, which impair the normal function of the eyelids.

Metal and engineering trades have a higher incidence of corneal abrasions and penetrating injuries, because industrial machines can propel foreign materials into the eyes of nearby personnel. Because of the risk of significant eye injury while working, safety glasses and other safety precautions, such as the designation of restricted areas and the provision of ocular irrigation fountains, are now mandatory in a number of industrial settings. Contusions to the eye are more prevalent in people whose occupations or leisure activities involve physical contact, such as athletes.

Sports injuries, especially those from racket sports (tennis, squash, and racketball), cause an increasing number of eye injuries each year. Hyphema is the most common eye injury. It is usually temporary, and normal vision is restored after the clot is absorbed in approximately 4 to 7 days. However, it may affect vision permanently if glaucoma or retinal detachments develop. Corneal abrasions and lacerations are also possible. Ear infections from water sports such as swimming and diving are common. Since some of the balls used in racket sports can travel more than 100 mph when hit with force, extensive injury to the eye or ear can occur. With hockey and lacrosse, blows to the eye and ear, as well as cuts and lacerations, are common.

Workers in some occupations incur exposure to radiant energy (ultraviolet light, infrared light, and other electromagnetic waves) at higher levels than normal. These occupations include welding, glassblowing, and any other jobs with prolonged exposure to the ultraviolet rays of the sun. Exposure to radiant energy may cause photophobia, superficial corneal lesions, and cataracts.

Many occupations now require the frequent or lengthy use of video display terminals (VDTs). At the request of labor unions, the National Institute for Occupational Safety and Health (NIOSH) has conducted an investigation to determine the potential health hazards associated with use of VDTs. The study indicates that the potential for visual alterations is practically nil.

Hazardous noises in the workplace cause hearing loss. Industrial workers exposed to the loud sounds of jet engines and heavy machinery, military personnel exposed to gunshots, and entertainers exposed to amplified music are especially vulnerable to noise-induced hearing loss. Unfortunately, workers—especially older workers—may be afraid to reveal their hearing loss to employers lest they lose their jobs. They may stay in environments that increase hearing loss.

Environmental Factors

Environmental influences may also adversely affect the function of the eye. These effects, which are usually temporary, include conjunctival irritation, tearing, blurred vision, and superficial infections. Smog, the prevalence of toxic chemicals, and water pollution are some of the contributing factors. Prolonged exposure to the sun without sunglasses can lead to photophobia and superficial lesions. Smokers frequently have conjunctival irritation, blurred vision, and difficulty seeing colors accurately. Some nonsmokers, because of high sensitivity, experience the same symptoms by just being in a room with a smoker.

The environment influences and affects blind or visually impaired people differently than it does sighted people. Activities usually taken for granted, such as grocery shopping, driving a car, or walking across a busy street, become more difficult, more dangerous, or impossible for the visually impaired.

Community noise is a major problem in contemporary society. Increased noise from vehicular traffic is one aspect of the problem. Another is the growing number of noisy labor-saving devices used in most homes, which exposes residents to levels of noise as hazardous as those in many industrial environments. The tendency of some young people to wear stereo headsets for long periods may also have some damaging effects. Pollution of lakes, rivers, and other waterways can also lead to hearing damage because of infections.

Chapter Highlights

The eyes, the sole means by which people gather visual data, are crucial sensory organs.

Protection is provided to the eye by the orbit, eyelids, tears, and conjunctiva.

The eye consists of three layers: The sclera and cornea make up the outer layer; the choroid, iris, and ciliary body constitute the middle layer; and the retina is the innermost layer.

The retina contains photoreceptors (rods and cones) that, when stimulated, send impulses to

the brain via the optic nerve. Cones are specialized for visual acuity and color discrimination, whereas rods are concerned with peripheral vision and vision under dim light.

The refractive media consist of four transparent structures: the cornea, lens, vitreous humor, and aqueous humor.

The regulatory process of the eyes that provides binocular vision involves refraction, accommodation, regulation of pupil size, and convergence.

The ears are special sensory organs whose major functions are hearing and maintaining equilibrium.

The ear can be divided anatomically into three structures: The auricle and the external auditory canal make up the external ear; the ossicles are contained within the middle ear; and the cochlea, organ of Corti, and semicircular canals are the major structures of the inner ear.

Hearing is a complex process that involves the external ear, middle ear, inner ear, the cochlear division of CN VIII, and the brain.

Hearing loss can be classified as conductive (resulting from defective transmission of acoustic energy or sound from the auricle to the hair cells of the organ of Corti), sensorineural (resulting from dysfunction occurring anywhere in the neural pathway from the organ of Corti to the auditory cortex of the brain), or mixed.

The inner ear provides information about the movement and position of the head and is responsible for maintaining equilibrium.

Alterations in other body systems may adversely affect the eye or the ear.

Loss of vision or hearing impoverishes human relationships and affects psychosocial development.

Culture and lifestyle may influence the function of the eye and the ear and the normal processes of vision and hearing.

Bibliography

Bateman HE, Mason RM: *Applied Anatomy and Physiology of the Speech and Hearing Mechanism.* Springfield, IL: Thomas, 1984.

Brookes E, Morrison AW: Vitamin D deficiency and deafness. *Brit Med J* (July) 1981; 283; 273–274.

Collins F: *Handbook of Clinical Ophthalmology.* New York: Masson Publishing USA, 1982.

Danino J et al: Tinnitus as a prognostic factor in sudden deafness. *Am J Otolaryngology* 1984; 5(6):394–396.

DeWeese D, Saunders W: *Textbook of Otolaryngology,* 6th ed. St. Louis: Mosby, 1982.

Dickman R: *A Vision Impairment of the Later Years: Macular Degeneration.* Washington, DC: Public Affairs Committee, 1982.

Garner A, Klintworth GK: *Pathobiology of Ocular Disease: A Dynamic Approach.* Marcel Dekker, 1982.

Goodhill V: *Ear Diseases, Deafness and Dizziness.* Hagerstown, MD: Harper & Row, 1979.

Keidel WD et al: *The Physiological Basis of Hearing.* Thieme, 1983.

Lohle E: The influences of chronic vitamin A deficiency on human and animal ears. *Arch Otorhinolaryngol* 1982; 234(2):167–173.

Marshall K, Attia E: *Disorders of the Ear.* Boston: John Wright-PSG, 1983.

McLaren DS: *Nutritional Ophthalmology,* 2nd ed. London: Academic Press, 1980.

Moses R: *Adler's Physiology of the Eye.* St. Louis: Mosby, 1981.

National Advisory Eye Council of the National Eye Institute. *Visual Research: A National Plan. 1983–1987.* Washington, DC: National Eye Institute, 1983.

Porcino J: *Growing Older, Getting Better.* Menlo Park, CA: Addison–Wesley, 1983.

Smolin G, O'Connor G: *Ocular Immunology.* Philadelphia: Lea & Febiger, 1981.

Spence AP, Mason EB: *Human Anatomy and Physiology,* 3rd ed. Menlo Park, CA: Benjamin/Cummings, 1987.

Spencer WH: *Ophthalmic Pathology.* 3rd ed. Philadelphia: W. B. Saunders, 1984.

US Department of Health and Human Services: *Potential Health Hazards of Video Display Terminals.* Washington, DC: US Government Printing Office, 1981.

US Public Health Service: *Vital and Health Statistics. Hearing Ability of Persons by Sociodemographic and Health Characteristics: United States.* PHHS Pub. No. (PHS) 82–1568. US Government Printing Office, Series 10, No. 140, 1982.

Vaughan D, Asbury T: *General Ophthalmology.* 9th ed. Los Altos, CA: Lange, 1980.

Voke J: Eye hazards in industry. *Occup Health* (Feb) 1982; 34–36.

CHAPTER 51

The Nursing Process for Clients With Visual or Auditory Dysfunction

Objectives

When you have finished studying this chapter you should be able to:

Specify the major components of the health history to be obtained from clients with visual or auditory dysfunction.

Explain specific assessment approaches in evaluating clients with visual or auditory impairment.

Identify the nursing implications of diagnostic studies commonly used to evaluate clients with visual or auditory dysfunction.

Determine appropriate nursing diagnoses for clients with disorders of the visual or auditory systems.

Develop, with the client, realistic goals of care.

Anticipate the psychosocial/lifestyle implications of visual or auditory dysfunction for clients and their significant others.

Develop a nursing care plan for a client with visual or auditory dysfunction.

Implement nursing interventions specific to clients with visual or auditory system disease.

Evaluate the effectiveness of the nursing care plan and modify it as necessary to meet client needs.

Care of clients with a loss of, or the threat of losing vision or hearing, is a major nursing challenge. The nurse can make a significant impact in the prevention and early detection of problems affecting the eyes and ears, as well as in the rehabilitation of clients with these disorders. This chapter discusses the nursing process as applied to clients with visual and auditory dysfunction.

SECTION 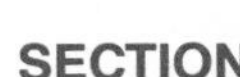

Nursing Assessment: Establishing the Data Base

Subjective Data

Clients With Visual Problems

The nurse begins assessment of a client with a visual disorder by determining the client's perception and feelings about the illness. Documentation of the client's primary concern is fundamental in making an accurate diagnosis, so a careful history is essential.

Determine the following in regard to symptoms: time of onset, duration, and whether the symptoms occur when the client is in certain positions or situations. It is important to determine whether the client has had treatment and is currently taking medication. Inquire about all medications the client takes because many drugs used for conditions unrelated to the eye have potential ocular side effects. Ask clients when they last had an eye examination and whether they wear corrective lenses and if so what kind. The nurse also will need to know the answers to such questions as:

- Has a decrease in visual acuity occurred?
- Has the client noted it in one eye or both?
- What exactly does the client see (or not see)?
- Does the client have pain?

DISTURBANCES IN VISION The client may experience *halos,* which are rainbow-colored rings encircling bright lights caused by an alteration in the ocular media. An incipient cataract is the most common cause, but rapidly increased intraocular pressure (IOP) from acute angle-closure glaucoma also may cause halo symptoms.

Photopsia, or the appearance of flashing lights, can disturb the client despite the short duration (less than a fraction of a second). It seems to worsen after dark and may be a warning signal of impending retinal detachment.

Floaters, small moving spots seen before the eye because of fine vitreous opacities, are visualized only when the eye is open. They are particularly apparent when viewed against an evenly illuminated bright background (such as a blue sky). Floaters are often due to the aging process; the vitreous degenerates and releases tissue deposits or sloughs off tissue. Floaters also may be due to hemorrhagic diseases (eg, diabetic retinopathy and hypertension) or to retinal tears, where small hemorrhages release red blood cells into the vitreous. Numerous or conspicuous floaters may help locate a retinal hole (indicating a vitreous hemorrhage). Most floaters do not warrant treatment or cannot be treated.

Diplopia (double vision), a common visual disorder, can be confused with vertigo because of certain similarities between the two, such as the inability to focus the eyes and a subsequent lack of equilibrium. It is important to determine the time of onset and duration of this symptom, as well as whether it occurs in certain positions or situations. Diplopia involves a weakness or paralysis of one or more of the extraocular muscles, and the visual axes of both eyes are not directed at the same object. Unilateral diplopia can occur with corneal opacity and cataracts by reflecting split light rays. Diplopia is often also seen in myasthenia gravis, thyroid exophthalmos, transient ischemic attacks, and orbital injuries with globe displacement.

PAIN AND IRRITATION Ocular pain takes many forms and necessitates careful investigation to determine its cause. Determine whether the pain occurs after extensive use of the eyes. Such pain is often **asthenopia**—ocular discomfort related to an uncorrected refractive error. The term *eyestrain,* commonly used to describe this condition, is actually misleading; strain connotes damage, but prolonged use of the eyes does not damage them.

Pain can range from aches (from accompanying fatigue, frontal sinusitis, or muscle imbalance) and stabbing pain (from penetrating injury or corneal ulceration) to sensations of pressure usually resulting from an abrupt increase in IOP (from angle-closure glaucoma). Severe pain can occur with inflammations of the iris and ciliary body, scleritis, and herpes zoster ophthalmitis. Other causes of pain include chemical irritants and blepharitis. Severe eye pain always requires examination by a physician.

In evaluating the client's pain, consider his or her anxiety level. A fear of blindness (the most dreaded sensory loss) or any alteration in the function of the eye may be paramount in the client's mind, possibly affecting not only the client's response but also the degree of discomfort experienced.

Headaches are a common discomfort associated with the eyes; they have numerous possible causes, many of them unrelated to the visual system. Assess the type of headache and its history of onset, relationship to eye use, location, duration, and associated symptoms. A refractive error seldom causes a headache. Should the client experience eye fatigue, the associated headache will probably be frontal, and refraction testing may indicate the need for corrective lenses. Other eye examinations can rule out an ocular basis for the headache, and a more complete physical assessment then becomes necessary.

Severe deep ocular pain usually indicates an increase in IOP, as is found in glaucoma. In severe acute glaucoma, the pain may be intense enough to precipitate nausea and vomiting. Untreated, a severe attack of acute glaucoma can cause permanent blindness within a few days.

Acute localized pain aggravated by movement of the eye or eyelid suggests a foreign body or corneal abrasion. Misdirected eyelashes rubbing on the cornea (*trichiasis*), **entropion** (inversion of the eyelid margin), conjunctivitis, and keratitis can cause considerable discomfort and require ophthalmic treatment.

Burning and itching generally do not indicate serious eye disease. The most frequent cause is inflammation of the eyelids or conjunctiva from irritation or infection. Smoke, smog, wind, and allergic reactions from hay fever or eye makeup can precipitate such symptoms. Prolonged use of the eyes (eg, long periods of time sitting at a computer terminal) also can cause mild irritation.

Dryness of the eyes occurs for many reasons ranging from conditions characterized by hypofunction of the lacrimal glands to excessive evaporation of tears to mucin deficiency. As dry spots appear on the corneal and conjunctival epithelium, vision may become slightly impaired, the client may feel burning or smarting, and secondary bacterial infections may occur. Early preventive treatment can reduce these complications.

Epiphora, excessive watering of the eye, is a common condition; it occurs when any portion of the lacrimal system is blocked or when the lower eyelid is displaced due to congenital, traumatic, inflammatory, or degenerative causes.

Lacrimation is the overproduction of tears; apart from emotion, it is caused by local irritation of the conjunctiva, cornea, or iris or by photophobia. Facial nerve paralysis (Bell's palsy) may cause unilateral lacrimation. Abnormal regeneration of the facial nerve fibers and an invasion of the salivary gland secretory fibers into the lacrimal glands (as occurs in Bell's palsy) results in increased tear secretions (crocodile tears) while eating. The origins of emotional, or psychogenic, tearing (crying) are in the hypothalamus. Emotional tearing is always bilateral.

Photophobia, an abnormal intolerance to light, is most often caused by corneal inflammation, iridocyclitis (inflammation of the iris and the ciliary body), and **aphakia** (absence of the lens). Photophobia can sometimes be associated with emotional distress and needs careful assessment. Regardless of its cause, the sudden appearance of severe photophobia may indicate a serious eye condition. The nurse should respond by darkening the room and providing supportive therapy. Some medications may produce photophobia. All mydriatic ophthalmic medications produce photophobia.

CHANGE IN THE EYE'S APPEARANCE *Red eye* is due to congestion of blood in the conjunctival or ciliary blood vessels. The eye displays a diffuse redness, the extent of which depends on the etiology and may alarm the client. Red eye is a cardinal sign of ocular inflammation and provides a detectable warning signal of many diseases. Conjunctival **injection** (congestion of blood vessels) is uncomfortable but does not compromise visual function. Because a red eye is the most obvious symptom nurses can recognize, they should also give serious attention to accompanying symptoms such as loss of vision, pain, visible loss of transparency of normally clear parts of the eye, irregular pupils, and a definite circular pattern around the cornea. These symptoms may indicate vision-threatening disorders such as acute angle-closure glaucoma, uveitis, and keratitis; or systemic diseases such as Sjögren's syndrome, hyperthyroidism, polycythemia vera, and gout.

Hyphema, or blood in the anterior chamber between the cornea and iris, results from a tear in the ciliary body. Hyphema is easily detected by a penlight. A subconjunctival hemorrhage is a localized, patchy area of bleeding from the rupture of a small blood vessel beneath the conjunctiva. Yellow sclera are commonly associated with jaundice. The sclera also may appear yellow from the use of antimalarial drugs (a normal side effect) or from their toxicity. The sclerae of blacks and other dark-skinned people are often yellowish in the normal state. A tumor beneath the sclera may cause discoloration.

Mucopurulent drainage from the eyes usually indicates a bacterial infection. The nurse should note the character and amount of discharge, when it occurs, and whether chronic crusting of the eyelid margins occurs. A specimen for microscopic identification, culture, and sensitivity testing may be required.

PERSONAL/SOCIAL AND FAMILY HISTORY Lifestyle considerations are important in gathering subjective data for clients with ocular dysfunctions. Assess nutrition because ocular pathology can be related to vitamin deficiency. Avitaminosis A has been associated with corneal ulcers and xerophthalmia (dryness of the conjunctiva and cornea). In avitaminosis C (scurvy), hemorrhages may develop in the eye as well as the skin, mucous membranes, and other parts of the body. Finally, people with poor nutritional habits may develop nutritional amblyopia (dimness of vision).

The client's age is important in determining degenerative changes and appropriate treatment. Loss of vision is often attributed to the aging process when, in fact, a condition may exist that can be corrected by medical attention.

The client's occupation can affect eye health. Does the client's job involve video display terminals, working with small objects, exposure to machinery, or exposure to chemicals, all of which can cause eye fatigue or visual loss? Decreased job performance may be a clue to blurred vision or intrusive symptoms such as headaches.

A careful family history will document congenital disorders of the eye or glaucoma within the client's blood relatives. A history of other diseases in the family that have ocular complications, such as hypertension and diabetes mellitus, is also significant.

Impaired vision or complete loss of vision can be devastating, causing depression, anxiety, and feelings of helplessness and isolation. Without visual aids, the formerly independent client may abandon hobbies, reading, and writing. Clients cut off from these activities of daily living and from visual stimuli may experience sensory deprivation, become depressed, and even suicidal.

Determine the client's home situation. Is the client living alone? Are family or friends in the area, and how do they feel about the client's visual loss? How is the client managing activities of daily living? What transportation is available? What is the client's economic status? Can the former job be resumed, or will the client have to seek another career direction? If the client requires medication such as insulin how will it be administered? Has the client been through a rehabilitation program to relearn mobility with a cane or to learn to use other aids to assist with activities of daily living? These and similar questions help the nurse assess the client's potential adjustment to visual loss.

Clients With Auditory Problems

The health history should begin with an exploration of the client's chief concern, whether it is hearing loss, pain (otalgia), discharge (otorrhea), tinnitus, or vertigo.

HEARING LOSS Careful questioning about any decrease in hearing is critical to the evaluation of the client with ear dysfunction. The client may not report a hearing loss until it is quite extensive. Family members or significant others are usually the first to recognize the loss. Obtain information relating to impaired hearing through questions such as:

- Is the hearing loss in one or both ears?
- Was the onset sudden or gradual?

- Is hearing more problematic in particular situations (eg, large groups)?
- Are all sounds or just certain sounds diminished?
- Is there a family history of hearing loss?

For the client with a known hearing loss, information specific to aural rehabilitation should be obtained. For example, does the client communicate manually or use speech reading? Usually, younger clients have been taught these skills, but older clients may need considerable assistance. Does the client use a hearing aid? Is it effective? Often clients have purchased a hearing aid but do not use it. Find out why it is not being used. Many clients are reluctant to accept their hearing disability, so they may reject the use of a hearing aid because it then becomes obvious that they have a hearing impairment. Some may not take the time to adjust to its use, and others may not have the financial resources to purchase a hearing aid and batteries and to provide for repairs. Also, many elderly clients do not have the manual dexterity to use or clean hearing aids.

PAIN AND DISCHARGE *Otalgia* may be caused by a specific disorder of the ear itself or by referred pain from other diseases of the head and neck. Differentiating between the two in the history is important for accurate care planning. Referred pain to the ear may be associated with temporomandibular joint disorders, malocclusion, or nocturnal teeth grinding (bruxism). Carious teeth; lesions of the mouth, tongue, hypopharynx, or larynx; or calculi in the parotid or submaxillary duct also may cause referral pain to the ear. Otalgia directly related to the ear may be secondary to trauma, infection, allergies, the presence of foreign bodies, impacted cerumen, or benign or malignant growths. Therefore, the history should elicit information about sports activities, particularly swimming and diving. Direct trauma to the ear can be caused by many contact and racket sports. Swimmer's ear (diffuse bacterial external otitis) is a common cause of ear pain. Barotrauma, which results from excessive ear pressure due to rapid or extensive altitude changes, can cause rupture of the tympanic membrane.

The nurse should ask questions about recent infections. For example, the client may have pain from enlarged cervical or auricular lymph nodes secondary to an upper respiratory tract infection that is referred to the ear. However, the client may also have an inflammation of the eustachian tube (eustachian tube salpingitis). The inflammation creates a vacuum in the inner ear with unilateral or bilateral middle ear effusion and retracted tympanic membrane(s), causing discomfort and a feeling that the ear needs to pop or crack.

An allergy history is important to document any seasonal allergies causing ear symptoms and nasal congestion, such as hay fever. Often the symptoms of seasonal allergy are similar to those of a viral upper respiratory tract infection. Medication allergies are also important to consider because the client may be using something topically on the auricle for pruitus or discomfort (eg, around a bothersome pierced ear opening) that is causing weeping, flaking, and inflammation rather than curing the problem.

One of the most common trauma and foreign body problems in adults is related to care of the ears. Many people dig in their ears with paper clips and cotton swabs. Clients come to ambulatory care facilities with trauma to the auditory canal or tympanic membrane, or with foreign bodies in their ears, because of improper cleaning with small, sharp objects. Clients might be advised facetiously that nothing smaller than their elbows should enter their ears.

Cerumen is problematic for many clients because it may cause scaling, pruritus, discomfort, and a decrease in hearing. Proper mastication normally takes care of cerumen by moving it to the external ear, where it flakes off unnoticed or is easily washed off. Therefore, a history of dental or jaw problems is significant. Clients with ill-fitting dentures or those who do not wear their dentures at all chew poorly, which interferes with normal cerumen removal. Clients who work in areas where there is considerable dust and dirt also may build up more cerumen, because the wax, in trapping this foreign material, tends to become harder and thicker. These clients need health education regarding safe ways to loosen and remove cerumen.

Otorrhea is an annoying symptom for many clients. Discharge may accompany external otitis or otitis media, or it may indicate the presence of a foreign body. Question clients about the color, odor, and amount of the discharge. Certain organisms causing otorrhea have characteristic odors. For example, drainage from the ear caused by *Pseudomonas* often smells sweet. (See Table 51–1 for characteristics of otorrhea.)

Table 51–1
Otorrhea: Color and Usual Cause

Appearance of Discharge	Usual Cause
Yellow	Soft cerumen
Green	Acute external otitis
Serous	Eczematous lesions of auditory canal wall; early acute otitis media; cerebral spinal fluid from fracture of middle cranial fossa
Purulent	Acute or chronic otitis media; tuberculous otitis media; cholesteatoma
Bloody	Trauma to auditory canal walls; rupture of tympanic membrane; fracture of middle cranial fossa

TINNITUS AND VERTIGO The nurse should also ask the client about **tinnitus.** Tinnitus is a sensation of noise such as ringing, buzzing, or hissing in the ear or head. This can accompany other symptoms such as otalgia and otorrhea secondary to impacted cerumen, the presence of a foreign body, or inflammation. It may also occur alone, can be extremely annoying and uncomfortable, and can interfere with sleep and normal daily activities.

Specific data to be collected include the perceived site of the tinnitus, its loudness and pitch, and its disappearance in the presence of other sounds. Tinnitus may be louder at night or certain times of the day or week. It may vary with the position of the head or body. Obtain information about noise exposure on the job and in the home. High-pitched tinnitus can be associated with an ototoxic reaction to drugs such as propranolol, caffeine, salicylates, quinidine, and indomethacin. A drug history is essential and should include all OTC drugs as well as prescription drugs that the client is taking or has taken in the past. The drug history also should include any history of drug allergies or side effects that the client has experienced.

Vertigo is a spinning sensation: Clients feel as if they are spinning or that the room is whirling around them. It is frequently associated with nystagmus, nausea, and vomiting. Vertigo is the most common symptom of a vestibular disorder. The health history can assist in differentiating between true vertigo and dysequilibrium. Vertigo may accompany diseases of the middle or inner ear. *Dysequilibrium* is a nonvestibular symptom of spacial disorientation. It is related to changes in cerebral oxygenation, changes in blood pressure, drugs, visual or emotional disturbances, and various metabolic disorders. Dysequilibrium is often described as an unsteadiness, queasiness, faintness, lightheadedness, or a blacking-out sensation. It usually is not accompanied by nystagmus.

PERSONAL/SOCIAL HISTORY Identify any lifestyle changes that have occurred as a result of the hearing impairment by asking about the client's activities during a 24-hour period. The client's role and responsibility in the family may be altered and diminished. An inability to participate in family discussions becomes frustrating for the client. Family members or significant others also become frustrated in trying to communicate and begin to ignore the client when the communication becomes difficult. Communication difficulties can also occur in social groups. The hearing-impaired person finds it difficult to enjoy meetings, parties, or lectures, or even to follow normal dinner table conversation. These difficulties result in client withdrawal from everyday activities and eventually isolation, which can result in depression. The acceptance of the hearing loss helps motivate the client to overcome communication difficulties through rehabilitation programs, the use of a hearing aid, or both.

The nurse should gather additional health history information about health risks. Both smoking and lack of exercise can affect ear disorders. Smoking irritates the mucous membranes in the upper respiratory tract, which can alter the function of the eustachian tube and lead to infections in the middle ear. Nicotine also causes blood vessel constriction. Auditory and vestibular functions rely on good circulation to the structures of the ear.

Eliciting information about the client's resources and support systems will aid in the planning of care. The elderly person living alone often has no support systems. The nurse should identify the availability of health and emergency services for the client. A social work referral for assistance with meeting the costs of rehabilitation programs may be needed.

Individuals with hearing loss function effectively in many professions and vocations, but they may experience difficulty in areas of employment that depend on sensory perception for safety, such as some assembly line positions. Through the history, the nurse may identify a need for vocational counseling. Vocational counselors assist clients in job relocation or suggest adaptations in the existing workplace for the hearing impaired. For example, a client who is gradually developing a noise-induced hearing loss that may be exacerbated by working in a noisy environment may be helped to find a similar position in a quieter environment or to find ways to reduce the noise in the present job.

Objective Data

Assessment of the Eyes

Physical examination of the eyes consists primarily of inspection with and without specific ocular tools. Before inspecting the eyes, look at the client. Note posture that may be compensating for a lack of clear vision. Evaluate the expression on the client's face; a wrinkled forehead might indicate eye pain, photophobia, or an attempt to elevate the upper eyelid in ptosis. Squinting may indicate strabismus. Look to see whether there is symmetry between the eyes, noting the presence of ptosis, exophthalmos, or facial nerve paralysis.

Ask the client to remove glasses or contact lenses for the examination. Pre-examination medication such as local anesthetic eyedrops are generally not necessary until tonometry is performed. Dilation of the pupils is desirable for examinations and will be discussed later in this chapter.

A systematic approach to the physical inspection is helpful. In good illumination, the examiner assesses the superficial parts, progressing to the ocular fundus with the use of the ophthalmoscope. Gentleness and reassuring the client are of utmost importance in ocular examinations.

Check the position of the eyelids, noting ptosis or drooping of the lower lid (**ectropion**). The closed eyelids should fit snugly without exposing the cornea. The eyelids are highly elastic, and any degree of swelling should be noted, along with redness and other signs of inflammation. The inward surfaces of the eyelids are examined for foreign bodies, defects, discharge, and other abnormalities. The eyelashes are examined to determine if they are rubbing on the cornea or crusting because of discharge.

The conjunctivae should be inspected for color; they should be a pale glistening pink. Note conjunctival injection, **chemosis** (edema of the conjunctiva around the cornea), and excessive discharge. Look for evidence of hemorrhage and the presence of foreign bodies.

The sclera may change color in disease states. A blue sclera occurs in disorders of the connective tissue; an icteric sclera (yellow sclera) is observed in jaundice. The sclera is normally smooth, and inflammation, abnormal growths, or bulging should be noted.

The cornea is checked for clarity, noting cloudiness or spots. The cornea's surface should be smooth and regular. Broken areas are examined by staining the surface of the eyeball with sodium fluorescein. Corneal sensation is tested by touching a wisp of sterile cotton to each corneal surface; decreased sensitivity (a decreased blink response) can indicate CN V lesions or a herpes keratitis. On the other hand, persons who have worn contact lenses for a long period of time may have diminished corneal reflexes without neurologic damage.

The iris may be examined directly. Compare its color in the two eyes; differences can indicate a uveal inflammation, tumor, or retained foreign body. Abnormalities of the iris may distort the shape of the pupil. Note each pupil's shape, size, reaction to light, and whether they are equal. The pupil's light reflex is then examined under darkened conditions by shining a penlight from the side of the eyeball inward. The light reflex is a neuromuscular response to light stimulus that constricts the pupil according to the amount of illumination falling on the retina. This response progresses to the optic nerve along the optic tract to the midbrain. CN III is then stimulated and innervates the sphincter muscle of each iris. For this reason, illumination of one eye constricts the opposite pupil simultaneously (consensual light reflex). An optic tract lesion could be the cause of dissimilar constrictions during unilateral illumination.

A dilated pupil can be caused by dimmed light, acute glaucoma, myopia, the use of sympathomimetic drugs, and old and new eye injuries. A constricted pupil will be seen with bright illumination, iris inflammation, glaucoma with pilocarpine treatment, and morphine and heroin use. Aging also can cause constricted pupils, but pupillary reflexes normally remain intact. Irregularly shaped pupils invariably indicate an abnormality such as iritis, central nervous system syphilis, injury, previous eye surgery, or congenital defects. Sphincter muscle tears can give the pupil border a scalloped appearance, and tears at the base of the iris produce a D-shaped pupil. A normal pupil and some of the alterations in various conditions are illustrated in Figure 51–1.

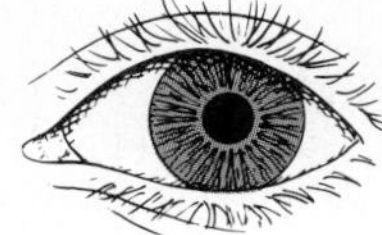

A Normal pupil

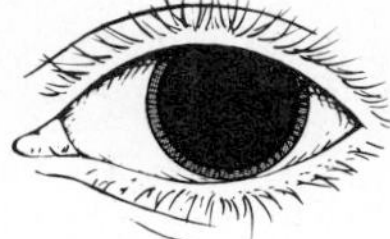

B Fixed, dilated pupil

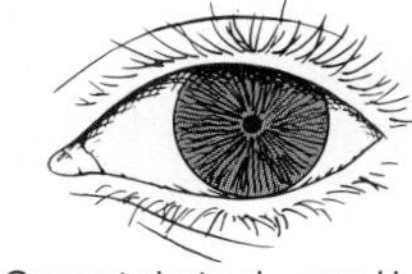

C Constricted pupil

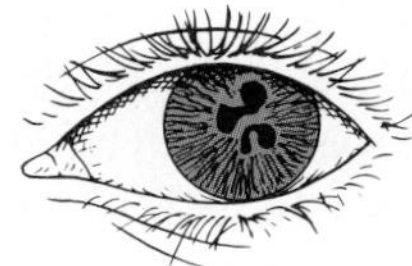

D Cloverleaf pupil (from adhesion of the iris to the lens)

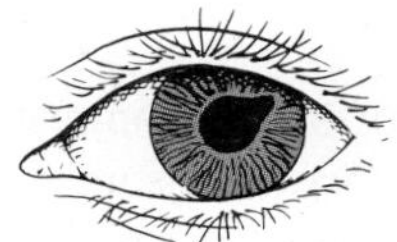

E Peaked, pear-shaped pupil (from perforation of cornea)

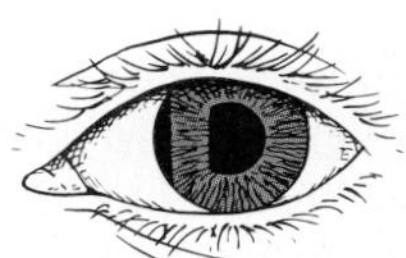

F D-shaped pupil (from a tear at the base of the iris)

Figure 51–1

Pupil signs.

When the normally transparent avascular lens becomes opaque (cataract), vision is reduced and surgery is often indicated. Cataract formation is often a degenerative change but can be seen in young people as a congenital defect. Trauma and diabetes also may be associated with the formation of cataracts.

Full movement of the eyeball is regulated by the integrity of CNs III, IV, and VI. Diplopia often results when only one eye is directed at the intended object (strabismus). Measurement of deviation is necessary to determine the treatment of choice.

The **visual field** is the area within which stimuli produce sight when the eye is looking straight ahead. By performing peripheral and central visual field tests, the examiner can assess the functions of the retina, optic nerve, and optic pathways. The confrontation test is an easy way to determine a decrease in peripheral vision. The examiner sits opposite the client and, with the directly opposite eye closed on both client and examiner, holds up a finger as far to the side as possible and slowly moves the finger inward into the line of vision. The client with normal vision visualizes the finger simultaneously with the examiner with normal vision.

The retinal area, the *ocular fundus,* is viewed with the ophthalmoscope. This is generally done by a physician or a nurse practitioner. The direct ophthalmoscope visualizes the optic disk, the macula, and the retinal vessels. If the ocular fundus cannot be easily inspected, the pupil may be dilated with a short-acting anticholinergic such as tropicamide (Mydriacyl 11%) or phenylephrine hydrochloride (Neo-Synephrine). The client's total systemic status must be assessed before dilating the pupils, because some mydriatics and other ophthalmic medications can interact with other medications or diseases and produce adverse effects, such as exacerbating glaucoma. After the eyes have been examined, a miotic such as pilocarpine hydrochloride can be used to reverse the effect of mydriasis. Usually, however, the client wears a pair of sunglasses until dilatation wears off (approximately 4 hours).

The slit lamp, a biomicroscope used by the physician in combination with a hand-held contact lens to flatten the corneal surface, can visualize the anterior part of the eye with great detail. It illuminates the cornea and lens up to 50 times. The light beam itself can be varied from a full circle beam to a narrow slit of light for examining a small section of the cornea or lens.

The ophthalmoscope and slit lamp examinations are always conducted in a darkened room. Explain all tests to the client to obtain accurate responses and reduce anxiety. Most eye examinations take 10 minutes, and the initial moments of bright light can be uncomfortable. Fortunately, the client usually overcomes this discomfort as the examination proceeds.

INTRAOCULAR PRESSURE Normal IOP is 12 to 20 mm Hg. Tonometry can determine the pressure by measuring the amount of corneal indentation produced by a given weight. Schiotz's tonometer, shown in Figure 51–2, is one instrument that may be used. A topical anesthetic is instilled, and the supine client fixates on a spot on the ceiling. The examiner places the tonometer on the apex of the cornea. The attached scale measures the amount of indentation made in the cornea by the weight of the tonometer, thus determining the pressure in the eye. The noncontact (or air-puff) tonometer is rapidly replacing Schiotz's tonometer as a screening tool in vision care facilities. It does not touch the eye. Rather, a puff of pressurized air is directed at the cornea. The deflections of the cornea in response to the puff of pressurized air are measured. Caution clients that the release of pressurized air results in an audible sound and a slight but nonpainful fleeting pressure on the cornea. Unprepared clients are often startled by the sound and sensation and become apprehensive over testing of the second eye.

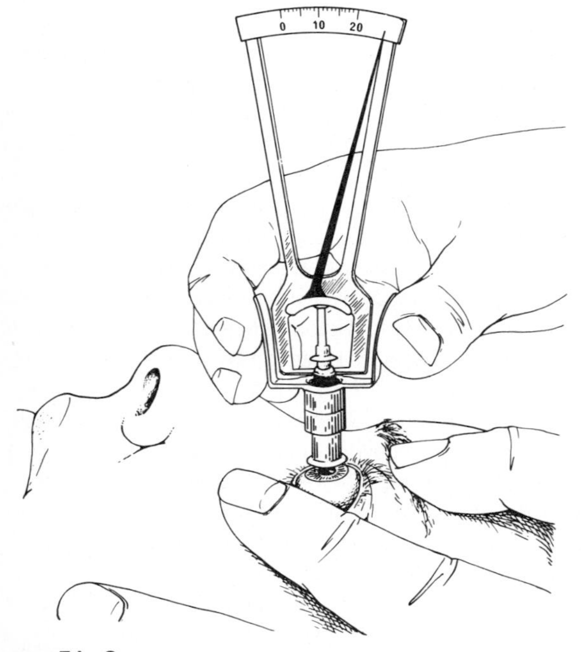

Figure 51–2

Schiotz's tonometer.

Since the symptoms and signs of glaucoma are insidious and often missed, encourage anyone over 40 years old to have regular ophthalmologic examinations, which should always include an IOP measurement.

REFRACTION The eye that sees a focused object at a distance of 20 ft is said to be normal (in a state of emmetropia). Farsightedness (hyperopia) is a failure of the light rays to converge at the retina; instead, the rays focus posterior to the retina, and vision consequently is blurred for distant objects and even more blurred for nearer objects. Vision cannot be improved by stepping farther away from the object, but the hyperopic condition can be resolved by the placement of convex lenses to neutralize the abnormal eye focus.

Nearsightedness (myopia) is caused by too strong a lens system for the distance of the retina behind the lens. In other words, the light rays focus before they reach the retina; by the time they do reach the retina, they have spread apart again, causing an unfocused object. Myopics see close objects without difficulty (the image can be brought closer to the eyes to focus the light rays on the retina) but cannot focus on distant objects. A concave lens corrects this refractive error.

Astigmatism is more complex to resolve and involves an irregular cornea or egg-shaped rather than spherical lens. Light rays cannot focus a clean image because of a dissimilarity in the cornea's north–south and east–west curves. A lens with more curvature in one direction than the other can correct astigmatism.

Visual acuity is the degree of detail that the eye can discern in an image; it is determined primarily by the function of the cones at the fovea centralis. The examiner can measure the ability to distinguish shapes or identify symbols to determine myopia, hyperopia, accommodation function, and the presence of clear transparent structures and an intact fovea centralis. If the client normally wears corrective lenses, the following tests should be conducted with and without the lens aid.

Snellen's chart is a group of letters that become smaller from top to bottom (Figure 51–3). The client has one eye occluded with an opaque card while the other eye is tested. At a distance of 20 ft, the client reads the line that he or she sees most clearly and continues to read each line in order of diminishing size until the letters are incorrectly identified. Acuity is recorded as a fraction; the numerator represents the client's distance to the chart, and the denominator represents the distance at which a normal eye can read the line. For example, 20/40 means that at 20 ft the client can correctly read a line that the normal eye is able to read at 40 ft. Legal blindness is defined as visual acuity of 20/200 or less in the better eye with best correction.

The pinhole test is a simple, useful test for determining decreased acuity that is due to retinal disease. With one eye occluded, the client looks at Snellen's chart through a pinhole punched in an opaque card. This prohibits all but the central rays from passing on to the macula. If the client has a refractive error, the pinhole will improve vision. Organic loss of vision, in contrast, cannot improve with a pinhole.

COLOR VISION Color blindness is inherited in 7% of men and 0.5% of women and is known to be an abnormality of the X chromosome. Central retinal degeneration and optic nerve disease also can cause loss of color vision in one eye from decreased cone function. Malnutrition and some drugs—for example, digoxin, quinidine gluconate, and hydrochlorothiazide—can affect color vision bilaterally. Color vision problems also may be associated with systemic disturbances (eg, yellow vision in jaundice).

Color vision testing is performed under good illumination, as the client is asked to identify items in color plates. The examiner determines the type of color blindness (red-green, blue-yellow, or violet blindness) according to the plates used.

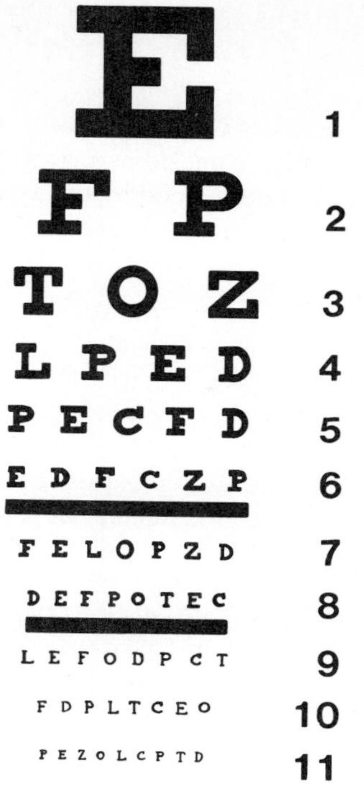

Assessment of the Ears

Examination of the ears begins by looking at the position of the auricle. An auricle that is absent, asymmetrical, or abnormal in configuration, as well as ears set low, are indications of congenital defects. Normally, the position of the ears does not vary or varies slightly from a horizontal line drawn across the inner and outer canthus of the eyes to the tip of the helix. The anterior and posterior surfaces of the auricle, the external auditory canal, and the mastoid areas are carefully inspected for skin changes, redness, swelling, or evidence of lesions or nodules. Observe clients wearing hearing aids for signs of irritation form ill-fitting molds. Palpation is useful in assessing for tenderness, heat, swelling, deformities, and crepitation. Areas palpated should include the auricles; the mastoid process; and the preauricular, postauricular, occipital, and cervical lymph nodes. Referred pain from the temporomandibular joint may be identified by crepitation in the joint. Palpate the joint by placing a finger in the joint space anterior to the ear while the client opens and closes the jaw or by placing the finger within the ear and pressing downward while the client opens and closes the jaw. Normally, a click may be heard or felt.

The examiner uses an otoscope to inspect the auditory canal for cerumen, foreign bodies, inflammation, swelling,

E 1
F P 2
T O Z 3
L P E D 4
P E C F D 5
E D F C Z P 6
F E L O P Z D 7
D E F P O T E C 8
L E F O D P C T 9
F D P L T C E O 10
P E Z O L C P T D 11

Figure 51–3

Snellen's chart.

bleeding, discharge, lesions, and growths. Removal of the cerumen may be necessary for an unobstructed view and is discussed later in this chapter. The amount, color, odor, and consistency of any otorrhea should be noted at this time.

An otoscope is also necessary for observing the normal landmarks of the tympanic membrane. Accentuation of the landmarks suggests a retracted membrane. Inability to visualize any of the landmarks suggests a bulging or thickened membrane. Other abnormalities include changes in color, scarring, increased vascularization (injection), perforations, and discharges.

The examiner can evaluate the mobility of the tympanic membrane with a pneumatic otoscope. A rubber squeeze bulb with tube is attached to the otoscope by a connecting tube. Squeezing the bulb pushes air into the canal, causing the membrane to move inward. Removing the air causes the membrane to bulge outward. No movement or jerky movement of the tympanic membrane suggests middle ear disease or an obstructed eustachian tube. Tympanometry, discussed in the section on diagnostic studies, is another more accurate assessment of tympanic membrane mobility.

AUDITORY FUNCTION Nurses should be alert for clues of hearing loss in all client interactions. Clues include turning of the head, cupping of the ears, or leaning toward the speaker. Nurses might suspect hearing loss if the client's voice is unusually loud or has a monotonous or unvaried tone, if word endings are omitted, or if certain types of words need to be repeated. Consider hearing loss if clients do not answer questions when they cannot see the nurse's mouth or if they answer questions inappropriately. Gross hearing screening is performed by the voice, watch tick, and tuning fork tests. More accurate testing requires an audiometer.

VOICE TEST The voice test provides a gross assessment of the client's ability to hear the whispered or normally spoken word. Each ear is tested separately. The client or examiner masks or occludes one of the client's ears by placing a finger within the ear. This does not prevent all hearing by this ear, so better results are obtained when the occluding finger is rapidly but gently moved back and forth in the ear while the examiner whispers numbers or words to the other ear at a distance of 30 to 60 cm (1 to 2 ft). The examiner then asks the client to repeat numbers that have two equally accented syllables, such as nine–four. To prevent lip reading, the client is asked to look away from the examiner, or the examiner stands behind the client. Normally, softly whispered words are heard bilaterally. If the client cannot hear the whisper, the examiner increases the intensity of the voice to a medium and then a loud whisper, then to a soft, medium, and loud voice.

WATCH TICK TEST In performing the watch tick test, the examiner observes the client's ability to hear the ticking of a watch at a distance of 2 to 5 cm (1 to 2 in.). Use of the watch tick test is limited, however, because it only tests high-frequency loss. A sound perceived as a low tone in pitch has a low frequency, whereas a sound perceived as a high tone in pitch has a high frequency. Hearing is most sensitive in frequencies of 500 to 4000 Hz. Higher frequencies are usually affected first with sensorineural hearing loss. Choose a watch carefully, because many watches today do not have a discernible tick.

TUNING FORK TESTS The client's response to a vibrating tuning fork helps evaluate the type of hearing loss. Common tests are the Weber's and Rinne tests. Tuning forks with vibrating frequencies between 512 and 1024 Hz fall within the functional level of speech frequencies, 300 to 3000 Hz. *Weber's test* differentiates between conductive and sensorineural hearing loss. The examiner places the handle of a softly vibrating tuning fork on the midline of the client's skull. If there is no difference in sensitivity between the ears, the tone will be heard equally in both ears. The client with conductive hearing loss, however, hears the tone as louder in the poorer ear; the client with sensorineural loss hears the tone as louder in the better ear.

The *Rinne test* also helps evaluate conductive and sensorineural hearing loss. A softly vibrating tuning fork is placed on the mastoid process (bone conduction), and when the client can no longer hear the sound, the fork is placed in front of the ear (air conduction). The client normally hears the tone twice as long in front of the ear; this is recorded as air conduction greater than bone conduction, or AC>BC. Abnormal hearing is recorded as bone conduction greater than air conduction, or BC>AC.

VESTIBULAR FUNCTION Labyrinthine disorders are evaluated by checking for nystagmus, for falling (the Romberg test), or for past pointing. To evaluate past pointing, the client sits facing the nurse with the eyes closed and the arms extended. The nurse touches the client's extended index fingers with his or her own fingers. Maintain this position while the client raises the hands above the head and then attempts to reassume the initial position (touching the fingers). The client's eyes remain closed. Past pointing is interpreted as the client deviating to the right or left of the target fingers and indicates inner ear stimulation or loss of position sense.

Vestibular assessment also includes cerebellar testing, including evaluation of gait. Since causes of vertigo are related not only to the vestibular system but also frequently to the central nervous system, an examination of all the cranial nerves is also indicated.

Diagnostic Studies—Eye

OCULAR CULTURE Obtaining a specimen to determine the organism present in an ocular infection involves taking a sterile swab and gently brushing the conjunctival surface to obtain possible pathogens. Transfer the specimen to the appropriate medium to favor the growth of either aerobic or anaerobic microbes, viruses, or fungi. Do not instill antibiotic drops or ointments until after the specimen has been collected. Culturing the eye is illustrated in Chapter 9, Figure 9–1.

CONJUNCTIVAL SCRAPING A conjunctival scraping may assist in the diagnosis of a disease; the histology can be studied under the microscope to identify abnormalities. In this procedure, the eye is topically anesthetized, and a conjunctival scraper (an aluminum rod with flattened ends) is gently brushed over the exposed conjunctiva by an ophthalmologist to obtain a surface scraping. The specimen is spread evenly on glass slides, dried, and sent to the laboratory for staining and examination.

FLUORESCEIN STAINING OF THE CORNEA Breaks in the cornea can be identified by applying a moist paper strip impregnated with sodium fluorescein to the inferior conjunctival cul-de-sac. Tears distribute the dye over the cornea. Irrigating the surface of the cornea will wash away excess dye, leaving only areas in which the corneal epithelium is absent stained green. Fluorescein staining may be combined with a slit lamp examination. A blue filter on the slit lamp highlights the fluorescein-stained cornea.

GONIOSCOPY Gonioscopy is a test used to examine the angle of the anterior chamber. The device looks much like a jeweler's loupe and has a contact lens containing a mirror. When it is placed on the eye it facilitates the detection of a narrow angle (Figure 51–4).

COMPUTED TOMOGRAPHY Computed tomography (CT) of the orbit can detect abnormalities such as intraocular foreign bodies, orbital disease, and retinoblastoma better than conventional roentgenography. Contrast dye is injected, and the eyeball is then scanned through 180° in a path from 0.9 to 1.0 cm wide. Tumors can be correctly determined in pictures that are 100 times more accurate than conventional x-ray films.

ULTRASONOGRAPHY Ultrasonography plays a useful role in determining pathologic conditions of the eye, especially the lens, retina, and choroid. Both intraorbital and orbital tumors, retinal detachment, and fibrous tissue proliferation can be documented easily. In this noninvasive procedure, a probe is simply placed on the eyelid to reflect back to the sound probe and form an echogram. Ultrasonography is a useful adjunct to the ophthalmoscope when opacities deter visualization.

FLUORESCEIN ANGIOGRAPHY Photographs of the ocular fundus, including the retina and retinal blood vessels, may be obtained through fluorescein angiography. This diagnostic test is probably the most frightening to the client because of its invasiveness and discomfort. The nurse can provide explanations and reassure the client as the ophthalmologist performs the procedure.

The fluorescein is injected into the antecubital vein and should appear in the retinal arterioles in 10 seconds. Rapid-sequence photographs are taken through the predilated pupil, and the presence of vascular obstructions, neovascularizations, microaneurysms, abnormal capillary permeability, and defects of the retinal pigment epithelium may be noted. The client needs a complete explanation of the procedure, including warning of the hot sensation experienced when the dye is injected (it lasts about 10 seconds and is similar to stepping into a hot shower) and the potential for an allergic reaction (itching and hives). The client's urine turns a bright yellow color for 18 to 24 hours after the procedure.

RADIOACTIVE PHOSPHORUS (^{32}P) NUCLEAR STUDIES Radioactive phosphorus is injected into the antecubital vein when a malignant intraocular tumor is suspected. Approximately 36 to 48 hours later, the ocular area is scanned using a special probe to determine the extent of phosphorus uptake. An elevated reading signals the presence of an intraocular tumor. The test differentiates between a melanoma (which requires enucleation) and a nevus, preventing unnecessary enucleation. Clients need to be prepared for what to expect when this study is performed. Inform clients that ^{32}P has a short life span and quickly passes out of the body. There is no discomfort other than that from the insertion of the IV needle.

Diagnostic Studies—Ear

CULTURE AND SENSITIVITY Common tests related to otologic infections include smears and cultures of secretions plus an antibiotic sensitivity test. Cultures are usually indicated when the client has a long history of an infection or does not respond to prescribed therapy.

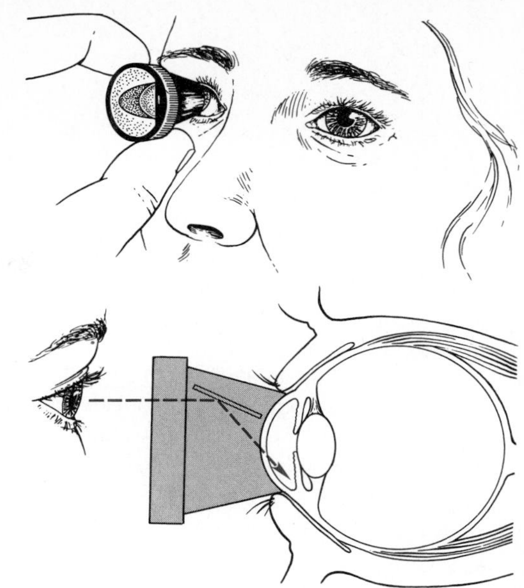

Figure 51–4

Gonioscopy. The mirror inside the lens facilitates detection of a narrowed angle.

Sterile cotton-tipped applicators used through a sterile speculum collect specimens from the external ear. For middle ear specimens, it may be necessary for the physician to perform needle aspirations through the tympanic membrane (tympanocentesis) or aspirations with a sterile suction tip through a tympanic perforation or small incision in the membrane (myringotomy). Cultures are examined for the presence of bacteria, fungi, or yeasts. If allergies are suspected, skin testing is done.

RADIOGRAPHIC STUDIES Radiographic views of the temporal bone aid in the diagnosis of inflammatory disease and other conditions leading to hearing loss. Tomography allows visualization of the desired structure while the areas in front of it or behind it are obscured. The tomographic examination of the temporal bone consists of a series of exposures taken 1 or 2 mm apart in different positions. Although total x-ray exposure to the client is an important consideration in using this technique, 30 tomograms expose the client to less radiation than a single routine chest x-ray. Before exposing a client to radiographic studies, obtain information about allergies (especially to iodine) and the date of the last menstrual period to be sure the client is not pregnant.

AUDIOMETRIC TESTING The *audiometer* is an electronic instrument that generates pure tones of different frequencies and intensities. Audiometric tests differentiate between conductive and sensorineural hearing loss and provide information about the amount and degree of hearing loss. Most audiometric tests are administered by audiologists, although nurses in community settings often perform screening (pure tone) audiometry. Audiometric testing should be conducted in a quiet, preferably soundproof, room. The two most common screening tests are pure tone and speech audiometry. *Pure tone audiometry* tests each ear separately for air conduction (via earphones) and bone conduction (via a vibrator placed on the mastoid bone). The examiner varies the intensity (decibels) at tested frequencies of 125, 250, 500, 1000, 2000, 4000, and 8000 Hz. The faintest point at which the client hears the tone is called the *hearing threshold level* (HRT). Thresholds are recorded on a graph called an audiogram. A hearing range of 0 to 20 for the tested frequencies is considered normal.

Speech audiometry tests the client's ability to understand and discriminate sounds. The speech audiometry test is administered via a monitored live microphone or recorded test material. Spondee words (two-syllable words with equal accents, such as *hotdog* or *airplane*) are presented. A speech reception test measures how loud speech must be before it is heard. The *speech reception threshold* (SRT) is the minimum intensity required for a client to understand speech. The SRTs are usually consistent with the pure tone averages. The lowest level at which the client correctly repeats 50% of the words is the speech discrimination level and is also recorded on the audiogram.

Speech discrimination testing measures the client's ability to distinguish phonetic elements of speech and thus understand what is heard. Using a live monitored microphone or recorded material at levels above the SRT, the examiner presents lists of single-syllable words, such as *day* or *jam,* selected in approximately the same proportion as they occur in spoken English. Clients with normal hearing usually have a discrimination score of 90% to 100%. Less than 90% usually indicates sensorineural hearing loss.

Impedance audiometry helps differentiate ear disorders. The impedance test battery involves three separate evaluations: tympanometry, static impedance, and acoustic reflex tests. Tympanometry measures the mobility of the tympanic membrane as air pressure is varied in the external ear. It works in a way similar to pneumatic otoscopy. The objective is to determine the impedance (resistance) or compliance (flexibility) of the tympanic membrane to sound waves. The test exposes the ear to a constant sound and measures the percentage of sound reflected back from the tympanic membrane with an electroacoustic impedance meter. This measurement is the drum compliance at a particular pressure. The more rigid the membrane, the less the compliance and the higher the impedance. The test is repeated with varying pressure, and a compliance curve, or tympanogram, is plotted. This curve varies with different ear disorders. The static impedance test measures the compliance of the middle ear at rest. The acoustic reflex test measures the changes in compliance caused by the contraction of the middle ear muscles in response to pure tone signals. In clients with normal hearing, the threshold level for the pure tone signals is usually 95 dB. Absence of the acoustic reflex provides helpful diagnostic information.

VESTIBULAR TESTS *Electronystagmography* (ENG), a clinical test of vestibular function, evaluates the status of the semicircular canals by measuring their effect on the ocular muscles. The nystagmus is electrically recorded on a graph. The ENG test battery includes a series of ocular, positional, and bithermal caloric tests used to assess clients with symptoms of dysequilibrium, vertigo, and other forms of imbalance. The battery also can be used to monitor vestibular function in clients at high risk for vestibular damage, such as those receiving gentamicin and streptomycin. The results are viewed as a whole, with certain abnormal findings suggestive of peripheral vestibular dysfunctions and others suggestive of CNS disorders (Zarnoch, 1982).

In preparation for the test, advise the client to avoid alcohol, sedatives, tranquilizers, or antivertigo drugs for at least 48 hours prior to the examination; the drowsiness produced by such drugs can reduce or weaken the response. An otoscopic examination and removal of cerumen prior to the examination is necessary, because impacted cerumen reduces the response. The skin around the eyes is cleansed, removing all makeup and skin oil. The client is placed supine on a table or in a chair with the head elevated 30°. Electrodes are attached to the skin with electrode paste. A ground electrode is attached to the forehead, and electrodes are placed above, below, and at the outer canthus of each eye to record horizontal and vertical nystagmus. The ENG is performed in a dark room and takes approximately 1 hour.

The *bithermal caloric test* compares the nystagmus produced by warm and cold stimulation in each ear. An ear is irrigated with warm (44°C) and then cold (30°C) water with a 5-minute interval between each irrigation. During the procedure, mental alerting tasks such as counting backward from 100 are used to prevent the suppression of responses (Zarnoch, 1982).

A simple caloric test, the *Kobrak caloric test,* stimulates the vestibular labyrinth by directing ice water into the external auditory canal through a Luer-Lok syringe with a 22-gauge needle. Ten to 12 seconds of stimulation will normally induce mild vertigo, nystagmus, and a tendency to fall toward the side of the stimulated ear. Sometimes it also induces vomiting. No response indicates that the labyrinth is nonfunctional.

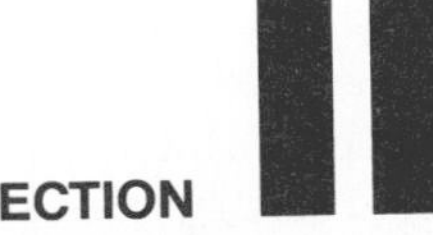

SECTION II

Nursing Diagnosis/Planning and Implementation/Evaluation

Information gathered from the client's health history, physical examination, and diagnostic studies is used to determine nursing diagnoses and the plan of care. Not every client will have the same needs. The Nursing Diagnoses box lists diagnoses **directly related** to visual or auditory dysfunction along with **potential** nursing diagnoses for clients with visual or auditory problems. The most common nursing diagnoses for clients with visual or auditory system dysfunction include knowledge deficit, sensory/perceptual alteration, impaired social interaction, self-care deficit, ineffective client coping, altered family processes, fear, potential for injury, and disturbance in self-concept. The sample nursing care plan in Table 51–2 focuses on self-care deficit related to visual and auditory impairment, disturbance in self-concept: self-esteem, altered role performance, ineffective individual coping, altered family processes, fear related to vision loss, and potential for injury. The narrative content discusses knowledge deficit, visual and auditory sensory/perceptual alteration, and impaired social interaction.

If the goals of care have not been met, re-evaluation is required. The nurse and client should jointly review the nursing care plan. New objectives may need to be formulated; other nursing interventions may be added or modified; or the evaluation may show that more time is required to meet the objectives.

Knowledge Deficit Related to Vision

Many people have limited knowledge about approaches they can take to preserve their vision, such as regular eye examinations and personal eye care. Clients with eye problems who are using prescribed eye medications often do not understand the desired effect of the drug, and consequently, may not use it as prescribed for maximum effectiveness. Clients needing eye patches or shields may not understand the purpose of the shield or how to apply it. Nurses in any setting need to be alert to opportunities to teach clients this care.

Planning and Implementation

EYE EXAMINATIONS In early adulthood, clients should have thorough eye examinations approximately every 5 years. At about 35 to 40 years of age, when many adults begin to experience vision problems, regular eye examinations every 2 years are recommended. Advise clients who have diabetes, glaucoma, or a family history of these disorders to contact a health care provider for an eye examination more frequently. An eye examination should be done whenever the client experiences any of the following:

- Disturbances of vision such as blurring, loss of peripheral vision, seeing halos around lights, or diplopia
- Pain
- Redness
- Sudden appearance of floaters
- Photophobia
- Persistent watering
- Purulent discharge
- Lesions of the eye or eyelid
- Trauma to the eye or eyelid
- Pupil irregularities

A number of health care providers are specialists in eye care. The client should know what services each provides to determine the appropriate person to consult. An *optician* grinds and fits corrective lenses and adjusts frames. An *optometrist* assesses refractive errors and eye muscle disturbances; adjusts lenses to changes in refraction and accommodation of the eye; prescribes corrective lenses, low-vision aids, and eye muscle exercises; and performs screening tests for glaucoma and color blindness. An *ophthalmologist* is a physician who specializes in the diagnosis and treatment of disorders of the eye, performs surgery, and prescribes corrective lenses and medication.

PERSONAL EYE CARE Because they are exposed organs, the eyes are especially vulnerable to infection and trauma. Caution clients to keep their hands away from their eyes, faces, and hair to reduce the likelihood of introducing bacteria. If the eyes must be touched, the hands should be washed thoroughly first. Eye makeup is a frequent source of infection and irritation. It should be used by one person only, not shared with others. Old eye makeup should be discarded, since it provides a good culture medium for bacteria.

The same rationale applies to discouraging clients from using someone else's eyedrops or eye ointment: Infection can be spread through contaminated materials. Proper methods for instillation of ophthalmic medications is shown in Figure 51–5. In addition, this practice may be harmful in other ways. One person's eye medication may be contraindicated for another person because of allergies, other health conditions, interaction with other medications, or the nature of the eye disorder causing the symptoms (eg, cycloplegics and mydriatics are contraindicated in glaucoma).

Encourage clients to be alert to work, school, and hobby situations in which the potential for eye injury is high. Encourage them to wear eye protection when working with caustic chemicals or when exposed to dust and dirt, wood, metal, or glass fragments. Caution clients against rubbing their eyes; rubbing can spread infection or, if a foreign body has entered the eye, can cause corneal abrasions or lacerations. The nozzle of spray products should be directed away from the eyes. Leisure and recreational activities such as racket sports or games in which sticks or flying objects are used are also potentially dangerous. In addition to helping clients assume responsibility to protect their eyes, nurses as citizen activists can support legislation outlawing the sale of dangerous toys and fireworks and promote the use of shatterproof glass, safety goggles, and protective sports equipment.

The client can prevent or reduce eye fatigue by following a few guiding principles:

NURSING DIAGNOSES IN
Visual or Auditory Dysfunction

DIRECTLY RELATED DIAGNOSES

- Coping, ineffective individual
- Family processes, altered
- Fear
- Injury, potential for
- Knowledge deficit
- Role performance, altered
- Self-care deficit
- Self-concept, disturbance in: self-esteem
- Sensory/perceptual alterations: visual, auditory
- Social interaction, impaired

OTHER POTENTIAL DIAGNOSES

- Adjustment, imparied

- Use adequate illumination. The lamp or light should not cast shadows on the work or reading area. Table lamps should be about 24 in. high and placed on the nondominant side (eg, to the left for someone who is right handed).
- Rest the eyes often during prolonged use. Looking away to focus on other objects in the distance or closing the eyes helps rest them.
- Individualize the work area that contains a VDT. Screen glare can be avoided by using a tilt table or turntable, adjusting the lighting or the location of the VDT (if possible), applying a nonglare coating to the screen, or purchasing eyeglasses specifically designed to ease eye fatigue from VDT work.

Discourage the practice of using old (and no longer accurate) or secondhand eyeglasses. Although they may improve vision, the refraction correction can be off considerably. Purchasing over-the-counter reading glasses that magnify print may be a very brief solution when reading glasses are lost or broken, but these lenses are not individualized and should not be used for a long period of time.

EYE MEDICATIONS Drugs prescribed by the ophthalmologist are usually applied to the eye in the form of drops or ointments. The categories of ophthalmologic medications and the effects they produce are listed here:

- **Adrenergics.** These drugs release epinephrine from the sympathetic nerve fibers and produce mydriasis and vasoconstriction of the ocular vessels. Adrenergics may be used in conjunction with miotics when miotics cannot completely control the intraocular pressure of clients with open-angle glaucoma.
- **Anticholinergics.** These drugs block the passage of impulses through the parasympathetic nerves, resulting in mydriasis and paralysis of accommodation. They are relatively short acting, lasting only a few hours.
- **Antimicrobials.** These drugs are administered topically, subconjunctivally, or systemically to treat bacterial, fungal, or viral infections by destroying or inhibiting the organism's growth.
- **Beta-adrenergic-blocking agents.** These agents block the release of epinephrine and reduce both normal and increased IOP. Their exact mechanism of action is not yet clear; they are thought to reduce the production of aqueous humor but in some instances have been observed to increase its outflow.
- **Carbonic anhydrase inhibitors.** These drugs are thought to inhibit the activity of the enzyme carbonic anhydrase, which apparently plays a role in the control of ocular fluid formation. The result is a reduction in IOP. Carbonic anhydrase inhibitors are generally used on a short-term basis to treat glaucoma.
- **Cholinergics.** The cholinergics are parasympathomimetics that act directly to release acetylcholine from parasympathetic nerve fibers. They produce miosis, contraction of the ciliary muscles, dilation of blood vessels, and increased aqueous humor outflow.
- **Cholinesterase inhibitors.** These newer agents are more potent miotics than the cholinergics. They act

1. Wash hands carefully to protect client.
2. Remove drainage and crusts from eye and lashes using sterile cotton and saline. Wipe from inner to outer canthus once, then discard.
3. Ask client to tilt face upward and head back.
4. Instruct client to look up.
5. Gently pull down lower lid exposing conjunctiva, taking care not to apply pressure to the eyeball.
6. Prevent contamination of medication, eye dropper, or tube.

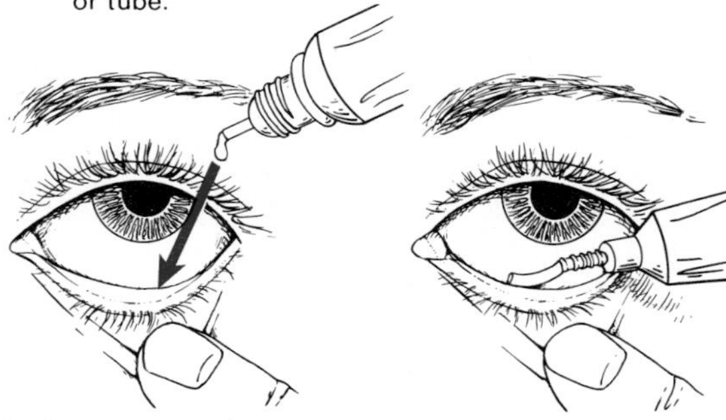

7. Squeeze the prescribed number of drops into the inferior conjunctival cul-de-sac, *not on the eye itself.*
8. Apply pressure at the inner canthus for 1 to 2 minutes, keeping the eyelid open.

7. Squeeze ointment onto the lid margin for ¼ to ½ in. Blinking and body temperature will distribute and melt the ointment.
8. Instruct client to close eyes gently for about 2 minutes.

9. Clean the client's cheek of any excess moisture or ointment.
10. Wash hands carefully to protect self from inadvertent systemic effects from client's medication.

Note: If client is to receive more than one type of eyedrop, instill the least viscous medication first, and wait at least one minute before instilling the second medication.

Figure 51–5

Instilling ophthalmic medications.

Table 51–2
Sample Nursing Care Plan for a Client With Visual or Auditory Dysfunction, by Nursing Diagnosis

Client Care Goals	Plan/Nursing Implementation	Expected Outcomes
Clients With Visual Dysfunction		
Self-care deficit related to visual impairment		
Maximize functional abilities and achievements	Encourage client to dress self, feed self, and ambulate (with degree of assistance necessary); encourage caretaker to consult client if uncertain whether help is needed; educate client about rehabilitation options related to mobility training and braille; reassure client that some dependency is necessary, such as in transportation, reading menus, and selecting clothes	Client will resume prior lifestyle as appropriate; will demonstrate ability to care for self; is aware of rehabilitative potential
Self-concept, disturbance in: self-esteem related to visual impairment		
Verbalize personal strengths; acknowledge impact of limitations on existing personal relationships and lifestyle	Encourage rehabilitation early in adjustment period; reassure client that dependence on support groups and significant others is warranted; encourage client to verbalize methods for coping, attitudes toward blindness, and anxiety	Will have resolution of feelings of loss, ability to cope with reactions, and support from significant others
Role performance, altered related to adjustment to new role		
Resume employment with acquired skills through career search and analysis of job skills; achieve or maintain finaincial security and independence	Educate client about legal blindness tax deductions and state and federal funding for rehabilitation; reassure client that qualified professionals can assist client in learning new skills	Will have financial security, satisfactory employment
Coping, ineffective individual related to personal vulnerability secondary to visual deficit		
Verbalize feelings about visual impairment; return to daily function as physically and socially active as possible; maximize achievements, functional abilities, and use of other senses	Provide opportunities to allow client to talk about shock of blindness or impaired vision; suggest counseling or psychotherapy to work out feelings of loss; encourage activities of daily living with visual aids for assistance as necessary; encourage independence as much as possible within a safe environment; emphasize remaining capabilities	Will cope with impaired vision in a healthy, realistic manner; will demonstrate normal psychosocial status and return to previous functional ability
Family process, altered related to disability of family member		
Normal relations with family; discuss loss with family member; maintain as much independence as possible; keep anxiety of family to a minimum to ease adjustment to blindness; keep perspective regardless of family interference	Encourage client and family to talk about grieving process (allow sufficient time); suggest that client and family seek counseling if developing guilty feelings become obsessive and interfere with client's rehabilitation; educate family about goals of rehabilitation; discourage dependency attitudes such as feeding client and inhibiting activities; encourage family to allow client to perform tasks; educate family to allow client to bump into objects in the rehabilitation period without excessive expressions of sympathy or overreaction; encourage family understanding and patience; educate family about potential of rehabilitated client; dissuade family from promoting unrealistic hopes for cures	Family will overcome grieving and promote client's rehabilitation; family will understand importance of allowing client to learn and develop skills and reason for client's frustrations; family will exhibit patience and understanding; family will accept reality of blindness in their loved one and assist positively in rehabilitation

(Continued)

Table 52–2
Sample Nursing Care Plan for a Client With Visual or Auditory Dysfunction, by Nursing Diagnosis (continued)

Client Care Goals	Plan/Nursing Implementation	Expected Outcomes
Fear related to vision loss		
Develop rapport with health care givers; perform activities of daily living without preoccupation with potential blindness	Educate client about disease process and expected level of visual function; develop client trust to assist in coping with disease process in healthy, effective manner; begin rehabilitative measures in timely manner so client will have confidence in management of activities of daily living; educate client about community groups that can provide support	Client will recognize that fear will interfere with a healthy outlook on life; client will understand the progression of disease without undue surprises; client will overcome fear and learn measures that allow maximum autonomy
Clients With Auditory Dysfunction		
Injury, potential for related to hearing deficit		
Prevent injury	Clients with hearing loss: Encourage use of other senses and hearing adaptive devices to identify hazards in the environment; provide client with information on adaptive devices and hearing guide dogs if appropriate; tag the hospitalized client's door, bed, and chart to alert other health care personnel to the client's special needs	Injury will be avoided
	Clients with vestibular problems: Instruct client to stop activities while experiencing vertigo; provide hospitalized client with call light and bed rails to prevent injury	Client will avoid hazardous situations until vertigo has diminished or been relieved
Social interaction, impaired related to withdrawal from socializations secondary to hearing loss		
Establish a satisfactory method of communication; maintain social interaction	Encourage client to express feelings; suggest alternative methods of communication; assist client with adaptive devices, hearing aids, etc; encourage seeking help from other health professionals if necessary (eg, audiologist, vocational rehabilitator, etc); support family and assist in adapting; encourage and assist client with family relationships and other social contacts	Client will demonstrate positive self-concept by accepting hearing loss; will begin learning other methods of communication; will begin using assistive hearing devices; will re-establish family and other social contacts; will establish plans for adjusting work situation or will seek alternative plans

indirectly by inhibiting the enzymatic destruction of acetylcholine. The acetylcholine then accumulates and acts on the iris sphincter and ciliary muscles, causing miosis. The short-acting compounds are used more often than long-acting compounds, which may actually decrease fluid outflow and increase IOP.

- **Corticosteroids.** Corticosteroids dramatically relieve ocular pain and discomfort. By suppressing ocular inflammation, they inhibit redness, swelling, capillary dilation, exudation, cellular infiltration, and collagen deposits.
- **Cycloplegics.** In addition to producing mydriasis, these drugs (usually anticholinergics) paralyze accommodation (cause **cycloplegia**) by blocking the action of acetylcholine on the iris sphincter and ciliary muscles. Cycloplegics are used for refractive purposes and when it is desirable to keep the pupil dilated (eg, for infectious conditions of the iris and ciliary body, in corneal diseases, and after certain operations). They should not be administered to clients with glaucoma.
- **Hyperosmotics.** These agents create a rapid increase in extracellular fluid osmolality, causing fluid to move

out of the eye and reducing IOP. They are used before or during surgery when it is desirable to reduce the intraocular pressure and to treat glaucoma. They may be administered parenterally or orally.

- **Miotics.** These drugs constrict the pupil (cause **miosis**). In addition, they produce accommodation and facilitate increased aqueous humor outflow, thus reducing IOP. Miotics are commonly used in the treatment of glaucoma. Both cholinergics and cholinesterase inhibitors can produce miosis.
- **Mydriatics.** Dilation of the pupil (**mydriasis**) can be produced by adrenergics and anticholinergics. Their use facilitates thorough examination of the fundus. Because they prevent the outflow of fluid and thus increase IOP, mydriatics should not be administered to clients with glaucoma. They do not interfere with accommodation and thus do not have a cycloplegic effect.

Most of these drugs are applied topically, although some may be administered orally or parenterally. Topical application, however, does not guarantee that unwanted systemic effects will be avoided. Cholinergic and miotic drugs (those that constrict the pupil) are most likely to cause systemic reactions. Scrupulously adhering to the prescribed dose helps avoid systemic reactions. Applying pressure at the inner canthus for 1 to 2 minutes after administration compresses the lacrimal duct, preventing systemic absorption through the mucous membranes of the nose. Ask the client to keep the eyelids apart for several seconds while applying pressure to allow the drug to act on the surface of the eye. People instilling miotics should wash their hands when finished to prevent systemic absorption from a drug-contaminated finger that comes in contact with the mucous membranes. Remember that whoever instills the eye medication—nurse, client, family member, or significant other—should begin only after careful handwashing; prevent contamination of the medication, eyedropper, or tube; and be gentle to avoid any injury to the eye.

A diffusional system is sometimes used to provide controlled consistent delivery of a drug for periods of up to a week. The system is a plastic device slightly larger than a contact lens, which is inserted into the conjunctival sac. The drug is contained in a reservoir between two membranes that allow it to diffuse into the eye. A diffusional system frees clients from having to administer multiple doses of eyedrops and is most commonly used for glaucoma, because the intraocular pressure can be controlled more consistently.

EYE PATCHES OR SHIELDS Eye patches are frequently used as protection for an affected eye. They also serve as bandages, to collect drainage, and to provide rest to limit eye movement. A tight pressure patch is occasionally used for corneal abrasions (to promote epithelial attachment) or after an enucleation (to prevent bleeding). Metal-pierced shields are common practice, placed over an eye patch to provide extra protection, particularly at night. Eye patches should be securely taped from the middle of the forehead outward to the cheekbone. They should be changed at least twice a day and more often when drainage is noted. It is important to dispose of the patches as warranted (drainage from infections requires that patches be separated from other refuse). Good handwashing is essential before and after changing patches, and cross-contamination from one infected eye to another is avoided by cleansing the hands between care of each eye.

Evaluation

Expected client outcomes following effective nursing interventions for knowledge deficit related to vision include statements by the client that indicate an understanding of good eye care, the importance of regular eye examinations, and the need to seek medical attention for any visual impairment. The client on eye medication is able to explain the effects of the drug and demonstrate proper drug instillation.

Sensory/Perceptual Alteration: Visual

The brain receives 90% of its sensory input through sight, so impaired or reduced vision obviously inhibits sensory perception. An infant born blind has no memory of objects, colors, the environment, or spatial relationships, making the learning process exceedingly difficult. Decreased vision or blindness that occurs later in life profoundly alters the client's lifestyle. The client will grieve for the vision loss and must develop new problem-solving abilities to fit altered communication patterns and sensory perception.

Planning and Implementation

Coping with changes in visual sensory perception is a long-term process facilitated by the client's new abilities to function in activities of daily living. Encourage the client to talk about the deteriorating vision and methods of coping. Preconceived attitudes about blindness may hinder the rehabilitative progress and thus should be identified at the onset.

The client care goals for those with sensory/perceptual changes are relearning independence through rehabilitation, education about visual pathology and treatment, and developing the ability to cope with impaired vision in a healthy, realistic manner. Finally, the client must re-examine how to continue to meet basic needs with a visual alteration.

The nurse should offer the client consistent encouragement and motivation throughout this difficult adjustment period. Encourage the client to discuss coping methods and evaluate his or her progress so that the health care program can be tailored to meet the most important psychosocial needs.

VISION AIDS Clients with problems of visual sensory perception can be helped by a variety of vision aids and other approaches. The most common aids to vision are corrective lenses (eyeglasses, contact lenses, and cataract glasses). Other aids to vision include intraocular lens implants, hand-held magnifiers, monocular telescopes, night vision magnifiers, visual field widening devices, enlarged print, and magnifying television screens.

Other approaches to assist people with visual loss to maintain optimal quality of life include:

- Talking books, magazines, and newspapers. Records or tapes of books, magazines, and newspapers are available on loan from agencies for the blind or public libraries. Tapes are also available for purchase.
- Braille. Agencies for the blind and correspondence courses will teach a client how to use the braille system of writing and printing by means of tangible points or dots. Specially designed braille watches, household devices, books, magazines, playing cards, and medical aids are available.
- Optical-to-tactile converters. These devices convert vision into tactile sensation. A miniature camera moved along a line of print reproduces the outline of a letter on a tactile screen by adjusting a series of tiny rods.
- Telephone aids. Special dials are available for telephones in both large print and braille.
- Canes. White canes with red tips help to identify the blind person who uses a cane to locate obstacles in the environment. Newly developed laser canes can not only locate objects, but can also identify changes in the terrain as far away as 20 feet.
- Guide dogs. Especially trained dogs help blind persons become mobile. Month-long training courses teach blind persons how to use this technique and how to care for the dog.

Evaluation

Expected client outcomes following effective nursing interventions for visual sensory/perceptual alteration include client ability to verbalize anxieties about visual impairment. There will be indications, through client verbalizations and actions and the reports of staff and significant others, that the client will be able to cope with the visual impairment. The client demonstrates continued efforts at becoming more independent.

Social Interaction, Impaired Related to Visual Loss

The visually handicapped person must make substantial adjustments to facilitate communication, or social isolation and its subsequent frustration will be almost inevitable. The client's inability to visualize body language and facial expressions of speakers can lead to unhappiness and misinterpretation for both sides. In addition, the client may find it difficult to verbalize frustrations and may withdraw rather than deal directly with the impairment.

Planning and Implementation

Clients with impaired vision because of disease or eye patches will have their anxiety lessened when care providers announce their presence and departure, letting clients know who they are and what they are doing. Remember to address clients directly when speaking to them and provide descriptions of people, places, and things. Avoid startling clients by touching them unexpectedly.

A trusting rapport can be initiated by taking time to introduce the hospital environment to the visually impaired client on admission. If placed in a two- to four-bed room, it is helpful to have the visually impaired client closest to the bathroom. The client should be walked around the room (and the bed), holding on to the nurse's elbow, to find his or her bearings. Descriptions such as "The nightstand is just to the right of the head of the bed as you're facing the bed" or "There is an armchair at the foot of the bed" are helpful (and important) information. Have the client touch the various pieces of furniture to understand the spatial scheme of the room. The call light and telephone should be within easy reach. The bedside table should be placed on the client's most visual side of the bed. Tissues and paper bags for refuse taped to the raised siderails are convenient for the visually impaired client. When assisting the client in unpacking personal belongings, allow the client to place any articles in the drawers to increase awareness of their location and promote independence in retrieving items as needed during the hospital stay.

When meal trays arrive, clients are often able to feed themselves provided the location of each food on the plate has been described. A common practice is to refer to each food on the plate by times on the clock (eg, "The potatoes are at 3 o'clock"). Assisting with the opening of condiment packages and milk cartons is helpful. The nurse may cut up the food and butter the bread. Warn the client of any hot beverages on the tray.

Discourage the newly visually impaired client from getting out of bed at night without assistance. Despite thorough orientations to the geography of the hospital, darkness may invite unsafe conditions, and clients with one eye patch or bilateral patches may have a different perception of their surroundings.

Evaluation

Expected client outcomes following effective nursing interventions for impairment of communication include observation and reports that the client is resuming prior communication efficacy and is attempting to cope in a healthy and realistic manner.

Knowledge Deficit Related to Hearing

Many people have limited knowledge about approaches they can take to preserve their hearing. Routine cleaning of the ear; keeping the ear dry; equalizing pressure in the middle ear; cerumen and foreign body removal; instilling drops, creams, or ointments; and preventing damage from noise are all related to prevention of injury and preservation of hearing.

Planning and Implementation

PERSONAL EAR CARE The external auditory canal is basically a self-cleaning structure. The muscles involved in chewing help work cerumen through the canal to the outer surface, where it can be readily removed with a washcloth in routine washing. Discourage clients from inserting objects such as cotton-tipped swabs, hairpins, safety pins, paper clips, or their own fingers into their ears to clean them. Not only is this likely to be unnecessary, but it is also *dangerous*. Even cotton-tipped swabs are relatively inflexible. A sudden movement of the head because the client has been startled or an accidental push by a person passing by can force the object deeper into the ear canal. This can push the cerumen further in and impair hearing, scratch or irritate the external auditory canal, or puncture the tympanic membrane. In general, it is safest to leave the outer ear alone.

The self-cleaning mechanism of the outer ear may not operate well under certain circumstances. When chewing is impaired, as occurs with a fractured jaw, malocclusion, or ill-fitting or no dentures, cerumen may build up. Cerumen removal by a knowledgeable health care provider may become necessary. The self-cleaning mechanism also may not be operating effectively in other less obvious situations. Consider checking for cerumen buildup in clients who are NPO, on a clear liquid diet, or receiving nourishment through intravenous infusions.

Tell clients to avoid washing their ears with strong soaps or shampoos that can irritate and dry the skin, causing itching. Scratching an irritated ear can result in a secondary infection. Clients who experience dry skin with aging may find this to be a particular problem.

Keeping water out of the ear is important, because moisture invites maceration that may result in infection. Thus, clients should try to avoid letting water run into the ears while showering. Using earplugs or Vaseline-impregnated cotton plugs will help. To make a cotton plug, unroll a cotton ball and apply Vaseline to its surface. Roll from one end to the other—Vaseline side out—ending with a cylinder that can be easily molded, cut to the desired length, and inserted into the ear. When swimming, it is best to use earplugs made especially for that purpose. Swimming should be limited to 4 to 5 hours at the most.

The external ear can be dried by using a hair dryer (taking care not to burn the external ear) or instilling a few drops of alcohol into the external auditory canal (being careful not to dry out the skin of the external ear).

Nursing Research Note

Magilvy J: Quality of life of hearing-impaired older women. *Nurs Res* 1985; 34(3):140–143.

Major variables were studied that influence the quality of life perceived by older hearing-impaired women. The study compared the quality of life experienced by women who were deaf before age 19 and those who developed hearing impairments in later life. The variables thought to influence quality of life were health, social support, age, financial adequacy, and social hearing handicap.

The results suggest that women who developed hearing impairments later in life had an overall lower perception of quality of life than the early-onset group. The older group perceived themselves as less healthy, lacking adequate social support, and experiencing greater social handicap. Financial adequacy and age of onset of deafness did not directly influence perceived quality of life in either group.

The findings indicate that quality of life is positively influenced by one's perception of health and by social support networks. Quality of life is negatively affected by perceptions of social handicap. Judging from these findings, nursing intervention with other hearing-impaired clients should focus on health promotion, enhancing social support systems, and facilitating adaptation to the hearing handicap.

EQUALIZING PRESSURE IN THE MIDDLE EAR Changes in altitude and inflammation of the eustachian tube from upper respiratory tract infections or seasonal allergies may cause discomfort when fluid or air is trapped in the middle ear. Clients can use a variety of self-ventilating techniques to help equalize the pressure; yawning, swallowing several times, chewing gum, and opening the mouth about 2 cm and protruding the jaw forward may help. The **Valsalva maneuver**—holding the nostrils shut and the mouth closed while gently blowing—may be used when the other measures are not helpful. However, clients with congestion from an upper respiratory tract infection should not use this maneuver, because it can force bacteria into the middle ear.

CERUMEN REMOVAL Clients prone to cerumen accumulation (people with a large amount of hair in the outer ear and those who work in dusty or dirty areas) should be taught how to soften and remove cerumen safely. Half-strength hydrogen peroxide solution instilled into the ear with a medicine dropper can help remove cerumen. The hydrogen peroxide should remain in the ear for 5 minutes and be irrigated out with clear water in a medicine dropper or while the client showers. Once a week is usually enough, although clients with a large accumulation may have to treat the problem more often. Commercial ceruminolytic agents such as Debrox (a combination of carbamide peroxide and glycerol) can be purchased OTC. Some people are allergic to OTC ceruminolytics with combined ingredients, however, and the nurse should caution them to avoid their use.

FOREIGN BODY REMOVAL Foreign bodies in the ear are a more common problem for children than adults. However, even adults insert foreign bodies into their ears for cleaning purposes and cannot get them out. Flying insects or debris blown into the ear by a strong wind are also common.

Instilling mineral, olive, or vegetable oil or alcohol into the ear will smother an insect and allow it to float to the top, where it can be easily removed. Water should *not* be used, because it will not kill the insect; in fact, the insect will cling to the canal wall, making it difficult to remove. If the insect has bitten or scratched the canal wall, the instillation of alcohol may be painful. Irrigation can flush out debris but should not be used if the foreign object is of vegetable origin, because it will tend to absorb the water and swell. Professional help in removing foreign bodies prevents additional damage to the ear. Surgery may be necessary to remove an object fixed within the canal.

EAR MEDICATIONS Drops or ointments should be inserted into the external auditory canal when the client is lying on his or her side with the affected ear up. Instruct the client to remain in this position for at least 5 minutes and to insert a cotton ball before assuming a sitting or standing position. This will allow the solution to drain into the cotton ball.

Creams can be carefully applied to the external ear with a cotton swab or cotton ball. Instruct the client to hold the swab close to its cotton-tipped end and to brace the fourth and fifth fingers against the face. This prevents inserting the swab too far and accidentally damaging the tympanic membrane.

Discourage clients from self-treatment with eardrops or oil when they have an earache. This not only delays effective treatment but may allow an infection to progress; keeping the ear canal continuously moist with eardrops or oil also may cause fungal infection.

PREVENTING NOISE DAMAGE The problem of noise pollution is increasing in the workplace, the home, and the city streets. Nurses should educate their friends, neighbors, and clients about the damage to the hair cells of the ears that can result from hazardous noise. Guidelines for protecting hearing are discussed in Box 51–1.

Hearing protectors can reduce and even prevent noise trauma. They can be purchased in sporting goods stores, medical supply stores, hearing clinics, and through audiologists. Hearing protectors should be available in work settings in which noise is a problem. If not, the client and nurse should bring the problem of noise to the attention of management.

Evaluation

Expected client outcomes following effective nursing interventions for knowledge deficit related to hearing include client descriptions and demonstrations of proper ear care, explanations of the dangers of excessive noise on hearing, and verbalization of the importance of seeking medical attention for any hearing impairment. The client on ear medication is able to explain the effects of the drug and demonstrate proper drug instillation.

Sensory/Perceptual Alteration: Auditory

Reduced hearing, regardless of its cause, affects all aspects of a client's life and impairs the client's ability to function normally. Tinnitus with or without hearing loss is another disruptive symptom with multiple effects on a person's life.

Planning and Implementation

Simple and inexpensive steps to alter the environment are often useful to people who do not hear well. For example, certain materials and furnishings help reduce echoes and muffle irrelevant noises that interfere with a hearing-impaired person's ability to hear. Movable furniture allows hearing-impaired people to sit where they can better hear and see the lips of speakers.

HEARING AIDS A hearing aid receives speech and environmental sounds through a microphone, converts them into electrical signals, strengths the electrical signals through amplification, and converts the amplified electrical signals back to sound. Hearing aids work by amplifying sound, not merely by intensifying it.

Many hearing aids can now be tailored to the client's specific needs. For example, rather than needing to have all sound made louder, a client with a sensorineural hearing loss may need to have low tones depressed and higher tones enhanced. In contrast, a client with a conductive hearing loss may benefit from amplification alone if it can overcome the blockage or damage that prevents sound from reaching the inner ear. Hearing aids are more likely to be helpful when the hearing loss is conductive rather than sensorineural. In consultation with an otologist and an audiologist, the client can make an informed decision about whether to attempt to use a hearing aid and what kind of hearing aid would be best.

Clients should understand that using a hearing aid does not guarantee perfect hearing and that not everyone is a good candidate. Because hearing aids increase sound, background sounds also are increased. Some people find this distracting and annoying. Also, although speech becomes louder, it may not be clearer. The hearing aid user may be disappointed to find that it may still be difficult to understand what others are saying. To take full advantage of the benefits of a hearing aid and learn to interpret speech more accurately, the hearing aid wearer may need auditory training or to learn speech reading.

Other approaches to assist people with hearing loss to maintain optimal quality of life include communication systems that can be installed in conference rooms, classrooms, theaters, and auditoriums or added to the radio, television, or telephone in the home or at work. Special headsets, devices that display subtitles or captions, telephone communication devices, and sign language interpreters are some examples. Hearing guide dogs are specially trained to alert the hearing-impaired person who lives alone to the sounds of the doorbell, telephone, alarm clock, and smoke alarm, as well as other sounds in the home or public places. The dogs are trained to protect their masters from danger and to assist them in carrying out daily activities that depend on sound.

Evaluation

Expected client outcomes following effective nursing interventions for auditory sensory–perceptual alteration include client ability to verbalize anxieties about hearing impairment. There will be indications, through client verbalizations and actions and the reports of staff and significant others, that the client will be able to cope with the auditory impairment. The client demonstrates continued efforts at becoming more independent.

Box 51–1
Guidelines for Protecting Hearing

Wear hearing protectors at home when working with power tools.

Run appliances one at a time to keep the noise level down, and do not use noisy appliances any more than absolutely necessary.

Be an informed consumer and select the quieter household appliances. Consumer guides often recommend appliances based on their decibel ratings.

Anticipate noise exposure at work, at home, or while engaging in recreational activities. Put on hearing protectors before starting up a motorcycle, a snowmobile, etc.

Avoid sitting close to loud music (either live or recorded).

Be cautious about any noise-making object close to the ears, including stereo headphones worn while jogging or mobile telephones.

Be a citizen activist and help reduce the noise levels in the community.

When caught unprepared by exposure to noise that cannot be controlled (an emergency siren, a malfunctioning automobile horn, a subway train, etc), cover the ears tightly with the hands.

Social Interaction, Impaired Related to Hearing Loss

Hearing loss may affect the development of verbal communication. The ears monitor speech, and the client's voice may be too soft or too loud when this ability is diminished because inflections cannot be heard; the client's voice also may become monotonous. Clients who do not hear themselves talk will be unaware when they have mispronounced words.

Planning and Implementation

When speaking with someone who is hard of hearing, attract the person's attention first. Gestures and touching are usually helpful ways to signal an intention to communicate verbally. Having attracted the person's attention, stand directly in front of the person and face the light. This gives the person the added advantage of being able to see formed words and to read lips. Speaking at a calm, relaxed pace lets the client know that the nurse understands and respects his or her limitation without increasing anxiety. The client who is relatively free from stress and anxiety probably will hear better.

Appropriate facial expressions and gestures help the hearing-impaired person comprehend what the nurse is saying more fully. It may be necessary to modify the tone or pitch of the voice so the person can hear better. If the client does not understand what has been said, try rephrasing it. If the nurse does not understand all the client has said, details can be filled in from the context of the communication. Be cautious, however, not to misunderstand without realizing it. A better approach might be to ask the client to repeat or rephrase what has not been understood.

The hospitalized hearing-impaired client should be identified by tags on the door, bed, and call system to alert all hospital staff to the hearing loss. Having a hospital room near the nurses' station helps decrease the client's feeling of isolation and increases the feeling of security. A pad and pencil should be handy in case the client finds it helpful. Write all important instructions for the client.

Encourage hearing-impaired clients to be assertive in asking others to repeat or rephrase what they have said, to speak louder, to face them directly, to move into the light, or to take any other action that helps clients better understand the verbal communication. Clients may be reluctant to ask others to accommodate them and need to know that most people are willing to be helpful when they understand what is being asked of them, and why. Clients with associated speech problems can anticipate situations in which they may have to repeat themselves or clarify a verbal communication.

When stress is a factor in hearing impairment or anxiety makes communication difficult, stress reduction exercises are often helpful. The nurse can teach these exercises to the client and encourage their use.

Some clients may find it necessary to learn speech reading. This helps clients identify spoken words even though they may not hear them. Auditory training is often a helpful adjunct to speech reading. In auditory training programs, people learn to discriminate between sounds and enhance their listening skills. Hearing centers, otologists, audiologists, and the organizations listed at the end of this chapter can direct clients to speech reading and auditory training classes in the local community.

Evaluation

Expected client outcomes following effective nursing interventions for impairment of communication include observation and reports that the client is resuming prior communication efficacy and is attempting to cope in a healthy and realistic manner.

Chapter Highlights

Assessment of the client's lifestyle and social support systems is an important component of subjective data collection.

The nurse should be alert to clinical clues of visual or hearing loss in any client, because clients are often sensitive and do not admit having sensory losses.

Families and significant others play an essential role in providing social support for visually or hearing-impaired clients.

Diagnostic approaches to evaluation of a client's vision include use of the ophthalmoscope, slit lamp, Snellen's chart, pinhole test, tonometer, color vision tests, computed tomography, fluorescein angiography, ultrasonography, and laboratory studies.

Diagnostic studies for clients with auditory dysfunction include radiographic studies, audiometric testing, and vestibular tests.

Teaching people how to protect and preserve their vision and hearing is a critical nursing role.

In planning and implementing care for the client with a visual or auditory impairment, the nurse must consider job factors, home maintenance, child care, financial security, transportation, self-care deficits, and independence.

Clients and their families should be instructed in the safe and effective administration of ophthalmic and otic medications.

Loss of vision or hearing can have major psychosocial/lifestyle consequences for the client and significant others.

Bibliography

American Council of Otolaryngology—Head and Neck Surgery: *Otologic Referral Criteria for Occupational Hearing Conservation Programs.* Washington, DC: American Council of Otolaryngology, 1981.

Belmont O: Some common visual symptoms: What they mean and what to do about them. *Occup Health Nurs* (June) 1981; 29:21–24.

Boyd–Monk H: Practical methods of how to examine the external eye. *Occup Health Nurs* (June) 1981; 29:10–14.

Clark JL: Otalgia: Identifying the source. *Postgrad Med* 1981; 70(4):99–103.

Cluff GL: After the hearing test: What then? *Occup Health Saf* (March) 1983; 14–21.

DeBlase R, Kucler M: Assistive hearing device aids patient-staff communication. *Ger Nurs* 1985; 64(4):223–224.

Franks JR, Bechmann NJ: Rejection of hearing aids: Attitudes of a geriatric sample. *Ear and Hearing* 1985; 6(3):161–166.

Gillin SL: Simple nursing procedures for the occupational health nurse. *Occup Health Nurs* (June) 1981; 29:18–20.

Hanawalt A, Troutman K: If your patient has a hearing aid. *Am J Nurs* 1984; 84:900–901.

Holder L: Hearing aids: Handle with care. *Nursing 82* (April) 1982; 12:64–65.

Hurvitz J, Carmen R: *Special Devices for Hard of Hearing, Deaf, and Deaf-Blind Persons.* Boston: Little, Brown, 1981.

King RC: Taking a close look at the eye. *RN* (Feb) 1982; 47:49–56.

Koch KH: Hidden handicaps: The deaf and hard of hearing. Some hints. *Nurs Times* 1981; 77(32):19–20.

LoGrasso BA: Using words without sound. *Am J Nurs* 1980; 80:2186–2187.

Magilvy J: Quality of life of hearing-impaired older women. *Nurs Res* 1985; 34(3):140–143.

Norman S: The pupil check. *Am J Nurs* 1982; 82:588–591.

Osguthorpe NC: If your patient has contact lenses. *Am J Nurs* 1984; 84:1255–1256.

Oyer HJ, Oyer EJ: Social consequences of hearing loss for the elderly. *Allied Health Behav Sci* 1983; 2(2):123–137.

Pesci BR: When the patient's problem is really poor vision. *RN* (Oct); 1986:22–25.

Ross T: Deafness: Breaking through the sound barrier. *Nurs Mirror* 1981; 152(21):20–23.

Smith JF, Nachazel PP: *Ophthalmic Nursing.* Boston: Little, Brown, 1980.

Stein HA, Slatt B: *The Ophthalmic Assistant: Fundamentals and Clinical Practice,* 4th ed. St. Louis: Mosby, 1983.

Tabor M: "Video display terminals: The eyes have it!" *Occup Health Safety* (Sept) 1981; 50:30–39.

Walsh C: Commonsense nursing care for the patient with poor vision. *RN* (Oct) 1986:24–25.

Watkins S, Moore TH, Phillips J: Clearing impacted ears. *Am J Nurs* 1984; 84(9):1107.

Zarnoch JM: Hearing disorders: Audiologic manifestations. In: *Speech, Language and Hearing.* Loss N et al. Philadelphia: Saunders, 1982.

Resources—Eye

SELF-HELP GROUPS AND OTHER ORGANIZATIONS

American Foundation for the Blind, Inc.
15 W. 16th St.
New York, NY 10011
Phone: (212) 620–2000

A national research and service agency for the blind. Publishes books, pamphlets, and professional reports including the *Directory of Agencies Serving Blind Persons in the United States.* Sells aids and appliances (kitchen, medical, sewing) for the visually handicapped.

Bold, Inc. (Blind Outdoor Leisure Development)
533 E. Main St.
Aspen, CO 81611
Phone: (303) 925–8922

Over 20 clubs nationwide are dedicated to providing outdoor recreational opportunities for the blind. They promote a more active life through skiing, swimming, rafting, camping, fishing, horseback riding, and golfing.

North Carolina Eye and Human Tissue Bank, Inc.
3195 Maplewood Ave.
Winston–Salem, NC 27103
Phone: (919) 765–0932

Provides corneas, sclerae, and vitreous humor without charge.

Eye Bank for Sight Restoration, Inc.
210 E. 64th St.
New York, NY 10021
Phone: (212) 980–6700

Receives donated eyes for distribution where needed to ophthalmologists.

Guide Dog Users
Box 174, Central Station
Baldwin, NY 11510
Phone: (304) 471–1490

This is an organization of persons who use guide dogs. Promotes education of its members and the public on guide dog training and supports the development of mobility aids for blind persons.

Hadley School for the Blind
700 Elm St.
Winnetka, IL 60093
Phone: (312) 446–8111

Provides tuition-free correspondence courses for the blind including vocational and university-level courses.

Library of Congress
Division for the Blind and Physically Handicapped
Washington, DC 20540
Phone: (202) 882–5500

Provides books in braille and talking book and magazine records and reproducers for these records. Distributes and maintains talking book machines through their 34 regional distributing libraries.

Local and/or state libraries

Supply books, magazines, and newspapers in large print as well as records and games.

National Retinitis Pigmentosa Foundation
1401 Mount Royal Avenue
Baltimore, MD 21217
Phone: (800) 638-2300 (toll-free)

An organization with over 40 chapters that supports research into retinitis pigmentosa and allied retinal degenerative diseases. Educates professionals and the public and trains self-help leaders.

National Society for the Prevention of Blindness, Inc.
79 Madison Ave.
New York, NY 10016
Phone: (212) 684–3222

Specializes in programs to eliminate preventable blindness through education, research, and prevention services.

New Eyes for the Needy, Inc.
549 Millburn Ave.
Short Hills, NJ 07078
Phone: (201) 376–4903

This nonprofit group of volunteers solicits used metal eyeglass frames and sells them to scrap refineries to raise money to buy prescription eyeglasses or prosthetic eyes for those who cannot afford them.

Recording for the Blind, Inc.
545 Fifth Avenue
New York, NY 10017
Phone: (212) 557–5720

A nonprofit organization that provides records or tapes of textbooks and other educational material. Will record books at the specific request of borrowers.

In Canada:

Blind Organization of Ontario with Self-Help
Tactics (BOOST)
100 Richmond St. E., Suite 408
Toronto, Ontario, Canada M4S 1E9
Phone: (416) 364–4639

Helps obtain employment for the blind and works toward improved legislation. Also provides a speakers bureau.

Canadian Council of the Blind
96 Rideout St. S.
London, Ontario, Canada N6L 3X4
Phone: (519) 434–4339

Promotes employment, public education, prevention of blindness, and social bonds between blind and sighted persons.

Canadian National Institute for the Blind
1931 Bayview Ave.
Toronto, Ontario, Canada M4G 4C8
Phone: (416) 486–2636

Offers counseling, education, social service, employment opportunities, and mobility training. Permanent resident accommodations (at a fee) are available.

John Milton Society for the Blind in Canada
40 St. Clair Ave. E., Suite 201
Toronto, Ontario, Canada M4T 1M9
Phone: (416) 921–4152

Founded by Helen Keller and church leaders from major denominations, this organization facilitates the spiritual development of the visually handicapped and assists them in participating in church and community work.

GUIDE DOG SERVICES

There are several centers that provide guide dog services for legally blind persons. Most programs are 4 weeks long and require full-time residence at the training facility where clients are matched and trained with a guide dog. There is no charge for the guide dog or the training program; however, not all training facilities cover travel expenses. Training services are provided by the following organizations.

Guide Dogs for the Blind, Inc.
P.O. Box 1200
San Rafael, CA 94902
Phone: (415) 479–4000
Training facilities in San Rafael, California.

Guiding Eyes for the Blind
611 Grant Springs Rd.
Yorktown Heights, NY 10598
Phone: (212) 683–5165
Training facilities in Yorktown Heights, New York.

International Guiding Eyes, Inc.
13445 Glenoaks Blvd.
Sylmar, CA 91342
Phone: (818) 362–5834
Training facilities in North Hollywood, California.

Leader Dogs for the Blind
1039 South Rochester Road
Rochester, MI 48063
Phone: (313) 651–9011
Training facilities in Rochester, Michigan.

(The) Seeing Eye, Inc.
P.O. Box 373
Morristown, NJ 07960
Phone: (201) 539–4425
Training facilities in Morristown, New Jersey.

HEALTH INFORMATION MATERIAL

The following resources provide helpful information about the eyes and vision:

Hammond RE: *Human Vision.* Raleigh, NC: Carolina Biological Supply Co., 1980.

This colorful 25-page booklet describes the structure and function of the eye, common disorders, and suggests activities for clients and students such as determining the size of the blind spot, color vision, and after images among others.

International Education Committee of the American Academy of Ophthalmology. *The Athlete's Eye.* San Francisco: Academy of Ophthalmology, 1983.

The 56-page booklet is written for athletes and those people responsible for their health and safety—coaches, athletic trainers, team physicians, and nurses. Includes color photographs.

Schulman J: *Cataracts: The Complete Guide from Diagnosis to Recovery for Patients and Families.* New York: Simon & Schuster, 1984.

Printed in large easy-to-read type, this book by an eminent eye specialist explains cataracts and every step of cataract surgery. Written in a conversational tone, the book is directed toward clients and their families.

SPECIALTY ORGANIZATION

American Society of Ophthalmic Registered Nurses
655 Beach
San Francisco, CA 94109
Phone: (415) 561–8500

Membership in this organization is composed of RNs working in ophthalmic nursing. The goal of the organization is to maintain excellence in client care through education of its members.

Resources—Ear

SELF-HELP GROUPS AND OTHER ORGANIZATIONS

American Academy of Otolaryngology—
Head and Neck Surgery, Inc.
1101 Vermont Ave. NW, Suite 302
Washington, DC 20005
Phone: (202) 289–4607

This association's members are physicians who specialize in treating people with disorders of the head and neck, especially disorders related to the ear, nose, and throat. The organization provides information and public service pamphlets.

American Athletic Association for the Deaf
3916 Lantern Dr.
Silver Spring, MD 20902
Phone: (301) 942–4042

This is an organization of deaf athletes and individuals interested in promoting competitive sports programs for hearing-impaired persons. They sponsor softball and basketball tournaments throughout the United States. Publish a quarterly bulletin.

American Humane Association
5351 S. Roslyn St.
Englewood, CO 80110
Phone: (303) 779–1400 (voice number)
(303) 287–6230 (TTY number)

Guide dogs trained to alert their masters to sounds such as alarm clocks, doorbells, telephones, or an infant's cry are available free of charge through this organization's Hearing Dog Program. Clients are also instructed in their use.

American Speech, Language, Hearing Association
10801 Rockville Pike
Rockville, MD 20852
Phone: (301) 897–5700

Information on hearing loss, as well as speech and hearing centers in locations across the country, is provided by this organization. Write or call (see Hot Line below) for information packet on cochlear implants, their risks and benefits, and the centers that provide this surgery.

Gallaudet College
Seventh St. and Florida Ave. NE
Washington, DC 20001
Phone: (202) 651–5000

This is the world's only liberal arts college for deaf persons.

Hearing and Tinnitus Help Association
32-A S. Main Street
New Hope, PA 18938
Phone: (215) 862–3475

An association that provides information and self-help to persons with tinnitus.

National Association of the Deaf
814 Thayer Ave.
Silver Spring, MD 20910
Phone: (301) 587–1788

This organization provides information on local chapters of interpreters.

Self-Help for the Hard of Hearing (SHHH)
7800 Wisconsin Ave.
Bethesda, MD 20814

Formed for people with hearing problems and their significant others, this organization provides education on hearing loss, remedial aids, and alternative communication skills. It also counsels members on the detection, management, and possible prevention of hearing loss.

Teletypewriters for the Deaf, Inc.
814 Thayer Ave.
Silver Spring, MD 20910
Phone: (301) 588–4605

This is an organization for deaf individuals who communicate through teletypewriters and for other persons and institutions interested in this form of communication. It encourages the development of networks and the installation of TTYs (teletypewriters) in public facilities, and distributes used equipment to deaf persons at a substantial discount. Publishes a quarterly newsletter and a directory of teletype terminals currently operated by deaf persons.

In Canada:

Canadian Deaf Sports Association
17512 86th Ave.
Edmonton, Alberta, Canada T5T 0L4
Promotes athletics for the deaf.

Canadian Speech and Hearing Association
Suite 1202
181 University Ave.
Toronto, Ontario, Canada M5H 3M7

Provides information on hearing loss and speech difficulties, and referrals to specialty centers throughout Canada.

Purple Cross Deaf Detection and Development Program
B. P. O. Elks of Canada
3420A Hill Ave.
Regina, Saskatchewan, Canada S4S 0W9

This organization raises funds for programs and research for hearing and speech services in Canada.

HOT LINES

AT&T
Phone: (800) 233–1222 (voice)

Hard-of-hearing people can obtain information on special telephone equipment for the hearing impaired at this number.

Phone: (800) 833-3232 (TTY)

People who use special telephone communication devices for the totally deaf can call this number to obtain assistance in placing person-to-person, third-number, collect, and credit card calls.

Hearing Helpline
Phone: (800) 424-8576 (9 AM to 5 PM Eastern Time)

This hot line operated by the Better Hearing Institute answers questions about hearing loss, hearing aids, and hearing aid services.

Kresge Hearing Research Laboratory of the South
Phone: (301) 897–8682

Call this number collect for information on help for people who can hear at only very high frequencies.

National Hearing Aid Society Helpline
(Mon–Fri, 9 AM to 5 PM)
Phone: (800) 521–5247 (nationwide)

Call this hot line for hearing aid information, consumer advice on hearing aids, and the names and locations of 2000 member dealers.

White House Hotline for the Hearing-Impaired
Comments Office
Phone: (202) 456–1414 (voice number)

Two White House offices have installed teletypewriter units so that hearing-impaired citizens can comment on presidential policies.

HEALTH INFORMATION MATERIAL

For helpful information about the ears and hearing, write to the following:

American Academy of Otolaryngology—
Head and Neck Surgery, Inc.
1101 Vermont Ave. NW, Suite 302
Washington, DC 20005

Bureau of Consumer Protection
Federal Trade Commission
Pennsylvania Ave. at Sixth St., NW
Washington, DC 20580

Conference of Executives of American Schools for the Deaf
5034 Wisconsin Ave., NW
Washington, DC 20016
Phone: (202) 363–1327

The April issue of American Annals of the Deaf includes a state-by-state listing of resources and services for the deaf that can be ordered.

National Association for Hearing and Speech Action
10801 Rockville Pike
Rockville, MD 20852

People with impaired hearing can obtain a national directory of public places that have devices specially designed to help them. The directory contains the names, addresses, and telephone numbers of more than 4,000 theaters, municipal buildings, houses of worship, and museums that have assistive hearing devices. The price of the 223-page "Directory of Assistive Listening Devices" is $12.95 for institutions and $7.95 for consumers. For a free listing for a particular state, call this organization's toll-free number listed under Hot Lines (voice or TDD).

NURSING ORGANIZATIONS

Otorhinolaryngology Head/Neck Nurses
℅ Warren Otologic Group
3893 East Market St.
Warren, OH 44484
Phone: (216) 856–4000

Members are RNs who promote continuing education and enhanced quality of client care in this specialty area, along with a strong sense of professional identity and an open forum for the exchange of ideas, information, and interests in the field.

CHAPTER **52**

Specific Disorders of Vision and Hearing

Other topics relevant to this content are: Administering ophthalmic medications, **Chapter 51;** Communicating with the hearing impaired client, **Chapter 51;** Communicating with the visually impaired client, **Chapter 51;** Personal ear care, **Chapter 51;** Personal eye care, **Chapter 51;** Personal eye care, **Chapter 51;** Removal of foreign bodies in the eye or ear, **Chapter 51;** Technique for equalizing pressure in the middle ear (Valsalva manuever), **Chapter 51.**

Objectives

When you have finished studying this chapter, you should be able to:

Identify common disorders affecting vision, hearing, and equilibrium.

Explain why psychosocial support of the client and family is a critical component in the nursing care of clients with eye and ear dysfunction.

Discuss the health education role of the nurse in preventing or limiting the effects of retinal detachment, glaucoma, motion sickness, and Meniere's syndrome.

Describe the nursing interventions in the detection and prevention of physiologic changes such as cataracts, macular degeneration, and presbycusis occurring in the eyes and ears of elderly clients.

Apply an understanding of the physiologic and psychosocial/lifestyle considerations of eye and ear surgery to the nursing care of the client.

Discuss the nursing implications of caring for these clients in the preoperative and postoperative periods.

Explain the complications of eye and ear surgery and the related nursing interventions.

Discuss alterations in body image encountered by clients having surgery of the eye or ear.

Teach clients and their families measures to avoid injuries and subsequent vision and hearing loss, thus limiting the effects of trauma to the eye or ear.

Many disorders of vision and hearing can be diminished in effect or prevented completely with early detection, prevention of injury, and appropriate treatment. The nurse plays an important role in all aspects of care and prevention. Emotional support is of primary importance in the nursing care of clients with visual, auditory, or vestibular dysfunction.

Ocular and aural surgery usually offer the client a chance for improved vision or hearing, pain relief, and a new outlook on life. Because of advances in technique, the frequency and number of available surgical procedures for the restoration or preservation of vision or hearing have greatly increased. Clients depend on health care professionals for their comfort and safety in the perioperative period. Many consider these surgeries frightening because of the importance of vision and hearing in daily life as well as the profound fear of blindness or deafness and lifestyle changes that accompany it.

SECTION 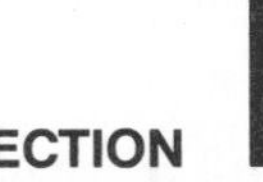

Congenital Disorders

Retinitis Pigmentosa

Retinitis pigmentosa, a hereditary disorder, involves the degeneration and clumping of the retinal pigment. This pigment lines the sensory retina (where the rods and cones lie) and serves a role in the physiologic function of the rods and cones essential for vision. Degeneration of the retinal pigment curtails the physiologic activity of the sensory retina, and it, too, begins to degenerate. Retinitis pigmentosa is primarily a disease of the rods; the cones are affected only late in the disease. The disorder may be mild or progress to total blindness, depending on the cause and duration of the disease. Other problems, such as deafness and mental retardation, can be associated with retinitis pigmentosa.

Transmission patterns of retinitis pigmentosa vary. Sex-linked retinitis pigmentosa seems to be the most disabling and rapidly progressive form. Approximately 55% to 60% of all reported retinitis pigmentosa cases affect males.

Clients with retinitis pigmentosa have a higher incidence of vitreous opacities, glaucoma, cataracts, retinal detachment, and myopia than the normal population.

Clinical Manifestations

The first signs of retinitis pigmentosa are usually seen by age 10. Night blindness is often the initial symptom, progressing to complaints of tunnel vision (even in the daylight) and, finally, total blindness, often by age 30 (Figure 52–1). Some cases remain stable instead of progressing. The final outcome for vision is better if the symptoms develop at an older age.

Medical Measures

No curative treatment of retinitis pigmentosa exists. The administration of vitamin A has been attempted without significant effects. Treatment should emphasize genetic counseling. Clients with the disease should be told that the chance of having an affected child is one in two and that the child may be more or less affected than they are themselves. The genetic background of the other parent does not influence the evaluation unless the family history also indicates the presence of retinitis pigmentosa.

Clients with retinitis pigmentosa should be treated for complications (eg, myopia or retinal detachment). Low-vision aids may provide slightly more vision. Low-vision aids for clients with retinitis pigmentosa include (1) field-widening devices for constricted peripheral fields (eg, Fresnel Press-On prisms applied to the spectacles); (2) hand-held magnifiers; and (3) night vision microscopes, which provide sufficient light amplification to allow the impaired cones to function. Rather than use such devices, many clients opt to deal with their progressing disease by learning early the rehabilitation methods used for the blind. Using a cane, learning braille, or possibly changing to a career that the client will be able to continue as vision deteriorates are a few rehabilitation methods that may be suggested.

Specific Nursing Measures

Emotional support of the client and family or significant others becomes the most important nursing intervention. Encourage the client to contact the National Retinitis Pigmentosa Foundation for counseling, reassurance, and information regarding testing for carriers and new lines of therapy (see resources section of Chapter 51).

Otosclerosis

Otosclerosis (otospongiosis) is a dystrophy of the temporal bone that begins as a softening of the bone because of resorption and increased vascularity. This spongy bone gradually becomes a dense sclerotic mass. It affects the bony labyrinth of the inner ear and usually invades the ligament around the stapes footplate, causing conductive hearing loss. The progressive involvement of the footplate causes its immobilization, preventing the transmission of sound through the oval window. Occasionally, the lesion invades the cochlear or vestibule of the inner ear and causes sensorineural hearing loss.

Although no definite cause of this bony growth has been established, heredity is a significant factor; 40% to 50% of cases report a family history of otosclerosis. This disease is common in whites but rare in blacks, Orientals, and Native Americans (Jerger & Jerger, 1981). Women have a greater incidence of otosclerosis than men. Puberty, pregnancy, and menopause often exacerbate it, and birth control pills can heighten the effects of the disease (Shambaugh & Glasscock, 1980).

Clinical Manifestations

The onset of otosclerosis usually occurs between 15 and 45 years of age but may occur as late as 70 to 80 years. A slowly progressive, bilateral conductive hearing loss is the primary clinical manifestation. The disease progresses slowly, with periods of inactivity. The client frequently can hear better in a noisy environment, and mild tinnitus often accompanies the hearing loss. When the disease progresses to the cochlea, mild vertigo may be present.

Medical Measures

Although there is no definitive medical treatment for otosclerosis, sodium fluoride has proven successful in arresting the process for some people. Florical, a combination of calcium carbonate and sodium fluoride sold as a dietary supplement, stops the progression of hearing loss in some clients. Hearing aids combined with a program of rehabilitation usually enable the client to hear. Surgical intervention involving the stapes also usually improves the hearing loss.

Specific Nursing Measures

Because the onset of otosclerosis usually occurs during the young adult period, affected clients may be anxious about whether the hearing loss will have an effect on their future. Reassure clients that if they use a hearing aid or

NURSING DIAGNOSES IN
Visual or Auditory Dysfunction

DIRECTLY RELATED DIAGNOSES

- Coping, ineffective individual
- Family processes, altered
- Fear
- Injury, potential for
- Knowledge deficit
- Role performance, altered
- Self-care deficit
- Self-concept, disturbance in: self-esteem
- Sensory/perceptual alterations: visual, auditory
- Social interaction, impaired

OTHER POTENTIAL DIAGNOSES

- Adjustment, impaired

undergo surgery, career plans usually need not be altered. The nursing care of a stapes surgery client is discussed below.

Tympanoplasty and Stapedectomy

Tympanoplasty designates a group of reconstructive procedures for repairing the tympanic membrane and the sound-conducting structures in the middle ear so hearing can be improved or maintained. Defects in the sound-transmitting apparatus can be caused by a congenital defect, trauma, otosclerosis, a cholesteatoma, or chronic suppurative otitis media.

Tympanoplastic surgery is individualized for each client according to the cause and amount of the defect in the sound-conducting apparatus. The simplest tympanoplastic procedure is the *myringoplasty,* a reconstruction of the tympanic membrane using a fascia graft taken from the temporal muscle behind the ear. Allograft tympanic membranes with or without attached ossicles also are used successfully for reconstruction.

Plastic or ceramic prostheses are used for partial or total ossicular replacements; however, human bone replacements are desirable, because they are rarely rejected (Hough, 1982). Other surgical procedures depend on whether the ossicles are fixed, whether they are partially or completely eroded, and whether any discontinuity, or gap, exists in the ossicular chain.

In the past, a stapes that was ankylosed, or fixed, because of otosclerosis was mobilized by removing the otosclerotic lesion around it. This procedure (stapes mobilization) is seldom performed today because the active otosclerotic lesion usually grows back. *Stapedectomy* is the current procedure of choice for an ankylosed stapes caused by otosclerosis. This procedure removes the head, neck, and crus of the stapes and connects a prosthesis from the footplate to the incus. This connects the incus to the oval window, bridging the gap between the incus and the inner ear.

Some surgeons perform tympanoplasty in stages. During the first stage, they generally perform a modified radical mastoidectomy to remove diseased tissue (eg, a cholesteatoma or otosclerosis) and then reconstruct the tympanic membrane. About 6 months later, they perform the second stage to inspect the cavity for recurrence of the cholesteatoma or otosclerosis and to perform any ossicular reconstruction that may be necessary. Client implications of tympanoplasty are summarized in Table 52–1.

Nursing Implications

Nursing implications for tympanoplasty are similar to those for mastoidectomy. Postoperatively, the head of the bed is elevated. Monitor the vital signs, observe for signs of bleeding and drainage, and report excessive bleeding to the physician. Outer dressings can be reinforced. If the client is feeling dizzy, the nurse assists in ambulation and uses siderails while the client is in bed. Dizziness may occur for a few hours after a stapedectomy. Be alert for signs of facial paralysis. Loss of taste or facial weakness due to trauma to CN VII should be reported immediately.

Medications administered may include analgesics, sedatives, and antibiotics as ordered. Occasionally, antiemetics are administered for nausea. Health teaching should include (1) warnings against nose blowing and keeping the mouth open when sneezing to prevent dislocation of the

Table 52–1
Tympanoplasty and Stapedectomy: Implications for the Client

Physiologic Implications	Psychosocial/Lifestyle Implications
Precautions to decrease bleeding during surgery	Hearing improvement after edema reduced and debris absent, if surgery successful
Need to change dressing three times a day after bulky dressing removal for 3 to 4 weeks	Need to report hearing decline
Possible dizziness	After stapedectomy, return to activities in 1 to 3 weeks
Avoidance of rubbing or scratching ear, sneezing or nose blowing with mouth shut, and water in ear until healed	After tympanoplasty with mastoidectomy, return to activities in 6 weeks
Possible broad-spectrum antibiotic administration	Slight clicking or popping of prosthesis heard in wind
Discharge evening of surgery or in 1 to 2 days	Yearly hearing tests
	Possible need for hearing aid

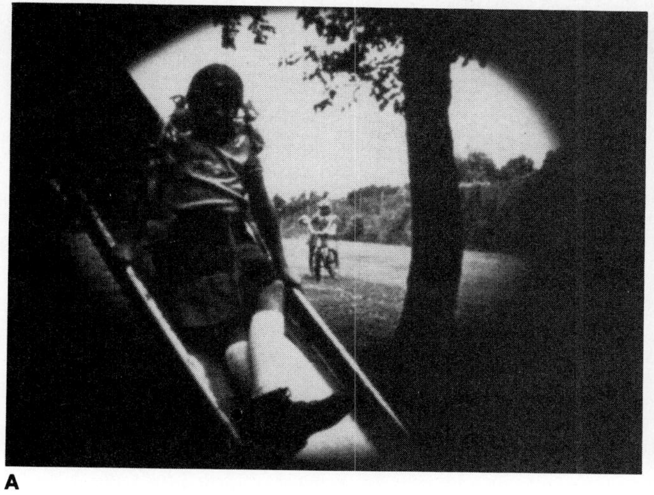

A

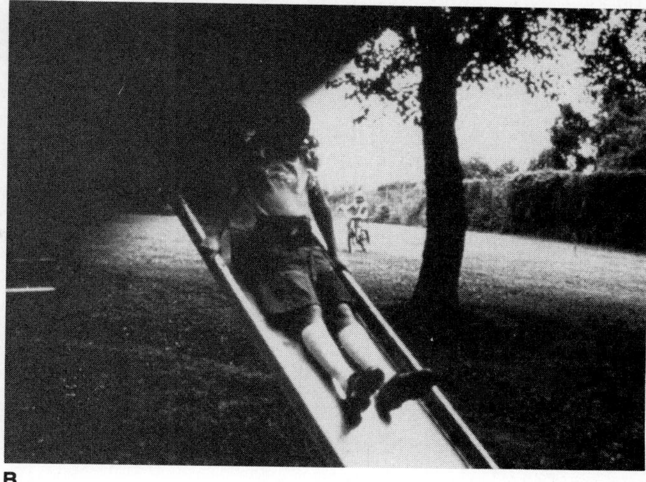

B

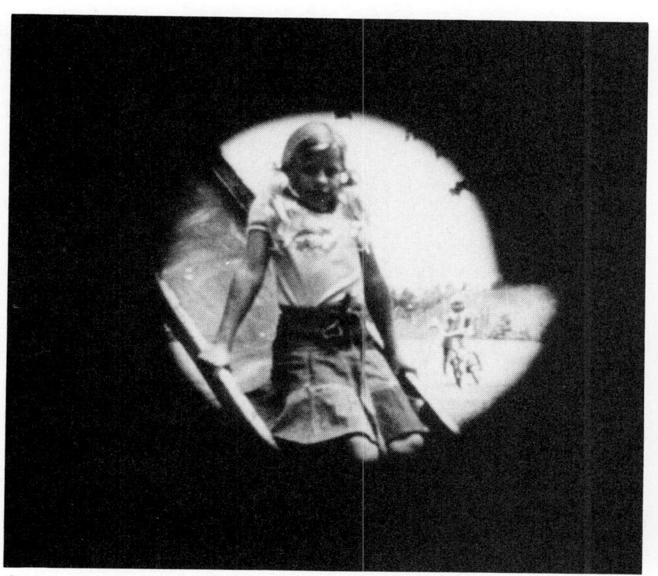

C

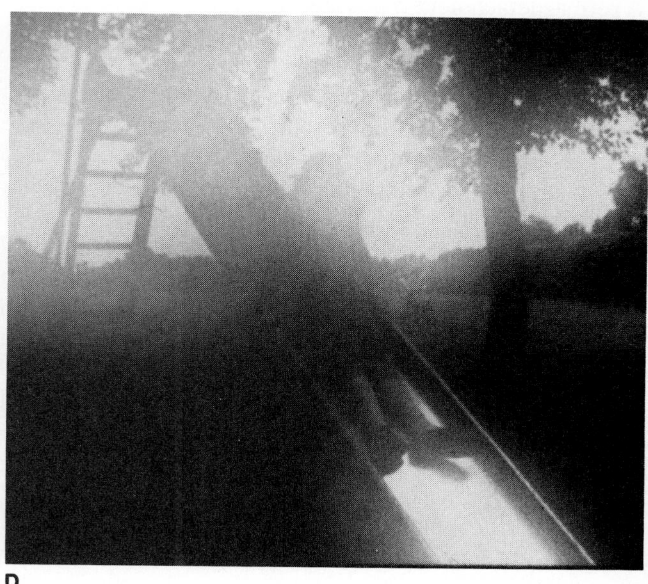

D

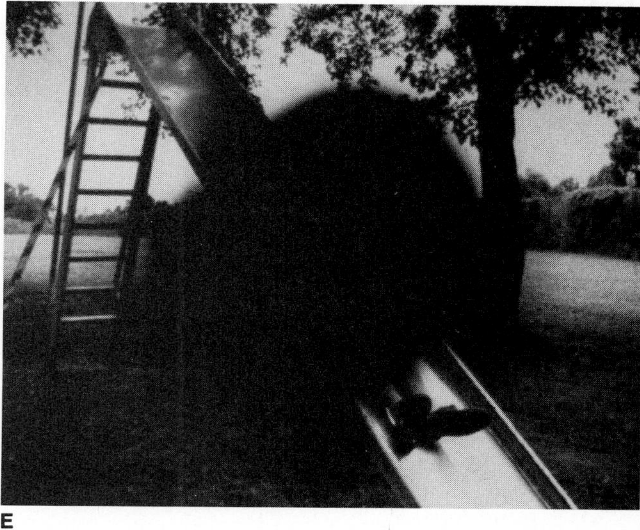

E

Figure 52–1

Visual changes in eye disorders. *Courtesy of National Eye Institute, Bethesda, MD.*

A. Retinitis pigmentosa.

B. Retinal detachment.

C. Advanced glaucoma.

D. Cataract.

E. Senile macular degeneration.

prosthesis and (2) instructions for changing the cotton ball in the external auditory canal. Also include instructions related to the client implications in Table 52–1.

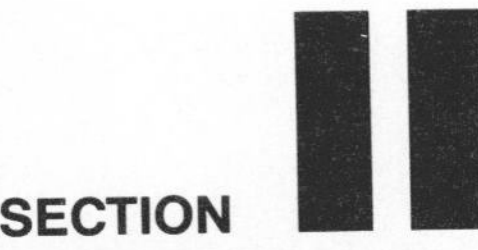

SECTION II

Disorders of Multifactorial Origin

Retinal Detachments

A retinal detachment is possible because the retina is physically attached to the inside of the eye (the choroid) in only two places: at the very back (the optic nerve) and at its front edge (the ciliary body). The remaining retina is held in position by the gentle pressure of the vitreous. A hole or tear can develop in any part of the retina but is most frequent near the front edge, where it is thinnest (Figure 52–2A).

When a tear occurs, vitreous leaks through the retinal hole, seeps behind the retina, lifts it from the choroid in a progressive fashion, and enlarges the detachment. Vision becomes compromised as the rods and cones are deprived of their choroidal nutritional supply. Untreated retinal detachment often eventually results in massive fibrosis of the retina and vitreous cavities; this frequently is complicated by uveitis and cataract formation. The eye may eventually become glaucomatous or atrophic and blinded.

Retinal detachments may have a variety of causes. Both severe myopia and aphakia have been implicated. A contusion or penetrating injury also can cause retinal detachment; in fact, detachment occurs in about 80% of ocular contusions. Racket sports are becoming major culprits in trauma-induced retinal detachments, and safety goggles are finding new clients as athletes recognize this danger. *Neovascularization,* commonly seen in diabetic retinopathy (discussed in Chapter 32), can extend into the vitreous. Traction along these vessels can cause severe vitreous hemorrhage and retinal detachment (Figure 52–2B).

Clinical Manifestations

The symptoms of retinal detachment include a "shadow" or "curtain" spreading across the field of vision (Figure 52–1B). The client may notice the sudden appearance of photopsia or floaters in one eye, followed eventually by a loss of a portion of the visual field. These floaters are caused by shadows cast by pigment or blood cells freed into the vitreous at the time the retina tears. Vision is at first blurred and becomes progressively worse. Nontraumatic retinal detachments have a strong bilateral tendency.

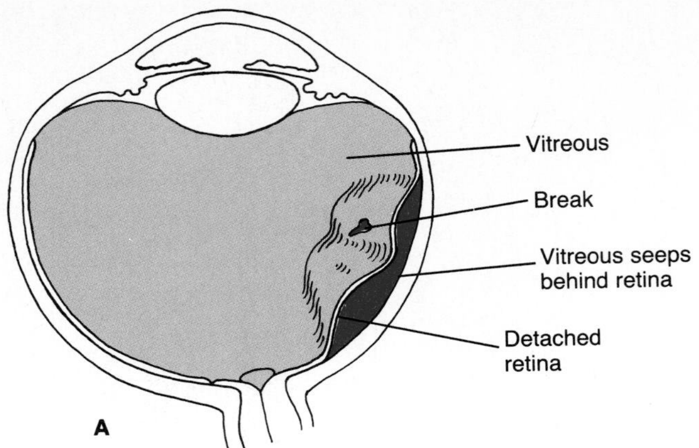

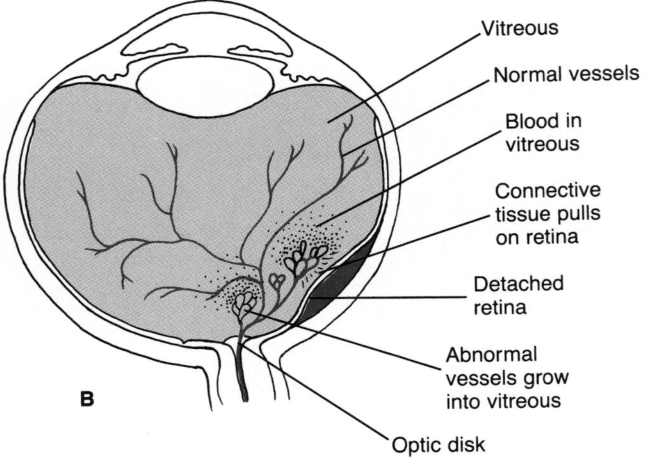

Figure 52–2

A. Retinal detachment. **B.** Traction retinal detachment because of neovascularization in diabetic retinopathy.

Medical and Specific Nursing Measures

The goal of treatment in retinal detachment is to seal holes and prevent their further development. Measures include cryotherapy, diathermy, photocoagulation, and surgery. In addition, panretinal photocoagulation, a "scatter treatment" with a wide band of laser spots, is sometimes performed to prevent neovascularization in diabetics. Client education in the symptoms of retinal holes and detachment is essential, because delay of repair may result in an uncorrectable injury to vision. Nursing care of the client undergoing surgery is discussed below.

Retinal Detachment Surgery

Sealing of a retinal break by the creation of a chorioretinal adhesion is accomplished by diathermy, cryotherapy, or photocoagulation. These procedures cause a chorioretinal scar to form around the lesion and hence prevent the leakage of vitreous fluid behind the retina. In diathermy, heat is applied directly to the sclera to create an adhesion. This

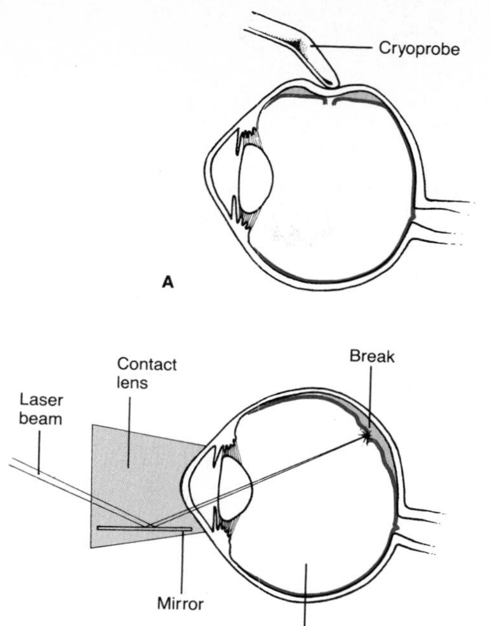

Figure 52–3

Retinal reattachment surgery. **A.** Using a cryoprobe. Scar tissue forms as the frozen area heals, reattaching the retina. **B.** Using a laser. Tiny laser burns weld the retina back together in a process called photocoagulation.

method is being abandoned in favor of cryotherapy and photocoagulation. Cryotherapy involves the use of a supercooled (−70°C) metal probe (cryoprobe) applied to the sclera opposite the borders of the retinal hole for a varying period of time (Figure 52–3A). The disruption of the pigment epithelium excites an inflammatory response, which leads to scar formation and retinal reattachment within about 1 week. Photocoagulation employs a bright light (eg, an argon laser or xenon lamp) focused through the refracting media (cornea, lens, vitreous, and aqueous humor) onto the retinal hole (Figure 52–3B). The heat generated by the light induces the retina and underlying retina to coagulate together. This procedure is often done on an outpatient basis for prophylactic treatment of predisposing peripheral degenerations of the retina. In all three procedures used to create a chorioretinal scar, local anesthetic is administered.

Scleral buckling techniques indent the sclera toward the vitreous by implanting various materials at the retinal break. Implants may be made of absorbable materials such as gelatin or nonabsorbable materials such as silicone rubber. Absorbable implants are used in uncomplicated cases of retinal detachment to create a temporary buckle. These implants are slowly broken down and absorbed by the host tissues and replaced by a layer of granulation tissue within 3 to 6 months. Nonabsorbable implants are used to create a permanent buckle and are indicated when there is a large break in the retina, multiple breaks, or signs of traction (eg, preretinal proliferation). An encircling element (a silicon rubber band that encircles the eye) is generally used in conjunction with silicone rubber implants and provides permanent relief of vitreous traction. Implications for the client with retinal detachment surgery are summarized in Table 52–2.

Nursing Implications

PREOPERATIVE CARE The client should have a thorough understanding of what to expect before, during, and after the surgery. A client information sheet such as the one in Box 52–1 will help reinforce the nurse's preoperative teaching.

Clients with a retinal detachment have usually had a sudden loss of sight. They are generally admitted to the hospital soon after the diagnosis has been made and often do not have time to prepare for surgery emotionally or physically. Recognize the intensity of their fear and apprehension. Explanations of the surgical procedure, reassurance, truthful answers to questions, and the provision of

Table 52–2
Retinal Detachment Surgery: Implications for the Client

Physiologic Implications	Psychosocial/Lifestyle Implications
Approximately 80% initial success for surgery; floaters may remain	Need for emotional support
Potential complications from prolonged bed rest (eg, thrombi and atelectasis)	Decreased physical activity (more so than any other eye surgery) for 6–8 weeks
Bilateral eye patches	Increased dependency on others while eyes are patched and activity is limited
Lid edema and chemosis	Concern and anxiety regarding amount of vision restored after surgery
Possible complications of general anesthesia	Fear of blindness (potential body image changes)
Postoperative complications, including infection, choroidal detachment, glaucoma, and vitreous hemorrhage	Potential sensory deprivation
	Possible adjustment to living with decreased vision
	Discouragement from potential for recurrence
	Financial strain if out of work for long period

Box 52–1
Client Information Sheet: Ophthalmic Surgery

Preoperative Phase

Become familiar with your surroundings because one or both eyes will be patched after surgery.

Blood and urine samples will be needed, as well as possibly an electrocardiogram (ECG) and chest x-ray.

There will be an order for you to have nothing to eat or drink after midnight the evening before your surgery. (The abbreviation for this is NPO.)

An intravenous line (IV) may be started before or during the surgery to give you fluids, avoid dehydration, and administer necessary medications.

Eyedrops will generally be given. There are many different kinds (eg, antibiotics, anti-inflammatory agents, and pupil dilators) to decrease eye movement and facilitate the surgery.

A tranquilizer will often be administered (either by pills or an injection). This will allow you to relax during the surgery.

Intraoperative Phase

A nurse will meet you upon your entrance to the operating room.

If you will be receiving local anesthesia, it will be important to hold your head still except when asked by the doctor to move.

Anesthetic eyedrops will be given to numb your eye.

Local anesthesia is often given (at the eyelids) to prevent blinking.

Eyelashes may be trimmed.

Sterile drapes will cover the rest of your face during surgery.

Postoperative Phase

You will return to your room after surgery. If you have had general anesthesia, you will go to the postanesthesia room first until you are fully awake.

One or both eyes may be patched for protection and rest, as well as to minimize movement.

If no nausea occurs, eating and drinking are usually allowed the day of surgery.

You will be encouraged to move your legs gently while in bed to prevent the formation of blood clots in your legs.

Postoperative Phase *(continued)*

Breathe deeply to expand your lungs and keep them free of secretions.

If you must cough, keep your mouth open to help decrease pressure inside the head.

Notify the nurse if you are nauseated or if you feel sharp pain or pressure in your eye.

Laxatives may be ordered to avoid straining with bowel movements.

Activity and position restrictions are important and should be followed to prevent complications. Each eye surgery and surgeon may have different requirements. Examples are: (1) head of the bed elevated; (2) bed rest; (3) avoiding putting the face down; (4) no lying on operated side to prevent pressure and contamination; (5) no leaning over or stooping (increases the pressure in your eye); and (6) no shaving, hair combing, or tooth brushing.

Be sure to clarify the specific instructions and postoperative restrictions regarding your surgery with your physician and nurse.

Activities that increase blood pressure in the head also increase eye (intraocular) pressure, which is undesirable. Thus, these activities may be restricted for several days to weeks. Examples are straining during bowel movements, heavy lifting, rubbing the eyes, squinting, and tightly closing the eyes.

Eye medications may be ordered, and patches may be changed daily by your physician or nurse. Instructions for taking medications at home will be given to you by the physician, nurse, and pharmacist.

Your family or friends are encouraged to visit and participate in your care as needed or desired.

Television watching and reading may be restricted by the physician.

Avoid eye cosmetics until given permission to use them by your physician.

Your specific surgery will be discussed with you by your physician. If you have any questions, do not hesitate to ask your physician or nurse.

realistic hope are nursing interventions that can significantly reduce the client's anxiety.

Upon admission to the hospital, the client is frequently limited to bed rest with bathroom privileges, and bilateral patches are often applied. Bed rest reduces eye movements, decreases the chance of the client's falling and causing further injury to the retina, allows a vitreous hemorrhage to clear, improves the position of the retina, and prevents macular detachment. The client is positioned so that the area of detachment is in the dependent position. Activity and position restrictions vary by surgeon and client. Therefore, the nurse must be familiar with the client's specific orders. Frequent reminders and explanations regarding which positions and activities are permitted encourage client cooperation. Evaluate whether the client needs a sedative to promote relaxation and comfort. For the client confined to bed, safety precautions, attempts to lessen sensory deprivation, and avoidance of potential complications are similar to those described at the beginning of the chapter.

POSTOPERATIVE CARE Many of the preoperative nursing measures are continued postoperatively. Specific position restrictions depend on the location and extent of the retinal detachment and on whether air was injected into the vitreous to help reposition the retina. If air was injected, position the client so the area of the retina that needs to be repositioned against the choroid is uppermost. Gravity then will cause the air bubble to rise and press against the retina. The surgeon should specify the position of the body (prone, supine, or on one side), the position of the head, and the elevation of the head of the bed.

Most clients are allowed bathroom privileges the day of surgery. Short walks in the hall and sitting in a chair for meals is generally permitted the day following surgery, depending on the severity of the case. The client on any degree of bed rest must resume leg exercises and deep breathing postoperatively. Expressions of empathy and reassurance are helpful for the client attempting to limit activity.

Bilateral patches are usually not indicated if the retina is flat at the end of the operation. Frequently check the dressing of the operated eye for drainage or bleeding but change it only if ordered to do so.

Discharge teaching is similar to that for any eye surgery. Emphasize that excessive eyestrain, constipation, straining, lifting heavy objects, contact sports, and stooping should be avoided for at least 6 to 8 weeks postoperatively. Nurses should address psychosocial implications such as fear of reinjury, fear that the repair will not work, or fear of potential blindness prior to discharge. Clients need and appreciate reassurance that these emotions are common in people having undergone retinal detachment repair.

Nursing Research Note

Hill BJ: Sensory information, behavioral instructions and coping with sensory alteration surgery. *Nurs Res* 1982; 31(1):17–21.

An experimental design was used to examine the relation between behavioral instructions, sensory information, and general information and their effect on the coping behavior of postsurgical cataract clients. The combination of behavioral instruction and sensory information decreased the time of the client's first venture from home. Explaining typical sensations to be expected by postsurgical cataract clients improved client outcome. Presurgical behavioral instructions for cataract clients (eg, how to reduce discomfort in the operative eye and appropriate self-care skills) are beneficial and should be instituted by nurses.

Vitrectomy

A vitrectomy is a microsurgical procedure in which the preretinal membranes are cut and abnormal vitreous is removed via suction and replaced by a balanced salt solution. This often prevents loss of vision from retinal damage.

A vitrectomy is performed when there is sufficient loss of vitreous or damage to the vitreous to cause a retinal tear or detachment or to block the light rays from the retina. Vitreous hemorrhage from trauma and retinal traction detachment from proliferative diabetic retinopathy are the main indications for a vitrectomy. Other indications include vitreous loss, vitreous opacity, and traction detachments from other causes such as vasculitis and sickle-cell disease. Implications for the client with a vitrectomy are summarized in Table 52–3.

Nursing Implications

PREOPERATIVE CARE Before caring for the client, be aware of the specific type of vitrectomy performed. Care of a client who has had a simple vitrectomy differs from care after retinal detachment surgery. Nursing care will be more complex if the retina was involved. (See nursing implications in the discussion of retinal detachment surgery.)

Often clients having vitrectomy surgery have such poor visual acuity (20/200) that they are considered legally blind. Therefore, safety precautions are imperative. Clients should be oriented to their surroundings and allowed to unpack their own belongings to avoid frustration; the nurse should avoid rearranging the belongings.

POSTOPERATIVE CARE One or both eyes will be patched upon the client's return to the room, so reorientation to the surroundings and safety precautions are important. Generally, no specific position must be maintained unless there was retinal involvement. A semi-Fowler's position is recommended if persistent bleeding exists to allow the blood to settle below the visual axis. Most clients are allowed bathroom privileges (with assistance) the day of surgery and slow walks in the hall the first postoperative day. The hospital stay of a vitrectomy client is from 3 to 7 days.

Table 52–3
Vitrectomy: Implications for the Client

Physiologic Implications	Psychosocial/Lifestyle Implications
Improved vision if no macular damage has occurred	Temporary curtailment of strenuous activities
Minimal postoperative pain	Temporary visual impairmentr with eye patch
Potential complications, including lens damage, retinal holes, delayed healing of corneal epithelium, and glaucoma	Return to work in 1–3 wk unless complications arise or manual labor is required
	Anxiety, fear, and concern

Glaucoma

Aqueous humor normally drains through the trabecular meshwork (located at the angle of the iris and the cornea) into Schlemm's canal and, finally, into the venous system (Figure 52–4A). In glaucoma, obstruction of the filtration system impairs the outflow mechanism, allowing the aqueous humor no exit. The subsequent accumulation of fluid causes a rise in intraocular pressure (IOP; normally between 12 and 20 mm Hg). The nerve fibers and blood vessels in the optic disk become compressed and are eventually damaged or destroyed.

Glaucoma is typically bilateral unless it occurs as a result of another disease. However, symptoms in one eye may be more pronounced than in the other eye. Visual impairment varies from blurred vision to complete blindness.

Glaucoma is one of the most common causes of blindness in North America. Approximately 2% of all people over 40 years old in the United States have glaucoma, and another 1 million cases have not yet been diagnosed.

Primary open-angle glaucoma, often referred to as simple glaucoma, is a chronic disease usually manifested in middle or late life. The most common form of glaucoma, it accounts for approximately 90% of the diagnosed cases. It results from a progressive narrowing in diameter of the trabecular meshwork openings (rather than from a narrowing or closure of the angle), which creates a resistance to aqueous humor outflow.

Primary angle-closure glaucoma, also called narrow-angle glaucoma, normally occurs in people who already have a narrow entrance into the filtration angle and a shallow anterior chamber (Figure 52–4B). Dilatation or forward displacement of the pupil causes the iris to push against the trabecular meshwork, thus blocking the exit of aqueous humor (Figure 52–4C). Conditions that would normally dilate the pupils, such as fear and dark adaptation, or medications that cause cycloplegia also may instigate this disorder. It may affect one eye at a time, and the extent of damage varies in relation to the severity and duration of ocular hypertension. Primary glaucoma—both open-angle and angle-closure—has no known basis other than genetic predisposition (Shields, 1982).

Secondary glaucoma results from other diseases of the eye that interfere with the outflow of aqueous humor. It may be of either the open-angle or angle-closure type. Secondary open-angle glaucoma may be caused by a blockage of the trabecular meshwork from debris or red blood cells (trauma), tumors, or iritis. Lens dislocation, scar tissue, or adhesions between the cornea and iris may give rise to secondary angle-closure glaucoma.

Congenital glaucoma is a very rare ocular disorder associated with congenital anomalies. Further information regarding this specific disorder may be obtained from an ophthalmology or pediatric text.

Absolute glaucoma is the end result of any uncontrolled glaucoma. Blindness always results, and the severe pain accompanying this form often necessitates an enucleation.

Clinical Manifestations

Primary open-angle glaucoma is a slowly progressive disease. Most clients are unaware they have glaucoma (or that they are at risk because of a shallow anterior chamber) unless it has been diagnosed on a routine eye examination, because there are no symptoms until visual impairment occurs. The earliest signs of visual impairment the client may detect include failure to perceive changes in color, blurred vision, premature presbyopia, decreased accommodation, and a persistent aching of the eyes. A decrease in peripheral vision over the years also may occur (Figure 52–1C).

Primary angle-closure glaucoma, in contrast, occurs suddenly. The client suffers intense pain and a sudden decrease or loss of vision. Nausea, vomiting, and diapho-

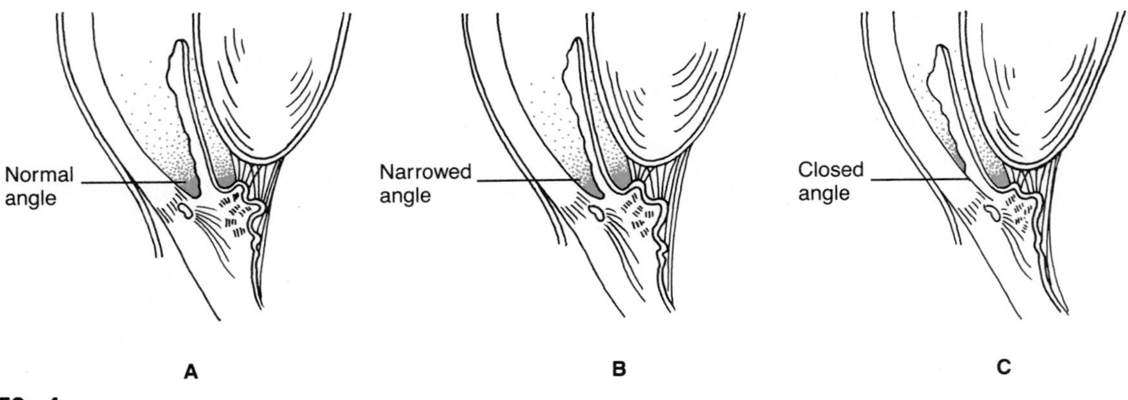

Figure 52–4

The anterior chamber angle in the normal eye and in glaucoma. **A.** Normal anterior chamber angle. **B.** Narrowed anterior chamber angle. **C.** Closed anterior chamber angle.

resis often accompany an acute attack because of the severe pain. The affected eye usually appears red, and the iris appears dull, gray, and patternless. The pupil is fixed, dilated, and unresponsive to light. Edema of the lids, cornea, and conjunctiva also may be present. IOP is frequently greater than or equal to 50 or 60 mm Hg. Over 50% of clients with angle-closure glaucoma experience transient subacute attacks. These generally last a few hours and increase in frequency prior to an acute attack. Clients often see halos of blue–violet and yellow–red rings around lights while experiencing a subacute attack.

The clinical manifestations of secondary glaucoma are similar to those of either primary open-angle or primary angle-closure glaucoma, depending on the etiology.

Medical Measures

Primary open-angle glaucoma is a chronic condition that cannot be cured; it can only be controlled to decrease visual loss. Treatment must be continued for the rest of the individual's life. It can often be controlled for long periods by miotic agents such as pilocarpine (1% to 6%), that constrict the pupil and allow opening of the outflow channel to facilitate aqueous humor drainage, thereby reducing the IOP. Pilocarpine can also be administered through a diffusional system, placed under the eyelid, that employs the principle of membrane-controlled drug release.

Epinephrine hydrochloride 0.5% to 2% (Epifrin) and timolol maleate (Timoptic) in concentrations of 0.25% to 0.5% also are used in the treatment of open-angle glaucoma.

When maximal medical management of open-angle glaucoma is not successful and there is progressive visual field loss, surgery is indicated. Filtering procedures such as trabeculectomy and sclerectomy, or procedures such as iridectomy or laser iridotomy are used most often.

Primary angle-closure glaucoma usually mandates immediate surgical management. Surgery is often curative if the duration of the attack is short and no scars have formed. Iridectomy or laser iridotomy are most commonly performed. Prophylactic surgery is recommended for the other eye to prevent a second acute attack.

An effort is made to decrease the IOP with medications prior to surgery. Pilocarpine (2% to 4%) instilled every 5 minutes for 30 minutes to 1 hour, then three to four times per hour until surgery, is often required. Sometimes cholinesterase inhibitors such as eserine and neostigmine are used alternately with pilocarpine in an attempt to open the angle. Hyperosmotic agents (mannitol or oral glycerin), which draw fluid from the eye, are also usually given. Carbonic anhydrase inhibitors such as acetazolamide (Diamox) may also be given IV in an attempt to decrease the intraocular pressure quickly. Pain and nausea must be controlled with narcotics and antiemetics.

Treatment of secondary glaucoma begins by treating the underlying cause. The disorder is then treated the same as open-angle or angle-closure glaucoma, whichever is present.

Marijuana is being used experimentally in some centers where it is available by prescription. Another experimental drug, levobunolol, is painless when applied topically.

Specific Nursing Measures

When clients are admitted to the hospital, assess their ability to see and orient them to their surroundings. Explain and assist with diagnostic procedures. Care of the client requiring surgery is discussed below.

PREVENTION Since glaucoma is a leading cause of blindness in North America, prevention is one of the nurse's most important functions. Mass screening of people over age 40 can be accomplished relatively easily. Temporary or mobile clinics may be set up to perform visual field tests, make tonometry readings, and provide general information regarding the disease. With practice, the nurse should be able to perform tests easily and accurately. Individuals with a family history of glaucoma should be encouraged to have regular tonometry tests well before they reach age 40. Making the public aware of glaucoma and its consequences often encourages people to seek early testing and treatment.

EMOTIONAL SUPPORT Those diagnosed as having the disease often are apprehensive about the threat to their sight and require emotional support. It is important to be honest and open with clients in as positive a manner as possible. Discuss information on disease progression and the steps that can be taken to prevent further damage:

- Routine eye examinations
- Compliance with the recommended medical regimen
- Prophylactic iridectomy
- Maintenance of general good health
- Avoidance of strenuous activities, which may increase IOP

Group sessions for individuals having difficulty dealing with their diagnosis of glaucoma often provide encouragement, new ways of coping, and peer support.

Client/Family Teaching

MEDICATION Another important function of the nurse includes assisting clients with their medication regimens. Instructions regarding the time, amount, side effects, and proper administration of medications are essential. For example, eyedrops are best placed in the lower fornix while occluding the tear duct to prevent excessive systemic effects. Inform clients of the inconvenience that miotics may cause, for example, increased difficulty seeing in the dark (see Chapter 51). Encourage all glaucoma clients to carry a card stating what medications they are taking and to wear an identification bracelet or necklace in case of an accident. This information not only alerts health care providers that an individual has glaucoma and that the prescribed glaucoma medications should be continued; it also prevents health care providers from using medications that cause pupil dilation (eg, atropine as a preoperative medication), which could precipitate an acute attack of glaucoma. Teach clients to wash their hands prior to instilling eye medications, and to take care not to touch the eyedropper to the eye.

Many glaucoma clients are elderly and may require additional teaching and support if their regimens are to be followed. Often the elderly live alone; are somewhat forgetful; have decreased vision, making it difficult to identify the proper eyedrops; or run out of medication before it is time for their appointments. Creative measures taken by the nurse often facilitate the elderly's adherence to treatment. For example, different bottles of medications can be identified by using small and large bottles or by placing a rubber band around one of them.

GENERAL HEALTH PRACTICES Urge all glaucoma clients or people at risk (those with a shallow anterior chamber) to establish and maintain general health practices. They should avoid constipation, heavy lifting and straining, and activities that increase the intracranial pressure and, hence, the IOP. Instruct clients to clean discharge with normal saline or warm water from the inside corner of the eye outward. In addition, caution clients against rubbing their eyes.

Clients at risk should not use some eye "whiteners" or antihistamines, because they may dilate the pupil and initiate an acute attack. Whiteners such as tetrahydrozoline hydrochloride (Visine) are vasoconstrictors that decrease ocular inflammation and redness.

Iridectomy and Iridotomy

An *iridectomy* is a simple, effective surgical procedure in which a small portion of the iris is removed. The procedure relieves the blockage of the trabecular meshwork by the periphery of the iris by creating a new channel between the chambers and allowing the iris to fall away from the trabecular meshwork (Figure 52–5). Drainage of aqueous humor via normal pathways is thus re-established.

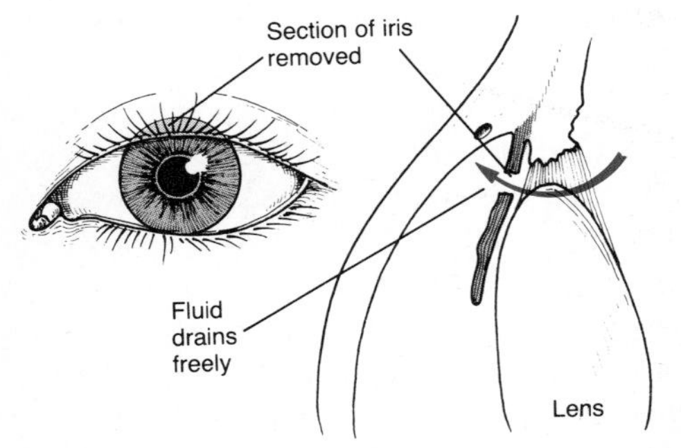

Figure 52–5

Iridectomy and iridotomy.

Laser *iridotomies* are increasingly frequent as experience with the procedure grows. They are performed on an outpatient basis using only a drop of topical anesthesia. The laser iridotomy is normally made in the upper quadrant of the middle to peripheral iris. The required number of laser applications for a successful iridotomy varies from individual to individual; the average falls between 60 and 90 applications in a single sitting. Implications for the client with an iridectomy or iridotomy are summarized in Table 52–4.

Nursing Implications

PREOPERATIVE CARE Clients with angle-closure glaucoma are usually admitted to the hospital during an acute attack of increased IOP. The nursing care has been discussed above.

POSTOPERATIVE CARE Orient the postoperative client to time and place upon return to the room. Encourage rest the first day to allow the wound to seal; however, the client may get up to go to the bathroom with assistance. Most clients resume a regular diet the first day.

Other important nursing interventions include the administration of prescribed medications and assessing the client for complications. Severe pain is uncommon and warrants an examination by the physician.

The client is generally discharged the day after surgery. Laser iridotomy clients may undergo same-day surgery. The nurse's discharge teaching should include information on prescribed medications (steroids and mydriatics), symptoms and signs of potential complications (persistent or intense pain, decreased or blurred vision, hyphema)

Table 52–4
Iridectomy and Iridotomy: Implications for the Client

Physiologic Implications	Psychosocial/Lifestyle Implications
Relief of pain	Minimal lifestyle changes
Cure of glaucoma if increased intraocular pressure was due solely to closed angle	Ability to resume activities of daily living the day after surgery
Rare postoperative complications, including hemorrhage, cataracts, persistent hypertension of the eye, and a flat or shallow anterior chamber	No adverse cosmetic effects (lid usually covers incisional site)
Complications of laser iridotomies are burns at the therapy site and retinal burns	No visual changes; freedom from glaucoma

and eye care. It should also emphasize the importance of follow-up care and routine eye examinations.

Filtering Procedures for Glaucoma: Trabeculectomy and Sclerectomy

Filtering procedures are used in the treatment of open-angle glaucoma when medical management is insufficient to prevent optic nerve atrophy. There are many types of filtering procedures; however, they all create a drainage channel from the anterior chamber through the sclera, allowing the aqueous humor to flow into the subconjunctival spaces, where it can be absorbed.

A *sclerectomy* creates a direct opening (fistula) through the sclera into the anterior chamber, allowing aqueous humor to drain freely. A *trabeculectomy* involves a partial-thickness scleral flap, under which lies the fistula to the anterior chamber. This surgical procedure removes a section of the blocked trabecular meshwork. A laser beam technique (trabeculoplasty) achieves the same effect. Client implications associated with filtering procedures for glaucoma are similar to those for iridectomy and iridotomy listed in Table 52–4.

Nursing Implications

PREOPERATIVE CARE A client having a filtering procedure for the treatment of glaucoma is usually admitted to the hospital the evening before surgery. The nurse should carry out routine admission procedures according to the institution's and surgeon's protocols. Take time to discuss the client's fears and misgivings and to clear up misconceptions. This often helps relieve the client's and family's anxiety, as well as fosters their cooperation and confidence.

POSTOPERATIVE CARE Postoperative nursing care of the client having a filtering procedure is similar to care after other eye surgeries. Discharge teaching is consistent with that discussed in the section on iridectomy.

Motion Sickness

Motion sickness is a temporary disturbance in the functioning of the semicircular canals. Little is known about its exact cause and nature. It happens to some but not all people exposed to repetitive, shifting movement such as riding in a boat, on amusement park rides, or in the back seat of an automobile for long distances. The constantly shifting head position, changes in acceleration, and conflicting vestibular and visual signals are thought to be responsible for motion sickness.

Clinical Manifestations

Symptoms are dizziness and nausea that often progresses to vomiting. Motion sickness may begin soon after the exposure to motion and may not subside until several hours after the stimulation has stopped.

Medical Measures

Some people are helped by taking steps to minimize changes in the visual field. It may help to hold the head in a fixed position and to focus the eyes on a single point. Dancers learn this early in their career; when twirling, spinning, or turning rapidly they keep their eyes fixed on one object and turn their heads rapidly to refocus as quickly as possible on the same object.

Antinauseants such as dimenhydrinate (Dramamine), meclizine hydrochloride (Antivert, Bonine), trimethobenzamide hydrochloride (Tigan), and cyclizine hydrochloride (Marezine) have been used successfully to prevent motion sickness as well as to relieve the symptoms. They may be taken by mouth ½ hour to 1 hour before the anticipated motion begins and then continued until the symptoms subside. If vomiting makes the oral route ineffective, intramuscular administration may be necessary.

Clients who anticipate long trips by air, sea, or car can use a transdermal system (Transderm-Scop), a flat disk with a drug reservoir containing scopolamine, applied to intact skin in a hairless area behind the ear. The disk delivers scopolamine at a relatively constant rate to the systemic circulation over a 3-day period. It should be applied approximately 4 hours before the antiemetic effect is needed.

Specific Nursing Measures

Clients should be taught measures to avoid or reduce motion sickness. Clients taking antinauseants should be cautioned about operating machinery or driving a motor vehicle. Sucking on hard candies will reduce the problems of dry mouth. Whoever applies or removes Transderm-Scop should wash the hands thoroughly with soap and water to prevent scopolamine from coming into direct contact with the eyes. The application site should also be thoroughly washed and dried.

Meniere's Syndrome

Meniere's syndrome (endolymphatic hydrops) is a disorder of the inner ear that results from an increased volume of endolymph with dilation of the membranous labyrinth that can progress to herniation and rupture of the membranous labyrinth. The disease is characterized by exacerbations of three symptoms (vertigo, tinnitus, and sensorineural hearing loss) and remissions until a complete remission occurs spontaneously. Meniere's syndrome usually begins between 40 and 60 years of age and is rare in children.

The exact cause of the increased volume of endolymph—whether excessive production or deficient reabsorption—is unknown. Deficient reabsorption suggests that the defect is in the function of the endolymphatic sac, but other factors also have been suggested, such as viral infections, allergies, endocrine disturbances, and paroxysmal vasomotor dysfunction. The disease seems to be exacerbated by emotional stress.

Clinical Manifestations

A client in the acute phase of Meniere's syndrome is in obvious distress and may be incapacitated and require hospitalization. Symptoms include severe vertigo with nausea and vomiting, tinnitus, nystagmus, and an uncomfortable full feeling in one ear progressing to hearing loss. The vertigo persists from 1 to 12 hours followed by a period of unsteadiness, fluctuating hearing loss, and tinnitus. The client may be anxious, irritable, and depressed. Future acute attacks can occur at any time from a few weeks to months after the initial attack. Remission between the acute attacks becomes longer until a complete remission occurs. The client is left with varying degrees of hearing impairment, especially for low tones.

Medical Measures

No treatment has been entirely successful in altering the course of Meniere's syndrome, but many drugs are useful for symptomatic relief. Vasodilation with histamine phosphate may control the vertigo. Other antivertiginous drugs include dimenhydrinate (Dramamine), meclizine hydrochloride (Antivert, Bonine), and diphenhydramine hydrochloride (Benadryl). Sedatives such as diazepam (Valium) and anticholinergic drugs such as atropine, propantheline bromide (Pro-Banthine), and glycopyrrolate (Robinul) help control nausea, vomiting, and perspiration.

Salt restriction and diuretics such as ammonium chloride may relieve fullness or pressure in the ear. Some clients show an immediate improvement on this regimen and are able to avoid taking high-risk drugs or having surgery. An essentially salt-free diet may benefit some clients. When allergy appears to be the cause, elimination diets to discover the source of the allergy, followed by desensitization injections, are used. Hearing aids can help with the hearing loss and mask tinnitus for some clients.

Surgical procedures include endolymphatic sac operations to preserve the residual hearing, or destruction of the inner ear to relieve the symptoms. The latter procedure is reserved for clients whose lives are intolerable because of severe attacks of vertigo or who have permanent hearing impairment in the affected ear.

Specific Nursing Measures

During the acute stage, bed rest with siderails to prevent falling is advisable. Support the client's head with pillows on each side to prevent movement, which usually aggravates the vertigo. The client will need assistance while vomiting. Reassure the client that the acute phase will soon end. Clear liquids as tolerated are encouraged to prevent dehydration, but usually an IV line is started for fluid and drug administration.

After the acute phase, encourage the client to lead as relaxed a lifestyle as possible, since stress appears to bring on the acute phase. Smoking and stress act as vasoconstrictors and can affect the absorption of endolymph. Encourage programs to reduce stress and to stop smoking.

Surgery to Correct Meniere's Syndrome

Clients with continued attacks of Meniere's syndrome despite medical treatment are candidates for a surgical procedure. Most are desperate for relief of vertigo. Surgical procedures for Meniere's syndrome are classified into two major groups: conservative and destructive. Conservative procedures are performed to reduce vestibular symptoms while preserving hearing. Destructive procedures eliminate vestibular symptoms but cause total hearing loss in the involved ear.

Ultrasound is a conservative technique for depressing vestibular activity in clients with Meniere's syndrome. An ultrasonic probe inserted through a tympanotomy directs energy at the round window. The effects of ultrasound are not yet well understood. An endolymphatic subarachnoid shunt is also a conservative technique that drains endolymph into the subarachnoid space in the brain. A shunt tube also can be inserted into the endolymphatic sac to drain it into the mastoid cavity. The most widely used conservative procedure to relieve attacks of vertigo is to section or cut the vestibular portion of CN VIII through a middle fossa approach (craniotomy approach), described in Chapter 29. This approach preserves hearing and provides permanent relief from vertigo.

Destructive procedures are used only for clients with minimal residual hearing in the involved ear. Destructive procedures remove contents of the vestibule, remove the membranous labyrinth, or section the cochlear nerve. Client implications of surgical procedures for Meniere's syndrome are summarized in Table 52–5.

Nursing Implications

See above for preoperative nursing care. Postoperative nursing care is similar to that for clients having a mastoidectomy. Nursing care after a craniotomy approach is discussed in Chapter 29. The nurse should assist the client until steadiness is regained. Help the client avoid moving quickly or becoming fatigued, which seems to exacerbate the unsteadiness.

Cochlear Implants

A cochlear implant is essentially an electronic inner ear. The cochlear implant is indicated for postlingually deaf adults (those who had learned to talk before losing their hearing) with nonfunctioning hair cells but viable auditory neurons.

Table 52–5
Surgical Procedures for Meniere's Syndrome: Implications for the Client

Physiologic Implications	Psychosocial/Lifestyle Implications
Relief from vertigo and tinnitus Risk of increased hearing loss, infection, spinal fluid leakage and CN VII paralysis with shunt operations Risks as above plus possible brain injury with middle fossa craniotomy approach Vertigo and nausea for 3 to 4 weeks, months, or (rarely) permanently after labyrinthectomy or nerve section Hearing loss in operative ear with destructive procedures	Hospital stay of 1 to 3 days (longer, if subarachnoid space entered) Usually can resume work about 4 weeks after discharge May have to modify lifestyle and continue to attend to safety precautions if unsteadiness or vertigo persist after surgery Depression and frustration if the symptoms are not relieved by surgery May need to learn speech reading or undergo auditory training when labyrinthectomy has been performed

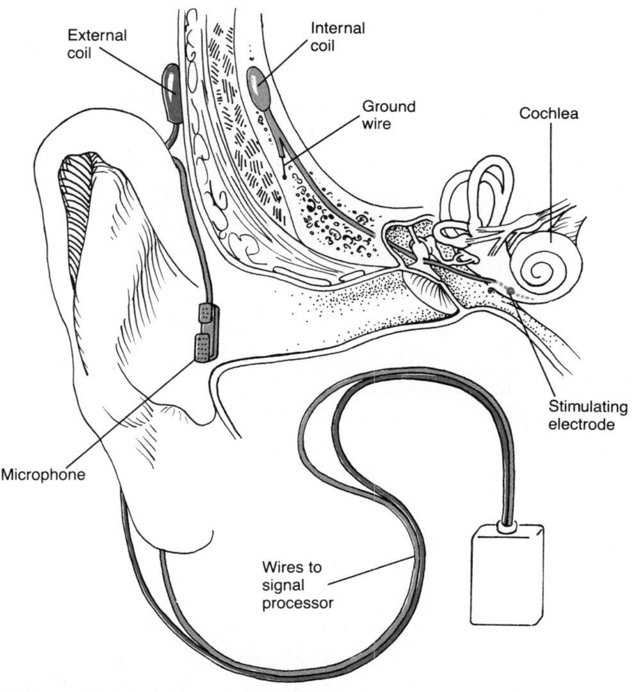

Figure 52–6

Cochlear implant.

In this procedure, an electrode is inserted into the scala tympani to the round window, and an inactive ground wire is placed in the middle ear. Both electrodes are attached to an internal coil embedded in the mastoid cortex (Figure 52–6).

After the incision has healed, an external coil is placed on the scalp directly over the internal coil. A small microphone placed on a shirt or blouse collar or on the ear picks up sound and carries it to a battery-operated signal processor, about the size of a deck of playing cards and worn on a belt, in a pocket, or attached to a brassiere. The processor converts the sound into an electrical signal and transmits it to the external coil and then to the internal coil to activate the electrode in the scala tympani, which stimulates the nerve fibers of CN VIII in the cochlea.

Clients with cochlear prostheses can detect their own voices and learn to detect other sounds in the environment, but normal hearing is still beyond the scope of cochlear implants. Although the prosthesis does not improve the client's ability to understand speech, it does provide acoustic cues that improve the tone, pace, and stress on words in the client's own speech. The ability to hear environmental sounds, such as doorbells and automobile horns, promotes safety and decreases feelings of isolation. Clients with implants describe an increased self-esteem and an increased sense of security. Client implications of a cochlear implant are summarized in Table 52–6.

Nursing Implications

Nursing implications for clients with cochlear implants are similar to those for mastoidectomy clients.

Table 52–6
Cochlear Implant: Implications for the Client

Physiologic Implications	Psychosocial/Lifestyle Implications
Ability to hear previously unheard sounds Possible dizziness Long-term effects of electrical stimulation unknown Long-term follow-up necessary	Improved client speech and improved ability to speech read Decreased feeling of isolation Increased self-esteem and sense of security and safety May be uncomfortable with visibility of microphone, wire, external coil, and signal processor

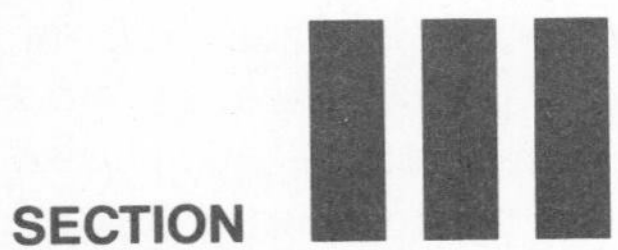

Degenerative Disorders

Cataracts

When the crystalline lens becomes opaque, it is called a cataract. This loss of transparency impairs vision. Many people believe cataracts mean blindness; in reality, however, cataracts develop slowly, and surgical extraction of a cataract can restore vision with little discomfort or risk.

Most cataracts (95%) are thought to be due to the aging process (senile cataracts). With age, the nucleus becomes dense, the cortex can opacify, and the lens becomes hard and unyielding. Furthermore, a gradual reduction in accommodative powers occurs. Cataracts of this degenerative type usually are evident at about age 50, although they may develop much earlier.

Other cataracts may be due to congenital factors (rubella in a pregnant woman during the first trimester can damage the developing lens), heredity, trauma (a penetrating wound or contusion), inflammation (long-standing uveitis or glaucoma), malignancy, metabolic factors (poorly controlled diabetes mellitus), radiation (prolonged exposure to infrared light), and long-term corticosteroid use.

Clinical Manifestations

Early stages of cataract development often go unnoticed, because many elderly people believe that old age brings a natural, unpreventable onset of blindness.

The primary symptom of cataracts is some degree of visual loss. Gradual blurring of vision is the most common symptom (Figure 52–1D). Glaring light such as bright sunshine constricts the pupil and makes vision seem worse. Double vision may occur in one eye (monocular diplopia), because the lens opacity splits light bundles, causing two parts of the sensory retina to be stimulated. Senile cataracts are often bilateral, although usually unequal in density. Cataracts cause no pain.

Ophthalmoscopy, biomicroscopy, or a loupe (a convex magnifying lens) can be used to identify a cataract. In advanced stages, a cataract is visualized as a white discoloration just behind the pupil that is easily observable by oblique illumination.

Medical Measures

The only effective treatment of a senile cataract is surgical removal. If the cataract is not removed, the client will eventually become blind. Extraction is usually postponed until vision in the better eye has fallen below 20/50 because functional vision is considered more desirable than the clear but distorted vision following cataract extraction. A senile cataract generally progresses slowly and may never attain a state in which extraction is necessary.

In the early stages, permanent dilation of the pupil with atropine (three times weekly) may improve vision. Medication to retard or inhibit the formation of cataracts has not proven effective except in the case of diabetic cataracts. In the early stages of a cataract, a change of glasses may be helpful. As the lens becomes more cloudy, however, glasses will not help.

Specific Nursing Measures

The nurse's primary responsibility to clients with degenerative disorders of the eye is health education.

Teach elderly clients with decreased vision not to rely on a driver's examination vision test for approval to drive. Snellen's charts are not infallible, and automobile accidents can be avoided if the visually impaired elderly client has ongoing care. Eyeglasses become increasingly necessary with age, and clients should be urged to be fitted appropriately.

Cataracts can occur simultaneously with other ocular disorders (eg, glaucoma), so the nurse should encourage clients to have a full ophthalmic examination when visual impairment occurs. They should be assured that cataract extraction, barring other health complications, is safe even for the very old and can improve vision considerably. The nursing care of the client having cataract surgery is discussed below.

Cataract Extraction

Cataract extraction removes the opaque lens, providing clear vision again (with corrective lenses). The procedure can be done with minimal risk in 60 minutes.

There are two types of cataract extraction: *intracapsular cataract extraction* (ICCE) and *extracapsular cataract extraction* (ECCE). The method is chosen according to the type of cataract, age of the client, and postoperative plan for refractive correction.

An ICCE removes the entire lens, including the capsule (Figure 52–7A). The procedure is done via a small superior corneoscleral limbal (the periphery of the cornea where it joins the sclera) incision. A cryoprobe inserted through the incision is placed on the lens to freeze it. The frozen lens is then gently withdrawn with the probe.

An ECCE removes the anterior capsule, lens nucleus, and lens cortex while retaining the posterior capsule (Figure 52–7B). The same superior corneoscleral limbal incision is made as for the ICCE. First, the lens nucleus is removed; the lens cortex is then removed by irrigation and suction. This type of cataract extraction is common with *intraocular lens* (IOL) *implantation* (a type of plastic artificial lens), because the remaining posterior capsule can provide support for the lens. ECCE with IOL is often done on a same-day surgery basis.

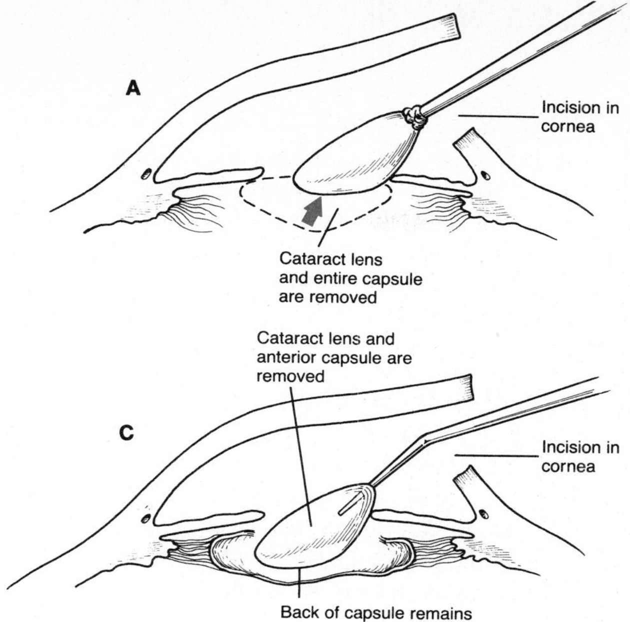

Figure 52–7

Types of cataract extraction. **A.** ICCE. **B.** ECCE.

A soft cataract involves the lens cortex and is often extracted via phacoemulsification. An ultrasonic needle inserted through a small incision fragments the lens, and the emulsified particles are then aspirated. This procedure is usually reserved for clients under age 50 with no nuclear sclerosis (hardness). Table 52–7 summarizes client implications for cataract extraction.

Table 52–7
Cataract Extraction: Implications for the Client

Physiologic Implications	Psychosocial/Lifestyle Implications
Restored vision, but aphakic eye Choice among cataract glasses, contact lenses, or intraocular lenses (IOLs) Possible complications of IOLs, including corneal endothelium damage, vitreous loss, intraocular infection, postoperative inflammation, and retinal detachment Three months needed for eye refraction stabilization Possible hemorrhage, retinal detachment, or posterior capsule opacification requiring repeat surgery Good success rate	Same-day surgery is done whenever possible Lifelong need for corrective lenses for refractive error Disadvantages of cataract glasses: weight and physical inconvenience, need for an adjustment process to tolerate a 25% magnification, inability to focus both eyes with monocular aphakia, limited side vision, expensive Contact lenses are a solution to magnification problem; however, conventional contact lenses require manual dexterity, can be expensive, and require scrupulous hygienic care Need for safety precautions in adjustment phase Possibility of IOL to relieve client from removable lenses and magnification problems Need for education to relieve fear and anxiety

Nursing Implications

PREOPERATIVE CARE Educating the client about cataract extraction and its typically successful outcome is only one part of the preoperative care provided by the nurse. Clarification about what a cataract is and how it will be removed must not be ignored. Same-day surgery clients need additional preoperative instruction. Teach them and their families about the postoperative care the client will require in the home.

Because of the nature of the disease, the client will have no depth perception. Clients with bilateral cataracts often are almost sightless. Thus, the nurse should orient the client to the hospital room and organize possessions within reach of the client's better eye.

POSTOPERATIVE CARE Postoperatively, the client depends on the family or the nursing staff for assistance in eating, bathing, and ambulating. Bed rest with bathroom privileges is usually allowed the day of surgery, but other activity should be discouraged. Instruct the client to lie on the unoperated side or back. An eye patch and metal shield will prevent trauma. The head of the bed is usually maintained at 30° to control IOP and minimize swelling. Clients who find themselves in an unfamiliar environment with monocular vision will appreciate reassurance from the nurse. Pain is nominal, and acetaminophen is usually sufficient to provide relief. Sharp, severe pain is unusual and could indicate a complication, so the physician should be notified if it occurs.

Reading may begin 24 hours (and light activity 24 to 72 hours) after cataract surgery and should be slowly increased as tolerated. Heavy work is usually not permitted for 4 to 6 weeks. Older people may have heard from friends who had cataract surgery many years ago before new techniques were developed that postoperative activity of any kind is contraindicated. Thus, reassurance and clarification of instructions are necessary before the client is discharged. The client ready for discharge may be required to take eye medication such as atropine sulfate (Isopto Atropine) to prevent posterior synechiae. The client and family or friends need instruction on the correct instillation of eyedrops, as well as on the application of eyepatches and shields. A case study of a client undergoing cataract extraction follows this chapter.

Macular Degeneration

The macula is more vulnerable to disease and degeneration than any other part of the retina. Senile macular degeneration (SMD) is the leading cause of new cases of blindness in the United States, accounting for 14% of the newly blind (Folk, 1982). It has been suggested that the aging of our population will make SMD an epidemic in 25 or 30 years. Degeneration in SMD is bilateral, but the progression in each eye usually occurs at different rates.

The cause of SMD is not known. Most cases are sporadic, and there seems to be a familial tendency. The disease process occurs because of an abnormality at the level of the retinal pigment epithelium and overlying photoreceptors. **Drusen,** yellow deposits on Bruch's membrane (beneath the pigment epithelium) are thought to represent secretory products from a "tired" retinal pigment epithelium (Folk, 1982). An abnormal fluid transfer then seeps through Bruch's membrane, promoting an elevation or "blistering" of the pigment epithelium and the neurosensory retina. In addition, an abnormal blood vessel from the choroid may grow through the defect in Bruch's membrane and lead to a subretinal hemorrhage, which usually leads to a subretinal scar. Recurrent scarring with decreased nourishment of the macula leads to destruction of the pigment epithelium and photoreceptors, as well as the permanent loss of central acuity. This degeneration of the macula can take years to run its course. Because of the typical client's age (greater than 50 years), arteriosclerotic vascular changes commonly coexist with the degeneration but are not responsible for it.

Clinical Manifestations

Macular degeneration spares peripheral vision. However, the client may experience blurred vision, and a central scotoma (blind spot) is inevitable (Figure 52–1E). Visual acuity is distorted. Visualization via ophthalmoscope will show a central retinal detachment and, in advanced cases, fibrosis with surrounding hemorrhage. Fluorescein angiography can help locate leaky vessels.

Medical and Specific Nursing Measures

Laser photocoagulation may help prevent further leakage of fragile vessels and result in transitory visual improvement.

Eventually, an unremitting macular degeneration blinds central vision. Reading is not possible, but the affected client may still have mobility without assistance. The nurse must remember that the difference between a loss of central vision and the loss of all vision is enormous and should reassure clients that unless other ocular disorders exist, they can perform activities of daily living independently.

Presbycusis

Presbycusis is a slowly progressive, bilateral hearing loss due to aging. It is usually more pronounced at frequencies above 2000 Hz. Hearing loss attributed to degenerative changes can be related to many factors, such as diet, exercise, smoking, noise, metabolism, arteriosclerosis, emotional stress, and heredity. The definitive cause remains unexplained.

Clinical Manifestations

A gradual progressive hearing loss, the major clinical symptom of presbycusis, is confirmed by hearing acuity tests and audiometry. The rate of progression varies with clients but usually accelerates with age. Some clients complain of tinnitus and dizziness, and families or significant others often notice personality changes in the client such as depression or irritability.

Medical Measures

No effective medical or surgical treatment has been found for presbycusis. Its management consists of aural rehabilitation including hearing aids, psychosocial counseling, and emotional support.

Specific Nursing Measures

Support and reinforce the programs instituted by the audiologist and discourage unproven cures. Safety is a concern whenever dizziness occurs; remind the client to keep safety measures in mind. The nurse's health teaching includes instructing the client and family or significant others about presbycusis and its effect on communication. The family or significant others should be taught how to communicate more effectively with the client and assist with the care of the hearing aid, if necessary. Caregivers should make a special effort to prevent client withdrawal and isolation; the nurse can encourage and even arrange for social contact with community groups or volunteers.

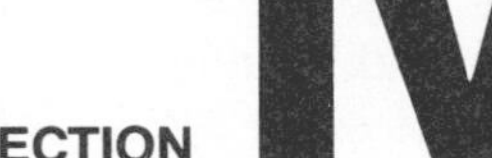

SECTION IV

Infectious Disorders

Most clients with localized infections are not hospitalized; therefore, nursing care consists of teaching the client and family or friends to care for the inflamed or infected eye.

Hordeola

A hordeolum (stye) is an acute benign abscess of the follicle of an eyelash or accessory gland along the eyelid margins. It may occur in crops as the infection spreads to adjacent hair follicles. The usual cause of a hordeolum is staphylococcal infection. Several hordeola may persistently recur in clients with chronic blepharitis or conjunctivitis or in debilitated people with compromised immune systems.

Clinical Manifestations

A hordeolum is characterized by a localized red, swollen, and acutely tender area. Pain is in direct proportion to the amount of eyelid swelling.

Medical Measures

Treatment in acute cases consists of the application of hot, moist compresses for 10 to 15 minutes four times a day. Gentle rubbing away from the eye will mechanically remove infected debris. An antibiotic ointment then may be applied. Incision and drainage are often indicated when the abscess becomes "pointed" and does not spontaneously drain.

Specific Nursing Measures

Good hygiene should be emphasized. Teach the client how to prevent the spread of the infection and demonstrate consistent clean technique by careful handwashing and use of individual towels and washcloths.

Urge the client not to squeeze the hordeolum, because the infection could be complicated by the development of cellulitis and can spread along the entire eyelid margin. Advise clients with persistent or recurring hordeola to see their health care provider.

Chalazia

A chalazion is a chronic sterile granulomatous inflammation of one of the meibomian glands. Often mistaken for a hordeolum, a chalazion is differentiated mainly by the fact that it tends to be on the conjunctival side of the eyelid and does not involve the eyelid margin. The cause of chalazia is unknown, and recurrence may require a biopsy to rule out malignancy.

Clinical Manifestations

Chalazia are characterized by gradual localized swelling of the meibomian gland and inflammation and tenderness not quite as severe as with a hordeolum. A small swelling at the conjunctival side of the eyelid feels like a small piece of buckshot. If the chalazion increases in size, astigmatism may develop as the globe is distorted.

Medical and Specific Nursing Measures

Asymptomatic chalazia do not require treatment. Short-term suppuration is treated with a topical antibiotic such as a sulfonamide. If vision is distorted, an excision of the chalazion is indicated. Chronic inflammations may require an incision and curettage. Apply hot, moist compresses to the affected eye q.i.d. for 15 to 20 minutes. A chronic chalazion is annoying and unpleasant for the client, and emotional support is helpful.

Conjunctivitis

Conjunctivitis is an inflammation of the conjunctiva characterized by hyperemia, cellular infiltration, and exudates. It may be caused by exposure to noxious elements such as bacteria, viruses, fungi, parasites, toxins, allergens, chemicals, and chronic irritation. Conjunctivitis is overwhelmingly the most common cause of an atraumatic red eye. *Pinkeye* is the acute contagious form of conjunctivitis common in children. Chronic conjunctivitis is the most troublesome, particularly in the elderly, since it is recurrent and of long duration. The type of exudate, degree of corneal complication, and severity of infection are influenced to a great extent by the hygiene, nutrition, and general health of the affected individual.

Conjunctivitis is most commonly caused by bacteria (eg, *Staphylococcus aureus,* alpha and beta streptococci, pneumococci, hemophilus organisms, *E. coli,* and *Pseudomonas*). Other causative organisms include viruses (eg, herpes viruses) and fungi (eg, *Candida albicans* and *Aspergillus fumigatus*). Endogenous diseases or syndromes that can cause conjunctivitis include Sjögren's syndrome, Reiter's syndrome, and Stevens–Johnson syndrome.

Noninfective causes of conjunctivitis include allergic responses; chemical and irritant responses to acids, alkalies, smoke, and wind; and chronic irritation, such as rubbing, entropion, or contact lens wear.

Clinical Manifestations

Signs of conjunctivitis include hyperemia, tearing, exudation, and pseudoptosis (drooping of the upper eyelid due to increased weight from cellular infiltration). The client experiences a foreign body sensation; a scratching or burning sensation; a sensation of fullness around the eyes; pruritus; and, when the cornea is involved, photophobia. Symptoms and signs of a more serious problem are significant pain, a change in visual acuity, an irregular cornea, and an abnormal pupil size or reaction.

A purulent discharge is noted in clients with bacterial conjunctivitis; even if untreated, it may subside within 2 weeks. Viral conjunctivitis is highly contagious and is manifested by a profuse watery discharge and diffuse redness. Fungal and parasitic forms of conjunctivitis are unilateral and often appear as localized inflammatory granulomas; fungal conjunctivitis is uncommon. Toxic or traumatic conjunctivitis also is unilateral. Allergic conjunctivitis may cause considerable swelling, marked pruritus, and a stringy discharge.

Medical Measures

Bacterial conjunctivitis can be treated with a broad-spectrum antibiotic until a culture and sensitivity test result has been obtained. Treatment of viral conjunctivitis is usually ineffective; it runs its course. Fungal conjunctivitis may respond to nystatin ointment. Topical corticosteroids and vasoconstrictors can relieve the congestion and pruritus associated with allergic conjunctivitis.

Specific Nursing Measures

To prevent the spread of infection, instruct the client and family or friends about the importance of good personal hygiene. For example, the use of individual towels and tissues instead of communal towels and handkerchiefs will decrease the spread of the organism. Teach the client and family how to instill eyedrops without touching the eye, and instruct them to instill medication in the unaffected eye first to prevent cross-contamination.

Eye patches are not used, because enclosure of the drainage would provide optimum conditions for the growth of bacteria and viruses. Irrigations may be ordered (always before instillation of the medication) to remove discharge. Use separate equipment for each eye and wash the hands between treatment of each eye to avoid cross-contamination. Finally, recommend dark glasses for photophobia.

Keratitis and Corneal Ulceration

The outer layer of the cornea, the epithelium, provides an adequate barrier against most microbes into the cornea. If the epithelium is traumatized, however, a variety of organisms can flourish within the inner layers and cause keratitis (inflammation of the cornea). Damage to the cornea usually leaves a permanent scar and may impair vision. The infection also may spread to other ocular structures. Corneal perforation and possible loss of the eye may occur.

Keratitis may be caused by pathogenic bacteria; viruses; fungi; facial nerve disorders such as Bell's palsy; traumatic insult (from chemicals, excessive ultraviolet exposure, and mechanical means); and exposure (from ptosis or severe ectropion). Despite the formidable corneal barrier, some bacteria are able to penetrate an intact cornea (eg, *Neisseria gonorrhoeae* and *Pseudomonas aeruginosa*). Clients with malnutrition, vitamin A deficiency, diabetes, or decreased resistance are more susceptible to a variety of microorganisms. Keratitis may be complicated by the formation of a corneal ulcer.

Clinical Manifestations

The predominant feature of keratitis is necrosis, often with resultant ulcer formation. Because the cornea has a rich nerve supply, clients may feel severe pain from seemingly minor irritations. Corneal lesions can cause blurred vision, with greater blurring if the lesion is centrally located. Since there are no blood vessels or mucous glands in the cornea, discharges are uncommon, except with a purulent bacterial ulcer. The client often has the sensation of a foreign body in the eye. Photophobia is not uncommon, and the eye may appear reddened (bloodshot).

Medical Measures

Broad-spectrum topical antibiotics are used until the results of culture and sensitivity studies are obtained. The instillation of atropine sulfate (Isopto Atropine) or scopolamine hydrobromide (Isopto Hyoscine) for pupil dilation keeps the ciliary body and iris at rest, thereby reducing pain. Nystatin or amphotericin B may be beneficial in the treatment of fungal corneal ulcers. Avitaminosis A corneal ulceration is treated with the intravenous administration of 10,000 to 15,000 units of vitamin A daily.

The corneal integrity can be maintained as long as the corneal surface is kept moist by the client's wearing a plastic wrap moisture chamber secured to the surrounding skin with adhesive tape. Another method for keeping the cornea moist is inserting a bandage soft contact lens. Sometimes taping or suturing of the lids is performed, or a conjunctival flap is surgically created to protect the exposed cornea. Surgical relief of exophthalmos can often cure exposure-induced corneal ulcerations.

Specific Nursing Measures

Hot, moist compresses should be used generously. Eye patches are not used on infectious or suppurative lesions, however, because they favor bacterial multiplication and prevent the free flow of discharge from the eye. Teach the client proper instillation of eyedrops, including the importance of washing hands before and after and methods of preventing contamination.

Corneal Transplant

A corneal transplant or keratoplasty can restore normal vision by transplanting a donor cornea in place of the diseased cornea. This procedure is indicated when inflammation or trauma to the cornea have caused scarring. Other conditions that may be helped by keratoplasty include corneal degeneration and subsequent corneal thinning, dystrophies, and recurrent infections.

There are two basic types of keratoplasties: lamellar (nonpenetrating) and penetrating. In *lamellar keratoplasty,* only the superficial (epithelial and subepithelial) layers are transplanted on the excised superficial opacity. *Penetrating keratoplasty* is indicated for pacification of the deeper layers of the cornea (beneath the two anterior layers). All five corneal layers are replaced, and a cataract extraction may be performed at the same time. In keratoplasty, either the entire diameter of the cornea or a partial (central or peripheral) section can be replaced.

The Donor Cornea

The donor tissue comes from a noninfected human cadaver and should be used ideally within 24 hours if a penetrating keratoplasty is to be done, because of the rapid endothelial death rate. For a lamellar keratoplasty, the cornea can be frozen, dehydrated, or refrigerated for up to 6 months before transplantation. The enucleated eye should come from a donor who died of an acute disease or injury. Some causes of death, such as leukemia, sepsis, central nervous system degenerative diseases, and previous eye disease, render a donor cornea unsuitable for transplantation. A young donor (25 to 35 years old) is preferable because of the large number of endothelial cells, which optimize transplant success. People wanting to donate their eyes for keratoplasty should contact an eye bank that is a member of the Eye Bank Association of America or their state's agency for the blind (see list of resources in Chapter 51). Client implications of keratoplasty are summarized in Table 52–8.

Table 52–8
Corneal Transplant: Implications for the Client

Physiologic Implications	Psychosocial/Lifestyle Implications
Rejection rate of 10% to 15% Months to years of healing; sutures remain in place 1 yr or longer Steroids to reduce inflammation and antibiotics to avoid infection Repeated transplant may be necessary	Activities limited until healing has occurred (from 1 mo to as long as 1 yr) Need for protection from mechanical trauma (protective glasses in industrial settings; use of metal eye shield at night) and from infection in postoperative period Fear of graft rejection

Nursing Implications

PREOPERATIVE CARE The keratoplasty is usually done as an emergency, but the client will have expected it and will be excited preoperatively. The nurse helping clients prepare for the procedure can educate them about it, answering questions and clarifying any misconceptions. Emphasize the goals of preventing postoperative trauma to the eye (an eye shield will be used) and avoiding coughing, bending, or straining. Reassure the client that little pain is experienced postoperatively but that analgesics and tranquilizers will be used as needed. The client's face is cleansed with an antibacterial soap.

POSTOPERATIVE CARE A keratoplasty heals extremely slowly, taking several months to years, because the cornea is avascular. Steroids are used to reduce the inflammatory process, and antibiotics are given postoperatively to avoid infection. Sutures are removed approximately a year or longer after the procedure.

Antiemetics and cough suppressants may be used postoperatively to avoid stress on the suture line. Because the keratoplasty heals slowly, the client must remember to curb activities that increase IOP to avoid stress on the suture line and subsequent leakage of aqueous humor. This period of time could be as brief as one month or as long as one year. The client who understands the inherent risks of unsafe care of the eye is often more willing to use protective measures to protect the delicate transplant.

Assess the client's occupation for potential trauma to the eye. For example, if the client cares for small children, cleans, and cooks, alternatives may be needed to avoid undue stress on the suture line of the cornea. In this case, a family member or friend might provide assistance, and a visiting nurse could provide health care supervision during home visits. The operated eye should be protected from mechanical trauma either by protective glasses (in industrial settings) or a metal eye shield (at night to avoid rubbing).

Promote good general hygiene of the client as needed to prevent infection. Washing the hands before and after care to the eyes is especially important. Avoidance of touching or rubbing the eyes is also essential to prevent infection.

Encourage follow-up visits to the physician so that possible corneal allograft reaction (graft rejection) can be closely monitored. Corneal allograft reactions may occur as early as 10 days, or as late as many years, after implantation of donor tissue into the recipient eye. Rejection is manifested by the donor cornea's becoming edematous and opaque. Clients experience little pain, but their vision is usually blurred. The mainstay of treatment for corneal allograft reactions is corticosteroid therapy.

Rejection of the donor transplant is a major disappointment for the client, especially one who made serious attempts to avoid it. The client may become discouraged and unwilling to undergo another transplant. He or she may withdraw from family and physician, developing mistrust in the health care system and the surgery itself. The client will need extra support at this time and reassurance that another transplant can be performed.

Uveitis

Uveitis, a general term for inflammatory disorders of the uveal tract, encompasses a number of diseases that affect part or all of it. The most frequent form of uveitis is iritis (acute anterior uveitis). Early diagnosis of iritis is important to prevent the formation of posterior **synechiae** (adhesions of the iris to the lens). In posterior uveitis, the retina is almost always secondarily affected (chorioretinitis). Uveitis is usually unilateral and is principally found in the young and middle age groups.

In addition to inflammation by pathogens, uveitis may also result from a hypersensitivity reaction such as arthritis or ankylosing spondylitis. Microorganisms are rarely identified, and only about one-third of all cases of uveitis have an identifiable cause; the other two-thirds are of unknown etiology.

Clinical Manifestations

Pain, photophobia, and blurred vision are common symptoms of uveitis. Depending on the cause, the onset can be from acute to insidious. Pathogenic invasion may cause a diffusely red eye. Pupils are usually small and irregular as posterior synechiae form.

Medical and Specific Nursing Measures

Because the tubercle bacillus and *Histoplasma capsulatum* have been known to be causative organisms in uveitis, skin tests may identify the probable cause and consequently aid in treatment. The pupil is kept dilated with atropine sulfate (Isopto Atropine) twice a day to prevent the formation of posterior synechiae. Steroids are helpful in the treatment of hypersensitivity-caused uveitis. Glaucoma is a common complication, and appropriate measures to decrease IOP are necessary.

Warm, moist compresses are applied for 10 minutes four times a day; analgesics also promote comfort. Dark glasses are recommended for photophobia.

External Otitis

External otitis (otitis externa) is basically an inflammation of the skin. Because of its location, its effect on hearing, and its complications, it is considered to be in the realm of otology even though it overlaps with dermatology.

External otitis can be localized or diffuse. Diffuse otitis includes the ear and surrounding face, neck, and scalp. Primarily dermatologic otitis, which includes herpes, warts, seborrheic dermatitis, and eczema, will not be discussed here. When these disorders occur in the ear, they are treated the same way as when they occur in other areas of the skin (see Unit 13).

A severe life-threatening external otitis, *malignant otitis externa,* occurs in elderly diabetics. It begins in the skin of the external auditory canal and, if not arrested, extends through the soft tissue to the temporal bone and the other bones that form the floor of the cranial cavity—the frontal, sphenoid, ethmoid, and occipital bones.

Furunculosis is a localized external otitis of the hair follicles in the cartilaginous part (outer half) of the external auditory canal (Figure 52–8). It begins as a red papule and develops into a pustule (furuncle), which usually erupts and drains spontaneously. Furuncles are caused by staphylococci, which are usually introduced into the skin by scratching with contaminated fingernails or other objects. Inflammation of multiple follicles is called a carbuncle. Recurrent furuncles occur more frequently in clients with diabetes.

Diffuse bacterial external otitis, commonly called swimmer's ear, affects 5% to 20% of clients seen in health care settings during the summer months. A combination of high temperature, high humidity, and contamination of the skin with gram-negative bacilli causes diffuse bacterial external otitis. Three stages of inflammation can occur; preinflammatory, acute, and chronic inflammation. In the preinflammatory stage, the cells become macerated because of moisture in the ear. Pruritus with scratching leads to traumatization and infection of the skin, which initiates the acute stage. This stage may be mild, moderate, or severe, depending on the clinical manifestations. Chronic inflammation is recurrent and does not respond to treatment.

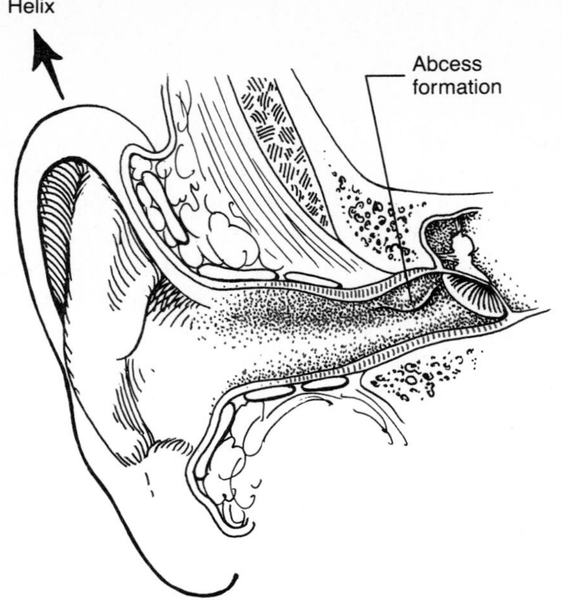

Figure 52–8

External otitis with furunculosis.

Otomycosis, an acute or chronic external otitis, is often found secondary to a bacterial infection, occurring after the extended use of topical corticosteroids and antibiotics. It is caused by fungi, most commonly *Aspergillus niger* and *Candida albicans.* The clinical course, usually occurring in hot weather, runs from a mild to a severe inflammation with frequent recurrences.

Clinical Manifestations

The first symptom of furunculosis is pruritus, which progresses to a persistent, excruciating pain in 24 to 48 hours. The nurse examining a client should be aware that pulling on the auricle, moving the jaw, or inserting a speculum causes extreme pain (Figure 52–8). Preauricular or postauricular adenopathy may be present. With the otoscope, an erythematous swelling is usually visible in the canal. Conductive hearing loss occurs only when the lumen of the canal is completely obstructed. A mild fever may be present until the furuncle erupts. Pain is relieved immediately after the furuncle erupts and drains. The drainage is a whitish-yellow, fetid exudate.

During the preinflammatory stage of diffuse bacterial external otitis, the client has severe pruritus, and scratch marks may be visible. Slight erythema of the skin in the external auditory canal and a dull (rather than shiny) tympanic membrane are observed during the acute mild stage. Occasionally, a clear odorless discharge may be present. Mild discomfort occurs when pressing on the tragus or pulling the auricle. During the acute moderate stage, the opening of the external auditory canal is partially occluded with seropurulent debris. Periauricular edema causes a moderate amount of pain, and preauricular and postauricular adenopathy may now be present. In the acute severe stage, the pain is so intense that the client is reluctant to move the jaw. Seropurulent bluish-gray or greenish secretions completely obstruct the canal. Severe periauricular edema is present. Cultures usually reveal *Pseudomonas,* and the client usually has a fever.

In chronic diffuse bacterial external otitis, there is a thickening of the skin and edema of the auricle. The skin may appear dry and scaly. A gray-brown or greenish secretion with a fetid odor is present in the canal. Pain is usually not as severe as in the acute stage. The tympanic membrane is thick and dull. Cultures reveal a gram-negative bacillus (usually *Proteus* or *Pseudomonas*) and fungal infections.

The client with otomycosis usually seeks care because of severe pain. Often there is a previous history of otomycosis. Otoscopic examination reveals the *Aspergillus niger* as a grayish or bluish membrane with black spots covering the external auditory canal and tympanic membrane. *Candida albicans* appears as a creamy white deposit. Removal of the membrane or deposit leaves a reddened area. A serous or serosanguineous otorrhea may be present.

Medical Measures

Conservative therapy is usually effective and preferable in treating furunculosis to prevent the possible spread of infection. The auditory canal is cleaned with an applicator or suction, and a cotton or gauze wick impregnated with an antibiotic ointment is inserted into the canal. Analgesics such as acetylsalicylic acid or codeine relieve pain. The wick is removed in 24 hours; if drainage has occurred, the area is cleansed with 70% alcohol and another wick is inserted (Senturia, Marcus, & Lucenti, 1980). If the furuncle has pointed, it may be drained by removing its head with an 18- or 20-gauge needle. Systemic antibiotics are sometimes given for 4 days. Prolonged therapy is required for carbuncles. Blood and urine are tested for sugar when infections are recurrent.

Early bacterial external otitis of the auditory canal can be treated with 3% hypertonic saline irrigations to remove debris and carefully drying the canal with cotton-tipped swabs or a hair dryer. Topical corticosteroids or antibiotic creams are usually effective early. If the auditory canal is obstructed, a gauze impregnated with an antibiotic and corticosteroid is packed into the canal. An oral broad-spectrum antibiotic also is administered. Analgesics and sedatives are necessary to relieve the pain. When the edema in the auditory canal subsides, antibiotic drops may be substituted for the gauze packing. This therapy usually continues for several days.

Added analgesics may be needed to control the pain. When the client cannot tolerate oral therapy because of nausea and vomiting, hospitalization becomes necessary for the administration of parenteral antibiotics and parenteral fluids. On rare occasions, an abscess may need to be incised and drained.

The treatment for chronic diffuse bacterial external otitis is similar to the treatment for the acute form. Aluminum acetate packs may also be applied to the periauricular eczematous areas. Failure of treatment may indicate a secondary fungal infection.

With otomycosis, careful cleaning of the auditory canal with suction or dry wipes is imperative for at least three consecutive days. Many topical antimycotic agents are available for treatment, such as nystatin (Nilstat) and clotrimazole (Lotrimin). Analgesics for pain also may be necessary. Treatment should be continued at least a week after the infection has cleared up.

Specific Nursing Measures

Heat applied to the ear of the client with furunculosis promotes eruption and drainage. Purulent drainage can cause the spread of the pathogens, however, so take care to prevent this spread by cleaning the discharge with a cotton ear swab.

Discourage clients from touching or scratching the ear, because staphylococci in the nares are often transferred to the ear by scratching the nasal mucosa and then the ears. Encourage frequent handwashing with a bactericidal soap. Tell the client to avoid inserting objects into the canal for removal of cerumen, an instruction that can be reinforced by information on the protective value of cerumen. All directions should be explained and written down. Include medication ordered, how it is administered, its side effects, and symptoms of allergic reactions.

Nursing management of the client with diffuse bacterial external otitis consists of cleaning the ear with cotton-tipped swabs and applying creams or drops as indicated. The client should be taught to administer ear drops and apply creams safely. Preventive measures are similar to those described for furunculosis. The client should be taught to keep water out of the ear (see Chapter 60) to prevent recurrence or chronicity. People who wear ear molds should pay special attention to cleaning and drying the ears.

Keeping the ear dry is the most important nursing measure for otomycosis. The client should wear earplugs or cotton plugs impregnated with a water-soluble jelly when showering. The nurse can help prevent otomycosis by discouraging self-treatment with ear drops for an earache.

Suppurative Otitis Media

Otitis media is an inflammation of the mucoperiosteal lining of the middle ear, including the eustachian tube, middle ear cavity, mastoid antrum, and mastoid air cells. The mucous membrane of the middle ear is continuous with the respiratory mucous membrane of the nasal cavity, sinuses, nasopharynx, eustachian tube, trachea, bronchi, and part of the larynx. Thus, otitis media may affect some or all of these structures. When associated with bacterial infection it is called suppurative otitis media. Inflammation of the middle ear without infection is called serous otitis media and is discussed later in this chapter.

Acute suppurative otitis media (acute purulent otitis media) is a bacterial infection of the middle ear lining. It occurs in people of all ages but especially in children, because their eustachian tubes are shorter and wider than adult eustachian tubes. In children, the condition affects both ears, whereas it usually affects only one ear in adults. *Chronic suppurative otitis media* is a continuous infection in the middle ear that lasts for at least 3 months. Severe cases can lead to an erosion of the ossicles.

The most common cause of acute suppurative otitis media is *Hemophilus influenzae* in children and pneumococci in adults. Beta-hemolytic streptococcus is usually the cause when otitis media occurs as a complication of the common cold. Suppurative otitis media can result from an upper respiratory tract infection, sinusitis, improper nose blowing, and the obstruction of hypertrophied adenoids.

In chronic suppurative otitis media, a permanent central perforation of the tympanic membrane exposes the middle ear lining to bacteria. Exposure of the middle ear lining also seems to make it more susceptible to infection via the eustachian tube.

Clinical Manifestations

Although acute suppurative otitis media is usually a self-limited disease, it runs through characteristic clinical stages depending on the virulence of the bacteria and the susceptibility of the host. A recent history of upper respiratory tract infection followed by an earache, fever, and sense of fullness in the ear is associated with the first stage. Hyperemic swelling beginning in the eustachian tube and extending to the middle ear causes the symptoms and signs. Hearing is usually normal at this stage. Otoscopy reveals a dull, thickened, injected tympanic membrane.

The second stage occurs 12 to 24 hours later. The formation of an exudate causes occasional vomiting (usually in children) and conductive hearing loss. Otoscopy reveals a bulging, red, lusterless, immobile tympanic membrane with loss of landmarks and cone of light. Superficial tenderness may occur over the mastoid process of the temporal bone. X-rays taken at this time may reveal air cells filled with fluid that appear cloudy; however, the bone cells are intact. Temperature also increases at this stage. If untreated, the tympanic membrane ruptures and expels a purulent discharge. Symptoms subside after the rupture.

A recurrence of pain with fever, deep mastoid tenderness, and an increase in foul purulent discharge indicate mastoiditis. However, this rarely occurs today with antibiotic therapy.

In chronic suppurative otitis media, the mucous membrane, seen through the perforated tympanic membrane, may appear edematous or pale and thin. Conductive hearing loss is present.

Medical Measures

Objectives of therapy are to resolve the infection and prevent its spread into the bone. The absence of fever indicates a viral or mild infection that will resolve spontaneously. When fever is present, antibiotic administration is started and continued for at least 7 to 10 days—even though symptoms subside—to prevent the recurrence of an incompletely resolved infection. Ampicillin, the drug of choice for adults, can be replaced by erythromycin in the case of allergy. Acetaminophen (Tylenol), aspirin, and occasionally codeine are used to relieve the pain. Decongestants may be used with inflammation of the eustachian tube to relieve pressure in the middle ear and eustachian tube.

With fever, extreme pain, and a bulging tympanic membrane, a myringotomy may be performed to release the exudate. Cultures and sensitivity of the exudate should be obtained if the drainage persists. Hearing should be tested after apparent resolution of the infection to be certain there is no residual hearing loss.

Treatment for chronic suppurative otitis media consists of cleaning the external ear with suction or dry wipes. A broad-spectrum antibiotic in boric acid powder is insufflated into the ear once or twice a week until the ear is dry.

Specific Nursing Measures

Care of clients with otitis media focuses on pain management and preventing the spread of the disease. Heat may be used to relieve pain. Cleaning the external ear with dry cotton swabs and placing cotton loosely in the ear prevents the drainage from spreading the infection to surrounding areas. Cold cream can prevent irritation of the skin of the external ear.

Provide the client with written instructions for the recommended treatment. Explain the cause of the disease and the rationale for taking the complete course of medication. Encourage fluids, adequate rest, and the use of earplugs or cotton impregnated with Vaseline during showering. When the tympanic membrane is perforated or a myringotomy has been performed, swimming is usually prohibited until the tympanic membrane has healed.

Clients should be aware that forceful nose blowing could force infected pathogens into the middle ear. Clients with an upper respiratory tract infection should not close their nostrils when blowing their noses; sniffing or just wiping the nostrils is safer.

Serous Otitis Media

Serous otitis media (middle ear effusion), a nonsuppurative otitis media, is an accumulation of serous fluid within the middle ear. Acute serous otitis media is a sudden accumulation of fluid. This occurs more frequently in adults, whereas the chronic form, a gradual accumulation, is more commonly found in children. The fluid can remain in the ear for months or years before it is detected.

The incidence of middle ear effusions seems to be increasing. Although it is technically not an infectious disorder, it is discussed here because it is thought to be related to the increased use of antibiotics for treating ear infections, which results in a residual sterile fluid. This condition is also associated with viral respiratory infections, allergies, or obstruction of the eustachian tube. Allergies cause hyperplasia of the secretory cells and increased secretions. An obstruction of dysfunction of the eustachian tube may result from upper respiratory infection, allergy, enlarged adenoidal tissue, trauma, or tumors. The eustachian tube clears secretions and replenishes oxygen to the middle ear mucosa. Thus, obstruction of the eustachian tube causes a negative pressure in the middle ear, resulting in removal of fluid from the cells and its accumulation in the middle ear.

Clinical Manifestations

The symptoms and signs of nonsuppurative otitis media are minimal. A history of allergies may or may not be present. Adult clients may complain of a feeling of fullness or bubbling and crackling in the ear. Usually, no pain is present. Mouth breathing may occur.

Medical Measures

Although decongestants have been the standard therapy, their efficacy in treating otitis media has not been proven. Often the client is observed for 3 to 4 weeks to allow normal absorption of the fluid with self-ventilating techniques. The client may be referred to an allergist for sensitivity testing and desensitization. Periodic audiometric testing to ascertain hearing loss is necessary.

A Mathes inflator can be used to inflate the eustachian tube. This device provides positive pressure through the nasopharynx while the client swallows, forcing air up the eustachian tube to the middle ear. Tympanocentesis or myringotomy with insertion of ventilating tubes may be performed to remove fluid. Other surgery includes adenoidectomy or removal of tissue obstructing the lumen of the eustachian tube.

Specific Nursing Measures

The client should be taught self-ventilating techniques and be encouraged to use them (see Chapter 51). When myringotomy has been performed, take precautions similar to those described previously. Nursing care for a client having a myringotomy is discussed below.

Myringotomy

A myringotomy is an incision of the tympanic membrane to release fluid under pressure and to insert ventilating tubes to aerate the middle ear (Figure 52–9). The drainage of purulent fluid from the middle ear prevents destruction of the ossicles, spread of infection to the mastoid cells, spontaneous rupture of the tympanic membrane, or a combination of these complications. A myringotomy is usually performed in an ambulatory setting (a physician's office, clinic, or day surgical center). The client implications of a myringotomy are summarized in Table 52–9.

Nursing Implications

PREOPERATIVE CARE Help alleviate anxiety by listening to the client, answering questions, explaining the procedures, and discussing postsurgical implications. A family member or significant other should participate in any discussions, especially if the client is very young or very old, to provide the support many clients need. A family member or significant other can also help interpret preoperative

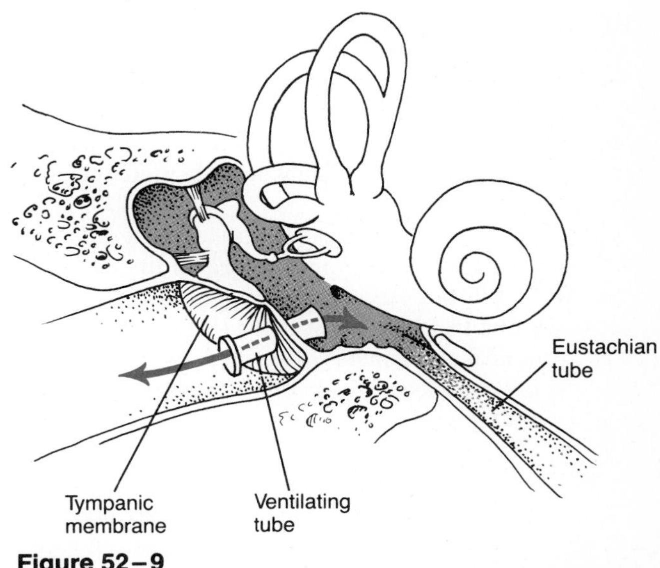

Figure 52–9

Myringotomy to release the exudate in chronic suppurative otitis media.

teaching to a client with hearing loss. Often, though, the nurse must find a method of communicating with the client. Writing all instructions may help the client understand them.

Home Health Care

POSTOPERATIVE CARE Postoperative instructions also should be written so the client can take them home. Health teaching should include:

- Instructions for washing hands before and after touching the ear to prevent the spread of infection
- Instructions for changing and disposing of the cotton ball placed within the external auditory canal to collect drainage
- Instructions for taking antibiotics or any other medications prescribed
- Encouragement to keep follow-up appointments
- Instructions for preventing water from entering the ear as long as a ventilating tube is in place or until the tympanic membrane heals

The client should use earplugs when showering and shampooing. The external ear should be cleaned with a washcloth. The client should avoid inserting applicators and going swimming. (These general instructions apply to the care of all clients having surgery of the ear.)

Table 52–9
Myringotomy: Implications for the Client

Physiologic Implications	Psychosocial/Lifestyle Implications
Relief from pain, fever, and possibly mild hearing loss	Marked increase in hearing (possibly uncomfortable at first)
Ventilating tubes extrude spontaneously after 3 weeks or may be removed after 6 weeks	Improvement in communication and cognitive skills
Need to keep water out of ear until tympanic membrane heals	Unable to engage in water sports until the tympanic membrane heals; must take precautions when showering and performing personal hygiene
Testing for reaccumulation of fluid in 6 to 12 months	

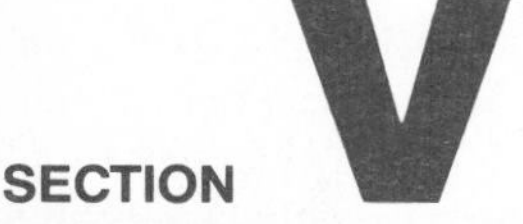

SECTION V

Neoplastic Disorders

Choroidal Melanomas

Choroidal melanomas are nonhereditary, unilateral tumors of the middle layer of the eyeball. Most ocular tumors are choroidal tumors in the posterior portion of the eye, making biopsy difficulty. They usually occur in white men over the age of 50.

The exact cause of choroidal melanomas is unknown. Malignant melanomas are found in 10% of the eyes blind from injury or inflammation, suggesting the possibility that irritation promotes malignancy. In the rare case that a metastatic choroidal melanoma is diagnosed, the probable origin is the breast or lung. The liver is the only organ known to be a site of metastasis.

Clinical Manifestations

Symptoms of choroidal melanomas often are not exhibited until the late stages of the disease process. A retinal detachment will cause visual distortion with an increase in choroidal volume. The loss of part of the visual field corresponds to the location of the tumor. Generally, the client has no pain unless glaucoma occurs.

Medical Measures

A diagnosis can be confirmed by indirect ophthalmoscopy, ultrasonography, fluorescein angiography, or computed tomography (CT). Often a small tumor will not change in size for a long time (months to years). When diagnosis is uncertain, therefore, regular examinations (every 3 to 4 months) are performed to watch for growth, which indicates the necessity for treatment because of the chance of metastasis. Metastatic spread of a uveal melanoma before the primary tumor has become symptomatic is virtually unknown.

A tumor less than 10 mm in diameter is associated with a client mortality of 13%, whereas a tumor greater than 12 mm in diameter has a 70% client mortality. The safest treatment is enucleation, with the age of the client and the size of the tumor being the major determinants. Recently, external proton beam irradiation has been used to treat eyes with tumors. Because this treatment requires the use of a linear accelerator, it is performed in only a few health care centers. Five- and 10-year survival rates are not as yet known.

Specific Nursing Measures

The loss of an eyeball can be a devastating experience for a client. With the decision of enucleation to save one's life, the client faces complex ramifications. The client will undoubtedly feel ambivalent about the choice of treatment; thus, psychologic support is greatly needed to help the client overcome confusion about the ultimate decision and to be able to cope with and accept the cancer and the treatment approach chosen. Alterations in lifestyle may be necessary, and assisting the client with necessary rehabilitative measures is an important aspect of the nurse's role. The nursing care of the client undergoing enucleation is discussed below.

Enucleation

An enucleation is a complete surgical removal of the eyeball. This procedure is indicated for a blind and painful eye; after trauma that caused irreparable harm; and in cases of infection, **sympathetic ophthalmia** (inflammation of the uveal tract of the uninjured eye), malignancy of the eye (eg, melanoma or retinoblastoma), and absolute glaucoma. An enucleation is usually the end result of a series of attempts to save the eyeball. The client's condition may have already been managed with cryotherapy, radiation therapy, chemotherapy, steroids, and other medications. When no other treatment is feasible, enucleation is done for palliative as well as lifesaving reasons.

A prosthesis, a removable artificial eye made by an oculist, can be fitted for the eye socket in approximately 1 month. Until then, a plastic shell (conformer) is placed in the socket to hold its shape while healing.

Sometimes only the intraocular contents of the eyeball are removed, and the sclera and cornea are retained in a procedure called an evisceration. Evisceration is seldom done today, however, because of the risk of sympathetic ophthalmia following it. Client implications of enucleation are summarized in Table 52–10.

Table 52–10
Enucleation: Implications for the Client

Physiologic Implications	Psychosocial/Lifestyle Implications
Possible complications (hemorrhage and infection) and need to avoid them by wearing a pressure dressing for 2 days and taking antibiotics	Relief from a painful, disfiguring, or blind eye
Use of a conformer initially to hold the shape of the socket during healing	Depression, withdrawal, and the need to grieve
Use of a prosthesis a month after enucleation	Change in body image
	Need to adjust to monocular vision
	Difficulties in prosthesis adjustment for client and significant others
	Fear of cancer

Nursing Implications

PREOPERATIVE CARE Routine preoperative nursing care is carried out for the client undergoing an enucleation. Emotional support and empathy help relieve some of the anxiety that clients experience.

POSTOPERATIVE CARE The postoperative client can move about without restrictions. Observe for bleeding, elevated temperature, and pain. After 48 hours, the instillation of antibiotics may be necessary.

Home Health Care

Before discharge, teach the client and family or friends the correct administration of medications and the proper hygienic care of the eye socket. The conformer is a temporary prosthesis and need not be replaced if it falls out. However, the client should learn the care and insertion of a prosthesis. It needs to be removed about twice a month for cleaning. Special polishing, usually done by an optician, is periodically required to remove dried protein secretions.

Prosthesis care should be carried out as follows:

- Wash the hands.
- Pull the lower lid down, and the prosthesis should slip out.
- Wash the prosthesis under running water.
- Reinsert the prosthesis by lifting the upper eyelid against the bony orbit and placing the prosthesis under the lower eyelid while it is pulled down. The prosthesis should slip into place.

Prosthesis care and placement may be trying for the client as well as family or friends. They may need time to accept the cosmetic effect of an artificial eye.

The client also must adjust to monocular vision. With monocular vision, the client loses approximately 50° of peripheral vision on the affected side (from a field of 180°), because the nasal fields of each eye overlap. Therefore, the loss of one eye does not mean a 50° loss of visual efficiency (Newell, 1982). With practice, the client can resume a normal lifestyle.

The loss of an eye can have a profound effect on clients. Although they may be relieved of a painful, disfiguring, or blind eye, they grieve the loss of the eye and experience a change in body image. Depression and withdrawal are often experienced. Psychotherapy or counseling may help the client overcome grief and to accept the lost eye, decreased vision, and a possible cancer diagnosis.

Cholesteatomas

A cholesteatoma is an ingrowth of epidermis (the squamous epithelium) from the external meatus into the middle ear attic. A *primary cholesteatoma,* the most common form, originates as an ingrowth through a perforation in the pars flaccida, the uppermost portion of the tympanic membrane. The cause of primary cholesteatoma is unknown; it is thought to be eustachian tube dysfunction that creates a vacuum within the middle ear, which causes the loosest part of the pars flaccida to invaginate. A *secondary cholesteatoma* is an ingrowth through a peripheral perforation of the tympanic membrane usually caused by chronic suppurative otitis media. A *congenital cholesteatoma,* which is seen in children and young adults, is presumably caused by

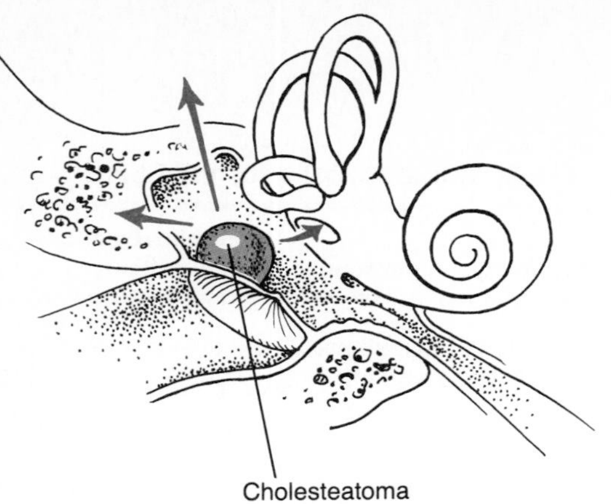

Figure 52–10

Cholesteatoma, which can erode into the inner ear, temporal bone, or epidural space.

epidermis congenitally left within the middle ear behind a normal intact tympanic membrane. It is not associated with perforation.

Epidermis in the middle ear produces keratin, which accumulates and destroys underlying tissue. As the disease progresses, it may destroy the ossicles and spread to the inner ear (Figure 52–10). Secondary infection often occurs at the site of the accumulated keratin.

Clinical Manifestations

An early cholesteatoma may be asymptomatic, and the perforation in the pars flaccida is usually detected during a routine otoscopic examination. The first symptom may be a conductive hearing loss in the affected ear. A painless, fetid otorrhea occurs when a secondary infection is present. As the disease progresses, facial paralysis and vertigo can occur.

Medical Measures

The treatment for a cholesteatoma is surgical removal. All the cholesteatoma must be removed to prevent further growth. If possible, a modified radical mastoidectomy followed by tympanoplasty is performed. Sometimes a radical mastoidectomy that removes all the mastoid air cells, the ossicles, and the tympanic membrane is necessary. After surgery, periodic lifelong follow-up to detect any new growth is essential (Marshall & Attia, 1983).

Specific Nursing Measures

Refer to the section on mastoidectomy, below, for a discussion of the nursing care of a client undergoing surgery for cholesteatoma.

Mastoidectomy

A mastoidectomy is the incision, drainage, and removal of diseased mucosa and bone from the mastoid process of the temporal bone. It may also be done to gain access to the middle or inner ear. There are three types of mastoidectomies: the simple (also referred to as complete) mastoidectomy, the radical mastoidectomy, and the modified radical mastoidectomy.

As a result of antibiotic therapy for acute otitis media, simple mastoidectomies are rarely performed today. A modified radical mastoidectomy is indicated for a cholesteatoma and for some carcinomas. The modified radical procedure is followed by a tympanoplasty (described later in this chapter) to restore hearing. A radical mastoidectomy is performed only when the preservation of hearing is secondary to preventing the spread of disease and is rarely used. Client implications of mastoidectomy are summarized in Table 52–11.

Nursing Implications

PREOPERATIVE CARE The client is instructed not to take aspirin or any other medication that may prolong bleeding before the mastoidectomy. Even a small amount of bleeding during aural surgery impairs the surgeon's ability to visualize the tiny structures, so every precaution is used to decrease bleeding.

POSTOPERATIVE CARE When the client returns from surgery after a mastoidectomy, the head of the bed is elevated at least 30°. Monitor the vital signs and observe for signs of bleeding or drainage. Excessive bleeding should be reported immediately to the physician. Be sure to check the dressing near the back of the head and the bed linens under the head for signs of bleeding. The outer dressing can be reinforced if necessary. Clients may be dizzy in the immediate postoperative period, so siderails are used while the client is in bed.

Because of its location, the facial nerve (CN VII) is vulnerable to injury during all types of surgery involving the middle or inner ear. The nerve enters the petrous

Table 52–11
Mastoidectomy: Implications for the Client 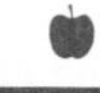

Physiologic Implications	Psychosocial/Lifestyle Implications
Precautions to decrease bleeding during surgery Discharge in 1 to 2 days and follow-up every week or until healing occurs Possible dizziness Possible facial nerve damage	Need to change dressing three times a day after bulky dressing removal for 3 to 4 weeks Return to activities in 6 weeks See Table 62–9 for implications following tympanoplasty, if performed

portion of the temporal bone through the internal auditory canal, winds around the ossicles, and exits through the mastoid process where it divides into many branches that course through the temporal bone to the lacrimal gland, the tongue, and the salivary glands (Figure 33–3). Watch for signs of facial paralysis, including sagging of the face, drooping of the mouth, drooling, or the inability to close the eyelid on the operative side. As soon as clients can respond, ask them to show their teeth, whistle, and wrinkle their foreheads. Clients who have injury to the nerve are taken back to surgery within 24 hours for decompression and repair of the injured nerve. Edema of the nerve also can cause paralysis, but this paralysis does not appear until several days postoperatively and usually resolves spontaneously.

Nausea and vertigo may be present following surgery, so always assist the client in getting out of bed. Administer medications for nausea, vertigo, and pain relief as ordered. Antibiotics are usually ordered to prevent infections. Encourage oral fluids as tolerated.

Prior to discharge instruct the client to:

- Report any change in drainage, pain, temperature, and weakness of the face.
- Wash hands before and after touching the ear and changing the dressing.
- Take medications as ordered. The nurse should write out the side effects of medications for the client.
- Prevent water from entering the ear for about 6 weeks.

Acoustic Neuroma

An acoustic neuroma (also called an acoustic neurilemoma or an acoustic schwannoma) is a benign tumor arising from the neurilemmal sheath of the vestibular branch of cranial nerve VIII (the vestibulocochlear nerve) and occurring within the internal auditory canal or in the region of the cerebellopontile angle. As the tumor grows, the cochlear branch of CN VIII becomes involved. The tumor can begin at any age and grows slowly. The specific cause of acoustic neuroma is unknown. A small number of tumors (usually bilateral) are a feature of von Recklinghausen's disease.

Clinical Manifestations

The most common first symptom is tinnitus, followed by an increasing high-frequency hearing loss with low speech discrimination. As the tumor progresses, symptoms of involvement of the cranial nerves V and VII (trigeminal and facial nerves, respectively) are present; these include an absence of an ipsilateral corneal reflex, facial hypesthesia, trigeminal pain, and loss of taste in the anterior two-thirds of the tongue. As the tumor progresses, nystagmus and ataxia may occur. Cerebellar pressure causing papilledema occurs late in the disease.

Diagnostic testing can include the examination of cerebrospinal fluid, which will show an elevation of protein. Tumors 2 cm in diameter or larger can be detected by a CT scan. If the CT scan fails to detect a tumor but symptoms are present, a myelogram may be performed. The response to the electronystagmographic caloric test is reduced or absent.

Medical Measures

The treatment for an acoustic neuroma is its surgical removal via craniotomy (discussed in Chapter 29). However, clients who are not safe candidates for surgery or have an extremely large tumor are treated with steroids. Gamma knife radiation has been successful for removing tumors less than 2 cm (Shambaugh & Glasscock, 1980).

Specific Nursing Measures

The nurse is responsible for preparing the client emotionally and physically for the diagnostic procedures and eventual surgery. Preoperative preparation and postoperative expectations should be discussed with both client and family or significant others. If the tumor affects the client's hearing, a method of communication should be established. Refer to Chapter 33 for surgical management of a client undergoing craniotomy.

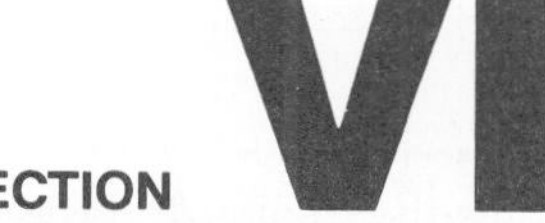

SECTION VI

Traumatic Disorders

Corneal and Other Abrasions of the Eye

Abrasions to the eyelid and conjunctiva rarely warrant medical attention, because they heal rapidly without treatment and cause little pain. Corneal abrasions, in contrast, disrupt the corneal epithelium and expose many nerve fibers, causing pain and prompting the client to seek medical treatment. Superficial abrasions normally heal without scarring or visual impairment. Two possible complications of corneal abrasions are delayed healing and recurrent corneal erosion. Infection as a result of an abrasion is rare.

Abrasions of the eye are traditionally found after the removal of foreign bodies and after injuries caused by such objects as paper, fingernails, or twigs of a tree catching the eye. Overwearing of contact lenses can also cause corneal abrasions.

Clinical Manifestations

Clients with corneal abrasions often feel as if they have foreign bodies in their eyes. These abrasions generally cause pain because of the exposure of nerve fibers in the epithelium; excessive lacrimation and photophobia are other symptoms. The use of a fluorescein strip aids in the diagnosis of corneal abrasions.

Medical Measures

The treatment of corneal abrasions centers around pain relief. Topical anesthetic eyedrops, such as 5% tetracaine, are routinely used. Systemic analgesics are rarely necessary. Continued and frequent instillation of anesthetic eyedrops delays healing and should not be permitted. Antibiotic eyedrops are also used to guard against infection.

A firm patch on the eye prevents movement of the eyelid, thereby promoting healing and relieving pain. The patch should be changed daily during the inspection of the eye. The client should wear the patch until healing occurs (usually within 24 to 72 hours). Rest and avoiding movements of the cheek, which loosen the eye patch and allow blinking, are recommended.

Specific Nursing Measures

The nurse working in ambulatory care, occupational health, or the emergency room has the most contact with clients having corneal abrasions. These nurses may flush foreign material from the eye, perform fluorescein staining procedures, administer the prescribed medications, and patch the eye firmly. Clients should be told they may experience pain as the anesthetic wears off, usually 1 to 2 hours after the initial treatment. Also instruct clients how to apply a firm eye patch in case it loosens or falls off.

Lacerations to the Eye

Lacerations to the eye may involve the eyelids or the globe itself and may be superficial or severe enough to damage the globe beyond repair. Lacerations of the cornea frequently lead to the loss of useful vision or prolapse of the iris, ciliary body, lens, or vitreous. The client with a laceration injury is predisposed to intraocular infection, cataract formation, and corneal scarring. Eyelid lacerations may be disfiguring and interfere with the normal flow of tears. Lacerations of either the cornea or eyelid are usually associated with penetration by sharp objects (eg, knives or scissors), explosive injuries, and automobile or bicycle accidents.

Clinical Manifestations

Pain, bleeding, tearing, and shock are common manifestations of eyelid lacerations. Clients with corneal lacerations may have mild to severe pain and symptoms of shock. Tissue prolapse may be evident upon examination. Iris prolapse causes the pupil to look like a teardrop. Other facial trauma often accompanies ocular lacerations.

Medical Measures

The treatment of lacerations depends on the structure injured and whether there is prolapse of tissue. Eyelid lacerations should be repaired as soon as possible, because a delay of 6 to 8 hours significantly increases the risk of infection.

Corneal lacerations without prolapsed tissue usually require suturing under an operative microscope. Cycloplegics and antibiotics are usually indicated. Bilateral patches are usually placed to ensure complete rest of the eyes. Bed rest also may promote healing. Tetanus prophylaxis is indicated in any injury that penetrates the eye. Measures to repair corneal lacerations with prolapsed tissue attempt to replace the prolapsed contents of the eye. If damage is severe and much of the intraocular content has been lost, evisceration or enucleation is indicated.

Small, clean lacerations of the cornea (3 to 4 mm) often seal spontaneously. A rigid eye shield and antibiotics are generally the only corrective measures taken.

Specific Nursing Measures

Eyelid lacerations and corneal lacerations without prolapsed tissue require little nursing intervention other than reassurance and instructions regarding the instillation of medications. If bleeding is present, application of pressure is contraindicated because this can damage the underlying globe.

Corneal lacerations with tissue prolapse generally require hospitalization of the client. Care of the client undergoing enucleation is discussed earlier in this chapter.

Foreign Bodies in the Eye

Foreign bodies in the conjunctiva and cornea are the most common cause of ocular trauma. They generally pose few problems unless laceration and tissue prolapse accompany them. Foreign bodies can also penetrate and perforate the intraocular contents and lodge in almost any structure. Intraocular foreign bodies carry a high risk of impairing sight to some degree. Frequently encountered foreign bodies include dirt, small metallic particles, eyelashes, and glass. Most clients who seek medical attention for known or suspected foreign bodies in their eyes have been hammering, welding, or standing next to an industrial machine that caused particles to blow into their faces and eyes.

Clinical Manifestations

A conjunctival foreign body is usually not painful unless the object is under the upper eyelid. Blinking then moves the particle over the cornea, creating irritation and pain. Corneal foreign bodies cause pain, tearing, and photophobia. The sensation that something is in the eye occurs with both conjunctival and corneal foreign bodies.

Symptoms of intraocular foreign bodies may not be commensurate with the seriousness of the injury. Immediate symptoms may be minimal if the foreign body enters the eye quickly and smoothly. Intraocular foreign bodies usually lodge in the vitreous cavity. Therefore, opthalmoscopic examination may reveal corneal lacerations, localized areas of conjunctival infection, a hole in the iris, hyphema, or disturbance of the lens. Retinal detachments may occur if the foreign body reaches the posterior portion of the eye.

Medical Measures

The client should not rub the eye because this may abrade the corneal tissue or cause the particle to become embedded. Eyes with penetrating injuries should be shielded from pressure. Attempts should not be made to cleanse the area of tears, discharge, and blood or to remove the penetrating object until an ophthalmologist has evaluated the client's condition.

Conjunctival foreign bodies frequently come out spontaneously with blinking. If this does not occur, they can be wiped out gently with a cotton swab moistened with normal saline. If the particle cannot be seen on the exposed conjunctiva, the examiner should evert and inspect the upper eyelid.

Foreign bodies embedded in the cornea must be removed by a physician, preferably an ophthalmologist. A local anesthetic, magnification, and the use of a slit lamp facilitate removal. Antibiotic ointments (eg, polymyxin B-bacitracin, gentamicin) should be instilled three times a day following removal of the foreign body. Eye patches may be used if a laceration results.

Ophthalmologic treatment of foreign bodies that have perforated the intraocular contents depends on the type of foreign body and the extent of damage to surrounding tissues. Some inert substances are left in place, whereas organic matter (eg, wood, copper, or iron) is normally removed. Because magnetic material can be removed relatively easily with the aid of a magnet, it creates fewer hazards than does penetration by nonmagnetic foreign bodies. The removal of nonmagnetic particles requires the use of forceps to grasp and remove the objects from the vitreous. Any other damage to the eye must be repaired. Evisceration or enucleation is indicated if trauma and loss of intraocular contents is severe. Any penetrating injury to the eye warrants tetanus prophylaxis as well as the administration of antibiotics and analgesics.

Specific Nursing Measures

The nurse often takes an active role in the care of clients with ocular foreign bodies. Remove conjunctival foreign bodies by using a moist cotton swab or gently irrigating the eye with normal saline. If corneal or intraocular foreign bodies are suspected, try to ensure that the client will be seen by an ophthalmologist as soon as possible. Meanwhile, shield the eye from pressure; try to provide a quiet, supportive environment; and obtain an order for analgesic medication. The nurse may assist the physician with removal of the foreign body or prepare the client for surgery.

Orbital Fractures

Two types of orbital fracture can occur. The first involves the bony rim of the orbit and is usually detected by x-rays. The second type, a blow-out fracture, involves the disruption of the thin inferior orbital wall, causing the orbital contents to herniate into the maxillary sinus. Approximately 15% of orbital fractures are associated with serious eye injury.

Almost all orbital fractures are caused by a direct injury usually from blunt blows to the eye from a golf ball, a piece of equipment, or a motor vehicle accident. Fractures also occur as an extension of fractures in adjacent bones. In a blow-out fracture, pressure from a direct blow pushes the eyeball back and increases the IOP. This sudden pressure increase causes the inferior orbital wall to fracture next to the air-containing sinuses.

Clinical Manifestations

The client with a blow-out fracture frequently has pain, nausea at the time of injury, and diplopia. Ecchymosis, swelling, and subcutaneous emphysema (if the ethmoid bone is involved) may be present in either type of fracture. Persistent diplopia and enophthalmos are the two complications frequently seen with orbital fractures.

Medical Measures

Surgical reduction of the fracture is undertaken if mobility of the eye is restricted or if endophthalmitis (extensive intraocular infection) is present. This procedure is not emergent and usually can be undertaken 7 to 10 days after the injury takes place to evaluate the indications fully. Simultaneous injury to the globe, however, may require immediate care.

Cold compresses applied during the first 24 hours help minimize swelling and bleeding into the surrounding tissues. Hot packs to speed the absorption of blood may be used after the first 24 hours. Analgesics are prescribed and administered.

Specific Nursing Measures

The nursing management of a client with an orbital fracture involves recognizing such an injury and urging prompt medical attention. The nurse may assist the ophthalmologist in examining the eye and carrying out therapeutic measures. Emotional support and teaching are the two most common and important nursing roles.

Burns to the Eye

Burns to the eye result from exposure to radiant energy, high temperatures, or chemicals. Radiant energy burns result from overexposure to ultraviolet rays, which most commonly occurs with the use of sunlamps or with carbon arc lamps used in welding. Overexposure can occur relatively quickly without a protective eye filter. Ultraviolet rays may also be absorbed by the eye when watching the sun or an eclipse, or when tanning in the sun with the face and eyes exposed. Reflections of the sun on snow or water constitute a greater hazard than the sun itself because the ultraviolet light concentrations are higher.

Thermal burns usually involve the eyelids rather than the globe. Flame, flare such as from a welding torch, or splashes of molten metal or other hot liquids are the most common causes.

Chemical burns occur in both home and work settings when a toxic substance comes in contact with the eye. The substance may be acidic (eg, sulfuric, hydrochloric, nitric, or acetic acid) or alkaline (eg, sodium hydroxide, ammonium hydroxide, lime, or calcium hydroxide). In general, alkali burns penetrate the tissue more quickly and are more serious than acid burns. The extent of damage to the eye depends on the concentration of chemicals, the duration of exposure, and the pH of the solution.

Severe burns to the eye may cause major ocular complications; poor rehabilitative prognosis; and, when bilateral, a life of dependency for the affected individual. Immediate first aid care of the burned eye often limits the amount of damage to the eye. Other organ damage may accompany burns to the eye (eg, extensive burns of the face, body, and upper airways). Care of these burns may supersede or coincide with eye care.

Clinical Manifestations

Radiant energy burns produce no immediate symptoms; they manifest themselves approximately 6 to 12 hours after ultraviolet exposure. The client experiences extreme pain from the development of superficial keratitis. Tearing, photophobia, and congestion of the globe are often present. Severe ultraviolet burns also may burn the macula, causing permanent visual impairment. Photophobia and blurred vision may be present for a week after the accident.

Thermal burns usually cause widespread tissue destruction. Depending on the extent of the burn, pain and shock may occur. Corneal sloughing may also be present if damage to the cornea has occurred.

The immediate manifestation of chemical burns is pain. After a chemical burn, the eyelids will be swollen and the conjunctiva reddened. The degree of corneal stromal whitening (marbleization) aids in determining the severity of the burn.

Medical Measures

Radiant energy burns usually cause significant pain and prompt the client to seek medical attention. A topical anesthetic reduces pain and facilitates examination. Patching the eye for 24 hours and applying cold compresses provide symptomatic relief. Recovery usually occurs within 12 to 36 hours without complications.

The treatment of thermal burns is similar to the treatment of skin burns elsewhere, because the eyelid tissue is usually involved. Skin grafts, mucous membrane grafts, or both may be required if eyelid contractures are present.

Chemical burns require the immediate dilution of the chemical, because the extent of damage to the eye depends on the concentration of the contacting solution and the amount of time it is in contact with the eye. Always flush the eye first, then seek medical attention. Copiously flush the eye with water for 20 to 30 minutes. Separate the eyelids well to allow the water to flush the cornea and conjunctiva. Do not try to neutralize the chemical with a buffering solution, because finding the correct solution often delays treatment. Industrial plants and research laboratories must have jet stream irrigating fountains or safety showers. Remove any particulate matter. After irrigation, the eye can be patched and the client sent to an ophthalmologist for examination. Corneal exposure resulting from eyelid edema and retraction or incomplete blinking must be treated quickly by artificial tears or moisture chambers.

The use of steroids for thermal or chemical burns is controversial, and most ophthalmologists avoid it. Instead, they usually order antibiotics to prevent or treat infection. If corneal damage from a chemical burn is severe, corneal transplantation may be undertaken approximately 18 months to 2 years after the accident.

Specific Nursing Measures

Nursing intervention with chemical burns to the eye involves immediate irrigation of the eye, as has been discussed, and calming the client.

Information regarding the type of chemical involved, its concentration, and the duration of probable exposure should be obtained. Occupational health nurses may be involved in ensuring that all employees follow safety regulations and that all irrigators function properly.

The incidence of ultraviolet burns can be decreased by public awareness. Inform the public formally and informally about the significance of ultraviolet burns and how to avoid them.

Ocular Contusions

An intraocular contusion is a bruising injury in which the exterior of the eye remains intact, but intraocular damage has occurred. This type of trauma most frequently results in a hemorrhage into the anterior chamber (hyphema) or the vitreous or surrounding tissues (ecchymosis). The consequences of such injuries vary and are often not immediately obvious. Contusions of the eyeball may be produced by a severe blow to the eye. The blow is usually blunt and comes from traumatic contact with a tennis ball, fist, golf ball, or baseball.

Clinical Manifestations

A client with an ocular contusion may have a large extravasation of blood under the skin that causes the tissue surrounding the eye to appear black and blue. Swelling of the surrounding tissues most often accompanies a black eye. Hyphema also may be evident and often can be observed by the naked eye. The client may experience impaired vision, pain, and fear. A sudden decrease in vision and complaints of floaters may indicate a hemorrhage into the vitreous. IOP almost always temporarily increases in a contusion of the eyeball.

Other complications that may develop immediately or weeks to months after the injury include lens dislocation, macular edema, retinal detachment, iridodialysis (splitting of the iris resulting in more than one pupil), and rupture of the sclera.

Medical Measures

Most immediate effects of an ocular contusion do not require immediate definitive treatment. Specific treatment depends on the location and extent of damage. Cold compresses and mild analgesics are used to treat ocular contusions. As the blood decomposes and is absorbed, the bruises change color and fade completely in 5 to 7 days.

Clients exhibiting signs of hyphema should have absolute bed rest with bilateral eye patches to minimize the risks of further bleeding. Diazepam (Valium) may be ordered to decrease anxiety and promote complete rest. IOP should be monitored.

Specific Nursing Measures

Clients with hyphema should have the head of the bed elevated. Change the eye patches daily and provide ongoing emotional support. Since clients have bilateral eye patches, the nurse must assist with many of the daily living activities, such as feeding and bathing. The nurse also may encourage family members or friends to assist with these tasks and to read to the client. Strongly encourage complete rest.

Injuries to the Auricle

Trauma of the auricle includes contusions, hematomas, abrasions, and lacerations caused by falls, vehicular accidents, blows to the ear, and foreign bodies. The ear's exposed position and the absence of subcutaneous tissue also predispose it to frostbite and burns.

Clinical Manifestations

Pain, numbness, paresthesia, tenderness, erythema, or ecchymosis of the auricle may be present. Repeated contusions may cause a thickening called cauliflower ear. Lacerations may be small and superficial, be deep into the cartilage, or involve a complete avulsion of the auricle. Burns can cause extensive blistering or destruction of tissue. Frostbite occurs on the upper and outer edges first, and its extent is often not apparent. The frozen area appears waxy and whitish-yellow and feels cold and hard.

Medical and Specific Nursing Measures

Mild analgesics are usually sufficient for easing pain of contusions and hematomas. Any fluid that accumulates should be aspirated; cotton impregnated with water-soluble jelly should be fitted into the contours of the auricle, and a pressure bandage should be applied for several days to prevent an accumulation of fluid. Antibiotics are recommended if there is evidence of infection.

Abrasions are cleaned thoroughly to remove any foreign matter. After an antibiotic ointment is applied, the wound can be left uncovered.

Surgical lacerations are sutured. When the laceration is contaminated or has been untreated for 24 hours, it may be debrided and treated with antibacterial preparations and wet dressings with aluminum acetate (Burow's) solution. Immediate reattachment of an auricle torn from the head is necessary to be successful; otherwise a prosthesis will have to be used. The treatment of burns is detailed in Chapter 12 and the treatment of frostbite in Chapter 55.

Be alert for any associated trauma to the skull or tympanic membrane. Any increase in pain or temperature is significant, because many injuries are prone to secondary infections.

Injuries to the External Auditory Canal, Tympanic Membrane, Middle Ear, and Inner Ear

Abrasions, small lacerations, insect bites, and hematomas can occur in the external auditory canal. The most common serious injury to the ear is perforation of the tympanic membrane. Fractured and displaced ossicles are often associated with a perforated tympanic membrane and fractures of the temporal bone. About 80% of temporal bone fractures are longitudinal (cross through the middle ear), and 15% are transverse (cross through the internal auditory canal, the optic capsule, or both) (Goodhill, 1979). A blow to the side of the head can cause a longitudinal fracture, whereas a transverse fracture is caused by a blow to the front or back of the head. Injuries are also caused by cotton applicators, pencils, paper clips, flying objects, and improper irrigation of the external auditory canal.

Clinical Manifestations

Abrasions, lacerations, or hematomas in the external auditory canal and perforations of the tympanic membrane are usually visible with careful otoscopic examination. Insect bites may cause wheals, vesicles, or ulcerations.

Longitudinal fractures of the temporal bone usually cause a perforated tympanic membrane and a bloody discharge in the external auditory canal. Facial paralysis is usually delayed, but conductive hearing loss may be present. Transverse fractures may occur bilaterally. Although the tympanic membrane is intact, injury to the inner ear can result from tearing of the membranous labyrinth and rupture of the oval and round windows (Jerger & Jerger, 1981). Vertigo, nystagmus, and sensorineural hearing loss may be present. Any facial paralysis will occur immediately.

Medical Measures

A topical antiseptic or antibiotic is applied to abrasions, small lacerations, or hematomas in the external auditory canal. If the canal's skin is torn and has an elevated skin flap, an absorbable gelatin sponge (Gelfoam) or a petroleum-jelly impregnated fabric (Adaptic) inserted into the canal for several days will hold the flap in place.

Foreign objects are removed with curets, suction, or irrigation. Removal of foreign bodies is discussed in Chapter 51.

Small perforations of the tympanic membrane are usually only observed for several days, and sterile cotton is placed in the external auditory canal. If the perforation remains dry after several days without signs of closing, patching with a paper moistened with 10% silver nitrate or a gelatin film promotes healing. Antibiotics prevent infection in the middle ear. When the perforation is large or patching is unsuccessful, surgery (tympanoplasty or myringoplasty) is necessary. Surgical exploration and repair of the ossicles may also be necessary.

For temporal bone fractures, the management of intracranial injuries with the establishment of ventilation and maintenance of vital signs takes precedence over the otologic problem. A sterile dressing is applied to the draining ear until the general condition has stabilized. Hearing may fluctuate during the first 6 months after temporal bone fractures, after which exploratory surgery may be necessary. Reconstructive surgery for the tympanic membrane or ossicles can be performed if necessary.

Specific Nursing Measures

The nurse's primary responsibility in caring for clients with injuries to the external auditory canal, tympanic membrane, middle ear, and inner ear may be emotional support and providing knowledge. Emotional distress because of hearing loss or fear of hearing loss is often the biggest problem these clients face. The removal of foreign bodies and the treatment of minor injuries are accomplished with little discomfort if the nurse reassures the client and explains the procedures.

If possible, elevate the head of the bed for clients with traumatic conditions of the middle or inner ear. Use sterile aseptic technique for all treatment to the ear. Establish a method of communication with the client until the hearing is improved. Instruct clients with perforated tympanic membranes to avoid putting water into their ears and to have regular examinations for evidence of cholesteatoma.

Barotrauma

Barotrauma occurs in clients during takeoff and landing in airplanes or underwater diving. It is caused by a failure of the eustachian tube to open sufficiently, causing an unequal pressure differential between the middle ear and the atmospheric pressure. Barotrauma is more common in clients with upper respiratory tract problems. This problem has increased today with the increased frequency of airplane travel and the popularity of scuba diving.

Clinical Manifestations

Clients with barotrauma usually complain of severe pain, fullness in the ear, and decreased hearing. The tympanic membrane can be retracted. With severe pressure differentials, fluid or blood may accumulate in the middle ear. Rupture of the tympanic membrane can occur. Occasionally, dislocation of the ossicles also may occur.

Medical Measures

Analgesics may be required for pain relief, and decongestants may be used to open the eustachian tube. It may be necessary for the otologist to catheterize through the nasopharynx to the eustachian tube to restore the pressure within the middle ear. With severe trauma, a myringotomy can be performed to release the pressure and aspirate any accumulated fluid. Clients with upper respiratory tract infections can take oral decongestants ½ hour before and periodically during flying to prevent barotrauma.

Specific Nursing Measures

Nursing management should concentrate on prevention. For example, instruct clients in self-ventilating techniques (described in Chapter 51) to use when flying. Sucking on hard candy and swallowing will open the eustachian tube. Discourage clients with upper respiratory tract infections from flying or diving. The client in whom barotrauma has occurred should avoid flying or diving for 2 weeks.

Noise Trauma

Noise-induced hearing loss is a sensorineural hearing loss that develops gradually over months or years from environmental or industrial noise exposure at or above 85 dB. Less intense sounds may cause fatigue or annoyance, but not hearing loss. The degree of hearing loss is proportional to the duration of exposure when the sound level is held constant. Table 52–12 illustrates the effects of common noises of daily life on hearing. The incidence of noise-induced hearing loss is higher in adults than in children, because adults are exposed to more of the conditions that predispose them to noise trauma. Acoustic trauma is an instan-

Table 52–12
Effects on Hearing of Common Noises in Daily Life

Sound	Decibel Level	Relative Sound Intensity	Effect
Rocket on launching pad	180	1,000,000,000,000,000,000	Hearing loss inevitable
Jet plane takeoff (close range)	150	1,000,000,000,000,000	Tympanic membrane rupture possible
Gunshot blast	140	100,000,000,000,000	Pain in the ear; possible tympanic membrane rupture; any length of exposure time is dangerous
Rock band concert in front of speakers, thunderclap, sonic boom, textile plant, sandblasting	120	1,000,000,000,000	Immediate danger to hearing
Snowmobile, auto horn at 3 ft, steel mill	110	100,000,000,000	
Chain saw, jackhammer, jet plane at 1000 ft, printing plant, pneumatic drill, boiler shop	100	10,000,000,000	Hearing damage after exposure for 2 hr; with every 5-dB increase, "safe time" cut in half
Heavy street traffic, power lawn mower, food blender, shop tools	90	1,000,000,000	Hearing damage in less than 8 hr
Telephone, garbage disposal, barking dog, clothes washer, average factory, dishwasher, subway	80	100,000,000	Hearing damage after more than 8 hr
Vacuum cleaner, noisy party	70	10,000,000	Critical level at which noise may begin to affect hearing after constant exposure
Average restaurant or office noise, crying infant	60	1,000,000	Intrusive; annoying
Ordinary conversation, quiet suburb (daytime)	50	100,000	
Library	40	10,000	
Quiet suburb or rural area (nighttime)	30	1000	
Rustle of leaves, whispering voices	20	100	
Breathing	10	10	

taneous hearing loss from brief exposure to a high-intensity sound at close range, such as gunshots or explosions.

Clinical Manifestations

The client with noise trauma may have hearing loss, a high-pitched tinnitus, and a feeling of fullness within the ear. Noise-induced hearing loss usually occurs bilaterally, whereas acoustic trauma may be unilateral. Vascular congestion of the tympanic membrane may occur with acute acoustic trauma. High-intensity noise can perforate the tympanic membrane and dislocate or fracture the ossicles.

Medical Measures

No medical or surgical treatment effectively restores the hearing loss after noise trauma. Therefore, prevention is most important. The control of noise exposure is the best means of prevention.

If noise trauma has occurred, rest and avoidance of further trauma is recommended. Aural rehabilitation may be necessary. The masking of tinnitus with special hearing aids or biofeedback with masking has been helpful for some clients. Surgery for repair of the tympanic membrane and ossicles may be necessary.

Specific Nursing Measures

The nurse's primary responsibility in dealing with noise trauma lies in prevention. Nurses can help inform clients about the health hazards of noise. Clients who work in noisy environments, for example, should be made aware of the potential risk to their hearing. Encourage periodic audiometric testing for those at risk, as well as the use of protective devices such as helmets, earplugs, or earmuffs.

Chapter Highlights

Early identification of visual or hearing impairment is important so a program of rehabilitation can be initiated. Emotional support is of primary importance.

Otosclerosis, which tends to run in families, is a common cause of conductive hearing loss in young adults.

The facial nerve, CN VII, is vulnerable to injury during surgery of the middle or inner ear. Check the postoperative client for signs of facial paralysis.

It is important to check the ear dressing near the back of the head and the bed linens under the head for signs of bleeding.

Dizziness or vertigo may be experienced to varying degrees by clients having otologic surgery; the nurse should be sure to assist the client in ambulating and provide safety measures such as bedrails.

A retinal detachment progressively impairs vision as the retina is pulled from the choroid, depriving the rods and cones of their nutritional supply. It may result from trauma, vitreous traction, or retinal degeneration.

Clients requiring eye surgery fear vision loss, discomfort, dependence on significant others and health care professionals, and possible lifestyle changes.

The nurse needs to assist the client in verbalizing fears, provide education on procedures and implications, and assist the client in regaining autonomy safely.

The nurse can promote an uneventful postoperative course by providing orientation of time and place to the client with an eye patch; preventing nausea with antiemetics; encouraging flexing and extending of the extremities to prevent thrombi; promoting deep breathing to expand lungs and prevent secretions; and discouraging coughing, bending, straining with bowel movements, and nose blowing to prevent increased intraocular pressure.

Retinal reattachment procedures often require stringent positioning for the immediate postoperative period to keep the retina and choroid in apposition.

Nurses can help prevent the disastrous effects of glaucoma through public education and mass screening of individuals over 40. Assisting clients with their therapy regimen and client education are other important responsibilities of the nurse.

Clients with Meniere's syndrome have extremely uncomfortable paroxysmal attacks of vertigo, tinnitus, and sensorineural hearing loss.

Surgical procedures are performed to eliminate the vestibular symptoms of Meniere's syndrome and preserve hearing, although some procedures do cause hearing loss.

Degenerative disorders such as cataracts and macular degeneration produce such changes as reduced visual acuity, loss of accommodation, loss of peripheral or central vision, and difficulty in color discrimination.

The aphakic client will have decreased refractive power and no accommodation ability after cataract extraction, so cataract glasses, contact lenses, or an intraocular lens will be necessary for adequate visual acuity.

Because there is no effective medical or surgical treatment for presbycusis, nurses should encourage the elderly to seek aural rehabilitation and amplification to improve hearing and prevent depression and isolation.

Benign and malignant tumors of the eye are usually not detected until a late stage of the disease. Of all ocular tumors 85% appear in the choroid. Enucleation is often the final outcome of ocular tumors.

Tinnitus and a gradual hearing loss may be the only early symptoms of neoplasms of the middle and inner ear.

Clients with perforated tympanic membranes should avoid getting water in their ears and should have regular examinations for evidence of cholesteatomas.

Bibliography

Alpiner J: Psychological and social aspects of aging as related to hearing rehabilitation of elderly clients. In *Aural Rehabilitation for the Elderly.* Henock M (editor). New York: Grune & Stratton, 1979.

Anderson RG, Meyerhoff WL: Otologic manifestations of aging. *Otolaryngologic Clin North Am* 1982; 15(2):353–370.

Armstrong BW: Prolonged middle ear ventilation: The right tube in the right place. *Annals of Otology, Rhinology, Laryngology* 1983; 92:582–586.

Balkany TJ: An overview of the electronic cochlear prosthesis: Clinical and research considerations. *Otolaryngology Clin North Am* 1983; 16:209–215.

Bloome MA, Garcia CA: *Manual of Retinal and Choroidal Dystrophies.* Norwalk, CT: Appleton–Century–Crofts, 1982.

Boyd–Monk H: Retinal detachment and vitrectomy: Nursing care. *Nurs Clin North Am* 1981; 16(3):383–477.

Chawla H: *Essential Ophthalmology.* Edinburgh: Churchill Livingstone, 1981.

Chignell AH: *Retinal Detachment Surgery.* New York: Springer–Verlag, 1980.

Ciolini N, Horowitz J: What diabetics need to know about their risk of blindness. *Sightsaving* 1983; 52:2–5.

Clayman H, Jaffe N, Galin M: *Intraocular Lens Implantation.* St. Louis: Mosby, 1983.

Folk J: Senile macular degeneration. *Primary Care* 1982; 9(4):793–799.

Girard L: *Corneal Surgery,* Vol. 2, St. Louis: Mosby, 1981.

Goodhill V: *Ear Diseases, Deafness, and Dizziness.* Hagerstown, MD: Harper & Row, 1979.

Grabham J: Vitrectomy surgery. *Nurs Times* 1982; 78:2113–2117.

Gruendemann BJ, Meeker MK: *Alexander's Care of the Patient in Surgery,* 7th ed. St. Louis: Mosby, 1983, pp. 593–612.

Hough JV: Experience in tympanoplasty: Avoiding revisions and complications. *Otolaryngology Clin North Am* 1982; 15:845–860.

Heller B, Gaynor E: Hearing loss and aural rehabilitation of the elderly. *Top Clin Nurs* 1981; 3(1):21–29.

Jerger S, Jerger J: *Auditory Disorders: A Manual for Clinical Evaluation.* Boston: Little, Brown, 1981.

Karmody C: *Textbook of Otolaryngology.* Philadelphia: Lea & Febiger, 1983.

Kaufman H et al: The ailing eye: treat, consult, refer? *Patient Care* (April 15) 1980; 14:16–69.

Kilroy J: Care and teaching of patients with glaucoma. *Nurs Clin North Am* 1981; 16(3):393–404.

Little H et al: *Diabetic Retinopathy.* New York: Thieme–Stratton, 1983.

Loeb GE: The functional replacement of the ear. *Sci Am* 1985; 252(2):104–111.

Marshall K, Attia E: *Disorders of the Ear.* Boston: John Wright-PSG, 1983.

Marta M: A guide to the posterior vitrectomy. *Today's OR Nurse* (March) 1983; 5:26+.

Mawson SR, Ludman H: *Diseases of the Ear: A Textbook of Otology,* 4th ed. Chicago: Year Book, 1979.

McCoy K: Cataracts and intraocular lenses: From cloudy to clear. *Nurs Clin North Am* 1981; 16(3):405–414.

Meltzer D, Drews R: Intraocular lens implantation. In: *Complications in Ophthalmic Surgery.* New York: Churchill Livingstone, 1983.

Miller D: *Ophthalmology.* Boston: Houghton Mifflin Professional Publishers, 1979.

Newell F: *Ophthalmology,* 5th ed. St. Louis: Mosby, 1982.

Niswander M: Making good "cents" out of hearing conservation. *Occup Health Safety* (March 1983):57–60.

Pfister R: Chemical injuries of the eye. *Ophthalmology,* 1983; 90(10):1246–1252.

Rados B: When motion sickness goes along for the ride. *FDA Cons* 1985; 19(2):6–9.

Sataloff J, Sataloff RT, Vassallo LA: *Hearing Loss,* 2nd ed. Philadelphia: Lippincott, 1980.

Saunders W et al: *Nursing Care in Eye, Ear, Nose, and Throat Disorders,* 4th ed. St. Louis: Mosby, 1979.

Schepens C: *Retinal Detachment and Allied Diseases.* Vol. 1. Philadelphia: Saunders, 1983.

Senturia BH, Marcus MD, Lucenti FE: *Diseases of the External Ear,* 2nd ed. New York: Grune & Stratton, 1980.

Shambaugh GE, Glasscock ME: *Surgery of the Ear,* 3rd ed. Philadelphia: Saunders, 1980.

Shields BM: *A Study Guide for Glaucoma.* Baltimore: Williams & Wilkins, 1982.

Smith JF, Nachazel DD: *Ophthalmic Nursing.* Boston: Little, Brown, 1980.

Theodure FM, Bloomfield SE, Mandine B: *Clinical Allergy and Immunology of the Eye.* Baltimore: Williams & Wilkins, 1983.

Tumulty G, Resker M: Eye trauma. *Am J Nurs* 84:740–745.

Vaughan D, Asbury T: *General Ophthalmology.* Los Altos, CA: Lange Medical Publications, 1980.

Warner GG (editor): *Emergency Care Assessment and Intervention,* 3rd ed. St. Louis: Mosby, 1983.

Whitton S: Penetrating keratoplasty. *Today's OR Nurse* (March) 1983; 5:20+.

Zach J, Smirnow J: IOL implantation. *Today's OR Nurse* (March) 1983; 5:13+.

Zimmerman L, McLean I: A comparison of progress in the management of retinoblastomas and uveal melanomas. In: *Ocular Pathology Update.* Nicholson D (editor). New York: Masson, 1980; pp. 191–210.

CASE STUDY

The Client With Cataract Extraction and Intraocular Lens Implant

I. Descriptive Data

Mrs Margaret Schwan, an 80-year-old retired librarian, was seen by her ophthalmologist because of blurred vision and subsequent difficulty reading. She had no pain other than occasional frontal headaches after long periods of reading.

II. Personal Data

Date and Time: March 2, 1988, 1 PM
Full Name: Margaret Louise Schwan
Social Security Number: 000-00-0000
Address: 2323 Lancaster Dr., Oakland, CA
Telephone: 000-0000
Sex: Female
Age: 80
Birthdate: 8-23-07
Marital Status: Widowed
Race: Caucasian
Religion: Lutheran
Occupation: Retired librarian
Usual Health Care Provider: Geraldine Drummond, MD; Michael Laski, RN, NP

III. Health History

Source of Information: Client
Reliability of Informant: Very reliable
Chief Concern: "For the past six months or so, I've noticed increasing difficulty reading fine print."

History of Present Illness: Mrs Schwan states she has noted a gradual deterioration in visual acuity (left eye more than right) over the last few years intefering with activities of daily living. No diplopia, eye pain, redness, halos, or floaters. She has no history of eye problems except for needing reading glasses since age 50; no eye trauma; no hx of DM, hypertension, cardiovascular disease, renal disease; no ⊕ F Hx of eye problems; has occasional headaches behind her eyes relieved by over-the-counter sinus medications; otherwise takes no meds except for acetaminophen for arthritic discomfort and psyllium and an occasional stool softener for constipation.

Past Health History:

Childhood: Usual childhood illnesses
Immunizations: Doesn't remember having any; never had dog bite or stitches requiring Td
Medical Problems: Chronic constipation X 25 years, currently managed with psyllium; osteoarthritis both hands, both hips, left shoulder
Surgeries: Bunionectomy rt foot, 1974; abd hysterectomy for fibroids, 1960
Pregnancies: None
Trauma: None
Allergies: Sulfa (urticaria)
Medications: Acetaminophen, gr X AM and PM
Psyllium 1 tbsp b.i.d.
Docusate sodium (Colace), 100 mg p.r.n.

Family History:

Father, died age 90, old age
Mother, died age 36, childbirth
Brother, died age 73, MI, also had Type II DM
Sister, age 82, A & W
Husband, died age 70, CVA

No known positive F Hx of TBC, cancer, glaucoma, cataract, or other eye problems

Personal/Social History:

Mrs Schwan has been widowed 11 years and lives alone in a one-story apartment; is a former smoker (1 PPD × 20 yr) and is accustomed to a glass of sherry after dinner; active in her church and volunteers 15 hours a week at the public library. She eats simple "convenience" foods, reassuring the interviewer that she gets proper nutrition; has no difficulty sleeping; no longer drives her own car because of her decreasing vision but has several close friends who take her shopping; is able to walk to church and to the library.

Review of Systems:

States her overall health is excellent

Eyes: See history of present illness

Ears: Has minor hearing difficulty in rt ear; was tested and told she had some nerve deafness; it does not bother her

Respiratory: No DOE, no cough

Cardiovascular: No chest pain; all past ECGs wnl; no ankle swelling

Gastrointestinal: No nausea, vomiting, change in bowel habits; stools brown; has daily BM with psyllium; eats whole grains and fresh fruits

Gynecologic: Was never able to become pregnant, which was a major disappointment in her life; had heavy bleeding with fibroids; no problems since hysterectomy

Musculoskeletal: Often has pain in fingers and hips on damp days and with overuse; joints rarely swell; uses acetaminophen for pain, which controls it well

IV. Physical Assessment

Weight: 152 lb

Height: 5 ft 5 in.

Vital Signs: Temperature 97.5 F (36.4°C); pulse 82; respirations 16; BP 130/84, rt arm, seated

Relevant Organ Systems:

Eyes:

- *VA using Snellen's chart* *PH (pinhole)*
  OD V (without corrective lenses) 20/80 → 20/80
  OS V (without corrective lenses) 20/20 → 20/200
  M (manifest: what a client can subjectively achieve when assessing for best acuity)
  M = OD no improvement; OS no improvement
- *External exam:*
  Lids: Normal, no ptosis, ectropion, or entropion noted
  Lashes: Scarce
  Lacrimal: nl; no swelling, erythema, epiphora, or dryness noted
- *EOMs:* Normal: Full movement OU; orthophoric (no strabismus)
- *Pupils:* Normal size; OD 3 mm → 2 mm (with light); OS 3 mm → 2 mm; round, regular, no defects
- *VFs:* Intact to finger confrontation
- *SLE (slit lamp examination):*
  Conjunctiva: White, no injection
  Anterior chamber: Deep without cells or flare (protein)

(continued)

CASE STUDY (continued)

The Client With Cataract Extraction and Intraocular Lens Implant

Relevant Organ Systems, (continued):

Iris: Nl
Lens: L > R cataract

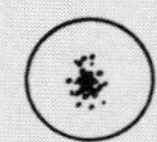

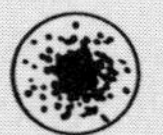

Frontal Cross-section Frontal Cross-section
OD OS
2+ nuclear sclerosis 3+ brunescent (brown) sclerosis

- *Fundus, using indirect ophthalmoscope:*
  OD (optic disk, vessels, macula, and periphery): No abnormality
  OS: Hazy view, probably nl optic disk, vessels, macula, and periphery
  Optical media: OD 20/80; OS 20/200

Respiratory: Sinuses, without tenderness; chest, clear to auscultation

Cardiovascular: Apical rate 78, regular; o m; S_1S_2 nl; ECG nl

Musculoskeletal: Heberden's nodes DIP joints of index, middle, and ring fingers both hands

Neurologic: CN II-XII intact; Romberg test negative

V. Diagnosis Bilateral cataracts

VI. Summary Physical examination revealed bilateral cataracts, and surgery was recommended. The ophthalmologist described the cataract extraction procedure and the potential surgery risks to Mrs Schwan. One week later, she was admitted to the hospital for cataract extraction and intraocular lens implant of her left eye, to be followed by extraction of the right cataract at a later date.

VII. Nursing Care Plan, by Nursing Diagnosis

Client Care Goals	Plan/Nursing Implementation	Expected Outcome
Self-care deficit related to loss of independence secondary to decrease in visual acuity and field		
Remain independent	Orient client to surroundings and organize possessions within reach of unoperated eye; explain use of an eyepatch postoperatively and the resultant loss of vision in that eye until patch is removed; reassure client that a degree of realistic dependency is necessary during healing process (ie, assistance with transportation, dressing)	Will resume previous lifestyle with improved vision
Knowledge deficit related to post-discharge instructions		
Understand temporary decrease in vision postoperatively	Educate about temporary period postoperatively when there will be less than desirable vision in the operative eye; allow client to be active; light reading and TV are ok; instruct client regarding contraindicated activities such as rubbing the eyes, straining at stool, bending over	Will understand and cooperate with visual limitations and contraindicated activities in postoperative period

Client Care Goals	Plan/Nursing Implementation	Expected Outcome
Mobility, impaired physical related to potential discomfort from osteoarthritic joints		
Experience minimal arthritic pain; maintain joint flexibility	Maintain activity patterns to retain flexibility of joints; use passive or active range-of-motion exercises; encourage self-care activities such as eating and bathing self; evaluate use of heat or cold for joint discomfort	Arthritis will not be exacerbated by decreased activity; able to resume full activity without limitation
Adjustment, impaired related to necessity for temporary lifestyle change		
Understand and tolerate the temporary period of inactivity postoperatively	Discuss with client what she is allowed to do, emphasizing activities of daily living; encourage verbalization about frustrations; encourage regular walks in hallways for stimulation; initiate discussion between client and physician regarding resumption of her work and rigorous reading schedule	Will not have change in behavior; remains interested in things around her and does not withdraw; actively plans for discharge and return home
Bowel elimination, altered: constipation related to decreased activity		
Achieve satisfactory nutritional pattern and daily bowel movement	Continue psyllium b.i.d. as is client's regular pattern; encourage 2000–3000 mL of fluids per day; obtain order for a stool softener if client is constipated despite previous measures; evaluate client's normal diet for fibrous foods such as fresh fruits, vegetables, and bran products; encourage regular walks (eg, 20 min walks 2–3 times/day); determine whether a support person is available to share meals and walks	Regular bowel movements without need for straining; states she feels good and has more energy with increase in exercise

UNIT

13

The Client With Integumentary Dysfunction

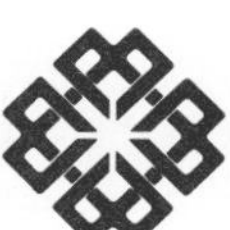

CHAPTER 53

The Integumentary System in Health and Illness

Objectives

When you have finished studying this chapter, you should be able to:

Identify the basic structures that form the integument.

Discuss the major functions of the integument.

Explain the physiologic mechanisms that regulate the activities of the skin.

Identify major factors that influence pathophysiologic alterations of the skin.

Describe general cutaneous effects that result from pathophysiology of the skin.

Link systemic disorders to their cutaneous manifestations.

Describe how psychosocial/lifestyle factors influence pathogenesis of skin disorders.

The integument, or skin, is the largest organ in the body, covering approximately 3000 sq in. of surface area in an average adult. One square inch of skin contains about 20 yards of blood vessels, 100 oil glands, 65 hairs and muscles, 650 sweat glands, and 78 yards of nerves with 19,500 touch nerve endings, 1300 pain nerve endings, 160 pressure nerve endings, 78 heat nerve endings, and 13 cold nerve endings. In all, there are almost 20 million cells of all kinds in one square inch of skin.

Because the skin is vital to the homeostatic balance of the body, it is essential for physical survival. It provides not only a protective barrier to the outside world, but it also, paradoxically, provides a major means of communicating with others and with the environment through touch and sensation. Therefore, the skin is essential not only for physical survival, but for the development of human behavior as well.

SECTION 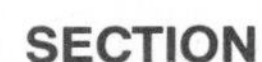

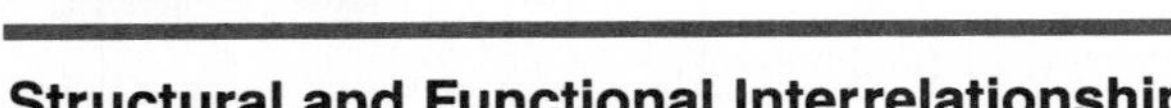

Structural and Functional Interrelationships

Structure of the Integumentary System

Two basic layers make up the integument: the epidermis and dermis. A bed of subcutaneous tissue (the hypodermis), although technically not considered skin, constitutes the innermost segment. These layers, although structurally different, are continuous with the mucous membranes at body openings of the gastrointestinal and genitourinary tracts. The thickness of skin varies; the thinnest layers are on the eyelids, eardrum, and penis, and the thickest are on the palms of the hands and soles of the feet. Hair, nails, and the sebaceous, eccrine, and apocrine glands are classified as cutaneous appendages. These structures are illustrated in Figure 53–1.

Epidermis

The epidermis, the paper-thin outermost cutaneous layer, is composed of epithelial cells, mostly of the type called *keratinocytes.* There are four major zones, the stratum germinativum (the growing layer where the keratinocytes reproduce), stratum granulosum, stratum lucidum, and stratum corneum (the horny layer consisting of dead keratinocytes that are eventually shed). The normal life cycle of epidermal cells lasts about 4 weeks. Any increase or decrease in the rate of keratinocyte production will alter the character of the skin.

The keratinocyte contains a waterproof, hard protein matter called *keratin* that is produced within the cell. Ker-

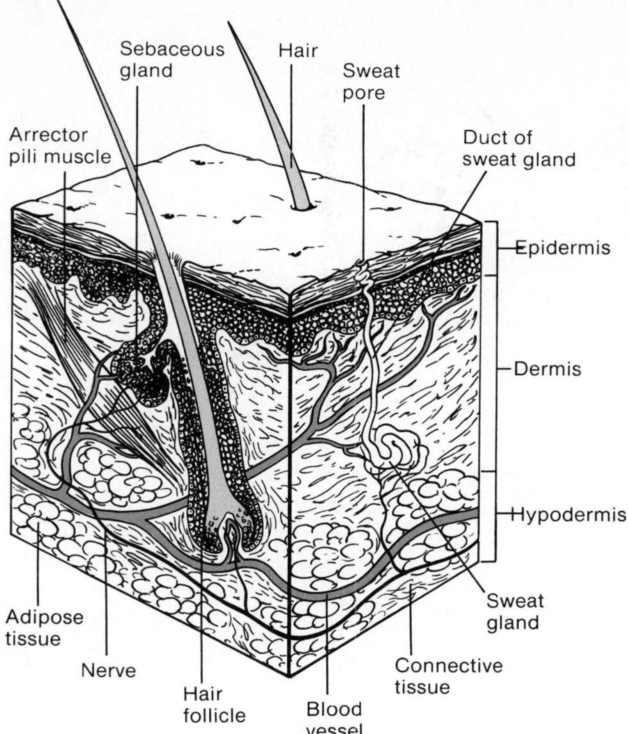

Figure 53–1

The skin and cutaneous appendages. SOURCE: *Adapted from Spence AP, Mason EB:* Human Anatomy and Physiology, *3rd ed. Menlo Park, CA: Benjamin/Cummings, 1987.*

atin is also responsible for the formation of hair and nails. Vitamin A is essential to the keratinizing processes and in the maintenance of normal epithelial structures.

The stratum corneum, through its relative imperviousness, protects the internal milieu. In addition, growth of infectious organisms is retarded by the dryness, constant shedding of the outermost layer of the epidermis, and the presence of an acid pH on most areas of the body except for the axilla, groin, and the skin between the fingers and toes (interdigital spaces).

Dermis

The dermis is denser than the epidermis and is primarily made up of connective tissue. A combination of fibers, water, and a gelatinous substance (collagen) makes it semisolid. The upper area of the dermis, known as the papillary layer, extends into the epidermis by means of projections or folds called *papillae.* Many of these protrusions contain capillary loops that nourish the epidermis, which has no blood vessels of its own. Curving parallel ridges created by these papillae are responsible for the development of fingerprint and footprint patterns within the epidermal layer of the palms and soles. Besides a network of blood vessels, the dermis also contains hair follicles, the glandular appendages, nerves, and lymphatics. These structures extend into the lower layer of the dermis (also called the *reticulum*).

The elasticity and resilience of the skin result from the presence of collagen, elastin, and reticular fibers in the dermis. Collagen is also important in maintaining durability of cutaneous blood vessels, healing of wounds, and increasing resistance to infection. Its formation requires adequate intake of vitamin C.

Subcutaneous Tissue (Hypodermis)

The hypodermis, also known as subcutaneous tissue or subcutis, is the third layer of the integument. This loose connective tissue is made up primarily of fat cells, but it also contains blood vessels, nerves, lymphatics, and protein fibers. The amount of subcutaneous tissue varies; it is absent from eyelids, penis, scrotum, nipple, areola, and the skin over the anterior surface of the tibia. The abundance and distribution of subcutaneous tissue is determined by sex hormones, heredity, age, diet, and disease states. The subcutis stores energy as fat (adipose tissue), which prevents loss of body heat through insulation and protects internal structures by cushioning mechanical shocks.

Hair

Hair covers most of the body surface except for the palms, soles, lips, nipples, and parts of the external genitalia. The millions of hair follicles, tubelike passages from which the hair grows, are formed during fetal development. Each hair is a column of keratinized cells that develops at the base of the follicle where the blood vessels within the papillae provide for circulatory and nutritional needs. The root is the part of the hair that forms in the follicle, and the shaft is the dead part of the hair that protrudes through the skin.

A smooth muscle (the arrector pili) is attached at the base of the follicle. When a stimulus such as cold or fright contracts the muscle, the follicle and hair are brought to an erect position, producing "goose pimples" or "goose flesh."

Hair grows in a cyclic pattern in which each follicle responds independently. Generally, each strand is shed when new growth begins pushing the old hair upward. Rates of hair regeneration on the various body surfaces differ. The scalp is most active.

Hair growth is basically influenced by blood supply and hormones. Excesses and losses of hair may occur at various times during the life cycle, in response to normal alterations in hormonal levels. Systemic illness, emotional stresses, drugs, chronic superficial irritation, cutaneous inflammation and infection, temperature extremes, and starvation may also influence hair growth.

Nails

Fingernails and toenails are formed from the strata corneum and lucidum. They appear as a dense layer of dead flat cells filled with keratin. The stratum germinativum provides an epithelial bed on which the nail plate rests, firmly attached along most of its length by the cuticle or eponychium. Growth is continuous from the nail matrix at the proximal end, also called the *lunula* because of its white crescent moon shape. Normal nails are transparent and durable; the proximity of capillaries accounts for the normal pink coloration. Nails protect the fingers and toes and assist in a variety of utilitarian activities.

Glandular Appendages

All three kinds of glandular appendages—sebaceous, eccrine, and apocrine glands—are formed from epidermal cells during fetal development. They excrete either through a duct that opens directly to the skin surface or into the hair follicle.

The sebaceous (oil) glands are located throughout the entire skin except for the palms of the hands and soles of the feet. They are abundant on the face, scalp, upper chest, and back. The duct of the sebaceous gland joins the hair follicle near the distal end, and the combined structure may be referred to as a *pilosebaceous unit.* The sebaceous gland produces a lipid substance known as **sebum,** which provides some lubrication of hair and epidermis, has an antibacterial–fungistatic action, and retards evaporation from the skin surface.

There are two kinds of sweat glands—eccrine and apocrine glands. Only the eccrine glands participate in heat regulation. Millions of eccrine glands are located over the body with the greatest distribution in the palms of the hands, the soles of the feet, and the forehead.

The apocrine (odoriferous) glands are found most significantly in the axillary, nipple, anal, and pubic areas. Their ducts empty into the upper portion of the hair follicle. These glands do not have a known physiologic role in humans, although water, salts, and organic matter are secreted. The decomposition of the excreta by bacteria on the skin causes body odor.

Skin and Hair Coloring

Melanin is a brown-black pigment that gives color to skin and hair. Melanin-forming cells (melanocytes) are interspersed among the basal cells of the epidermis but are derived from neural rather than epithelial tissue. The amount of pigment production in the melanocytes is regulated by melanocyte-stimulating hormone (MSH) from the anterior pituitary. Dendritic projections on the melanocytes transfer the pigment granules to the keratinocytes. Without melanin, skin looks pink or white depending on the degree of vascularity.

Because all humans have an equal number of melanocytes, it is the amount, size, and distribution of melanin granules produced that determine skin color. Caucasians have the least amount of coloring, with variances in Africans, Asiatics, and Native Americans. Blacks from Africa, New Guinea, and dark-skinned persons from southern India (tropical regions) have a high degree of pigmentation.

Function of the Integumentary System

The major biologic functions in which the skin and its appendages play a role are protection, thermoregulation, and sensory perception. The skin also has a significant role in metabolic activities.

Protection

The skin is the first line of defense against the external environment. It provides a barrier to a variety of noxious agents (including infectious organisms, parasites, radiant energy, and chemical substances) that could be harmful to internal structures and mechanisms. Because of its great durability, pliability, and adaptability, skin can serve as a buffer against trauma from physical objects and mechanical stressors. The waterproof quality of the outer layer of the skin prevents both excess water absorption and abnormal losses of body fluids. It also aids in maintaining a moist internal environment necessary for metabolism. Scalp hair and eyebrows are barriers against sunlight, and nasal hairs and eyelashes filter air.

The purpose of melanin is to protect living cells from damaging ultraviolet radiation. Cellular damage (sunburn, for example) occurs if the body is unable to defend itself against ultraviolet rays by synthesizing more melanin, which acts as a natural sunscreen. In dark-skinned people, protection is inherent. Those individuals who are capable of increasing melanin production will tan with exposure to the sun (see also Chapter 54 and Table 54–5).

Thermoregulation

The intense heat produced during cellular metabolism must be removed from the body's core. Heated blood from the interior flows to the skin, which is cooled by the air, and heat is transferred to the skin cells and from there to the air.

The flow of blood needed to nourish the skin is insignificant compared with the amount needed for thermoregulation. To accommodate this great variance, the skin contains a network of blood vessels that can adjust rapidly to increased or decreased demands. Venous plexuses, which are connected to arterioles by arteriovenous anastomoses, hold large volumes of blood during the cooling process. When heat must be conserved, or when large quantities of blood are needed elsewhere (as for digestion), the arterioles will constrict to allow only a minimum of blood into the veins. In a cold environment, skin and the adipose tissue in its deeper layers insulate the body's core to retain needed heat.

The nervous system controls thermoregulation by controlling blood flow to the skin. Temperature changes are registered in the hypothalamus, which in turn relays responses requiring vasodilation and activation of the sweat glands (for cooling) or vasoconstriction (for heat retention). These responses are mediated through the sympathetic portion of the autonomic nervous system.

Evaporative cooling takes place when the eccrine glands secrete sweat, a hypotonic mixture of water and sodium chloride (salt) with minute amounts of urea, sulfates, and phosphates, into ducts that empty to the surface of the skin. As the sweat evaporates, cooling takes place. Although heat is the primary stimulus for the production of sweat, emotional stress may also trigger increased perspiration.

Sensory Perception

The integument contains several types of receptor cells at various levels in the skin that perceive sensations of pain, pressure, touch, and temperature. Sensory receptors in the skin also play a direct role in the protective function of the skin. For example, the perception of an extreme temperature—dangerously hot or cold—causes an avoidance reaction almost before there is a conscious recognition of the danger. People with sensory receptor deficits (as a result of neurovascular disease, for instance) may fail to perceive the pain of a cut or burn and thus be unable to protect themselves from further damage.

Metabolism

The skin takes part in several metabolic functions. It assists in the regulation of fluids and selected electrolytes by eliminating water and small amounts of sodium chloride through the sweat glands. The amounts excreted are influenced by activity and by ambient temperature (the temperature of the surrounding air). When the kidneys and liver are not working properly, the skin may replace some of their function by excreting nitrogenous wastes and products of metabolism. Also, in the presence of sunlight or ultraviolet radiation, skin begins the process of forming vitamin D (cholecalciferol), a substance needed for absorbing calcium and phosphates from food.

SECTION 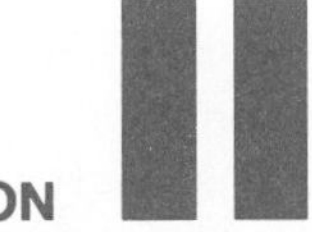

Pathophysiologic Influences and Effects

Few disorders have a single cause; many have several interrelated influences and for some, the cause is still unknown. Generally, the pathophysiology of the skin (or dermatoses) is correlated with one or more of the following factors: genetic and congenital factors, multifactorial or idiopathic causes, immunologic hypersensitivity, infections and infestations, neoplasia, or trauma.

Genetic and Congenital Factors

Factors such as skin color, thickness, hairiness, and glandular activity are all determined primarily by genetic makeup. Children may be born with "birthmarks." These congenital manifestations include any nonspecific localized skin malformation, usually vascular or pigmented. Mongolian spots (bluish spots in the sacral region), hemangiomas, and certain types of nevi (moles) may be evident. Although precursor cells for pigmented lesions may be present at birth, such lesions are more apt to appear with increasing age (usually after puberty). Freckles constitute an inherited type of alteration in pigmentation, even though they generally appear only as a result of sun exposure. Albinism (hypopigmentation) is caused by a genetic defect that prevents synthesis of melanin and results in the absence of color in the skin and hair. Heredity plays an important role in predisposition to the development of acne and atopic dermatitis (allergic tendency), although other factors are also implicated.

Skin loses water content from natural causes such as aging and low humidity (eg, desert air); however, there are people who tend to have chronic dry flaky skin. A child may be born with a condition called *ichthyosis,* which involves excessive scaling or thickening of the outermost layer of the skin. Such problems may continue into puberty and adulthood.

Multifactorial or Idiopathic Causes

Many dermatoses are classified as multifactorial because no outstanding factor can be linked with pathogenesis. A classic example is psoriasis. Although the disorder seems to have a familial tendency, there is no identifiable factor that causes an accelerated rate of cell proliferation. Seborrheic dermatitis (dandruff) is another common condition whose cause is unknown, although it has been associated with constitutional predisposition and with emotional and physical stress. Vitiligo (patches that lack pigment) and chloasma (patches darker than the surrounding skin) involve alterations in skin pigmentation that may be considered idiopathic in origin. Although familial tendency has been correlated with vitiligo, exactly why the skin becomes depigmented remains unknown. Chloasma, on the other hand, has been associated with pregnancy, chronic illness, and Latin American origin.

Immunologic Hypersensitivity

An allergic reaction, localized or general, triggers an inflammatory response. The alterations in the skin include erythema (reddening), rashes, urticaria (hives), and the onset of pruritus (itching) in varying degrees.

The cutaneous manifestations seen in autoimmune disease further illustrate the significance immunity has pathophysiologically. Although the basic reason for the phenomenon is unknown, the body produces antibodies against its own connective tissue. As a result, the skin may atrophy, harden, show changes in vasculature and pigmentation, develop rashes, or become edematous.

Immunity is also linked with the body's defense against cancer. Immune deficiencies have been noted in malignant melanoma.

Infections and Infestations

Infectious agents are responsible for much integumentary pathology. Problems occur when pathologic organisms gain entry beyond the protective epidermis, perhaps through natural openings such as the hair follicles and the eccrine ducts. More often, organisms invade the body through traumatic breaks in the cutaneous tissue (scratches, lacerations, punctures, bites), through areas damaged by excessive moisture, or by septic administration of parenteral substances.

Secondary infections may occur with stasis dermatitis (where impaired circulation damages skin cells of the feet and ankles), atopic dermatitis, or in pressure ulcers and leg ulcers. Skin damaged by any dermatosis, by diminished circulation, or by a disruption to neurologic controls is vulnerable to infection.

Skin may also become a site for clinical manifestations in systemic infections. Communicable diseases, such as measles, chickenpox, scarlet fever, and Hansen's disease (leprosy) produce classic skin symptoms and signs. Sexually transmitted diseases such as syphilis, genital herpes simplex, and condylomata acuminata (venereal warts) also present characteristic cutaneous lesions.

Infestations involve attacks on the skin by parasitic organisms, which are classified as protozoans, helminthoids (worms), and arthropods. The most common dermatoses involve bites by arthropods. Arachnids such as spiders, scorpions, ticks, and mites represent one group; insects such as lice, bedbugs, fleas, flies, mosquitoes, and bees are the other.

Neoplasia

Benign or malignant neoplasms may develop from every type of cell in the various layers and structures of the skin, but keratinocytes and melanocytes are the most frequently involved. Skin cysts are a form of abnormal mass, although most are not technically neoplasia. The growth usually contains some fluid or solid material (or both) and can occur for several reasons. Some are congenital; others arise from obstruction of the pilosebaceous duct.

Seborrheic keratosis, a hyperplastic epidermal lesion, is a common benign skin condition seen in middle-aged and other adults. Another type of benign tumor is the nevus or mole—a common malformation often considered a birthmark.

Several epidermal lesions are considered precancerous and require regular examination to detect malignant changes. They include senile keratoses, actinic keratoses, and arsenical keratoses. **Leukoplakia** (white plaques seen on mucous membranes) are also considered precancerous lesions.

Trauma

Physical injury to the skin is an ever-present hazard. Superficial lacerations, contusions, abrasions, and punctures occur frequently in accidents at home, in the streets, or at the workplace. Keloid formation and hypertrophic scarring involve excessive collagen formation after cutaneous injury. Exposure to extremes of temperature can cause injury; extensive burns or frostbite can cause loss of life or a limb. Everyday mechanical pressures or chronic irritation provokes the development of localized thickening of skin, or **lichenification.** Corns and calluses are good examples of the skin's attempt to adapt to these irritations.

A frequent cause of trauma to the skin is scratching to alleviate the discomfort of pruritus. Although scratching and rubbing of the irritated areas are defensive actions, too much can traumatize the protective layers of skin.

SECTION 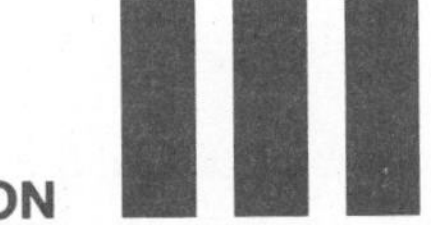

Related System Influences and Effects

Although the skin is not usually thought to be essential to life, without it, death would occur. Like other organ systems, however, the skin depends on proper functioning of the endocrine system, the heart and blood vessels, lungs, kidneys, and gastrointestinal tract.

Endocrine System

At puberty, hormonal changes trigger secretions from the apocrine glands, causing the redistribution of body fat and the development of axillary and pubic hair, and, in men, the development of chest, facial, and body hair. In addition, hormones stimulate secretion by the sebaceous glands, and the apocrine glands. Acne vulgaris, a common disorder in adolescence that may extend into adulthood, is related to the production of sebum. Testosterone decreases growth of hair on the scalp and may be responsible for some forms of alopecia in men. Estrogens, in turn, cause skin to become more vascular.

Pregnancy involves glandular activities that primarily result in the alteration of pigmentation, such as the presence of striae on the body (depressed atrophic stripes), the appearance of chloasma in a characteristic pattern called *pregnancy mask,* color changes to the vulva and nipples, and prominence of freckling and nevi. Pruritus is a fairly common discomfort, possibly resulting from excretion by cutaneous glands. **Hypertrichosis** (excess hair) may occur but in many cases disappears following delivery.

Menopausal changes involve the skin as a target area. Women experience "hot flashes," which entail cutaneous vasodilation and profuse perspiration. Alterations in hair growth and distribution (growth of facial hair) may also cause problems.

Endocrine system disorders such as Addison's disease, Cushing's syndrome, acromegaly, and hyper- and hypopituitarism cause significant changes in skin pigmentation and texture and in the amount and distribution of hair and subcutaneous tissue.

Cardiovascular and Respiratory Systems

Cardiovascular disorders often cause skin changes. For example, clients with peripheral vascular disease frequently have changes in the extremities including pallor, dependent rubor, cyanosis, dry scaly skin, cellulitis, ulcerations, and brittle toenails. Gangrene can be a long-term complication of peripheral vascular disease. Clients with chronic obstructive pulmonary disease or congestive heart failure are often cyanotic and have clubbing of the fingers. Blood dyscrasias often cause skin signs such as petechiae, ecchymosis, and pallor. Alopecia, skin eruptions, and pruritus are seen in some lymphomas.

Urinary System

Dysfunction in the urinary system may affect the integument in a number of ways. For example, chronic renal failure may result in pruritus, uremic frost, pallor, or a yellow cast to the skin.

Gastrointestinal and Hepatic–Biliary Systems

Clients who are malnourished may experience loss of subcutaneous tissue, alopecia, hyperkeratosis, or purpura. Persons who ingest excessively large amounts of vitamin A may have an orange color to the skin; this carotene pigmentation is the result of carotene toxicity. Biliary tract disease often causes jaundice, pruritus, and spider hemangiomas.

Musculoskeletal System

Connective tissue disorders may alter the appearance and function of the integument. For example, systemic lupus erythematosus has a characteristic butterfly-shaped rash on the face and causes small ulcerations of the fingertips. Scleroderma causes a leathery hardening of the skin. A joint disorder—rheumatoid arthritis—often coexists with psoriasis.

SECTION 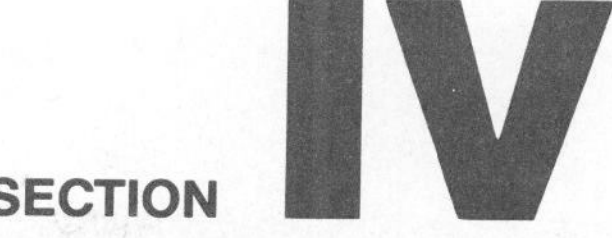

Psychosocial Influences and Effects

Skin disorders that can be attributed solely to psychologic or social causes are rare. However, many conditions show a correlation between emotional stress and the onset of exacerbation of the dermatosis; the skin may become the primary target.

Skin plays a significant role in the communication of feelings. The cutaneous blood vessels are affected by the emotional states of an individual, as are some of the glandular appendages. Fear may cause blanching, anger or embarrassment may produce a red face, and anxiety or stress may increase perspiration. Emotions can alter hormone production and circulation, which, in turn, can alter integumentary processes.

Some of the more common dermatoses known to be influenced by psychologic considerations include atopic dermatitis (eczema), alopecia areata, urticaria, and psoriasis. Flare-ups of atopic dermatitis are known to occur with emotional stress. Alopecia areata, in which loss of hair occurs suddenly, often follows a traumatic event, such as the death of a significant person. The onset or exacerbation of psoriasis is frequently preceded by some form of stressful or anxiety-producing situation.

Sex and Age

The aging process results in multiple effects to the skin for both men and women. Generally, there is an overall decrease in tissue mass, which results in a thinner, more transparent skin. Loss of collagen and adipose tissue results in sagging and wrinkling. As total body water decreases, skin becomes dry and scaly. Color changes and keratotic, vascular, and pigmented lesions appear with greater frequency. Increased fragility of blood vessels allows for easy bruising. Sluggish circulation leads to improper nourishment of the living portion of the integument. Finally, for a number of reasons (including all of the above plus, in many cases, years of chronic irritation), the elderly are predisposed to malignancies of the skin.

Developmental Factors

Tactile stimulation is the first means of communication. The physical closeness of mother and infant and the emotional messages that are relayed by touch through caressing, cuddling, holding, and stroking influence adult life as well as childhood.

Skin disorders that begin in infancy can influence personality development. Infantile forms of eczema can affect

Nursing Research Note

Randolph GL: Therapeutic and physical touch: Physiological response to stressful stimuli. *Nurs Res* 1984; 33(1):33–35.

Physiologic differences between groups reacting to stressful stimuli when treated by either therapeutic touch or physical touch were investigated. Physiologic responses measured included skin conduction, muscle tension, and peripheral skin temperatures. Physical touch consisted of placing one's hands on the subject's abdomen and lower back. Therapeutic touch consisted of the practitioner entering a meditative state, concentrating on the subject, and placing hands on the abdomen and back to transfer energy. Sixty healthy college female students were used in the sample. They viewed a stressful film and during the viewing received either therapeutic or physical touch.

There was no significant difference in the psychophysiologic measures between the groups. Both groups exhibited significant stress response to the film. Although therapeutic touch has received support in other research, this study failed to demonstrate its effectiveness in reducing stress. Additional research is needed on the effectiveness of therapeutic touch in stress reduction.

mother-child interactions and subsequent tactile communication. Disturbances in intimacy and self-image can be initiated in infancy that form barriers to normal adaptive processes in later life.

Dietary Habits

There are no known foods that cause or cure specific skin disorders. At one time, diet was considered relevant in the development of acne. Foods such as chocolate, nuts, cola, whole milk products, fatty meats, and spicy foods were to be avoided. Although these foods do not cause acne, their overconsumption by adolescents remains a general nutritional concern.

Poor nutrition, whether for economic or other reasons, may alter skin integrity. Nutritional deficiencies cause dryness, scaliness, inelasticity, decreased skin and hair pigmentation, edema, pallor, and dermatoses. Also, loss of subcutaneous tissue interferes with the protective and thermoregulatory functions of the skin. Xanthomas, yellow to brown skin deposits that are high in lipid content, are found on the eyelids in persons with hyperlipidemia, a condition associated with cardiovascular disease, or nutritional problems.

Of major concern is excessive intake of vitamin A. Excess vitamin A, besides being detrimental to the liver and to bone, causes such problems as dry, fissured skin; rashes; brittle nails; hair loss; and lip inflammation (cheilosis).

Climate

Exposure to excessive sun or humidity can influence the condition of the skin. For example, prickly heat or *miliaria,* a condition that involves blockage of sweat glands, is associated with hot and humid weather, as are cutaneous fungal infections. Premature aging, vitiligo, actinic keratosis, and skin malignancies all increase in body areas that have been exposed to a great deal of sunlight. Persons who live in geographic areas where the sun is strong are at increased risk for these skin disorders.

Sunlight has been considered therapeutic for some skin lesions but is known to aggravate psoriasis, herpes simplex, and atopic dermatitis. Protection must be given to persons with systemic illnesses who may develop photodermatoses. Adverse skin reactions may occur in persons with lupus erythematosus, scleroderma, pellagra, phenylketonuria, hypopituitarism, and albinism.

Some drugs can cause photosensitivity (increased redness on exposure to the sun, which can result in severe sunburn). The most common drugs involved are demeclocycline (Declomycin), doxycycline (Vibramycin), chlorpromazine (Thorazine), hydrochlorothiazide (HydroDIURIL), tolbutamide (Orinase), and nalidixic acid (NegGram). Oral contraceptives may also cause photosensitivity.

Body Image

Skin disorders that cause disfigurement alter the body image as well as one's self-view. The presence of extensive cutaneous lesions, particularly when inflammation or infection is obvious, may arouse fears of contagion in others. Rejection of a person for this reason, or because his or her appearance is repulsive, adds to the emotional stress and feelings of low self-worth the client may feel. In turn, the physiologic problem can be further compounded by the use of cosmetics intended to hide blemishes as the client attempts to present a more attractive appearance.

People whose sense of self-worth depends heavily on physical attractiveness often have great difficulty dealing with age-related alterations in appearance. When cosmetics fail to hide the natural changes, elective cosmetic surgery may be used to remove excess skin (sags or wrinkles) or to modify some body change (eg, sagging breasts).

Economic Factors

The poor may be exposed to skin problems as a result of unsanitary or crowded living conditions, unsafe heating (burns from open fires or unshielded portable heaters), community swimming pools where contagion may be a risk, and complications resulting from lack of (or inadequate) treatment. It would be an error to assume that skin disorders have economic boundaries, however. Outbreaks of infections and infestations may occur within any school or community.

Occupation and Avocation

Dermatologic problems have great significance in occupational health. They are the most frequently reported work-related disorders; 90% are the result of contact with substances causing inflammatory dermatitis. For instance, hand dermatitis is quite common among beauticians, photographers, and furniture refinishers. In addition, folliculitis, acne, pigment changes, neoplasms, ulcerations, and granulomas have been identified as occupationally related. Chronic exposure to sunlight has increased the incidence of skin malignancies in farmers, fishermen, and sailors. Insecticide makers, spray-rig operators, oil refinery workers, and smelter employees who work with arsenic face similar risks. Some of these same substances are used in the pursuit of leisure activities and may cause skin problems. Clients may need to limit, or even to give up, treasured leisure activities.

Some persons may lose jobs as a result of a dermatologic condition. Fellow workers may fear "catching" an illness; employers may be reluctant for the employee to have contact with the public. An employer may also be reluctant to retain an employee whose disorder is occupationally induced.

Sexual Expression

The skin plays an important role in how people express their sexuality since sexual arousal is facilitated by tactile stimulation of the skin's erogenous zones. In addition, insecurities and uncertainties about sexuality and sexual activity may be amplified by feelings of unattractiveness because of skin lesions. Contact with the skin may trigger unpleasant feelings in either partner. Even the anticipation that unpleasant feelings may be triggered can sometimes be reason enough to avoid sexual activity.

Roles and Relationships

One's interpersonal world is also strongly influenced by integumentary problems. For example, fear of being rejected by others may make it difficult to participate in usual socializing activities. Some conditions or symptoms (eg, severe pruritus) may actually interfere with or prevent a person from carrying out usual familial or social roles.

The development of chronic skin disorders whose treatment is exacting and unending may result in depression. Some individuals may withdraw, completely insulate and isolate themselves, or even consider suicide. Finally, fear, anxiety, anger, hostility, guilt, depression, loneliness, and denial may all accompany even a relatively mild skin disorder.

Chapter Highlights

The integument has a vital role in maintaining homeostasis.

The integument is composed of three distinct layers of skin, the dermis, epidermis, and subcutaneous tissue, and contains the cornified (hair and nails) and glandular (sebaceous, eccrine, and apocrine) appendages.

Skin is the first line of defense against noxious agents from the external environment and is also a key organ in thermoregulation, sensory perception, and metabolism.

General health and emotional state may be reflected in cutaneous manifestations.

In addition to primary disorders of the integument, cutaneous manifestations occur with systemic illness.

The cause-and-effect relationship of skin disorders must be viewed holistically because of the interactions and interrelations between physiologic and psychosocial/lifestyle factors.

The skin is often the primary target when the client is under emotional stress.

Normal alterations in skin and the appendages occur at significant times within the human life cycle.

Climate and occupation influence the condition of the skin.

Alteration in appearance of the skin has significant influence on body image and self-esteem.

Bibliography

Green ML, Harry J: *Nutrition in Contemporary Nursing Practice.* New York: Wiley, 1981.

Groër MW, Shekleton ME: *Basic Pathophysiology: A Conceptual Approach,* 2nd ed. St. Louis: Mosby, 1983.

Guyton AC: *Basic Human Physiology: Normal Functions and Mechanisms of Disease,* 3rd ed. Philadelphia: Saunders, 1981.

Larrabee, WF: The aging face: Why changes occur, how to correct them. *Postgrad Med* (Nov 15) 1984; 76:37–46.

Levy BS, Wegman DH: Environmental and occupational hazards. Pages 124–155 in: *Practice of Preventive Health Care.* Schneiderman LJ (editor). Menlo Park, CA: Addison–Wesley, 1981.

Luciano DS, Vander AJ, Sherman JH: *Human Anatomy and Physiology.* New York: McGraw–Hill, 1983.

Melamed E: *The Terror of Not Being Young.* New York: Linden Press/Simon & Schuster, 1983.

Montagu A: *Touching: The Human Significance of the Skin,* 2nd ed. New York: Harper & Row, 1978.

Muir BL: *Pathophysiology—An Introduction to the Mechanisms of Disease.* New York: Wiley, 1980.

Pillsbury DM, Heston CL: *A Manual of Dermatology,* 2nd ed. Philadelphia: Saunders, 1980.

Sauer GC: *Manual of Skin Diseases,* 4th ed. Philadelphia: Lippincott, 1980.

Spence AP, Mason EB: *Human Anatomy and Physiology,* 3rd ed. Menlo Park, CA: Benjamin/Cummings, 1987.

Wilson HS, Kneisl CR: *Psychiatric Nursing,* 3rd ed. Menlo Park, CA: Addison–Wesley, 1988.

CHAPTER **54**

The Nursing Process for Clients With Integumentary Dysfunction

Other topics related to this content are: Dermatologic and plastic and reconstructive surgery, **Chapter 55;** Phototherapy, including PUVA, **Chapter 55;** Skin disorders, **Chapter 55.**

Objectives

When you have finished studying this chapter, you should be able to:

Specify the major components of the health history to be obtained from clients with integumentary dysfunction.

Explain specific assessment approaches in evaluating clients with cutaneous lesions.

Identify the nursing implications of diagnostic studies commonly used to evaluate clients with integumentary dysfunction.

Determine appropriate nursing diagnoses for clients with disorders of the integument.

Develop, with the client, realistic goals of care.

Anticipate the psychosocial/lifestyle implications of integumentary dysfunction for clients and their significant others.

Develop a nursing care plan for a client with integumentary dysfunction.

Implement nursing interventions specific to clients with disease of the integument.

Evaluate the effectiveness of the nursing care plan and modify it as necessary to meet client needs.

The many types and complex causes of skin disorders require that the nurse use a thorough, systematic approach in assessing the client and developing the plan of care. Nurses must remember that the quality of their verbal and nonverbal communication skills with clients who may have disfiguring skin lesions is important in facilitating therapeutic nurse–client relationships.

SECTION 

Nursing Assessment: Establishing the Data Base

Subjective Data

The purpose of the interview is not only to obtain a dermatologic history, but to gather the total health picture. The nurse needs to know biographic data, the client's specific and general concerns, how the client sees the lesion or cutaneous manifestations, and how the client thinks the condition came about.

The client's age, sex, race, occupation, and environment (including climate) may be significant in assessing the problem and expediting the diagnosis. Information about lifestyle, recent travel, economic status, and living conditions may be helpful.

When questioning the client about the actual skin disorder, it is important to elicit the following information:

- The data of onset and duration of the problem
- The initial site of occurrence and progressive involvement of other areas
- Nature of the distribution of the cutaneous signs
- Skin texture, temperature, odor, drainage, and oil and water content
- Any change in cutaneous sensation (numbness, tingling, pruritus)
- Changes in color
- Specific alterations in hair texture, amount, color, distribution, and presence of dandruff
- Specific alterations in nail texture, color, and contour

- Factors that seem to aggravate or alleviate the problem
- Treatment prior to visit

Use terms or phrases that may be easily understood and helpful in facilitating descriptions. Accurate information is beneficial in identifying specific disorders that have characteristic onsets, locations, or symptomatology.

The dermatologic history must include an investigation into the following areas:

- Family or personal history involving allergic tendencies (hay fever, asthma, atopic dermatitis)
- Personal history of x-ray treatment for acne
- Family history of skin disorders
- Personal history of childhood diseases (measles, chickenpox, scarlet fever)
- Exposure to external allergens (soaps, deodorants, jewelry, metal, cosmetics, clothing, furs)
- Exposure to internal allergens (foods)
- Current medications, whether prescription drugs or over-the-counter preparations
- Occupational exposure to irritants or toxic substances
- Exposure to environmental factors, such as temperature extremes, excessive sunlight, or high humidity
- Seasonal influence on the condition
- Recent contact with animals, insects, or plants
- Involvement in out-of-door activities
- Menstrual history and sexual contacts
- Dietary and hygienic practices
- Alcohol or drug use
- Use of public swimming pools, restrooms, gym showers, or other facilities
- Recent travel
- Recent psychosocial stress

Information from client responses in these areas of concern will help to identify etiologic factors, appropriate treatment modalities, and preventive measures.

No history will be complete unless possible systemic influences are evaluated. Ask about general symptoms such as fatigue, anorexia, nausea and vomiting, weakness, weight loss, headache, fever, and chills. Also ask about the client's overall health with specific focus on each organ system.

Objective Data

Physical Assessment

Inspection and palpation are key in the next phase of data gathering. The sun provides the best light in which to view the skin, hair, and nails. Lamps containing 60-watt nonfluorescent bulbs are the recommended alternative. Oblique lighting in a darkened room may be used to determine subtle elevations or depressions. Variations in skin pigmentation may be seen better in subdued light.

Very dark skin may conceal certain skin problems. Nurses must learn to recognize the natural blend of pigmentation in various types of healthy skin and to examine the buccal mucosa, tongue, lips, nail beds, and sclera to supplement skin information.

The examining room should have a comfortable temperature to prevent both vasodilation and vasoconstriction that might affect the appearance of the skin. A relaxed supportive atmosphere is important to prevent errors such as mistaking an embarrassed blush for erythema.

After proper draping, begin the physical examination by viewing the overall appearance of the client to evaluate general health. Manifestations of systemic involvement should be recorded (such as yellowing that may indicate jaundice).

The examination is then conducted in a set sequence of careful inspection and palpation of all visible components of the integument. Beginning with the hair and scalp, progress from the head and neck to the upper extremities. Note the condition of the oral mucous membrane. If the client has a history of x-ray treatment for acne, palpate the thyroid. Move to the trunk and the lower extremities.

SKIN The skin should be assessed for color, temperature, texture, turgor, and the presence of edema. Then note the type, shape, arrangement, and distribution of lesions. It is important to be exact in the observations and to use the correct terms in recording the observations (see Tables 54–1 and 54–2). It will not be possible later to assess the progress of therapy without a clear and exact record of the initial condition.

COLOR Skin color is affected by pigmentation (melanin, carotene, hemoglobin) and vascularization. Alterations may be localized or general. Depending on the pathogenesis involved, more definite information can often be obtained by looking at the conjunctiva, the palms of the hands, the soles of the feet, the nail beds, and the lips. For example, the pallor of anemia in black clients is more readily visible in the conjunctiva.

Color may be *isochromatic* (uniform) or *versicolored* (a combination of shades). Observations may be documented by notation of the exact colors seen (pallor, rubor, cyanosis).

TEMPERATURE Warmth and coolness of the skin normally reflect adjustments in the circulatory system as it provides for thermoregulation in the body. Touch the skin so relative heat can be sensed by the fingertips. Localized heat may indicate the presence of an inflammatory process, whereas generalized hyperthermia reflects systemic involvement.

TEXTURE AND TURGOR To assess skin texture and turgor, gently grasp a small section of skin and evaluate it, then record the findings using the following terms:

- Consistency—May be smooth, rough, scaly, crusty, thin, thick, atrophied, firm, wrinkled, or nodular
- Accommodation—May be resilient, inelastic, pliable; may show increased or decreased tension
- Moisture and oil—May be dry, oily, moist, or weeping

Table 54–1
Primary Skin Lesions

Lesions	Characteristics	Examples	Illustrations
Macule	Small; circumscribed; less than 1 cm in diameter; flat; nonpalpable; brown, red, purple, white, or tan	Ephelis (freckling); purpura; rubeola; rubella; scarlet fever; lentigo; Mongolian and cafe-au-lait spots	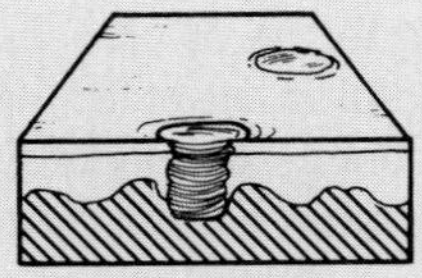
Papule	Circumscribed; elevated; less than 1 cm in diameter; palpable; firm; red, brown, pink, tan, or bluish-red	Mole; acne; pimple; angioma; wart; pityriasis rosea; actinic and seborrheic keratosis	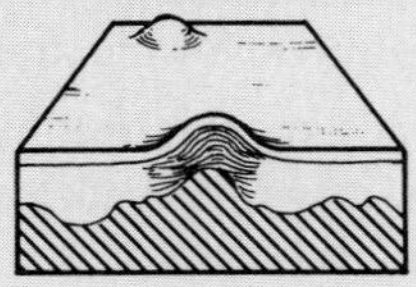
Vesicle	Superficial; circumscribed; less than 1 cm in diameter; elevated; filled with clear fluid	Blister; chicken pox; smallpox; herpes; poison ivy; contact and atopic dermatitis; insect bites	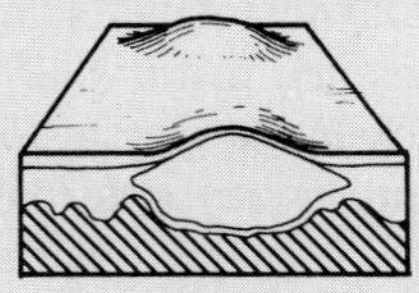
Bulla	Similar to vesicle but larger than 1 cm in diameter	Blister with second-degree burn; pemphigus vulgaris; drug eruptions	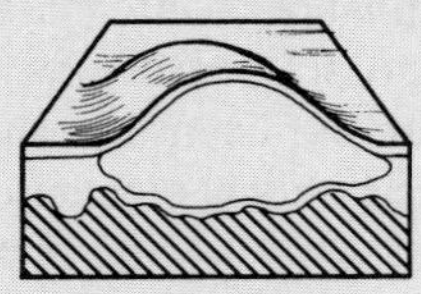
Pustule	Similar to vesicle and bullae but filled with pus; white or yellowish-cream	Acne; furuncle; variola; miliaria; impetigo; folliculitis	See vesicle (above)
Wheal	Flat-topped; elevated; variable diameter; irregular shape	Urticaria; insect bites; poison ivy	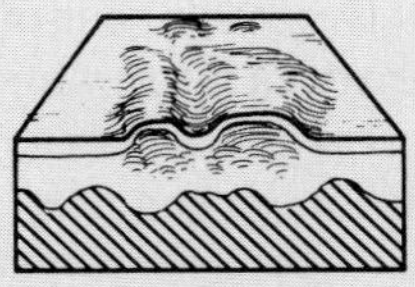
Nodule	Circumscribed; elevated; 1–2 cm in diameter; firm; deeper in dermis than papule	Tophi; Heberden's nodes; erythema nodosum; ganglion; dermatofibroma; acne	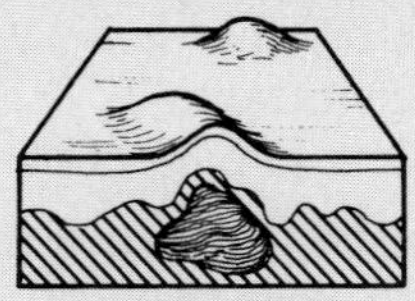
Tumor	Elevated; solid; greater than 2 cm in diameter; may or may not be clearly demarcated; may or may not vary from skin color	Epithelioma; fibroma; lipoma; cavernous hemangioma; melanoma	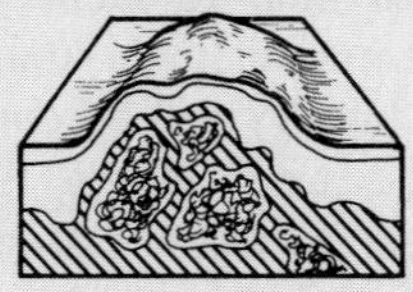
Patch	Flat; larger than 1 cm in diameter; irregular in shape	Vitiligo	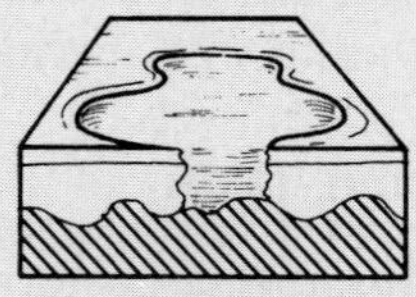
Plaque	Elevated; flat-topped; firm; rough; over 1 cm in diameter; may be coalesced papules	Psoriasis; seborrheic warts; discoid lupus erythematosus	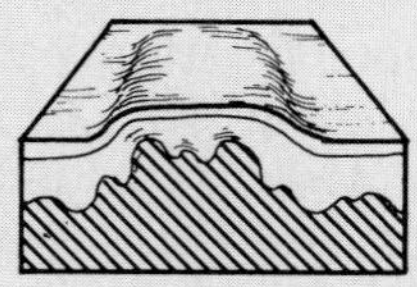
Cyst	Elevated, encapsulated mass in dermis or subcutaneous layer; fluid, semifluid, or solid content; may or may not appear raised	Epidermoid; sebaceous	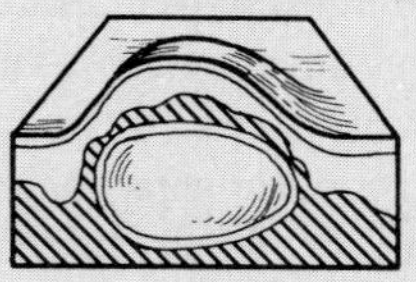

Table 54–2
Secondary Skin Lesions

Lesions	Characteristics	Examples	Illustrations
Crust	Slightly elevated areas of dried blood, pus, serum; size varies; color may be straw, tan, honey, brown, red, or black	Impetigo; eczema; scab on abrasion or laceration	
Scale	Irregular; dry or oily; thick or thin; flaky exfoliation; varied size; white, tan, or silver	Dandruff; psoriasis; exfoliative dermatitis	
Lichenification	Rough, thickened, hardened epidermis; increased skin markings due to chronic rubbing or irritation; not as clearly demarcated as a plaque	Chronic dermatitis	
Excoriation	Loss of epidermis; exposed dermis	Scratches; linear abrasions	
Fissure	Linear crack or break exposing dermis; small; deep; red	Athlete's foot; dishpan hands; cheilosis	
Erosion	Depressed; moist; glistening break in superficial epidermis; circumscribed; red; follows rupture of vesicle or bulla; larger than fissure	Smallpox; chicken pox; diaper dermatitis	
Ulcer	Depressed; involves total epidermis and all or part of dermis, may involve subcutaneous tissue; concave; varies in size; exudative; red or reddish-blue	Decubiti; stasis ulcers; third-degree burns; chancre	
Scar (cicatrix)	Thin line to thick irregular fibrous tissue; pink, red, or white	Healed wound or surgical incision	
Atrophy	Thin; shiny; translucent; paper-like; skin furrows obliterated	Striae; arterial insufficiency; aging skin	

EDEMA Increased fluid content may extend beyond the dermal levels into the subcutaneous tissue. Edema may be determined by looking and palpating to determine the extent or the degree of involvement. Record the presence and location of edema and use terms such as taut, tight, puffy, indented, or pitting to describe it further. Pitting edema is described according to stages in Chapter 5.

TYPE OF LESION The types of primary and secondary skin lesions that appear with disorders of the integument or disorders associated with systemic diseases are shown in Tables 54–1 and 54–2. The tables also describe characteristic features and provide examples of conditions in which the lesions are known to appear. Primary lesions represent the basic cutaneous responses to pathophysiologic influences or stressors. Secondary alterations develop from the initial manifestation.

After examining the lesions, record surface conformity, texture, mobility, presence of altered sensation (tenderness, pruritus), and depth of involvement. The skin must also be assessed for vascular lesions such as petechiae, purpura, ecchymoses, and telangiectasis. Any of these signs may aid in diagnosing disorders remote from the skin.

SHAPE OF LESION Configurations of individualized lesions should be described whenever feasible. Appropriate terms include round, oval, annular (ring shaped), elongated (tubular), or irregular. The lesions may also have sharp or diffuse (spreading) borders.

ARRANGEMENT The pattern of surface lesions should be recorded because it is of use in making the diagnosis. For example, in herpes simplex, the lesions appear in clusters, whereas in herpes zoster, they are linear and run along the course of a cutaneous nerve. Lesions may appear grouped, confluent (merging together), contiguous (touching or adjoining), disseminated (scattered), or symmetrical. Particular arrangements may be further described as being linear, serpiginous (snakelike), reticular (a network formation), or arcuate (arching).

DISTRIBUTION The extensiveness and location of the lesions are significant. The area of involvement should be classified as being isolated, localized, regional, or generalized. The nurse should learn characteristic distributions for common disorders and examine the sites accordingly. Certain problems may involve normally exposed skin, pressure points, or common sites on the body.

HAIR AND NAILS Hair should be examined for color and for dullness or sheen. Feel the hair to determine whether it is dry or oily, rough or soft, fine or coarse. A strand should be checked for brittleness or pliability. The distribution and amount should be evaluated in terms of the age and sex of the client.

The general appearance of the nails can show physiologic changes or disruptions and sometimes emotional stress, as when the nails have been bitten. The shape of nails may be altered from a normal convexity to a spoonlike or concave appearance, or clubbing may occur. Transverse furrows, called Beau's line, may appear as a result of a variety of cutaneous or systemic problems. Onycholysis, separation of the nail plate from the bed, is a common disturbance. The transparency of the plate may be impaired (stained or discolored). This transparent quality makes the nail bed ideal for assessing capillary filling and, ultimately, the adequacy of circulation to the distal portions of the extremities. The substance of the nail should be observed for bulk (thinness or thickness), smoothness, irregularities or pitting of the surface, and for flexibility or brittleness.

Diagnostic Studies

DIRECT EXAMINATION The use of a magnified hand lens is helpful in examining small lesions. A Wood's lamp may be used to determine the presence of fungal infections, which show a characteristic yellow–green fluorescence under black light. This ultraviolet long-wave light is also useful in identifying some bacterial infections and aids in the delineation of pigment disorders.

SKIN TESTING Skin tests are used to determine hypersensitivity and immune responses by the administration of allergens or antigens on the surface or into the dermis. The three types include patch, scratch, and intradermal tests.

Patch testing provides an accurate means for assessing contact sensitivity. One or more suspected allergens is placed on a hairless area of the body (often the skin of the forearm), one allergen per patch, and covered with an adhesive tape or patch-test dressing for 48 to 72 hours. During this time, the site must be kept dry. A positive reaction is shown by the appearance of redness, papules, vesicles, or edema.

Allergens may be introduced into the body through a superficial abrasion or intradermal injection. In the *scratch* test, a needle or special tool is used to scratch the skin. Scratches, 1 cm long and 2.5 cm apart, are made in rows on the client's forearm or back. Within 30 to 40 minutes after introduction of the allergen, the area is assessed for erythema, edema, or both.

Intradermal tests are usually performed to evaluate immunity from prior exposure or sensitization. Several antigens that may have relevance to the integumentary system include tuberculin, blastomycin, and coccidioidin. After inoculation with a tuberculin syringe into the layers of the skin, the reading takes place within 48 to 72 hours. Positive reactions will show signs of induration, or erythema, or both.

MICROSCOPIC EXAMINATION OF TISSUE OR A CULTURE The microscopic study of tissue or a culture allows a more decisive diagnosis to be reached. Bacteria, yeast, fungus, spirochetes, parasites, and many viruses can be recognized under a microscope. (For some viruses, an electron microscope is needed.)

Specimens for microscope study are obtained through several means. Scales, crusts, and exudate can be taken by gentle scraping. Smears can be taken of weeping lesions and are useful in diagnosing bullous diseases and vesicular eruptions. Gram's stains, potassium hydroxide (KOH) test, dark-field examinations, immunofluorescence, and various other preparations and methods may be used to facilitate microscopic visualization.

SKIN BIOPSY Skin biopsy is a valuable tool in diagnosis. Several methods of acquiring histologic samples are available. A *punch biopsy* usually provides sufficient tissue for examination and is a simple procedure to perform. The physician selects the area that is expected to be most informative, cleanses it gently, and administers a local anesthetic. A skin punch instrument specific for this type of biopsy can provide a 2 to 8 mm sample of tissue when it is pressed firmly into the lesion. Wound care following the biopsy may involve no more than a simple dressing, although suturing or application of adhesive strips may be necessary if a large sample is taken. Use of caustics or Gelfoam is not usually required.

A *shave biopsy* involves using a scalpel to remove the elevated part of a lesion. A biopsy sample may have to be scooped out from a flat or depressed area. A pedunculated lesion may be clipped off with scissors, as may a small fold of skin where the cosmetic appearance will not be disturbed. The use of pressure, caustics, or light electrosurgery may be necessary to stop bleeding after any of these procedures.

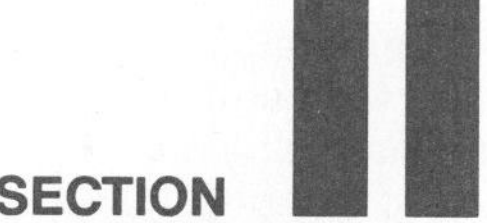

SECTION II

Nursing Diagnosis/Planning and Implementation/Evaluation

Information gathered from the client's health history, physical examination, and diagnostic studies is used to determine nursing diagnoses and the plan of care. Not every client will have the same needs. The Nursing Diagnoses box lists diagnoses **directly related** to integumentary dysfunction along with **potential** nursing diagnoses for clients with integumentary problems. The most common nursing diagnoses for clients with integument disorders include altered comfort, impaired skin integrity, potential for infection, knowledge deficit, and disturbance in self-concept: body image. The sample nursing care plan in Table 54–3 focuses on potential for infection, knowledge deficit, and disturbance in self-concept: body image. Altered comfort, impaired skin integrity, and potential for injury related to sun exposure are discussed in the narrative.

If the goals of care have not been met, re-evaluation is required. The nurse and client should jointly review the nursing care plan. New objectives may need to be formulated; other nursing interventions may be added or modified; or the evaluation may show that more time is required to meet the objectives.

Comfort, Altered

Pruritus is the most common problem of clients with dermatologic problems. Itching seems to demand scratching. Unfortunately, "one scratch is too many, and a thousand is not enough." An itch–scratch cycle can develop that damages the skin further and may lead to infection.

Planning and Implementation

Care of the client with pruritus should involve hydration of the skin by a cooling bath or use of compresses. The addition of antipruritic colloids such as oatmeal (Aveeno) or starches and use of bath oils are helpful when large body surfaces are involved. Keeping the skin relatively dry and cool is essential and usually requires climate and humidity controls. The application of local soothing emollients containing camphor, menthol, phenol, salicylic acid, or tars, alone or in combinations, may be prescribed (including some over-the-counter drugs). Topical anesthetics and antihistamines have not proven of value, although systemic antihistamines have some limited utility with histamine-mediated itching. (These drugs may also cause allergic responses that produce itching). Topical corticosteroids are effective, but long-term use may result in cutaneous side effects and adrenal suppression. Tranquilizers and sedatives may be prescribed when emotional disruptions accompany pruritus or when sleep patterns are disturbed. For most clients with pruritus, itching becomes more intense at night.

A major focus of care in treating severe pruritus is the avoidance of unnecessary stimulation from chemical agents that act as irritants or vasodilators (alcohol, coffee, spices); mechanical objects (rough clothing, long fingernails); heat; and psychic stress. The nurse should become aware of all factors that increase or stimulate discomfort and those that lessen or alleviate it. Diversion (reading, watching TV) should be actively explored.

Evaluation

Expected client outcomes following effective nursing interventions for alteration in comfort due to pruritus include observation and reports that the client is not itching, is comfortable, and is able to sleep. The client's skin is observed to be less dry, without excessive moisture. The client reports avoidance of situations that increase itching and appropriate use of any prescribed medications.

NURSING DIAGNOSES IN
Integumentary Dysfunction

DIRECTLY RELATED DIAGNOSES

- Comfort, altered: pruritus
- Infection, potential for
- Injury, potential for
- Knowledge deficit
- Self-concept, disturbance: body image
- Skin integrity, impaired: actual

OTHER POTENTIAL DIAGNOSES

- Skin integrity, impaired: potential
- Social interaction impaired
- Tissue integrity, impaired: oral mucous membranes

Skin Integrity, Impaired

Any break in the continuity of skin disrupts the protective mechanism of this organ system and predisposes the client to infection. The plan of care should provide defenses against infection and against external trauma. Intact skin areas must be protected from irritation and breakdown.

Planning and Implementation

Keeping the skin and its appendages healthy requires proper cleansing with soaps that do not cause drying or irritation. Intertriginous areas (where skin contacts skin) should be dried, particularly in the obese or where skin folds may prove problematic. Incontinent clients must be cared for quickly and efficiently. If the skin is dry (because of climate, disease, aging, or other reasons), it may be necessary to limit bathing and lubricate the skin. Body odors should be eliminated primarily by washing with soap and water, with sparing use of deodorants and perfumes. Therapeutic soaps, shampoos, powders, lotions, or selective agents may be required for any dermatologic problems.

Topical treatment for skin disorders usually involves the use of wet dressings or soaks or application of medications in an appropriate base. The type of skin disorder and whether the condition is acute, subacute, or chronic determine the basis of therapy, rather than the causative factors. Several guidelines are used by physicians to determine treatment, and nurses should also be aware of them. Moist, inflamed, and infected lesions are usually kept dry. Dry, scaling, lichenified lesions are covered with a medication, such as an ointment, to retard further drying. The skin must be closely observed during therapy because subsequent responses may require prompt changes in therapeutic modalities.

Open wet dressings are commonly used with inflammations that involve oozing, ulcers, erosions, or vesicular

Table 54–3
Sample Nursing Care Plan for a Client With a Dermatologic Problem, by Nursing Diagnosis

Client Care Goal	Plan/Nursing Implementation	Expected Outcome
Infection, potential for related to broken skin		
Prevent infection	Instruct client in daily hygiene of skin, nails, hair; observe for purulent drainage, increased redness, edema, tenderness; monitor temperature b.i.d.; instruct client in handwashing, avoidance of scratching, bumping, coarse clothing against affected area, temperature extremes	Absence of complications will be noted by no alterations in color, temperature, sensation, and fluid content; temperature within normal limits; no signs of malaise or fatigue; no signs of excoriations, bleeding, bruising
Knowledge deficit related to skin disorder		
Understand skin disorder	Discuss substances responsible for hypersensitivity reaction; instruct client to avoid use of those substances	Client demonstrates knowledge of problems such as contact dermatitis by identifying allergens responsible for reaction; will describe approaches to eliminate allergens
Self-concept, disturbance in: body image related to visible skin eruptions		
Decrease self-consciousness	Spend additional time with client; provide a specific time and place to discuss feelings; listen carefully; use touch appropriately; discuss implications of feelings and methods of coping; explore ways to facilitate coping; encourage client to socialize with client/family/significant others	Client demonstrates adjustment by expressing fears, concerns about rejection, alterations in lifestyle; identifies means to cope with feelings; client demonstrates ease in interacting with others; client has increased contact with staff and other clients; client derives comfort from supportiveness of others

skin conditions that do not cover a large surface area. The purpose of the dressing is to cause local vasoconstriction during the cooling and drying process and thereby reduce inflammation. Wound drainage, exudate, and crusts are removed when the dressing is changed.

Several solutions may be used to wet the dressing other than sterile water or saline solution. Aluminum acetate (Burow's) solution, which is commonly used, acts as an astringent and mild antiseptic. Acetic acid soaks reduce microbial counts in wound infections, particularly those containing *Pseudomonas* organisms. Silver nitrate solutions have been used effectively in the treatment of burns.

When a continuous wet dressing is required, sterile dressings (gauze, Kerlix) or clean cloths (soft toweling, linen, diapers) may be used to cover the lesion. Because dressings must not be allowed to dry, additional cover layers and frequent moistening may be needed. Nonporous wet or dry dressings should be avoided unless specifically ordered for the purpose of promoting hydration of the skin or penetration of a medication. Coverage with a nonporous wrap may cause heat retention, prevent evaporation, macerate the skin, and promote the overgrowth of bacteria.

Topical medications are suspended in a base that facilitates the penetration and absorption of the drug. The major types of bases or vehicles for therapeutic drugs are creams, lotions, ointments, and powders. Pastes, gels, and aerosols may also be used. Table 54–4 identifies the purpose, clinical indications for, and nursing implications associated with each modality. Medications incorporated into the base substance may act as anti-inflammatory agents, antipruritics, keratolytics, anti-infectives, antiseptics, antiparasitics, emollients, or protectants.

Each type of topical medication requires proper application. The nurse (or client giving self-care) should know the correct amount to use, whether to wear gloves while applying it, how and when to apply it, and how to recognize untoward effects. Information is readily available on package inserts, through pharmacists, and in drug textbooks.

Table 54–4
Types of Topical Agents

Type	Purpose	Clinical Indications	Nursing Implications
Creams	To provide cooling and increase moisture	Moist or dry lesions	Low penetration capacity and may be removed by perspiration or drainage; good for daytime use
Lotions (suspensions, solutions*)	To provide protective covering after facilitating a drying and cooling process	Acutely inflamed lesions; wet and oozing	Suspensions need shaking; preparations with alcohol may cause excessive drying
Ointments (water-in-oil, oil-in-water)	To lubricate and protect	Dry and scaly lesions	Ointments provide for greatest penetration and absorption because of their occlusiveness; water-in-oil is difficult to remove; may cause skin maceration if occluded; oil-in-water is relatively greaseless and easily absorbed; removable with soap and water
Powders	To promote dryness by absorption of moisture and protect by reducing friction	Intertrigo	Completely dry skin before application; easy removal may necessitate reapplication
Pastes	To protect and lubricate	Intertrigo, chronic skin ulcers	Useful in areas difficult to treat with wet compresses; difficult to remove with soap and water but responsive to mineral oil or vegetable oil
Gels	To provide a dry, greaseless, nonocclusive, nonstaining film	Before blistering, hairy areas	May be painful on application; cosmetically more favorable
Aerosols	To dry and protect skin	Peristomal hirsute areas and scalp	A substitute for lotions when direct application may be painful

*Suspensions contain insoluble powder in water. Solutions contain active ingredients in a fluid base.

Evaluation

Expected client outcomes following effective nursing interventions for impairment of skin integrity include observation and reports of a decrease in or absence of breaks in the skin and a decrease in discomfort. The client reports taking proper care of the skin such as use of appropriate soaps, lubricants, and topical treatments.

Injury, Potential for

In addition to injury related to infection, which is discussed in Table 54–3, skin injury from the sun is a major health problem. Protecting the skin from ultraviolet radiation is general good practice to avoid injury from sunburn, premature aging, and the development of neoplastic lesions. In recent years, classifications of sun-reactive skin types have been formulated. Table 54–5 lists these types and identifies high-risk individuals who need protective measures to minimize penetration of ultraviolet rays.

Planning and Implementation

Several means may be considered when establishing a protective plan, particularly for those whose skin typing is between I and III. Closer proximity to the equator and high altitude increase the exposure to ultraviolet radiation. It is critical to avoid peak hours of sunshine, even during cloudy days, unless protective clothing and wide brimmed hats are worn. Ultraviolet rays may also be reflected from snow, sand, and concrete. Sunscreens are of great assistance in absorbing or reflecting ultraviolet rays. Unfortunately, many people are more interested in tanning than protecting their skin, even though they may be aware of the aging and carcinogenic effects of sunlight.

Selection of an appropriate sunscreen should be based on a number of factors, which include:

- Skin typing and degree of photosensitivity
- Sun protection factor (SPF) offered
- Individual tendency toward drug sensitivity
- Cost

The three broad categories of sunscreens presently available are PABA or para-aminobenzoic acid (Presun, Pabanol); PABA esters and derivatives (Block Out, Pabafilm, Coppertone, Super Shade); non-PABA chemical agents (UVAL, Piz Buin); and physical sunscreens or sunblockers containing such substances as titanium dioxide or zinc oxide (A-fil, Shadow, Covermark). The purchaser may determine the length of time protection is being offered by multiplying the SPF shown on the bottle by the time required to obtain the minimal erythema dose (MED). Hypothetically, when a sunscreen with an SPF of 8 is used by a person who displays an MED in 30 minutes, a protection of 240 minutes or 4 hours is provided (8 SPF $\times$ 30 min $=$ 240 min).

These products must be applied one hour prior to sun exposure. All exposed areas should be covered. Reapplication is necessary when the sunscreen is removed by perspiration or water.

Evaluation

Expected client outcomes following effective nursing interventions for potential for injury related to sun exposure include observation and reports that the client is avoiding sun exposure and using appropriate sunscreens when the sun cannot be avoided. The client verbalizes the risks associated with overexposure of the skin to the sun.

Table 54–5
Classification of Sun-Reactive Skin Types

Skin Type	Risk	Response to MED*	Characteristics	SPF
I	Greatest	Always burns, never tans	Very light to light skin color (possible freckling); blue eyes; blonde or red hair	10 or more
II	Great	Always burns, sometimes tans	Blue eyes (some may have blue–gray eyes); red or blonde hair (some may have dark brown hair)	10 or more
III	Moderate	Sometimes burns, always tans	White skin; brown hair and eye color	8–10
IV	Low	Rarely burns, always tans	White or light brown skin (Mediterraneans, Orientals, Hispanics); dark hair and eye color	6–8
V	Very low	Rarely burns, tans easily	Heavily pigmented skin (Mediterraneans, Mongolians, American and East Indians, Hispanics)	4
VI	Negligible	Never burns	Black skin	0

*MED (minimal erythema dose) = 15–30 min initial exposure to the summer sun at peak hours, 11 AM–2 PM

Chapter Highlights

The complex cause-and-effect relationships of cutaneous manifestations require skillful use of the nursing process.

Nurses must learn to recognize the natural blend of pigmentation in various types of healthy skin and to examine the buccal mucosa, tongue, lips, nail beds, and sclera to supplement skin information.

Skin should be assessed for color, temperature, texture, turgor, and the presence of edema and the type, shape, arrangement, and distribution of lesions should be noted.

Hair should be examined for color, sheen, texture, pliability, distribution, and amount.

Nails are examined for shape, transparency, bulk, surface texture, and flexibility.

A hand-held magnifying lens and a Wood's light are useful in direct examination of the skin. Patch tests, intradermal skin tests, and skin biopsy with histologic study are also used.

Nursing care of clients with a cutaneous disorder focuses on the provision of care (general hygiene, skin and wound care, comfort and emotional support); protection (from further injury, secondary infection, the sun); and teaching self-care and health maintenance.

Skin disorders affect personal appearance and may affect self-image. Clients fear disfigurement, rejection, unemployment, and malignancy.

Client outcomes should demonstrate resolution of the skin disorder; a state of comfort and restfulness; an understanding of the problem, necessary therapy, and protective measures; proper self-care; and satisfactory coping.

Bibliography

Andberg MM, Rudolph A, Anderson TP: Improving skin care through patient and family training. *Top Clin Nurs* (July) 1983; 5:45–54.

Anders JE: Topicals. *RN* (Sept) 1982; 45:32–42.

Anders JE, Leach EE: Sun versus skin. *Am J Nurs* 1983; 83:1015–1020.

Arndt KA: *Manual of Dermatologic Therapeutics With Essentials of Diagnosis,* 3rd ed. Boston: Little, Brown, 1983.

Berliner H: Aging skin. *Am J Nurs* 1986; 86:1138–1141.

Berliner H: Aging skin: Part two. *Am J Nurs* 1986; 86:1259–1261.

Delancy VL: Skin assessment. *Top Clin Nurs* (July) 1983; 5:5–10.

Fitzpatrick TB, et al: *Dermatology in General Medicine.* 2nd ed. New York: McGraw–Hill, 1979.

Fitzpatrick TB, Polano MK, Suurmonch D: *Color Atlas and Synopsis of Clinical Dermatology.* New York: McGraw–Hill, 1983.

Fraser MC, McGuire DB: Skin cancer's early warning systems. *Am J Nurs* 1984; 84:1232–1236.

Grimes J, Iannopollo E: *Health Assessment in Nursing Practice.* Monterey, CA: Wadsworth, 1982.

Malkiewicz J: The integumentary system. *RN* (Dec) 1984; 44:55–60.

McKay M: Topical dermatologic therapy. *Primary Care* 1983; 10:513–524.

Neilley LK, DarEllis RA: Nailing down a diagnosis. *Nurs Pract* (May) 1984; 9:26–34.

Sauer GC: *Manual of Skin Diseases,* 4th ed. Philadelphia; Lippincott, 1980.

Turner ML: Skin changes after forty. *Am Fam Physician* (June) 1984; 29:173–181.

Resources

SELF-HELP GROUPS AND OTHER ORGANIZATIONS

Acne Research Institute
1587 Monrovia Ave.
Newport Beach, CA 92663
Phone: (714) 722–1805

Educational services to professionals and to persons with acne are provided through this organization.

Bald Headed Men of America
Morehead City, NC 28557
Phone: (919) 726–1855

Building self-pride and discouraging discrimination against persons who have lost their hair are the goals of this organization founded in 1973.

National Psoriasis Foundation
6415 S.W. Canyon Dr., Suite 200
Portland, OR 97221
Phone: (503) 297–1545

This organization provides services to both lay and professional persons through education, research, publications, and facilitating communication between persons with psoriasis.

Society for the Rehabilitation of the
Facially Disfigured
550 First Ave.
New York, NY 10016
Phone: (212) 340–5400

Clients with facial disfigurement from severe burns, congenital malformation, or cancer will find this organization useful in promoting self-esteem, providing surgical help and rehabilitation services for those unable to afford private care, and providing public education.

HOTLINE

American Academy of Facial, Plastic, and
Reconstructive Surgery
(800) 332-FACE

This 24-hour toll-free hotline can be called to obtain information and brochures about all facial plastic surgery procedures.

NURSING ORGANIZATIONS

Dermatology Nurses' Association
Box 56
Pitman, NJ 08071
Phone: (609) 582-1915

An organization for nurses with a special interest in dermatologic nursing. Membership is RNs and other interested health care workers.

CHAPTER **55**

Specific Disorders of the Integumentary System

Other topics related to this content are: Breast augmentation, breast reduction, and breast and nipple reconstruction, **Chapter 49;** Care of pruritic skin, **Chapter 54;** Care of the burned client, **Chapter 12;** Characteristics, examples, and illustrations of primary and secondary skin lesions, **Chapter 54;** Neurofibromatosis, **Chapter 29;** Rhinoplasty, **Chapter 15;** Skin lesions associated with STDs, **Chapter 49;** Sun-reactive skin types, **Chapter 54;** Topical treatment of skin disorders, including topical agents, **Chapter 54.**

Objectives

When you have finished studying this chapter, you should be able to:

Discuss common dermatoses that occur in adults.

Compare and contrast common dermatoses that may be prevented, cured, or become chronic.

Describe medical and surgical measures used to prevent and treat selected skin disorders.

Discuss the nursing implications of preoperative and postoperative care for clients having dermatologic or plastic and reconstructive surgery.

Explain the complications of surgery on the integument and the related nursing interventions.

Discuss alterations in body image encountered by clients having dermatologic, or plastic and reconstructive, survery.

Assume an active role in case finding for common dermatologic disorders.

Explain the therapeutic, comforting, teaching, and protecting roles of the nurse in the prevention and management of common dermatologic disorders.

Much of the monitoring of skin disorders will take place in community settings where the nurse may function in a variety of roles—professional health care provider, friend, or neighbor. Less frequently, the nurse will encounter clients with primary dermatologic problems in an acute care setting.

Understanding the pathogenesis of skin disorders allows nurses to teach clients to use measures that can avoid the onset of a disease state or prevent subsequent complications. Many skin diseases result in lifelong problems requiring frequent or intermittent medical supervision, periodic adjustments in treatment, and constant supportive care. Nurses who understand how and when to intervene effectively can assist a client with a dermatosis to attain problem resolution and restore skin integrity, or to control manifestations and prevent complications when a cure is not possible.

Surgery is a major therapeutic component in management of some skin problems. Surgery may range from a minor operation to a complex set of surgical procedures and may be performed by a dermatologist, a general surgeon, or a plastic surgeon. Procedures may be performed as an ambulatory care service in a physician's office or a clinic, or may require hospitalization for several days. For clients admitted to the hospital for traumatic injuries, such as burns, surgery is only a part of the treatment regimen.

Recent technologic advances have expanded the number of surgical approaches to dermatologic problems. For example, surgeons are able to transplant skin and tissue flaps using an operating microscope to reattach the finer blood vessels and increase success. Plastic surgery can reach beyond the cutaneous layers to include reconstruction of underlying musculoskeletal structures in repairing deformities and defects of the integument. The field of cosmetic or aesthetic surgery has grown as techniques have developed to remedy visible defects that often impose both an emotional and economic burden. All of the fine instruments used in this delicate surgery are small enough to fit into a teacup.

This chapter discusses both dermatologic surgery for the treatment of cutaneous lesions, as well as plastic and reconstructive surgery. Most dermatologic surgery for the treatment of cutaneous lesions can be carried out in an ambulatory care facility in a relatively brief period of time. Although often classified as "minor" surgery because of these factors, they may be anxiety provoking and not always perceived as minor by the client.

SECTION I

Congenital/Genetic Disorders

Acne Vulgaris

Acne vulgaris (common acne) is a frequent, chronic, inflammatory disorder affecting the pilosebaceous units of the integument. This disorder occurs predominantly in adolescence when the sebaceous glands are activated. Acne can extend into young adulthood, particularly in women. Males tend to be more severely affected than females, and Caucasians have a higher incidence than Orientals and blacks.

Many factors contribute to the cause or exacerbation of acne. Familial tendencies have been demonstrated, indicating a genetic linkage. Irritation has been attributed to a combination of increased sebum production and bacterial activity associated with the *Propionibacterium (Corynebacterium) acnes,* a normal organism of the hair follicle. Other contributing factors include endocrine imbalances; use of oral contraceptives; hormonal therapy (corticosteroids, androgens); other drugs (Dilantin, lithium); emotional stress; lack of cleanliness; exposure to comedogenic (lesion-producing) substances such as cosmetics, heavy oils, greases, and tars; and mechanical trauma of the lesions. Although some dermatologists cite dietary implications, no conclusive scientific evidence exists about the cause of acne. Flare-ups are seasonal and seen mostly in the fall and winter, although hot humid weather coupled with inadequate hygiene may also exacerbate the lesions.

Clinical Manifestations

Acne vulgaris is characterized by both noninflammatory and inflammatory skin lesions, primarily on the face and, to a lesser extent, on the neck, upper arms, and trunk (Figure 55–1). **Comedones** (blackheads and whiteheads), the classic noninflammatory lesions of acne, result from blockage of the follicle by lipid and keratin debris. An open comedo (blackhead) develops when the lipid oxidizes; its coloring comes from the presence of melanin. A whitehead is a closed comedo. Typical inflammatory lesions associated with acne vulgaris include papules and pustules. In severe cases, nodules and cysts may occur along with pitting and hypertrophic scarring. **Seborrhea,** an increase in the amount of sebum excreted (and possibly a change in the sebum itself), is commonly seen with acne, usually on the scalp and face.

Medical Measures

Regular atraumatic expression of comedones (removal of the plug) prevents lesions from becoming irritated and progressing to an inflammatory stage. A comedo extractor allows gentle removal without risk of trauma (and scarring) or further irritation. Abrasive cleansers may be used to remove surface debris.

Comedolytic (comedo dissolving) and peeling agents assist in the removal of the comedo plugs. Topical preparations containing a single drug or combination of sulfur, resorcinol, or salicylic acid have been used, although these substances are giving way to the use of retinoic acid.

The treatment of acne has been revolutionized by retinoids, analogues of vitamin A. Topical application of retinoic acid (tretinoin) is not only effective on existing lesions but ultimately prevents the formation of new comedones and the development of inflammation. Benzoyl peroxide may be included in the treatment plan—either alone or in combination with retinoic acid. In addition to its comedolytic effect, benzoyl peroxide provides a bacteriostatic action.

Systemic retinoids have been incorporated into the therapeutic regimen for severe inflammatory disease. Isotretinoin (Accutane), the newest synthetic drug, decreases the size and activity of sebaceous glands, reducing sebum production. If retinoid treatment is begun early, disfigurement from scarring can be largely prevented even in clients with severe cystic acne.

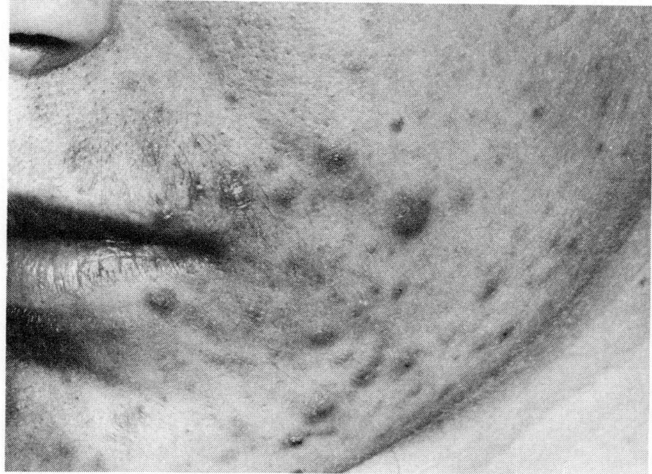

Figure 55–1

Acne vulgaris. Erythematous papules and pustules. SOURCE: *Binnick SA:* Skin Diseases: Diagnosis and Management in Clinical Practice. *Baltimore, MD: Williams & Wilkins, 1982.*

NURSING DIAGNOSES IN
Integumentary Dysfunction

DIRECTLY RELATED DIAGNOSES

- Comfort, altered: pruritus
- Infection, potential for
- Injury, potential for
- Knowledge deficit
- Self-concept, disturbance: body image
- Skin integrity, impaired: actual

OTHER POTENTIAL DIAGNOSES

- Skin integrity, impaired: potential
- Social interaction impaired
- Tissue integrity, impaired: oral mucous membrances

Clindamycin, erythromycin, and tetracycline are the antibiotics used in the presence of inflammation. Dilute triamcinolone acetonide (Aristocort, Kenalog) may be injected into lesions to manage severe acne in which cysts and nodules develop. Systemic corticosteroids such as prednisone or dexamethasone are reserved for cases refractory to all other modalities of treatment. Estrogen therapy and the use of anovulatory drugs may be selected for women, primarily postadolescents, who fail to show significant improvement from aggressive conventional acne treatment. The estrogens suppress the androgenic hormones that have activated the sebaceous glands.

Dermabrasion is a surgical procedure used to lessen the disfiguring effects that may have resulted from the inflammatory process.

Specific Nursing Measures

The greatest concern of the nurse is to encourage the client to make a major commitment to following the prescribed therapeutic plan. The client should understand the basic pathophysiology and the course of remissions and exacerbations involved in acne.

Client/Family Teaching

Instructions for treatment must be explicit and understandable. Clients must learn of potential problems and how to protect the skin from further injury. Sunlight, for example, may be used therapeutically but only if the skin is kept dry and exposure is not contraindicated by any of the drugs used. Irritation and subsequent inflammation may result from undue pressure, friction, rubbing, or squeezing of the affected areas. Clothing made from wool or roughly textured fabrics should be avoided. Athletes in contact sports or who perspire excessively under heavy clothing may need to stop playing temporarily. Undue pressure on the involved areas of the face, possibly caused by resting it against a hand while studying or listening to a classroom lecture, forceful expression (squeezing) of acne lesions, or a variety of other manipulations may activate the inflammatory process and lead to scarring. Anger or embarrassment over having blemishes may provoke squeezing that traumatizes the skin.

Hygiene is important to prevent external irritants from exacerbating the inflammatory process. Mild soaps and thorough drying of the skin should be encouraged when comedolytics are being used. Treatment may also require shampooing with a soap that controls the seborrhea. Clients whose work exposes them to oils, grease, and tars should be instructed to cleanse their skin frequently and particularly to wash off heavy perspiration.

Consideration must be given to avoiding substances that encourage comedones. Cosmetics containing heavy oil bases should be replaced with a thinner, water-based preparation. Cleansers, astringents, toners, and moisturizers should be selected that avoid excess oil but do not cause more dryness than desired. Major cosmetic companies perform comedogenic studies, and results are available upon request. Topical medications can be tinted so they do not have to be covered by cosmetics.

Provide clients receiving retinoic acid with directions for proper administration and information concerning side effects. Topical application will cause some feeling of warmth, redness, slight tingling, and scaling at the site. The client must be informed that the medication may have to be discontinued temporarily or the dosage readjusted if the reaction becomes severe. Other instructions must also be given. Use of strong or medicated cosmetics, soap, or skin cleansers should be avoided. The area must be thoroughly dry before retinoic acid is applied, avoiding contact with the eyes, mouth, and mucous membranes. Exposure to sunlight or ultraviolet rays must be minimized; treatment may have to be delayed if the skin receives a burn.

Clients receiving isotretinoin (Accutane) should know that the drug not only produces significant skin problems such as cheilitis (inflammation of the lip) and dry hair, but can cause conjunctivitis, hypertriglyceridemia, and musculoskeletal pain. Because toxic effects are increased by vitamin A, the client should avoid excessive intake of vitamin A. Isotretinoin causes embryonic deformities in animals, and sexually active women of childbearing age must use contraceptive measures during treatment and for a month after drug discontinuance.

Any person with acne needs to be able to express feelings freely to someone who is able to recognize the underlying dynamics the stress of acne may have triggered. Showing acceptance and sincere concern may encourage open communication and client trust that can enhance the relationship between nurse and client. (See the case study of a client with acne at the end of this chapter.)

Chemical Peeling/Dermabrasion

Chemical peeling (chemical planing, chemabrasion, or chemexfoliation) involves the use of caustics to destroy the epidermis and upper portion of the dermis by chemical coagulation. Cauterants such as liquid phenol, or Baker's formula (a 50% phenol solution); trichloroacetic acid (TCA); or Combes' formula, a combination of resorcinal, salicylic acid, and ethanol, may be used.

Dermabrasion (or surgical planing) involves the removal of the epidermis and the upper dermis by an abrasive instrument to eliminate superficial irregularities and discolorations. The face and scalp are most often treated because they contain more of the glands and follicles needed for re-ephithelialization.

The ultimate outcome of chemical peeling is a smoother skin and permanent lightening of pigmentation. Therefore, one of the major purposes of this procedure is to rejuvenate aging skin by removing fine facial wrinkles, lentigines (flat brown pigmented spots), and actinic lesions. Superficial scars from acne can be eradicated, and the discoloration from freckling or chloasma can also be effectively reduced. Chemical peeling is often used in conjunction with dermabrasion to obtain a more effective cosmetic improvement. The prime candidates for dermabrasion have been persons with shallow or moderate scarring, generally from acne vulgaris or a pox virus. The procedure may be used to remove fine facial wrinkles from aging skin. Traumatic or surgical scars may be flattened and made less conspicuous, and tattoos may be removed by dermabrasion.

Clients who demand perfection are not usually considered good candidates for either procedure. Also not considered good candidates are clients with a history of hypertrophic scarring or keloid formation, clients with an active skin infection, warts, or a prior severe or recurrent herpes simplex infection, and clients with highly pigmented skin.

In chemical peeling, the chemical is meticulously applied with cotton applicators, either to the entire face or to selected areas, avoiding contact with the eyes. Because of an increased tendency for scarring and hyperpigmentation on the neck, treatment of this location is contraindicated. Following application of the caustic agent, the treated area is taped with waterproof adhesive tape, which is left in place for 24 to 48 hours to improve the penetration process.

Dermabrasion is accomplished through use of a motor-driven rotary instrument consisting of fine stainless steel wires or coarse diamond burrs. The superficial layer of skin is sanded until irregular surfaces are minimized. The abraded area may be coated with an antibiotic ointment, left exposed or covered with petrolatum gauze, a non-adhering dressing (Telfa), or a pressure dressing. The outer dressing is usually removed after 24 to 48 hours. Because the wound exudes not only blood and serum but clotting substances such as fibrin and thromboplastin, excessive bleeding is not usually a major problem. Table 55–1 summarizes client implications for chemical peeling and dermabrasion.

Nursing Implications

PREOPERATIVE CARE The preoperative preparation should focus on reinforcement of teaching and client discussion regarding the aesthetic outcomes, description of the actual procedure, and self-care instruction. Thorough cleansing of the skin with a hexachlorophene-based liquid

Table 55–1
Chemical Peeling and Dermabrasion: Implications for the Client

Physiologic Implications	Psychosocial/Lifestyle Implications
Burning for 30–45 min after application of cauterant	Improvement in self-concept, self-esteem, and body image with successful treatment
Postoperative edema lasting for 3–4 wk after chemical peeling and 3–6 wk after dermabrasion	Edema, erythema, and crusting may be distressing and cause the client to limit social activities for 6–12 wk postoperatively
Postoperative discomfort and interference with sleep possible for the first 2 days from tightening of the exudate and during separation of the crust	Limitations on general activity as well as chewing, drinking, talking, and facial expressions, and alteration of diet until the crust resolves
Crust takes 7–10 days to loosen, sloughing spontaneously in about 2 wk; pruritus common at this time	Return to work in approximately 2 wk or after crust sloughs
Excess pigmentation, depigmentation, or brownish discoloration may occur	Complications may cause emotional distress and adversely affect self-esteem and body image
Potential complications are infection, development of milia, spread of existing warts or herpes simplex, hypertrophic scarring	Need to avoid direct exposure to sunlight for 3–6 months
Abraded skin is sensitive to sunlight	
Repeat treatments may be necessary	

soap for a few days prior to surgery will help prevent infection. Avoid any soap that produces an oily skin residue. Male clients must shave on the day of surgery.

A total chemical peel, or one-stage peel, may require hospitalization, or the surgery may be performed on an ambulatory basis. Dermabrasion may be performed in the physician's office or other outpatient health care facility, but extensive planing usually requires hospitalization.

POSTOPERATIVE CARE Elevating the head of the bed will decrease edema and is helpful in lessening discomfort during the first 2 postoperative days. Narcotic analgesics and hypnotics may be necessary to provide comfort and rest. Pain usually dissipates as the crust forms.

To promote a smoother epithelialization, instruct the client to avoid splitting the crust formed over the wound. A liquid diet minimizes chewing, and using written communication or hand signals limits talking. General activity is minimized to lessen movement.

Approximately 3 to 5 days after the crust has formed, it may be softened by gently washing the area with mild soap and water and applying an ointment containing 5% boric acid or vitamins A and D. Some surgeons prefer liberal coverage with petrolatum jelly or cold cream to facilitate crust removal and do not permit washing the face until 12 to 14 days after surgery. Encourage the client to allow spontaneous sloughing of the crust with whatever procedure is prescribed. Cool tap water compresses, steroid creams, analgesics, and tranquilizers may relieve the itching or burning sensation that occurs when the crust separates. Clients may also need to be instructed in how to avoid scratching and prevent infection from fingernail damage.

Remind clients to use sunscreen and avoid direct exposure to sunlight for 3 to 6 months. Water-based makeup may be used to cover the erythema when the wound area has healed.

Alopecia

Alopecia is the loss of body hair (primarily on the scalp) with the presence of bald spots or total baldness. Alopecia may be patchy or diffuse, scarring or nonscarring. In cases where scar tissue forms, regrowth of hair becomes impossible because the follicles have been permanently destroyed.

Causes for hair loss are multiple. The most common type of alopecia, *male pattern baldness,* is hereditary. Female pattern baldness occurs in a small percentage of women, usually around the age of 50.

Alopecia areata is a common disorder of asymptomatic, noninflammatory, nonscarring hair loss. The etiologic basis is unknown, although a family history has been implicated, as has autoimmune disease. Emotional stress, particularly a life crisis, has also been known to precipitate the loss. Alopecia areata affects both sexes equally, and the initial attack is frequently seen in clients under the age of 25.

Loss of hair may also occur from repeated friction; cutaneous infection; drugs and chemicals; trauma (frostbite, burns); skin disease and neoplasms; nutritional deficiencies (loss of large amounts of amino acids and trace elements); x-ray; endocrine imbalances; and acute and chronic systemic illness.

Clinical Manifestations

Male pattern baldness most often begins with receding of the hairline in front, followed by lessening of hair on the crown of the head and in the temporal areas.

The losses associated with alopecia areata appear gradually over several weeks and may be localized (areas on the scalp, eyelids, or cheeks) or extensive. Regrowth is often spontaneous but a less favorable prognosis exists when the onset occurs before puberty or if the losses are extensive. Recurrence is quite common.

Medical and Specific Nursing Measures

Topical, intralesional, or systemic corticosteroids, repeated applications of topical photosensitizers (DNCB), and prolonged photochemotherapy have been used to treat alopecia areata (phototherapy is discussed in the section on psoriasis). The major therapy may be directed toward assisting the individual in coping with any emotional disturbances caused by the alopecia, particularly if the condition becomes chronic with no possibility of inducing regrowth. Use of wigs or hair transplantation or replacement may be encouraged if at all possible. Artificial implants have not been successful to date, may cause infection and scarring, and should be discouraged. Research into the potential use of minoxidil, a vasodilator used as an antihypertensive, is ongoing.

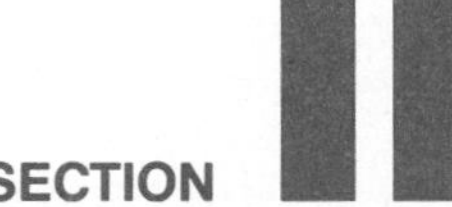

SECTION II

Disorders of Multifactorial Origin

Seborrheic Dermatitis

Seborrheic dermatitis is a chronic inflammatory condition characterized by red, scaling eruptions in areas where sebaceous glands are highly concentrated, such as the scalp, face, and trunk. The cause is basically unknown, although a familial tendency is suggested. Emotional and physical stress are also responsible for recurrence of the problem. Some individuals develop dandruff, a minor condition that involves excessive desquamation (shedding of dead cells), without any evidence of inflammation.

Clinical Manifestations

The onset of seborrheic dermatitis is gradual. The condition has a tendency to worsen in colder weather because of decreased indoor humidity and lack of summer sunlight. Pruritus is a common complaint. Varying-sized white or yellowish-red macules and papules may appear on the scalp, eyelids, eyebrows, paranasal area, ears, moustache, beard, presternal area, and in body folds (Figure 55–2). The lesions may be dry or greasy and may develop crusts or fissures.

Medical Measures

Shampoos that contain 2% selenium sulfide (Exsel, Iosel, Selsun Blue) are effective antiseborrheics. Similar responses may be obtained from preparations that contain 1% to 2% zinc pyrithione (Danex, Head & Shoulders, Zincon). Shampoos containing salicylic acid with sulfur (Ionil, Sebulex) or tar (Sebutone, Zetar) are less effective. Keratolytic gels may be applied overnight to remove thick crusts. Topical medications may include corticosteroids and sulfur-containing substances.

Specific Nursing Measures

Because seborrheic dermatitis is chronic, nursing care should help prepare the client to plan for long-term management and control. Shampooing schedules and techniques and the administration of topical medications in the prescribed vehicle should be explained and demonstrated. Because stress plays a major role in the exacerbation of this condition, the client needs to recognize the need to develop effective coping mechanisms whenever possible and to practice stress management techniques.

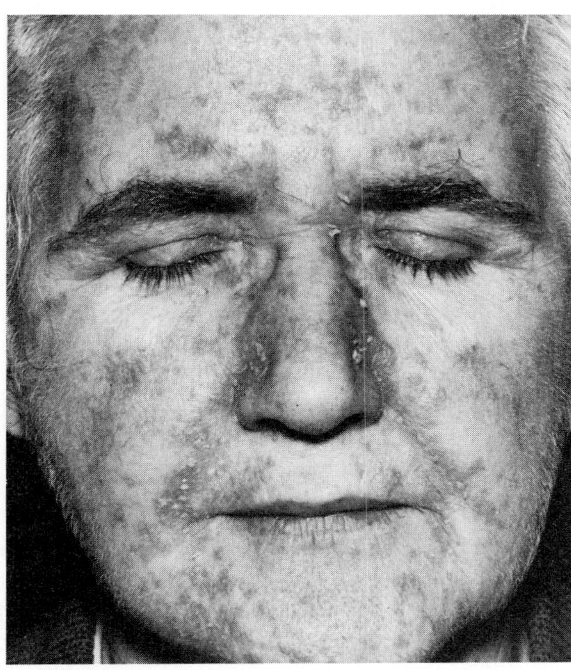

Figure 55–2

Seborrheic dermatitis. *SOURCE: Binnick SA:* Skin Diseases: Diagnosis and Management in Clinical Practice. *Baltimore, MD: Williams & Wilkins, 1982.*

Psoriasis

Psoriasis is a common recurring disorder indicative of an overly rapid proliferation of epidermal cells in which characteristic scaling, papules, and plaques appear, most frequently on the elbows, knees, and scalp. No cure exists.

Onset occurs generally during adulthood, although a significant number of cases are known to appear before the age of 20, with equal frequency in both sexes. Additionally, a significant number of people with psoriasis (5% to 10%) also have an associated arthritic condition to manage.

The reason why keratinocytes mature in 3 or 4 days in psoriasis instead of the normal 28 days remains unknown. Familial tendencies have been associated with approximately 30% of clients. Significant immunologic abnormalities have also been demonstrated. A form of acute psoriasis has also been known to follow several days after streptococcal pharyngitis. Exacerbations have been correlated with alcohol ingestion, excessive exposure to sunlight, stress, obesity, and use of certain drugs such as systemic corticosteroids, lithium, and chloroquine. Cutaneous trauma related to scratching, surgical wounds, and other superficial injuries may result in the formation of a new patchy lesion in clients with psoriasis.

Clinical Manifestations

The initial appearance of psoriasis usually is gradual and generally takes the form of elevated, sharply circumscribed lesions covered by white-silvery scales (Figure 55–3). The shape and arrangements of psoriatic lesions vary: they may be limited to one or a localized group of lesions, may be distributed over a region, or distribution may be general, including not only the skin but also the

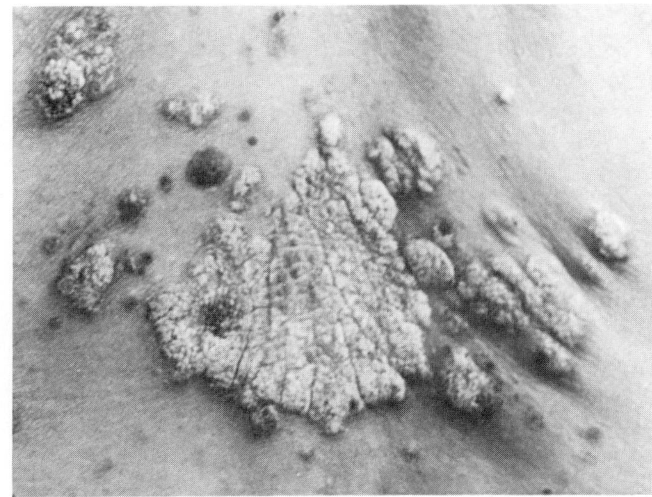

Figure 55–3

Generalized psoriasis. *Courtesy of Millard Fillmore Hospital, Buffalo, NY.*

nails. Cutaneous manifestations are most common over bony prominences and in intertriginous areas. Excoriation, lichenification, and oozing may occur with some cases. Psoriasis of the nails may cause crumbling, pitting, and distal detachment of the plates. Pruritus may be anticipated, particularly with scalp and anogenital involvement.

Medical Measures

The use of corticosteroids for management of psoriasis aims at inhibiting mitosis (formation of new cells), thereby reducing scaling and thickening of the skin. These drugs may be administered topically, systemically, or intralesionally.

Coal tar preparations, in the form of ointments, bath oils, emulsions, shampoos and lotions, have long had a significant role in the treatment of psoriasis. In addition to removing scales and plaque, these drugs inhibit DNA synthesis in both normal and hyperplastic skin. The preparation is usually used in conjunction with corticosteroids, other keratolytic agents such as salicylic acid and sulfur, or with phototherapy.

Phototherapy or actinotherapy provides a regulated exposure to ultraviolet light (UVL), either natural UVL (sunlight), or artificial sources of middle-wavelength UVL (UV-B), to reduce basal cell production in mild to moderate cases of psoriasis.

Photochemotherapy currently offers the most promising treatment for widespread, severe psoriasis. The mechanism involves administration of a chemical sensitizer followed by exposure to long-wave length UVL (UV-A) approximately 2 hours later. A group of drugs known as psoralens act as the photosensitizers and, in conjunction with UV-A, reduce the accelerated rate of cell production seen in psoriasis. This combination of a psoralen with UV-A is known by the acronym PUVA. Methoxsalen (Oxsoralen), the most commonly used psoralen derivative, is available for oral administration as well as topical application.

Effective treatment for widespread psoriatic lesions may be obtained from the use of anthralin (dithranol, Cignolin, Lassar's paste), a drug with cytotoxic and cytostatic actions. Cool tar baths, application of corticosteroid creams, UVL, or PUVA may be combined with the anthralin paste method.

Methotrexate (Amethopterin) or hydroxyurea (Hydrea) may be selected in the treatment of clients who have severe psoriasis that has become resistant to other forms of therapy. The purpose of using antimetabolites is to inhibit DNA synthesis and obtain remission of cell proliferation.

A new retinoid, etretinate (Tegrison) has been found to be useful in the treatment of psoriasis. Studies are continuing to measure its effectiveness alone and in combination with adjunctive therapy such as ultraviolet radiation and PUVA.

Specific Nursing Measures

Psoriasis is one of the few dermatoses that may require hospitalization, most likely because of a need for more intense or assisted therapy. Day care centers have also been established to provide closer supervision and aid with therapeutic measures without requiring 24-hour confinement.

Nursing care is directed at restoring skin integrity through the administration of the prescribed treatment. Be aware of and understand the responsibilities involved in drug therapy, particularly effective application and removal of topical drugs. Proper coverage of lesions is essential and usually requires airtight dressings or use of plastic wrap (Saran Wrap) so that penetration of lesions is effective. As each component of therapy is implemented, incorporate a teaching plan that will promote client self-care.

Client/Family Teaching

Potential for injury is always present. Clients with psoriasis should be cautioned to avoid rubbing or scratching the skin because trauma may initiate the development of new lesions. Excoriated areas may also be a port of entry for bacteria, and secondary infections may ensue.

Protection of the eyes and uninvolved skin is essential when artificial UVL is used. Teach the client to avoid overexposure to sunlight and additional cutaneous injury. Clients should always follow safety precautions in self-treatment and be certain that anyone administering UVL therapy, if not a physician, nurse, or recognized therapist, is experienced and technically competent. Commercial establishments offering UVL for tanning do not follow medically precise techniques and may be a source of injury.

Psoriasis is a classic example of a skin disorder that can be emotionally upsetting to the client. Whether generalized or local, lesions are usually visible and may cause feelings of humiliation and embarrassment. The chronicity and recurrent flare-ups; the tedious skin care; the staining of skin, nails, clothing, and bedding; and the financial drain may weaken coping mechanisms so that additional counseling may be required. As discouraged as someone may become with psoriasis, it is essential that treatments be continued and exacerbating factors avoided. The support that can be given by an individual, whether a lay person or professional, and by a mutual support group may prove highly valuable in motivating the client to persevere.

Vitiligo

Vitiligo is a disorder in which temporary or permanent depigmentation develops. It may involve the hair as well as the skin because of gradual melanocytic destruction. Although vitiligo occurs in all racial groups, an increased incidence has been recorded in India, Pakistan, and the Far East. Vitiligo has many psychosocial ramifications. In India, for instance, a woman with this condition is considered unmarriageable. Other psychosocial implications are discussed later in this section.

The pathogenesis is unknown, and vitiligo is classified as an acquired idiopathic disorder. Approximately 30% of persons with vitiligo have a family history of this skin disorder (Arndt, 1983). An associated depigmentation also occurs with systemic illnesses such as pernicious anemia, diabetes mellitus, and thyroid disease.

Clinical Manifestations

Lesions are macular, pure white, often symmetrical, and frequently develop over bony prominences (elbow, knee, ankle, wrist) and about body openings (Figure 55–4). Alterations are usually progressive and may be limited to an isolated lesion or become localized, generalized, or universal. Illumination from a Wood's light is useful in determining the presence of melanin within the area.

Medical Measures

Several methods are available to treat vitiligo, although none alters the pathophysiologic process. The prime objective, therefore, is to improve cosmetic appearance. Those with light complexions may not require treatment because depigmentation is not as obvious a problem as with dark-brown or black-skinned people.

The use of PUVA is the most effective therapy at this time. Depending on the degree of skin involvement, either a systemic or a topical psoralen preparation is administered. The unaffected skin should be covered with sunscreens to prevent excessive tanning. Re-establishing desired pigmentation may take as long as 2 years.

Depigmentation through chemical bleaching is recommended for clients over 40 years of age with more than 40% of their skin area showing vitiligo that has proved recalcitrant to PUVA. Monobenzone or hydroquinone ointment (Benoquin), applied topically, result in depigmentation.

Because treatment results are slow, cosmetics may be employed as a temporary camouflage. A solution of potassium permanganate has been used to paint vitiliginous areas in brown-skinned clients. Cosmetic coverups (Vita-Dye, Dy-O-Derm) and makeup (Covermark, Reflecta) are also available.

Specific Nursing Measures

Many clients may not know about or understand vitiligo and may have developed myths or unscientific rationales about the cause. Information that the pathogenesis is unknown must be made clear along with the chronic nature of the depigmentation. Options for treatment may need to be identified when clients have not received medical assistance, to prevent the search for a nonexistent cure. Clients should be cautioned to apply sunscreen to normal skin when exposed to the sun so that the contrast between the two areas is not increased.

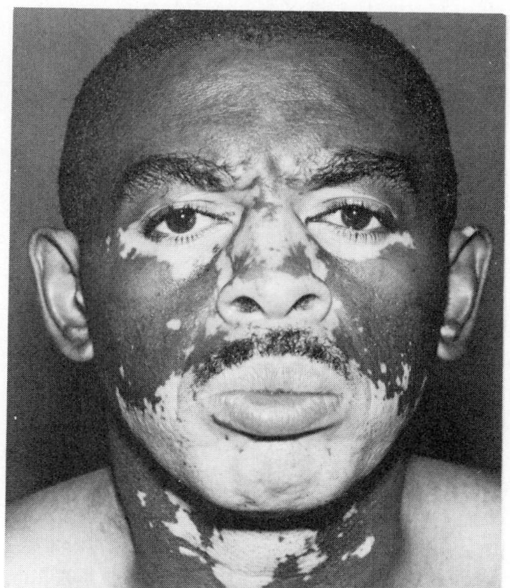

Figure 55–4

Vitiligo. SOURCE: *Binnick SA:* Skin Diseases: Diagnosis and Management in Clinical Practice. *Baltimore, MD: Williams & Wilkins, 1982.*

Serious disfigurement may already have deterred employment opportunities, interpersonal relationships, and personal growth. Support systems must be developed and strengthened so that the individual may adjust emotionally to the stresses imposed by vitiligo. Offer the client the opportunity to discuss fears and concerns.

Pressure Ulcers

Pressure ulcers are localized areas of cellular necrosis that result from ischemia because of vascular insufficiency in an area under pressure. Unrelieved external pressure that is greater than capillary pressure (32mm Hg; equivalent to one pound of pressure per square inch) damages the delicate capillary bed, eventually leading to tissue destruction. Pressure is higher at body sites where soft tissue overlies bony prominences. Areas such as the sacrum, greater trochanter, ischium, heel, and malleolus have a high incidence of pressure ulcers. The elbows, ears, breasts in women, genitalia in men, scapulae, or any bony prominence may develop a pressure ulcer depending on the clients' position. The term pressure ulcer is more appropriate than the older term, decubitus ulcer, because it correlates with the pathophysiology of these lesions.

A widespread and serious health problem, pressure ulcers are thought to develop in 3% to 5% of persons admitted annually to US hospitals, or between 1 and 2 million hospitalized clients per year.

Clinical Manifestations

Pressure ulcers are classified by appearance and tissue involvement as follows:

- Stage 1. Skin is red, but unbroken
- Stage 2. Epidermis broken by either a blister or superficial ulceration; dermis is intact; minimal bleeding, drainage, and granulation tissue; epithelium at wound margins; constitutes a partial-thickness wound
- Stage 3. Open lesion; epidermis and dermis are eroded; subcutaneous tissue and fat are exposed; crater formation with rubor, eschar, and drainage; wound base may be necrotic; granulation tissue may be present; constitutes a full-thickness wound
- Stage 4. Open lesion; epidermis and dermis totally eroded and/or lost; fat, muscle, tendon, fascia, or bone may be exposed; wound tunnels and osteomyelitis may be present; wound base usually necrotic; granulation tissue present; epitheliazation present at wound margins

These stages are illustrated in Figure 55–5.

Medical Measures

The treatment of pressure ulcers involves frequent position changes, skin care, the use of pressure relief devices, the provision of nutrients and protein as necessary, and wound care depending on the stage of involvement. Whirlpool baths and physical therapy are often prescribed. Antimicrobials may be used in the presence of infection. Surgical reconstruction through direct closure, the removal of underlying bursa or bone, skin grafting, or the creation of a skin flap or myocutaneous flap may be necessary to achieve healing.

Specific Nursing Measures

The single most important nursing measure is *prevention.* Although pressure is the primary cause of pressure ulcers, a number of risk factors predispose a client to the development of these lesions. Clients are at risk when:

- Activity is reduced
- Mobility is limited
- Mental status is impaired
- Nutritional deficiencies are present
- Incontinence is present
- Chronic illness exists

Examples of clients who may fit into these categories are persons with diabetes, spinal cord injury, multiple sclerosis, arthritis, renal failure, respiratory problems, depression, cancer, negative nitrogen balance, malnutrition, and those who undergo surgery on a conventional operating room table for 2 or more hours. The risk of pressure ulcer is twice as high in persons 85 years of age and older. Determining whether the client is at risk and taking steps to prevent the development of pressure ulcers are critical nursing responsibilities.

If a client is determined to be at risk, the most basic nursing intervention is pressure relief. Pressure relief can be achieved by frequent changing of position (at least every two hours), and by placing an alternating pressure or air mattress under the client. The pressure exerted by contact with the ordinary hospital mattress is great and will lead to tissue damage in the client at risk. Although sheepskin and foam pads provide comfort, they do not offer adequate pressure relief. Use extra precautions with the heel areas that are not adequately protected by any of the pressure relief devices available.

The nursing care specifics for a client who has developed a pressure ulcer, in addition to pressure relief interventions, include skin care and wound care. A comprehensive plan according to the four stages of pressure ulcer is outlined in Table 55–2. This plan includes instructions for client self-care, family involvement, and home care.

A pressure ulcer is both a physiologic and a psychosocial burden. Clients with pressure ulcers may have pain, and body image and self-esteem alterations. They, their caretakers, and family and friends may find the sight or smell of a pressure ulcer offensive. Provide clients and their significant others with the opportunity to discuss their psychosocial concerns and their reactions, and explore the physical and emotional ways in which they might manage their responses. A psychiatric-mental health nurse can often be helpful in this regard.

SECTION 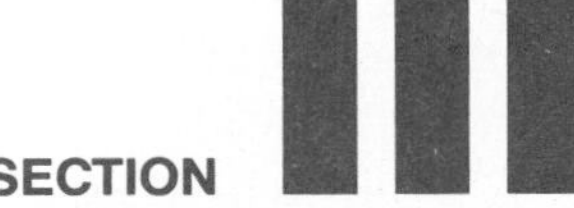

Immune Hypersensitivity Disorders

Eczematous dermatitis or eczema is a general term covering various forms of eruptive inflammatory disease of the integument that result from an immediate or delayed hypersensitivity reaction after exposure to an exogenous, endogenous, or unknown substance. One-third of the clients who seek the help of a dermatologist are troubled with eczematous dermatitis (Fitzpatrick, 1979).

These disorders occur readily within occupational, household, and recreational settings. Within the hospital, drug reactions are a leading cause for seeking a dermatologic consultation. The various forms of eczematous disease have proven costly in the loss of time and productivity, lost wages, medical expenses, and human suffering.

Contact Dermatitis

Contact dermatitis, a common inflammatory dermatosis seen in acute, subacute, and chronic forms, involves the epidermal and dermal layers of the skin. Causative agents responsible for the reaction act either as a primary irritant

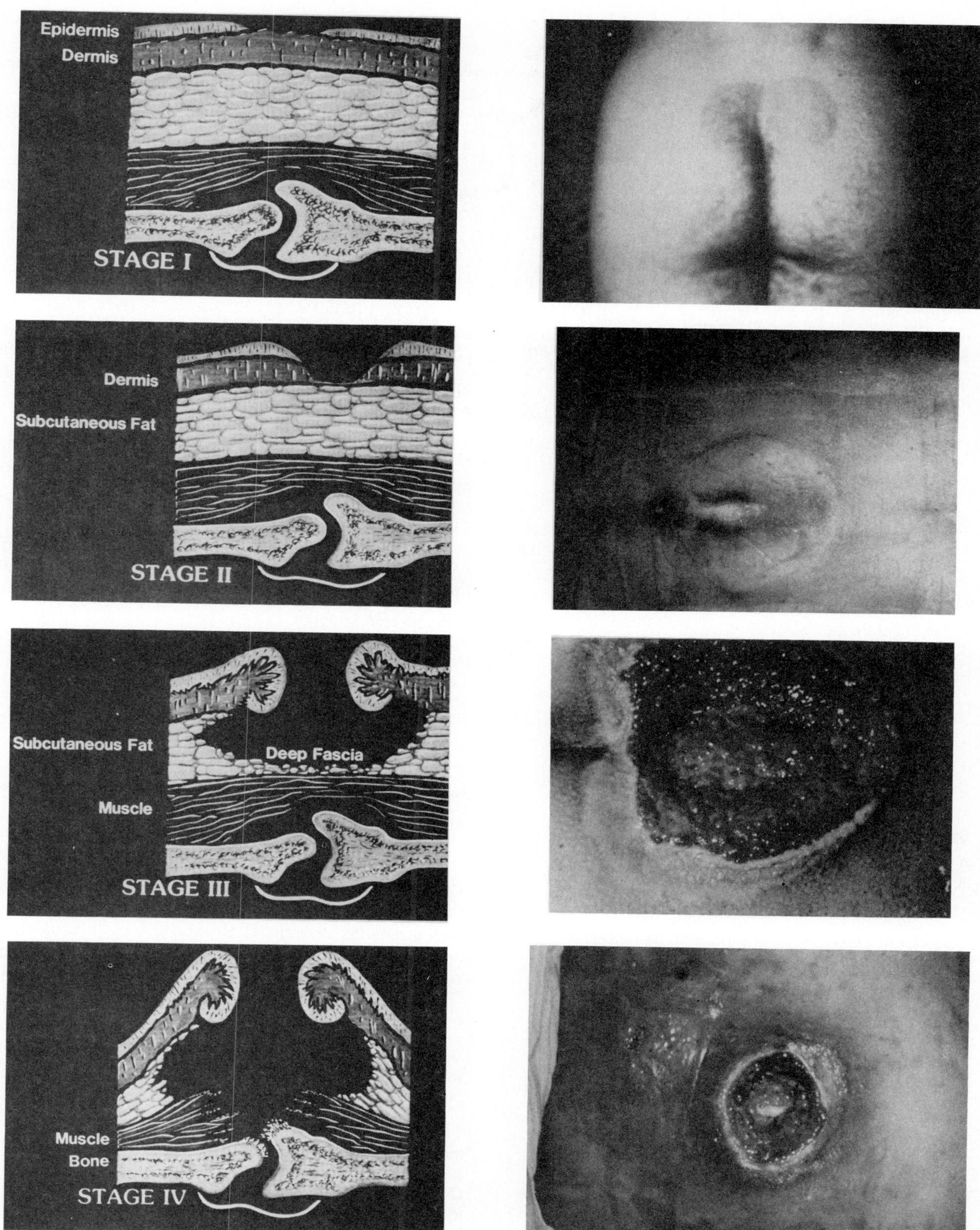

Figure 55–5

Pressure ulcer. **A.** Stage 1. **B.** Stage 2. **C.** Stage 3. **D.** Stage 4. *Courtesy of Gaymar Industries, Orchard Park, NY.*

Table 55–2
Nursing Care Plan for the Client With Pressure Ulcer

Intervention	Goal Rationale
Stage 0	
A. Identify clients at risk	
B. Skin care	Maintain skin integrity
1. Inspect skin daily. Identify high risk areas	
2. Bathe with mild soap (ie, Dove, Dial)	
3. Massage skin gently with lotion paying special attention to bony prominences	
4. Cover absorbent pad (eg, Chux) with towel or sheet if used	
5. Teach client to turn q2h or more frequently. If unable to turn self, implement turning schedule every 2 hours or more frequently as needed	Involve client in own care and provide education
6. While sitting on a chair, teach the client weight shift q1h, or lift client off the chair for 5 sec if unable to do for self	Repositioning allows for normal capillary refill and facilitates adequate circulation
C. Pressure relief: Place client on alternating pressure or fluid-filled or gel mattress for trunk involvement	Alleviate pressure
1. Pull sheet to lift and turn	Alleviate friction and shear.
2. Keep linen loose over air mattress	*Note:* Sheepskin should not be placed under buttock as it increases moisture, resulting in tissue breakdown
3. Use heel and elbow protector pillows for positioning. Use pillows or positioning devices to keep heels off bed	
Stage 1	
A. Skin care—see Stage 0	Maintain skin integrity
B. Pressure relief—see Stage 0	Alleviate pressure
C. Consult: Physical therapy—screening for ROM, mobility, and positioning	Physical therapy screening complements nursing measures to facilitate mobility and pressure relief
D. Cleansing	pH compatible products do not compromise the skin's "acid mantle." Will enhance healing and prevent drying of skin
1. Cleanse affected red areas with pH compatible soap (ie, Periwash, Uniwash)	
2. Massage skin gently with small amount therapeutic concentrated moisturizer that is pH compatible (ie, Sween cream, Uniderm)	
Stage 2	
A. Skin care—see Stage 0	
B. Pressure relief—see Stage 0	
C. Consult—see Stage 1	
1. 24 hr dietary intake Nutritional Consult (R.D.)	Optimal protein intake with positive nitrogen balance is a prerequisite for healing
2. Check weight and compare to ideal body weight. Continue to monitor weight weekly	
D. Request order from physician: Vitamin C, Zinc sulfate, and multivitamins	Vitamin C necessary for collagen formation Zinc sulfate facilitates healing
E. Lab values: Serum protein, albumin levels, CBC	Lower than normal levels of protein and albumin inhibit wound healing. In the presence of increased WBCs, nutritional requirements increase
F. Cleansing—see Stage 1	
G. Wound care	
1. Skin sealant (skin prep) over concentrated moisturizing cream (ie, Sween, Uniderm). Let dry	Increases adhesive capacity of occlusive dressing and seals in cream
2. Thin film polyurethane dressing (flat surfaces) or hydroactive dressing (Duoderm)	Occlusive dressing provides optimal moist environment for healing. (Should be changed only if leaking to avoid bacterial colonization and contamination.)
3. Continually moist normal saline (NS) dressing may also be utilized. NS may be prepared in home. Add 1 tsp salt to 1 qt of water in a closed qt container. Boil	Normal saline is compatible with body fluids

Table 55–2
Nursing Care Plan for the Client With Pressure Ulcer, continued

Intervention	Goal Rationale
in "water bath" 20 min and allow to cool to room temperature 4. Keep blisters intact	
Stage 3	
A. Skin care—see Stage 0 B. Pressure relief—see Stage 0 C. Consult—See Stage 1 (P.T.) See Stage 2 (R.T.)	
Infection Control: Consult individual acute care facility infection control nurse from discharge hospital	Infection control consult enhances treatment protocols and advises on need to isolate
1. Start 24 h intake and output	
2. Check laboratory values—see Stage 2. Add electrolytes, BUN, glucose	Stage 3 lesions are highly secreting and may result in electrolyte imbalance
3. Supplemental feedings (P.O. or enteral tube) may be necessary	Adequate nutritional balance, positive nitrogen status
D. Cleansing Necrotic tissue—irrigate with ¼ strength H_2O_2/NS. Follow with thorough rinse with NS. Clean tissue—irrigate with NS only. Suggest use of 10–12cc syringe with a 20 or 21 gauge needle for irrigation. *Break off needle* at hub & proceed with a forceful irrigation on *necrotic* tissue; *gentle* irrigation on clean tissue. Use of syringe/broken needle easily maintained with *clean* technique. Replace p.r.n.	H_20_2 is a debriding agent. Necrotic tissue must be removed to heal
E. Wound care 1. Necrotic wound: a. Surgical debridement b. Chemical debridement with Elase–Travase–Santyl or Biozyme C. Apply thin layer of enzyme to necrotic tissue only. Protect peri-lesion skin with skin barrier or petroleum product. Use moist NS dressing with fluffed 4 × 4 contact gauze. Change q6–8h	Leukocytes are ineffective in the presence of overwhelming necrotic material. This tends to harbor bacterial material and leads to sepsis For enzymes specific to different types of necrotic material, check literature
c. Dressings—wet to moist dressing. Use contact gauze 4 × 4; open and pack lightly into wound to rid "dead space."	
d. Whirlpool—portable whirlpool may be used for accessible extremities; physical therapy may be necessary for trunk involvement	Whirlpool provides gentle stimulation & helps debride wound. Prolonged use may dehydrate wound and remove new cells
2. Absorption of drainage: Use of wound absorption compounds (ie, Debrisan, Duoderm granules, Bard flakes, fluffed 4 × 4's moistened with NS)	Contain wound exudate, reduce odor and prevent wound dehydration
3. Antimicrobials: Acetic acid 0.5%, Betadine, Dakins solution, H_2O_2	Arrests growth of microorganisms
4. Antibiotics—used only in presence of symptoms and signs of infection (elevated temperature, elevated WBC, positive blood cultures, increased pain and redness, foul odor)	Are specific to certain organisms; check with wound culture and sensitivity
Stage 4	
A. Skin care—see Stage 0	
B. Pressure relief—see Stage 0 Use of Sof • Care® bed cushion, Clinitron, Mediscus or other bed if available.	Clients with impaired movement may need increased pressure relief offered by these beds. Use of these beds may be restricted by insurance coverage
C. Cleansing—see Stage 3	

(continued)

Table 55–2
Nursing Care Plan for the Client With Pressure Ulcer, continued

Intervention	Goal Rationale
D. Consult: 1. Physical therapy—see Stage 1 2. Nutritional—see Stage 2 3. Infection control—see Stage 3	
E. Wound care	
1. Protective skin sealant (ie, Skin prep) applied to peri-lesion. May be necessary to also apply Gelatin skin barrier (Stomahesive) to intact skin	Stage 4 lesions may be highly secreting and cause further skin deterioration. It is essential to protect peri-lesion skin
2. Low grade suction and pouching p.r.n. to collect and quantitate exudate	

SOURCE: Courtesy of Barbara Oot–Giromini, RN, ET. Lourdes Hospital, Binghamton, NY.

or an allergic sensitizer. Primary irritants are external or exogenous agents that cause an immediate inflammatory reaction when direct contact is made with the integument. Examples include chemicals, clothing, shoes, rubber, metals (nickel), dyes, preservatives, plants, solvents, topical medications, soaps, insect sprays, industrial oils, perfumes, cosmetics, and toiletries.

Allergic sensitizers involve a cell-mediated reaction that results in a delayed hypersensitivity response. Lymphocytes, specifically the T-cells, become sensitized when contact is made with allergens such as poison ivy or poison oak. An initial response may develop within 5 to 21 days, or a latent period may occur. Upon subsequent exposure, skin eruptions appear within 12 to 48 hours, depending on the potency of the allergen, duration of exposure, permeability of the skin, and the development of immunity.

Certain topical and systemic medications are known to be sensitizing agents and therefore, should be prescribed and used with caution. Unfortunately, some of the products may be sold over the counter, and the user may not be aware of the precautions. One such drug is benzocaine, a substance found in hundreds of compounds and used to produce local anesthesia. Neomycin and ethylenediamine are also common sensitizers. Ethylenediamine is a component of frequently used medications such as aminophylline and hydroxyzine hydrochloride (Vistaril, Atarax). Some antihistamines must be monitored for their own cutaneous side effects even though they may be ordered for allergic responses that involve skin manifestations. A client who is receiving diphenhydramine (Benadryl) and tripelennamine hydrochloride (Pyribenzamine) may develop urticaria, whereas use of promethazine (Phenergan) may evoke photosensitivity. A pharmacology textbook will give an extensive list of drugs that may cause sensitization.

Clinical Manifestations

Generally, the client will complain of pruritus (which varies in intensity), pain, and burning. Mild reactions will display erythema, microvesicles, and oozing. In an acute contact dermatitis, the degree of redness increases, and lesions may progress to the size of bullae, become eroded, or develop into ulcerations. The extent of the cutaneous lesion may be localized to the exact area of contact or generalized if an allergen was internalized. Edema in various parts of the body may become evident, as well as signs of systemic involvement (fever, general malaise, weakness).

Chronic exposure to irritants and allergens causes areas of skin to redden, dry, scale, lichenify, fissure, and at times to become hypopigmented and hyperpigmented (Figure 55–6).

Medical Measures

The primary objective in all cases is to identify and remove the irritant or allergen. Acute contact dermatitis may take several weeks to resolve and may require rest along with the prescribed therapeutic measures. Wet dressings soaked with aluminum acetate (Burow's) solution may be applied several times a day until vesiculation and oozing cease. Corticosteroids may be given systemically using prednisone, triamcinolone, or betamethasone if the allergic response or inflammation is severe; otherwise, topical application of fluocinonide, triamcinolone, or fluocinolone is started when vesicles have disappeared. Balneotherapy using Aveeno baths to soothe and protect the skin may be ordered if the problem is generalized and severe. Antibiotics may be necessary to combat any superimposed infection.

In chronic conditions, the application of a nonwater-soluble emollient (petrolatum) is used to prevent dryness and soften the skin, possibly in conjunction with topical corticosteroid ointments. Medical supervision may be required for a lengthy period of time to control the manifestations.

Specific Nursing Measures

Care of the client with contact dermatitis, beyond the prescribed medicinal treatment of the lesions and subjective symptoms, should center on teaching of preventive

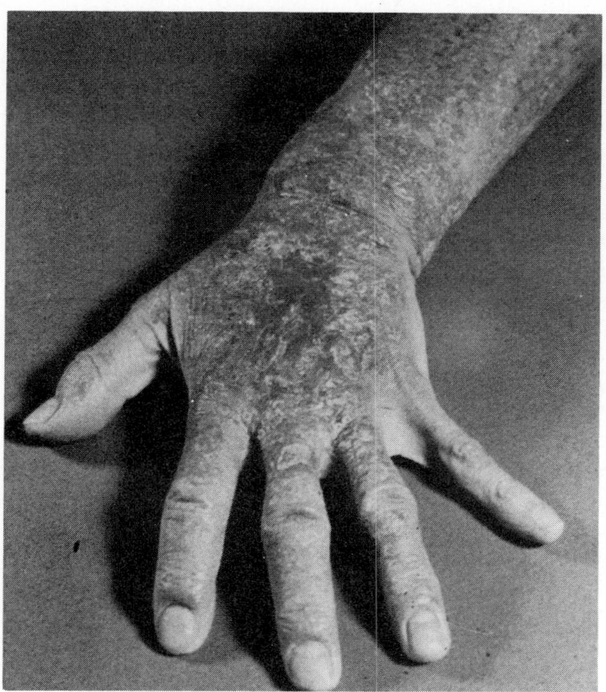

Figure 55–6

Contact dermatitis. *Courtesy of Millard Fillmore Hospital, Buffalo, NY.*

measures. The goal will be to increase the knowledge base so that the client can directly control his or her skin integrity. Specific points to be included in the instructions to the client are listed in Box 55–1.

A concern that may have to be addressed involves contagion. Clients should be made aware that contact dermatitis is not transmissible, not even with poison ivy or poison oak, unless the oils of the plant are still on the skin or clothing.

Atopic Dermatitis

Atopic dermatitis is a common pruritic inflammatory dermatosis seen most often as a chronic, recurring problem in persons with a hereditary predisposition toward allergy. Although this disorder usually appears first during infancy or childhood, it often extends into adolescence and adulthood.

Atopic dermatitis has been attributed to an immunologic defect because a significant percentage of clients have a personal or family history of allergic disease such as hay fever, asthma, and allergic rhinitis.

Attacks of atopic dermatitis may be set off or made worse by several factors. An episode of pruritus may develop from irritating or occlusive topical medications, items of clothing such as wool or silk, rapid changes or extremes in temperature, or too much bathing. Approximately 10% of the clients with atopic dermatitis respond allergically to foods, inhalation of allergens, and direct contact with irritants. Emotional stress is a key factor known to precipitate symptom recurrence.

Clinical Manifestations

No distinct primary lesions may be apparent in adulthood. The skin is usually markedly dry and contains papular lichenified plaques, excoriations, erosions, and crusts. Areas of involvement include cubital and popliteal fossae, anterior and lateral aspects of the neck, forehead, face, wrists, and dorsa of the hands and feet. Hand dermatitis is common.

The most outstanding feature in atopic dermatitis is the presence of intense pruritus. A cycle develops, in which the client feels an itch, scratches it, a rash develops, and the rash itches. Lichenification, which results from repeated rubbing and scratching over an extended period, further reduces the skin's threshold to withstand irritation, and the cycle becomes more permanent.

Lesions are vulnerable to invasion by microorganisms. Bacterial infections from staphylococci and streptococci are likely, as is contamination by the herpes simplex virus.

Medical Measures

Treatment aims at eliminating precipitating factors and pruritus, suppressing the inflammatory process, lubricating the skin, and providing essential emotional support.

The mainstay of treatment for atopic dermatitis is the use of topical corticosteroids. Fluorinated corticosteroids may be used short term to initiate healing, but replacement by other anti-inflammatory agents is important to avoid untoward skin changes. Ointments and occlusive therapy are preferred because penetration is faster. Because of keratolytic actions, coal tar preparations may be used as adjuvant therapy along with the corticosteroids.

Box 55–1
Home Health Care Instructions for the Client With Contact Dermatitis

- Limit exposure to household or occupational irritants if possible
- Wear protective clothing or gloves when contact cannot be avoided
- Wash new clothing and bed linens before use
- Avoid clothing made from synthetics known to cause irritation and wear as many natural fabrics as possible
- Avoid any natural fabrics such as wool or silk if they are allergens
- Use hypoallergenic cosmetics, jewelry, etc.
- Avoid abrasive soaps
- Lubricate skin to prevent cracking
- Wear protective creams
- Become aware of drugs known to cause sensitization, and monitor contents of any medication being used
- Wash skin and clothing thoroughly after exposure to allergens

Antibiotic therapy is used whenever the presence of bacteria is confirmed. Wet dressings are prescribed when a draining lesion appears. Ultraviolet light has beneficial effects and may be used judiciously.

Dealing with the pruritus that accompanies atopic dermatitis may be difficult and may require a multidimensional approach to both physiologic and psychologic factors. Covering the affected areas has no value, and lesions often appear beyond the borders of the dressing. Emollients (petrolatum, Eucerin, Nivea) can lessen the dryness. Antihistamines such as hydroxyzine hydrochloride (Atarax, Vistaril) may be incorporated into the regimen, although the benefits are limited. Because of the effects of prostaglandin, a pathogenic factor in itching, acetylsalicylic acid (aspirin) may be administered on a full dosage scale (300–600 mg daily with increases to just below the level causing tinnitus).

Tranquilizers and sedatives may be prescribed to assist in the alleviation of psychic stress or emotional factors influencing the dermatosis. If drugs and normal emotional supports do not resolve problems, further professional counseling may be required to decondition the learned pattern of response to the pathologic cycle or to assist the client in recognizing and coping with emotional stressors.

Specific Nursing Measures

The instructions in Box 55–2 will facilitate the client's understanding and ability to prevent recurrence and complications. Clients with atopic dermatitis may need hospitalization to disrupt the pruritus or when self-care is not feasible.

Box 55–2
Home Health Care Instructions for the Client With Atopic Dermatitis

- Provide a climate and humidity-controlled environment to avoid overwarming, chilling, sweating, and excessive dryness
- Wear clothing that is absorbent and nonirritating
- Launder clothing with bland soaps
- Rest and relax
- Avoid excessive bathing and use of irritating soaps
- Avoid known allergens or sensitizers, especially topical anesthetics or antihistamines
- Protect skin from secondary infection
- Avoid vaccinations or contact with persons who have been vaccinated (Kaposi's varicelliform eruptions, a viral disease, may develop.)
- Avoid contact with persons who have herpetic lesions (Disseminated eruptions may occur from self-inoculation.)
- Practice stress management techniques

Supportive care is important because problems with atopic dermatitis may extend through a lifetime. There may be an inability to respond pleasurably to touch or to accept the appearance of the body. Sometimes people become preoccupied with their skin disorder or the potential for exacerbation. The appearance of skin manifestations may have affected occupation, finances, leisure activities, and interpersonal relationships. Identifying the needs and feelings of each client is important before adaptability can be fostered.

Drug Eruptions

The skin is frequently affected by adverse drug reactions. A cause for the cutaneous eruptions is basically unknown, but allergy, pharmacologic factors (overdosage, drug interactions), and unexplained idiosyncracies are considered possibilities.

Clinical Manifestations

Lesions may occur immediately after taking the drug or be delayed for several days. Initially, the reaction may begin in a localized area and progress to a generalized state, in which the total surface of the body is involved.

In addition to anaphylaxis, serious and life-threatening situations can develop in which multiple bullous lesions appear, although this is rare. Toxic epidermal necrolysis, in which the full thickness of the epidermis is detached, and exfoliative dermatitis, a generalized scaling eruption, are also major untoward effects. Table 55–3 lists selected cutaneous manifestations and the drugs known to produce these adverse reactions.

Medical and Specific Nursing Measures

The drug or drugs responsible for the eruptions must be discontinued. Administration of antihistamines is the other important component of therapy. Hydroxyzine hydrochloride (Atarax, Vistaril), chlorpheniramine maleate (Chlor-Trimeton), cyproheptadine hydrochloride (Periactin), or diphenhydramine hydrochloride (Benadryl) may be prescribed. Colloidal or tepid baths, cool or ice water compresses, and antipruritic lotions or emulsions (calamine) may be used to treat subjective complaints. If serious damage and losses of the integument occur, the focus of concern becomes preventing fluid and electrolyte loss, infection, and major metabolic alteration.

A careful history of drug allergies and idiosyncrasies elicited upon admission and clearly noted on the client's chart is an important preventive tool. The following questions should be answered: Have you ever developed any allergic reactions when using prescribed or over-the-counter drugs? Were they taken orally; used topically; or admin-

Table 55–3
Adverse Cutaneous Manifestations Associated With Drug Therapy

Cutaneous Manifestations	Drugs
Acneiform	ACTH Androgenic hormones Diphenylhydantoin Glucocorticoids Lithium
Alopecia	Coumarin derivatives Cytotoxics
Bullae	Barbiturates Bromides Iodides Phenylbutazone Sulfonamides
Exanthema (rash resembling measles or scarlet fever)	Allopurinol Para-aminosalicylic acid Penicillins and related antibiotics
Fixed drug reactions (circumscribed hyperpigmented or purplish-red lesions, macular to bullous, which recur at the same site with each readministration)	Barbiturates Phenolphthalein Phenylbutazone Sulfonamides
Photosensitivity	Chlorothiazides Demeclocycline Phenothiazines Psoralens Sulfonamides Sulfonylureas
Purpura	Indomethacin Phenylbutazone Quinidine
Urticaria (most common)	Acetylsalicylic acid Blood and blood products Codeine Diazepam Morphine Penicillins and related antibiotics Radiopaque media Serum Sulfonamides

istered by injection, inhalation, instillation, or suppository? What kind of reaction did you have? Can you describe the skin changes? If the allergic response occurred during the client's hospitalization, a list of drugs received on a routine, stat, or p.r.n. basis must be identified in addition to any anesthetic and diagnostic agents.

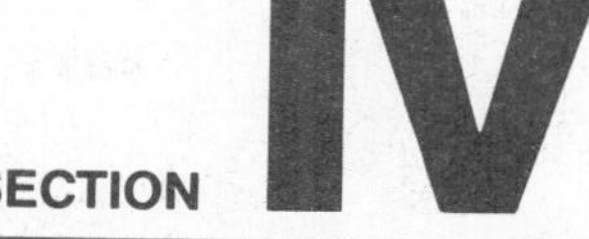

SECTION IV

Infections and Infestations

Specific Nursing Measures for Bacterial Skin Infections

The normal skin is inhabited by gram-positive cocci, primarily staphylococci *(S epidermidis, S albus)* and gram-positive diphtheroids or bacilli *(Corynebacterium acnes, Propionibacterium acnes)*. Gram-negative bacteria *(E coli, Proteus, Enterobacter, Pseudomonas)* are not commonly found on the skin surface except in the warm, moist intertrigenous areas. Most pyodermas are caused by staphylococci and a few by streptococci. These bacteria may penetrate as deep as the subcutaneous tissue (Figure 55–7). Specific bacterial skin infections and their incidence, causative agent, manifestations, duration, and treatment measures are described in Table 55–4.

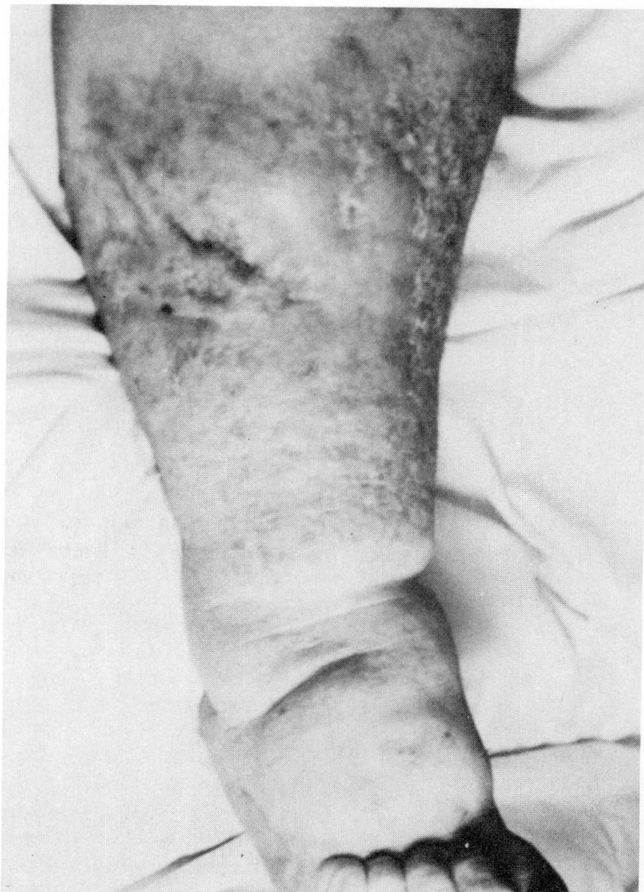

Figure 55–7

Cellulitis. *Courtesy of Millard Fillmore Hospital, Buffalo, NY.*

Table 55–4
Skin Infections and Infestations

Condition and Causative Agent	Incidence/Comments	Clinical Manifestations	Treatment Measures
Bacterial skin infections			
Carbuncle *(Staphylococcus)*	Collection of furuncles; commonly seen in thick inelastic skin	Similar to furuncles but with multiple points of drainage; usually appear on neck, back, and thighs; very painful; systemic signs such as fever, malaise; heal slowly and produce scarring	Similar to furuncles; surgical incision only if absolutely necessary
Cellulitis (gram-positive bacillus: *Streptococcus, Staphylococcus)*; (gram-negative bacillus: *Escherichia coli, Proteus, Klebsiella*)	Deep subcutaneous tissue involvement; usually a complication of ulcerations, decubiti, wounds, dermatitis	Dependent on causative organism; extensive erythema and tenderness with gram-positive; warmth and slight redness, brawny edema (increasing as infection progresses) with gram-negative; malaise, fever, chills, enlarged lymph nodes	Bed rest; systemic antibiotic specific for causative organism; surgical drainage; treatment of primary disease
Erysipelas (beta hemolytic *Streptococcus*)	Acute highly inflammatory infection involving subcutaneous tissue; uncommon; occurs in very young and elderly	Bright red, tender, hot, sharply defined bordered plaque, which may develop superficial vesicles and bullae; usually seen on face and around the ears; pain at the site of infection; lasts for 2–3 wks; recurrence common	Bed rest; oral or parenteral antibiotics (penicillin, erythromycin); local cool, wet dressing for comfort
Folliculitis *(Staphylococcus)*	Common infection of hair follicles; serious implications with scalp, nasal, and eye involvement	Superficial or deep pustules may be scattered or discrete; frequently seen on the face; also appears on trunk and extremities; pain; self-limited	Topical hygiene and antibiotics; remove predisposing factors (oils, tar)
Furuncle *(Staphylococcus)*	Deep follicular abscess; may have progressed from folliculitis; commonly found on hair-bearing skin where friction and sweating occur; seen in children, adolescents, and young adults	Firm, red, hard nodule that ruptures and discharges a purulent core; may ulcerate; usually seen on face, scalp, neck, buttocks, and axilla; highly tender and may cause throbbing pain; lasts for days	Moist heat; topical or systemic antibiotics sensitive to *Staphylococcus* (penicillin, erythromycin); recurrence may require long-term therapy and consideration for bacterial interference therapy
Impetigo (group A *Streptococcus, Staphylococcus*, or mixed)	Very common and contagious; seen primarily in children and young adults; approximately 5% of cases may be complicated by poststreptococcal glomerulonephritis	Erythematous macules, oozing vesicles; usually seen on face, arms, and legs; varying degrees of pruritus; lasts for days	Penicillin (long acting or divided doses); oxacillin for staphylococcal infection; erythromycin soak 3–4 times a day with warm water, saline, or soap solution to remove crusts
Viral skin infections			
Herpes simplex type 1 (cold sores, fever blisters, canker sores caused by *Herpesvirus hominis*)	Common disorder; primary infection occurs in young children; recurrence usually associated with adults; frequently seen in women; her-	Clusters of vesicles or vesicopustules on an erythematous base; may ulcerate or crust; appears on lips near mucocutaneous junction, cheek; burning, itching, tingling may develop; last 5–8 days; recurrent	Symptomatic treatment because of self-limiting nature; keep lesions dry (70% alcohol, Blistex); topical antibiotic; topical anesthetic

Condition and Causative Agent	Incidence/Comments	Clinical Manifestations	Treatment Measures
	pesencephalitis is a possible complication		
Herpes zoster (shingles) caused by activation of latent varicella-zoster virus	Majority over age 40; initially infected with varicella virus (chickenpox); organism resides in dorsal root of cranial and spinal nerve ganglia; 50% of clients develop ophthalmic involvement	Erythematous papules that progress into vesicles, pustules, and crusts; seen unilaterally, primarily on dermatomes of the thorax and less frequently in cervical, trigeminal, and lumbosacral areas; pain along the course of a peripheral sensory nerve can precede the eruptions; postherpetic neuralgia; lasts approximately 3 wks	Symptomatic treatment with analgesics; for vesicular stage use cool compresses with Burow's solution, drying lotion, splinting of area with dressing to relieve pain; systemic corticosteroids in selected acute cases; ophthalmic corticosteroids with keratoconjunctivitis involvement; immunosuppressed clients may receive cytosine arabinoside, interferon, acyclovir, zoster immune globulin (ZIG)
Herpetic whitlow or inoculation herpes (caused by *Herpesvirus hominis*)	Primary or recurrent; occurs on damaged or broken skin (burns, needle punctures, often seen in health personnel who come in contact with oral secretions or lesions of infected clients	Lesions of fingers, paronychia, and hands; erythema and edema develop with multiple discrete vesicles at the margins of the lesion; tingling sensation followed by intense, throbbing pain; lymphadenopathy and lymphangitis; possibility of fever, chills, and malaise; last 3–4 wks; recurrence possible	Analgesics for pain; topical acyclovir (Zovirax)
Verrucae (warts) caused by human papilloma virus	Benign epidermal tumors; spread by contact or autoinoculation	All warts manifest a local epidermal proliferation and keratinization; many warts are self-limiting to within a few weeks, months or years because of spontaneous involution	Common keratolytic therapy; painting of lesions with salicylic acid and lactic acid mixtures (SAL, Duofilm, Keralyt); cryosurgery; light electrosurgery; avoid treatment that scars; immunotherapy less common but used with resistive lesions (DNCB application); topical or oral vitamin A; topical 5-flourouracil; intralesional bleomycin
a. V. vulgaris (common wart)		Firm papules; hyperkeratotic surface with vegetation; isolated or clustered on hands, fingers, knees	
b. V. plantaris (plantar or palmar wart)	Often follows trauma	Small papules and plaques with a rough, hyperkeratotic surface; isolated; many (mosaic pattern) at pressure points, particularly on feet; may become painful	
c. V. planae (flat wart)		Flat-surfaced papules, usually numerous, closely set on face, dorsa of hand, shins, or knees	
Fungal skin infections			
Tinea (ringworm) caused by *Microsporum, Trichophyton, Epidermophyton*		All tinea infections involve an inflammatory process; pain and itching may be present; all, except those involving the nails, are of short duration when adequate treatment is given	Hygienic measures; topical antifungal solutions or creams treat most superficial fungal infections of the skin: clotrimazole (Lotrimin); miconazole (Monistat-Derm); haloprogin (Halotex); tol-

(continued)

Table 55–4
Skin Infections and Infestations (continued)

Condition and Causative Agent	Incidence/Comments	Clinical Manifestations	Treatment Measures
			naftate (Tinactin); may be combined with a keratolytic agent to soften and exfoliate skin; systemic griseofulvin for widespread or rapidly progressing infection, recalcitrant (hair, nails), or recurrent lesions
a. T. capitis (scalp)	Rare after puberty; highly contagious	Scaling patches with hair loss or breaking of the shafts	
b. T. barbae (beard)	Rare; seen in adult men, such as farmers in contact with contaminated cattle	Sharp scaling, loss of hair; kerion formation (inflamed purulent lesion) in a deeper infection	
c. T. cruris (groin)	Very common, mainly in men; may occur concomitantly with T. pedis	Scaly patches or plaques, usually symmetrical; may extend into gluteal folds and buttocks	
d. T. manuum (hands)	Usually seen with T. pedis and onychomycosis	Unilateral mild erythema with hyperkeratosis and scaling on palmar surface	
e. T. pedis (athlete's foot)	Most common fungal infection; generally seen in adults	Scaling, maceration, and fissures of toe webs; occasional vesicles and bullae; secondary bacterial infection; recurrent	
f. T. onychomycosis (nails)	40% of cases have fungal infection elsewhere	Whitish discoloration and thickening of nail plate with possible separation from nail bed; difficult to cure	
g. T. versicolor; caused by *Pityrosporon furfur*	Represents 5% of all fungal infection; common to young adults, usually in summer months	Lesions varying in color (white, pinkish-brown); macular scaling patches usually found on trunk and upper arms; light and dark pigmentary changes; recurrent; untreated conditions last for years	Wide range of treatment; topical application to affected areas with selenium sulfide (Selsun), 25% sodium hyposulfite, keratolytic creams (Keralyt Gel), imidazole creams and lotions (Lotrimin, Monistat-Derm, Halotex, Tinactin); hygienic measures
Candidiasis caused by *Candida albicans*			
a. Monilial paronychia (skin surrounding nails)	Occurs often in housewives from frequent water immersion of hands	Painful swelling around nail plate	Gloves and cotton liner to protect hands; wet Burow's solution soaks for inflammation
b. Monilial intertrigo	Common	Pruritus, burning; red eroded patches with axillary, inframammary, umbilical, anogenital, or interdigital involvement	Topical antifungal agents; amphotericin B (Fungizone); nystatin (Mycostatin)
c. Perlèche (may also be caused by streptococci or staphylococci)	A form of cheilosis	Cracks or erythematous fissures at corners of mouth	Carbol-fuchsin solution (Castellani's paint)

Condition and Causative Agent	Incidence/Comments	Clinical Manifestations	Treatment Measures
Skin Infestations			
Pediculosis (lice infestation)	Incidence has increased. Life cycle: Adult female lives approximately 1 month, laying up to 10 eggs daily; incubation 7–9 days; grows to adult louse in 1 wk	Extreme pruritus	Shampoos or topical application of pesticide (Kwell, Gamene), pyrethrins (RID Liquid)
a. Pediculosis corporis (body) caused by *Pediculus humanus corporis*		Scratch marks; eczematous changes; reddened papules	
b. Pediculosis capitis (head) caused by *Pediculus humanis capitis*		Ova (nits) visible on hairs, above ears	After treatment, use fine-tooth comb to remove nits and dead lice
c. Pediculosis pubis (genital) caused by *Phthirus pubis*	Frequently coexists with other sexually transmitted diseases	Ova visible on pubic and thigh hairs; difficult to locate insect on skin; may be in seams of clothing	
Scabies (mites) caused by *Sarcoptes scabiei*	Children, young adults; epidemics in a 30-yr cycle, the latest occurring in the 1970s; associated with skin-to-skin contact and with crowded and poor living conditions, sexual intimacy, or a nosocomial outbreak. Life cycle: Female mite excavates into skin for 1–2 months laying 10–25 eggs; incubation 3 wks	Ridges, small linear threadlike lines; characteristic burrows; possible vesicles, nodules, or secondary infections; lesions appear on hands (interdigital webs), wrists, axillary folds, penis, scrotum, buttocks, nipples, abdomen; intense pruritus, especially when skin increases in warmth (eg, while sleeping)	Bathe or shower and apply the pesticide gamma benzene hexachloride cream or lotion (Kwell, Gamene) to entire skin from neck down for 8–12 h, then bathe; repeat application in another week; apply crotamiton (Eurax), scabicide and antipruritic agent; apply 5%–10% precipitated sulfur; antipruritics
Tick bite from Argasidae (soft-bodied ticks) and ixodidae (hard-bodied ticks)	Large mites attach to human skin and engorge on blood; transmit several rickettsial and viral diseases. Tick may drop off spontaneously; lesions persis 1–2 wks	Pruritus after several days of attachment; presence of tick may resemble wart or vascular tumor; bite appears as a small nodule surrounded by a necrotic ring; fever, headache, abdominal pain, malaise occur from secreted toxins from female tick; granulomas may form.	Ensure removal of entire tick; remove by touching with a hot nail, extinguished match head or applying a few dops of chloroform, gasoline, or turpentine

A plan of care involves preventive measures as well as therapy to prevent recurrence and to protect others. Staphylococci colonize more readily in moist cutaneous lesions; therefore, maintenance of dry skin is an important nursing consideration. Contagion is associated with impetigo, and contamination of other family members is not uncommon. Removing crusts associated with impetigo is critical because beta hemolytic organisms thrive under semiaerobic conditions.

Home Health Care

Bacteria may arrive on the skin from sites that normally harbor potential pathogens, such as the upper airways. Antibiotic creams or ointments may be instilled into the anterior nares daily until the problem is resolved. Hygiene is important so bathing and shampooing with bactericidal (providone–iodine) or bacteriostatic (hexachlorophene) soaps are necessary, especially for family members who may have direct contact with the infected person or may be at high risk because of immunosuppression or breaks in the continuity of the skin.

Use of separate towels, washcloths, and bed linens and daily laundering are recommended. Handkerchiefs should be replaced by disposable paper tissues. Because those who work with oils and greases show an increased incidence of follicular infections, they should be informed that drying of the skin and avoidance of irritating and occlusive clothing may help avoid problems.

Specific Nursing Measures for Viral Skin Infections

Cutaneous viral infection develops below the stratum corneum and depends on the ability of the virus to adapt within the host cell. If the virus interferes with normal cellular structure and function, a local inflammatory process along with the formation of lesions and cell destruction may develop. The disorder need not become manifest and could remain latent if the organism is not sufficiently virulent to produce pathologic alterations in the host cells. Viral skin infections, their incidence, causative agent, clinical manifestations, duration, and treatment measures are discussed in Table 55–3.

Contagion is a prime nursing concern with viral skin infections. Protective efforts become critical when a client has a medical disorder or is receiving drugs that interfere seriously with the immune response. Prevention of contact is essential because exposure to infected individuals may prove life threatening, particularly to immunocompromised persons.

Inoculation herpes (herpetic whitlow) should be a concern for dental, medical, and nursing personnel because herpetic lesions may develop through direct hand or finger contact with the vesicular fluid of the area of involvement or by contamination from oral—pharyngeal—tracheal secretions. Use of gloves is recommended when caring for or treating clients with suspected lesions or those who have a potential to develop herpetic lesions.

Prevention of recurring herpes simplex should be incorporated into a treatment plan. Emotional stress, exposure to sunlight, illness, menstruation, and fatigue have been identified as precipitating factors. Proper use of sunscreens and maintenance of healthful living are basic to avoidance of recurrence.

With increased frequency, herpes zoster (Figure 55–8) is being complicated by postherpetic neuralgia in the elderly. Pain becomes chronic and difficult to alleviate. Use of antipsychotic drugs and transcutaneous electrical stimulators may be necessary in severe cases.

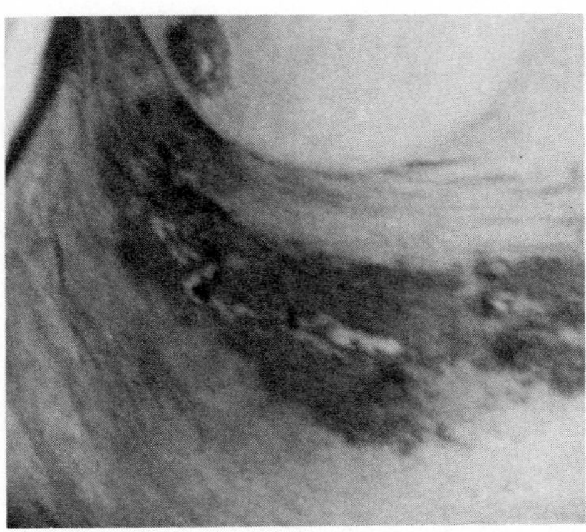

Figure 55–8

Herpes zoster showing distribution along nerve. *Courtesy of Millard Fillmore Hospital, Buffalo, NY.*

Plantar warts are known to occur more readily on surface areas that are moist and sustain friction. The importance of drying the feet and cushioning these areas should be stressed. Many people apply keratolytic agents to warts with or without the direction of a health care provider. Drugs that destroy cutaneous lesions may also be injurious to healthy skin, and users need to know this. Instruct clients to protect the surrounding skin with petroleum jelly and to make sure that a small amount of the keratolytic has been applied to the lesion only.

Specific Nursing Measures for Fungal Skin Infections

Superficial mycoses or fungal infections of the skin are among the most common types of dermatoses. Mycoses are caused by vegetative cellular organisms known as *dermatophytes,* which can survive on the dead horny layers of the skin and some of the appendages such as the nails (Figure 55–9). Because of strong host resistance in a healthy integument, the overall incidence of fungal infection is kept relatively low.

Predisposing factors include a hot and humid environment that allows unaerated skin surfaces to become excessively moist; macerated skin from occlusive dressings or clothing; systemic use of antibiotics, corticosteroids, or contraceptives; pregnancy; diabetes, Cushing's disease; and poor general health. Fungal skin infections, their incidence, causative agent, clinical manifestations, duration, and treatment measures are discussed in Table 55–4.

Prophylactic measures are the first line of defense against fungal infections and become more important when

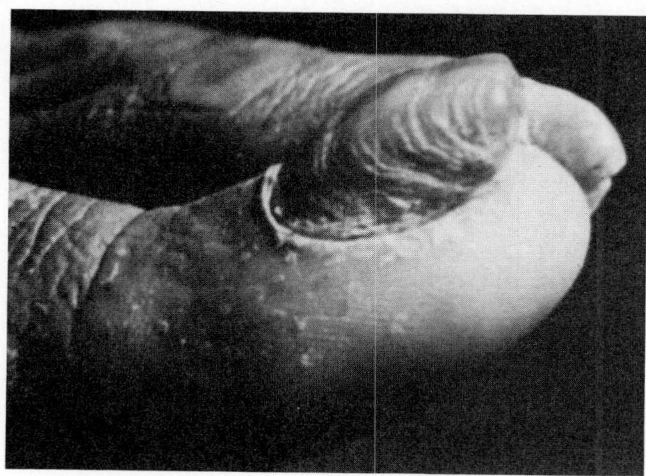

Figure 55–9

Fungal infection of the toenail (onychomycosis). The nail is thick, ridged, and brown. *Courtesy of Millard Fillmore Hospital, Buffalo, NY.*

the predisposing factors are numerous. Intertriginous and interdigital areas must be kept clean and dry. Bathing and application of a simple talc or antifungal powder at least once a day may prevent initial irritation. Shoes and clothing should allow for proper aeration and not build up moisture as plastic footwear, sneakers, wool, and synthetic fibers do. Advise clients to wear nonocclusive shoes and absorbent socks, preferably made of cotton. Wool socks worn by hikers and skiers tend to trap moisture. Frequent changes of apparel along with proper laundering in hot water are also important.

Use of griseofulvin (Fulvicin-U/F, Grifulven V), a fungistatic and fungicidal antibiotic, has been effective in the treatment of dermatophytes, especially when topical antifungals fail to resolve the condition. Although griseofulvin is used to treat tineal infections, onychomycosis is rarely cured by this drug or other therapy. Several cutaneous fungal infections have a tendency to recur. Clients should understand their role in prevention and continuance of prescribed care.

Specific Nursing Measures for Parasitic Infestations

Dermatologic parasites are an extensive problem around the world because of bites and skin invasion by protozoans, helminths, and arthropods. The focus in this discussion will be on scabies, pediculosis, and tick bites because they are a common cause of dermatologic problems. The parasitic skin infestations, their incidence, causative agents, clinical manifestations, duration, and treatment measures are discussed in Table 55–4.

As much as possible, transmission of pediculoses and scabies must be halted once the problem has been identified. Pesticides must be used to destroy the parasites. In addition, clothing, bed linens, and toweling require washing in boiling water, dry cleaning, ironing, or dusting with appropriate pesticides to prevent reinfestation from parasites and their ova. Those who have come in intimate contact with an infested client or who share clothing, hair brushes, combs, or bed linens may need treatment as well.

Protection against ticks may be obtained by applying insect repellents containing diethyltoluamide (Mosquitone lotion, Off liquid, Cutter Insect Repellent Cream) to skin and clothing. Wearing protective clothing in wooded areas is also a preventive measure. Proper removal of ticks is discussed in Table 55–4.

SECTION V

Neoplasia

The abnormal proliferation of cells within the various layers of skin is a common dermatologic problem. Many integumentary lesions are benign, with a few classified as precancerous. The three major types of malignancies originate either in the epidermal layer of skin or the melanocyte.

Skin cancer is the most frequent malignancy estimated at more than 500,000 new cases per year (American Cancer Society, 1987). Malignant melanoma is expected to account for 26,000 of these cases. Although the mortality is minimal compared to the death rate from primary tumors of other organs, and the systemic involvement is proportionately limited, the lesions cause their own set of physiologic and psychosocial stressors. Malignancies of the skin increase with age and are the most common dermatosis that bring the elderly to the dermatologist. Adults should practice skin self-examination once a month because early detection is critical.

Seborrheic Keratosis

Seborrheic keratosis is a common benign epidermal growth of keratinocytes and melanocytes and is most frequent in persons over 40. Aging skin characteristically contains an isolated lesion or several scattered lesions.

Seborrheic keratoses are genetically transmitted as an autosomal dominant trait. Individuals with oily acne or seborrheic-type skin may also be more likely to develop these lesions. Heavily pigmented people have a low incidence of occurrence.

Clinical Manifestations

The growth initially appears as a small, slightly elevated papule or plaque, possibly containing some pigmentation. Enlargement takes place slowly with the surface becoming rough or warty. Color varies from yellow to brown or may even be black. Keratotic lesions generally appear on the face, scalp, trunk, and upper extremities. The most common complaint involves cosmetic disfigurement.

Medical Measures

Simple curettage provides the easiest removal and causes the least cosmetic defect. Electrodesiccation also allows for easy removal but may result in minor scarring. Ethyl chloride, carbon dioxide, or liquid nitrogen may be used to freeze the lesions and facilitate easier scraping or allow sloughing.

Keloids/Hypertrophic Scarring

A **keloid** is a benign proliferative growth of fibrous tissue at the site of an injury or incision that extends beyond the confines of the wound. Hypertrophic scarring, which is the more common scarring problem, results in a much smaller dermal lesion. Both lesions represent a disequilibrium between the anabolic and catabolic phases of wound healing. A normal balance is usually reached at about 3 to 4 weeks after the injury. With abnormal scar formation, collagen is produced faster than it can be assimilated into the wound.

Although the basic etiology is unknown, the increased production of connective tissue has shown a correlation with trauma, a higher degree of inflammation, and infection. Wounds with excessive or poorly aligned tension because of location or suturing, burns, and the introduction of foreign substances into the skin are also considered to be some of the provocative factors. Young adults, particularly blacks and others with highly pigmented skin, show a predisposition for keloids and hypertrophic scarring.

Clinical Manifestations

Hypertrophic scars appear to correspond in size and shape to the underlying wound but become more raised, wider and thicker than anticipated, and remain reddened. Keloids may take several months to extend beyond the hypertrophic stage and develop into larger, smooth, hard, irregularly shaped, hyperpigmented lesions. The presternum, shoulders, upper back, lower legs, head, and neck are the most frequent areas of involvement. Problems may also develop in ear lobes following piercing for cosmetic purposes. Both types of lesions usually cause minimal sensory effects, although pruritus and pain may be noted on occasion with keloid formation. Both keloids and hypertrophic scars are illustrated in Figure 12–4 in Chapter 12.

Medical Measures

Treatment of lesions may result in additional problems with cellular proliferation, especially when simple surgical excision is used. The most important therapeutic step for persons at high risk is to avoid injury or incisions that would stimulate unchecked cell growth. When surgery must be performed, problems are less apt to develop in early childhood or in late adulthood. When surgery is necessary in a high-risk period, the direction of a scar may be changed by use of a Z- or Y-shaped incision line to reduce tension.

Hypertrophic scars may resolve spontaneously within 1 year of formation. Intralesional injections with corticosteroids (such as triamcinolone acetate or diacetate), coupled with cryosurgery, have been recommended. Precautions must be taken to deter atrophy, telangiectasia, and depigmentation of healthy tissue when intralesional steroids are used. A combination of x-ray therapy and surgical excision may be elected for large keloids. Pressure dressings and garments (see Figure 12–8 in Chapter 12 for an example) have been helpful; the continuous force can prevent collagen fibers from abnormal development.

Epithelial Cyst

Several types of cystic lesions may develop within the various layers of the skin; they consist of a sac or capsule that contains lipid and keratinous materials. Although the more common growths may be termed *sebaceous cysts,* the actual histologic classification further identifies the lesions as epidermoid or pilar cysts (wens). They have an unknown etiology. *Milia* are firm, pinhead-sized, asymptomatic, white globular lesions that develop spontaneously after trauma to the skin (burns, incisions, dermabrasion) or following dermatosis. They are normal in newborns. *Dermoid cysts* occur in the subcutaneous tissue and are congenital, originating from embryonic tissue. Besides epithelial cells and cutaneous appendages, dermoid cysts may also contain bone and cartilage.

Clinical Manifestations

Sebaceous cysts appear to be globular, elevated, and firm. Lesions may range from 0.2 to 5 cm, and any enlargement may be attributed to an increase in soft, yellow-white material that fills the sac. These cysts commonly appear on the scalp, face, neck, and back. Milia, in addition to forming in traumatized areas, also appear around the eyes and on the forehead. Dermoid cysts have more diversified locations and may develop at the lateral ends of the eyebrows; sublingually; on the neck; and in the sternal, perineal, scrotal, and sacral areas. These cysts grow as large as 10 cm.

Medical Measures

Complete surgical excision is the treatment of choice. Regrowth may be possible in some cases if the cystic capsule is not entirely removed. Milia and small cysts may be treated by simple incision and expression of the contents.

Lipoma

Lipomas, common benign tumors generally encapsulated in the subcutaneous layer of skin, are composed of adipose tissue. An individual may have one or several lesions on the body that vary in size and often feel rubbery or compressible. Lipomas are seen most frequently on the buttocks, thighs, back, forearms, and neck of adults. Surgical excision is limited to cases in which functional interference or obvious disfigurement develops.

Pigmented Nevus Cell Tumor

Pigmented nevus cell tumors (also referred to as moles) involve cellular proliferation of melanocytes. A junctional nevus, the most superficial lesion, arises from melanocytes above the basement membrane at the dermal–epidermal border. Because of the high activity level of these cells, this type of nevus is considered to be potentially malignant. Danger signals that indicate malignant changes in pigmented nevi are listed in Box 55–3. Compound nevi contain cells from both the deep dermis and the lining of the epidermal junction. Intradermal or resting nevi arise solely in the dermal layer of skin and are unlikely to become cancerous. Specific examples of these lesions include the giant hairy nevus, blue nevus, halo nevus, and juvenile nevus.

Studies have indicated that pigmented growths show a hereditary tendency (Fitzpatrick, 1983). Nevi arise from cells present since embryonic life, with only a small percentage being apparent at birth. These lesions may appear across the life span of an individual but usually become evident in early childhood with an increasing occurrence during puberty and pregnancy. Melanocytic nevi are common among Caucasians and are seen less frequently in highly pigmented people.

Box 55–3
Danger Signals That Indicate Malignant Changes in Pigmented Nevi

- Color and uniformity (red, white, or blue areas)
- Pigmentation (mottled shades of black or brown)
- Diameter (sudden enlargement)
- Border (development of irregular border or extension of lesion)
- Surface characteristic (presence of erosion, bleeding, ulceration, inflammation, blistering, and serous drainage)
- Sensation (onset of pain, itching, tingling)
- Consistency (softening or friable consistency)
- Shape (uneven elevation)

Clinical Manifestations

Nevi that appear in childhood tend to be flat and only slightly elevated compared to the more distinct conformations that develop in adulthood. Lesions vary considerably in size, color, surface appearance, and form. Dimensions may range from 1 or 2 mm to a growth that covers a large portion of the body surface. Color may vary from a normal skin tone through a spectrum of browns to black and depends in some degree on the exact depth of origin. Surface appearance may be smooth or rough, slightly to markedly elevated, hairy, or hairless. The shape may be round, domelike, polypoid, or papillomatous. Increased or decreased pigmentation around the periphery of the lesion presents a halo effect. Nevi can appear anywhere on the body. Those located on the palms, soles, and genitalia are most likely to be junctional and should be closely observed for significant changes.

Medical Measures

Biopsy is critical before any major decisions are made. Once the diagnosis is confirmed, subsequent therapy may involve total surgical excision with possible skin grafting or the use of electrosurgery.

Removal of all pigmented nevi to prevent the development of malignant melanoma is not practical because the skin may contain many lesions. Prophylactic surgery may be elected when a nevus develops in an area where malignant melanoma has an increased likelihood of occurrence, if the lesion is biologically active, or if chronic irritation is a problem.

Actinic Keratosis

Considered a precancerous growth, actinic, senile, or solar keratosis is a common disorder involving the development of single or multiple cutaneous lesions from chronic exposure to sunlight. Susceptible persons include those with skin types I to III. Rarely is the neoplastic disorder seen in people who tan easily. Farmers, ranchers, sailors, and those who participate in outdoor sports have an increased likelihood of actinic lesions—more so if they are genetically predisposed. Actinic keratosis occurs predominantly in middle and later years, but solar lesions may develop earlier when risk factors and exposure are high.

Clinical Manifestations

Actinic keratoses usually appear as flat, hard, dry, scaly, firmly attached lesions. The color may range from skin tone to yellow, brown, or black and are contingent on the amount of horny materials that adhere. Sites of predilection include the face, ears, neck, forearms, and dorsa of the hands.

Medical Measures

Use of 5-fluorouracil cream or solution (Efudex, Fluoroplex) in prescribed strengths has proven to be an effective treatment. An experimental antimitotic drug, cycloheximide (Acti-dione), may become an alternative. Cryosurgery, electrosurgery and curettage, dermabrasion, and/or chemical peeling have also been used to treat actinic keratoses. Nodules should be excised surgically.

Specific Nursing Measures

When fluorouracil has been prescribed, instruct the individual about appropriate and safe application of the drug. If gloves are not worn, hands must be washed immediately after fluorouracil has been handled to avoid effects on uninvolved skin and mucous membranes. The involved area must never be occluded, and the medication must be applied cautiously near the eyes, nose, and mouth. In addition, inform clients that the treatment may make the area unsightly because of erythema, scaling, hyperpigmentation, dermatitis, suppuration, and swelling. Complete healing may not occur for 1 or 2 months after chemotherapy has ended. Leukopenia, thrombocytopenia, bleeding stomatitis, and gastrointestinal ulcerations may occur with systemic absorption.

Prevention of actinic keratosis is the most important component of care whether by sunscreens, protective clothing, change in occupation, or an alteration in lifestyle and climate. The ultimate goal would be to markedly decrease sun exposure through client education.

Basal Cell Carcinoma

Basal cell epithelioma, the most common form of skin cancer, arises from the germinative layer of the epidermis or the appendages. This lesion carries the most favorable prognosis because cellular proliferation is slow, detection and treatment frequently occur in the early stage, and metastasis is extremely rare. Basal cell carcinoma is seen in adults, usually after age 40, and with a slightly higher prevalence in males (Fitzpatrick, 1979).

Basal cell carcinoma is closely linked with chronic exposure to strong solar ultraviolet radiation, particularly in those with skin types I and II. Incidence is highest in regions where sunlight is most abundant and intense, such as the southern and southwestern United States and Australia. X-ray irradiation, scars, and chemical carcinogens can also be implicated as causative agents.

Clinical Manifestations

Nodular–ulcerative basal cell carcinoma is the most common type. The lesion begins as a papule, progresses to the nodular stage, and can develop a depressed ulcerated center. The borders of the tumor are raised, appear waxy or pearly, and may contain fine telangiectatic vessels (Figure 55–10). Basal cell carcinomas characteristically invade the subcutis, bone, and other underlying tissue. Areas of predilection include the nose, eyelids, and cheek (that is, exposed parts of the head). Superficial basal cell carcinoma appears frequently on the trunk, often involving multiple tumors. These lesions appear to be barely elevated plaques whose centers are crusted and erythematous.

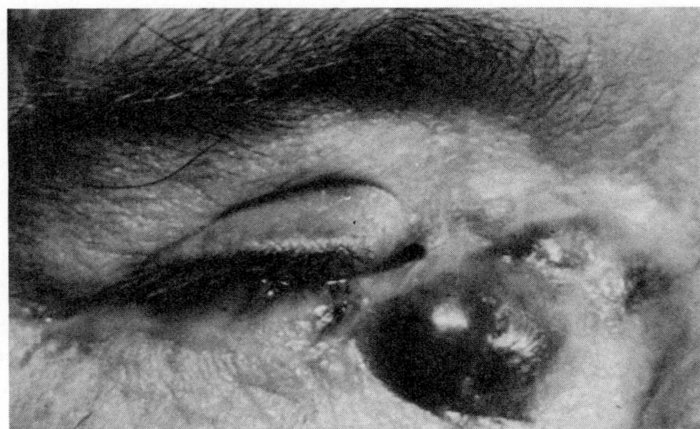

Figure 55–10

Basal cell carcinoma. *Courtesy of Millard Fillmore Hospital, Buffalo, NY.*

Medical Measures

Surgical excision, curettage and electrodesiccation, radiation therapy, cryotherapy, and microscopically controlled excision (Mohs' procedure, MCE) are all used. The primary aim is to eliminate the tumor and prevent irregular local extension of the lesion into the deeper tissues, but without destroying healthy cells and causing major cosmetic defects.

Specific Nursing Measures

The nurse plays a major role in the prevention and case finding of basal cell lesions. Many clients are treated on an outpatient basis, and the role of the nurse is often limited to preoperative teaching and immediate postoperative care. Health teaching should stress the need for regular health care follow-ups.

Squamous Cell Carcinoma

The second most common malignancy of the skin involves the prickle or squamous cell, cells which evolve in the maturation process of the keratinocytes. This neoplasm grows more rapidly than a basal cell carcinoma, is much more invasive, and carries a higher mortality rate because of its metastatic nature. Squamous cell epitheliomas are seen predominantly in males over 55.

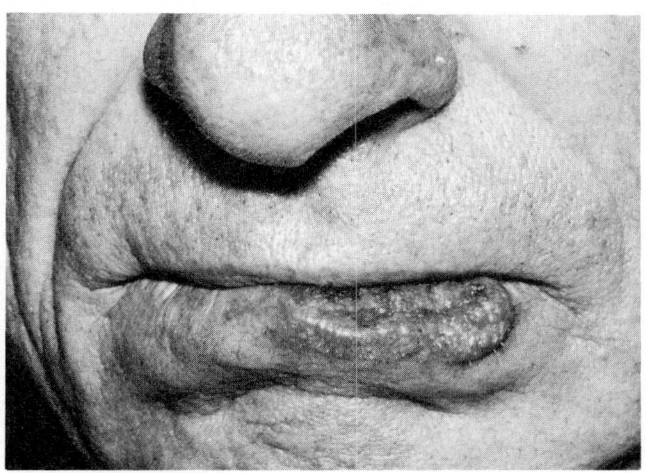

Figure 55–11

Squamous cell carcinoma. *SOURCE: Binnick SA:* Skin Diseases: Diagnosis and Management in Clinical Practice. *Baltimore, MD: Williams & Wilkins, 1982.*

Like basal cell carcinoma, squamous cell malignancies develop in proportion to excesses in sunlight exposure and inherent genetic tendencies (skin type and color). This type of neoplasm has frequently developed from other lesions. In addition to actinic keratosis, unstable thermal burn scars, ulcerations, chronic sinus tracts (draining a suppurative cavity to the skin surface or between cystic or abscess cavities), therapeutically irradiated skin, and discoid lupus erythematosus can develop squamous cell carcinoma. Chronic exposure to coal tar derivatives, arsenicals, and some other chemicals may also be contributory.

Clinical Manifestations

The lesion may appear as a papule, plaque, or nodule. Crusts, erosions, or ulcerations are characteristic, as is an irregular border (Figure 55–11). Lesions appear mostly on the exposed area of the head (cheek, lip, ears) but may frequent the neck, forearms, and backs of the hands, or appear on the legs. Regional lymph nodes may enlarge because of the metastatic process.

Medical and Specific Nursing Measures

Treatment of squamous cell carcinoma is basically similar to the method used for basal cell epitheliomas. Prevention of recurrence requires the elimination or minimization of exposure to carcinogens. The nursing measures are similar to those for basal cell carcinoma.

Malignant Melanoma

Melanoma, a malignancy arising from melanocytes, is the least frequent of primary skin cancers but the most serious. Because of a high degree of metastasis generally involving major organs, the 5-year survival rate for Caucasians (80%) is lower than the survival rate (95%) for clients with other types of skin cancer (American Cancer Society, 1987). Rates for blacks could not be calculated because of an insufficient number of cases. Malignant melanomas are responsible for 5800 of the 7800 deaths from skin cancer annually (American Cancer Society, 1987).

Exposure to intense sunlight, even intermittently, plays a key role in pathogenesis, especially with skin types I to III. Although it is rare, melanoma may develop in those with more highly pigmented skin—Asians, American Indians, blacks, and persons who tan easily.

Congenital or acquired nevi may be labeled as precursors to malignant melanomas, but because of inconclusive evidence, this remains controversial. Familial tendencies have been found in 2% to 5% of cases (Fitzpatrick, 1979).

Clinical Manifestations

The lesional changes identified in Box 55–3 are indicative of malignant melanomas. Color changes may include a variety of browns, black, blue-black, white, pink (amelanotic), red, purple, or gray. The lesion may be slightly raised, or may have a marked elevation.

Melanoma can occur on any part of the body. A small percentage of lesions appear on the palms, soles, or subungually (nail bed).

Any melanoma has the potential to metastasize through the lymphatic and vascular channels or to develop satellite extensions. The lungs, liver, bone, heart, stomach, small intestine, brain, and kidney may be invaded and result in the appropriate symptomatology for the organ. Added concern for metastasis exists when a melanoma develops on the hands, feet, and anogenital area.

Medical Measures

Surgical removal offers the best chance of cure. A wide and deep excision is usually performed to remove all cancerous cells. A regional lymph node dissection is included when findings are positive for lymphatic metastasis but is still considered controversial as an elective component of treatment. More extensive surgery such as amputation of a digit or a limb, abdominal perineal resection, or vulvectomy may be performed because of the extent and location of the malignant melanoma.

Radiation therapy may be used with other modalities to treat the primary tumor, but melanomatous cells have not proven radiosensitive to any great degree. Radiation may be instituted for management of metastatic lesions.

Chemotherapy is useful in adjuvant treatment and when dissemination of melanoma has occurred. Decarbazine (DTIC) has proven to be the most beneficial chemotherapeutic agent, although the nitrosoureas (BCNU, CCNU, MeCCNU) may also be used. Isolated regional limb hyperthermic perfusion (RLHP) has a 5-year survival rate of 75% to 80% compared to a 21% to 33% rate associated with the use of amputation to treat in-transit metastic disease (Loescher & Leigh, 1984). Malignant melanomas are considered in-transit when tumor cells arise between the primary site and regional lymph nodes. Although several chemotherapeutic agents have been used, phenylalanine mustard (L-PAM, or Melphalan) has proven effective in RLHP.

Research has also demonstrated that melanoma cells are destroyed by high temperatures and that a synergistic effect is obtained when L-PAM and hyperthermia are used in combination with RLHP. The procedure requires 1 to 2 hours and is performed under general anesthesia. Vascular cannulation provides for arterial inflow and venous outflow. A tourniquet is applied to the involved limb to prevent systemic leakage, allowing higher doses of the drug to be administered. The perfusate is oxygenated by pump oxygenator and heated to 41°C (105.8°F) while the temperature of the extremity is raised to 39°C (102.2°F) by use of heat lamps or Aquamatic K-pad. When the desired temperatures are reached, the drug is introduced into the venous outflow line. The residual cytotoxic drug is washed out from the system and the appropriate amount of blood replaced before the procedure is completed.

Immunotherapy has also been used in adjuvant therapy for advanced disease. It has not proven to be significantly effective, however. At present, no one treatment is the answer to eradicating a melanomatous lesion, and the trend is toward a combined approach.

Specific Nursing Measures

Emotional support is a critical part of nursing care. A client with malignant melanoma may be fully aware of the overall prognosis associated with the disorder but may need opportunities for expression of feelings and more information to facilitate a realistic adjustment. Coping mechanisms need to be assessed and assistance given to both client and family during the initial adjustment period and when further admissions are necessitated. Anxiety and fears may become evident as the client considers the following possibilities: loss of body parts, mutilation, recurrence of disease, and lifestyle and economic constraints.

Because surgical excision is usually involved in the initial treatment and may be used for metastatic lesions, nursing care will revolve around the operative procedure. Some clients may need minimal assistance, whereas others may become totally dependent on the nurse for maintenance of physiologic needs and emotional support, particularly when the melanoma has metastasized.

Clients who have received RLHP must be closely monitored for disruption in arterial and venous circulation to the involved extremity. Heparin is administered both during the perfusion procedure and postoperatively to prevent clotting problems. The involved limb should be kept elevated and the client should wear antiembolic elastic stockings. Blood and Doppler studies monitor the potential problems. Transient neuropathy may develop in the perfused limb from tourniquet pressure, causing the client to experience numbness and tingling. Instruct the client to protect the extremity from potential trauma such as burns and lacerations that result from sensory loss. Using L-PAM with RLHP may cause mild edema, erythema, reversible limb hyperpigmentation, alopecia, and a rare occurrence of blistering or ulceration. Clients may also develop myelosuppression and nausea or vomiting if systemic leakage occurs. High doses of L-PAM may prolong wound healing.

Clients should be reminded of the need for regular checkups to monitor remission and recurrence of melanoma.

Cryosurgery/Electrosurgery

Cryosurgery freezes tissue, either superficially or at a deeper level, to produce necrosis. It is a simple, safe, and fast procedure that has been effective in the treatment of superficial basal cell carcinoma, seborrheic and actinic keratoses, leukoplakia, and warts. The lesion is frozen using solid carbon dioxide (dry ice), liquid nitrogen, or Freon 114. Depending on the agent, administration involves direct application by a large loosely wound cotton swab, a spray, or a closed cryoprobe system.

Electrosurgery involves the use of electrical currents to destroy tissue selectively by thermocauterization. Electrosurgical instruments containing a wire loop, blade, needle, or ball can be used for cutting, cauterizing, and coagulating. A local anesthetic is administered unless the procedure can be done quickly. Small basal cell and squamous cell epitheliomas, actinic and seborrheic keratoses, leukoplakia, skin tags, cutaneous horns, warts, and hypertrichosis are a number of dermatologic conditions that can be treated by some form of electrosurgery. Electrosurgery is contraindicated in clients who have demand pacemakers because it could deactivate the pacemaker cycle.

The rate of healing depends on the depth and extent of the procedure as well as on the site involved, Facial wounds heal the fastest, taking from 1 to 6 weeks. Wounds in other areas may take longer to heal. Repeated treatment may be required. Table 55–5 summarizes client implications for cryosurgery and electrosurgery.

Nursing Implications

PREOPERATIVE CARE Because most cryosurgery and electrosurgery on skin is performed in a physician's office or outpatient health care facility, many nurses may have limited opportunity for direct client contact. The client should be prepared for the surgery and know what to expect during and after the surgery. The nurse's role is supportive and educative.

POSTOPERATIVE CARE Because hemorrhage and infections are rare, wound coverage is often not necessary, but the area must be kept clean and dry. If dressings are used, they should be nonadherent. The client may be required

Table 55–5
Cryosurgery and Electrosurgery: Implications for the Client 

Physiologic Implications	Psychosocial/Lifestyle Implications
Marked to moderate pain during the freezing-thawing process and first 24 h postoperatively	Improvement of body image
Edema and erythema at operative site usually subsides in 2–3 days	Reduction of anxiety associated with presence of lesion
Blister formation during thawing; dries, crusts, and sloughs off in 10–14 days	Minimal wound care and little or no restrictions on usual activity or lifestyle
Complications are rare	Embarrassment in regard to blister or crust if highly visible
May need to be repeated if lesion not completely eradicated	Anxiety or frustration if repeat procedure is necessary or malignant lesion not completely removed
Potential for severe scarring when the lesion is deep	Severe scarring may adversely affect body image

to return in 2 weeks for an evaluation to determine whether further surgery is necessary and to evaluate healing. Inform clients about edema, erythema, and healing requirements.

Surgical Excision

Surgical excision involves the sharp dissection of an abnormal cutaneous growth with immediate closure of the wound so primary healing can occur. Aesthetics are considered, but removing enough tissue to prevent regrowth is the most important goal.

Many types of benign and malignant skin lesions are removed by excision, including basal cell and squamous cell carcinomas, melanomas, sarcomas, nevi, lipomas, fibromas, and cysts. In select cases, scars and keloids are also treated by this approach. Tissue is also excised from the integument for biopsy.

Some minor lesions may be resected on an ambulatory basis. Hospitalization is warranted for more complex procedures, clients at risk because of age or health status, and when there is need for postoperative supervision. Table 55–6 summarizes client implications related to surgical excision.

Nursing Implications

PREOPERATIVE CARE Although the preoperative care is often routine, the client should be prepared for the experiences that may be foreign and frightening. Additional psychologic support may be required no matter how minor the procedure appears to be.

POSTOPERATIVE CARE Excised areas will probably be covered and should be observed for bleeding. Compression dressings, tissue drains, or wound suction will be

Table 55–6
Surgical Excision and Microscopically Controlled Excision: Implications for the Client

Physiologic Implications	Psychosocial/Lifestyle Implications
Surgical excision:	
Potential for bleeding and infection, other complications, and rate of healing contingent on anatomic site involved and extent of surgery	Because aesthetic considerations are secondary, disfigurement may result
Further surgical procedures for reconstructive purposes may be required	Potential alteration of body image
	Anxiety over reconstructive surgery if needed
	Apprehension while awaiting biopsy results
Microscopically controlled excision (MCE):	
Precision of anatomic mapping preserves healthy tissue	May need to be repeated if the lesion is not completely removed
Wounds that heal by secondary intention may take longer	Fear of disfigurement, especially if lesion is located in a highly visible area although disfigurement is less than with surgical excision in certain instances
Complications such as infection and bleeding are rare	Need to have frequent health checkups
Soft tissue sloughing occurs in 7 d	

employed to prevent the accumulation of blood, serum, or other drainage from interfering with the healing process. The wound may be closed with sutures, skin tape, or clips. How long the sutures remain depends on the rate of healing and the intent to prevent undue scarring in visible areas.

Microscopically Controlled Excision

Microscopically controlled excision (MCE) involves the removal of a precisely mapped epithelioma in serial fashion and the careful examination of the entire undersurface of each segment for malignant cells. The classic method, Mohs' technique, used a chemical fixative as part of the procedure. A more recent approach to MCE that eliminates the fixative is called the *fresh tissue technique.*

The types of tumors for which MCE is recommended include resistive or recurrent squamous cell or basal cell carcinomas, tumors greater than 2 cm in diameter (Robinson, 1982), and epitheliomas around the nose, ear, and eye. MCE can be performed under either general or local anesthesia, in the hospital or on an ambulatory basis.

The excision involves removing segments of the lesion in layers. A finely detailed anatomic map of the removed tissue, with number and color codes allows careful microscopic determination of the exact location of any remaining malignant cells. If malignant cells are found on the undersurface of any segment, the procedure is repeated as often as necessary to remove the entire tumor. Wounds may be surgically closed or allowed to heal by secondary intention, depending on size. Table 55–6 summarizes the client implications related to MCE.

Nursing Implications

PREOPERATIVE CARE The uniqueness of this surgery should have been explained by the surgeon, but the nurse may need to clarify aspects of the procedure the client hasn't understood. The client is likely to be under stress, which may become more evident during preoperative interactions. The presence of a malignancy, particularly on the face, provokes fears of disfigurement. Fears of a negative prognosis must also be addressed prior to treatment.

Home Health Care

POSTOPERATIVE CARE Clients who have been treated on an ambulatory basis should be given oral and written instructions for dressing change and cleansing of the wound. Dressings are usually changed twice daily and the wound cleansed with half-strength hydrogen peroxide. Although secondary infection is rare, topical antibiotic ointments may be prescribed for prophylaxis.

Laser Surgery

Selected skin lesions have been treated primarily by argon and carbon dioxide lasers. Argon lasers cause thermocoagulation in the dermal layer of the skin without removing or destroying overlying tissue and have proven useful for vascular lesions and removal of tattoos. Vascular lesions treated with the argon laser include spider ectasia, ectatic vessels associated with rosacea, telangiectasia, port-wine stains, and selected vascular tumors. The carbon dioxide laser affects the superficial layer of the skin and has been used in the treatment of warts, malignant skin tumors, leukoplakia, and actinic keratosis. Burns and pressure ulcers have also been debrided by this surgical approach. Both the carbon dioxide and argon lasers can be focused on the skin lesion with millimeter accuracy, and the depth can be controlled to minimize damage to surrounding tissue and the skin's glandular appendages. Table 55–7 summarizes client implications of laser surgery.

Nursing Implications

PREOPERATIVE CARE Alleviation of preoperative fear associated with laser therapy and health teaching regarding postoperative care are prime responsibilities of the nurse. Clients who are having laser surgery for port-wine stains

Table 55–7
Laser Surgery: Implications for the Client 

Physiologic Implications	Psychosocial/Lifestyle Implications
Skin effects ranging from mild erythema to blistering or charring	Must care for wound until it heals
Edema for several hours or days postoperatively	Use of cosmetics and shaving delayed until site is healed
Faster healing with carbon dioxide laser	Direct exposure to sunlight without sunscreen protection should be avoided for at least 10 wk; sunscreen should not be applied until healing has taken place
Eye damage is a hazard to both client and operating room personnel; protective safety gear should be worn	Altered body image and emotional distress if scarring and discoloration occur
Atrophic and hypertrophic scarring and pigmentation changes are potential complications	Lightening, flattening, and smoothing of skin, especially in visible areas, reduces emotional distress and improves self-esteem and body image

are requested to avoid direct exposure to the sun for 3 weeks preoperatively because the erythema could inhibit the treatment effects. Drugs containing aspirin or other anticoagulating agents are contraindicated for a week prior to surgery to lessen postoperative bleeding.

POSTOPERATIVE CARE The wound must be kept clean and dry, and covered with nonadherent dressings or Band-Aids to prevent trauma to the site or premature separation of the crust. Although infection is uncommon, precautions may be taken by topical application of antibiotics until the wound is healed.

SECTION VI

Trauma

A traumatic injury involves disruptive or destructive damage to the various cutaneous layers and appendages of healthy skin because of direct physical force, external penetration by objects, extreme heat, or extreme cold.

Trauma to the skin and underlying tissue is a common disorder that frequently brings a person to the hospital for emergency treatment. Minor problems may be cared for at the site of injury, but extensive wounds may require hospitalization for more involved therapy and rehabilitation.

Trauma to the skin, whether accidental or purposeful, as in surgical incision, often results in scarring. Hypertrophic scarring and keloids have been discussed earlier in this chapter in the section on neoplasia. Burns are discussed in Chapter 12.

Frostbite

Several types of dermatologic problems may result from exposure to freezing and near-freezing temperatures. Damage from cold injury may be minor or extensive enough to cause loss of a body part. The hands, feet, nose, and ears are the most commonly involved structures.

Individuals with a history of peripheral vascular disease have a higher susceptibility to cold injury. Persons who smoke or drink excessive amounts of alcohol are also at high risk. Alcohol causes heat loss from vasodilation, and the warmth generated may prevent adequate body coverage during inclement weather. Nicotine, on the other hand, causes vasoconstriction, thus diminishing peripheral circulation.

Frostbite is an injury in which tissue is damaged by freezing, either superficially or sufficiently deep to cause death to the skin and underlying muscle, bone, nerves, and blood vessels. Frostbite may be accompanied by hypothermia, a generalized cooling of the body below the core temperature of 37°C (98.6°F).

Degrees of tissue trauma caused by cold may be used to describe the severity of the effects. A *first-degree* injury results in erythema after rewarming, whereas patchy blistering characterizes a *second-degree* involvement. *Third-degree* penetration causes necrosis of the skin and may progress to *fourth-degree* injury where soft tissue loss and gangrene of digits or an extremity may result.

Clinical Manifestations

The symptoms in frostbite depend on the depth of involvement. Initially, a frostbitten part may appear blanched or actually frozen, and the person may experience a sharp aching pain or have no sensation except at the edge of the affected area. During thawing from ice crystallization, the affected area may become erythematous, deep purple, or black. Within 48 hours after warming of the superficial injury, plasma and intracellular fluid extravasate into the interstitial spaces causing blistering, bullae formation, or edema. A resultant hemoconcentration and decreased lumen of the blood vessels cause vascular sludging, increasing the likelihood of thrombosis in the smaller capillaries. Larger blood vessels may remain in a state of spasm and further decrease distal circulation. Another fluid shift occurs within 5 to 10 days when reabsorption takes place and the formation of eschar becomes evident. Viable tissue will appear as the eschar begins to separate during the subsequent weeks of the healing process.

It is difficult to assess the degree of injury until the remaining blood supply has been fully established. If an area remains unchanged, with persistent blanching, anesthesia, lack of edema, and cyanosis, necrosis may develop. In the presence of a dry gangrene that has resulted from a very deep frostbite, autoamputation is possible.

Medical Measures

The most immediate treatment for frostbite is to rewarm the affected area gradually. Shelter the person and avoid refreezing once first aid measures are begun. Treatment for hypothermia takes precedence over localized involvement, and warm clothing and beverages may prove helpful.

The involved area should be immersed in a water bath with a temperature ranging between 100° and 108°F (17.7° and 42°C) until the part is entirely flushed (DeLapp, 1980). Nonsubmergible structures such as ears and areas on the face should be treated with a warm moist cover. Rewarming causes a great deal of pain. The involved area should be protected from hitting the sides of warming tubs, and the administration of sedatives or analgesics may be required. To prevent further injury by tissue destruction or refreezing, *avoid* the application of snow, cold water, excessive heat, and rubbing or vigorous massages.

The injured part is carefully dried, an antibacterial agent applied, digits individually separated, and the entire area dressed similarly to a burn to protect it from infection and further tissue destruction. Elevation of the extremity is maintained. If an open method of treatment is elected, reverse isolation is required.

In addition to daily wound care, whirlpool hydrotherapy may be used to aid the natural debridement process, stimulate circulation, and provide buoyancy so that joints can be exercised. The physician may need to incise the eschar longitudinally to ensure adequate circulation to the surviving tissue. Surgery may be required to assist with debridement when the natural process is retarded and infection threatens. Other surgical interventions are used only when amputation or grafting is required.

Arteriograms, Doppler studies, and plethysmographic determinations may be needed to measure the vascular response to the injury. A vasodilator such as reserpine (Serpasil) may be injected into a vasospastic artery to cause a local medical sympathectomy. Anticoagulent therapy has some value but is not ordered routinely.

Specific Nursing Measures

Prevention is a foremost nursing concern with cold injuries. Industrial and school nurses may have the greatest occasion to provide information about how to avoid overexposure. Nurses who care for the elderly or for clients with peripheral vascular diseases or alcohol dependency should incorporate a list of precautions in a teaching program. The instructions for all susceptible persons include:

- Minimizing exposure to excess cold, wet, and high altitudes
- Dressing warmly with several layers of clothing
- Changing to dry clothing at once whenever necessary
- Wearing mittens, caps, and boot liners
- Avoiding alcohol and tobacco
- Inspecting the skin for color changes
- Being aware of altered sensations

Protecting the wound from infection is important because of the altered circulation and ultimate loss of nonviable tissue. Medical and surgical asepsis should be maintained, not only during dressing changes, but when bathing, turning, or touching the client. Comfort is of prime importance during the warming phase and may cause concern during tissue repair. Usually, clients who have sustained frostbite develop a high sensitivity to colder temperatures because of a resultant ischemic neuritis and tend to experience pain in the hands and feet.

When the limbs are involved, active and passive motion of the joints is essential, and the care plan should include a daily exercise program. When injuries are extensive and body function is adversely affected or parts have been lost, physical and occupational therapists may join the health team to provide rehabilitation services.

During the days when the extent of damage is uncertain, clients may require a great deal of emotional support. Initially, the client may be relieved to have survived. However, when the ultimate outcome is more obvious and loss of a body part becomes inevitable, the grieving process may begin. It is important to encourage expression of feelings and to provide an atmosphere in which acceptance and independence are fostered. Planning for the future may also require vocational counseling when loss of body function or loss of a body part prevents the client returning to his or her job.

SECTION VII

Plastic and Reconstructive Surgery

Contrary to the tendency to think of plastic and reconstructive surgery as purely cosmetic, most plastic surgical procedures are done to improve body function. The defects being treated often involve more structures than the skin alone. This section includes procedures to improve body function as well as procedures to improve body appearance.

Skin Grafting

Skin grafting entails the surgical removal of varying depths of cutaneous tissue from its vascular, nervous, and lymphatic connections and its transfer to a designated area without direct attachment to the underlying surface. The graft may be either a split-thickness or full-thickness graft (Figure 55–12). A split-thickness graft includes the entire epidermis and a portion of the dermis. A full-thickness graft includes the epidermis and the entire dermal layer. Grafts are also classified by source:

- *Autograft,* from the same person
- *Isograft,* from a genetically identical person (identical twin)
- *Allograft* or *homograft,* from the same species but genetically dissimilar, as from a cadaver
- *Xenograft* or *heterograft* from a different species, as from a pig (porcine graft)

New techniques of cloning the client's skin in vitro are under development, as are techniques of making artificial skin and culturing allograft skin cells in ways that reduce the likelihood of rejection. Except for autografts and isografts, skin from other sources provides only temporary wound coverage and in time will be rejected by the client's immune system.

Many clients who receive skin grafts have sustained trauma producing an acute or chronic skin loss—generally, thermal and chemical burns. Grafts are also performed when insufficient skin is available during excision of cutaneous tumors or to repair wound dehiscence. Skin ulcerations caused by infection, inadequate arterial or venous circulation, and pressure may also require skin grafts.

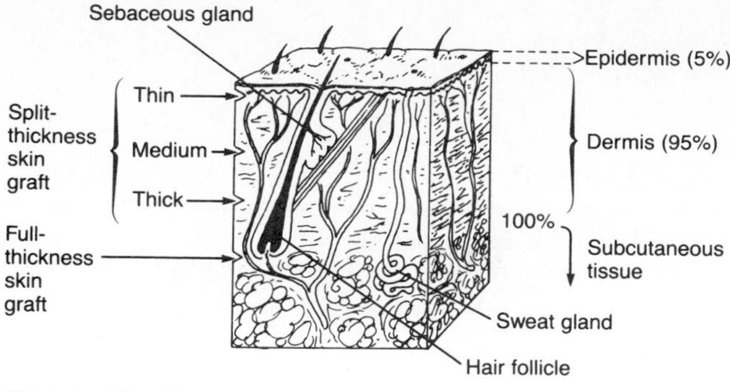

Figure 55–12

Skin graft thickness. A split-thickness graft includes the epidermis and a portion of the dermis. A full-thickness graft includes the entire epidermis and dermis.

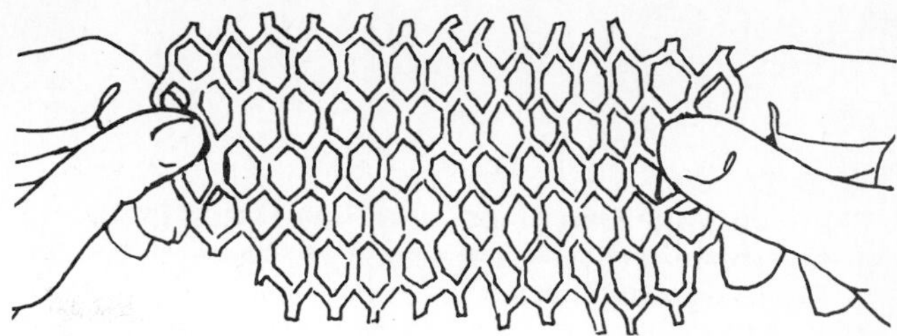

Figure 55–13

Meshed or expanded graft.

Because a vascular bed and healthy underlying tissue are essential, skin grafts are not indicated over denuded bone, tendon or cartilage; on heavily irradiated tissue; or for chronically ulcerated lesions. In these instances, other techniques such as skin flaps or free flap transfers may be indicated (these are discussed later in this chapter).

Most skin grafts are split thickness because vascularization occurs much more successfully. Full-thickness grafts, which allow closer matching of skin color, texture, and hair growth, are used when full-thickness loss has occurred and may be selected when cosmetic appearance is the prime consideration. Donor sites from which full dermal layers have been harvested usually require split-thickness grafts because the denuded areas lack the regrowth powers normally generated from the epithelial cells found in the lining of the sebaceous glands, sweat glands, and hair follicles extending into the dermis. Common donor sites include the thighs, abdomen, buttocks, arms, and chest, but the selection is always contingent on the availability of viable skin.

Grafts are harvested by several methods and are usually acquired after the client has received local or general anesthesia. *Pinch grafts,* no longer common, are "islands of skin" approximately 1 cm in diameter that have been transplanted to the denuded area. *Sheet grafts* are solid pieces of skin obtained usually by using an electric dermatome that allows for precise regulation of thickness and faster procurement of skin, thus reducing anesthesia time. *Meshed* or *expanded grafts* may be used to: (1) allow hematomas, seromas, and air to escape without need for disturbing the transplant; (2) cover large areas when donor sites are limited; (3) conform to irregular surfaces; and (4) decrease skin contractures (Figure 55–13). A major disadvantage is the initial cosmetic effects of the lack of uniformity in the appearance of the skin.

Immediately after the graft is placed on the recipient bed, a fluid exudate with a fibrin network develops between the two surfaces, anchoring the graft and providing nourishment. This plasmatic stage lasts for 24 to 48 hours. Its disturbance by blood clots, serum, air pockets, or presence of fatty tissue may result in partial or total loss of the graft.

Within 4 to 7 days, anastomosis of blood vessels begins as vascular channels from the recipient bed connect with the vessels in the graft. Simultaneously, a new vascular network forms on the recipient bed, and capillaries grow into the donated skin. At the completion of this biologic process, effective vascular and lymphatic circulation should be established. This process of successful vascularization is called a "take."

To promote successful transplantation, the graft must be immobilized to prevent any dislodgment that would disrupt the take. Fixation may be accomplished by suturing (running, interrupted, multiple quilting) and use of metal staples, self-adherent tape (Steri-strips), tie-over dressings (stinting), and numerous other means. If the client is not being treated by the open method, the graft site may be covered with petrolatum gauze (Xeroform), antibiotic gauze (Furacin), or a single layer of fine- or coarse-mesh gauze followed by additional wet (warm saline) or dry dressings and roller bandage to protect the area. Ace bandages or Elastoplast may be used for the outer layer. Regional immobilization may be required by splinting, casting, wiring of joints, or use of skeletal traction. Restriction of movement is especially important when the hands, axillae, neck, ankles, and extremities have been grafted.

The donor site may be similarly covered with a fine-mesh gauze or parachute silk and then dressed with multiple layers of moist or dry gauze to absorb blood and serum that ooze from the wound. A transparent polymer membrane such as OpSite allows the wound to be seen. Table 55–8 summarizes the client implications of skin grafting.

Nursing Implications

PREOPERATIVE CARE The nurse is actively involved in the preparation of the recipient skin graft bed. If wet-to-dry dressings are used, cover the wound with 8 to 12 layers of gauze, moisten them adequately with normal saline or a prescribed pharmacologic agent, and allow normal evaporation. Dressings must be changed dry every 4 to 6 hours to aid the debridement process, and premedication of the client may be required to diminish any pain. Sutilains ointment (Travase) may also be applied to digest necrotic tissue.

Table 55–8
Skin Grafting, Skin Flaps, and Free Flaps: Implications for the Client 

Physiologic Implications	Psychosocial/Lifestyle Implications
Skin grafting:	
Pain, especially in donor site Length of healing varies; split-thickness grafts heal faster, sometimes as early as 10 d Successful takes depend on a variety of factors such as proper preparation of recipient bed, absence of high bacterial count or streptococcal infection in wound, control of bleeding, immobilization of graft, prevention or elimination of hematomas and seromas, adequate venous circulation, prevention of infection Vascularization more successful with split-thickness grafts Long-term problems may exist: skin contractures; hypertrophic scarring; keloid formation; dryness and itching; altered pigmentation; hair loss or decrease; loss of sweating ability; loss of sebaceous glands; alteration in sensations of pain, touch, and temperature	Aesthetic considerations may not always be possible (eg, when extensive burns are involved) Body image disturbances from disfigurement or need to wear unsightly garments or appliances Disruptions in education, career, or interpersonal relationships with family and friends when extensive or multiple grafting is required Absence from the home for treatment may result in role change Emotional energy directed toward survival and coping; little is left over for others
Skin flaps:	
Vascularization takes 4–6 wk Original skin color and texture usually maintained if flap is local Hair growth and sebaceous gland secretion continue Loss of sensation and sweating ability may be temporary Flap growth occurs in proportion to body growth Flap necrosis is a possible complication for as long as 3 yr	Aesthetic effects considered whenever possible A number of operations may be necessary Lifestyle disruptions, body image disturbances, and coping patterns similar to those discussed above
Free flaps:	
Surgery is lengthy, requiring 3–8 h; increased potential for postoperative complications Success depends on immediate vascularization Potential vascular complications are arterial and venous thromboses and leaking at the site of an anastomosis; require immediate surgical correction Graft survival threatened by hematoma formation and external compression Postoperative pain in donor site; no pain in recipient site Sensory deficits in grafted area for several months	Smoking and substances containing caffeine must be restricted for 1 wk preoperatively and several months postoperatively Fewer restrictions on activity and positioning; shorter period of immobilization Performed in one stage Reduction in hospitalization time, cost, and morbidity Lifestyle disruptions tend to be less serious Initial bulkiness and loss of contouring at recipient site can be disruptive to body image Debulking and shaping the flap may be necessary 3–4 mo after tissue transplant Donor site can usually be hidden by clothing Body image ultimately improved

The client should be made aware preoperatively of the degree of immobilization that will be required after surgery so that informed and full participation can be anticipated. The emotional implications can be dealt with early in treatment, and discussion of cosmetic and physiologic effects should be considered critical.

POSTOPERATIVE CARE The most immediate postoperative nursing concerns are the restoration and maintenance of vital body functions. The age of the client, area of involvement, and presurgical health status contribute to the intensity of care involved. The nurse will also be concerned with two wounds (donor and recipient) when the client returns from surgery.

RECIPIENT SITE The ultimate aim for the recipient site is revascularization. A successful take is accomplished when the graft turns from pale white-yellow to pink. This goal may be aided by preventing any movement of or pressure on the graft, therapeutic management of any hematomas or seromas that may form, and by inhibiting infection.

If an open method of treatment or meshed grafts are not employed, the recipient bed should be inspected within 24 to 72 hours for the presence of hematomas or seromas that would interfere with vascularization if any salvaging of a disturbed skin transplant is likely. The dressing must be removed carefully by a qualified physician or nurse. Hematomas or seromas are removed by the physician by gently rolling a cotton-tipped applicator over the area, or creating a fish-mouth opening with fine scissors and either flushing with saline or aspirating the fluid.

In addition to avoiding any movement of the graft, the client must avoid continuous pressure on the graft site. Elevation of the involved part will facilitate venous circulation, and elastic bandages may also be prescribed. Whenever the arms and legs are bandaged, it is essential to assess the digits for color, temperature, and swelling to determine the circulatory status. If bed rest is prolonged when the legs have received grafts, problems related to immobilization must be actively deterred. Elastic stockings are not generally used because they may disrupt the graft. Ambulation should be performed slowly and carefully to prevent venous engorgement of grafted dependent areas.

Infection is prevented by maintaining good asepsis during wound management. An increase in temperature and an odor emanating from the graft around the fourth postoperative day may indicate infection. With sepsis, the blood pressure may drop and blood cultures will be positive. Early treatment with soaks and debridement may be necessary to preserve portions of the graft and decrease scarring. The treatment of sepsis is described in Chapter 12.

DONOR SITE Proper care of the donor site is also imperative; the site should be treated as a partial or full-thickness burn. The nursing goals are to promote healing and to prevent infection. The outer dressing may be removed within 24 to 72 hours after surgery. The fine-mesh gauze or innermost covering is allowed to fall off spontaneously, usually within 2 weeks.

Donor sites may be more painful than recipient areas because the donor sites have exposed nerve endings. Until the crust forms, wound coverage lessens the discomfort by preventing contact with air currents, clothing, and bedding. Bed cradles will help, and analgesics should be administered accordingly.

If donor sites become infected, treatment may incorporate topical antimicrobials such as those used in burn care. These include mafenide (Sulfamylon), silver sulfadiazine (Silvadene), silver nitrate, gentamicin (Garamycin), nitrofurazone (Furacin), povidone–iodine (Betadine), or polymyxin B-bacitracin (Polysporin).

Healing of the graft and donor sites, which varies with the depth of the transplanted skin, may be complete in as few as 10 days if a thin split-thickness graft has been used. The client's nutritional status, premorbid condition, and present homeostatic balance have a great influence on the repair process. Maintenance of a positive nitrogen balance is critical for fast and effective healing.

LONG-TERM SKIN ALTERATIONS Long-term problems associated with skin grafting should be addressed, and the client should be taught how to treat the alterations. Skin lotions, lanolin-containing ointments, vaseline, or any lubricating product should be applied to the cutaneous surface regularly to avoid or reduce dryness and itching when sebaceous glands are lost.

Contraction of grafts and the development of hypertrophic scars or keloids are potential problems. An active program of prevention is usually undertaken when the likelihood of scarring is increased because the client is younger or has highly pigmented skin, joints or high-risk areas on the body are involved, infection has occurred, or split-thickness grafts have been used. Braces, splints, pressure dressings or garments, or orthotic devices may have to be worn to prevent contracture for a number of years until the scars have matured.

Pigmentation may be altered by reduction or increase in color, although the grafted skin usually maintains its original characteristics. Hair growth depends on the thickness of the graft. Loss of hair follicles with split-thickness grafts may result in an absence of hair or a decrease in amount. The ability to sweat is lost in most skin grafts, although some return is possible. Sensations of pain, touch, heat, and cold return in proportion to the nerve potential of the recipient bed. The replaced skin should be actively protected until the client is aware of what new or restored sensations can be perceived. Active protection consists of avoiding temperature extremes and physical injury. If physical injury does occur, the skin surface must be closely

Nursing Research Note

Kravitz M, Green J, Langston L, Epstein B, Worden G: Improperly sterilized fine-mesh gauze associated with donor site infections in skin-grafted burn patients. *Am J Infect Control* 1985; 13(3):178–182.

An increased number of donor site infections during a 4-month period motivated a team of investigators to examine the cause. Ironically, neither the skin grafts themselves nor the ungrafted burn sites became infected. Many factors were examined. Ultimately, it was found that the strips in the inner half of the fine mesh gauze roll were not affected by sterilization procedures. When cultured, the strips were found to be contaminated by *Staphylococcus*.

In some cases, only exhaustive, repeated review of basic procedures can uncover reasons for some hospital infections. Nurses must follow basic infection control practices in all routine aspects of nursing care as well as isolation procedures when appropriate. Policy manuals for infection control in individual hospitals should be read and followed by all personnel.

monitored for untoward changes indicating interruption of vascularization or healing.

PSYCHOSOCIAL CONCERNS Emotional responses to skin grafts vary. A person highly influenced by physical attributes is likely to find the alterations in color and texture of the grafted skin upsetting. Clients who have been traumatized and close to death may respond positively despite the cosmetic alterations. Whatever the response, major disfigurement that requires reconstructive surgery may leave the client in need of intense psychologic support.

Behavioral maladjustments may become more apparent when the client has been discharged since most hospital environments support unusual behavior. After discharge, the stressors may be related to inabilities to adjust socially and an inability to cope with the long-term treatment of skin contracture and scarring. Whenever any emotional problems can be alleviated through verbal communication, the creation of a therapeutic milieu, and family support, the nurse should become a major facilitator. However, the nurse must also recognize the need for professional counseling and refer the client when appropriate.

Skin and Myocutaneous Flaps/Free Flaps

One of the greatest challenges in plastic surgery is developing a method to reconstruct a deformity in order to restore function and achieve an aesthetically pleasing result. Skin flaps are indicated to achieve the following goals:

- Providing bulk or padding when tissue has been lost over bony prominences through trauma or disease, such as a fingertip injury or a pressure ulcer
- Closing defects that cannot be effectively sutured or when vascularization is poor, such as tissue losses with head and neck cancer, radiated tissue, or avulsion wounds
- Covering wounds that will require later surgery, such as bone, cartilage, tendon, or nerve repair
- Reconstructing normal body contour after surgical excision, as for the breast, eyelid, nose, or face
- Protecting underlying structures such as carotid arteries that may have become surgically exposed during head and neck surgery or because of tumor erosion
- Restoring the lumen of the food and air passages

Reconstruction requires replacement of the missing body parts, insofar as possible. Some clients may require replacement of skin, muscle, tendon, fascia, or bone. Small defects may have nearby tissue that can be shifted to repair the wound. If the tissue needed is not nearby, it will need to be moved into the defect with an intact blood supply, or a new blood supply will have to be created.

Skin, myocutaneous, and free flaps are commonly used in reconstruction. The major difference in the flaps is their blood supply. *Skin flaps* consist of skin and subcutaneous tissue that is moved from one part of the body to repair a defect in another part of the body. The skin flap has a pedicle, or foot, which remains attached to the original site in the body to nourish the flap. The blood supply for a skin flap is random. *Muscle flaps* are entire muscles moved with the muscle's feeding artery and vein intact. The muscle can be moved only as far as the artery will reach. *Myocutaneous flaps* (also called musculocutaneous) are the same as muscle flaps with a piece of overlying skin; the skin gets its blood supply from vessels exiting from the muscle. *Fasciocutaneous flaps* are fascia and overlying skin without muscle. The skin obtains its blood supply from vessels running along the fascia to the muscle.

Free flaps are sections of skin, fascia, muscle, and sometimes bone, lifted from their origin, and moved to a defect without a pedicle. The blood supply to the flap is re-established by joining the original feeding vessels to vessels in the wound with the use of an operating microscope and microvascular techniques. The same technique is also used to reattach severed limbs. The blood supply to the flap is critical for its survival, and nursing care centers around this aspect.

Flaps also may be described by the distance they are moved to repair a defect. Adjacent flaps are those moved into a nearby area (Figure 55–14). They have a similar appearance to the missing tissues. An example of an adjacent flap is the moving of surrounding facial skin to repair a defect following the excision of a skin cancer on the face. Tubed pedicle flaps are skin flaps that are transferred to a defect by rolling a pedicle of skin into a tube shape and using the tube to bring skin from a distance to a defect. For example, a defect of the face could be repaired with a tubed pedicle flap from the chest or arm. Tubed pedicle flaps are rarely seen today since the advent of the operating microscope and microvascular techniques that allow free flaps. Free flaps can be moved anywhere because the blood supply is surgically re-established in the donor area.

Table 55–8 summarizes the client implications of skin and myocutaneous flaps and free flaps.

Nursing Implications

PREOPERATIVE CARE Survival of the skin flaps begins with the preoperative teaching program. Clients need a clear explanation of the nursing care involved in the perioperative period and the eventual self-care to be attained. After the surgeon has explained the surgical procedures and the expected outcomes, the nurse should discuss with the client any puzzling points, and any questions about the immediate and long-term physiologic effects. Provide a supportive environment that will help bring to the surface any psychosocial difficulties. Client anxieties will be intensified when gross disfigurement is involved.

The long surgical procedure makes the client more vulnerable to pneumonia, pulmonary emboli, wound infection, and pressure ulcers. Therefore, the preoperative preparation of the client includes a thorough assessment to detect any covert health problems that could increase the hazards as well as a thorough assessment of the vascular supply. Clients should be taught the necessary ventilatory measures and exercises and should be prepared to expect the necessary postoperative neurovascular assessments.

POSTOPERATIVE CARE The most immediate focus of care will be on avoiding or dealing with life-threatening problems related to pulmonary and cardiovascular sequelae. Frequently, flaps involve head and neck surgery on an elderly client with major health problems involving the lungs, heart, blood vessels, or metabolism.

Two key nursing objectives with this type of surgery involve (1) maintenance of circulation to and from the flap and (2) prevention of infection. Because a baseline reference point is critical, the nurse must begin an immediate assessment of flap color, temperature, skin appearance, and capillary filling. Observations are required every 2 hours for the first 72 hours and then every 4 hours. Free flaps should be assessed every 15 minutes for the first 48 hours, and then according to the schedule above. The major portion of the transplanted tissue is usually visible, facilitating assessment. Initially, the surgeon and recovery room nurse simultaneously evaluate color, capillary refill, and tissue turgor to establish a mutual baseline and to ensure minimal variance in the subjectivity of subsequent assessments. Temperature readings, a source of objective data, are provided by a digital telethermometer. A surface probe on the flap and a second probe on a surface area distal to the flap provide a control measure. Simultaneous assessments should also be made whenever the responsibility for monitoring the flap is transferred from one nurse to another.

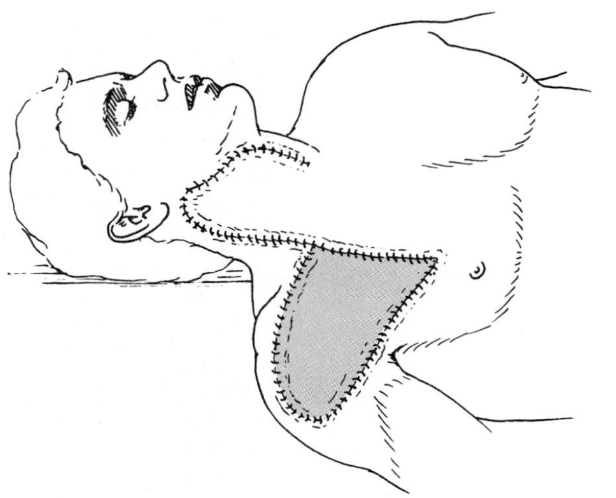

Figure 55–14

Direct transfer of a skin flap.

Distinctions can be made between arterial and venous problems. Arterial complications will be indicated by a pale or white color and a decrease in tissue turgor (shallow depression or concavity), temperature (a 2° deviation from baseline is abnormal), and capillary refill (normal is 1 to 3 seconds). Venous difficulties cause cyanosis, flap distention or fullness (slight edema may be normal), minimal temperature change, and a rapid capillary refill. Because alterations may be subtle, any uncertainties should be brought to the surgeon's attention immediately, along with overt manifestations. Nurses have a crucial role in the early detection of these postoperative complications. Bonavita (1985) has reported that these vital nursing observations were crucial in salvaging 4% of the free flap transfers at her facility.

Care must be taken to prevent any tension, overstretching, twisting, kinking, or pressure on the flap. Avoid placing tape, tracheostomy collars, ties, or tubes on any portion of the flap. Sometimes, tracheostomy tubes are sutured in place instead. For correct positioning, body parts, particularly the head and neck, should be supported by towel rolls or sand bags.

The promotion of venous circulation is an important nursing concern. Because edema will be a normal postoperative occurrence, gravity drainage should be instituted. Although a semi-Fowler's position will assist upper body involvement, prolonged periods of elevation without attention may also cause the flap to pull on the suture line or against a rigid bony surface. Drainage catheters should be monitored frequently to be sure they are functioning properly and the tubings gently milked (or Hemovacs emptied) as needed so internal pressures are reduced.

In addition to sluggish circulation, any inflammatory process in the area of the flap may potentiate a wound infection and possible flap necrosis. A program of incisional care is usually instituted to remove crusts and dried exudate. Half-strength hydrogen peroxide is applied with cotton applicators to the incision and completely swabbed off with normal saline or sterile water to prevent any chemical irritation. Antimicrobial ointment may also be applied. If areas of necrosis develop, treatment with acetic or boric acid soaks and wet-to-dry dressings promotes debridement. Sutures may be removed in 10 days if healing progresses smoothly.

Maintenance of an optimum nutritional intake for the client is important, and a high protein and high calorie diet may be helpful. An alteration in the consistency of the food or the route of delivery (such as tube or intravenous feedings) may also be necessary if the client is undergoing surgery of the head or neck.

Clients should be informed about the characteristics the skin flap will possess (refer to physiologic implications in Table 55–8). Instruct the client to take precautions to protect the grafted area until the sensory nerve endings are re-established.

Emotional responses to flap surgery are individual, especially when gross disfigurement is involved. Surgery on the head and neck can result in extensive losses of tissue with the need for major reconstruction and use of prosthetic devices. Some clients will undergo an emotional crisis because of the disfigurement or because of a long period of immobilization. Nurses need to be keenly perceptive of the psychosocial adaptive mechanisms each client employs. Elderly clients may need additional support and time to re-establish independence or to return to their premorbid level of activity.

Incorporate the appropriate nursing care into the preoperative regimen if a split-thickness graft or full-thickness graft was required at the donor site (see earlier discussion).

Rhytidoplasty

Rhytidoplasty is the use of plastic surgery to remove wrinkles from the face. The procedure, referred to as a "face lift," is performed primarily because of the degenerative effects of the aging process on the skin, particularly the face and neck.

Several approaches may be used, but a C-shaped incision extending from the temporal area of the scalp downward and posterior to the earlobe is most common. The skin is undermined and dissected, creating a facial flap that is raised upward and backward. Excess tissue is removed so the desired tautness can be achieved, or facial contour restored, especially in the area of the chin (mentoplasty). Blepharoplasty or chemical peeling may be performed concurrently. Table 55–9 summarizes the client implications of rhytidoplasty.

Nursing Implications

PREOPERATIVE CARE Each client will be individually evaluated and the desired outcome carefully plotted by the plastic surgeon before hospitalization. A preoperative weight reduction program may be essential so that later weight losses do not markedly alter the repair. Because clients are in an age range where medical problems are frequent, a complete physical examination must be performed to identify any difficulties, particularly hypertension or bleeding and clotting disturbances.

The face and neck are usually washed with hexachlorophene (pHisoHex) and the hair shampooed for several days before the operation. Men are required to shave on

Table 55–9
Rhytidoplasty and Blepharoplasty: Implications for the Client

Physiologic Implications	Psychosocial/Lifestyle Implications
Rhytidoplasty:	
Facial edema	Enhanced self-esteem and improved body image
Ecchymosis of conjunctiva and operative site lasting for weeks	Improvement not permanent because of aging
Hematoma formation and facial nerve (CN VII) damage are potential complications	Body image difficulties if scarring or hair loss occur
Hair loss if hair follicles destroyed	Activity limitations and diet alteration temporary and minimal
Temporary sensory deficits in operative site	Excessive weight loss after surgery can have untoward effects
Blepharoplasty:	
Ecchymosis and edema of eyelids for about 10 d	Increased anxiety because of occlusive dressing
Occlusive dressing for 12–24 h	Enhanced self-esteem and improved body image
Corneal injury, temporary or permanent ptosis, ectropion, asymmetry, and conjunctival injury are potential complications	Alteration in body image and increased emotional discomfort if complications occur

the morning of surgery. Any necessary cutting or removal of hair from the scalp will usually be carried out in the operating room.

POSTOPERATIVE CARE Clients return from the operating room with a firm dressing in place. They may have cotton padding around the ears to minimize discomfort and to protect the auricular cartilage from trauma.

Use of tissue drains and slight pressure exerted by roller gauze or Ace bandage help to prevent hematomas and limit edema. Edema can be decreased by keeping the upper body elevated in a semi-Fowler's position. Any abnormal increase in the anticipated swelling around the eye or mouth, specifically asymmetrical swelling, should be reported to the surgeon immediately, as should heightening discomfort from tightening of the skin. They may indicate hematoma formation. Ecchymosis in the conjunctiva and in the operative area is normal and will not resolve for a number of weeks.

Limitation of activity for at least 2 days will reduce stress on the surgical site. To reduce facial movement, the client should receive a liquid diet and limit talking. The client should also avoid tipping the head forward.

The bulky dressing is removed after approximately 48 hours. Preauricular sutures may be removed in 3 to 5 days; incisions in hair-bearing areas require 2 weeks for healing.

Discharge from the hospital may be allowed after the pressure dressings are removed. Showering may be allowed to help cleanse the area of drainage and the operative antiseptic. Instruct the client to exercise care in combing and brushing hair in the area of the incision and to avoid excess jaw movements until wound healing is complete. Shampooing, hair coloring, and makeup may also be restricted. Hair dryers and earrings should be used with caution until sensation returns.

Blepharoplasty

Blepharoplasty is the excision of redundant eyelid tissue. Anyone who develops an excess of skin in the eyelids or protrusion of periorbital fat may become a candidate for blepharoplasty. Normal aging produces a loss of elasticity and a relaxation of the eyelid skin. (Tissue excess seen in young and middle-aged persons can be the result of a hereditary tendency.) Because periocular manifestations occur with allergies and are associated with cardiovascular and thyroid disease, a complete medical evaluation is essential before surgery is decided on. Besides aesthetic reasons, surgery may be indicated because a drooping eyelid obstructs the client's vision.

Nursing Implications

PREOPERATIVE CARE The face is cleansed preoperatively as prescribed. The client may require additional emotional support because of a fear of injury to the eyes.

POSTOPERATIVE CARE An occlusive dressing may be maintained for 12 to 24 hours to minimize swelling, bleeding, or hematoma formation, and to rest the eyes. Subsequently, the area may be left exposed or covered with small dressings. The application of cold or iced saline dressings may also help to control the extent of swelling and bleeding. Precautions should be taken to prevent drying, irritation, and injury to the cornea because the edema will hinder complete closure of the lids. Skin sutures may be removed as early as the third or fourth postoperative day, depending on the area of involvement.

Chapter Highlights

Clients with skin disorders are frequently seen in schools, occupational health settings, clinics, summer camps, and other ambulatory care settings where the nurse may be closely involved with diagnosis and treatment.

Each dermatosis has a characteristic set of cutaneous clinical manifestations that include various changes in vasculature, pigmentation, configuration, density, texture, turgor, sensation, and temperature, with gains or losses of skin or hair and the appearance of fluid excesses and drainage.

Skin disorders may cause disfigurement and affect the emotional well-being of an individual.

A variety of surgical approaches including plastic and reconstructive surgery may be used to treat dermatoses and disfigurement from alterations of the integument, and to transplant skin.

Select surgical approaches may be contraindicated in clients who are young, highly pigmented, readily scar, have an active dermatosis, or have unrealistic expectations regarding the results of the surgery.

The rate of wound healing involving the skin primarily varies with the type of surgical approach and the blood supply to the anatomic area being treated.

Appropriate wound closure, drainage equipment, and dressings have a significant influence on the prevention of postoperative complications such as hematomas, seromas, infections, and scarring.

Alterations in the color, texture, configuration, and sensory perception of the skin may result from surgery involving the integument.

The nurse plays an important role in the viability of skin and tissue transplants by monitoring

and maintaining circulation and preventing infection.

Long-term exposure to the sun is responsible for alterations in the skin that may precede or result in serious disorders or cause the exacerbation of some dermatoses.

Anti-infectives, anti-inflammatory agents, anti-histamines, comedolytics, keratolytics, retinoids, pesticides, antipruritics, photosensitizers, immunosuppressants, and cytotoxics represent major classifications of drugs used to treat skin disorders.

Personal hygiene, climate and humidity control, appropriate clothing, cleaning agents, toiletries, cosmetics, and sunscreens should be considered in the prevention or treatment of skin disorders.

A teaching program for clients includes the identification of postoperative manifestations such as ecchymosis, erythema, drainage, edema, discomfort, sensory deficits, the anticipated duration of any physiologic or psychosocial alterations, self-care requirements, and measures to prevent injury to the skin.

Chronic skin conditions require heavy expenditures of time, human resources, and costly supplies.

Bibliography

Acres C, Kraft ER: Skin transplantation. *Am J Nurs* 1981; 81:1466–1467.

American Cancer Society. *Cancer Facts and Figures 1987.* New York: American Cancer Society, 1987.

Arndt KA: *Manual of Dermatologic Therapeutics With Essentials of Diagnosis,* 3rd ed. Boston: Little, Brown, 1983.

Barrett BM (editor): *Manual of Patient Care in Plastic Surgery.* Boston: Little, Brown, 1982.

Binnick SA: *Skin Diseases: Diagnosis and Management in Clinical Practice.* Baltimore, MD: Williams & Wilkins, 1982.

Bonavita L: Free tissue transfer. *Am J Nurs* 1985; 85:384–387.

Cassell BL: Treating pressure sores stage by stage. *RN* 1986; 49:36–41.

Conlee D: Cosmetic surgery patients. *Nurs 81* (Nov) 1981; 11:90–95.

Converse JM (editor): *Reconstructive Plastic Surgery: Principles and Procedures in Correction, Reconstruction, and Transplantation,* 2nd ed. Philadelphia: Saunders, 1977.

DeLapp TD: Taking the bite out of frostbite and other cold weather injuries. *Am J Nurs* 1980; 80:56–60.

Dixon JA: *Surgical Application of Lasers.* Chicago: Yearbook Medical Publishers, 1983.

Domonkos AN, Arnold HL, Odom RB: *Andrew's Diseases of the Skin; Clinical Dermatology,* 7th ed. Philadelphia: Saunders, 1982.

Dorr RT, Fritz WL: *Cancer Chemotherapy Handbook.* New York: Elsevier North Holland, 1980.

Emmett AJ, O'Rourke MG: *Malignant Skin Tumors.* Edinburgh: Livingstone, 1982.

Fidler JP: Debridement and grafting of full-thickness burns. In: *Clinical Burn Therapy: A Management and Prevention Guide.* Hummel RP (editor). Boston: John Wright PSG, 1982.

Fitzpatrick TB et al: *Dermatology in General Medicine,* 2nd ed. New York: McGraw–Hill, 1979.

Fitzpatrick TB et al: *Update: Dermatology in General Medicine.* New York: McGraw–Hill, 1983.

Fitzpatrick TB, Polano MK, Suurmond D: *Color Atlas and Synopsis of Clinical Dermatology.* New York: McGraw–Hill, 1983.

Grabb WC, Smith JW: *Plastic Surgery.* 3rd ed. Boston: Little, Brown, 1979.

Grant HD, Murray RH Jr, Bergeron JD: *Emergency Care,* 3rd ed. Bowie, MD: Brady, 1982.

Gumport SL: The diagnosis and management of common skin cancers. *CA* 1981; 31:79–90.

Hibbs P: Taking off the pressure. *Nurs Mirror* (March 27) 1985; 160:iii–vi.

Larrow L, Noe JM: Port wine stain hemangiomas. *Am J Nurs* 1982; 82:786–790.

Lawlis GF, Achterberg J: Acne: The disease and stress. *Top Clin Nurs* (July) 1983; 5:23–31.

Loescher LJ, Leigh S: Isolated regional limb hyperthermic perfusion as treatment for melanoma. *Cancer Nurs* 1984; 7:461–467.

Lucey J, Baroni M: Herpetic whitlow. *Am J Nurs* 1984; 84:60–61.

Lucke K, Jarlesberg C: How is the air-fluidized bed best used? *Am J Nurs* 1985; 85:1338–1340.

Lyons RJ: Promoting healing of skin flaps and grafts. *AORN J* 1982; 35:1174–1183.

Maddin S (editor): *Current Dermatologic Therapy.* Philadelphia: Saunders, 1982.

Maklebust J, Mondoux L, Sieggreen M: Pressure relief characteristics of various support surfaces used in prevention and treatment of pressure ulcers. *J Enterostomal Ther* 1986; 13:85–89.

McIntire SN, Cioppa AL: *Cancer Nursing: A Developmental Approach.* New York: Wiley, 1984.

Miaskowski C: Potential and actual impairments in skin integrity related to cancer and cancer treatment. *Top Clin Nurs* (July) 1983; 5:64–71.

Robinson JK: Mohs' surgery for skin cancer. *Am J Nurs* 1982; 82:282–283.

Sauer GC: *Manual of Skin Diseases,* 4th ed. Philadelphia: Lippincott, 1980.

Sklar CG: Pressure ulcer management in the neurologically impaired patient. *J Neurosurg Nurs* 1985; 17:30–36.

CASE STUDY

The Client With Acne

I. Descriptive Data

This is Mary Dixon's first visit to the Adolescent Outpatient Clinic. She was initially referred by a school nurse and is accompanied by her mother. Mrs. Dixon was present during the first part of the health history and then left the room. Additional information was sought from Mary alone, as is clinic policy. Mrs. Dixon was not present during the physical examination.

II. Personal Data

Date and Time: Jan 5, 1988
Full Name: Mary Therese Dixon
Social Security Number: 000-00-0000
Address: 920 Kings St., Apt. #110, Los Angeles, CA 90715
Sex: Female
Age: 15 years, 6 months
Birthdate: 6-3-72
Marital Status: Single
Race/Culture: Caucasian
Occupation: Student
Usual Health Care Provider: Has no regular health care provider; was assigned to Martha Donovan, RN, NP, at the Adolescent Clinic

III. Health History

Source of Information: Client and mother
Reliability of Information: Reliable
Chief Concern: "I want to get rid of these pimples."

History of Present Illness:

This is a 15½-year-old, white adolescent female with a 1-year history of acne that has gradually worsened. Client has sought no previous medical care, initially believing the pimples would go away with a proper diet and face washing. Six months ago began reducing intake of chocolate and fried foods without any noted improvement in complexion. In addition to a daily shower, began to wash face twice a day with Dial Soap followed by "lots" of rubbing alcohol applied to all pimples. Around that same time, she noted that the whiteheads and blackheads on her face were becoming larger, more reddened in appearance, and were spreading to her neck and shoulders. Four weeks ago, Mary started "picking" at the pimples on her forehead, resulting in some hard pus-filled whiteheads.

No past problems with skin rashes. Uses no lotions (prescription or OTC), creams, or cosmetics (except lipstick and eye shadow) on her face. Denies any relationship between acne and menstrual periods. Has a "best" boyfriend but is not sexually active. Mother had a "bad case" of acne as a teenager resulting in some facial scarring. Mary relates that she is now becoming embarrassed by her acne and is self-conscious about her "ugly face."

Past Health History:

Pregnancy/Labor/Delivery: Product of a normal, spontaneous vaginal delivery at term; birth weight, 7 lb, 8 oz; no neonatal complications
Childhood Illnesses: Mumps, age 4 yr
Immunization: Booster Td, age 14 yr; primary DTP and TOPV series completed; measles and rubella vaccine, age 2

(continued)

CASE STUDY

The Client With Acne (continued)

Past Health History, *(continued)*:

Hospitalizations: Four-day stay for dehydration due to gastroenteritis, age 4 mo

Surgeries: T&A, age 5

Allergies: Mold and cats (skin-testing positive) manifested by allergic rhinitis

Medications: Multivitamin 1 q.d.; chlorpheniramine (Chlor-Trimeton) sustained-release tabs, 8 mg q. 8–12 h p.r.n. for allergy symptoms, ASA for dysmenorrhea

Family History: Father, age 36, living; alcoholic (divorced from mother, 1983)
Mother, age 35, A&W; acne as a teenager, bronchial asthma
Sister, age 14, A&W
Brother, age 11, A&W; bronchial asthma, heart murmur
MGM, maternal aunt, both with history of asthma
No other significant family health problems

Personal/Social History: Lives with mother, sister, and brother in a two-bedroom apartment. Close-knit family. Generally gets along well with her sister and brother, although they do fight on occasion. Feels that she needs to help her mother more as she is the oldest child. No extended family members live close by. Mother employed as a clerk in a grocery store and is gradually working off debts incurred by ex-husband. Parents divorced 3 years ago. Mary says she loves her dad but fears his drinking. He has moved out of state, sends no support money, and has not been in touch with them for the last 2 years.

Mary is a sophomore in high school; maintains a C + average in required math, English, and biology courses. Does B work in social sciences and history. Mary asked the school nurse for help with her acne, and a referral was made to the clinic because Mrs Dixon's health insurance does not cover outpatient physician visits. Mrs Dixon had wanted to seek medical help for Mary earlier but felt she could not afford care and did not know that Mary could be seen on a sliding-scale payment basis.

Habits: Sleeps average 8 hours a night; runs at least 2 to 4 miles per day for girl's track team training; bites nails; drinks no alcohol; denies cigarette smoking and marijuana use (has tried smoking cigarettes twice); denies nonprescription and "street" drug use; uses car seat belts regularly.

Sexual History: Feels fairly comfortable talking about sex with her mother. Shares information with "best" girlfriend. Knowledgeable about sexual intercourse, conception, and some contraception practices. Has no plans to become sexually active in the near future.

Nutrition: Eats from basic four food groups with a three-meal pattern plus frequent snacking on cookies and diet soft drinks. Favorite meal—hamburger, coke, and fries. Average 16 to 24 oz of milk per day.

Review of Systems: States her overall health is excellent; has high energy level; only health concern is acne

Skin: See HPI

Eyes: Vision just tested at school, 20/20 OU; no history of infections, eye pain, or decreased vision

Ears: External otitis media 6 months ago, no further problems; passed school audiometric testing this year

Nose/Throat: Allergic rhinitis three to four episodes per year; responds well to chlorpheniramine; dental visit 2 months ago

Respiratory: Occasional cold; denies dyspnea/wheezing on exercising

Gynecologic:	Menarche: 14 yr, 3 mo; cycle regular 28 days; mild cramping first 24–36 h, responds to ASA, 650 mg q. 4–6 h p.r.n.; never had pelvic examination
Musculoskeletal:	Has no leg or joint pain; screened annually in school for scoliosis, no curvature noted
Psychologic:	No recent major changes in mood or behavior; generally feels positive about self except for "acne"; normal adolescent concerns noted

Physical Assessment:

Height:	5 ft, 5 in. (45th percentile for age)
Weight:	114 lb (6th percentile for age)
Vital Signs:	Temperature 98°F (36.7°C.); pulse 72; respirations 20; B/P 100/60 right arm, sitting
General Appearance:	Well-developed, well-nourished, smiling adolescent female with obvious facial acne
Skin:	Numerous open and closed comedones over face, neck and shoulders; occasional nodules and inflammatory papules on shoulders; several small pustules on forehead; no cysts; no scarring noted; no excessive oiliness noted
HEENT:	Conjunctiva clear, no redness, no exudate; left tympanic membrane slightly retracted but movable on pneumatic otoscopy, landmarks visible; light reflex normal; nasal turbinates with slightly bluish and boggy appearance, nostrils patent bilaterally; pharynx without exudate or redness; teeth, good hygiene and in good repair
Respiratory:	Lungs clear to auscultation, no rales, no rhonchi
Breasts:	Tanner Stage 5; no masses palpable, equal size bilaterally
Cardiovascular:	PMI at 5 LICS, slightly medial to MCL; S1, S2 normal, no murmurs; femoral pulses strong and equal bilaterally
Genitourinary:	Tanner Stage 5 pubic hair; normal external female genitalia
Musculoskeletal:	Spine straight; no thoracic hump, no sacral tilt, scapulae level, flank angles equal on scoliosis screening examination

IV. Diagnostic Data

Routine initial examination/laboratory screening showed a normal CBC, urinalysis, and negative tine test

V. Summary

Mary was placed on tetracycline, 500 mg PO, once daily plus the following topical keratolytic agents: Tretinoin (Retin-A) 0.05% cream in the morning and benzoyl peroxide gel 5% at bedtime. The purpose, action, and side effects of each drug were outlined, and a drug information sheet was given to Mary. Additional information was presented on proper skin hygiene and avoidance of squeezing the lesions. Common myths surrounding acne were also addressed. Issues of increasing sexual identity/awareness and body image concerns were discussed at this first visit. Mary was scheduled to return to the Adolescent Clinic to see her primary health care provider for on-going care of her acne and any other health care needs.

VI. Nursing Care Plan, by Nursing Diagnosis

Client Care Goals	Plan/Nursing Implementation	Expected Outcomes
Skin integrity, impaired related to broken skin secondary to acne		
Involve self actively in skin care regimen; ask questions freely	Instruct regarding skin hygiene and practices that worsen the skin problem (eg, squeezing pimples, oil-based cosmetics, rubbing alcohol); assess knowledge of the	Assumes responsibility for skin hygiene measures and taking medications as prescribed; reduces practices that are irritating to the skin (eg, squeezing pimples,

(continued)

CASE STUDY (continued)

The Client With Acne

VI. Nursing Care Plan, by Nursing Diagnosis, (continued)

Client Care Goals	Plan/Nursing Implementation	Expected Outcomes
	prescribed pharmacologic management plan: tetracycline, 500 mg, once daily, application of tretinoin 0.05% cream in AM and benzoyl peroxide gel 5% at bedtime; give personal medication profile sheet covering purpose, side effects (including teratogenic), and contraindications; discuss plan for long-term follow-up care necessary for acne control	using creams, rubbing alcohol); continues to use cosmetics sparingly; reduction in numbers of pustules and inflammatory papules within 1 to 2 months; describes correctly the rationale behind pharmacologic and hygiene treatment plan
Self-concept, disturbance in: body image related to obvious facial acne eruptions		
Express feelings of frustration over physical appearance due to acne	Assign primary health care provider to coordinate medical and psychosocial care; encourage attendance at clinic-sponsored adolescent group meetings where adolescents come to discuss various developmental concerns; encourage to share feelings with peers	Reduction in number of negative comments about complexion; continues to maintain friendships with peers and normal activities (no drastic change in behavior pattern)
Knowledge deficit related to emerging sexuality issues		
Understand the physical and psychosocial changes occurring during adolescence; readily discuss these issues	Facilitate discussion of sexuality issues and sex education; encourage reading of clinic pamphlets and booklets on sexual issues relevant to adolescence	Seeks out information and readily brings up concerns regarding sex education and sexual identity

Common Abbreviations and Acronyms

Acronym or Abbreviation	Definition
AAL	anterior axillary line
AC	air conduction
ADL	activities of daily living
AIDS	acquired immune deficiency syndrome
AP	anteroposterior; anterior and posterior
ARDS	adult respiratory distress syndrome
ASA	acetylsalicylic acid (aspirin)
ASHD	arteriosclerotic heart disease
ATN	acute tubular necrosis
A:V ratio	artery to vein ratio
AVM	arteriovenous malformation
A&W	alive and well
BC	bone conduction
BCG	Bacillus Calmette-Guerin (TBC vaccine)
BDR	background diabetic retinopathy
BGM	blood glucose monitoring
BM	bowel movement
BP	blood pressure
BPH	benign prostatic hyperplasia
BS	bowel sounds or breath sounds
BSE	breast self-examination
c̄	with
Ca	cancer
CAD	coronary artery disease
CAPD	continuous ambulatory peritoneal dialysis
CAT	computed axial tomography
CC	chief concern
CHF	congestive heart failure
CM	costal margin
CN	cranial nerve
CNS	central nervous system
COPD	chronic obstructive pulmonary disease
CSF	cerebrospinal fluid
CT	computed tomography
CTT	computed transverse tomography
CV	cardiovascular
CVA	costovertebral angle; cerebrovascular accident
CVP	central venous pressure
D/C	discontinued
DES	diethylstilbestrol
DIC	disseminated intravascular coagulation
DIP	distal interphalangeal
DJD	degenerative joint disease
DKA	diabetic ketoacidosis
DM	diabetes mellitus
DOE	dyspnea on exertion
DRGs	diagnosis-related groups
DTRs	deep tendon reflexes
Dx	diagnosis
ECG	electrocardiogram
EENT	eye, ear, nose, and throat
EOMs	extraocular movements
ESRD	end-stage renal disease
ETOH	alcohol
EUA	exam under anesthesia
FB	foreign body
FH	family history
Fx	fracture
G	gravida
GI	gastrointestinal
GU	genitourinary
gyn	gynecology
HDL	high density lipoproteins
HEENT	head, eye, ear, nose, and throat
HHNK	hyperglycemic hyperosmolar nonketotic
HJR	hepatojugular reflux
HMO	health maintenance organization
H or E	hemorrhages or exudates
HPI	history of the present illness
HTN	hypertension
Hx	History
I & D	incision and drainage
I & O	intake and output
ICP	intracranial pressure
ICS	intercostal space
IDDM	insulin-dependent diabetes mellitus
IOP	intraocular pressure
IPPB	intermittent positive pressure breathing
IU	international unit
IUD	intrauterine device
IVP	intravenous pyelogram

JVD jugular venous distention
JVP jugular venous pressure

KUB kidney, ureter, bladder

LBCD left border of cardiac dullness
LDL low density lipoproteins
LICS left intercostal space
LLQ left lower quadrant
LMP last menstrual period
LOC level of consciousness
LP lumbar puncture
LSB left sternal border
LUQ left upper quadrant

MAL midaxillary line
MCL midclavicular line
MGF maternal grandfather
MGM maternal grandmother
MI myocardial infarction
MSL midsternal line

NAD no acute distress
NIDDM noninsulin-dependent diabetes mellitus
nl normal limits
NPO nothing by mouth
NSAIDS nonsteroidal anti-inflammatory drugs
NSR normal sinus rhythm
N&V nausea and vomiting

ō none
OB occult blood
OC oral contraceptives
OD right eye
OR operating room
OS left eye
OTC over-the-counter
OU both eyes

PA posteroanterior
PAL posterior axillary line
Pap smear Papanicolaou smear
PCA patient-controlled analgesia
PDR proliferative diabetic retinopathy
PE physical exam; pulmonary embolism
PERRLA pupils equal, round, reactive to light and accommodation
PGF paternal grandfather
PGM paternal grandmother
PH past history
PI present illness
PID pelvic inflammatory disease
PIP proximal interphalangeal
PMD private medical doctor
PMI point of maximal impulse
PMP previous menstrual period
PND paroxysmal nocturnal dyspnea; post nasal drip
POR problem oriented record
PPD packs per day (cigarettes); purified protein derivative (tuberculin)
PPDR preproliferative diabetic retinopathy
PPO preferred provider organization
PTA prior to admission

RICS right intercostal space
RLL right lower lobe
RLQ right lower quadrant
RML right middle lobe
R/O rule out
ROM range of motion
ROS review of systems
RSB right sternal border
RSR regular sinus rhythm
RUL right upper lobe
RUQ right upper quadrant
Rx treatment

s̄ without
S_1 first heart sound
S_2 second heart sound
S_3 third heart sound
S_4 fourth heart sound
SC subcutaneous
SI systems international
SLE systemic lupus erythematosus
SOAP subjective, objective, assessment, plan
SOB shortness of breath
S/P status post
S&S symptoms and signs

T&A tonsillectomy and adenoidectomy
TBC tuberculosis
Td tetanus diptheria
TIA transient ischemic attack
TM tympanic membrane
TMJ temporomandibular joint
TPN total parenteral nutrition
TSE testicular self exam
TSS toxic shock syndrome

URI upper respiratory infection
UTI urinary tract infection

VA visual acuity
VD venereal disease
VFs visual fields
VLDL very low density lipoproteins
VS vital signs

WD well developed
WN well nourished
wnl within normal limits
w/fe white female
w/m white male

⊕ positive
⊖ negative
ō none
ⓜ murmur

abiotrophic diseases diseases which are not present at birth, but manifest themselves later in life
accommodation the process by which the eye adjusts for distance, maintaining a clear visual image with a shift in gaze
acholic (clay-colored) stools stools absent of brown coloration; indicative of biliary dysfunction
acini the terminal respiratory units of the lungs formed by the respiratory bronchioles, alveolar ducts, and alveoli
action potential the process of cardiac depolarization and repolarization
active immunity occurs when the host produces antibodies in response to antigenic stimulation
active transport the movement of small particles across cell membranes from an area of greater to lesser concentration
adenohypophysis the anterior lobe of the pituitary gland
afterload the tension the ventricles must develop in systole to pump against pressure in the aortic valve and aorta
agnosia the inability to recognize familiar objects in the environment through the senses of touch and vision
allergens substances capable of inducing hypersensitivity
allergy an altered bodily state in which an exaggerated response occurs with exposure to an antigen
alopecia the loss of body hair (primarily on the scalp) with the presence of bald spots or total baldness
amaurosis fugax a transient loss of vision in one eye
amenorrhea the absence of menstruation
anabolism building up of the system by changing simple compounds into complex substances; constructive phase of metabolism
angina chest pain that results from myocardial ischemia
anhidrosis the absence of sweat
anosmia loss of smell
antigen a foreign protein or protein complex capable of stimulating a specific immune response when present in the body
anxiety state of uneasiness, discomfort; feeling of apprehension
aphagia inability to swallow
aphakia the absence of the lens of the eye
apheresis the process of separating whole blood into its four major components and removing one for use
apraxia the inability to carry out a learned, voluntary act when motor function is intact
arcus senilis a peripheral corneal opacity common in clients over age 60
arteriovenous (AV) fistula the internal anastomosis of an artery to a vein
arteriovenous (AV) shunt the external connection of an artery to a vein using two pieces of synthetic tubing and a connector
arthroscopy the examination of a joint through a special fiberoptic endoscope (an arthroscope)
ascites the accumulation of protein-rich serous fluid in the peritoneal cavity
asterixis a flapping tremor of the hand characteristic of ammonia toxicity
asthenopia ocular discomfort related to an uncorrected refractive error
astigmatism irregularities in the surface of the lens or cornea
ataxia lack of muscle coordination
athetosis slow, twisting, snakelike movements in the upper extremities
atrophy a wasting away
auscultatory gap a silent interval between the systolic and diastolic pressure in some hypertensive clients
autodigestion digestion of tissues (especially in the stomach and pancreas) by their own secretions
azotemia the accumulation of urea and other nitrogenous substances (uric acid and creatinine) in the blood

B-lymphocytes (B cells) cells which mature in the bone marrow and, when triggered by an antigen, differentiate into antibody-producing cells
ballottement a palpatory technique used when the presence of fluid is suspected
band keratopathy calcium deposits in the cornea
bitemporal hemianopia the loss of the peripheral visual fields
body image a person's concept of the size, shape, and functioning of the body and its parts
borborygmi hyperactive bowel sounds
bradycardia a pulse rate below 60 beats per minute
brawny induration edema which acquires a "woody" feeling because of increased connective tissue in the subcutaneous tissue
bruit an audible murmur in a blood vessel secondary to turbulent blood flow
bulbar paralysis paralysis of the lips, tongue, mouth, pharynx, and larynx
bunion inflammation and thickening of the bursa on the medial side of the first metatarsal head of the great toe

cachexia the "wasting away" associated with chronic disease and cancer characterized by anorexia, weakness, and emaciation
café au lait spots spots of light brown patchy skin pigmentation
calculi stones
carcinoma in situ noninfiltrating carcinoma
cardiac output the amount of blood the heart pumps per minute
cardiac reserve the difference between cardiac output at rest and cardiac output when the physiological limit is reached
cardiac tamponade an accumulation of fluid in the pericardial sac which prevents the heart from filling and reduces cardiac output
cardinal directions of gaze the six directions in which the globe of the eye can move depending on which muscle is acting predominantly
cardiopulmonary bypass the use of a heart-lung machine during surgery, which allows the heart to be stopped and maintains a bloodless surgical field
cardiopulmonary resuscitation (CPR) artificial respiration combined with external cardiac compression to provide for oxygenation of vital tissues until cardiac function is restored
carpopedal spasm a spasm of the hands and feet associated with tetany
catabolism breaking down of the system by changing complex substances into simple compounds; destructive phase of metabolism

cavitary seeding the inadvertent transfer of tumor cells to a new site during surgery
cell-mediated immunity immunity depending on the local action of the T-lymphocyte after becoming sensitized by contact with a specific antigen
cerumen a yellowish-brown wax formed by secretions from the sebaceous and apocrine glands
cheilosis fissures and dry scaling of lips and at corners of the mouth
chemosis edema of the conjunctiva around the cornea
cholecystectomy a resection of the gallbladder
cholecystitis inflammation of the gallbladder
cholecystostomy the surgical formation of an opening in the gallbladder
choledochostomy incision of the common bile duct for removal of biliary calculi and insertion of a T-tube
choledocolithiasis obstruction of the common bile duct by gallstones
cholelithiasis gallstones
chondrocalcinosis calcification of the articular cartilage
chorea involuntary twitching of the limbs or facial muscles
Chvostek's sign twitching of the facial muscles when the facial nerve is percussed; seen in tetany
chylomicrons particles of lipids
chyme the food bolus after being mixed with gastric juices and churned by the stomach's musculature
circadian rhythms diurnal variation; a pattern based on a cycle consisting of 24 hours
climacteric the period of premenopausal changes
clinical death determination of death according to medical standards usually linked to irreversible cessation of circulatory and respiratory function or neurologic function
clonus a series of involuntary muscle contractions precipitated by a sudden passive stretch of muscle
cogwheel rigidity rhythmic jerking fluctuations in the intensity of muscle tone on passive range of motion
colic intermittent fluctuating pain caused by smooth muscle spasm
comedones blackheads and whiteheads
compromised host a client whose host defenses against infection are impaired
confabulate to fill memory gaps with imagined experiences
contracture the shortening and fixing of muscle fibers which limits a joint's range of motion
convergence the medial movement of the two eyeballs so they are both directed toward the object being viewed
crepitation a coarse, crackling sensation with palpation of the subcutaneous tissue caused by escape of air from the lungs into the tissue; also the grating sound and sometimes a palpable vibration when a joint is moved, produced by the roughened synovium in arthritic disease
cretinism a condition of severe congenital hypothyroidism marked by retardation of both growth and mental development
cross-tolerance the tolerance to one pharmacologic agent which then requires larger doses of similar drugs to achieve the desired effect
cyanosis a blue tinge to the skin that appears when hemoglobin oxygen saturation is reduced
cycloplegia paralysis of the ciliary muscle causing paralysis of ocular accommodation

debridement the removal of tissue or eschar prior to healing or any skin-grafting procedure
decerebrate posturing the hyperextension of both the upper and lower extremities
decorticate posturing hyperflexion of the upper extremities and hyperextension of the lower extremities
dehiscence disruption of the superficial layers of a wound
depolarization the flow of electrical impulses that leads to contraction of the heart muscle
dialysate a solution composed of water, glucose, sodium, chloride, potassium, calcium, and acetate or bicarbonate that passes through the semipermeable membrane in dialysis
dialysis removal of elements from the blood through a semipermeable membrane
diapedesis the passage of leukocytes through the unruptured wall of a capillary
diastasis recti a separation of the two rectus abdominis muscles
diffusion the mixing of molecules caused by their tendency to move continuously and randomly in a solution or gas
diplopia double vision
diverticuli a pouch or sac created by herniation of lining mucous membrane through the muscular coat of a tubular structure such as the large intestine
drug dependence a condition in which a person requires the effects of a specific drug to function
drusen yellow deposits visualized as mounds on Bruch's membrane
dysarthria poorly articulated speech
dyskinesias defects in voluntary movement resulting in fragmentary or incomplete movement
dysmenorrhea painful menstruation
dysmetria the inability to measure distance properly in muscular acts
dyspareunia pain associated with intercourse
dyspepsia indigestion
dysphagia difficulty swallowing
dyspnea difficult breathing
dysrhythmias disturbances in the heart's rhythm
dystonia intense, irregular torsion muscle spasms

ecchymoses irregular hemorrhagic areas larger than petichiae that can be dark purplish, brown, yellow, or greenish in color; bruises
echolalia the parrotlike repetition of words spoken by others
ectopic beats cardiac impulses originating outside the SA node
ectropion turning outward of the eyelid margin; usually of the lower eyelid
edema a local or general accumulation of excess fluid in the body tissues
effector T cells killer cells, helpers, and suppressors; essential in regulating the body's fight against invasive organisms
effusion swelling of a joint caused by an increase in synovial fluid or the presence of blood in the joint capsule
egophony a change from an "ee" to a long "a" sound heard when auscultating over an area of lung consolidation
ejection fraction the percentage of left ventricular end-diastolic volume that is pumped
electromyogram (EMG) a test to measure the electric currents produced by muscles, both at rest and during contraction
endotoxins part of the outer cell wall, usually of gram-negative bacteria, and released only upon its destruction
enophthalmos recession of the eye within the orbit; characterized by a drooping upper eyelid
enterotoxins exotoxins that impair intestinal absorption and provoke secretion of electrolytes and water
entropion inversion of the eyelid margin
epicritic (discriminating) pain sharp, localized, pricking pain produced by A-delta fibers

epiphora excessive watering of the eye
eructation belching; usually associated with the swallowing of air
erythropoietin a protein produced in the kidneys that stimulates red blood cell production
eschar necrotic burned skin
euthanasia mercy killing
euthyroidism a normal state of thyroid functioning
evisceration complete disruption of the surgical wound, with protrusion of the viscera
exophthalmos bilateral protrusion of the eyeball; often indicates a thyroid disorder
exotoxins particularly lethal toxins, usually produced by gram-positive bacteria, released by the bacteria itself
extra-anatomic bypass (EAB) the extension of a Dacron graft from one femoral artery to another
extravasation the leakage of a fluid (IV solutions, drugs) into surrounding tissues

fasciculations fine, rapid, twitching movements originating in small groups of muscle fibers
fecalith a hard mass of dry stool
feedback mechanisms a closed-loop mechanism driven by plasma concentrations of a specific hormone which, in turn, regulates its secretion
festination a shuffling and propulsive gait
fetor hepaticus a sweet breath odor resembling acetone or old wine
first-degree burn a burn which damages only the epidermal layer of skin
flaccidity decreased or absent muscle tone
flank the part of the body between the ribs and the ilium of the pelvis
floaters deposits of protein or cells suspended in the vitreous humor that float across the visual field
fortification a visual aura which includes colored patterns with a dark center and jagged edges
fracture a break in the continuity of a bone
full-thickness burn the equivalent of third-degree burns
fundus (of the eye) the retinal area

gallop rhythm an S_3 or S_4 heard along with S_1 and S_2, causing triplets of heart sounds resembling a horse's gallop
genogram a diagram of the family tree
glycemic index the blood glucose levels produced by various foods
glycogen stored carbohydrate
glycogenesis the synthesis of glycogen from glucose
glycogenolysis the conversion of glycogen to glucose
glycosuria glucose in the urine
goiter the enlargement of the thyroid gland
graft-versus-host disease (GVHD) a tissue incompatibility syndrome in which competent T-lymphocytes from the donor circulate and attack host tissue
gynecomastia enlarged, feminine-appearing breasts in males

habitus physical appearance
health risk appraisal (HRA) quantitative measure estimating an individual's probability of dying from a particular cause within a specified time
heart rate the number of strokes per minute
hematemesis bloody vomitus
hematochezia passage of stools containing bright red blood that originates high in the GI tract
hemodialysis dialysis in which an artificial kidney contains the semipermeable membrane
hemoptysis purulent, bloody, or blood-tinged sputum
hepatomegaly enlargement of the liver
heterozygous denotes two different alleles at the same locus
hirsutism excessive hair growth, especially of male hair patterns in women
HLA antigens a complex of antigens related to susceptibility to certain diseases and rejection of transplanted tissues
homonymous hemianopia the loss of half of the visual field
homozygous denotes two identical alleles at the same locus
hormone a chemical substance synthesized by an endocrine gland, secreted directly into the bloodstream, and carried to other sites where its physiological actions are exerted
hormone-receptor binding the process by which certain hormones bind to specific target cell receptors
hormone-target cell specificity the capability of certain cells to respond to a specific hormone
hospice a facility that specializes in caring for the terminally ill and their families
humoral immunity immunity mediated by antibodies that circulate in the blood and are present in the body fluids
hypercapnia above-normal levels of carbon dioxide in the blood
hyperopia farsightedness
hyperorality an insatiable need for oral stimulation by chewing or tasting objects
hyperplasia an increase in the number of cells
hypersensitivity an altered bodily state in which an exaggerated response occurs with exposure to an antigen
hypertonic (solution) a solution with a greater osmolality than blood plasma, causing a rapid influx of water from cells into the plasma
hypertrichosis excess growth of hair
hypertrophy an increase in the size of an organ or structure due to an increase in the size of its cells
hyphema blood in the anterior chamber between the cornea and iris resulting from a tear in the ciliary body
hypoacusia a hearing loss
hypotonia flaccidity of muscle
hypotonic (solution) a solution with a lower osmolality than blood plasma, causing water to move from the plasma into the cells
hypoxemia below-normal levels of oxygen in the blood

iatrogenic a condition or disorder induced by medical treatment
icterus jaundice
idiopathic a condition without recognizable cause
immunoglobulin (Ig) a specialized plasma protein (antibody) produced by the B-lymphocytes in response to the presence of an antigen
impotence an impairment of penile erectile function
injection congestion of blood vessels
interferon a protein produced by T-lymphocytes and many other cells in response to the presence of viruses and other parasites that stimulates noninfected cells to produce an antiviral protein that inhibits viral multiplication
intermittent claudication a cramping pain in a muscle brought on by exercise and relieved by rest
intertriginous areas apposed surfaces of the skin, such as the creases of the neck, breasts, groin, or buttocks
ischemia deficiency of blood because of a constricted or obstructed blood vessel
isometric contraction occurs when a muscle becomes tense while remaining the same length

isotonic (solution) a solution with the same osmolality as blood plasma
isotonic contraction occurs when a muscle shortens during contraction

jaundice yellow coloration of skin and sclerae

Kayser-Fleischer ring a rusty-brown corneal accumulation of copper characteristic of hepatolenticular degeneration
keloid a benign proliferative growth of fibrous tissue at the site of an injury or incision extending beyond the wound itself
ketosis accumulation of ketones
kwashiorkor protein malnutrition resulting from a protein-poor diet or protein loss because of physiological stress
kyphosis an increased convex curve of the thoracic spine (hunchback)

lacrimation the production of tears
laser a device that transforms light of various frequencies into a finely focused beam capable of great heat and power
leukoplakia white thickened plaques that form on mucous membranes
LeVeen shunt peritoneal-jugular shunt which provides a route for reinfusion of ascitic fluid into the venous system
lichenification localized thickening of skin resulting from everyday mechanical pressures or chronic irritation
lipolysis the breakdown of fat
living will a document stating a person's desires about care and intervention to prolong life artificially if he or she becomes unable to communicate
lordosis an increased concave curve of the lumbar spine (swayback)
lymphadenitis inflamed lymphatic vessels coupled with inflamed lymph nodes
lymphadenopathy lymph node enlargement
lymphangitis inflamed lymphatic vessels
lymphedema edema resulting from improper function or obstruction of the lymphatics

macrophages cells of the reticuloendothelial system that can engulf foreign particles
malnutrition the reduced intake or utilization of nutrients, particularly protein and calories, in relation to requirements
malocclusion imperfect alignment of teeth that affects how they meet during chewing (the "bite")
marasmus protein and calorie malnutrition resulting from a chronic reduction of protein and calorie intake
mastication (chewing) the initial preparation of food for the digestive process, when it is ground into a pulp and mixed with saliva
melanin a brown-black pigment that gives color to skin and hair
melena (tarry stools) usually associated with bleeding of the upper GI tract; the natural red color is lost during passage through the bowel
memory cells a subgroup of B cells which signal the immune system that previous exposure to an antibody has occurred
menarche the onset of menstruation
menopause the cessation of the menstrual cycle
menorrhagia excessive menstrual flow of greater than usual duration
metastasis spread of disease when malignant cells detach from the parent tissue and migrate to other body tissues
metrorrhagia bleeding between menstrual periods
microaneurysms minute aneurysms
micrographia handwriting which is cramped and small with signs of tremor
micturition urination
miosis the constricting of the pupil
mittelschmerz ovulatory pain
morbidity illness
mortality death
murmurs sounds resulting from vibrations produced by turbulence of blood flow in the heart
muscle tone the tension in the resting muscle or the response of a limb to movement
mydriasis the dilation of the pupil
myelosuppression the suppressive alteration in the function of the bone marrow; a side effect of most antineoplastic agents
myoclonus spasm of a muscle or muscle groups
myopia nearsightedness
myxedema hypofunction of the thyroid

neoplasm tumor
neovascularization the formation of new blood vessels
nephrolithiasis renal calculi
neuralgia an uncomfortable, painful, burning sensation that extends along the course of one or more nerves
neuritis pain and tenderness along the course of the nerve resulting from inflammation, trauma, or infection
neurohypophysis the posterior lobe of the pituitary gland
nociceptive impulses impulses giving rise to sensations of pain
normal sinus rhythm (NSR) the orderly rhythm of the healthy heart, whose rate at rest is between 60 and 100 beats per minute
nutrient deficiency specific vitamin and mineral deficiency states
nystagmus an abnormal involuntary movement of both eyes either horizontally, vertically, diagonally, or circularly

obesity an excess of relative body fat
obtunded lethargic, drowsy
oligomenorrhea markedly diminished menstrual flow
oncogenes genetic material that can spur malignant transformation and is thought to be latent in the chromosomes of some
opportunists normally harmless organisms which, under certain circumstances, can become pathogenic
orthopnea difficulty breathing when not in an upright position
osmol measures the amount of work dissolved particles can do in drawing fluid through a semipermeable membrane
osmolality the number of osmols per liter of solvent
osmolarity the number of osmols per liter of solution
osmosis the movement of water through a semipermeable membrane from an area of lesser to greater particulate concentration
osmotic pressure the force exerted by particles in solution to stop osmosis
ossification the process by which rapidly forming cells in the epiphyseal plates are gradually replaced by bone cells
overweight an excess in body weight
ovulation the rupture of an ovarian follicle and release of the ovum

pacemaker a device that supplies electrical impulses to the heart muscle to stimulate heartbeat
pallalia the involuntary repetition of sentences
palpitation an unpleasant awareness of a rapid or irregular heartbeat

papilledema edema and inflammation of the optic nerve at its point of entrance into the eyeball
paraplegia the paralysis of both legs and possibly other areas of the trunk
paresthesia an abnormal sensation such as numbness, tingling, burning, or prickling
paroxysmal nocturnal dyspnea (PND) a sudden attack of dyspnea that awakens the client from sleep
partial-thickness burn the equivalent of first- and/or second-degree burns
passive immunity acquired when antibody and complement are transferred to a person without the body's active participation
pericardial effusion an accumulation of fluid in the pericardial sac
peritoneal dialysis dialysis in which the client's peritoneal lining serves as the semipermeable membrane
perseveration the repetition of a motor or verbal action
petechiae red to brownish pinpoint hemorrhages in the skin or mucous membranes
phagocytosis the engulfing of foreign particles by macrophages
phlebothrombosis the formation of a blood clot in a vein, usually in the legs
photophobia ocular discomfort induced by bright light
photopsia the appearance of flashing lights
physical dependence occurs when a person experiences physiological symptoms of withdrawal when use of a drug is discontinued
pinguecula yellow raised fatty plaques on the bulbar conjunctiva usually seen nasally
plasma osmolality the concentration of particles (electrolytes and nonelectrolytes) in the plasma
plethoric round and full, with congestion of blood vessels; a red florid complexion
pleural friction rub leathery, grating sound produced when inflamed or roughened pleural surfaces rub together
pleximeter in indirect percussion, the middle finger of the nondominant hand
plexor in indirect percussion, the tip of the middle finger of the dominant hand
pneumoperitoneum air or gas in the peritoneal cavity
point of maximal impulse (PMI) the systolic thrust of the cardiac apex, which is sometimes visible and/or palpable
Poiseuille's law the flow rate of a fluid through a tube is proportional to pressure differences and the diameter of the tube in relation to the length of the tube and the viscosity of the fluid
polyp a pedunculated growth found on the mucosal surface of vascular organs
postural hypotension a drop in blood pressure when moving from a lying or sitting to a standing position
precordium the area of the anterior chest overlying the heart
preload the degree of stretch of myocardial fibers before contraction
premature ejaculation the inability to exert any voluntary control over the timing of the ejaculatory reflex
presbycusis a slowly progressive bilateral hearing loss related to aging
presbyopia a loss of ability to focus clearly on objects close to the eye
primary intention the healing of approximated and closed surgical wounds with minimal formation of granulation or scar tissue
Prinzmetal's angina angina that occurs at rest
prognathism the lengthening, thickening, and protruding of the mandible
proinsulin a precursor to insulin
proptosis a downward displacement, as with the eyeball in exophthalmos
prostaglandins compounds synthesized from unsaturated fatty acids with an apparent role in acute and chronic inflammatory reactions
protopathic (undiscriminating) pain slow, diffuse, burning, aching, poorly localized pain produced by C fibers
pruritus itching
psychological dependence occurs when a person has a compulsion to continue using a drug in order to maintain self-esteem and well-being
ptosis the drooping or dropping of an organ or a part, as in the drooping of the upper eyelid
pulmonary edema engorgement of the pulmonary vasculature with accumulation of fluid in the interstitial spaces and alveoli
pulmonary surfactant a fluid produced by the secretory glands of the alveolar wall which reduces its surface tension
pulse pressure the difference between the systolic and diastolic blood pressures

quadriplegia the paralysis of all four extremities

rales sounds heard on ausculation over the smaller bronchi or alveoli and caused by the passage of air through bronchi containing fluid
rebound a palpatory technique often used for assessment of peritoneal inflammation with appendicitis
rebound tenderness pain felt after withdrawal of pressure during palpation; a reliable sign of peritoneal inflammation
recombinant DNA the artificial introduction of DNA into a cell to alter it and the subsequent replication of the new and natural DNA
reflux backward or return flow
reflux nephropathy the directing back of urine from the bladder toward the renal pelvis through the ureters during voiding
refraction the passage of light rays from a transparent medium into a second transparent medium with a different density
renal osteodystrophy a serious bone pathology resulting from chronic disease of the kidneys
repolarization the return to the resting membrane potential resulting from the presence of potassium ions in the cardiac cell membrane
resting membrane potential the electrically negative charge of the inside of the cardiac cell membrane in relation to the outside
retinopathy pathological changes in the retina of the eye
retrograde ejaculation the backflow of ejaculate into the bladder
rhonchi gurgling sounds originating in the larger air passages and heard on auscultation; also called coarse rales
rigidity a pronounced increase in muscle tone
root pain pain caused by disease of the dorsal roots of the spinal nerves and felt in the cutaneous areas supplied by the affected roots

scanning speech speech that is slow and deliberate, punctuated with pauses between syllables
scoliosis a lateral curve of the spine
scotomas blind gaps in the visual fields
sebum a lipid substance produced by the sebaceous gland which provides some lubrication of hair and epidermis

seborrhea excess production of sebum
secondary intention the healing of an infected incision or one purposely left open, with greater formation of granulation or scar tissue
second-degree burn a burn which damages the epidermal layer and part of the dermal layer of skin
self-concept the total set of beliefs and feelings one holds about one's self
self-esteem the personal value placed on oneself
semen the collective product of the male accessory sex glands
sialolithiasis formation of salivary calculi; may cause parotitis if a stone lodges in the parotid gland
singultus hiccups
skin turgor the normal fullness and elasticity of the skin
smegma the cheesy secretion of sebaceous glands found chiefly beneath the prepuce
spasticity increased resistance of muscles to passive stretch with rapid extension or flexion of a joint
spermatogenesis the formation of sperm
splenic sequestration the trapping of sickled erythrocytes by the spleen
station the manner in which one stands
steatorrhea (fatty stools) frequent, frothy, foul, and floating stools; caused by altered digestion and absorption of fat
steatosis fatty infiltration of the liver which often precedes cirrhosis
striae streaks or lines
stroke volume the amount of blood the heart pumps with each stroke
substance abuse the continued use of chemical agents despite the emotional, social, legal, and health problems their use creates
sulcus (of the prostate) a midline groove that separates the two lobes of the prostate
superinfection a secondary infection resulting from overgrowth of normal flora during antibiotic treatment
sympathetic ophthalmia inflammation of the uveal tract of an uninjured eye
syncope a transient loss of consciousness associated with muscle weakness and an inability to stand; fainting
synechiae adhesions of parts, especially the iris to the lens or the cornea

T-lymphocytes (T cells) a heterogeneous group of cells that mature in the thymus gland and differentiate into a variety of effector T cells (killer cells, helper cells, and suppressor cells)
tachycardia a pulse rate greater than 100 beats per minute
tactile fremitus a palpable vibration of air through the airways as a person speaks
target cells cells that are sites for the physiological effect of specific hormones
teichopsia a visual aura which includes flashing lights zigzagging across the visual fields
tertiary intention healing which involves debridement of large infected or contaminated wounds followed by mechanical skin closure
third-degree burn a burn which damages both the epidermal and dermal layers of skin
thrills palpable vibrations over the precordium similar to those felt on the throat of a purring cat
thrombophlebitis inflammation of a vein with thrombus formation
tinnitus a ringing, buzzing, or hissing in the ear or head
tolerance the need for increasingly large amounts of a drug to produce the same effects; comes with repeated exposure
torticollis twisting of the head to one side in response to muscle contraction; wryneck
torus palatinus a midline bony outgrowth on the hard palate
total parenteral nutrition (TPN) the intravenous infusion of all necessary nutrients
toxins poisonous substances
traction pulling force applied to a fractured limb to overcome muscle spasm and realign the fracture
trigone an area of the posterior wall of the bladder defined by the urethra and the two ureteral slits
Trousseau's sign carpopedal spasm with inability to open the hand when a blood pressure cuff is placed on the arm, elevated over the systolic reading, and left in place for 2 to 3 minutes
twitching localized, spasmodic contraction of a single muscle group

universal donor type O blood, which can be transfused into clients without causing reactions because it lacks antigens
universal recipient type AB blood, which has both A and B antigens and can accept transfusions of any blood type
uremia azotemia with clinical symptoms
uremic fetor a urinelike breath odor
uremic frost the crust of urate crystals that can accumulate on the skin as a result of uremia
ureteral stent a hollow tubelike device made of silicone placed within a ureter to maintain ureteral flow

vertigo a sensation of disturbed motion as if the person was revolving in space
visual field the area within which stimuli produce sight when the eye is looking straight ahead
vitiligo skin patches that lack pigment

wheezes whistling sounds resulting from the narrowing of respiratory passages
whispered pectoriloquy whispered syllables heard clearly when auscultating over an area of lung consolidation

xanthelasmas (xanthomas) flat or slightly raised yellowish lesions on the upper or lower eyelids in the elderly; often associated with elevated cholesterol levels
xerostomia dryness of the mouth

NOTE: A page number followed by *(i)* indicates an illustration; a page number followed by *(t)* indicates a table.

D

E

F

G

O

T

U

W

X

Y

Z

Some SI Units Applicable to Health

Quantity	SI Unit	Symbol	Customary Unit	Typical Application
Length	kilometer meter centimeter millimeter micrometer	km m cm mm (10^{-3} m) μm (10^{-6} m)	mile, yard, foot, inch	Distance, distance in visual acuity, body linear measurement, size of bacteria
Surface area	square centimeter square meter	cm^2 m^2	square inch square foot	Surface area Body surface area
Mass	kilogram gram milligram microgram	kg g mg μg	lb, oz	Body mass, pharmaceutical and chemical products
Temperature	degree Celsius*	°C	°F or degree Fahrenheit	Body temperature, clinical thermometer
Time	day hour minute second	d h min s		Expression of point in time in a health record, 24 h clock, time of medication
Volume and capacity	liter milliliter	L mL	qt cc or fluid oz, teaspoon	Fluid or gas, measuring vessel, baby formula, oral dosage
Power	watt	W	horsepower	Mechanical power, bicycle ergometer tests

* ***The degree Celsius:*** Note that the unit of temperature is the degree Celsius (not degree centigrade). This has been accepted because the kelvin has limited application in medicine. The symbol for degree Celsius is °C. Although the scale origins of kelvin and Celsius differ, the degree Celsius equals the kelvin in magnitude, thus, a rise in body temperature of 1.0 k is equivalent to a rise of 1.0 °C. 0 °C is defined as 273.15 K, 98.6 °F-37 °C-310.15 K.

† Not yet an approved SI unit